Textbook of
MEDICINE

Textbook of
MEDICINE

Sixth Edition

Volume I

KV Krishna Das
BSc FRCP (E) FAMS DTM&H
Retired Director and Professor
Department of Medicine
Government Medical College
Thiruvananthapuram, Kerala, India

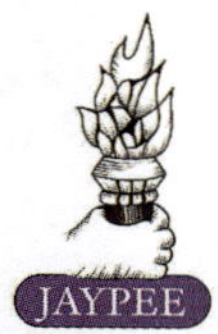

JAYPEE BROTHERS MEDICAL PUBLISHERS
The Health Sciences Publisher
New Delhi I London

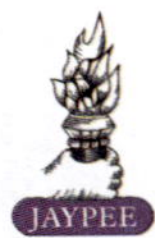 **Jaypee Brothers Medical Publishers (P) Ltd**

Headquarters
EMCA House
23/23-B, Ansari Road, Daryaganj
New Delhi 110 002, India
Landline: +91-11-23272143, +91-11-23272703
+91-11-23282021, +91-11-23245672
E-mail: jaypee@jaypeebrothers.com

Corporate Office
Jaypee Brothers Medical Publishers (P) Ltd.
4838/24, Ansari Road, Daryaganj
New Delhi 110 002, India
Phone: +91-11-43574357
Fax: +91-11-43574314
E-mail: jaypee@jaypeebrothers.com

Overseas Office
JP Medical Ltd.
83, Victoria Street, London
SW1H 0HW (UK)
Phone: +44-20 3170 8910
E-mail: info@jpmedpub.com

EU GPSR Authorised Representative
Logos Europe, 9 rue Nicolas Poussin
17000, La Rochelle, France
Phone: +33 (0) 6 67 93 73 78
E-mail: Contact@logoseurope.eu

Website: www.jaypeebrothers.com
Website: www.jaypeedigital.com

© 2017, Jaypee Brothers Medical Publishers

The views and opinions expressed in this book are solely those of the original contributor(s)/author(s) and do not necessarily represent those of editor(s) of the book.

All rights reserved. No part of this publication may be reproduced, stored or transmitted in any form or by any means, electronic, mechanical, photocopying, recording or otherwise, without the prior permission in writing of the publishers.

All brand names and product names used in this book are trade names, service marks, trademarks or registered trademarks of their respective owners. The publisher is not associated with any product or vendor mentioned in this book.

Medical knowledge and practice change constantly. This book is designed to provide accurate, authoritative information about the subject matter in question. However, readers are advised to check the most current information available on procedures included and check information from the manufacturer of each product to be administered, to verify the recommended dose, formula, method and duration of administration, adverse effects and contraindications. It is the responsibility of the practitioner to take all appropriate safety precautions. Neither the publisher nor the author(s)/editor(s) assume any liability for any injury and/or damage to persons or property arising from or related to use of material in this book.

This book is sold on the understanding that the publisher is not engaged in providing professional medical services. If such advice or services are required, the services of a competent medical professional should be sought.

Every effort has been made where necessary to contact holders of copyright to obtain permission to reproduce copyright material. If any have been inadvertently overlooked, the publisher will be pleased to make the necessary arrangements at the first opportunity.

Inquiries for bulk sales may be solicited at: jaypee@jaypeebrothers.com

Textbook of Medicine (Sixth Edition, Volume I)
First Edition   :   1986
Second Edition :   1990
Third Edition :   1996
Fourth Edition :   2002
Fifth Edition :   2008
Reprint   :   2014
Sixth Edition :   2017
Reprint   :   2023, 2024, **2025**

ISBN: 978-93-86056-10-8

Printed at: Samrat Offset Pvt. Ltd,

This book is dedicated to my alma mater
Medical College and Hospital, Thiruvananthapuram
*where I started learning the first principles of medicine and
thereafter; had the honor to serve as its staff and
continue my close association with the college
even several years after my retirement*

Contributors

A George Koshy MD (Med) DM Cardiology FACC FSCAI FRCP
Professor and Head
Department of Cardiology
Government Medical College
Thiruvananthapuram, Kerala, India

AG Unnikrishnan MD DM
Formerly, Professor of Endocrinology
Amrita Institute of Medical Sciences
Kochi, Kerala, India
Consultant in Diabetology
Chellaram Diabetes Institute
Bavdhan, Pune, Maharashtra, India

Anand Kumar MD DM
Professor and Head
Department of Neurology
Amrita Institute of Medical Sciences
Kochi, Kerala, India

Anjali Bhatt MD-Medicine Fellowship in Diabetology
Consultant in Diabetology
Chellaram Diabetes Institute
Bavdhan, Pune, Maharashtra, India

Arun N Babu MD DM
Assistant Professor
Department of Neurology
Amrita Institute of Medical Sciences
Kochi, Kerala, India

AS Girija MD DM
Retd Professor and Head
Department of Neurology
Government Medical College
Kozhikode, Kerala, India
Professor
Department of Neurology
Christian Medical College
Vellore, Tamil Nadu, India
Consultant Neurologist
Malabar Institute of Medical Sciences
Kozhikode, Kerala, India

Aswini Kumar MD
Professor and HOD of Medicine
Government Medical College
Parippally, Kollam, Kerala, India

B Jayakumar MBBS MD DM
Professor and Head of Department of General Medicine
Chief of Endocrinology and Diabetology
Government Medical College
Thiruvananthapuram, Kerala, India

B Krishna Swamy MD
Professor and Head
Department of Geriatric Medicine
Madras Medical College
Chennai, Tamil Nadu, India

Balu Vaidyanathan MD DNB DM FACC
Clinical Professor
Pediatric Cardiology
Fetal Cardiology Division
Amrita Institute of Medical Sciences
Kochi, Kerala, India

Binoy J Paul MD PhD DNB
Formerly Professor of Medicine
Government Medical College
Professor of Medicine and In-charge of Rheumatology
KMCT Medical College
Kozhikode, Kerala, India

C Sudheendra Ghosh MD (Med) MD (Resp) Dip NB MPH (USA)
Formerly Joint Director of Medical Education
Government Medical College
Professor of Respiratory Medicine
Sree Gokulam Medical College
Thiruvananthapuram, Kerala, India

CG Bahuleyan MBBS MD DM FRCP FSCAI
Formerly Professor and Head
Department of Cardiology
Government Medical College
Consultant Cardiologist
Ananthapuri Hospitals and Research Institute
Thiruvananthapuram, Kerala, India

CP Murali MD
Associate Professor of Chest Diseases
Government Medical College
Thrissur, Kerala, India

CV Soumya MD DM
Neurophysician
AKG Hospital
Kannur, Kerala, India

Davis Paul MD
Professor and HOD of Chest Diseases
Government Medical College
Thrissur, Kerala, India

George Kurian MD DM
Professor of Nephrology
Amrita Institute of Medical Sciences
Kochi, Kerala, India

Gomathy S MD DM
Additional Professor of Nephrology
Government TD Medical College
Vandanam, Alappuzha, Kerala, India

Jacob George MD DM FRCP (Glasgow) FICP (India)
Professor and Head
Department of Nephrology
Government Medical College
Thiruvananthapuram, Kerala, India

Jaisy Mathai MBBS Dip in Blood Transfusion
HOD-Transfusion Medicine
SCTIMST
Thiruvananthapuram, Kerala, India

Jayant Thomas Mathew MD DM
Professor of Nephrology
Amala Institute of Medical Sciences
Amalanagar, Thrissur, Kerala, India

Jigy Joseph MD DM
Associate Professor of Nephrology
Sree Gokulam Medical College
Thiruvananthapuram, Kerala, India

K Sreekanthan MD
Professor and Head
Department of Medicine
Azeezia Medical College
Meeyannoor, Kollam, Kerala, India

K Suresh MD DM
Formerly, Professor and Head
Department of Cardiology
Government Medical College
Consultant Cardiologist
KIMS Hospital
Thiruvananthapuram, Kerala, India

KA Kabeer MBBS MD DM
Additional Professor
Department of Neurology
Government TD Medical College
Alappuzha, Kerala, India

Kapilamoorthy MD DMR
Professor and Head
Department of Imageology
SCTIMST
Thiruvananthapuram, Kerala, India

Karru Venkata Ravi Teja MBBS PhD ICMR Fellowship
Senior Resident
NIMHANS
Bengaluru, Karnataka, India

Kasim Salim MD FRCP FRCP (Ed) FRCPath (Hematology)
Retd HOD–Medicine
Government Medical College
Consultant Hematologist
Kozhikode, Kerala, India

KE Elizabeth MD PhD
Professor and Head
Department of Pediatrics
Sree Mookambika Institute of Medical Sciences
Kulasekharam, Kanyakumari District, Tamil Nadu, India

KE Rajan MD
Professor–Respiratory Medicine
SUT Academy of Medical Sciences
Vattappara, Kerala, India

KP Poulose BSc MD FRCP
Retd Professor of Medicine
Government Medical College
Kottayam, Kerala, India
Consultant
Sree Uthradom Thirunal Group of Hospitals
Thiruvananthapuram, Kerala, India

KR Vinaya Kumar MD DM MRCP
Former Professor
Department of Gastroenterology
Government Medical College
Thiruvananthapuram, Kerala, India
Professor of Gastroenterology
Travancore Medical College Hospital
Kollam, Kerala, India

M Thomas Mathew MD DM
Formerly Professor
Government Medical College
Consultant-Nephrology
Baby Memorial Hospital
Kozhikode, Kerala, India

M Zulfikar Ahamed MD DM
Professor of Pediatric Cardiology
SAT Hospital
Government Medical College
Thiruvananthapuram, Kerala, India

Manu G Krishna MD DM
Assistant Professor
Pushpagiri Medical College
Thiruvalla, Kerala, India

Mathew John MD DM
Former Faculty
Department of Endocrinology
Christian Medical College
Vellore, Tamil Nadu, India
Chief Consultant
Providence Endocrine and Diabetes Specialty Centre
Murinjapalam, Thiruvananthapuram, Kerala, India

Mathew Thomas MD
Professor and Head
Department of Medicine
Dr Somervell Memorial CSI Hospital and Medical College
Karakonam, Thiruvananthapuram, Kerala, India

Mirza Masoom Abbas MBBS MD DM
Consultant in Neurology, currently in Singapore

Textbook of Medicine

N Krishnan Kutty MD (Psych)
Currently Consultant Psychiatrist
Formerly Professor and HOD–Psychiatry
Government Medical College
Thiruvananthapuram, Kerala, India

N Sudhaya Kumar MD DM
Consultant Cardiologist
Formerly HOD–Cardiology
Government Medical College
Kottayam, Kerala, India

Nethravathi M MD DM
Additional Professor
Department of Neurology
NIMHANS
Bengaluru, Karnataka, India

Noble Gracious MD DM
Associate Professor of Nephrology
Government Medical College
Thiruvananthapuram, Kerala, India

PK Jabbar MD DNB DM
Additional Director–Endocrinology
Indian Institute of Diabetes
Pulayanarkotta, Thiruvananthapuram, Kerala, India

PK Sasidharan MD
Ex-Professor and Head
Government Medical College
Consultant–Internal Medicine
PVS Hospital
Kozhikode, Kerala, India

R Jayachandran MBBS MD DM
Staff of NIMHANS on training in USA

R Kasi Visweswaran MD DM FRCP
Retd Professor and HOD
Department of Nephrology
Government Medical College
Consultant in Nephrology
Ananthapuri Hospital
Thiruvananthapuram, Kerala, India

R Sajith Kumar MD
Professor of Infecious Diseases
Government Medical College
Kottayam, Kerala, India

Ramdas Pisharody MBBS MD DM MSc (Clin. epidemiology)
Formerly Professor of Nephrology
Government Medical College
Hon Sr Consultant–Nephrology
KIMS Hospital, Thiruvananthapuram, Kerala, India

Ranjit Sanu Watson MD DNB (Neurology)
Additional Professor
Department of Neurology
Government Medical College
Thiruvananthapuram, Kerala, India

Reena Thomas MD DM
Associate Professor of Nephrology
Pushpagiri Medical College
Thiruvalla, Kerala, India

Rita Christopher MBBS MD
Professor and Head
Department of Neurochemistry
NIMHANS
Bengaluru, Karnataka, India

RK Shenoy MD
Retd Professor and Head
Government TD Medical College
Vandanam, Alappuzha, Kerala, India

RV Jayakumar MD DM FRCP MNAMS
Former HOD–Medicine
Government Medical College
Kottayam, Kerala, India
Professor of Endocrinology
Amrita Institute of Medical Sciences
Kochi, Kerala, India

S Bhasi MD
Professor–Medicine
Sree Gokulam Medical College
Thiruvananthapuram, Kerala, India

S Pradeep Nair MD
Professor and Head
Department of Dermatology and Venereology
Government Medical College
Thiruvananthapuram, Kerala, India

Sajan Z Ahmed MD
Resident
Department of Cardiology
Government Medical College
Thiruvananthapuram, Kerala, India

Salim Shafeek MD FRCP FRCP (Ed) FRCPath (Hematology)
Consultant Hematologist and
Clinical Director of Hemato-oncology
Worcestershire
Honorary Sr Lecturer in Clinical Hematology
University of Birmingham
United Kingdom

SR Chandra MD DM
Professor and Head
Department of Neurology
NIMHANS
Bengaluru, Karnataka, India

SR Srinivasa Kannan MD DM
Director
Vivek Laboratories
Nagercoil, Tamil Nadu, India

Sreelatha M MD DM
Professor of Nephrology
Government Medical College
Kozhikode, Kerala, India

Suhail Mohammed PT MBBS MD FCD DND (Cardiology)
ALMAS Hospital
Kottakkal, Malappuram, Kerala, India

Susan Uthup MD DM
Assistant Professor
Department of Nephrology (Pediatric)
SAT Hospital and Medical College
Thiruvananthapuram, Kerala, India

Swaraj Sathyan MD DM
Consultant Nephrologist
ALMAS Hospital
Kottakkal, Malappuram, Kerala, India

Thomas Gregor Issac MBBS MD PhD (Clinical neurology)
Resident
Department of Psychiatry
NIMHANS
Bengaluru, Karnataka, India

Thomas Iype MD DM
Professor and Head
Department of Neurology
Government Medical College
Thiruvananthapuram, Kerala, India

TK Suma MD
Professor of Medicine
Government TD Medical College
Vandanam, Alappuzha, Kerala, India

Usha Samuel MD DM
Professor of Nephrology
Government TD Medical College
Vandanam, Alappuzha, Kerala, India

Usha Vaidhyanathan MBBS DNB
Consultant in Dermatology and Cosmatology
KIMS Hospital
Anayara, Thiruvananthapuram, Kerala, India

Vidhya Annapoorni CS MBBS MS MCH
SAT Hospital
Government Medical College
Thiruvananthapuram, Kerala, India

Vimala A MBBS MD DM (Nephrology), FRCP (London)
Professor and Head–Nephrology
Dr Somervell Memorial CSI Hospital and Medical College
Karakonam, Thiruvananthapuram, Kerala, India

Vinu Thomas MD DM
Professor of Medicine
Government Medical College
Thrissur, Kerala, India

VN Unni MD DM
Consultant in Nephrology
Aster Medcity Hospital
Kochi, Kerala, India

VP Gopinathan MD MNAMS
Professor of Chest Diseases
Amala Institute of Medical Sciences
Amalanagar, Thrissur, Kerala, India

Preface to the Sixth Edition

During the past 6 years, the quantum and quality of a textbook in internal medicine to be used by a wide range of readership—undergraduates, primary care physicians, practitioners, teaching staff of medical colleges and first, second year postgraduate students in medicine and allied subjects in the Indian Universities and under the National Board of Exams, have grown enormously due to the results of studies under new scientific equipment, biologicals, genetic and molecular studies, and molecular tools employed in both research and treatment, especially monoclonal antibodies and others. This has made the volume grow in size, and subject has become more complex and difficult to comprehend by students and practitioners. I along with my contributors have taken all pains to make the subjects up-to-date, reader-friendly and authentic. Most of the contributors, particularly the section editors, are chosen among the best teachers and researchers with wide hands-on experience in the subject. They have made their contributions clear and understandable for the young students as well as postgraduates and practitioners.

All chapters have been thoroughly scrutinized with the addition of newer information and removal of redundant material. Tables, figures, flowcharts and other study aids have been introduced wherever necessary. Reference to the source has been included wherever new information has been added.

This volume mainly deals with the theoretical and clinical aspects of health and diseases. Its companion volume, (4th edition of clinical medicine) published by Jaypee Brothers Medical Publishers in 2013, edited by me, gives hands-on clinical information of examination of patients, planning the investigations and interpreting the results.

I hope these two volumes will serve to give the necessary information for learning the theory and practice of medicine needed by medical personnel in our country and abroad. I consider my mission fulfilled if my purpose is achieved.

The publishers, Jaypee Brothers Medical Publishers, headed by Shri Jitendar P Vij, has also encouraged us to bring out a full textbook which may evolve to be the flagship of the publishers.

The contributors have done their job. It is hoped that the 6th edition of *Textbook of Medicine* serves the purpose, it is intended to perform.

I would also like to thank Dr Archith Boloor, MBBS MD (Internal Medicine), Associate Professor of Medicine, Kasturba Medical College, Manipal University, Mangaluru, Karnataka, India for his contribution in the book.

KV Krishna Das

Preface to the First Edition

This book is written to fulfil a long-felt and widespread need among the undergraduate students. A questionnaire sent to several hundreds of clinical students revealed that majority of them rely on class notes and handbooks written on the subject by several authors. Many had no access to textbooks in the subject and the big volumes available were beyond their understanding. Comprehensive textbooks catering to the need of undergraduates written by Indian authors are only a few. Books published in other countries are quite freely available to our students, but naturally their emphasis is on conditions prevailing in their lands.

The medical problems of India are unique in that the disease-spectrum is a blend of what is seen in the affluent countries with what is seen in developing countries. This book has been written with this picture in mind. The section on 'tropical diseases' which usually gets a separate deal in most of the textbooks has been dovetailed into the other sections such as infections, physical agents, nutrition, etc. It is my feeling that with modern jet travel and the rapidly changing life-styles of Indian subjects, all diseases—the most modern and the most ancient are likely to be encountered by the clinical students in this country. Moreover, the so-called tropical diseases which used to be confined to the tropical belt, are now seen widely all over the world as a result of free and fast migration of population.

I consider my purpose fulfilled if the undergraduates in this country find this book useful.

KV Krishna Das

Acknowledgments

I acknowledge the support given to me by my wife Smt LN Kamalam, who stood with me and encouraged me to complete the task of editing the sixth edition, despite all her heavy domestic commitments and my strenuous schedule to complete this heavy task.

I thank to all my section editors and contributors who prepared the manuscript and periodically updated the material, due to the delay in bringing out the edition.

I thank Dr Archith Boloor, MBBS MD (Internal Medicine), Associate Professor of Medicine, Kasturba Medical College, Manipal University, Mangaluru, Karnataka, India, who was commissioned by the publishers for helping me to provide charts and tables which have made the material more reader-friendly.

I express my thanks to Shri Jitendar P Vij (Group Chairman), Mr Ankit Vij (Group President), Ms Chetna Malhotra Vohra (Associate Director–Content Strategy), Dr Madhu Choudhary (Content Strategist), Ms Payal Bharti (Project Manager), Ms Neelam Kakriya (Proofreader), Mr Akshay Thakur (DTP Operator) and staff of Jaypee Brothers Medical Publishers (P) Ltd, New Delhi for prompt execution of the work required for this rather voluminous textbook.

I express my humble *Pranam* to The Almighty, to have allowed me to complete this task of editing the sixth enlarged edition, with my section editors and contributors.

Editorial Committee

Section Editors	Sections	Titles	Chapters
KV Krishna Das	Section 1	General Topics	Ch 1–8
KV Krishna Das	Section 2	Diseases due to Arthropods, Marine Animals and Snakes	Ch 9–11
KV Krishna Das	Section 3	Disorders due to Physical Agents	Ch 12–21
KV Krishna Das	Section 4	Toxicology	Ch 22–26
KV Krishna Das	Section 5	Nutrition	Ch 27–33
S Bhasi Usha Vaidhyanathan	Section 6	Diseases caused by Infections	Ch 34–71
R Kasi Visweswaran	Section 7	Fluid and Electrolytes	Ch 72–74
KR Vinaya Kumar	Section 8	Gastroenterology	Ch 75–81
KR Vinaya Kumar	Section 9	Hepatobiliary System and Pancreas	Ch 82–90
AG Unnikrishnan	Section 10	Diabetes Mellitus, Other Metabolic Disorders and Inherited Disorders of Connective Tissue	Ch 91–95
KP Poulose	Section 11	Endocrinology	Ch 96–105
Binoy J Paul	Section 12	Rheumatology	Ch 106–118
K Suresh A George Koshy	Section 13	Cardiology	Ch 119–137
C Sudheendra Ghosh	Section 14	Respiratory System	Ch 138–157
Mathew Thomas KV Krishna Das	Section 15	Hematology	Ch 158–178
R Kasi Visweswaran	Section 16	Nephrology	Ch 179–192
SR Chandra	Section 17	Neurology	Ch 193–218
Usha Vaidhyanathan S Pradeep Nair	Section 18	Dermatology	Ch 219–234
N Krishnan Kutty	Section 19	Psychiatry	Ch 235–251
B Krishna Swamy KV Krishna Das	Section 20	Geriatrics	Ch 252–253

Contents

Volume I

SECTION 1 — GENERAL TOPICS

1. **Introduction to Medicine** — 1
   KV Krishna Das
2. **Medical Genetics** — 5
   KV Krishna Das
3. **Defense Mechanisms of the Host and Clinical Immunology** — 23
   KV Krishna Das
4. **Principles of Drug Administration** — 40
   KV Krishna Das
5. **Antimicrobial Agents** — 47
   KV Krishna Das, S Bhasi
6. **Therapeutics of Glucocorticoids** — 63
   S Bhasi
7. **Principles of Oncology** — 67
   KV Krishna Das
8. **Imaging Sciences and Interventional Radiology** — 80
   Kapilamoorthy

SECTION 2 — DISEASES DUE TO ARTHROPODS, MARINE ANIMALS AND SNAKES

9. **Myiasis** — 90
   KV Krishna Das
10. **Arthropod Bites and Stings, and Injuries due to Marine Animals** — 91
    KV Krishna Das
11. **Snake Bite** — 96
    KV Krishna Das

SECTION 3 — DISORDERS DUE TO PHYSICAL AGENTS

12. **Disorders caused by Heat** — 102
    KV Krishna Das, TK Suma
13. **Injuries due to Cold** — 107
    TK Suma, KV Krishna Das
14. **Disorders due to Alterations in Barometric Pressure** — 109
    TK Suma, KV Krishna Das
15. **Diseases due to High Altitude** — 111
    TK Suma, KV Krishna Das
16. **Drowning** — 113
    TK Suma, KV Krishna Das
17. **Injuries due to Ionizing Radiations** — 115
    TK Suma, KV Krishna Das
18. **Electrical Injuries and Lightning** — 116
    TK Suma, KV Krishna Das
19. **Dangers of Nuclear Explosion** — 118
    TK Suma, KV Krishna Das
20. **Adverse Effects due to Noise and Vibrations** — 119
    KV Krishna Das, TK Suma
21. **Motion Sickness, Problems due to Air Travel and Road Accidents** — 121
    TK Suma, KV Krishna Das

SECTION 4 — TOXICOLOGY

22. **Acute Poisoning: General Considerations** — 124
    KV Krishna Das, TK Suma
23. **Common Poisons** — 130
    KV Krishna Das, TK Suma
24. **Food Poisoning** — 142
    TK Suma, KV Krishna Das
25. **Endemic Fluorosis** — 147
    TK Suma, KV Krishna Das
26. **Therapy of Chronic Tobacco Addiction** — 149
    KV Krishna Das, KE Rajan, TK Suma

SECTION 5 — NUTRITION

27. **Nutrition: General Considerations** — 154
    KV Krishna Das
28. **Starvation** — 162
    KV Krishna Das, KE Elizabeth
29. **Protein-energy Malnutrition** — 163
    KV Krishna Das, KE Elizabeth
30. **Fat-soluble Vitamins** — 167
    KV Krishna Das
31. **Water-soluble Vitamins** — 174
    KV Krishna Das
32. **Minerals** — 179
    KV Krishna Das
33. **Obesity** — 186
    KV Krishna Das

SECTION 6 — DISEASES CAUSED BY INFECTIONS

34. **Infections: General Considerations** — 192
    S Bhasi
35. **Fever of Unknown Origin** — 197
    S Bhasi

xviii

36. **Sepsis and Septic Shock**   202
    S Bhasi
37. **Systemic Diseases caused by Cocci**   206
    KV Krishna Das
38. **Common Bacterial Infections of Childhood**   223
    KV Krishna Das
39. **Salmonella Infections**   228
    S Bhasi, KV Krishna Das
40. **Gram-negative Bacterial Infections**   234
    S Bhasi
41. **Anthrax, Plague, Brucellosis, Melioidosis**   239
    S Bhasi, KV Krishna Das, R Sajith Kumar
42. **Diarrheal Diseases of Infective Origin**   245
    KV Krishna Das, VP Gopinathan
43. **Bartonellosis, Legionellosis, Listeriosis, Yaws, Pinta, Relapsing Fevers, Lyme Borreliosis**   253
    KV Krishna Das
44. **Leptospirosis**   260
    R Sajith Kumar, KV Krishna Das
45. **Rickettsial Diseases, Q Fever, Human Ehrlichiosis and Anaplasmosis**   263
    KV Krishna Das, VP Gopinathan
46. **Anaerobic Infections: Tetanus and Gas Gangrene**   268
    KV Krishna Das
47. **Sexually Transmitted Diseases**   273
    KV Krishna Das, Usha Vaidhyanathan
48. **Sexually Transmitted Viral Diseases**   284
    KV Krishna Das, Usha Vaidhyanathan, R Sajith Kumar
49. **Mycobacterial Infections Tuberculosis, Nontuberculous Mycobacteria and Leprosy**   298
    KV Krishna Das, Usha Vaidhyanathan
50. **Chlamydial Respiratory Infections: Psittacosis and Primary Atypical Pneumonia**   319
    KV Krishna Das
51. **Viral Infections**   321
    KV Krishna Das, R Sajith Kumar
52. **Viral Infections of the Respiratory Tract**   323
    R Sajith Kumar, KV Krishna Das
53. **Exanthems and Enanthems**   328
    KV Krishna Das
54. **Mumps**   338
    KV Krishna Das
55. **Viral Hepatitis**   339
    KV Krishna Das, KR Vinaya Kumar
56. **Enteroviruses**   352
    KV Krishna Das
57. **Adenovirus Infections**   357
    KV Krishna Das
58. **Arenavirus Infections, Filovirus Infections and Hemorrhagic Fevers**   358
    KV Krishna Das, R Sajith Kumar

59. **Rabies**   361
    KV Krishna Das, K Sreekanthan, Aswini Kumar
60. **Arboviruses**   365
    K Sreekanthan, KV Krishna Das, R Sajith Kumar
61. **Other Viral Infections**   374
    KV Krishna Das
62. **Systemic Fungal Infections**   377
    KV Krishna Das, R Sajith Kumar
63. **Actinomyces and Nocardia**   382
    KV Krishna Das, R Sajith Kumar
64. **Disease caused by Protozoa**   384
    PK Sasidharan, KV Krishna Das, VP Gopinathan
65. **Amebiasis, Giardiasis, Balantidiasis, Toxoplasmosis and Cryptosporidiosis**   405
    KV Krishna Das, VP Gopinathan
66. **Helminthiasis: General Considerations**   413
    RK Shenoy, KV Krishna Das
67. **Intestinal Nematodes**   415
    RK Shenoy, KV Krishna Das
68. **Cestodiasis**   423
    RK Shenoy, KV Krishna Das
69. **Trematode (Fluke) Infections**   428
    RK Shenoy, KV Krishna Das
70. **Tissue Nematodes**   432
    RK Shenoy, KV Krishna Das
71. **Rare Helminthic Infestations**   441
    KV Krishna Das, RK Shenoy

SECTION 7   FLUID AND ELECTROLYTES

72. **Abnormalities of Water and Electrolyte Balance**   442
    R Kasi Visweswaran
73. **Abnormalities of Acid-base Balance**   452
    R Kasi Visweswaran
74. **Disturbances of Osmotic Equilibrium**   464
    KV Krishna Das, R Kasi Visweswaran

SECTION 8   GASTROENTEROLOGY

75. **Digestive Organs: General Considerations**   470
    KR Vinaya Kumar, KV Krishna Das
76. **Diseases of the Mouth and Tongue**   480
    KR Vinaya Kumar, KV Krishna Das
77. **Diseases of the Esophagus**   484
    KR Vinaya Kumar, KV Krishna Das
78. **Diseases of the Stomach**   489
    KR Vinaya Kumar, KV Krishna Das
79. **Diseases of the Small Intestine**   499
    KR Vinaya Kumar, KV Krishna Das
80. **Diseases of the Colon**   511
    KR Vinaya Kumar, KV Krishna Das
81. **Diseases of the Peritoneum**   518
    KR Vinaya Kumar, KV Krishna Das

SECTION 9 — HEPATOBILIARY SYSTEM AND PANCREAS

82. **Hepatobiliary System: General Considerations** — 521
KR Vinaya Kumar, KV Krishna Das

83. **Jaundice** — 523
KR Vinaya Kumar, KV Krishna Das

84. **Cirrhosis of the Liver** — 528
KR Vinaya Kumar, KV Krishna Das

85. **Hepatic Failure** — 536
KR Vinaya Kumar, KV Krishna Das

86. **Liver Transplantation** — 543
KR Vinaya Kumar

87. **Portal Hypertension** — 545
KR Vinaya Kumar, KV Krishna Das

88. **Other Hepatic Disorders** — 551
KR Vinaya Kumar, KV Krishna Das

89. **Diseases of the Gallbladder and the Major Bile Ducts** — 562
KR Vinaya Kumar, KV Krishna Das

90. **Diseases of the Pancreas** — 565
KR Vinaya Kumar, KV Krishna Das

SECTION 10 — DIABETES MELLITUS, OTHER METABOLIC DISORDERS AND INHERITED DISORDERS OF CONNECTIVE TISSUE

91. **Diabetes Mellitus** — 577
AG Unnikrishnan, Anjali Bhatt

92. **Complications of Diabetes Mellitus** — 601
AG Unnikrishnan, Anjali Bhatt

93. **Fibrocalcific Pancreatic Diabetes and Other Causes of Meliturias** — 615
KV Krishna Das, KP Poulose, RV Jayakumar

94. **Other Metabolic Disorders** — 618
KV Krishna Das, TK Suma

95. **Inherited Disorders of Connective Tissue** — 628
KV Krishna Das

SECTION 11 — ENDOCRINOLOGY

96. **Endocrinology: General Considerations** — 631
KP Poulose, B Jayakumar

97. **Hypothalamus, Pituitary and their Disorders** — 641
KP Poulose, B Jayakumar

98. **Pineal Gland and its Disorders** — 657
KP Poulose, B Jayakumar

99. **Thyroid and its Disorders** — 658
KP Poulose, B Jayakumar

100. **Parathyroids and their Disorders** — 676
KP Poulose, B Jayakumar

101. **Disorders of the Adrenal Cortex and Adrenal Medulla** — 684
KP Poulose, Mathew John, AG Unnikrishnan

102. **Gonads and their Disorders** — 696
Mathew John, KP Poulose, KV Krishna Das

103. **Miscellaneous Endocrine-related Conditions** — 711
B Jayakumar, KP Poulose

104. **Multiple Endocrine Neoplasia** — 715
PK Jabbar, KP Poulose

105. **Polyglandular Autoimmune Syndromes** — 717
PK Jabbar, KP Poulose

SECTION 12 — RHEUMATOLOGY

106. **Disease of Locomotor System** — 719
Binoy J Paul, KV Krishna Das

107. **Rheumatoid Arthritis and its Variants** — 727
Binoy J Paul, KV Krishna Das

108. **Systemic Lupus Erythematosus and Antiphospholipid Antibody Syndrome** — 739
Binoy J Paul, KV Krishna Das

109. **Progressive Systemic Sclerosis** — 748
KV Krishna Das, Binoy J Paul

110. **Systemic Vasculitis** — 752
Binoy J Paul, KV Krishna Das

111. **Polymyositis and Dermatomyositis** — 760
Binoy J Paul, KV Krishna Das

112. **Miscellaneous Rheumatic Syndromes** — 762
KV Krishna Das, Binoy J Paul

113. **Seronegative Spondyloarthropathies** — 763
Binoy J Paul, KV Krishna Das

114. **Metabolic Arthropathies** — 769
Binoy J Paul, KV Krishna Das

115. **Osteoarthritis** — 777
Binoy J Paul, KV Krishna Das

116. **Other Bone Diseases** — 780
KV Krishna Das, Binoy J Paul

117. **Rheumatological Manifestations of Systemic Diseases** — 784
Binoy J Paul, KV Krishna Das

118. **Newer Diagnostic and Therapeutic Modalities in Rheumatology** — 787
Binoy J Paul

Volume II

SECTION 13 — CARDIOLOGY

119. **Cardiology: General Considerations** — 791
   K Suresh, CG Bahuleyan
120. **Heart Failure (Cardiac Failure)** — 803
   CG Bahuleyan
121. **Shock** — 814
   N Sudhaya Kumar
122. **Congenital Heart Disease** — 817
   M Zulfikar Ahamed, Balu Vaidyanathan
123. **Chronic Valvular Heart Disease** — 838
   N Sudhaya Kumar
124. **Infective Endocarditis** — 855
   K Suresh, Suhail Mohammed PT
125. **Cardiac Arrhythmias** — 861
   K Suresh
126. **Systemic Hypertension** — 881
   K Suresh
127. **Ischemic Heart Disease** — 895
   CG Bahuleyan
128. **Diseases of the Myocardium** — 916
   K Suresh, CG Bahuleyan
129. **Diseases of the Pericardium** — 921
   CG Bahuleyan, K Suresh
130. **Pulmonary Embolism** — 924
   A George Koshy, K Suresh
131. **Diseases of the Aorta** — 928
   N Sudhaya Kumar
132. **Cardiac Manifestations of Systemic Diseases** — 933
   A George Koshy, Sajan Z Ahmed
133. **Pregnancy and Heart Disease** — 939
   N Sudhaya Kumar, K Suresh
134. **Cardiac Tumors** — 942
   A George Koshy, Sajan Z Ahmed
135. **An Introduction to Interventional Cardiology** — 945
   A George Koshy, Sajan Z Ahmed
136. **Cardiac Surgery** — 948
   A George Koshy, CG Bahuleyan
137. **Preventive Cardiology** — 951
   K Suresh, CG Bahuleyan

SECTION 14 — RESPIRATORY SYSTEM

138. **Respiratory System: General Considerations** — 953
   C Sudheendra Ghosh, CP Murali
139. **Respiratory Failure** — 968
   C Sudheendra Ghosh, CP Murali
140. **Diseases of the Upper Respiratory Tract** — 973
   KE Rajan
141. **Pneumonias** — 977
   C Sudheendra Ghosh, CP Murali
142. **Lung Abscess and Pleuropulmonary Amebiasis** — 981
   C Sudheendra Ghosh, Davis Paul
143. **Allergic Disorders of the Lung** — 984
   KE Rajan
144. **Diseases of the Lower Airways** — 996
   C Sudheendra Ghosh, Davis Paul
145. **Occupational Lung Diseases** — 1005
   KE Rajan
146. **Sarcoidosis** — 1008
   KV Krishna Das
147. **Pulmonary Fibrosis** — 1010
   C Sudheendra Ghosh, Davis Paul
148. **Circulatory Disturbances in Lungs** — 1012
   C Sudheendra Ghosh, Davis Paul
149. **Obstructive Sleep Apnea Syndrome** — 1015
   C Sudheendra Ghosh, CP Murali
150. **Neoplasms of the Lung** — 1019
   C Sudheendra Ghosh, CP Murali
151. **Pulmonary Cysts** — 1026
   C Sudheendra Ghosh
152. **Pulmonary Involvement in Systemic Diseases** — 1027
   C Sudheendra Ghosh, Davis Paul
153. **Diseases of Pleura** — 1028
   C Sudheendra Ghosh, Davis Paul
154. **Diseases of the Chest Wall** — 1034
   KE Rajan
155. **Diseases of the Diaphragm** — 1036
   KE Rajan
156. **Diseases of the Mediastinum** — 1039
   C Sudheendra Ghosh, Davis Paul
157. **Pulmonary Rehabilitation and Respiratory Physiotherapy** — 1041
   KE Rajan

SECTION 15 — HEMATOLOGY

158. **Hematology: General Considerations** — 1044
   KV Krishna Das
159. **Anemias: General Considerations** — 1057
   KV Krishna Das
160. **Nutritional and Other Anemias** — 1063
   KV Krishna Das
161. **Hemolytic Anemias** — 1072
   KV Krishna Das
162. **Anemias Characterized by Defective Erythrocyte Production** — 1089
   Mathew Thomas, KV Krishna Das
163. **Blood Transfusion** — 1096
   KV Krishna Das, Mathew Thomas, Jaisy Mathai

xx
Textbook of Medicine

164. Leukemias: General Considerations 1103
Salim Shafeek, Kasim Salim,
KV Krishna Das, Mathew Thomas

165. Acute Leukemias 1113
Salim Shafeek, Kasim Salim,
KV Krishna Das, Mathew Thomas

166. Chronic Leukemia 1122
Salim Shafeek, Kasim Salim, KV Krishna Das

167. Myelodysplastic Syndrome 1131
Mathew Thomas, KV Krishna Das

168. Agranulocytosis (Severe Neutropenia) 1135
PK Sasidharan, KV Krishna Das

169. Plasma Cell Dyscrasias 1137
Salim Shafeek, Kasim Salim,
Mathew Thomas, KV Krishna Das

170. Malignant Disorders of Lymphoid Cells 1147
Salim Shafeek, Kasim Salim,
KV Krishna Das, Mathew Thomas

171. Myeloproliferative Disorders 1160
PK Sasidharan, KV Krishna Das

172. Spleen and its Disorders 1167
KV Krishna Das, PK Sasidharan

173. Hemostasis: General Considerations 1169
Mathew Thomas, KV Krishna Das

174. Platelet and Vascular Disorders 1174
Mathew Thomas, KV Krishna Das

175. Defects of Coagulation 1185
Mathew Thomas, KV Krishna Das

176. Therapeutics of Anticoagulants 1194
Mathew Thomas, KV Krishna Das

177. Fragmentation Hemolysis 1199
Mathew Thomas, KV Krishna Das

178. Thrombophilia 1204
Mathew Thomas, KV Krishna Das

SECTION 16 NEPHROLOGY

**179. Structure and Function of the Kidneys
and Urinary Tract** 1207
R Kasi Visweswaran, Susan Uthup

**180. Clinical Approach:
Evaluation and Investigations** 1212
Jacob George

181. Glomerulonephritis 1220
Jacob George, Noble Gracious

182. Acute Kidney Injury 1230
Jigy Joseph, Vimala A

183. Chronic Kidney Disease 1236
Ramdas Pisharody, Gomathy S

**184. Diseases of Renal Tubules
and Interstitium** 1242
VN Unni, Manu G Krishna

185. Urinary Tract Infection 1250
Sreelatha M, Swaraj Sathyan

186. Nephrolithiasis 1256
Ramdas Pisharody, Vinu Thomas

187. Kidney in Systemic Diseases 1260
M Thomas Mathew

188. The Kidney and Hypertension 1266
R Kasi Visweswaran, Reena Thomas

**189. Renal Involvement in Systemic Diseases
with Special Reference to Pregnancy** 1270
Jacob George, Usha Samuel

190. Urinary Tract Obstruction 1274
Jayant Thomas Mathew, M Thomas Mathew

191. Renal Replacement Therapy 1276
VN Unni, George Kurian

192. Drugs and the Kidney 1284
Jacob George

SECTION 17 NEUROLOGY

193. Nervous System: General Considerations 1288
SR Chandra, Vidhya Annapoorni CS

**194. Neurological Examination
and Investigations** 1294
SR Chandra, SR Srinivasa Kannan

195. Cranial Nerves 1316
SR Chandra, Karru Venkata Ravi Teja

196. Coma and Brain Death 1333
SR Chandra, CV Soumya

197. Headache 1339
AS Girija

**198. Nutritional Disorders of the
Nervous System** 1344
Thomas Gregor Issac, SR Chandra

**199. Infections of the Central
Nervous System** 1351
SR Chandra, Nethravathi M,
Thomas Gregor Issac

200. Dementias and Metabolic Encephalopathy 1365
AS Girija

201. Prion Disease and Related Encephalitis 1373
SR Chandra, Thomas Gregor Issac

202. Epilepsies 1379
AS Girija

**203. Parkinson's Disease and
Related Disorders** 1391
SR Chandra, R Jayachandran

**204. Extrapyramidal Disorders other than
Parkinsonism and Related Syndromes** 1398
SR Chandra, Thomas Iype

205. Cerebrovascular Diseases 1406
SR Chandra, Ranjit Sanu Watson

206. Intracranial Space-Occupying Lesions 1417
Anand Kumar, Arun N Babu

**207. Multiple Sclerosis and other
Demyelinating Lesions** 1425
Anand Kumar, Arun N Babu

208. Motor Neuron Disease 1430
SR Chandra, KA Kabeer

209. Diseases of the Cerebellum 1435
Anand Kumar, Arun N Babu

**210. Diseases of Spinal Cord, Nerve
Roots and Plexuses** 1439
SR Chandra, Vidhya Annapoorni CS,
Thomas Gregor Issac, KV Krishna Das

xxii

211. **Diseases of the Vertebral Column Causing Neurological Lesions** 1448
Anand Kumar, KV Krishna Das

212. **Diseases of the Peripheral Nervous System** 1453
Anand Kumar, Arun N Babu

213. **Disorders of the Autonomic Nervous System** 1460
SR Chandra

214. **Myasthenia Gravis** 1466
SR Chandra, KA Kabeer

215. **Diseases of Muscles** 1472
SR Chandra

216. **Rehabilitation in Neurology** 1481
SR Chandra

217. **Investigation of a Child with a Suspected Neurometabolic Disorder** 1483
Rita Christopher

218. **Central Nervous System Manifestations in Systemic Disorders** 1489
SR Chandra, Mirza Masoom Abbas

SECTION 18   DERMATOLOGY

219. **Skin: General Considerations** 1496
Usha Vaidhyanathan

220. **Infections of the Skin and Appendages** 1500
Usha Vaidhyanathan

221. **Skin Infestations** 1507
Usha Vaidhyanathan

222. **Acne and Rosacea** 1509
Usha Vaidhyanathan

223. **Papulosquamous Disorders** 1511
Usha Vaidhyanathan

224. **Eczema** 1517
Usha Vaidhyanathan

225. **Vesiculobullous Disorders** 1523
S Pradeep Nair

226. **Urticaria and Angioedema** 1526
S Pradeep Nair

227. **Cutaneous Drug Reactions** 1528
S Pradeep Nair

228. **Disorders of Blood Vessels and Lymphatics** 1531
S Pradeep Nair

229. **Disorders of Pigmentation** 1533
S Pradeep Nair

230. **Disorders of Hair and Nails** 1534
S Pradeep Nair

231. **Disorders of Elastin and Collagen Fibers** 1537
S Pradeep Nair

232. **Cutaneous Manifestations of Systemic Disorders** 1539
S Pradeep Nair

233. **Skin Tumors** 1542
S Pradeep Nair

234. **Pregnancy and Skin** 1544
Usha Vaidhyanathan

SECTION 19   PSYCHIATRY

235. **Basic Concepts** 1546
N Krishnan Kutty

236. **Organic Mental Disorders** 1552
N Krishnan Kutty

237. **Schizophrenia and Delusional Disorders** 1554
N Krishnan Kutty

238. **Mood Disorders: Mania, Depression, Dysthymia** 1557
N Krishnan Kutty

239. **Anxiety Disorders** 1560
N Krishnan Kutty

240. **Obsessive Compulsive Disorders** 1562
N Krishnan Kutty

241. **Conversion Disorders, Dissociative Disorders, Somatoform Disorders, Cultural Bond Syndromes, Reaction to Stress and Adjustment Disorders** 1563
N Krishnan Kutty

242. **Torture** 1566
N Krishnan Kutty

243. **Disorders of Adult Personality** 1567
N Krishnan Kutty

244. **Psychoactive Substance-use Disorders and Alcohol-related Disorders** 1568
N Krishnan Kutty

245. **Behavioral Syndromes Associated with Physiological Disturbances and Physical Factors** 1571
N Krishnan Kutty

246. **Psychological Factors Affecting Systemic Medical Disorders** 1574
N Krishnan Kutty

247. **Mental Retardation** 1575
N Krishnan Kutty

248. **Behavioral and Emotional Disorders Occurring in Childhood and Adolescence** 1576
N Krishnan Kutty

249. **Psychiatric Emergencies** 1577
N Krishnan Kutty

250. **General Principles of Management of Psychiatric Disorders** 1579
N Krishnan Kutty

251. **Psychological Methods of Treatment (Psychotherapy)** 1583
N Krishnan Kutty

SECTION 20   GERIATRICS

252. **Principles and Practice of Geriatric Medicine** 1586
KV Krishna Das

253. **Clinical Aspects of Geriatric Diseases** 1590
B Krishna Swamy, KV Krishna Das

Index .... I-i

Textbook of Medicine

Volume I

Volume 1

CHAPTER 1

Introduction to Medicine

KV Krishna Das

Chapter Summary

- History of Medicine
- Medicine as a Profession
- The Final Diagnosis
- Progress in the Millennium Development Goals (MDGs)
- The Concept of Global Burden of Disease
- Recording of Medical Data
- Evidence-based Medicine
- Computers in Medicine

HISTORY OF MEDICINE

The practice of medicine existed even in the earliest periods of recorded human history.

Medical knowledge existed in folklore, local health traditions, verbal testimony and other sources. It is their periodic systematization and improvement that led to medical progress.

The fifth century BC was the golden age of Greek medicine and it was during this period that Asclepid Hippocrates (born around 460 BC), introduced scientific system of administering medicine, which till then was dominated by religious and mystic practices.

Hippocrates embodied the ideal virtues of a physician such as knowledge, readiness to help, purity of life, compassion, skill and patriotism. Hippocratic medicine was based on practice as well as theory with little emphasis on anatomy.

The history of Indian medicine dates back to 3000 BC and excavations of *Mohanjodaro* and *Harappa* throw light on medical practices that flourished at that age, which consisted mainly of religious, magical and empirical procedures.

Ayurveda (the science of life) arose as an offshoot of *Atharva Veda* which is the fourth Veda. *Atharva Veda* is dated to belong till 1500 BC. It consists of 6000 verses and 1000 prose lines. There are several pieces of evidence and statements that *Ayurveda* is very closely associated with *Atharva Veda*. In any case the science of life (*Ayurveda* means knowledge of life sciences) originated in India along with the *vedas*. It laid emphasis not only on healing, but also on the prolongation of life, preservation and promotion of health and prevention of illness. The ancient sages recognized health as the very basis of virtue, wealth, enjoyment and salvation. From very early times, *Ayurveda* had developed independent of religious precepts. *Agnivesa*

has been credited with the authorship of *Ayurveda*. *Agnivesa* composed *Agnivesa tantra*. Great names in *Ayurveda* include *Charaka, Susruta, Vagbhata* and several others. *Charaka* edited his encyclopedic text '*Charaka samhita*' between the 2nd century BC and 1st century AD (post Buddhist period) during the reign of the *Kusanas*. *Charaka samhita* is a creative revision of *Agnivesa tantra*. *Charaka samhita* is still in vogue as a basic test used by practitioners of *Ayurveda*. *Susruta,* who was a medical teacher in Varanasi during the Buddhist period, practised surgery. *Vagbhata*, another Buddhist physician living in the Indus region (second century AD) wrote two classics in *Ayurveda*—*Astanga Sangraha* and *Astanga Hridaya*. *Charaka* emphasized on therapeutics, *Vagbhata* focused on the principles and practice of medicine and Susruta dealt mainly with anatomy and surgery. The yoga concept of physical and mental culture to preserve the health of body and the mind developed in India. Even when the *Aryan* influx into India brought in *Ayurveda*, other systems of medicine such as *Siddha* and *Chintamoni* existed in this subcontinent, especially in the south from pre-Aryan times. The Buddha (sixth century BC) and his disciples practiced medicine and consequently healing of the sick was given great importance.

Arabic and Middle Eastern countries share the tradition of Arabic folk medicine and the *Unani* adopted Greek medicine. It was essentially taken from *Galenic* teachings during the early Islamic period. Several names stand out prominently among those who developed this system; lbn Sina of Andalusia in Spain, Al-Mansur of Baghdad, Avicenna, Razi, Rhazes and others. The backbone of the theoretical instruction was the Alexandrian Canon, which summarized a few books compiled by *Galen*. The major works in *Unani* were *Al Qanun fi al-Tibb* by lbn Sina, *Continend* by *Rhazes, Kitab Al-Shifa* by Avicenna, *Al-Tarsiff by* Abu-Qasim-Az-Zahrawi and several others. Hospitals were established from the tenth century AD in several towns. Surgery and ophthalmology were practiced during this period and the works of *Unani* surgeons paved the way for development of surgery in Europe. In India the Muslim rulers popularized the *Unani* system side by side with *Ayurveda*. The golden age of *Unani* medicine was possibly the twelfth century AD.

The Chinese system of medicine had great sway over the far east from very ancient times. Several of its tenets and the herbal pharmacopeia have percolated into other systems of medicine far and wide. Though all these systems of medicine flourished during various periods in their countries of origin and the neighboring regions, many of them suffered from want of continuing research. The homeopathic system of medicine which was founded by Dr SCF Hahnemann in 1796 in Philadelphia grew into a very popular therapeutic system which continues to grow and attract large sections of people all over the world even now.

In modern times it is common to include all these traditional systems of medicine as the ***alternate systems***. These flourish along with the system of allopathic medicine in almost all the countries including the developed nations and they provide healthcare services to large sections of the population. The Government of India has accepted many of these systems as part of the healthcare delivery agencies. There are also several institutions imparting teaching in these various systems.

The growth and development of the allopathic system (modern medicine) have been much more rapid and prolific compared to the other systems. Whereas, the alternate systems are most accepted in their countries of origin, the allopathic system has gained global acceptance. The term allopathy literally means 'treatment of disease by measures which contrast the effect of the disease', in contrast to homeopathy which literally means 'treatment of disease by drugs that produce symptoms like those of the disease'. In homeopathy the doses of drugs are minute.

The sixteenth and seventeenth centuries witnessed the growth of modern physical sciences and scientific methods of study and analysis. Andreas Vesalius, born in 1514, in Brussels made extensive dissections of the human body and produced his classic in anatomy '*De humani corporis fabrica libri*' on September 1, 1543. William Harvey, a British physician, published his monumental work on circulation of blood, *de Motu Cordis* in 1628. It was Harvey who established the scientific basis of medicine. Harvey is often credited with the invention of medical research, i.e. the search for factual evidence about bodily functions and structure.

Starting in the late eighteenth century and developing with a great rapidity in the nineteenth century, the modern medical theory and practice made great progress. Discovery of the microscope by Leeuwenhoek, three hundred years ago led to the identification of the cell as the basis of biological existence. Koch's postulates laid firm basis for establishing the etiology of microbial diseases. Gregor Mendel published his observations in 1865 and laid the foundations of modern genetics. Molecular diseases were also identified in the early part of the nineteenth century. From the middle of this century the development of knowledge has been explosive. The discovery of the structure of deoxyribonucleic acid (DNA) and the advances in the study of chromosomes and the study of genetic loci which confer susceptibility to disease were of great help in understanding the nature of molecular diseases. Studies of genes, availability of techniques such as polymerase chain reaction (PCR) which helps to identify the presence of nucleic acids [DNA and ribonucleic acid (RNA)] enabled great advances in genetic medicine. Completion of the ***human genome mapping project*** made available the blueprint of the human genome. Further genomic studies which aim at identification of the effect of different genes in causing and preventing diseases have helped to understand the genetic basis of several diseases including prediction of diseases such as cancer. With the passing of every decade, the explosion of medical knowledge adds newer informations. There have been great advances in accurate genetic and molecular identification of cells, gene based therapeutics, organ transplantation and several others. More details are included in respective chapters.

Availability of monoclonal antibodies have enabled specific diagnosis of heterogenous diseases such as lymphomas and breast cancers. They are also used in targeted therapy of malignancies, immune mediated diseases and several others for which treatment used to be unsatisfactory.

Even with all the developments in various technologies aimed at unraveling the disease process and instituting treatment, often surprises do occur. This is because, unlike as in the case of other forms of engineering and technology where blueprints of all machines are available and troubleshooting is also laid out, with regards to the molecular structure and basic functions of almost all organ systems in humans and other animal species, the exact blueprint and individual peculiarities are not yet fully available. Therefore, the physician may meet with difficult situations when employment of accepted therapeutic practices or surgical interventions are followed. Severe adverse reactions such as allergy, resistance to drugs or drug reactions may be encountered. All these add to the responsibility of the physician to envisage all the possibilities and take decisions based on available evidence, but still be prepared to meet an unexpected result, if it occurs. This is the art to be played by the treating physician, despite all the science at his disposal.

Though in early periods, medicine was practiced as an art, at present it is a harmonious blend of scientific practices generously tempered with human warmth, kindness and above all, sound common sense. What is spoken of as a clinical picture is not just the photograph of a man sick in bed, it is the sum total of the patient's condition, his home, his work, his relations, friends, joys, sorrows, hopes and fears. A good physician honours his patient and his time—sympathy and understanding are lavishly dispensed and the reward is to be found in that joy of personal bond which forms the source of the greatest satisfaction in the practice of medicine.

MEDICINE AS A PROFESSION

The word 'doctor' is derived from the Latin word 'docere' which means to teach since the doctor has the function of instructing the patient and his relatives regarding treatment. Medicine, moreover is a technique (an art or a craft of a special kind) with a broad philosophy. The medical profession is supported by a plethora of scientific knowledge which is continuously growing. It is also guided by the norm of conduct termed 'ethics'. Ethics deal with the principles of morality of right and wrong. Over the centuries the ***Hippocratic Oath*** has been handed down from one to the next generation of practitioners of medical science. Though generally, the code of ethics has been attributed to Hippocrates, it is quite likely that in its present form it came into existence much later. The ethics were laid down to be followed by the students and practitioners so as to command veneration from the public and to prevent misuse of the medical knowledge and exploitation of the society. In modern times in addition to high cost of patient care, availability of invasive investigations and treatment, prenatal diagnosis of the gender of the fetus, organ transplantation and several others have contributed to unethical use of medical knowledge. This led to the creation of *ethical committees* in all institutions for controlling research on humans and animals and ensuring proper treatment to all types of patients without causing harm and subjecting the patient to exploitation. In all developed countries, governmental agencies and professional bodies have laid down clear guidelines to be followed by the medical practioners.

The progress and achievements in the field of medical sciences have been phenomenal. But in comparison to several other fields such as engineering or technology the safety margin and success rate in techniques requiring precision and skills are considerably less. For example, a failure rate of 1–2% in a major surgical procedure is still acceptable, whereas in modern industrial process this would be the same.

The position of the doctor in society was an exalted one from the early stages of human civilization. It continues to be so even in modern times since, his role in relieving human suffering has been accepted in all cultures, especially in India. To perform his task ideally, the physician should combine knowledge, skills, empathy and a readiness to serve his fellow men at all times.

The term 'service' has been defined by the Gold Foundation which promotes the program on humanism to be integrated into the medical course in the United States of America (USA). This defines service as the 'sharing of one's talent, time and resources with those in need, giving beyond what is required. This is fundamental to the physician's role'.

In India, the medical profession has come under the *Consumer Protection Act* in which the doctor is accountable for his actions. This law empowers patients to exert their right to receive proper care and consideration from the physician. The patients and their relatives can implicate the doctor for malpractice and negligence. The law requires the doctor to use the appropriate skills and care in discharging his duties to the public.

UNIVERSAL HEALTH COVERAGE

Medical treatment has become very expensive since the drugs, instrumentation, laboratory investigations, use of devices such as heart valves, pace makers, arterial stents and others are exclusive and costly. In India, there is still no universal health cover by insurance, though on a small scale insurance for medical services is available in some government and private insurers. Most countries, both rich and poor, are trying to establish universal health cover for their citizens. Such an attempt has to be established in India too.

Disparity in Medical Care among Different Parts of the Globe

The term neglected tropical diseases (NTDs) include 10 diseases affecting mostly the poorest groups in the global community. These include lymphatic filariasis, trachoma, soil transmitted helminths, onchocerciasis, schistosomiasis, leprosy, guinea worm, visceral leishmaniasis, South American trypanosomiasis (Chagas' disease) and African trypanosomiasis. They affect more than 1 billion of the global population, 50% of them being children. These are preventable and treatable, but attention towards these diseases has been suboptimal. Efforts are afoot at present to tackle these diseases on a global scale by governments, non-governmental organizations (NGOs) and the academia.

Source: Neglected tropical diseases: becoming less neglected. Lancet. 2014;383(9925):1269.

THE FINAL DIAGNOSIS

The physician approaches the patient with the total picture of the patient in mind and with the determination and skill of a detective to unravel the disease and its cause. While ascertaining the history and conducting the physical examination, an experienced observer forms an impression about the probable diagnosis and the immediate differential diagnosis. The clinical diagnosis should be supported by investigations whenever required.

The purpose of investigations may be summarized as:
- Confirmation of the clinical diagnosis, e.g. sputum for acid fast bacilli in tuberculosis or blood culture in typhoid fever.
- Assessment of the severity of affection or damage to organs, e.g. liver function, renal function, etc.
- Assessment of prognosis, e.g. biopsy in malignancy.
- Differentiation of the condition from the closest resembling disease, e.g. liver biopsy in hepatomegaly or rheumatoid factor in subacute arthritis.
- Planning the therapeutic modality, e.g. determination of acetylator status to decide on the dose of isonicotinyl hydrazine (INH) therapy.
- Follow-up of the treatment and to detect early recurrence.

The planning of investigation has to be done according to evidence-based principles, depending on their sensitivity, specificity, adverse effects, cost and usefulness.

In general, invasive procedures include biopsies of vital organs, catheterization of vital structures, angiography, contrast radiography and endoscopies. These may cause temporary or permanent morbidity and even mortality in a small number. Hence, the decision to employ them should be taken after evaluating non-invasive methods and only if the risks involved are justifiable. Over-investigation should be avoided and this is possible only if the interrogations and physical examinations are properly done. Moreover, results of the investigations should be interpreted in the light of the clinical findings, otherwise they may be misleading and may result in administering inappropriate therapy.

PROGRESS IN THE MILLENNIUM DEVELOPMENT GOALS

The Millennium Development Goals (MDGs) adopted by the United Nations in 2000 AD with the participation

Introduction to Medicine

Textbook of Medicine

Table 1.1: Progress report for different countries*

		Countries on the track to achieve the target
MDG 4	Reduction of mortality of children younger than 5 years by 2/3 by 2015 compared to mortality figure in 1990	17
MDG 5	Reduction of maternal mortality by 3/4 in 2015 in comparision with data from 1990s	13
	Achievement of targets both 4 and 5	9

* Data quoted by Bhutta ZA, Black RE. Global maternal, newborn, and child health—so near and yet so far. N Engl J Med. 2013;369(23): 2226-35.

of over 189 countries has been working at different rates of progress in different countries. The main purpose of the MDGs was to eliminate healthcare inequalities across the globe and to make health related interventions—the key factor in economic and overall development of the countries. It has now been recognized that elimination of health disorders are essential to achieve overall progress of nations and therefore, the need for adequate investments to eliminate health related problems has been universally accepted—MDG 4, 5 and 6 are healthcare related. Assessment of progress made by different countries are given in Table 1.1.

The others are in different stages of progress. MDG 6 deals with the elimination of infectious diseases—acquired immune deficiency syndrome (AIDS), tuberculosis and malaria. Many countries including India have made considerable progress even though the targets are still far away.

At present, other components have been added to the MDGs and the strategies such as to sustain the achievements have also been included.

THE CONCEPT OF GLOBAL BURDEN OF DISEASE

Prevalence of selected major risk factors in different regions of the world has been studied by international agencies such as the World Health Organization (WHO) and others, both governmental and non-governmental. This information has been utilized to estimate the global prevalence of disease and disability adjusted life years (DALY). Maternal and childhood underweight, tobacco smoking, alcoholism, unsafe sex practices and hypertension account for the majority of the leading causes of global burden of disease. In the poor regions of the world, maternal and childhood underweight, unsafe sex practices, unsafe drinking water, poor sanitation and hygiene, indoor air pollution by smoke from burning solid biofuels and various micronutrient deficiencies were the main contributory factors.

In both the developed and poor countries alcohol, tobacco, hypertension and high cholesterol levels were equally prevalent.

THE CONCEPT OF CHRONIC NON-COMMUNICABLE DISEASE BURDEN

Since 1950, this problem has been recognized. Diseases related to lifestyles, which are slowly progressive such as obesity, diabetes mellitus, cardiovascular diseases (ischemic heart disease, hypertension, cerebrovascular diseases), chronic respiratory diseases [especially tobacco and other smoke related chronic obstructive pulmonary disease (COPD)] and various forms of cancer are increasing all over the world. This problem is more prevalent in the developing countries. In them non-communicable diseases (NCDs) occur at an earlier age and lead to mortality of younger individuals. Hence, this problem is more serious in developing countries. Developed nations have initiated measures to bring down the incidence and prevalence of these diseases, whereas the developing nations has yet to take remedial measures. NCDs contributed to 34.5 million deaths out of the total 52.8 million that occurred worldwide in 2010. The world health assembly has endorsed the goal to reduce NCD deaths by 25% by the year 2025 (25 by 25 goal). The key intervention for achieving this goal should be:

- Cessation of tobacco use
- Reduction of salt intake from 2 to 3 g/day to lower the blood pressure
- Care of patients with cardiovascular diseases and hypertension
- Improvement of financial resources and good primary care
- Universal health insurance to take care of medical expenses
- Reduction in use of alcohol.

RECORDING OF MEDICAL DATA

Recording of data is important and the method of recording has been considerably improved in recent years. The ***problem-oriented medical record (POMR)*** is a generally accepted form, which greatly helps data retrieval and also helps the physician to make decisions on the spot.

Flowcharts giving the design of management have been constructed for many of the common ailments. These help the physician to plan investigations and institute sequential therapy. Customized computer softwares designed for use in doctors' clinics and hospitals are available commercially. The doctor of the future will have to use them in order to keep up with modern progress and to guide him in his day-to-day work.

Many professional associations have produced consensus statements for the diagnosis, management and prognosis of several common diseases. These have to be strictly complied with by the doctors of the future, since such consensus statements are based on evidence based information. Though the doctor has freedom to decide on management strategies in individual cases under special circumstances, in general, consensus statements come up as ready and reliable data sources. This also will help as safeguards against litigations which may come up.

In India, the Association of Physicians of India and several specialist association have brought out such documents.

The electronic case record has been adopted in many institutions. These facilitate proper recording, updating and retrieval. It also facilitates analysis of data, transfer of data to other institutions for consultation and regular follow-up. One disadvantage is the infringement on the privacy of the patients' medical status.

EVIDENCE-BASED MEDICINE

This branch of medicine has developed during the past five decades. Several modern investigative and therapeutic modalities are very expensive, invasive and are liable to legal scrutiny. The doctors have great responsibility in recommending such procedures. Evidence-based medicine (EBM) gives the status report on

- The efficiency of the modality
- Risks involved regarding mortality and morbidity
- Cost-benefit analysis
- The improvement in the quality of life.

Collection and regular updating of objective evidence of the efficacy and safety of invasive investigations, therapeutic modalities such as drugs, surgery, invasive interventions, implanted equipment like coronary stents, organ transplantations and several others are systematically done by the process of meta-analysis of published data, multi-center and international prospective studies, reviews, seminars, international consensus conferences and other communications through the internet. There are several accepted bodies such as the Medline, Pubmed, Cochrane library, Embase and others which collect, analzse and store data for reference by scientists. This data is available on the internet. Decisions taken by the doctor have to be supported by such evidence based consensus.

Availability of the evidence-based consensus is a firm basis for doctors to take decisions in complex and difficult situations and to defend themselves in legal matters. All modern medical men have to follow the guidelines based on evidence and justify their action if it is at variance from evidence based norms.

COMPUTERS IN MEDICINE

Computers are integral equipment for the physician's profession. Patient's data, investigations, prescriptions, consultations, referrals, can all be stored by the computer and readily retrieved. Modern information available through the internet, textbooks, prescription guides and abstracts from journals can be stored in the computer and readily accessed. There are different software designed for assisting the doctor in his clinic and office, including financial matters, drug informations, drug interactions and incompatibilities, safety information on drugs and several other facilities. Many libraries have computerized their procedures and knowledge of computer methods is absolutely essential to retrieve information from libraries and other data sources.

Transplant associations, matching of donor and recipient for transplantation, cancer registries, blood banking data, population data, epidemiological studies, genetic information of population and multicentric and multinational clinical studies have all to depend on computing methodology for performing their tasks. It will not be an exaggeration to state—computer incompetence is even more serious 'a handicap rather than total illiteracy'.

Availability of the iPad, Facebook, internet facilities on mobile phones and other similar facilities have added further innovations in the field of information technology. Most of the accredited medical journals have their websites and publications on the internet which comes out earlier than the printed edition. These can be assessed by the subscribers through these online journals. Research work and other journal articles appear in the electronic version earlier than in the printed version.

CHAPTER

2

Medical Genetics

KV Krishna Das

Chapter Summary

- General Considerations
- Human Genome Project
- Brief Account on Proteomics
- Epigenetics
- Pharmacogenetics and Pharmacogenomics
- Types of Inheritance
- Chromosomal Disorders
- Autosomal Disorders
- Down's Syndrome
- Edward's Syndrome
- Patau's Syndrome
- Sex Chromosomal Disorders
- Klinefelter's Syndrome
- Turner's Syndrome
- Trisomy of Sex Chromosomes
- Chromosomal Translocation Syndromes
- Methods Employed in Studying Genetic Disorders
- Newer Developments in Genetics Prenatal Diagnosis
- Mitochondria and Mitochondrial Genetics
- Mitochondrial Inheritance
- Mitochondrial DNA Related—Respiratory Chain Diseases
- Genetic Counseling
- Gene Therapy
- Genetic Epidemiology
- Glossary of Terms used in Genetics

GENERAL CONSIDERATIONS

Many diseases develop as a result of the interaction between genetic and environmental factors. Some diseases are predominantly genetic, e.g. achondroplasia and Turner's syndrome, other cases are predominantly environmental, e.g. typhoid fever and tuberculosis, while

Textbook of Medicine

in others, genetic and environmental factors play similar roles, e.g. diabetes and hypertension.

The observations of genetics in modern biological sciences are credited to Gregor Mendel, an Augustinian monk and a naturalist at the monastery at Brunn, Bohemia. He observed the results of breeding experiment on peas planted in his garden, for over eight years and published his paper in 1865, on inheritance patterns. He also postulated mathematical laws of inheritance, generally known as Mendel's laws. **Cytogenetic** is the genetic analysis of cells using chromosome banding techniques, designed to demonstrate the number and structural integrity of the chromosomes. Several genes are contained in each chromosome and almost all of them have been mapped. The adult human cell nucleus contains 22 autosomes and one pair of sex chromosomes. The latter contains either two X chromosomes (female) or X-and Y-chromosomes (male) respectively. Chromosomes can be studied by karyotyping, rapidly dividing tissues like the bone marrow or by growing the cells in culture media and examining them during mitosis.

Gene is that length of deoxyribonucleic acid (DNA) which acts as a functional unit. It is also termed as cistron. One gene produces one polypeptide, which may combine with other polypeptides produced by other genes to form biologically active proteins like hormones or enzymes. The term **genome** refers to the total genetic information in the cell. This information is contained in the DNA content of the cells which is distributed between the nucleus and the mitochondria. The nuclear genome is large (3×10^9 base pairs) and the mitochondrial genome is small consisting of 16.6 kilobases.

The size of fragments of double-stranded DNA is indicated by their length in base pairs (bp) or nucleotides. Each chromosome carries several thousand genes. The DNA from all the human chromosomes exceed 3 billion nucleotide base pairs.

Genetic disorders may be classified as:

- Single gene disorders
- Polygenic disorders
- Chromosomal disorders.

Single gene disorders are those involving a mutation or change in a single gene, e.g. achondroplasia, thalassemia, sickle cell disease, hemophilia and others. In these the genetic change is sub-microscopic and hence, these have to be demonstrated by other methods. Polygenic disorders are those which arise from the combined influence of multiple small genetic defects. Chromosomal disorders are those in which a change or alteration of the chromosomal number or pattern can be demonstrated, e.g. Down's syndrome, Klinefelter's syndrome or Turner's syndrome. In these the genetic alteration involves large portions of the chromosomal structures so as to become demonstrable microscopically.

Genetic information is contained in DNA. It has a double stranded structure, twisted in the form of a helix, and distributed along the chromosomes. The strand consists of deoxyribose residues linked by phosphate bonds (covalent phosphate diester). Each strand is connected with one of the four bases—adenine, thymine, cytosine or guanine. The bases on the opposite sides in the two strands are aligned together as base pairs by hydrogen bonds. Adenine always pairs with thymine and cytosine with guanine.

The role of the DNA is to contain and transmit genetic information. This information is encoded by the sequence of bases. DNA transmits this genetic information by unraveling its two strands and exposing previously paired bases, thus forming a template for assembly of a new strand of nucleic acid. If the information is to be propagated to daughter cells, the new strand of nucleic acid synthesized is more DNA. This process of propagation is called **replication**. If the information is to be used by the cell, the new strand is ribonucleic acid (RNA). This process is called **transcription**.

RNA differs from DNA in having ribose as its sugar and the base uracil instead of thymine. Uracil, like thymine forms base pair with adenine.

The 'transcribed' RNA acts as a **messenger RNA** (mRNA), which travels from the chromosome on which it is synthesized to the cytoplasmic ribosomes, where it directs the assembly of amino acids into proteins. This process is called **translation**. The amino acids are carried to the ribosomes by small RNA molecules called transfer RNAs (tRNAs). Each of the 20 amino acids has one or more specific tRNAs.

Common Terms used in Genetic Studies

Diploid cells: These are somatic cells having two sets of chromosomes, each set derived from either parent, totalling 23 pairs in each cell.

Haploid cells: These are cells containing only half the number of chromosomes that are seen in somatic or body cells. These are germ cells of the ova and sperms.

Autosomes: These are the chromosomes other than sex chromosomes. X and Y are the sex chromosomes— the female pattern being X-X and male pattern being X-Y.

Alleles: These are one of two or more different genes containing specific inheritable characteristics that occupy corresponding portions (loci) on paired chromosomes. If the alleles are identical, either dominant or recessive, such an individual is termed homozygous for that particular gene. If one of the alleles is abnormal and the other is normal, such an individual is heterozygous for that particular characteristic.

Aneuploidy: This is the condition in which the chromosomal number is abnormal for the particular species.

If one of the pair of genes is altered in such a fashion that it manifests itself in a clinical disorder even when present in a single dose, it is called a **dominant gene**. If the mutant gene has to be present in double dose to express itself as a disorder, it is termed as **recessive gene**. Thus, both the genes of that pair are abnormal, one derived from each parent.

In general, it is seen that single gene disorders occur with a frequency of 10 per 1000 births. Of these, 6 are autosomal dominant, 3 are autosomal recessive and 1 is X-linked recessive. Autosomal dominant disorders are mild and variable in manifestation due to the presence of the other gene (allele) which may be normal. On the other hand autosomal recessive disorders are more severe and uniform in pattern since, both the genes are abnormal. The X-linked recessive disorders are intermediate in severity.

General Characteristics of Chromosomes, Nucleoproteins and Genes

Chromosomes

Chromosomes appear as colored bodies when stained with suitable dyes. They carry the genes which transmit hereditary characteristics. Gene carrying chromosomes are mainly found in the nucleus of the cell.

Morphology

- **During rest:** When the cell is not dividing, the individual chromosomes cannot be distinguished.
- **During cell division:** During cell division (mitosis or meiosis), the individual chromosomes **become shorter and thicker** (rod-like) and assume **x-shape**. The two identical strands called **chromatids** are held together by narrow region known as **centromere**. The centromere divides the chromosome into two arms. The **short arm** labeled the 'p arm' (p, from French, petit) and the **long arm** of the chromosome is labeled the 'q arm' (queue). The position of the centromere differs from chromosome to chromosome and gives each chromosome its unique shape.

Components of chromosome (Fig. 2.1)

Chromosomes consist of:

- **DNA:** Double-stranded, helical chain of nucleotides which consists of
  - Nitrogenous base
    - Purines: adenine (A) and guanine (G)
    - Pyrimidines: cytosine (C) and thymine (T)
  - Deoxyribose sugar
  - Phosphate molecule
    } Chromatin
- **Protein** which consists of approximately equal parts of
  - Basic core protein namely **histone**
  - Acidic **non-histone** protein
- **Small amount of RNA**.

Each chromosome consists of a single, enormously long, linear deoxyribonucleoprotein fibre, consisting of

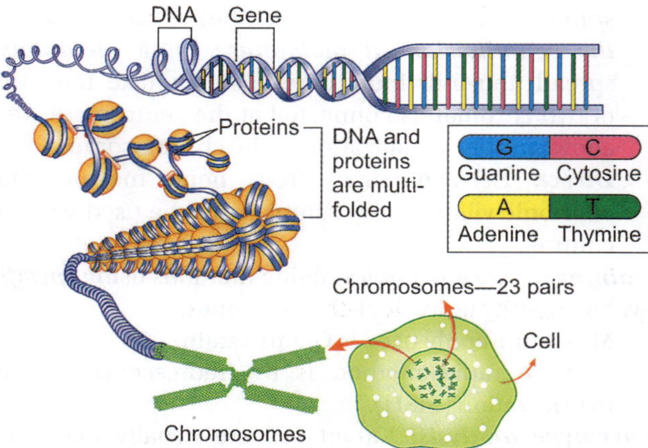

Fig. 2.1: *Structure of chromosome, DNA and gene*. Strands of DNA are wound and packed tightly into chromosomes located within the nucleus of a cell. The basic units of heredity consist of segments of DNA called genes

mixture of DNA and protein (histones and non-histone). This folds in a specific manner and pack the DNA into a more tightly packed (compact) complex structure called **chromatin. Thus, chromatin consisting of** complex of DNA and protein forms the basic unit of a chromosome structure.

Types of chromosomes

With the exception of germ cells (sperm and eggs) and highly specialized cells that lack DNA entirely (such as red blood cell), each human somatic cell contains chromosomes arranged in two sets of 23, each per cell (total 46 chromosomes). One set is inherited from the father and the other from the mother. The maternal and paternal chromosomes of a pair are called homologous chromosomes. Each set of 23 chromosomes have two types namely: **autosomal and sex chromosomes**.

- **Autosomal chromosomes (autosomes):** Each set of chromosomes have 22 autosomes and are identified by numbers from 1 to 22. The corresponding individual autosomes in each set are identical to one another in shape and size and are named as **homologous pair**.
- **Sex chromosomes:** The X and Y chromosomes are known as the sex chromosomes because they determine sex. The human cells contain one pair of sex chromosomes. Females have two X chromosomes (46XX) and males have one X and one Y chromosome (46XY). Morphologically, Y chromosomes is smaller than X chromosome.

Types of nucleic acids

Nucleic acids are of two types namely the DNA and RNA.

Location of DNA

- **Nuclear/chromosomal DNA:** Most of the DNA is inside the nucleus
- **Mitochondrial DNA (mtDNA):** Mitochondria contain small amount of DNA.

Structure of DNA

The structure of DNA was first described by James D Watson and Francis Crick in 1953 for which they received Nobel Prize (1962). The majority of chromosomal DNA is **double-stranded helix** comparable to a twisted ladder. But, it is single-stranded at the end of chromosomes, where it is called telomeres.

Nucleotides

Each DNA (and also RNA) strand consists of **chain of nucleotides**.

Structure of nucleotide unit: Each **nucleotide chain** is made up of three main components namely: (1) Nitrogenous base, (2) deoxyribose (ribose in case of RNA) sugar and (3) phosphate molecule.

- **Nitrogenous base:** These bases include purines and pyrimidines
  - **Purines:** The purine bases are adenine (A) and guanine(G)
  - **Pyrimidines:** The pyrimidine bases are thymine (T), cytosine (C) and uracil (which usually takes the place of thymine in RNA).

Textbook of Medicine

Pairing of nitogenous bases: Adenine (A) pairs with thymine (T) and cytosine (C) with guanine (G) to form a base pair.

- ***Deoxyribose sugar moiety:*** It is a pentose sugar with five carbon atoms
- ***Phosphate molecule.***

Bonds between nucleotides: The ***two nucleotide chains*** of DNA are ***held together*** by two types of molecular forces.

1. ***Hydrogen bonds:*** These are formed between the nitogenous bases on opposite nucleotide strands. They are always between a purine and pyrimidine nitogenous base only.
   - Adenine base on one strand always pairs with thymine on the other strand (A-T or T-A).
   - Guanine base on one strand pairs with cytosine on the other (G-C or C-G).
2. ***Phosphate diester bonds:*** These bonds are between sugar molecules.

Genes

Gene is defined as a ***segment of DNA*** which carries the genetic information. Gene is basic physical and functional unit of heredity. DNA also has segments which do not contain genes.

The human genome contains about ***30,000–40,000 genes*** and each gene varies in size.

Structure of gene (Fig. 2.2)

Each gene consists of a specific sequence of nucleotides. Genes may be silent or active. When active, the genes direct the process of protein synthesis. Genes do not code for proteins directly but by means of a genetic code. The ***genetic code*** consists of a sequence codeword called ***codons***. A codon for an amino acid consists of a sequence of three nucleotide base pairs called a ***triplet codon***.

Regions of gene

- ***Initiator and stop codons:*** The boundaries of a gene are known as start and stop codons. The start codon tells when to begin protein production and stop

(termination) codon tells when to end the protein production.

- ***Coding region:*** The nucleotide sequence between the start and stop codons is the core region known as ***coding region***. This region is divided into two main segments namely exons and introns
  - ***Exons:*** This region codes for producing a protein
  - ***Introns:*** These are regions between exons do not code for a protein (non-coding region).

Most genes contain both exons and introns, the number of which varies with different genes.

- ***Regulatory regions:*** These are also non-coding regions which control gene expression
  - ***Promoters*** are regions which bind to transcription factors, either strongly or weakly
  - ***Enhancers*** is the regions which can enhance the effect of a weak promoter
  - ***Silencers*** are regulatory regions that can inhibit transcription.

Karyotyping

The chromosomal constitution of a cell or individual is known as the ***karyotype***. The normal human karyotypes contain 22 pairs of autosomal chromosomes and one pair of sex chromosomes. Normal karyotype for females is denoted as 46,XX and for males as 46,XY. Study of ***structural patterns*** of the chromosomes in a sample of cells is known as ***karyotyping***. This includes both ***the number and appearance (photomicrograph) of complete set of chromosomes***. In karyotyping, the chromosomes in pairs are arranged in according to the decreasing order of size and is numbered 1–22. The 23rd pair is the sex determining (X and Y) chromosomes (Figs 2.3A and B).

Source of chromosome: Karyotyping requires cells capable of growth and division. The dividing cell is arrested at the metaphase of cell cycle. Cells for chromosomal study may be obtained from either by culture or directly.

- ***Culture:*** Peripheral blood lymphocytes are the more commonly used cells for chromosomal study. They are ***cultured in a media***. The cell is stimulated to produce cell division, through the addition of a mitogen (e.g. Phytohemagglutinin). Culture is treated with ***mitotic spindle inhibitors*** (e.g. colchicine) which will ***arrest the cell division at metaphase***. In a ***metaphase*** spread, the individual chromosomes take the form of two chromatids connected at the centromere. This allows proper visualization of the chromosomes.
- ***Direct:*** Cells obtained from bone marrow and chorionic villus biopsy samples may be used without culture.

Staining: There are many staining methods using ***specific dyes*** to identify individual chromosomes.

- Most commonly used is Giemsa stain.
- A more rapid method is by fluorescence in situ hybridization (FISH).

Karyotype analysis: Karyotypes are usually described using a standard short hand format in the following order:

- ***Total number of chromosomes:*** Deletion or addition of a chromosome is designated by a '+' or '–' sign. For example, Down's syndrome has one extra-autosomal

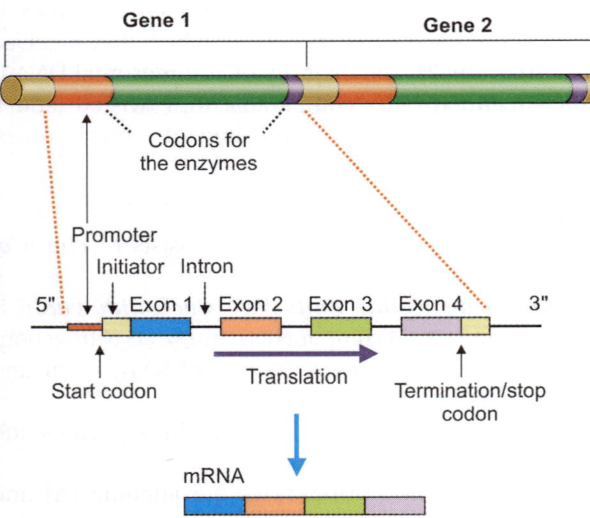

Fig. 2.2: Diagrammatic structure of gene and its mRNA product. Start and termination codons mark the limits of the gene. The coding portion of the gene is exons (four in this example) and interspersed with introns which do not appear in the mRNA product

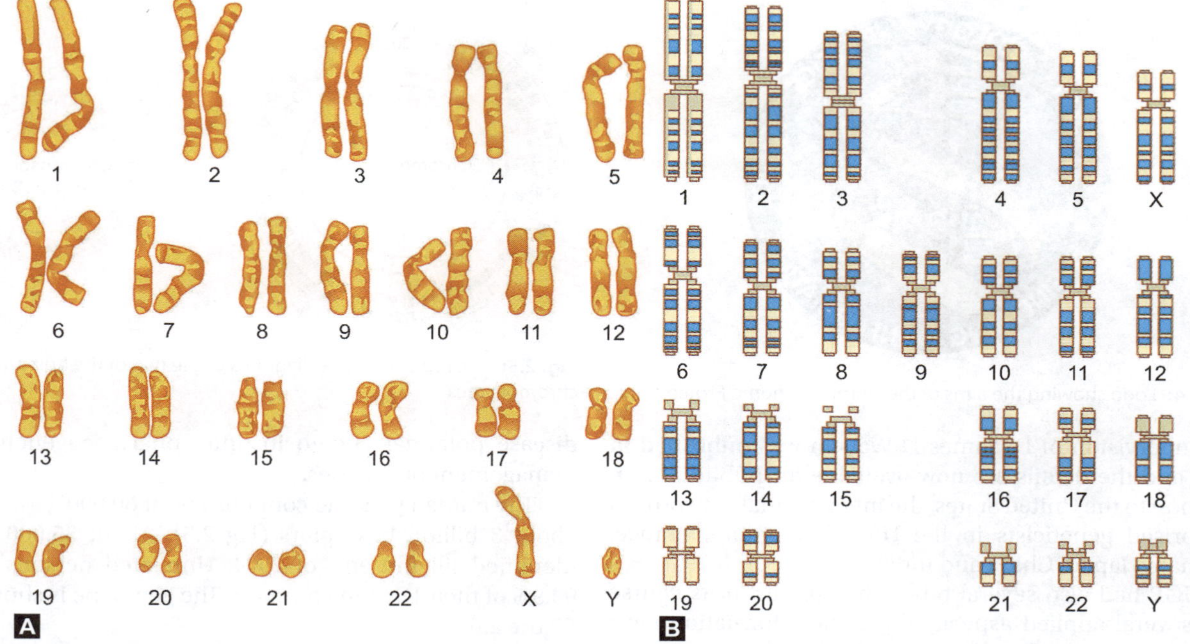

Figs 2.3A and B: A. Normal karyotype of human chromosomes—male G banding; **B.** An ideogram showing the G banding pattern

chromosome number 21 and in a male it represented as 47 XY, +21 (indicates one extra chromosome number 21).

- **Sex chromosome constitution.**
- **Description of abnormalities in ascending numerical order.**
- **Short arm or long arm:** Each chromosome has a short arm designated as 'p' (petit) arm and a long arm designated as 'q' (queue) arm. If a part of one arm is missing, it is indicated by '-ve' sign following the chromosome and arm in which it is missing. For example, in Cri-du-chat syndrome, it is designated as 46 XY, 5p- (indicating deletion of short arm of chromosome number 5).
- **Region:** Each arm of the chromosome is divided into two or more regions. The regions are numbered (e.g. 1, 2, 3) from the centromere outward.
  - Bands and sub-bands: Each region is further subdivided into bands and sub-bands and these are ordered numerically as well. This will help for precise localization of the gene. Example: The notation Xp21.2 refers to a chromosomal segment located on the short arm of the X chromosome in region 2, band 1 and sub-band 2.
- **Structural changes in chromosomes.**

Several alteration may occur on the chromosomes by natural and pathological processes and due to injury by chemical and external agents. These include deletion, translocation, re-duplication and several others, which all can lead to disease processes.

HUMAN GENOME PROJECT (HGP)

Genome: A genome is the entire DNA in an organism, including its genes. The human genome is estimated to contain 80,000 genes with about 3 billion base pairs, divided among the 23 chromosomes (Table 2.1). Out of the

Table 2.1: Comparative sizes and genome numbers of a few common organisms

Organism	Genome size (base pairs)
• Epstein–Barr virus	0.172×10^6
• Bacterium (*E. coli*)	4.6×10^6
• Yeast (*S. cerevisiae*)	12.1×10^6
• Roundworm (*C. elegans*)	95.5×10^6
• Thale cress (*A. thaliana*)	117×10^6
• Fruit fly (*D. melanogaster*)	180×10^6
• Human (*H. sapiens*)	3200×10^6

23 different chromosomes, 22 are **autosomes** (numbered 1–22) and 1 pair forms the **sex chromosomes** (X and Y). Even today functions of majority of the discovered genes are unknown.

Gene mapping: It is the process of identifying and sequencing each and every human gene of the human genome. The map of the human genome provides a picture of locations and structures of genes. There are two different types of mappings: **physical mapping** and **genetic mapping**. These maps are interdependent and complementary.

1. **Genetic mapping (linkage analysis):** A genetic map describes the order of genes and defines the position of a gene relative to other loci on the same chromosome.
2. **Physical mapping:** Physical mapping indicates the position of genes in a chromosome, which is determined by physical distances (measured in base pairs) between genes.

HGP (Fig. 2.4) is a highly ambitious project to map the genes and understand the genomes of humans and other organisms. It was undertaken by the National Institute of Health (NIH), Bethesda (USA) with active participation from many other laboratories internationally and was completed ahead of schedule. The project was started in 1991 and the first draft sequence of the human genome was published in 2001. The completed work done under

Textbook of Medicine

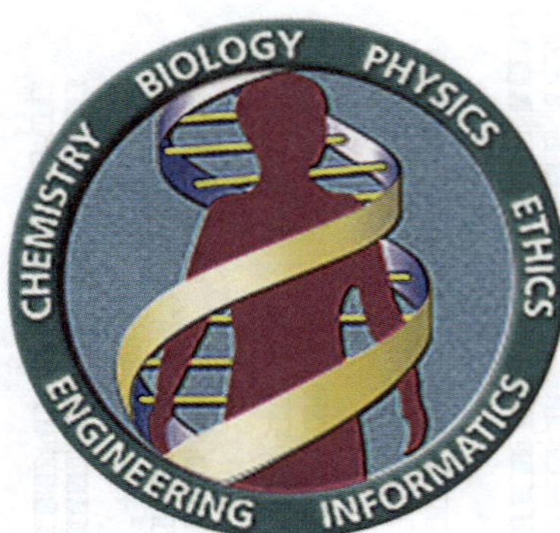

Fig. 2.4: Logo showing the aims of the Human Genome Project

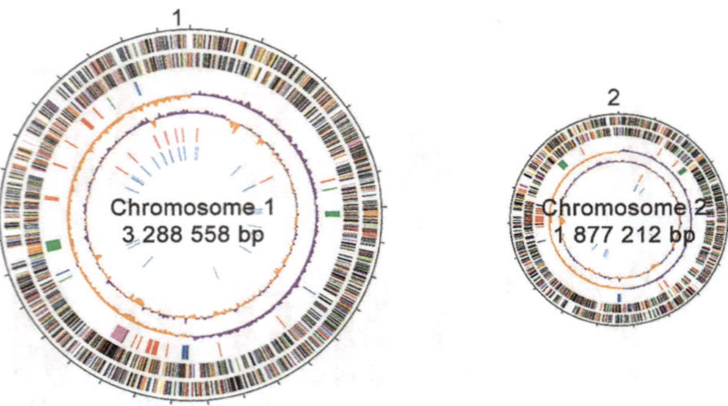

Fig. 2.5: The representative diagrams of the two of the human chromosomes

the supervision of Dr James D Watson was published in 2003 and the details are now available for public use. In addition to the United States, the international consortium comprised geneticists in the United Kingdom, France, Germany, Japan, China and India.

HGP had also several other sub-studies in its course and several applied aspects of genetic information have been published. Genetic maps giving many thousands of genetic variations (polymorphisms) throughout the genome are available. In addition to the original observations, more than four million single nucleotide polymorphisms (SNPs) have been identified. The work is still in progress to unravel the specific relationship to disease processes, detailing newer genes and their effects and applying genetic information for clinical use. The HGP also acts as a nodal agency to define ethical aspects of human genome research.

Studies on genome constitution of several other living organisms ranging from microbes to amphibians and mammals have progressed. Many of the genes in several other living organisms show similarity in the position and structure of the genes as seen in humans (homology—meaning similarity in position and structure, but need not be similar in function). Experimental work on such genes is being carried out with a view to further genetic studies in human health and disease.

Several subspecialties of genomic studies have evolved, such as:

Structural genomics	Study of structure of human genome
Functional genomics	Study of functions of the genes at cellular, biochemical and organismal levels including gene–gene interaction and influence of the environment
Transgenic animals	Animals produced either naturally or experimentally, which carry particular genes of interest
Knock-out animals	Animals in which gene of interest is knocked off (absent) or mutated
Transcriptomics	Study of total mRNA of the cell
Proteomics	Study of protein expression structure and protein interaction which help to study the functions and interactions of genes. It has become a major discipline in genetic studies at present
Metabolomics	Study of metabolites and metabolic networks involving genes

Genomic medicine aims at improving our understanding the ways to adopt healthy lifestyles, predict disease potential and to institute pharmacogenetics in management of diseases.

The human genome contains about 80,000 genes with about 3 billion base pairs (Fig 2.5). About 35,000 were identified till the end of 2004. Unrelated persons have 99.9% of their DNA in common. The genotype is shown in Figure 2.6.

Ninety eight percent of the genome does not code for any protein. Genes which code for proteins control metabolic functions. Several genes may code for the same protein or the same protein may be controlled by different genes. While the genes are responsible for determining the inherited characteristics, the environment is equally important in determining their expression.

Identification of genetic variations will help clinicians to subclassify diseases and tailor therapy to fit in with the genetic pattern. On an average one boy in every 100 and one girl in every 150 has a major congenital abnormality, some of which are genetically related. Less serious congenital abnormalities are at least 10 times more frequent.

Benefits of HGP

HGP will shed light on a wide range of basic questions, to identify the number of genes in humans, how cells work, how living things evolved, how single cells develop into complex creatures and what exactly happens when we are sick. The understanding of the genome provides clues for:

- Etiology of several diseases such as cancers, Alzheimer's disease mental subnormality, metabolic diseases and so on.
- Defining the pathogenesis of a disease and to study the disease processes at molecular level.

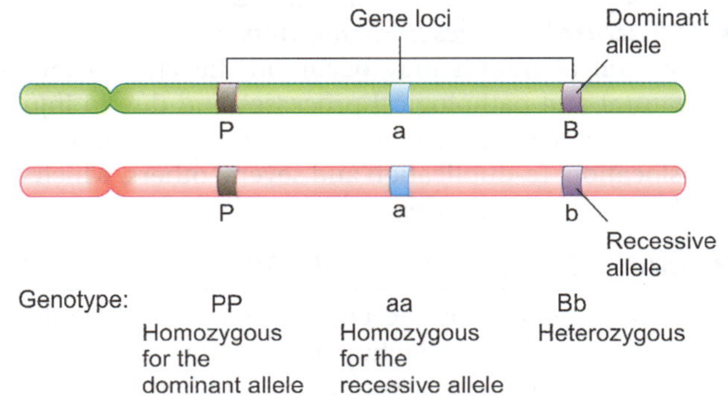

Fig. 2.6: Genotype of chromosome

- Susceptibility of an individual to a variety of illnesses, e.g. carcinoma breast, disorders of hemostasis, liver diseases, cystic fibrosis and help to take preventive measures and arrest transmission.
- Precise new ways to prevent a number of diseases that affects the human beings.
- To diagnose and treat disease. Target genes for treatment and management of diseases.
- Human development and anthropology: analysis of similarities between DNA sequences from different organisms helps to study evolution.
- Researcher: providing references about various publications required for researchers.

Ethical Issues

HGP helps to identify disease-causing genes, thereby can lead to improvements in diagnosis, treatment and prevention. It is estimated that most individuals harbor several serious recessive genes. However, completion of the human genome sequence and determination of the association of genetic defects with disease has raised many new issues with implications for the individual and mankind:

- Fairness in the use of genetic information
- Privacy and confidentiality
- Psychological impact and stigmatization
- Genetic testing
- Reproductive issues
- Education, standards and quality control
- Commercialization
- Conceptual and philosophical implications.

A Brief Account on Proteomics

Proteins are the functional units in all living tissues. The term proteome is derived from proteins expressed by a genome. It refers to all the proteins produced by an organism and thus proteome represents full sets of proteins produced by the body and it is similar to the term genome used for the entire set of genes. Human body contains more than 2 million different proteins, each having different function.

Proteomics is the study of the proteome (full set/entire library of proteins in a cell type or tissue) and its variation/relationship to disease. Various technologies of large-scale protein separation and identification are being used for this study. Study of proteomics is important because proteins represents the functioning units. Amino acids are the basic units of proteins and are very small. Each amino acid consists of atoms ranging from 7 to 24 and they are submicroscopic.

Uses: Proteomic technologies play an important role in drug discovery, diagnostics and molecular medicine. When a defective protein causing a particular diseases is detected, new drugs can be developed to either alter the shape of a defective protein or mimic a missing one.

Epigenetics

Epigenetics is a reversible, heritable change/alteration in gene expression which occurs without mutation and is unrelated to gene nucleotide sequence. Epigenomics is the study of epigenetics. Epigenetic alterations are associated with cancers and other diseases unlike genetic changes in cancer, epigenetic changes are reversible. In normal cells, the majority of the genome is not expressed. Some portions of the genome are silenced by DNA methylation and histone modifications. In some tumors epigenetic changes may directly contribute to tumor development. Epigenetic changes involve post-translational modifications of histones and DNA methylation, both of which affect gene expression. In cancer cells there is global DNA hypomethylation and selective promoter-localized hypermethylation. Such as:

- Silencing genes by hypermethylation (epigenetic mechanism)
  - Tumor suppressor genes:
    - The p 53 can be indirectly inactivated through silencing ARF by hypermethylation. This hypermethylated ARF prevents inhibition of the MDM2 oncogenic protein and the enhancement of p 53 degradation.
    - BRCA1 in breast cancer
    - VHL in renal cell carcinomas
  - DNA repair genes: Mismatch-repair gene MLH1 in colorectal cancer.

Hypomethylation: The genome of cancer cells may also undergo global DNA hypomethylation. Gene hypomethylation can cause chromosomal instability, depression of growth regulatory genes and overexpression of anti apoptotic genes which may induce tumors.

Clinical Applications

- Use of epigenetic tumor markers
- Use of epigenetic therapeutic agents (e.g. azacitidine, decitabine, vorinostat) in the treatment of myelodysplastic syndromes (MDS) and lymphoma.

Pharmacogenetics and Pharmacogenomics

Pharmacogenetics or pharmacogenomics is the study of interaction between genetics and therapeutic drugs.

Pharmacogenetics is the study of unexpected drug response resulting from genetic cause.

Pharmacogenomics is the study of identifying genetic differences within a population that explain certain observed responses to a drug or susceptibility to a health problem.

Applications

- To develop a drug that has maximum therapeutic effect and produce least damage to adjacent healthy cells.
- To prescribe drugs depending on the patient's genetic profile so as to reduce the adverse reactions.
- To determine the accurate dosage.
- To determine drug responses in the treatment of cardiac, respiratory and psychiatric conditions.

Targeted therapy can be applied by testing the abnormal gene to the influence of specific drug. This method is in vogue for the treatment of chronic myeloid leukemia, lymphomas, other hematological malignances, lung cancer, breast cancer and several others.

Prevention of Genetic Disease

- *Preimplantation diagnosis:* Before conception (i.e. when one or two of the parents are carriers of a certain trait). The human embryos can be produced using assisted reproductive techniques such as *in*

Medical Genetics

vitro fertilization (IVF). IVF involves removing egg cells from a woman's ovaries and fertilizing them with sperms outside the body and culture to blastomeric stage. One cell is then studied by polymerase chain reaction (PCR) or gene probe technique to detect genetic markers of diseases.

- **Prenatal testing:** These tests are performed on fetus or embryo before it is born to detect changes in a fetus's genes or chromosomes
  - Amniocentesis
  - Biochemical, cytogenetic and DNA studies
  - Transcervical chorionic villous biopsy [chorionic villous sampling (CVS)].
- **Newborn or neonatal, childhood screening**
- **Screening test in adolescence and adulthood**
- **Genetic counseling.**

TYPES OF INHERITANCE

The laws of inheritance are referred to as Mendelian inheritance forms, after Gregor Mendel, the 19th century monk whose experiments led to the laws of *segregation of characteristics, dominance* and *independent assortment*. He did hybridization experiments in garden pea and proposed laws which were known as Mendelian law of genetics.

- Autosomal recessive
- Autosomal dominant
- X-linked recessive
- X-linked dominant.

The pattern of inheritance is determined by taking a family history to cover three generations in full and constructing a pedigree.

Autosomal Recessive Inheritance (Figs 2.7 and 2.8A to E)

- Both parents are carriers of the disease. In the affected offspring one mutant gene comes from one parent, the other mutant gene in the pair is from the other parent.
- The affected individuals are in one generation. This is, therefore, called the horizontal transmission.
- Males and females are equally affected.
- There is a 25% chance of recurrence in siblings, if both parents carry the abnormal gene. In other words, on an average, one-fourth of the children manifest the disease. Another 50% become carriers, 25% may be normal.

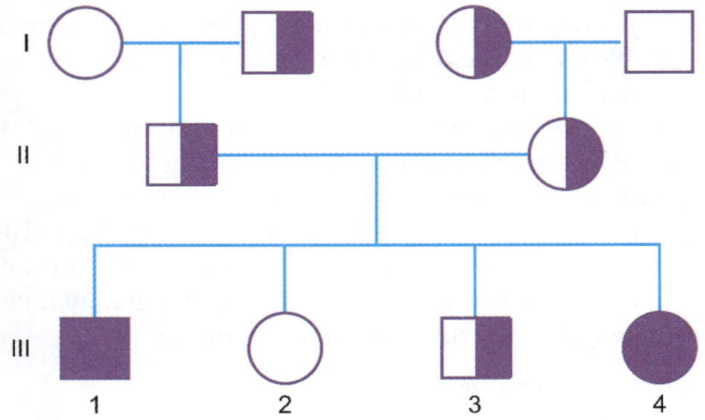

Fig. 2.7: Pedigree of a disorder with autosomal recessive inheritance (horizontal transmission). Roman numerals I-III indicate generations. The number 1–4 indicate siblings. Blacked out symbol means an affected individual. Those with one-half blackened indicate carriers

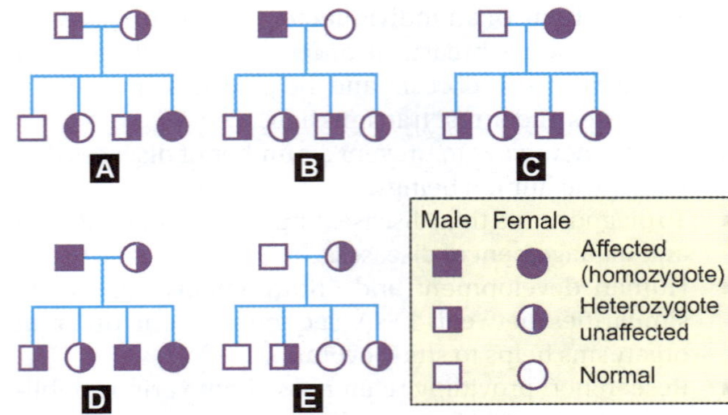

Figs 2.8A to E: Pedigree illustrating mechanism of autosomal recessive transmission. **A.** Both parents are unaffected heterozygotes; **B and C.** One parent is sufferer (homozygous) and other is normal; **D.** One parent is sufferer and other is unaffected heterozygote; **E.** One parent is normal and other is an unaffected heterozygote

- There is often consanguinity in the parents. The more rare the disorder in question, the more likely it is that the parents are consanguineous. Each individual is the carrier of 6–8 harmful autosomal recessive genes. In a consanguineous marriage, there is a greater likelihood that the offspring would inherit the same mutant gene from the parents, as a proportion of the genes are common in consanguineous parents, e.g. Friedreich's ataxia, phenylketonuria, Fanconi's syndrome. Autosomal recessive diseases are common to skip generations and appear in subsequent generations. Absence of disease manifestation should not be taken to mean disappearance of the abnormal gene from the kindred. Healthy siblings of an affected person have a two-third risk of being carriers.

Examples of autosomal recessive disorders: hemoglobinopathies, beta thalassemia, autosomal recessive polycystic disease of the kidney, Wilson's disease, cystic fibrosis, pyruvate kinase deficiency.

Pseudodominant Inheritance

Pseudodominant inheritance refers to the observation of apparent dominant (parent to child) transmission of a known autosomal recessive disorder. This occurs when a homozygous affected individual has a partner who is a heterozygous carrier, e.g. sickle cell anemia or congenital deafness due to *connexin 26* gene mutation.

Autosomal Dominant Inheritance (Figs 2.9 and 2.10A to C)

- The affected individuals are in more than one generation and if in the pedigree one draws a line through the affected individuals, it will be a vertical line. Hence, it is also called 'vertical transmission.'
- Males and females are equally affected.
- There is a 50% chance of recurrence in siblings, irrespective of sex. In other words, on an average, one-half of the children are affected.
- A male-to-male transmission provides evidence that the disease is not X-linked but is autosomal dominant.
- Occasionally, both parents of an affected child are normal. In such cases, it is presumed that the offspring has acquired the disease by a new mutation in the gametes of one of the parents. The more an autosomal

Textbook of Medicine

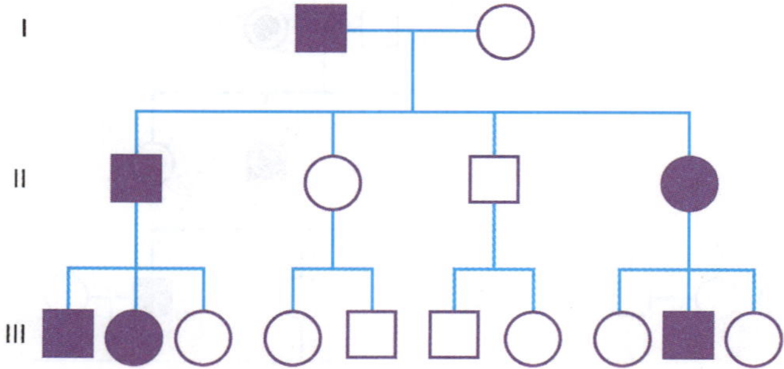

Fig. 2.9: Pedigree of a disorder with autosomal dominant inheritance (vertical transmission). Normal persons do not pass on the trait to their offspring

disorder limits reproduction, the higher is the rate of new mutation for that disorder. Where the disorder arises by a new mutation, the risk of recurrence in future siblings is negligible.

- Occasionally, an offspring affected by an autosomal dominant disorder is born to normal parents, while one of the grandparents is affected. In such cases it is presumed that the parent on the side of the affected grandparent has the gene but is not manifesting the disease. Such genes are considered *nonpenetrant*.
- The clinical manifestations in an autosomal dominant disorder vary considerably in the same family. This is partly explained by the fact that only one of the genes of a particular pair is abnormal, while the other gene is normal. The degree to which the presence of a gene is expressed clinically is termed as the *expressivity*. If the expressivity is reduced to an extreme extent so that there is no clinical manifestation, such a gene becomes *nonpenetrant*, e.g. achondroplasia, Huntington's disease and Marfan's syndrome.

Risk of recurrence in subsequent children in couples with one carrying the abnormal gene is 50%. If both the parents carry the abnormal gene the risk is 75%. In 25% of children both the abnormal genes may be inherited from the parents and the disease manifestations can be severe and even lethal.

Examples of autosomal dominant inheritance are depicted in table (Table 2.2).

Achondroplasia, autosomal dominant polycystic disease of the kidney, Huntington's disease, neurofibromatosis type 1 and 11, hereditary hemorrhagic telangiectasia, hereditary spherocytons and several others.

Pleiotropy

This term denotes the various and different effects caused by a gene in different organ systems, e.g. the various manifestations of neurofibromatosis type 1. It may be seen that different members of the same family carrying the abnormal gene may show different manifestation of the disease in differing degrees. This variability is due to the effect of interaction between different genes, by which the phenotype manifestations are modified. This type of genetic interaction is known as *epistasis*.

Sex Chromosome Related Disorders

In all females, one of the 'X' chromosome derived from either parent undergoes inactivation at the early period of gestation, in a random manner governed by the laws of probability *Lyon's hypothesis* (1961). Females, therefore contain a mosaic of tissue cells containing either the maternal or the paternal X chromosome. Inactivation of the X chromosome is effected by the action of a gene called the X-inactivation specific transcript, which is located in the long arm of the X chromosomes. Since 50% of the X chromosomes in carrier females are normal, they do not manifest signs of the disease, but male offspring's suffer from the disease.

X-Linked Pattern of Inheritance

Almost all sex-linked Mendelian disorders are X-linked. Males with mutations affecting the Y-linked genes are usually infertile. *Expression of a X-linked disorder* is different in males and females. Though X-linked disorders may be inherited either as dominant or recessive, almost all X-linked disorders have recessive pattern of inheritance.

- *Females:* They inherit one X chromosome from each parent (46, XX). The clinical expression of the X-linked disease in a female is variable, depending on whether it is dominant or recessive. Females are rarely affected by X-linked recessive diseases. However, they are affected by X-linked dominant disease.
- *Males:* They inherit only one X chromosome from mother and Y chromosome from father (46, XY). Males have only one X chromosome and gene mutation affecting X chromosome is fully expressed even with one copy, regardless of whether the disorder is dominant or recessive.

Characteristics of X-linked Inheritance

- Males are more commonly and more severely affected than females.

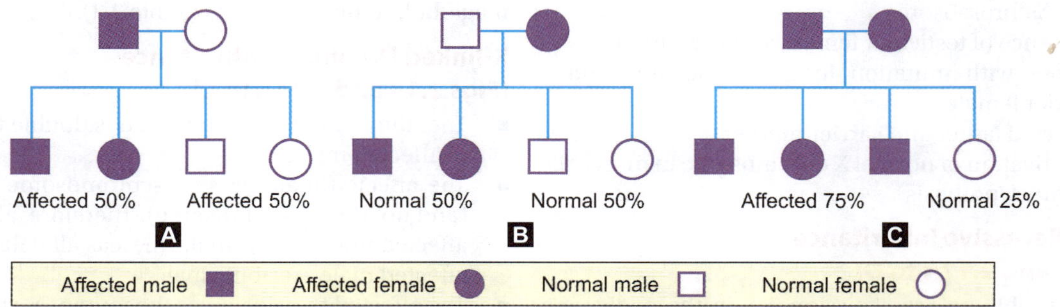

Figs 2.10A to C: Pedigree illustrating autosomal dominant transmission. **A.** Male parent is affected; **B.** Female parent is affected; **C.** Both parents are affected

Table 2.2: Examples of autosomal dominant and autosomal recessive disorders

System	Related autosomal dominant disorder	Related autosomal recessive disorder
Nervous	Huntington disease, neurofibromatosis	Neurogenic muscular atrophies, Friedreich ataxia, spinal muscular atrophy
Skeletal	Marfan syndrome, achondroplasia	Alkaptonuria
Metabolic	Familial hypercholesterolemia	Cystic fibrosis, phenylketonuria, lysosomal storage diseases, galactosemia, hemochromatosis, glycogen storage diseases
Hematopoietic	Hereditary spherocytosis, Von Willebrand disease	Sickle cell anemia, thalassemia
Renal	Polycystic kidney disease	
Gastrointestinal	Familial polyposis coli	

- Female carriers are generally unaffected, or if affected, they are affected more mildly than males.
- Affected males will have only carrier daughters.
- Carrier women have a 25% risk for having an affected son, a 25% risk for a carrier daughter, and a 50% chance for a child that does not inherit the mutated X-linked gene.

X-linked recessive traits

- This pattern of inheritance constitutes a small number of clinical conditions.
- ***Location of mutant gene:*** Mutant gene is on the X chromosome and there is no male to male transmission.
- ***Required number of defective gene:*** One copy of mutant gene is required for the manifestation of disease in males, but two copies of the mutant gene are needed in females.
- ***Sex affected:*** Males are more frequently affected and manifest disease than females; daughters of affected male are all asymptomatic carriers. In many diseases, males do not survive.
- ***Pattern of inheritance:*** Transmission is through female carrier (heterozygous). Mothers are always carriers and all their sons are affected. The disease is never passed from father to son.
- Very rarely, a female can develop the disease due to:
  - Female having Turner's syndrome (XO) with only one X chromosome.
  - Presence of testicular feminization syndrome.
  - Father with mutation in X chromosome and a carrier female.
  - Affected father and carrier mother.
  - Inactivation of normal X chromosome in most cells (Lyon Hypothesis).

X-linked Recessive Inheritance
(Figs 2.11 and 2.12A to D)

- There is 'oblique' transmission, i.e. in the pedigree a line drawn through the affected persons is oblique.
- Only males manifest the disease, females act as carriers.

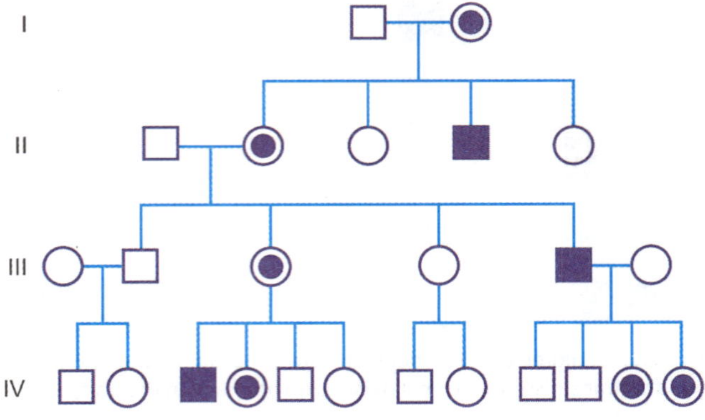

Fig. 2.11: Pedigree of a disorder with X-linked recessive inheritance (oblique transmission). Circles with dots in the center represent carrier females

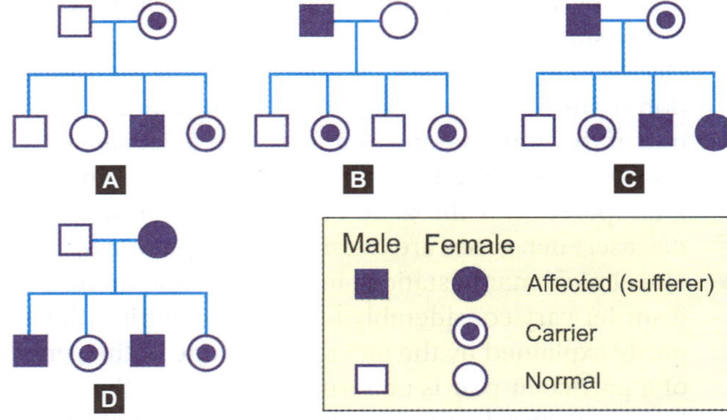

Figs 2.12A to D: Mode of X-linked recessive transmission. Note the absence of male-to-male transmission. **A.** Male is normal and female is a carrier; **B.** Male is sufferer and female is normal; **C.** Male is a sufferer and female is a carrier; **D.** Male is normal and female is a sufferer

- For the offsprings of a carrier female there is a 50% chance of sons being affected and a 50% chance of daughters being carriers.
- Among offsprings of an affected male, none of the sons will carry the trait, while all the daughters will be carriers.

A female may manifest an X-linked trait if the normal X chromosome is inactivated during early fetal life or if she is the offspring of a carrier female and affected male, or if the unaffected X chromosome is structurally abnormal, as in Turner's syndrome.

X-linked recessive inheritance, e.g. hemophilia, christmas disease, pseudohypertrophic muscular dystrophy, G6PD deficiency, X-linked ichthyosis, X-linked agammaglobulinemia and others (Table 2.3).

X-linked Dominant Inheritance
(Figs 2.13 and 2.14A to C)

- The number of females affected is double the number of affected males.
- The affected male passes Y-chromosome to his sons (and not the X-chromosome). Therefore, all sons of an affected male are normal, whereas all daughters of an affected male are abnormal.
- The affected female passes the mutant X-chromosome to half her daughters and to half her sons and therefore, half the daughters and half the sons are affected.

Table 2.3: Examples of X-linked recessive disorders

System	Related X-linked recessive disease
Musculoskeletal	Duchenne muscular dystrophy
Blood	• Hemophilia A and B • Glucose-6-phosphate dehydrogenase deficiency
Immune	Agammaglobulinemia
Metabolic	Diabetes insipidus
Nervous	Fragile-X syndrome

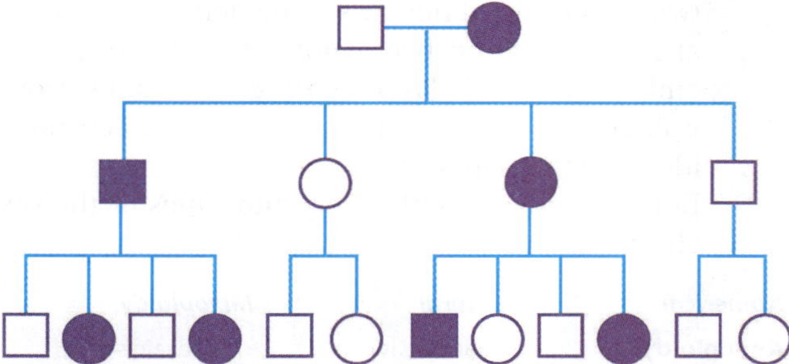

Fig. 2.13: Pedigree of a disorder with X-linked dominant inheritance. Double the number of females than males are affected

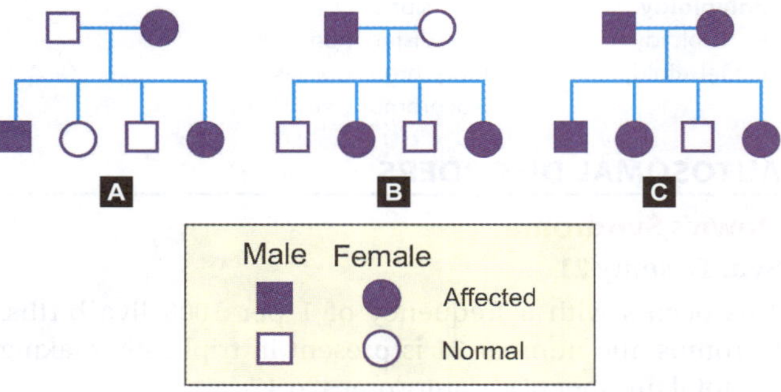

Figs 2.14A to C: Typical pedigree of X-linked dominant transmission. Only females are affected. Usually males who inherit the mutant allele die in utero. **A.** Normal male and female affected (sufferer); **B.** Affected male and normal female; **C.** Both male and female are affected

The disease is usually milder in the female, because of the normal gene on the other X-chromosome, examples of X-linked dominant inheritance include hypophosphatemic type of vitamin D resistant rickets and other rare disorders.

Y-linked Diseases

These are characterized by:

- Only males are affected
- An affected male transmits the disorder to all his sons but not to his daughters
- Most Y-linked genes are related to male sex determination and reproduction and are associated with infertility. Therefore, it is rare to see familial transmission of a Y-linked disorder.

Eg: Leri-Weill dyschondrosteosis, Langer mesomelic dysplasia.

Digenic Inheritance

Digenic inheritance explains the occurrence of *retinitis pigmentosa* (RP) in children of parents who each carry a different RP-associated gene. Both parents have normal vision, but the offspring who were *double heterozygotes* developed RP. Digenic pedigrees exhibit characteristics of both autosomal dominant (vertical transmission) and autosomal recessive inheritance (1 in 4 recurrence risk).

Polygenic Disorders

Polygenic disorders (or disorders due to multifactorial inheritance) are caused by the additive effect of several minor abnormal genes and environmental factors. These are some of the commonest disorders encountered in clinical practice, e.g. anencephaly, spina bifida, talipes equinovarus, congenital dislocation of the hip, diabetes mellitus, essential hypertension, coronary artery disease, and asthma, etc.

In such disorders the environmental factors also play a major part in the development of clinical abnormality. Inheritance of genetic traits goes a long way in the genetic makeup, physical and mental characteristics, propensity to develop diseases and response to therapy. With the acquisition of considerable knowledge of human genetics great stress is laid on taking genetic history and identifying genetic defects and providing gene based therapy.

Triplet Repeat Expansion Disorders

This disorder is caused by expansion in the number of three-base-pair repeats. An error in replication can result in expansion of that number, referred to as premutation. There is a clinical correlation to the size of the expansion, with a greater expansion causing more severe and/or earlier age of onset for the disease. The observation of increasing severity of disease and early age of onset in subsequent generations is termed *genetic anticipation* and is a defining characteristic of triplet repeat expansion disorders. Examples of triplet repeat expansion disorders are:

- Huntington—CAG
- Myotonic dystrophy—CTG
- X-linked spinal and bulbar muscular atrophy—CAG
- Spinocerebellar ataxia type I—CAG
- Fragile X syndrome (FRAXA)—CGG
- Fragile site FRAXE—CGG
- Machado-Joseph diseas—CAG
- Friedreich's ataxia—GAA

CHROMOSOMAL DISORDERS

These are disorders in which abnormalities in the number or pattern of chromosomes are demonstrable. The abnormality may involve the autosomes or sex chromosomes. Characteristics of autosomal disorders are:

- Mental retardation
- Retardation of physical growth
- Congenital malformations
- Dysmorphic features.

Sex chromosome disorders are characterized by:

- Abnormalities of body configuration
- Gonadal abnormalities
- Abnormalities of the genitalia and secondary sexual characters
- Disturbances of sexual and reproductive function.

Several chromosomal disorders are associated with higher incidence of other congenital abnormalities or neoplasms, e.g. congenital heart disease in Turner's syndrome, acute leukemia in mongolism.

Classification

Chromosomal aberration may be grouped into three broad classes:

1. *Structural*
2. *Numerical chromosomal aberrations*

   Normal cells are diploid containing 46 chromosomes, 22 pairs of autosomes and 1 pair of sex chromosomes. The 23 chromosomes (22 autosomes and one sex chromosome) constitute a haploid. Any exact multiple of the haploid number is called euploid. The total number of chromosomes may be either increased or decreased. The deviation from the normal number of chromosomes is called as numerical chromosomal aberrations.

   Types of numerical aberrations

   - *Aneuploidy:* It is defined as a chromosome number that is not a multiple of 23 (the normal haploid number). It is caused by either loss or gain of one or more chromosomes. Aneuploidy may result from nondisjunction or anaphase lag.
     - *Trisomy:* Numerical abnormalities with the presence of one extra chromosome are referred to as trisomy (2n + 1). It may involve either sex chromosomes or autosomes. For example in Down's syndrome patients have three copies of chromosome 21(47 XX, +21), hence Down's syndrome is often known as trisomy 21. This criteria is also in Patau syndrome (trisomy 13; 47 XY, +13) and Edward's syndrome (trisomy 18; 47XY,+18).
     - *Monosomy:* Numerical abnormalities with the absence or loss of one chromosome (2n–1) are referred to as monosomy. It may involve autosomes or sex chromosomes. Monosomy of autosomes is almost incompatible with survival because of loss of too much genetic information. Example for monosomy of sex chromosomes is Turner syndrome, in which the girl is born with only one X chromosome (45 XO) instead of normal XX (46 XX).
   - *Polyploidy:* Polyploidy is chromosome number that is a multiple greater than two of the haploid number (multiples of haploid number 23). Triploidy is three times the haploid number (69), tetraploidy is four times the haploid number (92). Polyploidy is incompatible with life and usually results in spontaneous abortion.
3. *Mixoploidy*
   - *Mosaicism*
     - Defined as the presence in an individual, or in a tissue, of two or more cell lines that differ in their genetic constitution but are derived from a single zygote, i.e. they have the same genetic origin.
     - Usually results from non-disjunction in early embryonic mitotic division with persistence of more than one cell line.

- Seen in 1–2% cases of Down syndrome.
- Also seen in Duchenne muscular dystrophy.

- *Chimerism:* Defined as the presence in an individual or in a tissue, of two or more cell lines that are derived from more than one zygote, i.e. they have different genetic origin. Chimera—mythological Greek monster that had the head of a lion, body of a goat and tail of a dragon. Chimeras are further divided into two types: (1) *Dispermic chimeras:* result of double fertilizations, whereby two genetically different sperms fertilize two ovas and the resulting two zygotes fuse to form one embryo and (2) *Blood chimeras:* results from exchange of cells, via the placenta between non-identical twins in utero.

  Both may involve either the autosomes or the sex chromosomes.

Numerical	Structural	Mixoploidy
Aneuploidy	• Translocations	• Mosaicism
• Monosomy	• Deletions	• Chimerism
• Trisomy	• Duplication	
• Tetrasomy	• Insertions	
Polyploidy	• Inversions	
• Triploidy	• Non disjunction	
• Tetraloidy	• Ring chromosomes	
	• Isochromosomes	

AUTOSOMAL DISORDERS

Down's Syndrome

Syn: Trisomy 21

This occurs with a frequency of 1 per 1000 live births. Chromosome number 21 is present in triplicate, making the total number of chromosomes to 47.

Maternal age: It has a *strong influence* on the incidence of trisomy 21. Children of older mothers have much greater risk of having Down syndrome.

The risk for mothers less than 25 years of age to have the trisomy is about 1 in 1500 births. At 40 years of age, 1 in 100 births. At 45 years 1 in 40 births.

Other factors: Increased incidence may be associated with exposure of mother to pesticides, electromagnetic fields, anesthetic drugs, alcohol and caffeine.

The clinical features include: (i) Marked hypotonia: easily appreciated by lifting the infant up in one's arms, (ii) Poor Moro's reflex, (iii) Flat facies, (iv) Upward slant of eyes, (v) Small circular and dysplastic ears, (vi) Loose folds of skin near the neck, (vii) Clinodactyly of little finger (short and incurved), (viii) Dysplastic middle phalanx of little finger and (ix) dysplastic pelvis (Fig. 2.15).

Radiologically the iliac bones appear wide and flat with absence of projection of the posterior superior iliac spine.

Diagnosis in the older child is fairly easy. The flat facies, the upward slant of the eyes, the flat occiput, the rough and dry skin, mental and physical retardation, clinodactyly, short and broad hands with simian crease (transverse creases) and wide gap between the big toe and other toes are some of the common features. About 40%

Textbook of Medicine

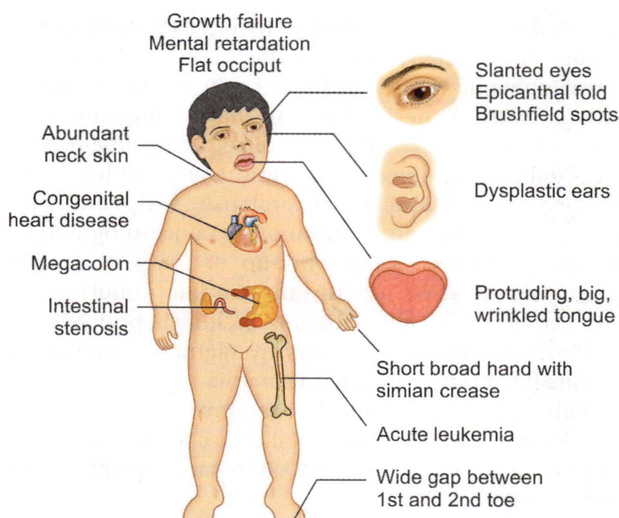

Fig. 2.15: Clinical features of Down's syndrome

have associated congenital heart disease, most commonly ventricular septal defect, endocardial cushion defects or Fallot's tetralogy and these may prove fatal in the third or fourth decades. Other adverse effects include duodenal atresia, thyroid dysfunction and early onset Alzheimer's disease. Males have reduced fertility.

Maternal serum markers are available for diagnosis of pregnancy with a Down's syndrome fetus. The alpha-fetoprotein level at 9–12 weeks of gestation is lower than normal. Other markers include maternal human chorionic gonadotropin, free beta subunit of human chorionic gonadotropin and pregnancy-associated protein A.

The incidence of Down's syndrome increases with increasing maternal age, being 1–2% in the age group of 38–45 years and 5% above this age. There is a twenty-fold increase in the incidence of acute leukemia (both acute lymphatic and acute non-lymphatic leukemia's) in Down's syndrome. Birth of an affected baby is preventable by maternal serum screening, imaging studies and selective termination of pregnancy.

Other common trisomy syndromes involve chromosomes 18, 13 and 8 and show characteristic morphological abnormalities. Deletion syndromes are those in which a part of a chromosome is lost. Common deletion syndromes involve chromosomes 4, 5 and 13.

Trisomy 18 (Edward's Syndrome)

This is the next autosomal trisomy after Down's syndrome with a frequency of (1/3000 live births). Incidence increases with increasing maternal age. Several congenital abnormalities manifest. These include lesions of the heart, central nervous system (CNS), kidneys, gastrointestinal tract and others. External features may include hypertelorism, low-set malformed ears, cleft palate, thumb abnormalities, clenched hands, joint contractures and rocker-bottom feet. Death in early life is common.

Trisomy 13 (Patau's Syndrome)

Compared to the other autosomal trisomies, this is rarer (1/10000 live births). Major congenital abnormalities involving the brain include holoprosencephaly, micro-

cephaly, microphthalmia, spinal defect, omphalocele, hand abnormalities (polydactyly and overlapping fingers), feet abnormalities (rocker bottom feet) and facial abnormalities cleft palate may be present. Many of these babies die within a few months of birth.

SEX CHROMOSOMAL DISORDERS

These constitute 50% of the chromosomal disorders seen at birth. Acquisition of extra X chromosomes in the male leads to Klinefelter's syndrome. Deletion of one of the X chromosomes gives rise to Turner's syndrome which is common in females. Males also may be affected rarely.

Klinefelter's Syndrome (Fig. 2.16)

It accounts for 1–3% of infertile males and 1/1000 of live male births with the karyotype XXY. It is characterized by tall stature and small atrophic testes (less than 2 cm in length or 6 mL in volume), scanty facial, pubic and axillary hair, X-chromatin positive buccal smear and XXY chromosomal constitution. The span (the distance between finger tips of outstretched hands) is greater than the height and lower segment greater than upper segment (lower segment is the distance from heels to the upper end of pubic bone and upper segment from top of the skull to the upper end of pubic bone). The testosterone level in the blood is low or normal and follicle-stimulating hormone (FSH) and luteinizing hormone (LH) levels are increased. Almost half the patients have gynecomastia. The testes show atrophic and hyalinized seminiferous tubules and hypertrophic Leydig cells on biopsy.

In some cases the number of extra X chromosomes may be more than one, i.e. more than two X chromosomes.

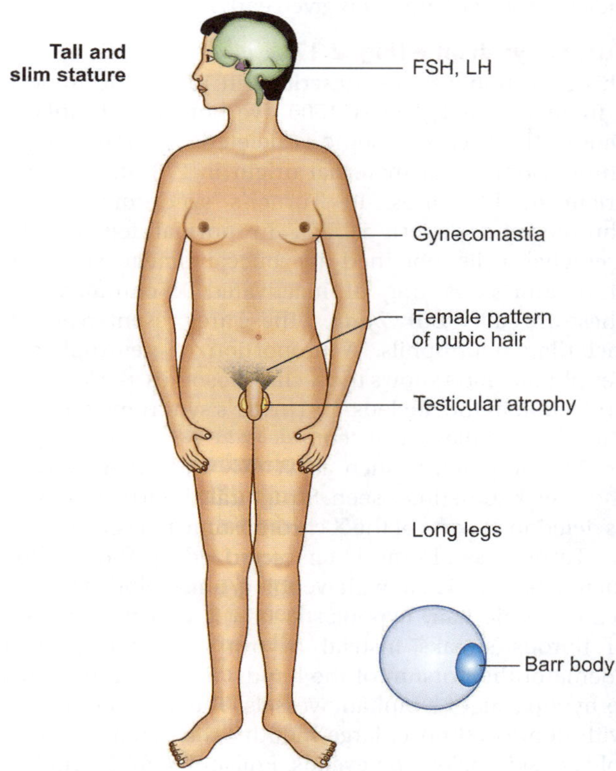

Fig. 2.16: Features of Klinefelter's syndrome
Abbreviations: FSH = Follicle-stimulating hormone; LH = Luteinizing hormone

Textbook of Medicine

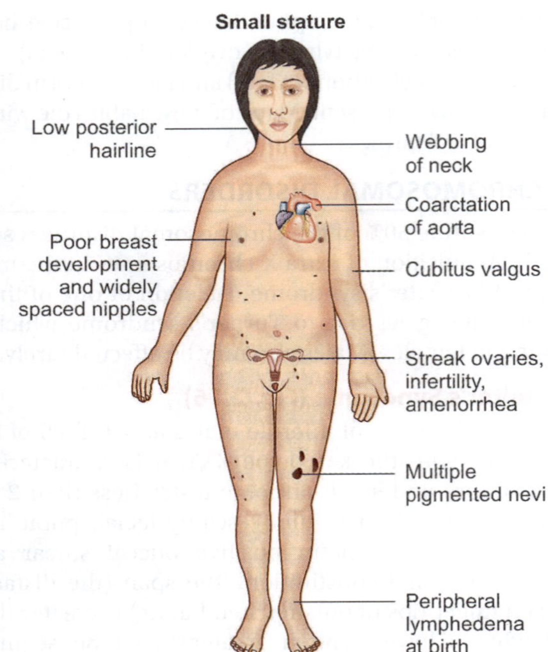

Fig. 2.17: Features of Turner syndrome

Increase in the number of X chromosomes increases the chance of mental retardation, as well as skeletal and somatic defects.

Treatment consists of administration of long acting testosterone to induce male secondary sexual characteristics during puberty. The dose has to be varied from 25 to 250 mg given IM once in three weeks. Azoospermia does not improve, though the physical features of the patient may change, if treatment is given early.

Turner syndrome (Fig. 2.17)

This condition was first described in 1938. It occurs with a frequency of 1/2500–1/1500 live born female infants. One of the X chromosome is deleted. The remaining X chromosome is of maternal origin in 2/3 and paternal origin in 1/3 cases. In Turner's syndrome the sex chromosome pattern is XO. In normal females, the epithelial cells obtained by buccal smear show sex chromatin consisting of inactivated X chromosomes. These are called ***Barr bodies***. These are present in all cells including neutrophils. A proportion of neutrophils in peripheral blood shows the X chromosomes as a knob like projection in the nucleus. In Turner's syndrome these sex chromatin bodies are absent.

Mosaic patterns such as XO/XX and others such as short neck sometimes seen. Structural abnormalities such as deletion of parts of the X chromosome may occur.

Turner's syndrome is characterized by short stature (height below 141 cm with webbing, undeveloped breasts, scanty pubic hair, hypoplastic uterus and the presence of fibrous streaks instead of ovaries. Often there is edema of the dorsum of the hands and feet at birth due to hypoplasia of lymphatic vessels. The face is triangular with depressed nose, large mouth, small chin and loose folds of skin below the eyelids. Epicanthic folds and high arched palate may be seen. The chest is shield shaped with widely separated nipples and pectus excavatum. Large

pigmented nevi, hyperconvex or hypoplastic nails, cubitus valgus, clinodactyly, short metacarpals and increased dermatoglyphic ridges on fingers may occur. 17–40% of patients with Turner's syndrome have congenital heart defects. Coarctation of the aorta, bicuspid aortic valves and left sided cardiac defects occur in the order of frequency. Hypertension, mitral valve prolapse and conduction defects are also more common. Echocardiography is mandatory in the initial work-up of cases of Turner's syndrome, so as to identify the cardiac abnormalities. Other concomitant abnormalities include hypothyroidism (15–30%), strabismus, cataracts, nystagmus, sensorineural hearing loss and recurrent otitis media.

Other stigmata include renal anomalies such as horse-shoe kidney. There is no mental retardation. Verbal IQ is lower than the performance IQ. The carrying angle of the elbow is increased.

Most patients are amenorrheic though some may show scanty periods. Replacement therapy with estrogens and progesterone after the age of 15 helps to maintain secondary sexual characters, though the height does not improve.

Therapy with human growth hormone initiated at about 5 years of age when growth retardation becomes manifest helps to restore the height partially. Supplementation of estrogens helps to retard osteoporosis. Assistance for pregnancy may be needed.

Patients with Turner's syndrome have a higher prevalence of diabetes mellitus.

Trisomy of Sex Chromosomes

XYY male—Karyotype XYY boys (also referred to as super males) present with increased growth velocity, learning difficulties and excessive acne at puberty. Testosterone levels and fertility may be normal.

XXX females (triple X females)—frequency may be 1/1000 live females births. Due to lyonization of one X chromosome, they may not show phenotypic abnormalities, other than menstrual disorders, early onset of puberty and early menopause.

Chromosomal Translocation Syndromes

These are caused by abnormal rearrangement of chromosomal parts between chromosomes, caused by fusion of parts between different chromosomes leading to abnormal phenotypic manifestations. They may lead to congenital malformations, infertility and cancers. Miscarriages and abortion are frequent complications.

Chromosomal breakages and damages have become important in modern times, since therapy employing DNA disrupting agents such as irradiation, ultraviolet light rays and alkylating agents (used in cancer, immunosuppression and others) may lead to chromosomal breakages—especially in the growing fetus. Such breakages can also occur spontaneously at times, e.g. Fanconi anemia, ataxic, telangiectasia and xeroderma pigmentosum.

METHODS EMPLOYED IN STUDYING GENETIC DISORDERS

Genetic studies are undertaken in all cases of morphological and biochemical abnormalities which may be prenatal, perinatal, postnatal or undetermined. Several techniques are employed in genetic analysis.

- **Karyotyping:** Humans have 22 pairs of autosomes and one pair of sex chromosomes. Each chromosome has a constriction along its length, called the centromere which divides the chromosomes into two arms of equal or unequal length. The short arm is called 'p' and the long arm is called 'q' for descriptive purposes. During gametogenesis the chromosome number is halved, and therefore, gametes are said to be haploid, whereas the somatic cells are called diploid. In the laboratory, chromosomal pattern is studied by arresting mitosis in a dividing cell, separating the chromosomes by suitable methods, arranging them in order and photographing them. Study of this pattern (karyotype) helps to identify deletion, addition, translocation, etc. (Figs 2.3A and B).

  Chromosomes are present in pairs. One chromosome of each pair comes from the mother and one from the father. As genes are located on chromosomes, it follows, therefore, that genes are also present in pairs.

- **Banding techniques:** By special staining techniques subtle abnormalities in individual chromosomes can be detected. The stained preparations take the form of alternate dark and light bands and the patterns are highly diagnostic. Fluorescent quinacrine (Q banding) giemsa (G banding) or R banding are generally used.

- **Gene mapping:** For gene mapping, hybrids between human and mouse cells are created *in vitro*. These hybrids progressively lose human chromosomes, until at last only one human chromosome persists. The genes on this chromosomes can be identified by studying the protein synthesis pattern of such a cell.

- **Fluorescence in situ hybridization (FISH):** Is employed to analyze chromosomes. FISH is a molecular cytogenetic technique used to detect and localize the presence of a specific DNA sequence on chromosomal and nuclear DNA. Fluorescent probes which are labelled nucleic acid sequences are used. These bind to DNA that have sequence homology. This helps to identify the test sample. FISH has contributed to great advances in molecular lab work.

- **Microarray analysis:** Is a mean to probe the expression of thousands of genes simultaneously. This method was introduced into clinical practice in the mid 1990s and it has gained wide popularity for the analysis of several genetic problems.

NEWER DEVELOPMENTS IN GENETICS

Human genes were first cloned and sequenced about the end of the seventies. From then, newer knowledge and techniques have developed explosively. The human genome has been almost completely mapped and the blueprint of the human genome is available at present. Prenatal diagnosis of genetic diseases is available for many diseases. Normal genes can be introduced into the cells of patients with genetic disorders in an attempt to correct the metabolic abnormality through complicated procedures.

Diseases such as severe combined immunodeficiency, phenylketonuria, galactosemia, hemophilia and diabetes mellitus, may lend themselves to such therapy.

Diagnostic techniques have reached an advanced stage of development at present. Some common terms used in genetic methodology are discussed later.

Restriction endonuclease: Several enzymes are used for cutting the double stranded DNA at specific nucleotide sequences. These enzymes are highly specific and give rise to predictable and uniform end products. Such enzymes are called restriction endonucleases. They are commonly used to identify the presence of the particular nucleotide sequence and to produce DNA fragments for the PCR.

DNA polymorphism: This is the inherited condition in which one or two different but normal nucleotide sequences can exist at a particular site in the DNA. Identification of DNA polymorphism can be made use of to identify the inheritance of abnormal genes that produce the disease.

Restriction site polymorphism: This is a specific type of DNA polymorphism in which the sequence of one form of polymorphism contains a recognition site for a particular endonuclease while the sequence in the other form is devoid of such a site.

Study of DNA polymorphisms is particularly useful to identify the genetic cause for metabolic defects which do not show chromosomal abnormalities. Particular DNA sequences can be identified using DNA probes. DNA probes are fragments of DNA that contain nucleotide sequences specific for the gene or chromosomal region near the region of interest.

The process by which specific DNA probes are made to bind to complementary DNA sequences is called **hybridization**. Isolation and identification of DNA and RNA are done by blotting studies. If the material being isolated and identified is DNA, the method is called **Southern blotting**, in honour of EM Southern who developed the method. If the material being identified is RNA, the method is called **Northern blotting**. Correspondingly the method used for isolation and identification of proteins is called **Western blotting**, e.g. human immunodeficiency virus (HIV) proteins.

Polymerase chain reaction: A common procedure employed in genetic analysis is the PCR by which portions of DNA that carry a particular gene are made to replicate and provide large quantities of the particular gene which is then identified by using biochemical methods. By this technique a particular portion of the genetic material can be multiplied several million folds within a short time and this can be further submitted for analysis. This method is widely used in genetic studies to analyze genes.

Other non-genetic uses of PCR are in the diagnosis of microbial infection. The nuclear material (DNA or RNA) of the microbe can be detected and quantified. In addition to perfect specificity, PCR studies can detect the infective organism early in the disease even before antibodies develop, thereby helping in early diagnosis.

PRENATAL DIAGNOSIS

Many genetic and other disorders can be diagnosed *in utero*. Biochemical tests in pregnant women provide evidence for abnormal pregnancy, e.g. rise in serum alpha-fetoprotein in spina bifida and anencephaly, reduction in

Textbook of Medicine

urinary estriol in fetal malformations. Direct evidence of fetal abnormality can be provided by imaging techniques such as ultrasonography or genetic analysis of fetal tissues. Materials for prenatal genetic diagnosis include fetal blood cells obtained by amniocentesis and fetoscopy done at 15–16 weeks of pregnancy under ultrasonographic control and chorionic villus biopsy done towards the end of first trimester by the cervical route. Such procedures are widely undertaken in many parts of the world including a few centers in India. Establishment of major genetic disorder gives the chance for parents to accept abortion. With the availability of assisted reproduction techniques like *in vitro* embryo transfer, pre-implantation genetic investigations are done in order to eliminate genetically defective embryos.

MITOCHONDRIA AND MITOCHONDRIAL GENETICS

Mitochondria (MC) are the only organelles in the cell besides the nucleus, that contain their own DNA called mtDNA and their own machinery for synthesizing RNA and proteins. There are numerous mitochondria per cell and each contains approximately five mitochondrial genomes. The MC is a 16569 base pair double stranded circular molecule containing 37 genes. 24 genes are needed for mt DNA translation and 13 genes code subunits of the respiratory chain. Approximately 900 gene products in the organelles are encoded by nuclear DNA (n DNA) and are imported from the cytoplasm. Structurally MC have four compartments—the outer membrane, the inner membrane, the inter membrane space and the matrix (the region inside the inner membrane). MC perform numerous tasks such as pyruvate oxidation, Kreb's cycle and metabolism of amino acids, fatty acids and steroids. The most crucial function is the production of energy as adenosine triphosphate (ATP) by means of electron transport chain and the oxidative phosphorylation system, the respiratory chain.

The mitochondria are present in the cells of both sexes, but mitochondrial diseases are transmitted exclusively through females. The exclusively maternal transmission is explained by the fact that the contribution of the ovum in forming the cytoplasm of the zygote is far more than that of the sperm. Both sexes suffer from the mitochondrial diseases. They exhibit extensive phenotypic variability. Offsprings of affected male does not suffer from the disease whereas, all the children of affected female have chance of developing the disease.

Mitochondrial Inheritance (Fig. 2.18)

An individual's mitochondrial genome is entirely derived from the mother. Mitochondrial disorders exhibit maternal inheritance, a woman with a mitochondrial genetic disorder will have only affected offspring of either sex, while an affected father will have no affected offspring. Examples include **MELAS** (myopathy, encephalopathy, lactic acidosis and stroke like episodes), **MERRF** (myoclonic epilepsy associated with ragged red fibers) and **Kearns-Sayre syndrome** (ophthalmoplegia, pigmentary retinopathy and cardiomyopathy).

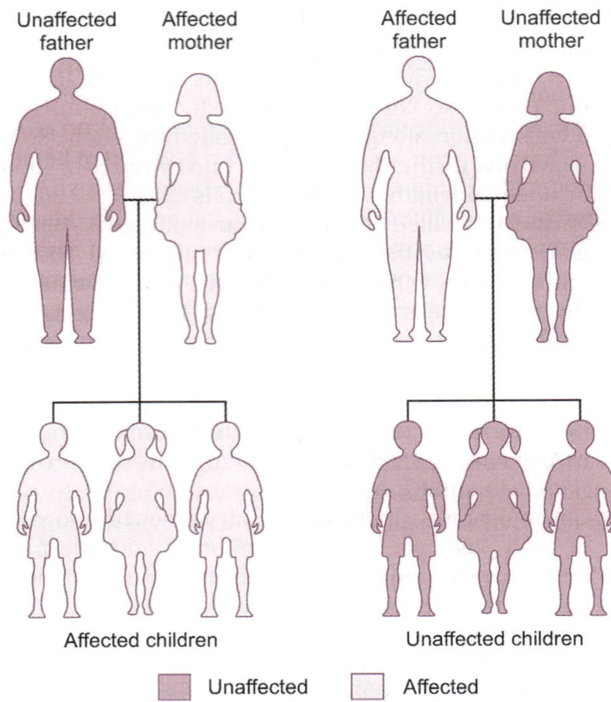

Fig. 2.18: Mitochondrial Inheritance

In MC diseases, some MC may have pathogenic mutations of mtDNA, others may be normal. This situation is known as **heteroplasmy**. The random distribution of organelles at the time of cell division can change the proportions of mutant mtDNA obtained by daughter cells and when the pathogenic threshold in a previously unaffected tissue is surpassed, the phenotype may also change. If all the mitochondrial DNA is of the same type in all mitochondria (either normal or abnormal) it is called **homoplasmy**.

Mitochondria have a crucial role in cellular bio-energetics and apoptosis and are thus important in determining support of cells and their deaths. Inherited mitochondrial diseases can be caused by mutations of mitochondrial DNA or nuclear genes that encode mitochondrial proteins. Many mitochandrial diseases are multisystemic but some are tissue specific such as optic neuropathy, sensorineural deafness and type 2 diabetes mellitus. The mitochondria are also the target of therapeutic interventions that encompass small molecules, transcriptional regulators and genetic manipulation offering treatment to a wide variety of diseases. Since the cardiovascular system and nervous system depend heavily on oxidative phosphorylation, these systems are more frequently affected in mitochondrial disease.

Mitochondrial DNA Related—Respiratory Chain Diseases

These share 2 features: Lactic acidosis and massive MC proliferation in muscle giving rise to ragged-red fiber in muscles, MC being present in all cells, many of the MC disorders produce widespread multisystem effects. Several distinct syndromes have been described depending upon the genetic alterations. Many more are being described.

Clinical features include symptoms pertaining to all systems. Some of them are listed below:

- **Nervous system:** Seizures, ataxia, myoclonus, psychomotor retardation, hemiparesis, cortical blindness, headache, dystonias, peripheral neuropathy and muscle weakness
- **Eyes:** Ptosis, retinopathy, optic atrophy
- **Blood:** Sideroblastic anemia
- **Endocrinology:** Diabetes mellitus, short stature, hypoparathyroidism
- **Heart:** Conduction defects, cardiomyopathy
- **Gastrointestinal system:** Exocrine pancreatic dysfunction
- **Kidney:** Fanconi's syndrome
- **Ear:** Sensorineural deafness.

Some examples of diseases due to mitochondrial abnormalities are:

- Mitochondrial myopathy with enecepthlopathy, lactic acidosis and MELAS syndrome
- Hereditary optical neuropathy (Leber's optic atrophy)
- Ophthalmoplegia pigmentary degeneration of retina and cardiomyopathy, Kearns-Syre syndrome
- Myoclonic epilepsy and ragged red fibres (MERRF syndrome)
- Failure of bone marrow and pancreatic function (PEARSON'S syndrome).

Management of Disease with Mitochondrial DNA Mutations

Guidelines have been published, co-enzyme Q is of benefit to patients with deficiency of this enzyme and creatine supplementation (10 g/day) is beneficial in creatine deficiency. Disease associated with abnormalities of mitochondrial genes include parkinsonism, Alzheimers disease, Huntington's disease, and several other neurodegenerative diseases–especially Leber's hereditary optic atrophy, myopathies and others. Diabetes mellitus is a recognized feature of mitochondria associated disease, mitochondria play a crucial role in glucose signaling and insulin release.

Mitochondria as Therapeutic Targets

Compounds like coenzyme Q_{10} which is an electron carrier and anti-oxidant in a dose of 1200 mg/day, slow progression of Parkinson's disease. Coenzyme Q_{10} seems to slow progression of Huntington's disease and Friedreich's ataxia and others.

Huntington's disease may benefit by the administration of creatine 10 g/day. Perioxisome proliferator activated receptor (PPAR) gamma trans-activates target genes. Drugs such as pioglitazone, rosiglitazone and others activate the (PPAR) gamma system.

Resveratrol which is a natural polyphenolic compound found in the skin of grapes substantially increases SIRTI which is an enzyme taking part in mitochondrial activity and which is used in Parkinsonism, Alzheimer's and Huntington's disease.

Indications of Cytogentic Analysis

Prenatal diagnosis of fetal abnormalities in pregnancies at risk.

Material employed: Chorionic villi of first trimester pregnancies or amniotic fluid of second trimester fetuses. Among infants and children the peripheral blood can be used. There are several other indications for genetic tests which are required under specific situations.

GENETIC COUNSELING

Genetic counseling is the process of communication which deals with the human problems associated with the birth of an abnormal child or possibility of similar incident to the concerned parents.

The steps involved are:

- Making a precise diagnosis and administering appropriate treatment.
- Reducing anxiety and guilt in the patient or parents and helping them to cope realistically with the affliction.
- Explaining the relevant genetic facts, informing them about diagnostic facilities and risk of recurrence in subsequent children.
- Helping the couple to make rational decisions regarding children in future.

Conclusions: From the days of Charles Darwin 140 years ago, genetics has made great progress so as to become a major subspecialty in medicine. It is likely to play a major role in the prediction, prevention, diagnosis and treatment of several major diseases:

Study of common diseases help to understand their mechanisms better and provide better care	Alzheimer's disease, asthma, breast cancer, heart disease, migraine and others
Re-defining disease	This helps to identify the mechanism, genotype and phenotype which will ultimately help to classify more objectively and manage more efficiently
Targeting treatment	Genetic studies help to reveal genetic makeup predisposing to disease, drug metabolism, effectiveness of drugs, etc. This helps to plan treatment more effectively
Discovering newer targets and effective treatment	In many cases the present day treatment, is the management of the final effect of the disease, e.g. diabetes, asthma, cardiac failure. Understanding the genetic pattern will help to target therapy to the basic abnormality and tackle the cause more effectively.
Providing effective preventive care.	

GENE THERAPY

Gene therapy is the insertion of genes into an individual's cells and tissues to treat a disease, such as a hereditary disease in which a deleterious mutant allele is replaced with a functional one.

The first successful attempt at transferring the normal gene for adenosine deaminase to a girl suffering from deficiency of this enzyme was performed on 14th September, 1990. Subsequently, several persons have been given normal genes in order to replace defective genes with a view to cure the metabolic defect. The procedure involves isolation of the healthy gene along with the sequences controlling its expression, incorporation of the gene on a carrier or vector as an expression cassette and finally the delivery of the same to the target cells. Gene therapy may be positive or negative. The former is the introduction of a gene whose protein product is necessary for the curative effect. Negative gene therapy implies the inhibition of the 'sick' or over expressed gene function. Though gene therapy is largely beneficial, insertion of a defective gene may lead to adverse effects in future, e.g. lymphatic leukemia in children treated with single gene therapy for severe combined immunodeficiency.

The other modality of treatment which has been successful in some of the genetically determined diseases is bone marrow transplantation, e.g. thalassemia, hemoglobinopathies.

In the gene therapy, functioning gene is introduced into cells in order to produce a protein product that is missing or defective or to supply a gene that has a novel function.

To be effective, the gene therapy requires methods that ensure the safe, efficient and stable introduction of genes into human cells.

Problems/Limitations of Gene Therapy

- *Short-lived nature of gene therapy:* Patients will have to undergo multiple rounds of gene therapy.
- *Immune response:* Gene therapy may stimulate the immune response against introduced gene and reduce the effectiveness of gene therapy.
- *Problems with viral vectors:* Viral vectors may sometimes cause potential problems to the patient like 'toxicity and inflammatory responses'. In addition, the viral vector, once inside the patient, may recover its ability to cause disease.
- *Multifactorial disorders:* Genetic disorders due to single gene mutations usually show best response to gene therapy. Unfortunately, some of the most commonly occurring disorders (e.g. atherosclerosis, hypertension, diabetes, Alzheimer's disease and rheumatoid arthritis) are multifactorial and are difficult to treat effectively using gene therapy.
- *Risk of inducing a tumor (insertional mutagenesis):* If the gene is integrated in the wrong place in the genome (e.g. in a tumor suppressor gene) it could induce a tumor.
- *Risk of death:* Deaths have occurred due to gene therapy. Therapeutic applications of gene therapy has not been approved for clinical use.

GENETIC EPIDEMIOLOGY

Genetic epidemiology which is a developing discipline is closely related to traditional epidemiology. It particularly focusses on the familial and in particular, the genetic determinants of diseases and the joint effects of genetic and non-genetic determinants.

The fusion of epidemiology and genetics provides the foundation for genetic epidemiology. Genetic epidemiology can contribute in establishing the causative role of environmentally modifiable risk factors and help in planning preventive measures in future. Pharmacogenomics is that branch of genetic study in which the appropriate dosing with maximum cost effectiveness can be selected, based on genetic information.

GLOSSARY OF TERMS USED IN GENETICS

Allele: One of two or more different genes containing specific inheritable characteristics that occupy corresponding positions on one or other (loci) of paired chromosomes.

Alternative splicing: A regulatory mechanism by which variations in the incorporation of a gene's exons or coding regions, into mRNA lead to the production of more than one related protein or isoform.

Autosomes: All of the chromosomes other than sex chromosomes and the mitochondrial chromosome.

Centromere: The constricted region near the center of a chromosome that has a critical role in cell division.

Codon: A three-base sequence of DNA or RNA that specifies a single amino acid.

Conservative mutation: A change in a DNA or RNA sequence that leads to the replacement of one amino acid with a biochemically similar one.

Missense mutation: Substitution of a single DNA base that results in a codon that specifies an alternative amino acid.

Nonsense mutation: Substitution of a single DNA base that results in a stop codon, thus leading to the truncation of a protein.

Epigenetic: A term describing non-mutational phenomena, such as methylation and histone modification, that modify the expression of a gene.

Frame-shift mutation: The addition or deletion of a number of DNA bases that is not a multiple of three, thus causing a shift in the reading frame of the gene. This shift leads to a change in the reading frame of all parts of the gene that are downstream from the mutation, often leading to a premature stop codon and ultimately, to a truncated protein.

Gain-of-function mutation: A mutation that produces a protein that takes on a new or enhanced function.

Genomics: The study of the functions and interactions of all the genes in the genome, including their interactions with environmental factors.

Genotype: A person's genetic makeup, as reflected by his or her DNA sequence.

Phenotype: The physical make up and appearance of an individual which gives the clinical picture.

Haplotype: A group of nearby alleles that are inherited together.

Heterozygous: Having two different alleles at a specific autosomal (or X chromosome in a female) gene locus.

Homozygous: Having two identical alleles at a specific autosomal (or X chromosome in a female) gene locus.

Exon: A region of a gene that codes for a protein.

Intron: A region of a gene that does not code for a protein.

Linkage disequilibrium: The non-random association in a population of alleles at nearby loci.

Loss-of-function mutation: A mutation that decreases the production and/or function of a protein.

Monogenic: Caused by a mutation in a single gene.

Motif: A DNA sequence pattern within a gene that, because of its similarity to sequences in other known genes, suggests a possible function of the gene, its protein product, or both.

Multifactorial: Caused by the interaction of multiple genetic and environmental factors.

Nonconservative mutation: A change in the DNA or RNA sequence that leads to the replacement of one amino acid with a very dissimilar one.

Penetrance: The likelihood that a person carrying a particular mutant gene will have an altered phenotype.

Point mutation: The substitution of a single DNA base in the normal DNA sequence.

Regulatory mutation: A mutation in a region of the genome that does not encode a protein but affects the expression of a gene.

Repeat sequence: A stretch of DNA bases that occurs in the genome in multiple identical or closely related copies.

Silent mutation: Substitution of a single DNA base that produces no change in the amino acid sequence of the encoded protein.

Single-nucleotide polymorphism (SNP): A common variant in the genome sequence, the human genome contains about 10 million SNPs.

Stop codon: A codon that leads to the termination of a protein rather than to the addition of an amino acid. The three stop codons are TGA, TAA and TAG.

Translation: This is the production of protein via mRNA. Most genes contain alternating regions with exons and introns.

Source:

1. WP Munjal, et al. API Textbook of Medicine. 9th edition Vol 1. Printed by Jaypee Brothers Medical Publishers (P) Ltd. 2012, Section-6, Chapter 1–10.

2. Schapira AH. Seminar. New Eng J Med. 2012;379:825-34.

CHAPTER 3

Defense Mechanisms of the Host and Clinical Immunology

KV Krishna Das

Chapter Summary

- Nonspecific Defense Mechanisms
- Specific Mechanisms
- Complement System
- Antibody Dependent Immunity
- Autoimmune Diseases
- Diagnostic Procedures in Immunology Serum Sickness
- Immunodeficiency States
- Compromised Host
- Fever in Immunocompromized Host
- HLA System in Humans
- Immunization

Nonspecific defense mechanisms		Specific defense mechanisms (immune system)
First line of defense	Second line of defense	Third line of defense
• Skin • Mucus membranes • Secretions of skin and mucus membranes	• Phagocytic white blood cells • Antimicrobial proteins • The inflammatory response	• Lymphocytes • Antibodies

Fig. 3.1: Systems of defense in sequential order

Immunology is that branch of science which deals with the immune mechanisms of the host which is concerned with the defense against microbial infections and several disease processes mediated by the immunological tissues in animals and humans. Immunology has developed and reached a high level of achievement in the past few decades. Immunological principles have helped in understanding the mechanisms of several disease processes and their management. Using immunological principles, several vaccines and therapeutic agents such as antibodies, monoclonal antibodies and similar specific tools have been developed for prevention, cure and diagnosis of several diseases which were at best only palliated till the recent past. Man has several defense mechanisms to protect him against microbial invasion. These may be nonspecific and specific (Fig. 3.1).

NONSPECIFIC DEFENSE MECHANISMS

- The skin and mucus membranes form protective barriers against bacteria. The stratum corneum which is a desiccated layer of the epidermis is impermeable to microbes. If microbes enter through wounds, the organisms are killed by neutrophils and macrophages through the mechanism of oxygen intermediates. Antimicrobial substances such as defensins and cathepsins act against bacteria, viruses and fungi. In atopic dermatitis these antimicrobial peptides may be deficient and this predisposes to bacterial infections, especially *Staphylococcus aureus*.

- Lactic acid in sweat and fatty acids in the sebaceous secretions inhibit growth of pathogenic flora. Fungal infections are common in parts devoid of sebaceous glands, e.g. interspaces between toes, the soles and the sides of the feet.

- Ciliary movement helps to carry bacteria along with mucus secretions in the respiratory tract and helps them to be expectorated. Organisms such as *Pseudomonas aeruginosa* colonize in the lungs, especially in cystic fibrosis. They form biofilms in the respiratory tract and thrive within the biofilm in a free-living planktonic state (a free-living drifting state) which resists all defense forces of the host.

Textbook of Medicine

In the normal state, inhaled pathogens are cleared by mucociliary action and natural defenses. If the bacterial population exceeds a threshold number they produce sensors which monitor the defense forces of the host and in turn, develop virulence genes which protect them against phagocytosis.

■ Mucus of respiratory and urogenital tracts possesses bactericidal properties due to the enzyme lysozyme which lysis the cell wall of the invading bacteria. Moreover, the neuraminic acid content of the mucus competitively inhibits the myxoviruses.

■ Normal commensals of the skin and gastrointestinal tract inhibit the proliferation of pathogenic bacteria.

■ Phagocytosis is the most important nonspecific mechanism by which body tries to eliminate invading organisms. Cells with phagocytic properties are:

- ***Neutrophil leukocytes:*** These are the first cells to reach the site of infection by microbes and inflammation caused by foreign matter. They engulf the microbes and foreign matter and digest them by enzymes in their intracytoplasmic vacuoles known as phagolysosomes. This reaction may be oxygen dependent or independent.

- ***Eosinophils:*** These are also phagocytic. Their role is mainly in allergic responses. Allergens and parasites (particularly helminths) stimulate antibody production of immunoglobulin E (IgE) which coats the antigen (allergen). The IgE-coated antigen is engulfed by the eosinophils which have receptors for the fragment crystallizable (Fc) portion of the IgE molecule and the eosinophils destroy the parasites by enzymic action.

- ***Monocytes:*** These (mononuclear phagocytes) are present in the circulation and also as specialized phagocytic cells in several tissues such as Kupffer cells in hepatic sinusoids, alveolar macrophages in the lung and microglia in the central nervous system (CNS). They bear large number of receptors for the Fc portion of the antibodies and therefore, they actively engulf antibody coated particulate matter. Ingested pathogens are broken down in phagosomes and the components are transported to the cell surface in a form which can be recognized by the antigen specific lymphocytes.

These macrophages carry specialized plasma membrane glycoprotein called major histocompatibility complex (MHC) molecules. When activated, the density of MHC molecules on the surface increases.

- ***Histiocytes*** in tissues.
- ***Sinus lining cells*** in the liver (Kupffer's cells), spleen and bone marrow.
- ***Reticulum cells*** in lymph nodes.
- ***Microglia*** in the CNS.
- ***Dendritic cells (DCs):*** These cells so called because of the presence of membrane or spine like projections on their surface are located in several tissues (most organs except the brain), particularly in T-cell rich areas of lymph nodes and spleen. Immature DCs are seen particularly in tissues exposed to microbes such as skin, pulmonary alveoli, gut mucosa and others. On meeting antigens they ingest the antigens, undergo maturation, lose their phagocytic capacity and become antigen presenting cells.

Foreign materials are ingested by the phagocytes and later digested intracellularly. The myeloperoxidase present inside the phagocytes also destroys viable bacteria. When the phagocytic function is reduced, generalized infections like septicemia develop leading to high mortality. Several processes aid in phagocytosis. These are:

■ Chemotaxis by complement breakdown products

■ Opsonization by specific antibodies which neutralize the negative surface charges of bacteria

■ Cytokines, such as macrophage activating factors and macrophage migration inhibition factors released by the T-lymphocytes, lead to local accumulation of active macrophages (Table 3.1).

Colloidal substances, high molecular weight substances and dyes may saturate phagocytic capacity and increase the susceptibility to infection, e.g. carbon particles in heavy smokers and silica particles in mine workers. Some organisms (e.g. *Mycobacterium leprae*) are not destroyed by the macrophages. On the other hand they multiply in the protected environment of the cell.

Components of the blood coagulation pathways interact with other defense mechanisms of the host to arrest microbial invasion and facilitate recovery.

Table 3.1: Cytokines of importance

Cytokine	Primary source	Other	Target	Effects
Interleukins Interferons factor (TNF)	Macrophages Leukocytes		Macrophages Granulocytes Tissue cells	Activation of cytotoxic cell activity, cachexia, adherence of leukocytes to endothelium
Interferons	Leukocytes T-lymphocytes natural killer (NK) cells	Fibroblast Epithelium	Tissue cells Leukocytes	Antiviral, macrophage activation
Macrophage (M) Colony stimulating factor (CSF)	Monocytes	Endothelium Fibroblast	Stem cells	Stimulation to divide and differentiate
Granulocyte (G) CSF	Macrophages	Fibroblast	Stem cells	-Do-
Migration inhibition factors (MIF)	T-lymphocytes	—	Macrophages	Migration inhibition
Chemotactic factors	Lymphocytes, macrophages, granulocytes	Tissue cells and their components	Leukocytes	Attract to site of infection or tissue damage

SPECIFIC MECHANISMS

The Immune Response

Any substance which evokes an immunological reaction is an ***antigen***. Certain components of the cell membranes act as ***specific antigens***. They differ from person to person in their chemical composition and three dimensional structure. The immunocompetent T-cells can recognize itself from the non-self. Moreover, the body can recognize one antigen from another leading to specificity of immunological reaction. Some substances are strongly antigenic, e.g. dinitrochlorobenzene, while others are weakly antigenic, e.g. bacterial capsular antigen. ***Antibody response*** is usually selective against certain important regions of the antigen, which are termed the antigenic determinant sites. A ***hapten*** is a small molecule which by itself cannot elicit antibody production, but when combined with a carrier molecule, can do so. The antibodies can combine with the hapten directly, without the help of the carrier. The presence of haptens in tissue proteins is one of the reasons for the development of autoimmunity.

The main cells involved in immune reactions are the lymphocytes. They originate from the totipotent cells of the bone marrow. Some of them pass through the thymus from where they develop to become T-lymphocytes with their specific antigens and functional capacities. They are then specialized for cell-mediated immune reactions and are recognizable by thymus specific antigens on their surface. These T-lymphocytes are found mainly in the paracortical areas of lymph nodes and periarteriolar sheaths in the spleen. On the other hand, the stem cells passing through gut and lung associated lymph nodes (bursa equivalent) are transformed into B-lymphocytes. They eventually occupy germinal centers of lymph nodes and spleen. Upon antigenic stimulation, they transform into plasma cells which synthesize the immunoglobulins which form mediators of humoral immunity. In peripheral blood, 80% of lymphocytes are T-cells, 15% are B-cells and 5% are K-cells (killer).

T-lymphocytes form spontaneous rosettes with sheep erythrocytes (*E. rosette*) at 4°C. These receptors are identified as the cluster of differentiation 2 (CD2) molecules on T-cells. They are also recognized by the presence of specific antigens on their cell surfaces, identified by monoclonal antibodies. CD3 marker is present on T-cells. T-cells include many subsets, most important ones are TH (T helper or CD4 +ve) cells carrying CD4 antigen and TS (T suppressor or CD8 +ve) cells carrying CD8 antigen. The term CD stands for 'cluster of differentiation' which refers to the monoclonal antibodies that react with particular membrane molecules, which help to group the lymphocytes, depending on the membrane molecules on them.

All T-cells have the T-cell antigen receptor (TCR) on their surface. TCR-2 contains alpha and beta chains. TCR-1 consists of gamma and delta polypeptides. Both are further associated with a set of 5 polypeptides, to form the CD3 complex or TCR complex. In human peripheral blood, 90% T-cells are TCR-2 and the remaining are TCR-1. TCR-2 cells are further divided into two groups, depending on the presence of CD4 or CD8 markers on their cell surface. The subset, which carries the CD4 marker, helps the B-cells to divide, differentiate and make antibody response, these are therefore called TH cells. CD4 T-cells recognize their specific antigens in association with MHC class II molecules. CD4 positive TH cells also carry CD29 antigen.

The CD4 positive cells are further subdivided into two subsets, depending on their capacity to produce cytokines. The TH-1 subset secretes TNF alpha, interleukin-2 (IL-2) and interferon-gamma—induces cytotoxic T-cells, enhances delayed hypersensitivity and activates macrophages. On the other hand TH-2 subset produces IL-4, IL-5, IL-6 and IL-13, which stimulates B-cells, enhances humoral immunity and activates eosinophils. A small number of CD4 cells belong to a third group, they are the memory cells (TH-M).

The second TCR-2 subset, which carries the CD8 marker, is responsible for suppressing antibody response and so they are termed as T-suppressor (TS) cells. CD8 T-cells recognize antigens in association with MHC class I molecules.

The CD8 positive cells are also subdivided into 2 subclasses. The subset that expresses CD28 molecule secretes IL-2 and is mainly suppressor in function. The other subset that carries CD18 antigen does not produce IL-2, but responds to IL-2 and is mainly cytotoxic. This group is responsible for the destruction of host cells that are infected by viruses or intracellular pathogens, they are therefore also called as T-cytotoxic (TC) cells.

B-lymphocytes are identified either by the rosette formation with sheep erythrocytes coated with antibodies and complement (*EAC rosette*) or by demonstration of surface immunoglobulins by fluorescent antibody technique. Immunoglobulins are classified into G, M, A, D and E. All B-cells carry CD19 and CD20 markers and MHC II marker. Pre-B-cells (immature B-cells) carry CD9 and CD10 markers. CD5 carrying B-cells are responsible for autoantibody production.

NK cells: These are large and granular lymphocytes, which are CD16 and CD56 positive. They do not have the membrane markers of T-cells such as CD4 or CD8 or B-cells with surface immunoglobulin molecules. They can kill and lyse a large variety of tumor cells and some viruses. They are the cells which are known as antibody-dependent cytotoxic lymphocytes (ADCL). They participate in antibody-dependent cell mediated cytotoxic reactions. Activation of innate immunity and antibody production are prerequisites for this type of reaction.

The NK cells have stimulatory and inhibitory receptors on their surface. Body's own normal cells are protected from the killing action of NK cells since the ligands for the inhibitory receptors which are MHC class 1 molecules are present in all nucleated cells in the body.

Alterations in the cellular characteristics on tumor formation make them susceptible to the destructive action of NK cells. NK cells mediate cytotoxicity through perforins which are enzymes contained in their granules. Perforins assemble within the membrane of the target cells and produce transmembrane perforin-channels. Granzymes

Textbook of Medicine

which are also enzymes of NK cells enter through the perforin channels and activate caspases. Caspases are proteolytic enzymes which initiate the programed cell death pathways known as apoptosis. In this process signaling occurs through various 'death receptors' on the surface of cells (e.g. TNF receptors). This results in the activation of the caspase family of molecules which leads to cleavage of deoxyribonucleic acid (DNA), resulting in cell death.

There are several 'death receptors' on cell surface, the most important being the tumor necrosis factor receptor (TNF receptor).

Once the antigens enter the body, they are processed by macrophages and then recognized by the antigen sensitive lymphocytes. Antigens synthesized within a cell, such as viral polypeptides are externalized and associated with MHC Class I molecules and beta-2 microglobulin. Class I molecules are present on all nucleated cells. The complexed antigen is then presented to the CD8 T-cells. By contrast, antigens that have been endocytozed are associated with MHC Class II molecules and these are then presented to the CD4 T-cells. The lymphocytes recognize the antigen by means of the receptors present on their surface. The T-cell antigen receptor (TCR) is part of the CD3 complex. Antigen recognition receptors on B-cells are made up of partly by surface immunoglobulins. When the antigen is recognized by receptor, the lymphocytes undergo morphological alterations (blast transformation) and after a series of divisions form a clone of cells which react against the specific antigen. These committed cells differentiate into plasma cells which secrete specific antibodies. Some of the remaining cells are responsible for immunological memory. Many infections and vaccinations lead to prolonged immunity due to persistence of immunological memory.

Most animals start producing specific antibodies within 10 days of injection of antigen. Initially these antibodies are mainly of IgM variety. This is the ***primary response***. When the same antigen is again introduced, the ***secondary immune response*** is elicited. The reaction occurs at a faster and augmented rate and lasts longer. This time IgG antibodies predominate. Sometimes even large quantities of antigen may not produce immune response. This is called *tolerance*, which again will be specific to that particular antigen. Tolerance acquired in postnatal life usually fades away with the passage of time. However, tolerance induced *in utero* tends to be permanent.

The effect or mechanisms involved in the immune response are as follows:
- Cell-mediated immunity
- Humoral immunity
- Antibody dependent cell mediated immunity
- NK cells mediated immunity
- Macrophage-mediated immunity.

Cell-mediated Immunity

This is mediated by the T-lymphocytes which form T-helper cells, T-suppressor cells and NK cells.

- ***Immunity against infections:*** Effective immunity against bacteria such as mycobacteria and listeria, certain viruses and almost all parasites is mediated by T-cells. T-cells from sensitized individuals lyse the target cells bearing the viruses.

- ***The rejection of allograft and destruction of tumor cells:*** These are also mediated mainly by T-cells, although other mechanisms are also involved.

- ***Helper function:*** The T-cells which express CD4 antigen on their cell surface. These are called CD4 positive cells or TH cells. They also carry receptors for the Fc portion of IgM. They form about 50% of the T-cells of peripheral blood. They are necessary for the optimal antibody production by plasma cells and for generation of cytotoxic T-cells. Moreover, they produce cytokines needed to stimulate immune response. These cytokines act in an autocrine manner on the CD4 cells themselves and in a paracrine manner on other cells. Human immunodeficiency virus (HIV) specially infects CD4+ cells with consequent destruction of these cells leading to acquired immunodeficiency syndrome (AIDS).

- ***Suppressor function:*** The suppressor cell (TS) subgroup which carry CD8 +ve antigen constitute 10% of the total lymphocyte pool. They can be distinguished by the presence of surface receptors for Fc portion of IgG. They regulate the activities of both T-and B-cells. The TS activity is depressed in many autoimmune diseases and in some of the human malignancies.

- ***Production of soluble mediators:*** Cytokines are biologically active molecules released by specific cells that elicit a particular response from other cells on which they act. T-cells stimulated by antigens liberate certain soluble substances called ***lymphokines***. These molecules produced in an antigen specific manner can act in an antigen nonspecific manner to recruit, activate and regulate effector cells with the potential to combat infectious agents. Several lymphokines and monokines (products of monocytes) are known.

Lymphokines include macrophage migration inhibition factor (MIF), macrophage activation factor (MAF), leukocyte migration inhibition factor (LMIF), leukocyte adherence inhibition factor (LAIF), chemotactic factor, interferons (IF) and interleukins (IL). The MIF and MAF help in accumulation of macrophages at the site of reaction. The resulting erythema and induration form the basis of skin tests. Administration of transfer factor to nonsensitized individuals leads to specific sensitization.

Chemokines (chemotactic cytokines) mediate inflammatory reaction. The attraction of leukocytes to the site of inflammation is central to the process. More than 40 cytokines have been identified. These are grouped mainly into 4 families. Alpha-chemokines attract neutrophils, while beta-chemokines act on monocytes, eosinophils and lymphocytes with variable selectivity. C5a (complement activation product) and leukotriene (LTB4) are generated at the site of bacterial infection and they attract macrophages and mast cells. Chemokines induce cell migration by attachment to specific G-protein controlled cell surface receptors on target cells. These chemokine receptors also act as co-receptors for infective agents such as *Plasmodium vivax* and HIV to get entry into host cells.

Interferons (IF) inhibit viral multiplication in host cells, modulate cell differentiation and inhibit oncogene expression.

The major types of IF are alpha, beta and gamma derived from leukocytes, fibroblasts and activated T-lymphocytes respectively. Gamma interferon is anti-viral in activity. It also increases cytotoxic activity of T-cells, enhances B-cell differentiation and induces respiratory burst in macrophages. Interferon is useful in the treatment of hairy cell leukemia and chronic myeloid leukemia in addition to several viral infections especially viral hepatitis C. Diagnostic tests for infections especially mycobacteria, viruses and others based on alterations in the interferon pattern are also available.

Interleukins (IL) are growth factors secreted by lymphocytes, monocytes and macrophages. There are several more than 15 different interleukins described so far. They are biological mediators which control the amplitude and duration of immune response. IL-1 stimulates production of receptors for IL-2 on lymphocytes. Moreover, IL-1 induces production of acute phase proteins, such as C-reactive protein from liver, which in turn produce fever and leukocytosis. IL-2 stimulates T-cells and NK cells so as to become lymphokine-activated killer (LAK) cells. Such specific LAK cells are being used for immunotherapy in cancer patients with promising results. IL-3 is colony stimulating factor for T-and B-cells. IL-4, 5, 6 and 7 are produced by TH cells; all of them help in B-cell differentiation. IL-5 stimulates eosinophil, IL-6 enhances myeloid cells and IL-7 increases platelet production. IL-8 is produced by monocytes and is chemotactic for neutrophils. IL-9 and 10 are general growth factors for lymphocytes.

Leukotrienes (LTs) are derivatives of arachidonic acid. The arachidonic acid may be converted to (A) cyclooxygenase products (prostaglandins and prostacyclin) and (B) 5-Lipooxygenase products (leukotrienes and lipoxins). In myeloid cells, leukotrienes A4, B4, C4, D4 are formed—the last mentioned two are components of the slow reacting substance (SRS) of anaphylaxis. LTs are chemical mediators of allergy and inflammation. LTs play important role in increasing vascular permeability and diapedesis of leukocytes. They produce bronchoconstriction, bronchial mucosal edema and mucus secretion in asthma. They have a role in pathogenesis of acute respiratory distress syndrome (ARDS) and ulcerative colitis.

- *Delayed hypersensitivity:* When tuberculin or a similar antigen is injected intradermally in a sensitized individual, an erythematous indurated lesion develops slowly, reaching its maximum within 48–72 hours. This is called delayed type of hypersensitivity. Hypersensitivity is the abnormal over-reaction of the immune system and it usually results in unwanted tissue destruction. This is responsible for caseation in tuberculosis, granulomatous skin lesions in tuberculoid leprosy, rashes in smallpox and measles, skin lesions in herpes simplex and contact hypersensitivity to chemicals and plants. Hypersensitivity reaction mediated by T-cells is called Type IV reaction.

Humoral Immunity (Fig. 3.2)

Antibodies are produced by plasma cells. These are immunoglobulins belonging to the class IgG, IgA, IgM, IgD, and IgE (Table 3.2). All except IgA are present in plasma mainly. IgA is also present in body secretions and hence, present in mucosal surfaces as well. The immunoglobulins consist of specific heavy chains and light chains. IgG is present in maximal amounts in plasma. It is mainly responsible for humoral immunity against microbial infection. Primary response produces antibodies of IgM type, while IgG antibodies predominate in secondary response. During the initial acute phase of infections IgM antibodies are formed which are replaced by IgG antibodies as the disease becomes subacute and chronic. IgG can cross placental barrier. Natural antibodies (e.g. antibodies against ABO system of RBC) are of IgM variety. They cannot cross placental barrier and so the fetus is protected. Anti-Rh antibodies, being IgG type, can cross the placenta, leading to Rh iso-immunization and consequent fetal distress.

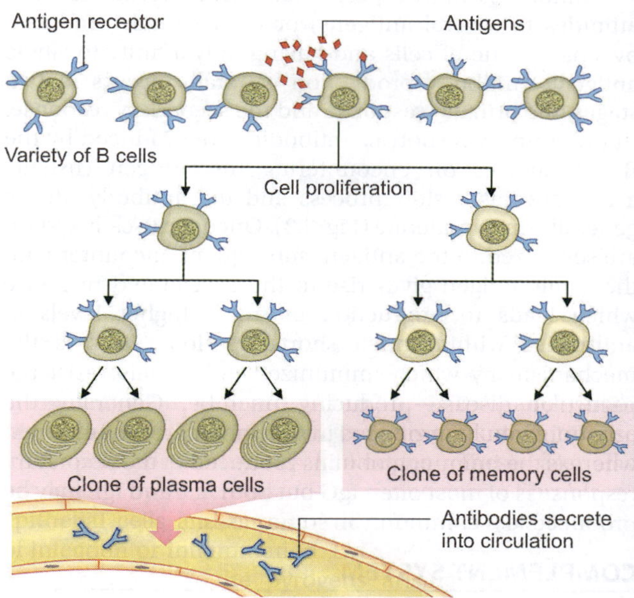

Fig. 3.2: Immune function performed by B-lymphocytes and plasma cells

Table 3.2: Characteristics of immunogiobulins					
Class	**IgG**	**IgA**	**IgM**	**IgD**	**IgE**
Heavy chain	Gamma	Alpha	mu	Delta	eta
Molecular weight	150,000	400,000	900,000	180,000	200,000
Ultracentrifuge value [S. value (Svedberg's units)]	7	11	19	7	8
Mean serum concentration (mg/dL)	1250	250	125	3	0.03
Antibody activity	+	+	+	–	+
Primary response	–	–	+	–	–
Secondary response	+	+	–	–	–
Placental crossing	+	–	–	–	–

Table 3.3: Characteristic features of various immunological arms

	T-cells	B-cells	K-cells	NK-cells	Macrophages
Cell surface marker receptor	Sheep RBC receptor surface	Complement receptor and immunoglobulins	Fc receptor surface Ig	Fc receptor	Fc receptor and complement receptor
Identification	E-rosette	EAC rosette	EA rosette	K 562 rosette	Adherence to glass surface
Mechanism of action	Direct cell mediated lysis; lymphokine production	Antibody dependent complement mediated cytolysis; agglutination	Antibody dependent cell mediated cytolysis	Direct cell mediated cytolysis	Phagocytosis
Activity against debris	Virus, parasites bacteria, cancers, transplanted organs	Bacteria, viruses	Cancers, parasites	Cancer cells	Bacteria, tissue
Hypersensitivity reaction	Type IV	Types I, II, III and V	Type VI		Type III

Humoral immunity plays a great role in conferring resistance to bacterial infection. The antibodies destroy the target cells by several mechanisms.

- Classical complement pathway
- Antibody dependent cell-mediated cytotoxicity
- Agglutination
- Opsonization of target cells, thereby making them more susceptible to phagocytosis.
- Characteristic features of various immunological effector arms are shown in Table 3.3.

Antibodies maybe polyclonal (with specificities and affinities to several antigens) or monoclonal (produced by single clone of cells and having only affinity to single antigen). Antibody production generally occurs in two stages, the primary response and the secondary response. In the primary response, antibodies are produced by the B-lymphocytes on encountering the antigen (usually a microbe) as a slow process and the antibody titre is generally only moderate (Fig. 3.3). Once the B-cells system are sensitized to the antigen, subsequent encounter with the same antigen gives rise to the accelerated response which leads to production of much higher levels of antibodies within much shorter periods. This is the mechanism by which immunized individuals resist the particular disease producing microbe. Generally the immunoglobulin produced in the primary response is IgM whereas the immunoglobulins produced in the secondary response is of most often IgG but both IgA and IgE may be produced less commonly in some cases.

COMPLEMENT SYSTEM

This consists of plasma and membrane proteins (globulins) that play a major role in host defense against microbes and in several other immunological processes such as hemolysis. They function in two major ways: (1) Opsonization of microbes and alteration in their surface membrane leading to disruption and (2) promotion of inflammatory response by altering vascular permeability and attracting inflammatory cells to the site of injury. Several of them have been named. These are C1q, C1r, C1s, and C2 to C9.

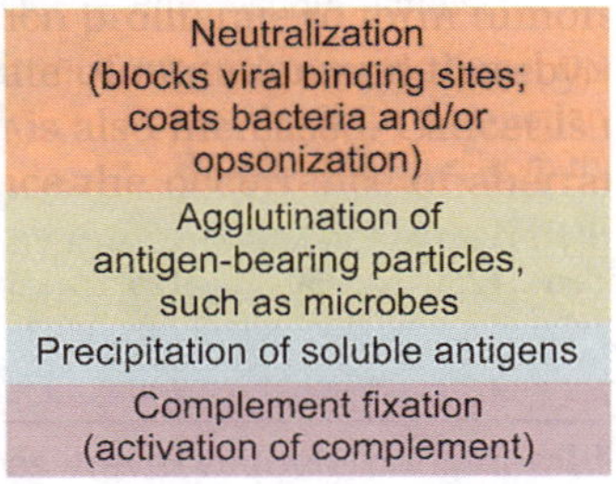

The complement system is an important component of innate immunity mechanism and it consists of about 20 different proteins present in the serum and which act sequentially with amplification at every stage leading to the production of thousands of effector molecules starting from a single molecule. The three different pathways of complement activations are listed below.

- Classic pathway activated by antigen—antibody complexes
- Alternate pathway activated by polysaccharides from yeasts and gram-negative bacteria
- Mannose binding lectin pathway activated by mannose containing proteins and carbohydrates in microbes.

Activation of any of these pathways leads to activation of C3 to C3 convertase. This leads to the formation of membrane attack complexes (MAC) which are formed from C5 to C9 complement components. Normal cells contain a number of complement regulatory proteins which inhibit the activation of the complement cascade. Microbes and pathologically altered human cells which lack the complement regulatory proteins will be subjected to lysis, whereas the normal cells will not be affected.

Abnormalities in the function of the complement pathway or absence of any of the components of the system lead to susceptibility to severe infections by pyogenic organisms, and gram-negative bacteria especially meningococcus.

Different pathways of activation and functions of the complement system. All pathways of activation lead to cleavage of C3.

Fig. 3.3: Mechanisms by which antibodies inactivate antigens (microbial and otherwise)

Complement System and Disease
Complement inefficiency:
- It results in immune deposition and inflammation, which in turn may lead to autoimmune diseases.
- Increased susceptibility to infection: Main role of complement system is defense against infection. Defective functioning of the complement system leads to increased susceptibility to infections (particularly *Neisseria meningitidis*).

Complement deficiencies: It may be acquired or congenital deficiencies of specific complement components. C1 inhibitor deficiency is associated with hereditary angioedema.

Table 3.4: Characteristics of complement components

	Serum concentration (µg/mL)	Thermal reaction	Site of synthesis	Functions
C1q	100–200	Labile	Epithelial cells of small intestine	$Clqc_2$ $c4c_3$ participate in classic pathway
C1r	—	Labile	-Do-	
C1s	20–120	Labile	-Do-	
C2	20–40	Labile	Reticuloendothelial cells (RE cells)	$C3b$, C_3b_8, $C3bBb$ (p)
C3	1200	Stable	Hepatocytes	
C4	250–400	Stable	RE cells	C_3a – participate in alternate pathway
C5	75–100	Labile	Macrophages	
C6	20	Stable	Hepatocytes	
C7	—	Stable	-Do-	
C8	10	Labile	-Do-	$(C_5b + C_8)$ C_7, C_8 and C_9 form the membrane
C9	2	Labile	-Do-	

Inflammation and necrosis: The complement system amplifies the inflammatory response. It may play a role in many diseases with an immune component, such as asthma, lupus erythematosus, membranoproliferative glomerulonephritis, multiple sclerosis, inflammatory bowel disease.

Their properties and functions are given in Table 3.4.

Acquired and inherited abnormalities of the complement system predispose to microbial infections and autoimmune disorders. For example, when antigen-antibody complexes are deposited in kidney glomeruli, complement components are activated, inflammatory cells are attracted and immune mediated glomerulonephritis develops. Complement components are used up differentially in several immune mediated diseases and therefore, measurement of serum levels of complement components gives diagnostic and prognostic information, e.g. systemic lupus erythematosus (SLE).

The complement system is activated sequentially when antibody attaches to antigen components on the cell surface. The final products create microscopic holes on the cell membrane. Osmotic entry of water through these holes results in lysis of the target cells. The complement products also activate phagocytosis, chemotaxis and immune adherence. Capillary permeability is also increased. Inhibitors of the complement are present naturally, which check the uncontrolled activity of the complement.

Apart from the **classical sequential complement pathway**, some microbial polysaccharides can activate an **alternate system (properdin system)**, thereby bypassing the initial complement components. Since this does not require specific antibodies, the alternate pathway acts as a first line of defense against invading microorganisms. However, the nonspecific nature may sometimes prove disadvantageous as in the case of complement activation by immune complexes leading to widespread tissue destruction as in type III hypersensitivity reaction.

The alternate pathway (APC) of the complement system is innate to the system. It is always active and its activity does not depend on specific sensitization. Unlike the classic pathways of complement which requires specific antibody for activation, the alternate pathway is in continuous activation.

Since the APC is always active, several inhibitors co-exist in blood which prevent their activation and lysis of normal cells. APC cascade can be divided into 2 functional units. The first is activation of C3 and C5 convertases which lead to formation of MAC which is cytolytic component of the complement system. Normal cells in the body resist the cytolytic effects of the complement system, e.g. CD55 and CD59 block the cytolytic MAC and thus protect normal RBC from lysis. Absence of these protective substances lead to hemolysis by the action of the complement system, e.g. paroxysmal nocturnal hemoglobinuria (PNH) results from absence of CD55 and CD59.

ANTIBODY DEPENDENT IMMUNITY

Hypersensitivity reactions mediated by antibodies fall into different types which are described below:

Type I Anaphylactic reaction: Introduction of the antigen (e.g., penicillin) leads to the production of cytophilic antibodies (mainly lgE) in sensitive persons. These are attached to the surface of mast cells. Unlike the other immunoglobulins which circulate in the plasma, IgE is bound to receptors especially to Fc receptor which is a distinctive receptor for beta chain, present more on basophils and mast cells and probably on eosinophils as well. Cross linking of cell-bound IgE with the multivalent antigen excites cellular processes which culminate in the liberation of chemical mediators such as histamine and serine proteins into the circulation. This brings on the anaphylactic reaction.

On subsequent exposure, the antigen reacts with the preformed antibodies causing mast cell degranulation and release of histamine, serotonin and slow reacting substance of anaphylaxis (SRS-A). This may lead to asthma due to bronchoconstriction or anaphylactic shock due to widespread capillary dilatation.

Allergens such as pollens, house dust and fungi react with cell bound lgE of the respiratory tract leading to bronchial asthma or hay fever. Allergens from food may cause urticaria.

Type I hypersensitivity reaction occurs within 30 minutes of exposure to the allergen. Such reaction can be abolished by drugs like adrenaline and sodium cromoglycate which prevent the release of histamine. Antihistamines compete with the released histamine for effector sites. Repeated introduction of the allergen in small doses results in hyposensitization.

Type II Cytotoxic hypersensitivity: Certain drugs may complex with membrane proteins of blood cells leading to production of autoantibodies. These antibodies can lyse the blood cells through the action of complement. Hemolytic anemia caused by alpha methyldopa, agranulocytosis produced by amidopyrine and thrombocytopenia induced by chlorothiazides are examples of this mechanism.

Type III Immune complex mediated tissue damage: The continued presence of antigen causes persistent antibody production. Antigen-antibody complexes form and circulate in the blood. These heavy molecules are entrapped in blood vessels, renal glomeruli, lungs, skin and joints. Complement system is activated through the alternate pathway. The complement degradation products attract polymorphs and macrophages and an inflammatory reaction sets in with resultant damage to the tissues.

Platelet aggregation occurs and these microthrombi leads to vascular occlusion and ischemia.

If the antibody is in excess, the complexes are rapidly precipitated and tend to be localized at the site of entry of antigen. This leads to Arthus type reaction. If an antigen is injected intradermally into a hyperimmunized animal, erythema and edema occur at the site of injection. This reaction reaches a peak in 3–8 hours and is referred to as intermediate type skin reaction. Farmer's lung is the classical example of localized type III reaction. On the other hand, if antigen is excess, soluble complexes are formed which precipitate in all tissues giving rise to the serum sickness type of reaction. The lumpy granule precipitates seen in renal glomeruli in post-streptococcal glomerulonephritis are due to systemic type III reaction.

Type IV T-cell-mediated hypersensitivity reaction: This is mediated by T-lymphocytes and it has been described earlier.

Type V Stimulatory hypersensitivity: Thyroid cells are normally stimulated by TSH through a membrane associated receptor. The long acting thyroid stimulator (LATS), otherwise known as thyroid stimulating immunoglobulin (TSI) is an antibody against some components of the receptor for TSH. The LATS produces TSH like activity, but the action is more prolonged. The continued stimulation by LATS leads to hyperthyroidism. Similarly, antilymphocyte globulin (ALG) is stimulatory to lymphocytes in appropriate conditions. It is used therapeutically in immune mediated aplastic anemia.

Type VI Antibody dependent cell-mediated cytotoxic mechanism (ADCC): This mechanism does not require complement activity. The effector cells are neither T-cells nor B-cells but are called K-cells. The specificity of this reaction resides in the antibody molecule. Only very small amounts of antibody are required to produce this reaction and therefore, this mechanism is effective in areas where antibody concentration may be minimal, e.g. at the site of solid tumors. The full significance of this mechanism is not known.

In certain circumstances, more than one mechanism may be operating. Thus in autoimmune damage to endocrine glands, e.g. type I diabetes mellitus, type II and IV hypersensitivity reactions are involved. Autoantibodies against insulin secreting cells, insulin molecules and insulin receptors were described. The clinical features of the hypersensitivity reactions are shown in Table 3.5.

Table 3.5: Common hypersensitivity disorders

	Skin diseases	Kidney diseases	Lung diseases	Diseases of other sites	Skin test
Type I					
Anaphylactic, IgE mediated, histamine dependent	Urticaria and rashes due to bacteria, viruses, parasites, food and drugs, atopic dermatitis		Rhinitis and asthma due to pollen dust, feathers, etc.	Penicillin reaction, food allergy	Wheal and flare reaction within 30 minutes, immediate type
Type II					
Cytotoxic antibody mediated complement dependent	Bullous pemphigoid (basement membrane), pemphigus vulgaris (desmosomes)	Goodpasture's (anti GBM) syndrome	Goodpasture's syndrome	Transfusion reactions, isoimmunization (Rh), drug-induced hemolytic anemia, thrombocytopenia, leukopenia	
Type III					
Immune complex mediated complement and dependent	Systemic lupus erythematosus (SLE)	Post-streptococcal glomerulonephritis, nephrosis of renal glomeruli	Farmer's lung due to dusts from hay, bagassosis	Arthus reaction, serum sickness, SLE	Erythema and edema, polymorphs predominate, maxiphagocyte intermediate group
Type IV					
T-cell mediated cytotoxic	Contact allergy to chemicals, granuloma in leprosy	Chronic and membraneproliferative glomerulonephritis	Granuloma and caseation in tuberculosis	Hashimoto's thyroiditis	Erythema and induration, lymphocytes predominate maximum
Type V					
Stimulatory antibody mediated				Thyrotoxicosis due to long acting thyroid stimulator	

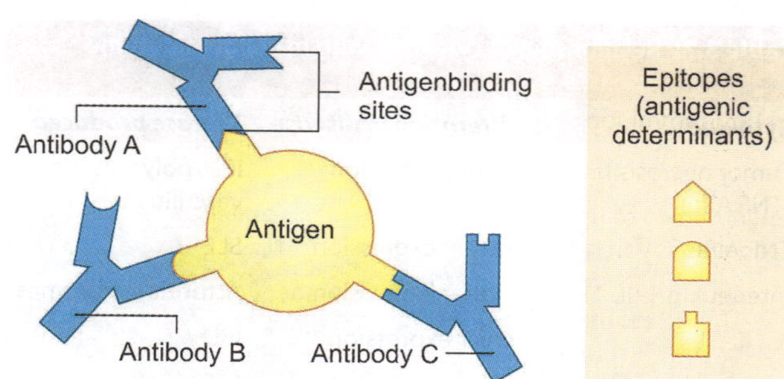

Fig. 3.4: Relationship between antigen, epitopes and different antibodies

Haptens: These are small foreign molecules that are not antigenic. They have to be coupled with a carrier molecule to become antigenic. Antibodies can recognize haptens.

Epitopes (Fig. 3.4):
- These are small part of an antigen that interact with antibodies.
- Any given antigen may have several epitopes.
- Each epitope is recognized by a different antibody.

AUTOIMMUNE DISEASES

The autoimmune diseases resulting from immunologically mediated tissue destruction where the antigens involved are autologous. These are broadly classified into two:

1. ***Organ specific diseases:*** The antibodies associated with Hashimoto's thyroiditis react only with thyroid tissue, so the lesion is highly localized. Another example of organ specific diseases is pernicious anemia.
2. ***Non-organ specific diseases:*** *e.g.* rheumatological diseases. The serum from such patient reacts with many tissues in the body—the dominant antibody is directed against cellular double stranded DNA. This is the reason why a wide range of organ involvement is common in systemic lupus erythematosus. Although not organ specific, some autoimmune diseases preferentially involve certain organs, such as rheumatoid arthritis (joints), scleroderma (skin) and dermatomyositis (skin and muscle). Removal of pre-formed antibody by plasmapheresis is a therapeutic tool in the management of some of these disorders.

Several mechanisms have been proposed to explain the pathogenesis of autoimmune diseases.

- ***Forbidden clone theory:*** All the clones which react with self-antigens are destroyed during intrauterine life, but such a clone may be generated by somatic mutation in later life.
- ***Sequestered antigen theory:*** Antigens exposed to lymphoid system during intrauterine life are recognized as self. But some tissues (e.g. lens, thyroid, CNS) are anatomically sequestered or guarded from the lymphocytes. In adult life, when such antigens are exposed, the immune system reacts against them.
- ***Suppressor cell deficiency:*** Small quantities of thyroglobulin (and other antigens) are seen in circulation even in normal persons, but they are below the threshold level for immunostimulation. The suppressor cells also inhibit sensitization. In persons with deficient T-cell activity, inappropriate immune reactions are produced.
- ***Genetic effect:*** Autoimmune diseases show familial distribution and female preponderance. Many of them are associated with particular human leukocyte antigen (HLA) types. These suggest that genetic predisposition may play a role in their pathogenesis.
- ***Cross reacting antibodies:*** Antibodies produced against exogenous antigens can cross react with tissue proteins, e.g. post-rabies vaccine encephalitis and post-streptococcal rheumatic fever. In any given instance one or more of the above mechanisms may be operative. Some of the immune-mediated disorders are listed in Table 3.6.

Table 3.6: Some important immune-mediated disorders

Diseases	Autoantigen	Diagnostic test
I. *Organ specific diseases*		
Pernicious anemia	Parietal cells of stomach, intrinsic factor	Neutralization
Ulcerative colitis	Lipopolysaccharides of mucus membrane of colon	IFT
Acute post-streptococcal nephritis	Streptococcal antigen	CFT and IFT
Sympathetic ophthalmia	Uveal protein	Skin test
Bullous pemphigoid	Basement membrane	IFT
Pemphigus vulgaris	Desmosomes	IFT
Hashimoto's thyroiditis	Thyroglobulin microsomes	CFT
Thyrotoxicosis by LATS	Cell surface receptor proteins	Bioassay
II. *Affecting two or more organ systems*		
Goodpasture's syndrome	Glomerular and lung basement membranes	IFT
Autoimmune hemolytic anemia	Membrane proteins of RBC	Coombs' test
Immune thrombocytopenia	Platelet components	Demonstration of antibody
Primary biliary cirrhosis	Acetylcholine receptors in nerve ending	IFT
Rheumatic fever	Liver and kidney mitochondria	IFT
	Streptococcal antigen cross reacting with heart and joint tissues	IFT
III. *Systemic or generalized diseases*		
Rheumatoid arthritis	Immunoglobulins, especially IgG	Latex agglutination
Sjögren's disease	Ducts, mitochondria of glands	IFT
Systemic lupus erythematosus	Nuclear DNA and nucleoproteins	IFT
Systemic sclerosis (scleroderma)	Nuclear proteins	IFT

Abbreviations: IFT = Immunofluorescence test; CFT = Complement fixation test

Textbook of Medicine

Autoimmune Diseases and Molecular Mimicry

This is one mechanism by which infecting agents or other exogenous substances trigger an immune response against host antigens. When an organisms, which has antigen immunologically similar to the tissue antigens of the host, but different significantly, induce an immune response when presented to T- cells. This results in loss of tolerance to the host's antigens.

Moreover, there is a pathogen specific immune response which cross reacts with host's structures to cause tissue damage and disease. Molecular mimicry play a great role in triggering autoimmune diseases, such as multiple sclerosis (polymerase of EBV) Guillain-Barre Syndrome *(C. jejuni)*, chronic inflammatory and demyelinating polyneuropathy (melanoma).

Other Examples of Molecular Mimicry

Rheumatic fever

Epitopes present in cell wall, cell membrane and the ABC repeat region of streptococcal. M protein show immunological similarity to molecules of human myosin, tropomyosin, keratin, actin, laminin, vimentin and n-acetylglucosamine. The type group A (beta-hemolytic) streptococcus (GABHS) cross-reacts with myocardial tissue. These lead to rheumatic fever and carditis.

Pediatric autoimmune neuropsychiatric disorders

They may be associated with streptococcal infection. Group-A beta hemolytic streptococcus antibodies cross reacts with the cellular components of the basal ganglia. Diseases in this class include Sydenham's chorea, Turette syndrome, dystonias, myoclonus, parkinsonism, paroxysmal dystonic choreoathetosis, motor stereotypes and encephalitis lethargica.

Lyme arthritis

B. burgdorferi spondyloarthritis and Reiter's syndrome are also related to HLAB27.

Type 1 diabetes mellitus and coxsackie virus

For example: The enzyme coxascke virus P_2-C shows some similarity to enzyme glutamate decarboxylase (GAD_{65}) present in β cells of the pancreas. Coxsackievirus infection may lead to interactions with the pancreatic beta cells and predispose to the development type 1 diabetes mellitus.

Autoimmune polyglandular syndrome

Molecular mimicry causes immune mediated damage to several endocrine organs.

Primary billary sclerosis may have a causative role with *E. coli* and its structural components.

Role of Cytokines in Autoimmune Disease

Several cytokines are implicated in the causation of auto-immune diseases. Some examples are listed in Table 3.7.

Immunological (Immune) Tolerance

It is the phenomenon in which there is no immune response to specific (usually self) antigens. It is the result of exposure of lymphocytes to that specific antigen from early life.

Self-tolerance is absence of immune response to an individual's own antigens. Absence of response to self is a

Table 3.7: Relationship of cytokines with major autoimmune diseases

Cytokine	Alteration in disease	Disease produced
Tumor necrosis factor (TNF Alfa)	Over expression	IBD, polyarthritis, vasculitis
TNF Alfa	Under expression	SLE
Interleukin 1 (IL-1)	Under expression	Arthritic syndromes
IL_2, IL_7, IL_{10}	Over expression	IBD
Interferon delta	Over expression	SLE
IL_{10}	Under expression	Type 1 diabetes and thyroid disease

Note: Several other examples of this relationship are known.

Abbreviations: IBD = Inflammatory bowel disease; SLE = Systemic lupus erythematosus

fundamental property of the normal immune system and this helps to maintain tissue integrity of the host. Several different mechanisms operate to establish immune tolerance.

Immune tolerance may be established by central or peripheral mechanisms:

- Central mechanisms
  - Deletetion of T and B-lymphocytes which react against self-tissues by apoptosis in early life
  - AIRE (autoimmune regulator) is a protein product which leads to destruction of offending lymphocytes and this is controlled AIRE gene
  - Some B-cells rearrange their receptors, so that the destruction of self-tissues is abolished.
- Peripheral mechanism is to eliminate or silence the offending T or B-cells.

DIAGNOSTIC PROCEDURES IN IMMUNOLOGY

The tests used in immunology range from simple tests such as agglutination, flocculation, precipitation, hemagglutination, reverse passive hemagglutination, complement fixation and immunofluorescence to the more advanced tests such as immunoelectrophoresis, enzyme-linked immunosorbent assay (ELISA), immunoblotting, e.g. Western blot and the use of specific monoclonal antibodies.

Enzyme-Linked Immunosorbent Assay (ELISA) Test

This is one of the most frequently performed immunological tests in most of the laboratories in India to detect antigens and antibodies. The test is useful even when they are present only in minute quantities. Specific pre-prepared antibody or antigen is employed to fix the corresponding antigen or antibody, respectively, present in the patient's serum. The antigen-antibody complex is detected by appropriate colour developing techniques. Though the original test was a complicated one, at present, test kits are available for most of these estimations. Therefore, ELISA tests are available even in laboratories which do not undertake high level work, e.g. detection of antibody—hepatitis B and C, HIV and detection of antigens—alpha fetoprotein, carcinoembryonic antigen.

Principles of Treatment of Autoimmune Diseases

Glucocorticoids and immunosuppression: Several cytokines specifically helping to reconstitute the immune system immunoglobulins, specific monoclonal anti-bodies against T and B lymphocytes and bone marrow transplantation to replace the deranged immunological apparatus are all employed for many of the autoimmune diseases at present. Use of monoclonal antibodies specific to several immunologically medicated diseases has become very popular in view of their specific beneficial effect and predictability.

Chemotherapy using drugs such as cyclophosphamide, azathioprine, ciclosporin, micophenolate mofetil and several others synthetic drugs available to inhibit particular processes in the disordered immune system is in vogue for several decades.

SERUM SICKNESS

Syn: Systemic Immune Complex Disease

This is produced as a result of circulating immune complexes. The biological and inflammatory potential of circulating immune complexes depend on the nature of the antibodies and antigens as well as the molar ratio of the two reactants. The magnitude and duration of antigen exposure is also important. The manifestations are transient if the exposure to the antigen is short, but if supply of the antigen is continued, immune complexes are continuously formed and serum sickness like reaction follows. Main lesions are in the glomeruli, choroid plexus, synovium, skin and uveal tract, which are the sites of inflammation due to deposition of immune complexes.

Apart from the introduction of external protein antigens and viral infections, drugs like penicillin and other drugs are more often responsible for this condition in man.

The antibodies are initially of IgG type and a Type III reaction occurs. Later IgE antibodies are formed and a Type I reaction may also occur.

Clinical features: About 7–14 days after the injection of serum or exposure to the offending drug, the disease starts with fever, arthralgia, periarthritis, urticarial or morbilliform rashes and lymphadenopathy. Myocarditis may occur rarely. Glomerulonephritis is rare in humans. Peripheral neuropathy is a late sequel. The condition generally is self-limiting.

Treatment: Withdrawal of the offending agent gives relief in mild cases. Prednisolone in a dose of 1 mg/kg body weight may be required in severe cases. Prednisone or other corticosteroids are indicated, if there is myocarditis and peripheral neuropathy.

Serum sickness may be partially prevented by giving large doses of cyproheptadine (0.7 mg/kg/day) or hydroxyzine (5 mg/kg/day) along with the serum.

IMMUNODEFICIENCY STATES

What is Immunodeficiency?

Failing of one or more of the body's defensive mechanisms results in morbidity or mortality. Any part of the immune system can be deficient; cells, proteins signaling mechanism. The body is susceptible to infection by organisms that receive little or no resistance.

In certain cases, other homeostatic systems in the body will be disrupted by the defect.

Severity is variable according to nature of infectious organisms. Immunodeficiency can be primary or secondary.

Immunodeficiency may be congenital or acquired. In many of these cases, the defect may differ and the susceptibility to get infection also varies.

Severe forms of immunodeficiency states are so incompatible with life that they are rarely seen in clinical practice. The disorders are classified as:

- ■ **Combined immunodeficiency states:** There is deficiency of both cellular and humoral immunity. This is produced as a result of block of maturation of the stem cells which give rise to immunocytes. Severely affected children are incapable of limiting bacterial, viral and fungal infections and they die in childhood. Several subtypes have been described, e.g. sex-linked recessive types (thymic type) and autosomal recessive (Swiss) types. Relatively benign types are the Wiskott-Aldrich syndrome (sex-linked) and ataxia telangiectasia (autosomal recessive). In both, lymphoreticular malignancies are more common. *Adenosine deaminase* (purine catabolizing enzyme) deficiency, an autosomal recessive disorder leads to severe combined immunodeficiency. Gene transfer therapy has been tried recently with promising results in a few of such cases. Adenosine deaminase gene from normal lymphocytes was introduced by gene splicing and recombinant technology into the defective lymphocytes. The cells are grown in culture and reintroduced into the patient.

- ■ **Deficiency of humoral immunity:** This may be a selective primary deficiency affecting only one of the G, M or A classes of immunoglobulins. In IgG deficiency, the affected persons suffer from repeated pyogenic infections, especially by encapsulated organisms such as *Haemophilus influenzae* and *Streptococcus pyogenes*. In IgA deficiency, respiratory and atopic allergies are also common. IgA deficiency also lowers the resistance to gut commensals leading to malabsorption syndrome. Congenital hypogammaglobulinemia may be sex linked (Bruton type) or autosomal dominant. In these cases, severe depletion of B-cells and circulating immunoglobulins are noticed with consequent severe bacterial infections. Incidence of autoimmune diseases such as hemolytic anemia are high in primary agammaglobulinemia. Immunodeficiency may occur in presence of normal quantity, but functionally deficient immunoglobulins, e.g. Job's syndrome.

- ■ **Deficiency of cellular immunity:** Primary deficiency of T-cells leads to severe viral and monilial infections and affected children usually succumb within the first few years of life. The lymphocytes of the patients are unable to respond to mitogens *in vitro*. The thymus may be almost absent **(Nezelof's syndrome)** or aplastic **(DiGeorge syndrome)** or in some cases it may be normal, e.g. chronic mucocutaneous candidiasis.

- ■ **Deficiency of phagocytes:** Chronic granulomatous disease is a sex-linked inherited condition where hydrogen peroxidase is deficient inside the phagocytes, leading to decreased microbicidal activity. Recurrent suppurative granulomas due to catalase positive and peroxidase negative organisms *(Staphylococcus aureus and Proteus)* are common in this condition. In myeloperoxidase deficiency, infections by peroxidase positive bacteria such as hemophilus are common. In Chédiak-Higashi syndrome, the neutrophils show defective degranulation and sluggish motility with consequent predisposition to pyogenic infections.

- ***Deficiency of complement system:*** Hereditary angioedema is inherited as an autosomal dominant disease. It is characterized by absence of the enzyme which normally inhibits the activity of C_1 esterase. This results in unrestrained C_1 esterase activity which activates the complement cascade reactions leading to liberation of kinin and vasoactive peptides. Recurrent attacks of edema of skin and mucosa are very common and edema of glottis may sometimes be life-threatening.

  Deficiency of C_3 is inherited as an autosomal recessive character. Deficiencies of other complement components, though reported, are very rare. Generally, the clinical conditions mimic immunoglobulin deficiency states.

- ***Secondary immunodeficiency states:*** The trans-placental transfer of immunoglobulins takes place mostly in the last few weeks of pregnancy. Premature infants, therefore, may suffer from mild hypo-globulinemia. Secondary defects in lymphocyte functions are seen in many conditions such as burns, malnutrition, leukemias, lymphomas and uremia. In multiple myeloma, though total immunoglobulins are increased, the biologically active ones are depressed, leading to functional deficiency. Acquired immunodeficiency may be due to primary causes such as infections (especially HIV), drugs or malignancies. These are listed in Table 3.8.

- ***Primary immunodeficiency states:*** These are a group of more than 200 clinically and immunologically defined diseases of varying degrees of severity (Box 3.1). In about 150 of them, molecular genetic diagnosis identifying the disease related genes is available. Allogenic stem cells transplantation and gene modified autologus stem cells transplantation have become a treatment option for them.

Treatment of immunodeficiency states as a whole is unsatisfactory. Immunoglobulin injection (0.25 g/kg/week) may abort recurrent pyogenic infections in hypo-gammaglobulinemia. Treatment of cell mediated immune deficiency states is still more difficult.

Immunocompetent cells can be restored by bone marrow transplantation.

Immunodeficiency and Genetic Defects of Pattern Recognition Receptors

Genetic factors can increase susceptibility to infection apart from the classic immunodeficiency states involving T-cell and B-cell defects. Defects in ***pattern recognition receptors (PRRs)*** have been identified which predispose to recurrent infections. PRRs allow for semi-specific recognition of invading pathogens by cells of the innate immune system. These receptors recognize pathogen associated molecular pattern. Among these Toll-like receptors (TLRs) are very frequently involved.

Source: Mihai G Netea, et al. New Eng J Med. 2011;364-1, 60-69.

Toll-like Receptors (TLRs)

Several distinct classes of PRRs have evolved in phagocytic cells to induce various host defense pathways. For example, secreted PRRs bind to microbial cells and mark them for destruction. Another class of PRRs function exclusively as signalling receptors. These receptors are known as TLRs. The TLRs recognize and bind unique pathogen-associated molecular patterns (PAMPs) of different microbes and subsequently communicate that finding to the host cell molecules to initiate appropriate gene expression and host response. There are at least 10 different proteins in the family of TLRs which identify different proteins. Binding of TLR triggers a signalling pathway resulting in expression of a variety of genes including those for cytokines, chemokines and co-stimulatory molecules which play crucial roles in calling forth and directing adaptive immune response later in the infection. Binding of microbial components to phagocytic receptors is an important first step in phagocytosis. Once bound, the microbe or its components can be internalized as part of a phagosome that is united with a lysosome to facilitate microbial killing and digestion.

Mainly there are four classes of pattern recognition receptor. These include:

- TLRs, which recognize microbial structure and activate coordinated activity of T-and B-cells
- C-type lectin receptors (CLRs) recognize microbial polysaccharides

Table 3.8: Acquired immunodeficiency		
Predisposing cause	***Effect on immune system***	***Types of infections***
Immunosuppression by drugs	Humoral and cellular immunity diminished	Infections of lung, urinary tract, bacteremias, fungal infections
Viral infections, measles, EB virus, HIV	Impaired T-helper activity	Secondary bacterial infections, opportunistic infections
Tumors of immune system, e.g. lymphomas, myeloma, leukemias	Replacement of immune competent cells	Bacteremia, pneumonia, urinary tract infections
Malnutrition	Lymphoid hypoplasia, decreased lymphocyte and phagocyte activity	Measles, tuberculosis, respiratory infections, Gastrointestinal infection
Breakdown of tissue barriers, burns, wounds, injury, foreign body, etc.	Local effect	Local and systemic infections

Box 3.1: Warning signs for suspicion of primary immunodeficiency disorders

- Four or more new ear infections within 1 year
- Two or more serious sinus infections within 1 year
- Two or more months on antibiotics with little effect
- Two or more pneumonias within 1 year
- Failure of an infant to gain weight or grow normally
- Recurrent, deep skin or organ abscesses
- Persistent thrush in mouth or fungal infection on skin
- Need for intravenous antibiotics to clear infections
- Two or more deep-seated infections including septicemia
- A family history of primary immunodeficiency disorders

- Nucleotide–binding oligomerization receptors (NOD). NOD_1 and NOD_2 recognize muramyl peptide receptor molecules of the peptidoglycans of gram-positive and gram-negative bacteria
- Retinoic acid-inducible gene 1 (RIG-1) protein helicase receptor.

These patterns resemble constituents of microbial cell wall, microbial nucleic acids or metabolic products. Defects in pattern recognition lead to disturbances in cytokine mechanisms.

TLR defects leads to bacterial, candidal, mycobacterial and trypanosoma infections.

CLR defects leads to infections by fungi, candida and micobacteria.

NLR defects lead to several bacteria, both gram-positive and gram-negative and flagellate bacteria.

Defects of RIG-1 receptors predispose to several viral infections. Whereas, immunodeficiencies caused by classic immunocytes persist lifelong, those caused by pattern recognition defects are worse during childhood and they tend to recover with increasing age.

THE COMPROMISED HOST

A compromised host is defined as a patient with a defect in the normal defense mechanisms, which makes him vulnerable to infection. He is not only liable to get severe or recurrent infections with the usual pathogens, but also liable to attack by 'opportunistic' microbes which otherwise have minimal pathogenic potential. Particular infections are common in the different types of immune defects.

- ***B-cell defect:*** *Streptococcus pneumoniae, Staphylococcus aureus, Neisseria meningitidis, Haemophilus influenzae, Escherichia coli, Giardia lamblia.*
- ***T-cell defect:*** *Listeria monocytogenes, Mycobacterium sp, Candida sp, Aspergillus sp, Cryptococcus neoformans,* cytomegalovirus (CMV), herpes simplex, herpes zoster.
- ***Combined B- and T-cell defect:*** Combination of (A) and (B).
- ***Neutrophil defects:*** This includes, neutropenias, defects of adhesion, defects in signalling, defects of intracellular killing and defects in the formation of cytoplasmic granules—gram negative bacilli, candida, *Staphylococcus aureus, Streptococcus pyogenes.*
- ***Complement defects:*** *Staphylococcus aureus, Streptococcus pneumoniae, Pseudomonas sp, Proteus sp, Neisseria sp, Salmonella sp.*

- Present day chemotherapy for cancer with anticancer drugs and several immune mediated diseases with immunosuppressant, monoclonal antibodies and others lead to severe immunodeficiency and susceptibility to opportunistic infections. They also increase the risk of development of secondary neoplasms such as lymphomas. Infection with HIV leads to gradual depletion of CD4 T-lymphocytes and profound immunodeficiency when the patient develops AIDS. Several opportunistic infections and specific neoplasms like Kaposi's sarcoma and lymphomas may develop.

In addition to systemic chemotherapy, an alteration or breach in the skin or mucosal defense barriers that permit micrograms to cause a local or systemic infection also makes the patient immunocompromised, e.g. burns, indwelling catheters, intravenous lines and others.

The type of immunosuppression and the duration of immunodeficiency partly determine the type of nosocomial or superinfection they acquire. Among the acquired causes of immunocompromise, cancer chemotherapy, use of corticosteroids and immunosuppressants, organ transplantations (both solid organ and bone marrow) splenectomy and AIDS from the major bulk.

Several systemic diseases like diabetes mellitus, chronic liver diseases, chronic kidney diseases, hematological malignancies, old age and HIV infection are associated with immune deficiency and increased susceptibility to specific infections. They have to be considered as immune compromised from the point of management.

FEVER IN IMMUNOCOMPROMISED HOST

At times fever may be the principal or even the only manifestation in the immunocompromised patient. The pattern of fever in such patients is nonspecific despite different pathogenic agents. In severely immunocompromised state, fever may even be absent. Fever is the result of the release of pro-inflammatory cytokines, such as IL-1α, IL-1β, IL-4, IL-6 and tumor necrosis factor. Endogenous pyrogens are known to arise from polymorphonuclear leukocytes. These are also produced by macrophages, lymphocytes, fibroblasts, epithelial cells and endothelial cells, as a consequence of infection or inflammation. Even in severe neutropenia fever may occur, the pyrogens arising from alternate sources.

Immunosuppressed patients rapidly deteriorate and die, if infection is allowed to establish. Therefore, empirical antimicrobial therapy may have to be started depending on the clinical state. In general neutrophil counts below 500 mm^3 predispose the patient to life-threatening infections. The clinical signs of infections may be minimal and therefore, misleading. Presence of multiple factors such as breaches in the epithelium, neutropenia, reduction in CD4 '+ve' lymphocytes and concurrent cytotoxic or immunosuppressant drugs worsen the condition. Neutropenia occurring after cytotoxic chemotherapy is much more dangerous compared to neutropenia occurring in aplastic anemia or following viral infection. Prolongation of neutropenia beyond 10 days adds to the risk of infection.

Textbook of Medicine

Severe depression of CD4 cell counts also predispose to infection. Reduction of CD4 cells to < 1500 mm³ in the first year of life, < 750 mm³ in children between 2 and 6 years of age and < 200 mm³ in children above 6 years is associated with risk of life-threatening infection with *Pneumocystis carinii*, *Toxoplasma gondii* and cytomegalovirus. Patients with AIDS are susceptible to tuberculosis irrespective of the CD4 counts, whereas *Mycobacterium avium* complex affects those with CD4 count < 50 mm³. The infective agents affecting the immunocompromized host vary widely. Virtually all organisms including avirulent ones can become pathogenic.

Acute infections are commonly due to *Staphylococci*, *Pseudomonas aeruginosa*, *Escherichia coli* and *Klebsiella*. Infections lower the immunity further. Infections such as *respiratory syncytial virus*, *Adenovirus*, *Parainfluenza virus* and *Cytomegalovirus* are common. Multiple infections by bacteria, fungi, viruses and protozoa may occur. Fungal infection by *Pneumocystis carinii*, *Cryptococcus*, *aspergillus*, *Candida* and *Mucor* are common. Protozoal infections include toxoplasmosis, Amebiasis, Cryptosporidiosis and others.

Patients who had splenectomy or autosplenectomy in sickle cell disease are susceptible to develop infection by capsulated organisms such as *Pneumococcus*, *Haemophilus influenzae* or *Neisseria meningitidis*.

Management: Fever and infection in the immunocompromized host are managed based upon the nature of the host's disability such as neutropenia, defective cellular immunity or mucosal disruption. The guiding principle has been to treat severely immunocompromized febrile patients empirically for the major pathogens to which they are susceptible. Broad spectrum antibiotic therapy is given with a view to cover gram-positive and gram-negative aerobic organisms. Combination antibiotic therapy or monotherapy with third generation cephalosporins or carbapenems is given.

HUMAN LEUKOCYTE ANTIGEN (HLA) SYSTEM IN HUMANS

Several diseases are known to have intimate association with disease susceptibility shown by distinctive HLA types (Tables 3.9 and 3.10). HLA system stands for human leukocyte antigen system which is the human version of the MHC.

MHC

- All human cells express a series of molecules on their surfaces that are recognized by other individuals as foreign antigens. It was observed that the rejection of transplanted organs was due to important antigens called major histocompatibility antigens. These antigens are encoded by a segment of chromosome 6 (6p21.3) known as the MHC.
- The MHC molecules were named so because they were responsible for tissue compatibility between different individuals. MHC/HLA system plays a central role in intercellular recognition and discrimination between self-and non-self-tissue rejection is a type IV immune reaction that leads to the destruction of a transplant by a recipient who is genetically non-identical to the

Table 3.9: Association of HLA system with diseases—global data

Diseases	Associated HLA type	Relative risk
Ankylosing spondylitis	B-27	81
Reiter's syndrome	B-27	48
Coeliac disease	B-8	9.5
Rheumatoid arthritis	DW4	8
Addison's disease	B-8	6.4
Chronic active hepatitis	B-8	6
Myasthenia gravis	B-8	5
Multiple sclerosis	DW2	5
Psoriasis	B-13	4.3
Pemphigus	A-IO	4.3
Sjögren's syndrome	B-8	3.2
Graves' disease	B-8	2.5
Hodgkin's disease	B-18	2
Diabetes mellitus (insulin dependent)	B-8	1–9

Note: Relative risk is the chance of developing the disease compared to controls who do not possess the particular HLA types.

Table 3.10: HLA association with diseases commonly seen in India

Ankylosing spondylitis	HLA B-27
Reiter's disease	HLA B-27
Acute anterior uveitis	HLA B-27
Rheumatoid arthritis	HLA DR4
Juvenile RA	HLA DR5, DR8
Insulin dependent diabetes	HLA B-8, B-21, DR3
Graves' disease	HLA DR2, DQ2
Rheumatic heart disease	HLA DR3
Myasthenia gravis	HLA B-21, B-8
Tuberculoid leprosy	HLA DR2, DR6
Lepromatous leprosy	HLA DQW1
Pulmonary tuberculosis	HLA DR2, DR6

Note: HLA association have been found for infections such as malaria, schistosomiasis and leishmaniasis.

donor. Here the recipient lymphoid system recognizes foreign (non-self) antigens in the donor tissue. These cell-surface antigens that evoke rejection of transplants are called MHC. MHC is also known as HLA complex because in humans MHC-encoded proteins were first identified on leukocytes and are expressed in high concentrations on lymphocytes.

- The MHC molecules are products of MHC gene. MHC is a general term used for all species.
- The best known of these genes are the HLA class I and class II genes. Their products are important for immunologic specificity and transplantation histocompatibility, and they play a major role in susceptibility to a number of autoimmune diseases.

Function of MHC Molecules

- MHC molecules are required for the recognition of antigens by antigen-specific T-cells. It is required for many of the important cell to cell interactions of the immune response.
- These MHC molecules are major immunogens and are targets in transplant rejection.

HLA system plays a role in very different situations such as:

- Transplant rejection
- Chronic inflammatory diseases such as rheumatoid arthritis and ankylosing spondylitis
- Coma in cerebral malaria
- Immunodeficiency states
- Advanced hepatic cirrhosis with iron overload.

HLA complex is mainly represented on chromosomes 6 and it contains over 200 genes. More than 40 of them encode leukocyte antigens. The HLA genes that are involved in the immune response fall into classes—I and II which are structurally and functionally different. The class I genes code for the alpha polypeptides of the class I molecule. The beta chain of class I molecule is encoded by a gene on chromosome 15—the beta 2 microglobulin gene. There are about 20 class I genes in the HLA region. Three of them—HLA-A, B and C functions mainly in the immune response. These are called the classic or class I genes. The class I genes code for both the alpha and beta polypeptide chains of the class II molecules.

Their position on chromosomes 6 is identified by the three letters given below:

- D—this indicates the class
- M, O, P, Q or R—this represents the family
- A or B—the chain that is affected.

The three main class II molecules are HLA, DP, DQ and DR. The individual genes of the HLA system are represented by Arabic numerals.

Class I genes are expressed by most somatic cells. In contrast class II genes are expressed selectively on a subgroup of cells concerned with immunity such as B-cells, activated T-cells, macrophages, dendritic cells and epithelial cells of the thymus.

The A, B and C loci can be identified by serologic tests. The D locus which controls lymphocyte antigens is detectable by mixed lymphocyte culture. The products of HLA genes are proteins which are found on all tissues including leukocytes and platelets but not on erythrocytes. HLA molecules are dimers of two different polypeptide chains, designated as alpha and beta. The variable amino acid sequences in these chains produce distinct three dimensional structures which will allow the identification of foreign cells. HLA typing of A, B and C loci is done by ***complement mediated cytotoxic test*** utilizing a panel of reference antisera. The D locus is typed by the mitogenic effect using a panel of lymphocytes. Inheritance of certain alleles confer susceptibility to particular diseases when exposed to suitable environment. Table 3.9 gives the association of HLA system with some of them.

The HLA antigens play a central role in cell-to-cell interaction in the immune process. The MHC molecule interacts with antigens and presents them to T-cell receptors for recognition and further action.

The HLA antigens play a great role in identifying self from non-self and in giving rise to rejection, when HLA incompatible tissues are transplanted into an individual. Histocompatibility is defined as the similarity between tissues of two different individuals. Organ transplantation can be successfully carried out only if the donor and recipient are at least partially, if not completely matched. Since identical twins have identical HLA loci, they are the most suitable for tissue transplantation. Next in order of compatibility are parents and siblings, near blood relatives and others. Since exact HLA matching is not available in the vast majority of cases, one has to satisfy with as close a match as possible.

The difference in HLA constitution between a donor and recipient results in immunological reactions against the graft (***host vs graft disease—HVGD***) or the graft against the host (***graft vs host disease—GVHD***). This can be suppressed to a great deal by continuous use of immunosuppressants like corticosteroids, cyclophosphamide, cyclosporine and anti-lymphocytic serum.

The role of HLA system has been recognized in many other infections, in non-communicable diseases and neoplasms. New information is pouring in from time-to-time on this subject which is always expanding.

IMMUNIZATION

Immunity in the human body against disease can be induced by several methods.

- ***Active induced immunity:*** This is induced by immunization with toxoid or killed and attenuated organisms.
- ***Active natural immunity:*** This is the immunity produced by exposure to clinical or subclinical infections
- ***Passive induced immunity:*** Temporary protection against the infecting organism can be conferred on the susceptible host by giving preformed antibodies obtained by immunizing heterologous or homologous hosts. Such passive immunization is recommended for the post-exposure prophylaxis in conditions as defined in Box 3.2 and Table 3.11. Along with the induction of passive immunity to tide over the incubation period, active immunization using vaccine should also be started simultaneously for conferring lasting immunity.

Box 3.2: Therapeutic use of preformed antibodies

Infective conditions	*Non-infective conditions*
Tetanus	Myasthenia gravis
Botulism	Guillain-Barré syndrome
Diphtheria	Immune thrombocytopenia
Anthrax	Some cases of aplastic anemia
The dose of IgG given is moderate	The dose of IgG in these conditions is very large

Table 3.11: Passive immunization by preformed antibodies

Hepatitis A	Human hyperimmune serum 0.02 mL/kg IM. Protection for < 3 months; and 0.06 mL/kg IM protection for 3–5 months
Hepatitis B	Hepatitis B immunoglobulin (HBIG) 0.5 mL IM–0.06 mL/kg single or multiple doses
Varicella	Varicella zoster immunoglobulin (VZIG) 125–625 units IM -125 units per 10 kg to be given upto 10 days after exposure
Tetanus	Tetanus immunoglobulin human 500–3000 units IM 250 IU for prophylaxis and 2500–5000 IU for treatment
Rabies	Rabies immunoglobulin-human (HRIG) 20 IU/kg. 50% IM as much as possible infiltrated around the wound and the rest deep IM (gluteal) and the rest infiltrated around the wound
Measles	Human immunoglobulin 0.25 mL/kg IM, 0.6 mL/kg

- ***Passive natural immunity:*** Transfer of immuno-globulins (especially IgG) to fetus takes place *in utero*. These antibodies remain in the circulation of the child for 3–6 months of postnatal life.

Immunization for Indian subcontinent patients is given in Table 3.12. Figure 3.5 presents the immunization schedule for adults by the Advisory Committee on Immunization Practices (ACIP).

Vaccinology

It is the science of vaccine production, preservation of vaccine efficiency and their appropriate use in clinical and epidemiological situations and their follow-up.

Among the most effective interventions to prevent infective disease on epidemiological scale vaccines have been the most potent with predictable results. Since, after use of vaccine against small pox by Edward Jenner in 1796, vaccinology has developed over the centuries and vaccines are the most effective tools for prevention and eradication of infection. Table 3.13 lists some of the commonly used vaccines in modern times.

The most consistent biomarkers for vaccine efficiency has been the presence of antibodies that neutralize the pathogen. Modern methods of vaccine production utilize information about the structure of the glycoprotein of the

Table 3.12: Immunization schedule for Indian conditions			
Vaccine		**Description**	**Route**
• Obligatory			
▪ DPT	1st dose—6–12 weeks 2nd dose—17–21 weeks 3rd dose—36–38 weeks	Tetanus toxoid Diphtheria toxoid Pertussis-killed organisms	IM or SC
Booster DT	1st dose—18–24 weeks 2nd dose—5–6 weeks	Purified components of B. pertussis (acellular vaccine) is available either singly or in combination as DTaP. The DTaP is safer in children who have febrile convulsions	
▪ Polio			
– Oral Polio Vaccine (OPV-Sabin)	1st dose—3rd month Thereafter 3–4 doses at 2–6 week intervals. Fifth dose later	Live attenuated human diploid cell vaccine oral	
Booster	Booster doses in the 2nd and 5 years		
– Inactivated Polio Vaccine (IPV Salk)	1st dose 3–4 months The next two at 4–6 weeks interval 4th dose 6–12 months later	Killed organisms This is rarely used in selected situations	SC
Booster	At 4–6 years		
▪ Measles (Solid immunity occurs when vaccine is given after the 1st birthday. If the vaccination is done earlier, booster dose is necessary)	12–15 months	Live attenuated	SC
• Advisable			
▪ BCG	During neonatal period or	Live attenuated any time during childhood	Intradermal
▪ Mumps Rubella	Along with measles vaccine Booster not required if given after first birthday	Live attenuated	SC
▪ Rota virus (**Note:** Combined MMR vaccines are available)	2, 3, 4 months	Live attenuated	Oral
• Vaccination necessary under special circumstances HEPATITIS-B vaccine vaccine (rDNA)	Pre-exposure prophylaxis: Special healthcare professionals, hemodialysis patients, hemophiliacs Travellers going to endemic areas, homosexual individuals, contacts of HBV carriers	Dose: 1 mL IM over deltoid 3 doses—2nd dose one month and 3rd dose six months after the 1st dose	
	Post-exposure prophylaxis: Infants of HBV carrier women, contacts of HBV hepatitis, victims of needle stick injuries from HBsAg positive patients or recipients of blood products	Give Hepatitis B Vaccine and Hepatitis B immunoglobulin at birth	
Rabies vaccine Human or others Diploid cell vaccines (Killed vaccine)	Pre-exposure prophylaxis: lab workers, veterinarians, etc.	1 mL IM over deltoid on days 0, 7, 28 Booster depending on serology	
	Post-exposure prophylaxis: (a) Those previously immunized	2 doses 1 mL over deltoid (IM) on days 0 and 3. Rabies immunoglobulin (RIG) should not be administered	

Contd…

Vaccine		Description	Route
	(b) Those not immunized	1 mL over deltoid (IM) on days 0, 3, 7, 14 and 28 RIG 20 IU/kg bw half infiltrated at bite site and rest IM if the risk is severe	
Japanese encephalitis (Killed vaccine)	To be given to communities exposed to risk of encephalitis	0.5–1 mL SC. Two doses at 7–14 days interval, and booster within 12 months Revaccination at 3 yearly intervals	

Vaccinations Desirable under Special Circumstances
(For detail see appropriate sections)

Enteric fever	Phenol and heat killed. 2 doses 0.5 mL SC. 4 weeks apart, or live oral vaccine, 4 oral doses, boosters every 4 years
Cholera	0.5 mL IM or SC. Phenol killed vibrio vaccine, 2 doses 1 week to 1 month apart, at least 10 days before travel
Yellow fever	Immunized before going to endemic areas of Africa and South America
Tetanus	In immunized persons, 2 doses of 0.5 mL toxoid, boosters every 10 years
Influenza	*H. influenzae* type B polysaccharide conjugated to diphtheria toxin, primary 1 dose 0.5 mL
Meningitis	Meningococcal polysaccharide vaccine, tetravalent, primary 0.5 mL SC given before going to endemic area
Pneumococcus	Polyvalent vaccine
Varicella	Live attenuated
H. influenzae	a b c d e f strains
Hepatitis A	rDNA vaccine
Japanese Encephalitis	During epidemics

Vaccine/age group	19–26 years	27–49 years	50–59 years	60–64 years	≥ 65 years
Tetanus, diptheria, pertussis (Tdap)	Substitute one time dose of Tdap with Td, then booster with Td every 10 years				Td booster every 10 years
Human pappiloma vaccine	3 doses				
Varicella	2 doses				
Zoster				1 dose	
Measles, mumps, rubella	1 or 2 does		1 dose		
Influenza		1 dose annually			
Pnemococcal (polysaccharide)		1 or 2 doses			1 dose
Hepatitis A	2 doses				
Hepatitis B	3 doses				
Meningococcal	1 or more doses				

- ▇ Recommended if some risk factor is present
- ▇ All persons who meet the age criteria
- ▇ No recommendation

Fig. 3.5: ACIP Adult Immunization Schedule, Age-Based Recommendations, India

Table 3.13: Commonly used vaccines in modern times

Type of vaccine	Date of Introduction
Diphtheria	1923
Tetanus toxoid	1926
Pertussis	1926
Tuberculosis (BCG)	1927
Influenza	1936
Polio	1955
Mumps live	1967
Anthrax	1970
Pneumococcus	1977
Hepatitis B plasma derived	1981
Hepatitis B surface antigens recombinant	1986
Typhoid live vaccine (type21a)	1989
Japanese encephalitis inactivated	1992
Cholera–recombinant toxin B vaccine	1993
Varicella	1995
Hepatitis A inactivated	1996
Lyme disease outer surface protein A vaccine (OSPA)	1998
Pneumococcal heptavalent vaccine	2000
Meningococcal quadrivalent vaccine	2005
Zoster live vaccine	2006
Rota virus	2006
Japan encephalitis vero cell	2009
Human papilloma virus-recombinant	2009

microbes (especially) viruses and specific interactions of the antibodies that inactivate them. The envelopes of virus contains specific sites that represent potential targets for the design of immunogen capable of inducing an immune response. The structure of viral and bacterial glycoproteins and their role in invasion of the host have been made use of in designing vaccines against them. e.g. HIV, influenza and meningococcus.

The introduction of therapeutic monoclonal antibodies has facilitated the identification of the effective targets and led to strategies for their successful use in humans. Modern vaccionology techniques employ methods including structure based vaccine design. Immune stimulation can be achieved by increasingly complex methods of antigen presentation and other techniques in which it enhance the immune process. The effectiveness of vaccines tested for field trials.

In future, vaccionology will employ procedures such as cell based recombinant methods including production from insect and plant cells, use of monoclonal antibodies for passive prevention and also for production of vaccines.

Many vaccines produce mild to moderate fibrile reactions and local pain at the site of injection. Prophylactic administration of paracetamol reduces the inflammatory and fibrile reactions but also reduces immunogenicity.

Source: Nabel GJ. Designing tomorrow's vaccines. N Engl J Med. 2013;368(6):551-60.

Acknowldgement: Valuable suggestions have been received from Professor R Sajith Kumar, Professor of Infectious disease, Medical College, Kottayam, for preparing this chapter.

Defense Mechanisms of the Host and Clinical Immmology

CHAPTER
4

Principles of Drug Administration

KV Krishna Das

Chapter Summary

- Routes of Drug Administration
- Drug Metabolism
- Pharmacogenetics
- General Principles of Drug Administration
- Drug Administration in Special Groups
- Drug Related Adverse Effects
- Drug Interaction and Prevention of Drug Interaction
- Medical Errors
- Suggestions to Reduce Adverse Drug Effects (ADEs)
- Prescription of Drugs

INTRODUCTION

Drug therapy has been in existence from the earliest recorded period in the history of all forms of medicine. At present drug formulation, manufacture, transport and prescription to the patient—form important activities leading to nationwide progress in wealth. Seldom it has been realized by the medical students and the public at large, that potent drugs are essential for relief and cure of many diseases, at the same time their dosages and administration have to be closely monitored in order to ensure optimum benefit, at the same time avoiding the toxic effects which may lead to considerable morbidity and mortality. About 25% of morbidity and about an equal proportion of deaths occurring in patients receiving drug therapy and other treatment modalities such as surgery, irradiation etc. are partly or even whole due to one or other of the therapeutic modalities. If not used for the correct indication and if not employed in the correct dosage frequency and duration, all drugs may lead to adverse effects. It is therefore necessary to follow proper guidelines and precautions in administrating drug therapy.

The word drug is derived from the French word 'drogue' a 'dry herb'. Drug is defined as any substance used for the purpose of diagnosis, prevention, relief or cure of disease in man or animal. According to World Health Organization (WHO), a ***drug*** is any substance or product that is used or intended to be used to modify or explore physiological systems or pathological states for the benefit of the receipent.

Drugs are generally employed as replacement therapy, as agonists or as antagonists. Drugs are used as replacement for conditions in which there is deficiency of a natural substance endogenous, e.g. hormones or exogenous, e.g. nutrients.

Agonist drugs produce a pharmacological effect, e.g. hypotensives, analgesics.

Antagonist drugs prevent the action of natural substances like anticholinergics or counteract the action of other drugs, e.g. anticholinergics blocking parasympathetic activities and nalorphine acting as an antidote to opiate sedatives.

The ***therapeutic index*** also known as ***therapeutic ratio*** or ***therapeutic window*** is a measure of the safety margin between the effective dose and toxic dose of the drug. Relatively safe drugs have a large therapeutic ratio and relatively toxic drugs have a narrow therapeutic ratio. Drugs like penicillin have a wide therapeutic ratio whereas, digoxin has a narrow therapeutic ratio. It is essential to know the therapeutic ratio of the prescribed drug so as to anticipate adverse effects promptly and take remedial measures early.

Drugs produce their effect by interacting with specific receptor sites on the cell membrane. At the receptor sites the action may be positive (e.g. agonists) or opposite to those of agonists (e.g. antagonists). Initially there is physical interaction between the drug and the receptor and this drug receptor complex produces the ***therapeutic response***.

ROUTES OF DRUG ADMINISTRATION

This may be oral, sublingual, topical or parenteral. ***Orally administered*** drugs are absorbed in different parts of the gastrointestinal tract (GIT). They pass through the portal circulation into the liver, undergo partial metabolism and pass into the systemic circulation to reach all tissues.

Drugs that are absorbed rapidly from the ***sublingual*** mucosa are administered by putting the drug under the tongue. The effect is immediate, e.g. glyceryl trinitrate (GTN) and in angina pectoris. Sublingual route is also preferred for drugs that may be partially or fully destroyed by the gastric juice.

Topical sites where drugs are administered for absorption are the skin, mucous membranes of the mouth, rectum, vagina, nasal mucsa (e.g. salmon calcitonin), respiratory tract (inhalers) and others. In addition several locally acting drugs are applied over the site of disease on the skin, e.g. antifungals in cutaneous and mucosal mycoses. Absorption of these drugs may occur in smaller quantities, but local effects are more pronounced.

Parenteral routes are subcutaneous, intramuscular (IM), intravenous (IV), intra-arterial, intrathecal, intraventricular (cerebral ventricles), intra-articular, intracavitary (into viscera like pleura or peritoneum or abscess cavities) and intra-amniotic.

DRUG METABOLISM

Absorption of Drugs

The amount of drug that reaches the systemic circulation intact and is available to the target tissues for effective

Table 4.1: Bioavaibaility of drugs based on the route of administration

Route	Bioavailability (%)	Characteristics
Intravenous (IV)	100 (by definition)	Most rapid onset
Intramuscular (IM)	75 ≤ 100	Large volumes often feasible; may be painful
Subcutaneous (SC)	75 ≤ 100	Smaller volumes than IM; may be painful
Oral (PO)	5 < 100	Most convenient; first-pass effect may be significant
Rectal (PR)	30 < 100	Less first-pass effect than oral
Inhalation	5 < 100	Often very rapid onset
Transdermal	80 ≤ 100	Usually very slow absorption; used for lack of first-pass effect; prolonged duration of action

function is called the ***bioavailability*** of a drug (Table 4.1). The rate of absorption and the metabolic processes which tend to eliminate or inactivate the drug determine the bioavailability of the ingested drugs. Absorption from the GIT depends upon lipid solubility, degree of ionization and molecular weight of the drug. Low molecular weight substances and alcohol are absorbed passively, while other drugs are absorbed by active processes requiring energy, e.g. alpha methyldopa. Lipid-soluble drugs are absorbed easily. Since, drugs have to be in solution to facilitate absorption, formulations which disintegrate rapidly, are more easily absorbed. Due to the variability of physical properties, bioavailability of the same drug may vary when administered in different formulations and therefore, it is important to avoid frequent changes in formulations from time-to-time. Other factors influencing GI absorption are the availability of surface area for absorption, motility of the gut, pH within the gut, local blood flow and presence of other substances such as food materials and other drugs in the gut lumen.

Drug interactions in the gut may alter absorbability. For example, antacids reduce the absorption of iron by changing the pH and anticholinergic reduce the absorption of other drugs due to delay in gastric emptying. Absorption of drugs may be altered by the presence of food in the stomach. In many instances the absorption is delayed, whereas it is facilitated in the case of others. It is important to know this aspect in order to optimize the timing of drug administration. For several drugs, administration with water on an empty stomach ensures maximum absorption. In malabsorption states drug absorption is erratic. In congestive heart failure, venous stasis occurring in the intestines impairs absorption. Drug absorption is unpredictable in the elderly.

Drugs which are better absorbed from the buccal mucosa are preferably given sublingually. Some drugs like nitroglycerin and isoprenaline are destroyed by the gastric acid and hence, sublingual administration is ideal. Usually, the clinical effect is evident within minutes. Another advantage of sublingual administration is that drug toxicity can be avoided by removing the drug from the mouth or swallowing it as soon as the desired effect is achieved.

Topical routes include the skin and the mucus membranes of the nose, rectum and lungs. Preparations for topical application include injunctions (e.g. nitroglycerine), suppositories into the rectum (e.g. pitressin) and aerosols which are inhaled. Rate of absorption of topically applied drugs depends on the concentration, lipid solubility and local blood flow. Absorption is lower from keratinized epithelium. The size of the particle is important when drugs are applied as aerosols. Only particles below 2 nm in size reach the alveoli. Absorption from the respiratory epithelium is rapid and the effect is immediate. The portion deposited in the oropharynx is later swallowed and absorbed to produce mild and delayed effect. Considerable attention to details is necessary for ensuring proper administration of the aerosol.

Parenteral administration is resorted when more rapid action is desired and when patient's cooperation cannot be relied upon. Local vascularity influences absorption from sites of IM or subcutaneous injections. Aqueous formulations are absorbed rapidly, whereas oily preparations are absorbed slowly. Local warmth and massage favor absorption.

IM injections are usually given into the deltoid, rectus abdominis or gluteal muscles. Certain drugs like diazepam and phenytoin may be erratically absorbed, so that oral administration may be more reliable than IM doses.

The subcutaneous route is to be preferred when the volume of drug is small and the drug is non-irritant. The rate of absorption is slightly lower than the IM route. When the peripheral circulation is insufficient, as is seen in shock, subcutaneous and IM routes are unreliable. IV route should be resorted to when the drug action has to be immediate or large volumes of drugs have to be given. Since, the onset of action is immediate, the pharmacological effect can be adjusted by controlling the rate of IV infusion. At present several devices such as programmable infusion pumps which can deliver the required quantity over prolonged periods are available and these are employed in critical care departments and intensive care areas. For management of conditions like diabetes where insulin has to be administered round the clock at varying rates, implantable devices are available. Certain drugs like digoxin take several minutes to exert their full effect even after IV administration. Even highly irritant drugs like nitrogen mustards can be given into a rapidly flowing drip. Since, the drug is diluted and the venous walls are relatively resistant. Local damage to vein can be avoided by releasing the drug into more central portions of the circulation, e.g. inferior vena cava. Intra-arterial infusions are indicated when a large dose of drug has to be given in a high concentration to a particular organ.

At present, the pharmaceutical industry is bringing newer forms of drug presentation and delivery systems in order to reduce the toxic effects, acceptability, absorbability and timed release in the body. Encapsulation within a lipid vesicle (liposome) or attachment to a polymer greatly increases safety profile and permits the use of higher dosage. Newer degradable materials which act as vehicles for drugs, intelligent drug delivery systems and newer routes of drug administration are all being actively pursued.

Drugs are transported with the aid of transport proteins and they exert their effects through specific receptors. Genetic factors modify the absorption, transport, receptor mechanisms, distribution, therapeutic effects, toxicity and the elimination of drugs. At the blood-brain barrier, P-glycoprotein in the choroid plexus limits the accumulation of several drugs in the brain.

Drug Distribution

In the circulation, the drugs are reversibly bound to plasma proteins. Entry into the tissues depends upon the blood flow and the ability of the drug to enter the tissues. Easy entry into the tissues depends upon lipid solubility and the concentration gradient across the cell membranes. Major proportion of any drug is distributed to the tissues, where it has no pharmacological action. In conditions like *shock* when tissue perfusion is poor, the drug remains in the plasma in high concentrations without entering the tissues and this leads to toxicity. Specialized tissues take up drugs selectively. Most tissues of the central nervous system (CNS) restrict the entry of polar (ionized) compounds. Lipid soluble substances enter easily down a concentration gradient, while sugars and amino acids are actively transported. This blood-brain barrier breaks down when there is meningeal inflammation. At conditions of equilibrium the drug is distributed among the plasma water, plasma proteins and tissues. Since, lipid soluble drugs enter cells more readily, their concentration in the plasma is lower compared to water soluble drugs. By hemodialysis water-soluble compounds can be removed from circulation, but this is not effective for lipid-soluble drugs. Magnitude of response of any drug depends on the level of free drug available at the receptor site. The level of free drug in the plasma depends upon two factors: plasma protein binding and ease of distribution to other tissues.

Liver: Since most of the absorbed drugs pass through the liver, they are either bound, metabolized or excreted in the bile. Hepatic metabolism of drugs occurs in two stages—stage I reactions include oxidation, reduction and hydrolysis and stage II reactions involve conjugation of the original compound or its metabolites by acetylation, sulphation, O-methylation and glycine conjugation. These products are water-soluble and hence are excreted.

The metabolism of drugs in the body is governed by enzymes belonging to the class cytochrome P450 (CYPS, CYP1, CYP2 and CYP3) which play important roles in the biosynthesis and degradation of endogenous compounds such as steroids, lipids and vitamins. There are more than 30 families of drug metabolizing enzymes in humans. All have several genetic variants which determine the functions of the proteins encoded. They metabolize drugs and several chemicals found in foods and environment. They also participate in their elimination. In humans more than 57 cytochrome P450 enzymes have been identified, each with substrate specificity. Liver is the major site of cytochrome P450 metabolism, next in importance is the enterocytes lining the small intestine. Enzyme CYP3A7 is an important enzyme present at both these sites. It is involved in the metabolism of more than 50% of the drugs administered.

Lungs: Basic compounds are selectively taken up and sequestered from the general circulation.

Transplacental transfer: The placenta behaves like a selective barrier. Lipid soluble drugs of molecular weight lower than 1000 diffuse freely from the maternal to fetal circulation, while water soluble drugs diffuse only slowly. Since, the drug elimination systems of the fetus are immature, serious toxicity will ensue. The mechanism to remove the drug from the fetal circulation is diffusion back to the maternal side. Direct approach to the fetus by surgical techniques is feasible in a few hospitals.

Plasma Protein Binding

Plasma proteins, especially albumin forms reversible complexes with drugs in circulation. The degree of absorption depends upon the plasma pH and affinity of the drug to the protein. When many drugs compete for absorption, the high affinity drug displaces the ones with weak affinity. Acidic drugs will be displaced from protein complex when acidosis develops.

Factors that alter Protein Binding Include

- Hypoalbuminemia
- Last trimester of pregnancy
- Renal failure
- Displacement by other drugs.

Elimination of Drugs

Drugs are eliminated from the body by (1) metabolism in the liver and kidney and (2) excretion as the parent drug as such or its metabolites by the kidneys predominantly, but also by the gut, skin, lungs, sweat glands, breasts and salivary glands. Urinary excretion depends upon the processes of (1) glomerular filtration (2) active tubular secretion and reabsorption and (3) passive diffusion.

PHARMACOGENETICS

The influence of genetic factors in drug effects was recognized as early as the 1950s. Enzyme defects may give rise to arrested metabolism of drugs, thereby leading to unexpected drug effects.

For example, cytochrome P4502D6 (CYP2D6) influences the metabolism of codeine, dextromethorphan, metoprolol and nortriptyline.

Deficiency of the enzyme N-acetyl transferase leads slow acetylation of isonicotinylhydrazide (INH), hydralazine and procainamide. At present genetic tools are available for identifying such genetic alterations.

Pharmacogenomics is the study of genes encoding the drug metabolizing enzymes and genome-based approaches to drug-behaviour in different persons.

Molecular diagnostic methods to determine the genotypes of individuals are becoming more freely available. At present, it is possible to get genotype analysis from single blood samples and about 5000 genes and 20,000 single nucleotide polymorphisms can be studied in a single assay. It can help more individualized selection of drugs with better efficiency and safety. This is much more useful for selecting drugs for cancer, infections such as tuberculosis, anticoagulants, antiretroviral drugs and others. Development of severe drug reactions such as Stevens-Johnson Syndrome due to carbamazepine therapy is related to association with HLAB 1502. Use of genetic studies in therapy is taking roots in India, despite its high cost and problems of availability.

GENERAL PRINCIPLES OF DRUG ADMINISTRATION

The effective and safe dose of any drug should be determined by considering the body mass or surface area. Though general instructions regarding dose are available, each dose should be tailored to the individual patient, based on his weight, status of vital organs like kidneys and liver, the severity of the infection and the immune status of the host. Though, a long course of therapy is ideal for an effecting cure, yet chances for toxicity limits the total dose.

Seriously ill patients should be treated by injection since, this ensures predictable serum levels. IV injection is more effective in giving peak serum levels and is less painful than IM or other routes. This is the route of choice when large volumes of drugs have to be given and that too continuously. Though polyethylene cannulas are handy and convenient for use, steel needles are better to avoid infection. Ideally, the needles have to be re-sited at least every 48 hours to avoid venous thrombosis and infections.

Parenteral preparations are more likely to produce anaphylactic reactions than oral preparations. Topical application of drugs for general antibacterial action except to the eye and ear should be discouraged, since they produce local reactions and also give rise to emergence of resistant strains. Intrathecal injection of antibiotics is potentially hazardous and is often unnecessary except in the case of resistant meningitis, unresponsive to systemic therapy. It is seen that several drugs pass into the cerebrospinal fluid (CSF) from blood when the meninges are inflamed, due to disruption of the blood-brain barrier.

Chemoprophylaxis: Use of antibiotics for chemoprophylaxis is controversial. Bacteria resistant to the antibiotics may be selected out to multiply and the possible toxicity of drugs may also occur. Chemoprophylaxis does not guarantee prevention of infection. The aim of chemoprophylaxis is to prevent a known organism from reaching a target tissue and if it reaches the aim shifts toward aborting infection. Chemoprophylaxis is employed in special situations such as prevention of active tuberculosis in special groups, prophylaxis against *Pneumocystis carinii* in acquired immune deficiency syndrome (AIDS) patients, accidental needle stick injuries in laboratory workers, newborns of human immunodeficiency virus (HIV) positive mothers and other similar circumstances. If an antibiotic is intended to give coverage during a surgical procedure, it should be given IM 30 minutes before an operation or IV during the surgery and for a short period thereafter.

Severe infections: Life-threatening infections such as septicemia, pneumonia, peritonitis, meningitis and others have to be treated even before microbiological results are available, especially so, if the patient is neutropenic. Helpful investigations include microbial identification, determination of antibiotic sensitivity and serum levels of the drug.

Factors Affecting Drug Metabolism

■ ***Age:*** Impaired metabolism in premature babies, infants and young adults, eliminate drugs more rapidly than adults.

- ***Children:*** The action of drugs differs quantitatively and qualitatively in children compared to that in adults. Before embarking on therapy it is absolutely essential to take into consideration the following points:
  - Is the drug absolutely essential?
  - Is it safe for the age group?
  - Which preparation is best, most palatable and convenient for administration?
  - Which is the best drug with least side effects? The absorption, distribution, breakdown and elimination of drugs depends upon the maturity and relative size of body tissues. Other than age and size, genetic constitution, maturity of the kidneys, enzyme development in the liver, protein binding of the drug, organ sensitivity, distribution of the drug in the body and development of the CNS affect drug response and toxicity in infants and children. Changes in body composition, development of blood-brain barrier with increasing age and metabolic disturbances such as acidosis affect the distribution of drugs. The rate of drug elimination is greatly diminished in neonates, especially premature infants. Topically applied drugs are significantly more absorbed in infants and children, particularly in prematures. Drugs excreted in breast milk during the early postnatal period may influence the baby. Proper education of the parent and child is important to ensure drug compliance.

- ***Drug administration in the elderly:*** Old subjects are likely to have multiple pathological lesions and hence, they are susceptible to the cumulative adverse effects of several drugs which are concurrently administered. Elderly persons behave erratically to drugs. Since, their weight is low, the ordinary doses may prove to be toxic. Absorption from the alimentary tract may not be predictable. Moreover, impairment of functions of the liver and kidney lead to their accumulation in the body. In addition, the organ systems may also show increased sensitivity, e.g. aged persons are more prone to develop cardiotoxicity of digitalis and ototoxicity of the aminoglycosides. In elderly persons above 60 years the renal function normally falls, even without specific kidney disease. This fall is much more pronounced in the presence of chronic kidney disease (CKD). Persons above 80 years may have a glomerular filtration rate (GFR) of $60\ \text{mL/m/1.7 m}^2$ body surface, just enough to carry on normal renal function, if undisturbed. Drugs such as nonsteroidal anti-inflammatory drugs (NSAIDs), drugs which raise serum potassium such as angiotensin receptor blockers (ARB) may lead to rapid fall in renal function and tip them into acute renal failure.

Adverse effects of drugs constitute a major cause for morbidity in old persons and therefore, great care is required for prescribing drugs to them. Aged women with history of allergic diathesis are particularly susceptible to develop drug toxicity. An early sign of drug toxicity is mental confusion and disorderly behavior which should not be ignored. Drug compliance is generally poor in the older age groups due to their physical disability, mental confusion and economic dependence. Particular care, therefore, is to be taken to ensure that drug schedules are followed. Hospitalization should be avoided as far as possible since, older persons cannot adapt to the hospital environment. As a consequence they develop confusion and dis-orientation. Moreover, hospitalization and immo-bilization lead to complications like respiratory infection, urinary retention, fecal and urinary incontinence, falls, venous thrombosis, embolism, and strokes. Confinement to bed should be kept to the minimum and the patient should be ambulated as early as possible.

- **Liver disease:** Oxidation reactions are less efficient in presence of severe liver disease and malnourished patients. Conjugation preserved.
- **Drug-drug interactions**
- **Diet and environmental factors**
- **Pharmacogenetics:** Drug metabolism that varies on genetic basis is often called polymorphic drug metabolism. Most common source is single nucleotide polymorphism.
- **Drug administration during pregnancy:** The fact that the drugs may harm the mother, fetus or both should be borne in mind. The main dangers to the growing fetus include:
  - Destruction of the embryo and abortion, e.g. quinine, cytotoxic drugs
  - Congenital defects and disorders of organ develop-ment are particularly common with drugs like thalidomide, radioactive drugs, anticonvulsants and anticancer drugs. Almost all drugs including large doses of some vitamins are associated with embryotoxicity in varying degrees at specific periods of gestation
  - Incorporation into the tissues of the fetus, e.g. tetracycline into the teeth
  - Pharmacological effects on the fetus by drugs which cross the placenta, e.g. antithyroid drugs may cause thyroid dysfunction in the newborn. Hormone administered to the mother may affect the fetus. Apart from the damage caused to the embryo, the mother is more susceptible to the toxic effects of several drugs during pregnancy, e.g. tetracyclines are more likely to produce hepatic damage during pregnancy. In general it is a golden rule to withhold medication to a pregnant woman unless absolutely indicated.

DRUG RELATED ADVERSE EFFECTS

Definition: An unwanted or harmful reaction experienced following the administration of a drug or combination of drugs under normal conditions of use and suspected to be related to the drug.

Adverse drug reactions are extremely common in present day medical practice. There are two types of adverse drug reactions: A and B. **Type A** is the result of an augmented or exaggerated pharmacological action of a drug given in the therapeutic doses (Table 4.2). These are primarily dependent upon the intrinsic biodynamic properties of the drug, often host-independent, dose-dependent and usually reproducible in animals. They are sometimes called predictable reactions which include overdosage, side effects, drug-caused disease and drug interactions, e.g. beta-adrenergic blockers produce bradycardia. Ephedrine causes tachycardia and insomnia.

Type B reactions causes totally bizarre unpredictable or aberrant effects that are not to be expected from the known pharmacological effects of a drug when given in usual therapeutic doses and with no alteration in pharmacokinetic processes. They are 'idiosyncratic', host-dependent, often apparently dose-independent and difficult to reproduce in animals.

Type A reactions: The factors involved in Type A reactions are divided into pharmaceutical, pharmacokinetic or pharmacodynamic causes.

Pharmaceutical causes: Factors that affect drug dose and release from the formulation
Pharmacokinetic causes: Factors which alter absorption, distribution, metabolism and elimination
Pharmacodynamic causes: Factors which depend on dose-response relationship, drug receptor status, homeostatic mechanisms and disease state of the individual.

Type B reactions: They are characterized by the existence of some qualitative difference either in the drug or in the patient or possibly in both, are classified as intolerance, idiosyncrasy and allergy. The causes of type B reactions could be pharmaceutical, pharmacokinetic or may lie in a target organ response.

Some of the serious and life threatening forms of idiosyncrasy caused by drugs are hematological compli-cations. These include agranulocytosis, bone marrow aplasia, hemolytic anemia, thrombocytopenia and distur-

Table 4.2: Types of adverse drug reactions

	Type A	Type B
Drug response	Augmented	Bizarre
Pharmacologically predictable	Yes	Bizarre
Dose-dependent	Yes	No
Dependence on host	Often independent	Usually dependent
Incidence	High	Low
Morbidity	High	Low
Mortality	Low	High
Treatment	Dose adjustment	Stop and antidotes

Textbook of Medicine

bances in the coagulation cascade. These may occur abruptly without warning and these have to be specially looked for. Early withdrawal of the drug and proper management results in recovery. The other two organs most commonly affected are the kidney and the liver.

In general adverse drug reactions may involve several systems and many present as systemic illness (e.g. serum sickness) or particularly affect any organ system (no organ is spared) and it is duty of the prescribing physician to be aware of these side effects and take steps to prevent these complications, detect them early if they occur and manage the events suitably to prevent deterioration and bring about recovery. It is also the duty of the physician to inform the patient and his relatives about the adverse reaction in order to prevent recurrence. Any error on the part of the physician in anticipating the adverse effect and managing it will be liable for legal actions.

Table 4.2 shows the salient differentiating features between the two types of adverse drug reactions.

Rational therapeutics is defined as the use of the least number of drugs to obtain the best possible effect in the shortest time and at a reasonable cost. In general about 25% of hospitalized patients suffer from DRAs which may prove fatal. Risk of adverse events increases at the rate of 6% for every additional day of hospitalization. It is likely that about 5 million persons may suffer from serious adverse drug reactions (ADRs). Aggressive drug therapy, particularly polypharmacy (concurrent use of several different classes of drugs) increases the risk, 50% of these are preventable, if the physician and his staff are careful to avoid DRAs and to take early remedial steps.

Suggestions to Reduce the Frequency of Adverse Drug Events (ADEs)

- Use of check lists, protocols and computerized aids for writing prescriptions
- Improved access to information using computerized programs
- Error proofing using customized computer software so that overdose, suboptimal drug doses, improper duration and allergic reactions can be avoided
- Training of doctors, nurses and other staff on safe prescribing practice
- Informing the public on adverse drug reaction and their remedy.

It is a golden rule to use a limited number of drugs, about which the doctor has full information as far as possible. The Government of India has accepted an essential drug list containing 279 drugs which are adequate to manage most of the common ailments.

The adage ***there are no biologically safe drugs; there are only safe physicians*** holds good even now and it will continue to be so forever.

The WHO has Suggested Core Interventions—To Promote Rational use of Medicines

- Formation of a mandated multidisciplinary national body to co-ordinate policies on medicine use
- Popularize evidence-based guidelines
- Essential medicines list to be adopted for drug procurement and distribution

- Drugs and therapeutic committees in all major institutions to monitor drug use, procurement and others
- Better training of medical students in the undergraduate courses
- Continuous medical education to practicing doctors should be compulsory for renewing the license
- Supervision and audit of prescribing doctors and sending feedback to them
- Provide unbiased information to the doctors on drugs from the central source
- Educate the public on rational use of drugs
- Avoid and discourage financial and other influences undertaken by commercial interests to influence doctors
- Governmental control on the pharmaceutical industry, particularly concerning promotional activities and to avoid 'across the counter' sales of particular drugs without prescription
- Sufficient governmental organization to provide adequate supervisional staff and essential drugs.

MEDICAL ERRORS

Adverse event (AE): A definable injury caused at least in part by medical management, the injury must have prolonged during the hospital stay or caused disability at the time of discharge.

Adverse drug event (ADE): AE related to the administration of drugs.

Negligent adverse event: An injury caused by failure on the part of the doctor to meet standards expected of an average doctor in his settings.

Drug related problem (DRP): An event or circumstance that involves patient's drug treatment that actually or potentially interferes with achievement of an optimal outcome.

The spectrum of ADEs include following types:
- Wrong choice of drug
- Wrong dose, frequency and route of administration
- Drug-drug interaction
- Inadequate instruction to nursing staff
- Allergic reactions.

Failure to use a life-saving drug when indicated, also amount to negligence on the part of the doctor. While prescribing antimicrobial agents the full duration of therapy should be insisted upon even though symptomatic relief is achieved early. In India, the most common causes of medical errors arise from inadequate information for the doctor (29%), wrong diagnosis (18%), wrong administration and failure to recognize ADEs early.

The need to monitor ADRs and to prevent them has been realized by the medical fraternity in India. The common defects in prescription detected by limited surveys included:

No mention of the dose of the drug	60%
Absence of information on the route and method of administration	99%
Administration of antibiotic for inadequate duration	60%
Information of the dose was given but partly	11%

Some of the State Governments in India including the Government of Kerala supply drug formularies to their doctors which provide factual data on drugs.

DRUG INTERACTION

Definition: A measurable modification (in magnitude and/or duration) of the action of one drug by prior or concomitant administration of another substance, including pre-scription, non-prescription (including complementary medicines) drugs, food, alcohol, cigarette smoking or diagnostic tests.

Outcomes of Drug Interaction

- Loss of therapeutic effect
- Toxicity
- Unexpected increase in pharmacological activity
- Beneficial effects, e.g. additive and potentiation (intended) or antagonism (unintended)
- Chemical or physical interaction, e.g. IV incompatibility in fluid or syringes mixture.

Mechanism of Drug Interaction

Pharmacokinetics: Involve the effect of a drug on another from the point of view that includes absorption, distribution, metabolism and excretion.

Pharmacodynamics: Are related to the pharmacological activity of the interacting drugs, e.g. synergism. Antagonism, altered cellular transport, effect on the receptor site.

Prevention of Drug Interaction

- Monitoring therapy and making adjustments.
- Monitoring blood level of some drugs with narrow therapeutic index, e.g. digoxin, anticancer agents etc.
- Monitoring some parameters that may help to characterize the early events of interaction or toxicity, e.g. with warfarin administration, it is recommended to monitor the prothrombin time to detect any change in the drug activity.
- Increase the interest of case report studies to report different possibilities of drug interaction.

PRESCRIPTION OF DRUGS

- Medicines should be prescribed only when absolutely indicated. Once prescribed, the dose, route of administration, relationship with food and duration of therapy should be clearly specified. The total quantity of each drug to be dispensed should be separately specified.
- As far as possible generic names should be specified. Proprietary names should be used only when it is unavoidable.

- Avoid decimal points as far as possible, e.g. 3 mg instead of 0.03 g or 3.0 mg.
- Quantities below 1 mg should be given as micrograms (mcg or μg) or smaller units, e.g. instead of 0.1 mg write as 100 mcg.
- When decimals are unavoidable, use the format as 0.5 mL and not as ·5 mL.
- The prescription should be authenticated by legible signature of the prescriber and his address. The legal responsibility of a prescription rests on the prescriber.

The drugs and cosmetics ACT of 1945 has included drugs into different schedules.

- Drugs in schedule G should be administered only under the supervision of a registered medical practitioner (RMP).
- Drugs in schedule H should be dispensed only on the prescription of RMP.
- Drugs included in schedule X include psychotropic drugs and all prescriptions should be made in duplicate and authenticated by the full signature, address and registration number of the practitioners.

Patient education is a very important responsibility of the prescribing doctor. He should include information on the following aspects:

- Drug
- Time
- Dose
- Intervals
- Duration of treatment
- Cost.

The patient should be instructed to report adverse reactions promptly after stopping the drug. On no account should the doctor turn away from the responsibility of having prescribed the drug. He should view the situation with empathy and confidence. Almost all the ADRs are remediable, if detected early. Prompt handling of the situation will increase the confidence of the patient. Irresponsible behavior on the part of the prescriber often leads to legal complications.

It should also be remembered that any doctor prescribing medicines should confine to the system, he is qualified in. Cross system medical practice which involves prescription of drugs or procedures from other systems of medicine in which the physician has no qualification is considered as ***medical negligence***.

Source:

1. API Textbook of Medicine, 9th edn, Section 4, pp 126-36.
2. Paul Y, Tiwari S. Issues to settle-cross system medical practice. J Assoc Physicians India. 2014;62(3):244-7.

Textbook of Medicine

Antimicrobial Agents

KV Krishna Das, S Bhasi

> **Chapter Summary**
>
> - Antibacterial Agents
> - β-lactam antibiotics
> - Antiviral Drugs
> - Antifungal Drugs
> - Drug Resistance of Microbes
> - The Problem of Superbugs
> - Rational use of Antibiotics

INTRODUCTION

The initial specific antibacterial drugs, sulfonamides were introduced in the early part of the 20th century. Discovery of penicillin and its introduction into therapeutics in the first half of the 20th century leading to dramatic cure of infections, acted as a stimulus for intense research to discover further antimicrobial drugs. As a result, many types of antibiotics were introduced in succession.

After the initial rapid spurt of production of newer and newer antibiotics (antibacterial, antifungal and antiviral) till the eighth decade of the previous century, there was a lull in the production of newer drugs and the main activity of the drug industry was to modify the molecules to increase potency and effectiveness and to increase their effectiveness against resistant microbes and also to make synergistic combinations.

With the turn of the twenty first century, after getting success in the manufacture of antiretroviral drugs and drugs for viral hepatitis and others there is again a very active revival of production of antiviral, antifungal and also antibacterial drugs belonging to several classes. Due to the rapid addition in the number of antimicrobials, a full list tends to become outdated within a short time. As far as possible these newer drugs are included in the appropriate sections.

Table 5.1 gives the site of action of the commonly used classes of antibacterial drugs.

ANTIBACTERIAL AGENTS

Penicillin

Penicillin, discovered by Alexander Fleming, in 1928 was the first effective antibiotic to be produced commercially, marketed widely and accepted with great zeal all over the world on account of its efficacy, safety and affordable cost. Introduction of penicillin ushered in the 'antibiotic' era in the therapy of infective diseases.

The basic nucleus is 6-aminopenicillanic acid which contains a thiazole ring linked to β-lactam ring. Further derivatives of penicillin contain the β-lactam

Table 5.1: Principal types of antibacterial agents and their mechanism of action

Drug	Antibacterial action on the susceptible microbes
Penicillin	Inhibits cell wall synthesis
Other β-lactam antibiotics	Inhibits cell wall synthesis
Cephalosporins	Inhibits cell wall synthesis
Aminoglycosides	Inhibits protein synthesis acting on ribosomes
Tetracyclines	Inhibits protein synthesis acting on ribosomes
Tigecycline	Inhibits protein synthesis acting on ribosomes
Macrolides	Inhibits protein synthesis acting on ribosomes
Ketolide, e.g. telithromycin	Inhibits protein synthesis
Chloramphenicol	Inhibits protein synthesis acting on ribosomes
Sulfonamide, trimethoprim, diaminopyrimidines, e.g. pyrimethamine	Inhibit folate metabolism of microbes
Glycopeptides, e.g. vancomycin	Inhibits cell wall synthesis
Lincosamides, e.g. clindamycin, lincomycin	Inhibits protein synthesis acting on ribosomes
Clindamycin	Inhibits protein synthesis
Oxazolidinone, e.g. linezolid	Inhibits protein synthesis
Daptomycin	Disruption of cell wall and cell lysis
Quinupristin/dalfopristin	Inhibits protein synthesis
Nitrofurans, e.g, nitrofurantoin, nifurtimox	DNA strand breakages in bacterial cells
Quinolones and nalidixic acid	Inhibits DNA metabolism of microbes
Nitroimidazoles, e.g. metronidazole, tinidazole	Damage to DNA in bacterial cell
Fusidic acid	Inhibits protein synthesis acting on ribosomes
Rifamycin and rifampicin	Inhibits transcription of DNA to RNA
Bacitracin	Inhibits cell wall synthesis
Polymyxin and colistin	Disrupt the permeability of the outer and cytoplasmic membrane
Gramicidin A	Cause pores in the lipid layer
Daptomycin	Cause channels in cell membrane
Vancomycin	Inhibits cell wall synthesis
Streptogramins	Blocks proteins synthesis
Mupirocin	Inhibits RNA synthesis

Abbreviations: DNA = Deoxyribonucleic acid; RNA = Ribonucleic acid

ring and all such members are included under the term β-lactam antibiotics. Many bacteria develop resistance by producing β-lactamase. Penicillin and its derivatives block the synthesis of the bacterial cell wall peptidoglycan. Penicillin and its derivatives hold their pride of place among the most powerful antibiotics against susceptible bacteria. They are the drugs of choice in the appropriate situations on account of their proven bactericidal activity, wide availability, safety profile and relatively lower cost.

Susceptible organisms: *Streptococcus pyogenes,* pneumococci, susceptible gonococci and meningococci, spirochetes such as *Treponema pallidum, T. pertenue* and *Leptospira,* anaerobes such as *Clostridium tetani, Clostridium botulinum, Clostridium perfringens, Peptococcus, Peptostreptococcus, Bacteroides, Bacillus anthracis* and staphylococci which are sensitive, respond well to penicillin. *Staphylococcus,* the organism causing infective endocarditis is susceptible in many cases.

Safety: Penicillin is generally safe. Most important adverse side effects are allergy and Jarisch-Herxheimer reaction. Anaphylactic shock and cardiac arrest may occur in unexpected situations. So any history of allergy to penicillin, however mild, is an absolute contraindication to even testing for drug sensitivity. In the absence of any history of allergy, allergy can be tested by a scratch test on the forearm using a weak solution (1000 units/mL) of penicillin. Negative scratch test is not an absolute safeguard against a major anaphylactic reaction. While testing for penicillin allergy, a resuscitation kit containing 1/1000 solution or adrenaline, hydrocortisone vials and intravenous (IV) drip glucose saline should be ready at hand in addition to syringes, needles and IV infusion sets.

Antacids reduce the absorption of orally administered penicillin. Penicillin is mainly eliminated in the urine. Probenecid reduces the urinary excretion when given in a dose of 250–500 mg bd orally along with penicillin. It helps to keep the blood levels of penicillin higher for longer periods.

Resistance to penicillin: Several microbes such as staphylococci, gonococci, meningococci, pneumococci and others have developed resistance in a big way and this has posed major problems in the management of life-threatening infections.

Mechanisms of Resistance

- Production of β-lactamases, e.g. staphylococci, gonococci. This can be overcome by the concurrent use of β-lactamase inhibitors such as clavulanic acid, sulbactam or tazobactum.
- Reduction in the permeability of the outer membrane, e.g. gram-negative bacteria.
- Alteration in the binding sites for β-lactams, e.g. methicillin resistant staphylococci.

Dosage of Benzylpenicillin Congeners

	Dose
Benzylpenicillin-penicillin G	4–6 lac units 6 hour
Phenoxymethylpenicillin-penicillin V	4–6 lac units 6 hour oral tablets (250–500 mg 6 hour) tablets
Procaine penicillin	6–12 lac units once or twice a day intramuscular (IM) injection
Benzathine penicillin	12–24 lac units IM (1.2–2.4 mega units once in 3 weeks)

β-lactamase resistant penicillin: These are less potent than benzylpenicillin, but they are effective against penicillinase producing staphylococci and other mixed infections. Cloxacillin, methicillin and nafcillin belong to this group.

Cloxacillin

It is available as capsules of 250 and 500 mg and as injections of 0.5 and 1.0 g.

Dose: Oral—500 mg 1 g 6 h; later maintenance dose of 250–500 mg 6 h, given one hour before or 2 hours after food. Parenteral—IV or IM injections 250–500 mg 6 hour.

Cloxacillin is available as combination preparations along with ampicillin or amoxicillin.

Other members of this group are methicillin and nafcillin which are not freely available in India.

Broad spectrum penicillins: The antimicrobial activity covers gram-negative organisms such as *Haemophilus influenzae. Escherichia coli* and β-lactam antibiotics in addition to the spectrum of penicillin. These are also inactivated by β-lactamase.

Ampicillin

Preparations available include capsules of 250 and 500 mg, injections containing 250 mg–1 g and pediatric syrup and drops.

Dose: Oral—250–500 mg 6 h. Parenteral—0.5–2 g IM or IV 6 hour, depending upon the severity of the infection.

Cross sensitivity with penicillin may occur but allergic reactions are generally milder. In patients with infectious mononucleosis, ampicillin worsens the clinical condition. Administration of probenecid or sulbactam helps to maintain blood levels higher for longer periods. Vials containing ampicillin 1 g and sulbactam 0.5 g are available.

Amoxicillin

This drug resembles ampicillin in actions and antimicrobial spectrum. When given orally the blood levels are twice as high as that of ampicillin. Addition of clavulanic acid prolongs the action of amoxcyillin.

Preparations available: Capsules 125, 250 and 500 mg 30 minutes before or 2 hours after food every 4–6 hourly, injections containing 250 and 500 mg. Ampicillin and amoxicillin in combination with cloxacillin (250 mg of each drug) are available in the Indian market for oral use.

Dose: 250–500 mg oral or IM or IV 8 h.

Other members of this group include bacampicillin, pivampicillin and talampicillin. These are not freely available in India.

Extended spectrum penicillins: The additional spectrum includes *Pseudomonas, Klebsiella, Enterobacteriaceae* and *Proteus.* Carbenicillin, ticarcillin, azlocillin, piperacillin and mezlocillin come under this group. Piperacillin and mezlocillin are active against *Klebsiella* also. Dose of pre-piperacillin 2 g 8 hourly IV. The preparation should not be mixed with aminoglycosides since, the latter may be inactivated.

Carbenicillin

Preparations available include injections of 1 g and 5 g.

Dose: 2–6 g 6 h IM or slow IV infusion.

Mixed infections including *Pseudomonas* and *Proteus* especially in immunocompromised hosts are special indications for carbenicillin.

Special risk: Due to the high sodium content it may precipitate cardiac failure in susceptible subjects.

Ticarcillin in combination with clavulanic acid is active against *Pseudomonas* and *Proteus* species as well. Available preparation is 1 g vials dose is 3 g IV every 6–8 hours.

β-LACTAM ANTIBIOTICS

Imipenem (Carbapenem)

This is a very powerful bactericidal antibiotic with a very broad spectrum including gram-positive and gram-negative aerobic and anaerobic organisms. It is enzymically inactivated in the kidney and therefore concurrent administration of cilastin which inhibits the enzyme helps to potentiate the antibacterial activity. Adverse effects include allergic reactions, gastrointestinal disturbances, pseudomembranous colitis, elevation of liver enzymes, hemolysis, seizures, dysgeusia, jaundice and mental disturbances.

Dose: 500–1000 mg 8 hour IM or IV upto 2 g/day in divided doses.

Meropenam: 500 mg IV or IM 3–4 times a day. It has action against aerobic and anaerobic, gram-positive and gram-negative organisms.

Aztreonam

This is a monocyclic β-lactam antibiotic. It is active against gram-negative aerobic bacteria including *Pseudomonas aeruginosa*. It is particularly useful to treat hospital acquired infections arising from the urogenital tract, biliary system, respiratory system and female genital tract. Adverse effects include local pain and inflammation and seizures.

Cephalosporins

These are among the most popular and widespread antibiotics at present. They contain 7-aminocephalo-sporanic acid (ACA) nucleus, which bears structural resemblance to 6-aminopenicillanic acid (APA) and the β-lactam ring. They are listed arbitrarily as first, second, third and fourth generation mainly on the basis of their antimicrobial activity and also on the period of their introduction as well as structure.

The first generation members resemble penicillin in antibacterial activity. Successive inclusion in the second, third and fourth generations depends upon their wider antimicrobial coverage and effectiveness on resistant strains.

The list is very long and several newer drugs are being added from time to time. The important and easily available members are listed in Table 5.2.

The bacterial spectrum includes gram-positive cocci, gram-negative bacilli, gram-positive bacilli and gram-negative cocci in decreasing order of sensitivity. Main

Table 5.2: List of cephalosporins and their route of administration

Oral	Parenteral
First generation	
Cephalexin	Cefazolin
Cefadroxil	Cephalothin
Cefradine	Cefapirin
	Cephaloridine
Second generation	
Cefaclor	Cefuroxime
Cefuroxime axetil	Cefoxitin
	Cefamandole
	Cefotetan
Third generation	
Cefixime	Ceftizoxime
	Cefoperazone
	Ceftazidime
	Cefotaxime
	Ceftriaxone
	Cefsulodin
Fourth generation	
	Cefepime and Cefpirome

indications include skin and soft tissue infections with *Staphylococcus aureus* and *Staphylococcus pyogenes*.

Boxes below show details of the drugs, their dose, route and available preparations.

First Generation

They resist β-lactamase. They do not penetrate into cerebrospinal fluid (CSF). This group includes:

Drug	Route	Dose	Frequency	Available preparations
Cephalexin	Oral	250–500 mg	6 h	Tab or cap 150, 250, 500 mg
Cefadroxil	Oral	1–2 g	12 h	Tab or cap 125, 250, 500 mg
Cefradine	IV or oral	1–2 g	4–6 h	Vials 1, 2 g
Cefazolin	IV or IM	0.5–2 g	8 h	Vials 125, 250, 500 mg
Cephalothin	IV	1–2 g	4–6 h	Vials 1, 2 g
Cephaloridine	IV	0.5 g	6 h	Vials 0.5, 1 g

Bacterial spectrum includes gram-negative cocci, gram-negative bacilli, gram-positive cocci and gram-positive bacilli in decreasing order of sensitivity these drugs are used for upper respiratory infections (URI), urinary infections, soft tissue infection, meningitis and gonorrhea.

Second Generation

They have expanded spectrum of activity against gram-negative bacilli, especially ampicillin resistant *Haemophilus influenzae*. Penetration into CSF is poor. Activity against gram-positive cocci is less than that of the first generation.

Textbook of Medicine

Drug	Route	Dose	Frequency	Available preparations
Cefaclor	Oral	150–500 mg	8 h	275 or 350 mg tablets
Cefuroxime axetil	Oral	250 mg	12 h	125, 250, 500 mg tablets
Cefuroxime	IM or IV	750 mg–1.5 g	8 h	250, 750 or 1500 mg vial
Cefoxitin	IM or IV	1–2 g	4–8 h	1, 2 g vial
Cefamandole	IM or IV	1–2 g	4–6 h	1, 2 g vial
Cefotetan	IM or IV	1–3 g	12 h	1, 2 and 10 g vial

Third Generation

The bacterial spectrum in order of decreasing sensitivity include gram-negative cocci, gram-negative bacilli and anaerobes, gram-positive cocci and gram-positive bacilli. Main clinical indications include cellulitis, meningitis, septicemia, respiratory and urinary tract infections (UTIs) and intra-abdominal infections.

Drug	Route	Dose	Frequency	Available preparations
Cefixime	Oral	200–400	12–24 h	Tablet of 200 mg and 400 mg
Ceftizoxime	IM or IV	1–2 g	8–12 h	0.5, 1 g vial
Cefoperazone	IM or IV	1–2 g	8–12 h	0.5, 2 g vial
Ceftazidime	IM or IV	1–2 g	8–12 h	0.5, 1 g vial
Cefotaxime	IM or IV	1–2 g	8 h	0.5, 1 g vial
Ceftriaxone	IM or IV	1–2 g	12–24 h	0.5, 1 g vial
Cefsulodin	IM or IV	0.5–1 g	6 h	0.5, 1 g vial

Fourth Generation

This include drugs which have got extended spectrum of activity compared to the third generation drugs. They are also more resistant to the action of β-lactamase. The bacterial spectrum in order of decreasing sensitivity are gram-negative cocci, gram-negative bacilli resistant to third generation cephalosporins. They are not effective against gram-positive bacilli and anaerobes. Their special use is in the treatment of aerobic gram-negative bacilli resistant to the other drugs, such as hospital acquired pneumonia, UTIs, septicemia and intra-abdominal infections.

Drug	Route	Dose	Frequency	Available preparations
Cefepime	IV	2 g	12 h	1 g and 2 g powder with diluent
Cefpirome	IV/IM	1–2 g	12 h	1 g and 2 g powder with diluent

Aminoglycosides

These are bactericidal antibiotics. They derive their name on account of the presence of amino sugars in glycoside linkage in their structures. They have to be given parenterally, since they are not absorbed from the gut. Their distribution is mainly in the extracellular fluid (ECF), higher concentrations in renal cortex and endolymph and perilymph of the internal ear. These organs are more liable to suffer from toxic effects, especially in the elderly. At both extremes of age and in the presence of renal insufficiency

Table 5.3: Therapeutic details of aminoglycoside

Drug	Route	Dose	Preparation
Streptomycin	IM single dose	15–25 mg/kg/day	1 g or 0.75 g vials
Gentamicin	IM or IV	2–5 mg/kg/day 80 mg or 60 mg divided doses 8 h	80 mg vials
Amikacin	IM or IV	15 mg/kg/day 8 h	50 mg–500 mg vials
Kanamycin	IM	15 mg/kg/day 8 h	500 mg–1 g vials
Tobramycin	IM	3 mg/kg/day 8 h	40 mg and 80 mg vials
Netilmicin	IV/IM	5 mg/kg bw 8 h	Vials of 10–200 mg/mL

the dose has to be modified to avoid toxicity. Diffusion into CSF and ocular structures is poor. Bacteria develop resistance rapidly, especially if administered singly. Administration along with other antibacterial agents reduces the chances for development of resistance. When combined with β-lactam antibiotics such as penicillins or cephalosporins the action is synergistic. The important members in this group are streptomycin, gentamicin, amikacin, kanamycin, tobramycin, netilmicin, neomycin, framycetin and paromomycin (Table 5.3).

Antibacterial Spectrum

Streptomycin: Gram-negative bacteria, *Streptococcus viridans, Yersinia pestis, Francisella tularensis, Brucella, Mycobacterium tuberculosis.* Until four decades ago this was among the first line drugs for the treatment of tuberculosis. With the availability of rifampicin, streptomycin has been moved down to be a second line drug due to its lower efficacy, need for IM administration and likelihood to develop bacterial resistance.

Gentamicin: Gram-negative bacteria especially *Escherichia coli* and *Proteus, Pseudomonas aeruginosa, Klebsiella, Acinetobacter, Mycoplasma,* group A *Streptococcus* and *Staphylococcus* are susceptible. It is very effective in mixed infections such as peritonitis, empyema, UTIs and others. It is one of the very reliable and powerful bactericidal antibiotics to be used in combination in serious life-threatening infections, even before the microbiological results are available. Preparations for topical use are available, e.g. eyedrops. In view of the risk of development of resistance it is advisable to minimize their use. It is contraindicated in pregnancy. Adverse side effects include nephrotoxicity and irreversible ototoxicity.

Amikacin: *Serratia, Proteus, Pseudomonas, Klebsiella, Enterobacteriaceae, E. coli.* Nosocomial gram-negative infections and atypical mycobacteria are susceptible. This is one of the very powerful antibiotics available for use in life-threatening conditions. This may also be used as a second line drug for *Mycobacterium tuberculosis.*

Kanamycin: Gram-positive and gram-negative organisms causing UTIs, septicemia, meningitis, bacterial endocarditis and pelvic infections respond to the drug. It is an 'add-on' drug with other broad spectrum antibiotics. It is used as second line drug for resistant *Mycobacterium tuberculosis.* Dose is 15 mg/kg/week (0.5–1 g IV or IM twice or thrice a week). It amplifices the neuromuscular block caused therapeutically by muscle relaxants given during anesthesia and this has to be borne in mind when the drug is used for surgical patients.

Tobramycin: It is more active against *Pseudomonas*. It is usually given along with ampicillin or ceftazidime. The dose is 3 mg/kg/bw/day given as IM injection 8 hour.

Netilmicin: This drug is effective in serious infections of the respiratory tract and other locations such as intra-abdominal infections. It is also used as a prophylaxis for bacteremias in a dose 5 mg/kg bw 8 h. It is available as IV injection vials in strengths ranging from 10 mg–200 mg/mL. Adverse side effects include neurotoxicity and nephrotoxicity. It is very effective in serious infections by *Enterobacteriaceae, Klebsiella* and *Staphylococci*.

Tetracyclines

These are in existence for over six decades. They are bacteriostatic. They act by inhibiting protein synthesis in the microbe. Though they are not considered as the first line of drugs for the common bacterial infections, they retain their pride of place for several infections such as *Rickettsia, Mycoplasma, Borrelia* and *Chlamydia* and others. They are active against a wide range of micro-organism. Their popularity has come down due to their adverse side effects, tendency to confer resistance and the availability of safer and equally or even more effective antibacterial in the market.

Antimicrobial Spectrum

They are the drugs of choice for *Rickettsia, Mycoplasma, Ureaplasma* and *Chlamydia*.

They are effective against gram-positive cocci, gram-negative bacteria, *Haemophilus influenzae, Klebsiella, Lyme borrelia, E. coli, Brucella, Yersinia pestis, Francisella tularensis, Borrelia recurrentis, Campylobacter jejuni* and *Helicobacter pylori*. Their adverse side effects include diarrhea, drug rashes, photosensitization and hepatic and renal damage in susceptible individuals, especially in pregnant women. Tetracycline orthophosphate gets deposited in the developing teeth of fetuses and young children, and also in bones. The teeth may become permanently discolored yellow. In patients on marginal nutritional status, destruction of the colonic bacterial flora may give rise to overt deficiency of the B-complex vitamins. It has therefore been a practice to prescribe B-complex vitamins along with tetracyclines. Tetracyclines can be given orally on an outpatient basis. Absorption is better if given on an empty stomach. Parenterally they can be given IM or IV. The popular preparations in this group were tetracycline, oxytetracycline and chlortetracycline which are short acting (6 hours) and doxycycline and minocycline which are long-acting (up to 24 hours). Doxycycline is excreted by the liver.

Dose	Oral	Parenteral	Preparations
Tetracycline	250–500 mg 6 h	250–500 mg IM or IV 8–12 h	Tablets and capsules 250 mg and 500 mg Injections 100–500 mg vials
Doxycycline	Oral	200 mg first day 100 mg/day for 5–10 days	Capsules/tablets 100 mg
Minocycline	Oral	100 mg bd	7–10 days

Chlortetracycline and oxytetracycline resemble tetracycline in dose, efficacy and toxicity. Tetracycline, chlortetracycline and oxytetracycline are not freely available in the Indian market for human use.

Doxycycline: 200 mg oral on first day followed by 100 mg once or twice a day for 5–10 days. Capsules and tablets of 100 mg are available. At present the freely available tetracycline in the market is doxycycline. It is used for the treatment of nongonococcal (chlamydial) urethritis, rickettsial diseases, nocardia, actinomyces, *C. jejuni, H. pylori* and as an 'add on drug' for *Plasmodium falcipuram*. Demeclocycline which is a tetracycline is used as a drug in the management of the **syndrome of inappropriate antidiuretic hormone secretion (SIADH)**.

Minocycline: Monocycle is available as oral tablets or capsules. The dose is 100 mg bd for 7–10 days.

Tigecycline: It is a derivative of tetracycline which is an alpha glycylcycline. It is active against tetracycline resistant bacteria since it is not removed from the bacterial cell and it can bind to altered ribosomes. Tigecycline is used in septicemias and life-threatening infections, especially in patients with neutropenia. The drug is eliminated in the bile.

Macrolides

These antibiotics derive their name due to the presence of many numbered lactone ring in the nucleus. They are very popular and safe drugs which can be given orally. Macrolides inhibit protein synthesis in the bacteria by binding to 50s ribosomal sub unit. The important members in this group are erythromycin, roxithromycin, azithromycin, clarithromycin, oleando-mycin and spiramycin (Table 5.4). Antimicrobial spectrum includes gram-positive cocci, gram-negative bacilli, *Corynebacterium diphtheriae, Campylobacter, Legionella, Leptospira, Borrelia, Nocardia, Mycoplasma* and *Chlamydia* (trachoma). Side effects include gastrointestinal upsets, allergy and hepatic damage and Stevens-Johnson syndrome (SJS). Erythromycin estolate may give rise to hepatitis more frequently. Macrolides interact with several drugs and therefore great care has to be taken when prescribing them along with other drugs. Drug interactions leading to increase in plasma levels of digoxin, cisapride, theophylline and anticoagulants are reported for erythromycin.

Table 5.4: Dosage of macrolides

	Dose	Route	Preparation
Erythromycin	250–500 mg 6 h	Oral	Tablets and capsules of 100 and 500 mg
Roxithromycin	150 mg bd or 300 mg od (once a day)	Oral	150 and 300 mg tab, capsules
Azithromycin	250–500 mg od	Oral on empty Stomach	100 and 250 mg tablets or capsules
Clarithromycin	250–500 mg bd or tds (thrice a day)	Oral	250 and 500 mg tablets
Spiramycin	3 MIU bd	Oral	Tablets 3 MIU

Textbook of Medicine

Main indications for macrolides are infection of the respiratory tract, skin, soft tissues and sexually transmitted diseases (STDs).

Clarithromycin is useful for the prophylaxis and treatment of atypical mycobacteria, eradication of *H. pylori* and as an add-on drug for treating resistant malaria. It is available as 250 mg capsules for oral use and creams, ointments and gels for topical use.

Spiramycin is the antibacterial spectrum resembles that of erythromycin. This drug is particularly effective against *Toxoplasma gondii*. It is indicated in respiratory infections, prostatitis, urethritis, skin infections and toxoplasmosis occurring during pregnancy. Dose 6–9 million IU (4–6 tablets/day) in 2–4 divided doses for three weeks and repeated at 2 weekly intervals till delivery. The drug is better absorbed when given in empty stomach since food reduces absorption. Adverse effects include nausea, vomiting, abdominal pain, urticaria and benign hepatitis. Drug interaction occurs with theophylline, carbamazepine warfarin and digoxin.

Ketolides such as telithromycin. These are drugs with spectrum of action similar to macrolides. They inhibit protein synthesis in the microbe. Though the antibacterial spectrum resembles that of other macrolides, it is more potent than erythromycin. It is active against multi-drug resistant pneumococcus, *H. influenzae, M. catarrhalis, N. gonorrhoeae* and *N. meningitidis*. It is not active against *Enterobacteriaceae, Acinetobacter* and *Pseudomonas aeruginosa*.

Dose: 800 mg oral od for 7–10 days for community acquired pneumococcus. The course is for 5 days for other respiratory pathogens. Adverse effects include gastrointestinal upsets, elevation of liver enzymes and prolongation of QT interval in the electrocardiography (ECG). Mitochondrial damage has been reported.

Chloramphenicol

It is a bacteriostatic drug active against gram-positive and gram-negative organisms, *Rickettsia, Chlamydia* and *Mycoplasma*. Since it diffuses into CSF, it is an excellent drug for the treatment of meningitis especially due to meningococci, pneumococci and *H. influenzae*. It held its pride of place as the antibiotic of choice for treatment of enteric fevers till four decades ago. Development of resistance by salmonella against chloramphenicol and other drugs has been rapid and widespread and therefore at present it is used as a second line drug for the treatment of enteric fevers only under special circumstances. Major toxic effects include allergy, peripheral neuropathy, optic neuritis, dose related reversible anemia, fatal bone marrow depression and permanent aplastic anemia (in 1/30,000). When chloramphenicol is given to newborn infants whose hepatic and renal functions are still immature, a toxic state may develop in which the baby becomes listless, pale and gray in color. This is called 'gray baby syndrome'. Continuation of the drug may lead to death due to circulatory failure.

Dose	Route	Dose	Frequency	Preparations
250–500 mg	Oral/parenteral IV or IM same	125–500 mg	6 h	Tablets or capsules 500 mg and 1 g vials

Due to the possibility of fatal bone marrow depression, chloramphenicol should be used with caution.

Sulfonamides

These were the first group of antibacterial drugs introduced for the therapy of infections. The commonly used sulfa-drugs, in vogue from time to time include sulfadiazine, sulfaguanidine, sulfamethoxazole, sulfafurazole, sulfadoxine, sulfacetamide, silver sulfadiazine and salicylazosulfapyridine (salazopyrin). Sulfonamides are bacteriostatic. Sulfamethoxazole in combination with trimethoprim (co-trimoxazole), salazopyrin, sulfadoxine and silver sulfadiazine are currently in wide use. The other members in this group have been largely replaced by newer drugs, on account of the greater efficacy and safety of the latter. The bacteriostatic action is due to the sequential block of folinic acid synthesis.

Co-trimoxazole

This is a combination of 1 part of trimethoprim with 5 parts of sulfamethoxazole 80 mg and 400 mg respectively. The action is bactericidal. The antimicrobial spectrum includes gram-positive cocci, *Proteus, Brucella, Yersinia, E. coli, Klebsiella, H. influenzae, Shigella, Salmonella, Pneumocystis carinii* and others. Adverse side effects include allergy, leukopenia, megaloblastic anemia and bone marrow suppression.

Dose: 160 mg trimethoprim with 800 mg sulfamethoxazole twice a day orally for the usual infections.

For the treatment of *Pneumocystis carinii* pneumonia and its prevention in immunocompromised hosts, larger doses have to be employed. IV preparation is available. This may be combined with carbenicillin for the management of infections in neutropenic patients.

Trimethoprim

This is structurally a diaminopyrimidine. This has antibacterial property of its own. It is active against *E. coli, Proteus, Klebsiella, Enterobacter* and *Staphylococci*. The antibacterial action is by enzymatic inhibition of folic acid, metabolism, inhibiting the reduction of dihydrofolic acid to tetrahydrofolic acid.

Dose: 100 mg oral bd or 200 mg od.

Toxic effects include rashes, gastrointestinal upsets and bone marrow suppression.

Sulfadoxine

It is a dihydropteroate synthetase inhibitor, acting as a folate antagonist

This has a serum half-life of six days. It is used as an antimalarial against resistant *P. falciparum* infections. The compound Fansidar tablets containing sulfadoxine 0.5 g and pyrimethamine 25 mg are given in a dose of 3 tablets orally as a single dose.

Salazopyrin

This is used as an anti-inflammatory and immunomodulatory drug in ulcerative colitis, rheumatoid disease and reactive arthritis. It is not used as an antimicrobial drug.

Silver sulfadiazine: Is used as 1% drops or cream for topical use, especially in burns to prevent bacterial colonization.

OTHER ANTIBIOTICS

Vancomycin

It is a glycopeptide antibiotic used for the treatment of *Methicillin-resistant Staphylococcus aureus* (MRSA) and pseudomembranous colitis caused by *Clostridium difficile*. It has action on staphylococci and its action is inhibition of cell wall synthesis of susceptible organisms. It is bactericidal. It can be given orally or parenterally.

Dose: Oral 125–500 mg 6 hour (7 mg/kg bw) for pseudo-membranous colitis.

Parenteral IV infusion of 500 mg–1.0 g over one hour at 1 hour intervals. It is available as 50 mg tablets and vials of 0.5 and 1 g.

Teicoplanin

This is a glycopeptide antibiotic, inhibiting microbial cell wall synthesis. It is similar to vancomycin in action, but with a longer duration of activity. This drug is active against potentially serious gram-positive infections including MRSA. The drug is available as Targocid (Aventis) as vials containing 200 and 400 mg. The dose is 400 mg IM or IV single dose on the first day followed by 200 mg daily. In severe infections the dose is 400 mg IM/IV 12 hourly for the first 3 days followed by 400 mg daily.

Newer glycopeptide antibiotics having bactericidal activity against vancomycin-resistant enterococci (VRE) have been developed. These include oritavancin, dalba-vancin and telavancin.

Dose: They are highly protein bound in plasma therefore their elimination half-life is long.

Lincomycin

It is a lincosamide antibiotic active against organisms which are penicillin resistant. Action is inhibition of protein synthesis in bacteria. Its use is limited to acute and chronic osteomyelitis, respiratory infections, septic arthritis and endocarditis.

Dose: Oral 500 mg 6–8 h or 600 mg IV or IM 12 h.

Preparations available: Capsules of 500 mg and injections of 600 mg in 2 mL.

Clindamycin

It is a semisynthetic derivative of lincomycin useful in infections caused by mixed bacterial flora, malaria and toxoplasmosis. It can be given orally or parenterally. It inhibits bacterial protein synthesis. The action is bacteriostatic at low concentration and bactericidal at high concentrations.

The drug is effective against penicillinase producing staphylococci, pneumococci and some types of streptococci. *Corynebacterium diphtheriae* and *Bacillus anthracis* are moderately sensitive. Adverse effects include nausea, vomiting, abdominal pain and diarrhea. At times it leads to pseudomembranous colitis and monilial superinfection. The main indications include acute and chronic osteomyelitis, anaerobic infections, pus collections such as empyema, and brain abscess and infection by penicillin resistant streptococci, pneumococci and staphylococci.

Dose: Oral 150–300 mg 6 h. Parenteral 600 mg to 2.7 g as IV infusion or IM over 24 hours in divided doses. This drug is available as 150 mg capsules and vials containing 150 mg/mL.

Oxazolidinones

Linezolid: These are synthetic antibacterial antibiotics which inhibit protein synthesis in the microbes. Linezolid is 100% bioavailable on oral administration. The antibacterial spectrum is wide against gram-positive bacteria. It is especially useful against MRSA and vancomycin resistant *Enterococcus faecium.*

Dose: Oral 600 mg 12 h or IV 600 mg 12 h for 10–14 days. When giving IV, linezolid should not be mixed with other drugs. Adverse side effects include pain at the site injection, elevation of liver enzymes, renal impairment and thrombocytopenia.

Linezolid Optic Neuropathy

This drug is used as one of the 'add-on' drugs for multidrug-resistant tuberculosis (MDR TB) at the dose of 300 mg bd oral. On long-term it causes optic atrophy which starts with fall in visual acuity bilaterally. Funduscopy shows peripillary retinal fiber swelling. Optic disk appears hyperemic and swollen. Later, telangiectatic microangiopathy and vessel tortuosity ensue. The mechanism seems to be mitochondrial respiratory function defect.

Source: Khadilkar SV, Yadav RS, Rajan S. Linezolid optic neuropathy: be careful and quick. J Assoc Physicians India. 2013;61(11):866-7.

Daptomycin: It is a cyclic lipopeptide antibiotic that is rapidly bactericidal for most of the gram-positive bacteria including *S. aureus*. Its action is disruption of the cell wall and cell lysis.

Dose: 4–6 mg/kg bw given once a day by IV infusion over 30 minutes for 7–14 days. It has been tried to treat MRSA bacteremia with encouraging results. Main indication include complicated skin infections by staphylococci, streptolococci and enterococci and for anaerobic gram-negative infections. Main toxic effects are myositis and myopathy with accompanying elevation of serum creatine phosphokinase (CPK) levels.

Fusidic Acid

Sodium Fusidate (Fucidin) is obtained from the parasite fungus *Fusidium coccineum*. It has a steroid structure and it is active against gram-positive organisms. All strains of staphylococci are sensitive. Streptococci and pneumococci are relatively resistant.

Dose: 500–1000 mg oral 8 h. Milk reduces the absorption of this drug. The available parenteral preparation is Diethanolamine fusidate 580 mg IV 8 h. Sodium fusidate is also a general purpose local antiseptic, available as ointment. Fucidin shows bactericidal synergism with penicillin and erythromycin.

Spectinomycin

This is effective in gonococcal urethritis.

Dose: IM or IV 2–4 g single dose or 2 g bd for 3–5 days.

Quinupristin-Dalfopristin

This group of drugs belongs to the class of streptogramins. These are naturally occurring compounds isolated from

Textbook of Medicine

Streptomyces pristinaespiralis. They inhibit protein synthesis in bacteria. The antibacterial spectrum resembles that of vancomycin. Indications include infections by gram-positive organisms, MRSA, resistant enterococci and atypical organisms.

Dose: Quinupristin/dalfopristin mixture (30/70%) is given IV 8 h at 7.5 mg/kg bw. Adverse effects include arthralgia, myalgia, local phlebitis and conjugated hyperbilirubinemia.

Nitrofurantoin

This is a synthetic nitrofuran with activity against gram-negative bacteria of the urinary tract. Action of the drug causes deoxyribonucleic acid (DNA) strand breakages in the bacteria. It is used for the prophylaxis and long-term treatment of UTIs.

Dose: Oral for prophylactic use 50–100 mg at night (HS).

For therapy of established infection 200–400 mg/day is divided doses.

The drug has to be used with caution in the presence of renal impairment.

Quinolones

The fluoroquinolones are synthetic bactericidal agents related to the parent drug nalidixic acid. They inhibit DNA gyrase in a wide variety of bacteria. They are all well absorbed when given orally. The popular drugs in this group are norfloxacin, ciprofloxacin, pefloxacin, ofloxacin, lomefloxacin, sparfloxacin, levofloxacin, gatifloxacin and moxifloxacin, less popular members of the group include gemifloxacin. The parent drug nalidixic acid is still in use. The antimicrobial spectrum is wide including gram-negative cocci and bacilli such as *Enterobacteriaceae, H. influenzae, Shigella, Campylobacter, Neisseria gonococcus, Pseudomonas* and others. They have antimicrobacterial activity and therefore they are used as second line reserve drugs in the treatment of resistant tuberculosis.

Side effects of quinolones include QT prolongation in ECG, cardiac arrhythmias, hepatic impairment, tendon inflammation and polyneuropathy. These drugs are generally contraindicated in children and pregnant-lactating women.

Details of the popular quinolones are listed below:
Ciprofloxacin, one of the most potent among the quinolones, is bactericidal for salmonella and at present this is the drug of choice for enteric fevers. It is also used to eradicate the carrier state for meningococci and *Salmonella typhi.* It is particularly active against *Pseudomonas.*
Ofloxacin has action against multidrug resistant *Staphylococci, Chlamydia* and *Legionella.*
Lomefloxacin has action similar to ciprofloxacin.
Sparfloxacin has action against anaerobic organisms. Lomefloxacin and sparfloxacin are long-acting and therefore once a day dosage is adequate. Some of quinolones are available for local application such as eyedrops. Quinolones are generally contraindicated during pregnancy and lactations.
Levofloxacin: This is available as tablets of 250–500 mg to be given orally once or twice a day for up to 14 days. It is also available as an IV infusion containing 5 mg/mL,

100 mL vials, to be given as a slow infusion over 60 minutes, once or twice a day for up to 14 days.

Gatifloxacin and ***moxifloxacin*** are newer fluoro-quinolones and are powerful antibacterial drugs. They act by inhibiting the enzyme DNA gyrase (topoisomerase: II and IV) which are required for DNA replication, transcription, repair and recombination. Both are active against a wide spectrum of gram-positive and gram-negative bacteria, *Chlamydia pneumoniae, Mycoplasma pneumoniae* and penicillin resistant pneumococcus. They are less effective than ciprofloxacin against *Pseudomonas aeruginosa.*

Adverse effects include dizziness, nervousness, precipitation of seizures, erosion of cartilage in weight bearing joints in young subjects and prolongation of QT interval in the ECG. Gatifloxacin may produce hypoglycemia and at times, hyperglycemia with symptoms requiring urgent attention.

Dose: 400 mg daily orally for 5–10 days. The drug has to be given with caution in diabetes (Table 5.5).

Quinolones have become popular antibacterial agents on account of their powerful action, free availability, ease of administration and reasonable cost.

The Imidazole Derivatives

Metronidazole and its analogue tinidazole are synthetic imidazoles. They cause DNA damage in their susceptible organisms. Both of these drugs originally developed as antiamoebic drugs, and have potent antibacterial properties against anaerobic organisms and therefore they are used widely for that purpose as well.

Metronidazole: This drug has antiprotozoal actively against amebae, giardia and trichomonas. It has wide antibacterial activity against the anaerobic organisms *Bacteriodes, Clostridium, Fusobacterium, Peptococcus, Peptostreptococcus* and *Eubacteriacea.* In combination with clarithromycin and a proton pump inhibitor it is bactericidal to *Helicobacter pylori.* Mitronidazole is available as tablets of 200 and 400 mg, suspensions

Table 5.5:	Dosage of quinolones		
Norfloxacin	400 mg bd	Oral	Tablets 100–800 mg
Ciprofloxacin	250–750 mg bd 200–400 mg bd	Oral IV infusion	Tablets 100–750 mg
Pefloxacin	400 mg bd 400 mg	Oral IV infusion 1 hour	Tablets 400 mg IV infusion 4 mg/mL 100 mL
Ofloxacin	200–400 mg/bd 200-mg infusion	Oral IV in 30 minutes	Tab 100 and 200 mg infusion 2 mg/mL 100 mL
Lomefloxacin	400 mg od	Oral	Tab 400 mg
Sparfloxacin	400 mg first day Then 200 mg/day	Oral	Tab 200 and 400 mg
Levofloxacin	250–500 mg	Oral IV infusion	Tab 250 and 500 mg 500 mg vials
Gatifloxacin	400 mg od	Oral	400 mg tablets
Moxifloxacin	400 mg od	Oral	400 mg tablets
Nalidixic acid	1 g qid	Oral	Tab 250 mg–1 g

containing 200 mg/5 mL and vials of 100 mL containing 500 mg of the drug for IV use. The drug is effective both for intestinal and tissue lesions caused by protozoa, especially by *Entamoeba histolytica*.

Dose: Amebiasis 400–800 mg tds po × 5–10 days.

For trichomoniasis, giardiasis and others 400 mg tds × 5 days. For anaerobic infections, loading dose of 15 mg/kg bw IV infusion over 30–60 minutes followed by maintenance dose of 7.5 mg/kg bw 6 h for 7–10 days. Metronidazole can be used as a primary drug for *Clostridium difficile* in dose of 400 mg tds oral for 5–7 days.

Tinidazole: It is available as tablets containing 500 mg and 1 g. It is effective against protozoa such as amebae, giardia and trichomonas.

Dose: Amebic dysentery—2 g/day/po in single or divided doses for 3–5 days.

- Amebic liver abscess—2 g/day in divided doses for 5 days or more.
- Giardiasis and trichomoniasis—2 g/day for 1 day as single or divided doses.
- Anaerobic infections-treatment and prophylaxis—2 g initially, followed by 500 mg bd po for 5–7 days.
- For preoperative sterilization—2 g single dose po 12 hours prior to surgery.
- Ulcerative gingivitis and bacterial vaginosis 2 g po single dose.

Adverse side effects include nausea, metallic taste in the mouth, peripheral neuropathy, encephalopathy seizures, ataxia and severe discomfort (similar to that caused by disulfiram) when alcohol is consumed while on treatment.

Rifampicin

This is a bactericidal antibiotic with a wide antibacterial spectrum. Rifampicin group of drugs bind to the beta subunit of the DNA dependant ribonucleic acid (RNA) polymerase, thereby inhibiting the transcription of DNA to RNA and nucleic acid synthesis. Rifampicin is very effective against *Mycobacterium tuberculosis* and *Mycobacterium leprae* and therefore is used for treating them. They are active against other organisms as well.

Dose: 10 mg/kg bw orally daily as a single dose. Capsules of 150–600 mg and tablet of 450 and 600 mg are available. Absorption is best when given an empty stomach. Any food or drink should be given only an hour later. Resistance develops very rapidly if given alone. All forms of tuberculosis respond. The course of treatment should continue uninterrupted for six months or more as per fixed protocols. For the treatment of leprosy supervised monthly doses of 450–600 mg are given depending upon the clinical status evidence protocols have been developed.

Other indications include infections by *Staphylococcus*, *Legionella* and gram-negative bacilli. It is effective as a prophylactic agent against *H. influenzae* and meningococcal meningitis in contacts.

Rifabutin

It is an antimycobacterial antibiotic, used for the prophylaxis and treatment of *Mycobacterium avium* complex (MAC).

Dose: 150 mg/day oral for 6 months. In acquired immune deficiency syndrome (AIDS) patients the dose is 300 mg/day to be given indefinitely. For MDR TB, rifabutin is effective in a dose of 300–450 mg/day.

Rifapentine: This is a rifamycin derivative with excellent activity against *M. tuberculosis*. Compared to rifampicin, its half-life is longer (10–15 hours versus 2–3 hours). Therefore, it can be given at longer intervals. Regimens such as rifapentine 600 mg once a week with isoniazid (INH) 900 mg weekly have been tried in non-cavitating pulmonary tuberculosis in human immunodeficiency virus (HIV) negative persons with success.

OTHER ANTIMYCOBACTERIAL DRUGS

Several antimycobacterial drugs have been developed and are undergoing clinical trials. Two of them diarylquinoline-bedaquiline and nitroimidazole-delamanid—are both being tried in phase 3 trials.

Dose bedaquiline: Oral 400 mg/day/2 weeks followed by 200 mg three times a week for 22 weeks taken with food.

Bedaquiline: 100 mg bd oral for 24 weeks. A mild adverse side effect is prolongation of QTC intervals for both drugs.

POLYENE ANTIBIOTICS

These are all polypeptide antibiotics. These include bacitracin, polymyxin B and colistin.

Bacitracin

This drug inhibits cell wall synthesis of bacteria. The antimicrobial spectrum includes gram-positive organisms—*Meningococcus, Gonococcus, Treponemes* and *H. influenzae*. For systemic use it has to be given IM or IV.

Dose: 1000 units/kg/day in divided doses. For local use it is available as eye ointment of 500 units/g and powder in combination with polymyxin B and neomycin.

Polymyxin B

Specific antimicrobial action is to disrupt cell membrane permeability. The drug is active against gram-negative organisms, especially *Pseudomonas aeruginosa*. It is used systemically as well as for topical use in the eye and skin. It is available as injections (vials containing 5,00,000 units), eyedrops (5000 u/mL) and ointment (5000 u/g).

Dose: IM injection 15–20,000 units/kg bw/day in divided doses.

Colistin

It is a member of the polymyxin family (polymyxin E) colistin (polymyxin E). It is powerful against hospital acquired gram-negative bacilli resistant to other drugs, especially *P. aeruginosa* and *Acinetobacter* species. It is used in life-threatening infections.

Dose: 100 mg 12 hour IV for the minimum period to get a clinical response in *P.* aeruginosa and other organisms.

General Note: In many life-threatening infections, powerful bactericidal drugs such as meropenem, piperacillin, imipenem, colistin, tigecycline and others may have to be used early in the disease to save life, especially in immunocompromised patients. Delay in the administration of antibiotics in immunodeficient individuals leads to fatal outcome.

ANTIVIRAL DRUGS

Several specific antiviral drugs are entering the market in recent years. Their mechanism of action varies and depending upon this, combination of antiviral drugs have been introduced in the management of diseases such as infection by HIV and AIDS, hepatitis viruses, respiratory tract viruses and several others. Since, newer and newer drugs are entering the market at short intervals and many of them have had only short periods of clinical use, it has not been attempted to include them in this section. Wherever, major innovations have been made they have been referred in appropriate chapters dealing with the infections (Tables 5.6 to 5.8). For further details on them reader may refer to more detailed literature on virology.

The antiviral drugs can be classified based on their pharmacological action as given below.

Drugs interfering with nucleic acid synthesis in the virus	Acyclovir, ganciclovir, penciclovir, valacyclovir, famciclovir, ribavirin, idoxuridine, trifluridine, adenine-arabinoside, azidothymidine
Inhibitor of viral attachment and penetration	Amantadine, rimantadine, zanamivir, oseltamivir
Inhibitor of reverse transcriptors	Zidovudine, lamivudine, zalcitabine, nevirapine, efavirenz and several other antiretroviral drugs
Drug acting through immune mechanism	Interferons, gamma globulins and monoclonal antibodies

Several newer drugs are being added on for the treatment of HIV infection, viral hepatitis and other viral diseases. These are dealt with in the appropriate chapters.

Table 5.6: Mode of action of antiviral agents	
Acyclovir	Nucleoside analogue
Amantadine and rimantadine	Viral uncoating and assembling
Foscarnet	Inhibition of polymerase
Ganciclovir	Nucleoside analogue
Idoxuridine	-Do-
Ribavarin	-Do-
Trifluridine	-Do-
Vidarabine	-Do-
Zidovudine	-Do-
Inosine pranobex	Immunomodulator
Inosiplex	Nucleoside analogues interrupt viral nucleic acid synthesis

Table 5.7: Site of action of antiviral drugs	
Stage of viral replication	*Effective drug*
Attachment	Antibody to virion-binding Antibody to cell receptors
Penetration/uncoating	Amantadine
Viral macromolecular synthesis	Nucleoside analogues
	Vidarabine, acyclovir, ganciclovir, ribavirin, zidovudine, foscarnet, interferons

Note: The details of antiviral drugs are given in Table 5.8.

Acyclovir (Acycloguanosine): This is a potent drug which inhibits the multiplication of herpes simplex virus types 1 and 2, varicella zoster virus (VZV) and Epstein-Barr (EB) virus. Acyclovir is given IV in a dose of 5 mg/kg as an infusion running over 1 hour and repeated every 8 hour for 5 days. Side effects include allergy, renal impairment, local necrosis of tissues and hepatic dysfunction. The dose should be reduced in patients with impaired renal function. This is one among the most effective and widely used antiviral drugs. It inhibits replication of herpes viruses. Infected cells concentrate the drug 40–100 times higher than uninfected cells. It is the most active agent in herpes simplex virus (HSV1), HSV2 and VZV. Preparations for topical use are also available for herpes simplex and herpes zoster lesions.

	Dose
Genital herpes curative	200 mg oral 5 times a day—10–12 days or IV 5 mg/kg 8 h for 5 days
Suppression	400 mg bd for long periods.
HSV encephalitis	10 mg/kg IV 8 h for 10–14 days
Neonatal HSV	IV 10 mg/kg 8 h for 10–14 days
Varicella zoster	800 mg qid or tds for 10–14 days

Gancyclovir: This drug is effective against cytomegalovirus (CMV) and is indicated for the treatment of life-threatening lesions such as colitis and pneumonias in immunocompromised host and for retinitis which may lead to blindness. The dose is 5 mg/kg given as IV infusion within one hour, repeated twice daily. The initial course extends for three weeks after which the maintenance dose is 5 mg/kg/day for several weeks. Drug toxicity includes neutropenia and thrombocytopenia. It is available in vials of 500 mg.

Phosphonoformate (foscarnet): This is a pyrophosphate analogue that inhibits DNA polymerase of all herpes viruses and RNA polymerase of influenza viruses. Topical application is found to be beneficial in herpes labialis and herpes genitalis. It is being used parenterally in AIDS and CMV infections.

Vidarabine: This is a derivative of adenine-arabinoside. It inhibits DNA synthesis and is active against several herpes group viruses. It is used therapeutically in HSV, VZV and CMV infections. For the treatment of herpes simplex encephalitis and neonatal herpes simplex infections, vidarabine has to be given IV as a 12 hours infusion in a dose of 5–15 mg/kg/day for 10 days. Toxicity occurs in a few cases and this includes nausea, vomiting, diarrhea and tremors. Adenine-arabinoside is available as a 3% ointment for topical use in herpetic keratoconjunctivitis.

Idoxuridine: This is effective against herpes simplex infections, although the organisms develop resistance rapidly. The drug is given as local application to the eye as 0.1% drops and as 0.5% ointment. Toxic effect includes irritation and local allergy. ***Trifluridine*** is an alternative used for the same indication.

Amantadine hydrochloride (Symmetrel): It is active against RNA viruses such as myxoviruses, paramyxoviruses and togaviruses. The drug is effective particularly against influenza A virus, but not against influenza B. The drug is mainly used for the prophylaxis against influenza A in

Textbook of Medicine

Table 5.8: Antiviral drugs, their antiviral activity, preparations and toxicity

Name	Antiviral activity	Preparation	Indication	Main toxicity
Idoxuridine	HSV	0.1% solution or superficial lesions	HSV keratitis 0.5% ointment for eye	Local irritation
Trifluridine	HSV keratitis	1% eye drops	-do-	
Vidarabine	DNA viruses espcially herpes group, HSV, VZV, CMV	Eye ointment, IV infusion 5–15 mg/kg/day for 10 days	HSV keratitis, HSV encephalitis, disseminated varicella zoster, CMV infections	GI toxicity, tremors
Acyclovir (Zovirax)	HSV, VZV-BB virus	Local cream 5% IV 15–30 mg/kg/day	Herpes labialis, Herpes encephalitis oral tablets 800 mg 4 h	Allergy, renal and hepatic damage EB virus infection
Ganciclovir (Cymevene)	CMV infections	IV 7.5 mg/kg/day	Systemic congenital or acquired CMV infections	
Zidovudine (Azidothymidine)	HIV	250 mg oral 6 h	AIDS and AIDS related disorders	Bone marrow suppression
Ribavirin	Lower respiratory tract viruses especially syncytial virus, Lassa fever virus hepatitis B and C virus	Aerosolized ribavirin, oral tablets 600–1200 mg/day	Influenza, respiratory syncytial virus, Lassa fever HBV, hepatitis C virus	Hemolytic anemia neoplasia
Amantadine and rimantadine	Influenza A virus	200 mg/tablets orally	Prevention of influenza A	Neurotoxicity
Zanamivir and oseltamivir	Influenza A and B	Zanamivir 5 mg inhalation oseltamivir 75–100 mg bd oral	Do treatment	—
Phosphonoformate (foscarnet)	Herpes viruses and influenza virus	Topical and IV	Recurrent herpes labialis, CMV retinitis	
Fomivirsen (oligonucleotide)	CMV	330 mg IV 2 weeks apart	CMV retinitis	Ocular inflammation
Sorivudine (pyrimidine nucleoside analogue)	Herpes zoster			
Alpha interferon	Rhinoviruses HBV, non A non B hepatitis, delta virus hepatitis	Nasal spray parenteral preparation up to 20 mega units/day	Prevent rhinovirus infections, Hepatitis B, C, D	Fever

Note: Several newer antiretroviral drugs and antihepatitis virus drugs are being developed in recent times. These are described in the appropriate chapters.

Abbreviations: HSV = Herpes simplex virus; DNA = Deoxyribonucleic acid; VZV = Varicella zoster virus; CMV = Cytomegalovirus; IV = Intravenous; GI = Gastrointestinal; EB virus = Epstein-Barr virus; HIV = Human immunodeficiency virus; AIDS = Acquired immune deficiency syndrome

vulnerable groups. There is a 50–60% reduction in attack rates. For prophylaxis after exposure it should be given within 24–48 hours. It is given orally 100 mg twice a day. Toxic effects include confusion, hallucinations, anxiety and insomnia. It may produce embryopathy when given in pregnancy. This drug is also used in Parkinsonism. **Rimantadine** is an analogue, it is 4–10 times more potent than amantadine.

Ribavarin: It is a synthetic triazole nucleoside with wide spectrum of activity both against DNA and RNA viruses. It is useful in the treatment of influenza and respiratory syncytial virus (RSV) when given as an aerosol. When given orally or IV the drug is effective against Lassa fever, hepatitis B and C, viral hemorrhagic fevers caused by hantavirus and Argentine and Crimean-Congo hemorrhagic fever.

Lamivudine has also suppressive action on hepatitis B virus (in a dose of 100 mg oral daily). Several others antiretroviral drugs have also been produced and they are under different stages of trial.

Neuraminidase inhibitors: They are powerful inhibitor of viral neuraminidase. They inhibit the growth and release of influenza virus from the infected cell. The available drugs are zanamivir and oseltamivir. They inhibit both influenza types A and B. They are used for chemoprophylaxis and curative treatment.

Adefovir: This drug is available as adefovir dipivoxil which is a prodrug. It is active against hepatitis B, HIV and herpes viruses.

Entecavir: This is a guanosine nucleoside. It competitively inhibits HBV, DNA polymerase. It is orally absorbed.

Telbivudine: This is a thymidine nucleoside analogue orally absorbed and not affected by food. It is active against HBV.

Tenofovir: This is a nucleoside/nucleotide reverse transcriptase (NTRI) antiretroviral drug effective against HBV as well.

Interferons

Interferons are cytokines produced by host cells in response to viral infection or other stimuli. They are glycoproteins in structure.

Three types of interferons are available, **alpha interferon** produced by lymphocytes and monocytes, **beta interferon** produced by fibroblasts and **gamma interferon** produced by sensitized T-helper (TH1) lymphocytes. Alpha interferon has two subtypes 2a and 2b, which slightly differ in activity. Interferons are commercially produced by ribosomal DNA (rDNA) technology and they are widely used for a large variety of unrelated conditions. Alpha interferon is the most widely used. The antiviral spectrum includes hepatitis B, C and D, herpes zoster, EB virus and juvenile laryngeal papillomatosis. Interferon exerts its action possibly by interfering with the translation function in the host cell.

Neoplastic conditions such as chronic myeloid leukemia, hairy cell leukemia and multiple myeloma respond well to alpha interferon.

Alpha interferon is given SC, IM or IV in doses of 5 million units daily or on alternative days for prolonged periods depending upon the indications. Adverse side effects include flu-like symptoms, somnolence, confusion, paresthesia, motor neuropathy, alopecia, leukopenia and thrombocytopenia. ***Pegylated interferon*** is available. Adverse side effects are less and the preparation is more acceptable. It is more expensive too. A single dose costs Rs. 1500–2000 and therefore the treatment becomes very expensive.

Beta interferon is used to reduce the frequency and severity of relapses in multiple sclerosis. Gamma interferon is immunomodulatory in action. It takes part at different stages of the immune mechanisms of the host, including activation of macrophages and natural killer (NK) cells and regulation of antibody production by lymphocytes.

Inosiplex (Inosine pranobex): This drug stimulates B-lymphocytes to produce antibodies, promotes the differentiation of T-lymphocytes and increases macrophage and interleukin activity. It is indicated in hepatitis, subacute sclerosing panencephalitis (SSPE) and HSV infections.

At present specific antiviral drugs should be considered for the treatment of the following conditions:

- Herpes simplex infections—severe mucocutaneous or generalized forms in an immunocompromised host, ophthalmic forms, genital herpes, lesions in neonate, meningitis and encephalitis
- Varicella zoster infections in immunocompromised host
- CMV
- EB virus
- Hepatitis B, C and delta virus
- Respiratory viruses—influenza A, RSV, rhinoviruses, corona virus
- AIDS and HIV infection
- Lassa fever and other viral hemorrhagic fevers.

ANTIFUNGAL DRUGS

Fungal infections may take the form of superficial or deep systemic infections. With the increase in number of immunocompromised individuals as a result of disease or its treatment, systemic fungal infections have assumed more serious proportions. Several drugs are available for their treatment. Refer Table 5.9.

Systemic Antifungal Drugs

Several groups of drugs have antifungal properties. These include:

- Antibiotics, e.g. amphotericin B, nystatin, hamacin, griseofulvin.
- Antimetabolites, e.g. flucytosine which impairs synthesis of fungal DNA.
- Azoles, e.g. ketoconazole, fluconazole, itraconazole, voriconazole and others (see description below).
- Other topical agents, e.g. tolnaftate, terbinafine.

Table 5.9: Antifungal drugs

Drug	Dose	Main toxicity
Amphotericin B	0.5 mg/kg/day intravenous infusion daily or 0.8–1 mg/kg intravenous infusion in 5% glucose over 4–6 h	Phlebitis, vomiting, nephrotoxicity, anaphylaxis, hypomagnesemia, hypokalemia
Flucytosine	150 mg/kg/day in 4 divided doses orally for 6 weeks 200 mg/kg iv infusion daily	Nausea, vomiting, leukopenia, thrombocytopenia, hepatic dysfunction
Griseofulvin	125–250 mg qid oral with meals for 2 weeks-1 year	Photosensitivity, urticaria, gastrointestinal disturbance, hepatotoxicity
Itraconazole	100–200 mg oral/day	Photosensitivity, urticaria, gastrointestinal disturbance, hepatotoxicity
Ketoconazole	200–400 mg orally daily	Rashes, hepatotoxicity, gynecomastia
Miconazole	• Oral gel 125–250 mg 6 h • Parenteral IV 8 h; intrathecal 20 mg; topical 2% cream or 100 mg pessary	Mild local reaction, anaphylaxis, nephrotoxicity, hyponatremia, hyperlipidemia, acute psychosis
Fluconazole	50–200 mg/day oral or 200–400 mg/IV day	Mild local reaction, anaphylaxis, nephrotoxicity, hyponatremia, hyperlipidemia, acute psychosis
Voriconazole	4–6 mg/kg bw IV bd oral 200 mg bd	
Posaconazole	IV 200 mg qid, later 400 mg bd	
Nystatin	Oral 50,000 U 6 h; topical 10,000 U/g ointment or vaginal tablet	Rash, lymphadenopathy, parotitis, lacrimation, dermatitis
Clotrimazole	1% cream or 100 mg vaginal tablet for 6 days	Mild local effects
Econazole	1% cream or powder	Nil
Miconazole	Oral 250 mg daily	
Terbinafine	Cream for local use 10 mg/g	

Most important among them are amphotericin B and the azole drugs.

Mechanism of action: Antifungal drugs, especially the azoles are targeted against ergosterol which is the main sterol in the fungal cell membrane. The synthesis of ergosterol is inhibited. Ergosterol is required for the membrane integrity and growth of fungi. Respiration of the fungi is also inhibited in body tissues.

Amphotericin B: The drug is both fungistatic and fungicidal depending upon the dose. It attaches to ergosterol of the fungus and causes poses and channels increasing membrane permeability and destruction. This is active against *Cryptococcus, Aspergillus, Histoplasma, Coccidioides, Blastomyces* and *Candida*. This drug is indicated in systemic infections by these fungi. The drug is contraindicated in renal failure.

Liposomal formulations are available. These permit higher dosage. Toxicity is less, but cost is higher.

Azoles: They are active against most of the organisms that cause systemic and deep-seated fungal infections. The sensitive spectrum includes: *Cryptococcus neoformans, Candida albicans, Coccidioides immitis, Histoplasma capsulatum, Blastomyces dermatitides* (miconazole is not effective against this organism), *Paracoccidioides brasiliensis* and *Sporothrix schenckii.*

The ***azole drugs*** include a wide spectrum of therapeutic agents consisting of—metronidizole and tinidazole active against protozoa and anerobic bacteria, anthelmentics mebendazole and albendazole, and the antifungals-imidzoles and triazoles.

Systematically administered drugs in this class include clotrimazole, ketoconazole, miconazole, itraconzaole, fluconazole, voriconazole and posaconzole.

Voriconazole: This is a broad spectrum triazole compound active against *Aspergillus* species. Dose is 4–6 mg/kg bw IV bd for 7 days followed by 200 mg oral bd for maintenance.

Posaconazole is another analogue with action against invasive *Aspergillus*. Dose is 200 mg qid, IV initially to be followed by 400 mg IV bd for varying periods. Compared to amphotericin B the results are superior. Action against *Candida* and related yeasts and *Torulopsis glabrata* is weaker.

Ketoconazole inhibits cytochrome p-450 enzyme which is necessary for adrenal and gonadal steroids synthesis, thereby leading to inhibition of these glands in experimental animals, though this action is very weak. Azoles are embryotoxic and therefore contraindicated in pregnancy.

Terbinafine is an orally and topically effective fungicidal agent. It is an alkylamine. Its spectrum of activity includes mainly dermatophytes and to a lesser extent, candida and pityriasis ovale. The drug is lipophilic and keratinophilic. Adult dose is 250 mg orally daily given for periods varying from 2–6 weeks depending upon the indication.

Echinocandins

Over 50% of *Candida* species isolated from blood stream is formed by *Candida albicans.* They inhibit the cell wall synthesis of *Candida* species. *Candida* species which are resistant to azoles may be susceptible to echinocandins. Drugs in this class include:

- ***Caspofungin (Candide Merck)*** dose 70 mg IV 1st day thereafter 50 mg IV daily.
- ***Micafungin (Mycamine/Funguard, Fujisawa)*** dose 100 mg IV daily.
- ***Anidulafungin (Eraxis, Pfizer)*** dose 200 mg IV initially, followed by 100 mg IV daily.

These drugs are not absorbed orally in effective doses. Adverse side effects include histamine like reactions, thrombophlebitis. These drugs are expensive. The dose for 20 days costs $7000–8000. These drugs should be considered in *Candida* bacteremia not susceptible to amphotericin B or fluconazole.

Source: Bennett JE. Echinocandins for candidemia in adults without neutropenia. N Engl J Med. 2006;355(11):1154-9.

Flucytosine is a prodrug converted into 5-fluorocytosine in the fungal cell and it inhibits DNA and RNA synthesis. Dose is 150 mg/kg/day in four divided doses orally for six weeks. It can also be given IV 200 mg/kg as infusion daily. Side effects include nausea, vomiting, leukopenia, thrombocytopenia and hepatic dysfunction.

Treatment of Specific Fungal Infections

Systemic candidiasis: Amphotericin B is the drug of choice. Combination of amphotericin B with flucytosine may be synergistic. Fluconazole given orally is almost as effective as amphotericin B.

Cryptococcosis: For cryptococcal meningitis, the conventional treatment is to give amphotericin B. Fluconazole is an attractive alternative, since it penetrates into CSF. Both the drugs are equally effective in cryptococcal meningitis complicating AIDS. Due to the chance of recurrence such patients should receive life-long maintenance therapy. A common regimen is to give amphotericin B in a dose of 1 mg/kg IV once a week and 200 mg fluconazole orally once everyday.

Endemic mycosis: Blastomycosis, coccidioidomycosis and histoplasmosis. Amphotericin B is very effective. Azole drugs are effective alternatives. Itraconazole is the drug of choice due to ease of administration and effectiveness, in these infections.

Invasive Aspergillosis: Amphotericin B, itraconazole, voriconazole, posaconazole and echinocandins are effective.

Antifungal prophylaxis: This may become necessary under special situations like neutropenia, organ transplantation and others. The orally administered antifungal drugs are being tried for this purpose.

Antifungal drugs used for superficial mycoses: Superficial mycoses are treated generally by surface applications of the drug. These are described in Ch 219.

Since, many of the superficial infections tend to persist locally after local therapy, for considerable periods and tend to recur many dermatologists include systemic therapy with appropriate antifungal drugs for eradicating the infection.

DRUG RESISTANCE OF MICROBES

Failure to attain optimum response to a drug may be:

- Due to wrong diagnosis of the disease and choice of the antimicrobial agent.

Textbook of Medicine

- Inadequate dose and inappropriate route of administration.
- Impotency of the drug due to several factors.
- Resistance developed by the microbes against the therapeutic agent.

Drug resistance is a major problem encountered in present day clinical practice, and at present several microbes are highly resistant to drugs which were very effective, when they were introduced. Though some degree of development of resistance is an inescapable biological process evolved by the microbes, a great deal of this problem has been brought about by the widespread and often inappropriate use of the drug over prolonged periods. The magnitude of drug resistance is given below:

- *S. aureus*—80% of strains resistant to β-lactam antibiotics.
- *N. gonococci*—more than 50% resistant to penicillin.
- *S. typhi*—more than 50% resistant to chloramphenicol.
- *S. shigae*—more than 80% resistant to tetracyclines.
- *P. falciparum*—more than 50% resistant to chloroquine.

Mechanism of Resistance

It is almost a universal phenomenon that when microbes are exposed to antibiotics or other antimicrobial agents, they develop resistance to the original drug. This makes the organisms insensitive to further doses of the same drug, sometimes also to other related drugs. This has caused very serious problems in the management of infective diseases in modern times. The capacity to develop resistance by different organisms varies. Some develop resistance to single agents, while others develop resistance to multiple drugs. The exposure of the drug to the microbe may be direct through therapy or indirect, by contamination of the environment by the drug. Several of the drugs used for human disease are also employed for poultry farming, dairy industry, and agriculture and so on. So also, the widespread distribution of the microbes as well as the antibiotics in the hospital environment has resulted in widespread development of drug resistance in hospitals leading to nosocomial infections which are very difficult to manage.

Microbes can develop resistance *de-novo* by exposure to the drugs or transmit the developed resistance to other microbes by several methods in a polymicrobial environment. Hence, it is quite likely that even at the first encounter the patient is harboring drug resistant microbes. This has posed serious problems in modern times in infections with *Staphylococci, E. coli, Klebsiella, Proteus, Pseudomonas, Salmonella, Falciparum malaria* and several others. Once a colony of organisms becomes resistant, this resistance is transmitted to the successive generations. It is essential that the prevalence of resistant strains in the environment is taken into account before prescribing antibiotics in life-threatening situations. It is also seen then some of the resistant organism may lose their resistance, if exposure to the offending drug is withdrawn for sufficiently long periods, e.g. *Salmonella typhi* resistant to Chloromphenicol and *P. falciparam* resistant to chloroquine have been observed to become sensitive to these drugs after varying periods of withdrawal.

At present, problem of MDR TB and extensive drug resistance tuberculosis (XDRTB) are posing major problem in the containment of TB. Hospital acquired pneumonias, UTIs, leprosy, HIV infections, influenza and other disease are becoming increasingly resistant to treatment.

Different processes adopted by microbes to cause resistance (Table 5.10):

Table 5.10: Major mechanisms of microbial resistance against commonly used antibiotics

Drug class	Main mechanism of resistance	Organisms
β-lactam antibiotics	Production of β-lactamase which inactivates the drug	Gram-positive and gram-negative bacteria
Vancomycin	Enzyme inhibition and alteration of the targets for vancomycin binding by plasmid mediated gene transfer and through transposons	*Enterococci*
Aminoglycosides	• Inactivation of the drug by inactivating enzymes encoded on plasmid • Inhibition of uptake of the drug, e.g. pseudomonas • Alterations of the target of action of the drug, e.g. ribosomal RNA	*Pseudomonas aeruginosa*
Chloramphenicol	Enzyme mediated inactivation of the drug through plasmid encoded gene transfer	*Salmonella*, gram-negative organism
Tetracyclines	• Removal of antibiotic from the cell–plasmid mediated mechanism • Reducing the binding of the antibiotic to the target in the cell	Gram-negative bacteria Gram-positive bacteria
Macrolides, ketolides, lincosamides and streptogramins	• Plasmid mediated enzymic alteration of ribosomal RNA which is the target for the drug • Promote efflux of the antibiotic from the cell	Gram-positive bacteria *Streptococci* and *Staphylococcus*
Quinolones	• Mutation in the target DNA gyrases and topoisomerase IV that interfere with drug action • Remove the drug from the cell	Gram-positive and gram-negative bacteria Gram-positive bacteria
Sulfonamides and trimethoprim	Alter the sensitivity of the target by plasmid-encoded genetic mechanism	Gram-positive and gram-negative bacteria
Rifampicin	Mutation in the β-subunit of RNA polymerase which renders the enzyme unable to bind the antibiotic	*Staphylococcus*
Resistance to multiple antibiotics	• Multiple unrelated genetic mechanisms • Some of them tend to eliminate the drug from the cytoplasm	Hospital acquired bacteria, e.g. gram-negative bacteria *Enterococci, Staphylococci, Salmonella, Pneumococci, Gonococci*

- Reduced permeability of outer membrane of the bacteria restricts access of the antibodies
- Cell wall efflux pumps drives out the antibiotic
- The target site for the antibiotic is altered
- Antibiotic resistance gene develops
- Through mechanisms of plasmids antibiotic inactivating enzymes spread and antibiotic is inactivated
- Antibiotic modifying enzymes develop.

Biofilm formation is a common feature of chronic airway infections in cystic fibrosis. Bacteria growing in biofilms are embedded in a matrix of endopolymeric substances including exopolysachride DNA and proteins. They are more resistant than bacteria growing planktonically. The biofilm has a negative charge which binds to positively charged antibiotics, e.g. aminoglycosides and prevent diffusion. Bacteria living in biofilm have slower rates of growth. Additionally, bacteria might interact through ***quorum sensing (QS) signals*** which are part of cells to cell signaling system that allows bacteria to communicate when growing in polymicrobial cultures.

Role of anaerobic bacteria: These can contribute to the development of resistance by the pathogen by different mechanisms such as—1) producing beta-lactamases, 2) contribute to QS signaling or activate resistance of the pathogen and 3) help in biofilm formation.

Future strategies in antibiotic resistance:
- Disruption of biofilm formation—iron chelating agent help to chelate iron and disrupt the biofilm barrier.
- Azithromycin has been used as a long term quorum sensing inhibitor (QSI).
- Agents that improve host immunity—β-carotene, garlic and supplementation of zinc.

Resistance analysis: This is the study of resistance mechanisms in microbes using molecular methods to identify the resistance inducing gene. In chronic infections the microbes change their genetic structure when exposed to antibiotics. Study of this phenomenon helps to institute effective antibiotic therapy. Examples of resistance inducing genes are β-lactamase genes and genes that promote efflux of the drug from the bacterial cell.

Source: Sherrard LJ, Tunney MM, Elborn JS. Antimicrobial resistance in the respiratory microbiota of people with cystic fibrosis. Lancet. 2014;384(9944):703-13.

THE PROBLEM OF SUPERBUGS

Microbes resistant to several antibiotics were identified in New Delhi as early as 2008–2009 and the mechanism of resistance was found to be the production of New Delhi metallo-beta-lactamase (NDM-1) which is a transmissible multiple resistance gene, originally found in a strain of *Klebsiella* isolated in a patient. Subsequently *Enterobacteriaceae* containing NDM-1 was identified in many parts of India, Pakistan, Bangladesh and later, several other countries. The resistance factor confers resistance against almost all antibiotics except polymyxins. Genes encoding the enzyme ***methlylase*** that alters ribosomal binding of the antibiotics were responsible for this phenomenon. Transmission of this gene was through plasmids. Resistance to beta-lactam antibiotics, cephalosporins, erythromycin, carbapenam, rifampicin, chloramphenicol, clindamycin, linezolid and streptogramin B was observed. Subsequently other organisms containing NDM-1 were also identified in several countries. These include *E. coli, Enterobacter* species *Morganella morganii* and others. This problem of MDR is causing serious concern at present.

Source: Moellering RC Jr. NDM-1—a cause for worldwide concern. N Engl J Med. 2010;363(25):2377-9.

RATIONAL USE OF ANTIBIOTICS

Selection of Antibiotics

The drug has to be tailored to the need of the individual patient, site of infection and organism causing the infection. The following points are important:
- Efficacy—to be given top priority
- Cost—must be affordable to the patient
- Toxicity—potentially toxic drugs like aminoglycosides, chloramphenicol and others are to be used only when definitely indicated
- Availability
- Least disturbance to normal flora whenever possible
- Prevent development of drug resistance and super infections
- As far as possible try to get culture and sensitivity results to select the appropriate antibiotic. However, in special situations the laboratory results should not be the only criteria for deciding the treatment, clinical judgment may also have to play its role. If the specimens are obtained from closed sites that are normally sterile, e.g. CSF, blood and pleural, peritoneal and joint fluids, isolation of a microorganism is definitely pathological. Isolation of a pathogen from areas such as skin, mucosa and the respiratory, alimentary and lower genitourinary tract should be interpreted on the basis of the clinical picture as well.

Overuse of Antibiotics—Common in the Following Situations
- Higher specialties—all branches
- General specialists
- General practitioners
- Quacks
- Chemists who dispense over the counter drugs
- Patients who resort to self-medication.

Misuse of Antibiotics
- Use without evidence of bacterial infection
- Prophylactic antibiotics without indication
- Combination of drugs when single agent is sufficient
- Use of unscientific combinations
- Use of parenteral agents when oral medication is sufficient
- Use of expensive and newer drug—when simple and cheaper agents are equally effective
- Improper selection of antibiotics
- Duration and dose—not conforming to the standard recommendation
- Using single drugs when combinations have to be used, e.g. TB.

Overuse and misuse of antibiotics are commonly seen in the treatment of fever, upper respiratory tract infections (URTI), viral infections, poisonings, asthma, chronic respiratory diseases (CRD), amebic liver abscess, indwelling urinary catheters and the like.

Antibiotics are employed empirically without evidence of bacterial infection.

More than 75% of antibiotic prescriptions are without indication.

Fever: Short febrile illness is most commonly produced by self-limiting viral infections with no indication for antibiotics, but extensively used.

URTI: Almost always they are viral in etiology and there is no role for the routine use of antibiotics. The common adage: ***'If common colds are left alone they clear over the course of a week, whereas, if treated vigorously they disappear within 7 days'*** holds true even now.

Influenza: Routine antibacterial drugs are not indicated, but they have to be used in selected patients with severe chronic obstructive pulmonary disease (COPD) or heart disease.

Poisoning: Routine use of prophylactic antibiotics is not recommended, but extensively overused. Appropriate antibacterial drugs are indicated only in selective situations.

Asthma: Usually the precipitating factor is viral infection. Parainfluenza and RSV in young children and rhinovirus and influenza virus in older children and adults. Bacterial infection may supervene and then the sputum becomes purulent. Rarely yellow sputum may be due to the presence of eosinophils even without secondary infection. Therefore the routine use of antibiotics is not indicated.

Indwelling catheter: Prophylactic antibiotic during the first 4 or 5 days reduces the risk of infection. Beyond 5 days there is no benefit, and hence antibiotic prophylaxis fails when the catheter is kept for longer periods. Infections have to be treated when they occur.

Prophylactic Antibiotics

Indications for Chemoprophylaxis

- When there is a high risk of infection, e.g. wound infection after colonic surgery.
- Risk is low, but consequences are severe if infection results, e.g. insertion of prosthetic heart valves and prosthetic joints.

Observe the Following Principles

- Risk of severe infection should be greater than the adverse effects of antimicrobials.
- Antibacterials should be given only for the minimum period necessary to prevent infections.
- The drug should be given before the onset of risk such as before starting surgery or as soon as possible after exposure to infection.

Common Clinical Situations Requiring Prophylactic Antibiotics

- Rheumatic fever
- Infective endocarditis
- Meningococcal meningitis
- Recurrent cystitis
- Surgical prophylaxis in selected situations
- Recurrent cellulitis in conjunction with lymphedema especially in lymphatic filariasis
- Severely neutropenic patients
- HIV infected person harboring tubercle bacilli—INH prophylaxis
- Trimethoprim prophylaxis in HIV positive individuals to HIV positive individuals to prevent *Pneumocystis jiroveci.*

Note: Several other infections in normal and immuno-compromised hosts may require prophylactic antibiotics under special circumstances.

Improper Selection of Antibiotics

This leads to poor clinical response, increased cost of treatment and adverse side effects.

Use of Parenteral Route When Oral Administration is Effective

The route of administration should be preferably oral if the drug in suitable for oral use and the patient can tolerate oral medication. Since, parenteral administration ensures quicker and more reliable bioavailability, parenteral route should be preferred in severe infections such as meningitis, infective endocarditis or severe pneumonias. IV route is preferable in patients with hypotension and circulatory depression. In those in whom repeated large doses are required for prolonged periods, an IV line or central venous line is the ideal route. When the patient improves, change to the oral route. Parenteral therapy is inherently more expensive, inconvenient and predisposing to the risk of nosocomial infection. Drugs which are effective when administered orally as single daily doses have better patient acceptance and compliance.

Use of Combination Drugs When Single Agent is Effective and Using Unscientific Combinations

Infections are to be treated with single drugs if they are definitely effective. Combinations are definitely indicated in some situations.

- ***When antimicrobial synergy is clearly advantageous:***
  - *Pseudomonas aeruginosa*—aminoglycoside + β-lactam (ceftazidime/piperacillin) more effective
  - Enterococci—ampicillin + aminoglycoside like (gentamicin)
  - Brucellosis—aminoglycoside + doxycycline or doxy-cycline + rifampicin
  - Mycobacteria—combination of 3 or more anti-tuberculosis drugs for preventing the development of drug resistance.
- ***To broaden the spectrum of antibacterial action***, e.g. peritonitis following perforation—mixed infection is common. This may require a combination of β-lactam antibiotics + aminoglycoside + metronidazole.
- ***Neutropenic patients with sepsis.***

Combination therapy may lead to increased cost, change in microbial ecology and chances of superinfection.

Combination of amoxicillin/ampicillin with cloxacillin is marketed by many pharmaceuticals and extensively prescribed. Such fixed drug combination should be avoided as for as possible.

Use of Costly and Newer Agents When Cheaper Conventional Agents are Effective

When many drugs with equal efficacy and toxicity are available, one should choose the least expensive drug. When an expensive drug is more effective and absolutely indicated, its use is justified. Newer agents generally cost more and they are promoted more vigorously. Older agents like penicillin G, amoxicillin, co-trimoxazole and doxycycline are relatively cheap, but quite effective against several organisms.

Duration of Therapy

Therapy has to be continued until cure is achieved as assessed by clinical and laboratory parameters. Most acute infections require treatment for 5–10 days. The key factors include—type of infection, location of infection and immunocompetence of the patient. The duration may vary from single oral dose for gonococcal cervicitis to 4–6 weeks of IV therapy for infective endocarditis. Most acute infections of the respiratory tract, ear, paranasal sinuses and GIT should be treated for 5–10 days.

For streptococcal pharyngitis/tonsillitis, 10 days treatment is indicated to ensure eradication.

Prolonged therapy is not only more expensive, it can also lead to adverse side effects and emergence of bacterial resistance.

Consequences of overuse and misuse:

- Emergence of drug resistance
- Increased cost of treatment
- Unwanted side effects
- Disturbance of the normal flora and risk of super-infection.

The modern trend is to de-escalate the intensity of therapy once the infection is controlled, rather than to adopt the same duration and dosage for all subjects. This should be done under close specialist supervision.

CHAPTER 6

Therapeutics of Glucocorticoids

S Bhasi

Chapter Summary

- General Considerations
- Common Indications
- Adverse Side Effects
- Management of Patients on Glucocorticoid Therapy
- Inhibition of Hypothalamo-pituitary-adrenal Axis and Steroid Withdrawal

GENERAL CONSIDERATIONS

The initial therapeutic use of glucocorticoids in 1948 resulted in dramatic clinical improvement in a patient with severe rheumatoid arthritis. Today, glucocorticoids are extensively used in therapeutics to manage a wide variety of conditions. Presently available corticosteroid preparations are mainly synthetic.

Cortisol (hydrocortisone) is the natural glucocorticoid produced from adrenal cortex. The normal rate of endogenous cortisol production as evidenced by recent studies is only about 20 mg/day. Adrenocorticotropic hormone (ACTH) controls normal secretion. In healthy unstressed persons normal secretion shows a diurnal pattern—plasma cortisol is highest in the early morning hours and lowest in the evening. Less than 10% is in the free form which is biologically active. In stressful situations like sepsis, trauma, burns, surgery and others, cortisol secretion is increased 2–6 times in proportion to the severity of the stress. The diurnal variation is also lost.

Several formulations of corticosteroids are available for therapeutic use (Table 6.1). They differ in their gluco-

Table 6.1: Comparison of commonly used glucocorticoids

Compound	Anti-inflammatory potency	Minera-locorticoid potency	Duration of action (hours)	Equipotent dose (mg)
Short acting				
Cortisol	1	1	8–12	20
Intermediate acting				
Prednisolone	4	0.25	16–36	5
Methyl-prednisolone	5	<0.01	18–40	4
Triamcinolone	5	<0.01	12–36	4
Long acting				
Betamethasone	25	<0.01	36–54	0.75
Dexamethasone	25	<0.01	36–54	0.75

corticoid and mineralocorticoid activities. Preparations available for systemic use include hydrocortisone, prednisolone, methylprednisolone, betamethasone, dexamethasone triamcinolone and deflazacort. The synthetic agents have the following properties:

- Higher affinity for glucocorticoid receptors
- Less binding with cortisol binding globulin and therefore, more of the drug remains in the free form. Dexamethasone least bound
- Higher potency
- Longer duration of action
- Less salt-retaining property.

Textbook of Medicine

Therapeutic Effects

- Anti-inflammatory effect—suppress inflammatory activity
- Immunosuppressive action
- Membrane stabilizing effect
- Modulates vascular responsiveness and permeability
- Surfactant production in the lung.

COMMON INDICATIONS

Replacement therapy: Primary and secondary hyper-adrenocorticism.

Hydrocortisone is ideal from 15 to 20 mg/day. Prednisolone is the convenient alternative—dose 5 mg/day. Its two-third dose is given in the morning and one-third in the evening. Doubling the dose is needed during concurrent minor acute illnesses. Further increase is required in severe stressful situations. Maximum hydrocortisone dose in severe stress in 50 mg IV (intravenously) q6 hourly.

Hypoadrenalcorticism due to primary adrenal damage may require addition of mineralocorticoid like fludrocortisone acetate 0.05–0.3 mg daily or every other day.

Nonendocrine indications: Steroids are given in pharmacological doses which are larger.

- ***Allergic diseases:*** Anaphylactic shock, atopic dermatitis, drug reaction, urticaria and others.
- ***Autoimmune diseases:*** Systemic lupus erythematosus (SLE), rheumatoid arthritis, systemic vasculitis, temporal arteritis, myasthenia gravis, mixed connective tissue disease and others.
- ***Hematological diseases:*** Autoimmune hemolytic anemia, immune thrombocytopenia, leukemia, lymphoma, multiple myeloma.

Gastrointestinal disorders: Ulcerative colitis, Crohn's disease, autoimmune chronic active hepatitis.

Ocular conditions: Acute uveitis, choroiditis, optic neuritis.

Respiratory diseases: Asthma, interstitial lung disease, chronic obstructive pulmonary disease (COPD), tuberculous pleural effusion.

Neurological conditions: Cerebral edema especially due to tumor, demyelinating disorders like multiple sclerosis, acute disseminated encephalomyelitis, chronic inflammatory demyelinating polyneuropathy, tuberculous meningitis, central nervous system (CNS) vasculitis.

Severe infections with overwhelming toxicity: Corticosteroids may be life-saving, if applied along with appropriate antimicrobial therapy.

Prevention of graft rejection: In organ transplantation.

Metabolic homeostasis: Acute hypercalcemia.

Miscellaneous conditions: Septic shock, thyroid storm, myxedema coma and several others.

ADVANTAGES OF GLUCOCORTICOIDS

In several life-threatening and serious diseases such as severe asthma, fulminant ulcerative colitis and systemic vasculitis, the relief brought about by glucocorticoids is dramatic. Maintenance dose helps to prevent exacerbation. Glucocorticoids produce mild euphoria and offers better quality of life. They are relatively cheap and widely available. Due to all these advantages glucocorticoids have been used extensively and also misused for prolonged periods, often empirically, even as self-medication.

Glucocorticoids have several adverse effects. Therefore, it is necessary to assess the benefits and adverse effects before starting therapy. In medical emergencies, often high doses may have to be administered for short periods even in the presence of minor contraindications, e.g. severe asthma in diabetic patients. However, they should never be administered for more than a few days in such patients without full evaluation and review.

ADVERSE SIDE EFFECTS

- Iatrogenic Cushing's syndrome
- Growth retardation in children
- Flaring up of infection—especially tuberculosis and fungal infections
- Hyperglycemia/new onset diabetes—more common in patients with prediabetes or risk of developing diabetes. Pre-existing diabetes worsens
- Osteoporosis—especially in elderly and post-menopausal women, leading to compression fractures
- Hypertension
- Increased appetite, polyphagia, obesity and dyslipidemia
- Delayed wound healing, dehiscence of scars, striae over the skin, thinning of skin, purpura and easy bruisability
- Acid peptic disease—hyperacidity, ulceration of the upper gastrointestinal tract (GIT), exacerbation of peptic ulcer and precipitating complications like hemorrhage and perforation. Concomitant nonsteroidal anti-inflammatory drugs (NSAIDs) use increases the risk
- Ocular problems—cataract, glaucoma
- Myopathy—mainly proximal muscles
- Mood change (euphoria or depression)—delirium, sleep disturbances and rarely frank psychosis. Greater risk in older patients and those with pre-existing behavioral changes. Psychosis is rare and occurs with prednisolone doses exceeding 20 mg/day.
- Hypothalamo-pituitary-adrenal (HPA)-axis suppression—some features are more common with iatrogenic Cushing syndrome compared to endogenous Cushing syndrome, e.g. worsening of glaucoma, posterior capsular cataract, benign raised intracranial tension and osteonecrosis of femoral/humeral head, pancreatitis and panniculitis.

Timing of Side Effect

Insomnia, euphoria, glucose intolerance and increased appetite may develop within hours. Psychotic symptoms may occur within hours or may develop later. Osteoporosis takes weeks to months to develop.

Preventing/Minimizing Side Effects

- Use lowest dose for the shortest duration to achieve treatment goal
- Use only when absolutely indicated
- Monitor side effects

- Treatment of pre-existing conditions that may increase the risk of side effects, eg. diabetes mellitus (DM), hypertension, dyslipidemia, heart failure, peptic ulcer, presence of infection, low bone density/osteoporosis
- Avoid co-administration of NSAIDs whenever possible
- Exercise program to reduce the risk of myopathy and osteoporosis.

Evaluation of Patient Prior to Glucocorticoid Therapy

Look for the following

- Presence of tuberculosis (TB) or other chronic infections
- Evidence of glucose intolerance or frank DM
- Evidence of osteoporosis
- History of peptic ulcer, esophagitis or gastritis
- Evidence of hypertension or cardiovascular disease (CVD)
- History of psychiatric disorder.

MANAGEMENT OF PATIENTS ON STEROID THERAPY

- Diet with calorie restriction to avoid weight gain, high protein, low sodium and rich in potassium and calcium.
- Regular exercise to prevent myopathy and osteoporosis.
- Patients with acid peptic disease to be given H_2 receptor antagonists or proton pump inhibitors.
- Growing children should have regular monitoring of growth.
- Monitor blood pressure (BP), weight and blood sugar periodically. If hyperglycemia/diabetes develop, consider withdrawal or at least substantial reduction of dose of the glucocorticoid. If the glucose does not come to normal start antidiabetic therapy. If the glucocorticoid cannot be withdrawn, give it with concurrent antidiabetic therapy—preferably insulin.
- Supplement vitamin D 60,000 IU weekly × 6–8 doses followed by monthly once or 2000 IU daily and calcium salts (gluconate, carbonate and others) 500 mg bd (twice a day) orally and bisphosphonates to prevent osteoporosis.

Routes of Administration

- ***Oral:*** This is the most commonly used route for systemic effects. Prednisolone is the commonly recommended drug.
- ***Parenteral:*** IM (intramuscular)/IV—acute severe asthma, craniospinal trauma, brain tumor with cerebral edema, transplant rejection, fulminant presentation of autoimmune diseases, septic shock with corticosteroid deficiency and acute adrenal crisis.
- ***Inhalation:*** For long-term prophylaxsis of asthma and selected patients with COPD.
- ***Intralesional:*** Tenosynovitis, enthesitis, keloids, local painful inflammatory lesions and others.
- ***Intra-articular:*** Inflammatory joint disease such as oligoarticular rheumatoid arthritis in 1 or 2 joints.
- ***Topical to skin:*** Many steroid responsive dermatoses.
- ***Retention enema:*** Ulcerative colitis.
- ***Ophthalmic indications:*** Topical application in the form of eye drops or ointment is indicated for condi-

tions like allergic conjunctivitis and other inflammatory conditions.

Topical preparations of corticosteroids, especially betamethasone and its analogues may be absorbed from normal and inflamed skin, joints and the large intestine to produce systemic adverse effects if continued for long. Aerosol preparations also can give rise to systemic side effects, if used regularly over several months in high doses.

Live Vaccine and Glucocorticoids

Live vaccines can be given to patients on glucocorticoid therapy, if they come under the following categories:

- Prednisolone < 20 mg or equivalent for < 14 days
- Taking replacement dose only
- Topical steroids only.

ADVERSE SIDE EFFECTS OF CORTICOSTEROID THERAPY

Suppression of Hypothalamo-pituitary-adrenal Axis

Glucocorticoids give rise to suppression of the HPA-axis leading to reduction in corticotrophin releasing hormone (CRH) and adrenocorticotrophic hormone (ACTH). The degree of suppression depends on duration of treatment and the dose. There is inter individual variation due to variation in metabolism. Subjects who metabolize steroids slowly have increased risk of side effects. Clearance in older individual is less than in the young. Patients are categorized into 3 groups based on HPA suppression:

1. ***Not suppressed***
   - Any patient receiving any dose of nonparenteral steroid for less than 3 weeks.
   - Alternative day therapy with physiological dose.
2. ***Suppressed***
   - Any patient who receive more than 20 mg of prednisolone per day for more than 3 weeks.
   - Any patient who has clinical features of Cushing syndrome.
   - Anyone who have received bed time dose of prednisolone for more than few weeks.
3. ***Uncertain suppression***
   - Patient taking prednisolone 10–20 mg for more than 3 weeks.
   - Less than 10 mg/day prednisolone for more than few weeks other than as bed time dose.

These patients need ACTH stimulation test to assess function of adrenal gland.

Steroid Withdrawal Following Long-term Therapy

The following problems occur:

- Worsening of underlying disease
- Slow recovery of HPA-axis with secondary adrenal insufficiency.

In the early stages of drug withdrawal, though adrenal cortical function may recover to be adequate at ordinary times, it may fail during stress. Complete recovery may take 6–9 months or even more. Many patients may remain steroid dependent.

Steroid withdrawal syndrome: This develops in persons receiving prolonged glucocorticoid therapy with HPA-axis suppression on rapid withdrawal of the drug. It is characterized by lethargy, anorexia, vomiting, malaise,

Textbook of Medicine

weight loss, arthralgia, myalgia, headache and sometimes fever. Since aldosterone secretion is not ACTH dependant, its level is maintained. Therefore, BP level and electrolytes remain normal unless dehydration occur due to poor intake and vomiting.

Protocol for corticosteroid withdrawal: These should be followed for all cases where steroid therapy is given in doses above the equivalent of 20 mg of prednisolone daily for more than 3 weeks and HPA-axis is suppressed.

Step 1: Taper steroid dose gradually to physiological level, i.e. 5 mg/day.

Step 2: Change to alternate day therapy for prednisolone and single morning dose for cortisone when possible.

Tapering Regimen

- When duration of therapy is less than 3 weeks and HPA not suppressed tapering is not mandatory, if the basic disease is stable and do not require tapering.
- When duration of therapy is longer with expected HPA-axis suppression, tapering is recommended. Goal of tapering is to use a rate of change that will prevent recurrence of activity of the underlying disease and also symptoms of cortisol insufficiency. Aim at a relatively stable decrement dose of 10–20% at a time. Guidelines for dose decrement of prednisolone is given below:
  - 5–10 mg/day for every 1–2 weeks from an initial dose of 40 mg
  - 5 mg/day every 1–2 weeks from an initial dose of 20–40 mg
  - 2.5 mg/day every 2–3 weeks from an initial dose of 10–20 mg
  - 1 mg/day every 2–4 weeks from an initial dose of 5–10 mg
  - 0.5 mg/day every 2–4 weeks from an initial dose of 5 mg/day (alternate day change of 1 mg is acceptable).

Testing for Recovery

Estimate the morning plasma cortisol. Normal value is 7–20 mcg/dL (7–13 borderline, 13–20 definitely normal). If test result is less than 13 and symptoms of cortisol deficiency is present Synacthen test is advised. Estimate cortisol at 30 and 60 minutes. One value must be greater 18 mcg to ensure recovery of HPA-axis.

Glucocorticoid Resistance in Inflammatory Diseases

Even when glucocorticoids are given in full dose of 40 mg prednisolone daily for 2 weeks or more, 10% of patients fail to get relief from the inflammatory process, e.g. asthma, rheumatoid disease, inflammatory bowel diseases and other immune mediated diseases. Despite absence of beneficial results adverse effects do occur.

Tobacco-smoking is a common cause for resistance to glucocorticoids. Major action of glucocorticoids as anti-inflammatory drugs is to activate genes which encode cytokines, chemokines, adhesion molecules, inflammatory enzymes and receptors.

Mechanisms of glucocorticoid resistance:

- Genetic factors—a familial gene concerned in the process is bone morphogenetic protein receptor type-II (BMPR-II)
- Defective glucocorticoid receptor binding and translocation
- Increased expression of glucocorticoid receptor β
- Transcription factor activation
- Abnormal histone acetylation
- Reduction of regulatory T-cells. Vitamin D is an important regulator of the immune system particularly in the control of regulatory T-cells
- Increase in the level of permeability glycoprotein (P-glycoprotein)—170 transports several drugs including glucocorticoids out of the cells.

Management

Alternative Drugs

Calcineurin inhibitors such as cyclosporine A and tacrolimus may be useful. Several p38 mitogen-activated protein kinases (p38 MAP) inhibitors are in the process of development for glucocorticoid resistance.

P-glycoprotein inhibitors—drugs like theophylline, vitamin D and powerful antioxidants may be tried to counter glucocorticoid resistance.

Points to Remember

- Glucocorticoids are life-saving drugs in many serious clinical conditions.
- On no account fear of side effects should result in withholding the drug when there is absolute indication for use.
- Use lowest dose for the shortest duration to reduce side effects.
- Monitor therapy and take measures to reduce side effects.
- When duration of therapy is more than 3 weeks with greater than 20 mg prednisolone or equivalent suppression of HPA-axis is likely and tapering is necessary.

Source: Barnes PJ, Adcock IM. Glucocorticoid resistance in inflammatory diseases. Lancet. 2009;373(9678):1905-17.

7

Principles of Oncology

KV Krishna Das

Chapter Summary

- General Considerations
- Genetic Aspects of Cancer
- Etiological Factors
- Tumor Markers
- Paraneoplastic Syndromes
- Metastasis
- Tumor Kinetics
- Prognosis in Cancer
- Therapy
- Radiotherapy, Chemotherapy, Immunity-based Therapy
- Cancer Screening Programs
- Palliative Care and Pain Management

GENERAL CONSIDERATIONS

Historic Landmarks in Oncology

1863—Rudolf Virchow deduced the cellular origin of cancer
1809—Ephraim McDowell removed ovarian tumor by surgery
Turn of the 20th century—Paul Ehrlich developed chemicals against cancer
1950—Standard radiation therapy for cancer
2000—Human Genome Project and Cancer
4th of February every year is termed the World Cancer Day

The International Union against Cancer has defined cancer as a disturbance of growth characterized primarily by excessive proliferation of cells without apparent relation to the physiological demands of the organs involved. Oncology deals with the prevention, diagnosis, treatment and research aspects of cancer. Cancer is a leading cause of death all over the world, 7 million deaths occurred during 2001. Globally 35% of these are attributable to 9 potentially modifiable factors. 1/3 of cancer deaths occur in affluent and 2/3 in developing countries. Among these 2/3 are men and 1/3 are women. The modifiable risk factors include tobacco smoking, alcoholism, unsafe sex practices, urban air pollution, indoor air pollution by burning biofuels and sharing of contaminated needles obesity, low consumption of fresh vegetables and fruits, physical inactivity. The life expectancy in India is 64 for male and 67 for females at present (2013 AD).

As the life expectancy increases, the incidence of cancer also increases. In many countries of the world cancer has become the second or the third most common cause of death and the number of patients with cancer are steadily increasing. The modalities for diagnosis and treatment of cancer are steadily increasing and more and more cases are detected and the disease also have been detected at earlier stages compared to previous years. Several newer drugs including monoclonal antibodies have been introduced for treatment.

Tumors depend on their microenvironment for their survival and growth. The stromal cells and extracellular matrix play the supportive role. Drugs acting on the microenvironment such as thalidomide are showing promise as anti-neoplastic drugs. Studies are in progress.

The pattern of cancer has changed over the past decade in many parts of India. Figures of the hospital-based tumor registry from Regional Cancer Centre (RCC), Trivandrum for the years 2010 and 2011 reveal the following. Oral cancers related to tobacco chewing habit still constitute the single largest group. Among the other leading cancers, the frequency is given in Table 7.1. The statistics of prevalent childhood cancers in Regional Cancer Centre (RCC), Trivandrum is listed in Tables 7.2 and 7.3.

Table 7.1: Number and relative proportion of 10 leading sites of cancer for males and females- Data RCC- 2010

	Males			*Females*		
	Site	**No.**	**%**	**Site**	**No.**	**%**
1	Lungs	839	14.5	Breast	1737	29.8
2	Oral cavity	823	14.2	Thyroid	731	12.5
3	Leukemia	496	8.6	Cervix uteri	448	7.7
4	Lymphoma	386	6.7	Oral cavity	392	6.7
5	Stomach	306	5.3	Leukemia	363	6.2
6	Pharynx	297	5.1	Ovary	303	5.2
7	Esophagus	222	3.8	Lymphoma	206	3.5
8	Larynx	221	3.8	Corpus uteri	179	3.1
9	Prostate	211	3.6	Lung	148	2.5
10	Thyroid	208	3.6	Rectum	135	2.3

Source: www.rcctvm.org, www.rcctvm.gov.in
Abbreviation: RCC = Regional Cancer Centre, Trivandrum

Table 7.2: Number and relative proportion of childhood cancers (0–14) years seen in RCC, Trivandrum

Males			*Females*		
Site	**No.**	**%**	**Site**	**No.**	**%**
Leukemia lymphoid	118	37.5	Leukemia lymphoid	82	34.5
Brain	41	13	Brain	32	13.4
Leukemia myeloid	21	6.7	Leukemia myeloid	21	8.8
Hodgkin's disease	18	5.7	Bone of limbs	12	5
Diffuse NHL	17	5.4	Connective tissue	11	4.6
Adrenal gland	12	3.8	Kidney	10	4.2
Bone of limbs	11	3.5	Hodgkin's disease	8	3.4
Connective tissue	11	3.5	Leukemia, unspecified	7	2.9
Leukemia, monocytic	8	3	Liver	7	2.9
Leukemia, unspecified	7	2.2	Other bones	6	2.5
			Adrenal gland	6	2.5

Abbreviations: RCC = Regional Cancer Centre; NHL = Non-Hodgkin lymphoma

Textbook of Medicine

Table 7.3: Pediatric oncology—fresh cases seen in 2010

	Males		
	Site	No.	%
1	Leukemia	245	39.7
2	Brain tumors	86	14
3	Neuroblastoma	38	6.2
4	Lymphoma	34	5.5
5	Bone tumor	27	4.4
6	Kidney tumor	21	3.4
7	Germ cell tumor	20	3.3
8	Rhabdomyosarcoma	15	2.4
9	Retinoblastoma	11	1.8
10	Hepatic tumors	10	1.6
11	Others	105	17

Note: Total number of new cases = 612

Table 7.4: Results of examination of patients at cancer camps

Number of camps	80
Number of people screened	6634
Oral cancer	13
Breast cancer	15
Cervix cancer	1
Others	17
Oral pre-cancer	191
Cervical pre-cancer	115

This clearly shows that as the health conditions improve there is a change in the pattern of malignancy as well. Moreover, with improved facilities for early cancer detection and the mass education programs launched by the RCC, Trivandrum and a considerably higher proportion of cancer patients are seeking treatment at an earlier stage when chance for cure is much higher. The present concept is that by positive measures like education of the population on cancer prevention and early detection the disease should be diagnosed at the early stages in order to achieve maximum cure rate with minimal residual morbidity and expense. The RCC, Trivandrum and several other institutions conduct cancer detection camps.

Findings at cancer detecting camp or source of RCC. Table 7.4 showing the results of examination of patient seen at organized cancer detection camps.

Etiology: Several factors operate to bring about carcinogenesis. These are genetic, hormonal, metabolic, physical, chemical and other environmental factors. During the course of cell division malignant mutants may be formed which proliferate to form tumors. Carcinogens increase the rate of mutation and thereby, the possibility of malignancy is also increased. Cancer is more frequent in old age, since the occurrence of aberrant mutation is increased. Many mutants are destroyed by immunological mechanisms of the body.

GENETIC ASPECTS OF CANCER

Genetic studies have yielded considerable information on the genesis, pathology, behavior, response to therapy, follow-up and prediction of cancer in near relatives.

Genetic factors: Many neoplasms show evidence of genetic predisposition. For example:

- Retinoblastomas, multiple polyposis of the colon and carcinoma breast run in families.
- Mongolism is associated with a ten-fold increase in the risk of leukemia.
- Blood group A is associated with a higher risk of gastric carcinoma, compared to blood group B and O.
- Hodgkin's disease is more frequent in subjects with HLA B18.

Breast cancer shows a strong familial predisposition. Women with BRCA1 or BRCA2 mutations have a 60–85% cumulative lifetime risk of invasive breast cancer up to 70 years of age and 15–65% cumulative life time risk of invasive ovarian cancer. Prophylactic mastectomy reduces the risk of breast cancer. Salpingo-oophorectomy reduces the risk of both breast cancer and tubo-ovarian cancer.

Colonic epithelial cancers, also increased in patients with BRCA1 and 2 mutations.

Several chromosomal changes have been demonstrated in malignant cells. Many of them are characteristic to be of diagnostic help, while others are not. For example, Ph1 chromosome is diagnostic of chronic myeloid leukemia. When chronic myeloid leukemia transforms into the acute phase diagnostic chromosomal rearrangement occurs. Myelodysplastic syndrome is characterized by specific chromosomal patterns. Several examples of chromosomal abnormalities in cancers are known at present.

Genetic studies have yielded rich dividends in understanding the initiation and progress of cancer. These include the identification of oncogenes, proto-oncogenes, onco-suppressor genes, genetic changes caused by retroviruses and several others.

Oncogenes and oncoproteins: Oncogenes are altered forms of normal genes called proto-oncogenes. Oncogenes have the ability to promote cell growth in the absence of normal growth-promoting/mitogenic signals. Products of oncogenes are called oncoproteins, which resemble the normal products of proto-oncogenes. Oncoprotein production is not under normal regulatory control. Cells proliferate without the usual requirement for external signals and are freed from checkpoints, therefore growth becomes autonomous. Growth becomes autonomous.

More than 80 human proto-oncogenes are known. For example, erb-B is located in chromosome number 7, and it produces the receptor for epidermal growth factor (EGF). The sis gene, located in chromosome 22 produces platelet derived growth factor (PDGF). The abl, located in chromosome no. 9 and src, in chromosome no. 20 produce proteins with tyrosine kinase activity. The protein products of proto-oncogenes have essential roles in cell growth and differentiation. But the proto-oncogenes are under the control of other regulatory genes. When proto-oncogenes are activated there will be continuous expression of the gene leading to uncontrolled cell division and malignant transformation. A proto-oncogene may be activated by the following mechanisms:

Chromosomal translocation: In all cases of Burkitt's lymphoma, translocation of chromosome 8 to 14 takes place with consequent activation of C-myc. In non-

Hodgkin's lymphoma, translocation of chromosome 14 to 18 is very common. The breaks on chromosome 18 occur either in major break point region (MBR) or at the major cluster region (MCR), both involving the bcl-2 oncogene. The bcl-2 product suppresses programed cell death, leading to tumor formation.

Promoter insertion: Virus promoter genes may be integrated upstream to the oncogene so that continuous expression of the oncogene takes place.

Mutation of proto-oncogene: The ras gene produces a protein termed p-21 (mol. wt. 21,000), which suppresses the activity of adenyl cyclase and thereby, cell division. In human bladder cancers, a mutated p-21 is demonstrable, leading to continuous activity of adenyl cyclase. In many cases particular mutations leading to the formation of oncogenes have been identified.

Oncogenes are generally coded with a combination of three small letters, e.g. myc, L-myc, N-ras, C-abl, etc. while onco-suppressor genes are coded by two capital letters, e.g. RB-1 for retinoblastoma, WT-1 for Wilms' tumor, NE-1 for neurofibromatosis.

Onco-suppressor genes present in normal cells usually prevent cancer formation. For example, when both alleles of the RB gene are deleted, retinoblastoma results. An onco-suppressor gene called p-53 produces a phosphoprotein with molecular weight 53,000. It can complex with proteins generated by other oncogenes.

Most tumors have a complete absence of p-53 while others show mutant non-functional p-53.

Several different mechanisms may activate oncogenes. Thus viruses, chemical carcinogens, chromosome translocation, gamma rays and spontaneous mutation may activate oncogenes to produce malignancy.

Growth factors: These are humoral factors which generally cause mitosis or differentiation to target cells. More than 100 such growth factors are described. EGF produced by fibroblasts stimulates growth of epidermal and epithelial cells. PDGF produced by platelets, accelerates wound healing and stimulates growth of mesenchymal cells. Nerve growth factor (NGF) produced by salivary glands stimulates growth of sensory and sympathetic neurons. Oncogene activation leads to imbalance in such growth factors.

Apoptosis: Programed cell death is known as apoptosis. During the normal growth, old cells are to be removed, so that new cells can replace them. Hypoxia, reactive oxygen species, chemicals, irradiation, DNA damage, immune attack, malnutrition, tumor necrosis factor, and many other signals activate the apoptotic pathway. The final effectors of this pathway are a group of enzymes known as caspases (cysteinyl peptidases with aspartate specificity). They are named 1 to 14 according to their order of identification. They activate nucleases and cause DNA to be fragmented into small fragments (step ladder pattern of DNA in agar gel electrophoresis). The apoptotic cells show chromatin condensation, shrinking of the cells, and finally disintegration. In normal organs, the number of cells produced by cell division will be equal to the number of cells undergoing apoptosis. If the regulation of apoptosis is altered the cells in that tissue accumulate leading to neoplasms. Apoptosis promoting (suicidal) genes are c-fos, P53 and Rb: they are oncosuppressor genes. On the other hand, apoptosis inhibiting genes are cancer promoting genes, e.g. Bcl-2.

Clonal origin of neoplasms: It is widely accepted that most of the tumors arise from a single clone of altered cell, the clone having the potential to multiply and form the tumor. The biological history of a tumor shows several steps of progression. In the normal individual the aberrant cells tend to be destroyed by immune mechanism. When this breaks down, cells with malignant potential survive and proliferate. Initial progression of the tumor is very slow and it takes several years for an abnormal clone to multiply and become clinically recognizable. The early changes indicating dysplasia of the cells, can be identified and treatment at this stage can lead to arrest of the neoplasm and cure in many cases.

The Human Genome Project has given information about molecular markers which predict the development of tumors. By tests such as fluorescence *in situ* hybridization (FISH), polymerase chain reaction (PCR), DNA microarray, Southern blot hybridization and detection of tumors markers, reliable predictions can be made and appropriate surveillance and preventive measures can be adopted, e.g. hematological neoplasms; chronic myeloid leukemia (Ph(t 9:22) chromosome), N-myc in neuroblastoma, erb B_2 in breast cancer, gene-1 (RB-1) in retinoblastoma and others such as colorectal cancer and cervical cancer. Detection of these molecular abnormalities help in diagnosis, prognosis, predicting the disease in close relatives and appropriate use of the therapeutic modality.

Immunological changes: Malignant cells show different degrees of dedifferentiation. Several functional genes are present which are active in fetal life, but which are repressed in later life leading to the disappearance of several fetal antigens from the surface of the adult cells.

In malignant cells, embryonal antigens reappear on the cell surface due to depression of these genes, and these are termed onco-fetal antigens, e.g. carcino-embryonic antigen (CEA) in colon cancer and alpha-fetoprotein (AFP) in liver cancer.

ETIOLOGICAL FACTORS

Chemical carcinogens: These act cumulatively to bring about carcinogenesis. Food additives, coloring agents, aflatoxins and n-nitroso compounds are common carcinogens. The incidence of lung cancer is about 11 times more in cigarette smokers compared with non-smokers. Cancer may be produced: (a) at the site of exposure to the carcinogen, e.g. skin cancers in tar workers and buccal cancer in tobacco chewers; (b) at the site of metabolism, e.g. liver cancer in aflatoxicosis or (c) at the site of elimination, e.g. bladder cancer in workers using aromatic amines.

Diet: Some dietary factors or aspects of life-styles are significantly associated with certain malignancies. Thus salt-cured and smoked foods are related with cancer of esophagus and stomach; high fat diet with cancer of breast and colon; alcohol with cancer of liver and esophagus; tobacco with cancer of lung and oral cavity. Vegetable

Principles of Oncology

Textbook of Medicine

Table 7.5: Important etiological agents of cancer

Agent	Associated cancer
Physical agents	
Sunlight (UV)	Skin cancers
Chemical agents	
• Tobacco smoking	• Lung, mouth, esophagus, larynx, bladder
• Tobacco chewing	• Oral cavity
• Alcohol	• Oral, esophagus, liver
• Polycyclic aromatic hydrocarbons (produced during deep frying)	• Liver colon
• N-nitroso compounds	• Stomach, esophagus, bladder, liver
• Aflatoxins (fungal contamination)	• Liver
Microbial agents	
• *Helicobacter pylori*	• Stomach
• *Schistosoma hematobium*	• Urinary bladder
• Viruses	
• Epstein-Barr virus	• Burkitt's lymphoma; nasopharyngeal carcinoma
• Hepatitis B virus	• Hepatocellular carcinoma
• Hepatitis C virus	• Hepatocellular carcinoma
• HTLV-1	• T-cell leukemia
• HPV (human papilloma)	• Uterine cancer
• HSV-2 (herpes simplex)	• Uterine cancer
• HHV-6 (human herpes)	• Lymphomas
• HHV-8	• Kaposi's sarcoma

fibers in the diet increase the intestinal motility and so reduce the incidence of colon cancers. Fresh vegetables, beans and fruits in the diet will reduce cancer incidence, especially of gastrointestinal tract cancers. Some of the important etiological agents are shown in Table 7.5.

Initiation and progression: It is postulated that a carcinogen produces a mutation, but it remains dormant unless acted upon by a promoter. Benzopyrine or croton oil applied alone will not produce skin cancer. But when benzopyrine is followed by croton oil, tumor develops. The benzopyrine acts as a carcinogen to produce a mutation. But the promoter (croton oil) gives the drive for unchecked cell division, which is the characteristic feature of malignancies.

Antimutagens are substances which will inhibit with tumor promotion. Vitamin A and carotenoids are shown to reverse precancerous conditions, especially oral leukoplakia. Butylated hydroxyanisole (BHA), vitamin E and vitamin C are antioxidants, which prevent the damage made by free radicals and superoxides. Curcumin, the yellow substance in turmeric is known to prevent mutations in experimental systems.

Viruses: Several viruses have been implicated in many cancers. Epstein-Barr virus has been identified as the causative factor for Burkitt's lymphoma in African children and for nasopharyngeal carcinoma in Chinese population. Papilloma viruses (different types) and herpes virus type 2 have been shown to be associated with carcinoma cervix, hepatitis B and C viruses with primary carcinoma of liver, herpes virus type 6 with lymphomas and herpes virus type 8 with Kaposi's sarcoma. This virus is also associated with multicentric lymphoma and multicentric Castleman's disease.

Physical agents: Ionizing radiation cause a marked increase in cancer incidence in later life. Exposure to X-rays in fetal life increases the risk of developing leukemia in later life. The risk of developing cancer in a population exposed to ionizing radiation in a dose of 1 rad/year is 40 per million annually. Indiscriminate use of diagnostic X-rays constitutes a health hazard, and has to be avoided. Chronic irritation by heat (*kangri* in Kashmir and lighted cigarettes inside the mouth in Andhra Pradesh) lead to cancer of the abdominal wall and the palate in different populations. Bilharziasis is associated with higher risk of bladder neoplasms.

The four processes involved in tumorigenesis are:

1. ***Initiation***—a brief exposure to the causative agents induces changes in the tissue.
2. ***Promotion***—this is the process by which the induced abnormal tissue is made to proliferate and grow. Several substances, may act as promoters. Dietary fat has been implicated as a promoting agent for colon cancer.
3. ***Conversion*** involves induction of growth of all the abnormal tissue.
4. ***Progression*** refers to the later stages of tumor growth and proliferation—which are irreversible.

Characteristics of neoplastic cells which promote tumorigenesis and spread.

- Loss of differentiation and dedifferentiation to stem cells phenotype
- Genetic instability
- Enhanced response to growth factors
- Insensitivity to natural growth inhibitors
- Absence of contact inhibition
- Neovascularization to create abnormal blood vessels
- Evasion of immune mechanisms
- Invasion of natural limiting structures
- Ability to get seeded and proliferate in other locations
- Production of abnormal cytokines, hormones and other metabolic products with natural or abnormal metabolic effects, e.g. paraneoplastic syndromes.

TUMOR MARKERS

Tumor markers or tumor index substances are factors released from the tumor cells; these could be detected in blood and therefore indicate the presence of the tumor. They are useful: (A) For follow-up of cancer and to monitor the effectiveness of the therapy, (B) to detect the recurrence of the tumor, (C) for prognosis; serum level of tumor marker usually indicates roughly the tumor load, which in turn indicates whether the disease is advanced or not and (D) to facilitate detection of cancer. The presence of high levels of tumor marker suggests the diagnosis, but caution is to be taken to rule out other nonmalignant conditions. The levels of tumor markers are increased in inflammatory and other conditions as well but drastic elevation is suggestive of malignancies. The following are some of the commonly employed tumor markers:

- ***Alpha-fetoprotein (AFP):*** It is a fetal albumin. It is increased in hepatocellular carcinomas, germ cell tumors, teratocarcinoma of ovary and in pregnancy with fetal malformations of neural tube.

- ***Carcino-embryonic antigen (CEA):*** It is increased in colorectal and other gastrointestinal (GI) tumors.
- ***CA-125 (ovarian cancer antigen)*** is a glycoprotein and is increased in ovarian cancers of epithelial origin.
- ***CA-199*** is another glycoprotein seen in circulation in cancers of stomach and colon.
- Alkaline phosphatase (ALP) level is increased in bone and liver diseases; high level of heat-labile isoenzyme (bone isoenzyme) is seen in bone secondaries.
- ***Placental isoenzyme of ALP*** (heat stable and inhibited by phenyl alanine) is found in normal pregnancy. It is also seen in certain cases of carcinoma of lung, liver and gut and testicular seminomas, then it is called Regan isoenzyme.
- ***Acid phosphatase*** (tartrate labile isoenzyme) is increased in prostate cancers.
- ***Prostate specific antigen (PSA)*** is produced by secretory epithelium of prostate. It is normally secreted into seminal fluid, where it is useful to liquify the ejaculate. It is a protease, and in serum it is seen complexed with alpha-1 antitrypsin. The PSA level, especially the complexed form is increased in prostate cancers.
- ***Neuron specific enolase (NSE)*** level is raised in nervous system tumors.
- Beta-chain of human chorionic gonadotropin (hCG) is elevated in choriocarcinoma.
- Big ACTH is seen in pulmonary oat cell carcinomas.
- Vasoactive intestinal polypeptide (VIP) is elevated in apudomas (amine precursor uptake decarboxylaseomas).
- Tissue polypeptide specific antigen (TPS) measures an antigenic determinant associated with human cytokeratin. TPS level is elevated in almost all solid tumors. It is a marker of tumor cell activity, in contrast to all other markers related to tumor burden. Although non-specific with reference to the site of origin of tumor, it is very useful in assessing the efficacy of the treatment, and also for early detection of recurrence.
- Immunoglobulin levels are increased, and are seen as a monoclonal peak in electrophoresis, in multiple myeloma and in Waldenström's macroglobulinemia.
- Vanillyl mandelic acid (VMA), metabolite of catecholamines, is excreted in increased quantities in urine of patients with pheochromocytoma and neuroblastoma.
- Hydroxy indole acetic acid (HIAA), metabolite of serotonin, is raised in urine of patients with carcinoid syndrome.
- Hydroxy proline excretion in urine is elevated in bone metastasis.

Malignant cells show several biochemical abnormalities compared to normal cells. Some of them have been beneficially exploited in cancer chemotherapy, e.g. use of L-asparaginase for acute lymphatic leukemia.

PARANEOPLASTIC SYNDROMES

Tumors may produce signs and symptoms distant from the tumor site of metastasis; this is referred to as paraneoplastic syndrome. This is due to the production of hormones or metabolically active factors by tumors arising from non-endocrine tissues. The substances produced by the neoplasms are analogues of the natural hormones or their precursors. Several neurological manifestations may develop, such as neuropathies, myopathies, myasthenic reaction, myositis, and brainstem encephalitis. Antibodies against neuronal proteins may be demonstrable. These lesions may precede the overt manifestations of the tumor in many cases. Some of the important paraneoplastic syndromes are listed below:

- ***Ectopic adrenocorticotropic hormone (ACTH) syndrome*** is seen in small cell carcinoma of lung, medullary cancer of thyroid and cancer of pancreas. These malignant cells may produce ACTH, leading to Cushing's syndrome.
- ***Syndrome with inappropriate antidiuretic hormone*** (SIADH), where arginine vasopressin is synthesized by the tumor cells, leading to clinical manifestations of hyponatremia. It is seen in non-small cell lung cancers, lymphomas, leukemias, and head and neck cancers.
- ***Ectopic parathyroid hormone*** (PTH) is produced by thoracic and intestinal solid tumors.
- ***Oncogenous osteomalacia*** is seen in calcitonin secreting malignancies, usually cancers on thyroid and mediastinum.
- ***Human placental lactogen*** (HPL) is commonly elevated in bronchial cancers and thyroid cancers.
- ***Polycythemia*** is occasionally noticed in hypernephroma.
- ***Acanthosis nigricans*** (brown plaques in neck, axilla and flexor regions) are seen in adenocarcinomas, especially of gastrointestinal origin.
- ***Hyperpigmented palms*** are seen in some cases of gastric and lung cancers.
- ***Acrokeratosis*** (acral hyperkeratosis) in toes, ears and nose is seen in squamous cell carcinomas.
- ***Hypertrophic osteoarthropathy*** (digital clubbing) is noted in non-small cell cancers of lung and metastatic malignancies.
- Symptoms of ***limbic and brainstem encephalitis*** may occur at times in testicular tumors.

It should be remembered that many typical or atypical endocrine manifestations can develop as a result of paraneoplastic manifestations of several neoplasms. It should be the endeavour to detect such lesions if the clinical manifestations are not classic.

METASTASIS

Cell membrane of the malignant cells show qualitative and quantitative changes resulting in an increase of the negative charge on the surface. This leads to mutual repulsion of the cells and increases the tendency to disseminate. Tumor cells secrete matrix metalloproteinases (MMPs) which help metastatic cells to permeate into blood vessels and reach distant sites. Another phenomenon noted in malignant cells is loss of contact inhibition. When two normal cells come into contact this inhibits further cell multiplication. This property is lost in malignant cells which continue to multiply and grow. The tissue in which the metastasis

Textbook of Medicine

develop is also conditioned to favor the growth of the metastatic cells. Therapeutic attempts to inhibit MMPs as an adjunct to cancer therapy are in progress.

Tumors and Angiogenesis

Both primary and metastatic tumors secrete vascular endothelial growth factor (VEGF) which signals normal blood vessels to proliferate and grow, in order to sustain the abnormal tissue. Efforts to suppress the angiogenic factors as aids to tumor therapy are in progress. Thalidomide with its immune-modulatory and anti-angiogenic properties is used in the treatment of multiple myeloma and other tumors.

TUMOR KINETICS

Growth of the tumor depends on the balance between cell proliferation and cell loss. Cellular proliferation depends on: (1) The proliferation coefficient, i.e. the ratio of active to resting cells and (2) the cell cycle interval.

Cell loss depends upon: (1) Cell death by apoptosis aging, lack of oxygen and nutrition, (2) abortion, i.e. incapability of the cells to multiply, (3) escape, detachment of cells from the tumor mass and (4) specific cell destruction by immunological mechanisms. All these parameters are important in deciding 'tumor doubling time' (i.e. the time taken by a tumor to exactly double its mass), which will be constant for a particular growth over a long period. The tumor doubling time in human cancer varies widely between 10 and 450 days, with a median of about 100 days. In the case of a tumor with doubling time of 100 days, the time taken for the growth to reach 1 g from the initial mutation is about 8–10 years. It naturally follows that the tumor is present in the system for a considerable period before clinical detection. The same reason can explain the development of the secondaries several years after the treatment of primary growth. Modern treatment aims at reducing the tumor growth by increasing the cell loss coefficient. When this is achieved, the patient may remain apparently normal for many years. When referring to the management of cancer, the term 'control' is more appropriate than 'cure'. Five-year survival figures are usually taken for comparing the results of different forms of treatment in several neoplasms. It should be remembered that 5-year survival is not synonymous with cure of the lesion.

Precancerous lesions: Precancerous or preinvasive lesion is a stage where individual cells are abnormal but cancer cells have not yet invaded the surrounding normal tissues. About 5–10% of such cases develop invasive tendency within a few years, e.g. leukoplakia of oral cavity, hyperkeratosis of skin, papillomas of the urinary bladder, polyps of bowel, and stage 0 cancer of cervix.

PROGNOSIS IN CANCER

- The most important factor determining survival is early detection. The earlier the diagnosis, the better is the curability. Mass screening of susceptible groups of persons by Pap smear and other methods can lead to early diagnosis.
- Prognosis is better for slow-growing tumors.
- Well-differentiated tumors have a better prognosis than undifferentiated ones.
- If the host can effectively mount an immunological attack against cancer cells, the outcome is more favorable. Prognosis is better in neoplasms where the immunological status of the individual is not depressed.
- For several cancers modern treatment protocols are available, which are highly effective. In such lesions early diagnosis and proper therapy are curative.

THERAPY

The aim of therapy is to reduce the tumor mass within the shortest possible time and to destroy the remaining cells and prevent them from multiplying and disseminating. This ideal is possibly achieved only in the case of very few cancers but in the majority of cases this is not possible due to: (1) Late diagnosis, (2) presence of secondaries early in the disease, (3) surgical risk and (4) toxic effects of radiation and chemotherapeutic agents. Cancer has emerged as one of the curable diseases among the serious chronic diseases. Modern radiotherapy has reached a high level of effectiveness in eradicating tumors, with minimal damage to normal tissues. In the management of solid tumors, multimodal therapy, combing irradiation with chemotherapy is employed, except in the case of very early tumors.

Surgery and radiotherapy are most effective to reduce the initial tumor load. These are the prime modalities of treatment in solid tumors. In the case of disseminated neoplasms like leukemia and myeloma and in the case of some rapidly growing tumors like trophoblastic tumors, chemotherapy has to be employed as the first line of treatment. The technical perfection and complexity of management of malignant neoplasms have resulted in the achievement of successful results in many case if detected early. Several subspecialities such as radiation oncology, solid tumor oncology, hemato-oncology and others have developed.

Radiotherapy

Tumor cells are more radiosensitive as they proliferate faster than normal cells. Radiotherapy may be given as the only modality of treatment or combined with surgery and chemotherapy. With the advent of highly sophisticated equipment such as the linear accelerator, large doses may be focused on deep seated tumors with only minimal injury to adjacent tissues. Therapeutic efficacy of radiation is enhanced by exposure to hyperbaric oxygen and radiosensitizing drugs such as metronidazole.

Radiation produces ionization in its path. This causes physical and/or chemical changes. The nucleic acid in the cell is damaged, so as to arrest the next cell division. Radiotherapy mainly affects cells in the dividing phase. X-rays produce breaks in DNA. Break of two single strands of DNA lead to disruption of the integrity of the chromosomes and tissue destruction.

Depending on the sources of radiation, the radiotherapy may be: (a) Unsealed sources, (b) sealed sources or brachytherapy and (c) teletherapy. Unsealed

Table 7.6: Widely used radioisotopes

Element	Isotope	Half-life	Major radiation	Important applications
Carbon	^{14}C	5600 years	Beta	Research in metabolism
Phosphorus	^{32}P	14 days	Beta	Polycythemia treatment
Chromium	^{51}Cr	28 days	Gamma	RBC kinetics in diagnosis
Iodine	^{125}I	60 days	Gamma	Radioimmunoassay
Iodine	^{131}I	8 days	Gamma	Thyroid cancer treatment
Radium	^{226}Ra	1600 years	Gamma	Implantation in Tumors
Tantalum	^{182}Ta	115 days	Gamma	Implantation, bladder cancer
Gold	^{198}Au	2.5 days	Beta	Instillation into serous cavities
Cobalt	^{60}Co	5.3 years	Gamma	Teletherapy for cancer
Cesium	^{137}Cs	30 years	Gamma	Teletherapy for cancer

sources are radioactive substances kept in liquid form. The beta rays are the main effective radiation in these sources. For treating primary and metastatic thyroid cancer, ^{131}I (dose 50-100 mCi) is administered. Since, iodine is preferentially concentrated in thyroid cells, the radioactivity is specifically taken up by these cells and so they are destroyed. ^{32}P (dose 5 mCi) is given intravenously to treat polycythemia vera. Phosphorus is an essential constituent of DNA and so rapidly dividing cells take up the radioactive phosphorus. The dose may be repeated after 3 months, if necessary. Radioactive gold (^{138}Au) (75–150 mCi) may be instilled into serous cavities to reduce malignant pleural and peritoneal cavities. Commonly used radioisotopes are listed in Table 7.6.

Brachytherapy: The radioactive source is covered by platinum alloy to absorb alpha and beta radiation, so that only gamma rays are allowed to penetrate into the tissue. Alpha and beta rays if allowed to come out, will produce necrosis of tissue around the source within a short time. The sources are packed as needles inside small tubes with a length of about 2 to 5 cm and a diameter of about 2 mm. ^{137}Cs with a half-life of 30 years, is the preferred sealed source. Intracavitary application (for cancer of body of uterus, cancer of cervix uteri, cancer of vagina) and interstitial applications (for buccal cancer, tongue cancer) are very commonly used.

Teletherapy: Here the source of radiation is kept at a distance from the patient. The high penetration power of the gamma rays has an advantage. Maximum dose is received not on the skin, but on the underlying tissues, which reduces unwanted skin reactions.

Gamma rays from ^{137}Cs (Cesium) or ^{60}Co (Cobalt) are used for teletherapy. Here the energy equivalent is in the order of 2 MV (megavolt or million volts). Usual diagnostic X-ray works in the region of 80–150 KV (kilovolt or thousand volts). Since, penetration power is dependent on the energy of the ray, better machines, called linear accelerators with energy levels of 5–12 MV are now being used. The present machines are able to provide programmed doses of radiation at specific targets in high doses, with minimal damage to surrounding tissues. The aim of radiotherapy in general, and teletherapy in particular, is to provide maximum destruction of tumor tissue, while retaining the regenerative capacity of surrounding normal tissues.

The art of radiotherapy is to decide the most beneficial risk-benefit ratio. Radiation fields can be designed, using shielding blocks, computerized planning and automated tracking techniques.

Radiosensitivity: The effectiveness of radiotherapy varies with different tumors. In general, lymphomas, Hodgkin's disease and neuroblastoma are highly radiosensitive. Epithelioma, cancer of oral cavity, cancer of cervix, cancer of breast and lung cancer are moderately radiosensitive. Poorly radiosensitive tumors are osteosarcoma, and malignant melanoma.

Fractionation of doses: Radiation given in a single dose is not optimally effective, because only 5–10% of cells are in the dividing phase at any one time and the radiation kills only this fraction. If divided doses are given at programed intervals which coincide with the cell division, fresh cells are killed successively. Fractionation also helps to reduce the toxic effects of radiation. In general a total dose for many cancers is 5,000 to 6,000 rads (also called centigray-cGy) given in 15–20 fractions, administered over a period of 25–35 days. Recovery from radiation damage is quicker in normal cells than in cancer cells.

Adverse effects: The adverse effects of radiotherapy are due to the damage caused to normal tissues; some degree of which is inevitable. These are described below:

- ***Skin*** Epilation, damage to sweat glands, erythema and blisters. These constitute the syndrome of acute radiation dermatitis. These reactions are generally mild and acceptable in most cases, but overdosage may produce burn and sloughing of superficial tissues. Long-term effects include minor degrees of ischemia, atrophy, hypopigmentation, fibrosis and loss of elasticity.
- ***Mucous membranes:*** Mucosal surface cells are replenished very rapidly, about a third being formed every day. Since radiation damages the dividing cells most, gastrointestinal problems are very common during radiotherapy. Minor manifestations include nausea, vomiting, and diarrhea. In severe cases, ulceration and bleeding may occur. Late sequelae such as adhesions, fibrosis, stenosis and luminal obstruction may develop several months after radiotherapy.
- ***Blood cells:*** Bone marrow and lymphoid tissues are highly radiosensitive because of the higher rate of cell division in the organs. Cytopenias are the most

Textbook of Medicine

common adverse effects. Platelets, granulocytes and erythrocytes are frequently reduced. Continuation of the dose may lead to marrow aplasia. Leukopenia leads to infections and thrombocytopenia leads to hemorrhage. It is important to repeat blood counts before each successive dose of irradiation and modify therapy accordingly.

- ■ ***Reproductive organs:*** Complete sterility may result, if 1000 rads are given over the pelvic region. Smaller doses of radiation may produce genetic effects in the offspring.
- ■ ***Radiation sickness:*** This depends on the radiation dose and the tissue volume irradiated. 100–150 rads given as a total body irradiation will cause severe illness which can be fatal, if untreated.

The maximum permissible dose (MPD) of radiation for whole body among radiation workers including doctors, is 5 mRem/year, and for general population is 0.5 mRem/year.

In may cases surgery or radiation is used as the first modality to reduce tumor bulk. This can be followed or preceded by chemotherapy. Various chemotherapeutic drugs can be used in combination in various malignancies Table 7.7.

Chemotherapy

Chemotherapy is the sheet anchor of therapy in leukemias, advanced lymphomas, choriocarcinoma and other widely disseminated malignancies (Table 7.8). It is combined with surgery in embryonal tumors and used as the primary treatment in advanced cancers not amenable to surgery or radiation. The effectiveness of cytotoxic drugs is directly proportional to the doubling time of the tumors and is inversely proportional to the number of cancer cells. Prior reduction of tumor mass by surgery or radiotherapy augments the effectiveness of chemotherapy. Cytotoxic drugs are non-selective and affect all cells which are in certain phases of their proliferative activity.

Cell destruction by a cytotoxic drug follows the first order kinetics, i.e. it reduces a constant percentage and put in larger values not a constant number of cancer cells. Thus the same dose which reduces the cancer cells from 10^8–10^7

is required to reduce them from 10^3–10^2. It is difficult, therefore, to eradicate the last portion of any tumor by chemotherapy alone without serious toxicity. Surgery, radiation and chemotherapy leave residual tumor tissue even after completion of therapy. These cells are generally destroyed by the immunological system of the body, but if the immune mechanism is weak, the residual cancer cells rapidly multiply and produce recurrence. It should be remembered that both radiotherapy and chemotherapy depress the immune status of the individual. From time to time attempts have been made to stimulate the immune status of the individual by nonspecific immunostimulants such as levamisole or specific immunizing agents such as tumor antigens or modified tumor tissue. Tumor infiltrating cells and LAK (lymphokine activated killer cells) specifically active against tumor antigens were used with limited success in advanced solid tumors. Monoclonal antibodies (immunoglobulin of known specificity produced by single clone of hybrid cells) conjugated with toxins or radioactive isotopes were used in hematological malignancies.

Human interferon obtained by recombinant DNA technology has been successfully used in hairy cell leukemia, chronic myeloid leukemia, cutaneous T cell lymphomas and Kaposi's sarcoma. Interleukin-2 has been tried in advanced cancers, especially in renal cell cancers with success. Interferons and interleukins are described in Chapter 3.

Newer Immunity-based Therapeutic Innovations in Cancer

Anti-idiotype Therapy

Idiotype is the unique protein structure in the combing site of antibody seen on the cell surface of neoplasms—especially some forms of B-cell lymphomas. The idiotype can be used as an antigen to develop an antibody and this antibody acting on the idiotype can be used therapeutically.

Radioimmunotherapy

This is the method of delivering irradiation specifically to the tumor site by producing radio-labelled antibodies against the tumor cells , to which the antibody attaches and delivers irradiation with only minimal damage to normal tissues, e.g ibritumomab and tositurnomab for non-Hodgkin's lymphoma. Attempts to perfect the technique are being pursued.

Therapy with Immunotoxins and Fusion Toxins

This method employs the combinations of cytotoxic toxins with specific antibodies against the surface antigens of tumor cells. The toxins at present derived from plant or bacteria include pokeweed antiviral protein, ricin-A, diphtheria toxin, pseudomonas exotoxin-A and others. These potent toxins enter the tumor cells, inhibit protein synthesis and destroy both resting and dividing cells.

Bispecific Antibodies

These are antibodies constructed to bring about two effects: (1) Recognition of tumor associated antigen and (2) activate effector cells of the immune system to start antitumor action and eliminate the tumor cell when they come into contact. This study is in progress.

Table 7.7: Common malignant conditions in which combination chemotherapy is administered

Acute lymphatic leukemia	:	Vincristine + prednisone + adriamycin + L. asparaginase
Acute myeloid leukemia	:	Doxorubicin + 6-thioguanine + cytosine arabinoside
Hodgkin's lymphoma	:	Nitrogen mustard + vincristine + prednisone + procarhazine
Non-Hodgkin's lymphoma	:	Cyclophosphamide + vincristine + prednisone
Multiple myeloma	:	Melphalan + vincristine + prednisone
Ewing's tumor	:	Vincristine + actinomycin D + cyclophosphamide
Embryonal tumors	:	-do-
Breast cancer	:	5-Fluorouracil + adriamycin + mitomycin
Oral cancer	:	Mitomycin + methotrexate + bleomycin

Table 7.8: Commonly used anti-cancer drugs

Group of drug and mechanism of action	Name of drug	Dose and route	Most important side effects	Indications
Alkylating agents				
They form electrophilic ions making covalent bonds (alkylation) with guanine residues leading to cross-linking of DNA strands and interference in DNA replication	Cyclophosphamide Endoxan Cytoxan	100–150 mg oral daily or 1 g/m² every 3 weeks	Cystitis and marrow suppression	Acute and chronic lymphatic leukemia (ALL, CLL) and lymphomas carcinoma of breast, ovary lungs and cervix
	Nitrogen mustard (Mustargen)	6 mg/m² infusion intravenous	Local inflammation	
	Phenylalanine mustard Alkeran (Melphalan)	6 mg/m²/day oral for 5–10 days every 4–6 weeks	Marrow suppression	Several tumorus Multiple myeloma
	Chlorambucil (Leukeran)	0.1 mg/kg/day oral	-do-	CLL, lymphoma
	Busulfan (Myeleran)	4–12 mg/day oral	Pulmonary fibrosis marrow suppression	CML
Antifolates				
Inhibit dihydrofolate reductase; tetrahydro-folate is not produced; one carbon units are not available for DNA synthesis	Amethopterin Methotrexate	5 mg/day oral or 30 mg/m² intravenous twice weekly	Marrow suppression; hepatic and renal toxicity, painless nodules over fingers	All, carcinoma of breast, lung, head and neck sarcomas choriocarcinoma
Antipyrimidines				
Inhibit thymidylate synthetase and thus DNA synthesis Inhibit deoxycytidine and DNA synthesis	5-Fluorouracil Cytosine arabinoside Cytosar, Ara-C Cytarahine Gemcitabine (Difluorodeoxy cytidine)	15–20 mg/kg/week intravenous: maximum dose is 1 g 100–200 mg/day intravenous 1000 mg/m² IV infusion	Gastrointestinal disturbance; marrow suppression -do- Hyperuricemia Myelosuppression hepatotoxicity	Carcinoma of breast, colon, stomach, ovary, head and neck AML, ALL Advanced adenocarcinoma of pancreas
Antipurines				
Interfere with purine biosynthesis and interconversions	6-Mercaptopurine Purinethol (Hypoxanthine analogue)	2.5 mg/kg/day oral	Hepatotoxicity marrow suppression	AML, ALL, CML
	6-Thioguanine (Guanine analogue)	2 mg/kg/day oral	Marrow suppression	AML, ALL
Vinca alkaloids				
Derived from periwinkle (vinca rosea) plant Interfere with microtubule assembly in mitotic spindle formation	Vinblastine (Velban)	5–15 mg/m² every 1–2 weeks intravenous	Mental depression, local inflammation, marrow suppression.	ALL, neuroblastoma Wilms' tumor lymphomas, Carcinoma lung
	Vincristine (Oncovin)	0.5–2 mg/m² every 1–2 weeks intravenous	Peripheral and autonomic neuropathy; alopecia	
Taxene group				
Inhibits microtubule assembly; mitotic block in metaphase/anaphase boundary	Paclitaxel (Taxol)	175/m² IV infusion repeated every 3 weeks	Hypersensitivity Myelosuppression	Breast cancer Ovarian cancer
	Docetaxel	60 mg/m² IV infusion	Hypersensitivity fluid retention	Advanced Breast carcinoma
Podophyllotoxins				
Semisynthetic drugs Selective inhibition of DNA topoisomerase, G2 phases of cell cycle	Etoposide (VP-16) and inhibition of S and Teniposide	100–200 mg/m² IV on alternate days 3–4 weeks	Marrow suppression Late development of leukemia	Carcinoma of lung, breast and testis lymphomas, AML, Kaposi's sarcoma
	(VM-26) Irinotecan	125 mg/m² IV infusion 1.5 mg/m²	Diarrhea Myelosuppression Myelosuppression	Advanced cancers of colon and rectum Ovarian carcinoma
	Topotecan	IV infusion × 5 days		

Contd...

Contd...

Group of drug and mechanism of action	Name of drug	Dose and route	Most important side effects	Indications
Antibiotics				
Inhibiting DNA directed RNA synthesis	Actinomycin Dactinomycin Cosmegan Bleomycin	12–15 mcg/kg/day 5 d for 2–4 weeks intravenous 1–5 mg/d intravenous or intramuscular. maximum 300 mg/m^2	Marrow suppression local inflammation Pulmonary fibrosis with minimal myelosuppression. Cardiotoxicity	Wilms' Tumor Rhabdomyosarcoma Carcinoma of head and neck, skin, lung, gut and git
Inhibiting DNA synthesis	Daunomycin Daunorubicin Rubidomycin Adriamycin	60 mg/m^2 intravenous 3–4 weeks 60 mg/m^2 intravenous (Doxorubicin) weeks. Maximum total dose 500 mg	Cardiotoxicity once in 5 days for 3–4	AML, ALL Soft tissue tumor, lymphomas, ALL, carcinoma of breast and gut
	Mitomycin-C Mutamycin	20 mg/m^2 intravenous every 4–6 weeks	Local inflammation, marrow suppression.	Carcinoma of stomach, cervix, colon, breast
Enzymes				
L-asparaginase depletes asparagine availability: inhibits protein synthesis	L-asparaginase	6000 IU/m^2 intravenous	Allergy; coagulation defects. Pancreatitis	ALL
Nitrosoureas				
Inhibit nucleic acid synthesis	Cyclohexyl chloroethyl nitrosourea (CCNU) Bis chloroethyl nitrosourea (BCNU)	100 mg/m^2 oral every 4–6 weeks 200 mg/m^2 intravenous every 4–6 weeks	Delayed marrow suppression -do-	-do-
Hydrazine derivatives				
Damage DNA through peroxide formation	Procarbazine (Methylhydrazine derivative)	50–100 mg/m^2 daily orally for 10–14 days	Myelosuppression CNS depression	Hodgkin's
Imidizole derivatives				
Mechanism uncertain, probably alkylation	Dimethyl triazenomidazole carboxamide (DTIC dacarbazine)	150–250 mg/m^2 intravenous for 5 days repeated every 3 weeks	Myelosuppression Hepatotoxicity	Malignant melanoma Hodgkin's sarcoma
Platinum complexes				
Inhibit DNA synthesis by intrastand crosslinking	Cis-diamino dichloro platinum. Cis-platin Carboplatin Oxaliplatin	100 mg in 500 mL intravenous once a week in 3–4 weeks 300 mg/m^2 IV infusion every 28 days 130 mg/m^2 IV infusion	Renal toxicity, Ototoxicity Peripheral neuropathy Thrombocytopenia GIT toxicity Myelosuppression	Carcinoma of head and neck, lung, cervix, ovary Advanced ovarian carcinoma Colorectal and liver cancers
Hormones				
Androgens	Testosterone	300 mg weekly deep intramuscular	Virilization	Carcinoma of breast
Antiandrogen Estrogens Estrogen linked to nitrogen mustard	Flutamide Diethylstilbesterol Estramustine	750 mg oral daily 5–15 mg oral daily 140 mg oral	Feminization	Advanced prostate cancer carcinoma of prostate Advanced prostate cancer
Progestogens	Medroxy progesterone acetate (Provera)	300 mg daily orally	Withdrawal bleeding	Carcinoma of breast and endometrium
Antiestrogens Adrenocorticoids Thyroxine	Tamoxifen (Nolvadex) Prednisone L-thyroxine sodium	20–30 mg daily orally 40–60 mg/m^2 orally/day 0.1–0.3 mg daily orally	Vomiting Cushingoid features Hyperthyroidism	Breast cancer ALL Carcinoma thyroid
Biological response modifiers				
Interleukin-2		6 lakhs IU/kg, IV every 8 hr × 5 days	Hypotension fever	Advanced renal cancer, AML
Interferon-Alpha		1–2 million U/day		Hairy cell leukemia CML, Kaposi's sarcoma
GMCSF (Granulocyte macrophage colony stimulating factor)		250 mcg/m^2 IV daily	Fever, bone pain, hypotension	

Contd...

Textbook of Medicine

Group of drug and mechanism of action	Name of drug	Dose and route	Most important side effects	Indications
Adjuvants used in cancer therapy				
Levamisole (immunostimulant)		150 mg/d/oral		Useful in 5-FU treatment
Amifostine (Radioprotector)		900 mg/m² IV	Hypotension infusion	Prevents hepatotoxicity of cis-platin; reduces mucosal toxicity of radiation
Pamidronate (Bone resorption inhibitor)	IV infusion	60–90 mg	Fever Paget's disease of bone	Osteolytic bone lesions;
Dexrazone (Radioprotector)		500 mg/m²	Myelosuppression IV infusion	Prevents cardiotoxicity of doxorubicin
All trans retinoic acid (ATRA) (Vesanoid)		45 mg/m² daily oral	Hypervitaminosis	Induced cytodifferentiation; adjuvant in acute promyelocytic leukemia, germ cell tumors
13-cis retinoic acid		1–2 mg/kg daily oral for 3 months		Oral leukoplakia, basal cell carcinoma, T cell lymphomas

Signal Transduction

Cells control many of their biological functions via signals delivered from the cell membrane through transmembrane receptors. These signals are needed for the nucleus of the cell to control gene expressions, macromolecule production and cellular proliferation. The transmembrane receptor can be controlled by circulating growth factors. The intracellular domain of transmembrane receptors contain protein kinases, which, when stimulated, leads to initiation of a phosphorylation cascade which promotes tumor growth. Manipulation of these protein kinases has been utilized in devising therapeutic agents such as tyrosine kinase inhibitors like *imatinib* and *dasatinib* used in chronic myeloid leukemia and gastrointestinal stromal tumors. Other examples include *geftinib* used in lung cancer and *sorafenib* and *sunatinib* used in renal cancer.

Use of Antibodies in Cancer Therapy

Attempts to employ monoclonal antibodies to inhibit tumor growth are progressing fast and at present antibodies are employed for several tumors along with other modalities, e.g anti-CD20, antibody in B-cell lymphomas, transtuzumab in breast cancer, cituximab in colorectal cancer and several others. Development of specific monoclonal antibodies acting against the cancer tissue has reached a high-level of therapeutic success and at present several monoclonal antibodies are available for use singly or in protocols in standard regimens (Table 7.9). This area is rapidly developing.

Table 7.9: Source and examples for early monoclonal antibodies introduced among this group		
Structure	**% Human**	**Example**
Mouse	0	Tositumomab, Ibritumomab
Chimeric	65	Cetuximab, Rituximab
Humanized	95	Trastuzumab
Human	100	Panitumumab

Monoclonal antibodies directed against cell surface antigens of malignant cells have been introduced as therapeutic tools in treatment of cancer, along with other modalities. Several newer products are being produced with specificity against different tumors monoclonal antibodies (MAb) are directed against tumor cell surface antigens, e.g. rituximab is a chimeric monoclonal antibody targeted against the cell surface receptor CD20 (antiCD20 surface antigen) present in many B-cell-NHL subtypes. It produces lysis of tumor cells by both complement and antibody dependent cellular cytotoxicity. Monoclonal antibodies may be produced from several sources such as animals and humans.

Targeted therapy of cancer makes use of identification of specific receptor to which the drug can be targeted, e.g. breast cancers, gastrointestinal stromal tumors and others.

Many cancer cells are transformed by the activity of the oncoproteins (products of oncogenes) that act on growth factor receptors. They produce growth signal by phosphorylation of tyrosine residues on the intracellular portion of growth factor receptors.

Example of tyrosine kinase inhibitor (TKi)—imatinib inhibits the BCR-ABL gene product, tyrosine kinase that is responsible for chronic myeloid leukemia. TKi is a very effective drug for the treatment for chronic myeloid leukemia. The same drug can be used in gastrointestinal stromal tumor (GIST) that has overexpression of another cell surface tyrosine kinase, c-kit.

- *Inhibitor of Her2:* Lapatinib inhibits human epidermal growth factor receptor 2 (HER2) and increases the survival in breast cancer.
- *Inhibitor of signalling by EGFR and VEGFR:* TKIs sunitinib and sorafenib inhibit signalling by EGFR and VEGFR in metastatic renal cancer. Erlotinib and gefitinib are effective in lung cancer.

Proteasome inhibitors

- The proteasome is an organelle that physiologically degrades and recycles damaged proteins by a process called ubiquitination. Examples of such proteins include cyclins and cyclin-dependent kinases and factors in the NFκB pathway. Inhibition of the proteasome leads to apoptosis in cancer cells. **Bortezomib** is the proteasome inhibitor used in relapsed/refractory multiple myeloma and in some types of non-Hodgkin's lymphoma.

Estrogen which is required for growth of breast cancer has been targeted for control of tumor growth. Therapy targeted at the receptor for estrogen has been invogue over several years. Examples:

Tamoxifen
Toremifene }   Selective estrogen receptor modulators (SERMs)

Fulvestrant   Estrogen receptor inhibitor and destroyer

Anastrozole
Letrozole }   Estrogen synthesis inhibitors—aromatase inhibitors (AIs)
Exemestane

Cancer Screening Programs

Based on longitudinal observations of predisposing factors for cancer in various sites, standardized screening programs have been evolved. In many precancerous conditions and cancers which have been treated, protocols for screening have been evolved by consensus.

- Repeated colonoscopy in intestinal polyposis, ulcerative colitis and others
- Repeated mammography and /or magnetic resonance imaging (MRI) in breast lesions
- Cancer surveillance in prostatic lesions
- Tumor markers.

Tumor markers are biochemical substances or products of malignant tumors that can be detected in the cells themselves or in serum or other body fluids. They may be normal endogenous products produced in excess by cancer cells or products of newly switched on genes that remained quiescent in the normal cells. They include diverse molecules such as serum proteins, oncofetal antigens, hormones, metabolites, receptors and enzymes. Their levels increases with tumor progression, highest levels occur when tumors metastasize. They are useful in screening populations at risk. Even though they are generally reliable, exceptions occur and therefore each case has to be dealt with individually. Several substances have been studied in this group, carcinoembronic antigen (CEA) and alpha fetoprotein are the most time honored ones.

PALLIATIVE CARE AND PAIN MANAGEMENT

WHO Definition on Palliative Care

WHO defines palliative care as 'an approach that improves the quality of life of patients and their families—by means of early identification and impeccable assessment and treatment of pain and other problems, physical, psychological and spiritual'. Specialized palliative care teams enact their approach through the holistic care of patients dying of cancer or other terminal illness.

Source: WHO definition of palliative care, www.who.int/cancer/palliative/ definition.

Palliative care is the active total care of the patient and their families by a multiprofessional team at a time when the patient's disease is severe, distressing, prolonged, involving heavy financial burden and severe stress on the family members and carers. At least many of them may be non-responsive to curative treatment and life expectancy may be relatively short. Worst symptom is intractable pain which is distressing and demoralising.

The care for moderate to severely advanced cancer patients include: (a) Control of symptoms, (b) control of pain, (c) treatment of psychological disturbances, (d) maintenance of quality of life, and (e) preparation for a decent death. 80–90% of advanced cancers are associated with moderate to severe pain. The pain may be somatic (soft tissue origin; dull, aching localized type) in 40% cases; visceral (due to compression of tissues; deep and poorly localized) in 20% cases; neuropathic (due to infiltration of nerve; severe burning type) in 10% cases; or a combination in the rest of the cases.

Symptom Management

Pain

'Pain is what the patient says hurts'.

Pain is an unpleasant **sensory** and **emotional** experience associated with actual or potential tissue damage or described in terms of such damage. In other words, pain is a somatopsychic phenomenon.

The aim of management of pain in terminal cancer cases is to render freedom from pain. Treatment of cancer pain includes: (a) Treatment of the underlying cause, if possible; (b) analgesic drug therapy; (c) anesthetics; (d) neurosurgery and (e) psychiatric consultations. Out of this, analgesic drug therapy is the main choice. Here, the aim is to make adequate pain relief with minimum side effects. Drug dose is to be titrated to individual needs. The basic principle is summarized as 'by the clock, by the mouth, by the ladder'. Drug doses are titrated to individual needs, and doses are given every 4–6 hours, by the clock. Oral administration of drugs is preferred wherever possible.

Factors affecting pain threshold	
Threshold lowered	**Threshold raised**
Discomfort	Relief of other symptoms
Insomnia	Sleep
Fatigue	Sympathy
Anxiety	Understanding
Fear	Companionship
Anger	Creative activity
Sadness	Relaxation
Depression	Reduction in anxiety
Boredom	Elevation of mood
Mental isolation	Analgesics
Social abandonment	Anxiolytics
	Antidepressants

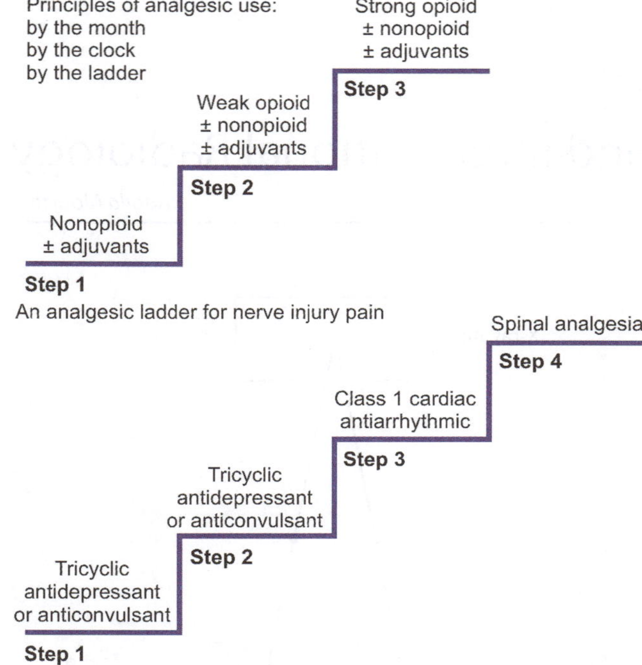

Fig. 7.1: The World Health Organization 3-step analgesic ladder

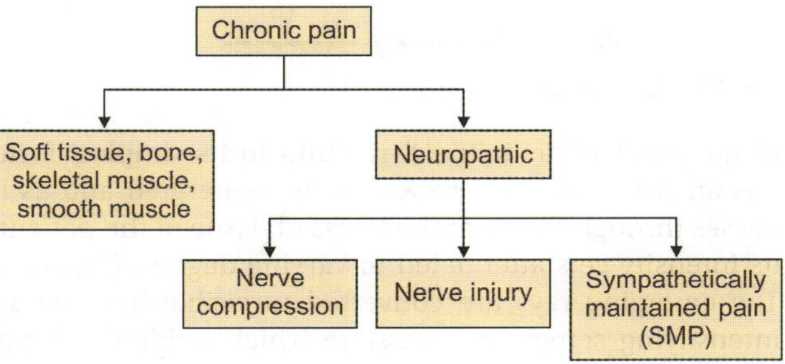

The WHO three-step analgesic ladder is briefly shown (Fig. 7.1 and Table 7.10):

- Start with nonopioid drugs individually or in combination. If necessary, adjuvant drugs may be added. This form of therapy produces no tolerance or physical dependence. The first step will be sufficient in about 20–40% patients.
- If pain persists, as the second step, mild opioids are started, along with nonopioid drugs, with or without adjuvant drugs. Taper the opioid dose slowly, reduce by 25% every 2 days, until a suitable dose is reached. This strategy will be useful for another 20-40% patients.

Table 7.10: Drugs used to control pain in palliative care

Nonopioid drugs (oral administration)
- Paracetamol, up to 4 g/day in divided doses
- Naproxen, up to 1 g/day in divided doses
- Ibuprofen, maximum 2 g/day in divided doses
- Diclofenac, 50 mg 6 hourly
- Ketorol, maximum 100 mg/day in divided doses
- Aspirin, 500 mg 4 hourly (maximum 4 g/day)

Mild opioids (oral administration is preferred)
- Codeine, 200 mg 6 hourly
- Propoxyphene, 100 mg 6 hourly
- Oxycodone, 30 mg 6 hourly
- Tramadol, 50 mg 6 hourly
- Buprinorphine (sublingual, not freely available)

Strong opioids
- Morphine 30 mg/dayorally, in divided doses
- Methadone, 10 mg orally (useful in morphine dependence)
- Fentanyl, 25–100 mcg/hour, transdermal patch
- Pethidine (Meperidine) 75 mg intramuscular

Adjuvant drugs
- Antidepressants:
  Amitriptyline, 50 mg at night
  Bensodiazepines, diazepam, 10 mg at night
- Antiemetics:
  Domperidone, 30 mg/day
  Metaclopromide, 3–5 mg/kg/day
  Ondansetron, 8 mg/4 hourly
- Anticonvulsants:
  Carbamazepine, 200–400 mg/8 hourly
  Sodium valproate, 200 mg/8 hourly
- Corticosteroids, prednisolone, 15–30 mg/day or higher doses

Anesthetics
- Local anesthetics
- Nerve block (peripheral, epidural, intrathecal
- Lumbar sympathetic/stellate ganglion block
- Nerve root ablation (rhizotomy)

- If pain still persists, as the third step, strong opioids are used, along with non-opioids and adjuvants. Oral route is preferred, but severe pain may need continuous subcutaneous or intravenous administration.
- As a last resort, as the step four, anesthetic drugs may be employed. Further, nerve block or even nerve root ablation may be tried. Metastasis in bone may produce severe pain, which may be treated by osteoclast inhibitors such as biphosphonate compounds (etidronate, 60 mg biweekly; pamidronate, alandronate), gallium nitrate, strontium and calcitonin (25 IU per day). Corticosteroids are used especially in pain associated with spinal cord compression.

Textbook of Medicine

CHAPTER
8

Imaging Sciences and Interventional Radiology

Kapila Moorthy

Chapter Summary

- Scope of the Specialty of Radiodiagnosis
- Instrumentations
  - X-ray Unit for Radiography with Facility for Fluoroscopy
  - Current Scenario of Conventional Imaging
  - Ultrasound Scanner and Ultrasonography
  - CT Scanner and Scanning
    - Spiral CT, Multidetector CT and Indications for CT
  - MRI Scanner and Scanning
  - Special Applications of MRI Scan
    - Diffusion Weighted Imaging
    - Functional Images
    - Diffusion Tensor Images
    - Digital Subtraction Angiography
  - Nuclear Medicine Techniques
    - Single Photon Emission Tomography
    - Positron Emission Tomography
  - Hybrid Techniques
- Interventional Radiology
- Contrast Media used in Radiology Techniques
- Radiation Issues
- Choice of Modalities

SCOPE OF THE SPECIALITY OF RADIODIAGNOSIS

The speciality of radiology has totally transformed in the past two decades. It is partly due to the technical advancements and partly due the utilization of this advancements for better diagnostic and treatment capabilities. The specialty is aptly now known as imaging sciences and interventional radiology. A good radiologist should be equipped with a good clinical knowledge and should be able to design and suggest the best sequential algorithm for a given problem. The speciality caters to all systems in the human body. Hence several subspecialties have developed from the parent discipline and at present radiodiagnosis have reached a very high state of perfection. It is one of the most sought after investigational methods. The vastness of the subject can be compared to that of general medicine with its various subspecialties. Apart from diagnosis, the radiologist has an important role in treating patients in the subspecialty of interventional radiology. In interventional radiology, patients are offered minimally invasive treatment. Hence all the skill needed for patient care is mandatory if one chooses this subspecialty. Interventional radiology is a part of each subspecialty in radiology.

INSTRUMENTATIONS

X-ray Unit for Radiography with Facility for Fluoroscopy

Ever since the discovery of X-ray by the German physicist Wilhelm Röntgen in 1895, one of its major uses has been

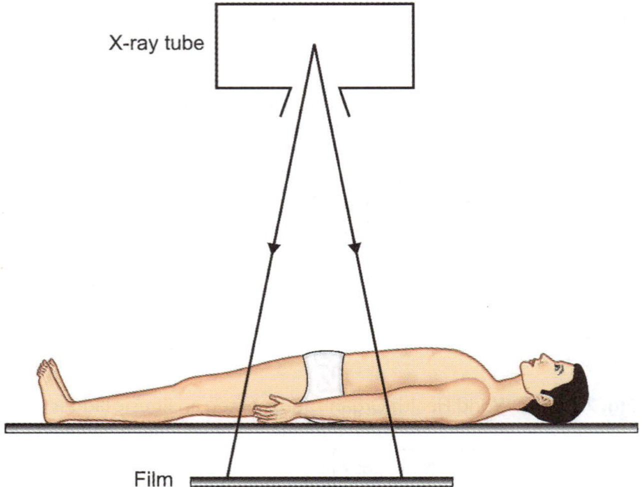

Fig. 8.1: Basic design of X-ray unit

in the medical field. The X-ray unit in its simplest form has an X-ray tube where X-rays are generated and as it passes through different thickness of tissue of the patient, its intensity gets attenuated to varying degrees (Fig. 8.1). The emerging rays are converted to visible light by an intensifying screen in a cassette which holds the X-ray plate. Digital systems are available at present to process the final image. There are two parameters viz—kilovoltage (kV), milliampere seconds (mAs), employed in X-ray machine. kV will decide the penetrating capacity of X-rays and mAs will decide the current passing through the X-ray tube. For soft tissue radiography like mammography, one has to employ low kV and high mAs and for bones high kV. Thus, different density of tissues caste different intensity shadow in the film, which can be interpreted as in X-ray chest. Portable systems are also available to take the images at bedside for ill-patients. About 30–40% reduction in quality of the images occur in these machines and hence it is always advisable to reduce the use of portable X-rays as far as possible.

The following investigations can be done in X-ray unit with fluoroscopy facility:

- Plain X-rays, e.g. chest, abdomen and other regions
- Special investigations like barium meal, intravenous urogram (IVU), myelogram and several others.

Current Scenario of Conventional Imaging

All the plain X-ray studies including the conventional contrast studies like barium meal and IVU; even though have lost their charm in the present era, their role as a primary investigative step in diagnosis needs stressing. These investigations are relatively affordable, freely

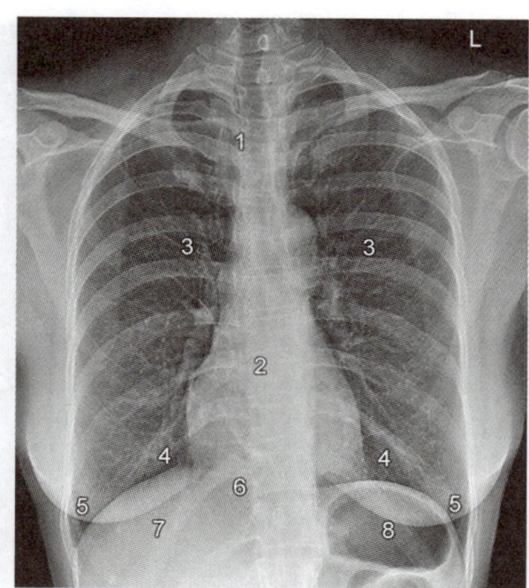

Fig. 8.2: X-ray chest

Keys: 1. Trachea, 2. Mediastinum, 3. Lung fields, 4. Cardiophrenic angles, 5. Costophrenic angles, 6. Diaphragm above abdominal organs, 7. Liver, 8. Gas bubble in the stomach

available and clings the diagnosis quickly. Some of the common clinical indications are given below:

- ***Chest X-ray posteroanterior (PA) view (Fig. 8.2):*** For consolidation of lung and pleural effusion. Minimal pleural effusion can be made out in decubitus views with patient lying down on the side of interest and employing a horizontal X-ray beam towards chest.
- Erect views of abdomen to show gas under diaphragm.
- Radio-opaque foreign bodies in respiratory tract/ gastrointestinal system.
- Small bowel enema in case of small intestinal diseases like Crohn's disease, etc. Here a special tube is inserted through mouth under fluoroscopic guidance and kept at the duodenum and dilute barium sulphate solution is instilled under fluoroscopic guidance to opacify the jejunum and ileum. Pathologies like fistulous communications, ulcers in jejunum/ileum divericulae, inflammatory pseudopolyps and others can be made out. Small bowel is an area beyond the reach of endoscopy and hence the importance of this investigation. The motility pattern of the intestine also can be studied under fluoroscopy.
- Barium enema for diagnosing diseases such as colonic diverticulae where double contrast barium enema is superior to endoscopy in detection of the same.
- Barium swallow under fluoroscopy can study the motility pattern of esophagus and can differentiate organic versus structural causes of obstruction, e.g. carcinoma esophagus vs achalasia cardia.
- In IVU, apart from structural abnormalities, it will also give functional status of kidneys. After injection of iodinated contrast media, the initial films are taken at 5 minutes (to see the contrast with in the tubules of kidney called nephrogram), 15 minutes for the pelvicalyceal system and 30 minutes for the urinary bladder and post void film for the residual urine. Even though, ultrasound (US) scan has replaced to make out structural lesions, the function of kidney can be qualitatively assessed by IVU.

- Lymphangiography where an oily (poppy seed oil) iodinated contrast media is injected into the web space of foot and later taken up by lymphatics, is a tedious procedure and has mostly replaced by nuclear study coupled with computerized tomography (CT)-positron emission tomography (PET).
- Cholecystography is obsolete now and is totally replaced by ultrasound scan were one can make out gallstones, gallbladder wall thickness and contraction of gallbladder after giving fat rich diet.

Ultrasound Scanner and Ultrasonography

Sound waves in the frequency range of 1–20 MHz (100–1000 times greater than audible range) are used to produce the image as reflected from the various structures of body. The basic component of US probe is the piezoelectric crystal (lead zirconate titanate). When it is electrically excited acoustic energy is produced (piezoelectric effect). The piezoelectric crystal is used both for transmitting and receiving the sound waves. The received sound wave from the body are processed by a computer and displayed as an image. There are 3 modes of display—A (amplitude) mode, B (brightness) mode and M (motion) mode. High frequency probes (low penetration) are used for superficial structures like thyroid and low frequency probes (high penetration) are used for deeper structures of abdomen. Highly reflective tissues are termed as hyperechoic, e.g. fat and tissues with low reflectivity are called hypoechoic, e.g. water (Fig. 8.3).

Indication for Ultrasonography

It can be broadly divided into those for soft tissues like thyroid (for nodules), breast (for masses) and those used to survey internal organs, e.g. liver and biliary tree (as a part of investigation of jaundice), spleen, retroperitoneal structures like kidneys, pancreas and uterus. In chest, it is used to make out pleural effusion. In echocardiography (ECG), low frequency pencil probes are used in imaging the heart with its various valves and chambers. As mentioned elsewhere, superficial structures like scrotum, thyroid are outlined by high frequency probes and deeper structures like pancreas by low frequency probes. In general, sonography differentiates between cystic and

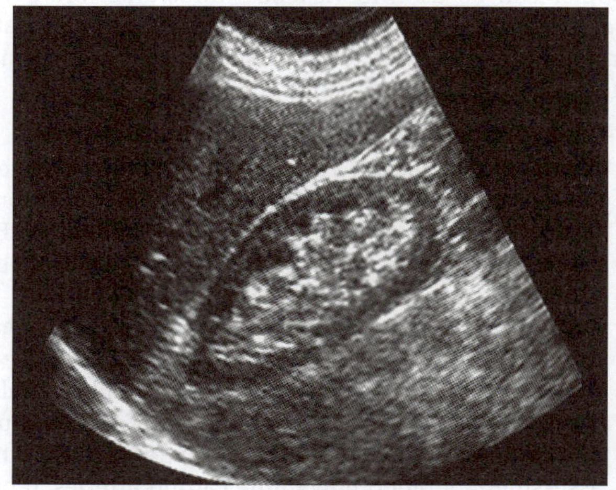

Fig. 8.3: Ultrasound image of Kidney

Textbook of Medicine

solid swelling. As real time motion mode is available it can make out motion of heart valves, abdominal aorta and other blood vessels. Transcranial sonography (TCS) can be used to see through fontanel of infants, the parenchymal changes in brain secondary to hypoxia and hemorrhage. The thin temporal bone and posterior occipital region can be used to view the branches of internal carotid artery around circle of Willis and branches of vertebral arteries and basilar trunk in the posterior fossa in skull. In pelvic US, organs like urinary bladder, uterus and adnexa can be made out well and pathologies like uterine fibroid urinary bladder growth, prostate enlargement can be made out. In obstetrics, it has wide application in making out lie of fetus, age and maturity of fetus. Standard norms are available for age matched values of maturity in relation to biparietal diameter (BPD) of head and femoral length measured by sonography. Placental anomalies as to its position and structure can be made out and it is useful in cases like uterine bleeding that occurs in placenta previa.

Many ultrasound guided procedures are available like percutaneous nephrostomy, drainage of liver abscess, pleural tap and are included under interventional radiology which is described in detail elsewhere. Hence, in these situations ultrasound can guide the needle track to the target. Special facilities are available along with the probe for needle attachment.

Preparation of Patient for Sonography

A gas free abdomen is best for abdominal sonography. The gas can be minimized by doing the procedure in a fasting state in the morning itself. Air and fat (as in obese individuals) are enemies of ultrasound and these will reflect the sound waves back and the structures under them will not be well-visualized. An apprehensive patient swallows air and hence it is mandatory to do the test in the morning itself in an empty stomach. In case to see the pelvic structures like uterus and prostate, it is mandatory to do sonography in full bladder.

Advantages: Absence of ionizing radiations, repeatability, portability and relatively low cost.

Disadvantages: Experienced operator required. Bowel gas and bone because of their high reflectivity, hinders imaging of deeper structures like pancreas. However, Doppler can be used to visualize intracranial branches of carotid artery, intracranial hemorrhage if appropriate window is available, e.g. fontanel and thin squamous part of temporal bones (transcranial).

Other Added Advancements in Sonography

- ***Doppler ultrasound:*** Here Doppler effect has been applied for imaging. Flowing blood causes alterations to the frequency of returning echoes from blood. By calculating this frequency, shift blood flow can be quantified and can be displayed as a graph.
- ***Duplex ultrasound:*** Refers to a combination of real time ultrasound and Doppler ultrasound.
- ***Color Doppler*** is an extension of this principle. Usually blood flows towards transducer is colored as red and away from transducer as blue. It is very useful in the assessment of blood flow in the carotid arteries, renal vessels and other peripheral vessels (Fig. 8.4).

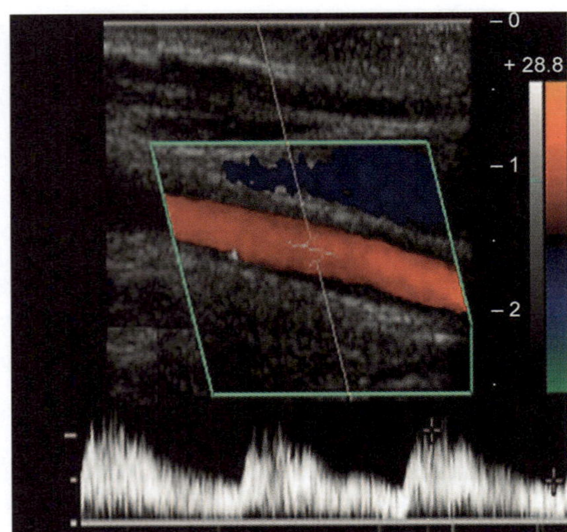

Fig. 8.4: Color Doppler of normal carotid artery

- ***Power Doppler:*** It is highly sensitive to flow regardless of direction and is used in areas of minimal flow due to occlusive vascular diseases.
- ***Elastography:*** Transducer is used to apply a distorting force, producing a stress on the tissue. This can produce a very high contrast between tumors and adjacent normal tissue. This principle can be used either with ultrasound scan or with magnetic resonance imaging (MRI) scan. The ultrasound scan has the advantage of seeing in real time. The elastograms created by this method are more sensitive, especially to deeper structures and the information gained can be compared to that obtained by clinical palpation. This method is widely used in the studies of breast, prostate and liver.
- ***Use of contrast agents:*** Sonovue is a recent ultrasound contrast agent which is a phospholipid and polyethyl-ene glycol with an innocuous gas in a saline solution. It can be used to confirm diagnosis of hemangioma of liver. Uptake by myocardium is a measure of the viability of ischemic/infracted myocardium.
- ***Transesophageal echo:*** This is mainly used to view the posterior most structures of heart like left atrium to see atrial myxoma attachment site, anomalous drainage of pulmonary veins.
- ***Intravascular ultrasound:*** Special small probes are attached to catheters to view the interior of arteries to see the adequacy of angioplasty in coronary arteries. The recurring expense is huge and as such it is confined only to special cardiac centers.
- ***Three dimensional (3D) imaging:*** It is especially useful in seeing fetal anomalies and heart valves.
- ***Other special probes:*** Probes attached to endoscopes can view the stomach wall during gastroscopy. Also transvaginal probes can make out adnexa better including ectopic tubal pregnancy.

Instrument technology in ultrasonography has progressed to a high level and at present cardiac events (ECG can be performed by the clinician at the bedside using a handheld ultrasonography instrument).

CT Scanner and Scanning

In 1969, GN Hounsfield developed the first clinically useful CT head scanner. He along with Allan M Cormack shared the Nobel Prize in Physiology and medicine in 1979.

In CT scan, cross-sectional images are obtained using X-rays and detectors on opposite sides with patient in between. The X-rays are attenuated to varying degree by the tissues of varying density in the body. The data acquired is processed in a computer to get a final image. The term hypodense is used to a low attenuated tissue like water or hyperdense for tissues like bone. Hounsfield unit (HU) is used to represent the linear attenuation coefficient of a tissue relative to water. Thus, air has a HU of –1000, bone +700 to 3000, blood is 35 to 55 HU, calcium +130 to +500 and fat –100 to –50 HU. By altering the window setting one can visualize the mediastinum, lung and bone separately in the same section (Figs 8.5 and 8.6).

Spiral CT: Here during continuous rotation of X-ray tube and detectors, the patient table also moves through the gantry aperture allowing examination of a spiral volume of tissue.

Multidetector CT (MDCT): Subsecond MDCT scan uses a rapidly rotating X-ray tube and several rows of detectors. Using the slip ring technology, the X-ray tube and the

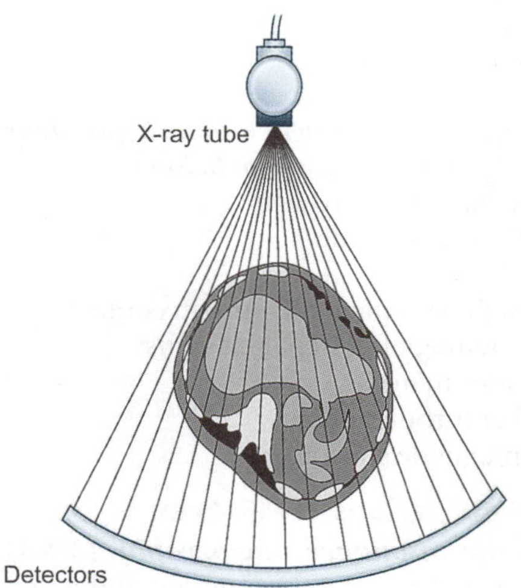

Fig. 8.5: Basic structure of CT scanner

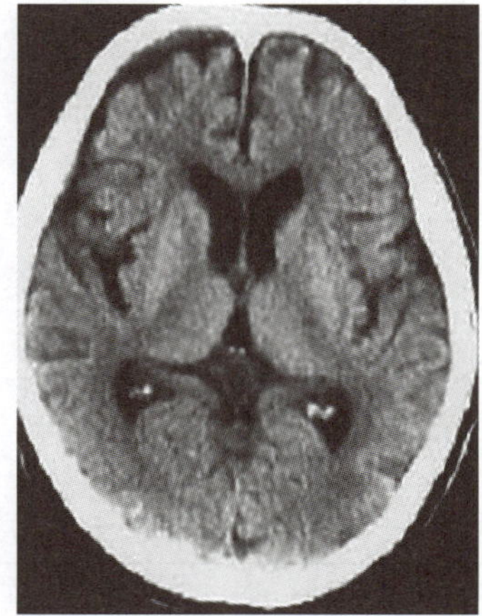

Fig. 8.6: Axial CT scan brain

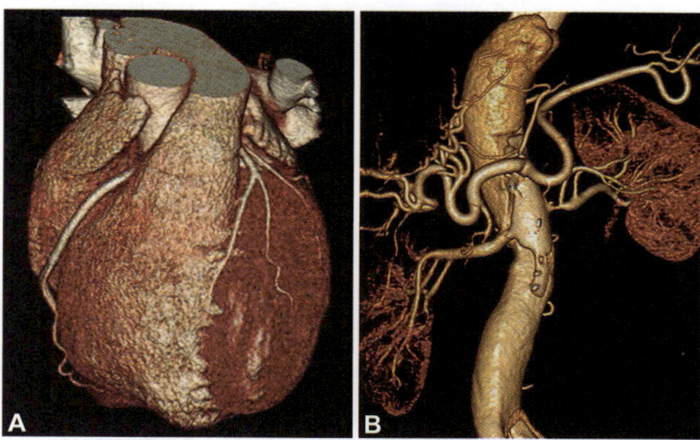

Figs 8.7A and B: Multidetector CT 3D reconstruction. **A.** Coronary arteries; **B.** Abdominal aorta

detectors continuously move through multiple 360° rotations. Current generations of MDCT systems allows a 360° rotation in about 300 ms and are capable of acquiring 64 slice, 256 slice and 320 slices by different manufacturers. Scanning can be done with ECG gating also which is useful in imaging of coronary arteries. The data acquired can be processed as a 3D volume rendered image (Figs 8.7A and B).

- *Advantages:* Rapid scanning (useful in uncooperative patients), reconstruction retrospectively at any level (useful in reconstructive surgeries) and performing coronary and peripheral vessel angiograms.
- *Disadvantages:* Radiation dose and contrast media injections.

Indications for CT scanning:

- Traumatic injuries to head, chest and abdomen. In the present MDCT scanners, as scanning is over in a few seconds, it is best suitable for unconscious patients.
- Early subarachnoid hemorrhage can be made out.
- Cerebral perfusion study can be done in case of acute cerebral infarct.
- Coronary angiogram can be done in a less invasive way by injecting contrast intravenously (IV).
- All abdominal viscera and their vascularity can be assessed for lesions like hepatoma, pancreatic and renal tumors which are not clearly made out in ultrasound.
- Abdominal aorta and its branches can be made out well for diagnosing conditions like aortic aneurysm, dissection.
- Multiplanar 3D reconstructions are possible which aids in planning surgery in fracture of facial bones.

Though MRI has several advantages over CT, there are specific situations where CT still stands out as the investigation of choice. Bones are better made out in CT scan unlike in MRI scan. A comparative chart of the strengths and weakness of MRI scan versus CT scan given in the Table 8.1.

MRI Scanner and Scanning

MRI is a non-invasive method of imaging internal structure. The basic principle of MRI was independently described by Bloch and Purcell in 1946 and was awarded jointly Nobel Prize for Physics in 1952.

Textbook of Medicine

Table 8.1: Relative merits of CT and MRI scans

No.	Parameters	CT	MRI
1.	Energy	X-Ray	Magnet
2.	Slices	Axial	Multiplanar
3.	Time	Fast	Slow
4.	3D	Yes	Yes
5.	Angiogram	Yes	Yes
6.	Moving Parts	Yes	No
7.	White matter disease	+	++++
8.	Resolution	++	++++
9.	Number of lesion detected	+++	++++
10.	Involve adjacent structures	++	++++
11.	Location	+++	++++
12.	Spine and spinal cord	++	++++
13.	Previous surgery/metal	++++	+
14.	Bone disease	++++	+
15.	Calcification	++++	++
16.	Edema	++	++++
17.	Guidance	+ –	Yes

MRI portrays the distribution of hydrogen nuclei and their parameters of motion with in a given tissue. MRI requires superconducting clinical magnet providing strong and uniform magnetic field. The field strength of the magnet is measured in Tesla (T) and at present 1.5T and 3T is available in commercial systems, most which requires liquid helium for cooling the magnet. The lower field strengths can be achieved with permanent magnets (open MRI scanners) which is useful for claustrophobic patients. When a patient is kept inside a gantry within the magnetic field, most of the hydrogen nuclei in the tissue align parallel to the magnetic field. When a second magnetic field, i.e. radio frequency (RF) pulse is applied perpendicular to the main magnetic field, an extra energy is added to the protons and they flip into a transverse plane. Also, the RF pulse brings the protons in phase, i.e. the protons are in synchrony. On removal of this RF pulse, the protons relax back to their original longitudinal state releasing the extra energy acquired. This relaxation of protons from transverse magnetization to longitudinal magnetisation is called T_1 relaxation. The time taken for the same is called T_1 relaxation time. The corresponding reciprocal decay of the transverse state is called T_2 relaxation. The signal emitted, when the RF pulse is switched off, is collected and analyzed by a computer to get a final image (Fig. 8.8).

The signal converted to image obtained during T_1 relaxation is called T_1 weighted image. Similarly image obtained during T_2 relaxation is called T_2 weighted image (Figs 8.9A and B).

The relationship between intensities of image and T_1 and T_2 sequences can be understood by the following Table 8.2.

Contrast agents used in MRI (gadolinium) shortens the T_1 of tissue and shows increased signal intensity.

Tissues and substances which show hyperintensity (bright areas) in T_1 weighting is given below:
- Fat (biological/oil-based contrast agent)
- Very high non-paramagnetic protein content
- Paramagnetic or iodinated contrast agent
- Calcification
- Paramagnetic ions (associated with liver disease, hyperalimentation, calcification, necrosis)
- Mucinous material
- Intraluminal melanin
- Hypermyelination
- Paramagnetic artefact
- Slow flow.

Tissues and substances which show hypointensity (black areas) in T_2 weighting is given below:
- Iron without hemorrhage
- Calcification or bone
- Air
- Very high paramagnetic protein content
- Deoxyhemoglobin in patent veins
- Mucinous material
- Rapid or turbulent flow
- Ferromagnetic substances.

Special Applications of MRI Scan
- ***Magnetic resonance angiography (MRA):*** Rely on flow-related signal enhancement and a flow sensitive

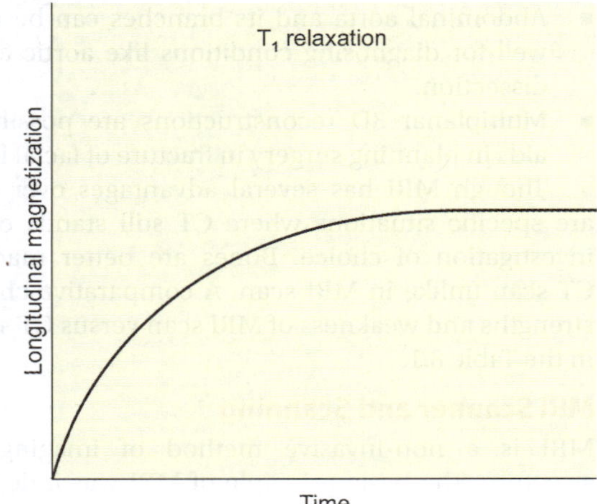

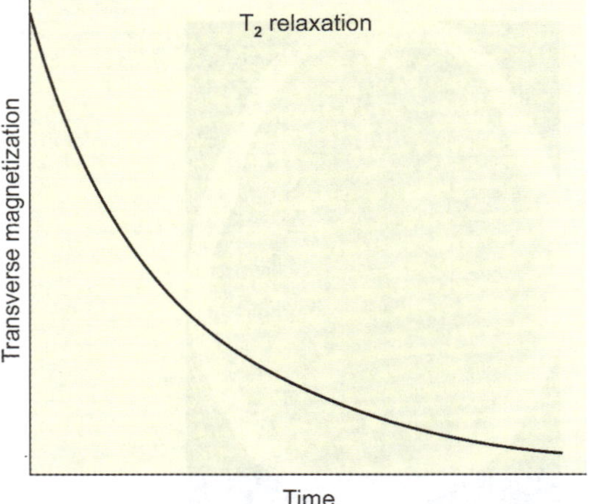

Fig. 8.8: T_1 and T_2 relaxation (signal intensity) curves

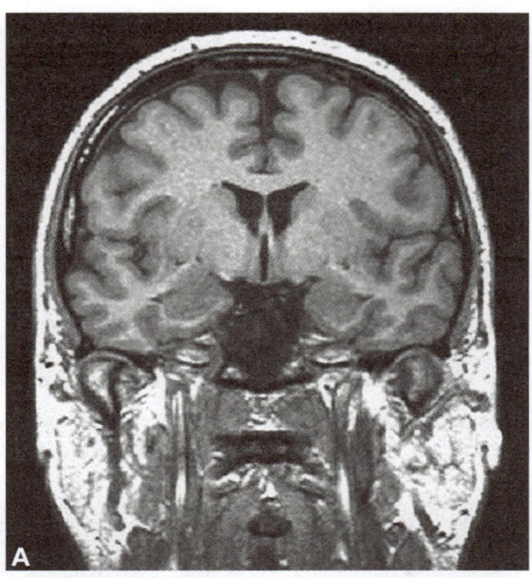 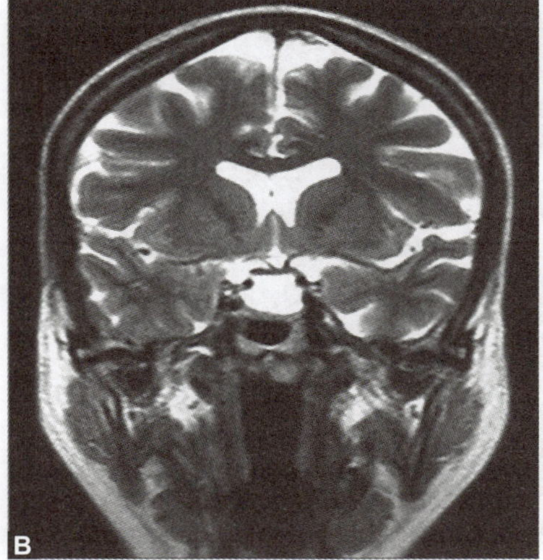

Figs 8.9A and B: A. T_1 weighted; **B.** T_2 weighted coronal MRI of brain

Table 8.2: Intensities of image and T_1 and T_2 sequences

MRI sequence	Intensity of image: Dark	Intensity of image: Bright
T_1 weighted image	Long T_1	Short T_1
T_2 weighted image	Short T_2	Long T_2

image is acquired with suppression of signal from the background. Best results are obtained with contrast injection of gadolinium. Both arterial and venous phase can be taken separately.

- ***Magnetic resonance spectroscopy (MRS):*** This is a metabolic imaging to get the concentration (in parts per million) of choline, N-acetylaspartate (NAA), lipid, lactate, creatine and others (major and minor metabolites). Choline increases in membrane turnover and NAA reduction signifies cell death. This will be useful in characterizing and grading tumors in brain, prostate, etc. A metabolic mapping of the various metabolites with respect to creatine can be done (Figs 8.10A and B).

- ***Diffusion weighted imaging (DWI):*** Visualizes the microscopic motion of water in biological tissues. 'Diffusion gradient' will alter MRI signal intensities proportionally to the water tissue diffusion. In vasogenic edema (as in chronic infarct, tumors, infection), there is free diffusion of water molecules and the area appears hypointense in DWI and bright in apparent diffusion coefficient image. In cytotoxic edema (as in acute brain infarct) there is restriction of water molecules and the area appears as hyperintense in DWI and hypointense in apparent diffusion coefficient (ADC) map. Thus, vasogenic edema can be distinguished from cytotoxic edema which is useful in evaluation of stroke patients (Fig. 8.11).

- ***Functional imaging:*** This is a most exciting application of MRI scan. This depends on the activation of certain specific cortical areas of the brain, e.g. motor cortex by an appropriate task, e.g. hand movement. The blood flow to the hand area increases by 20–40% and thereby blood O_2 level also increases. The signal from the activated area is subtracted from the background

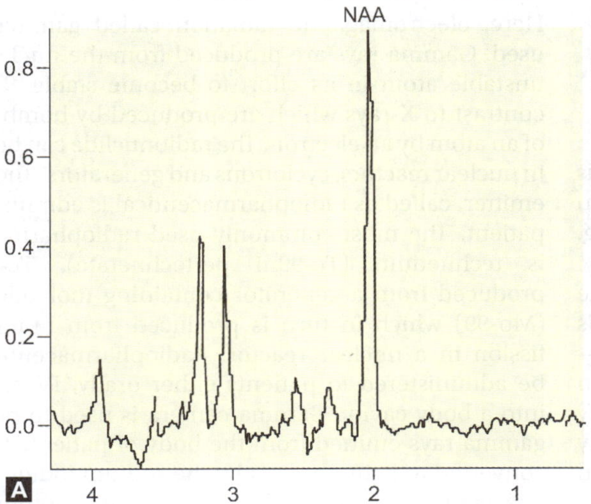

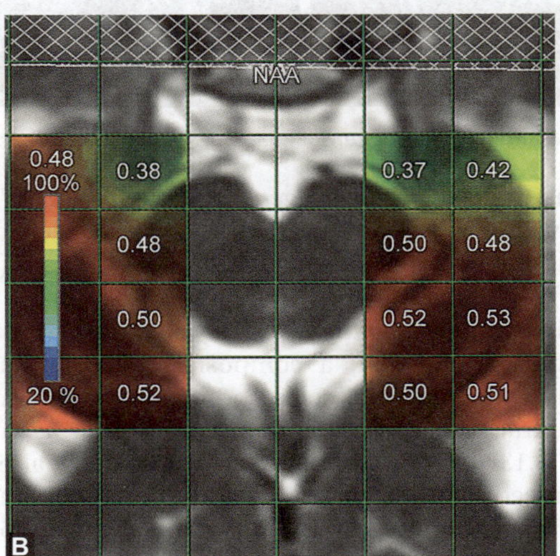

Figs 8.10A and B: A. Magnetic resonance spectroscopy metabolite spectrum; **B.** Metabolite mapping-hippocampus

Abbreviation: NAA = N-acetylaspartate

Textbook of Medicine

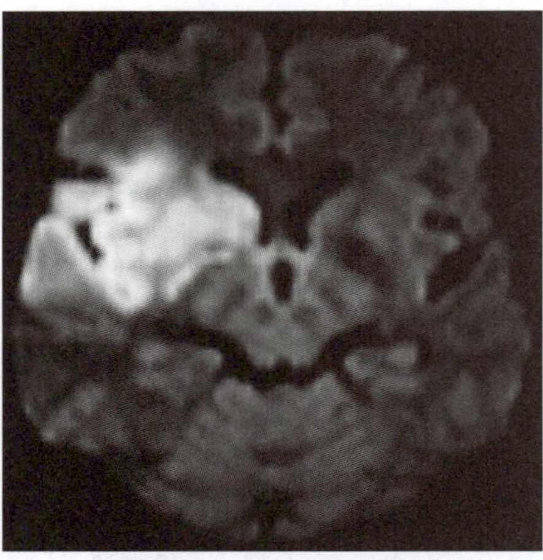

Fig. 8.11: Diffusion weighted imaging showing restriction of diffusion (bright)

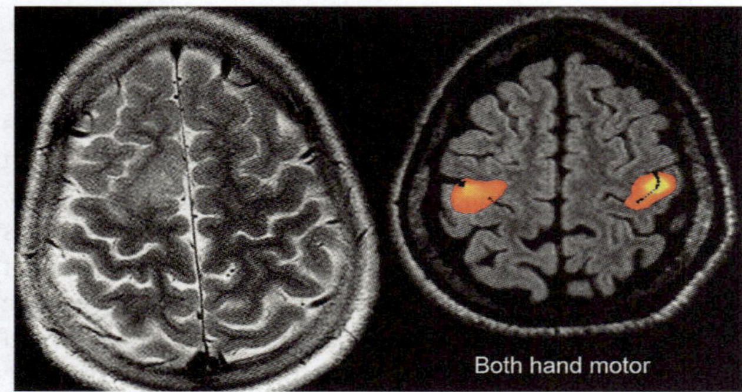

Fig. 8.12: Activation of hand knob in functional imaging

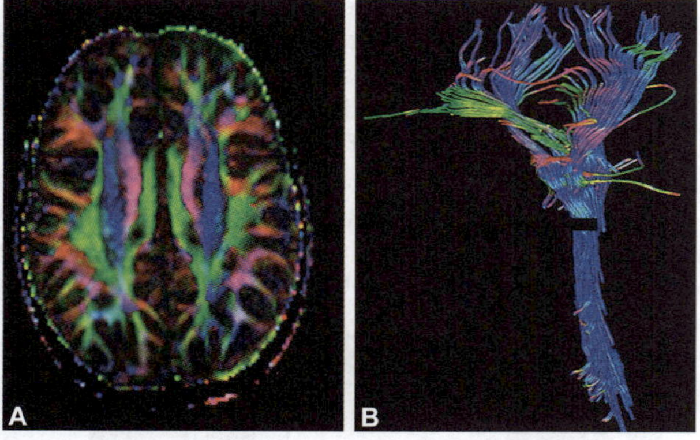

Figs 8.13A and B: Diffusion tensor imaging. **A.** Brain; **B.** Motor tract

tissue to get a ***blood oxygen dependent image***. This has wide practical applications in brain especially in planning area of resection in vital areas of brain (Fig. 8.12).

■ ***Diffusion tensor imaging (DTI):*** According to the pattern of diffusion, a composite color pattern is made with a definite color coding. Superoinferior—blue, transverse as red and anteroposterior as green (Fig. 8.13B). DTI and fiber tractography have already advanced the scientific understanding of many neurologic and psychiatric disorders and have been applied clinically for the presurgical mapping of eloquent white matter tracts before intracranial mass resections (Fig. 8.13A).

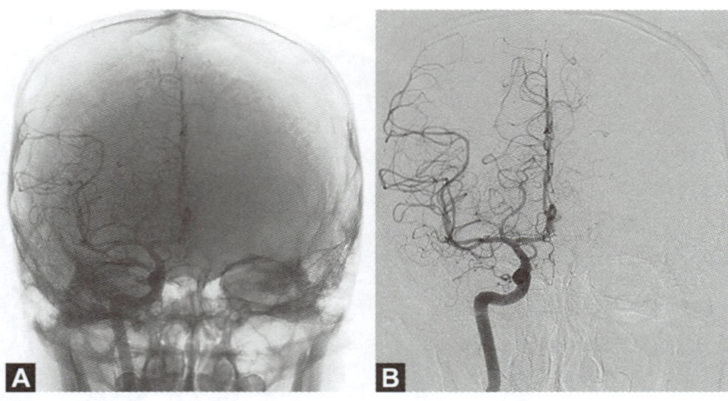

Figs 8.14A and B: Digital subtraction angiography—carotid angiogram. **A.** Unsubtracted image; **B.** Subtracted image

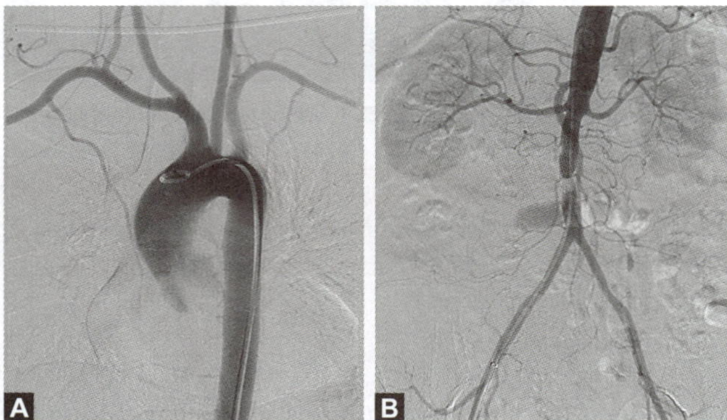

Figs 8.15A and B: Aortogram. **A.** Thoracic part; **B.** Abdominal part

■ ***Digital subtraction angiography (DSA):*** It refers to the technique of subtracting images taken before and after injecting the contrast media in an angiogram. Here, the depiction of blood vessels are clear as the bone and other soft tissues are subtracted in the final image (Figs 8.14A and B). Injections are given intra-arterial mostly and rarely IV. Presently 3D rotational angiography is also available for better localization of vascular lesions like aneurysms. All intracranial and peripheral vessels can be delineated precisely by this technique (Figs 8.15A and B).

Nuclear Medicine Techniques

Here, electromagnetic radiation called gamma rays is used. Gamma rays are produced from the nucleus of an unstable atom in its effort to become stable. This is in contrast to X-rays which are produced by bombardment of an atom by an electron. The radionuclide can be created in nuclear reactors, cyclotrons and generators. The gamma emitter, called as radiopharmaceutical is administered to patient. The most commonly used radiopharmaceutical is technetium (Tc-99m pertechnetate). Tc-99m is produced from a generator containing molybdenum-99 (Mo-99) which in turn is produced from uranium 235 fission in a nuclear reactor. Radiopharmaceuticals can be administered to patients either orally, IV or directly into a body cavity. Gamma camera is used to detect the gamma rays emitted from the body of patient. These are converted to light photons by the sodium iodide crystals. The light photons are detected by the photomultiplier tube which converts them into electrical voltage and later a computer circuitry converts them into a final dot image.

Radioisotopes of Tc (half-life 6 hours), [67]galliuum (half-life 78 hours), [201]thallium (half-life 3 days) and [131]iodine (half-life 8 days) are commonly used.

Single photon emission computed tomography (SPECT): Here gamma camera rotates around patient as in CT scan and 2D/3D image is produced which improves localization of radiopharmaceuticals and results in better localization of the lesion.

Positron emission tomography (PET): Positrons are positively charged electrons and are emitted by the decay of proton rich radionuclides like [11]carbon, [13]nitrogen, [15]oxygen, [18]fluorine and others. The protons encounter electrons and are annihilated releasing energy as two 511 KeV gamma rays in opposite directions. Most of the PET isotopes are made in cyclotrons and have very short half-life (a few minutes to hours). The commonly used PET chemical is glucose labelled with fluorine-18 (F-18) fluorodeoxyglucose (FDG), called FDG-PET. Tissues actively metabolising glucose like brain, heart and tumors take up this isotope and hence can be actively imaged depending on the turn over. PET scans have higher resolution than SPECT scan.

Advantages:
- Produce excellent physiological and functional information
- Localizes a lesion much before anatomical disruption
- Scan can be repeated for seeing the movement/uptake of radionuclide tracer.

Disadvantages:
- Lacks the high resolution offered by other imaging modalities
- Involves ionizing radiation and for longer half-life isotopes patient continues to radiation for a few days
- Isotopes of PET scan are expensive and they have to be produced by on-site cyclotron because of their extremely short half-life.

Hybrid Techniques

Radionuclide images depict organ function rather than structure. This limitation is addressed in hybrid imaging where PET scans are superimposed on either CT scan (PET CT) or MRI scan (PET MRI). The color images of PET are superimposed onto CT/MRI scan so that the anatomical image is superimposed on functional image. This is very useful for the survey of metastases, lymphoma and postsurgical evaluation of residual and/or recurrent tumors. Accurate co-registration is possible as the two image data sets are acquired using the same imaging system within a short time interval (Figs 8.16A to C).

Advantages: Useful in radiotherapy planning as radionuclide image data can be incorporated into CT-based radiotherapy planning systems. Aids in differentiation between malignant and inflammatory causes of uptake of positron emitting radiopharmaceutical F-18 FDG with accurate morphological study.

INTERVENTIONAL RADIOLOGY

In this branch of radiology, the radiologist is involved not only in diagnostic aspect of disease but also in subsequent treatment of the condition, e.g. intracranial aneurysm

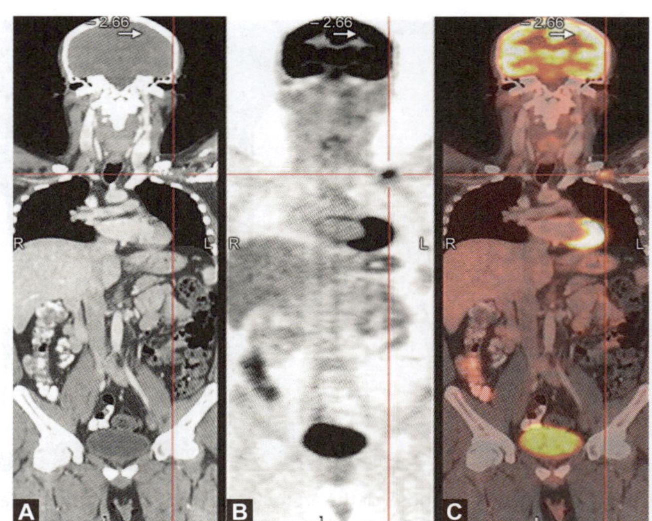

Figs 8.16A to C: **A.** CT scan; **B.** PET scan; **C.** Hybrid image

coiling and peripheral angioplasty. It demands a good clinical knowledge and patient management in ICU set up. Interventional radiology can be divided into percutaneous image guided procedures and intra-arterial/venous route studies. The latter include procedures like CT/US guided biopsy or fine needle aspiration cytology (FNAC). The vascular route interventions can be further subdivided into vascular interventions and neurointerventions. Vascular interventions include bronchial artery embolization (BAE), uterine artery embolization (UAE) for arrest of bleeding from branches of the corresponding vessels and aortic and peripheral angioplasty and stenting for occlusive vascular disease (Figs 8.17 and 8.18). Neurointerventions include coiling of intracranial aneurysms and cerebral arteriovenous malformations (AVMs) and other vascular abnormalities (Figs 8.19A and B). Broadly, most of the procedures are either opening procedures (e.g. angioplasty) of occluding procedures (e.g. coiling of pseudoaneurysm) (Figs 8.20A and B).

Advantages:
- Minimally invasive percutaneous procedure
- Minimum hospital stay—only for few days
- Suitable for high risk surgical patients.

In this context, one has to remember that intervention procedures are technically challenging like open surgery. They also carry considerable risk of mortality and morbidity in high risk cases, even though to a lesser extent than surgery. This has to be explained to the patients and relatives and informed consent obtained beforehand. In addition, some of these procedures are expensive due to the cost of the materials used like stents and technical expertize required.

CONTRAST MEDIA USED IN RADIOLOGY TECHNIQUES

They are used in investigations involving:
- In X-rays (including CT scan)
- In MRI scan
- In ultrasound scan.

Textbook of Medicine

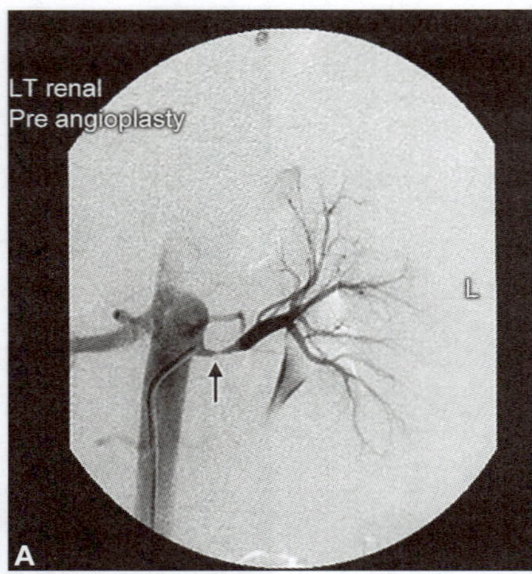
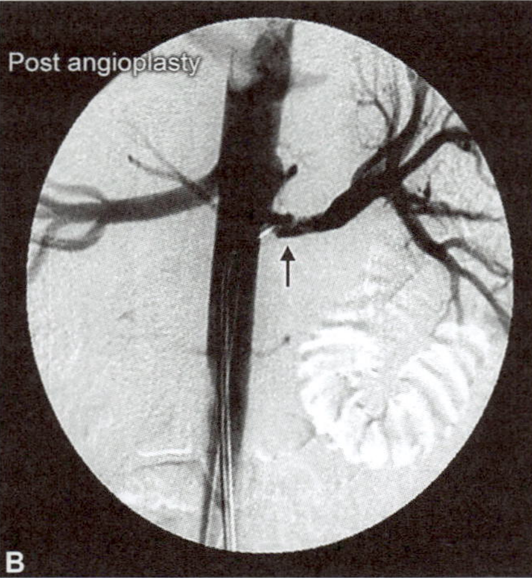
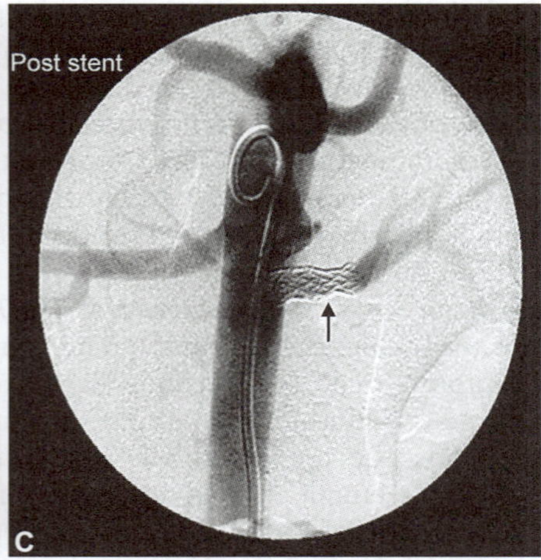

Figs 8.17A to C: A. Stenosis of the artery (arrow); **B.** Stenosis dilated (arrow); **C.** Stent introduced (arrow)

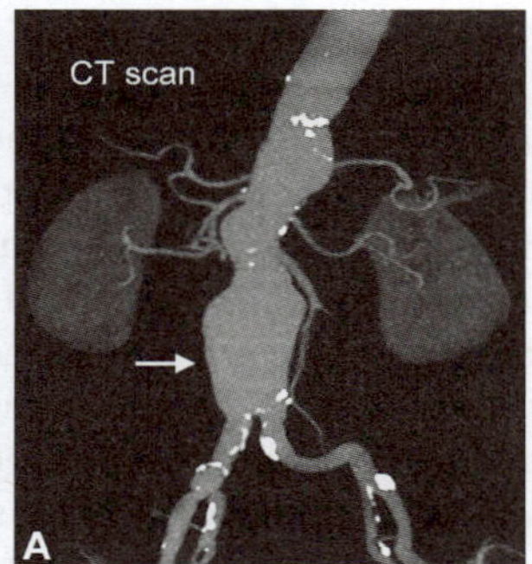
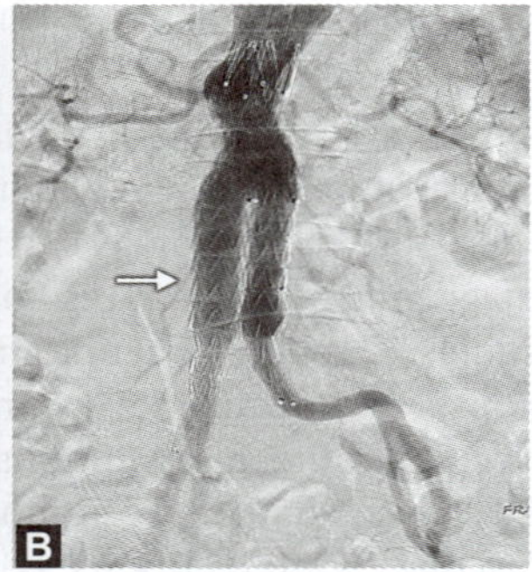

Figs 8.18A and B: Interventional radiology. **A.** Aortic aneurysm before repair (arrow); **B.** Aneurysm repaired with stent (arrow)

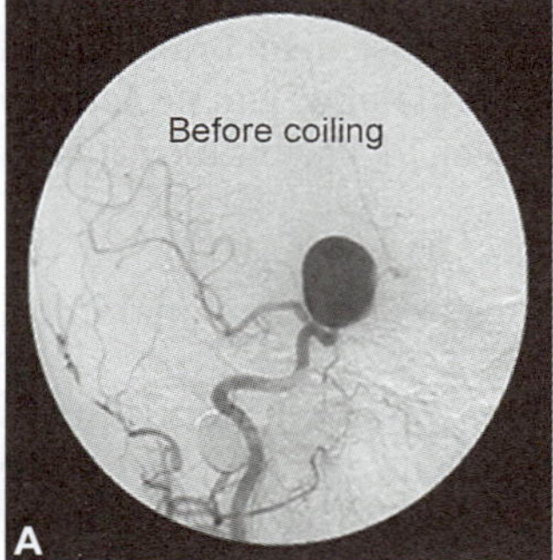
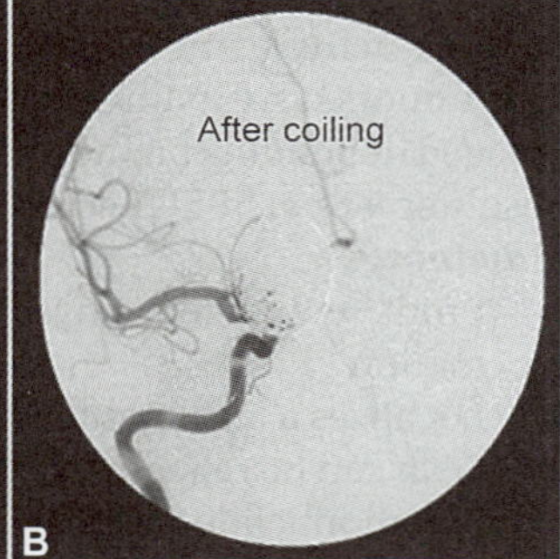

Figs 8.20A and B: A. Middle cerebral artery aneurysm; **B.** Disappearance of the aneurysm after coiling

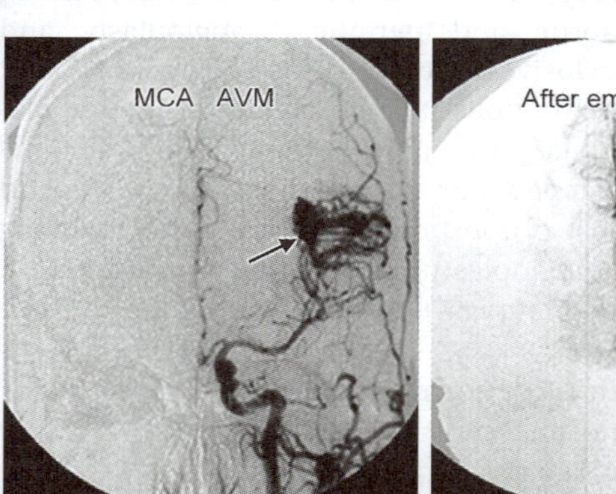
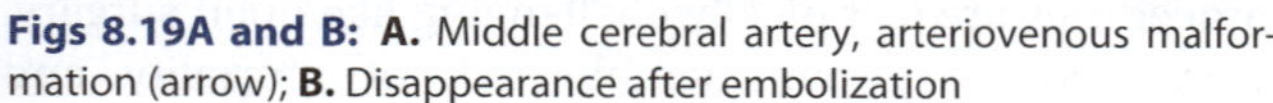

Figs 8.19A and B: A. Middle cerebral artery, arteriovenous malformation (arrow); **B.** Disappearance after embolization

X-rays (including CT Scan)

Contrast media are of 2 types: Negative contrast media like air used in double contrast study of bowel and positive contrast media. The latter includes barium sulphate suspension (used in barium meal study, barium enema, small bowel enema), iodinated media (used in IVU, CT angiography and similar procedures).

According to the route: It may be oral, IV/intra-arterial or local instillation. Example of oral route is barium sulphate suspension given in barium meal study. Air is a negative contrast media used along with barium suspension in barium meal/barium enema double contrast study.

Parenteral contrast media include iodinated dyes given intra-arterially (in digital subtraction angiography), IV (in IVU/CT scan contrast study) intrathecally (to demonstrate leak in CSF rhinorrhea) and into lymphatics (Lipiodol injection for lymphangiography).

Iodinated media (CT scan, catheter angiography and others): Iodine with an atomic weight of 127 has good radio-opacity and is widely used as a contrast media. Following types are recognized:

- Ionic monomers (high osmolar contrast media with 3 iodine atoms—sodium iothalamate, e.g. Conray)
- Nonionic monomers (low osmolar contrast media—iohexol, e.g. Omnipaque)
- Ionic dimers (with 6 iodine atoms—sodium ioxaglate, e.g. Hexabrix)
- Nonionic dimers (iodixinol, e.g. Visipaque).

On IV injection, these are distributed readily into the extravascular, extracellular space. Over 90% of the contrast is eliminated by glomerular filtration rate (GFR) by the kidneys within 12 hours. Nonionic dimers like Visipaque are safer to use especially in aged patients and infants.

Adverse reaction to contrast media:

- Anaphylactic reaction to iodine which is not dose dependent. It is more severe and common in asthmatics and atopic patients.
- Nonidiosyncratic reactions which are dose dependent and related to the chemical composition, osmolality and concentration of the contrast. ***Clinical features***

include symptoms related to vasodilatation and hypovolemia. Asthmatics, cardiac patients with decompensating, diabetic nephropathy, patients on metformin, very ill and underweight infants and elderly patients have higher risk of developing this type of reaction.

MRI Scan

The commonly used contrast media is gadolinium diethylenetriaminepentaacetic acid (Gd-DTPA) which is a paramagnetic substance. It produces enhancement by reducing the T_1 relaxation time of the tissue. Hence all contrast images in MRI scan are T_1 weighted images.

Adverse reactions: Gadolinium is relatively safe and adverse reactions are only a few. Its safety in pregnancy is not yet known and it is better avoided unless it is highly essential. In 3–5% of patients with GFR less than 30 mL/mt, it can produce nephrogenic systemic fibrosis. The onset varies from a few days to 3 months and is characterized by scleroderma-like skin changes affecting the limbs and trunk leading to flexion contracture of joints.

In contrast-enhanced MR imaging of the liver and pancreas, nonspecific extracellular gadolinium chelating agents can be used. In imaging of the liver other than non-gadolinium based agents, manganese based agents (Mangafodipir trisodium—Teslascan) and iron oxide based agents (superparamagnetic iron oxide particles—Endorem) are also used.

Ultrasound Contrast Agents

Microbubble agents are used to enhance ultrasound signals and these agents are injected IV. The size range of these ultrasound agents is 2–7 µm and it resonates in an ultrasound frequency of 2–10 MHz. As they tend to collapse because of their high surface tension, stabilization is achieved by encapsulating them in a membrane of denatured albumen or phospholipid. This has wide application in myocardial perfusion studies and in studies of liver lesions.

Picture archiving and communication system (PACS): It is a computerized electronic network in which digital images are viewed on monitors along with clinical details of the patient and radiological report displayed in electronic format. Image retrieval is infinitely quicker from PACS and all previous images of a given patient can be viewed at anytime anywhere in the hospital. This leads to film—less practice in hospital with direct cost savings. Apart from a local area network (LAN), PACS also sets the stage for teleradiology over a wide area network (WAN). Teleradiology offers a centralized reporting service to remote areas.

RADIATION ISSUES

The worldwide standard for radiation protection is set by the International Commission on Radiological Protection (ICRP) in 1928. Radiation hazards produce mitotic inhibition, chromosome damage leading to genetic effects/mutations and cell death. Actively dividing cells in the fetus, bone marrow, gonads intestinal epithelium

Table 8.3: Radiation doses

Imaging procedure	Effective dose
X-ray chest	0.02 mSv
Lumbar spine	1 mSv
X-ray skull	0.06 mSv
X-ray pelvis/abdomen	0.7 mSv
Barium enema	7.2 mSv
Barium meal	2.6 mSv
Intravenous urogram	2.4 mSv
CT scan head	2.0 mSv

Table 8.4: Relationship between present and past units in radiation dosimetry

SI units	Historical dosimetry
1 Gray	100 R
1 Sievert	100 rem = 100 rad
io10 mGy	1 roentgen
10 mSv	1 rem = 1 rad

and others are more vulnerable. The nature and degree of damage depend on the tissue, dose and duration of exposure. The doses of irradiation obtained to the patient in various common investigations are given in Table 8.3. In the SI system, a millisievert (mSv) is defined as the average accumulated background radiation dose to an individual for 1 year. 1 mSv is the dose produced by exposure to 1 milligray (mG) of radiation. In the historical system of dosimetry, exposure to 1 roentgen (R) of X-rays results in absorption of 1 rad (radiation-absorbed dose), which had the effect of 1 rem [roentgen-equivalent (in) man]. The unit equivalences between the systems are given in Table 8.4.

The dose equivalent of radiation dose is expressed as FtaSievert (Sv). Table 8.3 gives the cumulative radiation obtained with different imaging procedures.

Radiation doses that exceed a minimum (threshold) level can cause undesirable effects such as depression of blood cell-forming process (threshold dose = 500 mSv) or cataracts (threshold dose = 5,000 mSv). Radiation also can cause an increase in the incidence of malignant disease. Epidemiologic studies have found that the estimated lifetime risk of dying from cancer is greater by about 0.004% per mSv (0.04% per rem) of radiation dose to the whole body. The radiation dose obtained for more investigations tend to cumulate with increasing age and if sufficient care is not taken to avoid unnecessary radiological investigations, they may predispose to the development of neoplasms. This risk is more so in children and to fetus.

CHOICE OF MODALITIES

In the scenario of changing technical advancement in radiology, algorithms for each disease entity and survey has to be revised in consultation with a radiologist. This will reduce unnecessary investigations with full benefit transferred to the patient care.

CHAPTER 9

Myiasis

KV Krishna Das

Chapter Summary
- General Considerations
- Cutaneous Myiasis—Ectoparasitic
- Deep Tissue Myiasis
- Ophthalmic Myiasis
- Intestinal Myiasis
- Urinary Myiasis

GENERAL CONSIDERATIONS

Invasion of tissues or body cavities by the larvae (maggots) of dipterous flies is called myiasis. Myiasis maybe of either primary or secondary type.

In *primary myiasis,* the human infection occurs as part of the obligate lifecycle of the parasite and in secondary myiasis the human infection is accidental. Primary myiasis affects people in good general health, whereas *secondary myiasis* supervenes on dead or necrotic tissues. The flies lay eggs in the necrotic tissues in secondary (or healthy tissues in primary) myiasis of humans. These eggs hatch from larvae, feeding on the necrotic and living tissues which are devitalized and they hatch into adult flies. Myiasis affects several animals species—both living and after death.

Classification

In general, the infection is of two types:
1. *Ectoparasitic and Auchmeromyia luteola*
2. *Endoparasitic*
   - Cutaneous, e.g. caused by *Dermatobia hominis* and *Cordylobia anthropophaga*
   - Tissues or cavities, e.g. caused by *Sarcophaga, Wohlfahrtia, Fannia, Oestrus, Chrysomya* and *Callitroga.*

The maggots are dull white or pink in color, actively motile and have spines on their body. The body is tapered and segmented, the narrow anterior end bears the mouth parts, the thicker posterior end bears the opening of the spiracles which are dark colored and useful in identifying the genera. Their length varies from 0.5 to 3 cm. The larvae feed voraciously on tissues or discharges and in 2–4 weeks develop and fall off to the ground to pupate.

Final identification of the species can be done by allowing the larvae to complete the lifecycle *in vitro* and examining the adult flies.

CUTANEOUS MYIASIS—ECTOPARASITIC

Auchmeromyia luteola (Congo maggot fly): This fly lays eggs on soil and crevices in the floor. The larvae hatch out in 2 days. They can survive without food and water up to one month. Once hatched out, they attach themselves to the skin of the humans who sleep on the floor unprotected, suck blood for 20 minutes and drop off leaving maculopapular lesions. This process is repeated several times before the larva pupates in 2–12 weeks. Bites can be prevented by protective clothing or insect repellents like dimethylphthalate or N, N-diethyl-benzamide.

Localized Cutaneous Myiasis

Dermatobia hominis (Human bot fly or warble fly): The adult fly lays eggs on hematophagous insects like mosquitoes, stomoxys and ticks or others such as housefly *(Musca).* When the latter alights on man, the larvae hatch out and wriggle on to the surface. They enter through the wound, produced by the insect or penetrate the unbroken skin and develop in the subcutaneous tissues.

The initial lesion is papular and pruritic. It becomes furuncle-like and painful later. The posterior end of the actively motile larva may be seen in the lesion through the opening. In 2–3 months, the larvae mature and fall off to the ground. Lesions are seen on the exposed parts. The disease is distributed worldwide.

Cordylobia anthropophaga (African tumbu fly): The adult flies lay eggs on clothes spread out for drying or in dirty soil.

The larvae develop in 24–48 hours and penetrate the human skin either from the clothes or through the bare feet.

The lesion is initially papular and pruritic and becomes painful in a short time. Secondary infection may occur. Unlike the former, lifecycle is shorter and is completed in 2–3 weeks.

Treatment: The maggots may be extracted surgically. A drop of mineral oil placed on the lesions suffocates the larvae which wriggle out and can be extricated. Penicillin in usual doses should be used to prevent secondary infection.

Migrating lesions resembling cutaneous larva migrans are produced by the larvae of genus *Gasterophilus (horse bot flies)* and *Hypoderma (cattle bot flies),* which develops from eggs laid on the hair. Man is an accidental host and the larvae penetrate the skin, enter the subcutaneous tissues and wander producing eruptions similar to larva migrans of *Ancylostoma braziliense,* but more painful. They survive for a few weeks and die. Application of mineral oil over the lesions helps to visualize the underlying larvae. Tissues of the eye may be affected. In addition to surgical removal, symptomatic relief may be obtained by antihistamines.

DEEP TISSUE MYIASIS

Larvae of the flies belonging to the families *Callitroga (Cochliomyia), Chrysomya, Sarcophaga, Wohlfahrtia, Fannia* and *Oestrus* invade tissues extensively when the eggs are laid on open wounds, damaged tissues or discharging surfaces, by the adult flies. The larvae of *Wohlfahrtia* can penetrate even unbroken skin.

The lesions are commonly seen in the nasal cavities, paranasal sinuses, middle ear and orbit. Cartilage and bone may also be destroyed by the screw-shaped larvae which may extend intracranially leading to fatal meningitis. The lesions are very painful and the larvae may be discharged from these sites.

Treatment is manual removal of larvae or extraction after spraying the area with chloroform. Repeated sessions may be necessary.

Secondary infection has to be treated with broad spectrum antibiotics like ampicillin.

OPHTHALMIC MYIASIS

Flies of the genus *Chrysomya* and *Oestrus* may lay their eggs in the conjunctival sac. The larvae hatch out and produce lesions resembling acute conjunctivitis with severe irritation. Rarely corneal ulceration and loss of sight may occur.

Removal of the maggot after anesthetizing the eye and application of topical antibiotic drops will relieve the condition.

INTESTINAL MYIASIS

The larvae or pupae of *Musca, Fannia, Sarcophaga* and *Tubifera* may be passed in stools or appear in vomitus. The eggs may be laid by the flies around the lips or anus while sleeping, especially if there are foul smelling discharges around these orifices.

The larvae hatch out from a few hours to two days and are swallowed to reach the upper gastrointestinal tract (GIT) or they may crawl up into the rectum and large intestine. They develop in the stomach or in the intestines. Sometimes larvae may be swallowed along with infested foodstuffs. The larvae cause symptoms of gastritis or colitis which may persist from weeks to months. If reinfection does not occur, the condition is self-limiting.

Treatment consists of administration of purgatives and reassurance about the self-limiting nature of the illness.

URINARY MYIASIS

Larvae of *Musca, Fannia* or *Sarcophaga* may enter the bladder, when the eggs are laid around the external genitalia and produce symptoms of lower urinary tract infection (UTI) with proteinuria, pyuria and hematuria. The larvae may pass in urine. Rarely urinary system may be involved by maggots eroding their way from the GIT.

CHAPTER 10

Arthropod Bites and Stings, and Injuries due to Marine Animals

KV Krishna Das

Chapter Summary

- Spider
- Scorpion
- Bees, Wasps and Hornets
- Centipedes
- Ants
- Lice
- Ticks
- Chigoe Flea
- Leech Infestations
- Injuries due to Marine Animals

SPIDER

Nearly 40,000 species of spiders have been identified worldwide. A few are poisonous and aggressive. Reliable information can be obtained from local inhabitants. Several species of spiders bite man accidentally. Some species like *Latrodectus mactans* (black widow spider) attack man

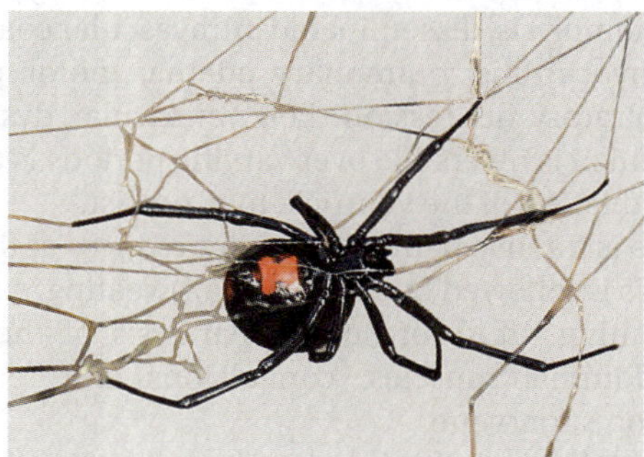

Fig. 10.1: Black widow spider

(Fig. 10.1). Females are more aggressive and venomous compared to males. The venom is generally neurotoxic, sometimes, also hemolytic. The bite is followed by intense local pain and the part becomes tender and spastic. Generalized muscular rigidity especially marked over the abdomen, pupillary constriction, salivation, excessive sweating and cardiovascular collapse may follow. Death may occur in children and debilitated subjects. Spiders of the genus *Loxosceles* seen in the tropical regions of several countries cause necrotic ulcers at the sites of bite.

Treatment consists of washing the area of bite with soap and water. Administration of 20 mL of calcium gluconate intravenously (IV) relieves muscle spasm. Muscle relaxants like mephenesin in a dose of 1 g orally and anticholinergics like atropine (0.5 mg given IV) give symptomatic relief. Supportive measures are indicated if shock supervenes.

Specific antivenins are available in different countries depending upon the different toxic effects of the prevalent spiders in severe cases the antivenins is indicated.

SCORPION

Scorpions are nocturnal in habits and they come out at night to catch insects as their prey. They kill by injecting the poison by the sting arising from the poison gland situated at the posterior end of the tail like abdomen. Nearly 1000 species of scorpions belonging to six families are known. Among these some species belonging to the family buthidae, especially the red scorpions are capable of inflicting toxic sting which could be fatal. In India, *Mesobuthus tamulus* is one among the dangerous scorpions. Scorpion venom contains short chain peptides that affect the mechanisms of sodium and potassium channels in excitable tissues. The toxins are classified into alpha and beta toxins. The peptide beta toxin opens the sodium channels. In addition, the alpha toxin inhibits deactivation of sodium channels. By acting on sodium potassium channels, they lead to intense persistent depolarization of the cell membranes and autonomic nerves with massive release of neurotransmitters from adrenal medulla.

The neurotoxic effects leads to a cholinergic stimulation followed by adrenergic stimulation resulting in tachycardia, hypertension, cardiac failure and pulmonary edema in 1–2%. Electrocardiogram (ECG) abnormalities may develop which clear up on recovery. Cerebral and cerebellar infarcts may develop. Other major effects include hemolysis, disseminated intravascular coagulation (DIC), myocarditis, pulmonary edema, motor paralysis and respiratory depression. Left ventricular dysfunction (LVD), which is reversible over varying periods is a sequel. At times dilation of the ventricle may persist.

There is intense pain, edema and redness at the site of sting. This is followed by tachycardia, sweating, salivation, and vomiting. In severe cases, paralysis of the tongue and abdominal muscles, convulsions and respiratory depression supervene.

Myocarditis manifesting as tachy or brady arrhythmias and cardiac failure may occur not unusually. Rarely, hemorrhagic states due to DIC may develop. Pancreatitis may develop in stings of *Tityus serrulatus* (scorpion seen more in Trinidad).

Treatment: For local treatment, the affected part is immersed in ice cold water and washed. Infiltration of 5 mL of 2% xylocaine around the sting gives relief to pain.

General treatment consists in the management of anaphylactic shock, ventilatory support and prevention of cardiac death. The use of prazosin, an alpha blocker has revolutionized the management of scorpion stings. Oral prazocin given in a dose of 250–500 µg/kg in children and 500–1000 µg/kg in adults at 3 hours intervals is life-saving. Scorpion antivenom is available and it may be given in doses of 10–20 mL IV. This neutralizes the circulating venom. Acute pulmonary edema responds to general resuscitative measures and sodium nitroprusside given IV. Another drug which is also reported to be effective is captopril given in doses of 12.5–25 mg thrice daily orally. Physical activity should be permitted only after adequate convalescence and normalization of the ECG.

Source:

1. Bawaskar HS, Bawaskar PH. Utility of scorpion antivenin vs prazosin in the management of severe Mesobuthus tamulus (Indian red scorpion) envenoming at rural setting. J Assoc Physicians India. 2007;55:14-21.
2. Krishnan A, et al. Ibid. pp 22-6.

HYMENOPTERA STINGS

Bees, Wasps, Hornets and Fire Ants

Hymenoptera commonly causing injuries to humans belong to three families:

1. Apidae—honeybees and bumblebees
2. Vespidae—hornets, wasps and yellow jackets
3. Formicidae—fire ants.

The sting apparatus is the modified ovipositor and only the females sting. The venom is used for defence and also can be used for capturing the prey. The quantity of venom delivered at a sting varies from 50 ng (fire ants) to 50 µg (bees). The venom sac may remain detached from the insect's abdomen and continue to squeeze out venom even after the insect escapes. This can be avoided by removing the venom sac manually, thereby reducing the severity of envenomation.

The venom from the different insects varying in composition, relative content and antigencity even though some degree of cross reactions may occur within families.

Action of Venom on the Humans (Table 10.1)

The venom binds to venom specific immunoglobulin E (IgE) receptor on mast cells and leads to rapid release of mast cells mediators such as histamine, leukotrines, prostaglandins and platelet activating factor. These lead to a spectrum of allergic reaction varying from small (1 cm) or large (10 cm) local urticaria and swelling, anaphylactic shock and death. Stings on the neck and face are

Table 10.1: Contents of the venom and their action

Biological effects	Type of venom	Clinical effects
Histamine, dopamine, norepinephrine and kinins	Vasoactive amines	Pain, erythema swelling, pruritus at the site and may be generalized
Protein enzymes: Phospholipase hyaluronidase phosphatase	Allergens	Allergy in sensitive persons varying in degree and extent
Toxic alkalodis particularly in fire ants	Toxins	Vesiculation of skin

associated with rapid swelling of the oral mucosa, tongue and larynx which may be fatal abruptly unless attended to in time. Multiple stings are much more serious than single sting and the risk is additive. All persons who get local reactions may not get systemic manifestations and in them even subsequent stings may not cause systemic illness (only in < 10%). But in those who had systemic reactions the risk of developing severe systemic reactions is high if sting occurs again (> 30–60%).

Epidemiology

In India, hymenoptera stings are frequently seen among persons working in agriculture, forestry, timber operations who are all occupationally exposed to it and also in children who are stung by ants. The flying insects build nests on trees and other areas whereas some members of Vespidae and fire ants live in holes on the earth. Some varieties of these insects positively attack and effect the sting in groups and more than 3–4 stings effected above the neck and face are highly dangerous and demand emergency intensive care to save life.

Clinical Features

Local Reactions

Following the bite, there is intense pain with transient local swelling over areas varying from small to large. In the case of fire ant bites—vesiculation may occur, lymphangitis may develop and secondary infections are generally unusual.

Systemic Reactions

These may occur abruptly after the sting or after a particular periods. If the stinger is left behind at the site of sting, envenomation is likely to be more severe and systemic effects more serious. Biphasic reactions in which an initial reaction is followed by recurrence of symptoms several hours later (typically 8 hours) are not unusual. It is essential that patients are observed for this period so that the late recurrence is not missed. ***Factors that are associated with severity of the reaction include:***

- Type of the insect—honeybee is more dangerous than the other hymenoptera
- Number of stings—multiple stings being proportionately more severe
- Underlying mast cell disorders with elevated serum tryptase levels at baseline
- History of previous systemic reactions to insect bite
- Pre-existing cardiovascular disease
- Concomitant therapy with beta blockers, angiotensin converting enzyme inhibitors (ACEIs), angiotensin converting enzyme (ACE) inhibitors or both.

β-blockers potentiate the negative inotropic and chronotropic effects of mast cell mediators and inhibit the beta agonist effects of epinephrine which is the sheet anchor of emergency therapy. ACE inhibitors prevent the break down of neuropeptides and bradykinin which are released as a result of mast cell degranulation.

Anaphylaxis gives rise to the spectrum of reactions leading to affection of several organs systems especially skin, gastrointestinal tract (GIT), upper and lower respiratory tracts, cardiovascular system (CVS) and nervous system. The hallmark of severe anaphylaxis are the development of hypotension and multiorgan system involvement.

Organ systems symptoms include the following:

Nervous system—depression, fear, headache, dizziness, and seizure.

Eyes, nose, mouth—pruritis, angioedema rhinitis, lacrimation and metallic taste.

Respiratory system—dysphagia, hoarseness, asthma, asphyxia, cyanosis.

CVS—tachycardia, arrhythmia, hypo-tension, myocardial infarction (MI) and cardiac arrest. Death occurs due to upper air way obstruction and/or cardiovascular collapse.

Treatment

Local

Removal of the stinger, washing the part and application of antihistamine or corticosteroid creams.

Systemic Treatment

- Management of the airway and maintenance of respiration/ventilation.
- Maintenance of blood pressure (BP) and prevention of shock by giving IV fluids.
- Specific therapy which is most effective is to give injectable epinephrine at a dose of 0.01 mg/kg bw in a 1:1000 (1 mg/mL) solution—intramuscular (IM) injection into the muscles of the lower or upper limb—as early as possible.
- In an average adult, 0.3–0.5 mg (0.3–0.5 mL) of the drug may be required as the initial dose. Delay in administration of epinephrine may lead to worsening of the condition.

The dose of epinephrine can be repeated 5–15 minutes later if symptoms tend to persist or worsen. H_1 antihistamines given orally or IM can relieve cutaneous swelling and purities. Pain relief can be achieved by oral paracetamol or injectable paracetamol.

Corticosteroid (hydrocortisone 100 mg) given IM or IV gives symptomatic relief and improvement in the general reaction in most cases, though evidence base for this measure is lacking. Still many physicians give glucocorticorids as the improvement is encouraging.

Long-term Follow-up

Prevention of exposure to the offending insects.

Provision of epinephrine auto-injector (available as Auvi-Q from Sanofi—to be procured from abroad by special request) containing 0.15 mg or 0.3 mg or vials of epinephrine for self injection by the patient. If this not available, hydrocortisone 100 mg IV can be used as an emergency measure.

Immunotherapy

Skin tests for detecting the insect specific IgE are available and these are done as routine practice by allergist immunologists in several countries. This facility is not generally available in India.

Subcutaneous (SC) immunotherapy can be done for those who have clinical disease and positive skin testing. Venom immunotherapy is available in several countries against the hymenoptera insects either specific or mixed. The duration of venom immunotherapy is generally for

3–5 years after which systemic reactions to further stings do not occur. Persons who have only cutaneous reactions are not required to take immunotherapy.

Source: Casale TB, Burks AW. Clinical practice. Hymenoptera-sting hypersensitivity. N Engl J Med. 2014;370(15):1432-9.

CENTIPEDES

Syn: Chilopoda

Several species of centipedes are seen in warm climates. They vary in length from a few centimeters up to 20 cm, the larger ones can affect painful bites on man. The poison glands are situated at the anterior end and the poison is injected through the claws on the mandibular legs during the bite. Centipedes hide under clothes or bedding and bites are accidental. Bite mark may be visible as a pair of tiny red spots separated by a few millimeters. Symptoms consist of local pain lasting for 2–4 hours, edema, redness and enlargement of the draining lymph node. Headache, vertigo, vomiting and fever may follow. Centipede bites are usually not fatal.

Treatment: Consists of antihistamines, analgesics and reassurance. Infiltration of 2% xylocaine locally gives immediate relief from pain.

ANTS

Certain species of fire ants belonging to the genus *Solenopsis* inflict bites on the skin and also introduce the poison through the stinger situated at the posterior end of the abdomen. Local irritation and allergic reactions follow.

Ants may colonize in the bed clothes of debilitated patients, newborn babies and comatose subjects and eat away superficial tissues producing shallow ulcers. When large numbers are involved, tissue loss may be considerable. This can be avoided by exerting care in nursing chronically bedridden patients and dusting 10% dichlorodiphenyltrichloroethane (DDT) powder under the cot and bed.

LICE

Lice, belonging to the family *Pediculidae* cause pediculosis in man. Their bodies are flattened and their mouth parts which are retractile are intended for piercing and sucking. The legs are provided with single claws which enable the insect to cling to hairs or clothes. The posterior end of the male is rounded and that of the female is notched. Lice are found all over the world.

Head louse *(Pediculus humanus capitis)* is found on the head; the body louse *(Pediculus humanus corporis)* is found all over the body and clothes; the pubic louse *(Phthirus)* is seen over the pubic hair, eye lashes and sometimes all parts of the body as well. The eggs (nits) are glued to the hairs. The nymphs hatch out within 7–10 days. They reach adulthood after three moultings in two weeks and the fertilized females start laying eggs within a month. Each female lays a total of about 300 eggs. Lifespan is 4–6 weeks. Pediculosis leads to local irritation, pruritus, secondary infection and local lymphadenopathy of the posterior cervical group. Chronic infestation leads to pigmentation—***Vagabond's disease***.

Spread from person to person by close contact, sharing of clothes or sleeping in the same room. Pubic louse may spread through sexual contact.

Lice leave the body when it cools down after death or when there is rise of temperature due to fever or physical exercise and seek new hosts. By this process the body louse transmits typhus, trench fever and relapsing fever.

Treatment: Benzyl benzoate 25% emulsion, applied to the scalp or other infested areas for a period of three hours, followed by a bath serves to kill the lice and nits. Alternatively, DDT powder 10% applied over the surface once a week for 3 weeks eliminates the infestation. Reinfestation from bedding and clothes should be avoided. Lice and nits on clothes can be killed by immersion in boiling water or use of a hot iron. All affected members should be treated simultaneously.

Topical insecticides such as permethrin, synergized pyrethrin and malathion are effective for preventing reinfestation. Resistance to the insecticide may develop. Ivermectin applied as a 0.8% weight to volume solution is highly effective if applied overnight.

The local custom of wet-combing of hair practiced in several communities is an effective and safe method of delousing.

TICKS

Medically important ticks belong to the families ixodidae (hard ticks) and argasidae (soft ticks) (Figs 10.2A and B). *Dermacentor, Amblyomma, Rhipicephalus, Hemaphysalis* and *Ixodes* are the hard ticks which are vectors of rickettsiae, borrelia, viruses and bacteria. Among the soft ticks, *Ornithodoros* is the most important. It transmits *Borrelia recurrentis* and *Pasteurella tularensis*. Ticks crawl up and attach themselves to skin folds, insert their mouth parts into the skin and feed for 24–48 hours after which they fall off and undergo moulting. The site of bite may develop into an eschar which is an indolent necrotic ulcer.

Borrelia recurrentis and *Coxiella burnetii* can be transmitted transovarially to the subsequent generations of ticks and hence, an infected colony can act as reservoir of infection for prolonged periods. Ticks live for two years or more.

Tick Paralysis

This is a neurologic syndrome caused by a potent neurotoxin produced by female ticks which attach themselves to host for feeding purpose, particularly in the upper parts of the body, especially on the scalp, face or neck. *Dermacenter variabilis* and *Dermacenter andersoni*

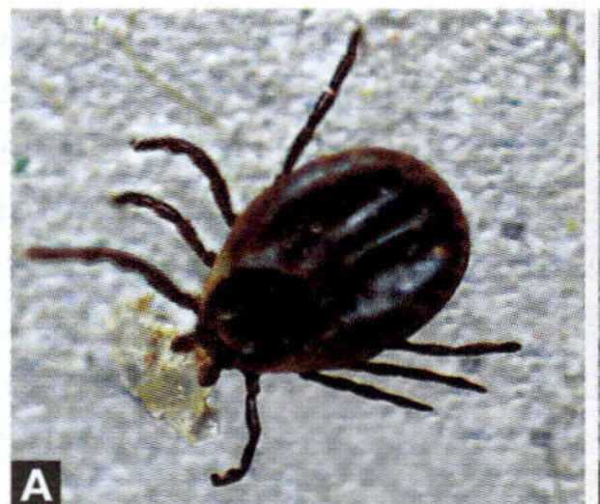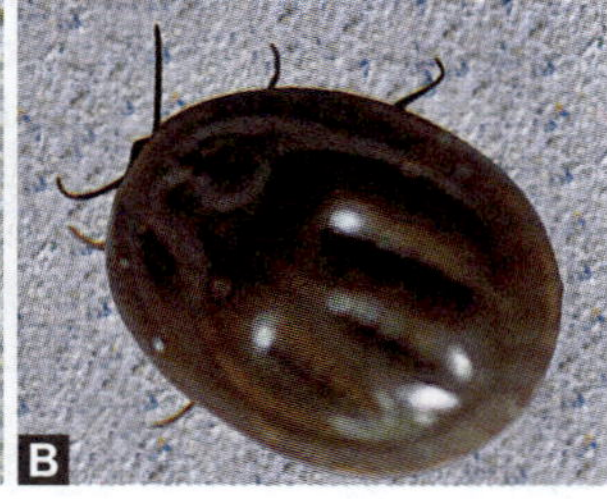

Figs 10.2A and B: **A.** Hard tick; **B.** Soft tick

Textbook of Medicine

have been described from North America. In Australia the main offender is *Ixodes holocyclus*. The ticks take 4–5 days to engorge fully and drop off. Mating with male may occur during this process and this leads to acceleration of the engorgement of the tick, fertilization of the ova and oviposition after falling off. The toxin of the tick is called ixovotoxin.

The neurotoxic venom causes impairment of nerve conduction, reduction of muscle action potential, inhibition of terminal nerve conduction and acetylcholine release at the presynaptic neuromuscular junction of muscle fibres. It may lead to total blockage of transmission at myoneural junctions.

Clinical Features

Children are more affected mainly on account of their lower body weight and greater susceptibility to tick infestation. Symptoms start with tingling sensations of extremities and weakness of limbs and trunk, ataxia of limbs and trunk and flaccid paralysis closely resembling Guillain-Barré syndrome (GBS). If the tick continues to feed this may progress to total flaccid paralysis demanding ventilatory support to maintain life. With the removal of the tick rapid resolution of symptoms occur and recovery may be complete within hours to days. Untreated, the condition can be fatal. Differential diagnosis includes GBS, paralytic poliomyelitis, other forms of paralytic viral diseases, botulism, myasthenic reactions and others. Electrophysiology tests show reduced nerve conduction, reduction in muscle action potentials and neuromuscular block. The cerebrospinal fluid (CSF) is normal unlike as in GBS and encephalomyelitis.

Diagnosis: Strong clinical suspicion and careful search of the scalp and other parts of the body for attached ticks help to establish the diagnosis (Figs 10.2A and B). Its removal and supportive care during the period of paralysis are most rewarding. In Australia, *Ixodes holocyclus* antitoxin is available for administration before the tick is removed.

CHIGOE FLEA

Tunga penetrans (Chigoe flea or jigger): This is found in the feet or other exposed parts of body in people who walk bare-footed and with poor hygiene. The fertilized female burrows into the skin and produces painful itchy lesions. Secondary infection is common. ***Treatment*** consists of immersing the part in lysol baths, surgical removal of the fleas and antibiotics to combat secondary infection.

LEECH INFESTATIONS

Leeches are annelid worms that attach to their hosts by their chitinous cutting jaws and actively suck blood. They produce anticoagulant hirudin which helps them to suck relatively large amount of blood (milliliters). When fully engorged they drop off, but the bite wound continues to bleed for varying periods. Leeches grow in grassland, wet and marshy areas and aquatic environment. They attack fishes, frogs, turtles and big mammals with whom they come into contact with.

Application of alcohol, lime, tobacco, salt, insect repellants or heat help to detach the leech. Forcible pulling out of an attached leech leads to trauma at the bite site and continuous bleeding.

Leeches may be occasionally encountered in body cavities such as nose, paranasal sinuses, mouth, nasopharynx, vagina and so on, where bleeding may be initiated. It is doubtful whether leeches transmit diseases apart from non-healing ulcers and sepsis.

Special types of leeches (*Hirudo medicinalis*) have been employed in *Ayurvedic* system of medicine and also in modern medicine to reduce venous congestion in inflammatory lesions and postoperative edema in surgical flaps.

INJURIES DUE TO MARINE ANIMALS

Seabathers, fishermen or persons working underwater may be stung by marine animals. Among these, the most important are jellyfish, cone shells and stinging fish.

Jellyfish belonging to the class *Hydrozoa* (Portuguese men of war) and *Scyphozoa* which are frequently found in coastal water in the sea, backwaters and riverine estuaries in all parts of India especially the eastern coast. These animals (included under the term cnidaria) secrete specialized living stinging organelles called **cnidae**. Within each of these organelles, a living stinging organism (called the 'third tube') with its venom is present. These organisms are released and discharged on mechanical and sensory stimulation. They get attached to the surface of the host and continue to discharge the venom which is a mixture of proteins, carbohydrates and other constituents.

Some of the marine animals possess tentacles which may be several meters long and these bear nematocysts which contain poison and on contact with the human skin the contents are injected over a period of time. There is intense irritation followed by formation of wheals, vesicles and anaphylactic reaction. Sweating, abdominal pain and vasomotor collapse may occur. Rarely, the stings may be fatal due to cardiac and respiratory failure. Treatment is to give IV calcium gluconate, adrenaline and glucocorticoids to combat the allergic reaction. If tentacles are left on the surface, the nematocysts must be inactivated by the application of dilute acetic acid (vinegar), concentrated sugar or salt solution for 30 seconds before pulling out the broken tentacles. In some countries (Australia), specific antisera are available. The dose is 20,000 IU given IV slowly. ***Cone shells or conidae*** are large marine snails found in the bed of lakes, coral reefs and similar regions. The venom is neurotoxic and in severe cases death results from respiratory paralysis. Treatment is symptomatic. The spines on sea urchins may cause painful injuries.

Stinging fishes: Many species of fishes are capable of inflicting painful stings. Their dorsal fins contain spines connected to poison sacs. The spine may be broken and remain embedded in the victim. Intense local irritation occurs. In a few neuroparalytic symptoms may develop. Rarely respiratory paralysis may lead to death. Treatment is symptomatic and supportive. Immersion of the part in hot water may give relief of pain. In some countries, specific antiserum is available.

Sting rays: These are common around the sea coasts and river mouths in tropical countries. Venom secreting tissue is situated in the grooves and sheaths of barbed horny spines seen on the dorsum of the tail. Stings are inflicted when these animals are trodden upon. Treatment is symptomatic.

Several animals inhabiting the sea have dangerous and painful stings with poison.

Poison of different marine animals constitute the following:	
Sting rays	Neurotoxic venom
Scorpion fish	Neurotoxic venom

Coelentrates including hydroids, jellyfish and anemones	Local effects and systemic toxicity
Sponges	Local pruritus
Sea urchins, starfish	Myotoxicity
Bristle worms	Local pruritus
Molluscs and others	Curare like effect (paralysis)

Treatment consists in measures to relieve pruritus, antihistaminics and supportive measure.

Textbook of Medicine

CHAPTER
11

Snake Bite

KV Krishna Das

> **Chapter Summary**
> - Identification of Poisonous Snakes
> - The Venom
> - Clinical Features
> - Management
>   - Adverse Reactions to Anti-snake Venom (ASV)
>   - Steroid Therapy
> - Treatment of Complications
>   - Neurological Complications
>   - Renal Failure
>   - Late Serum Sickness
> - Prevention

GENERAL CONSIDERATIONS

Snake bite is a common emergency seen in almost all parts of India. Most of the time snake bites occur with people who are engaged in agricultural operations or while walking in darkness. Snakes are found more frequently around dwelling houses, embankments, cultivated fields and in bushes. They tend to go to places where they get their prey—rodents and frogs. Most of the bites take place in the rural areas though they do occur in towns also. About 35–50 thousand deaths occur in India due to snake bite annually. Most of the poisonous bites (80%) are due to vipers (*Vipera russelli* and *Echis carinatus*), cobras (*Naja naja*) cause 10% and kraits (*Bungarus caeruleus*) 4%. Rarely, poisoning due to sea snakes is encountered (1%). Majority of bites are inflicted by nonpoisonous snakes. The incidence of snake bites varies with the season in different regions. More than 2010 species of snakes are present in India.

Poisonous snakes belong to three families on the basis of poison secreted:
1. ***Elapidae:*** Neurotoxic
   - Common cobra/*Nag* or *Kalsap* or *Naja naja*
   - King cobra—*Raj Nag* or *Naja hanna* or *Naja bangarus*
   - Krait: Subgrouped into:
     - Common krait or *Bangarus caeruleus*
     - Banded krait or *Bangarus fasciatus*
     - Coral snake
     - Tiger snake
     - Mambas
     - Death adder
2. ***Viperidae:*** Vasculotoxic
   - ***Pitless vipers:*** They are:
     - Russel's viper
     - Saw-scaled viper
   - ***Pit vipers:*** They are:
     - Pit viper—crotalidae
     - Common green pit viper
3. ***Hydrophidae:*** Myotoxic
   - 20 types of sea snakes found in India
   - All are poisonous
   - They are myotoxic.

IDENTIFICATION OF POISONOUS SNAKES

- They have large ventral scales covering the whole of the ventral aspect.
- The mouth contains only one pair of poison fangs in the upper jaw, placed anteriorly (krait and cobra) or posteriorly (viper).
- Presence of rows of small teeth is characteristic of non-poisonous snake.

Viper: The head is triangular with a narrow neck. The scales on the body and neck are small and of uniform size. *Vipera russelli* is larger, often grows to one meter in length and shows three rows of oval rings on the body, running along the whole length. *Echis carinatus* has overlapping saw-shaped scales covering its body and a broad arrowmark on its head and two rows of wavy bands running longitudinally.

Pit vipers belonging to the family crotalidae are less common in India. They show a depression between the nose and eye 'the loreal pit'. Vipers have larger fangs which are tunneled and the bite marks are more prominent. Often the snake hangs on to the limb and it has to be disentangled by violent movements.

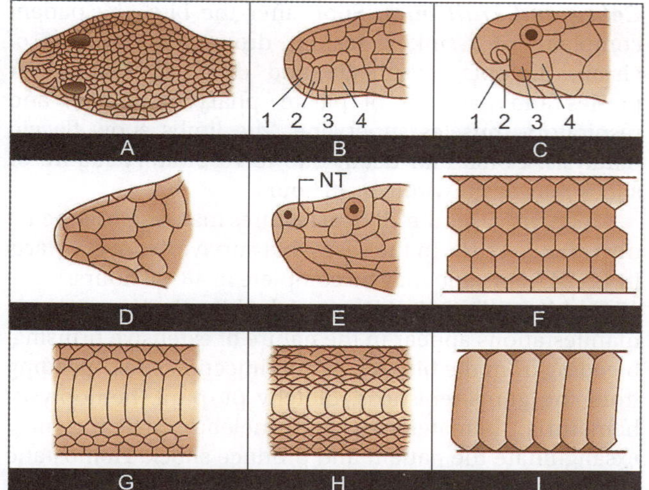

Figs 11.1A to I: Identification of snakes. **A.** Small uniform head scale, narrow neck—viper; **B.** Undersurface of mouth, the 4th inferolateral shield is largest—krait; **C.** Third supralabial shield larger than the rest and touches the shields of the nostril and eye—cobra or coral snake; **D.** Large head shields; **E.** Deep pit midway between the nostril and the eye (Loreal pit)—pit viper; **F and G.** Under surfaces of nonpoisonous snakes—small belly scales and moderately large transverse scales which do not reach the entire length; **H.** Hexagonal row of spinal shields on the dorsum of krait; **I.** Large ventral shields reaching the entire width of the body—poisonous or nonpoisonous

Cobra: Cobra has an expandable neck and the head shows a single (monocellate) or double (binocellate) dark ring on the dorsum. The third supralabial shield touches the eye and nostril. When provoked, the head and neck are raised to form the hood. The fangs are small and anteriorly grooved.

Rarely, King cobras *(Ophiophagus hannah* or *Hamdyard)* may be seen in thick forests but bites by these deadly snakes are very uncommon. They grow to large size (often 3-4 meters) and unlike the cobra, they are unhooded.

Krait: Kraits show white bands on the body—those in the posterior part being more definite. The dorsal scales on the body are hexagonal. The head and sides of the lower jaw are covered with large shields, the fourth shield on the lower jaw being the largest.

Sea snakes: They are found in good numbers in the coastal waters of India. They show laterally compressed and flattened tails. The two common genera seen in the western coast are *Enhydrina* and *Hydrophis* (Figs 11.1A to I).

Snakes bite when they are inadvertently trodden upon. Rarely, cobras may attack but they usually do so only during the mating season.

THE VENOM

Venom is modified saliva and 0.25–1 mL of it is injected into the victim when the snake bites. Snake venom is a toxin (hematotoxin, neurotoxin or cytotoxin). It is modified saliva injected through the fangs from the modified parotid salivary gland located on each side of the skull, behind the eye through a pumping mechanism from the venom sac which stores the venom. Snake venoms contains 90% protein by dry weight and most of these are enzymes

Table 11.1: Components with pathological effects of the venom	
Component	**Action**
Serine proteases	Hemolysis
Other proteases	Hemolysis
Phospholipase A$_2$	Myotoxic, cardiotoxic, neurotoxic, increases vascular permeability
Hyaluronidase	Local tissue destruction
Neurotoxins	Acting on peripheral and autonomic nervous system
α-bungarotoxin, cobrotoxin	Postsynaptic inhibition
β-bungarotoxin, crotoxin	Presynaptic inhibition

which vary from 10–25 in number. Often their action is synergistic.

Composition of Snake Venom (Table 11.1)

Enzymes

- Phospholipase A$_2$ (lecithinase), 5'-nucleotidase, collagenase, L-amino acid oxidase, protinases, hyaluronidase, acetylcholine, phospholipase B mostly in elapidae
- Endopeptidases, kininogenase, factor-X, prothrombin activating enzyme mostly in vipers.

Non-Enzyme Peptides

- α-bungarotoxin, β-bungarotoxin, crotoxin, crotamine, cardiotoxin
- Peptide—pyroglutamyl peptide
- Nucleoside—adenine, guanine, inosine
- Lipid—phospholipid, cholestrol
- Amine—histamine, serotonin, spermin
- Metals—copper, zinc, nickel and magnesium.

The most common enzymes are proteolytic, phospholipases and hyaluronidase.

- Proteolytic enzymes—digestive properties
- Phospholipases—degrade lipids
- Hyaluronidases—facilitates venom spread throughout the body.

Cobra venom is mainly neurotoxic and to a lesser extent cardiotoxic, hematotoxic and cytotoxic. It also blocks the acetylcholine receptors giving rise to myasthenia like features.

The viperine venoms contain hemorrhagic, necrotic, coagulant and hemolytic substances leading to extensive damage to several tissues. Lesions are due to intravascular coagulation, fibrinolysis, damage to the vascular endothelium and extensive necrosis. Involvement of the kidneys and renal failure are common and may be fatal.

Venom of sea snakes is neurotoxic, myotoxic and hematotoxic. This leads to paralysis including respiratory paralysis, severe myalgia and muscle tenderness, myoglobinuria and hyperkalemia. Acute renal failure (ARF) may develop. Local lesion may be minimal or even absent.

The speed of action of the venom depends upon the site of injection and the amount of venom injected. If the venom directly enters the bloodstream, the effect may be rapid and lead to sudden death. In most of the cases, the absorption of venom is slower and especially in viperine bites with extensive local reaction, considerable amount of venom may remain locally to be absorbed into circulation in due course.

Most of the elapid snakes (e.g. cobra) inject 10% of the contents of the poison sac during each bite, whereas the Russell's viper injects most of its content during each bite accounting for severe envenomation by this snake. Venom is of large molecular size and it passes up mainly through the lymphatics. Proximal lymphadenopathy is not uncommon.

The severity of envenomation depends upon the circumstances of the bite. Bites sustained during the early part of the night are generally more serious since, the poison sacs of the snake are full at this time. Bites through clothes are less dangerous. Children and underweight persons suffer more than normal adults since, the concentration of the venom is relatively higher in them. Violent physical activity helps to disseminate the venom rapidly and this worsens the prognosis.

The contents of the venom change between seasons and metabolic activities of the snake.

CLINICAL FEATURES

Immediate response: Severe fright and mental agitation leading to tachycardia, sweating, hypotension and even vascular collapse are prominent features soon after the bite. These nonspecific symptoms may be seen in all snake bites.

Local reactions: They are more prominent in the case of viper bites and less so in others. Intense pain, swelling and violaceous discoloration develop within minutes and often serosanguinous fluid exudes from the fang marks. The edema and discoloration spread proximally and in a few hours vesicles and hemorrhagic blebs may appear. Rarely, gangrene may supervene (Fig. 11.2).

General effects: These vary with the type of snake. Cobra and krait venom are predominantly neurotoxic, while those of vipers are histotoxic and hemorrhagic. Some degree of overlap does occur, especially during certain seasons of the year, cobra bites producing moderate or severe tissue necrosis and viperine bites leading to mild neuroparalysis.

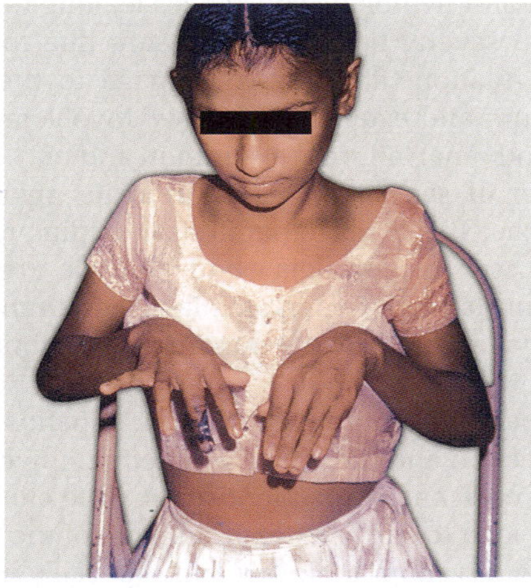

Fig. 11.2: Viper bite. ***Note:*** Gangrene of middle finger right

Cobra and krait bites: Soon after the bite, the patient complains of a sinking feeling, drowsiness, blurring of vision, diplopia, dysphagia and dyspnea. Extraocular palsies and paralysis of palate, pharynx, tongue, and respiratory muscles supervene. The limbs show flaccid paralysis. Coma and death due to respiratory failure or shock may occur within 6–48 hours.

In many cases the clinical features may resemble acute myasthenic crisis. In the cases that survive, recovery starts in 12–24 hours and may be complete in 48–96 hours.

Viper bites: Within 3–4 hours of the bite, the hemorrhagic manifestations appear in the nature of extensive bruising, bleeding from the bitten part and injection sites, bleeding from the gums, epistaxis, blotchy purpura, hemoptysis, hematuria, hematemesis and melena. Bleeding may exsanguinate the patient and produce shock. Hemostatic failure is due to the action of procoagulant contents of the venom which initiates massive thrombosis leading to consumption coagulopathy especially hypo-fibrinogenemia. The clotting time may be prolonged more than 20 minutes and this is a reliable indication of moderately severe envenomation. Platelet count may be reduced.

The blood is uncoagulable when taken in a test tube and estimation of coagulation time provides a fairly reliable side room test for the severity of envenomation and requirement of antivenin. Cardiac manifestations include tachycardia, myocarditis and cardiac failure. Electrocardiogram (ECG) may show abnormal T waves and disturbances of conduction. Pulmonary edema and hemorrhage may develop.

Rarely, optic neuritis may develop leading to partial or complete blindness in 2–7 days. Delayed onset of optic atrophy has also been recorded. Blindness may also result from intraocular bleeding.

Renal changes: Proteinuria and hematuria may develop within a few hours after the bite. In the majority of cases, these subside with treatment. ARF may develop in 50–60% of cases with severe envenomation. This manifests in 3–7 days of the bite. The most frequent and dreaded complication is anuric renal failure developing as a result of direct nephrotoxicity of the venom, hypotension, disseminated intravascular coagulation (DIC), hemoglobinuria and reactions to the antivenom administered therapeutically. Lesions include acute tubular necrosis (ATN), hemorrhagic interstitial nephritis and even glomerulonephritis. Shock aggravates the renal damage. In 10%, anuria may supervene and persist demanding peritoneal or hemodialysis. In survivors, renal sequelae are rare but salt losing nephritis, renal parenchymal calcification and membranous glomer-ulonephritis (MGN) have been reported.

Neurological features such as ptosis, bulbar palsy, ophthalmoplegia and respiratory paralysis may occur in viperine bites as well.

Death in viperine bite is due to shock, hemorrhages, secondary infection, renal failure or cardiac failure.

Long-term sequelae like panhypopituitarism may manifest 3–5 years after severe viperine envenomation. Pituitary apoplexy has been noted. Myxedema may develop rarely.

Table 11.2: Interval between the snake bite and time of death

	Range	Mean
Cobra	30 minutes–60 hours	8½ hours
Krait	3–68 hours	18 hours
Russell's viper	2 hours–9 days	2 days
Echis carinatus	1–41 days	5 days
Sea snakes	12–24 hours	Variable

Krait venom is the most lethal on weight by weight basis. Manifestations are similar to that of a cobra bite but the local reaction at the site of bite may be minimal.

Since, kraits are prone to come into dwelling houses and hide under clothes or other material, bites acquired during sleep and paralysis manifesting on waking up are more likely to be due to krait bites. Careful search of the premises may reveal the offender.

Sea snake bites are identified by the victims as sharp pricks. The local reaction may be insignificant. Signs of envenomation occur within one hour and initial symptoms consist of pain and stiffness of the muscles of the neck, back and proximal parts of the limbs but rapidly becoming generalized. Trismus, ptosis, external ophthalmoplegia and paralysis leading to respiratory failure may follow. Proteinuria and myoglobinuria are seen 3–6 hours after the onset of symptoms. Death is due to respiratory paralysis or renal failure. If the victim survives, muscle weakness may persist for months.

The overall mortality of the poisonous bites is 10–15% (Table 11.2).

Death in snake bites is due to: (1) Paralysis of respiratory muscles, (2) upper airway obstruction, (3) cardiac arrest, (4) hypotension and shock, (5) severe bleeding including intracranial bleed, (6) renal failure and (7) septicemia.

Note: Symptoms produced by snake bites may not always run true to type and there may be overlap in symptoms (Table 11.3). Snakes bites in children are more lethal and those in adults. Since, the amount of venom injected in both is similar.

Table 11.3: Comparative clinical picture in bites caused by common poisonous snakes in India

Feature	Cobras	Kraits	Russell's viper	Sas scaled viper	Hump nosed viper
Local pain/ tissue damage	Yes	No	Yes	Yes	Yes
Ptosis/ neurological signs	Yes	Yes	+/–	No	No
Hemostatic abnormalities	No	–/+	Yes	Yes	Yes
Renal complication	No	No	Yes	No	Yes
Response to neostigmine	Yes	No	No	No	No
Response to ASV	Yes	Yes	Yes	Yes	No

Abbreviation: ASV = Anti-snake venom

Panic and violent movements such as running or attempts to find the snake favour rapid dissemination of the venom. Bites sustained on arms soles, scrotum and face are more dangerous since, the envenomation is more effective. Bites on naked skin are more dangerous than bites through protective clothing or shoes. Since the venom sacs are full in the early hours of the night before the snake catches its prey, bites sustained at that time are more dangerous.

MANAGEMENT

The most important step is to start first aid, reassure the victim and to decide upon the need for specific antivenom. Information from the local inhabitants can be very helpful from distinction between poisonous and nonpoisonous bites.

Poisonous	Nonpoisonous
Only two fang marks	Multiple teeth marks
Local reaction present	No local reaction
Evidence of systemic envenomation present	Only fright reaction

Proper first aid is vitally important to reduce envenomation and this plays a major role in subsequent treatment. The bitten part should be immobilized using an improvised splint, washed well with soap and water and a proper tourniquet applied nearest to the site of bite where there is only a single bone. This tourniquet should occlude the lymphatics and veins but not the arteries. Chilling the limb in ice reduces the rate of absorption of venom. Immediate hospitalization is required.

General treatment consists of reassurance, sedation with diazepam, treatment of shock, antibiotics to cover the infection and immunization against tetanus and gas gangrene. Corticosteroids may be necessary to combat shock. Metronidazole in a dose of 500 mg intravenously (IV) every 8 hours is very useful in treating anaerobic sepsis which invariably accompanies the snake bite.

Specific Treatment

Specific treatment is to administer anti-snake venom (ASV) which should be given only if signs of envenomation are definite or if the snake is identified to be definitely poisonous. The ASV available in India is made by Haffkine Bio Pharmaceutical Corporation Ltd, Bombay and the Central Drug Research Institute, Kasauli. It is polyvalent. One mL of reconstituted ASV can neutralize 0.6 mg each of Cobra, Krait, Russell's viper and saw scaled viper venoms. It is prepared from serum of horses hyperimmunized with the venom and is available as the lyophilized product with the diluent.

Once reconstituted, the ASV has to be used immediately as it rapidly loses its potency. Being made from horse serum, it has to be tested for anaphylaxis by intradermal and IV methods before administration and the product instructions should be carefully followed. ASV neutralizes the venom and it is the most effective antidote to abolish the hemorrhagic manifestations of viperine bites.

The total dose of ASV depends on the severity of envenomation.

Dose of ASV	
Mild envenomation	3–5 vials
Moderate envenomation	5–10 vials
Severe envenomation	10–20 vials
Very severe envenomation	20–40 vials

ASV is given IV as a drip or slow push doses. Many authorities recommend higher doses of the order of 50-100 mL as initial dose. Several studies and publications have appeared on the total dose and timing of administration of ASV. In general, the consensus is to use moderate doses that are effective, without over dosing the patient since the latter is associated with immediate complications such as anaphylaxis and delayed side effects such as serum sickness and prolonged disability.

Children and underweight persons require the same dose of ASV as for the normal adults.

In cases allergic to horse serum, ASV may have to be withheld. In such cases, desensitization may be done by injecting small quantities of ASV under cover of corticosteroids, before administering the full dose.

The tourniquet if applied proximal to the bite should be released after systemic administration of antivenom. Wound toilet and protective dressings must be done. Incisions, suction, drainage and local instillation of ASV which used to be in vogue earlier are not undertaken. With adequate dosage of systemic ASV such aggressive measures can be avoided.

Guidelines for repetition of ASV: Recurrence of the signs of envenomation and presence of non-coagulability of blood after initial improvement are indications for repeating the ASV. Clotting and clot retraction can also be employed to assess the adequacy of ASV in viparine bites.

Antivenom administration is adequate if the clotting time is within 20 minutes, the clot retraction is complete within 6 hours and the serum is straw colored.

If clotting time is prolonged beyond 20 minutes a further 10 vials may be needed.

If clotting time is below 20 minutes but clot retraction is poor after 6 hours, a further 5 vials of ASV are needed.

If clotting and clot retraction are normal, but the serum is red, two vials have to be given further.

For neurotoxic bites, since there is no laboratory parameter to monitor treatment, higher doses are often used. ASV should be given if signs of envenomation are present even if the patient is seen 1–2 days after the bite. Trials employing regimen containing higher and moderate doses of ASV have shown that the latter is quite adequate, if laboratory monitoring is possible and the clinical condition is stable. Cases which have received smaller doses of ASV have quicker recovery and shorter hospitalization. Therefore, overdose of ASV should be avoided. The cost of 1 vial of ASV ranges around Rs. 300.

Adverse Reactions to ASV

These may occur in 20% of cases. They may be mild, moderate or even severe and therefore, the physician should anticipate them and be prepared to take remedial measures. Usually they start along with the injection or within 20 minutes of the dose or delayed even beyond 3 hours. Initial symptoms include utricaria, itching, fever, chills, nausea, vomiting. diarrhea, abdominal cramps, angioedema, tachycardia, hypotension, bronchospasm.

Management of Adverse Reactions

Stop the infusion of ASV, give adrenaline, 1/1000 solution, 1 mL intramuscular (IM). This can be repeated after 5 minutes if necessary. Many cases may also require injectable antihistaminics and/or hydrocortisone 100 mg in bolus and 300 mg added to 500 mL glucose saline to run slowly. In most of the cases, the panic may have to be controlled by anti-anxiety drugs such as alprazolam (1 mg). Pain has to be controlled by analgesics such as nonsteroidal anti-inflammatory drugs (NSAIDs) or paracetamol.

Some cases do not tolerate even small doses of ASV, these have to be managed by supportive therapy in an acute care unit or intensive care unit (ICU) taking care of the pain, anxiety, metabolic and fluid requirements, status of the vital organs and treatment of infection at the bite wound and other infective complication. Intensive treatment without antivenom can safe quite a number of patients and therefore these should be instituted in institutions where facilities are available.

Steroid Therapy

In a few cases, methylprednisolone given in a dose of 1 g IV daily for 2–3 days may be life-saving. The indications include: (1) Hypotension persisting after fluid and electrolyte correction before the administration of antivenin (2) periorbital puffiness, (3) chemosis of conjunctiva, (4) acute respiratory distress and (5) edema due to capillary leak.

TREATMENT OF COMPLICATIONS

Neurological complications: Since cobra and krait bites may lead to acute myasthenic reaction with respiratory paralysis, prompt administration of neostigmine can be life-saving (Fig. 11.3). IV doses of 2.5 mg repeated at suitable intervals brings about prompt relief. Premedication with atropine abolishes the troublesome side effects. Respiratory failure has to be managed with artificial ventilation, if injection of neostigmine does not work.

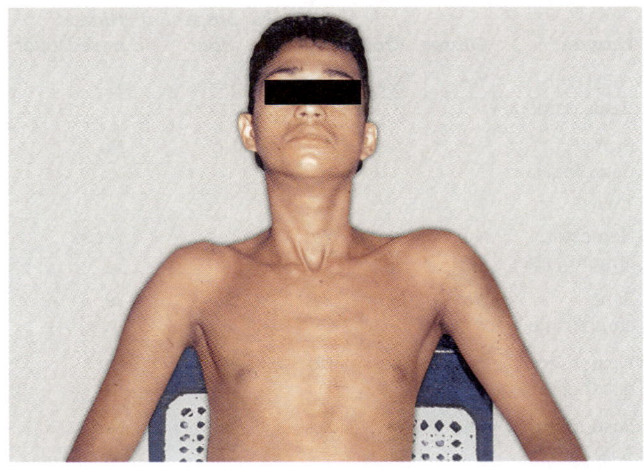

Fig. 11.3: Cobra bite with myasthenic reaction

Renal failure has to be anticipated in all cases of viperine bites. Urine volume has to be regularly monitored. Early institution of hemodialysis and careful management of renal failure in an institution with facilities for renal support have helped to save many patients, who would otherwise have died. Extensive local sloughing may demand skin grafting.

Late serum sickness like reaction: This manifests 1–12 days after the ASV treatment. It ushers in with fever, nausea, vomiting, diarrhea, arthralgia, renal symptoms, myoglobinuria and others. Treatment consists of fluid management, supportive care and glucocorticoids.

Long-term complications of viper bites include—panhypopituitarism either florid or in different degrees the target endocrine glands being affected selectively, they may require continued endocrine replacement.

PREVENTION

Snakes should not be indiscriminately killed since, they play a major role keeping the rodent population under check. Snake bites can be avoided by:

- Carrying a torch while walking in the snake infested areas
- Wearing shoes and other protective clothing
- Using a stick which if tapped on the ground, scares away most of the snakes.

Potent antivenin in sufficient quantity should be readily available in all the hospitals situated in snake-infested areas.

Source: HS Bawaskar-snake bite poisoning. In API Textbook of Medicine 9th edition, 2012, p. 955-59, edited by YP Munjal. Jaypee Brothers Medical Publishers (P) Ltd.

CHAPTER 12

Disorders caused by Heat

KV Krishna Das, TK Suma

Chapter Summary

- General Considerations
- Heat Stroke
- Anhidrotic Heat Exhaustion
- Heat Syncope
- Water Depletion Heat Exhaustion
- Salt Depletion Heat Exhaustion
- Heat Cramps
- Skin Lesions caused by Exposure to Sun and Hot Environment

GENERAL CONSIDERATIONS

Man has a remarkable ability to withstand physical stresses and strains, and adapt to varying environment. When changes in climate are abrupt, adaptation may not be possible in some individuals and this leads to adverse effects. Ill-effects of heat are seen in tropical conditions either among the natives or the new entrants. Heat is dissipated from the human body by conduction, convection and radiation, through breathing and by evaporation of the sweat, which is the most effective way. Radiation accounts for 65% of body heat loss under normal conditions. But at high temperatures evaporation becomes the major mechanism for dissipation of heat. Heat disorders result from the breakdown of heat regulatory mechanisms. The clinical picture may be acute or chronic.

On a very hot day, the total loss of water in the form of sweat may reach 5–6 L with a salt loss of 10–12 g. When acclimatization occurs there is increase in extracellular fluid volume, which is accommodated by expanded vascular bed. This results in reduction of the pulse rate and increase in the cardiac output. The sweat glands start producing more sweat even at lower temperatures. Excretion of salt is reduced by lowering the levels of salt in the sweat (2 g/L) and urine, mainly due to activation of renin-angiotensin system (RAS) and increased production of aldosterone. Acclimatization to hot environment by proper training occurs in 10–14 days. Acclimatized individuals are capable of performing well in hot climates, provided the intake of water and salt are adequate (5–6 L and 15–20 g/day, respectively).

There is evidence that the global temperature is going up steadily due to various factors such as increase in population, burning of fossil fuels, denudation of forest cover, irrigation schemes and the effect of heat-trapping gases which produce a greenhouse effect. The major greenhouse gases are water vapor, carbon dioxide, methane, nitrous oxide and ozone. The Intergovernmental Panel on Climate Change (IPCC) has predicted that the global temperature may go up by 2.5°C by 2100 AD. In addition to the direct effects of warming it may also increase the incidence of natural disasters and vector transmitted diseases. It is estimated that the sea level will rise by an additional 19 inches by 2100, due to increased ocean warming and increased loss of mass from glaciers and icesheets. Heatwaves will be more frequent and more intense. Droughts and wildfires will occur more often. Disease-carrying mosquitoes will expand their range. More than one million species could be committed to extinction by 2050 if global warming pollution is not curtailed.

Despite wide variations in ambient temperatures, humans and other mammals can maintain a constant body temperature by balancing heat gain with heat loss. When heat gain overwhelms the body's mechanisms of heat loss, the body temperature rises and a major heat illness ensues. Excessive heat denatures proteins, destabilizes phospholipids and lipoproteins, and liquefies membrane lipids, leading to cardiovascular collapse, multiorgan failure and ultimately death. Management of heat related disorders is closely linked with that of fluids and electrolytes.

HEAT STROKE

Syn: Heat hyperpyrexia

Definition, Etiology and Pathogenesis

Heat stroke follows exposure to heat and is characterized by hyperpyrexia owing to deranged heat regulatory mechanism. Heat stroke is defined clinically as a body temperature than 41.1°C (106°F) associated with neurological dysfunction. Heat stroke occur in two forms— from exposure to a high environmental temperature especially heat waves (classic or non-exertional heatstroke) or from strenuous exercise (exertional heatstroke). Heat stroke generally occurs at temperatures ranging from 40 to 45°C, but may also occur at temperatures as low as 30–35°C, especially if the humidity is high. The external temperature at which heatstroke occurs varies between individuals and therefore is not a reliable parameter for diagnosis. Elderly individuals and infants, patients with skin disease and those with cardiac dysfunction are more prone for heatstroke. Precipitating factors include lack of acclimatization, unaccustomed and sustained heavy work at high temperatures, alcoholism, infections, dehydration, use of drugs like atropine, antihistamines, phenothiazines, antidepressants and diuretics, and obesity.

The systemic and cellular responses to heat stress include thermoregulation, an acute-phase response whereby various cytokines and acute-phase proteins are liberated and the production of heat-shock proteins (HSP). Increased levels of HSP in a cell induce a transient state of tolerance to heat stress, allowing the cell to survive. Thermoregulatory failure, exaggeration of the acute-phase response and alteration in the expression of HSP contribute to development of heatstroke.

Flowchart 12.1 showing the effects of heat on the human system and the contributory factors which worsen the ill-effects.

Predisposing Factors

- Increased heat production
  - Hyperthyroidism
  - Exercise
  - Sepsis
- Impaired heat loss-impaired sweating
  - ***Drugs:*** Anticholinergics, antiparkinsonian drugs, antihistamines, butyrophenones, phenothiazines, tricyclics
  - Abnormal sweat glands
    - Sweat gland injury following acute heatstroke, barbiturate poisoning
    - Cystic fibrosis
    - Healed thermal burn salt and water depletion
    - Diuretic induced
  - Hypokalemia

Flowchart 12.1: Effects of heat on the human system

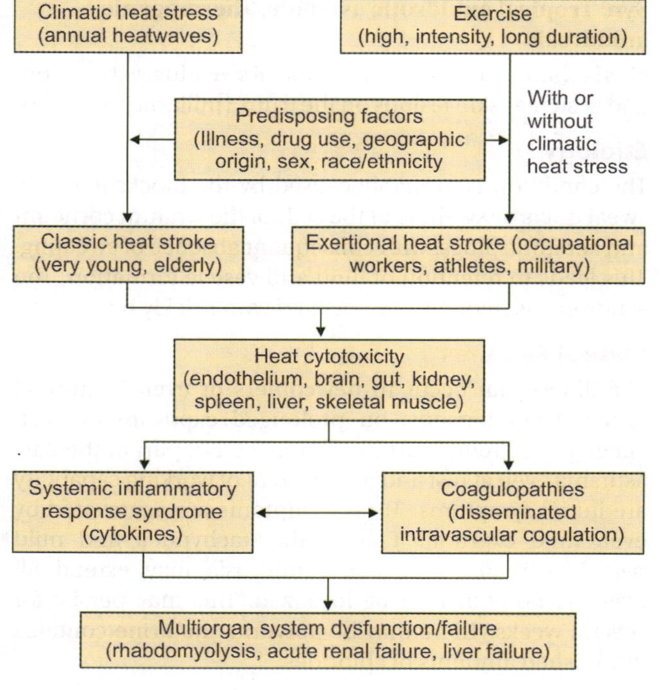

- Impaired voluntary mechanisms
  - Coma
  - Physical disability
  - Mental illness
- Impaired delivery of blood to peripheral circulation
  - Cardiovascular disease
  - Hypokalemia (decreased muscle blood flow)
  - Dehydration
- Others
  - Elderly
  - High ambient temperature and humidity, poor ventilation
  - Lack of acclimatization
  - Obesity
  - Fatigue
  - Diabetes mellitus (DM)
  - Malnutrition
  - Alcoholism.

Clinical Features

The onset is sudden or even abrupt with a rapid rise of body temperature to 41°C or more with acute neurological features such as confusion, restlessness, delirium, agitation, convulsions and coma. In few patients, there may be prodrome such as headache, giddiness, thirst, irrational behavior and restlessness, and onset is gradual.

The cardinal diagnostic features are hyperpyrexia, neuropsychiatric disturbances and a hot and dry skin (hot dry man). The temperature varies from 41.5 to 44°C. It is preferable to take the rectal temperature in these cases. The patient will have tachycardia and tachypnea. Twenty five percent of patients may have hypotension due to peripheral vasodilatation. Electrocardiogram (ECG) shows T wave changes suggestive of myocardial involvement.

Complications

The most serious complication of heatstroke is multi-organ dysfunction. This includes encephalopathy, rhabdomyolysis, acute renal failure (ARF), acute respiratory distress syndrome, myocardial injury, hepatocellular injury, intestinal ischemia or infarction, pancreatic injury and hemorrhagic complications, especially due to disseminated intravascular coagulation (DIC). Untreated, the condition is fatal owing to circulatory, hepatic or renal failure.

Diagnosis

Diagnosis should be suspected in the presence of the three cardinal features, viz. hyperpyrexia, neurologic disturbances and a hot and dry skin in a subject exposed to high ambient temperature. It is important to rule out falciparum malaria and sometimes malaria may coexist with heatstroke. Other conditions like septicemia, pyogenic meningitis, encephalitis, pontine hemorrhage and closed head injuries have to be excluded.

Laboratory Features

It include neutrophil leucocytosis, thrombocytopenia, elevation of blood urea bilirubin, uric acid and reduction of plasma bicarbonate, potassium, sodium, calcium and phosphorus. None of these are diagnostically specific. Therefore, diagnosis has to be clinical. The following records

Textbook of Medicine

have to be maintained and periodically updated to monitor the progress of the patient.

- Temperature recording, complete hematology including platelets, urine output and urinary abnormalities particularly myoglobinuria
- Electrolytes, urea, creatinine, calcium
- Liver function tests (LFT)
- Fasting blood glucose, clotting time, fibrinogen, fibrinogen degradation products (FDP), D-dimer.
- Creatine phosphokinase (CPK)
- Arterial blood gases (ABG)
- ECG monitoring.

First Aid for Heat Stroke or Sunstroke

- Remove victim to cooler location, out of the sun.
- Loosen or remove clothing and immerse victim in very cool water if possible.
- If immersion is not possible, cool the victim with water, or wrap in wet sheets and fan for quick evaporation.
- Use cold compresses especially to the head and neck area, also to armpits and groin.
- Seek medical attention immediately—continue first aid to lower temperature until medical help takes over.
- Do not give any medication to lower fever—it will not be effective and may cause further harm.
- It is not advisable to give the victim anything by mouth (even water) until the condition has been stabilized.

Treatment

Heat stroke is a medical emergency. Treatment aims at the reduction of the core temperature to 39°C within one hour (Box 12.1), restoration of circulating blood volume and support of various organ system functions.

The patient is covered with wet sheets or towels and sprayed with cold water while air is blown or fanned over him to promote evaporative cooling. The patient should preferably be in the lateral recumbent position or hands and knees position to expose as much of skin as possible to the air. As an alternative the patient may be immersed in cold water. Immersion in ice water is not preferred because of the possibility of shivering and hypotension. The limbs are gently massaged to promote circulation. When the rectal temperature falls to 39°C the patient is transferred to a cool room and watched for further rise of temperature. Recurrence is quite common and temperature regulation may remain unstable for weeks. Rapid cooling to rectal temperatures below 38–39°C may precipitate convulsions, vomiting and hypotension.

Prompt and effective cooling restores neurological functions in the majority of patients. Recovery of central nervous system function is a favorable prognostic sign.

Box 12.1: Commonly employed cooling methods

- Cooling by evaporation—swabbing the body with lukewarm water and exposing to fan breeze
- Immersion in cold water
- Ice packs applied strategically—torso and limbs
- Cooling blankets
- Cooled intravenous (IV) fluids administered carefully
- Gastric lavage with cold water
- Treating in an air-conditioned environment with temperature control.

Chlorpromazine was the mainstay of therapy in the past but better avoided due to its deleterious effects such as reduction in seizure threshold and interference with thermoregulation. Antipyretics like acetaminophen, aspirin or other nonsteroidal anti-inflammatory drugs (NSAIDs) have no role and are contraindicated. Aggressive fluid resuscitation is not recommended even in the presence of hypotension since it may lead to pulmonary edema.

If there is suspicion of malaria, antimalarials are given parenterally. Shock and cardiac failure have to be treated appropriately. The patient should also be observed and treated for renal failure due to rhabdomyolysis, DIC and hepatic failure. Maintenance of hydration and electrolyte balance are important to prevent renal failure.

Sequelae: It include headache, insomnia, giddiness, cerebellar dysfunction and even coma. Most of these clear up in the course of weeks or months.

Prognosis: If left untreated, 50–70% of subjects die of heatstroke. Early treatment reduces the mortality to 15-20%. Shock also carries a bad prognosis. Presence of other systemic diseases and extremes of age worsen the prognosis.

Prevention: Heat stroke is a preventable disease. To prevent heatstroke, people should acclimatize themselves to heat, schedule outdoor activities during cooler times of the day, reduce level of physical activity, drink additional water and consume extra amounts of salt (12–15 g/day).

Points to Remember

- Heat stroke, which is preventable, occurs at temperatures ranging from 40 to 45°C.
- Heat stroke could be exertional or non-exertional.
- Neuropsychiatric manifestations are prominent.
- Multiorgan dysfunction is the usual cause of death.
- Shock, extremes of age and systemic diseases are bad prognostic features.

ANHIDROTIC HEAT EXHAUSTION

Syn: Tropical anhidrotic asthenia, Thermogenic anhidrosis

This is characterized by depression of sweating, exhaustion, and vesicular skin lesions on the trunk (miliaria profunda).

Etiology

The condition is probably caused by the blockage of the sweat ducts by swelling of the cells of the stratum corneum and keratotic plugs, with consequent absence of sweating. This leads to retention of fluid and vesicle formation. The syndrome is frequently associated with prickly heat.

Clinical Features

The illness can occur in newcomers or even in normal acclimatized persons, on prolonged exposure to heat. Feeling of extreme warmth during the hot part of the day, asthenia even at rest and impairment of working capability are initial symptoms. These symptoms are aggravated by even mild exertion. Tachycardia, tachypnea and mild pyrexia (38–40.5°C) occur. Anhidrosis may extend all over the body or may be localized. This may persist for several weeks. There may be polyuria, the urine contains diminished amounts of chlorides.

Skin lesions superficially resemble prickly heat, but in miliaria profunda there is no erythema around the lesions and these are seen most commonly in the proximal parts of the limbs and on the trunk.

Diagnosis

Clinical diagnosis is based upon the symptoms.

Treatment

The patient should be transferred to cool surroundings. Recovery is generally rapid. Resumption of work in hot environment may lead to relapse.

Points to Remember
- Anhidrotic heat exhaustion is caused by blockage of sweat ducts
- Frequently associated with prickly heat
- Asthenia even at rest and impairment of work capacity are early features
- Diagnosis is based on symptoms.

HEAT SYNCOPE

Syn: Heat collapse

Heat syncope may occur in a hot environment in the absence of demonstrable water and salt depletion. Heat syncope may occur in a wide range of temperatures, not necessarily the highest. The condition may affect new-comers or the natives in the locality doing excessive physical exertion.

Syncope results from cutaneous vasodilatation and resultant systemic and cerebral hypotension, pooling of blood in the blood vessels of the muscles and skin, especially of the lower limbs, during or after physical activity.

Clinical Features

Syncope or collapse occurs either during or immediately after heat exposure on prolonged standing or sudden change of posture. Giddiness, vertigo and nausea are common. The patient is pale with shallow breathing and frequent yawning. The blood pressure (BP) is low and the pulse is slowed as in vasovagal syncope. The symptoms may pass off in a few minutes after lying down. Rapid recovery occurs if the patient is transferred to cool environment.

Diagnosis

Syncope with postural changes during or immediately after heat exposure, without demonstrable water or salt depletion and the rapid recovery of the patient are diagnostic.

Treatment

The patient should be transported to a cool room and put to bed. Adequate fluids in the form of simple beverages should be given and urine output maintained at 1.5 L per day. The patient should be encouraged to take adequate amounts of salt (15–20 g/day) to avoid recurrence.

Points to Remember
- Heat syncope occurs in the absence of demonstrable water and salt depletion.
- Syncope is secondary to cutaneous vasodilatation.
- Rapid recovery results when patient is transferred to cool environment.
- Intake of adequate quantity of water and salt are to be ensured for recovery.

WATER DEPLETION HEAT EXHAUSTION

This type of dehydration is caused from prolonged strenuous activity in a hot environment with inadequate intake of water and other fluids. This is usually preceded by a period of prolonged sweating which leads to considerable loss of water. Children are more susceptible to this disorder than adults.

Etiology and Pathogenesis

The major factor is water deprivation, which may be due to insufficient provision of water at the place of work or voluntary avoidance of fluids in between meals. Negative water balance develops in persons doing heavy manual work in hot environment due to excessive sweating; 6–8 L of sweat may be lost in a day. Loss of water leads to increase in the osmolarity of the extracellular fluid (ECF) and then intracellular water moves into the extracellular compartment. Salt depletion and hyponatremia occur if salt intake is inadequate. Heat exhaustion is characterized by dehydration, sodium depletion or isotonic fluid loss with associated cardiovascular changes.

Clinical Features

Severe thirst is experienced in the early stages. The patient sweats even when the extremities are cold. Other early symptoms are nonspecific such as dryness of the mouth, irritability, restlessness and weakness. Hyperventilation secondary to heat exhaustion can lead to respiratory alkalosis. In the fully established case dysphagia, hoarseness of voice, tachycardia, hypotension, oliguria and anuria follow. Untreated, mental changes such as delirium and coma supervene, and the condition may end fatally.

Diagnosis

The circumstances under which this syndrome occurs viz. the high environmental temperature and the clinical picture, especially with intense thirst, are diagnostic in a conscious patient. Difficulties arise in comatose patients who are also febrile. Distinction from salt deficiency may be difficult but the high sodium content of urine and plasma help to distinguish pure water depletion state.

Treatment

Patient should be kept at rest in a cool room. In mild cases, oral fluids and flavored drinks are adequate. In severe cases, the oral intake should be 5–8 L on the first day with 15–20 g sodium chloride. In an unconscious patient, 5% dextrose solution is given intravenously in the first 24 hours with close monitoring of urine output. The levels of serum sodium, urinary sodium and chloride should be estimated, and deficiencies should be corrected. Increasing urine output, rise of BP and return of weight to normal are indications of clinical recovery.

SALT DEPLETION HEAT EXHAUSTION

This condition is characterized by asthenic symptoms, because of salt depletion caused by prolonged sweating without sufficient intake. The symptoms are fatigue, nausea, vomiting, giddiness, insomnia and cramps, but these patients do not complain of thirst.

Textbook of Medicine

Etiopathogenesis

Unacclimatized subjects engaged in hard work in a hot environment are affected. There is considerable variation in susceptibility. Salt depletion has been proved to play a major role in the pathogenesis. There is a fall in osmolarity of extracellular fluid leading to movement of water intracellularly and consequent reduction in ECF volume. Plasma sodium and chloride levels fall.

Clinical Features

A wide spectrum of symptoms may occur. In many patients, there is a prodromal phase with vague symptoms like anorexia, nausea, giddiness and headache. Even at this stage the patient sweats profusely and the urine output is reduced. Diagnosis at this stage may not be very clear in the absence of cramps. The severe illness is characterized by asthenia and painful cramps. As the condition progresses, tachycardia, hypotension, dehydration, oliguria and even shock ensue. Postural syncope is common. Coma and pulmonary edema precede death.

Laboratory Findings

Plasma sodium and chloride levels are proportionately reduced. Volume and salt content of urine are low. Severe dehydration leads to prerenal azotemia.

Diagnosis

The salt depletion heat exhaustion has to be differentiated from the water depletion type by the absence of thirst, the presence of muscle cramps and oliguria with low levels of sodium and chloride in urine.

Treatment

In mild cases, oral replacement with 4–5 L of normal saline in 24 hours may be adequate. Ten or twenty g of salt can be added to food and drinks as supplement. Severe cases require IV fluids. Two L of isotonic saline are given in the first four hours rapidly with monitoring of urine volume and urinary chloride. IV 3% saline may be necessary if sodium depletion is severe. Recovery is rapid. Consumption of extra salt in food and drinks helps to prevent recurrence.

Points to Remember

- In salt depletion, heat exhaustion asthenic symptoms occur due to salt depletion.
- Usually there is a prodromal phase with vague symptoms.
- Asthenia and painful cramps, and absence of thirst are characteristic features.
- With severe sodium depletion, IV 3% saline infusion may be required.

HEAT CRAMPS

This occurs in persons who sweat excessively in hot environment without having normal or supplementary salt intake. This is a milder form of salt deficiency heat exhaustion. Severe cramps develop in the voluntary muscles. These are painful and may last from a few seconds to several minutes. The cramps are precipitated by heavy work, are very painful and commonly involve the extremities. Muscle cramps recur at intervals. Laboratory evaluation may show low serum sodium, hemoconcentration and elevated urea and creatinine. Oral supplementation of 10–15 g of salt relieves the cramps in mild cases. In more severe cases, administration of 600 mL normal saline gives dramatic relief. The patient has to take rest for 1–3 days with continued dietary salt supplementation before returning to work.

SKIN LESIONS CAUSED BY EXPOSURE TO SUN AND HOT ENVIRONMENT

Direct exposure to sun leads to sunburn and solar keratosis. Prickly heat develops in persons exposed to hot environment even without direct exposure to the sun.

Sunburn: It is caused by direct exposure to ultraviolet (UV) light. Fair-skinned persons, especially newcomers are more commonly affected. Symptoms start with erythema and pruritus and proceed to acute painful edema, vesiculation and bullae formation. Prolonged and repeated exposure results in increased pigmentation and improved tolerance. Local application of calamine lotion containing 0.5% crystal violet or any antihistaminic cream gives relief. Para-amino benzoic acid, which absorbs ultraviolet light, gives some protection and this can be applied as a cream (5%) or lotion. Prevention consists of avoidance of direct exposure and the use of protective clothing and umbrella.

Solar keratosis: Repeated exposure to direct sunlight causes patchy hyperkeratosis. The neck, back, dorsum of the hands and forehead are affected maximally. Albinos suffer more. These lesions may predispose to melanoma.

Miliaria rubra (prickly heat): These are papular lesions seen in persons exposed to hot environment, especially if humidity is high. This condition results from blockage of sweat glands by the prickle cell layer of the epidermis, escape of sweat in to the epidermis and further inflammatory changes. Areas covered by clothing are more severely affected. Papular lesions develop which may become vesicular or pustular with surrounding erythema. These may be associated with pruritus and a prickly sensation. Secondary infection may develop later.

Treatment: Local application of calamine lotion gives soothing relief. Excessive washing of the skin with strong soap should be avoided. Use of bland soaps and regular use of gingeli oil (sesame oil) over the skin applied for one hour weekly prevents this lesion in the native population. In established cases, stay in a cold environment and use of loose clothing brings about relief in 2–3 weeks.

CHAPTER
13

Injuries due to Cold

TK Suma, KV Krishna Das

Chapter Summary
- Freezing Cold Injury
- Non-freezing Cold Injury
- Hypothermia

FREEZING COLD INJURY

Syn: Frostbite

It is defined as the freezing and crystalizing of fluids in the interstitial and cellular spaces as a consequence of prolonged exposure to freezing temperatures. This is seen in persons exposed to temperatures below –10°C, such as mountaineers, explorers, war casualties or victims of natural disasters. This can also occur in winter seasons especially in diabetics with compromised vascularity of extremities. The fingers, toes, ears, nose and lips are the areas susceptible to frostbite. There is freezing of extravascular fluid with formation of ice crystals in tissues leading to damage of vascular endothelium, microvascular thrombosis, ischemia and superficial necrosis. Paresthesia and stiffness occur with involvement of deeper tissues. The skin looses its elasticity and becomes immobile. Blisters, edema, necrosis and gangrene may set in (Fig. 13.1). In mild cases where only the skin and subcutaneous tissues are involved numbness, prickling and itching are possible.

Management

The goal of treatment is to salvage as much tissue as possible, to achieve maximal return of function and to prevent complications.

Rewarming: General warming of the body to elevate core temperature should be undertaken before local warming of the affected limb. After restoration of the core temperature, the affected limb should be warmed in a moving water bath preheated to 40–42°C. During thawing, re-establishment of circulation may result in intense pain due to release of multiple inflammatory mediators. Analgesics and antibiotics are given if indicated. Protection of the affected part by avoiding friction or pressure is important. Tetanus prophylaxis has to be considered as there is increased susceptibility. Antiplatelet agents, hemodilution, peripheral vasodilators and hyperbaric oxygen are other therapies used with varying results. Early sympathetic blockade may reduce symptoms, but use of sympathectomy is controversial. The condition can be prevented by covering the body with proper clothing, protection of the affected part, avoidance of local pressure, frequent changes of position and smoking.

Points to Remember
- Frostbite occurs when exposed to temperature below freezing point.
- Damage to vascular endothelium caused by the ice crystals is the main pathology.
- In mild cases, only the skin and subcutaneous tissue are involved.
- Severe cases produce paresthesia, weakness and gangrene.

NON-FREEZING COLD INJURY

Syn: Trench foot, Immersion foot

Exposure to cold damp environment above freezing point for long periods leads to tissue ischemia. This is seen in warfare, people marooned in floods, cases of shipwreck and other natural calamities. Initially, the limb is cold, numb and pale (prehyperemic phase). During the hyperemic phase, they become hot with intense pain and burning. The posthyperemic phase is the vasospastic period where the skin becomes pale or cyanotic. Movements may not be possible. Arterial pulses may be undetectable. The limbs are especially susceptible to trauma and infection leading on to gangrene and maceration. In many cases, permanent sequelae like sensorimotor defects may result. Secondary complications are lymphangitis, cellulitis and thrombophlebitis.

Management

The body is gradually warmed by exposure to air at room temperature, keeping the limb elevated and taking care to avoid overheating of the part. Analgesics and antibiotics should be given as indicated. Chilblains result from minor forms of cold injury. This manifestation is reversible if the environment is altered.

Points to Remember
- Trench foot occurs on exposure to damp environment above freezing point.
- Three phases—prehyperemic, hyperemic and posthyperemic.
- Permanent sequelae like sensorimotor defects may occur.
- Gradual warming of the part without overheating reverses lesion.

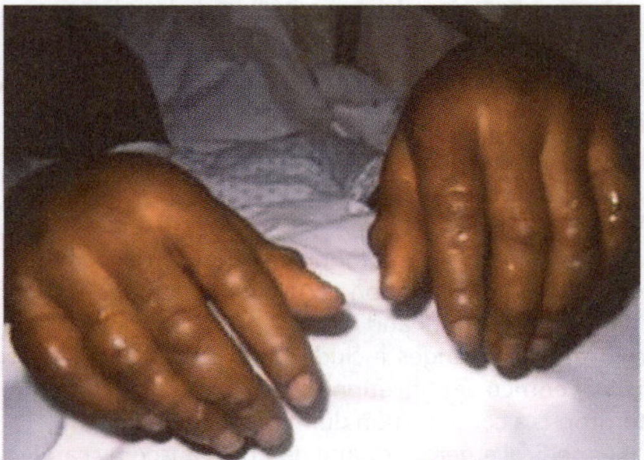

Fig. 13.1: Blisters of fingers due to frostbite

HYPOTHERMIA

When the core temperature falls below 35°C (95°F), condition is called ***hypothermia*** (HT). It may be induced for therapeutic purpose or may be accidental. The latter is serious and it affects persons at extremes of age with disturbed thermoregulatory mechanisms or may be caused by disease, starvation or injury. It can occur in fit subjects when subjected to extreme cold without protection.

Accidental Hypothermia

This condition develops during cold-water immersion, shipwreck, mountaineering, etc. HT may be rapid or slow depending upon the rate of cooling. When cooling is slow, compensatory mechanisms set in. Starvation, alcoholism and drugs like phenothiazines aggravate the ill-effects of cold environment. Diseases like hypothyroidism, hypopituitarism, hypoadrenalism and cirrhosis of the liver predispose to HT. Physiological functions such as oxygen consumption, myocardial repolarization, peripheral nerve conduction, gastrointestinal (GI) motility and respiration will be slowed down due to systemic HT.

Clinical Features

HT can be staged from 1 to 4 (Table 13.1) based on symptoms, higher the grade, worse is the prognosis for recovery. The appearance of a patient with accidental HTs is characteristic. The skin is pale, cold and cyanotic. Initial manifestations include lethargy, drowsiness, irritability, confusion and impaired coordination. As the core temperature falls below 35°C, there is progressive slowing down of cerebral functions resulting in mental stupor and subsequently leads to coma.

Shivering may occur if the temperature is above 30°C but below this level the muscles become spastic and resemble rigor mortis. Respiration is slow and shallow. Tissues suffer from hypoxia, since the oxygen dissociation curve of hemoglobin shifts to the left at low temperatures. Cardiovascular signs include bradycardia, hypotension and cardiac arrhythmias like atrial fibrillation and ventricular fibrillation.

Cardiac arrest is likely to occur when the core temperature drops to 25°C. Electrocardiographic (ECG) changes such as prolongation of PR and QT intervals and J waves (positive deflection at the end of QRS complex) may occur. Biochemical abnormalities include hypoglycemia, metabolic acidosis, hyperkalemia and mild azotemia. Thyroid function may be depressed.

Complications

The core temperature usually continues to drop further for 10–20 minutes even after removing the patient from the cold environment. This phenomenon is called 'afterdrop'. Respiratory infections are common in cases of HT.

Differential Diagnosis

This includes myxedema coma which closely resembles HT, poisoning, starvation, hypoglycemia and neurological disorders.

Treatment

Accidental HT has to be managed as a medical emergency to save life, if possible in an intensive care room. As in all comatose patients attention should be given to the maintenance of patent airway, proper ventilation, blood volume and levels of electrolytes.

External re-warming is effective in the mildly hypothermic patient. External re-warming is done in a moving water bath heated to 40–42°C. When the core temperature has reached 34–35°C, the patient is placed on a warm bed and insulated against further heat loss. Antibiotics are required in many patients. In severe cases, it is advisable to increase core temperature by hemodialysis or repeated peritoneal dialysis using 2 L of warm potassium, free dialysate warmed to 37°C, wherever facilities are available.

Prognosis

The prognosis depends upon the duration and severity of HT and the underlying disorder. Aged patients are at a higher risk. In general, majority of deaths occur within 30 minutes of rescuing the victim. Death is caused by cardiac arrest or ventricular fibrillation. In a few patients with apparent absence of vital signs on admission, these appear when the body is warmed. ***Hence, all cases should be resuscitated irrespective of the initial findings and they should not be pronounced dead until they have been observed for at least 30 minutes, after warming to 36°C or above.*** In persons who are susceptible to chronic HT, preventive measures like domestic heating and visits by social workers should be arranged. In all cases of HT, underlying medical conditions such as hypothyroidism, hypopituitarism and poisonings should be excluded by early investigation, since specific management for these conditions is absolutely essential to save life.

Table 13.1: Stages of hypothermia (HT)

Stage 1 HT-I: Normal mental status with shivering (core temperature 32–35°C or 90–95° F). Symptoms include normal mental status amnesia, dysarthria, ataxia, tachycardia and tachypnea.

Stage 2 HT-II: Moderate severity (core temperature 28–32°C or 82–90°F). Shivering may be absent bradycardia, atrial fibrillation, hypotension, dilation of pupil and slowing of respiration may occur.

Stage 3:

- ***Severe HT-III:*** Patient appears to be more moribund (core temperature 24–28°C or 75–82°F). Unless vigorously treated the condition may be fatal.
- ***Severe HT-IV:*** Apparently dead (core temperature 13.7–24°C or 56.7–75°F). Characterized by coma, corneal and oculocephalic reflexes are absent, blood pressure may not be recordable, heartbeat may be slow or in asystole or ventricular fibrillation. Breathing may be slow or absent, patient is areflexic, pupils are dilated, the electroencephalogram (EEG) will be flat, shows the rhythm.

  Note: Even such a severely moribund patient can be revived by intense resuscitatory measures at times.

Stage 4: Death—due to irreversible HT (core temperature 9–13.7°C or 48.2–56.7°F). Resuscitation is not possible.

Points to Remember

- Accidental HT is more common and serious in extremes of age.
- Slowing of cerebral function occurs at body temperatures below 35°C leading to stupor and coma.
- Cardiovascular changes include bradycardia, hypotension and atrial or ventricular fibrillation.
- 'Afterdrop' is a complication during management.
- HT is a medical emergency and death is caused by cardiac arrest or ventricular fibrillation.

CHAPTER 14

Disorders due to Alterations in Barometric Pressure

TK Suma, KV Krishna Das

Chapter Summary

- Exposure to Increased Barometric Pressure
- Effects of Sudden Reduction in Barometric Pressure
- Caisson Disease

The standard atmospheric pressure of 760 mm Hg exerted at mean sea level may fluctuate by 15–20 mm Hg under normal weather conditions. Lowering of barometric pressure is generally associated with lowered oxygen content of inspired air. If the oxygen supply is maintained adequately, humans can tolerate lowering of atmospheric pressure for prolonged periods. The volume of gases held in closed body cavities changes inversely with the external pressure.

EXPOSURE TO INCREASED BAROMETRIC PRESSURE

Syn: Barotrauma

This may occur in deep-sea divers, tunnel workers and patients under hyperbaric therapy chambers. The volume of gases held in the middle ear, paranasal sinuses, lungs, intestines, dental cavities, etc. diminishes under the high pressure and transudation occurs into these cavities. Severe rise of pressure leads to distortion and damage to tissues. Three major manifestations of barotrauma include sinus or middle ear effects, decompression sickness and arterial gas emboli. In the middle ear, it may lead to transudation and in severe cases even rupture of the tympanic membrane—***otitic barotrauma***. Changes in the volume of air in the paranasal sinuses lead to headache, nasal discharge or epistaxis. In decompression sickness, gas bubbles, nitrogen or other inert gases may form bubbles in blood vessels and tissues. Arterial gas embolism result from rupture of pulmonary capillaries or expanded alveoli. Pre-existing pulmonary emphysema predisposes to this condition.

Barotrauma has also been reported with both tracheal intubation and fiberoptic endotracheal intubation. Airway pressure is increased by the insufflated oxygen used during fiberoptic endotracheal intubation leading to alveolar rupture with pneumothorax and subcutaneous emphysema. Compressed air, used for breathing at depths by sea divers, is generally safe but the increased partial pressure of nitrogen can cause nitrogen narcosis. This is characterized by euphoria, error of judgment and intellectual impairment. Oxygen toxicity may occur if pure oxygen is administered at a pressure of 2.8 bar (equivalent to a depth of 18 m water), especially when the individual is engaged in vigorous activity. Confusion, convulsions and damage to the lungs may result from oxygen toxicity.

EFFECTS OF SUDDEN REDUCTION IN BAROMETRIC PRESSURE

Syn: Dysbarism

Those who live in high altitudes, passengers in unpressurized aircrafts, divers and workers in pressure chambers who are decompressed without proper supervision are susceptible to the ill-effects of sudden reduction in ambient pressures. Slow and graded decompression allows the gases contained in body cavities and dissolved in the blood and tissue fluids to be liberated gradually without producing untoward effects. Normally Eustachian tube functions to equalize middle ear and ambient environment pressures. In persons suffering from upper respiratory infection, sinusitis or Eustachian blockage, symptoms like ear pain, vertigo, giddiness or deafness may occur. Expansion of gas in the alimentary tract results in abdominal distension and dental pain which results from increase in the volume of gases within dental cavities. Aseptic necrosis of bone may occur in some cases. As a result of rapid decompression, more serious consequences occur due to formation of bubbles from liberation of nitrogen dissolved in the blood and tissues fluids. Acute decompression sickness follows rapid reduction of environmental pressure sufficient to cause the formation of bubbles from dissolved gases in the tissues. The bubbles act as emboli. In decompression illness, gas bubbles (nitrogen and other inert gases) may form in blood vessels and tissues. Aterial gas embolism results from rupture of pulmonary capillaries of expanded alveoli. Pre-existing pulmonary emphesema and blebs predispose to gas embolism. Twenty to thirty percent of apparently healthy adults have patent foramen ovale. Therefore, paradoxical embolism is also not rare. This disease is seen in divers and those working underwater in harbors, ports, naval installations, offshore oil drilling and mining industry. In patients with airway obstruction, expansion of air in the lungs leads to pulmonary rupture with resultant pneumothorax or surgical and mediastinal emphysema.

Factors, which influence clinical manifestation are obesity and physical activity during the compression phase and individual susceptibility. In addition to the mechanical effects due to the liberated gases, secondary phenomena also develop. These are fat embolism, sludging of erythrocytes in the microcirculation, platelet activation and disseminated intravascular coagulation (DIC). Formation gas bubbles themselves may be transient, but the effects they induce are prolonged. Increased permeability leads to fluid loss into tissues, hypovolemic shock, hemoconcentration and hyperviscosity states. The classical form of decompression sickness occurs in

Caisson disease. Caisson is pressurized equipment used to take divers underwater for work. Safety rules have been laid down for surfacing such workers from depths. Noncompliance with the rules results in development of decompression sickness.

Points to Remember
- Increase in volume of gases in body cavities produces symptoms when there is sudden reduction in barometric pressure.
- Nitrogen bubbles liberated during decompression result in serious problems like embolism.
- Pulmonary rupture, pneumothorax and mediastinal emphysema are other complications.
- Fat embolism, DIC, hypovolemic shock and hemoconcentration are secondary phenomena of decompression sickness.

CAISSON DISEASE

Syn: Bends, Acute decompression sickness, Compressed air illness

Caisson is a large water tight chamber open at the bottom in which workers can work underwater for long periods. A high air pressure is maintained within the Caisson to keep water out. Persons who work in deep underwater surroundings have to follow strict safety precautions to avoid ill-effects of rapid changes in barometric pressure. Caisson disease occurs in divers who have been brought to the surface rapidly without conforming to the safety precautions. Under high barometric pressure much of the air dissolves in blood and tissue fluids. When the barometric pressure is lowered, the nitrogen comes out of the solution as bubbles which lead to pathological consequences. Nitrogen being more lipid soluble, more bubbles are formed in the nervous tissue and hence, neurological symptoms predominate. The spinal cord is most commonly affected, the brainstem and cerebral hemispheres are affected to a lesser extent. Autopsy shows hemorrhages and micro infarcts in the white matter. Other tissues involved include the joints, skin and lungs.

Clinical Features

Symptoms start within three hours of surfacing, but rarely may be delayed by several hours. Mild cases show pain and cutaneous lesions. Cutaneous rash (livedo reticular) may develop. More serious features are pulmonary decompression. In the severe types, neurological and pulmonary lesions are prominent. An apparently mild case may rapidly become severe and hence the initial presentation may be misleading. Early cutaneous manifestations include pruritus, erythematous skin lesions and cyanotic patches, and these should alert the physician of the impending disease. The most common presenting symptom is joint pain (bends) felt over the knees, shoulder, hips and elbows. Sickness (chokes) presenting with retrosternal pain, cough and dyspnea, and neurologic manifestations. Tachypnea, hypotension and shock may follow the onset of chest pain and the patient may die. The neurologic symptoms include paresthesia, girdle pains, varying degrees of motor and sensory deficits, headache, blurring of vision, diplopia, pupillary abnormalities, dysarthria and vestibular dysfunction characterized by vertigo, nystagmus, nausea and vomiting (staggers).

Diagnosis

The condition is likely to be missed by the unwary physician. History, the circumstance of the case and physical manifestations should suggest the possibility of decompression sickness. Delay in onset of symptoms should not go against the diagnosis if other features are suggestive. Chest X-ray may show pneumothorax. Other imaging procedures such as computed tomography (CT) and magnetic resonance imaging (MRI) are generally unhelpful.

Course and Prognosis

The course is unpredictable since mild cases may rapidly become serious and die. Prognosis depends upon the promptness and adequacy of recompression and graded decompression. This measure should be instituted without delay even in hopeless cases. Many a time the recovery is remarkable. Neurological deficit tend to persist if treatment is delayed. Early recompression can prevent the development of neurological lesions. In suggestive cases, valuable time should not be wasted by undertaking detailed clinical examination before recompression is instituted.

Treatment

First aid is to give 100% oxygen inhalation for several hours. Nonsteroidal anti-inflammatory drugs (NSAIDs) such as piroxicam given early during resuscitation may help symptomatically. Perfluorocarbon preparations given intravenously (IV) have been tried with beneficial effects in some.

Specific treatment is to institute immediate recompression in a pressure chamber, as an emergency measure. Respiratory depressants like morphine should be avoided. The pressure equivalent and the duration of recompression have to be decided by personnel trained in recompression techniques. Usually, a pressure of 2.8 atmospheres (283.7 kPa) is beneficial. ***Hyperbaric oxygen*** helps to improve oxygenation of ischemic tissues.

In patients with neurological deficits, shock or cerebral edema, corticosteroids are beneficial. Low molecular weight dextran (dextran 40) helps to reduce vascular sludging. Infusion of appropriate fluids helps to restore blood volume, improve the circulatory state and mobilize trapped bubbles.

After suitable recompression, the patient should be carefully decompressed, allowing sufficient periods at each stage to prevent recurrence of bubble formation. Susceptible persons should refrain from diving till recovery is complete.

Points to Remember
- In Caisson disease, nervous system involvement is more predominant-spinal cord being commonly affected than the brainstem or cerebral hemispheres.
- Joint pain (bends) involving knee, elbow, hip and shoulder are common. Skin rashes may develop.
- Pulmonary symptoms (chokes) are retrosternal pain, cough, dyspnea and tachypnea.
- Immediate recompression in a pressure chamber is the treatment.

Diseases due to High Altitude

TK Suma, KV Krishna Das

Chapter Summary

- Acute Mountain Sickness (AMS)
  - High Altitude Pulmonary Edema
  - High Altitude Cerebral Edema
- Chronic Mountain Sickness

INTRODUCTION

Twenty-five percent of the earth's land mass is mountainous, at heights 2500 m above sea level. Ten percent of the world's population lives in mountains. More than 80% of them are poor without basic medical facilities. Iodine deficiency is common. Natural calamities such as land slides, avalanches, floods, thunder and lightning, and earthquakes are more common in these regions since mountains are sites of continental plate collision in the natural evolution of the planet. Many people from other regions of the world visit the mountainous regions for occupation, sport or adventure. ***The term high attitude illness refers to the total clinical picture occurring in unacclimatized entrants into high attitude regions shortly after their entry***.

In India, in the Himalayas alone more than 2 lakh persons undertake trekking annually. Many of the Indian troops are deployed at high altitudes. Constant vigil and unexpected combats have to be performed by our troops to protect our northern borders, in very adverse conditions such as altitude above 3000 m, temperature below 5°C, atmospheric pressures far below normal and inadequacy of communication are built-in handicaps. Peoples inhabiting heights above 2000 m are smaller in size, have a higher hemoglobin level in health and are adapted to the environment. Features such as koilonychia have been detected in them, even in the absence of iron-deficiency anemia (IDA). Incidence of tobacco-smoking and alcoholism is high among the mountain tribes. Mountaineering and trekking by holiday makers are popular sports in India.

High altitude illness describes the cerebral and pulmonary syndromes developing in unacclimatized persons shortly after ascent to high altitude. These include acute mountain sickness (AMS), high altitude cerebral edema and high altitude pulmonary edema (HAPE). Usually 2500 m has been used as the threshold for high altitude illness, but rarely mild illness can occur in people who have ascended to heights above 2000 m but below 2500 m.

ACUTE MOUNTAIN SICKNESS (AMS)

Syn: Soroche

Sudden exposure to heights above 2500 m may lead to headache, hyperventilation, increased heart rate and palpitation resulting from lowered oxygen tension and this is known as AMS. The symptoms typically develop within 6–12 hours after ascent. Ten to twenty five percent of unacclimatized persons develop AMS at 2500 m altitude. Cold weather and intense physical activity predispose to this condition but good physical fitness is not a protection from AMS. The exact process of AMS is not known. Hypoxia elicits neurohumoral and hemodynamic responses in brain and lungs and this result in over perfusion of microvascular beds, elevated hydrostatic capillary pressure, capillary leakage and edema. Newer evidence suggests that all people develop swelling of the brain on ascent to high altitudes. Those with a greater ratio of cerebrospinal fluid (CSF) to brain volume are better able to compensate for swelling through displacement of CSF. These people may not develop AMS.

Clinical Features

Three clinical patterns are seen as follows:

1. The ***pulmonary form*** is characterized by cough, dyspnea, chest pain and basal rales. Cheyne-Stokes respiration may be observed. During the apneic phases, the patient may be cyanosed. There is peripheral vasoconstriction. Appearance of basal rales may precede the onset of HAPE.
2. The ***cerebral form*** presents with headache, giddiness, irritability, forgetfulness, insomnia, drowsiness and convulsions. Vertigo, tinnitus, visual and auditory disturbances can also occur. Papilledema may be observed in severe cases. Headache increases with increase in cerebral edema.
3. The ***hypoxic form*** is vague in its clinical picture. Symptoms include muscle cramps, anorexia, gastrointestinal disturbances and epistaxis.

In the majority of cases, the onset is within 6–24 hours after arrival. Symptoms subside spontaneously, but recur everyday for 3–4 days till acclimatization occurs. A few cases may develop acute pulmonary edema. Altitude proteinuria is a common finding, which tends to disappear with oxygen therapy or on returning to the lower altitudes.

Treatment

Definitive treatment is immediate descent to lower altitude. Rest and administration of oxygen 1–2 L/min often relieves acute symptoms. If immediate descent is not possible portable hyperbaric chambers may be useful. Other recommended therapies are acetazolamide 125–250 mg every 12 hours and dexamethasone injections 8 mg initially followed by 4 mg every 6 hours. Trials have shown that ibuprofen reduced headache significantly in affected persons.

Prevention

Slow ascent and avoidance of physical exertion for 72 hours help to prevent AMS. Acetazolamide in a dose of 250 mg four times a day is beneficial if started a day prior to the travel and continued for 2–3 days. Dexamethasone 4 mg every 12 hours beginning the day of ascent, continued for three days at high altitude and then tapering off over 5 days is another alternative.

> **Points to Remember**
> - AMS occurs on rapid ascent to above 2000 m.
> - Symptoms usually start within 6–10 hours after ascent and subside within 48 hours.
> - Hypoxia and its effects result in edema in brain and lungs.
> - Oxygen inhalation, acetazolamide and dexamethasone recommended for treatment.
> - Slow ascent and avoidance of physical exertion help to prevent AMS.
> - If not treated properly will result in life-threatening HAPE or cerebral edema.

HIGH ALTITUDE PULMONARY EDEMA

This is a more serious complication compared to AMS. Young subjects in apparently good health are more affected. It may manifest in newcomers and also in subjects acclimatized to high altitudes, if they ascend the heights rapidly after long periods of stay at lower altitude. Most of the cases occur at heights above 3000 and symptoms develop 2 or more days after exposure to this altitude. Heavy meal, physical exertion and too rapid an ascent precipitate the condition. The risk increases in persons with a history of HAPE and the rate of recurrence is about 60% in such individuals.

Pathophysiology

HAPE is a noncardiogenic pulmonary edema associated with pulmonary hypertension and elevated capillary pressure. The pulmonary hypertension is secondary to the exaggerated pulmonary vasoconstriction induced by hypoxia. Sympathetic overactivity, endothelial dysfunction and hypoxemia are the proposed mechanisms. An immunogenetic basis also has been suggested because of higher incidence of human leukocyte antigen (HLA)-DR6 and HLA-DQ4 antigens in susceptible individuals.

Clinical Features

Many cases follow AMS, but in some, pulmonary edema develops abruptly. Early symptoms are cough, tachypnea, dyspnea and chest pain. These are soon followed by hemoptysis, cyanosis, frothy expectoration and intense chest discomfort. Oliguria may develop.

The course is variable. In some, the pulmonary edema worsens while in others it may become sub acute and persist for a few days. In severe cases, right-sided heart failure may follow and this may precede death. Radiographic abnormalities include prominence of the pulmonary arteries, irregular patchy infiltration of one lung or bilateral nodular densities (Fig. 15.1). Electro-cardiogram (ECG), reveals acute right ventricular strain due to pulmonary hypertension.

Diagnosis

HAPE should be anticipated in healthy subjects who develop vague cerebral and respiratory symptoms on

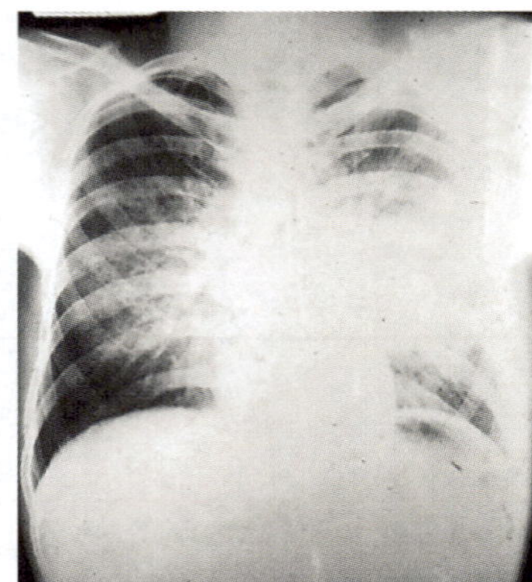

Fig. 15.1: **Chest X-ray:** High altitude pulmonary edema. **Note:** The bat-wing like opacities arising from the hilum

reaching high altitudes. Early recognition and treatment are necessary to avoid rapid deterioration or cardiac failure. Malingering has to be differentiated from this condition.

Treatment

Immediate treatment under field conditions is rest and administration of 100% oxygen at a rate of 4–6 L/min for 15–30 minutes. Recompression using a portable hyperbaric bag will reduce symptoms if immediate descent is not possible. If oxygen is not available the patient should be evacuated to a lower camp, hospitalized and administered oxygen. Nifedipine 10 mg initially followed by 20 mg repeated every 12 hours gives symptomatic relief. Physiological venesection by applying tourniquets proximally to the limbs helps to reduce pulmonary edema. There is no role for diuretics in treatment of HAPE. Precipitating factors such as respiratory infection have to be looked for and treated appropriately.

Cases, which do not respond to the resuscitatory measures, should be evacuated to lower altitude urgently to prevent death.

Prevention

Proper training and conditioning for 1–2 weeks should be undertaken before reaching high altitudes. Ascent should be gradual to permit acclimatization. On reaching high altitudes, all unacclimatized persons should avoid physical exertion for 48–72 hours. Randomized controlled trials (RCTs) have shown that recurrence can be prevented by use of drugs that lower the high pulmonary artery pressure in susceptible individuals. Slow release nifedipine 30 mg twice daily, the phosphodiesterase inhibitor tadalafil 10 mg twice daily and dexamethasone injections 8 mg twice daily were found to be effective in reducing risk from 70% to 10% or less. Salmeterol inhalation 125 µg every 12 hours beginning 24 hours before the ascent is recommended to reduce incidence of HAPE. Those planning to ascent 3000 m should carry supply of oxygen and equipment sufficient for several days.

> **Points to Remember**
> - HAPE is a serious complication occurring at heights of > 3000 m.
> - Pulmonary hypertension and elevated capillary pressure secondary to hypoxia form the basic pathology.

- Radiographic abnormalities vary from patchy opacities in one lung to bilateral nodular opacities.
- Immediate descent and hospitalization are required in severe cases.
- Drugs lowering the elevated pulmonary artery pressure like nifedipine, tadalafil and dexamethasone are useful in preventing recurrence.

HIGH ALTITUDE CEREBRAL EDEMA

This disorder is less common than pulmonary edema. Cerebral edema may follow AMS at least 2 days after reaching altitudes of above 4000 m. Vasodilatation, impaired cerebral autoregulation and elevated capillary pressure are the pathogenic mechanisms. Alteration of blood brain barrier secondary to hypoxia also contributes to the symptoms. The mediators are endothelium derived vasodilator growth factor, bradykinin and nitric oxide. Early clinical features consist of lethargy, insomnia, dreamy state and irritability. Truncal ataxia, decreased consciousness and mild fever ensue and if not treated properly progresses to coma and death from brain herniation within 24 hours. Headache not responding to nonsteroidal anti-inflammatory drugs (NSAIDs) and vomiting may indicate progression from AMS to high altitude cerebral edema. Magnetic resonance imaging (MRI) has shown vasogenic edema and microhemorrhages especially in the corpus callosum.

Treatment

The patient should be administered oxygen (2–4 L/min) and evacuated to a lower camp. Dexamethasone given intravenously (IV) or intramuscularly (IM) in a dose of 4–8 mg every 6 hours gives relief.

CHRONIC MOUNTAIN SICKNESS

Syn: Monge's disease, Chronic soroche, High altitude disease

Some persons living at high altitudes lose their acclimatization and develop symptoms. Most of such reports have come from South America. Males are affected more than females. The mechanism is not fully understood. Features include somnolence, hypoxemia, cyanosis, clubbing, polycythemia, mental depression and evidence of right ventricular failure. Angiotensin-converting enzyme inhibitors (ACEIs) such as enalapril in doses of 5 mg daily have been shown to reduce polycythemia. It is advisable to remove affected individuals to low altitudes and this reverts to normal on reaching low altitudes.

Source: Bärtsch P, Swenson ER. Clinical practice: Acute high-altitude illnesses. N Engl J Med. 2013;368(24):2294-302.

CHAPTER
16

Drowning

TK Suma, KV Krishna Das

Chapter Summary

- General Considerations
- Pathology and Clinical Features
- Management

GENERAL CONSIDERATIONS

According to World Health Organization (WHO) drowning is defined as a process of experiencing respiratory impairment from submersion/immersion in liquid; outcomes are classified as death, morbidity and no morbidity. There are an estimated 388,000 annual drowning deaths worldwide and account for 7% of all injury-related deaths. Twenty five percent of drowning accidents occur in seas and 75% occur in inland waters.

Drowning usually occurs silently and rapidly. Previously two types of drowning have been recognized—**dry drowning** and **wet drowning**. During the sequence of drowning, laryngeal spasm occurs by water entering the upper airways. Subsequently spasm relaxes and water enters the lungs and this was known as wet drowning. In 10–20% of cases, the laryngeal spasm does not relax and no water enters the lungs and this was termed as dry drowning. It is now felt that there is no clinical difference between wet and dry drowning and the distinction does not affect patient treatment or outcome. The term ***immersion syndrome*** refers to sudden death occurring due to cardiac arrest or fibrillation caused by rapid immersion into severely cold water.

The term ***secondary drowning*** used to denote the fatal consequences of complications such as pulmonary edema, pneumonia, pneumothorax and other complications. This may occur in 25% of persons after initial resuscitation.

Drowning may be further classified as ***cold-water*** or ***warm-water injury***. Warm-water drowning occurs at water temperatures of 20°C or higher and cold-water drowning occurs at water temperatures of less than 20°C. Additional classification is based on the type of water in which submersion occurred such as fresh water and salt water. In fresh water drowning, water entering the lung is quickly absorbed, leading to hemodilution and hemolysis with release of potassium from the red blood cells (RBCs). In addition to hypoxia and ventilatory failure, hyperkalemia precipitates ventricular arrhythmias, which may prove fatal. In salt water drowning, the fluid in the lung is hyperosmotic. It absorbs more fluid into the

Textbook of Medicine

alveoli causing pulmonary edema and respiratory failure. Hypernatremia follows later when the salt is absorbed into the circulation. In addition to the metabolic and local effects, impurities and contaminants give rise to local infection.

PATHOLOGY AND CLINICAL FEATURES

The main factors responsible for morbidity and mortality from drowning are hypoxemia and acidosis, and its further effects. Depending upon the degree of hypoxemia and acidosis the person may develop myocardial dysfunction and electrical instability, cardiac arrest and central nervous system (CNS) ischemia.

Lungs: Pulmonary vasoconstriction and hypertension develops following aspiration of fluid into the lungs. Disruption of alveolar surfactant produces alveolar instability, atelectasis and decreased compliance of the lungs. Bronchospasm induced by fluid also aggravates hypoxia. Aspiration of foreign particles worsens the atelectasis. Bacterial infection leads to pneumonia or lung abscess. Acute respiratory distress syndrome (ARDS) from altered surfactant effect and neurogenic pulmonary edema are common complications.

Heart: Arrhythmias such as ventricular fibrillation and cardiac asystole may occur. Electrocardiogram (ECG) may show nonspecific changes due to hypoxia. Hypovolemia occurs primarily due to fluid loss from increased capillary permeability. Profound hypotension may occur during and after the initial resuscitation period, due to vasodilatation.

Kidneys: Acute tubular necrosis (ATN) may develop in near-drowning in fresh water due to hemolysis and prolonged hypotension.

CNS: Asphyxia leads to loss of consciousness, cerebral edema and convulsions. Sequelae of anoxic encephalopathy such as transient hemiparesis, quadriparesis, choreoathetosis, aphasia and faciobrachial weakness may develop.

MANAGEMENT

First Aid

- Clear the airway of water and foreign bodies by putting the patient head low and by suction
- Institute mouth-to-mouth breathing as early as possible
- Closed chest cardiac massage should be instituted if heart sounds are absent
- All cases must be hospitalized to prevent death from secondary drowning.

Hospital Treatment

This aims at (1) maintenance of adequate oxygenation, (2) correction of metabolic and electrolyte imbalance and (3) prevention of secondary effects. Adequate oxygenation is achieved by the use of controlled ventilation with 100% oxygen, later to be reduced to 40%. If the patient remains dyspneic on 100% oxygen or has low oxygen saturation, use continuous positive airway pressure (CPAP) if available. If not, intubation and application of positive end-expiratory pressure (PEEP) respiration should be resorted to. The PEEP increases the functional residual capacity, thereby minimizing intrapulmonary shunts and ventilation perfusion abnormalities and promotes better oxygenation. If bronchospasm is present, inhalation of salbutamol 200 μg should be administered. Acidosis is to be corrected with sodium bicarbonate given IV in a dose of 0.7–1 mmoL/kg. Proper correction of electrolyte imbalance and acidosis should be monitored.

Constant observation and appropriate management of pulmonary edema, pneumonia and pneumothorax serves to prevent secondary drowning. Prophylactic antibiotics have to be used to prevent respiratory infections. Chest X-ray is necessary in all cases to detect complications. Atelectasis has to be managed with bronchoscopic aspiration. In severe cases of pulmonary edema, dexamethasone given in a dose of 0.5–1 mg/kg in 24 hours IM or IV has been successful. If signs of intracranial hypertension develop, it is treated with IV infusion of 200 mL of 20% mannitol.

Prognosis

This depends on the extent and duration of hypoxia and the first aid. Patients presenting with coma and cardiac irregularities have higher mortality and morbidity. Immersion in cold-water causes death earlier due to rapid cooling, but survivors show less tendency to develop neurological sequelae. Residual complications of near drowning include convulsive disorders, intellectual impairment, cardiac neurosis and pulmonary atelectasis leading to bronchiectasis. In general, duration of submersion for more than 5 minutes, unavailability of resuscitation within ten minutes, Glasgow Coma Scale (GCS) < 5 (comatose), arterial blood pH < 7 and nonrecovery after vigorous efforts for 25 minutes are all poor prognostic factors.

Prevention

Education of the public on the hazards in water and first aid measures to save drowning victims should be available in places of water sports, holiday resorts and beaches. Trained lifeguards should be available at public swimming places.

Points to Remember

- In dry drowning, laryngeal spasm is the cause of death.
- In fresh water drowning hemodilution, hemolysis, ventilatory failure and ventricular arrhythmia may occur.
- Pulmonary edema and respiratory failure are the features in salt water drowning.
- Maintenance of adequate oxygenation, correction of metabolic and electrolyte imbalances, and prevention of secondary effects are the mainstay of management.

Injuries due to Ionizing Radiations

TK Suma, KV Krishna Das

Chapter Summary
- General Considerations
- Acute Radiation Syndrome
- Damage to Embryo by Irradiation in Fetal Life
- Local Radiation Injury

GENERAL CONSIDERATIONS

Ionizing radiations are either electromagnetic or particulate in nature. They are derived from natural or artificial radioactive isotopes, nuclear reactors, diagnostic and therapeutic equipment [e.g. X-rays, computed tomography (CT) scan] and the complex shower of particles from the outer space, the cosmic rays. The radiations include alpha, beta and gamma particles, and electromagnetic waves.

Radiation injury is seen in survivors of nuclear war, after radiotherapy, persons engaged in industries involving radioactive materials, radiologists and radiotherapists. In some parts of the world, radioactive sand accounts for low dose continuous radiation, e.g. the mineral beaches of Kerala. Radiation is harmful at all doses, the danger increasing with the rate and dose of exposure (Table 17.1). The age group 10–19 years is most susceptible. The maximal permissible radiation exposure for occupationally exposed workers is 0.1 rem/week for the whole body. Critical targets are the cellular nuclei. The damage caused to the biological systems is of two types:

1. Direct absorption of radiation energy results in the formation of H^+ ion, OH^- ion and hydrogen peroxide which all interfere with enzyme systems.
2. Direct injury to chromosomes lead to chromosomal breaks and abnormal cross links in the deoxyribonucleic acid (DNA) or between the DNA and cellular proteins. Dividing cells are more susceptible to radiation injury.

The effects may be—(1) delay in mitosis, (2) reduction in the number of dividing cells and (3) chromosomal changes.

The effects of radiation vary according to the degree and nature of exposure. Massive radiation exposure causes immediate effects, while small repeated exposures induce response that may not be perceived even for years. Large dose and extensive exposure, results in the acute radiation syndrome. Excessive dosage delivered locally gives rise to localized damage, e.g. radiation dermatitis, radiation nephritis, etc.

Pathological Changes

Radiation leads to arrest of mitotic activity, which progresses to cell damage and death. Tissues, which have a high rate of cell division such as bone marrow, intestinal epithelium and germinal cells of gonads, suffer most. Secondary complications include infection, hemorrhage and fibrosis. Loss of epithelium, neutropenia and depression of immune response favor bacterial invasion and septicemia. Infective lesions are most evident in the oropharynx and intestines. The brain and spinal cord are more sensitive to radiation than peripheral nerves.

ACUTE RADIATION SYNDROME

Acute exposure of the whole body to 300 cGy is fatal. Lethal doses produce maximal effects on the bone marrow and the intestinal epithelium. With high doses, intestinal lesions predominate over marrow toxicity. With still

Table 17.1: Clinical response to different doses of whole body irradiation

Dose centigray (cGy)	Clinical effects	Mortality
0–100	Men may develop temporary azoospermia	Nil
100–200	Nausea and vomiting starts in 3–6 hours and may persist for a whole day or so. In some cases, this starts after a latent period of even two weeks	Nil
200–600	Nausea and vomiting lasts for 1–2 days, there may be a latent period of 1–4 weeks, symptoms may recur for up to 8 weeks, and severe leukopenia, purpura, hemorrhage, infections and loss of hair may develop	Up to 90% in 2–12 weeks from hemorrhage or infection
600–1000	Nausea and vomiting start within 30 minutes and last for 2 days. There is a latent phase of 5–10 days followed by severe leukopenia, purpura, hemorrhage, infections and death	90–100% in 6 weeks from hemorrhage or infection
1000–3000	Nausea and vomiting start within 30 minutes and last for 1 day. The latent phase is for 7 days or less. This is followed by gastrointestinal syndrome with diarrhea, fever and disturbed electrolyte balance. These last for 2–14 days	100% with 14 days from toxemia and circulatory collapse
More than 3000	Nausea and vomiting start almost immediately followed by respiratory convulsions, tremor, ataxia and lethargy	100% in 48 hours from failure or brain edema

Note: X-ray and gamma rays used to be measured in rads. Exposure to 1 roentgen results in an absorption of about 1 rad equivalent to 100 ergs/g. At present, the unit of measurement used is the gray. 1 rad = 1 centigray (cGy).

higher doses neurological features such as disorientation, convulsions and shock predominate. Except in the fulminant neurological type of injury, the classical form occurs in four phases:

Phase 1 prodrome: This phase occurs within minutes of exposure and is characterized by nausea, vomiting, diarrhea abdominal cramps and dehydration. Reduction in lymphocytes may occur in 24–30 hours due to direct destruction of these cells.

Phase 2 clinical latency: There is a latent period of about a week after which the third stage develops.

Phase 3 manifest illness: During this critical phase, there is marrow failure leading to neutropenia and thrombocytopenia, which result in secondary infection and hemorrhage. Fever, vomiting, diarrhea, oropharyngeal ulceration and purpura may be seen.

Phase 4 recovery: The survivors enter the fourth (recovery) phase in which the symptoms subside.

Temporary sterility may develop and persist for up to one year. Risk of developing malignancies such as chronic myeloid leukemia (CLL), carcinoma of breast, thyroid, lungs and digestive organs is considerably increased in such persons.

Treatment

It is supportive and aims at:

- Correcting toxemia and infections
- Correcting fluid and electrolyte imbalances
- Treating hemorrhagic manifestations, profound anemia and neutropenia.

These patients are preferably managed in an aseptic environment. Adequate antibiotic therapy and transfusion of neutrophils and platelets are life-saving. Hematopoietic factors such as *filgrastim* and *sargramostim* help in the recovery of blood cells. Blood stem cell transplantation and bone marrow transplantation may be needed later.

Points to Remember

- The extent of damage due to radiation depends on the dose, rate and type of radiation and organ exposed.
- Tissues with high rate of cell division such as bone marrow, gastrointestinal epithelium and gonads are affected mostly.
- Acute exposure of >300 cGy may be fatal.

DAMAGE TO EMBRYO BY IRRADIATION IN FETAL LIFE

Irradiation during stage of implantation results in fetal death. During the stage of organogenesis, fetal malformation or abortion may result. After three months, by which time, the main organs would have formed, gross deformities are not produced, but stunting of growth, reduction of lifespan, sterility and tendency to develop leukemias and cancers have been noted. Radiation dose as low as 5 cGY can injure the growing fetus. The irradiation given out by modern X-ray machines for Chest X-ray is only 1/100 cGY.

LOCAL RADIATION INJURY

Erythema develops over the area of exposure within days or weeks after acute exposure and this may progress to epidermolysis. Late complications are atrophy of the skin, subcutaneous fibrosis, telangiectasia and later hyperkeratosis. These hyperkeratotic lesions may develop malignancy later.

CHAPTER

18

Electrical Injuries and Lightning

TK Suma, KV Krishna Das

Chapter Summary

- Electrical Injuries
- Lightning

ELECTRICAL INJURIES

The risk of electrical injuries is often overlooked due to over familiarity. In most cases, accidents occur from faulty domestic electrical apparatus, rarely it may be from high tension lines or other installations. Classification of electrical injuries generally focus on the power source (lightning or electrical), voltage (high or low voltage) and type of current (alternating or direct), each of which is associated with certain injury patterns. Electrical characteristics of the exposed part, conductivity of tissues, extent of grounding and the duration of the contact determine the amount and the path taken by the current. The type and severity of injury depends upon the strength of the current, its type and duration of exposure and the path taken by the current. Individuals vary in susceptibility to the effects of electricity. Injuries associated with electricity may be due to either direct electrical shock or burns resulting from electrothermal effects and flames. Alternating current (AC) is more damaging than direct current (DC). A current of 100 mA flowing from hand to feet can induce ventricular fibrillation. Following the passage of the current, myocardium is vulnerable and highly excitable. Fatal ventricular arrhythmias may occur.

Clinical Features

Burns develop at the sites of entry and exit of the current. When the current is high, instantaneous ignition of clothing or nearby objects add to the injury. Electrical current may produce three distinct types of burns. *Arcs*—deep thermal burns where the current contacts the skin; *flame* (clothing) burns, ignition of clothing causing direct burns from flame and the direct effect of the current (*Joule burn*). Burns get secondarily infected in 2–3 days.

The nervous system is highly sensitive to electrical injury. Spinal cord may develop lesions leading to paraplegia and urinary retention. Convulsions, cerebral edema and cerebral thrombosis may develop. Current passing through the skeletal muscle can cause muscle necrosis and contractions severe enough to result in bone fracture. Peripheral nerve involvement can cause acute or delayed peripheral neuropathy. Cardiac symptoms include tachycardia, which may be persistent, shock, cardiac arrhythmias including ventricular fibrillation and cardiac failure. Pneumonia, pleural effusion and disorders of ventilation, and hypoxia are the common respiratory findings. Secondary hemorrhage from blood vessels and acute upper gastrointestinal (GI) bleeding may develop in a few days. Acute renal failure (ARF) is a common sequel. Current passing through the abdomen may be complicated by damage to the viscera. Cataracts may form as late sequelae. If current passes through the heart or brainstem death is immediate.

Treatment

First aid includes immediate disconnection of the live contact and cardiorespiratory resuscitation. Due to muscle spasm, the limb holds on to the live wire. This prolongs the injury and this is the main cause of death. Urinalysis, serum creatine kinase (CK) and CK-MB and an electrocardiogram (ECG) should be done immediately. Administration of intravenous (IV) saline or Ringer lactate solution helps to combat shock. Dexamethasone 8 mg and 20% mannitol 250 mL given IV help to reduce cerebral edema. Furosemide 40–80 mg IV is given to overcome pulmonary edema and prevent renal shutdown. Sodium bicarbonate is given to prevent acidosis as an early measure. The prognosis is monitored by estimating the hematocrit, urine volume and arterial pH serially. Suspicion of visceral damage calls for imaging studies and surgical management.

Prevention

Proper insulation is necessary while handling electrical equipment. Low plug sockets should be protected from the reach of children. While rescuing an electrocuted person the rescuer should take enough care in first insulating himself properly. Many deaths have occurred among rescuers who have failed to observe proper precautions.

LIGHTNING

Injuries due to lightning are encountered commonly in the tropics. Lightning induces a high electrostatic charge on the victim. Identically charged particles repel each other, giving rise to disruptive forces, which lead to damage of organs. Organ damage may occur even without external injury. The high current produces violent muscular contractions and severe burns, and ignites inflammable objects on the body.

Clinical Features

The patient is usually restless, disoriented and may be comatose. Retrograde amnesia is common. Later on, patient may show psychiatric and hysterical manifestations. Severe vasoconstriction produces manifestations like cold limbs and transient ischemic palsies. Arterial spasm may result in absence of pulse in the affected limb. Increased vascular permeability results in massive edema of the affected part.

Cardiovascular manifestations: It include tachycardia, extrasystoles and electrocardiographic abnormalities such as elevation of ST segment and inversion of T waves. Sudden death may occur on account of respiratory center paralysis or cardiac asystole. Intracranial hemorrhage (ICH) may develop.

Treatment

If the vital signs are absent, immediate resuscitatory measures should be started. Management of survivors consists mainly of supportive measures and treatment of the complications. Vasodilators and low molecular weight dextran help to prevent gangrene. Tetanus prophylaxis must be given if tissue injury has occurred. Major burns are best managed in a surgical burns unit with experience of similar cases.

> **Points to Remember**
> - Lightning usually involves high voltage.
> - Organ damage occurs even without external injury.
> - Multisystem involvement is common.
> - Death is usually due to cardic asystole rather than ventricular fibrillation.

CHAPTER
19

Dangers of Nuclear Explosion

TK Suma, KV Krishna Das

Chapter Summary

- General Considerations
- Blast Wave
- Thermal Injury
- Ionizing Radiations
- The International Physician for the Prevention of Nuclear War (IPPNW)

GENERAL CONSIDERATIONS

The present day warfare makes use of nuclear explosion to increase destructive power. Many nations on the globe are having sophisticated nuclear weapons, the explosive powers of which exceed the power of several thousand tons of trinitrotoluene (TNT). Nuclear explosions may result from deliberate actions of warring nations or accidents in high power nuclear reactors. It is estimated that among the nuclear powers like the United States of America (USA) and Russia, the destructive power that can be generated by nuclear armament may be far in excess of that required to annihilate life totally from the surface of the globe. Many physicians all over the world consider a nuclear war as the worst and the last disaster that can happen to mankind and all other living organisms.

A nuclear explosion results when the fission of uranium or plutonium proceeds in a rapid and relatively uncontrolled manner. The tremendous release of energy can produce severe explosive shock and temperatures exceeding one million degrees celsius. The explosion is associated with several destructive phenomena.

BLAST WAVE

It is also known as shock wave or pressure wave is transmitted to the surrounding medium with a highly destructive force. The blast arising from an ordinary nuclear bomb will destroy most of the commercial buildings, apartments and houses, within a radius of 1 km.

THERMAL INJURY

The high temperature produced by the explosion converts the materials of the explosive nature into a ball of very hot gases. This ball expands rapidly engulfing and incorporating the air it meets, becoming larger in the process and this progress centrifugally. This causes severe burns, maximal at the center and reducing towards the periphery. At Hiroshima, during the explosion of the atom bomb in the second world war almost all persons within a radius of 1.6 km were burnt to varying degrees. Another consequence of thermal injury is flash blindness, which is transient blindness (which may become permanent) that results from too powerful a flash.

IONIZING RADIATIONS

Nuclear explosion emits large amounts of ionizing radiations which themselves are highly injurious to life and health. In addition, they can make other objects also radioactive, so that these objects act as sources of long-term radioactivity in that area, with consequent health hazards. Large areas may be made unfit for human existence for several decades. Long-term ill-effects include higher incidence of several cancers, genetic mutations and congenital malformations. Since the radioactive fall out spills over a much wider area from the target of attack, these phenomena also involve neighboring countries. Radioactive materials may go up into the atmosphere to form radioactive clouds, move to other regions and cause *radioactive rain*. The radioactive particles may remain in the troposphere (layer of atmosphere extending up to 11 km from the earth) and stratosphere (layer above troposphere) for up to 30 days or more.

The very high temperatures produced by the explosion will ignite all inflammable materials and lead to large urban fires and forest fires. Liberation of soot and smoke into the atmosphere block sunlight reaching the earth's surface and lead to a precipitous fall in temperature to well below minus 20°C which may persist for several months. This phenomenon is referred to as *nuclear winter*.

Other consequences of a nuclear explosion are common to all mass scale accidents, but on a much higher scale. These include total disruption of communication, breakdown of all rescue and medical facilities, disruption of essential services such as protected water and electricity, and occurrence of severe environmental pollution. These, in their turn start off problems such as starvation, widespread epidemic and famine.

Medical men from several countries have joined to form an international organization—***The International Physician for the Prevention of Nuclear War (IPPNW)*** with a view to educate governments and public on the possible ill-effects of a nuclear war and to use the moral and social position of the doctors on public and government to adopt nuclear disarmament.

India is a participant in this movement. It is the duty of every doctor to uphold and promote these aims. The National Association of Indian Doctors for the Prevention of Nuclear War (NAIDPNW) which was later changed to

Textbook of Medicine

Indian Doctors for Peace and Development (IDPD), has its office at 139-E, Kitchlu Nagar, Ludhiana-141001 (Punjab) India.

Points to Remember

- Release of energy during nuclear explosion produces severe shock and high temperature.
- Thermal injury causes severe burns and flash blindness.
- Ionizing radiation from nuclear explosion results in long-term effects like development of cancers, genetic and congenital abnormalities.
- Nuclear winter is a complication of nuclear explosion.
- Physician have a great role in preventing nuclear warfare and 'The International Physician for the Prevention of Nuclear Warfare is a Worldwide Organization spreading the message of Nuclear Disarmament'.

CHAPTER 20

Adverse Effects due to Noise and Vibrations

KV Krishna Das, TK Suma

Chapter Summary

- Noise
  - Systemic Diseases Contributed by Unwanted Noise Pollution
  - Effects of Impulse Noise on Middle Ear and Eardrum
- Vibration

NOISE

It is unwanted sound and produces adverse effects on man. With the progress in industry and transport, noise pollution is increasing in all countries. Continuous loud noises lead to impairment of hearing, irritability and accelerate fatigue. Noise disturbs sleep.

Noises occur in various forms. They may be pure tones (siren), narrowbands of frequencies (hiss of escaping stream), broadbands of frequencies (radio), impulses (explosive release of gas in gunfire) or impacts (hammer striking a steel plate). The stimulus may be continuous or intermittent and the intensity also varies. The unit of sound is the decibel (dB). Decibel is 1/10 of a bel. Bel is the unit of sound pressure intensity and is measured as the logarithmic ratio of the particular sound to that of a reference sound, which has an intensity of 0.002 dynes/cm² at 1000 cycles per second.

Exposure to noise levels greater than 85 and 95 dB for months to years can lead to cochlear damage. In the early stages, there is loss of hearing at or near frequencies of 3000–4000 cycles per second. Later, the damage extends to both higher and lower frequencies. Higher tones are affected early, later extending to lower tones as well. The subject may not be aware of the hearing loss until it is severe. Speech reception is not altered seriously until the loss of hearing is greater than 30 dB in the speech frequencies (500, 1000, 2000 cycles per second). Children are more susceptible for noise-induced hearing impairment than adults.

Noise-induced loss of hearing has two phases. In the initial phase, there is a rise in threshold of sound, which is temporary and in the latter phase this defect becomes permanent. Further a temporary threshold shift can be superimposed on permanent defect of hearing.

Persons vary in their sensitivity to the effects of noise. The factors, which influence the final outcomes are:

- Overall sound pressure levels of the noise
- Frequency bands of which the noise is composed
- Daily distribution and total duration of noise exposure
- Susceptibility of the ear exposed to the noise.

The most striking finding in noise-induced loss of hearing is injury or degeneration of the sensory cells, mainly the outer hair cells of the organ of Corti. After exposure to noise the cilia in the inner and outer hair cells of the cochlea become fused and bent. After more prolonged exposure, there is degeneration of the outer and inner hair cells related to transmission of high-frequency sounds.

In old age, there is a general tendency to develop hearing loss (presbycusis) = due to degeneration of the stria vascularis of the cochlea. Presbycusis starts with loss of high frequency sound. Exposure to heavy background noise, smoking and high lipid diet accelerates this hearing loss.

Epidemiology

The information of the ill-effects of noise on the human system and the damage it causes on the hair cells of the cochlea and damage to nerve endings at the molecular level and the ill-effects on health and performance have all substantially improved. The non-auditory ill efforts of unwanted noise are also becoming evident.

Noise exposure leads to annoyance, sleep disturbance, day time somnolence, affects patient's outcomes and staff performance in hospitals, increased occurrence of hypertension and cardiovascular disease and impairment of learning and cognitive skills in school children. Adequate regulatory measures are necessary to prevent noise pollution.

The Global Burden of Disease (GBD) 2010 identified noise-induced and other causes of hearing loss as the 13th cause of disability globally (19.9 million person every year and prevalence 2.5%). In 50% of them, the cause of auditory damage is exposure to intense noise. Noise-induced hearing loss may be due to occupational factors, social causes or age-related phenomena.

World health organization (WHO) estimated that 45000 disability-adjusted life years (DALYs) are lost annually in children aged 7–19 years in high income Western European countries. The effects manifest as communication difficulties, impaired attention, increased arousal, frustration, noise annoyance, learned helplessness, sleep disturbances and its consequences. Sleep disturbances form the most important among these factors since a sufficient period of undisturbed sleep is needed to maintain day time performance, alertness, quality of life and health.

Systemic Diseases Contributed by Unwanted Noise Pollution

Unwanted arousals of the autonomic nervous system and endocrine system lead to rise in systolic and diastolic blood pressure (BP), changes in heart rate and excessive release of catecholamines and glucocorticoids—manifesting clinically as hypertension, ischemic heart disease (IHD), stroke and peptic ulcer.

Ill-effects of noise during pregnancy may affect fetal development. Hospital noise caused by gadgets used in intensive care rooms, medical devices like alarms, telephones, pagers, beeps and others add to the noise pollution and lead to ill-effects on staff performance and patient outcomes. Table 20.1 gives the average noise levels and their health consequences.

Effects of Impulse Noise on Middle Ear and Eardrum

Impulse noise can be defined as an acoustic event associated with sudden changes in pressure. The pressure wave initially travels faster than the speed of sound. Very high intensity impulse noises from explosions are known to damage the eardrum, middle ear and inner ear structures. The body reacts to impulse noise by increasing BP, heart rate and respiration. Muscles become tense and there will be increased secretion of catecholamines. These changes can occur even during sleep and continuous exposures during the night may affect person's general health producing irritability and fatigue. Studies have shown that children studying in schools near airport subjected to chronic aircraft noise exposure have impaired reading

comprehension, intellectual performance and long-term memory.

Mortality in relation to noise pollution: Probably death due to cerebrovascular accidents (CVA), cardiovascular disease and cirrhosis of liver increases with increasing noise pollution. There is also increasing incidence of stroke, hypertension and peptic ulcer. It may affect fetal development.

Prevention of noise-induced loss of hearing involves regular audiometric screening of workers exposed to industrial noise and reducing the noise levels to the minimum and protection of exposed personnel. The recommended noise level at night is a maximum of 35 dB. For hospital wards, an ambient level of 40 dB has been recommended.

Points to Remember
- Exposure to noise levels more than 85–90 dB can lead to cochlear damage.
- Children are more susceptible for noise-induced hearing impairment than adults.
- Noise-induced hearing impairment may be permanent.
- Impulse noise damages the eardrum, middle ear and inner ear structures.

VIBRATION

Vibratory tools and machines of various types including pneumatic hammer and drills are in common use at present. Frequencies of 250 Hz with an amplitude of 1 mm are most likely to cause damage. The group of symptoms and signs produced by exposure to vibration is known as ***hand-arm vibration syndrome (HAVS)***. This depends on—(a) the amount of vibration the tool produces, (b) the length of time the tool is used each day, (c) the total number of hours or days or months the tool has been used and (d) the way in which tool has been held. HAVS results in vascular damage, neurological and musculoskeletal dysfunctions. Due to vascular damage, episodic blanching of one or more fingers occurs, which will be well demarcated and is known as the ***white finger***. This is usually triggered by cold. The latency period for development of ***white finger*** may vary from 6 months to 20 years. Neurological symptoms are tingling and numbness, reduced strength of grip and impaired dexterity. Musculoskeletal damage caused by vibration includes:
- Decalcification or cyst formation of carpal bones
- Injuries to the soft tissues of hand
- Arthritis of wrist, elbow and shoulder
- Spasm of the arteries and ***Raynaud's phenomenon— the white hand*** or ***dead hand.***

Bone cysts rarely produce pathological fractures. Injuries to the soft tissues often involve the palmar aponeurosis and may produce adventitious bursae, which fill the palm. Arthritic symptoms are attributable to active damage of joint surfaces, caused by the large pneumatic tools. Once established, the damage persists. Very recently, HAVS has been reported following prolonged use of vibrating computer games especially in children.

Table 20.1: Impact of noise intensity on health	
Noise intensity (dB)	**Effects**
Below 30	No adverse effects
30–40	Sleep disturbances, especially in children and elderly
40–55	Adverse effects occur on exposed persons, vulnerable groups are affected more
More than 55	Increasingly dangerous for public health, adverse effects on health are common, annoyance in insomnia and increase in risk of cardiovascular disease occur

Textbook of Medicine

Motion Sickness, Problems due to Air Travel and Road Accidents

TK Suma, KV Krishna Das

Chapter Summary

- Motion Sickness
- Medical Problems of Air Travel
  - Problems due to Reduction in Barometric Pressure and Partial Pressure of Oxygen
  - Problems in Apparently Healthy Travelers
  - Problems in Chronically Ill Patients
- Deep Vein Thrombosis
- Road Accidents Injuries caused by Road Accidents
- Management at the Site of Accident

MOTION SICKNESS

The term motion sickness refers to the clinical picture resulting from movement of an individual on land, sea or air when journeys are undertaken. Repetitive irregular movement as in a swing, a lift or even dancing, may bring on such symptoms.

It is mainly a disorder of gastric and intestinal functions brought on in susceptible subjects while traveling. Irregular and unaccustomed stimulation of the labyrinth causes nausea and vomiting and also disorders of function in the viscera innervated by the vagus or parasympathetic system. During sea voyage, the roll and pitch of the ship causes excessive stimulation of the labyrinth. In the case of car and aeroplane travel, labyrinth is subjected not only to the effects of rotation of the body through planes to which it is not accustomed, but also to rapid acceleration, deceleration and altitude changes. Angular acceleration of train and the linear-angular acceleration of turbulent flights are important causes of motion sickness. Visual stimuli from moving objects and proprioceptive stimuli from muscles and joints contribute to the final outcome. Fear and anxiety make the condition worse. Early infancy is immune from this affection, since the orienting mechanism has not attained full physiological activity and old age is relatively immune, probably because of the lessened sensitivity of the nervous system. The signs and symptoms of motion sickness occur when sensory information about the body's position in or movement through space is contradictory to prior experience. Susceptibility and tolerance to motion sickness vary widely among individuals. Motion sickness is more common in women, especially during pregnancy or menstruation, in children aged 2–12 years and in persons who have migraine headaches.

Clinical features: The initial symptoms include loss of usual sense of wellbeing, abdominal and visceral discomfort, salivation, nausea and yawning. The patient becomes pale and respiration becomes irregular. These symptoms are followed by retching, vomiting and desire to defecate. The vomiting may be mild and transient in some, while in others this may be violent, distressing and recurrent. Headache, giddiness, continued pallor, apathy, lassitude, weakness, dehydration and prostration follow. The skin may become cold and clammy, tongue coated, both breath and urine may contain acetone bodies, pulse and respiration become rapid and the blood pressure (BP) drops.

Diagnosis: It is easy when the symptoms are related to travel, but other causes of abdominal disorders must not be overlooked.

Course and prognosis: The symptoms usually subside when the travel or the movement causing the condition comes to an end, but in some cases dizziness, headache and gastric symptoms persist for a long time. In cases of long voyages by seas, the symptoms may subside in a few days but may sometimes persist.

Prophylaxis and treatment: Reclining posture, avoidance of visual stimuli and reduction in head movements to the minimum help to minimize the condition. Mental distraction may help to allay the symptoms.

Antihistamines given in small doses 30–60 minutes before starting the travel prevent motion sickness, e.g. diphenhydramine 25–50 mg oral, phenothiazines such as trifluoperazine 10 mg or hyoscine (0.3 mg) are good alternatives. To treat motion sickness higher doses of the same drugs have to be given. The choice of drug should be based on the underlying conditions if any.

MEDICAL PROBLEMS OF AIR TRAVEL

The long hauls and undue delay *en route* are matters of great concern to the severely ill patients. Psychological stress caused by frequent dislocation of connecting flights and fear of skyjacking adds to the problem. Travel by modern aircrafts is safe and comfortable on account of the appropriate adjustment of cabin pressure, cabin atmosphere, air conditioning and oxygen supply. Many modern aircrafts fly at altitudes of 7,000–13,000 m.

Problems due to reduction in barometric pressure and partial pressure of oxygen (PaO₂): The commercial transport aircrafts are pressurized, but cabin pressure is subject to fluctuations. At 2,600 m, the ambient pressure is about 560 mm Hg, the partial pressure of inspired oxygen is 118 mm Hg and that of alveolar oxygen 65 mm Hg. In patients with ischemic and hypertensive heart diseases, this degree of hypoxia can cause angina or cardiac failure. Cerebral ischemia may manifest in atherosclerotic individuals. Sickle cell crises may be precipitated in susceptible patients. There are many airports situated at altitudes more than 1800 meters above sea level and relative hypoxia at these levels can cause problems of high altitude in such individuals. Decreased barometric pressure results in expansion of gas trapped in body cavities. Blocking of sinuses and Eustachian tubes lead to severe facial or middle ear pain. Dental pain may develop due to expansion of air trapped in badly filled cavities. In pneumothorax and pneumoperitoneum, the entrapped air expands and can cause rise in tension. The gas in the stomach and intestines (about 1 to 1.5 L) can expand as much as 25%. This may cause a feeling of fullness and discomfort, acute abdominal colic, lower central chest pain and collapse resembling myocardial infarction (MI). The risk of gastrointestinal hemorrhage is increased. Unsupported hernias strangulate more readily.

Problems in apparently healthy travelers: Long flights result in rapid changes in climate and time zones. Rapid geographical transitions around the world disturb the natural biological rhythms of the individual. Motion sickness, sleeplessness, tension, headache, pain in the neck, shoulders and back, nausea, dyspepsia, urinary frequency and constipation are not unusual accompaniments of the flying stress. More serious symptoms such as cardiac arrhythmias, manic excitement, hallucinations and paranoid delusions may develop in a few. As a result of long flying sessions and rapid changes of climate and time zones, symptoms like physical exhaustion, spurious sensation of mental alertness and mild euphoria may persist for one or two days after reaching the destination. Some passengers find it difficult to adapt quickly to the new climatic environment and they may develop sleep disturbance, intellectual underfunctioning and psychosomatic symptoms. Reduction in fatty food and alcohol intake during flights help to reduce the symptoms to a great extent. Immobility during long flights may predispose to deep vein thrombosis (DVT).

Problems in chronically ill patients: Facilities in commercial aircraft make it possible to airlift even acutely ill and seriously injured persons, although isolation facilities may not always be available. Oxygen delivered by nasal masks is available in all modern aircraft for emergency use.

- ***Cardiovascular diseases:*** In view of the lower PaO_2, it is advisable to avoid flying for six weeks following acute MI. Treated cardiac failure, occasional angina, old infarction, hypertension and chronic valvular diseases, do not carry any added risk. During 'check-in', patients with implanted pacemakers should avoid electronic and magnetic devices used for screening the passengers. Many major airports are equipped with emergency resuscitation equipment and trained volunteers who can attened to sudden cardic events.

- ***Cerebrovascular accidents (CVA) and epilepsy:*** Flying is contraindicated for six weeks following stroke. Flying at more than 3000 m altitude may precipitate epileptic attacks if proper medication is not given.

- ***Pulmonary diseases:*** Persons with pulmonary decompensation at rest or on mild exertion should undertake air travel only when there are facilities for therapeutic oxygen. Patients with acute asthmatic episodes not relieved by self-medication and status asthmaticus should avoid air travel till such attacks are well controlled. Rupture of emphysematous bullae producing tension pneumothorax is a possible risk on board the aircraft.

- ***Hematological diseases:*** It would seem wise to restrict air travel if the hemoglobin level is less than 9 g/dL. Patients with sickle cell disease should undertake air travel only if the ambient oxygen tension can be maintained at 150 mm Hg. Splenic infarction and serious sickle cell crises can be precipitated if the oxygen tension is low.

- ***Pregnancy*** beyond the 35th week may pose the risk of labor during flight.

DEEP VEIN THROMBOSIS

Many long distance travellers who sit crammed up in aircraft for flights exceeding eight hours may develop DVT in the lower limbs particularly so in obese and elderly persons. Presence of thrombophilia adds to the risk. In addition to the mechanical obstruction to venous drainage and inactivity during the flight, there is evidence that continuous flights exceeding 8 hours may activate the coagulation cascade in predisposed individuals.

Fighter aircrafts: Modern fighter aircrafts exceed human physiological limits to withstand head to foot acceleration forces (positive G2 forces). This may lead to sudden syncope with prolonged periods of incapacitation, especially in vagotonic individuals. Psychomotor performance may be impaired. All these adverse effects can be avoided by proper conditioning of the individuals during training.

All commercial airlines provide information on the facilities available with them for transportation of invalid passengers. All airports have facilities for attending to emergencies that may develop during air travel.

Points to Remember

- Hypoxia may aggravate angina or cardiac failure in a hypertensive or patients with coronary artery disease (CAD).
- Atherosclerotic individuals may develop cerebral ischemia.
- Expansion of gases in body cavities produces various symptoms.
- Healthy individuals may be prone to motion sickness, cardiac arrhythmias and manic excitement.
- Chronically ill patients should take sufficient precautions before undertaking air travel.
- DVT may occur in susceptible individuals during long flights.

ROAD ACCIDENTS

General Considerations

In modern times, mortality and morbidity caused by road accidents is on the rise. This is common in all countries of the world where fast traffic on the road is increasing.

In India, 30 persons out of 100,000 die annually due to road traffic accidents. The accidents may involve the vehicles or the pedestrians using the road. The major types of accidents are collision between vehicles, loss of control of the vehicle and collision with hard objects or overturning. The other type of accidents involves knocking down pedestrians or occupants of lighter vehicles such as two wheelers and light motor vehicles. In general, the major damage and passenger injury occurs to the lighter vehicle.

The major factors contributing to road accidents can be classified as given below:

- Causes attributable to the vehicles:
  - *Speed of the vehicle:* The rate and severity of the accident increases with increasing speed of either vehicle. With the introduction of modern highways speed-related injuries have become much more common.
  - *Mechanical defects in the vehicle*, which lead to failure of the controls.
  - *Exceeding the safety limits* prescribed for the vehicle in terms of speed, loading and maintenance.
- Causes attributable to the driver:
  - *Fatigue and sleep:* Long driving exceeding 6 hours of continuous driving leads to driver fatigue, delay in the reflexes and tendency to sleep.
  - *Drunkenness:* Consumption of alcohol and less commonly other narcotic drugs impairs the efficiency of the driver.
  - *Inattention, non-compliance with signals and rash driving.*
  - *Inexperience of the driver.*

Most of the major collision accidents occur on highways, especially in the early hours of the morning when driver fatigue and somnolence are maximal. Rarely accidents may occur due to organic disease in the driver such as epilepsy, cardiovascular disease, strokes and others.

Injuries to Pedestrians

Walking on highways and fast traffic roads is associated with injury to the pedestrians. Elderly people, obese individuals, persons with movement disorders, alcoholics and children are involved more.

INJURIES CAUSED BY ROAD ACCIDENTS

Vehicular Accidents

Trauma to the driver and passengers due to the impact and damage and deformation to the vehicle are usually serious. This leads to injuries which may be instantaneously fatal. In motor car accidents, the luggage kept unsecured in the passenger compartment fly out and cause further missile-like injuries to the passengers. Trauma to vital parts such as head, chest cage, spine, bones, abdomen and major blood vessels, intracranial injuries, intracranial bleeding, tension pneumothorax, rupture of major blood vessels like aorta, injuries to the heart, rupture of solid organs and hollow viscera in the abdomen and pelvis and exsanguinating bleeding (both external and internal) are the causes of death at the site of accident or within a few hours. Pedestrian injuries cause death due to damage to vital structures, especially intracranial bleeding, chest injuries, intra-abdominal injuries and exsanguination.

MANAGEMENT AT THE SITE OF ACCIDENT

Effective first aid helps to save life and reduce morbidity and delayed mortality. Mainly this consists of maintenance of the airway and attention to ventilation, tourniquets to arrest external hemorrhage, immobilization of parts of the body such as the neck and spine to avoid further damage to the vital neural structures, covering open chest injuries which interfere with ventilation and rapid transport to the nearest hospital with adequate facilities. ***It is the duty of all medical men to give first aid in such a situation.*** It is to be remembered that an obvious injury may distract the attention of the doctor from other invisible injuries such as internal bleeding or rupture of viscera which can cause death.

When major accidents involving buses occur, a large member of persons will be simultaneously affected and this may cause a heavy strain on the medical facilities. In this situation, a senior medical officer has to inspect the victims and using the principles of 'triage', arrange for appropriate management. In such an emergency all medical personnel have to participate in the emergency management.

All road traffic accidents invite legal procedures which have to be complied with.

GENERAL GUIDELINES TO REDUCE ROAD TRAFFIC ACCIDENTS AND THEIR CONSEQUENCES

- Education of the public on the safe use of roads and motor vehicles
- Strict compliance with road traffic rules
- Avoidance of alcohol and drugs before driving
- Avoid driver fatigue and somnolence
- Avoid the presence of unsecured luggage in the passenger compartment
- Use the seat belts as prescribed
- Enforcement of traffic regulations by the appropriate authorities.
- Modern automobiles are providing safety equipment such as airbags which inflate automatically on the occurrence of a crash and prevent chest injury to the driver against the steering wheel and head injuries to the passengers.

Note: In all developed countries, well-coordinated emergency management teams attached to major hospitals are available, ready to render assistance at the site of accident, during transport to hospital and later. This team consists of trained ambulance personnel, anesthetists, trauma care surgeons, other physicians and specialists, trained nursing team and paramedics.

Points to Remember

- Road accidents are increasing to reach epidemic proportions.
- Main causes are over speed and driver fatigue.
- Proper first and specialized care help to save life and reduce morbidity.
- Road accidents are preventable to a great extent.

CHAPTER 22

Acute Poisoning: General Considerations

KV Krishna Das, TK Suma

Chapter Summary

- General Considerations
- Clinical Presentation
- General Management
  - Specific Measures
- Methods to Eliminate Poisons
  - Forced Diuresis
  - Dialysis and Hemoperfusion
- Indications for Treatment in Intensive Care Unit
- Prognosis of Poisoning

GENERAL CONSIDERATIONS

Acute poisoning accounts for 2–3% of admissions into major general hospitals in India. Poison is defined as a substance that causes injury, illness or death, when introduced into the body by ingestion, inoculation, inhalation or any other route which permits absorption of the substances into tissues. Poisoning may be suicidal, accidental or homicidal. The high incidence of poisoning is attributed to the widespread use and free availability of insecticides, pesticides and other harmful chemicals for use in agriculture and industry. Depending upon the cost and local availability, varied substances are used. In the order of frequency, the toxic agents include organophosphorus compounds, barbiturates, benzodiazepines, vegetable poisons, phenothiazines, corrosive acids and several others. The precipitating factors, which drive persons to commit suicide, are depressive illness, financial problems, domestic conflicts, and frustration in studies and jobs or incurable illness. Among epileptics and alcoholics the incidence of suicidal poisoning is high. Accidental poisoning is common in children. Persons engaged in the use of toxic chemicals in agriculture and in industry are liable to suffer if proper safety precautions are not adhered to.

Classification of Poisons

Based on the chief symptoms they produce are as follows:
- Corrosives—strong acids, strong alkalis, metallic salts
- Irritants—organic, inorganic
- Systemic—cerebral, spinal, peripheral, cardiovascular system (CVS), asphyxiants
- Miscellaneous—food poisoning and botulism.

Household poisons: Shampoos, toothpaste, lipstick, creams, shaving cream, toilet soaps, cosmetics, hair dye/oil.

CLINICAL PRESENTATION

Though poisoning by many chemicals lead to characteristic clinical features, in the majority of cases symptoms are nonspecific and may be mistaken for other acute illnesses. The presentations could be vomiting, convulsions, gastro-enteritis, acute psychosis, coma, circulatory collapse or pulmonary edema.

Corrosive poisons produce noticeable lesions at the points of maximum contact such as the mouth, esophagus and stomach. Other poisons affect specific organs maximally, e.g. liver damage in paracetamol poisoning, cardiac dysfunction in *Cerbera odollam* poisoning and renal damage in copper sulfate poisoning. Poisons consumed on an empty stomach are absorbed more rapidly than if taken on full stomach. Also, if taken along with alcohol, many poisons are quickly absorbed and their damaging effects become cumulative.

Diagnosis: It is rendered easy if proper history or evidence of the material is obtained, but in many cases such help is not available. A high index of suspicion on the part of the physician is absolutely necessary for arriving at an early diagnosis in such cases.

Abrupt occurrence of acute illness in a person who is in good health should suggest acute poisoning as a possibility. Smell of alcohol or kerosene, severe respiratory depression, circulatory collapse, convulsions, constricted pupils, cardiac arrhythmias, dystonic postures and muscle fasciculation add support to this diagnosis. The outcome depends upon factors like:

- The amount of poison and its mode of administration
- Presence of food in the stomach at the time of ingestion
- Delay in starting treatment
- Age
- General health and concurrent illness
- Availability of specific antidotes.

Patients who are comatose due to acute poisoning face the twin dangers of the toxic-effects of the chemical and the grave consequences of an obstructed airway.

Potential Complications

- Thrombocytopenia (about 30% reduction)
- Leukopenia (about 10% reduction)
- Loss of clotting factors
- Lowering of calcium, glucose
- Bleeding tendency due to heparinization

- Patient may disconnect shunt lines
- Air embolism
- Infection.

GENERAL MANAGEMENT

Irrespective of the clinical condition attempts to identify the poison should be started. These include: (1) Examining the container which may be left behind, (2) Odor, (3) Examining the gastric and intestinal contents obtained spontaneously or deliberately collected and getting clues from the clinical presentation.

An apparently mild case may sink into dangerous states when the unabsorbed poison gets absorbed.

Acute poisoning is a medical emergency and is best treated in a well-equipped hospital with teams specially trained to handle such cases. Since in many cases the nature of the poison will not be evident at first, the aim of treatment is to keep the patient alive with support of vital functions, eliminate as much of the poison as possible from the body and prevent further absorption of poison. Specific antidotes are to be given as soon as the nature of the poison is known. Selective antidotes are available only for 2% of such poisons. A detailed history particularly including the previous mental state and social status of the patient is very helpful. Specimens for analysis should be collected in appropriate containers for chemical and other tests. If a toxin is suspected its dose duration of action and progression of symptoms should be recorded. All forms of poisoning (homicidal, suicidal and accidental) invite medicolegal problems and therefore the appropriate personnel should be informed about the patient as early as possible.

Goals of Treatment

- Reduce absorption of the toxin (xenobiotic)
- Enhance elimination
- Neutralize toxin.

Emergency management: Most important is to clear the airway and ensure adequate ventilation by positioning, suction or by insertion of nasal or oropharyngeal airway. The respiration should be clinically assessed and if there is ventilatory impairment necessary support with supplemental oxygenation and mechanical ventilation should be instituted. Intermittent positive pressure respiration has to be started with endotracheal intubation, if conservative measures fail. The patient should be turned from side to side at four-hourly intervals to prevent aspiration and pneumonia. Frequent bronchial suction helps to prevent atelectasis and aspiration pneumonia.

Shock is managed on the usual lines. Maintenance of fluid and electrolyte balance is of utmost importance in all cases.

Reduce Absorption of the Toxin

Removal from surface skin and eye.

Decontamination of skin: Pesticides and other chemicals which are present on the clothes and skin get absorbed through the skin and worsen the condition. Similarly corrosive agents rapidly injure the skin and eyes. In these situations, washing the affected area with large quantities of water and soap prevents further systemic absorption of the toxin. Normal saline is preferred for irrigation of the eyes.

- Induction of emesis
- Gastric lavage
- Activated charcoal administration and cathartics
- Dilution—milk/other drinks for corrosives
- Whole bowel irrigation
- Endoscopic or surgical removal of ingested chemical.

General Measures

Intake of fluid and urine output should be monitored and a urine output of at least 1500 mL should be ensured. Replacement of electrolytes and correction of acidosis should be done with proper laboratory monitoring. Maintenance of nutrition is equally important. Diet containing 2000 calories should be given orally if the patient is conscious. In unconscious patients, nasogastric tube feeding should be given. Parenteral nutrition has to be started in severely affected patients.

Repeated examination of blood and urine for the level of the toxic agent helps to monitor the progress with treatment.

Specific Measures

Reduce Absorption

Ingested poisons: In many cases of ingested poisons, considerable amounts remain in the gastrointestinal tract (GIT) up to four hours; hence it is absolutely necessary to take appropriate measures for their removal. Induction of vomiting is safe in conscious patients. Vomiting is induced by tickling the pharynx or administration of gastric irritants such as concentrated common salt solution 200–400 mL. In case of corrosive poisons and highly irritant substances like kerosene, emesis and gastric intubation are contraindicated. Gastric lavage using a stomach tube is an effective method to empty gastric contents rapidly and this can be done even in unwilling patients. This is the method of choice in all conscious patients who have consumed noncorrosive poisons. However, it is risky in comatose patients due to the danger of aspiration into the respiratory tract. In such cases, aspiration through Ryle's tube is preferable. Gastric contents should be preserved in a sealed bottle for chemical examination and further medicolegal procedures. Use of activated charcoal, which absorb many toxins reduces gastric and intestinal absorption further. Activated charcoal 5 g/dose can be repeated 4 hourly and can also be given with sorbitol, a cathartic. The surface area of activated charcoal increases several folds and this large surface area adsorbs several substances non-specifically.

Gastric lavage

- It decreases absorption by 42% if done 20 min and by 16% if performed at 60 min
- Performed by first aspirating the stomach and then repetitively instilling and aspirating fluid
- Left lateral position better—delays spontaneous absorption
- Choice of fluid is tap water—5–10 mL/kg
- Preferably done on awake patients
- Presence of a tracheal tube does not preclude aspiration, though preferred if Glasgow coma scale (GCS) is low

Textbook of Medicine

- Contraindicated in comatose patients, in corrosive poisoning, kerosene poison and in patients with convulsions.

Enhance elimination: Purgatives such as magsulf 15–30 g or sorbitol 1 g/kg bw (maximum of 150 g) orally followed by bowel wash 2 hours later help to eliminate the poison from the intestine.

Multiple dose activated charcoal: Doses of activated charcoal 1–2 g/kg bw repeated every 2–4 hours hasten elimination of drugs by adsorption of drugs excreted into the gut lumen (gut dialysis).

- Increased elimination is possible only if—
  - The drug is distributed predominantly in the extracellular fluid (ECF)
  - Has a low protein binding
  - The induced rate of elimination is faster than the normal rate
  - Hazards of having a longer time of exposure to the drug mortality is increased.

METHODS TO ELIMINATE POISONS

- Forced diuresis
- Peritoneal dialysis
- Hemodialysis
- Hemoperfusion

Forced Diuresis

The kidneys can be made to eliminate poisonous drugs at a rate consistent with the urine output. Contraindications include congestive cardiac failure (CCF), renal failure, rhabdomyolysis and cerebral edema.

In an unconscious patient, a Foley's catheter should be introduced to facilitate uninterrupted flow of urine and for proper monitoring of output.

This is employed when the toxin is removable by the kidney and the metabolites are toxic to the system. A substantial proportion of the poison is excreted in the urine unchanged. For this, the poison should be distributed mainly in the ECF and only minimally bound or not bound at all to proteins.

Rationale: Elimination of the toxic substance is enhanced by manipulation of the urine pH so as to render the toxin in the ionized form. Forced diuresis should be considered and may be indicated, in poisoning due to the following substances.

Alkaline diuresis	Acid diuresis
Phenobarbitone or barbitone	Phencyclidine
Salicylates	Amphetamine
Phenoxyacetate herbicides	Fenfluramine

Potential Complications

- Fluid overload
- Pulmonary edema
- Cerebral edema
- Electrolyte and acid-base disturbances.

Diuresis is induced by giving 5% glucose continuously IV as drip and furosemide IV in dose of 20 mg/6 hours depending on the response. Proper estimation of electrolytes and acid-base states should be undertaken during and after the procedure.

Forced acid diuresis: The urine pH is adjusted to 5.5–6.5 by giving—10 g arginine or lysine hydrochloride IV over 30 minutes followed by ammonium chloride 4 g/2 hours, by mouth.

Forced alkaline diuresis: The urine pH is adjusted to 7.5–8.5 by giving boluses of 50 mmoL (approx 50 mL) of 7.5% sodium bicarbonate solution. Often 200–300 mmoL is required in the first 1–2 hours. Since a large sodium load is being given with the bicarbonate cardiac failure may be precipitated in susceptible individuals.

Dialysis and Hemoperfusion

Dialysis: Since most of the cases recover with forced diuresis, hemodialysis is indicated only in a few. Indications for hemodialysis are: (a) High blood levels of the drug, (b) renal failure, (c) nonresponsiveness to forced diuresis and (d) poisoning associated with deep coma, hypotension and fluid, and electrolyte disturbances. In the absence of facilities for hemodialysis, peritoneal dialysis should be undertaken. Hemodialysis is 6–10 times more efficient than peritoneal dialysis.

Hemoperfusion is the process of passing the patient's blood through cartridges packed with activated charcoal, which adsorbs drugs and toxins such as barbiturates, carbamazepine, glutethimide, meprobamate, methaqualone and several others. Cartridges ready for use are available commercially.

In hemodialysis, materials which are dialyzable including toxic materials, are dialyzed across a semipermeable membrane, using appropriate solutions, which will permit the removal of the toxic substance. This can be done even in secondary care hospitals. Hemoperfusion is the removal of the toxic material by perfusion of blood through a cartridge containing material, which will adsorb the particular substance.

Requisites for Instituting Dialysis Procedures

- The drug or toxic substance should diffuse easily through the peritoneum or dialysis membrane or be readily adsorbed to activated charcoal or uncharged resin.
- A significant proportion of the poison should be present in plasma or be capable of rapid equilibration with it.
- The pharmacological effect of the substance should be directly related to the blood concentration.
- Antidote is not easily available.

Indications for Dialysis and Hemoperfusion

- Severe clinical intoxication as shown by grade IV coma, hypotension, hypothermia and hypoventilation caused by hypnotic drugs.
- Progressive clinical deterioration, despite adequate supportive management.
- High plasma concentration of the toxic agents.

Drugs that can be effectively dialyzed includes barbiturates, phenytoin, primidone, paraldehyde, chloral hydrate, amphetamine, alcohols, methanol, ethylene glycol, salicylates, paracetamol, several antibiotics, isoniazid, quinine, quinidine, metallic salts including lithium, bromide, iodide and potassium, ergotamine, carbon tetrachloride toxic principles of mushrooms and others.

Contraindications

- The toxic substance is a rapid acting metabolic poison.
- The effect of the substance is irreversible, e.g. organophosphorus compounds.
- The drug is relatively nontoxic, e.g. benzodiazepines.
- The drug has a very large volume of distribution.
- Cardiogenic shock.
- Coagulopathy.

Antidotes: They are available for 2% of the poisonous substances. These may be chemical antidotes, which neutralize the action of the poison, or biological antidotes, which prevent their pharmacological response. They should be employed only after ascertaining the nature of the poison. In most cases, the antidote is indicated by the manufacturers on the packing of the toxic chemical (Table 22.1).

Many of the patients with suicidal poisoning attempt to repeat these episodes because of their psychiatric problems. Hence, it is necessary to instruct their relatives, also arrange for proper psychiatric assessment and treatment after the initial episode.

Types of elimination procedure ideal for specific toxic agents	
Salicylates	1, 2, 3
Phenobarbitone	1, 2, 3
Barbitone	1, 2, 3
Methanol/ethanol	1, 2, 3
Lithium	1, 2
Isopropanol	1, 2
Short and medium acting barbiturates	3
Glutethimide	3
Meprobamate	3
Methaqualone	3
Disopyramide	3
Theophylline	3

Key: 1. Peritoneal dialysis, 2. Hemodialysis, 3. Hemoperfusion

The choice of elimination technique should depend upon the plasma level of the substance.

INDICATIONS FOR TREATMENT IN INTENSIVE CARE UNIT

Respiratory Problem

- Airway protection
- Respiratory failure

Cardiovascular Problem

- Hypotension despite fluid challenge
- Heart block, arrhythmias, QTc prolongation [as in tricyclic antidepressant (TCA)]

Neurologic Problem

- Glasgow coma scale < 8
- Seizures

Metabolic

- Hypoglycemia
- Significant electrolyte abnormalities, metabolic acidosis
- Hepatic failure
- Coagulopathy with bleeding.

PROGNOSIS OF POISONING

Apart from the immediate acute situation whose prognosis depends on the following:

- Type, quality, mode of administration and availability of the specific antidote
- The clinical condition when first encountering the patient
- The availability of facilities in the treating institutions, many cases attempt to commit self harm repeatedly, often with better success rates, so it is essential to arrange counseling sessions for the survivor and the near relatives to avoid recurrence.

Table 22.1: Specific antidotes to poisons commonly consumed

Poison	Antidote	Dose
Organophosphates	Atropine	Loading dose 2 mg IV every 2–5 minutes until pupils dilate and salivation is reduced. Maintenance based on pupil size for hours to days
	Pralidoxime	Loading dose 1–2 g IV repeat after 3 hours
Opiates (opium, morphine, meperidine, propoxyphene, pentazocine, diphenoxylate)	Naloxone (nalorphine hydrochloride)	Loading dose 0.4–2 mg IV repeat in 2–5 minutes, as is required
Methanol, ethylene glycol	Ethanol	Loading dose 0.6–0.7 g/kg. Maintenance—sufficient ethanol to keep serum alcohol level at 100 mg/dL (approx 125 mg/kg/hour) and methanol concentration falls below 10 mg/dL
Cyanide	Amyl nitrate, sodium nitrite, sodium thiosulfate to be given sequentially	• Start with amyl nitrate inhalation 1 amp every 2–3 minutes • Then give sodium nitrite 10 mL of 3% solution IV over 5 minutes • Then give 50 mL of 25% sodium thiosulfate over 10 minutes
Acetaminophen	N-acetylcysteine	140 mg/kg oral, thereafter 70 mg/kg oral every 4 hours for 17 doses (72 hours)
Iron salts	Desferrioxamine	If the patient is hypotensive 10 mg/kg/hour IV for 4 hours, then 5 mg/kg/hour IV until serum iron level is less than 100 μg/dL. If patient is normotensive, 40 mg/kg IV every 4–12 hours. Total daily dose should not exceed 6 g.

Appendix 22.1: Elimination procedures for substances if their plasma level is high

Substance	Procedure
Salicylates	
500 mg/L + metabolic acidosis or 750 mg/L	Alkaline diuresis
750 mg/L + renal failure or 900 mg/L	*Hemodialysis or

Contd...

Substance	Procedure
All barbiturates except phenobarbitone and barbitone 50 mg/L	*Hemoperfusion
Glutethemide 50 mg/L	-do-
Meprobamate 100 mg/L	-do-
Methaqualone 40 mg/L	-do-
Trichloroethanol derivatives 50 mg/L	-do-
Phenobarbitone and barbitone	
75–100 mg/L	Alkaline diuresis
150 mg/L	Hemodialysis, hemoperfusion
Theophylline 60 mg/L	Hemoperfusion. Correction of hypokalemia is most important and this may obviate the need for hemoperfusion
Methanol, ethylene or glycol 0.5 g/dL	• Peritoneal dialysis • Hemodialysis • Dialysis is indicated if more than 30 g has been ingested or there is metabolic acidosis, mental, visual or funduscopic abnormalities. Many antifreeze solutions now contain methanol as well as ethylene glycol
Isopropanol 0.4 g/dL	Hemodialysis, significant hypotension is an important clinical indication for hemodialysis
Lithium 5 mmol/L (3470 g/L)	Peritoneal dialysis or hemodialysis. Forced diuresis is ineffective and an infusion of sodium chloride is dangerous as well

Note: *Hemodialysis and hemoperfusion are more efficient than forced diuresis.

Appendix 22.2: Clinical clues to identify the poison	
Odor	
Bitter almonds	Cyanide
Acetone	Isopropyl alcohol, methanol, paraldehyde, salicylates
Alcohol	Ethanol
Oil of Wintergreen	Methyl salicylate
Garlic	Arsenic, thallium, organophosphates
Ocular signs	
Miosis	Narcotics (except meperidine), organophosphates, muscarinic mushrooms, clonidine, phenothiazine's, chloral hydrate, barbiturates (late), PCP
Mydriasis	Atropine, alcohol, cocaine, amphetamines, antihistamines, cyclic antidepressants, cyanide, carbon monoxide
Nystagmus	Phenytoin, barbiturates, éthanol, carbon monoxide
Lacrimation	Organophosphates, irritant gas or vapors
Retinal hyperemia	Methanol
Poor vision	Methanol, botulism, carbon monoxide
Cutaneous signs	
Needle tracks	Heroin, PCP, amphetamines
Bullae	Carbon monoxide, barbiturates
Dry, hot skin	Anticholinergic agents, botulism
Diaphoresis	Organophosphates, nitrates, muscarinic mushrooms, aspirin, cocaine
Alopecia	Thallium, arsenic, lead, mercury
Erythema	Boric acid, mercury, cyanide, anticholinergics
Oral signs	
Salivation	Organophosphates, salicylates, corrosives, strychnine
Dry mouth	Amphetamines, anticholinergics, antihistamine
Burns	Corrosives, oxalate-containing plants
Gum lines	Lead, mercury, arsenic
Dysphagia	Corrosives, botulism

Contd...

Intestinal signs	
Cramps	Arsenic, lead, thallium, organophosphates
Diarrhea	Antimicrobials, arsenic, iron, boric acid
Constipation	Lead, narcotics, botulism
Hematemesis	Aminophylline, corrosives, acid and alkalines iron, salicylates
Cardiac signs	
Tachycardia	Atropine, aspirin, amphetamines, cocaine, cyclic antidepressants, theophylline
Bradycardia	Digitalis, narcotics, mushrooms, clonidine, organophosphates, β blockers, calcium channel blockers
Hypertension	Amphetamines, LSD, cocaine, PCP
Hypotension	Phenothiazines, barbiturates, cyclic antidepressants, iron, β blockers, calcium channel blockers or any type of severe poison
Respiratory signs	
Depressed respiration	Alcohol, narcotics, barbiturates, overdose of sedatives
Increased respiration	Amphetamines, aspirin, ethylene glycol, carbon monoxide, cyanide
Pulmonary edema	Hydrocarbons, heroin, organophosphates, aspirin
Central nervous system (CNS) signs	
Ataxia	Alcohol, antidepressants, barbiturates, anticholinergics, phenytoin, narcotics
Coma	Sedatives, narcotics, barbiturates, PCP, organophosphates, salicylates, cyanide, carbon monoxide, cyclic antidepressants, lead any severe poisoning
Hyperpyrexia	Anticholinergics, quinine, salicylates, LSD, phenothiazine's, amphetamines, cocaine
Muscle fasciculation	Organophosphates, theophylline
Muscle rigidity	Cyclic antidepressants, PCP, phenothiazines, haloperidol
Convulsions	Strychnine, any stimulant drug in high over dose
Paresthesia	Cocaine, camphor, PCP, MSG
Peripheral neuropathy	Lead, arsenic, mercury, organophosphates
Altered behavior	LSD, PCP, amphetamines, cocaine, alcohol, anticholinergics, camphor

Abbreviations: PCP = Phencyclidine; LSD = Lysergic acid diethylamide; MSG = monosodium glutamate

Appendix 22.3: Antidotes to commonly taken toxic substances	
Acetaminophen	N-acetylcysteine
Anticholinergics	Physostigmine
Calcium channel blockers	Glucagon, insulin + dextrose, calcium
Carbamate	Atropine
Cyanide	Thiosulfate, nitrate
Digoxin	Digoxin antibodies
Isoniazid	Pyridoxine
Methanol	Ethanol, fomepizole
Glycol	Ethanol, fomepizole
Opioid	Naloxone

Contd...

Contd...

Oral hypoglycemics	Glucose
Organophosphate	Atropine, pralidoxime (2-PAM)
Warfarin	Vitamin K
Iron	Desferroxamine
Copper	Penicillamine, dimercaprol, CaEDTA
Lead	CaEDTA, dimercaprol (BAL)
Mercury	DMPS, DMSA, BAL
Arsenic	BAL and derivatives
Antimony	BAL and derivatives

Abbreviations: CaEDTA = Calcium ethylenediamine tetracetic acid; BAL = British anti-Lewisite; DMPS = 2,3-Dimercapto-1-propanesulfonic acid; DMSA = Dimercaptosuccinic acid

Common Poisons

KV Krishna Das, TK Suma

Chapter Summary

- Organophosphorus Compounds
- Organocarbamates
- Organochlorine Insecticides
- Ethylene Dibromide Poisoning (EDB)
- Phosphide Poisoning
- Pyrethroid Poisoning
- Bipyridyl Herbicides
  - Paraquat and Diquat
- Rodenticides
- Cyanide Poisoning
- Methanol
- Barbiturates
- Sedative Drug Poisoning
  - Benzodiazepines Poisioning
- Alcohol Intoxication
  - Alcohol Withdrawal Syndrome
- Cerbera Odollam
- Cleistanthus Collinus Leaf
- Corrosive Acids
- Acetic Acid
- Formic Acid
- Alkalies
- Narcotics (Morphine and Opioids)
- Paracetamol
- Petroleum Products (Kerosene)

ORGANOPHOSPHORUS COMPOUNDS

These are the most widely used toxic agents for suicidal poisoning. Accidental poisoning occurs in workmen engaged in spraying the compound. Contamination of food materials during storage or transportation has led to dramatic outbreaks of food poisoning in Kerala and many other parts of India. A dose of 40–100 mg proves fatal.

The commonly available products are methyl parathion (Folidol, Paramer, Metacid, Paramet), malathion (Malathion Cythion) and phaolone (Zolone, Sumithion, Faithion, Timidan, Ekatkin).

Organophosphorus compounds irreversibly phosphorylate acetylecholinesterase (AChE) enzyme which usually degrades acetylcholine into choline and acetic acid. This leads to the accumulation of acetylcholine at the cholinergic nerve endings such as autonomic ganglia, parasympathetic nerve endings and motor end plates.

Clinical Features

Symptoms start within 15–30 minutes after ingestion of the toxin. Consumption on an empty stomach and along with alcohol favors rapid absorption. Gastrointestinal or neurological symptoms may predominate. Nausea, vomiting, diarrhea, involuntary defecation, blurring of vision, miosis, excessive sweating, lacrimation, salivation, and pulmonary edema constitute the muscarinic effects. Effects on central nervous system (CNS) include drowsiness, coma, convulsions and respiratory depression. Stimulation of preganglionic fibers leads to sympathetic over action and later paralysis, muscle twitching, fasciculation, weakness and flaccid paralysis (nicotinic effects) (Tables 23.1 and 23.2).

Clinical features take the pattern of a triphasic illness:

Acute cholinergic syndrome

- Cholinergic symptoms develop within the first 24 hours and persists due to blockade of ***AChE*** at all the receptors.
- Features include garlic like odor in the breath/vomitus and clothes, bradycardia (80%), miosis, fasciculations, twitching, convulsions, flacid paralysis of limbs and extraocular muscles and central depression of respiratory system.

Intermediate syndrome: This ushers in 24–96 hours after the cholinergic phase settles. Further details are given in page 33.

Diagnosis

In almost all cases, history circumstances and smell of the poison help to confirm the diagnosis. The chemical can be identified by examination of gastric contents and blood.

Table 23.1: Clinical features of poisoning by organophosphorus compounds

Time of manifestation	Mechanism	Manifestation
Acute (minutes to 24–h)	Nicotinic receptor action	Weakness, fasciculations, cramps, paralysis
	Muscarinic receptor action	Salivation, lacrimation, urination, defecation, gastric cramps, emesis, bradycardia, hypotension miosis, bronchospasm
	Central receptors	Anxiety, restlessness, convulsions, respiratory depression
Delayed (24-h to 2-week)	Nicotinic receptor action	Intermediate syndrome
	Muscarinic receptor action	Cholinergic symptoms— bradycardia, miosis, salivation
	Central receptors	Coma, extrapyramidal manifestations
Late (beyond 2-week)	Peripheral-neuropathy target esterase	Peripheral neuropathic process

Textbook of Medicine

Table 23.2: Specific clinical features due to action on different receptors

Muscarinic	Nicotinic	Central receptors
Cardiovascular	**Cardiovascular**	Anxiety
Bradycardia	Tachycardia	Restlessness
Hypotension	Hypertension	Ataxia
Respiratory	**Musculoskeletal**	Convulsions
Rhinorrhea	Weakness	Insomnia
Bronchorrhea/	Fasciculations	Dysarthria
spasm	Cramps	Tremors
Cough	Paralysis	Coma
Gastrointestinal		Absent reflexes
Increased salivation		Cheyne-Stokes
Nausea/vomiting		respiration
Abdominal pain		Respiratory
Diarrhea		depression
Fecal incontinence		Circulatory collapse
Genitourinary		
Urinary incontinence		
Ocular		
Blurred vision/miosis		
Increased		
lacrimation		

Diagnosis is clinical, supported by evidence of consumption of the poison. Estimation of serum levels of pseudocholinesterase enzyme is helpful. Normal level of pseudocholinesterase in serum is 1750–3500 µU/mL. Serum levels of the enzyme correlate inversely with the severity and this is a practical method to assess severity and response to treatment.

Reduction of serum pseudocholinesterase values below 50% of baseline suggests poisoning.
- Levels of 20–50% = mild poisoning
- 10–20% = moderate severity
- <10% = severe
- Levels < 200 IU are associated with ventilatory failure.

Treatment

The general measures for oral poisons should be instituted without delay.

Atropine

It is the pharmacological antidote and is the sheet anchor of treatment since it antagonizes the peripheral effects of acetylcholine. This drug prevents pulmonary edema and excessive secretions. The dose requirement varies widely. In general, large doses have to be used. The ideal way to administer the drug is through an intravenous (IV) 5% glucose drip. A dose of 2 mg is given initially and 1 mg or more is repeated every 10 minutes (or even at shorter intervals) till the pupils are dilated to normal size and pulmonary edema and bronchorrhea is cleared. In many cases, several hundred ampoules of atropine may be required within a few hours to tide over the crises. The patient has to be observed very closely to prevent deterioration and death.

Maintenance dose is continued to keep the pupils in mid-dilation. In many cases, pupillary dilation may be delayed. It is usually possible to withdraw atropine after 24–48 hours but in some cases it may have to be continued for up to 5 days. Release of the toxin from lipid tissues after an interval of 2–3 days may result in return of symptoms and death after a period of apparent recovery. Hence, all patients have to be closely watched for at least 7 days after onset of the symptoms. In such cases, repetition of massive doses of atropine and supportive measures are to be undertaken. It is not uncommon to use 200–300 ampoules of atropine for a moderately severe case.

Atropine toxicity is indicated by **absence bowel sounds, fever and confusion**. If this occurs stop atropine infusion for 60 minutes and restart infusion at 50% of initial rate, once the temperature comes down and the patient gets calm.

Pralidoxime Hydrochloride

Pralidoxime hydrochloride is the specific antidote. It is given IV in a dose of 1–2 g initially and repeated 2–3 hours later along with the use of atropine. It is available as 500 mg in 20 mL vials. Pralidoxime hydrochloride reactivates cholinesterase enzyme at the neuromuscular junctions by removing the phosphate group bound to the cholinesterase. It also binds to free organophosphate. The toxic effects of pralidoxime include tachycardia, cardiac arrhythmias, tachypnea, hypertension and relaxation of sphincters. The commercial preparation is 2 pyridine aldoxime (aldopam). Pralidoxime methane sulfate is also available in India. In addition to pralidoxime, atropine has to be continued for symptomatic therapy in the required doses till the enzyme levels reach normal.

A high dose regimen of pralidoxime consisting of a continuous infusion of 1g/h for 48 hours after a 2 g loading dose reduces morbidity and mortality in moderately severe cases of acute organophosphorus pesticide toxicity. This reduces the need for atropine, as well as duration of ventilatory support.

Source: Pawar KS, Bhoite RR, Pillay CP, et al. Continuous pralidoxime infusion versus repeated bolus injection to treat organophosphorus pesticide poisoning: a randomised controlled trial. Lancet. 2006;368(9553):2136-41.

Complications

Fatal bronchopneumonia may develop during convalescence. The neurological complications may take the form of **intermediate syndrome** occurring within 1–4 days of poisoning usually after resolution of acute symptoms. This syndrome is characterized by bulbar, nuchal and proximal muscle weakness including respiratory paralysis requiring mechanical ventilation. Distal muscle groups are usually spared whereas a distal sensorimotor polyneuropathy may occur 2–3 weeks later. Sometimes cranial nerves may also be involved. The onset of intermediate syndrome usually coincides with the time of atropine withdrawal. Therefore, oximes and atropine should be withdrawn carefully and gradually.

Prevention and first aid: Accidental poisoning can be prevented by taking adequate precautions detailed on the commercial packing. Persons spraying insecticides should wear protective clothing and masks, and wash their bodies with soap and water thoroughly after the work, before taking food or drink. Immediate first aid after accidental poisoning includes induction of emesis and removal of contaminated clothing and washing the body thoroughly with soap and water. The subject should be transported to a hospital without delay.

> **Points to Remember**
> - Organophosphorus compounds irreversibly phosphorylate AChE enzyme.
> - The symptoms include muscarinic and nicotinic features.
> - Atropine is the pharmacological antidote to be given till features of atropinization appear.
> - Pralidoxime hydrochloride reactivates cholinesterase enzyme by removing phosphate group.
> - Intermediate syndrome is a complication occurring 1–4 days after poisoning.
> - Precautions are to be taken for accidental poisoning.

ORGANOCARBAMATES

Organocarbamates (OC) are structurally similar to organophosphorus compounds and they inhibit AChE. The common preparations are aldicarb (Temik), aprocarb, bendigocarbonate, carbofuran (Furadan), carbosulfan (Marshal), N-methyl carbamate (carbamoyl), propoxur (Baygon) and others.

Duration of action of OC is shorter than that of organophosphorus compounds and therefore, generally the duration of symptoms in mild cases is shorter. This may not be true in severe cases. Amitraz which is used in agriculture and veterinary medicine as an acaricide, insecticide and antiparasite drug produces stimulation of alpha 2 effects on the nervous system leading to neurotoxic and preconvulsant effects. Multiple system failure occurs which could be fatal. This poisoning has been reported from India.

Treatment: Atropine is quite effective as in the case of organophosphorus poisoning.

Glycopyrrolate which is a quaternary ammonium compound is an effective antidote. It is available as 1 mL ampoules containing 2 mg of the drug. The dose is 0.05 mg/kg IV or intramuscular (IM), to be repeated to achieve symptom relief. It does not reach the CNS and therefore the CNS side effects of atropine such as delirium and involuntary movements are avoided.

> - Organocarbomates inhibit cholinesterase transiently and reversibly
> - Regeneration of enzyme occurs within minutes to hours, therefore the effect is short-lived
> - Symptoms of intoxication are similar to organophosphates, but are of shorter duration
> - Carbamates do not effective penetrate into CNS, so there is less of CNS toxicity and seizures
> - Atropine therapy is usually not needed for longer than 6–12 hours
> - Avoid 2- pralidoxime hydrochloride since irreversible binding does not occur, it may even worsen the clinical pictures in some cases.

ORGANOCHLORINE INSECTICIDES

These common chemicals, which are used as insecticides in houses, gardens and in agriculture, have different chemical structures.
- Chlorinated diphenyls, e.g. DDT, TDE, DFDT and DMC
- Chlorinated polycyclic compounds, e.g. Chlordane, Aldrin and Endrin
- Hexachlorobenzene compounds, e.g. lindane.

These are insoluble in water, but freely soluble in organic solvents and lipids. Their solutions in petroleum, kerosene or other organic solvents are used for spraying. Poisoning may be accidental or suicidal. Acute toxicity results from ingestion or inhalation of these substances. Variable amounts of these chemicals may be absorbed through the skin and can result in toxicity. They stimulate the CNS. When used in the form of solutions, the action of the solvent modifies the total effect.

The fatal doses of these compounds are:	
DDT	20 g
Lindane	3 g
Chlordane	1 g
Aldrin and Endrin	Less than 1g

Clinical features: Early manifestations are nausea, vomiting, irritant cough, headache and body aches. These are followed by nervous irritability, mental sluggishness, muscle twitching, tremors, incordination, convulsions, paralysis and coma. Acute pulmonary edema and shock may occur if the exposure is heavy. Liver dysfunction is a prominent feature in Endrin poisoning.

Treatment: The general measures are instituted without delay. Administration of activated charcoal and saline purgatives help to reduce absorption of the chemical. Convulsions have to be controlled with injection of 10 mg of diazepam. Calcium gluconate 1 g given IV has been found to reduce the convulsive tendency. Ventilatory assistance is required if respiratory failure sets in.

Widespread use of organochlorine compounds in agriculture has led to their slow absorption through food, milk and water and these chemicals accumulate in human and animal tissues. Chronic toxicity is a potential hazard.

ETHYLENE DIBROMIDE (EDB) POISONING

It is used as an insecticide against soil nematodes, insects and termites and also as a fumigant to protect stored products. It is a colorless volatile liquid with an ethereal odor, available as liquid, capsules or granules. Suicidal poisoning has been reported from Madhya Pradesh. Symptoms include vomiting circulatory failure, pulmonary congestion, liver damage leading to hepatic encephalopathy and renal failure. Mortality may go up to 50%. Treatment is symptomatic.

PHOSPHIDE POISONING

Both zinc phosphide and aluminium phosphide are freely available rodenticides. When ingested, they liberate phosphine gas on coming into contact with moisture. This toxic phosphine is lethal to cells by reacting with the enzyme cytochrome oxidase. Zinc phosphide produces early vomiting and diarrhea within 20 minutes when ingested and severe cough, breathlessness and pulmonary edema when inhaled. Metabolic acidosis, hypocalcemic tetany and hypokalemia follow. Organs affected include the heart (toxic myocarditis), pleura (effusion) and lung (respiratory distress syndome). Fatal shock may ensue. Magnesium sulfate infused IV at a rate of 3 g in the first 3 hours and then 6 g in the next 24 hours is being evaluated in treatment. The results are equivocal.

PYRETHROID POISONING

Pyrethroids are being used more frequently in modern times in the place or organophosphorus and organo-carbamates, several preparations are available, fatal toxicity is less compared to the former.

Classification of Pyrethrins and Pyrethroids

Pyrethrins			
Cinerin I	Pyrethrin I	Justmolin I	
Cinerin II	Pyrethrin II	Jusmolin II	
Pyrethrum extract			
Type I Pyrethroids			
Allethrin	Bioallethrin	Cismethrin	Kadethrin
Permethrin	Phenothrin	Resmethrin	Tetramethrin
Type II Pyrethroids			
Cyhalothrin	Cypermethrin	Cyphenothrin	Deltamethrin
Fenpropenthrin	Fenvalerate	Fluvalinate	

Effects of Pyrethroids Exposure

- Direct toxic
- Hypersensitivity
  - Allergic rhinitis
  - Bronchitis
  - Bronchial asthma
  - Anaphylactic shock
- Local irritation
  - Contact dermatitis
  - Corneal abrasion

Pyrethroid Poisoning: Insect

The type I syndrome (caused by type I pyrethroids):

- Fine tremor
- Reflex hyperexcitability
- Sympathetic activation.

The type II syndrome (caused by type II pyrethroids):

- Salivation
- Coarse tremor
- Choreoathetosia
- Reflex hyperexcitability
- Sympathetic activation and seizure.

Death from pyrethroid poisoning is rare.

Diagnosis

- Clinical diagnosis is important.
- There are no specific laboratory tests.

Management

Treatment of hypersensitivity adrenaline: 1/1000 solution 1 mL SC

- Corticosteroids
- Bronchodilators
- Antihistamines orally.

Direct toxic: Effects are managed symptomatically by supportive treatment.

BIPYRIDYL HERBICIDES

These chemicals are highly toxic and account for several deaths.

- Examples are paraquat and diquat
- In most cases, poisoning is by ingestion—the drug is absorbed rapidly

- Severe local irritant and devastating systemic toxicity follow
- Plasma concentrations peak within 2 hours of ingestion
- Distributed to most organs, with kidneys and lungs having the highest concentration
- Acute exposure causes liver and renal necrosis, that is followed within a few weeks by pulmonary fibrosis
- The toxin accumulates in the alveolar cells of the lungs, where it is transformed into a reactive oxygen species—a superoxide radical which is responsible for lipid peroxidation that leads to degradation of cell membranes, cell dysfunction and cell death. This occurs in two phases: (1) Initial destructive phase causes inflammatory cells and hemorrhage, but these changes may be reversible. (2) Second proliferative phase involves fibrosis in the interstitium and alveolar spaces. Myocardial injury and necrosis of the adrenals may occur.

Clinical Features

- Caustic effects produce local skin irritation and ulceration, as well as corneal injury in eye exposures
- Upper respiratory tract exposure may result in mucosal injury and epistaxis
- Inhalation may lead to cough, dyspnea, chest pain, pulmonary edema and hemoptysis
- Ingestion causes gastrointestinal mucosal lesions and ulcerations
- Hypovolemia occurs from gastrointestinal fluid losses and decreased oral intake of nutrients
- Cardiovascular collapse may occur early
- Seizures, gastrointestinal perforation and hemorrhage and hepatic failure may occur
- Massive ingestions lead to multisystem failure and death within a few days
- Renal and hepatocellular necrosis develop by the 2nd and 5th days, with pulmonary fibrosis leading to hypoxemia 5 days to several weeks later.

Diagnosis

- History is important.
- Qualitative and quantitative analyzes for paraquat in urine and blood can confirm the diagnosis.
- Nomograms are available to predict survival based on plasma paraquat concentration and time of ingestion.
- Level of plasma paraquat greater than 0.4 mg/L carries a high probability of death.

Treatment

- Early and vigorous decontamination.
- Any exposure to paraquat is a medical emergency with hospitalization indicated even if patient is asymptomatic.
- Attempt should be made to discourage superoxide radical formation by using low inspired oxygen to produce a hypoxemia to reduce pulmonary injury.
- Using oxygen mixtures (FiO_2 <21%) with positive pressure ventilation reduces pulmonary toxicity in ***experimental models*** and may be of therapeutic benefit.
- Gut decontamination is indicated.

- Charcoal (1–2 g/kg), diatomaceous Fuller's Earth (1–2 g/kg in 15% aqueous suspension) or bentonite (1–2 g/kg in a 7% aqueous slurry) are given and repeated every 4 hours.
- Sorbitol (70%) using 2 mL/kg cathartic should be administered initially.
- Charcoal hemoperfusion is known to remove paraquat and should be instituted as soon as possible and continued for 6–8 hours.
- Support includes attention to airway, maintaining intravascular volume, monitoring the vitals and arterial blood gasses pain relief, treatment of renal failure and treatment of infection.
- Immunosuppresive therapy to reverse lung fibrosis with cyclophosphamide has been tried with variable results.

RODENTICIDES

This groups contains nonanticoagulant and anti-coagulants. They are widely used in agriculture storage areas and several other places.

Nonanticoagulants rodenticides
- High toxicity
  - Arsenic
  - Barium
  - Phosphorous
  - Strychine
- Moderate toxicity
  - α-Naphthylthiourea
- Low toxicity
  - Red squill
  - Norbormide
  - Bromethalin

Anticoagulant rodenticides

Clinical Features

- Warfarin types and superwarfarin.
- They present with predominantly hepatic dysfunction and coagulopathy.
- In phosphorous poisoning, initial findings consist of perioral and mucosal burns, nausea, vomiting and diarrhea. A garlic odor on the breath may also be noted. The feces or vomitus may exhibit phosphorescence, called ***smoking stool syndrome.***
- Systemic toxicity involves multiple organ systems such as the gastrointestinal tract (GIT), liver, heart, kidneys and brain. Hepatotoxicity with jaundice and hypoglycemia and acute kidney injury (AKI) with renal failure are most common.
- Treatment consists of supportive measures.
- Use of parenteral vitamin K and fresh frozen plasma (FFP) is recommended based of coagulopathy.
- IV N-acetylcysteine (NAC) has shown promising results.

CYANIDE POISONING

Poisoning by the lethal chemical, potassium cyanide is rarely only seen in suicidal attempts committed by persons who have access to this chemical. Apart from chemical laboratories, cyanide is used in several industries—cottage industries, gold smithy and so on. Most of the cases are either accidental or suicidal.

In addition to cyanide occurring in pure state cyanogens are widely distributed in nature especially products of vegetable origin such as cassava (104 mg CN/100 g), bitter almonds (250 mg CN/100 g), wild cherries (140–150 mg CN/100 mg) and so on. By consuming these materials without suitable processing to remove the cyanide, the toxin may get into the system and produce either acute or chronic toxicity. Refer also acute cassava toxicity in (*See* Ch 24 , p. 166).

Routes of Entry of Cyanide

Inhalation as gas, aerosols, ingestion or skin contact or deliberate parenteral injection. When introduced parenterally or inhaled, the action is most rapid death occurring within 6–8 minutes. Lethal dose by inhalation is 2–5 mg/kg bw.

Cyanide leads to cellular hypoxia, metabolic acidosis and nonspecific symptoms.

Clinical Features

Other symptoms include dizziness, nausea, vomiting, drowsiness, tetany, trismus and hallucinations. Cardiac arrhythmias and hypotension supervene. Respiratory distress and depression follow leading to death.

Diagnostic laboratory parameters include estimation of blood cyanide levels and high anion gap metabolic acidosis. Arterial and venous oxygen saturation is usually normal and the defect in the utilization of oxygen by cells.

Treatment

It should be started as emergency before laboratory results are available.

Principles of treatment
- Assisted ventilation with supplementary oxygen.
- Removal of ingested toxin with activated charcoal.

Antidotes to cyanides
- Sodium nitrite IV, amyl nitrate as inhalation, sodium thoisulfate and hydroxocobalamin have been employed with varying results.
- Sodium nitrite is given in doses of 350 mg IV in 5% glucose solution over 5 minutes with care to avoid hypotension. For children, the dose is 0.12–0.33 mg/kg bw as slow infusion. Nitrites convert hemoglobin to methemoglobin with combines with cyanide to form cyanmethemoglobin which is nontoxic.
- Sodium thiosulfate in a dose of 25 g in 50 ce water can be given IV slowly, 12.5 g within 10–20 minutes and thereafter as slow infusion. Sodium thiosulfate detoxifies cyanide as it is released from cyanmeth-emoglobin. It also helps to convert cyanide to thiocyanate. Being too slow in its action it should be preceded by sodium nitrite which acts faster. Thiosulfate may lead to hypotension psychosis, coma and allergic manifestations.
- Hydroxocobalamin binds to cyanide and chelates it. The dose is 4–5 g IV. The drug is safe.

Prognosis: Even though most of the cases are seen late or brought dead, rapid resuscitatory measures have helped to prevent death and bring about recovery.

METHANOL POISONING

Poisoning with methanol may occur sporadically when industrial (methylated) spirit is consumed in the place of ethanol or epidemically when the supply of liquor is adulterated with methyl alcohol. Several outbreaks have occurred in closed communities from time to time. Minimum lethal dose is 30 g. Methanol is metabolized in the system to formaldehyde and formic acid by alcohol dehydrogenase enzyme. In addition, derangement of hepatic metabolism results in the accumulation of lactate. Severe metabolic acidosis results after a latent period of 8–12 hours. Optic neuritis develops as a specific toxic reaction.

Clinical Features

Within hours of consuming methylated alcohol, patients develop restlessness, irritability, confusion, epigastric pain, vomiting and rapid loss of vision followed by metabolic acidosis. Visual loss is concentric. Ophthalmoscopy shows pale edematous discs. Coma may develop, which may become deep. Mortality in a large series is about 20%.

Treatment

Aims of treatment are: (1) Correction of acidosis, (2) inhibition of methanol oxidation and (3) removal of circulating methanol and its toxic products.

Acidosis is corrected by sodium bicarbonate given IV in adequate amounts. Hemodialysis helps to remove circulating methanol. Hemodialysis should be started without delay if the blood level of methanol exceeds 0.5 g/L or the total quantity ingested exceeds 30 mL. Peritoneal dialysis is only one-eighth as effective as hemodialysis in removing methanol and therefore, this should not be relied upon.

Ethanol should be given if methanol level in blood exceeds 20 mg/dL. Blood ethanol concentration above 100 mg/dL inhibits the metabolism of methanol to formaldehyde and formic acid by competing for the enzyme alcohol dehydrogenase. The equivalent of 30–50 mL of ethanol is given orally at 2–4 hours interval for a few days. Once the optic nerve is affected, ethanol does not reverse the damage. IV ethanol is also available for treatment.

Fomepizole is a competitive inhibitor of hepatic alcohol dehydrogenase. Given early it reduces the need for hemodialysis. First a loading dose of 15 mg/kg IV (maximum of 1500 mg) is given and then the first maintenance dose of 10 mg/kg IV is given 12 hours later. Then repeat same dose every 12 hours up to 4 doses. Fomepizole induces its own metabolism, so after the fourth 10 mg/kg dose, increase the dose to 15 mg/kg IV every 12 hours. Treatment to be continued till the methanol level is < 20 mg/dL or patient is asymptomatic with normal pH. Fomepizole is removed by dialysis, so if the patient is already on dialysis the dosing interval must be decreased.

Points to Remember

- Lethal dose of methanol is 30 g.
- Severe metabolic acidosis occurs within 12 hours and optic neuritis is a specific toxic reaction.

- Treatment aims at correction of acidosis, inhibition of oxidation of methanol by giving ethanol and removal of the toxic products.
- Hemodialysis should be started if blood level of methanol is more than 0.5 g/L.
- Fomepizole is a competitive inhibitor of alcohol dehydrogenase used in treatment of methanol toxicity.

BARBITURATES

They are derivatives of barbituric acid (2,4,6-trioxo-hexa-hydro-pyrimidine) and were the popular sedative and hypnotics up to 1960s. They are nonselective direct CNS depressants which can produce effects ranging from sedation and reduction of anxiety to unconsciousness and death from respiratory and cardiovascular failure. They bind to gamma-aminobutyric acid (GABA) receptors and prolong the opening of chloride channels inhibiting excitable cells of the CNS. Till recently, barbiturates were the most common drugs used for suicide. Accidental poisoning is seen in epileptics, psychiatric patients and children who get regular prescription for these drugs.

Classification based on duration of action:

Long-acting (6–12 hours)

- Mephobarbitone
- Phenobarbitone

Intermediate acting (3–6 hours)

- Amobarbitone
- Aprobarbitone
- Butobarbitone

Short-acting (<3 hours)

- Hexobarbitone
- Pentobarbitone
- Secobarbitone

Ultrashort acting (<15–20 minutes)

- Thiopentone
- Methohexitone.

The most widely used barbiturate used to be phenobarbitone and it is used as an anticonvulsant. Absorption and metabolism of phenobarbitone are slow. About 10% of the drug is excreted in urine unchanged. The lethal dose for adult is about 5 g. Simultaneous administration of alcohol aggravates its effects.

Clinical Features

Central nervous, respiratory and cardiovascular system (CVS) are affected the most. Drowsiness, slowing of respiration and hypotension follow. Pupils are small and react to light. In severe poisoning when medullary centers are depressed, the pupils are dilated and fixed, which indicates a poor prognosis. Tendon reflexes are sluggish or absent. Necrosis of sweat glands and bullous lesions over the skin develop in a few as a hypersensitive reaction. These lesions heal slowly.

Diagnosis can be confirmed by detection of barbiturates in the gastric contents and estimation of barbiturate in blood.

Treatment

In addition to general measures, forced alkaline diuresis and dialysis are helpful. Bemegride (megimide) considered to be a specific antidote but subsequent research has disproved this assumption. Repeated doses of activated charcoal and hemoperfusion are the modalities described. Since pneumonia is a fatal complication, these patients should be observed for a week till recovery is complete.

> **Points to Remember**
> - The lethal dose of phenobarbitone, the most commonly used barbiturate is 5 g.
> - CNS and CVS are the most affected by overdosage.
> - Respiratory depression indicates poor prognosis.
> - Forced alkaline diuresis and hemodialysis are the treatment options.

SEDATIVE DRUG POISONING

Benzodiazepines Poisioning

History: Benzodiazepines (BZDs) are sedative-hypnotic agents that have been in clinical use since the 1960s.

The first benzodiazepine, chlordiazepoxide, was discovered serendipitously in 1954 by the Austrian scientist Leo Sternbach.

Mode of Action

BZDs exert their effect via modulation of the GABA receptor. GABA is the chief inhibitory neurotransmitter of the CNS.

Types

BZDs are commonly divided into three groups based upon half-life duration:
1. Short-acting (half-life of less than 12 hours).
2. Intermediate acting (half-life between 12 and 24 hours).
3. Long-acting (half-life greater than 24 hours).

Hypnotic	Antianxiety	Anticonvulsant
• Diazepam	• Diazepam	• Diazepam
• Flurazepam	• Chlordiazepoxide	• Lorazepam
• Nitrazepam	• Oxazepam	• Clonazepam
• Alprazolam	• Lorazepam	• Clobazepam
• Temazepam	• Alprazolam	
• Triazolam		

Kinetics

BZDs are rapidly absorbed in the GIT and most are highly lipophilic and highly protein-bound. The metabolism of BZDs is primarily hepatic. Within the liver, most BZDs are metabolized to a significant extent by the CYP2C19 and CYP3A4 enzymes.

Clinical Features

Oral BZDs taken in overdose without a coingestant rarely cause significant toxicity.

The classic presentation of a patient with an isolated BZD overdose consists of CNS depression with normal vital signs.
- Toxic symptoms—sedative action on the CNS.
- Large doses—neuromuscular blockade.
- IV injection peripheral vasodilation—fall in blood pressure (BP), shock.
- Decrease alveolar ventilation [↓ partial pressure of oxygen (PO_2), ↑ partial pressure of carbon dioxide (PCO_2)].

- Induce CO_2 narcosis in persons with chronic obstructive pulmonary disease (COPD).
- Respiratory depressant effect with sedative drugs-concomitantly taken.
- Death occurred in persons who concurrently injected ethanol/CNS depressant.
- IV dosing—hypotension and respiratory depression-death.

Of note, most intentional ingestions of BZDs involve a coingestant, the most common being ethanol.

Acute poisoning
- *Mild:* Drowsiness, ataxia, weakness.
- *Moderate to severe:* Vertigo, slurred speech, nystagmus, partial ptosis, lethargy, hypotension, respiratory depression, coma (stages 1 and 2).
- *Coma 1 (stage 1):* Responsive to painful stimuli but not to verbal or tactile stimuli, no disturbance in respiration or BP.
- *Coma 2 (stage 2):* Unconscious, not responsive to painful stimuli, no disturbance in respiration or BP.

Differential Diagnosis

- Altered mental status, a common finding in BZD overdose, is found in a wide range of medical and toxicologic conditions.
- Any number of sedative-hypnotic medications share clinical features with BZDs in overdose, including ethanol, barbiturates, gamma hydroxybutyrate (GHB), and chloral hydrate.

General Diagnostic Testing

- Fingerstick glucose, to rule out hypoglycemia as the cause of any alteration in mental status.
- Acetaminophen and salicylate levels, to rule out these common coingestions.
- Electrocardiogram (ECG), to rule out conduction system poisoning by drugs that effect the QRS or QTC intervals.
- Pregnancy test in women of childbearing age.

Life Supportive Procedures and Symptomatic/Specific Treatment

- Airway, breathing and circulation
- IV fluid administration for hypotension
- Endotracheal intubation
- Assisted ventilation
- Supplemental oxygen.

Treatment Principles

- Gastric lavage
- Activated charcoal is administrated orally or by nastrogastric tube
- Measures for removal of barbiturates
- Frequent doses of activated charcoal
- Forced diuresis with alkalization of urine
- Hemodialysis and hemoperfusion.

Decontamination

GIT decontamination with activated charcoal is usually of no benefit in cases of isolated BZD ingestion and increases the risk of aspiration.

Antidote Treatment: Flumazenil

- Flumazenil—reversing the coma induced by BZDs.
- Mode of action—competitive antagonism.
- Complete reversal of BZD effect with a total slow IV dose of 1 mg.
- Administered in a series of smaller doses beginning with 0.2 mg and progressively increasing by 0.1–0.2 mg every minute until a cumulative total dose of 3.5 mg is reached.
- Resedation occurs within half an hour to two hours.

Side effects: Nausea, vomiting, arrhythmias, convulsions, C/I status epilepticus.

ALCOHOL INTOXICATION

Alcohol is available in several forms commercially. The common forms are toddy (5%), beer (5%), wine (10%), arrack (40–60%), and gin, whisky and brandy (45–60%). Illicitly distilled liquor may contain several chemical impurities. One standard drink contains 12 g alcohol. It is made up by 180 mL wine, 360 mL beer or 45 mL 90% proof spirit.

Absorption of alcohol from the stomach and small intestine is rapid and detectable blood levels occur within five minutes of ingestion, reaching the highest levels in 30–90 minutes. The peak level is maintained for two hours. Fat in the food impedes absorption. Once absorbed, it is converted by alcohol dehydrogenase to acetaldehyde, which is then converted to acetate and then to acetyl coenzyme A (CoA), and ultimately carbon dioxide and water. Alcohol is widely distributed in tissues. It appears in the cerebrospinal fluid (CSF), urine, and alveolar air. Alcohol is metabolized primarily in the liver. It supplies energy like carbohydrates, though it has no nutritive value.

Consumption of alcohol is not a criminal offence till it leads to alcoholic intoxication and antisocial behavior. Both the physical and psychiatric disturbances caused by alcohol fall under the purview of the physician. Alcohol intoxication is common in modern society, largely because of its widespread availability. More than 8 million Americans are believed to be dependent on alcohol and up to 15% of the population is considered at risk. Studies have shown that more than half of all trauma patients are intoxicated with alcohol at the time of arrival to the hospital. India has been identified as the potentially third largest market for alcoholic beverages in the world. The mean age of initiation of alcohol use has decreased from 23.36 years to less than 19 years.

Alcohol produces acute and chronic gastritis, acute intoxication ranging from excitement to coma, various nutritional and nervous disorders, and hepatic damage. Long-term use of large amounts of alcohol results in parenchymal damage to several organ systems like the liver, heart and brain.

Acute gastritis: This occurs in people who consume spirits in large amounts. It is characterized by severe vomiting, abdominal pain and headache. The vomiting responds to any phenothiazine such as trifluoperazine hydrochloride. 10 mg. Oral antacids and IV fluids are required in cases with persistent vomiting.

The cerebral effects of alcohol start within minutes of ingestion. The amount of alcohol and the extent of habituation of the patient determine the clinical picture. Slurring of speech and loss of refined mental and physical capacities occur when the blood level is 0.5 g/L. At 3 g/L ataxia, double vision, tremor, incoherent speech and serious loss of mental capacity become evident. Blood levels above 5 g/L are fatal. Death occurs in coma and is caused by respiratory failure.

Diagnosis: Alcoholic intoxication should be suspected from the smell of alcohol, clinical picture and the circumstances. Estimation of the levels of alcohol in urine, blood or expired air help in confirming the diagnosis. Samples of 10 mL of urine and 2 mL of blood should be collected and sent in sealed bottles for chemical examination.

All other organic causes of coma, hysterical conversion reaction, psychiatric disorders and malingering should be excluded.

Treatment: Supportive treatment as in the case of coma is instituted without delay. The diuretic effect of ethanol may lead to dehydration. IV administration of dextrose solution (500 mL of 20% solution followed by 1 L of 5% solution) along with massive doses of vitamin B complex factors and vitamin C are beneficial. Early treatment improves the prognosis. Common complications include aspiration pneumonia and lung abscess. Psychiatric assessment and counseling with rehabilitation are required to avoid recurrence.

Points to Remember

- Symptoms of acute intoxication range from excitement to coma.
- Lethal blood level of alcohol is 5 g/L.
- Diagnosis is by clinical picture and estimation of levels in blood or urine.
- Correction of dehydration, dextrose IV and vitamin B are the treatment modalities.

Alcohol Withdrawal Syndrome

This occurs typically within 5–24 hours after withdrawal of alcohol, in alcohol dependent subjects. The signs and symptoms are largely due to autonomic overactivity. Three groups of symptoms may occur.

1. Signs of autonomic overactivity occurring within a few hours of the last drink and becoming maximal in 24–48 hours. These consist of tremulousness, sweating, nausea, vomiting, anxiety and agitation.
2. Signs of neuronal excitation such as generalized seizures occurring within 12–48 hours of abstinence.
3. ***Delirium tremens***, characterized by tremor, auditory and visual hallucinations, confusion, disorientation, clouding of consciousness, hypokalemia, hypomagnesemia and prolonged autonomic hyperactivity leading to tachycardia, hypertension and tachypnea. Death may occur at this stage due to cardiovascular and respiratory collapse in less than 5% of cases. In many cases, the symptoms are self-limiting within one week.

Management: It consists of supervised detoxifying regimes, sedation on demand, counseling, reassurance and social support. Large doses of diazepam 10–20 mg given at 2-hour intervals or chlordiazepoxide 25–50 mg every 4–6 hours may be needed to sedate the

Common Poisons

Textbook of Medicine

patient. Once sedated, the drug is stopped. Repeated dosage may be required in a few. Seizures are also controlled by diazepam given in doses of 5–10 mg oral or 2–5 mg IV slowly or as a slow IV infusion, the total dose not to exceed 1–2 mg/kg bw in 24 hours. In those with hepatic damage, sedatives such as oxazepam 30 mg or lorazepam 20–30 µg/kg IV should be given. They do not cause further damage to the liver. More serious complications such as Wernicke's encephalopathy, dehydration and electrolyte imbalance may develop. Prophylactic thiamine is given in a dose of 20 mg IM or IV bd.

Management of alcohol withdrawal syndrome and deaddiction are specialized procedures requiring the combined effects of the physicians, psychiatric and social workers.

Points to Remember
- Alcohol withdrawal symptoms develop typically within 5–24 hours after withdrawal.
- Predominant symptom is autonomic hyperactivity.
- Delirium tremens is a serious complication wherein cardio-vascular and respiratory collapse may occur.
- Management includes benzodiazepines and other supportive measures.

CERBERA ODOLLAM

Cerbera odollam belonging to the family Apocynaceae, a small tree found all over India, is a frequent cause of poisoning especially in Kerala. Many cardiac glycosides have been isolated from the plants belonging to this family, e.g. strophanthin, ouabain, oleandrine, cerberin and thevetine. The active principles seen in *Cerbera odollam* are cerberin, cerberoside and odollin, which are seen in highest amounts in the kernels of the seeds. The seeds taste very bitter. The contents of a single fruit can be fatal if ingested.

Cerberin, like digitalis, reduces the heart rate by inhibiting sinoatrial (SA) and atrioventricular (AV) conduction, mainly by a vagotonic action, which can be partially reversed by atropine. In higher doses, cerberin has a direct depressant action on the myocardium, which cannot be reversed by administering atropine. The majority of poisoning cases are suicidal.

Morbid anatomy: Autopsy studies are not very rewarding. Except for subepicardial and subendocardial hemorrhages, the gross anatomy appears normal. The conducting tissue of the heart is histologically normal.

Clinical features: Within an hour of taking the poison, retching, nausea, vomiting and abdominal pain occur. Later, the patient becomes weak and drowsy and may lapse into coma. Bradycardia, only partially responsive to atropine, is the most obvious finding.

The ECG may show various types of bradyarrhythmias like sinus bradycardia, AV dissociation and junctional rhythms. Different grades of AV block and SA block have been described. Ventricular extrasystoles may occur rarely. The changes in the ST segment, the T wave and the QT interval are similar to those produced by digitalis. 60% of the patients show hyperkalemia (Figs 23.1A to E).

Treatment: Management consists of the elimination of unabsorbed poison by stomach wash, purgatives, bowel wash and correction of bradyarrhythmias by IV atropine (0.5 mg). In severe cases, the drug has to be repeated even at 15 minutes intervals, or it has to be administered as a continuous drip. Hyperkalemia should be treated by appropriate measures (insulin glucose regimen). When bradycardia is not corrected by atropine, the patient may require cardiac pacing. The presence of hypotension, alteration of consciousness, bradyarrhythmias not responding to treatment, hyperkalemia, and significant electrocardiographic changes indicate severe poisoning and the prognosis in such cases is poor with an overall mortality of 20–25%. Management in a cardiac intensive care facility is certainly likely to improve results, although the experience is still limited. Once established, the cardiac phenomena persist for one to three weeks since the toxin is only very slowly eliminated. Hence prolonged observation is required.

Points to Remember
- Active principles of *Cerbra odollam* are cereberin, cereberoside and odollin.
- Cerberin has vagotonic action and direct depressant effect on the myocardium.
- Various types of bradyarrhythmias and hyperkalemia can occur.
- Treatment is with atropine, management of hyperkalemia and temporary cardiac pacing when required.

CLEISTHANUS COLLINUS LEAF

This is emerging as a common suicidal poison in Tamil Nadu. It is ingested in several forms. Main toxic effect is on the heart. Progressive bradycardia, sudden cardiac arrest and progressive respiratory failure follow. Hypokalemia occurs in over 70%. Prolongation of the corrected QT interval in the ECG above 0.45 second is associated with poor outcome. General measures, atropine and temporary cardiac pacing have been employed in treatment.

CORROSIVE ACIDS

Acids like hydrochloric acid, sulfuric acid and nitric acid are widely used in the laboratory. Cases of accidental and suicidal poisoning are not rare. Corrosive acids produce similar clinical picture, which is due to their direct chemical action on tissues.

Clinical features: Sites of intimate contact like the lips, throat, palate and posterior pharyngeal wall show scalding. They bleed easily and slough away leaving raw areas. Clinical features of acidosis occur if large amounts are ingested. Metabolic acidosis occurs as a result of cellular injury and from systemic absorption of acids. Complications like perforation of the esophagus and stomach, severe hematemesis, acute renal failure (ARF) and severe shock are fatal. Esophageal stricture is a common sequel.

Treatment: Emesis and gastric lavage are contraindicated. The acid in the stomach can be diluted by large volumes of water or milk. Pain is relieved by local anesthetics like xylocaine viscous and analgesics. Oral feeds should be avoided for a day or two after which swallowing of fluids like milk should be encouraged. Infection has to be prevented by the administration of ampicillin 1 g IV 6th hourly. If esophageal perforation is excluded, cortico-

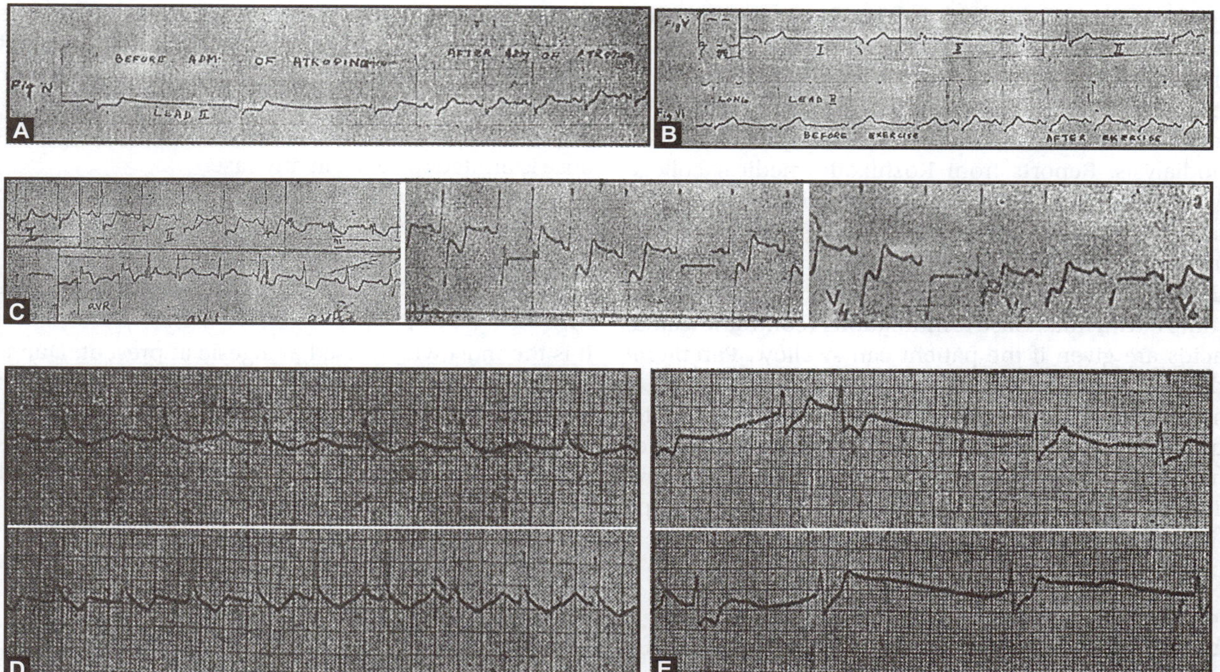

Figs 23.1A to E: ECG changes *Cerbera odollam* poisoning. **A. *Early stage:*** Sinus bradycardia, responding to atropinization; **B. *Mild case:*** Sinus bradycardia persisting for one week after recovery, responding normally to exercise; **C. *Moderately severe cases:*** Note (a) Tachycardia, (b) ST depression in leads I, II, III, aVF and V1-6, (c) ST elevation in lead aVR, (d) Biphasic T waves leads II, aVF and V1-6; **D. *First degree AV block*** (top) responding to atropinization (bottom); **E. *Severe toxocity:*** Idioventricular rhythm. Often this is fatal

Source:
1. Kunhali, et al. Ind Heart J.1970;22(4):373-7.
2. Narendranathan MA, et al. Ind Heart J.1975;27(4):283-6.

steroids may be given parenterally in doses equivalent to hydrocortisone 25 mg 6 hourly for 3–5 days. This may prevent the formation of esophageal stricture.

Metabolic acidosis develops in most of the cases. This has to be corrected by the administration of IV normal saline and sodium bicarbonate, depending upon the requirement.

Treatment of shock, perforation, peritonitis and acute renal failure should be undertaken when they occur. Early institution of oral feeds helps to reduce the occurrence of esophageal stricture. If stricture occurs, the treatment is surgical.

ACETIC ACID

It is used for coagulating rubber latex and, therefore, it is freely available to workers in rubber plantations. Poisoning is usually suicidal, rarely accidental. The fatal dose varies from 15 to 60 mL.

Clinical features: Intense scalding and burning of the lips, mouth, pharynx and throat occur over areas of direct contact. Dysphagia and burning pain along the esophagus and stomach follow. There is excessive salivation. The patient shows anxiety and there will be acidosis. Hemoglobinemia and hemoglobinuria develop within hours. Bronchitis, bronchopneumonia and aspiration pneumonia follow. Shock, severe acidosis, pneumonia, mediastinitis, perforation of the stomach or esophagus and renal failure result in death.

Treatment: Diazepam in a dose of 5–10 mg is given IV to sedate the patient. Gastric intubation is contraindicated. Demulcents like egg albumin or milk may be given if the patient can swallow. Oral intake of fluids should be encouraged early, since this helps to prevent stricture. Glucose saline drip is started early to provide nutrition, fluids and electrolytes. Acidosis is corrected by suitable doses of sodium bicarbonate. Furosemide 20 mg given IV may be beneficial to prevent the development of renal failure. Mortality ranges from 20 to 30%. Esophageal stricture may occur which will require surgical treatment.

FORMIC ACID

Formic acid and its salts are used in textile, leather and rubber industries. It is also a component in some descaling agents, disinfectants and preservatives. Suicidal attempts and accidental ingestion of formic acid are common in many rubber cultivating areas of Kerala and Tamil Nadu because of its free availability. Protoplasmic coagulation, precipitation or dissolution of proteins and exudation of fluid occur at the sites of intimate contact.

Since in most cases of accidental ingestion, the person tries to spit out the acid, burns occur in and around the mouth. However, if acid is consumed with suicidal intent, the attempt to swallow evokes reflex cough because of its irritant vapors. Acid enters not only the esophagus but also the respiratory tract. This results in ulceration, bleeding, sloughing and perforation of the esophagus and stomach, tracheitis, bronchitis, pulmonary edema and pneumonia.

Systemic effects of the acids are acidosis, intravascular hemolysis, hemoglobinuria and shock. Renal failure is common.

Hemoglobinuria and oliguria should portend the onset of renal failure, which demands early and repeated hemodialysis. Reports from Kozhikode medical college show that even superficial burns exceeding 20% of body surface caused by formic acid may lead to acute tubular necrosis (ATN) and renal failure.

First aid treatment is to dilute the acid with water or neutralize with milk. Gastric intubation is contraindicated, antacids are given if the patient can swallow. Parenteral fluids are given to hydrate the patient and acidosis is combated by the IV administration of sodium bicarbonate. Frequent feeding with milk, egg albumin and other demulcents helps to reduce the incidence of stricture. Antibiotics, analgesics and respiratory physiotherapy are indicated in all cases. Late occurrence of esophageal stricture has to be treated surgically.

Points to Remember

- Corrosive acids produce burns or scalding in the lips, throat and posterior pharyngeal wall due to chemical reaction.
- Ulceration and perforation of esophagus and stomach, pulmonary edema and pneumonia are the usual manifestations.
- Systemic effects include acidosis, intravascular hemolysis, hemoglobinuria and renal failure.
- Esophageal stricture is a common sequel.

ALKALIES

Strong alkalies are used in industry. Household cleaning materials contain alkaline substances. Ammonium hydroxide, potassium hydroxide, sodium hydroxide, potassium carbonate, sodium carbonate and sodium and potassium phosphates account for the vast majority of alkali poisoning. Strong alkalies lead to scalding and ulceration of tissue. On ingestion, patients experience severe pain in the mouth, throat, chest and abdomen. Tongue, oral mucosa and pharynx show areas of erythema and necrosis. Metabolic alkalosis develops as a systemic effect. Sodium and potassium phosphates may cause severe reduction in serum calcium leading to tetany.

Treatment: This consists of diluting the alkali by the administration of water or milk and maintenance of fluid and electrolyte balance. Local pain can be allayed partly by the use of xylocaine viscous. Tetany is managed by the administration of calcium gluconate IV. Prevention of secondary infection by the use of antibiotics and corticosteroids to prevent stricture of the esophagus have to be considered in selected cases. Endoscopy done within 24 hours of admission helps to assess the severity of lesions in the esophagus and stomach and institute surgical treatment when appropriate.

NARCOTICS (MORPHINE AND OPIOIDS)

Poisoning by morphine and its allied narcotic analgesics leads to initial excitement followed by a depression of the nervous system. The patient is stuporous or comatose with pin-point pupils, slow and shallow respiration, cyanosis and hypotension.

Treatment: In addition to supportive measures and gastric aspiration, ventilatory assistance is required in comatose patients. Specific antidote is nalorphine hydrobromide (Lethidrone) given IV 0.4–2 mg every 2–5 minutes till the respiration and BP become normal. In general, the total dose is limited to 40 mg in any case.

Toxic effects of nalorphine include respiratory depression, hypotension, drowsiness and hypothermia.

PARACETAMOL

Syn: Acetaminophen

It is the most widely used analgesic at present. Due to its free availability, paracetamol poisoning is becoming more frequent. Doses exceeding 8 g can produce toxicity. These tablets are pleasant to take, they dissolve rapidly and reach peak serum levels in 3–4 hours after ingestion unless delayed in the presence of other drugs such as antihistamines, anticholinergics, opiates and others. The half-life of the drug when taken orally is 1–3 hours. Half-life is delayed when excess doses are taken. Acute hepatocellular and less frequently renal tubular necrosis may follow ingestion of a single dose exceeding 10 g. A highly reactive metabolite of paracetamol, N-acetyl-p-benzoquinone imine (NAPQI), which is normally inactivated by hepatic glutathione is responsible for the hepatic failure. With overdosage of acetaminophen, hepatic glutathione is rapidly depleted and NAPQI binds to cellular proteins causing necrosis of cells. Hepatic levels of glutathione are increased by N-acetylcysteine and methionine thereby protecting the liver from injury. Factors influencing toxicity include— dose ingested, chronic alcoholism, concurrent use of drugs like carbamazepine, phenytoin, isoniazid, rifampin and others. Decreased capacity for glucuronidation or sulfation and depletion of glutathione stores due to malnutrition or chronic alcoholism predispose to severe toxicity.

Clinical Features

Early symptoms are nausea, vomiting and sweating. The most dangerous complication is hepatic damage.

This becomes manifest 1–2 days after onset with jaundice, bleeding tendency and hepatomegaly. A few cases progress to fulminant hepatic necrosis resulting in hepatic coma and this is associated with high mortality. Other serious but rare complications are acute tubular necrosis, pancreatitis, carditis, hypoglycemia, metabolic acidosis and hypersensitivity reactions.

Liver function tests (LFT) become abnormal and the maximum damage is reached within 72–96 hours. Serum glutamic-pyruvic transaminase (SGPT) levels go very high (even up to 10000 IU/L). Prothrombin time (PT) is prolonged. International normalized ratio (INR) above 6.5 portend the possibility of fatal liver failure. Blood lactate levels are raised due to over production and diminished excretion. Values above 3.5 mmol/L in arterial blood persisting after fluid replacement should alert the physician about the risk of hepatic failure and the need for hepatic replacement. Jaundice may occur. Recovery phase that usually begins by day 4 is complete by 7 days after overdose in those that are improving. PT and its INR if normal at 24 hours, indicate good prognosis for recovery.

In those with massive ingestion (massive ingestions 600 mg/kg: early onset metabolic acidosis occurs). Death is due to mitochondrial poisoning resulting in coma, hypotension, acidosis and less commonly due to hepatic failure.

Treatment: Correction of fluid and electrolyte imbalance should be started immediately. Gastric lavage should be performed to remove unabsorbed drug. Activated charcoal may help to adsorb the residual drug. In severe cases where the blood level of paracetamol is above 300 mg/L at 4 hours, hemoperfusion is the best method for rapid elimination of the drug. Forced alkaline diuresis is ineffective.

Specific management is to give the antidote N-acetyl cysteine (NAC). In patients who have reached the hospital within four hours of ingestion, gastric lavage and activated charcoal may help to prevent systemic effects. Serum levels of paracetamol should be estimated after 4 hours in order to assess the risk. Paracetamol levels above 100 mg/dL indicate high mortality and therefore demand the administration of NAC. It is given as IV infusion in Table 23.3.

Nomograms have been made to access paracetamol toxicity and institute treatment, e.g. Rumack-Matthew nomogram (Fig. 23.2).

Another prognostic standard if the King's College criteria which gives the following adverse factors for death pH < 7.30, PT > 100 seconds, creatinine > 3.4 mg/dL, grade III+ encephalopathy.

An oral preparation of NAC cysteine is also available. The dose is 140 mg/kg orally initially followed by 70 mg/kg 4 hourly for 72 hours. This should not be relied upon in an emergency.

Liver failure should be treated on the lines of fulminant hepatic failure. Paracetamol poisoning is one of the frequent causes of fulminant hepatic failure in western countries demanding emergency liver transplantation.

PETROLEUM PRODUCTS (KEROSENE)

Accidental poisoning with kerosene is common in India because of its free availability in the household. Children suffer more. Cases of poisoning with other petroleum products like petrol, diesel oil and paint thinners are encountered less commonly. Petroleum products are used

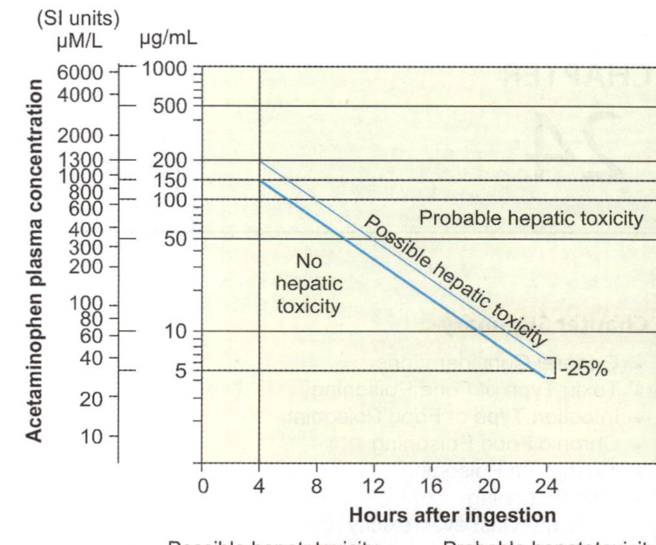

Fig. 23.2: Rumack-Matthew nomogram for acetaminophen toxicity

as solvents in the manufacture and application of polishes, paints and pesticides. Some persons develop the habit of sniffing paints and polish for the nervous effects produced by the solvents. They contain various amounts of aliphatic and aromatic hydrocarbons, which are mainly depressants of the CNS. They cause damage to the cells on direct contact on account of their ability to dissolve cellular lipids. The low surface tension facilitates their spread along mucosal surfaces and the lungs even when only small amounts are ingested or inhaled.

Poisoning usually results from ingestion but can also result from inhalation. The clinical features depend on the quantity and route of poisoning.

Clinical features: Symptoms pertaining to the CNS include headache, nausea, tinnitus, drowsiness, convulsions and coma. Severe vomiting occurs when the oral route is adopted. Kerosene reaching the trachea spreads widely throughout the respiratory tract resulting in the most common and potentially dangerous complications of pneumonia and pulmonary edema. Death may result due to respiratory embarrassment, ventricular fibrillation or severe chemical pneumonia.

Treatment: All suspected cases of kerosene poisoning should be hospitalized for 24 hours to watch for aspiration pneumonia. Simple gastric lavage is better avoided. If it is deemed essential, a cuffed endotracheal tube should be introduced prior to gastric lavage to protect the respiratory tract.

Chemical pneumonia is treated with oxygen inhalation, corticosteroids and ventilatory assistance when indicated. Antibiotics should be employed to prevent secondary infection.

	Table 23.3: Dosage of NAC		
Dose	**NAC mg/kg**	**Volume of 5% glucose**	**Duration of drip**
1.	150	200	15 minutes
2.	50	500	4 hours
3.	50	500	8 hours
4.	50	500	8 hours

Abbreviation: NAC = N-acetylcysteine

Food Poisoning

TK, Suma, KV Krishna Das

Chapter Summary

- General Considerations
- Toxin Type of Food Poisoning
- Infection Type of Food Poisoning
- Chronic Food Poisoning
- Mushroom Poisoning
- Fish Poisoning
  - Acute Cassava Toxicity
- Onyalai
- Hepatic Veno-occlusive Disease
- Aflatoxicosis
- Epidemic Dropsy
- Lathyrism
- Ergotism
- Lead Poisoning

GENERAL CONSIDERATIONS

Sometimes articles of food cause toxic reactions. This toxicity, in general, is caused by the following factors:

- The food may be naturally toxic, e.g. poisonous mushrooms, toxic fish, etc.
- Toxicity may be imposed upon the food material by the polluted environment, e.g. contamination of fish by mercury from industrial effluents, infection of oysters by *Salmonella* due to fecal contamination.
- Contamination of food during collection, transportation, storage, cooking or serving by:
  - Chemicals (accidental or by addition of adulterants)
  - Microbial agents—bacteria, viruses, protozoa
  - Preformed toxins contaminating the food articles.
- Allergy to the food materials.

Episodes of food poisoning are characterized by several distinctive features, which help to diagnose them and study their epidemiology.

- They occur in small outbreaks in several persons who have shared a common item of food.
- The symptomatology is similar in all cases, but severity varies depending on the quantity of the food ingested, age of the individual and weight. Children suffer more than the adults.
- The incriminated food material may show abnormalities such as putrefaction, distaste and altered consistency. Tinned food packed in vacuum shows bloating of the tins.

For preventing spread of the outbreak and to help in investigating the cause, the primary physician has to follow a set procedure. At the first suspicion of food poisoning, the incriminated food should be isolated and even small quantities should not be consumed further. Those who are apparently well and who would have consumed the food should be advised to induce vomiting by tickling the throat after drinking a glass of water and as much of the food as is possible should be removed, by repeated vomiting. This single measure reduces the risk considerably.

- The appropriate health authorities should be notified.
- Proper clinical records should be maintained.
- Remnants of food should be preserved for chemical and microbiological tests.
- Vomitus, urine and feces should be collected sealed, and sent for chemical analysis.
- If death occurs, medicolegal autopsy is indicated and the stomach, intestines, liver and other organs have to be sent for chemical examination.

The general principles of treatment are similar to those for chemical poisoning.

TOXIN TYPE OF FOOD POISONING

Preformed toxins present in food are responsible for this condition, e.g. organisms like *Staphylococcus aureus*, *Bacillus cereus*, *Clostridium botulinum*, *Clostridium perfringens* and *Salmonellae* are the common agents responsible for such outbreaks. The most dangerous among them are the soil *Clostridium* species which are gram positive *Cl. perfringens* causes food poisoning and necrotizing hemorrhagic enteritis. *Cl. botulinum* is capable of producing toxin-mediated food poisoning termed botulism, wound infection and intestinal infection. In all cases the absorption of toxin is the crucial pathogenic event. Staphylococcal contamination usually results from pustules in the udder of the cow or from the skin or nose of food handlers. *Bacillus cereus* is usually seen in contaminated fried rice.

Staphylococcal Food Poisoning

It is caused by the enterotoxin of *Staphylococcus aureus*. The common articles of food include stored cooked meat, milk and cheese. The onset is acute with vomiting, diarrhea and crampy abdominal pain developing 1–6 hours after ingestion of the food. Shock may supervene, but recovery in 24–48 hours is the rule. Treatment is symptomatic.

Botulism

This results from the ingestion of the toxin of *Cl. botulinum*. The organism grows under anaerobic conditions in contaminated meat foods like sausages, fish, etc. The organism is present in the soil and it spreads through the spores, which can resist boiling for considerable periods. The toxin, which can be separated into fractions A, B and E acts on the nervous system and it inhibits release of acetylcholine at the neuromuscular junction and blocks neuromuscular transmission in cholinergic nerve fibers.

The toxin rapidly fixes to the nerves and once endocytosis occurs, its effects cannot be reversed. The toxin consists of seven serologically distinct, but structurally similar components A, B, C, D, E, F and G of which only types A, B, E and F cause illness in humans. The paralysis persists for 2–3 months or even more. Botulism may occur in one of three forms, food borne botulism, infant botulism and wound botulism. In addition to its role as a cause of food poisoning, *Cl. botulinum* can contaminate wounds and also grow in the intestinal tract and elaborate toxins.

Symptoms start in 12–36 hours after ingestion with diplopia, blurring of vision and paralysis of cranial nerves. Other features are dry mouth, dysphagia and dysphonia. Progressive muscular involvement results in respiratory paralysis. Death is caused by respiratory failure or pneumonia (10–20%). Neurological sequelae in the form of motor paralysis may persist for several months in a few. *Diagnosis:* Other conditions leading to neuromuscular paralysis such as Guillain-Barré syndrome (GBS), myasthenic crises, cobra or krait bites and vascular accidents of the brainstem have to be differentiated. Myasthenic crises responds to Tensilon whereas in botulism this is not so.

Treatment: Adequate ventilatory support and general supportive measures should be instituted. Guanidine hydrochloride in a dose of 15–50 mg/kg/day has been used but without proven effect. A trivalent preparation containing antitoxin is available, it is given intravenous (IV) in doses of 50000 units stat and repeated after 2 hours. This vaccine is not freely available in India.

Infant Botulism

This is caused by *Cl. botulinum* colonizing in the colon of infants. They produce the toxin which is absorbed and leads to systemic effects. Infant botulism is defined as an illness consistent with paralysis typical of botulism toxin. The typical organisms are cultured from feces or enema material. Treatment consists of giving botulinum immunoglobulin (Ig) containing neutralizing antibodies.

Anaerobic Food Poisoning

Cl. perfringens food poisoning—usual source of contamination is meat. Heat resistant spores survive improper cooking. They germinate when the food is cooled. On reaching the intestine they sporulate and produce exotoxin which causes abdominal cramps and diarrhea.

INFECTION TYPE OF FOOD POISONING

In this group, organisms enter along with contaminated food and multiply in the gut to produce the lesions after an incubation period ranging from 24 to 72 hours. The organism may be noninvasive or invasive depending on their action on the intestinal mucosa. The organism may be noninvasive such as *Enterotoxigenic Escherichia coli* or *Klebsiella*. They produce diarrhea by locally acting enterotoxins, which stimulate adenylyl cyclase and cyclic antimicrobial peptides (AMP) mechanisms.

The intestinal mucosa is not destroyed. Stools are watery and generally devoid of inflammatory cells. Clinical features of severe dehydration predominate with relatively mild constitutional symptoms.

Invasive group includes organisms like *Shigella, Salmonella typhimurium, Salmonella enteritidis, Yersinia enterocolitica*, invasive strains of *E. coli* and *Vibrio parahaemolyticus*. They produce inflammatory lesions. They destroy the intestinal mucosa and the feces contain abundant inflammatory cells and erythrocytes. Constitutional symptoms of varying severity accompany this syndrome.

In the infection type of food poisoning antimicrobial therapy is indicated to arrest the multiplication of the organism in the gut. Systemic antibiotics are indicated in the invasive type. General measures of treatment of gastroenteritis are indicated.

CHRONIC FOOD POISONING

Some cases of chronic food poisoning, caused by repeated exposures to fish contaminated by industrial effluents, have been reported.

- *Haff disease* is produced by eating fish poisoned by toxic resinous acids from cellulose. This condition produces myoglobinuria in the affected persons.
- *Minamata disease* is caused by consumption of fish, which has ingested methyl mercury compounds. Outbreaks of mercury poisoning occurred in cats and people living in fishing villages in Japan.

Due to the rapid growth of industry and the present day tendency to interfere with natural ecosystems, such examples are likely to be on the increase, unless sufficient care is taken to prevent them.

Mushroom Poisoning

Mushrooms are delicacies on the table. In India, they are grown commercially in Himachal Pradesh and many other parts including the southern states. Many people eat wild mushrooms collected seasonally and some of them cause accidental poisoning. The common toxic mushrooms include *Amanita muscaria, Amanita phalloides, Amanita verna, Amanita virosa, Helvella esculenta* and *Galerina* species. All these species contain amatoxin, which is a potent cytotoxin. Deaths have resulted from the ingestion of even 50 g of mushrooms. The toxic principles vary in different species.

Amanita muscaria contains three toxic principles. (1) A parasympathomimetic alkaloid-muscarine, (2) a neurotoxic substance and (3) an alkaloid with atropine like action. The toxins of *Amanita phalloides* and related species are cytotoxic alpha-amanitin and phalloidin. These toxins inhibit protein synthesis. The toxic principles are thermostable and, therefore, resist cooking. *Pathogenesis:* The toxin leads to severe cholinergic overactivity similar to organophosphorus poisoning. Autopsy shows extensive cellular degeneration, necrosis, edema and hemorrhage in the liver, kidney, gastrointestinal tract (GIT) and brain. *Amanita muscaria:* Signs of toxicity develop sometime after the consumption of contaminated food. Symptoms may be atropine like including, excitement, delirium, flushed skin, dilated pupils and muscular twitchings. Other features include hypotension, convulsion, delirium and coma.

Textbook of Medicine

Early recognition and treatment give good results with complete recovery within 24 hours. In addition to general measures, specific treatment is with physostigmine 0.5–1 mg IV which corrects the anticholinergic effects of the poisoning.

Amanita phalloides: The clinical picture develops in two phases. The first phase starts after a latent period of 8–12 hours and essentially resembles acute gastroenteritis (belated mycetismus choleriformis) with muscle cramps, vomiting, profuse diarrhea, dehydration and circulatory collapse. The second phase sets in 2–3 days later even after apparent initial recovery. The features resemble acute yellow atrophy of the liver, progressing to hepatic and renal failure. The prognosis is poor. Mortality may exceed 50%. In those who survive recovery is slow.

Sometimes mushrooms belonging to *Coprinus* species produce an antabuse-like reaction if consumed with alcohol. *Panaeolus* produces atropine toxicity like picture and *Helvella* produces hemolytic reaction.

General Management

Stomach wash should be given early. Oral administration of 25–50 g of activated charcoal helps to bind amatoxin for which it has high affinity. This simple procedure is very helpful if instituted within 36 hours of poisoning.

Several drugs have been employed as possible antidotes, some of them are still experimental. These include massive doses of penicillin, vitamin C, silymarin and thioctic acid.

Thioctic acid (alpha lipoic acid) is given IV in doses of 200–300 mg twice daily. The results are encouraging. Hemperfusion over charcoal has been found to be beneficial in severe cases. All patients with suspected mushroom poisoning should be observed for at least 24 hours since in a few cases the onset of symptoms could be delayed.

> **Points to Remember**
> - There are different species of mushrooms with varied toxic principles.
> - Most of the very toxic species contain amatoxin, which is a potent cytotoxin and deaths have been reported within minutes of intake.
> - Symptoms vary from gastrointestinal irritation, anticholinergic effects, muscarinic or hallucinogenic effects depending on the species.
> - Hemoperfusion using charcoal is beneficial in severe cases and several antidotes have been tried.

FISH POISONING

In many parts of India, toxicity to fish is encountered seasonally from time to time. This may occur as small outbreaks confined to families or may be widespread. The term 'icthyotoxism' refers to poisoning by intrinsic toxins in fish. The toxic principles may be sarcotoxic (flesh and viscera are toxic), ootoxic (only the reproductive organs are toxic) or hemotoxic (where the toxicity is predominantly in the blood). Some varieties of fish become toxic to man only in particular seasons.

Several factors such as glandular activity during spawning season, consumption of toxic dinoflagellates or toxic plants in the sea and contamination by industrial effluents can make the fish toxic. Toxic principles may be confined to the liver in many fishes. During certain seasons, the livers of some fishes may contain very high levels of vitamin A (600,000 units/100 g). Ingestion of such livers leads to acute vitamin A toxicity characterized by headache, nausea, vomiting, prolonged sleep or drowsiness followed later by extensive exfoliative dermatitis. Another type of toxicity is related to the very high histidine content of scromboid fish. On storage, due to the action of marine bacterial flora, histamine and saurine are produced. These reach high levels causing an acute histamine intoxication syndrome with headache, flushing, urticaria, vomiting and circulatory failure (scrombotoxicity).

Dinoflagellate-induced toxins lead to neuroparalytic syndromes.

Acute renal failure following consumption of gallbladder of raw carp—*Ctenopharyngodon idellus* has been described from Manipur, India. This presented with vomiting and rapid onset of oliguric renal failure. The pathology is likely to be tubular necrosis due to direct nephrotoxicity. These cases responded well to conservative treatment including peritoneal dialysis.

Diagnosis of icthyotoxism can be made from epidemiological and clinical considerations. Bacterial food poisoning has to be excluded. Treatment is only symptomatic and in majority of cases, complete recovery is the rule.

Acute Cassava Toxicity

Cassava or tapioca (manioc) is a staple diet among the poor people in many parts of the world, especially in Africa and Southern States of India. Certain bitter varieties (Manioc utilissima) are toxic during particular seasons due to ***linamarin***, which contains cyanogenic glycosides and a glucosidase enzyme. The toxins are maximum in the outer coat, which can be removed by peeling. Bruising, soaking in water, cooking in insufficient quantity of water or prolonged storage serves to bring together the glycoside and the enzyme and liberate hydrocyanic acid. A lethal dose of hydrocyanic acid (60 mg) may be acquired from 300 G of partly damaged cassava.

Symptoms of acute poisoning: It include giddiness, headache, mental confusion, coma and collapse. Death occurs because of asphyxia. Convulsions and incontinence of sphincters may precede death, which usually occurs within 2 hours of the meal.

Treatment: Early gastric lavage with 1% sodium bicarbonate should be given. Specific measures are those for cyanide poisoning. These are as follows:

- Oxygen inhalation
- Specific antidote is amylnitrate, which is given by inhalation every 2 minutes. This is followed by IV administration of 10 mL of 3% sodium nitrite, taking 5 minutes for the injection and later 50 mL of 25% sodium thiosulfate over a period of 10 minutes.
- This course should be repeated if required. Blood level of methemoglobin should be estimated and this should be kept below 40%.
- Dicobalt-acetate in a dose of 300–600 mg given IV in one minute is a chelating agent used for removing cyanide.

Cassava toxicity should be prevented by avoiding bruised tubers and taking care in storage and cooking. Boiling the tuber in a large quantity of water and discarding the supernatant removes the toxic content. The increased content in cassava has been implicated in the causation of several conditions such as calcific pancreatitis, konzo—which is a form of tropical myelopathy first detected in Africa, and possibly other conditions as well.

In India, the Tuber Crops Research Stations have helped to develop newer less toxic varieties of cassava, which have become very popular. The occurrence of cassava toxicity has come down in recent times. Far from its original position as poor man's staple, at present cassava has gained the position of being a delicacy on the table.

> **Points to Remember**
> - The toxicity of cassava is due to linamarin which contains cyanogenic glycosides and a glucosidase enzyme.
> - Acute poisoning may produce giddiness, headache, mental confusion, coma and collapse.
> - Treatment is as for cyanide poisoning.
> - Cassava toxicity has been implicated in calcific pancreatitis, tropical myelopathy, etc.

ONYALAI

This is an acute purpuric disease, characterized by hemorrhagic bullae inside the mouth, seen in Africa. It is attributed to the mycotoxin of *Phoma sorghina* isolated from the cereals, millet and sorghum, though its etiology is not fully known.

HEPATIC VENO-OCCLUSIVE DISEASE

Syn: Veno-occlusive Disease of Jamaica

Though originally described from Jamaica, cases have subsequently been reported from all over the world. The toxic principles of **senecio** and **crotalaria** are responsible for this syndrome. These plants are taken as bush teas. Malnourished children in the age group 2–5 years are particularly vulnerable. The toxin causes proliferation of intimal cells and swelling of subintimal tissues. This leads to occlusion of centrilobular veins of the liver. Liver cells atrophy and are replaced by centrilobular fibrosis. Outbreaks have been reported from central and north India.

Clinical features: It varies in severity. In the acute form hepatomegaly, ascites and rapidly progressive hepatic failure develop. Many cases recover completely. Rare sequelae include asymptomatic hepatomegaly or gradual progression to cirrhosis liver and portal hypertension.

Treatment: It consists of prompt withdrawal of the offending materials and dietary supplementation with high quality protein. No specific antidote is available (*See* also Section 9, Chapter 87).

AFLATOXICOSIS

Aflatoxins are products of fungi particularly those of *Aspergillus flavus*. These are widespread in several articles of human and cattle food and, therefore, aflatoxicosis involves wide population groups. Groundnuts, cereals or pulses are invaded by the fungus, especially when stored in damp environment. The damaged grains show obvious abnormalities. The toxin contains several components (B_1 which is most toxic, B_2 and G_2). Acute toxicity occurs when mouldy cereals, pulses or nuts are consumed. Aflatoxin is hepatotoxic to many animals and birds. Fungus affected grains are likely to be consumed during periods of drought, famine and nonseasonal rains. Generally, the poor socioeconomic sections of the communities are affected. The clinical picture may be that of acute hepatitis, cirrhosis of the liver or hepatoma depending on the dose and duration of exposure. The outbreaks reported from western India and Rajasthan resembled viral hepatitis and mortality ranged from 10 to 25%.

Diagnosis: In all outbreaks of acute hepatitis, aflatoxicosis should be considered. Diagnosis is based on the clinical picture, exclusion of other conditions and the epidemiological evidence. Treatment is supportive with rest in bed, adequate supply of glucose and B-complex factors and maintenance of fluid and electrolyte balance. Complications have to be treated symptomatically as they occur. Chronic aflatoxin exposure is an important etiological factor in the production of hepatocellular carcinoma in India.

> **Points to Remember**
> - Aflatoxin is a product of fungus *Aspergillus fumigatus*
> - Aflatoxin is hepatotoxic and may produce hepatitis, cirrhosis liver or hepatoma.
> - Chronic exposure is an etiological factor for hepatocellular carcinoma.
> - Treatment is with symptomatic measures.

EPIDEMIC DROPSY

Syn: Toxicity due to Argemone Mexicana (Yellow Mexican Poppy)

Argemone mexicana grows wild in the cold season all over India and is known by different names as *Brahmadandi* or *Pildhatura* (Maharashtra), *Sialkanta* (Bengali), and *Satyanashi* (Gujarati). The seeds resemble mustard seeds. Argemone oil is used as an adulterant of mustard oil, more during times of famine and drought. The toxic principles are sanguinarine and dihydrosanguinarine, the former being more toxic. Poisoning occurs due to consumption of adulterated mustard oil used as cooking medium. Several outbreaks have occurred and are still being reported in Bengal, Bihar, Orissa, Madhya Pradesh, Uttar Pradesh, Gujarat and Maharashtra.

Clinical features: The onset is insidious with loss of appetite, diarrhea and pitting edema over the legs. Sometimes the edema may be massive and effusion into pleura and pericardium may occur. Cardiac enlargement and failure develop. The extremities are warm due to vasodilatation. Subcutaneous telangiectasia or even hemangiomata develop. These are seen on the mucus membrane of the cheek, gums, tongue and nose as fleshy dark red or warty growths (sarcoids). Tingling and numbness of the extremities and calf tenderness are present. About 10% cases develop glaucoma. Electrocardiogram (ECG) reveals nonspecific changes resembling myocarditis. Serum albumin is lowered and alpha-2-globulin is raised. Death is caused by cardiac failure. Withdrawal of the toxic oil leads to recovery in most cases.

Treatment: The treatment is supportive with nutritional supplements. Cardiac failure should be treated symptomatically. A simple method to detect the presence of argemone oil is to mix the suspected sample with an equal volume of nitric acid, when a crimson color develops in case of contamination.

LATHYRISM

Syn: Epidemic Spastic Paraplegia

Chronic ingestion of the toxic principles of *Lathyrus sativus* leads to spastic paralysis of the lower limbs. This pulse is known in various parts of India as *Kesari dal, Teora, Matra, Batura, Gharas, Lang, Lakh* and *Latri dal.* Lathyrism is more prevalent in Madhya Pradesh, Bihar and Uttar Pradesh in India. It has also been reported from Greece, Iran, Russia, Italy, Spain and parts of Africa. Men are more affected than women. The toxic principles are probably ***Beta-oxalylaminoalanine or alkaloids like B-aminopropionitrile.*** The latter is present in the weed akta, which contaminates lathyrus peas. Pathological lesion is demyelination of the pyramidal tracts in the lumbar region and some degeneration of the anterior horn cells.

Clinical features: The onset is acute or subacute in 90% of cases with muscular pain in the back followed by paraplegia or paraparesis within days to weeks or even after several months. In those with acute onset cramping pain in the calf muscles and muscles of the thigh may occur. This may be followed by rapid onset of paralysis of varying degrees. In those with subacute onset stiffness and heaviness of the lower limbs start after about a month and paralysis sets in and proceeds to varying severity. In the typical case, paralysis and spasticity progress to cripple the patient. Sensations and autonomic functions are normal. The paralysis tends to be permanent.

Treatment: It is symptomatic. There is no specific antidote.

Prevention: The toxin can be removed by steeping the cereal in four times its volume of hot water for one hour before cooking. Education of the public on the methods to identify *Lathyrus sativus* will help in wiping out this disease.

Points to Remember

- Chronic ingestion of toxic principles of *Lathyrus sativus* leads to lathyrism.
- Pathology is demyelination of pyramidal tract and degeneration of anterior horn cells at the lumbar level.
- In a typical case, paralysis and spasticity progress to crippling.
- No specific antidote is available.

ERGOTISM

This is caused by the toxin of the fungus *Claviceps purpurae,* which infects rye and other cereal grains. Ergot alkaloids are highly variable mixtures of toxins, the most important one being ergotamine. When ingested, the toxin produces either cardiovascular or neurological manifestations. The former includes vasoconstriction, mental confusion and convulsions. Ergot alkaloids and their derivatives are widely used in therapeutics for their various actions. One of the alkaloids lysergic acid diethylamide (LSD) is a hallucinogen.

LEAD POISONING

Lead poisoning may occur in households among children and in industrial workers. Lead is widely used in paints, storage batteries, petrol and several industries. Ingestion, inhalation or absorption from the skin may lead to acute poisoning. Workers engaged in printing, lead smelting, ship building, tank cleaning are at risk of developing chronic toxicity. Children may eat flaked paint as a form of pica. Lead accumulates in the body and it is deposited in bone and other tissues.

Acute lead poisoning: Initial symptoms are metallic taste, irritation of throat, salivation and intense thirst. These are soon followed by colicky abdominal pain, painful spasm of abdominal muscles, hematemesis and constipation. The stools are black due to the formation of lead sulphide. More serious cases develop drowsiness, headache, muscular cramps, convulsions, paralysis of lower limbs, hemolysis and renal failure.

Treatment: Calcium disodium versenate ethylenediaminetetraacetic acid (EDTA) in a dose of 1 g in 250–500 mL of 5% dextrose IV twice daily (50 mg/kg/d) for 8–10 days or longer helps to eliminate the lead. Symptomatic treatment is indicated as the condition warrants.

Chronic lead poisoning (Plumbism): The main symptoms are abdominal colic, constipation, hemolytic anemia, paralysis and cerebral, cardiac and renal damage. It manifests initially as tubular damage going on to chronic renal failure. There is no threshold level for lead to initiate toxicity. Severe intestinal colic and constipation may be mistaken for other alimentary disorders.

In chronic lead poisoning, the lead is deposited in cortical bone. Lead impairs the enzyme delta-aminolevulinic acid dehydrogenase which is needed for heme synthesis. Moderate to severe hemolytic anemia occurs. The peripheral blood shows punctate basophilia and reticulocytosis. In long-term lead poisoning, lead is deposited in cortical bone. Motor neuropathies manifest as wrist drop and foot drop. Shoulder girdle muscles may be affected rarely. Sensory symptoms are usually absent. Lead encephalopathy manifests as headache, loss of memory, epileptiform convulsions and coma. Optic neuritis may occur. Urine may show protein, delta amino levulinic acid and coproporphyrin III. Blood pressure (BP) is elevated. Deposition of lead in the gingival margins results in the formation of a black line in people with poor oral hygiene. In edentulous subjects, this lead line ***(Burtonian line)*** does not form. Chronic renal failure may develop. It manifests initially as tubular damage, later, tubular atrophy and interstitial nephritis. Exposure to lead during intrauterine life leads to erosion of cognitive skills with subclinical but permanent reduction in intelligence quotient (IQ). This may result is permanent impairment in performance standards in adult life.

Source: Grandjean P, Landrigan PJ. Developmental neurotoxicity of industrial chemicals. Lancet. 2006;368 (9553):2167-78.

Diagnosis: The clinical diagnosis is confirmed by the elevated levels of lead in blood. Levels above 80 mcg/dL are diagnostic. A test for chronic lead accumulation is

Textbook of Medicine

EDTA mobilization test. Urinary loss of >600 mcg of lead in 72 hours indicates lead poisoning.

Treatment: In severe toxicity EDTA is administered as described earlier. In less severe cases, other than EDTA an oral chelator, succimer (dimercaptosuccinic acid) has been used in a dose of 10 mg/kg orally every 8 hours for 5 days.

Prevention: Proper washing of the hands before eating and provision of protective clothing and masks reduce absorption of lead. Provision of 300 mL of milk to such workers may be helpful in reducing toxicity. Persons working in risky occupations should be periodically monitored. Pollution of the environment by lead salt is a major concern in recent years. The use of lead in automobile fuels has resulted in the discharge of appreciable amounts of lead into the atmosphere. In many states of India the use of leaded petrol is restricted.

Points to Remember

- Acute lead poisoning presents with predominantly gastrointestinal symptoms and in serious cases drowsiness-convulsions, hemolysis and renal failure may occur.
- Chronic lead poisoning is characterized by abdominal colic, constipation and basophilic stippling of red blood cells (RBCs).
- Motor neuropathies, optic neuritis and lead encephalopathy can also occur in chronic lead poisoning.
- EDTA is the mainstay of treatment.

CHAPTER 25

Endemic Fluorosis

TK Suma, KV Krishna Das

Chapter Summary

- Epidemiology
- Clinical Features
- Treatment
- Prevention of Endemic Fluorosis

Endemic fluorosis is caused by chronic fluoride intoxication acquired by ingestion of water containing high concentration of fluorides. It is characterized by dental and skeletal changes.

EPIDEMIOLOGY

The disease is present in many states in India where fluoride content of drinking water exceeds 2 ppm. Andhra Pradesh, Punjab and North Karnataka show high prevalence. Endemic areas have also been found in Tamil Nadu, Haryana, Rajasthan, Uttar Pradesh and New Delhi and its surrounding areas. In Kerala, three districts are affected. The disease is present in certain parts of China, Japan, South Africa, Saudi Arabia and USA.

The disease is more prevalent in males who are engaged in hard manual work because of their higher consumption of water. Total hardness of drinking water (calcium and magnesium hardness) has a protective role.

Presence of fluoride up to 0.5–0.8 ppm in drinking water is considered safe in India. With higher levels, fluoride accumulates in the skeletal system and teeth.

Pathophysiology: Ingestion of fluoride causes reduction of ionized calcium. This hypocalcemia leads on to secondary hyperparathyroidism and increased osteoclastic activity. Increased levels of lactic acid and citric acid are produced from the osteoclasts thereby increasing the hydrogen ion concentration and lysis of lysosomes. Lysosomal enzymes like protease, collagenase and hyaluronic acid produce disintegration of hydroxyproline and other ground substances of bone and other calcified tissues like teeth. This is responsible for the signs and symptoms of fluorosis like dental hypoplasia with areas of hypocalcification, hypomineralization and softening. The bones are heavier and irregular. There is excessive subperiosteal bone formation at the sites of muscular, fascial and tendinous attachments. Ligaments show various grades of calcification. The most advanced changes are seen in the spine. There is narrowing of the vertebral canal, which leads to compression of the spinal cord. Marked changes are seen in the ribs, pelvis, sternum, mandible and skull. Over a period of 10–20 years, the subject develops crippling deformities.

CLINICAL FEATURES

Dental fluorosis: Enamel and dentin of teeth have strong affinity for fluoride during the formation of teeth. Mottled enamel is an early, sensitive and easily distinguishable manifestation in children. This has been taken as an index of endemicity in epidemiological surveys. Dental fluorosis develops only if the child has lived in the endemic area during dentition. It can be graded depending on the severity.

Grade-I: White chalky opacities or patches on enamel without faint yellow lines.

Grade-II: Distinct brownish discoloration.

Grade-III: Besides pigmentation there is pitting of enamel surface, sometimes with chipping of edges (Figs 25.1 and 25.2).

Premature loss of teeth is not rare. Both permanent and deciduous teeth may be affected.

Skeletal fluorosis: It is not easily recognizable in the early stages. The initial symptoms are nonspecific such as

Textbook of Medicine

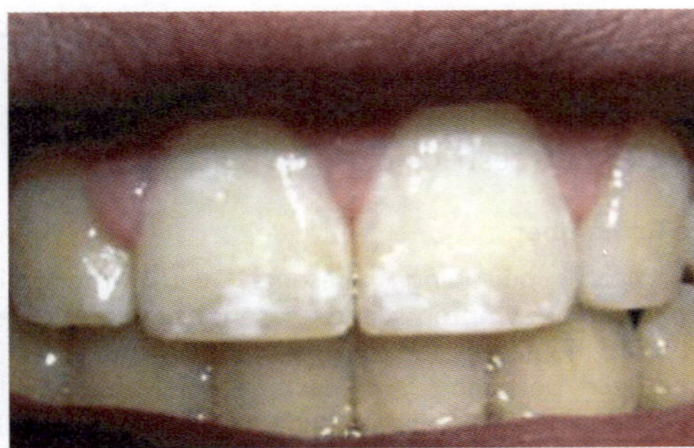

Fig. 25.1: White chalky opacities in mild dental fluorosis

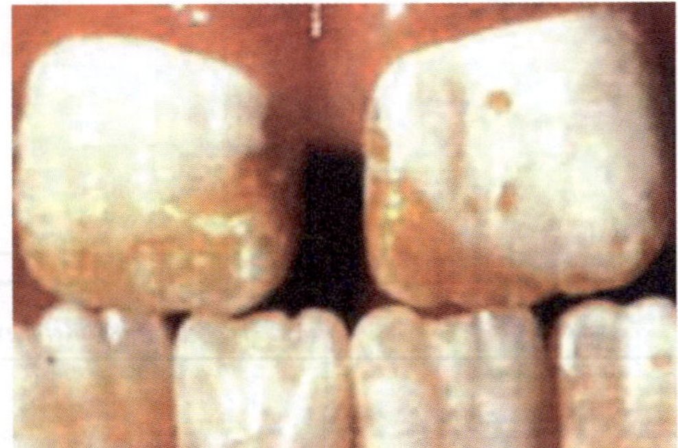

Fig. 25.2: Severe dental fluorosis

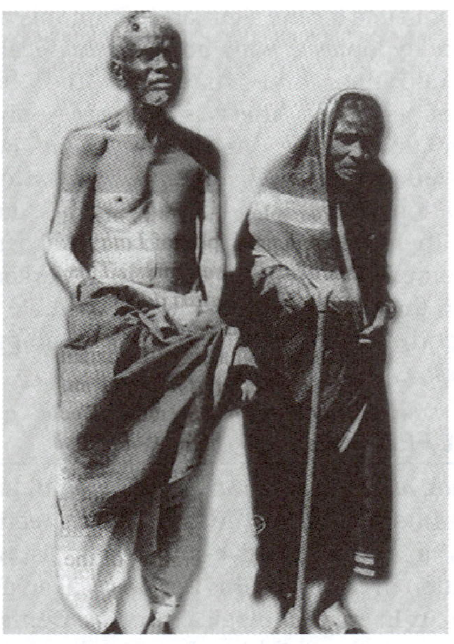

Fig. 25.3: Advanced skeletal changes in fluorosis

pain in the neck and back associated with rigidity, joint pains and paresthesia of the limbs. These cases may be mistaken for rheumatoid arthritis, ankylosing spondylitis or osteoarthritis.

The physical findings include kyphosis, limitation of movements of the spine and exostoses. Exostoses can easily be palpated along the anterior border of the tibia, over the olecranon, and along the medial border of the scapula. These are diagnostic. In advanced fluorosis, kyphosis, fixed flexion deformities of hips and knees and paraplegia, may develop (Fig. 25.3).

Nonskeletal manifestations: These include neurological manifestations like tingling sensation in fingers and toes, weakness and stiffness of skeletal muscles, nervousness and depression, gastrointestinal manifestations like nonulcer dyspepsia, abdominal pain, diarrhea and/ or constipation. The red blood cell (RBC) membrane becomes more pliable due to decreased calcium and forms into echinocytes. Early destruction of echinocytes results in anemia. Flouride has inhibitory effect on iodine uptake and so may cause enlargement of thyroid.

Complications: About 8–10% of cases show compression of spinal cord and the roots by protruding osteophytes. The vertebral arteries may also be occluded. The clinical picture may resemble cervical myeloradiculopathy, cervical myelopathy or radiculopathy, dorsal myelopathy and peripheral neuropathy. Bladder involvement manifests as precipitancy of micturition or retention of urine.

Occasionally, peripheral neuropathy manifests as acroparesthesia, but with only minimal sensory or motor defects. Cranial nerve involvement is rare.

Investigations: Radiologic and biochemical investigations should be carried out.

Radiology: The classic features are osteosclerosis, irregular osteophyte formation and calcification of ligaments, especially in the vertebral column. In advanced cases, the bones look chalky white. Irregular subperiosteal new bone formation may be observed along the muscular, fascial, and tendinous attachments. Interosseous membrane of the forearm shows calcification and this has been taken as a definite radiological index of skeletal fluorosis (Fig. 25.4).

Computed tomography (CT) and magnetic resonance imaging (MRI): CT of the bones may show prominent cortical thickening and increased density with irregular contours. Bony excrescences are detected in both the pelvic bones and the lower extremities. The sacroiliac joints may be narrowed. MRI may show reduction in the intervertebral disc spaces and multiple disc prolapse. The medullary canal may be narrowed by bony excrescences and by the ossified posterior longitudinal ligament.

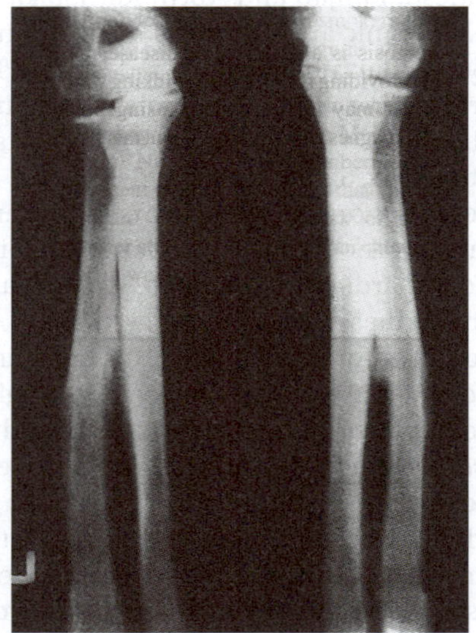

Fig. 25.4: Skiagram of forearm showing calcification of interosseous membrane

Biochemistry: Fluoride content is increased in the blood, urine and bone ash. Serum fluoride level varies from 0.05 to 0.8 mg/dL. Serum alkaline phosphatase is moderately raised (15–30 KA units). Serum calcium, phosphorus and magnesium are normal.

TREATMENT

Endemic fluorosis is a preventable disease, which can be eradicated by providing fluoride-free drinking water. Defluoridation of water may be affected by using bone meal and metasilicate of magnesium (serpentine) but this is not yet widely used. Vitamins and antioxidants have been tried in many cases. Changing the dietary habits by restricting use of fluoride-rich food is also important.

There is no effective treatment for the established case. Patients with skeletal fluorosis, when fed with fluoride-free drinking water, seem to improve over the years. Improvement in the dental changes is reported within weeks. Cases of spinal compression require laminectomy.

PREVENTION OF ENDEMIC FLUOROSIS

In endemic areas fluorosis can be prevented by reducing the fluoride content of water to less than 1 ppm. Two methods are available for defluoridation of water, the Nalgonda technology and the activated alumina technology. In Nalgonda technique alum and lime are used in various proportions depending on fluoride content of water. In activated alumina technology activated alumina is used in domestic filters. Encouraging the use of calcium, vitamin C and vitamin E may help to reduce the skeletal changes.

Points to Remember

- Ingestion of water having high fluoride content over several years results in fluorosis.
- Fluorosis leads to reduction in the level of ionized calcium. Osteoclastic activity increases.
- Dental fluorosis, skeletal fluorosis and nonskeletal manifestations occur.
- Established skeletal lesions tend to be permanent.
- Fluorosis can be prevented by defluoridation of drinking water.

CHAPTER
26

Therapy of Chronic Tobacco Addiction

KV Krishna Das, KE Rajan, TK Suma

Chapter Summary

- General Considerations
- Pathogenesis and Pathology
- Smoking
- Tobacco Control
- Occupational Health Problems among Tobacco Workers

GENERAL CONSIDERATIONS

Native American tribes are believed to have used tobacco (*Nicotiana tabacum*) as early as 1400-1000 BC. Jean Nicot (from whose name nicotine was derived) introduced tobacco to France, which later spread to England and Europe. The Portuguese introduced tobacco to India in the 17th century. At present, tobacco is consumed in the form of smoke (beedies, cigarette, pipe, cigar, hookah, vaporizer, etc.) or for chewing with or without other constituents such as betel, areca nut and lime or as snuff applied to the nasal or oral mucosa. All these habits are very much prevalent in all societies in India.

According to the World Health Organization (WHO), tobacco is the single greatest cause of preventable death across the globe. About a third of the world population use tobacco in one form or other. A billion people smoke globally. Tobacco kills up to half of its users. Every 6.5 seconds, someone on the earth dies from tobacco use. Annually, more than 5 million deaths result from direct use of tobacco. More than 600,000 nonsmokers die due to effects of second hand smoke every year. Annual mortality due to tobacco is likely to go up to 8 million by 2030 AD, if the tobacco epidemic is not controlled.

Smoking increases the risk of coronary heart disease (CHD) as well as cerebrovascular disease by 2–4 times. Lung cancer risk increases by 25 times. Smoking causes 9 out of 10 lung cancer deaths and 8 out of 10 chronic obstructive pulmonary disease (COPD) deaths. It increases the risk of type II diabetes by 40–50%. Tobacco-related morbidity will top the list of global burden of disease. Developed countries have been successful in reducing the prevalence of smoking while developing countries including India have not done so. Multinational tobacco manufactures are selectively targeting developing countries for sales promotion. One-third of the cancers reported from Western countries are probably tobacco related.

In India, tobacco consumption is responsible for half of all cancers in males and a quarter of all cancers in females. India is home to 275 million tobacco users. ***Global Adult Tobacco Survey (GATS)*** aimed at determining the magnitude of tobacco use in low income countries including India. This survey found 48.6% of men and 11.3% of women were tobacco users. The Indian Council of Medical Research (ICMR) estimates that about 1 million Indians die annually due to tobacco-related diseases. By 2020, tobacco will be responsible for 13% of all deaths in India. Here, men smoke more than women. In all countries, the prevalence of smoking in women is increasing.

Textbook of Medicine

Around 464,000 hectares are under tobacco cultivation in India, with an annual production of 650,000 tonnes of tobacco and contributing 7% to the total world production. More than 3.4 million persons are engaged in the tobacco cultivation and many more in tobacco-related industry and trade. Over 20 companies manufacture more than 100 brands of cigarettes. In addition, beedies are rolled in smaller establishments as cottage industry. Of the tobacco consumed in India, 24% is used for cigarettes, 40% go into beedies and the rest used for chewing.

PATHOGENESIS AND PATHOLOGY

Tobacco is the most important cause of cancer and cancer death, affecting several organ systems. Tobacco smoke contains several constituents, which irritate the respiratory tract and inhibit ciliary action. The tar is the resinous, partially combusted particulate matter produced by the burning of tobacco. Content of tar per cigarette vary from 7 to 22 mg. Tar is highly mutagenic and carcinogenic, especially to the respiratory tract. It contains several polycyclic aromatic hydrocarbons (PAHs). It is estimated that every gram of dried tobacco leaf contains more than 1 µg of nitrosamines and more than 5ng of benzopyrine. Tobacco cured using wood smoke has higher contents of the carcinogens. Depending upon the brand of cigarette and manner of smoking, the level of carbon monoxide (CO) in the smoke may vary from 1 to 5%. Rise in blood CO leads to intimal hypoxia, increase in the permeability of arterial intima and lipid deposition. Blood levels of carboxyhemoglobin are elevated in smokers. Oxygen-carrying capacity of blood is reduced in them.

Nicotine present in tobacco is responsible for the addiction. The nicotine content of an average cigarette varies from 2 to 4 mg. Beedies contain a third of the nicotine content of the cigarette. Sympathomimetic effects of nicotine give rise to higher heart rate, elevation of systolic and diastolic blood pressure (BP), increase in cardiac output and peripheral vasoconstriction. The threshold for ventricular tachycardia (VT) and ventricular fibrillation (VF) is lowered. By increasing platelet aggregation, platelet adhesion, plasma fibrinogen and viscosity of blood nicotine favors the intravascular thrombosis. There is reduction in platelet survival and clotting time. Atherogenesis is favored by the rise in total cholesterol, low-density lipoproteins (LDL) and free fatty acids (FFA), and also fall in high-density lipoproteins (HDL) brought about by nicotine. Addiction to tobacco use is mediated by nicotine. It acts on nicotinic-acetylcholine receptors to release neurotransmitters [dopamine, glutamate and gamma-aminobutyric acid (GABA)]. In India, oral cancer which is the most common cancer, shows a strong association with tobacco chewing or smoking habit. In those who practice the chewing habit, in addition to absorption of nicotine from the buccal mucosa the local irritation caused by the cud leads to precancerous and cancerous changes. See Table 26.1 for more ill-effects of tobacco use.

SMOKING

Tobacco smoke is a highly habit forming agent, because of nicotine. Addiction will occur even with the second or

Table 26.1: Tobacco-related diseases

- **General effects**
  - Diminished overall health
  - Reduced immunity
  - Increased absenteeism from work
  - Increased healthcare utilization and cost
  - Increased risk of death from all causes
- **Cancers**
  - Lung/larynx/nose/paranasal cavities
  - Oral cavity/nasopharynx/oropharynx/hypopharynx
  - Esophagus/stomach/pancreas/liver/colon/rectum
  - Kidney/urinary bladder
  - Breast/uterine cervix
  - Acute myeloid leukemia (AML)
- **Skin**
  - Premature ageing/wrinkling/drying/yellow color
  - Psoriasis
- **Bones and Joints**
  - Decreased bone density
  - Rheumatoid arthritis (RA)
- **Eye**
  - Premature cataract
  - Macular degeneration
  - Tobacco amblyopia
- **Ear**
  - Hearing loss
  - Increased susceptibility to middle ear infections
- **Mouth**
  - Excess plaque formation/yellowing of teeth
  - Periodontitis/increased teeth loss
  - Gum infection/bleeding
- **Fingers/toes**
  - Buerger's disease and amputations
  - Discolored fingers
- **Cardiovascular system (CVS)**
  - Tachycardia/arrhythmia
  - Hypertension/dissecting aneurysm
  - Atherogenesis
  - Coronary artery disease (CAD)
- **Endocrine**
  - Type II diabetes mellitus (DM) and worsening its control
- **Respiratory system**
  - Lung cancer
  - Chronic bronchitis
  - Emphysema
  - Pneumonia, pneumothorax
  - Tuberculosis, asthma
- **Gastrointestinal tract (GIT)**
  - Increased susceptibility to *Helicobacter pylori*
  - Impaired neutralization of acid
- **Central nervous system (CNS)**
  - Cerebrovascular disease and stroke
  - Anxiety and depression
  - Negative impact on cognition/dementia
- **Reproductive system**
  - Reduced sperm count/deformed sperm/damaged sperm DNA
  - Erectile dysfunction/Impotence
  - Infertility (male/female), premature menopause
  - Ectopic pregnancy/ miscarriage/stillbirth/ birth defects
  - LBW in babies/SIDS
  - Higher incidence of cancer in offspring

Abbreviations: LBW = Low birth weight; DNA = Deoxyribonucleic acid; SIDS = Sudden infant death syndrome

third smoke. Children of smoking parents acquire this habit more freely.

The harmful ingredients taken up by the smoker and exhaled by him depend upon several factors such as the number of cigarettes smoked and their frequency, depth of inhalation, smoking the cigarette only partially or fully and the environment in which the smoker smokes—whether open or confined space. Inhalation of the exhaled smoke by others nearby is termed passive smoking, which is also associated with adverse effects in various degrees.

Cigarette smoking is shown to be associated with airway obstruction and impairment of lung function in adolescents. Females are affected more. Heavy smokers suffer from tachycardia, palpitation, cardiac arrhythmias, hypertension, tremors, anorexia, agitation and insomnia. Smoking can damage every part of the body. There is irrefutable evidence that smoking is a major risk factor for chronic bronchitis, emphysema and cancers of lung, larynx, esophagus, bladder, kidney, pancreas and cervix uteri. CHD, hypertension, strokes, peripheral vascular occlusions, thromboangiitis obliterans, peptic ulcers and several other conditions are directly or indirectly attributable to tobacco. Both main stream and second hand smoke are group-1 carcinogens, i.e. included among the highest cancer causing agents in humans. Over 90% of bronchogenic carcinoma is related to smoking, either direct or passive. Smoking contributes to 50% of the death of cigarette smokers, with half of these deaths occurring in middle life. Smokers lose 10 years of their life expectancy, compared to nonsmokers.

Smoking and Women

Incidence of smoking among women is increasing all over the globe. More women die from lung cancer each year than from breast cancer in the West. Smoking among women leads to more deleterious results. It is estimated that a male loses 13.2 years of life due to smoking, while a female smoker loses 14.5 years of life. Smoking lowers the estrogen and HDL with resultant deleterious effects on the cardiovascular system (CVS). Premature menopause is a definite risk for women smokers. Postmenopausal smokers have lower bone density compared to nonsmokers and they are at greater risk for fractures. A prospective study involving 1.3 million UK women smokers showed a mortality ratio of 2.76 compared to nonsmokers. Mortality tripled in those who continued to smoke and proportionate reduction was seen in those who quit. Substantial reduction in mortality was seen for those who stopped smoking. The extent of improvement depended upon the age of quitting.

Smoking by parents has an adverse effect on their children. Smoking makes it harder for a woman to conceive and can affect her baby's health before and after birth. Smoking mothers have an increased risk of ectopic pregnancy, spontaneous abortion and preterm delivery. They are at higher risk of delivering babies with congenital abnormalities, longer lengths, smaller head circumferences, and low birth weight. Smoker's children have lower birth weights, higher perinatal mortality and a greater risk of sudden infant death syndrome (SIDS). Orofacial clefts are more common among babies born to smokers.

Passive Smoking

Passive smoking is the inhalation of smoke [second hand smoke, or environmental tobacco smoke (ETS)] by persons other than the smoker. Tobacco smoke permeates the surroundings, leading to passive smoking. Exposure to second hand tobacco smoke causes disease, disability, and death. Second hand smoke causes many of the same diseases as direct smoking, including cardiovascular diseases (CVD), lung cancer and respiratory diseases. Children are particularly susceptible to ETS.

Babies exposed to ETS are at increased risk for brain tumors, middle ear infections and carotid artery damage. They are also at risk of worsening of asthma and development of lung infections, including bronchiolitis. There is increased risk of developing tuberculosis among them. Impaired respiratory function, slowed lung growth, allergies and Crohn's disease are seen at higher rates among them. They are also at risk for learning difficulties, developmental delays and neurobehavioral effects. In the US, it is estimated that ETS leads to yearly incidence of 150,000–300,000 lower respiratory tract infections (LRTI) in children below 18 months of age. Babies exposed to ETS are more likely to suffer from respiratory ailments and atopic dermatitis during later life. They are also more likely to become smokers in adolescent age.

Smokeless Tobacco

Smokeless tobacco denotes tobacco used for chewing or as snuff. PAHs in these agents cause cancers of the oral/nasal cavity and pancreas.

Tobacco Chewing

There are recent reports from India that tobacco chewing is also associated with increased risk of cardiovascular morbidity. Further studies are needed. Betel chewing is a cause of oral cancer and it is well-known. Though officially banned, several brands of such proprietary preparations (pan masalas) are available in the Indian market. These are being used by a large number of persons, especially the youth. Their role in the genesis of oral cancer and other systemic diseases is not yet fully assessed.

TOBACCO CONTROL

Medical associations of several countries have urged their governments to undertake measures to restrict the spread of tobacco habit. These include restriction of sales of tobacco to those below the age of 18 years, ban on advertisement, education in schools and through public media, prohibition of smoking in public places and public transport, heavy taxation on cigarettes and withdrawal of aids to tobacco industry.

The role of the physician/dental surgeon/paramedical staff is paramount in controlling the smoking habit. Physician should set an example by giving up the habit of using tobacco. Smokers should be motivated to give up smoking by counseling and providing information on the ill-effects. Governmental measures to restrict sales by imposing penal taxes and statutory directions to exhibit the dangers caused by smoking on the cigarette packs have made only minimal impact. Many governments in Indian states have prohibited smoking in public places. ***The WHO has declared the 31st of May every year as the 'No tobacco day'. During 2005, WHO had developed a 'code of practice' on tobacco control for health professional*** *organizations (website:http://www.who.int/tobacco).* Despite all the vigorous efforts, reduction in smoking habit is coming down only slowly. More of youth and females are probably taking to the habit.

Therapeutic Assistance to Patients to Quit Smoking

Smoking cessation or quitting smoking is a process of discontinuing tobacco smoke and maintaining abstinence. Cessation of smoking leads to symptoms of nicotine withdrawal such as anxiety and irritability. Hence, it is necessary to address both nicotine addiction and withdrawal symptoms. It takes between 6 and 12 weeks after quitting before the nicotinic receptors in the brain return to the level of a nonsmoker.

Unassisted Methods

About 4–7% of people are able to quit smoking on any given attempt without medicines or other help. The methods adopted by those trying to quit include:

- ***Cold turkey:*** Abrupt withdrawal, leading to complete stoppage of all nicotine use. This method is advocated by several authors.
- ***Cut down:*** Involves gradual reductions, slowly reducing one's daily intake of nicotine. A Cochrane systematic review analysis of 2012 found no significant difference between these two modes of trying to quit. Those who want to stop smoking can choose between these two methods.

Assisted by Healthcare Personnel through Counseling

Increased abstinence rates are observed where physicians or other healthcare providers advocate and reinforce the need to quit. Dental professionals also play a key role in increasing tobacco abstinence rates in the community through counseling patients in conjunction with an oral examination.

Multicomponent interventions—***5 A's***: Combination of two or more of the following strategies of interventions (known as the 5 A's), increased quit rates. Reducing/eliminating the cost of cessation therapies for smokers increased quit rates.

- ***Ask***—Systematically identify all tobacco users at every visit
- ***Advise***—Strongly urge all tobacco users to quit
- ***Assess***—Determine willingness to make a quit attempt
- ***Assist***—Aid the patient in quitting (provide counseling support and medication)
- ***Arrange***—Ensure follow-up contact.

Biochemical Feedback

Here, a marker allows the smoker to see the impact of tobacco use on his body. Handheld breath CO monitor closely reflects the blood carboxyhemoglobin levels. It is useful to link smoking with the harm it causes to the body. Within hours of quitting, CO concentrations show a noticeable decrease, which is very encouraging for someone striving to quit. Breath CO monitoring has been utilized in smoking cessation as a tool to provide patients with biomarker feedback. Assessing cotinine (metabolite of nicotine) levels in urine, saliva or blood can serve as a reliable biomarker to determine smoking status. These methods can be used either alone or together, for helping the smoker to quit.

Medications

Nicotine replacement therapy (NRT): According to American Cancer Society, 25–33% of smokers who use medicines can stay smoke-free for over 6 months. Five medications approved by the US Federal Food and Drug Administration (FDA) deliver nicotine in a form that does not involve the risks of smoking (but still may have harmful effects of nicotine). NRT is meant to be used for a short period of time and thereafter tapered off. NRT medications increased the chances of stopping smoking by 50–70% compared to placebo (Cochrane review). NRTs include transdermal nicotine patches, gum, lozenges, inhalers and sprays. The patches are to be applied at reducing dosages usually at 6 weekly intervals, to taper off dependence on nicotine. Nicotine gum is supplied in 2, 4 and 8 mg strengths. ***Chew and park*** technique is advocated for use of gum. Dosage needs to be tapered off at convenient intervals, depending upon the individual patient and his addiction levels.

Antidepressants: Bupropion is an approved drug for aiding quitting. It is contraindicated in patients with seizures, or on monoamine oxidase (MAO) inhibitors. It helps in long-term smoking cessation, with few adverse events.

Nicotinic receptor partial agonists: These drugs act by blocking the pleasant effects of nicotine/tobacco smoke on the human brain. ***Cytisine*** is a plant extract that has been in use since the 1960s in former Soviet Union. It was the first medication approved as an aid to smoking cessation and has very few side effects in small doses. It is a partial agonist that binds with high affinity in the $\alpha4\beta2$ subtype of nicotine-acetylcholine receptor. This receptor subtype has been implicated to perpetuate nicotine dependence. The same receptor is the target for ***varenicline***, a drug synthesized as an improvement on cytisine, for aiding tobacco rejection. Varenicline is superior to cytisine in efficacy. Varenicline is used as oral tablets. For days 1st to 3rd of therapy, 0.5 mg is given once daily. This is followed by 0.5 mg twice daily for 4th to 7th day. During the continuing weeks, the dosage is 1 mg twice daily for 12 weeks. Common adverse effects include nausea, abnormal dreams, constipation, flatulence and vomiting. The patients are to be cautioned on driving or operating machinery while taking varenicline.

Therapies under trial: Moclobemide and nortriptyline are antidepressants which show some value in aiding the process of quitting smoking. Clonidine reduces withdrawal symptoms. It is shown to double abstinence rates among those who stopped smoking. Clonidine should not be withdrawn abruptly on account of hypertension and other side effects.

E-Cigarette

E-cigarette (electronic cigarette) or electronic nicotine delivery system (ENDS) is a battery-powered device which simulates tobacco smoking. In this device, a heating

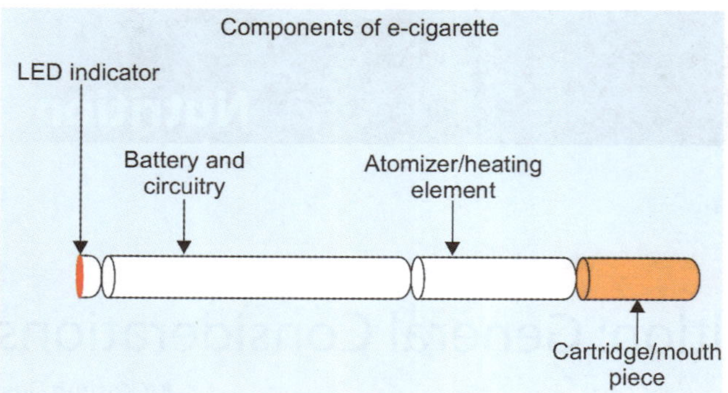

Fig. 26.1: Components of an electronic cigarette

element (atomizer) vaporizes a liquid mixture of nicotine and flavorings or flavored mixture without nicotine (Fig. 26.1).

The WHO has stated that the efficacy of e-cigarettes as an aid in smoking cessation has not been conclusively demonstrated. WHO strongly advised against ENDS till sufficient evidence accrues to support their utility and safety. A 2011 review found that e-Cigarette may aid in smoking cessation and are likely to be more effective than traditional pharmacotherapy. The tactile experience with the e-cigarette may be useful for improving short-term craving. There has been no study that directly measured the effectiveness of e-cigarettes in smoking cessation.

ENDS appears to deliver less nicotine than smoking. It remains to be demonstrated whether electronic systems can effectively substitute for tobacco smoking over long-term. There was no significant difference in smoking cessation rates between e-cigarettes with nicotine, e-cigarettes without nicotine and traditional NRT patches, according to a 2013 randomized controlled trial (RCT). There are some noncontrolled studies that reported possible benefit.

Evidence suggests that ENDS are safer than real cigarettes, possibly as safe as other NRT. There is no regulation of the contents of the different brands of e-cigarettes. Nicotine is a substance with potential for addiction and abuse. Hence, the Centre for Disease Control has issued warnings regarding the use of e-cigarettes.

In India, the use of electronic cigarettes is legal. Under the Indian Health Law of 2006, tobacco smoking has been banned in public. Since e-cigarettes avoid the use of tobacco, they do not fall under this law. However, their sale to minors must not be allowed. American Academy of Pediatrics (AAP), US Food and Drug Administration (USFDA), International Union Against Tuberculosis and Lung Disease (IUATLD), WHO and a number of other bodies are concerned that e-cigarettes might increase use/addiction to nicotine. They may encourage the use of tobacco products in children.

For psychiatric aspects of nicotine-related disorders (Refer to Section 19, Ch 244).

OCCUPATIONAL HEALTH PROBLEMS AMONG TOBACCO WORKERS

In India, tobacco is cultivated mainly in Gujarat and Andhra Pradesh. The varieties of tobacco include Virginia tobacco (cigarette tobacco) and non-Virginia tobacco. Persons may be exposed to tobacco during agricultural operations or curing processes. Ill-effects of tobacco are considered to be due to absorption of nicotine through the skin or respiratory tract. The levels of nicotine and its metabolic product cotinine are increased in urine.

Symptom

Complex occurring in the exposed workers is collectively known as *green symptoms*. These consist of neurological symptoms like headache, giddiness, nausea, vomiting, prostration and respiratory symptoms such as cough and dyspnea. Usually, these symptoms are transient. The occurrence of *these symptoms* is associated with raised urinary levels of nicotine and cotinine. Virginia tobacco is less toxic than the non-Virginia variety. The respiratory symptoms may be aggravated by aeroallergens such as pollen and fungi belonging to the species *Cladosporium* and *Alternaria*.

The nature of contact with tobacco also partly determines the clinical manifestations. Persons who pluck the leaves generally get headache and giddiness, while those carrying the leaves for curing get nausea and vomiting. In agricultural workers engaged in curing, entry of tobacco constituents is through the respiratory tract.

Treatment

The symptoms are usually mild and last only for a few hours. Removal from the surroundings is itself curative. The local practice among the workers is to take tea and jaggery followed by rest.

Points to Remember

- A nonsmoker lives 20–25 years longer than a smoker who starts smoking in his teens.
- It is estimated that 5.5 million deaths occur annually all over the world from tobacco-related diseases.
- ETS is as dangerous as mainstream smoke.
- Nicotine present in tobacco increases sympathetic activity, favors vascular thrombosis and atherogenesis.
- Smoking is a major risk factor for acute bronchitis, emphysema, carcinoma of lungs, larynx, urinary bladder and pulmonary tuberculosis. CAD, stroke and peripheral vascular disease are directly related to tobacco smoking.
- Nicotine replacement products and bupropion are being given as treatment for cessation of smoking.

CHAPTER 27

Nutrition: General Considerations

KV Krishna Das

Chapter Summary

- Assessment of Nutritional Status
- Malnutrition
- Functions of Food
- Standard Nutrition Tables
- Bioactive Phytochemicals in Food
- Prescription of a Balanced Diet

The term 'nutrition' came from the Latin Word 'nutrire' meaning—to suckle, nurse or nourish. In the English language it meant supplying or receiving nourishment. Hippocrates advised 'let your food be medicine and your only medicine be your food'. The close relationship between food, life and health has been amply stressed in the Indian Vedic texts. *Ayurveda* discusses the role of food and specifies elaborated dietary management of several diseases.

It is realized again and again all over the world that the most important single factor for human progress is food that qualitatively and quantitatively appropriate the basis for health in all societies. The Millennium Development Goals (MDGs) have laid stress on the role of health as the foundation for human progress in all fronts. The science of nutrition has gained great importance in the past decades. Food has become a medicine linked to a concept of beauty, harmony and equilibrium.

'*Aapo vai bheshajam. Annam vai bheshajam*'. These are two of quoted references in all vedas—meaning 'are not water and food medicines'?

MODERN CONCEPTS IN NUTRITIONAL SCIENCE

Nutritional science has been defined as the science of food and other substances, their use, actions, interactions and balance in relation to health and disease—the process by which the organism ingests, digests, absorbs, transports and utilizes nutrients and disposes their end products. A simpler definition will be 'the area of knowledge regarding the role of food (dietary inputs) in the maintenance of health'.

The essential requisites (dimensions) of health should include the following:

- Achieving optimal growth and development reflecting full expression of the genetic potential
- Maintenance of the structural integrity and functional efficiency of body tissues necessary for an active and productive life

- Mental wellbeing
- Ability to withstand the inevitable process of aging with minimal disability and functional impairment
- Ability to combat diseases such as:
  - Resisting infections
  - Retarding the progress of degenerative diseases and cancer
  - Resisting the effects of environmental toxins and cancers.

This newer concepts of nutritional science has come out as a result of the progress made in the studies of immunology, molecular biology, oncology, geriatrics, phytochemistry and similar others.

ASSESSMENT OF NUTRITIONAL STATUS

Nutrition of communities can be assessed by large surveys. These surveys are of epidemiological importance. The methods employed to assess the nutritional status in communities are listed below:

- Studies on food production or total food availability in relation to total food needs.
- Measurement of food and nutrition intake.
- Studies on dietary habits and practices.
- Special studies on food to assess biological values and prevalence of interfering substances like toxins and goitrogens.
- Studies based on socio-cultural parameters.
- Vital statistics like morbidity and mortality rates.
- Studies on health conditions indirectly related to the nutritional status of the population such as infections and parasitic diseases.

Nutrition in individuals can be assessed by clinical examination, anthropometric measurements, biochemical and other laboratory tests.

Clinical assessment forms an important part of all nutrition surveys (Table 27.1).

Anthropometry: It involves measure-ment of growth and physical development, is particularly useful in children. The most commonly employed measurements are: (i) Height (ht-linear growth), (ii) weight (wt-body mass), (iii) head circumference (HC-possible relationship to mental development), (iv) mid-arm circumference (MA-variations being mainly due to changes in muscle mass and fat calories), (v) chest circumference and (vi) skin fold thickness (fat calories). The measurements are related to expected standards for age. When the exact age of the

Table 27.1: Prominent clinical features in undernutrition

General signs	Apathy, loss of weight and recent emaciation, dependent edema, delayed milestones in children and delay in secondary sexual characters in adolescents and adults
Hair	Lack of lustre, sparseness or thinness, straightness, dyspigmentation, easy pluckability
Face	Diffuse pigmentation, nasolabial dyssebacia, moon face
Eyes	Pale conjunctiva, Bitot's spots, conjunctival xerosis, corneal xerosis, keratomalacia and angular palpebritis
Lips	Angular stomatitis and cheilosis
Teeth	Mottled enamel
Gums	Spongy and bleeding gums
Skin	Xerosis, follicular hyperkeratosis, pellagrous dermatitis, flaky paint dermatosis, scrotal and vulval dermatosis
Nails	Koilonychia
Muscular and skeletal	Muscle wasting, craniotabes, frontal and parietal-bossing, epiphyseal enlargement, beading of ribs, persistently open anterior fontanelle, knock-knees, bow-legs poor development of muscles
Systemic signs	Hepatomegaly, alteration in mental functions, peripheral neuropathy myelopathy, cardiac changes, reduction in immunity predisposition to infections especially tuberculosis

child is not known, age-independent indices are made use of. These are wt/ht, wt/ht², wt/HC, MA/HC, etc. The Indian Council of Medical Research (ICMR) has laid down norms for the Indian subjects.

The traditional gold standard to estimate the fat content in the body has been hydrodensitometry (underwater weighing)—which is not practicable universally. Fat is less dense than muscle and bone. Dual energy X-ray absorptiometry (DEXA) is now replacing densitometry on account of its precision and availability. Other methods used to assess body fatness are the circumference of the waist and the hip and their ratio, the body mass index (BMI), also known as quetelet index which is the weight in kilograms divided by the square of the height in meters. The BMI has gained popularity on account of its reliability, relationship with morbidity and mortality and ease of performance. BMI above 25 suggests fatness, values below 20 suggests underweight.

Laboratory examination: At present, sensitive methods are available for the accurate determination of vitamins and trace elements in body fluids and tissues, but these are expensive and cannot be employed universally. Moreover, the values of nutrients in blood and tissues show a wide range of levels in normal individuals. No test is specific for a particular kind of malnutrition. Conditions of collection, storage and technique of estimation can all introduce variations. Table 27.2 lists the main tests employed.

MALNUTRITION

Malnutrition results because of deviations from normal nutrition. Frank clinical signs and definite biochemical abnormalities occur in gross malnutrition, but only borderline changes occur in the majority of cases.

Malnutrition may be primary when it is caused by defective intake and secondary when it results from other disease processes. In clinical practice one seldom comes across isolated deficiencies. More often the malnutrition is generalized, but one or other nutrient deficiency predominates.

Malnutrition results basically from inadequate or improper food consumption. The abnormality may be quantitative, qualitative or both. In addition to poverty which is the main cause—social, cultural, agricultural and educational factors modify the form and extent of malnutrition. Diarrhea, helminthic infestations and other infections aggravate malnutrition resulting in high mortality and morbidity.

Table 27.2: Biochemical investigations in malnutrition

Nutrient deficiency	Tests
Proteins	Serum protein fractions, especially albumin, amino acid imbalance, hydroxyproline excretion. Urinary urea, urinary creatinine excretion/unit time
Vitamin A	Serum vitamin A, serum carotene
Vitamin D	Serum alkaline phosphatase (in young children), calcium, phosphorus, serum vitamin D metabolites (1, 2, 5 cholecalciferol)
Ascorbic acid	Serum ascorbic acid, leukocyte ascorbic acid, urinary ascorbic acid-load test
Thiamine	Urinary thiamine, blood pyruvate-lactate, red blood cell (RBC) transketolase load test
Riboflavin	Urinary riboflavin, erythrocyte riboflavin loading test
Niacin	Urinary N-methylnicotinamide load test
Folic acid	Hemoglobin, serum folate, RBC folate—'Figlu' test
Vitamin B$_{12}$	Hemoglobin, serum B$_{12}$, Schilling's test
Iodine	Urinary iodine tests for thyroid function, thyroid hormones, thyrotropin
Minerals	Calcium: serum calcium, bone calcium, calcium turnover studies, serum alkaline phosphatase. Iron: serum iron, iron binding capacity, tissue iron, serum ferritin
Trace elements	Analysis of hair

Note: Recently the importance of chemical analysis of the hair in determining levels of trace elements has been recognized. The advantages are (1) it reflects the variation in the level of trace element over a long period and (2) hair is easy to be preserved and transported. Trace elements are concentrated in the hair.

Textbook of Medicine

Social aspects of nutrition: In addition to the nutritive values of diet, food is a part of security, social behavior and civilization. Occurrence of malnutrition in an individual is only an index of the same disorder in the household and the community as well. So identification of an index patient should be the starting point for further case detection and the treatment should cover the entire community.

Etiological Factors

- Inadequate supply of food due to poverty
- Ignorance of dietary principles
- Wrong practices of cooking and storage of food
- Malabsorption of nutrients
- Parasitism
- Loss of nutrients through urine, stool, bleeding, etc.
- Increased demands due to pregnancy, intercurrent illness or repeated deliveries
- Interference with metabolism
- Other environmental factors like general insanitation, intercurrent illness, overcrowding, rapid population growth and political instability and urbanization which is becoming a universal phenomenon.

Nutritional disorders often present as multiple deficiencies and rarely as isolated entities. The most pronounced deficiency manifests clinically, the others remain subclinical. In such cases, supplementation of the missing nutrient without overall dietary correction leads to temporary improvement, but sooner or later another malnutrition becomes evident. Irrespective of the type of nutritional disorder, overall dietary correction is mandatory. The presenting symptoms should be treated with additional supplementation of the deficient factor.

Care should be taken to prescribe a proper diet suitable to the patient's cultural and economic state and providing articles that are cheaply and freely available in the locality. Prescription of a diet unsuitable to the sociocultural background of the patient is the most common cause for non-compliance.

In healthy state, many nutrients are stored in the body and therefore, dietary deprivation initially leads to depletion of the stores. This period may be asymptomatic or only mild symptoms may manifest, e.g. pica and cognitive impairment in iron deficiency and aches and pains in vitamin D deficiency. Symptoms occur only when the deficiency is far advanced. Hence, it is essential to continue nutrient therapy for at least 4–6 months after full correction of the clinical condition to replenish the stores. Natural food are more palatable, but they are slow in action and several factors influence their absorption and utilization. Therefore, therapeutic preparations are employed for immediate correction and thereafter dietary measures are continued. It is absolutely essential to detect the primary cause in each case otherwise many underlying serious diseases like cirrhosis of liver or malignancy may be missed, till the condition becomes advanced beyond treatment. All cases of secondary malnutrition should be fully investigated to detect the primary cause.

FUNCTION OF FOOD

Living organisms cannot create energy but can only transform energy. The food provides calories for energy needs, proteins to build and maintain the body tissues and vitamins and minerals to regulate the biochemical processes essential to maintain health and offer resistance against disease.

Carbohydrates, fats and proteins together are called the proximate principles. These substances share the common property of chemical degradation with the release of utilizable energy. Under normal dietary conditions. However, the contribution of proteins to energy supply is minor. The unit of energy used at present in nutrition is the joule, though till recently the unit was kilocalorie (kcal).

$$1 \text{ kcal} = 4.184 \text{ kJ}.$$

Basal metabolic needs for an adult male doing minimal physical activity is 2000 kcals $\equiv$ 8372 kJ.

Energy value of the proximate principles: The value of energy yielded by carbohydrates, proteins and fats are approximately 4.0 and 9.0 kcals respectively.

Carbohydrates

Carbohydrates are the main sources of energy. They are not indispensable, if other sources of energy are available, but in most parts of the globe carbohydrates are the most easily available and cheapest food sources.

Carbohydrates account for 45% of total energy in the western diets and over 80% in the diets of many communities in India. In India, most of the carbohydrates were in the form of unprocessed starch, along with dietary fibers, whereas in the West the starch have been progressively replaced by sugars. Even in India, over the past few decades processing industries are introducing more and more refined palatable and easy to cook products (flour vermicelli, noodles, pasta and others) increasing the glycemic index of the food articles and reducing the fiber content.

Glycemic index of carbohydrate relates to its rate of absorption and elevation of postprandial blood glucose levels. High-glycemic-index foods are characterized by rapid absorption, attainment of high postprandial blood-glucose level and insulin response. They are particularly harmful if given to diabetic patients.

Fats

Dietary fats are composed of triglycerides, phospholipids and sterols. Triglycerides which supply energy are made up of fatty acids and glycerol. Most of the fatty acids occurring in nature are carbon atom fatty acids.

Functions of Fat

- Source of energy
- Body building
- Vehicle for fat soluble vitamins A, D, E and K
- Source of antioxidants, e.g. carotene, tocopherols
- Addition to taste and acceptability of food.

Fatty acids are classified as saturated and unsaturated according to the presence and number of double bonds. Saturated fatty acids have no double bonds, e.g. myristic acid (14C), palmitic acid (16C) and stearic acid (18C). Unsaturated fatty acids may contain one or more double bonds. Oleic acid contains one double bond. Polyunsaturated fatty acids (PUFAs) contain two or more double bonds. They can be further divided into Omega

6 and Omega 3 families according to the position of the omega terminal double bond. Out of these, linoleic acid (10C-2), linolenic acid (18C-3) and arachidonic acid (20C-4) are named essential fatty acids (EFAs), since they have to be supplied at least in small quantities in the diet. The EFAs are the precursors of the prostaglandins and they are required for formation of cell membranes and phospholipids. Vanaspathies and margarines are prepared by hydrogenating oils with high content of PUFAs. In this process they are converted into saturated fatty acids.

In India, the poor section of the population derive only 10% of their energy needs from fats whereas up to 35% of the energy requirement should be provided by fats in the diets of the affluent groups. Visible fat comprises the oils and fats used for cooking, whereas invisible fat consists of lipids incorporated in articles of food such as cereals, spices, nuts, oil-seeds, coconut, vegetables and others. The invisible fat accounts for up to 10% of the total energy needs in all groups. ICMR has recommended the addition of visible fat at 5% of energy needs for adults and children, 12.5% for pregnant women and 17.5% for lactating women.

Consumption of fats has increased in affluent countries, since fats increase the taste and acceptability of food.

Vegetable oils with the exception of coconut oil and palm oil provide adequate amounts of PUFAs. Vegetable oils are devoid of cholesterol. Animal fat except fish liver oil are generally saturated, with very little of PUFAs. They contain varying quantities of saturated fats and cholesterol, e.g. butter, *ghee*, lard, meat and others. Fish liver oil contains good amount of PUFAs, eicosapentaenoic acid and docosahexaenoic acid (DHA) which lower very low density lipoprotein (VLDL) in plasma.

Functions Attributed to EFAs

- For cell membrane mechanisms and messenger actions.
- Immune response: PUFAs have antibacterial, antiviral and antifungal properties. They indirectly modulate T-cell response.
- Possibly anticancer activity.
- Inhibits the development of atherosclerosis.
- For normal brain development and neurological functions in the fetus and newborn.

Several beneficial effects of EFAs are being recognized and they have attained a place in modern therapeutics.

Increase in the total quantity of saturated fats in the diet above 25% of energy needs elevate serum cholesterol levels and also adversely affect the high-density lipoprotein (HDL)/low-density lipoprotein (LDL) ratio. Ideally at least 3% of the dietary fat should be polyunsaturated. Apart from the total quantity, the quality of the fat also plays a important role. Hydrogenation of vegetable oils convert the unsaturated fatty acids into saturated trans-fatty acids. Trans-fatty acids elevate LDL and reduce HDL, thereby promoting atherogenesis in arteries and increasing the risk of coronary and cerebral vascular occlusions.

By a regular process of dietary education in the community and the provision of health foods, most of the developed nations have brought down their per-capita consumption of dietary fat. The population has been rendered diet conscious. Even items of confectionary such as chocolates and ice-creams are made to contain less fat. Such measures have served to bring down the incidence of coronary artery disease and myocardial infarction. Attempts in this direction are on the way in India and a sizeable proportion of the population has been sensitized to healthy dietary practices. An increased dietary intake of n-3 PUFA is found to be of benefit in preventing atherosclerosis and arterial thrombosis. In man the minimum requirement of n-6 and n-3 fatty acids for cardiovascular protection is 1% and 0.2% of daily energy intake. Daily requirement of eicosapentaenoic acid is 0.25 g and DHA is 2.0 g. Marine animals and fish oils are rich sources of eicosapentaenoic acid and DHA.

Proteins

Proteins, together with water, form the basic building units of tissues. In addition, they function as enzymes and hormones and also take part in transport mechanisms. Of the twenty amino acids present in proteins, eight have to be supplied to a man through dietary sources almost continually. For adults the essential amino acids are lysine, methionine, valine, leucine, isoleucine, tryptophan, phenylalanine and threonine. For infants histidine is also essential. Animal protein is rich in essential amino acids, whereas vegetable proteins are deficient in one or more of them.

An ideal protein is one which contains all essential amino acids in optimal amount and is completely digestible and utilizable. For the human infant, mother's milk fulfils these requirements. Whole egg proteins are considered the next best and this is given a rating of 100 arbitrarily. Other proteins are compared with whole egg protein. Biological value (BV) and net protein utilization (NPU) are most popular indices used for comparison (Box 27.1). In addition, chemical method, i.e. chemical score (CS), is also widely employed to assess dietary protein quality.

Vegetable proteins have lower quality ratings than animal proteins. In the ordinary Indian diet, cereals, pulses and other vegetable sources also contribute proteins. The biological efficiency of such a mixed protein source is far higher than the average to be expected. The enhancement

Box 27.1: BV, NPU and chemical score of proteins			
Food	*BV*	*NPU*	*Chemical score*
Whole egg	96	91	100
Cow's milk	84	75	66
Liver	77	65	66
Meat	80	76	70
Fish	85	72	60
Rice	64	57	60
Wheat	58	47	42
Bengal gram	56	45	42
Groundnut	54	45	44
Coconut	67	56	52

Abbreviations: BV = Biological value; NPU = Net protein utilization

in protein quality resulting from a mixture of vegetable sources is known as the supplementary value of proteins.

Protein deficiency in the later part of fetal life and early childhood will lead to structural and functional derangements in the development of neural structures in the brain. This may lead to permanent impairment of cognitive and other higher functions. ***The most vulnerable period when qualitative and quantitative dietary deficiency leads to permanent or long-lasting damage are the first thousand days of the baby's life.*** The importance of the adequacy of protein supply to pregnant and lactating women cannot be overemphasized. Acute or even chronic episodes of malnutrition occurring in later life can be almost fully compensated by eliminating the primary cause and refeeding practices.

Protein deficiency leads to T-cell dysfunction and immunological deficiency. Malnutrition related diabetes mellitus (MRDM) has been attributed mainly to protein malnutrition. Normocytic anemia may occur rarely as a result of protein deficiency.

Well-balanced traditional Indian diets are quite adequate to supply the protein requirements. An important reason for protein deficiency in a sizeable proportion of the population in India is the availability of foods in amounts far too short to supply energy needs.

STANDARD NUTRITION TABLES

The ICMR has prescribed standard dietary allowances for the Indian people at different stages of life (Tables 27.3 to 27.6). Tables 27.7 and 27.8 lists the recommended dietary allowance (RDA) for energy, protein, fat, minerals and vitamins.

Table 27.9 gives the standard height and weight for Indian subjects.

BIOACTIVE PHYTOCHEMICALS IN FOOD

In addition to the proximate principles, several articles of food contains substances which alter cellular metabolism and thereby promote health and wellbeing, e.g. beta carotene, ascorbic acid, tocopherols and selenium. In addition to their primary nutritional roles, they help to promote health and prevent disease process. Nearly twenty such substances have been identified belonging to different classes.

- Phenolic compounds—indoles
- Flavonoids—anthocyanins
- Isoflavonoids—isothiocyanates
- Coumarins—diterpenes
- Lignans.

Food items such as cabbage, cauliflower, carrots, tomatoes, chillies, onions, garlic, citrus fruits, *amla*, guava, green leafy vegetables, ginger, cloves, sesame, tea, sunflower oil and palm oil contain them. Bioactive phytochemicals act as antioxidants, detoxifying agents and anticancer agents.

Substances such as carotenoids, ascorbic acid and tocopherols present in green leafy vegetables, fruits, palm oil and others act as antioxidants.

Normal cellular metabolic processes involve reactions requiring pro-oxidants and antioxidants. The former promote the release of O_2 for energy and cellular metabolism. The latter neutralize deleterious oxidants and free radicals generated during normal metabolism and environmental stresses such as smoke, carcinogenic chemicals, industrial effluents and food additives. Free radicals promote peroxidation of membrane lipids. They impair cellular function and damage cellular proteins and deoxyribonucleic acid (DNA). Peroxidation of circulating lipoproteins convert them into more harmful substances. Cumulative tissue injury caused by free radicals lead to aging, atherosclerosis, cancer and so on.

Toxic molecules are detoxified and converted into excretable forms by microsomal oxidase and conjugase enzymes, e.g. indole derivative present in various foods such as cabbage, tomatoes, strawberries, pineapple, green peppers and tea. Garlic can inactivate carcinogens present in food. The various dimensions played by food in addition to the nutritive value have led to the concept of ***total health value of food***. The present day recommendation is to consume 800–1150 g of fresh vegetables and fruits daily. This helps to reduce the incidence of ischemic heart disease, strokes and cancers.

The term 'functional foods' is coined by food processors, in order to promote their sales. Functional foods are those which exert beneficial effects beyond their nutritional effects on specific body functions which promote health and wellbeing and prevent disease. Some of the common examples include bran which relieves

Table 27.3: Balanced diet for pre-school children (2–6 years)				
	2–3 years		**4–6 years**	
Food item (g/day)	**Vegetarian**	**Non-vegetarian**	**Vegetarian**	**Non-vegetarian**
Cereals	150	150	200	200
Pulses	50	40	60	50
Green leafy vegetables	50	50	75	75
Other vegetables including roots and tubers	30	30	50	50
Fruits	50	50	50	50
Milk	300	200	250	200
Fats and oils	20	20	25	25
Meat, fish, eggs	—	30	—	30
Sugar or jaggery	30	30	40	40

Table 27.4: Balanced diet for school children (7–12 years)

Food item (g/day)	7–9 years		10–12 years	
	Vegetarian	Non-vegetarian	Vegetarian	Non-vegetarian
Cereals	250	250	320	320
Pulses	70	60	70	60
Green leafy vegetables	75	75	100	100
Other vegetables including roots and tubers	50	50	75	75
Fruits	50	50	50	50
Milk	250	200	250	200
Fats and oils	30	30	35	35
Meat, fish, eggs	–	30	–	30
Sugar or jaggery	50	50	50	50

Table 27.5: Balanced diet for adolescent boys and girls

Food item (g/day)	Boys 13–15 years		Boys 16–18 years		Girls 13–18 years	
	Vegetarian	Non-vegetarian	Vegetarian	Non-vegetarian	Vegetarian	Non-vegetarian
Cereals	430	430	450	450	350	350
Pulses	70	50	70	50	70	50
Green leafy vegetables	100	100	100	100	150	150
Other vegetables	75	75	75	75	75	75
Roots and tubers	75	75	100	100	75	75
Fruits	30	30	30	30	30	30
Milk	250	150	250	150	250	150
Fats and oils	30	40	45	50	35	40
Meat and fish	—	30	—	30	—	30
Eggs	—	30	—	30	—	30
Sugar and jaggery	30	30	40	40	30	30
Groundnuts	—-	—	50*	50*	—	—

* An additional 30 g fats and oils can be added in place of groundnuts.

Table 27. 6: Balanced diets for adult men and women (figures in brackets give the requirement for women)

Food item (g/day)	Sedentary work		Moderate work		Heavy work	
	Vegetarian	Non-vegetarian	Vegetarian	Non-vegetarian	Vegetarian	Non-vegetarian
Cereals	400 (300)	400 (300)	475 (350)	475 (350)	650 (475)	650 (475)
Pulses	70 (60)	55 (45)	80 (70)	65 (55)	80 (70)	65 (55)
Green leafy vegetables	100 (125)	100 (125)	125 (125)	125 (125)	125 (125)	125 (125)
Other vegetables	75 (75)	75 (75)	75 (75)	75 (75)	100 (100)	100 (100)
Roots and tubers	75 (50)	75 (50)	100 (75)	100 (75)	100 (100)	100 (100)
Fruits	30 (30)	30 (30)	30 (30)	30 (30)	30 (30)	30 (30)
Milk	200 (200)	100 (100)	200 (200)	200 (100)	200 (200)	100 (100)
Fats and oils	35 (35)	40 (35)	40 (35)	40 (40)	50 (40)	50 (45)
Meat and fish	—	30 (30)	—	30 (30)	—	30 (30)
Eggs	—	30	—	30	—	30

Contd...

Contd...

Food item (g/day)	Sedentary work		Moderate work		Heavy work	
	Vegetarian	Non-vegetarian	Vegetarian	Non-vegetarian	Vegetarian	Non-vegetarian
Sugar or Jaggery	30 (30)	30 (30)	40 (30)	40 (30)	55 (40)	55 (40)
Groundnut	—	— (40)	—	—	50* (40)	50*

* An additional 30 g of fats and oils can be added in place of groundnut.

Note: During pregnancy and lactation an allowance of 50–100 g cereals, 10 g pulses, 25 g leafy vegetables, 125 mL milk, 15 g fats and 10–20 g sugar is to be added.

Table 27.7: Recommended dietary allowance (RDA) for energy, protein, fat and minerals for Indians (2010) (ICMR) recommendations

Group	Particulars	Body weight (kg)	Net energy (kcal/day)	Protein (g/day)	Fat (g/day)	Calcium (mg/day)	Iron (mg/day)	Zinc (mg/day)	Magnesium (mg/day)
Men	Sedentary work	60	2320	60	25	600	17	12	340
	Moderate work		2730		30				
	Heavy work		3490		40				
Women	Sedentary work	55	1900	55	25	600	21	10	310
	Moderate work		2230		30				
	Heavy work		2850		30				
	Pregnant woman		+ 350	78	30	1200	35	12	
	Lactating woman								
	0–6 months		+ 600	74	30	1200	21	–	
	7–12 months		+ 520	68	30			–	
Infants	0–6 months	5.4	92/kg	1.16/kg	–	500	46 µg/kg/day	–	30
	6–12 months	8.4	80/kg	1.69/kg	19		05	–	45
Children	1–3 years	12.9	1060	16.7	27	600	09	5	50
	4–6 years	18.0	1350	20.1	25		13	7	70
	7–9 years	25.1	1690	29.5	30		16	8	100
Boys	10–12 years	34.3	2190	39.9	35	800	21	9	120
	13–15 years	47.6	2750	54.3	45	800	32	11	165
	16–17 years	55.4	3020	61.5	50	800	28	12	195
Girls	10–12 years	35.0	2010	40.4	35	800	27	9	160
	13–15 years	46.6	2330	51.9	40	800	27	11	210
	16–17 years	52.1	2440	55.5	35	800	26	12	235

Abbreviation: ICMR = Indian Council of Medical Research

Table 27.8: Recommended dietary allowance for vitamins for Indians

Group	Particulars	Body weight (kg)	Vitamin A (µg/day) retinol	β-carotene	Thiamin (mg/day)	Riboflavin (mg/day)	Niacin equivalents (mg/day)	Vitamin B$_6$ (mg/day)	Dietory folate (µg/day)	Ascorbic acid (mg/day)	Vitamin B$_{12}$ (µg/day)
Men	Sedentary work	60	600	4800	1.2	1.4	16	2.0	200	40	1.0
	Moderate work				1.4	1.6	18				
	Heavy work				1.7	2.1	21				
Women	Sedentary work	55	600	4800	1.0	1.1	12	2.0	200	40	1.0
	Moderate work				1.1	1.3	14				
	Heavy work				1.4	1.7	16				
	Pregnant woman		800	6400	+ 0.2	+ 0.3	+ 2	2.5	500	60	1.2
	Lactating woman		950	7600							
	0–6 months				+ 0.3	+ 0.4	+ 4	2.5	300	80	1.5
	7–12 months				+ 0.2	+ 0.3	+ 3	2.5			

Contd...

Group	Particulars	Body weight (kg)	Vitamin A (µg/day) retinol	β-carotene	Thiamin (mg/day)	Riboflavin (mg/day)	Niacin equivalents (mg/day)	Vitamin B_6 (mg/day)	Dietory folate (µg/day)	Ascorbic acid (mg/day)	Vitamin B_{12} (µg/day)
Infants	0–6 months	5.4	350	–	0.2	0.3	710 µg/kg/day	0.1	25	25	0.2
	6–12 months	8.4		2800	0.3	0.4	650 µg/kg/day	0.4			
Children	1–3 years	12.9	400	3200	0.5	0.6	8	0.9	80	40	0.2–1.0
	4–6 years	18			0.7	0.8	11	0.9	100		
	7–9 years	25.1	600	4800	0.8	1.0	13	1.6	120		
Boys	10–12 years	34.3	600	4800	1.1	1.3	15	1.6	140	40	0.2–1.0
	13–15 years	47.6			1.4	1.6	16	2.0	150		
	16–17 years	55.4			1.5	1.8	17	2.0	200		
Girls	10–12 years	35.0			1.0	1.2	13	1.6	140	40	0.2–1.0
	13–15 years	46.6			1.2	1.4	14	2.0	150		
	16–17 years	52.1			1.0	1.2	14	2.0	200		

Source: Nutrient requirements and recommended dietary allowances for Indians. A Report of the Expert group of the Indian Council of Medical Research, 2010

Table 27.9: Weight and height chart for males and females

Height (cm)		Normal weight (kg)		Overweight limit (+ 20%)		Underweight limit (– 20%)	
Males	**Females**	**Males**	**Females**	**Males**	**Females**	**Males**	**Females**
148	148	47.5	46.5	57.0	56.0	38.0	37.0
152	152	49.5	48.5	59.0	58.0	39.0	39.0
156	156	51.5	50.5	62.0	60.5	41.0	40.5
160	160	53.5	52.5	64.0	63.0	43.0	42.0
164	164	56.0	55.0	67.0	66.0	45.0	44.0
168	168	59.0	58.0	71.0	69.6	47.0	46.5
172	172	62.0	60.5	74.5	72.5	49.5	48.5
176	176	65.5	64.0	78.5	77.0	52.4	51.0
180	180	68.5	67.0	82.0	80.5	55.0	53.5
184	184	72.0	70.5	86.5	84.5	57.5	56.5
188	188	75.5	74.0	90.5	89.0	60.5	59.0
190		77.5		93.0		62.0	

constipation and low sodium high potassium foods which lower blood pressure.

Immunological competence and nutritional status are two of the most important determinants of morbidity and mortality. Malnutrition, immunodeficiency and infection create a vicious cycle in which each factor contributes to the adverse outcome. Primary immunodeficiency may also lead to secondary nutritional disorders.

Prescription of a Balanced Diet

Energy requirements are determined by: (1) Physical activity, (2) body size and composition, (3) age and sex, (4) physiological state and (5) climate and environment. Generally, the energy requirement of people living in tropical countries is lower than those in the colder climates.

Pregnancy, lactation and repeated infections and infestations are widely prevalent in India increases the need for protein. Since, the nutritive value for proteins varies widely, it is convenient to express the requirements of protein in terms of a reference protein with an assumed net protein utilization (NPU) of 100, which is fully digested and utilized. The reference protein can be converted into proteins of customary diets using the formula:

$$\frac{\text{Reference protein requirement}}{\text{NPU of dietary protein}} \times 100$$

The NPU of Indian diets is approximately 65.

KV Krishna Das, KE Elizabeth

CHAPTER
28

Starvation

Textbook of Medicine

Chapter Summary

- General Considerations
- Clinical Features
- Treatment
- Nutritional Support under Special Circumstances

GENERAL CONSIDERATIONS

Severe starvation on a mass scale occurs during special situations like prolonged war, drought and other natural or political calamities. Chronic starvation of different grades affects large number of people in the developing countries, even during normal times. Several famines have occurred during the 19th and early part of the 20th centuries. Famines were regular occurrence in many parts of the World and India in those days. Though acute and chronic food shortage occurred time to time in some parts of India as a result of floods, drought or earthquakes, widespread famine has not occurred in the latter part of this century. In addition to food shortage, inability to ingest or digest and absorb food also results in starvation. Individuals may resort to starvation voluntarily or this may result from psychiatric abnormalities.

Loss of weight amounting even up to 50% of bw is the most prominent feature. The weight loss is initially caused by the loss of fluid. Later on it is owing to catabolism of tissues to meet energy needs. The body stores of carbohydrate (liver and muscle glycogen) are depleted within two to three days and fat is mobilized in the form of free fatty acids which is used as fuel by the muscles. Glucose is spared for the brain. Tissue proteins are also broken down in order to meet the energy needs.

Protein synthesis is diminished and alanine is released by the muscles to the liver for conversion to glucose, which is made available to the brain. During prolonged starvation, brain metabolism can adapt to use β-hydroxybutyrate and acetoacetate also as fuel. Generalized emaciation results over a period of time. Liver and intestines are the first to loose tissue and this is followed by muscles and skin. The brain is preserved right till the end.

CLINICAL FEATURES

In starvation, the patient is apathetic and irritable. The loss of fat around the buttocks, thighs, back and buccal region gives the characteristic appearance with prominence of bones and dry, thin, inelastic, loose skin. A brownish, patchy pigmentation is generally encountered. The hair becomes characteristically dry and easily pluckable. During cold weather cyanosis of extremities may develop. *Systemic disturbances:* Cardiovascular changes include bradycardia, lowered systolic and diastolic pressure and reduction in venous pressure and cardiac output. The heart size is also reduced. Respiratory rate is lowered, so also the vital capacity. Growth hormone level is decreased. Basal metabolism is lowered. Corticosteroid is normal. In both sexes, sexual function is diminished leading to loss of libido in males and amenorrhea in females. Hypothermia may develop on exposure to cold. Though personality changes may manifest, the intellect usually remains clear till the end. Capacity for work is reduced due to loss of muscle mass. Mild normocytic normochromic anemia is not uncommon.

In some individuals, dependent edema appears even without lowering of plasma albumin. Nocturnal polyuria is common though the renal function is not grossly affected.

TREATMENT

The course of treatment should depend upon the severity of the disorder. Mild cases of starvation require only oral feeds. Overzealous dietary supplementation may lead to diarrhea and death. In the early stages, gradual introduction of easily absorbable and predigested food may be necessary till the alimentary functions return to normal. Fats and fatty foods have to be avoided to prevent diarrhea. Skimmed milk is superior to whole milk. Skimmed milk powder reconstituted to give 10–15% strength is well tolerated if given as small feeds (up to 100 mL) frequently. A daily intake of about 3,000 kcal and 100 g proteins should be aimed at. Severely debilitated patients should be fed using an intragastric tube in order to ensure adequate intake. After the initial rapid gain in weight due to correction of dehydration, a steady increase of 1–1.5 kg/week can be considered as adequate response.

In all cases of severe starvation, especially if complicated by intercurrent illnesses and diarrhea, parenteral nutrition should be resorted to without any delay. If starvation occurs on a wide scale, relief camps have to be organized to provide shelter, food, portable water and general sanitation.

Community kitchens may have to be set up to provide food. In these endeavors, the medical personnel have to work in close liaison with social service organizations and governmental agencies.

NUTRITIONAL SUPPORT UNDER SPECIAL CIRCUMSTANCES

When food cannot be ingested by the oral route, special methods should be resorted to ensure adequate nutrition intake. This includes *enteral* and *parenteral nutrition* methods.

Enteral feeding is providing the nutrients straight into the gastrointestinal tract (GIT) by tubes introduced through the nose, esophagus, stomach, intestines or by artificial stoma. This one is the simpler method out of the two since, it can be instituted with greater ease, cheap, preserves gut integrity, maintains the immunological function of the gut and decreases the likelihood of microbial translocation.

Parenternal nutrition consists of delivering nutrients in the form in which the tissue cells can metabolize them into peripheral or central veins depending upon the quantity to be delivered and the period for which the process has to be maintained. If large volumes have to be maintained and that too for periods exceeding a few days, central venous access has to be resorted to (jugular veins or vena cava).

Parenteral nutrition is more expensive, requires more care for maintaining patency and sterility of the venous line. The materials to be supplied have to be in appropriate forms for the cells to metabolize them. Central line is positioned in the superior vena cava. Strict aseptic precautions have to be maintained.

Indications

- Nonfunctioning GIT
- Functioning small intestine is less than 60 cm in length
- Gastrointestinal fistula
- Acute pancreatitis
- Short bowel syndrome
- Malnutrition with loss of 10–15% of body weight.

The fluid given parenterally should contain carbohydrates, amino acids, fats, fluids, electrolytes, vitamins, trace minerals and adequate fluids. Several commercially available preparations are in common use.

Complication

Unless the physician or the paramedics have experience of instituting parenteral nutrition, it leads to complications. These includes:

- Problems with catheter
- Fluid overload
- Imbalance of the nutrients
- Sepsis at the catheter site.

When severely malnourished patients are given supplementary nutrition vigorously they may develop refeeding syndrome. This is characterized by metabolic disturbances starting 3–4 days after onset of refeeding. Initial features may be non-specific, main features include rhabdomyolysis, leucocyte dysfunction, respiratory and cardiac failure, hypotension, arrhythmias, seizures, coma and sudden death.

Management

- ***Starting slowly:*** Start nutritional supplement at 5–10 kcal/kg/day and work up gradually. Supplement thiamine, multivitamins—trace elements and fluid balance and also treat the underlying causes.
- ***Parenteral nutrition*** is associated with severe life-threatening infections which demands close supervision, early diagnosis and treatment. Therefore, it should be instituted only in institutions where sufficient expertize is available.

CHAPTER
29

Protein-energy Malnutrition

KV Krishna Das, KE Elizabeth

Chapter Summary

- General Considerations
  - Underweight
  - Stunting
  - Wasting
  - Severe Acute Malnutrition
  - General Principles of Routine Care
  - Ready to use Therapeutic Foods (RUTF)
- Weight-length for Boys
- Marasmus
- Kwashiorkor
- Marasmic Kwashiorkor

GENERAL CONSIDERATIONS

Protein-energy malnutrition (PEM) has been defined by World Health Organization (WHO) and Food and Agriculture Organization (FAO) (1973) as a range of pathological conditions arising from coincident lack of protein and calories in varying proportions occurring most frequently in infants and young children and commonly associated with infections.

The changing profile of undernutrition and occurrence of severe acute malnutrition (SAM) and edematous SAM (E-SAM) are of great concern in this electronic era, 20 years after initiating 'Breastfeeding Policy' in 1992 and 10 years after initiating the global strategy for Infant and Young Child Feeding (IYCF) since 2002.

Ever since Prof Cicely Williams described kwashiorkor in 1933, similar cases have been observed in the stereotypic profile of poverty, ignorance and illiteracy or natural calamities like war, famine and other devastating situations. Currently, cases of SAM and E-SAM are noted in settings without the above said risk factors. The common causal factors identified were 'man-made perception' of lactation failure/breast milk withdrawal and early introduction of very dilute milk formula or dilute starch-based liquid diet without any good quality protein like arrow root/banana powder, rice/ragi/oats and other

Textbook of Medicine

locally available foods. Animal milk protein is often totally avoided, being branded as an allergen, especially as per the advice from complementary and alternate medicine. The imbalance in the dietary ratio of protein to energy has been clearly implicated in the pathogenesis of E-SAM.

Malnutrition can be undernutrition, micronutrient malnutrition or overweight and obesity.

TYPES OF UNDERNUTRITION

Underweight (Mild, Moderate and Severe)

When a child does not have expected weight for his age, then a child is categorized as underweight. Underweight is often used as a basic indicator of the status of a population's health, as weight is easy to measure.

Measurement: It is measured by evaluating weight and age. With the help of WHO growth charts children falling in yellow region are moderately underweight (MUW < –2 SD) and who fall under red region are severely underweight (SUW < –3 SD). Those who are < 1 SD are mildly underweight.

Cause: This condition can result from either chronic or acute under nutrition or both.

Consequences: The mortality risks of children who are even moderately underweight are increased and severely underweight children are at even greater risk.

Stunting (Severe Chronic Undernutrition)

When a child does not attain expected height for his age, then the child is known as stunted. It indicates past growth failure. This includes cases of chronic malnutrition, intrauterine growth retardation and also other causes of dwarfing.

Measurement: Length/height is measured along with age. Children who are below 2 years, their length is taken in recumbent position (or children with less than 87 cm) and children above 2 years their height is taken in standing position. With the help of WHO growth charts, children falling in yellow region are moderately stunted (< –2 SD) and who fall under red region are severely stunted (< –3 SD).

Causes: In the setting of malnutrition, this condition can result from failure to receive adequate nutrition over a long period or recurrent infections, sustained inappropriate feeding practices and poverty. It may be worsened by recurrent and chronic illness such as frequent respiratory infections, diarrhea, soil-transmitted helminths, tuberculosis, asthma and others.

Consequence: Stunting results in delayed psychosocial and cognitive development and poor school performance. This in turn affects economic productivity at national level.

Wasting (Mild, Moderate and Severe Acute Malnutrition)

When a child does not attain expected weight for his height, then the child is known as wasted. It indicates current or acute undernutrition.

Measurement: Weight is measured along with a child's length/height and plotted on weight for height charts (Fig. 29.1). Children who are below 2 years, their length is taken in recumbent position (or children with less than 87 cm) and children above 2 years their height is taken in standing position. With the help of WHO growth charts children falling in yellow region are moderately wasted (< –2 SD) and who fall under red region are severely wasted (< –3 SD), which is also known as SAM.

Causes: This condition can result from inadequate food intake, incorrect feeding practices, diarrhea and acute illness (acute respiratory illness, measles and malaria) or more frequently a combination of these factors.

Consequence: It results in child mortality.

Severe Acute Malnutrition (SAM)

- Very low weight-for-height/length (Z-score below –3 SD of the median/< 70% of the expected)
- A mid-upper arm circumference (MUAC) <115 mm, due to visible wasting
- Presence of nutritional bipedal edema.

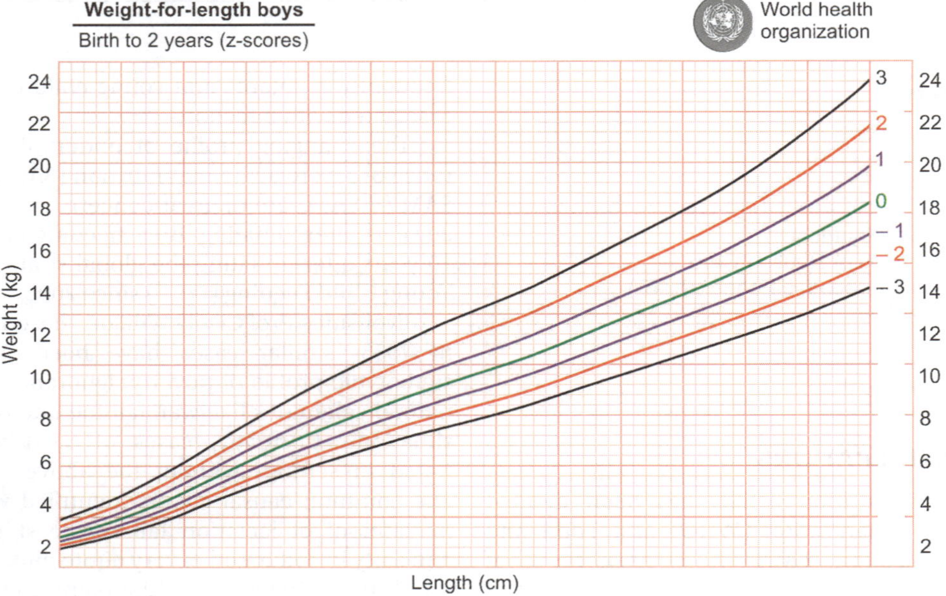

Fig. 29.1: Weight-for-length chart for boys

For infants below 6 months:
- Not gaining weight/feeding problem/too weak to suck
- MUAC < 110 mm as one of the criterion if length < 65 cm.

General Principles of Routine Care for SAM

Admit and manage the 10 steps:

Step 1: Treat/prevent hypoglycemia (< 54 mg/dL)

Step 2: Treat/prevent hypothermia (< 35 axillary/< 35.5 rectal)

Step 3: Treat/prevent dehydration [oral rehydration solution (ReSoMal)/in shock, 15 mL/kg 0.5 N saline with 5% glucose]

Step 4: Correct electrolyte imbalance (include K, Mg)

Step 5: Treat/prevent infection (amoxicillin/injection cefotaxime)

Step 6: Correct micronutrient deficiencies [vitamin A, folic acid (FA), Zn, multivitamin] iron supplementation (start in the 2nd week after stabilization). Severe anemia < 4 g blood/packed red cells (PRC).

Step 7: Start cautious feeding using F-75 supplying 75 kcal/100 mL and 1 g protein and change over to F-100 supplying 100 kcal/100 mL and 3 g protein

Step 8: Achieve catch-up growth using F-100, ready to use therapeutic foods

Step 9: Provide sensory stimulation and emotional support

Step 10: Prepare for follow-up.

Ready to use Therapeutic Foods (RUTF)

Children with SAM need safe, palatable foods with a high energy content and adequate amount of vitamins and minerals. RUTF are soft or crushable foods that can be consumed easily by children from the age of six months without adding water. RUTF have a similar nutrient composition to F-100, which is the therapeutic diet used in hospital settings. But unlike F-100, RUTF are not water-based, meaning that bacteria cannot grow in them. Therefore, these foods can be used safely at home without refrigeration and even in areas where hygienic conditions are not optimal. When there are no medical complications, a malnourished child with appetite, if aged six months or more, can be given a standard dose of RUTF adjusted to his/her weight. Guided by appetite, children may consume the food at home, with minimal supervision, directly from a container, at any time of the day or night. Because RUTF does not contain water, children should also be offered safe drinking water to drink at will. 100 g RUTF supplies 500 kcal and 15 g protein. 20 g RUTF is equivalent to 100 mL F-100. SAT mix 3 parts mixed with 1 part skimmed milk powder and 1 part coconut oil can be used as RUTF.

Children Above 6 Months of Age

- Early initiation of appropriate feeding is an important step in the management of SAM. Therapeutic feeding with F-75 composition can be used as starting formula in the acute phase, 130 mL/kg in SAM and 100 mL/kg in E-SAM and quantity can be scaled by 10 mL/kg.
- In transition phase, the same quantity that the child is accepting is replaced as F-100.
- F-100—volume up to 200 mL/kg and RUTF are given in the rehabilitation phase.
- Weight gain of 10 g/kg/day is ideal. Weight gain < 5 g/kg is non response and > 20 g/kg is overweight/fluid overload.

Infants Less than 6 Months

- ***Prospect of continuing or re-initiating breastfeeding:*** Breastfeeding should be encouraged in children (aged less than 6 months) and having SAM. Supplemental suckling technique (SST) can be used to support and enhance breastfeeding. These children should be monitored by determining weight gain and amount of supplemental feeding taken. The supplemental feeding can be slowly withdrawn as the breast milk output increases and baby shows weight gain. A baby showing consistent weight gain on exclusive breastfeeding can be discharged from the inpatient facility. The baby's growth can then be monitored on outpatient basis.
- These babies should be treated with F-100 diluted to 130 mL/kg in order to supply more fluid and protein in < 6 months-old-babies. But in E-SAM, F-75 is initially started 100 mL/kg.
- FA supplement is given as a single dose given before the baby is 6-month-old.
- Vitamin A is given beyond 2 months only. 50,000 U is given to 2–6 months babies.
- Weight gain 10 g/day is ideal.
- It is necessary to monitor the child and check for failure to respond to therapy. E-SAM cases initially lose weight leading to ***tick sign.*** Failure to respond to therapy should prompt a review of the case, assessment of actual intake and checking for untreated infection and biopsychological problems.
- Continuation of breastfeeding should be encouraged.
- Sensory stimulation in the form of tender loving care, cheerful stimulating environment, structured play therapy, initiation of physical activity as soon as the child is well and maternal involvement in comforting, feeding and play are important aspects of overall management.
- Target weight for discharge—15% of trough weight.
- Target weight for cure > 90% of expected/> 1 SD.

Prevention

- Follow the 10 steps of infant and young child nutrition (IYCN) for 1st 1000 days of life; minus 9 to plus 24 months (270 days *in utero* + 1st 730 days up to the age of 2 years).
- Timely initiation of breastfeeding within 1 hour of birth.
- Exclusive breastfeeding during the first six months of life.
- Timely introduction of complementary foods at six months.
- Age-appropriate foods for children six months to two years.
- Hygienic complementary feeding practices.
- Immunization and bi-annual vitamin A supplementation with deworming.
- Appropriate feeding for children during and after illness.
- Therapeutic feeding for children with SAM.

Table 29.1: Grades of protein-energy malnutrition (PEM)

Grade	Percentage weight to the reference standard (Harvard)
I	71–80%
II	61–70%
III	51–60%
IV	50% and below

Note: 'K' in front of a grade denotes kwashiorkor. Recommendation of the nutrition subcommittee of the Indian Academy of Pediatrics (IAP).

- Adequate nutrition and support for adolescent girls to prevent anemia.
- Adequate nutrition and support for pregnant and breastfeeding mothers.

The 10 essential interventions that can have the undernourished children over the next 10 years.

The clinical spectrum includes a variety of clinical syndromes, with 'marasmus' and 'kwashiorkor' at the two extremes and the intermediate forms (marasmic kwashiorkor) and nutritional dwarfism in between. Mild cases may present only with apathy and retardation of growth. Childhood malnutrition has been graded taking the weight for age as the criteria (Table 29.1).

Etiology and pathogenesis: PEM is an environmental disease, caused by deficient intake of protein and calories. It results from the combined influences of low food availability, poverty, ignorance, illiteracy and cultural taboos, frequent infections and poor environmental sanitation.

CLINICAL FEATURES

Marasmus (Fig. 29.2A)

Severe restriction of food in an infant, as in cases of gross inadequacy of breast milk, leads to arrest of growth. Due to starvation the subcutaneous fat and muscles are used up as energy sources. The baby becomes emaciated. Unlike as in kwashiorkor, there is no edema. Loss of the buccal pads of fat give the infant a withered and old man's look. The weight is below the 60th percentile. The height depends upon the onset and duration of undernutrition. In early stages, the infant eats well but appetite is lost as the condition progresses. Initially, inadequacy of food leads to constipation, but later on diarrhea sets in with green stools containing mucus. In the well-established form, the baby is apathetic. Moderate anemia may develop. The skin and hair are usually normal.

Kwashiorkor (Fig. 29.2B)

This name was coined by Dr Cicely Williams in 1933, to denote 'disease of the child deposed from the breast by the conception of a new fetus'. Children between the ages of 1 and 3 years are affected more. The disease starts when the baby is weaned from the breast.

Pathology: Main changes are seen in the small intestines, liver, pancreas and thymus. Small intestinal mucosa shows blunting of villi and atrophy of brush border, so that the columnar epithelium appears to become cuboidal. The total absorbing surface is reduced. Lactose intolerance is common because of disaccharidase deficiency. Liver

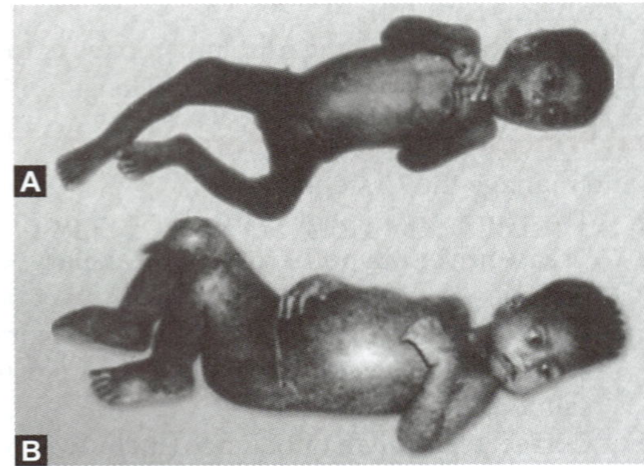

Figs 29.2A and B: **A.** Marasmus; **B.** Kwashiorkor

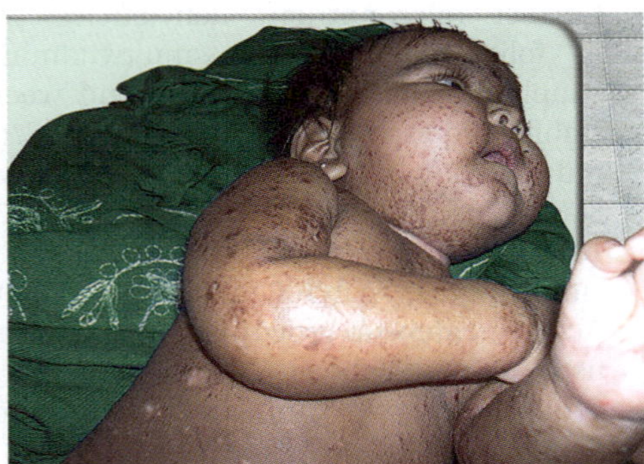

Fig. 29.3: Baby with kwashiorkor
Note: Edema and skin changes

shows fatty infiltration of the parenchymal cells. The pancreatic acini are atrophic and enzyme activity is reduced. Thymus is markedly atrophied and this may contribute to deficiency of cell mediated immunity.

Clinical features (Fig. 29.3): The child is stunted and skeletal muscles are wasted. The presence of fairly normal amounts of subcutaneous fat and edema give a deceptively plump appearance. Pitting edema is a prominent feature. The child is apathetic, irritable and drowsy. Characteristic skin changes occur in many and when present, these are diagnostic. These include flaky paint dermatosis seen over areas of pressure and trauma, fissuring and ulceration at the flexures and a mosaic like appearance (crazy pavement appearance). The hair becomes thin, sparse, brownish and lustreless. They may fall off. Regrowth of normal pigmented hair heralds nutritional recovery. Since, periods of nutritional deprivation and partial correction of nutrition alternate in many cases, the hair shows alternate bands of pigmentation and depigmentation (flag sign). The appetite is poor. Diarrhea is a frequent feature. There may be concomitant deficiencies of iron, folate, fat soluble vitamins and B complex factors. Hepatomegaly occurs in a third of the cases. This is due to fatty infiltration. With recovery the liver reverts to normal without sequelae.

Marasmic Kwashiorkor

In this condition, features of marasmus and kwashiorkor are present simultaneously. The body weight is less than 60% of the normal. Dependent edema is present. Mental changes, skin and hair changes and hepatomegaly are evident.

Secondary infection is very common in PEM. This is due to the fact that both humoral and cellular immunity are defective. The intestinal flora is altered and this may account for the diarrhea. Episodes of infection further jeopardize the nutritional status.

Laboratory investigations: The total protein content of the body is reduced and this is reflected most prominently as hypoalbuminemia. The plasma levels of essential amino acids are low, but the non-essential amino acids remain normal or even elevated. Basal metabolic rate is reduced. Hypoglycemia occurs commonly.

Total body water is increased and all the compartments show increase of fluid. The plasma osmolality is reduced. Renal plasma flow is diminished and this results in impairment of renal function. Plasma sodium is increased with reduction in potassium and magnesium. Gross reduction of serum sodium is associated with a poor prognosis.

Prognosis: Depends on the severity of the disease at diagnosis and promptness of treatment. Marked weight loss, severe infections, fluid and electrolyte imbalance, hypoglycemia, hypothermia, cardiac failure, elevation of serum bilirubin and liver enzymes, drowsiness and xerophthalmia indicate poor prognosis. In severe cases mortality goes up to 20%. The disease is entirely preventable by ensuring adequate caloric and protein intake to the growing child in the first three years of life. Proper management in the established case gives rise to full recovery, catch-up growth and restoration of normal parameters. Recurrence is likely if the adverse environment is not corrected.

Treatment

Treatment is aimed to supply a diet rich in calories, proteins and other essential nutrients. For success of treatment, supplementation should be with natural foods available locally. 150 kcal/kg of energy and 3.3 g/kg of proteins are optimally required to catch-up growth. Fats are administered to supply adequate calories without increasing the bulk. Children with lactose intolerance do not tolerate carbohydrates, but they tolerate fats. As the child gains appetite the frequency of feeding is increased. If there is severe anorexia, forced feeding has to be resorted to. Salt should be restricted to avoid congestive cardiac failure. The National Institute of Nutrition, Hyderabad has formulated an energy-protein rich mixture to treat PEM at home. It consists of whole wheat 40 g, bengalgram 16 g, groundnut 10 g, jaggery 20 g (total 86 g). This supplies 330 calories and 11.3 g proteins. Skimmed milk, eggs and cereals are added as the condition improves. In addition to nutritional correction, intercurrent infections have to be controlled simultaneously.

Initial recovery is heralded by the disappearance of edema. The major biochemical abnormalities are corrected within 2–3 weeks. Complete correction of all reversible changes, referred to as 'clinical recovery' occurs only in 2–3 months.

Prevention and Rehabilitation

PEM is a preventable disease. Three levels of prevention have been formulated. ***Primary prevention*** is achieved by nutrition education to prevent occurrence of PEM. ***Secondary prevention*** is aimed at early detection and proper treatment. ***Tertiary prevention*** consists of nutritional rehabilitation of an established case.

The importance of breastfeeding as a prophylactic against protein calorie malnutrition cannot be overemphasized. Correct feeding practices, both during health and disease, proper sanitation, deworming and family planning methods have to be employed simultaneously to achieve lasting benefit.

Nutrition rehabilitation is employed to prevent residual nutritional handicap and prevent recurrence of protein energy malnutrition. Even at the initial stages of treatment, the mother should be made to participate in the selection, preparation and administration of food. This measure helps to impart nutritional education to her, prevent recurrence and detect relapse early.

CHAPTER
30

Fat-soluble Vitamins

KV Krishna Das

Chapter Summary

- Vitamin A
- Vitamin D
  - Biological Actions of Vitamin D Metabolites
  - Rickets
  - Treatment
  - Osteomalacia
  - Hypervitaminosis D
- Vitamin E
- Vitamin K
- Hemorrhagic Disease of the Newborn
- Anticoagulant Therapy

Vitamins are organic substances which have to be supplied in food in minute quantities to maintain the biochemical and structural integrity of many cells and tissues. The human body cannot synthesize them. Most of them are integral parts of certain co-enzymes required for biochemical reactions at tissue levels.

The vitamins have been classified into fat-soluble and water-soluble groups based on their presence in natural foods. By synthetic processes water-soluble preparations of some of the fat-soluble vitamins have been produced, e.g. vitamin K. The fat-soluble vitamins are A, D, E and K. The water-soluble vitamins are C and B complex group consisting of thiamine, niacin, riboflavin, pyridoxine, biotin, cyanocobalamin, folic acid and pantothenic acid.

VITAMIN A

Syn: Retinol

Vitamin A has a crucial role in normal visual processes and the maintenance of health of epithelial cells. Deficiency of vitamin A is one of the major causes of preventable blindness occurring in many developing countries. This deficiency is widely prevalent in India and about 10% of school children are affected. Its prevalence is higher in the southern states.

- Vitamin A is a fat-soluble vitamin
- Required for vision, repair, reproduction, growth and tissue differentiation.

Two groups of compounds have vitamin A activity:

1. *Retinoids*
   - Vitamin A in the strictest sense, refers to retinol.
   - However, the oxidized metabolites, *retinaldehyde* and *retinoic acid*, are also biologically active compounds.
   - The term retinoids includes all molecules (including synthetic molecules) that are chemically related to retinol.

2. *Carotenoids*
   - There are more than 600 carotenoids in nature and approximately 50 of these can be metabolized to vitamin A.
   - *β-carotene* is the most prevalent carotenoid in the food supply that has provitamin A activity.
   - In humans, significant fractions of carotenoids are absorbed intact and are stored in liver and fat.

Source of intake: Vitamin A is found exclusively in animal foods. Rich sources of animal origin are liver, especially fish, liver, butter, *ghee*, cheese, egg yolk and milk. Vegetable sources contain the precursor for vitamin A, i.e. carotene especially *β-carotene*. Rich sources of carotene include dark green leafy vegetables such as spinach and *amaranth*, yellow vegetables like carrot and pumpkin and fruits like mangoes and papaya. Red palm oil is a very rich source of carotene. In the body carotene is converted into vitamin A. Six parts of carotene are equivalent to one part of vitamin A. Vitamin A is stable at temperatures below 100°C. Vitamin A is stored in the liver as retinyl esters and these stores can last for 6–9 months.

Causes of Vitamin A Deficiency

Primary vitamin A deficiency	Secondary vitamin A deficiency
• Prolonged dietary deprivation	• Sprue
	• Cystic fibrosis
• Vegetarians	• Pancreatic insufficiency
• Refugees	• Duodenal bypass
• Chronic alcoholics	• Chronic diarrhea
• Toddlers	• Bile duct obstruction
• Preschool children	• Giardiasis and cirrhosis

Mechanism of action: Vitamin A aldehyde is present as rhodopsin in the retina. The changes undergone by rhodopsin form the molecular basis of visual excitation. Vitamin A is required for growth, reproduction and maintenance of life. Synthesis of glycoprotein, essential for proper epithelial function, also may be a major function of vitamin A. Vitamin A is essential for proper metabolism and integrity of epithelial cells in many sites. In the absence of vitamin A, the epithelium undergoes squamous metaplasia and the flattened epithelial cells are heaped upon one another. Dryness of the eyes leads to xerophthalmia. Bitot's spots develop as whitish scaly plaques on the sclera and they consist of heaped up metaplastic epithelium. The cornea softens, opacifies, ulcerates and necrosis and this condition is called *keratomalacia*. This leads to blindness.

Even in subclinical vitamin A deficiency the conjunctival epithelium shows changes in 90–95% of cases. The conjunctiva is made up of epithelial and goblet cells. Conjunctival impression cytology using a multipore filter (pore size 0.45/µm) applied to the conjunctiva for 2–3 minutes is diagnostic. On staining this with periodic acid Schiff (PAS), the epithelial abnormality can be made out.

Normal serum vitamin A level is 0.7–2.8 µmol/L (10–20 µg/dL). Vitamin A absorption occurs in the ileum (distal small intestine) where vitamin B_{12} is also absorbed. The body is able to store vitamin A for only a few months whereas vitamin B_{12} stores lasts for several years. Hence, malnutrition of vitamin A manifests early.

Daily requirements	
Man	750 µg
Woman	750 µg
Infants	300–400 µg
Children	400–600 µg
Adolescents	750 µg

A dose of 1 µg of retinol is equivalent to 3 international units of vitamin A and 6 µg of carotenoids. An additional 400 µg should be provided during lactation.

Primary vitamin A deficiency generally results from inadequate intake of the vitamin or the carotenoids in the diet. Deficiency of other nutrients usually coexists. Secondary vitamin A deficiency occurs due to intestinal malabsorption, liver diseases like cirrhosis and enhanced renal excretion.

Clinical features: General symptoms include fatigue, anemia, diarrhea, reduced growth rate, frequent respiratory infection, decreased bone development and in adults, reduced fertility. Earliest symptom is night blindness, followed by degenerative changes in the retina. The bulbar conjunctiva becomes dry and rough grayish triangular-foamy-raised patches appear (Bitot's spots). A solution of 1% Rose Bengal instilled into the eye stains Bitot's spots dark pink and makes them stand out prominently. Both night blindness and xerosis of the conjunctiva readily disappear on administering vitamin

A. When the cornea also becomes dry and lustreless, it is called *xerophthalmia*. More serious complications are keratomalacia involving the cornea with ulceration and necrosis. These changes follow if xerophthalmia is left untreated. Keratomalacia is more common in children aged 1–5 years. It leads to perforation, prolapse of the iris and endophthalmitis leading to blindness. Skin changes include dryness and hyperkeratosis. A variety of infantile hydrocephalus has been attributed to vitamin A deficiency.

Vitamin A deficiency should be suspected in all malnourished children. Normal serum level of vitamin A is 20 µg/dL. Serum levels less than 10 µg/dL are indicative of deficiency.

Several secondary benefits are attributable to proper vitamin A nutritional status. Epidemiological studies report increased mortality due to diarrhea and measles in children who are deficient in vitamin A.

Treatment: A mixed diet with adequate amount of protein is recommended. Vitamin A may be administered orally as retinol, 30 mg (9,000–10,000 IU) for 3 days. In more advanced cases retinol acetate or palmitate may be given intramuscularly (IM) in a dose of 5000–10,000 units. The corneal lesions clear up within 48–72 hours. The vitamin preparation in a dose of 8–10 mg/day should be given for a month and thereafter maintenance dose of 1.5 mg/day should be continued regularly. Patients with ocular complications should be referred to the ophthalmologist.

Prevention: The diet should contain at least 100 g of green vegetables and adequate amounts of animal products. Occurrence of vitamin A deficiency in 5% or more of the population calls for mass treatment. In poor communities 60 mg retinol palmitate or acetate administered orally once in 6 months or 300,000 IU once a year under supervision has been found to be extremely useful. Vitamin A deficiency occurring during pregnancy and lactation leads to poor vitamin A stores in the fetus and low vitamin A content of breast milk. These can be prevented by adequate supplementation during pregnancy.

Treatment schedule for xerophthalmia for all age group children.

Time schedule	Vitamin A dosage
Immediately on diagnosis	
6 months of age	50,000 IU
6–12 months	1,00,000 IU
12 months	2,00,000 IU
Next day and two weeks later	Same doses to be repeated

High dose universal distribution schedule for prevention of vitamin A deficiency.

Age	Vitamin A dosage
Infants < 6 months	50,000 IU/orally
Infants 6–12 months	100,000 IU/oral once in 4–6 months
Children >12 months	200,000 IU/orally once in 4–6/months
Mothers	200,000 IU orally within 8 weeks of delivery

Overdosage of carotene: Excessive intake of carotene containing foods, principally carrots, leads to hyper-carotenemia. It is a cosmetic problem due to yellowish pigmentation of skin. The serum is yellow but sclera is white. The pigmentation disappears with the elimination of excessive carotene from the diet. Hypothyroid patients are very susceptible to hypercarotenemia. Hypercarotenemia does not lead on to hypervitaminosis A.

Vitamin A toxicity: This may be due to self-medication or large scale ingestion of livers of fish or polar bear having enormous quantities of vitamin A.

Acute toxicity: Symptoms include abdominal pain, nausea, vomiting, headache and desquamation of the skin. Recovery occurs spontaneously on removing the source of the vitamin from the diet.

Chronic toxicity: This is seen in people who take 40,000 units or more of vitamin A daily for a prolonged period. It is characterized by body aches, arthralgia, hair loss, anorexia, benign intracranial hypertension, weight loss and hepatomegaly. Chronic overdose of vitamin A may be associated with osteoporosis and increased incidence of hip fractures, have been reported in Scandinavian countries.

Clinical diagnosis can be confirmed by demonstrating raised vitamin A concentration in the serum and normal retinol binding protein. Withdrawal of the vitamin from the diet brings about prompt relief.

VITAMIN D

Syn: Calciferol

Vitamin D is required mainly for normal metabolism of calcium and phosphorus and for bone formation. It enhances the absorption of these minerals from the gut, their mobilization from bone and the reabsorption of phosphorus by the kidney. Vitamin D_1 is the essential precursor for 1,25-alpha-dihydroxy-vitamin D_1 (1,25-alpha-OH-vitamin D_1) which is the steroid hormone required for the development of bone, growth in children and maintenance of bone mass in adults and also for the retardation of osteoporosis and prevention of fractures in the elderly.

The two different forms of vitamin D active in man are vitamin D (calciferol) obtained by ultraviolet (UV) irradiation of ergosterol (also called ergocalciferol or provitamin D_2) which is of plant origin and vitamin D_3 (cholecalciferol) which is formed by activation of 7-dehydrocholesterol present in the epidermal cells of human skin as a provitamin D_2. This activation is effected by the UV rays ranging in wavelength from 296 to 310 Å obtained from sunlight naturally. Exposure to sunlight for 20–30 minutes daily ensures adequate supply of vitamin D. Excessive exposure does not lead to overdose of the vitamin. Skin damaged by burns will not be capable of producing vitamin D on exposure to sunlight. Dark skin produces vitamin D from ergocalciferol less efficiently than fair skin. Sunscreens reduce the formation of vitamin D from ergocalciferol. Continued exposure to sunlight does not lead to hypervitaminosis D. Maximum amount of cholecalciferol synthesized by skin is only 20,000 units/day, since excess sunlight breaks down the vitamin. Burns, scars, clothes, pigmentation and sunscreens retard vitamin D synthesis. At least 10,000 units of vitamin D are synthesized within 30 minutes. Over exposure to

Textbook of Medicine

sunlight breaks down the provitamin D_3 to lumisterol and tachysterol.

Vitamin D_2 is obtained from the diet and vitamin D_3 is formed endogenously. On an average the endogenous source supplies about 80% and diet about 20% of the total requirement. Vitamin D_2 and D_3 which are identical in potency, differ only in the configuration of the side chain. Vitamin D_3, though formed in the skin is also absorbed through the small intestine. Further metabolism of vitamin D_2 and D_3 is identical and these together are referred to as vitamin D.

In the liver vitamin D undergoes its first metabolic change, being hydroxylated to 25-hydroxyvitamin D (25-OH-vitamin D) which is the major component in circulation. In the plasma the vitamin remains bound to a protein called vitamin D-binding protein. In the proximal convoluted tubule of the kidney several metabolic changes occur and the most active end product 1,25-OH-vitamin D_2 is formed, which is about 1000 times more active than the parent substance. The enzyme 25-OH-vitamin D_3 1-alpha-hydroxylase present in the kidney is the key enzyme regulating the formation of the active product.

Vitamin D supply depends on the amount of exposure to sunlight and the dietary intake. Conversion of vitamin D to 25-OH-vitamin D is not rate-controlled and therefore the circulating level of 25-OH-vitamin D indicates the amount of vitamin available to the body. On the other hand conversion of 25-OH-vitamin D to $1,25\text{-}OH_2$-vitamin D is rate-controlled by several factors such as serum phosphate levels, concentration of parathormone and levels of other hormones such as prolactin and sex hormones. Fall in the serum phosphate levels and rise in parathormone stimulate the formation of $1,25\text{-}OH_2$-vitamin D. Vitamin D and its metabolites are all conjugated to form glucuronides and sulfates in the liver during enterohepatic circulation. Since, vitamin D is itself biologically inactive and have to be converted into active metabolites in the system, it is often referred to as a prohormone.

Vitamin D deficiency is defined as serum levels of 2.5 OH vitamin D < 50 nmol/L. It affects more than 1 billion people worldwide. At least 3, (probably 4) genes control vitamin D status in the body.

- 7-dehydrocholesterol (DHC) reductase responsible or availability of 7-DHC on the skin
- The liver 2.5 hydroxylated ($CYP2R_1$) which is involved in the conversion to 25 OH vitamin D
- $CYP24A_1$ which is a degradation enzyme, genetic defects of which leads to vitamin D malnutrition.

Biological actions of vitamin D metabolites:

- Increase the absorption of calcium and phosphate from the small intestine by promoting active transport.
- Increase mobilization of calcium from bone by promoting osteoclastic activity.
- Stimulation of reabsorption of calcium and phosphate at the renal tubules.

The overall result of all these processes is to increase serum calcium and phosphate. Deficiency of vitamin D results in impairment of mineralization of bone leading to nutritional rickets in children and osteomalacia in adults.

In addition to the direct nutritional benefits of vitamin D, several other systemic disorders have been linked to vitamin D. These include type 1 and type 2 diabetes, cardiovascular disorders, increased risk of falls and cancers of breast, colon and prostate and immunity.

Vitamin D binding protein is the primary carrier of vitamin D in the circulation. 85–90% of the circulating 25-OH-vitamin D is bound to this protein. 10–15% of total hydroxyvitamin D is bound to albumin and about 1% is in free form. Only free vitamin D is available to the target tissues. Vitamin D binding protein seems to inhibit some actions of vitamin D. The bound fraction is unavailable to the target tissues. Genetic polymorphism in the vitamin D binding protein gene produces variant proteins with differing affinities to vitamin D. The differences in the polymorphism leads to different levels of vitamin D binding protein in different racial groups.

Vitamin D levels in blood are estimated by high performance liquid chromatography (HPLC), radioimmunoassay (RIA) and chemiluminescence assay (CLIA).

The lab assessment of total 25-OH-vitamin D measures the total vitamin D without distinguishing between the bound and free forms. Mean levels of 25-OH-vitamin D in blacks and whites Americans were 15.6 ± 2 ng/mL vs 25.8 ± 0.4 ng/mL.

Dietary sources of vitamin D are milk, butter, cheese, egg yolk and fish liver oils. This vitamin is heat stable. One international unit (IU) is equivalent to 0.025 µg. The daily requirement varies depending on the age.

	Daily requirement
Infants and children	400 IU
Age 19–50 years	200 IU
51–70 years	400 IU
71 and above years	600 IU

Rickets

Prevalence: Rickets is prevalent in India, more so in the north than in the south. Premature babies are more vulnerable. The disease is more florid during winter months when exposure to sunlight is minimal. Prevalence is more among the poor and illiterate classes. Indians who have immigrated to affluent countries still show a higher prevalence of rickets. Osteomalacia is more common in multiparous women who have nursed their babies repeatedly. Rickets has been ranked among the most frequent childhood diseases affecting children in the developing world. There is evidence that dietary deficiency of calcium may also lead to rickets.

In rickets, the arrangement and normal regenerative processes of cartilage are abnormal. Subsequent calcification of the cartilaginous matrix and osteoid do not proceed normally. The osteoid and cartilage which remain uncalcified are deposited irregularly. This gives rise to a wide irregular frayed zone of non-calcified cartilage and osteoid termed rachitic metaphysis. These in turn account for many of the skeletal deformities. In the subperiosteal region also, while resorption of cortical bone continues normally, new bone is not laid down, resulting in softening and rarefaction of the bone shaft.

In vitamin D deficiency, since absorption of calcium and phosphorus from the gut is defective, serum calcium and phosphorus levels fall. Lowered level of serum calcium stimulates the secretion of parathyroid hormone which in turn, leads to mobilization of calcium from the bone. Thus, the serum calcium is usually maintained normal for considerable periods, tetany developing only rarely. Since, parathyroid hormone (PTH) decreases reabsorption of phosphorus by the renal tubule, the serum phosphorus falls. The serum alkaline-phosphatase is elevated due to increased osteoblastic activity.

Rickets may develop as a primary nutritional disease or may be part of other multisystem diseases. Causes of rickets are listed in Table 30.1.

Clinical Features

Florid rickets manifests by the age of 1–2 years.

Early manifestations: These include irritability, flabbiness of muscles, prominence of abdomen and delay in the appearance of milestones, except speech.

Skeletal manifestations: These are the most characteristic features. They develop several months after the deficiency is established. The bones which have the maximum rate of growth at the time of onset of the deficiency show gross abnormalities.

In children below the age of 1 year, the lesion is craniotabes, characterized by abnormal softening of the skull in the occipital region. In children aged 2 years or more epiphyses of the wrists and ankles are widened and costochondral junctions are enlarged and beaded.

In advanced rickets, deformities of bones are aggravated because of muscular action, gravity and weight-bearing.

Head: Craniotabes disappears by 1 year of age, but the excess of osteoid and non-calcified cartilage gives rise to frontal and parietal bossing giving the skull a 'hot cross bun' appearance. Due to softening of the skull bones the calvarium is asymmetric. The head may be larger in size and closure of the anterior fontanel may be delayed. The teeth erupt late; show defective enamel and are more susceptible to develop caries. Permanent teeth also show grooving, pitting and hypoplastic enamel.

Rib-cage: Costochondral junctions are thickened (rachitic rosary) and the sternum projects forwards (pigeon chest deformity). A horizontal groove (Harrison's sulcus) develops along the diaphragmatic attachment due to muscular pull of the diaphragm on the softened bone.

Spine: This shows kyphosis and scoliosis when the baby starts sitting and later lordosis in the erect posture.

Pelvis: In lordotic subjects the pelvis shows a corresponding deformity. The pelvis is small and deformed (triradiate pelvis) and in female subjects the obstruction caused to the pelvic outlet gives rise to dystocia during parturition.

Extremities: The femur, tibia and fibula bend producing deformities like knock knees, coxa vara and others. The thickened epiphyseal ends may be more prominent. Deformities of upper limbs develop if rickets sets in when the infant is crawling. Long bones may develop green stick fractures and pseudofractures. The sum total of bony deformities of the spine, pelvis and legs leads to rachitic dwarfism.

Other general manifestations include hepatosplenomegaly, tetany, laryngysmus stridulus, convulsions and frequent respiratory infections.

Diagnosis: Rickets should be suspected in any child showing deformities of skull, long bones and ribs and in those with apathy, flabbiness, delayed milestones of development, laryngysmus stridulus or convulsions.

The clinical diagnosis is supported by the history of inadequate vitamin D in the diet or chronic diarrhea interfering with absorption of vitamin D and it is confirmed by radiological investigations and biochemical tests.

X-ray findings in active rickets: Routine skiagrams of the wrists give clues in diagnosis and are helpful for following the progress. The distal ends of radius and ulna appear concave (cupping), widened (flaring) and irregular (fraying). The distance between the distal ends of the ulna and the radius and the metacarpal bones is apparently increased since, the uncalcified rachitic metaphyses is translucent to X-ray. Shafts of long bones show decreased density and prominent trabeculation. Subperiosteal osteoid may give a double contour to the shaft.

With treatment, the lesions tend to heal. A line of preparatory calcification (LPC) appears. This is separated from the distal end of the shaft by a zone of translucency caused by the uncalcified osteoid. As healing progresses, the osteoid becomes calcified and shaft apparently grows towards the LPC and unites with it.

Measurement of serum 25-OH-vitamin D gives a reliable indication of the adequacy of the nutritional status. Normal values are above 15 ng/mL. Values below 8 mg/mL indicate severe deficiency.

Biochemical changes: In florid cases the serum phosphorus is low (1.5–3.5 mg/dL). Serum calcium may usually be normal, but in advanced cases it is reduced especially in cases with tetany. Serum alkaline phosphatase is raised to 20–60 KA units/dL (normal 5–15). With correction of the lesion alkaline phosphatase level falls and serum phosphorus level goes up.

Normal serum vitamin D levels range from 35 ± 3.5 ng/mL (80 nmol/L) and $1,25\text{-OH}_2$-vitamin D is 35 ± 3 pg/mL. In active rickets these levels are lowered.

Prognosis: For growth and cosmetic recovery is excellent, if the condition is recognized early and treated before deformities develop. Intercurrent infections make the

Table 30.1: Causes of rickets	
Renal	**Non-renal**
• Renal osteodystrophy • Familial hypophosphatemic rickets • Renal tubular acidosis • Fanconi syndrome: Primary or secondary—cystinosis, Wilson's disease • Lowe syndrome, tyrosinemia • Vitamin D dependent type 1 rickets • Vitamin D independent type 2 rickets	• Nutritional insufficiency • Intestinal—malabsorption • Hepatobiliary disease • Metabolic—anticonvulsant therapy • Oncogenic-mesenchymal tumors • Rickets of prematurity

prognosis worse. If treatment is started after the bony deformities are established and the epiphyses are ossified, the deformities tend to persist.

Treatment: Oral administration of vitamin D in doses of 1500–5000 IU daily brings about rapid improvement in the vast majority of cases. Vitamin D_3 supplements are better absorbed than vitamin D_2 supplements. Vitamin D supplements available as pills, pressed powder tablets and oily capsules. Pressed powder tablets are better absorbed than oily preparations. Radiological improvement will be demonstrable in 2–4 weeks. A single dose of 600,000 units is preferable for advanced cases. The dose may be given orally or as in IM injection. An oily preparation is available for IM injection which is effective for 3 months. Three to four injections are given at intervals of two weeks. Parenteral administration is mandatory in cases showing malabsorption. If there is no improvement even after two parenteral doses of vitamin D, the case is considered to be resistant to vitamin D.

After complete healing of the lesion vitamin D should be given in doses of 400 units daily for preventing recurrence. ***Children should be encouraged to get exposure to sun for 20–30 minutes daily.*** Early bone lesions will be corrected with simple medical treatment. If treatment is started late and deformities are permanent, orthopedic correction is indicated.

Vitamin D-resistant rickets: This may be acquired, as in chronic renal failure or inherited as in congenital enzyme defects.

In chronic renal failure conversion of 25-OH-vitamin D_3 into the active metabolite 1,25-OH_2-vitamin D_3 becomes defective due to the progressive deficiency of the enzyme in the renal tubules. Such patients develop features of rickets (renal rickets) forming part of renal bone diseases.

Inherited forms of rickets: Pseudovitamin D deficiency— two types are known. Rickets develop early in life. Hypotonia, weakness, seizures and growth failure develop.

Vitamin D dependent rickets type I: This is an autosomal recessive trait in which the gene for expressing the renal enzyme 25-OH-vitamin D_3 1-alpha hydroxylase is defective and so this enzyme level is low or absent. Plasma levels of 25-OH-vitamin D_3 are normal, but 1,25-OH_2-vitamin D_3 are low. The gene is located on chromosomes X 12 q 13.3.

Vitamin D dependent rickets type II: Two forms exist. In one form, the gene for vitamin D receptor is mutated. Hypocalcemic rickets develops. In the second form, also known as X-linked hypophosphatemic vitamin D resistant rickets the phosphate regulating gene (PEX gene) with homology to endopeptidases on the X chromosome is defective. All these forms respond to 1,25-OH_2-vitamin D.

Osteomalacia

Definition: Osteomalacia denotes those disorders where mineralization of newly formed bone matrix (osteoid) is defective.

Etiology: Osteomalacia may be of two different types:
1. Nutritional inadequacy of vitamin D, calcium or both.
2. Vitamin D-resistant osteomalacia. The latter occurs in the following conditions:
   - In renal tubular defects which produce hypo-phosphatemia and chronic metabolic acidosis
   - Chronic administration of diphenylhydantoin which leads to excessive metabolism of vitamin D
   - Osteoporosis
   - After parathyroidectomy for osteitis fibrosa or hyperthyroidism in which rapid formation of new bone outstrips bone resorption.

Clinical features: Osteomalacia presents with vague pain which starts as aches and pains insidiously, in the lumbar spine and thighs and spreading later to the arms and ribs. The pain is frequently felt over the bones themselves and not at the joints. The pain is usually symmetrical and non-radiating and is accompanied by tenderness of involved bones. Proximal muscles are weak and there is difficulty in climbing up stairs and getting up from squatting position. Occasionally, localized acute bone pain develops rapidly. These sites correspond to the development of pseudofractures. Classical radicular pain may develop due to compression fracture of the vertebra.

Physical signs include deformities, which may be missed if not specifically looked for. The usual deformities are triradiate pelvis and spinal kyphosis (due to action of gravity). Pathologic fractures due to weight-bearing and avulsion of tendinous attachments may develop. Biochemical features resemble those of rickets.

Characteristic radiological features are the appearance of 'pseudofractures' (Milkman's lines and Loser's zones). These are loss zones of decalcification which tend to be symmetrical and extend perpendicular to the cortex. The common sites are the pubic ramus, ischium, the neck of the femur, the outer edge of the scapula, ribs and vertebra. Occasionally, Loser's zones may extend right across a long bone simulating complete fractures. They are called pseudofractures because the gap is bridged by uncalcified osteoid tissue. They do not reveal any discontinuity of bone clinically. The pseudofractures are caused by the decalcification along the course of the major arteries entering the bones especially in areas of muscular attachment, namely the adductor insertion in the pubic ramus and attachment of gluteal muscles to the trochanters of the femur.

Vertebral bodies show compression and widening of intervertebral spaces to produce biconcave or cod-fish vertebrae.

However, in patients who develop osteomalacia secondary to renal tubular disorders or chronic renal failure, there is marked cortical thickening and increased density of trabecula in spongy bone. The reason for this hyperostosis is not clear. Despite the radiological appearances the bone is abnormally brittle and prone to develop fractures.

Treatment: Nutritional osteomalacia responds well to daily administration of 2000–4000 IU of vitamin D (0.05–0.1 mg) for 6–12 weeks followed by maintenance doses of 400–600 IU daily.

Dietary supplementation of calcium in the form of milk 500 mL per day hastens recovery. Medicinal calcium in the form of calcium gluconate, lactate or carbonate can be given as tablets or suspensions orally in doses of 500–1000 mg daily. Supplementation has to be continued as long as the diet is deficient in calcium.

Table 30.2: Giving the details of calcium preparations and their details

Calcium carbonate: 1–2, 500 mg tablet taken oral 2–3 times/day with meals	Elemental calcium 40%	Acidity improves absorption
Calcium citrate: 1–2, 500 mg tablet taken 2–3 times a day	21%	Need not be taken with meals, can be used in patients taking long-term acid suppression
Calcium gluconate: 500, 642 or 972 mg	9%	
Calcium lactate: 300–325 mg tablet	13%	
Bone meal, oyster shell, dolomite Dose varies	30%	May contain lead as a contaminant

Note: In persons genetically predisposed to urinary stone formation dietary calcium supplementation may favor urolithiasis.

Adequate supplements of calcium are provided in the form of milk 500–750 mL per day or calcium salts tablets 1 g along with food (Table 30.2).

Hypervitaminosis D

Prolonged administration of massive doses of vitamin D results in vitamin D intoxication. Serum levels of vitamin D above 374 nmol/L are toxic. This causes hypercalcemia. Symptoms include nausea, vomiting, constipation, drowsiness and signs of renal impairment. Metastatic calcification occurs in several tissues including the kidneys, lungs, gastric mucosa and blood vessels. Renal function may deteriorate before other signs of toxicity are manifest. Subjects receiving high doses of vitamin D should have regular monitoring of serum calcium and if it is above 2.6 mmol/L (10.5 mg/dL), the intake of the vitamin should be stopped.

VITAMIN E

Syn: Anti-sterility vitamin

Vitamin E is a tocopherol. Among the tocopherols, alpha tocopherol is the most easily absorbed and biologically most active compound. All vegetable oils, wheat-germ, cotton seeds, egg yolk, butter and peas contain this vitamin and the average Indian diet contains the daily requirement which is 15 IU or 5 mg. Vitamin E which is a strong antioxidant prevents the peroxidation of cellular and subcellular membrane phospholipids. It is probably involved in preserving the integrity of cell membranes. In cattle and poultry, vitamin E deficiency may lead to infertility. Nutritional deficiency of vitamin E is rare. Excess of free fatty acids in the diet increases the requirement for vitamin E. In premature infants fed on artificial diets containing iron and high concentrations of fatty acids, conditioned deficiency may develop, leading to the production of hemolytic anemia.

In doses of 400–800 mg, vitamin E acts as an effective antioxidant, thereby retarding the development of atheromatous changes in arteries.

VITAMIN K

Syn: Coagulation vitamin

This vitamin which is chemically a substituted naphtho-quinone is present in adequate amounts in vegetable oils and green leafy vegetables as vitamin K_1 (phytomenadione). Vitamin K comprises of several molecular forms that have a common 2-methyl-l, 4-naphthoquinone ring, but different side chains at the third position. In green leafy vegetables and legumes and vegetable oils such as rapeseed oil and soyabean oil, vitamin K occurs as phylloquinone (old name K_1). Bacteria synthesize vitamin K which is named menaquinone (MK-n) which occurs in several molecular forms. Milk is a poor source. The colonic bacteria synthesize this vitamin (vitamin K_2) and this supplements the dietary source. Naturally occurring vitamin K is fat-soluble. The synthetic form of this vitamin is vitamin K_3 which is water-soluble. This can be given IM or intravenously (IV), unlike the oily preparations which can be given only IM. Daily requirement is not clearly known, but is probably 1 µg/kg bw. Body sources are limited and, therefore, signs of deficiency develop within 3–4 weeks of dietary deprivation.

Oxidative phosphorylation processes which take place in cellular mitochondria requires the presence of vitamin K. Vitamin K occurs in large amounts in liver and bone. In the liver it takes part in the synthesis of precursors for coagulation factors, protein C and protein S. Vitamin K-dependent coagulation factors (factors II, VII, IX and X) are produced in the inactive form by the liver and vitamin K is required for their biological activation. The inhibitors of coagulation—protein C and protein S are also produced in the liver and these are also vitamin K dependent. Coumarins inhibit the enzyme vitamin K epoxide reductase and thereby inhibit further actions of vitamin K.

Prothrombin (factor II) is synthesized in the liver as an inert precursor, termed protein induced by vitamin K absence (PIVKA). This is carboxylated to form prothrombin by the vitamin K dependent enzyme—gamma carboxylase. In the absence of vitamin K or after administration of vitamin K antagonists such as coumarin, PIVKA appears in the plasma.

Vitamin K is needed for the formation of several proteins concerned with calcium homeostasis. Vitamin K promotes the conversion of protein-bound glutamate residues to gamma-carboxyglutamate (Gla). Proteins containing Gla are present in several tissues such as bone, kidneys, placenta, pancreas, spleen and lungs.

Vitamin K also takes part in bone metabolism—both bone formation and resorption. Two of the important vitamin K dependent proteins are osteocalcin and matrix Gla protein.

Vitamin K Deficiency

Vitamin K deficiency occurs in conditions associated with malabsorption of fat such as obstructive jaundice and malabsorption states. Prolonged treatment with broad spectrum antibiotics destroys the colonic bacteria which synthesize this vitamin. Deficiency manifests as mild or severe bleeding tendency occurring from injection sites, mucous membranes and skin. Injections of vitamin K in doses of 5–10 mg corrects the defect, if hepatic parenchymal function is normal. In the presence of hepatic failure, vitamin K may not be effective.

HEMORRHAGIC DISEASE OF THE NEWBORN

Hemorrhage may develop in newborn infants occasionally. Prematurity predisposes to this condition. Vitamin K deficiency in the mother and anticoagulant medication aggravate this disorder. Hemorrhagic tendency develops on the second or third day of delivery. This is due to exaggeration of the physiological hypoprothrombinemia which develops before the colon is colonized by bacteria. A dose of 1 mg of vitamin K_1 given IM to the baby brings about relief. Synthetic vitamin K is also effective. Larger doses have to be avoided since this lead to hemolysis. Administration of 5–10 mg vitamin K to the mother in late pregnancy abolishes this risk in the newborn.

Anticoagulant therapy: Use of coumarin drugs or warfarin leads to alteration in the synthesis of coagulation factors. As a result proteins antigenically similar to factors II, VII, IX and X are produced but they lack the procoagulant properties. Excess of anticoagulants leads to hemorrhagic tendency.

Bleeding occurs from injection sites, urinary tract, gastrointestinal tract (GIT) and uterus. IM injection of 10 mg vitamin K is usually effective. When the bleeding tendency is severe, large IV doses (50–75 mg) may be required. For severe cases transfusion of fresh blood or vitamin K-dependent coagulation factors may also be necessary (*See* also Ch 176).

Water-soluble Vitamins

KV Krishna Das

Chapter Summary

- Thiamine
- Riboflavin
- Niacin
- Pellagra
- Pyridoxine
- Pantothenic Acid
- Biotin
- Cyanocobalamin
- Folic Acid
- Ascorbic Acid and Scurvy

THIAMINE

Syn: Vitamin B_1—Aneurine

Thiamine plays an essential part in the metabolism of carbohydrates by acting as a coenzyme required for the decarboxylation of pyruvate to acetyl coenzyme A. It also takes part in other steps of the ***Kreb's tricarboxylic acid cycle.*** Cereals contain vitamin, which is maximal subjacent to the brain. Thiamine content of rice is lost during milling and polishing. Parboiling allows the vitamin to penetrate the grain and conserves it to some extent. Other good sources of the vitamin are sprouting pulses, green leafy vegetables, liver, pork and legumes. Part of the vitamin is lost by washing or discarding the water used for cooking. The daily requirement is 0.4 mg/1000 kcal, i.e. 1.2 mg/day. Requirement is partially influenced by the intake of carbohydrates.

Deficiency States

These occur mainly due to deficiency of this vitamin in the diet as occurring during famine, refugee camps, psychiatric conditions, severe alcoholism and malabsorption states. Bariatric surgeries short circuiting the absorptive portions of the intestine give rise to thiamine and several other vitamin deficiencies.

Pathology of deficiency: In thiamine deficiency, the cells cannot utilize glucose aerobically. Nervous system is affected first. Pyruvic and lactic acids accumulate and this leads to vasodilation. The myocardium shows loss of striation, vacuolation of fibers, fragmentation and edema. Cardiomyopathy, encephalopathy and peripheral neuropathy may develop. Sensory, motor and autonomic nerves show demyelination and degeneration.

Clinical features: Cardiovascular involvement results in ***wet beriberi*** and nervous system involvement results in ***dry beriberi*** (*See* also Ch 198).

Cardiovascular system: Peripheral vasodilation leads to high output circulatory state, myocardial failure and retention of sodium and water leading to edema. The pulse is of high volume. The extremities are warm owing to vasodilation and tender owing to neuropathy. Acute fulminant cardiac failure may be rapidly fatal. ***Wet beriberi*** may occur in breastfed infants aged 2–8 months. The child presents with edema, oliguria and an aphonic cry. If not clinically suspected, this condition may be missed. Sudden death may occur.

Neurological involvement: This manifests as symmetrical sensorimotor polyneuropathy with muscle wasting. Foot-drop and wrist-drop are common. Deep hyperesthesia occurs and it manifests as calf tenderness.

Wernicke's encephalopathy: This is an acute neurological manifestation which is more common in alcoholics. Pathological changes occur in the upper part of the midbrain, hypothalamus and the walls of the third ventricle which show congestion and petechial hemorrhages, most marked in the mammillary bodies. The onset is sudden with vomiting, confusion, bilateral ophthalmoplegia, loss of consciousness, nystagmus, ataxia and psychological disturbances. Confusion proceeds to coma and death. Korsakoff's syndrome is characterized by retrograde amnesia, impaired ability to learn and confabulation. Wernicke's encephalopathy is associated with high mortality. Prompt administration of thiamine rapidly restores normalcy (*See* also Ch 198). 500 mg of thiamine intravenous (IV) tds for 2 days and thereafter once a day for 7 days cures most of the cases.

Diagnosis of thiamine deficiency: The condition has to be suspected clinically. It can be confirmed by demonstrating raised levels of blood pyruvate. Normal blood pyruvate is 62.5–125 mmol/L and it may rise to 375 mmol/L (3.3 mg/L). Measurement of erythrocyte transketolase activity, before and after the addition of thiamine pyrophosphate gives the most reliable diagnostic test.

Treatment: When beriberi is suspected or diagnozed, 50 mg thiamine should be given intramuscularly (IM) daily for several days. After controlling the acute symptoms, 2.5–5 mg should be given orally as maintenance. Wet beriberi and Wernicke's encephalopathy have to be treated as medical emergencies. A dose of 25–100 mg of thiamine should be given IV to save life. Dramatic recovery with diuresis occurring within hours of injection confirms the diagnosis.

Infants with beriberi should be given 10 mg thiamine IM followed by oral doses. The mother also should be treated with oral doses of 10 mg twice daily for several days. Since polyneuropathy and Korsakoff's psychosis are more resistant to treatment, the vitamin has to be given for prolonged periods. Once neuropathy is established, residual paralysis persists even after therapy. Adverse side effects to thiamine include sensitization and anaphylactic shock.

RIBOFLAVIN

Syn: Vitamin B$_2$

Riboflavin is essentially required in all oxidation reduction reactions involving the coenzymes flavin mononucleotide and flavin adenine dinucleotide which take part in tissue oxidation and respiration. It is moderately heat resistant, but boiling in alkaline media or exposure to sunlight destroys this vitamin.

Good dietary sources include liver, meat, eggs, kidney, milk, other dairy products, green leafy vegetables and sprouted cereals and pulses. Daily requirement is 0.60 mg/1000 kCal, i.e. a total of 1.5–2 mg.

- ***Signs of deficiency:*** Angular stomatitis, cheilosis, nasolabial seborrhea and possibly vascularization of the cornea are the characteristic features. Angular stomatitis may also occur in deficiencies of niacin and folic acid. Mucosa of the lips appears red and denuded in cheilosis. On taking hot and spicy food there may be soreness. Vascularization of the cornea has been described in some surveys. In glossitis the mucosa over the tongue is red, swollen and painful (Fig. 31.1).

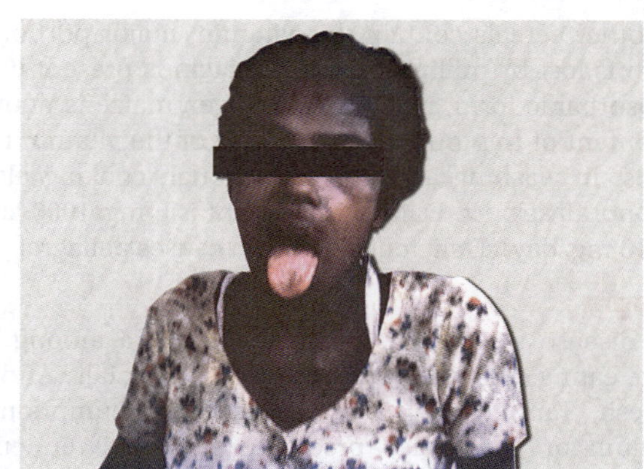

Fig. 31.1: Glossitis and angular stomatitis

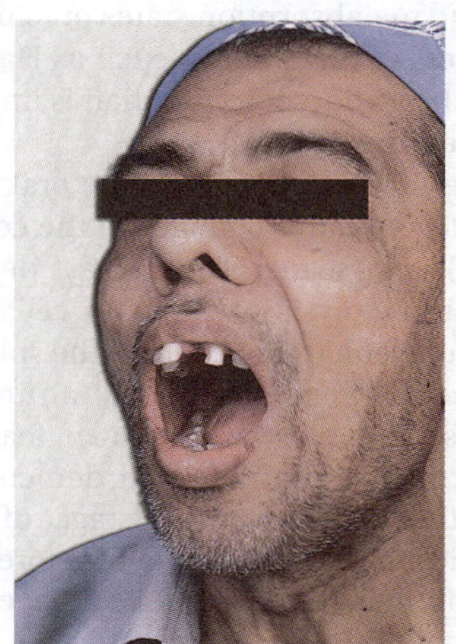

Fig. 31.2: Angular stomatitis

This responds to riboflavin therapy. Some cases show lesions in the oral mucosa, eyes and genitals (oculo-orogenital syndrome) (Fig. 31.2). The ***oculo-orogenital syndrome*** presents as blepharoconjunctivitis, angular stomatitis, bright red atrophic tongue and dermatitis of the pubic region. This syndrome may occur in pyridoxine deficiency as well.

- ***Treatment:*** Riboflavin in a dose of 2–5 mg thrice a day cures the condition in a few days. The drug can be given orally as tablets or syrup or by injections. Treatment of oculo-orogenital syndrome is to give riboflavin up to 100 mg/day and pyridoxine 150 mg/day. The lesions clear within 7–10 days.

NIACIN

Syn: Nicotinic acid, Nicotinamide, Anti-pellagra Vitamin, Vitamin B$_3$

Nicotinic acid forms an integral part of nicotinamide adenine dinucleotide (NAD) and its phosphate (NADP) which act as coenzymes in the metabolic pathways of glucose and proteins. Nicotinic acid and nicotinamide have equal biological potency and are together referred to as niacin. Tryptophan is converted into niacin in the body; 60 mg of tryptophan giving rise to 1 mg niacin. Dietary sources include liver, pulses, whole cereals, fish, meat, groundnuts, milk, eggs and to a smaller extent, vegetables. Coffee contains appreciable amounts of this vitamin. Rice and other cereals contain this vitamin, major portion of which is lost by milling. In maize niacin is present in an unabsorbable form 'niacytin.' Moreover, maize is poor in its content of tryptophan. One-fourth of the vitamin may be lost in washing and cooking, though cooking alone does not destroy it. Daily requirement is 6 mg/1000 kcals (15–18 mg/day). Deficiency of niacin causes pellagra.

Pellagra

This disease was widely prevalent in India among the maize eating communities in all states, especially Andhra Pradesh, Tamil Nadu and Rajasthan. Consumption of sorghum or *jowar* also predisposes to this tendency. Newer varieties of maize and sorghum with better nutritive value have helped to reduce the incidence of pellagra. Alcoholism and malabsorption states precipitate pellagra. Inborn disorders of metabolism such as Hartnup disease in which the absorption of tryptophan is impaired lead to pellagra in rare cases.

Pathology: Dermatitis, changes in the oral and intestinal mucosa and degenerative changes in the central nervous system (CNS) are seen. Ulcers may develop in the intestines. Chromatolysis of ganglion cells occur in the CNS. Patchy demyelination occurs in the spinal cord.

Clinical features: Generalized malnutrition is evident in most cases. The most well-known features are the three Ds—dermatitis, diarrhea and dementia, but these characterize the very advanced stage of the disease. Pellagra should be diagnosed much before this classical picture develops, since the advanced stage is associated with high mortality.

- *Skin changes:* These are seen over areas exposed to sunlight. These start with erythema which may resemble sunburn. This progresses to vesiculation, ulceration, secondary infection and crusting. In chronic pellagra the skin becomes rough, thickened, scaly and pigmented. In home-bound patients not exposed to the sun, pellagra may develop without the skin changes—*Pellagra sine pellagra*. Mucous membrane changes are evident in the mouth and vulva. Skin of the perianal region shows degenerative and inflammatory lesions. The tongue is raw and beefy in appearance. Angular stomatitis may be present.
- *Alimentary symptoms:* Vague alimentary symptoms like anorexia, nausea, vomiting and dyspepsia are invariably seen. Diarrhea is common but not always present. The stools may be watery or rarely dysenteric.
- *Neurological features:* Anxiety, depression, irritability and failure to concentrate are early symptoms. Advanced cases show delirium, dementia and psychiatric manifestation. Mental symptoms may be mistaken for primary psychiatric disorders.

Course and prognosis: Advanced cases are fatal due to diarrhea, secondary infections or other associated nutritional disorders. Early treatment reverses the symptoms completely.

Treatment: Well-balanced diet containing adequate supply of proteins should be instituted. Nicotinamide is well absorbed if given orally. It is given in a dose of 100 mg every 6 hour for 2–3 weeks. In the advanced cases 50–100 mg may be given IM or IV. Supplements such as the other B complex vitamins and iron should be concurrently administered. Local application of antihistamine creams and protective clothing gives relief to the skin lesions.

Prevention: In maize eating communities other sources of niacin should be provided along with. In non-endemic areas pellagra may develop in the elderly, inmates of mental homes, etc. Such groups require vitamin supplementation.

PYRIDOXINE

The active form of this vitamin is pyridoxal. Pyridoxal phosphate acts as a coenzyme in several reactions, especially in the metabolism of amino acids and biological amines such as catecholamines and 5-hydroxytryptamine. It takes part in the biosynthesis of gamma-aminobutyric acid in the brain. Yeast, liver, meat, whole grain cereals, peanuts, bananas and legumes are good dietary sources. Normal daily requirement is 1.25 mg and it is present in the ordinary Indian diets and hence, nutritional deficiency is rare. Drugs like isonicotinylhydrazide (INH), oral contraceptives and hydralazine may interfere with the metabolism of this vitamin and produce conditioned deficiencies.

Clinical features: Include dermatitis, cheilosis, angular stomatitis, glossitis, dizziness, vomiting and peripheral neuropathy. Infantile convulsions have been attributed to nutritional pyridoxine deficiency. Pyridoxine deficiency is known to produce one form of sideroblastic anemia which responds to high doses of this vitamin. Concurrent administration of 6 mg of pyridoxine prevents the development of neuritis in subjects treated with INH (*See* also Section 17, Ch 198).

PANTOTHENIC ACID

Pantothenic acid is converted to coenzyme A in the body. This vitamin is widely distributed in animal and vegetable foods and hence, dietary deficiency is very rare. Though the exact requirement is not clearly known, 10 mg may represent an adequate daily intake. Deficiency in experimental animals leads to dermal and hair changes, neuromuscular degeneration and fatal adrenal hemorrhage.

Calcium pantothenate has been used for other conditions like paralytic ileus and streptomycin toxicity based on empirical findings. There is no conclusive proof to support these claims.

BIOTIN

Syn: Vitamin B$_7$, Vitamin H

This is an organic acid functioning as a co-enzyme in several carboxylation reactions. Biotin acts as a cofactor for four carboxylases each of which catalyses an intermediate metabolism. It is present in several articles of food and is also synthesized by intestinal bacteria. Daily requirement is about 100 µg. Naturally occurring deficiency is rare, but conditioned deficiency may develop by overfeeding exclusively with white portion of egg. This is due to the presence of avidin which antagonizes biotin. Infants who are on parenteral feeding with biotin

Textbook of Medicine

deficient diets may develop symptoms such as lassitude, irritability, paresthesia, anorexia, rashes and hair loss. All these improve with the administration of biotin. Biotin deficiency can lead to more serious features such as ataxia, seizures and growth retardation. Normal levels of serum biotin are 6.5–12.3 nmol/L and urinary biotin is 1.9–11.6 μmol/moL of creatine.

Inherited disorders of biotin metabolism occur rarely. Two types are known. One type may present in the first few weeks of life with metabolic acidosis and a rash. Skin rashes due to biotin deficiency may be mistaken for allergic rashes in babies. The other presents in the first few months of life with rash, keratoconjunctivitis, alopecia, ataxia, hypotonia and metabolic and lactic acidosis. Both groups respond dramatically to large doses of biotin.

CYANOCOBALAMIN

Syn: Vitamin B_{12}

Deficiency of vitamin B_{12} or folates leads to abnormality in DNA synthesis, characterized by megaloblastic erythropoiesis and similar changes in many tissues in the body. Due to its fatal outcome in pre-vitamin B_{12}, it was called pernicious anemia.

Absorption of B_{12}: The dietary vitamin B_{12} which is bound to proteins has to be liberated from them to enable absorption. Cooking converts a part of these into dialyzable form. Low pH achieved in the stomach helps further liberation of this vitamin. After liberation, cobalamin is bound to the intrinsic factor (IF) which is a glycoprotein with a molecular weight of 44,000 present in the gastric juice. Proteolytic enzymes of the pancreas play a part in this process.

The vitamin B_{12}-IF complex is taken up by receptor sites present in the microvilli of the ileum by passive absorption. In the plasma 20% of cyanocobalamin remains bound to a polypeptide of molecular weight 38,000 known as transcobalamin II (TC II). This is the form in which cyanocobalamin is delivered to the cells. This complex passes into cells and its B_{12} is liberated by lysosomal enzymes. About 80% of cyanocobalamin circulates in combination with haptocorin. Liver can store up to 2 mg of vitamin B_{12} which is adequate for several years. The daily requirement of B_{12} is 2.5–4.5 μg. Meat, liver, eggs, dairy products and yeast contain adequate amounts of this vitamin. Purely vegetable sources are deficient in vitamin B_{12}. Therefore, vegans (persons who do not take any form of animal foods or dairy products) suffer from nutritional deficiency. Normal levels of vitamin B_{12} in serum ranges from 1200 to 900 pg/mL in Indian subjects. Both in normal and even in PA patients 0.5–4% of ingested vitamin B_{12} can be passively absorbed in the intestine. Vitamin B_{12} deficiency is less common than folate deficiency.

Etiology of vitamin B_{12} deficiency

- Malabsorption states—diseases of the ileum
- Dietary inadequacy—vegans
- Intrinsic factor deficiency—pernicious anemia. This is usually acquired, rarely this may be congenital
- Chronic disorders destroying the gastric mucosa and partial or total gastrectomy
- Blind loop syndromes—with colonization of the small intestine by bacteria
- Pancreatic insufficiency
- Familial deficiency of TC II
- Inherited disorders of vitamin B_{12} metabolism
- Interference with absorption of vitamin B_{12} by drugs, e.g. para-aminosalicytic acid (PAS), colchicine, phenformin, neomycin
- Long-term use of powerful antacids such as proton pump inhibitors which suppress gastric acid and bariatric surgical measures such as short circuiting the upper gastrointestinal tract (GIT) and ileum lead to therapeutically induced vitamin B_{12} deficiency, unless this vitamin is supplemented.

Effects of B_{12} deficiency: Megaloblastic anemia develops owing to diminished red cell production and dyserythropoiesis. Cobalamin is an essential co-factor in several metabolic pathways. Intracellular conversion occurs to form adenosocobalamin in the mitochondria and methylcobalamin in the cytoplasm. Adenosocbalamin is involved in the catabolism of odd chain fatty acids and some amino acids. Methylcobalamin is the co-enzyme for cytosolic methionine synthase which converts homocysteine to methionine. Further action includes methylation and deoxyribonucleic acid (DNA) synthesis—which are vital processes. In addition, cells from other organs with rapid cell turnover such as the GIT and cervicovaginal mucosa also show similar abnormalities. The CNS and peripheral nerves are also affected. The neurological lesions include subacute combined degeneration of the spinal cord, optic neuritis and demyelination of the cerebral white matter and peripheral nerves. Cognitive changes and psychiatric disturbances may develop which clear up completely if treated early.

Neurological damage occurs due to impaired DNA synthesis and myelin formation (*See* also Ch 198). The occurrence of neuropathy does not bear any direct relationship to the severity of anemia.

Treatment: Dietary deficiency can be corrected by giving 4 μg of vitamin B_{12} orally. If megaloblastic anemia has developed, larger doses are required (100 μg/day) oral, if absorption is reliable. Otherwise 1000 μg of hydroxocobalamin is given IM once a week for 3–4 weeks and thereafter the daily dietary supplementation of 4 mcg is continued. Deficiency of B_{12} should be corrected without delay before neurological features develop.

There is evidence that vitamin B_{12} can be absorbed from the buccal mucosa when applied sublingually. This route can be made use for therapy in mild deficiency states.

FOLIC ACID

Syn: Pteroylglutamic acid

Folic acid molecule consists of a pteridine ring, para-amino benzoic acid and l-glutamic acid. The free form does not occur commonly in nature. Foods and tissues contain several folate compounds (pteroyl polyglutamate). The main form present in human plasma and CSF is 5-methyltetrahydropteroylmonoglutamate. Rich dietary sources are yeast, liver, nuts, green vegetables and chocolate. Folic acid is lost by boiling the articles of food in a large volume of water. Average requirement is 200–300 μg/day. The vitamin is absorbed in the proximal small intestine after hydrolysis of polyglutamates. Human body can store about 6–10 mg, especially in the liver. Megaloblastic anemia has developed in volunteers after 10–20 weeks of dietary deprivation. Dietary deficiency is widely prevalent in India. It is seen most in pregnant women and children. A study conducted in Balrampur dist in UP, India by Anil Cheriyan, et al. 2002–2003 revealed neural tube defects in 6.57–8.2 children out of 1000 live birth. This figure is one of the highest in the world. The main reason was deficiency of folates, vitamin B_{12} and other deficiencies such as vitamin B_6 occur together or singly.

Source: Cherian A, Seena S, Bullock RK, Antony AC. Incidence of neural tube defects in the least-developed area of India: a population-based study. Lancet. 2005;366(9489):930-1.

Causes of folate deficiency:

- Dietary inadequacy of animal foods and green vegetables
- Malabsorption states
- Increased demands due to pregnancy, lactation, growth and intercurrent illnesses in children
- Alcohol intake increases folate requirements
- Accelerated erythropoiesis as in hemolytic anemia
- Other disorders like tuberculosis, rheumatoid disease and malignancy increase folate requirements
- Several drugs interfere with the metabolism of folates, e.g. amethopterin, pyrimethamine, trimethoprim, hydantoins oral contraceptives
- Folate losses may occur in several disorders of skin and the intestinal tract
- Inborn errors of metabolism may interfere with the utilization of folate.

Folate deficiency leads to megaloblastic anemia and similar changes in several rapidly proliferating tissues. In the body the metabolic pathways of folates and vitamin B_{12} are closely interrelated. In many cases of nutritional anemias, combined deficiencies of iron, folate and to a smaller extent B_{12} operate.

Normal serum folate levels are 4–10 ng/mL and red cell folate is above 100 ng/mL.

Folic acid deficiency occurring in the early period of gestation when the neural tube of the embryo develops, may result in the higher incidence of neural tube defects such as spina bifida and anencephaly. Supplementation of 400 μg of folate starting from 28 days before and continuing for 28 days after conception reduce the risks of neural tube defects substantially.

Treatment: Dietary deficiency can be corrected by giving 5–10 mg of folic acid orally, in addition to the dietary improvement. Pregnant and lactating women, children and alcoholics require prophylactic supplementation. In poor communities routine folic acid supplementation in pregnancy (1 mg/day) reduces the incidence of premature births. Premature infants should be given folate supplementation.

Folate and vitamin B_{12} deficiencies are known to elevate serum homocystein levels and this may lead to abnormal thrombotic tendency leading to arterial and venous thrombosis.

ASCORBIC ACID AND SCURVY

Syn: Antiscorbutic Vitamin—Vitamin C

James Lind, a Scottish naval physician, recognized the antiscorbutic properties of citrus fruits in 1753 and this was considered an important discovery with far-reaching effects. May 20th is declared as the *International Clinical Trials Day* in honor of James Lind who started the systematic study of the prevention of scurvy in sailors between six treatment schedules in 1747 AD.

Dietary sources: Ascorbic acid is present in a wide variety of foods. In the process of cooking about 50% of vitamin C passes into water and 20% gets destroyed. Fresh fruits, green leafy vegetables and germinating pulses are rich in ascorbic acid. The Indian gooseberry and guavas are particularly rich sources. Animal food like milk and meat contain only small amounts of this vitamin. The vitamin is present in potato in the layer just below the skin. If the potatoes are boiled whole with the skin, the vitamin diffuses into the deeper layers.

The minimum daily requirement for an adult is 30–40 mg and for infants 5 mg/kg bw. Normal plasma levels vary between 0.7 and 1.5 mg per dL. Leukocytes, platelets and adrenal glands contain large amounts of vitamin C. Deficiency of vitamin C causes scurvy. In scurvy the plasma levels are below 0.1 mg/dL.

Physiological actions: Vitamin C is a strong reducing agent. It takes part in biological oxidation-reduction reactions. Vitamin C is required for the formation of collagen by the hydroxylation of proline. It takes part in the formation of hemoglobin, erythrocyte maturation and the conversion of folic acid to tetrahydrofolate. Ascorbic acid reduces ferric iron to ferrous iron which is more easily absorbed. Body stores of ascorbic acid are small and therefore, dietary deficiency leads to the development of scurvy.

Major roles of vitamin C in health:

- Vitamin C (ascorbic acid) plays a role in collagen, carnitine, hormone and amino acid formation.
- It is essential for wound healing and facilitates recovery from burns.
- Vitamin C is also an antioxidant, supports immune function and facilitates the absorption of iron.
- Scurvy is caused by a dietary deficiency of vitamin C.
- The body's pool of vitamin C can be depleted in 1–3 months.

Risk factors include the following:

- Babies fed purely on cow's milk for more than 1 year
- Alcoholism, elderly who are on tea and toast diet, poverty, heavy cigarette smokers (smoking reduces vitamin C absorption and metabolism), pregnancy, thyrotoxicosis, anorexia nervosa, type 1 diabetes (increased requirement) malabsorption states and iron overload states.

Scurvy

Deficiency of vitamin C in the diet over a few weeks or months will lead to scurvy.

Textbook of Medicine

Clinical features of scurvy: Classic scurvy is seen only infrequently in India, since small amounts of vitamin C are obtained in vegetables and pickled berries which form essential items of the Indian diet. Cases do occur among inmates of mental homes, elderly persons and among the very poor.

Manifestations of scurvy vary in children and adults. Early symptoms include weakness, lassitude and normocytic normochromic anemia. In infancy and childhood subperiosteal hemorrhages occur, which lead to painful swellings over long bones. Scurvy in infancy produces pseudoparalysis owing to pain. This condition may mimic arthritis, osteomyelitis or poliomyelitis. X-ray abnormalities may develop over the sternal ends of ribs and ends of long bones. Bleeding from the gums occurs commonly at the sites of erupted teeth. Retrobulbar, subarachnoid and cerebral bleeding may develop in a few cases.

In adults early manifestation is follicular hyperkeratosis over the skin of the lower limbs. The lesions are papular with perifollicular hemorrhages which appear as purpura. Hemorrhage into the deep tissues of the thighs and legs cause tense induration (woody leg). Other sites of hemorrhage include joints, nail beds and viscera. The gums are hypertrophied and the interdental papillae are red and prominent (scurvy-buds). They bleed easily. Edentulous subjects do not get gingival abnormalities. The gum changes are aggravated by infection. The teeth become loose and may fall-off. The hair assumes cork-screw shape since, the follicles are obstructed by keratin plugs. Wound healing is delayed and resistance to infection is reduced. The condition is fatal if untreated.

Treatment: Scurvy is a potentially fatal disease and sudden death may occur unexpectedly. Treatment should be started without delay. In infants and children 25–50 mg of ascorbic acid given daily three times a day is sufficient to replete the body stores. In adults 500 mg is given daily in divided doses up to a total of 4 g. A diet rich in vitamin C should be given to prevent relapse.

Prevention: Infant foods should contain fruit juices or vitamin C supplements. Children, convalescent subjects and elderly people who are liable to be neglected, should receive 25 mg of vitamin C daily. As an alternative, 500 mg may be given once a month.

Adverse effects of vitamin C: Side effects like digestive upsets and hypoglycemia occur if the drug is given in doses exceeding 3 g/day. Oxaluria and oxalate stone formation in the urinary tract may result from prolonged overdosage.

Minerals

KV Krishna Das

Chapter Summary

- Calcium
- Phosphorus
- Iron
- Iodine
- Fluorine
- Copper
- Magnesium
- Zinc
- Selenium

Fourteen elements are absolutely essential for normal body metabolism. These minerals are sodium, potassium, calcium, magnesium, iron, iodine, copper, zinc, cobalt, phosphorus, sulfur, chromium, selenium and fluorine. Though several other elements are detectable in tissues, their role in nutrition is not clearly understood the term trace elements denote these elements whose concentration in biological fluids does not exceed 1 µg/mL.

CALCIUM

(*See* also Ch 72)

The total body content of calcium is 1200 g in an adult. This is present in the skeleton, teeth, plasma and all tissues.

Of the total body calcium, 98% is present in the bones as calcium phosphate (hydroxyapatite) held in a protein matrix (osteoid). Calcium gives the strength and rigidity to the skeleton. In the plasma, calcium is present as free ions, albumin-bound form and as complexes which are diffusible. In health, serum calcium level ranges from 9 to 10.5 mg% (2.2–3.6 mmol/L). Calcium and phosphorus levels vary inversely with each other and the product Ca×P is almost constant around 40. The normal function of cell membranes and the electrical activity of excitable tissues like the muscles, nerves and heart depend upon ionized calcium. Calcium ions facilitate the release of acetylcholine from the vesicles in the motor end plates. Coagulation processes require small amounts of calcium.

The main sources of calcium is the diet—milk, cheese, eggs, meat, peas, beans, certain leafy vegetables, dried fruits and nuts contain good amounts of calcium. Milk protein (casein) is the richest and most reliable source. One liter of milk contains about 1.2 g of calcium. An egg contains about 30 mg of calcium. Drinking water may also contain a variable, but significant amounts of calcium in many areas. Calcium from vegetable foods is not well absorbed since, it is present as oxalate. In cereals, calcium

Textbook of Medicine

is found in the form of phytates which are not absorbed and hence, except millets the cereals are poor sources.

Calcium is absorbed actively from jejunum and passively from the ileum. Intake of vitamin D, acidic pH and presence of proteins in the food favor absorption. In growing children, pregnant and lactating women absorption is increased. In older age groups, absorption falls. High fat diet, phytates, oxalates and alkaline pH impair the calcium absorption. Normally 70–80% of ingested calcium is lost in feces unabsorbed. In steatorrhea, calcium soaps are formed and excess calcium is lost in stool. Calcium is also lost in the urine.

Urinary calcium level depends on the blood levels. Normal adults excrete 300–400 mg of calcium in 24 hours. Lowering of dietary calcium does not lower urinary calcium correspondingly. As a result, very low calcium intake results in negative balance. Lowering of serum calcium stimulates the secretion of parathyroid hormone which mobilizes calcium from bones. The metabolism of calcium is intimately related to those of vitamin D, parathyroid hormone and calcitonin (*See* also Ch 100).

Recommended daily intake is 500 mg for adults, 1200 mg for pregnant and lactating women and 700 mg for adolescents. Postmenopausal women should have 500 mg of elemental calcium (available form 1250 mg of calcium carbonate or other calcium salts in suitable doses) as supplement to diet. Daily administration of 1000 mg of calcium carbonate with 400 units vitamin D_3 has shown to reduce hip fracture in postmenopausal women. There has been a slight increase in the incidence of urinary calculi. Since, it has been detected that vitamin D deficiency abnormalities, osteomalacia and demineralization of bone are widespread in India and several neighboring countries. The general tendency has been to prescribe higher dose of vitamin D and calcium salts to postmenopausal women and elderly persons. Up to 700–100 mg of elemental calcium and 1000 units of vitamin D have been recommended.

Hypercalcemia leads to anorexia, nausea, vomiting, constipation, hypotonia, mental depression, lethargy and even coma. Persistent hypercalcemia leads to calcification around joints, ligaments, gastric mucosa, cornea and kidneys. Hypercalcemia further depresses the renal function. Hypercalcemia is a medical emergency which may occur in osteoclastic conditions including bone tumors, hyperparathyroidism. Hypercalcemia arising from over ingestion of vitamin D and the milk alkali syndrome. Management of acute and chronic hypercalcemia is given in (*See* Section 11, Ch 100).

Hypocalcemia leads to tetany. Tetany can be relieved by giving calcium gluconate IV (intravenous) 10% solution, 20 mL as slow injection. Further follow-up is to give calcium supplements 1–1.5 g of calcium carbonate and vitamin D 500–1000 units orally daily.

PHOSPHORUS

(*See* also Chapters 72 and 100)

Most of the phosphorus (85%) in the body is present in bones and teeth. In all tissues, this element is present intracellularly as phosphates. The total body content of phosphorus is 800–900 g. In the plasma, it occurs as inorganic orthophosphate at a concentration of 2.8–4.5 mg/dL (0.8–1.5 mmol/L). Around 88% of phosphorus is in ionic form and the rest is present in the protein-bound form. Phosphorus is widely distributed in dietary articles and hence, dietary deficiency is rare. Though the exact requirement of phosphorus has not been determined, probably it is the same as calcium. Dairy products, eggs, cereals and meat are rich sources.

About 80–90% of ingested phosphorus is absorbed. The serum level is controlled mainly by the renal excretory mechanism. Around 85% of filtered phosphate is absorbed at the proximal tubule and only 10–15% is lost in urine. Negative phosphate balance is usually caused by the abnormalities of renal clearance. In renal failure, serum phosphate goes up and in renal tubular dysfunctions it may fall. Aluminum hydroxide binds phosphates and makes it unabsorbable so that in prolonged antacid therapy, phosphorus absorption may suffer.

Facts about phosphorus

- 85% in skeleton
- 15% in extracellular fluid and soft tissues
- Normal diet supplies 800–1400 mg/day
- Absorption from gut is passive. 60–80% absorbed, 1-25 $(OH)_2 D_3$ promotes absorption
- Normal plasma levels 2.8–4.5 mg/dL or 0.89–1.44 mmol/L
- Plasma levels are higher in children and they fall with age.

Hypophosphatemia

The serum level is below 2.5 mg/dL, i.e. 0.8 mmol/L.

Causes

- ■ ***Redistribution between internal compartments,*** e.g. respiratory alkalosis, recovery from star-vation, recovery stage of diabetic ketoacidosis, endocrino-pathies, avid uptake of phosphorus by bone (hungry bone syndrome).
- ■ ***Increased urinary losses,*** e.g. hyperparathyroidism vitamin D deficiency, renal tubular defects, alcoholism, metabolic and respiratory acidosis (*See* also Ch 100).
- ■ ***Diminished absorption,*** e.g. malabsorption states, fall in dietary phosphorus, vitamin D deficiency, antacid overuse.

Manifestations include proximal myopathy, dysphagia, intestinal ileus, rhabdomyolysis, thrombocytopenia, respiratory muscle weakness and encephalopathy.

Management: If the serum phosphorus level is near about 0.32 mmol/L, oral supplementation with sodium or potassium phosphate in a dose of 2–3 g/day is sufficient. Cow's milk contains 1 mg phosphorus per mL. In an emergency, sodium phosphate can be given IV as infusion in a dose of 2.5 mg/kg bw over a period of 6 hours. Infusion of phosphate leads to fall in plasma calcium level.

Hyperphosphatemia

Plasma level of phosphorus exceeds 1.5 mmol/L.

Causes

- ■ ***Increased exogenous load:*** IV infusion, heavy oral intake, feeding cow's milk to premature babies, vitamin D overdose, abuse of phosphate-containing enemas, acute phosphorus poisoning.

- ***Increased endogenous production:*** Tumor lysis syndrome, rhabdomyolysis, bowel infarction, hemolysis, malignant hyperthermia, lactic acidosis, diabetic ketoacidosis and respiratory acidosis.
- ***Reduction in urinary elimination:*** Renal failure, hypoparathyroidism, acromegaly, vitamin D intoxication, phosphonate therapy and magnesium deficiency.

Pseudohyperphosphatemia

This is the condition in which spuriously high blood levels are seen if colorimetry is adopted for estimation. This occurs in multiple myeloma, hypertriglyceridemia and if hemolysis occurs in the blood sample after collection.

Clinical features: Acute hyperphosphatemia depresses plasma calcium levels and precipitates tetany. Chronic elevation of the Ca×P level above 70 leads to metastatic calcification.

Treatment: Induce intestinal malabsorption of phosphate by administering phosphate binding salts of aluminum, magnesium or calcium. In the presence of renal failure, aluminium salts should be used with caution.

IRON

The total content of iron in healthy adults is 4.2 g. Out of these, 58–66% is present in hemoglobin. Part of the iron is present in myoglobin which is present widely in cardiomyocytes and skeletal myofibrils. It is a small monomeric cytoplasmic tissue hemoglobin which facilitates the transport of oxygen from erythrocytes to the mitochondria to maintain oxidative phosphorylation for myocardial contractility. Neuroglobin is a tissue hemoglobin discovered in vertebrate brains. It is likely that it may function during hypoxemic episodes and protect against damage.

Iron also exists in combination with the iron storage proteins such as ferritin and hemosiderin, in the macrophages seen in the muscles, liver and bone marrow. Stored iron is demonstrable by Prussian blue reaction histochemically. Stored iron available for erythropoiesis is about 1.2–2 g. Tissue iron is mainly present in enzymes, this amounts for 300 mg and is not available for erythropoiesis. Total plasma iron is 34 mg and the levels range from 80 to 120 µg/dL. Animal foods like meat, liver, kidney, fish and egg yolk are rich in iron. Vegetable sources are green vegetables and fruits, onions, cereals, pulses, oil seeds, jaggery, raisins, grapes, apricots and dates. The daily average intake of iron is 10–20 mg, out of which 1–2 mg is absorbed. Significant amounts of iron may be obtained from water sources and from iron cooking vessels (*See* also Chapters 158 and 159).

Absorption and Further Metabolism of Dietary Iron

Iron is one of the most highly conserved elements in the body. Dietary iron occurs in two forms:

1. Heme iron found in hemoglobin and myoglobin, obtained from animal foods.
2. Non-heme iron present in green vegetables, fruits and cereals. They are absorbed by different mechanisms. All forms of dietary iron are absorbed in the duodenum and upper jejunum where the contents are acidic.

Heme iron is bound to proteins released by acid and proteases in the stomach. Ferrous iron in the heme is oxidized to ferric iron and heme is converted to hemin which is absorbed as such without interaction with other dietary factors and without any regulatory mechanisms. The enterocytes—lining cells of the small intestine play a crucial role in iron absorption. Heme enters the enterocytes with the aid of heme receptors. It is degraded into free iron, bilirubin and carbon monoxide by the action of heme oxygenase.

Non-heme iron is present as green vegetables, fruits and cereals. Non-heme iron is released from food by the action of acid either in the ferrous or ferric state. Iron is absorbed only in the ionic state. In the alkaline pH of the duodenum, ferric iron salts are insoluble whereas ferrous iron is soluble. Therefore, most of the absorbed iron is in the ferrous form. Absorption of iron is influenced and moderated to a great extent by the availability of iron stores and the need of the body.

Passage into the Gut-epithelium and Circulation

The enterocytes which line the epithelium of duodenum and upper jejunum play a major role. Brush border cells of upper small intestine, divalent metal transporters receptors on the surface facilitating absorption of iron. Absorption occurs in 3 stages:

1. Entry of iron into the apical cell membrane
2. Intracellular processing of the iron and transfer to the basolateral membrane
3. Transfer of the requisite amount of iron through the basolateral membrane into the portal circulation.

The enterocyte regulates the entry of iron into it and transport across it to the portal circulation. When enterocytes are shed after their lifespan of 2–3 days the iron contained within them are lost in feces.

At the brush border of the enterocyte, the ferric iron is reduced to ferrous iron by a ***ferri reductase enzyme***. Iron in the enterocyte is transported to the basal region by the iron transporter ***ferroportin***. The function of ferroportin is controlled by ***hepcidin*** which is primary iron regulatory hormone which inhibits the action of ferroportin. Higher levels of hepcidin inhibit iron transport across the enterocyte and vice versa.

At the base of enterocyte, the iron is released into the circulation, it is oxidized to ferric form by a ferroxidase hephaestin, the iron is bound by transferrin for transport to iron utilizing tissues. Hephaestin has similarities to ceruloplasmin. Hephaestin levels in circulation are inversely related to the rate of iron release from the enterocytes.

Iron entering the enterocyte is either temporarily stored in the cell or transported across the basolateral membrane to the capillary network. The fate of the iron entering the enterocyte depends on the availability of body stores and the body's need for iron.

Factors Participating in Iron Metabolism

Hemoglobin: Each molecule of hemoglobin has a central ferrous iron to which oxygen is loosely attached. Each molecule of hemoglobin contains 0.34% iron by weight, i.e. 1 mL of packed erythrocytes contain 1 mg of iron. Major portion of the absorbed iron is used for the formation of hemoglobin.

Hemosiderin: It is a form of storage iron seen mainly in the monocyte-macrophage system in small amounts normally but in higher amounts in iron overload states. It is composed mainly of ferric hydroxide crystals which are deprived of their apoferritin coat. It contains 25–30% of iron by weight. It is demonstrable by Pearl's staining. Hemosiderin is not readily available for iron recycling even though smaller amounts of iron can be extracted for further use by reticuloendothelial cells. In large amount, as seen in iron overload phase it leads to tissue destruction and organ damage, e.g. hemosiderosis, hemochromotosis and others. Parenchymal tissues of the liver, heart, pancreas, testis and endocrine glands may be affected and this leads to organ dysfunction.

Ferritin: Free iron is toxic to cells. It has to be combined with apoferritin to form ferritin the form in which it is stored in cells. This iron is freely available for further utilization. Ferritin is an alpha-2-globin which binds iron. It is a compound formed from apoferritin and ferric hydroxide $[Fe(OH)_3]$. It is a very efficient storage form of iron. Ferritin contain two types of monomers—the light (L-monomer) and the heavy (H-monomer). The L-monomer which is basic, binds very readily and tightly to iron. This property makes it suitable for storing iron. L-monomer-rich ferritin is seen mainly in the liver, spleen and serum. L-monomer is in excess of H-monomer. H-monomer which is acidic takes up and releases iron readily. It is found in the heart, kidney, placenta, monocytes, lymphocytes and erythrocytes. There are 20 isofoms of ferritin. Apart from its storage function, ferritin has a role in metal detoxification and diversion of excess iron. Unbound iron is toxic to tissues, since it causes free-radical injury. The level of apoferritin in blood regulates the absorption of dietary iron.

Transferrin: It is the most dynamic part of the iron-metabolic chain. It is a glycoprotein which binds to ferric iron and can exist in monoferric or diferric forms. It is synthesized in the liver as apotransferrin. By combining with iron, it becomes transferrin. Its rate of synthesis is inversely proportional to the iron stores.

Transfer time from transferrin to erythyroid marrow cells is only 10–15 minutes in the presence of iron deficiency. Plasma iron is 80–100 μg/dL. Within the erythyroid cell, iron in excess of the quantity required for hemoglobin synthesis combines with apoferritin and is stored as ferritin. This happens in the liver parenchymal as well. This storage iron in the erythyroid cell is released into circulation only when the erythrocytes dies and its contents are released. This storage iron is made available for further hemoglobin synthesis. Inflammatory conditions can impair iron release from iron stores and therefore lead to iron deficiency anemia (IDA).

Transferrin receptor (TfR): These are transmembrane glycoproteins which exist in two forms TfR1 and TfR2. They both bind to transferrin. TfR1 has high affinity, TfR2 has only low affinity. TfR1 binds to plasma transferrin and delivers it to the erythroblasts. The TfR1 transferrin complex is internalized into the erythroblast via an endocytic vesicle. In the cell, the iron dissociates from the complex—the iron is delivered to the cytoplasm and the TfR1 goes back to the cell surface. All cells in the body have TfRs on their surface, but maximum number (80%) is on erythroblasts.

TfR2 which has low affinity to transferrin is seen mostly in hepatocytes and erythroid cells. It has also a role in regulating iron metabolism. Most tissues regulate their iron content by modulating TfR expression. Truncated portions of TfR are shed into the circulation. These can be estimated using laboratory kits as serum transferrin receptor (sTfR). Concentration of sTfR is directly proportional to the rate of erythropoiesis. In IDA, sTfR levels are high, whereas they are low in anemia of chronic disease.

Mobiliferrin: This is a cytosolic protein that transports iron across the enterocytes and other cells in the body. It is also responsible for receiving iron from transferrin which transports iron in the plasma.

Ferroportin and hephaestin: Ferroportin is the protein that helps to transport the iron that enters the terminal border of the enterocyte to the basal region. Hephaestin is a ferrioxidase which converts the ferrous iron transported by the enterocyte and released at the basal part of the cell into the ferric form to be bound by transferrin.

Hereditary Hemochromatosis Gene Product (HHGP): Human hemochromatosis protein (HFE) binds transferrin receptor with an affinity equaling that of transferrin and competes with transferrin binding. HHGP might facilitate the sensing of the need for iron absorption across the enterocyte. In hereditary hemochromatosis, there is decrease in the amount of functional HHGP protein.

Hepcidin: It is an iron regulating hormone which controls the passage of iron absorbed by the enterocyte to the basal part to be released into the circulation. Higher levels of hepcidin impairs the action of ferroportin and thus inhibits iron absorption. In iron deficiency states, hepcidin levels are low and therefore, iron absorption is accelerated. This is a newly identified iron regulator that appears to communicate the status of the body's iron stores and the demand for erythropoiesis to the enterocytes and thereby regulate iron absorption. Hepcidin levels are low in iron overload and high in iron deficiency.

The absorption and utilization of iron which are complex processes can be summarized as given below:

- Absorption of ferrous iron through the apical membrane of the enterocyte. The rate of absorption depends directly on the level of apoferritin in blood.
- Transport across the enterocyte. The iron that is absorbed is either stored in the enterocyte or transported across the basolateral membrane to the circulation as an active process. The cells lining the intestinal crypts (base of the villi) act as sensors of the iron status of the body.
- Transferrin transports the iron in ferric form in the circulation and delivers it to cells, with the aid of TfR.
- Most of the iron is utilized for heme synthesis in erythroblasts. Iron is also taken up by macrophages by the process of erythrophagocytosis. This iron in the macrophages does not re-enter the circulation.

- Excretion of iron occurs through shedding of enterocytes, exfoliation of skin, sweat and urine. Loss of blood from the body contributes to the major source of blood loss.

Development of Iron Deficiency

The bioavailability of iron in the average Indian diet is low. Milk is a poor source of iron and hence, babies fed solely on unfortified milk develop iron deficiency within 6–12 months. Iron from animal foods is absorbed better (11–22%) than that from vegetable sources (1–7%). Animal proteins and vitamin C enhance iron absorption, while phytates and phosphates retard it. Iron is absorbed from the duodenum and upper jejunum. Iron is lost in desquamated epithelial cells of the gastrointestinal tract (GIT), urinary tract and skin and through the loss of nails and hair. Menstruation, pregnancy, parturition and lactation account for further losses in women who suffer from iron deficiency more than men. Dietary requirement is higher for women. Daily requirement is 10–20 mg for men and 30–40 mg for women. Infants require 1 mg/kg bw.

Considerable periods elapse between the onset of iron deficiency and the clinical manifestations. Since, large stores are present normally, clinical symptoms do not occur till the stores have been depleted. Pure nutritional deficiency manifests clinically only a few years after institution of a diet poor in iron. In actual practice, anemia manifests much sooner since, in the vast majority of cases there is also concomitant blood loss.

In India, about 20–40% of pregnant women show iron deficiency. Depletion of iron in the mother during pregnancy results in diminution of iron stores in the fetus. Premature infants have lower iron stores and are vulnerable to develop iron deficiency states.

Effects of Iron Deficiency

Iron deficiency state manifests in different stages. The earliest stage is depletion of iron stores, during which time the condition is asymptomatic. The second stage is one of tissue iron deficiency. At this stage symptoms such as pica, sideropenic dysphagia and koilonychia may develop. Subtle disturbances of function of many organ systems can be detected.

At this stage, general symptoms such as fatigability disinclination for work, poor mentation in children and diminished performance at school are common. Often these are overlooked and therefore many cases go on to more severe forms of iron deficiency. The third stage is one of IDA. Microcytic hypochromic anemia occurs on account of diminished hemoglobin synthesis. Non-hematological manifestations include koilonychia, dysphagia, glossitis and rarely raised intracranial tension.

Iron deficiency is one of the most widespread nutritional disorders present all over the world.

Siderosis

Siderosis denotes excessive accumulation of iron which is seen in persons who have excessive intake of iron over prolonged periods. The iron is deposited in the liver, which may undergo fibrosis. Excessive dietary intake occurs in South African Bantus who ingest about 100 mg of iron derived from iron cooking and brewing pots. Iron overload can occur in persons having thalassemia, sickle cell disease or aplastic anemia, who are repeatedly transfused with blood (usually more than 100 transfusions). Iron absorption is very high in hemochromatosis and thalassemia and sickle cell disease. When excess of inorganic iron is ingested (as in excessive consumption of iron tablets or intoxicating drinks brewed in iron pots) the iron absorbed exceeds the capacity of transferrin saturation leading to deposition of iron in several parenchymal tissues such as cardiac myocytes (siderosis). Elimination of iron can be enhanced by chelating agents such as desferrioxamine.

Note: Refer to the topics nutritional anemias (Ch 160), hemochromatosis (Ch 94) and thalassemias (Ch 161).

Prevention

Vulnerable groups of persons require prophylactic iron supplementation. These include premature infants, persons after upper GIT surgery and bariatric surgery, pregnant and lactating women and those with chronic blood loss.

At the community level, iron deficiency can be prevented by fortifying food with iron. Several articles like bread and infant foods have been fortified in many countries. The Indian Council of Medical Research (ICMR) has suggested fortification of cooking salt with iron. Initial field trials are encouraging.

Trace elements in nutrition

- Those elements which occur or function in living tissues in concentrations most conveniently expressed in µg/L are included under this term.
- Arbitrarily, the term 'trace' has been applied to concentrations of element not exceeding 250 µg/g of extracellular matrix.
- Essential trace elements include iodine, zinc, selenium, copper, molybdenum, chromium, cobalt and iron.
- Trace elements that are probably essential include manganese, nickel, silicon, boron and vanadium.
- Some of the trace elements which are toxic when given in higher doses include fluoride, lead, cadmium, mercury, arsenic, lithium, tin and aluminum.

IODINE

(Also Refer to Section 11, Ch 99)

Iodine is widespread in nature and it is obtained especially from sea water, salt, sea fish, vegetables, drinking water and milk. The daily requirement is about 150–250 µg. Adolescents and adults require about 150 µg iodine daily. For pregnant and lactating women, the requirement goes up to 200 µg/day. Two billion individuals worldwide suffer from iodine deficiency. More than 400 million people are affected in Asia alone. In India, such goiter belts occur in the foothills of the Himalayas, several parts of northern India and midlands and highlands of Kerala. In man and animals, chronic iodine deficiency produces characteristic responses.

Iodide is rapidly and wholly absorbed from the stomach and duodenum. Seventy five percent of orally ingested iodide is absorbed intact. In conditions of adequate iodine nutrition, 10% or less of absorbed iodine is taken up by the thyroid gland. Vegetables produced in iodine deficient areas have lower levels of iodine. Iodine is concentrated by

Table 32.1: Iodine deficiency disorders

Fetus	Neonate	Infant/child/adolescent	Adult
Spontaneous abortions	Goiter	Goiter	Goiter and its compilations
Stillbirths	Overt or subclinical hypothyroidism	Subclinical or overt hypothyroidism	Hypothyroidism. Endemic mental retardation
Congenital anomalies	Cretinism	Mental retardation	Decreased fertility
Increased perinatal and infant mortality		Retarded physical development	Spontaneous hyperthyroidism in the elderly
Endemic cretinism		Increased susceptibility of the thyroid gland to nuclear radiation	Increased susceptibility of the thyroid gland to nuclear radiation

the thyroid gland for the formation of thyroid hormones. A healthy adult contains 15–20 mg iodine, 70–80% being in the thyroid [65% weight of thyroglobulin (T_4) and 59% of triiodothyronine (T_3) respectively]. Thyroid enlargement is the classic sign of iodine deficiency. Calcium retards absorption of iodine.

Iodine deficiency leads to inadequate production of thyroid hormones and these cause diseases. A wide spectrum of iodine deficiency disorders are seen depending on the age of onset (Table 32.1).

Goitrogens cause adverse effects on the thyroid in the presence of iodine deficiency. Commonly occurring goitrogens (seen mainly in cattle and other experimental animals) include vegetables like cabbage, broccoli, other leafy vegetables, cauliflower, cassava and others if consumed in large quantities over long periods. Zinc salts interfere with absorption of iodine in the duodenum.

Iodine deficiency is the single most important and prevalent cause of preventable brain damage. During pregnancy, the fetus does not produce thyroxine during the first trimester and it is entirely dependent on maternal thyroxine. During the subsequent two trimesters it derives thyroxine from its own thyroid and it is supplemented by maternal thyroxine. Maternal thyroxin constitutes 20–40% of the total thyroxin in cord blood. In endemic iodine-deficient areas, the maternal and fetal thyroid function is subnormal. Provision of iodine supplements to the mother even in the latter half of pregnancy persists the ill effects in fetus.

Assessment of iodine nutrition in the community is done by—urinary iodide, goiter, thyroid stimulating hormone (TSH) in the newborn and blood thyroglobulin levels.

World Health Organization (WHO) recommends that the total goiter rate can be used to define severity of iodine deficiency in populations using the following criteria:

Below 5%	—	Iodine sufficiency
5.0–19.9%	—	Mild deficiency
20.0–29.9%	—	Moderate deficiency
> 30%	—	Severe deficiency

Goitrous Cretinism

It is common in iodine deficiency areas. The cretinism take two forms—(1) neurological and (2) myxedematous. Prevention of iodine deficiency disorders has been achieved to some extent in India and other countries by fortification of common salt with potassium iodide at the rate of 60 ppm. The aim is to give 150 µg iodine daily.

Another intervention is to give an annual injection of iodized oil (IM) to susceptible population at risk. Poppy

Table 32.2: Results of 'iodine deficiency disorder survey' carried out in seven states in India from 1999–2006. Proportion of households consuming adequate amounts of iodized salts are given below

States	Given in percentage
Jharkhand	64.2
Bihar	40.1
Orissa	45.0
Goa	91.9
Tamil Nadu	18.2
Kerala	48.2
Rajasthan	42.1

seed oil and rapeseed oil have been used as vehicles. **Brassidol** which is derived from rapeseed oil contains 376 mg/mL of iodine. Early goiters will also recede with iodine supplementations.

Recommendation for iodine intake	
Infants (0–12 months)	110–130 µg
Children (6–12 years)	120 µg
Children (> 12 years and adults)	150 µg
Pregnancy	250 µg
Lactation	250 µg

At times, iodine supplementation in the community has been associated with adverse effects. These include hyperthyroidism autonomous thyroid nodules and possibly autoimmune thyroiditis.

Iodine induced hyperthyroidism (IIH) syn: Jod Basedow phenomenon. This is caused by the increased proliferation of thyrocytes and increase in the mutation rates of the cells. This leads to hyperthyroidism.

Despite minor adverse effects, iodine supplementation has served to reduce iodine-deficiency disorders, especially brain dysfunction in the young. Strong political lobbies working against the 'universal iodization of salt' program have resulted in slowing the progress in this direction (*See* also Ch 99). ***21st October is the WHO iodine deficiency disorders day***.

FLUORINE

Fluorine is present in small amounts in human bones and teeth. Fluoride is obtained from drinking water, tea and sea fish. Water sources are more important. Daily requirement is 1–2 mg. Fluoride is deposited in the enamel of developing teeth. Once the teeth are fully developed, fluoride is not further incorporated. Low levels of fluoride in drinking water are associated with higher prevalence of dental caries. In many countries, addition of 1 ppm fluoride to drinking water has served to reduce the incidence of dental caries. Such a legislation does not exist in India. On the other hand in many parts of India, drinking water contains higher amounts of fluoride and this leads to fluorosis. Increase in the content of fluoride in drinking water above 100–150 mg/L gives rise to acute toxic symptoms consisting of nausea, vomiting, diarrhea, abdominal pain and paresthesia. Death may occur at times.

Note: Refer Section—Fluorosis.

COPPER

Copper is widespread in all foods and hence, dietary deficiency of copper is very rare. Copper is necessary for the proper formation of hemoglobin and several enzymes. Normal serum copper levels range from 11 to 26 μmol/L.

Young children fed solely on milk may develop copper deficiency. The main features include anemia, neutropenia and retardation of growth and rarefaction of bones.

Daily requirement is 2–3 mg. Meat, liver, shellfish, nut seeds, legumes and whole grains contain copper. Copper takes part in the synthesis of hemoglobin in association with iron. It is an integral part of several oxidative enzymes.

Absorption and Metabolism

Copper is absorbed in the upper part of the small intestine and is transported into the epithelial cells through the medium of a copper transporting protein. The copper is incorporated into the intracellular enzymes such as superoxide dismutase, cytochrome oxidase and others. Excess copper is fixed to the Golgi apparatus and eliminated when the epithelial cell is shed.

Copper reaches the hepatocytes, bound to albumin. In the hepatocytes, copper is bound to ceruloplasmin and in this bound form copper circulates in blood. Excess copper, unbound to ceruloplasmin is excreted by the hepatocytes into bile. Both these processes are facilitated by the copper transporting protein.

Normal ceruloplasmin level in blood is 20–40 mg/dL. It is low in Wilson's disease in which the production is normal, but its degradation is accelerated. In Wilson's disease, the levels of plasma ceruloplasmin are below 20 mg/dL. Normal level of hepatic copper is below 55 mg/g of dry weight. In Wilson's disease, the hepatic copper level may exceed 250 mg/g. Other conditions in which ceruloplasmin levels are low include nutritional hypoproteinemia, nephrotic syndrome, hepatic diseases and congenital ceruloplasmin deficiency. The major regulating mechanism in copper homeostasis is the excretion of excess into bile, which is 1–2 mg/day.

Nutritional deficiency of copper may occur in premature infants, generalized malnutrition, malabsorption states and prolonged parenteral nutrition. Nutritional supplementation is by giving copper sulphate 2–3 mg tds orally.

Reduction or absence of ceruloplasmin is a genetic abnormality which leads to Wilson's disease. Wilson's disease is an autosomal recessive disorder.

Menkes disease is an X-linked disease affecting the copper metabolism. It is characterized by features resembling Ehlers-Danlos syndrome. Serum ceruloplasmin is low. ***Clinical features*** include mental retardation, abnormalities in bone formation, lability of temperature regulation, susceptibility to develop infections, cutis laxa and tendency to develop vascular rupture. Death occurs in early life.

Note: Refer to Wilsons' diseases (*See* Chapters 94, 203).

MAGNESIUM

(*See* also Ch 72)

This is the fourth most abundant cation in the body, next only to sodium, potassium and calcium. It is the second most prevalent intracellular cation. The importance of magnesium in health and disease has been bought out by recent studies.

- Total body content—1000 mmol (22.6 g)
- Distribution—50–60% in bone
- The rest is intracellular in all tissues
- Extracellular part 1%
- Serum levels 0.75–0.95 mmol/L, i.e. 1.7–2.2 mg/dL
- Dietary intake 300–350 mg/day
- Absorption from gut is by passive diffusion.

The total body content is determined by the balance between intestinal absorption and urinary loss. It is absorbed by a process of passive diffusion, which is a self-limiting process. The rate of absorption is inversely proportional to the intake.

Dietary sources include a wide range of food, especially cereals, animal food and water.

Functions of Magnesium

- Integral part of several enzymes participating in adenosinetriphosphate (ATP) and deoxyribonucleic acid (DNA) metabolism
- Stabilization of cell membranes
- Neural transmission
- Stabilizing calcium channel activity

Both hypomagnesemia and hypermagnesemia cause adverse effects. The former is more common. These are described in Section 7.

ZINC

Zinc is present in many enzymes. Highest concentration occurs in the liver, voluntary muscle, bone, prostate and occular structures. Foods such as meat, fish, peas and cereals contain zinc. Daily requirement is not clearly known, but is around 15 mg. Normal zinc levels in serum is 9.8–29.7 μmol/L. Dietary deficiency is very rare. Zinc deficiency leads to impairment of maturation and immunodeficiency. In malnourished subjects, zinc deficiency may result in thymic atrophy. A syndrome of dwarfism and hypogonadism seen in Egypt and Iran has been attributed to zinc deficiency. Oral zinc sulfate corrected this clinical picture. Acrodermatitis enteropathica is an inherited disorder resulting from the malabsorption of zinc, probably due to an enzymic defect. Administration of zinc sulfate 30–150 mg/day results in complete remission. Oral zinc sulfate 100 mg/day has been found to stimulate the growth of granulation tissue in chronic ulcers. Oral supplementation of zinc 10 mg (5 mg) in children less than 1 year of age for 16 months reduced overall cause mortality by 7%. This study is being pursued.

Source: Sazawal S, Black RE, Ramsan M, et al. Effect of zinc supplementation on mortality in children aged 1-48 months: a community-based randomised placebo-controlled trial. Lancet. 2007;369(9565):927-34.

SELENIUM

Selenium is a constituent of selenoprotein. It has structural and enzyme roles and it acts as an important antioxidant. Other functions include: (1) Proper functioning of the immune system, (2) sperm motility, (3) maintenance of proper mood and mental state and (4) resistance against cancer. Selenium retards the progress of acquired immunodeficiency syndrome (AIDS). It is a catalyst for the production of thyroid hormone. In the body, highest concentration of selenium is in the thyroid gland. Supplementation with 80–200 µg selenium per day protects against Hashimoto's thyroiditis. Daily requirement of selenium is 60 mcg/day for men and 52.3 µg/day for women. Dietary sources includes Brazil nuts, kidney, crab, liver, shellfish, fish, meat, poultry, wheat and some vegetables. In animal foods, selenium is present as selenocysteine. In vegetable sources it occurs as selenomethionine.

In infections, oral supplementation of selenium to raise serum selenium to 135 µg/L has led to better recovery rates and reduction of mortality.

Keshan disease which was described in 1935 as an outbreak of fatal cardiomyopathy in Keshan and neighboring counties of north eastern China and later in 1960 when the disease affected other parts of China showed extensive patchy necrosis and fibrosis of the myocardium, associated with low selenium levels. Selenium deficiency has been shown to exacerbate the cardiomyopathy of Chagas disease. Selenium deficiency has been implicated in disorders of the immune system.

Source: Loscalzo J. Keshan disease, selenium deficiency, and the selenoproteome. N Engl J Med. 2014;370(18):1756-60.

Probiotics and Prebiotics

Microorganisms especially bacteria can be used to improve health. A bacterium which confers specific health benefits in addition to nutritional improvement is known as probiotic. Yoghurt and butter milk are examples. They contain lactobacilli such as *Lactobacillus rhamnosus, L. reuteri, L. casei* and others which help to stop diarrhea, especially after rotavirus infection. Prebiotics are non-digestible food ingredients which selectively affect the gut flora and benefit the host.

CHAPTER
33

Obesity

KV Krishna Das

Chapter Summary

- General Considerations
- Etiology
- Clinical Features
  - Complications
  - Course and prognosis
- Diagnosis
- Treatment
  - Dietary Regulation
  - Drugs
- Total starvation
- Surgical measures
  - Bariatric surgical techniques

GENERAL CONSIDERATIONS

The term obesity has come from the Latin word ***'obesus'*** which means ***'stout or plump'***. Increase in body weight of 10–20% above the normal, caused by excess accumulation of fat is termed obesity. Healthy young men and women have a total body fat content below 20–25% respectively. When excess calories are supplied in any form, they are stored as fat. In addition to general appearance and weight, measurement of skin fold thickness over the biceps, triceps, subscapular and suprailiac regions is helpful in the assessment of obesity. The skin fold thickness over the triceps for normal Indian subjects is below 20 mm. The proportion of body fat can be assessed from the skin fold thickness using nomograms. Obesity has become the sixth common cause for disease burden worldwide. Adipose tissue in the body, in addition to its role as a source of stored energy, is emerging as an endocrine organ producing hormone and cytokines. In general, the ideal weight of an individual should be (height in cm minus 100) kg. For example, an adult male 175 cm tall should have a weight of 75 kg ± 5% owing.

Body Mass Index (BMI)

Body weight is only a crude indicator of obesity. A more reliable parameter is the BMI (Fig. 33.1).

$$BMI = \frac{(Weight\ in\ Kg)}{(Height\ in\ m^2)}$$ For Asians, separate norms have been proposed (Table 33.1).

In 2008, 1.46 billion people globally were overweight (BMI > 25 kg/m²) and 502 million were obese (BMI > 30 kg/m²). Furthermore, 170 million children were estimated to be

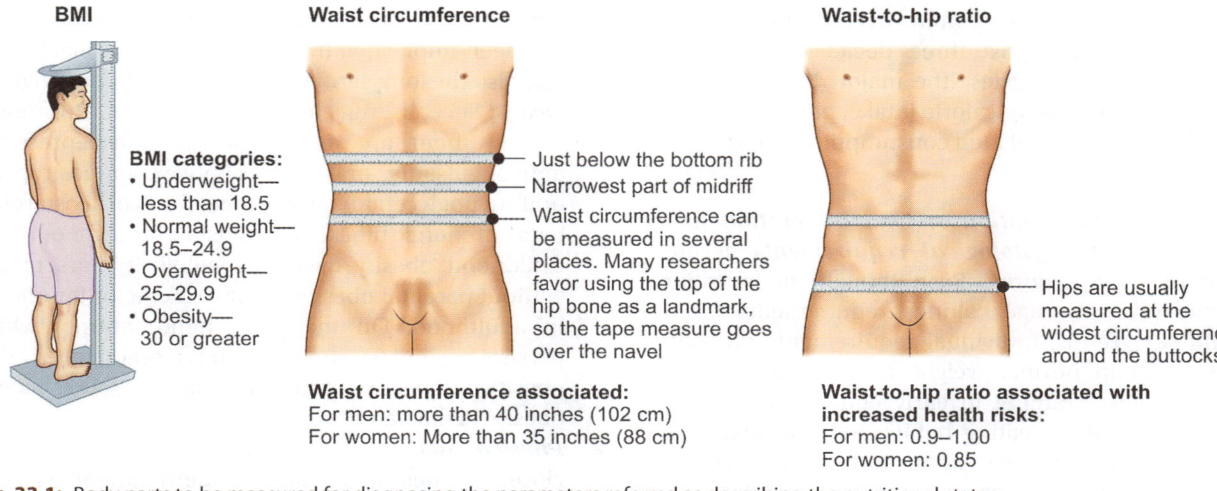

Fig. 33.1: Body parts to be measured for diagnosing the parameters referred as describing the nutritional status

Table 33.1: Shows the recommended values for BMI

Weight class	Global	Asians*
Normal	18.5–24.5	18.5–22.9
Overweight	25–29.9	23–24.9
Obese	> 30	>25
Severely obese	> 40	

*Note: Association of Physicians of India guidelines for Indian college of Physicians Jan 2009, Supplement.

overweight or obese. Obesity is increasing rapidly in the lower income groups. About 10% of the population in India is obese. Small community-based surveys done in several parts of the country give figures ranging from 17 to 38% BMI above 28 is associated with higher incidence of strokes, ischemic heart disease and diabetes mellitus (DM). The distribution of fat deposition in the body is also important. For this purpose, the circumference at the waist and the hip are taken as reference measurements. Waist is measured after an overnight fast at the midpoint between the lower costal margin and iliac crest. Hip is the widest part over the gluteal region. Waist hip ratio above 1.0 in men and above 0.9 in women is an independent risk factor for higher incidence of insulin resistance, hypertension, rise in low-density lipoprotein (LDL), lower levels of high-density lipoprotein (HDL), hyperuricemia, cardiovascular disease, type 2 diabetes, stroke and several cancers. Obesity has overtaken tobacco as a major preventable cause of disease burden. Less time to sleep or impaired sleep quality have important effects on weight gain. Heritability of BMI is generally cited as 40–70%. Obese persons have 30% more healthcare costs than non-obese persons. Ideal waist to hip ratio is below 0.85 in men and 0.75 in women. The waist circumference above 102 cm is an independent risk factor. Abdominal obesity with accumulation of fat in the abdominal viscera is more associated with metabolic complications. The waist/hip ratio shows a graded and highly significant direct relationship with the risk for myocardial infarction.

Health risk	Women	Men
Low-risk	Below 31.5 inches	Below 37 inches
Moderate-risk	31.5–35 inches	37–40 inches
High-risk	35 inches or more	40.2 inches or more

	BMI category		
Waist circumference	Normal 18.5–24.9 kg/m²	Overweight 25–29.9 kg/m²	Obese class I 30–34.9 kg/m²
Men: < 102 cm Women: < 88 cm	Least risk	Increased risk	High-risk
Men: < 102 cm Women: < 88 cm	Increased risk	High-risk	Very high-risk

Every additional gain of 5 kg /m² in BMI increase the risk of esophageal cancer by 52%, colon cancer by 24%, in women endometrial cancer by 59%, gallbladder by 59% and post-menopausal breast cancer by 12%. Other disorders more prevalent in obesity include benign prostatic hypertrophy, infertility, asthma, sleep apnea and risk of congenital abnormalities in fetus.

Global regional and national prevalence of overweight and obesity in children and adults during 1980–2013 a systematic analysis for the Global Burden of Disease Study 2013.

Source: Ng M, Fleming T, Robinson M, et al. Global, regional, and national prevalence of overweight and obesity in children and adults during 1980-2013: a systematic analysis for the Global Burden of Disease Study 2013. Lancet. 2014;384(9945):766-81.

The data figures for India subcontinent is given in the Table 33.2.

Obesity

Table 33.2: Prevalence of overweight and obesity

	Boys < 20 years		Men ≥ 20 years		Girls < 20 years		Women ≥ 20 years	
	Overweight and obese	Obese	Overweight and obese	Obese	Overweight and obese	Obese	Overweight and obese	Obese
India	5.3 (4.3–6.4)	2.3 (1.8–2.8)	19.5 (17.8–21.2)	3.7 (3.3–4.1)	5.2 (4.2–6.4)	2.5 (1.9–3.1)	20.7 (18.9–22.5)	4.2 (3.8–4.8)

Prevalence of obesity and overweight has risen substantially in the past three decades with marked variations across countries. The major determinants for this reason are excessive caloric intake, physical inactivity and active promotion of food consumption by industry.

Etiology

- **Excessive consumption of food in relation to the individual's physiological requirements** accounts for the vast majority. Even though the nutritional table gives average calories requirements for age and sex groups, individual requirements of calories to maintain normal weight varies widely between individuals. Training in early childhood and social factors influence eating habits. Both in anxiety and depression, excessive eating may be resorted to. It is not uncommon to develop obesity after recent bereavement or change of job. An increase of 0.5% in food consumption above the optimal caloric intake can lead to an annual rise in weight of 1 kg. Pregnancy and contraceptive pills tend to predispose to obesity. Persons show strong genetic predisposition to obesity and the amount of food leading to obesity varies widely between subjects. Therefore, prescription of dietary management has also to be individualized.

- **Hormonal and other factors:** Obesity may be part of the clinical pictures of well-known endocrine disorders such as type 2 diabetes, hypothyroidism, Cushing's syndrome, gigantism, acromegaly, insulinomas and others. In addition, several hormones regulate appetite and modulate intake of food and fat accumulation. Insulin and cholecystokinin acting on the central nervous system (CNS) retard the appetite regulating mechanism.

- **Genetic factors** do play a role. Metabolically, some individuals are more efficient in conserving energy and thus they put on fat, while others require more energy for the same amount of work performed. Moreover, obesity may run in families.

  Role of leptins: There is strong evidence that body fat is biologically regulated. Most cases of obesity probably reflect a multigenetic predisposition for excess intake of food, low level of physical activity and accumulation of excess amounts of fat. Leptin encoded by the Lcp gene is a cytokine–like molecule synthesized and secreted by adipose tissue in proportion to adipose tissue mass. It has several biological effects, an important one being reduction of food intake. Leptin deficiency leads to hyperphagia, obesity and several endocrine abnormalities such as infertility, diabetes, reduction in metabolism, impairment of somatic growth and elevated levels of glucocorticoids. Leptin deficiency and resistance to leptin may be genetically determined.

  Several other hormones also influence food intake and body weight. A gut hormone fragment peptide-Y3-36 (pYY) reduces appetite by acting on the appetite centers in the hypothalamus.

  Ghrelin: It is a hormone primarily secreted by the stomach and duodenum. Plasma ghrelin levels are higher before meals and their levels fall after meals. It has been implicated in causing hunger at meal times and also the long-term maintenance of body weight.

  Drugs: Several drugs lead to weight gain. Prominent among them are antipsychotics, anti-depressants anticonvulsants, oral contraceptives, progestrogens, oral hypoglycemic agents, insulin, corticosteroids, beta adrenergic blockers, antihistamines and others. Childhood obesity occurring below 3 years of age without parental obesity is not a risk factor for obesity in adulthood. On the other hand, obesity which persists beyond 6 years of age, it is a predictor of adult obesity irrespective of the parental status. Presence of obesity in the parents doubles the risk.

- **Physical activity** which causes loss of calories is closely related to obesity. Modern amenities such as automobiles and lifts which tend to minimize day-to-day physical exertion favor the development of obesity. Obesity is more evident when there is a sudden cessation of physical activity. Eating habits are also influenced by physical work. Moderate work is associated with optimal food intake whereas both physical inactivity and overexertion lead to overeating.

- **Alcohol** being a good source of non-diet calories tends to aggravate obesity in the mild and moderate alcoholics. Cessation of smoking leads to recovery of appetite and gain in weight.

- **Pathology:** Obese subjects have increase of both fat and non-fat mass. In obesity developing from childhood, there is probably increase in the number of fat cells and a generalized increase in adipose tissue.

  In others, there is hypertrophy of the fat cells. Distribution of obesity may be android (abdomen and shoulder predominantly) or gynoid (buttocks, thighs, breasts, arm and face predominantly). Obesity leads to impairment of carbohydrate tolerance, elevation of cholesterol level in blood and mild elevation of blood pressure.

  It predisposes to premature atherosclerosis. Obesity is associated with an absolute increase in energy expenditure, lower respiratory quotient and insulin-resistance. Though obese subjects have to spend more energy for the same amount of work done by their normal counterparts, they tend to restrict their physical activity further and accumulate more fat.

CLINICAL FEATURES

Only few children are born obese—obesity seen in early childhood commonly disappears later. Middle-aged persons are more affected though no age is immune. Women outnumber men and the male to female ratio is 1:5. Multiparity is associated with increasing grades of obesity. The patient may not complain of her obesity on account of its gradual development and therefore, it has to be identified during general examination. Common symptoms include exertional dyspnea, sluggishness, angina, arthralgias of knees and hips or any of the complications.

Complications: These develop invariably in all cases depending on the severity and duration of the disorder.

Textbook of Medicine

- ***Ill-effects of increased weight:*** Slowness of movement, proneness to falls and accidents, osteoarthritis of weight-bearing joints like knees, hips and spine.
- ***Skin:*** Abnormal skin folds develop and these give rise to fungal infection (moniliasis), recurrent bacterial infections and chafing of the skin of the thighs and axillae. In extreme obesity, striae may develop.
- ***Cardiovascular system:*** Atherosclerosis, hypercholesterolemia, angina, ischemic heart disease, hypertension, varicose veins, venous thrombosis and recurrent embolism. Hypertension is due to increase in cardiac output and heart rate. Increase of 10% of weight above the ideal weight leads to 30% rise in the risk of heart disease. Mortality is lowest between BMI of 20–24.9.
- ***Respiratory system:*** Exertional dyspnea, reduction in vital capacity due to restriction of diaphragmatic movements and the increased mechanical effort required to move the thoracic cage, recurrent bronchitis and in extreme cases, respiratory failure. 'Pickwickian syndrome' is the condition where obesity is associated with central depression of respiration and somnolence. Sleep apnea and the related complications are more common in them (Figs 33.2 and 33.3).

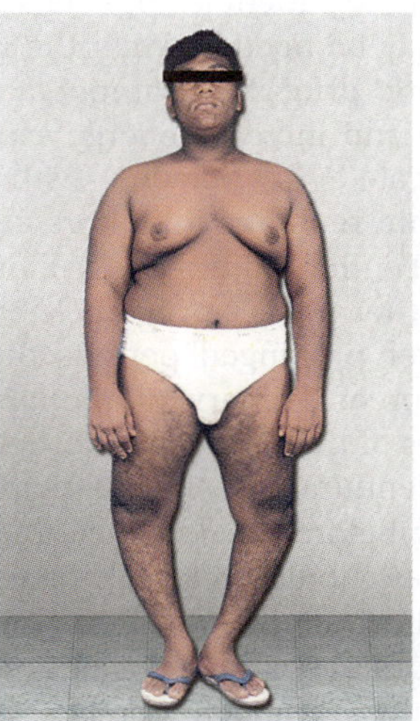

Fig. 33.2: Nutritional obesity boy aged 18 years

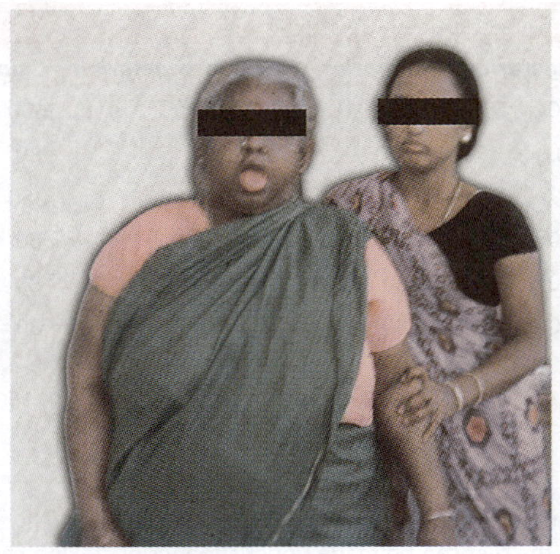

Fig. 33.3: Morbid obesity: Woman aged 50 years

- ***Abdomen:*** The skin over the anterior abdominal wall hangs down as a fold (abdominal apron). Hernias develop owing to the increase in the intra-abdominal pressure. Gallbladder lesions are more common.
- ***Metabolic complications:*** DM, hyperlipidemias, gout and cholesterol gallstones are more common. The deadly quartet of obesity is contributed to by: (1) Insulin resistance, (2) overweight and (3) dyslipidemias and hypertension, all forming part of the metabolic syndrome.

Central obesity or upper body fat distribution is more harmful than obesity of the other parts. Normally, adipose tissue undergoes lipolysis and release of free fatty acids (FFAs) and glycerol into the circulation which provides 50 to 100% of daily energy needs. This lipolysis is inhibited mainly by insulin and stimulated by catecholamines. Upper body obesity is associated with many abnormalities of adipose tissue lipolysis, most significant being increased concentration of FFA due to its increase in postprandial release.

- ***Psychological abnormalities:*** Obese persons may develop depression because of their unattractive physical appearance and mechanical disability. They tend to avoid company and become socially isolated.
- There is evidence that cancer of the colon, breast, uterus, ovaries and prostate may be more common in the obese. Obesity is the biggest preventable cause for cancer next after tobacco smoking.

Course and prognosis: The condition is gradual in its progress. Complications increase the mortality in them. Mortality rate is 30% higher in people 25–30% overweight and 50% higher in persons 35–40% overweight. Death is caused by cardiovascular, metabolic or respiratory complications. Obesity is an independent risk factor for higher mortality.

DIAGNOSIS

Clinical diagnosis is based on weight, physical appearance and measurement of skin fold thickness. Sophisticated methods are available to establish the diagnosis in a borderline case. Dual energy X-ray absorptiometry (DEXA) imaging gives a reliable assessment of the adipose tissue mass.

Increase in weight occurring during pregnancy, fluid retention, hypothyroidism, hypothalamic lesions and other endocrine disturbances should be differentiated from obesity due to nutritional causes. Therefore, overweight may be caused by excessive muscular development in wrestlers, weight-lifters and boxers. Estimation of BMI and the waist to hip ratio help to assess the risk of complications further. The aim of management is to reduce weight, achieve metabolic and physical fitness, reduce morbidity and achieve cosmetic results. A negative balance of 8000–9000 calories has to be achieved to clear 1 kg of adipose tissue.

Treatment

Dietary Regulation

An imbalance of energy intake and energy expenditure is accounted for by a gain or loss of body fat and lean tissue which run in parallel. Energy content per kg change of body fat is 39.5 MJ and it is 7.6 MJ for a kg of lean tissue.

Physical activity increases energy expenditure slightly more compared to an equivalent energy reduction in food intake.

Consumption of dietary protein elicits a substantially higher increment of energy expenditure for several hours after a meal than does dietary fat or carbohydrates. Low carbohydrates diet lead to greater weight loss at least in the short term.

Strong motivation of the patient is absolutely essential for successful management. Dietary regulation is the basis of modern therapy. Calorie intake should be reduced below the basal requirements and the patient has to be kept on negative energy balance over prolonged periods of time. The excess fat is catabolized and weight is lost.

The therapeutic diet should contain 500–1000 calories less than the energy expenditure of the individual. An ideal weight reducing diet should be:

- Deficient in calories
- Otherwise nutritionally adequate
- Acceptable socio-culturally
- The diet should be suitably timed to avoid long intervals between eating (Table 33.3).

Since, dietary fats account for the palatability of food and they provide the maximum amount of calories the first step should be to cut fat intake to the maximum. This is the most effective single step to bring down weight rapidly in the initial stages. Young and tall subjects lose weight more efficiently than older and shorter people. On an average, daily intake has to be limited to 800–1000 calories. More drastic cuts on foods are frequently resented and result in non-compliance. For optimal results, the diet should be acceptable, sufficient in volume and conforming to the general eating habits of the individual. Bulk is provided by adding moderate amounts of fresh vegetables (not curried) and low-calorie fruits. Vegetables when made into curries with coconut, oil, dal and condiments become very rich in calories. Clear instructions on the exact quantity of food and its timing are very essential. Regular follow-up is necessary for proper motivation and assessment. Patients put on the sub-calorie diets lose weight steadily after an initial latent period ranging from days to weeks. It is ideal to reduce the weight by 1 kg a week. Vitamin and mineral supplementation is advisable since, the restricted diet may fail to meet these requirements.

Obese persons do not generally comply with diets. The low caloric diet should be maintained indefinitely since the tendency to regain weight persists. Strong motivation of the patient is needed to achieve good results. Initial motivation to reduce weight may be easy, but persistent efforts to maintain the ideal weight are generally slackened, so a major proportion of patients regain their weight and may even overshoot the original levels. Even moderate reduction in weight such as 6–10% of the body weight is accompanied by reduction in metabolic risks and blood pressure.

Exercise: Moderate exercise augments the beneficial effect of dieting. Walking slowly up to 4–5 km/day, swimming or games are ideal, depending upon individual preferences. Prescription of the exercise regime should take into account the cardiovascular status and exercise tolerance of the patient. Preferably it should be supervised by traning staff.

Drugs: Several drugs are available which reduce appetite. These anorectic drugs have been employed on short-term basis when the patient is not able to resist the desire to eat. Drugs may be needed when the BMI exceeds 30. Sympathomimetic drugs with amphetamine-like action reduce appetite and increase energy expenditure. These are contraindicated in persons with cardiovascular disease. Serotonin reuptake inhibitors are good appetite suppressants. Fenfluramine and fluoxetine can be given on a short-term basis over weeks to a few months. When given over prolonged periods they may lead to the development of primary pulmonary hypertension. Acquired defects of the mitral and aortic valves may also develop. Dose Fenfluramine 20–120 mg twice a day given orally one hour before meals. Since, these drugs cause dependence, they should preferably be withdrawn after 3 months of administration. Side effects include dryness of the mouth, abdominal pain, drowsiness, alopecia, mental depression, confusion and impotence. These drugs are contraindicated in patients with psychiatric illness.

Table 33.3: Subcaloric diet for obesity for adults with moderate activity. Total allowances for a day are given				
Article of food	**Vegetarian**	**Calories**	**Non-vegetarian**	**Calories**
Cereals	150 g	600	150 g	600
Dal or lentils	50 g	200	20 g	80
Fish or lean meat not cooked in oil or fats	–	–	100 g	250
Milk or curd in any form	300 mL	180	100 mL	60
Green vegetables	150 g	80	150 g	80
Fruits: Very sweet fruits like grapes and mangoes are to be avoided. Papaya, melon, small bananas, guava and apples are preferable	150 g	80	150 g	80
Total calories		1140		1150

Note:

1. Sugar, sweets, honey and similar high-caloric articles of food and alcohol are to be strictly avoided.
2. Timing of the diet and the menu should be adjusted to conform to the occupation and dietary habits of the individual.
3. When the optimum weight reduction has been achieved, graded increases in the diet can be made under supervision, taking care not to restore the original weight and to ensure balanced nutrition.

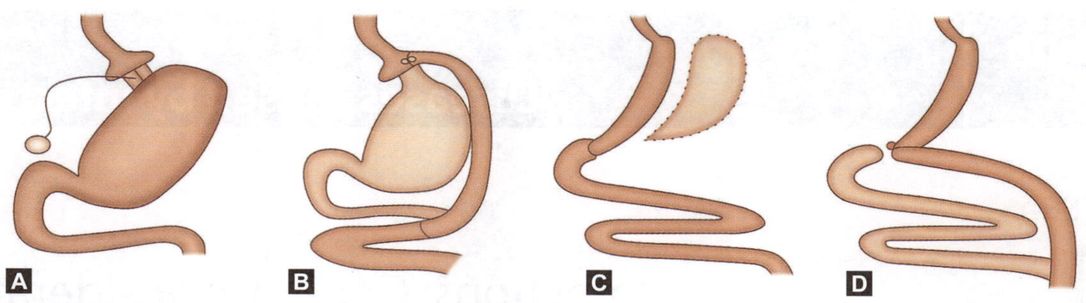

Figs 33.4A to D: Diagrammatic representation of the surgical techniques in current use. **A.** Adjustable gastric band; **B.** Roux-en-y gastric bypass; **C.** Vertical sleeve gastrectomy; **D.** Biliopancreatic diversion with a duodenal switch

Note: Though the bariatric surgical procedures are formidable when done by experts in the field they are still safe and are being done in large numbers including in India. With proper dietary and lifestyle adjustments by the patient, results for sustained weight loss, normalization of glucose and lipid levels and reduction of risks of cardiovascular events have been proved and therefore, in severe cases of obesity surgery should be resorted to if medical measures fail.

Sibutramine is an appetite suppressant which can be given in doses of 5–15 mg once a day. It produces loss of weight by reducing appetite and increasing energy expenditure. Side effects include dryness of mouth insomnia and constipation. Sibutramine should not be given to patients with ischemic heart disease or heart failure, arrhythmia and stroke. Sibutramine leads to a lean weight loss of 4–5 kg.

Orlistat is a lipase inhibitor which prevents absorption of dietary fat. The dose is 120 mg tid. Side effects include flatulence, fecal urgency and malabsorption of fat soluble vitamins. Orlistat leads to a mean weight loss of 3 kg.

Rimonabant is an endocannabinoid receptor antagonist. The dose is 20 mg given orally daily. It reduces body weight on an average of 4–5 kg. It improves the metabolic syndrome as well. Adverse effects include nausea, dizziness, diarrhea and depression. When obesity is extreme and rapid weight reduction is desired, more drastic measures are employed. These include total starvation program and surgical procedures.

Newer drugs in the pipeline include melanocortin-4, receptor agonist, leptin, neuropeptides Y antagonists, beta 3 adrenergic agonists (Amibegron, Solabegron) and glucagon like peptide agonists

Total starvation: This can be undertaken under strict medical supervision for 2–3 weeks. Only water, salts and vitamins are allowed during this period. Complications include starvation ketosis, ventricular arrhythmias and sudden death. Due to these risks, total starvation should be undertaken only under exceptional circumstances. Wiring of the jaw to prevent ingestion of solid foods has been practiced on persons unable to undertake starvation. Rapid weight loss is achieved by total starvation. Follow-up treatment consists of sub-caloric feeding.

Surgical measures (Figs 33.4A to D): Surgical measures done to produce short-circuiting of digestive and absorptive portions of the intestines may be required for severe cases. The procedures include jejunoileal bypass and gastric bypass. Gastric plication may be done with a view to reduce the capacity of the stomach. Extirpation of excessive fat and plastic surgical procedures to remove redundant skin folds remaining after achieving weight loss help to correct cosmetic disability and also to augment the effects of dietary treatment. Liposuction is a surgical technique which removes large amounts of fat from localized areas such as the abdomen, gluteal regions, breasts, arms and face. This procedure is gaining popularity, being safe and cosmetically rewarding. The surgical management of obesity, as a part of cosmetic surgery is known as ***bariatric surgery***.

Bariatric surgical techniques divided into two groups:

1. ***Malabsorptive procedures:*** Induce decreased absorption of nutrients by shortening the functional length of the small intestine.
2. ***Restrictive procedures:*** Reduce the storage capacity of the stomach and as a result early satiety arises, leading to a decreased caloric intake.

In general, loss of weight up to 5–10 kg is easy but further reduction and maintenance of the optimal weight demand great motivation on the part of the patient and skill on the part of the physician. Once the optimum weight is reached, the patient should slowly increase the diet to prevent further weight loss and try to adhere to the optimum weight. Even an occasional dietary excess results in rapid weight gain. All the complications of obesity can be arrested and may even regress if normal weight is maintained for long periods. Secondary obesity should be treated by adopting dietary measures and giving due attention to the primary cause.

CHAPTER 34

Infections: General Considerations

S Bhasi

Chapter Summary

- Infection
- General Symptomatology
- Pathogenesis of Fever
- Systemic Responses in Fever
- Approach to a Patient with Fever
- Laboratory Investigations

INTRODUCTION

Microbes are abundant in nature, the vast majority of them are harmless to man and many of them are essential to life. They are mostly commensals and a few are pathogens. Primitive ancestors of homosapiens and their colonizing bacteria have evolved over 500,000 years. Some experts have determined the total number of cells in the human body are 10^{13} and the total number of colonizing microbes are 10^{14}. The organisms capable of establishing themselves and multiplying in hosts are called parasites, which may be commensals or pathogens. All our body surfaces have an indigenous bacterial flora. This normal flora protects us from infection by multiple mechanisms such as: 1. Compete with pathogens in utilizing nutrients, 2. producing antibacterial substances inhibiting growth of pathogens, 3. inducing host immunity that is cross reactive and effective against pathogens (Table 34.1).

Pathogens lead to adverse effects on hosts while commensals cause no harm to their hosts and exist in harmony. Commensals may cause disease when host resistance is lost or when transferred to an inappropriate site, e.g. oropharyngeal commensals aspirated into lung.

Table 34.1: Approximate bacterial count in the human body	
Skin general	10^3/g
Skin groin/axilla	10^6/g
Bile, liver	Nil
Stomach	10^3/mL
Small intestine	10^4/mL
Large intestine	10^{10}/mL
Lungs	Nil
Nasal secretions	10^5/mL
Saliva	10^8/mL
Urine	10^3/mL

INFECTION

Infection is defined as entry and multiplication of microbes in the tissues of the host with or without producing disease. Infections without disease manifestations are called *subclinical infections*.

Infections remain one of the main causes of morbidity and mortality in man worldwide. Poverty and overcrowding in the underdeveloped countries increase this burden.

Infectious agents include bacteria, viruses, fungi, protozoa, helminths and prions.

Types of Infections

- *Exogenous infection:* Infection from external source.
- *Endogenous infection:* Infection by organisms harbored by the individual.
- *Primary infection:* Initial infection of a host by an organism.
- *Secondary infection:* Host suffering from an infectious disease invaded by another organism.
- *Re-infection:* Subsequent infection by same/different organism.
- *Focal infection:* Infections confined to one area/organ, e.g. tonsillitis.
- *Nosocomial infection:* Infections acquired after admission to hospital, not incubating/present at the time of admission.
- *Super infection:* Patient receiving broad spectrum antibiotics get colonized by resistant pathogens and infection produced by them.
- *Opportunistic infection:* Organisms that ordinarily do not cause infection in healthy individuals but do so in individuals with markedly reduced resistance (immunocompromised hosts).
- *Latent infection:* Pathogen remains in the tissue without producing disease but may lead to disease when host resistance is lowered.

Source of Infection

Infection may be obtained from human, animal or other sources. When the source of infection is man, the infectious agent may originate from patients or carriers.

A carrier who harbors the pathogenic organism without developing any disease due to it is called *healthy carrier*.

A *convalescent carrier* is one who harbors the organism for some period after recovering from the disease.

Zoonoses are infections transmitted from wild or domestic animals to man, e.g. plague, rabies.

Some infections are transmitted by insect vectors, e.g. *Anopheles* mosquito transmits malaria.

Direct contact is necessary for transmission of organisms like *Staphylococci*. Respiratory diseases such as influenza, tuberculosis, pneumonia and others spread by air-borne droplets. Food or water borne transmission occurs in typhoid, hepatitis A and E, cholera and others. Sexual transmission is the main route for syphilis, gonorrhea and human immunodeficiency virus (HIV). Vertical transmission, i.e. from mother to fetus, occurs in diseases like rubella and syphilis.

Pathogenesis

The pathological lesions, symptoms and signs may be produced by several mechanisms:

- It is caused by the organism directly, e.g. boils, abscesses, pneumonia, dysentery and tuberculosis.
- Organisms like *Corynebacterium diphtheriae* and *Clostridium tetani* multiply locally without entering the system and elaborate toxins (exotoxins) which are absorbed into the system producing the manifestations.
- *Vibrio cholerae* elaborates an exotoxin having local effect on the intestinal mucosa producing secretory diarrhea.
- Many gram-negative bacteria produce endotoxins by disintegration in the tissues producing direct effect on tissues and liberation of chemical mediators of inflammation like cytokines which are mainly responsible for the manifestations.
- Activation of immunological mechanism is one of the most important pathogenic mechanisms of tissue damage in several infections.
- Infections like HIV and syphilis suppress the immune mechanism of the host by acting upon the lymphocytes.
- Some infectious agents are oncogenic, i.e. giving rise to tumors, e.g. HIV, Epstein-Barr (EB) virus, hepatitis B and others.

Medical care itself increases the patient's risk of acquiring infection in several ways:

- Contact with pathogens in the hospital
- Breach of skin [e.g. incisions, intravenous (IV) devices] or mucous membranes (e.g. endotracheal tube, indwelling catheter)
- Alteration of normal flora by antibiotics
- Reduction of immunity by immunosuppressive drugs.

The body's mechanisms to prevent and overcome the infections are local defenses, phagocytic cells, antibodies (immunoglobulin), immunocytes and nonspecific defense aids such as lysozymes, complement and properdin.

Changing scenario of infection worldwide: The pattern of infectious agents and pathogenesis are changing due to several factors such as changes in environment, influence of polymicrobial therapy and alterations in host defense. The prevalence of immune deficiency either natural or iatrogenic has increased so that several infections have become more invasive and virulent. Classic infection such as *Streptococcus, Staphylococcus, E. coli, Salmonella, Pneumococci* which were all drug sensitive are giving

place to either drug resistant mutants or other types of organisms in their place.

Emerging and Re-emerging Infections

The pattern of infection is changing over the past few decades. Classic infections such as *Streptococcus, Staphylococcus, E. coli, Salmonellae, Pneumococcus* and others which were all drug sensitive are giving place to either drug resistant mutants or other types of organisms in their place. Viral infections have overtaken bacterial infections in number and severity. The prevalence of immunodeficiency either natural or iatrogenic has also increased, so that several infections have become more invasive and virulent, e.g. methicillin-resistant *Staphylococcus aureus* (MRSA), dengue viruses, herpes viruses, nosocomial infections and others. Several infections even though initially mild, suddenly becomes serious leading to multi-organ dysfunction and multi-organ failure with high mortality.

Newly recognized infections are acquired immunodeficiency syndrome (AIDS), severe acute respiratory syndrome (SARS), avian influenza, Middle East respiratory syndrome (MERS), Ebolavirus infection, Zika virus and others.

Rebound of diseases like malaria, tuberculosis, rheumatic fever and others thought to have been eradicated from developed countries.

Recognition of role of infectious agents in the causation of diseases previously thought to be non-infectious, e.g. *Helicobacter pylori* in the causation of peptic ulcer, *human papilloma virus* in carcinoma cervix.

Human Polymicrobial Infections

In the immunocompetent state, colonization by one organism inhibits colonization by another. This is known as microbial interference, e.g. *Streptococcus pneumonia* and *Streptococcus aureus*.

At present, due to the prevalence of different kinds of immunosuppressed states, polymicrobial disease caused by combination of viruses, bacteria, fungi and parasites are being recognized. In this situation, presence of one microorganism causes a niché for other pathogens to colonize and thrive, e.g. measles, tuberculosis and *S. aureus;* EB virus and retrovirus; hepatitis B virus and HIV; HIV and tuberculosis.

Immunodeficiency states may be congenital or acquired. The latter include malnutrition, extremes of age, loss of surface epithelium, diabetes mellitus (DM), cancer, cancer chemotherapy, chronic renal failure, chronic hepatic failure, immunosuppressant drugs, HIV infection and others. The resultant degree of immune suppression is the total effect of all the contributory factors.

Immunodeficiency may be general or specific towards specific pathogens. Neutropenia and reduction of other phagocyte cells predispose to infection by extracellular bacterial pathogens, both endogenous and exogenous. Suppression of T-cell mediated immunity predisposes to viral infections. Multiple intubations, hospitalization and management in intensive care facilities predispose to infections.

Clinical features of infection in the immuno-compromised host differ from those in immunocompetent hosts. Signs of infection in the immunocompromised hosts include:

- Confusion
- Faint erythematous rashes
- Lymphangiectatic streaks on the skin
- Dyspnea or cough with clear chest X-ray
- Minimal erythema with serosanguinous discharge at sites of insertion of catheters, surgical sites, abscess or drains
- Minimally elevated values of liver function tests and serum levels of lactic dehydrogenase (LDH) and creatine kinase (CK)
- Unexplained rise or fall of leukocyte and platelet counts.

Antimicrobial resistance: As we developed newer antimicrobial drugs, microbes developed the ability to elude our best weapon. Antibiotic resistance is developing at an alarming rate. Multidrug resistant pathogens such as *E. coli, Klebsiella, Pseudomonas, S. aureus, M. tuberculosis,* HIV and others are extremely common. Especially in the intensive care units (ICUs), these get disseminated.

Bioterrorism: Use of biological infectious agents such as anthrax spores, plague, smallpox and others may be resorted to as potential weapons for stealthy warfare.

***Eradication of infectious disease*s** like smallpox, totally from the world and polio from most countries has been achieved.

GENERAL SYMPTOMATOLOGY

Fever

Fever is perhaps the most common manifestation of ill health due to infection. It is an early and non-specific body response to many infectious and non-infectious causes. In humans, metabolic processes are critically temperature dependent. In a healthy individual, body temperature is kept constant around 37°C within a very small range despite larger difference in surrounding temperature.

Normal Temperature

In healthy individuals, normal body temperature varies from 36.6 to 37.2°C (98–99°F), usually 98.4°F (36.9°C). The normal diurnal variation is approximately 1°F with maximum between 4.00 and 8.00 pm and minimum between 2.00 and 6.00 am. In fever, this variation is exaggerated. In old age, body temperature may be lower due to low metabolic rate. Women in the reproductive period show elevation of body temperature 24–48 hours after ovulation due to increased progesterone level. Temperature may also increase after exercise if normal heat loss is prevented.

Recording of Temperature

In all conscious, cooperative adults and older children—oral temperature is ideal for clinical use. Equilibrium time with mercury-in-glass thermometer is a minimum of 90 seconds. Hot or cold liquid and even smoking can alter the recorded temperature. In these situations it is best to delay measuring the temperature for 10–15 minutes. Axillary temperatures are less reliable since they are considerably altered by environmental factors. On an average, axillary temperature is 0.3–0.6°C (0.5–1°F) less than oral temperature. Temperature of the inner tissues and viscera (core temperature) is about 0.6°C (1°F) higher than oral temperature. Rectal temperature represents the core temperature. Rectal temperature may be recorded in unconscious patients, undergoing intensive care and during major surgery. Due to breakage and mercury exposure, glass thermometer is being replaced by electronic thermometer in many hospitals. Reading can be taken after 10 seconds.

Tympanic membrane thermometer is increasingly used especially in the west. It is quick, safe and reliable if used properly; reading is closer to core temperature.

Normal temperature	36.6–37.2°C (98–99°F)
Fever	>37.2°C (>99°F)
Hyperpyrexia	>41.1°C (>106°F)
Subnormal temperature	<36.6°C (<98°F)
Hypothermia	<35°C (<95°F)
Note: 1°C = 1.8°F	0°C corresponds to 32°F

Abbreviations: C = Centigrade; F = Fahrenheit

Regulation of Body Temperature

Temperature is regulated by thermoregulatory center in the hypothalamus, which receives information from cold and warm receptors of peripheral nerves and temperature of blood perfusing the area. Heat is produced by metabolic process and muscular activity. Normal heat production by metabolic processes is in excess than is necessary to maintain body temperature and the same is dissipated by heat loss through lungs and skin. Rapid rise in temperature is effected by increasing metabolism, rapid muscle contractions (rigor) and conserving heat by peripheral vasoconstriction. Heat loss by radiation, convection and conduction from the surface is slow. Rapid loss of heat is achieved by evaporation of sweat. Presence of cold extremities and rigor precede rapid rise of temperature. Diaphoresis (excessive sweating) accompanies rapid fall of temperature.

Fever is defined as the elevation of body temperature above normal (regulated rise to a new set point of body temperature). This occurs as a result of increase in hypothalamic 'set point' for temperature. Once hypothalamic set point is raised, neurones in the vasomotor center are stimulated leading to peripheral vasoconstriction especially in the limbs, leading to decrease in heat loss from the skin. The person feels cold. Metabolic processes being slow, they elevate body temperature only gradually, but steadily. If there is need for rapid increase in temperature, shivering occurs. Due to vigorous muscle contraction with rapid heat production temperature rises sharply. When hypothalamic set point is reset downwards (either by reduction in pyrogen concentration or by antipyretics) heat loss occurs by vasodilatation and sweating. Exposure of the body to the environment leads to dissipation of heat.

In the vast majority of febrile states, temperature does not exceed from 104 to 105°F (40–40.6°C). Degree of

Textbook of Medicine

temperature elevation does not necessarily correspond to severity of illness.

Hyperpyrexia

This denotes temperatures above 41.1°C (106°F). This may complicate conditions such as malaria, septicemia, pontine hemorrhage, thyrotoxic crisis, heat stroke and neuroleptic malignant syndrome produced by drugs like phenothiazine.

Once the body temperature rises above 41°C, the thermoregulatory mechanism fails and the body behaves like poikilothermic organism. Diurnal variation disappears. Body temperature >41°C may produce irreversible protein denaturation and resultant brain damage. Unless managed as an emergency to lower the temperature, hyperpyrexia is fatal due to damage to vital cells.

PATHOGENESIS OF FEVER

Pyrogens are substances causing fever. These may be exogenous or endogenous. Exogenous pyrogens are molecules which interact with host cells to induce secretion of pyrogenic cytokines. Most of these are microbial products, microbial toxins or whole microorganisms. The best example is the lipopolysaccharide endotoxin found in the cell wall of gram-negative bacteria. Enterotoxin of *S. aureus* and group A and B streptococci are other examples. Endogenous pyrogens are cytokines which have small molecular weight proteins most important being interleukin-1 (IL-1), IL-6 and tumor necrosis factor alpha (TNF-α). The synthesis and release of pyrogenic cytokines are induced by a wide spectrum of exogenous pyrogens most of which are of bacterial, fungal or viral origin. In addition, inflammation, trauma, tissue necrosis and antigen–antibody complexes induce production of pyrogenic cytokines. Main source of pyrogenic cytokines are monocytes and macrophages and to a lesser extent neutrophils and lymphocytes.

Pyrogenic cytokines stimulate production of the prostaglandin—PGE2 from arachidonic acid near the hypothalamic thermoregulatory center. Arachidonic acid is released from cell membrane by the enzyme—phospholipase A2. PGE2 raises the set point in the thermoregulatory center. Pyrogenic cytokines also induce production of PGE2 in the periphery which is responsible for myalgia, arthralgia and malaise that accompany fever. Cytokine induced fever seldom exceeds 41.1°C. Unless there is structural damage to hypothalamic regulatory centers.

Fever as a Defense Adaptation

There is suggestive evidence that for some microorganisms at least, a febrile host response may assist in curtailing infection and speedy recovery. Experimental data support the notion that raised body temperature interferes with growth and/or virulence factors of some bacterial and viral pathogens. Fever, slightly increases immune reaction and increases chemotactic, phagocytic and bactericidal activity of polymorphonuclear leukocytes. In immunocompromised individuals and those at the extremes of age, a prompt febrile response may not develop even in the presence of severe infection. Such people are at greater risk of succumbing to the infection.

SYSTEMIC RESPONSES IN FEVER

- ***Increase in metabolic rate:*** Oxygen consumption increases by 13% for each 1°C rise of temperature. Hence, fever may aggravate or precipitate pre-existing cardiac, cerebrovascular or pulmonary insufficiency.
- ***Increase in heart rate:*** For every 1°C rise of temperature above normal, the heart rate increases by 18 beats/minute. In some fevers like pneumonia and rheumatic fever, heart rate may be disproportionately high (***rapid pulse fever-relative tachycardia***). In typhoid, some viral infections including dengue fever, meningitis, brucellosis, drug induced fever and many cases of leptospirosis; pulse rate may be disproportionately slow (***slow pulse fever-relative bradycardia***).
- ***Blood pressure:*** It may increase during the period of rise of temperature because of vasoconstriction and decrease during the period of defervescence because of vasodilation.
- ***Fluid loss increases:*** Due to evaporation and sweating. Average of 360 mL excess fluid is required for 24 hours/1°C rise in temperature (200 mL/1°F).
- ***Increase in respiratory rate*** occurs with fever. The usual ratio of 1:4 with heart rate is maintained except in the case of primary respiratory diseases such as pneumonia and pleural effusion.
- ***Chills occur*** in the initial phase because of peripheral vasoconstriction.
- ***Rigors*** accompany rapid increase in temperature. They are due to vigorous muscle contractions. Repeated occurrence of rigor is most typically seen in malaria, filariasis, urinary tract infections (UTIs) and abscess formation anywhere in the body. Rigor may occur in many types of continuous fever treated intermittently with antipyretics. When the effect of the drug wanes off rigor occurs in an attempt on the part of the body to resume the high temperature.
- When the high temperature falls to normal or subnormal within a few hours, it is called fall by ***crisis***, and when the temperature reaches normal slowly over several days, it is called fall by ***lysis***.
- ***Headache*** may accompany any type of fever but severe headache and photophobia are characteristic prominent features of intracranial infections and sinusitis. High temperature during 1st trimester of pregnancy may cause birth defects. Fever increases insulin requirement.
- ***Delirium:*** This is toxic confusional state. It is more common in the very young and very old. Fever may induce mental changes in those with organic brain syndrome. The cytokines TNF-α and IL-1 cause release of endorphins in the brain and may precipitate delirium.
- ***Excessive sweating*** is the regular accompaniment of defervescence. Particular patterns of sweating like 'night sweats' are more common in tuberculosis and lymphoma. In almost all fevers fall of temperature is accompanied by sweating.

Textbook of Medicine

- **Muscle pain (myalgia)** is the prominent feature of infections such as influenza, enterovirus, dengue fever, leptospirosis and others.
- **Herpes labialis:** Fever may activate the latent viral infection herpes simplex which causes vesicles at mucocutaneous junctions of the nose and lips. Pneumonia and meningitis are common to produce herpes labialis whereas typhoid is very rare to do so.
- **Feverishness:** This is a subjective feeling of fever which may be experienced even without rise in temperature. Therefore, it is essential to record the temperature to distinguish between the two conditions.

APPROACH TO A PATIENT WITH FEVER

In the diagnosis of the cause of fever, science and art of medicine come together. History is most important. History of travel to a malaria—endemic area may give a clue. Presence of nasal symptoms and sore throat suggest viral etiology. Severe myalgia may suggest influenza, dengue fever or leptospirosis. Eye congestion, subconjunctival hemorrhage and muscle tenderness may suggest leptospirosis. Skin rashes and mucous membrane lesions give diagnostic clue. Erythematous blanching rash indicates viral exanthematous fever as the most likely cause. Palatal petechiae along with posterior cervical lymphadenopathy and gray-white tonsil exudate suggest infectious mononucleosis. Enlarged tender tonsil lymph nodes with tonsil exudate and neutrophilic leukocytosis suggest streptococcal tonsillitis. Koplik's spots in the buccal mucosa indicate measles. Dysuria and loin pain with tenderness suggests pyelonephritis.

Duration of fever: This is an important point which helps in clinical diagnosis. Fever lasting for less than two weeks is called short fever and fever with duration of more than 3 weeks is prolonged fever. Regular recording of temperature, pulse rate and respiration rate are routinely done in all hospitals. Fever of more than 5–7 days with gastrointestinal symptoms with or without malena and just palpable soft spleen may suggest typhoid fever. Onset may be abrupt in infections like pneumonia or may show a step-ladder type of rise in typhoid. Fever with clubbing of fingers and splinter hemorrhages in the nail bed in a patient with congenital or rheumatic valvular heart disease suggest infective endocarditis.

Patterns of fever (Fig. 34.1): Recording the pattern of temperature is an important clinical clue to diagnosis. In the ordinary febrile patient, temperature is recorded thrice daily, but in special cases where large fluctuations occur and in acute care settings temperature has to be recorded more frequently, e.g. every 4 hours.

Continuous fever: Temperature is persistently elevated with diurnal variation of less than 1°C, e.g. typhoid in the 2nd week, typhus, viral infections and others.

Remittent fever: Temperature is persistently elevated with diurnal variation more than 1°C—typhoid in 1st week, brucellosis, leptospirosis and others.

Intermittent fever: Temperature is discontinuous, touching normal at least once in 24 hours. This may be seen in pyogenic infections, lymphomas, tuberculosis, bacteremias, malaria and others.

Periodic fever: These show a regular periodicity in their occurrence. Fever occurring on alternate days with one day interval in between is called **tertian periodicity,** e.g. vivax malaria (benign tertian). Fever occurring every 4th day with 2 days' afebrile period in between is known as **quartan periodicity**, e.g. quartan malaria. Continuous and remittent fevers may be converted to intermittent fever by repeated doses of antipyretics. Quotidian fever, i.e. one spike everyday occurs classically in mixed malaria. Quotidian fever is seen with visceral leishmaniasis, gonococcal endocarditis and adult onset Still's disease.

Drug induced fever: Several drugs can produce fever by various mechanisms. Drug induced fever becomes a diagnostic problem in patients receiving multiple drugs for long periods, especially in hospitals.

Of the medications that cause fever, antibiotics are the most frequent, especially penicillins, cephalosporins, sulfonamides, nitrofurantoin, antituberculous agents and others. Antiepileptic drugs especially phenytoin are also known to cause fever. Drug induced fever does not have specific characteristic features. Most often, it occurs 5–10 days after starting the drug, but can occur even after the first dose itself. During afebrile period, patient feels almost normal. Blood examination may show eosinophilia.

LABORATORY INVESTIGATIONS

Leukocyte Patterns

Neutrophilic leukocytosis and presence of juvenile or band forms of neutrophils and toxic granulations in neutrophils usually suggest bacterial infections. Leukocytosis is also common in the first day of many viral infections. Total leukocyte counts above 10,000/mm^3

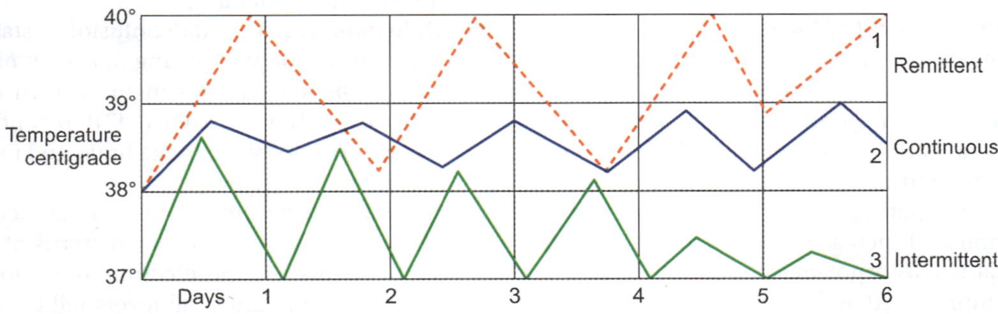

Fig. 34.1: Patterns of fever

with more than 70% as neutrophils are very suggestive of pyogenic infection. Leukemoid reaction may accompany severe leukocytosis.

Neutropenia, mild to moderate, is usually seen in many viral infections, about 25% of typhoid, brucellosis, leishmaniasis, tuberculosis, histoplasmosis and others.

Leukopenia with relative or absolute **lymphocytosis** occurs in several viral infections. Many viral infections show moderate or even severe thrombocytopenia with or without bleeding manifestations.

Atypical lymphocytes are seen in some viral infections especially EB virus, cytomegalovirus, HIV, dengue, rubella, viral hepatitis, varicella and others.

Monocytosis is commonly seen in typhoid and tuberculosis.

Eosinophilia occurs in parasitic infections, filariasis, tropical pulmonary eosinophila and hypersensitivity to drugs.

Specific diagnostic investigations:

- ***Isolation or identification of the infective agent in blood/urine/body fluids/pus and tissues specimens***
  - ***Culture:*** Proper collection of sample without contamination and transport to the lab is important, e.g. blood culture in sepsis, urine culture in UTI, cerebrospinal fluid (CSF) in meningitis, sputum in pneumonia, pus in abscess.
  - ***Gram stain*** of specimen may help, e.g. sputum, CSF, pus, urethral discharge and others. The findings on gram-stain should correspond to the results of culture to be diagnosed.

- ***Demonstration of parasites*** like malaria and microfilaria in blood, leishmania in bone marrow splenic aspirate and liver biopsy specimens, vegetative amoeba in stool or scrapings from abscess wall.
- ***Demonstration of antibodies to specific pathogen***, e.g. Widal in typhoid, IgM antibodies against many viruses like hepatitis A, E and dengue virus.
- ***Detection of bacterial/fungal/viral antigens*** in blood/body fluids even when cultures are negative or practically difficult, e.g. HBsAg in virus B hepatitis.
- ***Detection of very minute quantities of nucleic acid*** by techniques such as polymerase chain reaction (PCR) that allow amplification of specific DNA (deoxyribonucleic acid)/RNA (ribonucleic acid) sequences.
- ***Histopathology:*** Tuberculosis, histoplasmosis, sarcoidosis and others can be diagnosed by biopsy of lymph node, liver and other organs.

Points to Remember

- Infection is defined as entry and multiplication of microbes in the body.
- Antimicrobial resistance is on the increase.
- Fever is the most common manifestation of infection. Duration and pattern of fever may give a clue to diagnosis.
- Fever increases metabolic rate, heart rate (HR), respiratory rate (RR) and fluid loss.
- A properly elicited history followed by good clinical examination often suggests the diagnosis.
- Most short fevers are self-limiting. Avoid over investigation and over use of drugs.

CHAPTER

35

Fever of Unknown Origin

S Bhasi

Chapter Summary

- General Considerations
- Definition
- Etiology
- Diagnostic Approach
- Investigations
- Management

GENERAL CONSIDERATIONS

Syn: Pyrexia of Unknown Origin (PUO)

Fever of unknown origin (FUO) is the term used to denote fever that does not resolve spontaneously in the period expected for self-limited infections and whose cause could not be ascertained even after reasonable investigations.

This presents one of the most difficult diagnostic problems in medicine. Atypical presentations of common illnesses are responsible for majority of such cases.

DEFINITION

FUO was defined by Petersdorf and Beeson in 1961—temperature more than 38.3°C (101°F), lasts for more than 3 weeks and failure to reach a diagnosis, even after 1 week of inpatient investigations. A subsequent definition in 2003 stated that failure to get a diagnosis after 3 days of inpatient investigations or three outpatient visits should qualify for the term FUO. The interval specified in the criteria for diagnosis are arbitrary aimed at excluding patients with protracted but self-limiting viral infections and also to get time for usual serological, cultural and radiographic investigations to be done.

Classification of FUO

FUO are classified into four categories:

1. Classic
2. Nosocomial

3. Neutropenic
4. Human immunodeficiency virus (HIV) associated.

Classic FUO

Includes all cases of FUOs other than nosocomial, neutropenic and HIV associated FUOs.

Nosocomial

This term denotes fever above 38.3°C (101°F) lasting for more than 72 hours, developing in a hospitalized patient due to a process not present or incubated at the time of admission. Most common causes are pneumonia, urinary tract infection (UTI), catheter related infections, *Clostridium difficile* colitis, cytomegalovirus (CMV) infection, sinusitis, septic thrombophlebitis and pulmonary embolism.

Neutropenic

This is fever more than 38.3°C (101°F) lasting for more than 72 hours in a patient with absolute neutrophil count less than 500/mm^3 or expected to reach that level in 1–2 days. Most commonly this is produced by bacterial infections—bacteremias, pneumonia and soft tissue infections. Infection of the perianal area is also common. If neutropenia is prolonged, fungal and viral infections also supervene.

Human Immunodeficiency Virus Associated

Fever is a common accompaniment of HIV infection when it leads to immunodeficiency. The most common infective agents are *Mycobacterium tuberculosis, Mycobacterium avium* complex (MAC), *Pneumocystis carinii*, disseminated cryptococcosis, toxoplasmosis and nocardiosis. Uncomplicated HIV infection itself can be the cause of prolonged fever.

ETIOLOGY

Most cases represent unusual presentation of common diseases and are not rare diseases.

- **Infections:** In India about 50% cases are caused by infections. These include the following:
  - **Occult tuberculosis (TB):** Extrapulmonary TB affecting the lymph nodes, intestines, mesentery, vertebrae, joints, liver, pleura, pericardium and genital organs may remain latent without any local symptoms but causes fever. The local lesion may become evident only after several weeks or months.
  - **Intra-abdominal infections:** Renal, retroperitoneal, paraspinal, subdiaphragmatic and pelvic abscesses may remain silent and cause diagnostic problems. Complicated urinary tract infections UTIs and infections of the biliary tree may also present as FUO.
  - **Other infections:** Infective endocarditis, brucellosis, osteomyelitis, dental and sinus infections, enteric fever with atypical presentation, malaria, amebiasis, syphilis, leprosy, leishmaniasis and prostatitis may present as FUO.
  - **Viral infections:** Infectious mononucleosis and CMV infection may present as FUO.
  - **Fungal infections:** Examples are histoplasmosis and cryptococcosis.

- **Malignancy:** These form about 20% cases. Leading malignancies presenting as FUO are:
  - Leukemia, lymphomas and multiple myeloma
  - Solid tumors like renal cell carcinoma, liver (primary/metastatic), colon, stomach and pancreatic cancers.
- **Autoimmune diseases (about 15%):** Systemic lupus erythematosus (SLE), rheumatoid arthritis, rheumatic fever, polyarteritis nodosa, temporal arteritis, polymyalgia rheumatica, Wegener's granulomatosis, adult Still's disease and others.
- **Miscellaneous (about 20%):** Inflammatory bowel disease (IBD), cirrhosis of the liver, granulomatous hepatitis, sarcoidosis, atrial myxoma, thyroiditis, thyrotoxicosis, drug reactions, hemolytic anemias, hematomas, deep vein thrombosis (DVT) and pulmonary embolism.
- **Undiagnosed:** About 15% may remain undiagnosed.

Factitious Fever

This is elevation of temperature, self-induced by patients with psychological problems—mostly young women working in health profession. They may induce disease or may devise methods to make the thermometer record higher temperature even when they are normal.

Common Causes of Prolonged Fever

- **Infections (40% cases):** Most common infections causing pyrexia of unknown origin (PUO) are TB, malaria, typhoid and HIV. Other causes are:
  - **Bacterial**
    - **Abscesses:** Previous abdominal or pelvic surgery, trauma or history of diverticulosis or peritonitis increases the likelihood of an occult intra-abdominal abscess. Most commonly in the subphrenic space, liver, right lower quadrant, retroperitoneal space or the pelvis in women.
    - **TB:** Dissemination of TB may occur in immunocompromised patients, makes initial presentation more constitutional symptoms than localizing signs. Chest X-ray may be normal.
    - **UTIs** are rare causes. Perinephric abscesses occasionally fail to communicate with the urinary system resulting in a normal urinalysis.
    - **Infective endocarditis:** Culture-negative endocarditis occur in 5–10% of endocarditis. The HACEK (*Haemophilus* species, *Aggregatibacter* species, *Cardiobacterium hominis, Eikenella corrodens* and *Kingella species*) group are responsible for 5–10% of cases of infective endocarditis and are the most common cause of gram-negative endocarditis in individuals without any abuse of intravenous (IV) drugs.
    - **Hepatobiliary infections,** e.g. cholangitis can develop without local signs and with only mildly elevated or normal liver function tests especially in the elderly.
    - **Osteomyelitis:** Usually causes localized pain or discomfort at least sporadically.
    - **Brucellosis:** It should be considered in patients with persistent fever and a history of contact

Textbook of Medicine

with cattle, swine, goats or sheep or patients who consume raw milk products.

- *Borrelia recurrentis:* It is transmitted by ticks and is responsible for relapsing fever.
- *Other spirochetal diseases* that can cause PUO include *Spirillum minor* (rat-bite fever), *Borrelia burgdorferi* (Lyme disease) and *Treponema pallidum* (syphilis).

- **Viral**
  - *Herpes viruses:* Such as CMV and Epstein-Barr (EB) virus can cause prolonged febrile illnesses with constitutional symptoms without any significant organ manifestations, particularly in the elderly.
  - *HIV:* Prolonged febrile episodes are frequent in patients with advanced HIV infection.

- *Fungi:* Immunosuppression, the use of broad-spectrum antibiotics, the presence of intravascular devices and total parenteral nutrition all predispose individual to disseminated fungal infections.

- *Parasites*
  - *Malaria*
  - *Toxoplasmosis:* It should be considered in a febrile patients with lymph node enlargement.
  - *Trypanosoma, Leishmania* and *Amoeba* species may rarely cause PUO.

- ■ **Rickettsial organisms:** *Coxiella burnetii* may cause chronic infections—chronic Q fever or Q fever endocarditis may be identified in patients with a PUO.
- ■ **Psittacosis:** Infection by the causative organism, *Chlamydophila* should be considered in a patient with PUO, who has a history of contact with birds.
- ■ **Neoplasms:** Primary or metastatic neoplasms constitute 20% of cases of PUO (Table 35.1).
- ■ **Collagen vascular disease/autoimmune disease constitute 20% of cases of PUO (Table 35.1).**
- ■ **Psychogenic fevers**
  - *Habitual hyperthermia:* It is seen in young females, characterized by temperatures of 99°–100.5°F that occurs regularly or intermittently for years. No organic cause can be found.
  - *Afebrile FUO:* In this, patient always complaints of feverishness but the temperature recorded is always less than 38.3°C.

- **Exaggerated circadian rhythm:** Normal person usually have an evening rise of temperature which is not normally apparent. In this condition, it becomes evident.
- **Hysterical fever:** In this, the patient is thinking in subconscious mind that he is always having fever.
- **Malignant hyperthermia:** It is a rare life-threatening condition triggered by exposure to certain drugs used for general anesthesia (specifically all volatile anesthetics), nearly all gas anesthetics and the neuromuscular blocking agent succinylcholine.
- **Neuroleptic malignant syndrome (NMS):** It is a rare, life-threatening, neurological disorder most often caused by an adverse reaction to neuroleptic or antipsychotic drug. It presents with muscle rigidity, fever and autonomic instability.

- ■ *Periodic fevers,* e.g. familial mediterranean fever (polyserositis).
- ■ *Miscellaneous constitute 10% cases.*
- ■ *Undiagnosed FUOS (10% cases):* About 10–15% of patients remain undiagnosed despite extensive investigations and in 75% of these, the fever resolves spontaneously. In the remainder, other signs and symptoms make the diagnosis clear.

DIAGNOSTIC APPROACH

Most important parameter to be ascertained is whether there is a rise of temperature above normal (to be verified by proper measurement with a thermometer) or it is only the patient's feeling of feverishness (which is a vague subjective sensation by the patient which he interprets as fever even without raise of temperature). In most cases feverishness does not have the same significance as fever.

Careful attention to history and a complete physical examination is repeated when necessary. It may reveal the etiology in many cases. Enquire about possible recent exposure to sexually transmitted disease (STD), injected illicit drug use, which may predispose to hepatitis B and C, HIV and infective endocarditis. Travel history may give a clue. Occupational history may be significant and give evidence of exposure to birds (psittacosis) or animals (toxoplasmosis and brucellosis).

Examination of ocular fundi may reveal etiological clues—Roth spots in infective endocarditis, choroid tubercles in miliary TB and CMV retinitis. It is important to reasses the patient clinically at regular intervals. Look carefully for skin rash, skin nodules, conjunctival petechiae, clubbing and splinter hemorrhage. Digital rectal examination may suggest the cause occasionally. Perianal disease suggest IBD. Local sepsis, abscess, rectal carcinoma, prostatitis and prostatic malignancy may be suspected by per-rectal examination and examination of the perianal region.

Even though the first clinical examination may be negative, repetition at weekly intervals or more frequently will bring out diagnostic clues and therefore this is an important diagnostic procedure.

Investigations: Investigations must be individualized based on the most probable suspected diagnosis.

Table 35.1: Neoplasms and collagen vascular diseases causing PUO

Neoplasms—primary or metastatic (20% cases)	Collagen vascular disease/ autoimmune disease (20% cases)

• Hematological leukemias, lymphomas, plasma cell dyscrasias, bone marrow aplasia, Myelodysplastic syndrome
• Non-hematological
  ▪ Renal cell cancer
  ▪ Hepatocellular carcinoma
  ▪ Pancreatic cancer
  ▪ Colon cancer
  ▪ Sarcomas
  ▪ Atrial myxoma
  ▪ Malignant histiocytosis
	• Adult Still's disease
	• Polymyalgia rheumatica
	• Temporal arteritis
	• Rheumatoid arthritis
	• Rheumatic fever
	• Inflammatory bowel disease
	• Reiter's syndrome
	• Systemic lupus erythematosus
	• Vasculitides
	  ▪ Polyarteritis nodosa
	  ▪ Giant cell arteritis
	  ▪ Kawasaki disease

Differential diagnosis will depend upon the geographical area, age of the patient and comorbid conditions. In general non-invasive investigations should be done first before resorting to invasive investigations such as biopsy endoscopy and others.

A complete blood count and erythrocyte sedimentation rate (ESR) is to be done in all cases. ESR above 80 mm/first hour is seen in TB, malignancy, connective tissue diseases and temporal arteritis. A peripheral smear is to be examined for abnormal cells, malarial parasite and atypical lymphocytes.

Mid-stream urine is to be collected for microscopy and culture. Bacterial counts above 10^5 organisms/mL indicate UTI.

Isolation of Infective Agent

Blood culture should be done routinely in all fevers persisting more than a week. Many a time repeated blood cultures may have to be done to isolate the organism, e.g. infective endocarditis.

Polymerase chain reaction (PCR) is very valuable in detecting ribonucleic acid (RNA)/deoxyribonucleic acid (DNA) of infecting organisms early in the disease. It is also useful in estimating the viral load in infections due to hepatitis virus B and C. It is specific and reliable, but false positive results may occur.

Rise in serum uric acid level may suggest rapid cell turnover occurring in malignancies like lymphomas. Rise in alkaline phosphatase, especially the hepatic isoenzymes indicate liver cell involvement.

Mantoux test: This is a commonly done test to detect hypersensitivity to tuberculoprotein. Positive Mantoux test indicates the possibility of tuberculous infection—past or active. In active TB, the Mantoux test is generally hyperactive, but it may be misleadingly negative in miliary TB and immunocompromised persons. The specificity of this test is very low and diagnostic value is poor except in children.

Imaging Studies

X-ray imaging: This is the most time honored, almost universally available, relatively cheap and non-invasive imaging modality which is very helpful in the diagnosis of lesions in the chest (e.g. pneumonia and TB), paranasal sinuses, bones and joints and others. Plain skiagrams and specialized procedures are available to delineate almost all organ systems. Limited skeletal survey is useful in suspected multiple myeloma.

Ultrasound imaging: The morphology of several organ systems in the body can be imaged by ultrasound using appropriate probes and computer techniques. This modality has become a very useful and commonly used investigation to detect organomegaly in the abdomen, detection of fluid in the abdomen, plural cavities and pericardium. Examination of the abdomen may detect abnormalities in the liver (tumor, abscess), biliary system, kidneys, retroperitoneal nodes, pus and fluid collections, ascites and organomegaly. Thyroid and cervical axillary lymph nodes also can be assessed.

Echocardiography is useful in detecting cardiac vegetation, atrial myxoma and other cardiac abnormalities.

Therefore, this is a very valuable investigation to rule out or confirm a diagnosis of infective endocarditis. In infective endocarditis transesophageal echocardiograph yields better results.

Isotope bone scan is useful in detecting malignancy, osteomyelitis and septic arthritis.

Other imaging modalities: These include computed tomography (CT) scanning, magnetic resonance imaging (MRI) scanning, positron emission tomography (PET) scanning and their further modifications are appropriate to the organ and the disease to be studied.

Selected Serological Tests

- ***Infections:*** Examples are typhoid, leptospirosis, brucellosis, dengue fever, EB virus, CMV, chlamydiae, mycoplasma, Q fever, amebiasis, leishmaniasis, toxoplasmosis and others.

  Detection of specific antibodies against infecting organisms or their products, e.g. widal reaction detects antibodies against salmonella. Antistreptolysin-O (ASO) titer estimates the antibody to the toxin of streptococcus. Tests such as ESR and C-reactive protein (CRP) indicate the presence of an inflammatory process, nonspecifically. Once the infection is identified, serial determination of ESR or CRP helps to assess progress.

  Elevation of procalcitonin levels in serum is a fairly reliable test for bacterial infections. Normal level in serum is only less than 0.1 µg/L (0.1 ng/mL). Elevation to 2 ng/mL strongly suggests bacterial infection. Elevation above 10 ng/mL is almost conclusive. The test is expensive and available only in highly specialized centers. Still in conditions where the diagnosis is in doubt in a life-threatening illness, procalcitonin levels give helpful clue for diagnosis and follow-up.

- ***Autoimmune disease and vasculitis:*** Antinuclear antibody (ANA), anti-dsDNA helps in diagnosis of SLE. Rheumatoid factor and anti-CCP are useful in diagnosis of rheumatoid arthritis. Antineutrophil cytoplasmic antibody (ANCA) is useful in certain types of vasculitis (PAN and Wegener's granulomatosis).

  Selection of further investigations needs careful consideration of the likely benefit and the cost involved. Gastrointestinal endoscopy with biopsy is indicated, if symptoms or findings on imaging studies suggest diseases of the abdominal hollow viscera such as IBD, intestinal TB or cancer.

Bronchoscopy and bronchoalveolar lavage for Gram stain, culture of organisms and cytology for malignant cells may be considered in selected cases. Presence of more than 90% lymphocytes in bronchial lavage washing is suggestive of pulmonary sarcoidosis. If the relative proportion of CD4–CD8 lymphocytes is more than 3.5, it further strengthens the diagnosis. Estimation of angiotensin converting enzyme (ACE) levels in serum is helpful to diagnose sarcoidosis.

Sarcoidosis shows elevation of serum ACE levels. Normal levels are 9–67 U/L. High levels are seen in 50% of acute and only 20% of chronic cases. This test is not routinely

Textbook of Medicine

done at present due to unreliability. Sarcoidosis is better diagnosed by biopsy procedures done transbronchially or done on minor salivary glands (*See* Ch 146).

Role of biopsy in the diagnosis of FUO: All biopsy procedures are invasive and associated with some risks and hence, should be reserved for cases where diagnosis is not arrived at by simpler procedures. Biopsy specimen can be obtained either by open biopsy or fine needle aspiration cytology (FNAC). Biopsy specimen should also be sent for culture of the organisms and sensitivity studies as well.

Liver biopsy: This procedure may help to diagnose miliary TB, sarcoidosis, lymphoma, histoplasmosis and tumors. Guidance with ultrasound helps to reach the target precisely. Yield is generally low if liver function test and liver imaging are normal.

Bone marrow aspiration and biopsy: This is most useful in diagnosing hematological disorders such as leukemias, myeloma and marrow infiltrates. Among infections, visceral leishmaniasis is diagnosed by bone marrow examination. Typhoid, brucellosis, TB and other infections can be diagnosed by bone marrow culture and this is done when blood culture is negative.

Lymph node biopsy: This is useful when nodes are enlarged, as in lymphomas, TB, secondary malignant deposits and others. In generalized lymphadenopathy, it is better to take a node which is moderately enlarged. Since, the inguinal nodes are likely to show non-specific changes, they are preferably avoided.

MANAGEMENT

Symptomatic Treatment for Fever

Fever demands treatment on its own when it becomes uncomfortable or positively harmful as in hyperpyrexia.

Physical methods such as sponging with lukewarm or room temperature water and exposure to breeze, help to dissipate heat and lower the temperature rapidly, but the effect is transient.

Antipyretics

Paracetamol is a commonly used, reasonably safe and freely available antipyretic and analgesic drug, often obtainable even as a non-prescription drug.

Usually given in doses of 500–750 mg orally 3–4 times daily. The temperature starts falling within 10–15 minutes with sweating and it remains normal or elevated to a lower level for 3–4 hours after which the temperature shoots up again when the effect of the drug wanes. Adverse effects include allergy, gastrointestinal upsets. Maximum recommended dose per day in adult is 4 g in 4 or more divided doses. It should be remembered that though paracetamol is a common across the counter drug, overdose of this drug leads to very serious liver damage with high mortality. In persons with liver disease, paracetamol is better avoided. Aspirin and nonsteroidal anti-inflammatory drugs (NSAIDs) show potent antipyretic effect, but they are not recommended for routine use because of their common side effects like acute gastritis, hemorrhagic gastritis with upper gastrointestinal bleed and renal damage in some individuals. Many short viral fevers, especially dengue fever, leptospirosis, malaria

and sepsis may be associated with thrombocytopenia. NSAIDs and aspirin may aggravate bleeding in them. Since, renal involvement is common in dengue fever, leptospirosis, falciparum malaria and sepsis, NSAIDs which are nephrotoxic should be used with caution. There is no indication to give antipyretics if the fever is tolerated by patient comfortably and the fever itself does not rise to hyperthermic level. Indiscriminate use of antipyretics lead to the following disadvantages:

- Diagnostic clues from the pattern of fever are lost
- Beneficial effect of fever in infections is lost
- Response to specific treatment cannot be assessed
- The drug may induce rigors with return of fever—once antipyretic effect is over
- Excess sweating with fluid loss and occasionally hypotension may develop.

Definite indications for antipyretics

Hyperpyrexia is the most urgent indication to bring down the temperature. Other indications are:

- Significant somatic symptoms like headache and bodyache
- Coexisting symptomatic coronary artery disease and cardiac failure
- Cerebrovascular disease, nervous system dysfunction and head injury
- Epileptic patients
- Children with history of febrile convulsions.

Pregnancy and psychiatric illness are relative indications to lower the temperature, since there are some complications.

Diet in Fever

Since fever increases metabolism, high calorie diet is recommended. Adequate fluid and electrolyte are also important to avoid dehydration. Observe oral hygiene. Diet containing at least 1500 calories and 3.5–4 L of fluids in various forms should be administered. It is preferable to avoid food which produce a sense of bloating and discomfort.

Antibiotics

Fever is to be treated with antipyretics and not with antibiotics. It is a common practice to give a trial of empirical antibiotics in short febrile illness. Favorable response is not a proof of bacterial infection. Most of the short febrile illnesses are due to viral infections, which are self-limiting. In immunocompetent subjects, antibacterial antibiotics should not be used empirically. They are indicated only if there is clinical or investigation evidence of bacterial infection. There is no need for general use of prophylactic antibiotics except in special situations (Refer Ch 5). Glucocorticoids should not be used as general antipyretics since, they may lead to several adverse effects (Refer Ch 6). 'Shotgun mixtures of antibiotics and steroids are to be condemned, because they usually solve nothing, confuse the clinical picture and are not without hazards'.

- ***Treatment of classic FUO:*** If the condition is stable and no etiological diagnosis is arrived—avoid empirical therapy. However, if an undiagnosed patient is too ill to permit prolonged observation, empirical treatment

Textbook of Medicine

may be considered based on the best clinical judgment. It is also to be emphasized that 'initiation of empirical therapy does not make the end of diagnostic work up; rather, it commits the physician to continue thoughtful re-examination and evaluation' so that the empirical therapy does not cause further harm.

- ***Treatment of neutropenic FUO:*** After sending specimens for culture of organisms, empirical broad spectrum antibiotic coverage for pseudomonas such as ticarcillin/piperacillin/ceftazidime with gentamicin/amikacin is to be initiated. If clinical features point to fungal infection, antifungal drugs such as amphotericin in the usual dose has to be given.

- ***Treatment of HIV associated FUO:*** Acute onset fever with hypoxia in an HIV infected patient is often treated for *Pneumocystis carinii* infection after sending specimens to confirm the diagnosis. In undiagnosed prolonged fever investigation for TB and other opportunistic infection to be performed. Anti-TB treatment to be considered if there is evidence/strong suspicion of TB. Specific treatment for HIV should also be started simultaneously.

- ***Treatment of nosocomial FUO:*** Many patients may be critically ill. IV lines may have to be changed and cultured. Empirical antibiotics may have to be given depending on the microbial prevalence in the environment in critically ill patients.

Undiagnosed FUO: About 15% remain undiagnosed despite extensive evaluation. Of these patients, fever subsides in about 75% without a diagnosis, the remaining more classic manifestations of the underlying disease may appear overtime.

Prognosis: This depends on the success of the investigation to arrive at the specific etiological diagnosis and prompt therapy. The overall mortality in FUO is 20–30%. It is higher as age advances.

CONCLUSION

FUO is a common challenge to the practicing physician. Many patients are placed in FUO category because the attending physician overlooks, disregards or rejects an obvious clue. Physicians who care for febrile patients need to talk to them, observe them and think about them. There are no substitutes for these simple clinical principles.

Points to Remembers

- Majority of FUOs are due to atypical presentation of common diseases.
- In India about 50% are caused by infections. Other common causes are autoimmune diseases, malignancy and drug fever.
- A properly elicited history and good clinical examination and repeated re-evaluation give a clue about the diagnosis.
- Avoid empirical antibiotics except in life-threatening situations.

CHAPTER

36

Sepsis and Septic Shock

S Bhasi

Chapter Summary

- Epidemiology
- Etiology
- Pathogenesis
- Clinical Manifestations
- Diagnosis
- Treatment

INTRODUCTION

The clinical syndrome of sepsis is defined as ***infection with evidence of systemic inflammatory response***.

In 1992, the American College of Chest Physicians and the Society of Critical Care Medicine (ACCP/SCCM) developed a consensus statement on the definition of sepsis and its sequelae (details are given below). The definition as per new guidelines (2012) 'presence of infection (probable or documented) together with systemic manifestations of infection'.

Systemic inflammatory response syndrome (SIRS) may have an infective or non-infective etiology such as autoimmune disorders, pancreatitis, vasculitis,

burns, surgery and others. Sepsis can be classified as uncomplicated sepsis, severe sepsis and septic shock. ***Uncomplicated sepsis***, such as that caused by flu and other viral infections, gastroenteritis and others is very common, experienced by millions every year and majority self-limiting. When sepsis is associated with dysfunction of organs distant from the site of infection, it is termed as ***severe sepsis***. When severe sepsis is accompanied by hypotension which is not correctable by appropriate intravenous (IV) fluid infusion (30 mL/kg of crystalloid solutions), the condition is termed as ***septic shock***. Sepsis, severe sepsis and septic shock can be considered as a continuous process, depending on increasing severity of the condition (Fig. 36.1). Septic shock is a kind of vasodilatory or distributive shock.

EPIDEMIOLOGY

The incidence of severe sepsis is estimated to be about 90 million cases worldwide per year and is on the increase. About 10% of sepsis progresses to severe sepsis and 3% of severe sepsis develops septic shock. Advancing age,

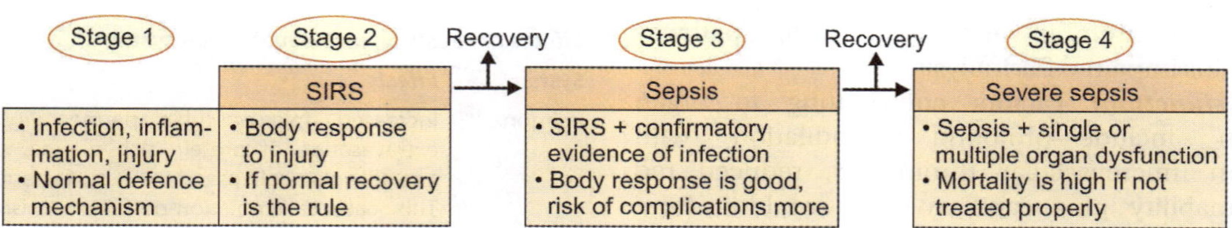

Fig. 36.1: Progress of events leading to severe sepsis

Abbreviation: SIRS = Systemic inflammatory response syndrome

diabetes mellitus (DM), malignancy, immunodeficiency and chronic organ failure predispose to the development of shock. Males are more prone than females to develop septic shock. Genetic factors may contribute.

ETIOLOGY

Severe sepsis occurs as a result of both community acquired and healthcare associated infections. Pneumonia is the most common disease accounting for about half of all cases, followed by abdominal and urinary tract infections (UTIs). Soft tissue infections may also be responsible in some. In the past, majority of cases were due to gram-negative bacterial infection. At present approximately 50% are due to gram-positive organisms as well. *Staphylococcus aureus* and *Streptococcus pneumoniae* are the most common gram-positive isolates. *Enterococci*, coagulase negative *Staphylococci* and *Streptococcus pyogenes* are responsible in some. *Escherichia coli*, *Klebsiella* species and *Pseudomonas aeruginosa* predominate among gram-negative isolates. *Enterobacter* and *Proteus* are less common causes. Less frequently *Bacteroides* and *Clostridia* may cause sepsis. Viruses, rickettsia and fungi are responsible at times. Incidence of fungal sepsis has increased over the past decade, but remains lower than bacterial sepsis. Polymicrobial infection is not uncommon. About 25% of the infections are multidrug resistant. Implanted foreign bodies, indwelling vascular appliances and indwelling urinary catheters may contribute to development of infection. Severity of disease appears to be increasing.

Definitions of commonly used terms in sepsis	
Term	**Definition**
Bacteremia	Presence of viable bacteria in the blood
SIRS	Severe inflammatory response characterized by 2 or more of the following: • Temperature ≥ 38.3°C or < 36°C • Heart rate > 90 beats/min • Respiratory rate > 20/minute • White blood cell count > 12000 cells/mm³ • < 4000/m³ or > 10 % band forms of neutrophils
Sepsis	Presence of SIRS with definitive evidence of infection
Severe sepsis	Sepsis associated with organ dysfunction, hypoperfusion or hypotension (systolic BP < 90 mm Hg) or a decrease of 40 mm Hg from baseline systolic BP or MAP < 70 mm Hg
Septic shock fluid	Sepsis with hypotension (systolic BP < 90 mm Hg) persisting despite adequate resuscitation and the development of abnormalities such as oliguria, altered mental status or lactic acidosis
MODS	Progressive organ dysfunction in an acutely ill patient such that homeostasis cannot be maintained without intervention

Source: American College of Contingency Planners (ACCP), Society of Critical Care Medicine (SCCM)

Abbreviations: SIRS = Systemic inflammatory response syndrome; MODS = Multi-organ dysfunction syndrome; BP = Blood pressure; MAP = Mean arterial pressure

PATHOGENESIS

Pathogenesis of sepsis is very complex. The host response of sepsis is characterized by proinflammatory responses and anti-inflammatory plus immunosuppressive responses. Activation of immune system during microbial infection is generally protective, properly regulated and contained, with a balance set between inflammatory and anti-inflammatory mediators.

Th_1 lymphocytes are proinflammatory. The proinflammatory reactions are needed in eliminating invading pathogens but also responsible for tissue damage in severe sepsis. Tumor necrosis factor alpha (TNFα), interleukins-1 (IL-1) and IL-2 and interferon γ (IFNγ) are proinflammatory. Th_2 lymphocytes and IL-4 and IL-10 help to restrain the inflammatory process and reduce tissue damage. In severe sepsis this balance is upset and the inflammation is uncontrolled, poorly regulated, self-sustaining, widespread and involving distant organs away from the site of infection as well.

The products of micro-organisms include lipoteichoic acid, endotoxins which are lipopolysaccharides (LPS), exotoxins and various microbial antigens. When liberated, these act directly on the host tissues. They stimulate the production of proinflammatory cytokines such as TNFα, 1L-1, and IFNγ and enzymes such as proteases. TNFα and IL-1 produce fever, vasodilation, hypotension, gluconeogenesis, lipolysis, myocardial depression, hypoxia and increased capillary permeability. This leads to extravasation of plasma with resultant low intravascular volume, hypoperfusion and shock. Nitric oxide is also released producing excessive vasodilation. Endotoxins also activate the alternate complement cascade. This results in the release of anaphylatoxins such as C3a and C5a leading to vasodilation, increased vascular permeability, aggregation of platelets and neutrophils.

Coagulation abnormalities: Severe sepsis is invariably associated with coagulation abnormalities leading to disseminated intravascular coagulation (DIC) especially microvascular thrombosis. This is caused by activation of coagulation, mediated by tissue factor, impairment of anti-coagulant mechanisms like reduced levels of activated

Textbook of Medicine

protein C, antithrombin and tissue factor pathway inhibitors plus impaired fibrinolysis.

Organ dysfunction: Factors contributing to organ dysfunction include—profound vasodilation with hypotension, microvascular thrombosis, reduced red cell deformability plus capillary leak resulting from endothelial dysfunction leading to interstitial edema, tissue hypoperfusion and reduced tissue oxygenation. In addition, mitochondrial damage caused by reactive oxygen species, IL-1 and TNFα impair cellular oxygen use. Injured mitochondria release alarmins into extracellular environment which will activate neutrophils and cause further tissue injury. Global tissue hypoxia leads to elevated serum lactate, a value of more than 4 mmol/L is correlated with increased severity of illness and poor outcome.

Immunosuppression: The immune system harbors humoral, cellular and neural mechanisms (mediated by vagus) that attenuate potentially harmful effects of proinflammatory responses. Phagocytes transform to anti-inflammatory phenotype promoting tissue repair. Regulatory T cells and myeloid derived suppressor cells reduce inflammation. Many patients with severe sepsis show evidence of immunosuppression.

CLINICAL MANIFESTATIONS

The clinical manifestations of sepsis are highly variable depending on the initial site of infection, causative organism, underlying health status of the patient and degree of acute organ dysfunction. These may be classified as: 1. Features of the primary disease and 2. Features of sepsis and septic shock.

1. ***Findings at the primary site of disease:*** These include the organ system which is primarily affected, e.g. pneumonia, cellulitis, pyelonephritis or intra-abdominal infection.
2. ***General effects of sepsis and septic shock:*** Varying degrees of fever occur in the vast majority, but in 15% of patients temperature may be normal or even subnormal/hypothermia. Tachypnea, tachycardia with weak thready pulse, hypotension, cold clammy skin, cyanosis, oliguria and alteration of sensorium are common. Cyanosis may be peripheral in shock or central in ventilatory failure. In the early stages of sepsis the mental state may be normal, urine output normal and extremities are warm due to hyperdynamic circulation. Tachypnea may produce respiratory alkalosis. Metabolic acidosis occurs in later stages. Critical illness polyneuropathy and myopathy are common in severe sepsis especially with prolonged intensive care unit (ICU) stay. Paralytic ileus, elevated transaminases, altered glycemic control, adrenal dysfunction and euthyroid sick syndrome (ESS) are all common with severe sepsis. Survivors of severe sepsis may show impaired physical or neurocognitive functioning and low quality of life.

If shock worsens and is prolonged multi-organ failure occurs and the condition becomes irreversible. At this stage mortality exceeds 80%. Death is often due to multi-organ failure and DIC.

Effects of sepsis on individual organ systems

System	Effects
Pulmonary	Increased microvascular permeability leads to extravasation of protein rich edema within lungs and alveolar collapse due to surfactant deficiency. This causes ventilation-perfusion mismatch, decrease in lung compliance and development of acute respiratory distress syndrome (ARDS). ARDS is defined as hypoxemia with bilateral infiltrates in the lungs of non-cardiac origin
Heart	Early in sepsis there is usually hyperdynamic circulation with increased cardiac output and increased heart rate. Later cardiac dysfunction may occur with global reduction in ejection fraction and elevated troponin level. There is usually diastolic dilatation of left ventricular and may require greater filling pressure to maintain cardiac output. This results in hypoperfusion, hypoxia and elevated serum lactate. Pulmonary vascular resistance may increase. Cardiac dysfunction in sepsis is usually reversible
Central nervous system (CNS)	Inadequate oxygen delivery leads to agitation, delirium, mental confusion and coma. Depression of the cough reflex predisposes to accumulation of secretions in the airway and respiratory infection
Bone marrow and blood	Hematopoiesis, particularly thrombopoiesis and myelopoiesis may be depressed. DIC and alteration in red blood cell (RBC) deformability lead to thrombosis and occlusion in the microcirculation
Renal	Acute kidney injury mainly due to ischemic tubular necrosis lead to oliguria (< 0.5 mL/kg/hr) and acute renal failure (ARF) (creatinine rise more than 0.5 mg/dL from baseline). Use of IV contrast dyes and aminoglycoside antibiotics may precipitate renal failure

DIAGNOSIS

A careful history, physical examination and appropriate imaging and laboratory studies are to be conducted in all cases.

Leukocytosis with shift to left with toxic granules in the neutrophils, thrombocytopenia and hyperbilirubinemia are present early in the course. Leukopenia may develop later. The primary site of infection—respiratory, intra-abdominal, urinary tract, soft tissues or IV line-related, should be identified. Elevated lactate indicates tissue hypoperfusion with hypoxia. Elevated serum procalcitonin suggests bacterial sepsis. C-reactive protein (CRP) test is elevated. With coagulopathy, activated partial thromboplastin time (APTT) can be increased more than 60. Prothrombin time (PT)/international normalized ratio (INR) may be prolonged. Appropriate investigations have to be done to find out site of infection. Culture of blood and other specimen to be sent before starting antimicrobials.

The circulatory state, hematological abnormalities, respiratory function, renal function and fluid—electrolyte status should be assessed from time to time in order to institute life-saving measures.

Course and Prognosis

Unless recognized early and managed with intensive care facilities, septic shock is invariably fatal due to circulatory and multi-organ failure. The risk may be evaluated from the onset and during the course by acute physiology and chronic health evaluation (APACHE) protocols. Higher scores indicate higher risk.

TREATMENT

Management of patient with severe sepsis and septic shock is complex, requiring multiple concurrent interventions with close monitoring and re-evaluation. The main principles are treating and eliminating the source of infection, timely and appropriate use of antimicrobials, hemodynamic optimization and organ support measures.

Antimicrobials: Early institution of specific antimicrobial therapy is life-saving and is to be started within 1 hour of recognition of severe sepsis/septic shock. Blood and other relevant specimens should be sent for culture before starting antimicrobials. The choice of the agent depends on knowledge of the likely pathogen, the specific site of infection, sensitivity pattern of organisms in the institution, immunocompetence of the patient and whether the infection is hospital acquired or community acquired. The empirical initial choice should be bactericidal, broad spectrum with activity against gram-positive and gram-negative organisms given IV in the maximum recommended dosage. Reassess after 48–78 hours on the basis of microbiological and clinical data, with the aim of changing to narrow spectrum to prevent the development of resistance, reduce toxicity and cost. Combination therapy is recommended only for sepsis caused by *Pseudomonas* species and neutropenic sepsis. Typical duration of therapy is 7–10 days guided by clinical response. Longer duration is recommended if response is slow. Consider coverage of anaerobes also when indicated.

Recommended antibiotics are:

- Inj. ceftriaxone 1–2 g IV bd (ceftazidime/cefepime in neutropenic patients to cover pseudomonas)
- Ticarcillin and clavulanate 3.1 g 4 times daily by IV or infusion
- Piperacillin-tazobactam 4.5 g 4 times daily IM or IV or infusion
- Imipenem cilastatin 500 mg 4 times day IM or IV or meropenem 1 g by IM or IV injection 3 times a day.

An aminoglycoside may be added to any of the above drugs in selected cases.

Patients allergic to β-lactamase be given ciprofloxacin (400 mg IV bd) or levofloxacin (500–750 mg IV od) with clindamycin 600 mg 3 or 4 times a day by IV infusion. Vancomycin 1 g IV bd or Q8H by slow IV infusion over 60 minutes may be added if methicillin-resistant *Staphylococcus aureus* (MRSA) is suspected. Antifungal therapy may be needed in immunocompromised neutropenic patients. The duration of therapy and alteration of the agent have to be based on microbiological investigations.

- ***Attention to the focus of infection:*** Drainage of abscesses, debridement of infected necrotic tissue and removal of potentially infected devices including intravascular devices and foreign bodies are necessary early in the disease.
- ***Fluid therapy:*** Begin goal directed fluid resuscitation during the first 6 hours (with documented benefit) in presence of hypotension and/or serum lactate ≥ 4 mmol/L (36 mg/dL). Initial fluid therapy is about 20 mL/kg—average 1000 mL of crystalloid like normal saline over 30 minutes. The target central venous pressure (CVP) is 8–12 mm Hg (12–15 mm in mechanically ventilated patients). Albumin may be added if very large volumes of crystalloids are required to maintain arterial pressure. Up to 5 L of crystalloids may be required in the first 6 hours. Continuation of less rigorous IV fluid is often needed in first 24 hours. Parameters suggesting adequacy of therapy are mean arterial pressure (MAP) ≥ 65 mm Hg, heart rate (HR) < 110, CVP > 8 mm, urine output > 0.5 mL/kg/hour, normal consciousness, apparent skin perfusion, central venous (superior vena cava) oxygen saturation ≥ 70% (or mixed venous oxygen saturation ≥ 65%). Fluid administration to be reduced when cardiac filling pressure (CVP and pulmonary capillary wedge pressure) increases without concurrent hemodynamic improvement. Monitor and avoid pulmonary edema.
- ***Vasopressors and inotropes:*** It is customary to use an arterial catheter to enable continuous arterial BP monitoring. Noradrenaline increases MAP due to vasoconstrictive effect with little change in heart and cardiac output and is the agent of choice. Dobutamine may be added to noradrenaline with better efficacy especially in patient with myocardial systolic dysfunction. The aim is to maintain systolic BP > 90 mm Hg, MAP > 65 (higher target to be aimed in patients with pre-existing uncontrolled hypertension). Low dose vasopressin (0.01–0.04 u/min) may be added in selected patients not responding to conventional vasopressors. Relative vasopressin deficiency is documented in some patients with septic shock.
- ***Blood glucose control:*** Patients with septic shock tend to develop glucose intolerance. Insulin therapy is to be started if 2 consecutive blood glucose values are > 180 mg to maintain a target of 140–180 mg/dL.
- ***Deep venous thrombosis (DVT) prophylaxis:*** Recommended because of higher incidence of DVT.
- ***Glucocorticoids:*** Low dose hydrocortisone—200 mg/day as IV in divided doses in septic shock patients and BP response to fluid resuscitation and vasopressor therapy is poor. This is to be continued for 5–7 days. This promotes more rapid shock reversal. Adrenocorticotropic hormone (ACTH) stimulation test is not recommended. Relative glucocorticoid deficiency is seen in some patients with septic shock and this forms the basis. Hydrocortisone may be tapered when vasopressors are no longer required.
- ***Ventilatory support:*** About 50% patients with severe sepsis will develop acute lung injury (ALI)/acute respiratory distress syndrome (ARDS). Diagnostic feature are bilateral patchy infiltrates on chest X-ray, low PaO_2/FiO_2 ratio (less than 300 for ALI, < 200 for ARDS). Ventilatory support is needed with adequate oxygen supplementation to maintain pulse oximetry saturation of more than 90%. Elevate head end of the bed unless contraindicated. Use conservative fluid therapy for established ALI/ARDS with no evidence

of tissue hypoperfusion. Assistance to ventilation in tachypnea patients reduces the effort for respiration and favors recovery. Non-invasive methods of ventilatory assistance is adequate in most cases.

- ***Blood and blood products:*** These are life-saving if used appropriately with care. Whole blood, packed red cells, platelets, plasma and coagulation factors have to be used when indicated. If the patient is hypovolemic and anemic with hematocrit < 30% it is appropriate to transfuse packed red cells. This helps in improving oxygen delivery to ischemic tissue beds and keeps CVP > 8 mm for longer periods than fluid therapy alone. In the absence of ischemic heart disease, severe hypoxemia, red cell transfusion is recommended only is Hb is < 7 g to a target of 7–9 g. In the absence of bleeding, prophylactic ***platelet transfusion*** is indicated when the count is less than 10,000, less than 20,000 if patient has significant risk of bleeding. Platelet transfusion to be given to patient with >50,000 count only if invasive procedures are needed. Fresh frozen plasma (FFP) not to be used to correct lab clotting abnormalities in the absence of bleeding or planned invasive procedures. Routine use of ***immunoglobulin*** is not recommended.
- ***Renal replacement therapy:*** This is needed in those who develop renal failure; best results are obtained with early dialysis or continuous venovenous hemofiltration.
- ***Stress ulcer prophylaxis:*** To be administered to prevent upper gastrointestinal tract (GIT) bleed which

may complicate the illness. Proton pump inhibitors, like omeprazole or pantoprazole 20–40 mg given bed time reduces the risk.

- ***Sodium bicarbonate:*** For patients with sepsis of any etiology and lactic acidosis, no benefit from giving IV bicarbonate therapy and hence not recommended.
- ***Nutrition:*** Sepsis is a hypermetabolic state. High calorie high protein diet with supplementation of micronutrients and maintenance of electrolyte balance is important. Oral or enteral feeding as tolerated is superior to parenteral feeding.
- ***Addendum (by editor):*** Several prospective trials have been conducted to study the effect of maintaining euglycemia and several protocol based studies instituted for the management of septic shock have not shown a distinct advantage in recovery and survival so far.

Source: Rhee C, Gohil S, Klompas M. Regulatory mandates for sepsis care—reasons for caution. N Engl J Med. 2014;370(18):1673-6.

Points to Remember

- Patients with severe sepsis and septic shock to be managed in ICU.
- Multidisciplinary approach is necessary in reducing mortality.
- Timely institution of antibiotics, fluid resuscitation, vasopressor agents with or +/– inotropes are main stay in the treatment.
- Ventilatory support and renal replacement therapy may be needed in severe cases.
- Blood and blood products to be used only when absolutely indicated.

CHAPTER 37

Systemic Diseases caused by Cocci

KV Krishna Das

Chapter Summary

- Streptococcal Infections
  - General Considerations
    - Pharyngitis
    - Scarlet Fever
    - Erysipelas
    - Impetigo
    - Cellulitis
    - Lymphangitic
    - Bacteremia
    - Necrotizing Fasciitis
    - Myositis
    - Pneumonia and Empyema
    - Toxic Shock Syndrome
  - Other Pathogenic Strains of Streptococci
    - *Streptococcus agalactiae*
    - *Streptococcus viridans*
    - *Enterococci*

- Acute Rheumatic Fever
  - Epidemiology
  - Pathogenesis
  - Pathology
  - Clinical Features
  - Course and Progress
  - Diagnosis
  - Differential Diagnosis
  - Treatment
  - Prevention
  - Post-streptococcal Glomerulonephritis
- Staphylococcal Infections
  - General Considerations
    - Epidemiology
    - Pathogenesis
    - Lesions Produced by Staphylococci
  - Superficial Lesions
    - Furuncle
    - Carbuncle

  – Impetigo
  – Ecthyma
  – Sycosis Barbae
  – Follicular Impetigo of Bockhart
  – The Scalded Skin Syndrome
- Staphylococcal Pneumonia
  – Osteomyelitis
  – Bacteremia
  – Food Poisoning
  – Toxic Shock Syndrome
  – Suppurative Infections
  – Tropical Pyomyositis
  – Diagnosis
  – Treatment
- Coagulase Negative Staphylococci
  – *Staphylococcus epidermidis*
  – Treatment
  – Prevention
- Pneumococcal Infections
  - General Considerations
    – Pneumococcal pneumonia
    – Pathology
    – Clinical Features
    – Laboratory Findings
    – Complications
    – Prognosis
  - Extrapulmonary Pneumococcal Lesions
    – Pneumococcal meningitis
    – Pneumococcal peritonitis
    – Treatment
    – Susceptibility Rates of Respiratory Pathogens to Antimicrobials
    – Prevention-Vaccination
- Meningococcal Infections
  - General Considerations
    – *Neisseria meningitidis*
    – Epidemiology
  - Pathogenesis and Pathology
  - Meningococcal Meningitis
  - Meningococcemia
    – Fulminant
    – Chronic
  - Diagnosis
  - Treatment
  - Course and Prognosis
  - Prevention
  - Vaccination

STREPTOCOCCAL INFECTIONS

GENERAL CONSIDERATIONS

Streptococci are among the most common pathogens in homosapiens. The lesions which are caused by direct streptococcal invasion include **pharyngitis** (sore throat), **tonsillitis, erysipelas, cellulitis, impetigo, scarlet fever, septicemia, necrotizing fasciitis, toxic shock syndrome** and **myositis (Table 37.1)**. Immunologically mediated post-infectious complications include acute rheumatic fever and acute glomerulonephritis.

Streptococci is gram-positive cocci 1 μm in diameter, non-motile and non-sporing. Many strains are capsulated. Majority are facultative anaerobes, but some are strictly anaerobic. Streptococci are classified on the basis of

Table 37.1: Lesions caused by *Streptococcus pyogenes* (group A streptococcus)

Lesions	Mechanism
Pharyngitis	Direct infection
Scarlet fever	Erythrogenic toxin
Impetigo	Superficial skin infection
Cellulitis	Infection of deeper layers of the skin
Necrotizing fasciitis, myositis	Invasive and toxigenic infection
Toxic shock syndrome	Virulent factor (M protein) of streptococcal cell wall acting as the triggering agent

the type of hemolysis. Beta-hemolytic strains possess **streptolysins O** and **S**. Majority of the pathogenic strains of streptococci are beta-hemolytic. These have been further subdivided into broad groups A-H and K-V by Lancefield, based on the group specific polysaccharide antigen of the cell wall. *Streptococcus pyogenes* belongs to group A. This strain is further subclassified by Griffith based on surface protein antigens—M, T and R. Out of these, M is the most important and it exists in approximately 60 different antigenic forms, each of which is present in a different serotype 1, 2, etc. Determination of serotype is important to trace source of infections during epidemiological investigation. Over 80 different serotypes of group A streptococcus have been identified. Based on the serotype and the ability to produce the bacterial products pathogenicity varies.

Principal types of streptococci and enterococci pathogenic to man are listed below.

Species	Lancefield group	Type of hemolysis on blood agar
Str. pyogenes	A	Beta
Str. agalactiae	B	Beta
Str. pneumoniae	None	Alpha
Str. mutans	None	None

Humans carry streptococci in the nose, throat, skin and mucous membranes. Common route of entry is the upper respiratory tract (URT) or direct inoculation into other sites. Nearly 5% of the population are carriers of pathogenic streptococci. Streptococci spread by inhalation of large droplets or intimate contact with contaminated secretions.

Various products secreted by streptococci, which aid in their pathogenicity, include **streptolysins O** and **S, deoxyribonucleases, hyaluronidase** and **erythrogenic toxins.**

Effects of streptococcal products on the host	
Erythrogenic toxins	3 types: Pyrogenic, cytotoxic, suppression of reticuloendothelial activity, immunosuppresssion and inducing susceptibility to endotoxin
Streptolysin O	Lysis of erythrocytes, cytotoxic action on neutrophils, platelets and cardiac tissue
Streptokinase	Fibrinolysis
Deoxyribonucleases	Hydrolyse nucleic acids and nucleoproteins. These are antigenic

| Hyaluronidase | Spreading factor, helps the organism to spread in tissues |
| Nicotinamide adenine dinucleotidase (NADase) | Antigenic |

Streptococcal Pharyngitis

The incubation period is 2–4 days. This presents with abrupt onset of sore throat, dysphagia, headache, malaise, anorexia and fever. The posterior pharyngeal wall is red and edematous. The tonsils are enlarged, red and covered with yellowish exudate, which can be easily removed with a swab. Anterior cervical lymph nodes are enlarged and tender. The disease runs a short course, lasting for about a week. Thirty to forty percent of tonsillitis and pharyngitis are streptococcal, the rest are viral or caused by mycoplasma. Rheumatic fever and glomerulonephritis (GN) are two major immunologically triggered complications of streptococcal infection of the upper oropharyngeal regions.

Pharyngitis responds readily to penicillin, erythromycin, cephalosporins (first generation given orally) or clindamycin 600–900 mg given in every 8 hours. Treatment has to be continued till the lesion subsides (3–5 days). Culture of throat swab will confirm eradication of the infection.

Scarlet Fever

This is characterized by the occurrence of an erythematous rash on the second day of illness. The primary lesion is in the throat. Erythrogenic toxin of the streptococcus is responsible for the rash. The rash is seen over the neck and trunk, the palms and soles are generally spared. The rash blanches on pressure. The rash subsides with extensive desquamation after 4–5 days.

Scarlet fever has to be differentiated from other exanthems, drug rashes, allergic dermatitis and infectious mononucleosis.

Diagnosis: It is established by isolating group A streptococci from the exudate obtained from the tonsillar crypts.

Treatment: Streptococcal lesions respond promptly to penicillin. A single intramuscular (IM) injection of benzathine penicillin G 600,000 units for children less than 25 kg and 1.2 million units for all others is enough to clear the infection. Phenoxymethylpenicillin (penicillin V) 250 mg orally four times daily for 7–10 days is also equally effective. Erythromycin 250 mg 6 hourly for 7–10 days is a suitable alternative for subjects allergic to penicillin. If suppuration develops, surgical drainage of the pus may be required.

Erysipelas

Erysipelas is an acute spreading infection of the skin and the subcutaneous tissue by streptococci. Face is commonly affected. The disease sets in abruptly with malaise, chills, headache and vomiting. The skin lesions are erythematous with clear advancing margins which may show vesicles. The part is tender and local lymph node enlargement may occur. If left untreated, the lesions rapidly spread. In immunocompromised individuals (e.g. diabetics) fatal septicemia may develop if the diagnosis is missed.

Treatment: Prompt treatment with penicillin 0.6–1 million units given IM or intravenous (IV) 4–6 hourly till the acute symptoms subside and thereafter continue with longer acting penicillin for 3–5 days. The underlying condition should also receive attention.

Streptococcal Impetigo

This is inflammation of the skin characterized by isolated pustules which become crusted. Sites of predilection are around the mouth and nostrils. If left untreated they may ulcerate to produce shallow ulcers with crusts or scabs, which may lead to pigmentation and scarring. This stage is called ecthyma.

Cellulitis

This is spreading inflammation of the subcutaneous tissue due to entry of the organism through the abrasions of the skin. There is pain, tenderness, erythema, fever and often regional lymphadenopathy.

Lymphangitis

Acute lymphangitis may follow local trauma. This condition presents in the form of linear red streaks radiating from the site of entry to the draining lymph nodes.

Streptococcal Bacteremia

Irrespective of the focus of entry and primary lesion, streptococcal bacteremia gives rise to metastatic foci of infection such as suppurative arthritis, osteomyelitis, peritonitis, endocarditis, meningitis or visceral abscesses.

Necrotizing Fasciitis

Syn: Streptococcal gangrene

This is a progressive destructive lesion of the subcutaneous tissue leading to necrosis of fascia and adipose tissue, but often sparing the skin. The organisms enter through trivial wounds, but within 24 hours the part is hot, swollen, tender and edematous. The edema and violaceous hue spread in all the directions. This condition is more common in diabetes, immunocompromised individuals and those with local conditions impairing the vitality of the part, e.g. vascular occlusions, chronic edema and infective lesions. Increase in the fascial compartmental pressure further jeopardises the vascularity. Within 48 hours bullae develop, which go on to gangrene within 4–5 days. The gangrenous area gets demarcated. General symptoms include severe prostration, toxemia, mental clouding and delirium. If the diagnosis is missed, mortality is high.

Differential diagnosis includes infection by *Cl. septicum*, *Cl. perfringens* and *Staphylococcus aureus*. Treatment consists of the administration of benzylpenicillin and gentamicin in usual doses and aggressive fasciotomy and surgical debridement. In severe cases with toxemia and rapid progression, clindamycin should be employed. This drug effectively arrests the growth and toxin-production of streptococci.

Streptococcal Myositis

This is an uncommon lesion. Infection reaches the muscles by the bloodstream. Onset is with severe pain and swelling of muscles. Muscle compartment syndromes may develop. If unrecognized, mortality is over 80%. Streptococcal myositis has to be differentiated from spontaneous gas gangrene. Presence of superficial crepitus favors the diagnosis of gas gangrene. Treatment includes administration of broad spectrum antibiotics and early surgical debridement.

Pneumonia and Empyema

Streptococcal pneumonia usually follows a viral infection and it manifests as bronchopneumonia. In many cases empyema develops as a complication.

Most of the strains of streptococci are sensitive to penicillin. Benzylpenicillin G (crystalline penicillin) given IM or IV in a dose of 600,000 units to 1 million units 6 hour for 5–10 days generally clears the infection. Some strains have developed resistance to penicillin. Such infections have to be treated with broad spectrum bactericidal antibiotics.

Streptococcal Toxic Shock Syndrome

Infection by group A streptococcus may lead to vascular collapse and organ failure. M protein which is a constituent of the cell wall is the virulence factor which plays a major role in the pathogenesis of toxic shock syndrome. It forms large aggregates with fibrinogen in blood and tissues. These activate polymorphonuclear leukocytes intravascularly and this leads to the production of toxic shock syndrome.

OTHER PATHOGENIC STRAINS OF STREPTOCOCCI

Group B Streptococcus

Syn: Streptococcus agalactiae

This is a major pathogen found in the female genital tract, rectum and also throat. Chorioamnionitis, septic abortion and puerperal sepsis may occur during pregnancy. Urinary tract infection (UTI) may occur in both sexes. Hematogenous spread may result in endocarditis, pneumonia, empyema, meningitis and peritonitis. Immunocompromised hosts and elderly subjects are more susceptible.

Neonatal infections are caused by group B streptococcus. The lesions include neonatal sepsis and meningitis. Early infection of the newborn leads to septicemia. Infection a few days after birth usually leads to purulent meningitis.

Streptococcus viridans

This is a heterogeneous group consisting of *Streptococcus mutans, Streptococcus sanguinis* and *Streptococcus mitis.* They produce either alpha hemolysis or no hemolysis in culture. They are normal inhabitants of the oral cavity. Viridans streptococci account for more than 40% cases of infective endocarditis. *Streptococcus mutans* which colonizes dental plaques is an important cause of dental caries.

Organisms closely related to streptococci are *Streptococcus pneumoniae* and *Peptostreptococcus.*

Enterococci

These are gram-positive cocci originally classified with streptococci. The name indicated its abundance in the gut. The most common species is *Streptococcus faecalis,* followed by *Streptococcus faecium.* In the mid-1980s, nucleic acid studies indicated that enterococci were not closely related to streptococci and therefore these are classified as a separate genus and the nomenclature of the species is *E. faecalis, E. faecium, E. durans* and others.

They colonize the intestines and vagina. They are pathogenic and the lesions include UTI, biliary tract infections, septicemia, peritonitis, infective endocarditis and abdominal suppuration. They are best known as antibiotic resistant, opportunistic pathogens especially in patients who have been treated with several antibiotics with prolonged hospitalization.

Treatment: Enterococci are notorious for developing multidrug resistance. Vancomycin is effective in many cases. Resistance against beta-lactam antibiotics, aminoglycosides and vancomycin is common. The prevalence of vancomycin resistance in tertiary care hospitals is around 10%. Teicoplanin, linezolid and quinupristin/dalfopristin are effective in vancomycin resistant cases.

Fluoroquinolones gatifloxacin and moxifloxacin and the antibiotic chloramphenicol are effective against some strains.

ACUTE RHEUMATIC FEVER

This is a not an uncommon sequel of recurrent and persistent group A streptococcal infection in humans, especially children and adolescents. With the general improvement of health awareness of the population and more prompt treatment of streptococcal infections—the incidence of acute rheumatic fever has come down. Even now new cases do occur at times in localized clusters in India and in several other countries as well. Rheumatic heart disease (RHD) is the most dreaded and disabling complication of rheumatic fever.

Epidemiology

Group A hemolytic streptococci may occur as commensals in the throat in a small proportion of people. Sometimes, these streptococci become virulent and produce outbreaks of URT infections, especially in children living in closed communities like schools and dormitories. Rheumatic fever occurs only in humans. Repeated infection by streptococci increases the chance of developing rheumatic fever. Spread of group A streptococcus occurs rapidly from person to person by contact.

World Health Organization (WHO) estimated that 15.6 million people have RHD globally. In India, 0.5 million develop acute rheumatic fever annually, out of which 300,000 may develop heart disease. Annual incidence is 54/100,000 population. Soman, et al. found that the prevalence of RHD in Ernakulum district in Kerala during 2000–2004 in children aged 5–16 years was 0.12/1000 population and the incidence was 0.08. RHD is the result of cumulative damage produced by repeated attacks of rheumatic fever. Prevalence of RHD increases with age, maximum is in the age group 25–34 years.

Source:

1. Padmavati S. Rheumatic fever and rheumatic heart disease in India at the turn of the century. Indian Heart J. 2001;53(1):35-7.

2. ICMR data unpublished, quoted by R Krishna Kumar. API Textbook of Medicine, 9th ed, p. 629.

Since overcrowding and poor living conditions predispose the spread of streptococcal infection, rheumatic fever is more common in the poorer socioeconomic groups. The risk of developing rheumatic fever after an attack of streptococcal tonsillitis is 0.3–3%. The most vulnerable age group is 5–15 years, though any age may be affected. In India, the mean age of affection is 6 years. Both sexes are affected and a familial predisposition is noticed in many cases. Rarely skin infection by streptococcus may lead to acute rheumatic fever, otherwise it may increase the susceptibility to it. After several decades of freedom from rheumatic fever, small outbreaks have been reported from many developed countries as well.

Pathogenesis

In 80% of cases the disease follows streptococcal tonsillitis. In 20–30% cases the episode of tonsillitis may go unnoticed. Over 80% of subjects with rheumatic fever show rise in antistreptococcal antibodies within two months. Extrapharyngeal streptococcus infection does not generally lead to rheumatic fever. The M protein of streptococci contain epitopes that cross-react with cardiac tissues and other tissues such as synovium and brain (molecular mimicry).

The antigens contained in streptococcus show similarity to several tissue antigens in the human body, especially myocardial sarcolemma. Antibodies produced against streptococcal antigens cross-react with tissue antigens resulting in a type II antigen antibody reaction and consequent inflammation. Lesions are most evident in the connective tissue.

The M serotypes 3, 5, 6, 14, 18, 19 and 24 have strong association with cardiac disease. Throat infection is more commonly caused by serotypes 12, 1, 25, 4 and 3. Antistreptolysin O (ASO) titer is more elevated in infections of the throat than in skin infections (Table 37.2). Strains of streptococci leading to rheumatic fever increase more of streptolysin O rather than streptolysin S. Strains giving rise to skin infections give rise to greater elevation of anti-deoxyribonuclease (ADNase) B titers. Rheumatic fever represents an autoimmune reaction triggered by pharyngeal infection by the appropriate strain of group A streptococcus and amplified by recurrent infection by the same or related group A streptococci.

Pathology

The pathological process consists of an exudative stage which is seen in the acute phase and a proliferative stage which is a more prolonged process. In the exudative stage, fibrinoid necrosis of the connective tissue is seen. There is edema of the collagen fibers which later undergo fragmentation. Immune response affects myosin in muscle leading to myocarditis. In the valves which lack myosin, the attack is against laminin which is present in the basement membrane and around the endothelium.

The hallmark of the proliferative phase is the formation of ***Aschoff's bodies***. These are small granulomas consisting of a central zone of fibrinoid necrosis surrounded by round cells, epithelioid cells, Aschoff's giant cells and fibroblasts. This histological appearance is similar in all tissues showing rheumatic lesions.

Heart: All the layers are involved to produce endocarditis, myocarditis and pericarditis (pancarditis). Endocarditis affects the valvular or mural endocardium. When the valvular endocardium heals, it results in scarring and deformity of the valves. Scarring alters mural endocarditis may be seen as the ***MacCallum's patch*** in the posterior wall of the left atrium. Affection of the myocardium may be mild or severe. Lesion in the pericardium is a fibrinous inflammation. The pericardium shows a ***bread and butter*** appearance microscopically. Pericardial effusion may develop. Adhesive pericarditis may follow rarely.

Joints: Rheumatic lesions involve large synovial joints producing acute synovitis. Effusions develop which clear up completely without any residual deformity.

Other organs: Rheumatic granulomas found in the subcutaneous tissues, are seen as ***subcutaneous nodules***. Respiratory involvement manifests as pneumonia with or without evidence of pleurisy. The basal ganglia of the brain are affected. The lesions take the form of aseptic focal encephalitis which clear completely. Autoantibodies to caudate and subthalamic nuclei are detectable in patients with rheumatic chorea. These antibodies can be absorbed by group A streptococcal membranes. These also cross-react with the sarcolemmal membrane of the heart. In India, the occurrence of cutaneous and neurological lesions is distinctly less when compared to the descriptions from the west.

Clinical Features

In some cases prodromal symptoms include epistaxis (bleeding from the nose), ***erythema nodosum*** and vague discomfort. Rheumatic fever starts abruptly as a remittent or intermittent pyrexia with characteristic sweating. In many cases other manifestations may not develop for considerable periods, so that the diagnosis may be unsuspected in them. In 20–25% of cases the fever is accompanied by polyarthritis and carditis. Sometimes these are mild and go unrecognized, especially in children.

Arthritis: Acute arthritis affecting the major joints is the characteristic involvement. The joints show signs of acute inflammation and exquisite pain which make the subject immobile. Knees and ankles are most often affected followed by hips, elbows, wrists and shoulders. Small joints of the hands and feet and axial joints are affected only rarely. The arthritis is migratory and fleeting and leaves behind no residual changes. Sometimes the manifestation may be subacute with arthralgia, pain and tenderness over the neighboring tendons and muscles. This may be mistaken for growing pains in children.

Jaccoud's arthritis: This is a benign chronic arthropathy without any functional impairment and no radiological

Table 37.2: Comparison to the streptococcal lesion in acute rheumatic fever (ARF) and glomerulonephritis (GN)

	ARF	**GN**
Site of lesion	Mostly throat	Throat or skin
Prior sensitization	Essential	Not necessary
Serotypes of streptococci	3, 5, 6, 14, 18, 19	12, 44, 2, 52, 55, 57, 4
Immune response	Marked	Moderate

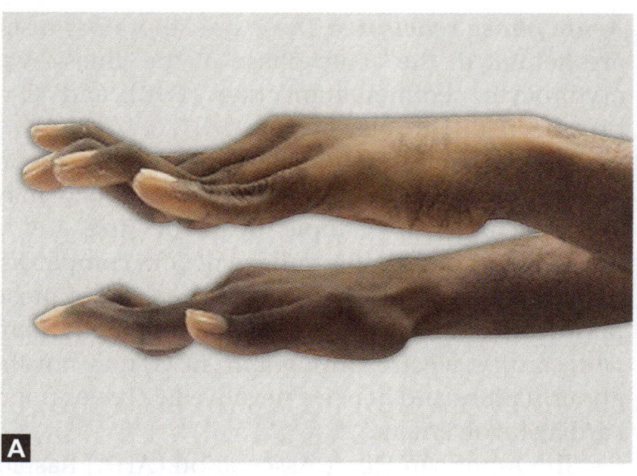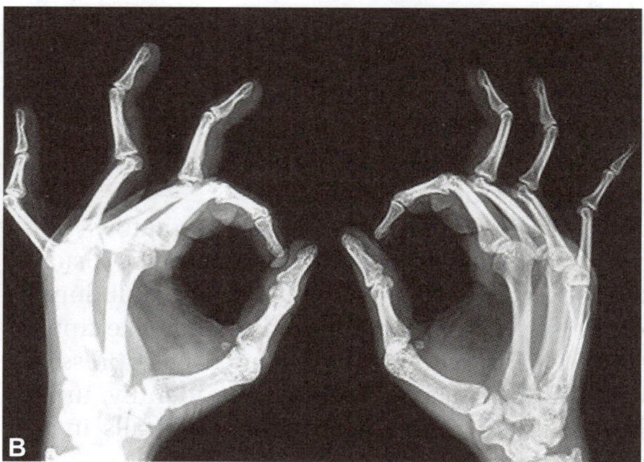

Figs 37.1A and B: Jaccoud's arthritis—deformity which can be easily corrected. X-ray shows no destructive lesions

abnormalities. Jaccoud's arthropathy may affect the hand in up to 50% of cases. It is characterized by reducible, non-erosive joint deformities with preservation of hand function. The pathogenesis of this condition is probably extra-articular, secondary to inflammation and shortening of the tendons. The condition clears up with treatment. It has to be differentiated from other joint lesions such as rheumatoid arthritis (RA) and systemic lupus erythematosus (SLE) (Figs 37.1A and B).

Carditis: There may be clinical features of endocarditis, myocarditis and pericarditis in varying combinations. Tachycardia out of proportion to fever, arrhythmias, gallop rhythm and congestive cardiac failure should suggest the presence of myocarditis. Mild cardiomegaly may be evident in the skiagrams. Arrhythmias include frequent ectopic, paroxysmal tachycardias, atrial fibrillation and heart blocks.

Presence of endocarditis is evidenced by the appearance of murmurs or change in the quality of the already existing murmurs. Mitral, aortic, tricuspid and pulmonary valves are affected in the order of frequency. Acute valvulitis may lead to mitral and aortic regurgitation. Sometimes a low pitched mid-diastolic murmur may be heard in the mitral area due to acute mitral valvulitis ***(Carey-Coomb's murmur)***. It is transient and disappears as the valvulitis subsides. With passage of time, fibrosis proceeds to produce varying degrees of deformities of the valve apparatus resulting in stenotic and regurgitant lesions.

Pericarditis is clinically manifested as chest pain, presence of pericardial rub or a small pericardial effusion.

A prospective study conducted at Kottayam Medical College revealed that echocardiographic studies including Doppler are of great value in detecting acute rheumatic valvulitis. Combination of arthritis and carditis occurred in 56.6% of cases of rheumatic fever. Carditis without arthritis occurred in 19.4%. Acute aortic regurgitation occurred in about 50% but most of them (43%) cleared-up on follow-up. Sequelae included mitral regurgitation, mitral stenosis, a few cases of aortic regurgitation and occasionally tricuspid regurgitation. Pericardial involvement is also easily detected by echocardiography (*See* also Section 13, Ch 123).

Rheumatic Chorea

Syn: Sydenham's chorea, St. Vitus dance, Minor chorea

Chorea generally occurs 1–6 months after the onset of rheumatic fever. Since chorea sets in much later than the other manifestations of rheumatic fever, in many cases it may be the only abnormality encountered. Chorea is more common in females and that too in children. It is characterized by involuntary movements which are quasi-purposive, non-repetitive, rapid and jerky and these involve mainly the distal joints. Upper limbs are mostly involved, but lower limbs, face and tongue may also be involved to a lesser extent. These movements may be mistaken for tantrums or fidgety behavior. Emotional disturbances are frequent and these aggravate the chorea. The limbs are hypotonic and when the hands are held outstretched they assume characteristic postures (choreic hand). The movements disappear during sleep.

Chorea gravidarum is the recurrence or first appearance of chorea in pregnancy during which there is a predilection for development of chorea. Almost always it is rheumatic and self-subsiding. At times there is recurrence during subsequent pregnancies.

Diagnosis of chorea is clinical and there is no pathognomonic investigation. The cerebrospinal fluid (CSF) is normal. Sydenham's chorea is almost always rheumatic in nature. For chorea and indolent carditis evidence of streptococcal infection need not be stressed upon for diagnosis (WHO Expert Consultation, Geneva, Oct-Nov 2001-WHO publication 2004).

Chorea is self-limiting and it completely disappears within weeks or months without leaving any neurological sequel. Subjects developing chorea have a higher incidence of cardiac involvement. Except during pregnancy, rheumatic chorea is rare in adults. Rarely chorea may be caused by SLE.

Treatment of chorea: Salicylates and steroids have no effect on chorea. The patient is put to bed in a quiet room. Involuntary movements can be controlled by diazepam, chlorpromazine or phenobarbitone, given in the usual doses. Haloperidol is very effective in controlling the chorea if given in a dose of 0.25 mg every 6 hour. Rarely intravenous immunoglobulin (IVIG) may be required in an intractable case (*See* Section 19, Ch 204).

Textbook of Medicine

Skin Manifestations

Subcutaneous nodules: They are firm, nontender, pea-sized nodules seen over the extensor aspects of the forearm, elbows, ankles, scalp and scapulae. These last for 1–2 weeks and disappear. The risk of carditis is high in those who develop rheumatic nodules.

Erythema marginatum: These are erythematous non-pruritic annular lesions with serpiginous borders, usually seen over the anterior aspects of the chest and abdomen and over the thighs. They spread peripherally like ripples with central clearing. The lesions blanch with pressure. In colored races this lesion is difficult to identify, unless carefully examined in good light. This rash falls in the category of toxic erythema.

Other Rheumatic Manifestations

Pleurisy and pneumonitis are not generally evident clinically, these are made out more often by investigations. Rheumatic fever tends to recur during pregnancy. Preterm labor, fetal loss and maternal death have been reported.

Course and Progress

Rheumatic fever tends to subside spontaneously over a period of weeks or months. The arthritis subsides but the cardiac lesion progresses and worsens with each rheumatic exacerbation; which is triggered by persistence or recurrence of streptococcal infections. Recurrence of streptococcal infection results in exacerbation of the rheumatic process and hence relapses invariably occur. The course of the disease extends over several months or even a few years with remission and relapses. The risk of developing fresh cardiac lesions and worsening of the existing lesions is increased with successive relapses. Mortality in the acute phase is due to sudden cardiac failure, fatal arrhythmias or heart block. In India, the course of the disease is accelerated when compared to the west, so that established valvular disease is seen even as early as 6–7 years of age.

Diagnosis

Clinically rheumatic fever should be considered in all cases of prolonged fever in India. Rapid pulse, arthritis, skin manifestations and carditis suggest the diagnosis.

Streptococcal infection may be demonstrable either by throat swab culture or by serological methods. Moderate neutrophil leukocytosis occurs in many cases.

Serodiagnosis: Several antibodies to streptococcal antigens have been identified.

- Antistreptolysin O titer (ASO)
- Antistreptokinase (ASK)
- Antideoxyribonucleotidase B (antiDNAse B)
- Anti-nicotinamide-adenine-dinucleotidase (antiNADase)
- Antihyaluronidase (AH)
- Antistreptozyme test (ASTZ).

ASO titer has been widely accepted as one of the more easily available diagnostic tests and any value above 250 Todd units in adults and 333 Todd units in children is suggestive. However, the diagnostic levels vary in different places and it is related to the prevalence of antibody levels in the local population. ASO titer does not correlate with the clinical severity.

ASTZ is a highly sensitive hemagglutination test.

Acute phase reactants: These are laboratory tests which are helpful in the acute phase of the illness. Values of erythrocyte sedimentation rate (ESR) and C-reactive proteins (CPR) are elevated.

The presence of carditis is suggested by the presence of electrocardiographic abnormalities which may show sinus tachycardia, ectopic beats or first and second degree heart blocks. The voltage of QRS complexes is low; ST elevation and T inversion are seen in the presence of pericarditis. It should be remembered that in many cases with carditis, electrocardiograph (ECG) may not show any abnormalities and hence a negative ECG does not rule out cardiac involvement.

The American Heart Association (AHA) has accepted the ***modified Jones criteria*** (1965) for diagnosis which are relevant in Indian conditions as well. The major criteria denote the more specific lesions, whereas the minor criteria are nonspecific. For the diagnosis of rheumatic fever two or one major and two minor criteria should be present. In any case there should be evidence of previous streptococcal infection. In Indian subjects polyarthralgia is also taken as a major criterion if supported by the evidence of streptococcal infection (Table 37.3).

The original Jones' criteria have been modified depending upon the present changes in clinical manifestation, diagnosis and management.

Modified Jones' criteria 2002–2003: WHO criteria for the diagnosis of rheumatic fever and RHD (based on the 1992 revised Jones criteria) (Table 37.4).

Exceptions to Jones Criteria

- Chorea alone, if other causes have been excluded
- Insidious or late-onset carditis with no other explanation
- Patients with documented RHD or prior rheumatic fever, one major criterion or fever, arthralgia or high CRP suggests recurrence.

Differential Diagnosis

Infective endocarditis may present with fever and heart lesions. Presence of clubbing, hepatosplenomegaly, absence of arthritis and development of embolic complications help to distinguish this condition. Henoch-Schönlein purpura may resemble rheumatic fever when purpura is insignificant. Acute leukemia may present with arthralgia and arthritis and produce difficulty in diagnosis

Table 37.3: Manifestations of modified Jones' Criteria (revised)*	
Major manifestations	**Minor manifestations**
Carditis	Previous rheumatic fever or history of RHD
Polyarthritis	Fever
Chorea	Acute phase reactants
Erythema marginatum Subcutaneous nodules and evidence of preceding streptococcal infection, i.e. ASO titer > 250 Todd units	Prolongation of PR interval in the ECG

* Duckett Jones

Abbreviations: RHD = Rheumatic heart disease; ECG = Electrocardiogram; ASO = Antistreptolysin

Table 37.4: 2002–2003 WHO criteria for the diagnosis of rheumatic fever and RHD (based on the 1992 revised Jones criteria)

Diagnostic categories	Criteria
Primary episode of rheumatic fever	One or two major and two minor manifestations plus evidence of preceding group A streptococcal infection
Recurrent attack of rheumatic fever in a patient without established RHD	One or two major and two minor manifestations plus evidence of preceding group A streptococcal infection
Recurrent attack of rheumatic fever in a patient with established RHD	Two minor manifestations plus evidence of preceding group A streptococcal infection
Rheumatic chorea Insidious onset rheumatic carditis	Other major manifestations or evidence of group A streptococcal infection not required
Chronic valve lesions of RHD (patients presenting for the first time with pure mitral stenosis or mixed mitral valve disease and/or aortic valve disease)	Do not require any other criteria to be diagnosed as having RHD
Major manifestations	Carditis polyarthritis, chorea, erythema marginatum, subcutaneous nodules
Minor manifestations	**Clinical:** Fever, polyarthralgia **Laboratory:** Elevated ESR rate or leukocyte count **ECG:** Prolonged P-R interval
Supporting evidence of a preceding streptococcal infection within the last 45 days	Elevated or rising ASO or other streptococcal antibody or a positive throat culture or rapid antigen test for group A streptococcus or recent scarlet fever

Abbreviations: RHD = Rheumatic heart disease; ESR = Erythrocyte sedimentation rate; ECG = Electrocardiogram; ASI = Antistreptolysin O

before the blood picture becomes diagnostic. Presence of severe pallor, bleeding tendencies, non-migratory arthritis, hepatosplenomegaly and fundal hemorrhages should alert the physician about the possibility of leukemia. Septic arthritis is usually monoarticular and the source of primary infection may be evident. Gonococcal arthritis, Reiter's syndrome, SLE, polyarteritis nodosa, allergic arthritis and serum sickness have to be excluded in atypical cases. Acute or subacute rheumatoid arthritis may cause genuine diagnostic difficulty especially in children.

Chronic RHD has to be differentiated from congenital heart diseases (CHD) and other acquired heart diseases.

Treatment

Treatment may be divided into: (i) Management of the acute stage, (ii) eradication of the streptococcal infection and (iii) prevention of recurrences (secondary prevention).

Acute Phase

Strict bed rest: It should be instituted, since it is absolutely essential to limit the carditis and reduce the incidence of chronic heart disease. It is to be continued till ESR comes down to normal.

Anti-inflammatory agents: The drug of choice is aspirin which has a dramatic effect. The antirheumatic dose of aspirin is 90–100 mg/kg/day, given in four divided doses after food, since in this high dose the drug may produce gastric irritation. Antacids, such as aluminium hydroxide or magnesium trisilicate may be given simultaneously along with an H_2 receptor blocker like ranitidine (150 mg bd) or a proton pump inhibitor like omeprazole 20 mg bd. The dose of aspirin is reduced when fever subsides and it should be continued in a small dose for 10 days after disappearance of all the symptoms. Adverse side effects of aspirin include nausea, dizziness, tinnitus, deafness, vomiting, hyperventilation, hemorrhagic tendency and psychosis. Idiosyncrasy to aspirin ingestion may lead on to asthma and nasal polyposis. Aspirin sensitivity can be allayed by desensitization using incremental doses under supervision.

Alternatively glucocorticoids may be given. Corticosteroids and salicylates are equally effective in the management of rheumatic fever. Corticosteroids are preferable in those with carditis, since it controls the cardiac lesion, whereas aspirin may not. The common preparation is prednisolone in a dose of 40–50 mg daily given orally. Withdrawal of steroids may result in exacerbation and hence it should be tapered off under the cover of aspirin. Rheumatic fever occurring during pregnancy is an indication for treatment with glucocorticoids

Streptococcal infection is controlled by giving benzathine penicillin 1.2 million units as a single dose IM. Erythromycin and cephalexin are suitable alternative drugs.

Primary prevention: It has been achieved very effectively in most of the developed countries by early diagnosis and prompt treatment of streptococcal infections. Sporadic cases occur when this policy is slackened. Attempts to produce antistreptococcal vaccine are also going on.

Secondary prophylaxis: Since rheumatic recurrence is invariably precipitated by streptococcal reinfection, benzathine penicillin 1.2 mega units is given once every three weeks to prevent streptococcal reinfection and rheumatic recurrence. As an alternative, oral penicillin 200,000 units twice daily may be given. Penicillin-sensitive individuals may be treated with erythromycin 250 mg/day. It is desirable to continue rheumatic prophylaxis lifelong but the chance of recurrence comes down with increasing age and the passage of time after the acute attack. It is mandatory to continue penicillin prophylaxis at least till the age of 25 years or for 5 years after the initial attack, whichever is later.

POSTSTREPTOCOCCAL GLOMERULONEPHRITIS (PSGN)

This may follow either cutaneous or pharyngeal lesion by group A streptococcus. About 10–15% of children getting recurrent skin infections may develop GN. Serotypes 12, 44, 2, 52, 55, 57 and 4 are more often nephritogenic. Latent period for the development of acute GN is 10 days after pharyngitis and 3 weeks after pyoderma. Streptococcal infection supervening on scabies is a common cause for acute GN in India. This described in Section 16, Ch 181.

STAPHYLOCOCCAL INFECTIONS

GENERAL CONSIDERATIONS

Staphylococci are the most ubiquitous organisms affecting man. Staphylococci are gram-positive cocci 1 μm in diameter, capable of aerobic and anaerobic metabolism. They produce lesions by direct invasion. Many strains are toxigenic and several syndromes result from toxic effects. Incubation period for local lesions is 2–3 days.

Staphylococcus aureus is coagulase positive. *Staphylococcus epidermidis* and *Staphylococcus sapro-phyticus* are coagulase negative. All are pathogenic, the most common type is *Staphylococcus aureus.*

Epidemiology

Healthy people carry staphylococci in the nose and to a lesser extent in the perineum. The organism is spread by direct contact, through fomites, dust or by airborne droplets. Large number of organisms are shed from superficial lesions and from the respiratory tract. Although initially staphylococci were sensitive to sulphonamides and penicillin, many strains have developed resistance to several antibiotics in common use. Penicillin is inactivated by penicillinase (beta-lactamase) and this is the basis of penicillin resistance. Resistance can be transferred from one strain to another by transduction through the mechanism of plasmids. At present most hospital strains of staphylococci are resistant to several antibacterial agents. Methicillin-resistant *Staphylococcus aureus* (MRSA) are resistant to several other beta-lactam antibiotics, fluoroquinolones, carbapenem and vancomycin. Therefore, resistance to methicillin is tested to identify such strains.

MRSA is endemic in hospitals worldwide. Healthcare associated resistant *Staphylococcus aureus* arise in individuals with predisposing risk factors such as surgery or indwelling medical devices. On the other hand community acquired-MRSA (CA-MRSA) occurs in otherwise healthy people who do not have such risk factors. CA-MRSA is more virulent and more transmissible than hospital acquired MRSA. MRSA circumvents natural immune mechanisms. Human immunodeficiency virus (HIV) positive patients are more susceptible to MRSA. Spread of MRSA is largely through physical contact.

Pathogenesis

Staphylococci invade hair follicles and sebaceous glands. Incidence of infection is higher in diabetics and obese subjects. Subjects recovering from influenza and measles are more susceptible to staphylococcal infection. The organism multiplies in the lesions and leads to suppurative inflammation.

Lesions Produced by Staphylococci

Staphylococcus aureus: Pyogenic lesions such as boils, carbuncles, wound infection, abscesses, impetigo, mastitis, osteomyelitis, pneumonia, septicemia and pyemia.

Coagulase negative staphylococci: Infection of cardiac and vascular prostheses, endocarditis, ventriculitis (cerebral), peritonitis in continuous ambulatory peritoneal dialysis, septicemia, cystitis.

Toxins of staphylococci: *Staphylococcus aureus* elaborates toxins like hemolysins, leukocidins, enterotoxin, hyaluronidases, fibrinolysin, nuclease, lipase and protease. In addition, nontoxic substances like coagulase, which facilitate invasion, are also produced.

Toxin-mediated lesions: Food poisoning, toxic shock syndrome, scalded skin syndrome, pemphigus neonatorum.

Toxins produced by strains of Staphylococcus aureus and the syndromes produced	
Enterotoxin A-E	Gastroenteritis
Epidermolytic toxin A and B	Blisters of skin, pemphigus neonatorum scalded skin syndrome
Toxin-1	Toxic shock syndrome

SUPERFICIAL LESIONS

Furuncle

A furuncle is an acute necrotic infection of a hair follicle. It presents as a small follicular inflammatory nodule, soon becoming pustular and then necrotic. It heals after discharge of the necrotic core to leave a violaceous macule and ultimately a permanent scar.

Carbuncle

It is a large furuncle or an aggregate of interconnected furuncles accompanied by intense inflammatory changes in the surrounding and underlying connective tissue. Sites of predilection are the back of the neck, the hips and thighs. It starts as a hard red lump, at first smooth and acutely tender. It slowly increases in diameter to reach 3 to 10 cm. Suppuration begins after 5–7 days and pus is discharged from multiple follicular orifices. Constitutional symptoms are usually severe. Carbuncles are particularly common in diabetics and those with lowered general resistance.

Impetigo

Bullous impetigo is purely staphylococcal. It usually occurs in newborns and infants. Face is more often affected although lesions may occur in the palms and soles. The lesions consist of multiple pustules.

Ecthyma

Both staphylococci and streptococci can cause ecthyma. The lesion is characterized by small bullae or pustules on an erythematous base, soon developing into a hard crust. Irregular ulceration is evident when the crust is removed. The sites of predilection are the buttocks, thighs and legs.

Sycosis Barbae

This is seen in males after puberty and the lesions are seen on the beard region. The lesion starts as an edematous,

Textbook of Medicine

red, follicular papule or pustule, centered by a hair. The individual papules remain discrete.

Follicular Impetigo of Bockhart

This is staphylococcal infection of the hair follicle seen commonly in childhood. It occurs mainly in the scalp or scalp margins.

The Scalded Skin Syndrome

Syn: Pemphigus neonatorum, Ritter's disease, Toxic epidermal necrolysis

This is a generalized exfoliative dermatitis caused by *Staphylococcus aureus.* It is characterized by generalized painful erythema and large bullae which can be easily disrupted by finger pressure. Newborns are commonly affected.

Staphylococcal Pneumonia

Staphylococcal pneumonia occurs as a complication of influenza, measles or other viral infections. It starts with high fever, chills, dyspnea, cyanosis, cough and pleural pain, sputum may be bloody or purulent. Scattered fine to coarse rales and rhonchi may be heard over the involved areas. Typical consolidation is rare. Primary staphylococcal pneumonia may occur in infants and young children and this causes pneumothorax, pneumatocele or empyema. Hematogenous secondary staphylococcal pneumonia is frequent in drug addicts who also develop endocarditis. Staphylococcal pneumonia carries a higher mortality, especially in the old and debilitated patients.

Osteomyelitis

Majority of cases of primary osteomyelitis are due to staphylococcus.

Staphylococcal Bacteremia

The primary source consists of local staphylococcal infections, urinary catheters, foreign bodies or infected IV shunts. The onset is marked by high fever, tachycardia, cyanosis and vascular collapse. Pyemic abscesses may form in the skin, bone, kidneys, brain or lungs. Fulminant sepsis may lead to death within 24 hours.

Other staphylococcal lesions include endocarditis, pericarditis, arthritis, polymyositis, parotitis and UTI.

Staphylococcal Food Poisoning

Staphylococcal food poisoning occurs as a result of ingestion of preformed enterotoxin in food contaminated by *Staphylococcus aureus.* Canned food, processed meat, milk, cheese and others account for the majority of cases. Symptoms start within 6–8 hours and the patients present with varying grades of gastroenteritis or dysenteric symptoms. There is mild fever.

Staphylococcal enterocolitis is due to direct invasion of the bowel mucosa, sometimes seen in surgical patients. Gram staining of feces reveals the organisms.

Toxic Shock Syndrome

This syndrome described first in 1978 consists of sudden development of shock associated with high fever, headache, sore throat, diarrhea and erythroderma. It was noted in young girls using certain brands of vaginal tampons during menstruation. This syndrome is caused by a diffusible toxin produced by staphylococci (phage type 1) which grows in such tampons. Blood cultures are negative. Mortality is high in untreated cases. This syndrome can develop even when the source of infection is different.

Treatment: Emergency measures to combat septic shock should be instituted. Beta-lactamase-resistant antibiotics should be used in full dosage from the onset. Corticosteroids have helped to reduce toxemia in some cases. Further use of such tampons should be avoided. Strong clinical suspicion is absolutely necessary to save life in such situations.

Suppurative Infections

These are seen at times. Staphylococci can produce suppurative lesions in all tissues in the body, if it reaches the site by direct inoculation or through the bloodstream. Systemic lesions such as staphylococcal pneumonia, meningitis, endocarditis or lesions in body cavities result in acute fulminant infections associated with severe morbidity and high mortality.

Tropical Pyomyositis

This is more commonly described from Africa, but cases occur in India too. Large abscesses develop in the muscles of the limbs or trunk in apparently healthy adults. The spread of the organism is probably hematogenous. In addition to systemic therapy surgical evacuation of pus is also necessary.

Diagnosis of Staphylococcal Infections

Clinical diagnosis should be confirmed by culturing the organism from the exudates. Phage typing is employed for identifying the strains in epidemics and tracing the carriers.

Treatment

Superficial skin infections respond to proper cleaning and application of topical ointments containing chlorhexidine or cetrimide. In systemic infections or when the lesions are deep, systemic antibiotics are required. Benzylpenicillin is the most effective antibiotic if the organisms are sensitive.

Infections acquired from the community may be sensitive to benzylpenicillin in usual dosage. Up to 90% of hospital acquired infections may be resistant to penicillin and other beta-lactam antibiotics due to the production of penicillinase. **Methicillin, cloxacillin, flucloxacillin, cephalosporin, clavulanic acid** and **sulbactam** resist **penicillinase** and therefore, these may be effective. Hence, it is ideal to get culture and sensitivity results where circumstances permit. Pending the result, **cloxacillin** or **flucloxacillin** may be started in a dose of 250–500 mg orally sixth hourly.

Antibiotics for MRSA include oral drugs like clindamycin, long acting tetracyclines (doxycycline), minocycline, cotrimoxazole, vancomycin, teicoplanin, linezolid, daptamycin, rifampicin and others. Rifampicin in doses of 400–600 mg daily orally acts synergistically with vancomycin. Some of the strains of MRSA are susceptible to colistin.

Textbook of Medicine

Two newly introduced antibiotics dalbavancin and oritavancin which are lipoglycopeptides (related to vancomycin and teicoplanin) have been introduced to treat gram-positive organisms. They are active against MRSA and their half-life is for two weeks. Dose of dalbavancin is 1 g IV infusion over 120 minutes on first day followed 1 week later by 500 mg IV infusion. Dose of oritavancin is 120 mg by IV infusion single dose. The effect is comparable to 1 week treatment with vancomycin. Adverse effects include nausea, diarrhea and pruritus. These drugs are not yet freely available in India.

Source: Chambers HF. Pharmacology and the treatment of complicated skin and skin-structure infections. N Engl J Med. 2014;370(23):2238-9.

- Antistaphylococcal antibiotics which can be hard in resistant cases—oxacillin (methicillin), first generation cephalosporins—cefazolin, cefalotin.
- Antistaphylococcal antibiotics of the second choice (for MRSA/vancomysin-resistant *S. aureus*): Lincosamides (e.g. clindamycin), gycopeptides (vancomycin, teicoplanin), quinupristin/dalfopristin, chloramphenicol, minocycline, rifampin, trimethoprim sulfamethoxazole, fosfomycin, linezolid, daptomycin, tigecycline, dalbavancin oritavancin, telithromycin, ceftobiprole medocaril.

LESIONS PRODUCED BY COAGULASE NEGATIVE STAPHYLOCOCCI

These produce localized lesions, the rate of progression is slow and toxemia is less.

Staphylococcus Epidermidis

This is present abundantly in the skin. It produces a biofilm which is an exopolysaccharide which facilitates adherence of the organism to foreign material and also protects it from phagocytosis. *Staphylococcus epidermidis* is a common infective agent in implanted prosthetic devices. Most of the infections are acquired from hospital.

Staphylococcus saprophyticus: It is a frequent cause of UTI in sexually active women.

Treatment

Quinupristin/dalfopristin which is a streptogramin antimicrobial agent is licenced in the UK and USA for the treatment of gram-positive organisms, coagulase negative *Staphylococcus aureus* with intermediate glycopeptide resistance (i.e. to teicoplanin), vancomycin resistant *Enterococcus faecium* and penicillin resistant and macrolide resistant *Pneumococci*. It is inactive against *Enterococcus faecalis*. It can be given as IV infusion, preferably though central venous catheter over a period of 60 minutes. Adverse side effects include rashes, gastrointestinal upsets and irritation at the site of injection.

Staphylococcus epidermidis cystitis responds to co-trimoxazole or norfloxacin.

Prevention

Patients with open staphylococcal lesions should be isolated. Surgeons and hospital staff should be periodically checked for carrier state and positive cases are treated by local application of neomycin and chlorhexidine. Topical application of antiseptics such as hexachlorophene are found useful in preventing staphylococcal infection in selected cases. The importance of proper hand washing by the attending staff cannot be overemphasized.

MRSA is found to colonize the nose, wounds and other parts in 30–40% of patients undergoing prolonged hospitalization. During an outbreak of MRSA infection in hospitals, application of mupirocin ointment to the nose helps to eradicate the nasal carrier state. The whole genome sequence of methicillin resistant *Staphylococcus aureus* has been unravelled by Japanese workers. About 70 genes have been identified to contribute to drug resistance.

Source: Kuroda M, Ohta T, Uchiyama I, et al. Whole genome sequencing of meticillin-resistant Staphylococcus aureus. Lancet. 2001;357(9264):1225-40.

PNEUMOCOCCAL INFECTIONS

Syn: *Diplococcus pneumoniae, Streptococcus pneumoniae*

GENERAL CONSIDERATIONS

Streptococcus pneumoniae is a leading cause of pneumonia, bacterial meningitis and sepsis in children. Seven lakhs to 1 million deaths occur annually worldwide due to *Streptococcus pneumoniae* (*See* Section 14, Ch 141).

Pneumococci are found in the URT of about half of the population. On the basis of capsular precipitation reactions using type specific antisera, about 84 serotypes have been identified. All are pathogenic to man but the most commonly encountered types are 1, 2, 3, 4, 7, 8 and 12. These are gram-positive, nonmotile, encapsulated ovoid or lanceolate organisms 1 μm in length occurring in pairs. Most strains are facultative anaerobes, some are strictly anaerobes.

Pneumococcus spreads by direct contact with contaminated respiratory secretions. About 10% of healthy adults and 20–40% of healthy children are carriers, usually one serotype is carried. Pneumococcal capsular antigen is the most important determinant for virulence. The pneumococcal capsule which is highly negatively charged helps in (i) transit of organisms to epithelial surface, (ii) inhibit phagocytosis, (iii) restrict autolysis and (iv) reduce exposure to antibiotics.

Route of entry in the respiratory tract is by droplet infection. The normal respiratory tract offers adequate resistance to invasion by pneumococcus. Patients with underlying lung diseases such as bronchiectasis, carcinoma or chronic obstructive airway disease and respiratory viral infections are predisposed to develop pneumonia. Aspiration of infected material, respiratory irritants, pulmonary edema and trauma to the chest reduces the local resistance and favors the growth of pneumococci. Large droplet size and close contact favors infection.

Alcohol intoxication and anesthesia impair leukocyte migration. The mucinous secretions of the respiratory tract protect the pneumococci and these multiply and lead to further outpouring of proteinaceous fluid.

Pneumococcal infection is predisposed by several conditions such as asplenia, sickle cell disease, celiac disease, extremes of age, chronic obstructive airway disease, chronic heart disease, diabetes and chronic kidney disease.

The normal defense mechanisms consist of migration of polymorphonuclear leukocytes and phagocytosis. These are enhanced by the presence of antibodies. Exotoxin of pneumococcal-pneumolysin which is pore-forming and lytic to host cells, is released by autolysis of the bacterium. Pneumolysins inhibit ciliary action of epithelial cells, activate CD4+ T cells, impair respiratory burst of phagocytic cells, induce production of chemokines and cytokines, stimulate complement fixation and activate inflammation.

Pneumococci are slowly killed inside phagolysosomes. Respiratory epithelial cells, in addition to ciliary action to remove pneumococci, produce pneumococcal binding protein known as **surfactant protein D**. Alveolar macrophages form the cells of defense which phagocytose and kill small number of pneumococci. Pneumococcal pneumonia is uncommon in adults with isolated neutropenia, without other immune defects. Clearance of pneumococci from the circulation depends on opsonization by complement components and phagocytosis by myeloid cells.

Cytokines such as tumor necrosis factor (TNF) alpha and interleukin-1 (IL-1) protect against pneumococcal dissemination. Anti-inflammatory cytokine IL-10 impairs the defense mechanism. Extensive cross talk occurs between components of the coagulation systems and innate immune system in response to microbial infection. These systems simultaneously activate and collaborate to contain and eradicate localized infection.

Pneumococci use the host derived receptor for platelet activating factor to cross from lung tissue into blood. Children genetically deficient in myeloid differentiation primary response gene 88 (MYD88) or IL-1 receptor-associated kinase 4 (IRAK4) are especially susceptible to invasive pneumococcal disease.

Breakdown of the defense mechanisms result in bacteremia and the development of metastatic lesions in the meninges, joints, peritoneum or the endocardium. Recovery from infection starts with the formation of type specific antibodies in the circulation and this is clinically marked by a fall in temperature by crisis. Treatment with antimicrobials reduces the bacterial population and enhances the host defense mechanism which is still important in the elimination of bacteria. Necrosis of lung parenchyma is uncommon.

Local spread of pneumococci from the nasopharynx to the adjacent structures results in the development of otitis media, mastoiditis, paranasal sinusitis or conjunctivitis. Pneumococci form surface adhesions which enable them to adhere to and colonize the nasopharyngeal areas and spread to contiguous sites.

PNEUMOCOCCAL PNEUMONIA

Syn: Lobar pneumoniae

Pneumonia is the most common pneumococcal lesion in adults. In adults, pneumonia is commonly segmental or lobar in distribution, but in children and the aged, the lesion may be bronchopneumonic.

Pathology: Invasion of the lung by pneumococci leads to the formation of an inflammatory exudate in several alveoli and this depends upon the virulence of the organism. Segmental boundaries are not preserved and the bronchi which are relatively uninvolved, remain patent. Cytokines IL-1β, TNF alpha and IL-6 are released by the action of pneumococcal cell wall constituents and complement activation. These lead to rapid influx of neutrophils at the site of inflammation. The pneumococcal capsule impairs the phagocytic action of the neutrophils. Pneumolysin damages membranes. An immunoglobulin A_1 (IgA_1) protease derived from the virulent pneumococci inhibits mucosal immunity. Recovery is facilitated by the formation of anticapsular antibody.

The inflammatory exudates contain a large number of neutrophils and red cells. In the initial stages the alveoli are filled with red blood cells and fibrin and the pulmonary capillaries are widely dilated (red hepatization). In the next stage neutrophil leukocytes predominate. They phagocytose the bacteria. The capillaries become less congested (gray hepatization). It is uncommon for the inflammatory process to proceed the necrosis. As resolution starts, the inflammatory exudate liquefies and it is absorbed through lymphatic and removed by the alveolar macrophages. It takes considerable period of time for complete recovery.

Clinical features: Pneumonia is often preceded by coryza or other URT infections. Incidence of pneumonia is higher in males. The onset is sudden with fever and chills in the majority of cases. There is marked tachycardia and tachypnea. The alae nasi are seen to move when the patient breathes. Severe pleuritic pain and cough with expectoration of pinkish or rusty mucoid sputum follows. The respiration becomes rapid and shallow and may be associated with grunting. Respiratory embarrassment results in cyanosis. The patient becomes very ill and toxic. In the untreated case fever persists continuously for 7–11 days after which it comes down by crisis. It is common to get a crop of labial herpes simplex during the fever.

Physical examination reveals rapid pulse fever and signs of consolidation over the affected lobe of the lung. As resolution starts, coarse crepitations develop. If pleurisy occurs, pleural friction rub may be elicitable. In uncomplicated cases, once the temperature comes down, the patient feels well and recovery starts. However, the pulmonary lesions resolve completely only after a few weeks.

Early institution of specific therapy can prevent the development of consolidation and the general symptoms, but if consolidation has been established, resolution takes time, depending on the body's natural defenses. The response to penicillin therapy is dramatic. With the widespread use of antibiotics from the start of fever, the classic picture of lobar pneumonia is seldom seen at present.

Laboratory findings: Skiagrams of the chest is one of the easiest and most reliable investigation to diagnose pneumonic consolidation and its further changes. Whenever pneumonia is suspected skiagram should be taken and repeated as is necessary to follow-up the progress. Skiagram of the chest shows a homogeneous opacity corresponding to the lobe or segment involved (Fig. 37.2).

Textbook of Medicine

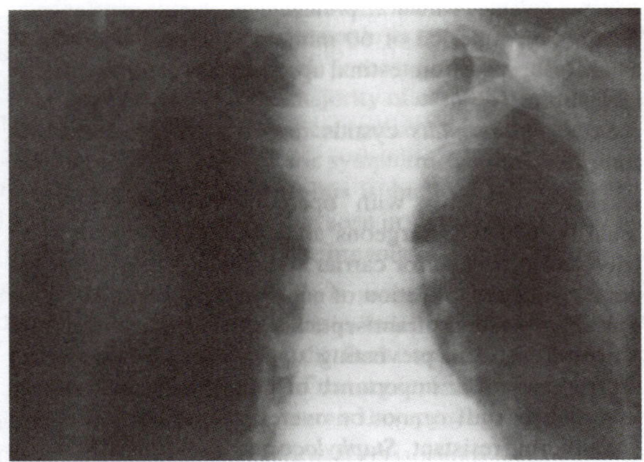

Fig. 37.2: Skiagram chest lobar pneumonia—right (pneumococcal). See well demarcated homogenous opacity right mid zone

Sputum is rusty in color. Pneumococci can be demonstrated by Gram staining. Blood culture is positive in 20–25% of cases in the early stage of the disease.

There is marked leukocytosis ranging from 12,000 to 25,000 cells/mm³ and neutrophils from 85 to 90% of the total. Absence of leukocytosis or even leukopenia may sometimes be observed in patients with overwhelming infection and bacteremia. The prognosis in such cases is very poor.

Bacterial organisms in respiratory infections (percentage of the total)			
	S. pneumoniae	*H. influenzae*	*M. catarrhalis*
Acute sinusitis	42	29	22
Acute otitis media	42	38	17
Acute exacerbation of chronic bronchitis	15	32	13
Community acquired pneumonia	20–75	3–10	–

Complications: Local complications include atelectasis, lung abscess and delayed resolution.

Spread of inflammation to adjacent structures leads to pleural effusion, empyema, pericarditis and peritonitis.

Hematogenous spread results in septicemia, meningitis and acute endocarditis. Gastrointestinal complications include paralytic ileus, gastric dilatation, impairment of liver function and jaundice.

Prognosis: In the vast majority of cases the lesion subsides and recovery is complete. Adverse prognostic signs include leukopenia, bacteremia, multilobar involvement, extrapulmonary involvement, circulatory collapse, presence of pre-existing systemic diseases and occurrence of the disease at both extremes of life (below 3 years and above 55 years). Recurrence of pneumonia in the same location should suggest a local endobronchial lesion. Recurrence in different bronchopulmonary segments should suggest immunocompromised state such as HIV, congenital B-cell disorders, ciliary dysfunction, myeloma, lymphoma and others. Infection with type 3 pneumococcus has a higher mortality rate (Tables 37.5 and 37.6).

Table 37.5: Assessment of severity index in community acquired pneumonias—algorithm	
Parameter	**Risk points**
Clinical points	
Age, men	age in years
Age, women	age minus 10
Co-existent disease	+10
Neoplasms	+30
Liver disease	+20
Congestive heart failure	+10
Cerebrovascular accident	+10
Renal disease	+10
Mental clouding	+20
Respiratory rate > 30/minute	+20
Systolic BP < 90 mm Hg	+20
Temperature < 35°C or	+15
> 40°C	+15
Pulse > 125/minute	+10
Pleural effusion	+10
Laboratory parameters	
Arterial pH < 7.35	+30
Blood urea nitrogen >30 mg/dL	+20
Serum sodium <130 mmol/L	+20
Blood glucose > 250 mg/dL	+10
PCV < 30%	+10
Arterial pO_2 < 60 mm Hg or oxygen saturation < 90%	+10

Abbreviations: BP = Blood pressure; PCV = Packed cell volume; pO_2 = Partial pressure of oxygen

Table 37.6: Prognostic significance based on risk factors			
Risk class	**Risk**	**Score based on algorithm**	**Mortality**
I	Low	< 70	0.1%
II	Low	< 70	0.6%
III	Low	71–90	0.9%
IV	Moderate	91–130	9.3%
V	High	> 130	27%

Source: Fine MJ, Auble TE, Yealy DM, et al. A prediction rule to identify low-risk patients with community-acquired pneumonia. N Engl J Med. 1997;336(4):243-50.

Pneumonia severity index (PSI) in community acquired pnuemonia

Scoring for deciding on hospitalization	
Clinical factor	**Points**
Confusion	1
Uremia (blood urea nitrogen) > or = 20 mg/dL	1
Respiratory rate > or = 30 breaths/min	1
Systolic BP < 90 mm Hg or diastolic BP < or = 60 mm Hg	1
Age > or = 65	1
A score of > 3 indicate for the need for hospitalization	

EXTRAPULMONARY PNEUMOCOCCAL LESIONS

Pneumococcal meningitis: Pneumococcal meningitis may develop primarily or this may be a complication of pneumococcal pneumonia, otitis media, mastoiditis or sinusitis. This is a serious illness associated with 20–30% mortality and up to 50% residual morbidity in survivors, if not treated in time.

Over 75% of community acquired meningitis is caused by *S. pneumoniae* and *N. meningitides*.

Early lumbar puncture on clinical suspicion and the promptness with which early specific antimicrobial treatment is started are the most important prognostic factors for recovery.

Pneumococcal peritonitis: This is a rare infection. It is more frequent in girls, patients with nephrotic syndrome, cirrhosis of liver and abdominal malignancies.

TREATMENT OF PNEUMOCOCCAL INFECTIONS

Pneumococci are generally susceptible to penicillin, but resistant strains are frequent. It is advisable to send the sputum for sensitivity tests before starting specific therapy. Benzylpenicillin is the drug of choice for uncomplicated pneumococcal infections.

Pneumonia: Crystalline penicillin is given IM in a dose of 0.5 mega units/8 hour till the temperature comes down to normal and till the patient is well on the road to recovery. In the ordinary case the antibiotic has to be administered for a total duration of 7–10 days. When resolution is delayed, the cause should be detected by investigations. An alternative to penicillin is ampicillin (250–500 mg) 6 h for 7–10 days.

The abnormal physical findings in the chest clear in 2–3 weeks. The skiagram may show abnormalities for up to 2 weeks after the temperature comes down to normal. Delay in resolution is due to bronchial obstruction or other underlying lung diseases.

Multiple-drug-resistant (MDR) pneumococci respond to vancomycin 2 g/day given IV in divided doses or cefotaxime or ceftazidime. Levofloxacin is also effective.

Symptomatic treatment includes analgesics (aspirin) for chest pain, oxygen inhalation, non-narcotic sedatives (diazepam) and expectorants for clearing the respiratory passages. Medicated steam inhalations containing tincture benzoin or eucalyptus oil provide symptomatic relief and assist expectoration. It is important to ensure adequate convalescence (at least 2 weeks) after lobar pneumonia and this helps in reducing the sequelae.

Note: *See* Section 14, Ch 141.

Since, *S. pneumoniae* has acquired resistance to penicillin, other antibiotics may have to be used. These include vancomycin and third generation cephalosporins.

SUSCEPTIBILITY RATES OF RESPIRATORY PATHOGENS TO ANTIMICROBIALS

Percentage susceptibility to various antibiotics using NCCLS (National Committee for Clinical Laboratory Standards) breakpoints (Table 37.7).

PREVENTION-VACCINATION

Specific prophylaxis is by vaccination: Pneumococcal vaccine contains a mixture of 23 polysaccharide serotypes giving protection against 90% of the infecting strains. The vaccine has to be given by SC or IM injection. A single

Table 37.7: Susceptibility of respiratory pathogens to antibiotics

	S. pneumoniae	H. influenzae	M. catarrhalis
Penicillin	76	–	8
Ampicillin	78	87	18
Amox-clavulanate	84	98	100
Ceftriaxone	85	100	100
Erythromycin	78	–	100
Clarithromycin	78	95	100
Azithromycin	78	100	100
Chloramphenicol	88	98	100
Doxycycline	78	100	100
TMP-SMX	69	88	100
Ofloxacin	96	100	100

Note: Percentage susceptible using NCCLS breakpoints
Abbreviation: TMP-SMX = Trimethoprim/sulfamethoxazole

dose gives protection for about 3–5 years or longer. Vaccination may have to be repeated after 5 years, if exposed to the risk of infection. Mass vaccination of children in a community produces herd immunity in the population, in addition to the individual benefits. This phenomenon is being studied further. It has been observed that individuals immunized against pneumococcus may be predisposed to colonization of the nasopharynx by *Staphylococcus aureus*. In adults, the vaccine efficiency after single vaccination is 50–70%.

Indications for vaccination: Asplenia, nephrotic syndrome, sickle cell disease, lymphomas and other immunodeficiency states. In children below 2 years of age and in immunocompromised individuals, vaccination is not effective. They have to be given orally phenoxymethylpenicillin on a long-term basis. Protein conjugate pneumococcal vaccine may be given to children > 2 years for protection. Multiple doses may have to be given.

General Measures to Increase Resistance

Studies from Dhaka, Bangladesh have shown that malnutrition predisposes to pneumonia. Oral supplementation of 70 mg of zinc acetate in 10 mL of syrupy base once a week was associated with substantial protection against pneumonia and suppurative otitis media. Mortality from pneumonia was also reduced.

Source: Brooks WA, Santosham M, Naheed A, et al. Effect of weekly zinc supplements on incidence of pneumonia and diarrhoea in children younger than 2 years in an urban, low-income population in Bangladesh: randomised controlled trial. The Lancet. 2005:366:999-1004.

MENINGOCOCCAL INFECTIONS

GENERAL CONSIDERATIONS

Neisseria meningitidis (meningococcus) is pathogenic exclusively to man. The clinical syndromes include meningitis, meningococcal septicemia and rarely lesions in the joints, ears, eyes, adrenal glands, lungs and heart.

Meningococci are gram-negative diplococci. Based on the capsular polysaccharide antigens, these are divisible into three main serogroups A, B and C. Group A

Textbook of Medicine

commonly produces epidemics and group C, localized outbreaks of meningitis. Other serogroups W_{135} and Y are also pathogenic.

Epidemiology: The organisms are found in the nasopharynx of 5–10% of humans who act as carriers. Before the onset of epidemics, carrier rate among the local population goes up above 20% and during an epidemic 90% of subjects may carry the organisms. Outbreaks usually occur in close-knit communities such as inmates of jails, ships, army camps or dormitories. Sporadic cases may also occur. In India, a clear seasonal prevalence is not seen. The organism commonly spreads through droplet infection and to some extent through fomites. In the majority of cases the infection is asymptomatic. In some, the only manifestation is an URT catarrh.

PATHOGENESIS AND PATHOLOGY

The major lesions are cerebrospinal meningitis and meningococcal septicemia. Bacteremia precedes the meningitis. The organism may reach the central nervous system (CNS) directly along the perineural sheath of the olfactory nerves or through the bloodstream. Bacteremia leads to endothelial damage and the organisms enter the CSF. Group C produces more serious disease compared to A and B. Meningococci have the capacity to exchange genetic material responsible for capsule production and interchange the serogroup between B and C and vice versa. In India, group A and C account for most of the infections, though serogroup B may also occur sporadically.

Once the CSF is reached, further multiplication is rapid as the humoral defenses are absent. Cytokines promote inflammatory processes and increase vascular permeability. Leukocytes adhere to endothelium. Vasogenic cerebral edema occurs which itself may lead to brain herniation. In the CNS, meningococci produce suppurative lesions of the pia-arachnoid. Inflammatory lesions are seen on the surfaces of the brain and spinal cord and the ependymal-lining of the ventricles. The whole of CSF becomes turbid and purulent. The base of the brain and the surface of the cerebral hemispheres show thick pus. This exudate may block the foramina leading to internal hydrocephalus and also compress the cranial nerves emerging from the base of the brain. Meningococci may invade the underlying cerebral cortex as well and cause encephalitis.

Susceptibility to infections is high in the following groups:
- Children from 6 months to 4 years
- Concurrent URT infection
- Tobacco-smoking
- Complement deficiency
- Asplenia (functional or post-surgical)
- Immunodeficiency and HIV
- Chronic diseases impairing antibacterial resistance such as cirrhosis liver, SLE, multiple myeloma and others.

Histologically the lesions show perivascular cuffing with polymorphs. Thrombosis of small blood vessels may occur. In severe cases, subdural effusions containing blood or exudate may occur.

Clinical pattern of meningococcal infections

Site of infection	Clinical syndrome	Outcome
Blood and CSF	Septicemia and meningitis with rash	Fatal in 14–50%
	Septicemia and meningitis without rash	Fatal in 2–6%
Blood	Fulminant septicemia Waterhouse-Friderichsen syndrome	Fatal
Blood	Septicemia purpuric rash	Fatal 14–50%
Blood	Chronic septicemia	Recovery with treatment
Metastatic lesions	Arthritis, osteomyelitis, pericarditis, endocarditis, local lesions, pneumonia	Recover with treatment
Eye	Purulent conjunctivitis	Clears with treatment

MENINGOCOCCAL MENINGITIS

Syn: Cerebrospinal fever

Infection of the leptomeninges by *N. meningitides* leads to meningococcal meningitis. This may occur in epidemic and sporadic forms. The most common age group is from 6 months of life to adolescence. Incubation period varies from 3 to 5 days and there may be a preceding URT infection. Onset is acute with fever and other constitutional features like severe headache, neck rigidity, vomiting and photophobia. Fever is usually high grade, intermittent and associated with rigor and chills. The pulse is slow. Herpes labialis may develop. The patient is irritable and prefers to lie curled in bed. Drowsiness, confusion, delirium and coma supervene. Convulsions are common at the onset, especially in children. In children, early signs such as leg pain, coldness of the extremities and abnormal skin color may develop even before the classic signs of meningitis. Recognition of the disease at this stage and institution of specific therapy are more beneficial.

In a large proportion, features of meningococcal septicemia are seen. These include maculopapular and purpuric skin rashes appearing over the axilla, flanks, wrists and buttocks and ecchymosis and peripheral gangrene (Fig. 37.3). Signs of meningeal irritation are evident from an early stage. These include neck rigidity, Kernig's sign and Brudzinski's signs. There is pain over the hamstrings when the knee is extended passively with the hip flexed to 90° and the extension is restricted (***Kernig's sign***). ***Brudzinski's leg sign*** is the flexion of the opposite knee when Kernig's sign is elicited on one side.

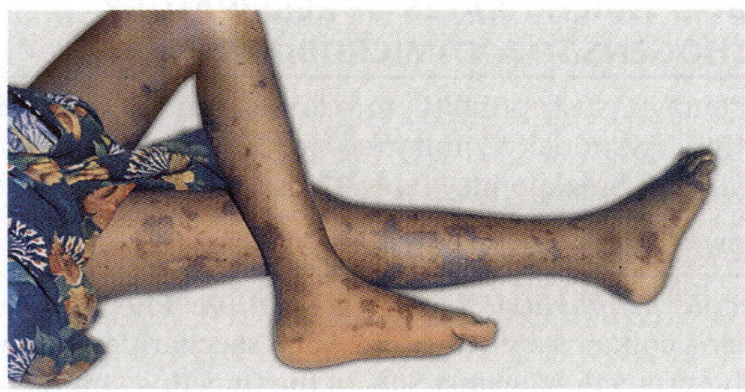

Fig. 37.3: Meningococcemia. *Note:* Blotchy ecchymosis

Brudzinski's neck sign is flexion of both legs when the neck is passively flexed. In severe cases, especially in children, the spasm of neck muscles may be so severe as to produce head retraction and opisthotonus.

Rise in intracranial tension may lead lo papilledema. In a small proportion of cases, blindness, deafness and hemiplegia may be found in the acute phase. Some of the patients recover within a month. A toxic encephalopathy may develop in some patients and this is probably due to diffusion of toxins or bacterial invasion.

It is characterized by the development of deep coma within a few days of onset. This condition is associated with a mortality up to 50%. The development of subdural effusion, internal hydrocephalus or brain abscess should be suspected from the development of localizing signs and progressive deterioration, despite adequate therapy. Most of the untreated patients die in a stage of deep coma within days or weeks, but a few may proceed to a chronic phase characterized by progressive emaciation, opisthotonus, paralysis, bedsores and hydrocephalus.

Meningococcemia

Meningococcemia may be fulminant or chronic: Meningococcal septicemia (meningococcemia) is characterized by hemorrhagic manifestations. The organisms can be demonstrated in the small blood vessels from all organs. Vascular damage occurs as an allergic phenomenon (***Schwartzman phenomenon)*** caused by the endotoxin of meningococci. In fulminant meningococcemia, hemorrhage occurs into the adrenal glands leading to adrenal failure and profound shock. Generalized hemorrhagic tendency may develop due to disseminated intravascular coagulation (DIC). Metastatic lesions occur in the joints, ears, eyes and lungs.

Fulminant meningococcemia: This is characterized by abrupt onset, severe constitutional disturbances, peripheral vascular collapse, shock and sometimes myocarditis. The skin rashes are extensive and may even ulcerate. Though in many cases there is associated meningitis, the signs of meningeal irritation may be absent due to shock. In some cases the illness may progress rapidly so that toxemia and shock may occur within hours. These features are collectively called ***Waterhouse-Friderichsen syndrome***. This syndrome is caused by hemorrhage into the adrenal glands resulting in acute adrenal failure. Toxic vasculitis aggravates the hypotension. Complications include endocarditis, allergic polyarthritis, pneumonia and osteomyelitis.

Chronic meningococcemia: It is characterized by intermittent fever lasting for several weeks, maculopapular rashes, erythema nodosum, arthralgia or arthritis and splenomegaly in 20%. If left untreated, the infection may either subside or progress to meningitis.

Other rare meningococcal lesions include ***pneumonia, genitourinary infection, endocarditis, osteomyelitis*** and ***purulent conjunctivitis***. In acute meningococcal infections, polymorphonuclear leukocytosis with total counts going up to 12,000–40,000/mm³ is common. In chronic meningococcemia, the leukocyte count may be normal.

Diagnosis

Clinically, meningitis is diagnosed when there is fever, severe headache and signs of meningeal irritation. This has to be distinguished from meningism which is seen in toxic febrile states where the signs of meningeal irritation are present but the CSF is normal. Meningitis has to be distinguished from encephalitis, subarachnoid hemorrhage and other causes of coma. Meningococcal meningitis has to be distinguished from other causes of purulent meningitis. At the slightest suspicion of meningitis, lumbar puncture should be done and the CSF should be examined to establish the diagnosis. ***Since early diagnosis and institution of specific antibacterial treatment is the most important single factor in determining the outcome, lumbar puncture should not be delayed.***

Differential diagnosis includes other bacterial meningitis, mainly caused by *H. influenzae* and pneumococci.

Laboratory diagnosis: Diagnosis of meningitis is confirmed by examination of CSF (Table 37.8). Lumbar puncture should be done at the earliest if there are no contraindications. If available it is better to do computed tomography (CT) before lumbar puncture to rule out increased intracranial tension. CSF culture is the gold standard for diagnosis. In 80–90% of cases, positive results are obtained. Molecular diagnostic methods such as polymerase chain reaction (PCR) in CSF are more helpful in getting positive results. Start antibiotic treatment as early as possible. Even after starting antibiotics PCR test may remain positive for about 2 hours. An immunochromatographic test is also available.

The following features predict bacterial meningitis in comparison to viral meningitis.

- CSF glucose concentration is 1.9 mmol/L
- Ratio of CSF/blood glucose less than 0.23
- CSF protein concentration > 3.2 g/L
- CSF cells > 2000/mm³ or > 1180 neutrophils/mm³
- CSF lactate levels are good markers of bacterial meningitis even superior to leukocyte counts

Table 37.8: Diagnostic findings in CSF for meningitis	
Rise in pressure	Opening pressure may exceed even 400 mm CSF
Physical appearance	Turbid or purulent
Pleocytosis	Leukocyte count is usually 500–10000/mm³ or even more. Over 95% are neutrophils. Rarely lymphocytes may be the predominant cells. In 5–10% of cases cell count may be only mildly elevated or be normal. This is associated with poor prognosis
Demonstration of organism	Gram staining of CSF shows meningococci in 60–90% of cases. PCR of CSF can detect the organism early
CSF glucose	It is less than 40% of the level of blood glucose estimated simultaneously
Culture of organism	Positive in a variable propostion. Organisms disappear rapidly on starting specific therapy
Detection of meningococcal antigen in CSF	Counterimmunoelectrophoresis

Abbreviations: CSF = Cerebrospinal fluid; PCR = Polymerase chain reaction

Textbook of Medicine

- Serum CRP levels ≥ 20 mg/L and serum procalcitonin levels of ≥ 0.5 g/L suggest bacterial meningitis.

Conditions which resemble meningitis include subdural empyema, brain abscess or necrotic temporal lobe in *herpes simplex* encephalitis. In patients with onset of seizures, signs of raised intracranial tension and moderate or severe impairment of consciousness, CT or MRI should be done to assess the intracranial pathology before performing lumbar puncture. Repetition of lumbar puncture is indicated when the progress with treatment is not satisfactory.

In patients with persistent elevation of intracranial tension lumbar picture and release of CSF may lead to transtentorial herniation of the temporal lobe of the brain and coning of the brainstem which can be fatal, if unrecognized. In such cases lumbar puncture should be done with precaution to monitor the patient and institute life-saving measures if coning occurs. Coning of the brainstem leads to drowsiness, coma and slowing of respiration and death. Emergency management consist of IV administration of 200 mL of 20% mannitol, elevation of the foot end of the bed and release of supratentorial pressure by surgical means. If in any case the lumbar puncture in likely to be delayed and the clinical suspicion is strong, antibiotic therapy should be started straight away, empirically.

Identification of the infecting agent:

- Meningococci may be seen in Gram stained CSF preparations. This is the most rapid method for diagnosis.
- The organism can be cultured from CSF, blood or material taken from skin rashes.
- Meningococcal antigen can be identified in CSF by counterimmunoelectrophoresis.
- Sera of convalescent patients show antibodies to meningococci and these can be demonstrated by complement fixation test, passive hemagglutination or by radioactive antigen binding tests. These tests are helpful in retrospective diagnosis.
- Carrier state is diagnosed by isolating the organisms from material collected from the nasopharynx using a West's postnasal swab. The swab has to be transported to the laboratory in a special medium (Sturt's medium).

Treatment

As early as possible, specific treatment should be started. Any delay in antibiotic treatment > 3 hours of diagnosis is associated with higher 3 month mortality and considerable morbidity. Penicillin G is the antibiotic of choice and should be administered IV in a dose of 24 million units daily in divided doses. In children the dose is 16 million units/m². Dexamethasone 10 mg IV should be started with the first dose of antibiotic and repeated 6 h for 4 days. Further doses should be determined, based on the patient's progress. Addition of glucocorticoids early in treatment favors prompt recovery and prevents complications considerably. Dexamethasone is to be started with or before the first dose of antibiotics, at a dose of 0.6 mg/kg/bw/day IV for children or 10 mg IV every 6 hourly for adults for 4 days.

Treatment should be continued for several days. Ampicillin in a dose of 200–400 mg/kg bw daily is also equally effective. Since penicillin and ampicillin enter the CSF through the inflamed meninges, intrathecal administration is not necessary. In penicillin-allergic patients, chloramphenicol in a dose of 4–6 g daily in divided doses can be used IV. The third generation cephalosporin, especially cefotaxime is quite effective when given in doses of 6–8 g/day. The exact dose can be calculated from the weight of the patient. 150–200 mg/kg IV daily in 6 hourly doses to a total of up to 12 g. An alternative is ceftriaxone in a daily dose of 75–100 mg/kg (up to 5 g) given in two divided doses.

The administration of antibiotics is continued at high doses till the CSF becomes clear and cell count comes down. Thereafter, the drug is continued at a lower dose till all symptoms subside and the CSF returns to normal. Return of the CSF sugar level to normal indicates full recovery.

Supportive treatment consists of the maintenance of nutrition, fluid and electrolyte balance, treatment of shock and the management of convulsions. Adrenal crisis should be managed with large doses of hydrocortisone.

Course and Prognosis

The disease was invariably fatal before the advent of specific antimicrobial therapy. At present the mortality is reduced to 10%. Prognosis for full recovery and avoidance of complications depends directly on the early institution of specific antimicrobial therapy with glucocorticoids and therefore, it is of utmost importance to make the diagnosis and start treatment without delay. Other poor prognostic factors include extremes of age, presence of rash, tachycardia (>120/minute), diastolic BP < 60 mm Hg, total leukocyte count < 1000/mm³ and platelet count below 180,000/mm³. Long-term sequelae include cranial nerve palsies, seizure disorders, various forms of paralysis and cognitive impairment.

Prevention

During epidemics, the aim should be to reduce the carrier state among the susceptible population. Rifampicin is given in a dose of 10 mg/kg once in 12 hours for 2 days for adults and children above 1 year. For children below 1 year the dose is 5 mg/kg bw 12 hourly for 2 days.

Alternate drugs include ciprofloxacin 500 mg oral or ofloxacin 400 mg oral single dose daily for four days. For pregnant women ceftriaxone 250 mg in single dose daily for a few days is the drug of choice.

Vaccination

Vaccines containing pure group specific capsular polysaccharides of meningococci A, C, Y and W135 groups are available. The vaccine is given subcutaneously. Immunity lasts for three years. At present this vaccine is available for persons going for *Hajj* pilgrimage.

Recommendation for general population:

- For children aged 11–15 years a single dose of conjugate vaccine on entry into school is recommended
- For persons aged 11–55 years at increased risk a single dose of conjugate vaccine
- Vaccination is not recommended for children below 2 years of age.

Common Bacterial Infections of Childhood
Diphtheria, Pertussis and *Haemophilus Influenzae*

KV Krishna Das

Chapter Summary

- Diphtheria
  - General Considerations
  - Pathogenesis and Pathology
  - Clinical Features
  - Diagnosis
  - Treatment
  - Prevention
- Pertussis Infections
  - General Considerations
  - Clinical Manifestations
  - Complications
  - Diagnosis
  - Treatment
  - Prevention
- *Haemophilus Influenzae* Infections
  - General Considerations
  - Clinical Syndromes
  - Treatment
  - Active Prophylaxis

DIPHTHERIA

General Considerations

Definition: Diphtheria is an acute infectious disease caused by *Corynebacterium diphtheriae*, clinically characterized by a membranous inflammation at the site of infection and deleterious effects on several tissues particularly on the myocardium and nervous system due to the exotoxin.

Corynebacterium diphtheriae is gram-positive rod 3×0.3 μm in size, pleomorphic, non-motile, non-sporing, non-capsulate, generally aerobic and facultatively anaerobic. Based on the colony morphology on tellurite medium, biochemical reactions and hemolytic property. *C. diphtheriae* is classified into three main types—gravis, intermedius and mitis. Virulent strains produce an exotoxin which is responsible for producing remote effects. Around 90–95% of the gravis and intermedius strains are toxigenic while 80–85% of mitis strains are so. The toxin is a labile protein of molecular weight 62,000 and it is inactive when released by the bacterium. Action of proteases present in infected tissue is necessary for its activation. The toxin inhibits protein synthesis and leads to fragmentation of deoxyribonucleic acid (DNA) and cytokines. Affected tissues undergo necrosis as an effect of the toxin. Absorption of the toxin from the local site of infection gives rise to systemic effects. Treatment with 0.2–0.4% formalin converts the toxin into toxoid. The toxoid is not harmful to the tissues, still it possesses antigenicity and hence is used for immunization.

Epidemiology: The disease has been almost wiped out from developed countries, but in India it is still prevalent. Diphtheria is more common in children, though all ages may be affected. The organism is harbored by carriers and cases. The disease is spread by droplets, contaminated vessels shared by children or by direct inoculation into skin abrasions or eyes. Unimmunized children in a partially immunized community are highly susceptible. Relaxation of immunization schedule has led to resurgence of outbreaks of diphtheria in some Asian countries. Untreated cases are infective for more than 2 weeks. Antibiotic therapy reduces the communicability to 2–3 days. During outbreaks, susceptible individuals can be identified by the Schick intradermal test, but this method is seldom used in practice.

Pathogenesis and Pathology

The organisms gain entry through the respiratory passage, eyes, middle ear, genitalia and skin. Incubation period is 3–4 days but it may vary from 2–7 days. The exotoxin causes tissue necrosis which favors further growth of the organism and toxin production. The epithelium degenerates and a serofibrinous exudate develops which contains inflammatory cells and fibrin. This forms a bluish white membrane over the involved area. The membrane is adherent and when removed forcibly it leaves a raw bleeding surface. Site of predilection for the primary lesions is the respiratory tract. Other sites of infection are the nose, ears, conjunctiva, genitalia and skin. Around the membrane there may be necrosis, ulceration or hemorrhage. Sometimes, the membrane may not be evident, but the pharynx may show hyperemia and edema.

Regional lymph nodes are markedly enlarged. The toxin is absorbed from the primary site and it causes damage to the myocardium, kidneys, adrenal glands and the cranial and peripheral nerves. Myocardium shows cloudy swelling, fatty change, minute hemorrhages and round cell infiltration. This may lead to cardiomegaly and conduction disturbances. Kidneys show cloudy swelling of the tubular epithelium and interstitial nephritis. The adrenal glands are enlarged with hemorrhages in the cortex. Liver cells show degenerative changes with scattered areas of focal necrosis.

Peripheral nerves may show degeneration of the myelin sheaths and axis cylinders, motor fibers being more affected. The posterior column of the spinal cord may be involved. Rarely cerebral hemorrhage, meningitis and encephalitis have been described. Respiratory obstruction by the membrane or toxic myocarditis may lead to death.

Textbook of Medicine

Clinical Features

These depend on the primary site of involvement, duration of the illness, systemic effects of the toxin and resistance of the host. Incubation period is 1–6 days. The disease starts with sore throat, low grade fever, headache, malaise, vague aches and pains and catarrhal symptoms. As the disease progresses, tachycardia, nausea, vomiting, pallor and weakness follows.

Pharyngeal diphtheria: It is the most common form and the membrane is present over the tonsils and pharynx. Gross cervical lymphadenopathy (described as bull neck) is evident and respiratory obstruction may develop, especially in children. In severe cases, circulatory collapse occurs. Local effects of the toxin lead to paralysis of the palate and pharynx. The term 'malignant diphtheria' is given to the condition characterized by marked edema of the submandibular areas and anterior part of neck. There is moderate leukocytosis (14,000–16,000/mm^3) with polymorphs forming 60–80%.

Laryngeal diphtheria: This forms 25% of the cases. It produces respiratory obstruction early, which may be fatal. The clinical features include barking cough, hoarseness, dyspnea, stridor and cyanosis. Infants with laryngeal diphtheria may refuse to suck the breasts due to choking.

Nasal diphtheria: It occurs in 2–3% of cases. The membrane is limited to the septum or turbinates and it is usually unilateral. The condition may present with a foul smelling serosanguinous nasal discharge or frank epistaxis.

Cutaneous diphtheria: *Corynebacterium diphtheriae* cannot penetrate the intact skin and it gains entry through wounds, burns or abrasions. It causes ulceration. The typical ulcer is usually punched out and 0.5 cm or more in size. Sometimes, it may resemble a nonspecific ulcer. In the early stage, the ulcer is covered by a grayish-yellow or brownish membrane. There may be coexistent pharyngeal diphtheria in 20% of cases.

Other sites of lesion are the conjunctiva, vulva, vagina, uterine cervix, bladder, urethra, penis, middle ear, buccal mucous membrane and esophagus. Sites of lesion are covered with purulent foul smelling discharge.

Complications: Mechanical obstruction of airway by the spreading membrane is a dreaded complication. The other complications are due to the systemic effects of the toxin. The incidence and severity of toxic manifestations increase in proportion to the extent of the membrane.

Toxic complications are most pronounced in the heart and motor nerves. Though 60% of patients have pathological lesions in the heart, only 10–12% manifest clinically. Myocarditis should be suspected if there is variation in the intensity of heart sounds, systolic murmurs, conduction defects, atrial fibrillation, ventricular ectopic beats or ventricular tachycardia. Sudden death may occur due to ventricular fibrillation. Congestive failure and cardiac dilatation are less common. In infants and young children vomiting may be an early symptom of cardiac involvement. Though electrocardiographic changes are nonspecific, the presence of abnormalities strongly suggests myocarditis.

Toxic peripheral neuritis develops 2–6 weeks after the primary lesion. Third, sixth, seventh, ninth and tenth cranial nerves are commonly affected. Palatal and pharyngeal paralysis may occur as early as the third day. External ophthalmoplegia and paralysis of accommodation are frequent. The autonomic neuropathy leads to paralysis of accommodation with preservation of light reflex. This pattern distinguishes diphtheritic paralysis from other conditions like botulism. Autonomic neuropathy involves the heart, vasomotor tone, urinary bladder and bowel. Motor weakness may involve the limbs or respiratory muscles. Ascending polyneuritic type of lesions may follow 2–3 months after the acute attack of diphtheria. Though there are pathological lesions demonstrable in the adrenals, most cases do not manifest clinically.

Diagnosis

The diagnosis of diphtheria is essentially clinical. Confirmation of the diagnosis depends on the demonstration of the organism in stained smears made from the membrane and by culture using Loeffler's medium. Fluorescent antitoxin staining provides a method for rapid diagnosis. Toxigenicity can be assessed by guinea pig inoculation, passive agar gel diffusion (Elek plate method) or counter immunoelectrophoresis.

Differential diagnosis: Acute follicular tonsillitis with exudate over the tonsils may resemble diphtheria. In follicular tonsillitis, the exudate is confined to the tonsils. It is yellowish and can be wiped off without being adherent. The fever is high in acute tonsillitis, whereas it is only mild in diphtheria. Regional lymphadenopathy is more marked in diphtheria than in acute tonsillitis. Infectious mononucleosis may lead to formation of exudate confined to the tonsillar surface. Herpetic lesions may give rise to vesicles and inflammation over the oral mucosa, including tonsils.

Agranulocytosis and acute leukemia may lead to necrotic ulceration of the tonsils. In these there is no true membrane. The tonsils are red, enlarged and necrotic or hemorrhagic. Hematological examination establishes the diagnosis. In all cases of reasonable clinical suspicion, the antitoxin should be given without delay.

Treatment

The aim of treatment is to neutralize the formed toxins and eradicate the organisms from the primary site to prevent further production of toxin. The formed toxin is neutralized by the administration of diphtheria antitoxin ***[(anti-diphtheritic serum (ADS)]*** in adequate quantities. It can be given intramuscularly (IM) or intravenously (IV). The dose can be roughly estimated from the extent of the membrane.

Only one tonsil involved	20,000 units
Both tonsils	40,000 units
Laryngeal and pharyngeal forms	80,000 units
Severe cases	120,000 units

The ADS is prepared in horses and so sensitivity to horse serum has to be tested by appropriate intradermal test using 0.1 mL of 1/100 solution. One centimeter erythema developing within 20 minutes indicates allergy. In allergic cases, ADS should be administered only after desensitization or after taking appropriate measures to combat anaphylactic shock. Usually one dose of ADS is sufficient.

Corynebacterium diphtheriae is sensitive to penicillin and erythromycin. Procaine penicillin 600,000 units IM bd or erythromycin 40 mg/kg body weight in four divided doses for 6 to 7 days is adequate to eliminate the organisms. Since there is the possibility of developing carrier state and spread of the infection, the child should be allowed to mix with other children only after ensuring that three repeated throat cultures are negative. General measures of treatment include rest in bed for 2 weeks and soft liquid feeds. Tetracycline, rifampicin and clindamycin are also effective against *C. diphtheriae.*

Since an attack of diphtheria may not lead to solid immunity, all cases should be followed up with regular vaccination with diphtheria toxoid, during convalescence. ***Treatment of complications:*** Myocarditis is managed with strict bed rest, use of antiarrhythmic drugs and supportive measures. Corticosteroids (betamethasone 8 mg four times daily) have been employed with beneficial results in some. Artificial pacing may be required if heart block develops.

Neuritis is usually self-limiting and does not respond to any specific treatment. Supportive care and physiotherapy are indicated. Nasogastric tube may be required to aid feeding, if there is palatal and pharyngeal paralysis.

Respiratory obstruction due to the presence of the membrane is an emergency indication for tracheostomy and maintenance of the airway. Respiratory paralysis is managed by artificial ventilation.

Prevention

(*See* also Section 1, Ch 3 for immunization schedule)

Prevention includes general active immunization and management of contacts. Active immunization is done with diphtheria, pertussis, tetanus (DPT) vaccine which is also known as triple antigen. The first dose should be given at 2 months and thereafter two more doses at 4 week intervals. Booster doses must be given at the second and fifth years. The DPT vaccine gives substantial immunity, but rarely the disease may occur even in immunized children. *Hemophilus influenzae* type b (Hib) vaccine can be combined with DPT vaccination for primary vaccination.

Immediate contacts should be given 2000 units of ADS. Throat swab culture should be done to identify the carrier state. Carriers should be given treatment. Penicillin or erythromycin is used to eradicate the infection. An alternative is rifampicin in a dose of 600 mg daily orally for 7 days.

A booster dose of DPT is required in previously immunized persons on fresh exposure.

Non-diphtheria corynebacterium: At times, coryne-bacterium other than *C. diphtheriae* may cause lesions as given in Table 38.1.

Table 38.1: Pathogenic non-diphtheria corynebacterium	
Immunocompetent hosts	
C. ulcerans	Acute pharyngitis
C. hemolyticum	
C. pseudotuberculosis (C. bovis)	Lymphadenopathy
C. minutissimum	Erythrasma
Immunocompromised hosts	
Opportunistic infections	
C. jeikeium	Infective endocarditis
C. xerosis	Infection of intravascular prosthesis
C. pseudodiphtheriticum	
C. equi	Necrotizing pneumonia

PERTUSSIS INFECTIONS

Syn: Whooping Cough

General Considerations

The term pertussis, which means intensive cough, is an acute respiratory infection, seen more commonly in young children. The disease is also much serious in them. The term 'whooping cough' is derived from the occurrence of progressive repetitive paroxysms of cough followed by inspiratory whoop. Natural pertussis infection and vaccination do not produce life-long immunity. The immunity wanes over a few decades. Since, there is almost complete coverage of DPT vaccination in children, adolescents and adults may become susceptible to infection increasingly. It is therefore possible that adults develop pertussis infection.

Pertussis is caused by *Bordetella pertussis* which is highly infective. *Bordetella parapertussis* and *Bordetella bronchiseptica* are members of the same genus, rarely causing disease in man. Maximum incidence is seen in children below 5 years and the mortality is highest for children below 1 year of age. The organisms spread by droplet infection and the route of entry is the respiratory tract. The infectious period is the catarrhal prodrome and for 3 weeks after the onset of illness. Bordetella is small gram-negative coccobacilli, exclusively pathogenic to humans. The genome of *B. pertussis* has been sequenced.

Pathology

The mucosal lining of the respiratory tract shows inflammation. Peribronchial lymphoid hyperplasia occurs initially and this is followed by necrosis of the midzonal and basilar layers of the bronchial epithelium. This leads to the accumulation of tenacious mucus, atelectasis and eventually bronchiectasis.

Clinical Manifestations

The incubation period is usually 7–14 days but may be prolonged to 20 days. Three stages can be distinguished—***catarrhal, paroxysmal*** and ***convalescent***—each lasting up to 2 weeks so that the course of the disease extends to 6–8 weeks.

The ***catarrhal stage*** manifests with rhinorrhea, mild fever and cough. During this stage, clinical recognition of the disease is difficult. This is the most infective stage.

In the ***paroxysmal stage,*** cough starts, increases in severity and becomes repetitive and explosive. Each paroxysm is followed by a whoop produced by a sudden massive inspiratory effort through a narrowed glottis. During the paroxysms of cough the infant develops facial congestion, distension of neck and scalp veins, lacrimation, cyanosis and clouding of consciousness. The paroxysm ends with the onset of vomiting. The whoop may not be distinctly made out in younger infants, but they may become asphyxiated and develop anoxic convulsions. Physical examination may reveal periorbital edema. In the uncomplicated cases lung signs are usually absent. Pertussis occurring in adults causes prolonged cough. With increasing age, the manifestations also become more severe.

Convalescence is marked by the decrease in frequency and severity of the paroxysms. Vomiting subsides and the patient's appetite improves. At this stage the child is very susceptible to develop superinfections by other respiratory pathogens and this may lead to recurrence of the paroxysms of cough. When this occurs it may last for several months.

Complications

Complications are common to develop.

- ***Respiratory***
  - Otitis media, especially in infants
  - Bronchitis
  - Bronchopneumonia
  - Atelectasis (segmental or lobar)
  - Interstitial or subcutaneous emphysema or pneumothorax due to rupture of alveoli
  - Bronchiectasis
  - Flare-up of tuberculosis
  - Sudden death of the infant may occur.
- ***Central nervous system (CNS):*** Convulsions may occur due to anoxia, encephalopathy or rarely intracranial hemorrhage.
- ***Gastrointestinal:*** Severe vomiting with dehydration, tetany, ulceration of the frenum of the tongue (due to biting during a paroxysm), prolapse rectum, hernia.
- ***Hemorrhages***
  - Epistaxis
  - Subconjunctival hemorrhage
  - Hemoptysis, hematemesis.
- ***Malnutrition:*** Severe emaciation occurs in most of the affected children. In poor communities it is the starting point for marasmus and kwashiorkor.

Diagnosis

The disease has to be suspected clinically, particularly in an unimmunized child with known contact with the disease. Total leukocyte count is elevated to 20,000–50,000/mm^3 with absolute lymphocytosis. A leukemoid reaction may sometimes occur. Chest X-ray may show perihilar infiltrates or segmental collapse. Bacteriological diagnosis is established by culturing the organism obtained from nasopharyngeal swab or cough plate culture. Fluorescent antibody staining of pharyngeal specimens provides a rapid and specific diagnosis. Polymerase chain reaction (PCR) using nasopharyngeal aspirate reveals the organisms. In cases with duration above 2 weeks IgG antitoxic antibody can be demonstrated in serum.

Differential diagnosis: Whooping cough has to be differentiated from other conditions in childhood causing spasmodic cough. These are acute bronchitis, bronchopneumonia, aspiration of foreign bodies, extrinsic compression of the trachea and bronchi by tuberculous glands or other masses, obstructive airway disease, cystic fibrosis and congenital malformations of the upper respiratory tract. Infections with *B. parapertussis, B. bronchiseptica* and adenovirus types 1, 2, 3 and 5 closely resemble whooping cough and cannot be clinically differentiated. Respiratory syncytial virus infection is becoming more widespread, accounting for a high proportion of respiratory morbidity in children. This has to be borne in mind. Postnasal drip caused by dripping of exudate from the nasopharynx may lead to spasmodic cough when the child lies in bed. This may mimic whooping cough.

Treatment

Supportive care is important to maintain nutrition, prevent aspiration into the respiratory tract and maintain the airway. Cough suppressants like dextromethorphan and pholcodine, bronchodilators such as a low dose of salbutamol (1–2 mg) and mucolytics such as bromhexine give relief to symptoms. Steam inhalations provide comfort and favor resolution of disease. The airway is cleared by suction of the exudates. Anoxic convulsions are managed by administration of oxygen and anticonvulsants. Small, frequent feeds are tolerated if given soon after a paroxysm of cough. IV fluids may be required if the child is dehydrated. In general, administration of antibiotics does not shorten the paroxysmal stage, once it is established. Erythromycin 50 mg/kg/day given for 5–7 days will reduce the period of communicability. It may even abort or prevent the progress of the disease if given in the catarrhal stage. Ampicillin, chloramphenicol and cotrimoxazole may also be used as alternative drugs. Azithromycin 250–500 mg po, od for 7–10 days is effective in controlling the infection if started early. Clarithromycin is a suitable alternative.

Antibodies are not transferred transplacentally in the case of whooping cough. In most patients, a single attack confers life-long immunity.

Prevention

Active immunization is achieved by the administration of the pertussis vaccine, usually given in combination with diphtheria, pertussis and tetanus toxoids (DPT). The vaccine contains killed *B. pertussis*. The initial dose is given at 2 months, with two more doses at 4 week intervals. The first booster is given 1 year later and the next one at school entry. Adverse reactions may develop after vaccination. These are local reactions, fever developing within 12–24 hours of injection and rarely post-vaccination encephalitis. The reported risk of encephalitis is 1 in 10^5–10^6 vaccinations. At present the benefits of vaccination far outweigh the risks and hence vaccination should be recommended for all infants. Contraindication to vaccination is severe adverse reaction to a previous dose. If a child has missed pertussis vaccination at the

Textbook of Medicine

ideal period, it is better to start the course as early as possible. Conventional pertussis vaccine produced in India contains products of whole organisms. It is cheap, but it is likely to cause more adverse reactions. With whole cell vaccines the immunity begins to diminish after 3–5 years and possibly vanishes by 10–12 years.

Source: Halperin SA. The control of pertussis—2007 and beyond. N Engl J Med. 2007;356(2):110-3.

Acellular vaccines containing up to five specific antigens of *Bordetella pertussis* are available in other countries. They produce less of adverse reactions, but are more costly. Adults exposed to risk of infection, such as doctors and nurses can also be protected by vaccination.

Since whooping cough leads to severe nutritional impairment in children, nutritional supplementation should be started during convalescence.

HAEMOPHILUS INFLUENZAE INFECTIONS

Syn: Hib Infection

General Considerations

Haemophilus influenzae type b (Hib) is a common cause of infection in children worldwide—most common lesions being pneumonia, meningitis, epiglottitis and soft tissue lesions in bones, joints and other sites. Three million cases occur annually and 38,600 childhood deaths occur (WHO 2006). For every case of Hib meningitis there are about five cases of pneumonia (vaccination prevents infections).

Haemophilus are pleomorphic gram-negative rods, which are generally aerobic, but can be facultatively anaerobic. *H. influenzae* is an exclusively human parasite, residing principally in the upper respiratory tract.

Haemophilus influenzae exists in coccobacilli form in cultures but shows bacillary morphology in cerebrospinal fluid of patients with meningitis. It is mainly aerobic but can also grow anaerobically. Culture yields capsulated and non-capsulated colonies. The capsulated forms are more virulent. The organisms have been classified into six types designated A to F based on the capsular polysaccharide. The polysaccharide capsule-polyribosylribitol phosphate (PRP) is an important determinant of virulence and the major target for specific immunity. Type B is responsible for most of the serious infections. Around 60–80% of children below 3 years harbor the organism in the upper respiratory tract. Maternal antibodies confer passive immunity to the child up to the age of 2 months. Children aged 2 months to 3 years are more susceptible to infection. Natural immunity develops due to subclinical infections after the age of 3 years.

H. influenzae is noted for its wide range of pathological lesions (Table 38.2).

Pathogenesis and Pathology

Haemophilus influenzae may act as the primary pathogen to cause meningitis in children, laryngoepiglottitis, otitis media, pneumonia, arthritis, endocarditis and pericarditis. It acts as a secondary pathogen in bronchitis, bronchiectasis and sinusitis in adults. Secondary infection is caused by non-capsulated strains. Development of antibodies to the capsule confers immunity. Immunocompromised and unvaccinated children are most susceptible to infection.

Table 38.2: Lesions caused by *H. influenzae*

Head and neck lesions	Cellulitis over the face and orbits, purulent conjunctivitis, sinusitis, otitis, epiglottitis cervical adenitis
Brain meninges	Meningitis, brain abscess, cerebral herniation
Respiratory system	Pneumonia, empyema
Cardiovascular system and childhood	Bacteremia, endocarditis, pericarditis
Neonatal infections	Bacteremia, sepsis, meningitis, hearing loss, developmental delay, cognitive impairment, seizures

Splenectomy acquired asplenia, sickle cell disease, human immunodeficiency virus (HIV) infection and presence of malignant disease predispose to Hib infection. *H. influenzae* is notorious for producing widespread lesions in several organs in the body.

Clinical Syndromes

Haemophilus influenzae meningitis follows an acute course and is fatal in 90% of cases, if left untreated. Clinical manifestations of Hib meningitis are similar to those of other purulent meningitides. Disease course may be fulminant with death occurring within hours or days. Mortality in India overall for treated Hib meningitis is 11% but in children it is 20%. Meningitis is the most serious infection caused by *H. influenzae*. Hib pneumonia also clinically mimics other forms of bacterial pneumonias, but the onset may not be explosive. Laryngoepiglottitis causes considerable edema and airway obstruction. Emergency tracheostomy may be necessary to save life. Infection of the lung and pleura lead to lobar pneumonia with empysema.

Haemophilus influenzae frequently causes pharyngitis in children. In adults during prolonged antibiotic therapy superinfection by *H. influenzae* may develop. The mucosa is red and may be covered by a soft yellow exudate. The local pain and discomfort are out of proportion to the appearance of the lesion. Systemic complications such as septicemia with arthritis, endocarditis and pericarditis may occur, especially in children.

Secondary infection by *H. influenzae* causes bronchopneumonia, exacerbation of chronic bronchitis and other suppurative pulmonary lesions.

Laboratory Diagnosis

The organism can be identified by Gram stain and can be cultured from materials such as cerebrospinal fluid (CSF), sputum, pus, etc. Since, the organism is highly susceptible to low temperatures, refrigeration during transit should be avoided. The capsulated strain shows Quellung phenomenon when added to type B antiserum. Tests such as counter-current electrophoresis latex particle agglutination and enzyme-linked immunosorbent assay (ELISA) tests help to detect the antibodies to the capsular material.

Treatment

The common antibiotics such as chloramphenicol, ampicillin and cotrimoxazole are effective. Resistant

Textbook of Medicine

strains have emerged. Tetracycline or chloramphenicol can be used for treating exacerbations of chronic bronchitis and emphysema. In milder nonfatal infections these drugs can be tried. Meningitis and epiglottitis are rapidly fatal if untreated. The intensity of antibiotic treatment has to be tailored to the severity and location of infection. Ampicillin does not cross the blood brain barrier in adequate concentration. Third generation cephalosporins are the drugs of choice. For children, cefotaxime 200 mg/kg bw in divided doses IV has to be administered. For adults, the daily dosage may reach up to 12 g. Ceftriaxone in a dose of 100–150 mg/kg bw/day is an effective alternative.

In severe cases meropenem may have to be employed. The duration of treatment has to be 7–14 days depending on the clinical condition.

Active Prophylaxis

In many parts of the world a purified capsular polysaccharide vaccine is used. Vaccines have been developed through covalent linkage of the PRP to carrier protein. Four different types of vaccines are available. Hib polysaccharide tetanus protein conjugate vaccine (PRP-T) contains tetanus toxoid as the carrier protein. This can be given along with DTP vaccination in the second, third and fourth month. A booster dose may be required after 2 years. Routine vaccination has almost eliminated the infection in many countries.

In household contacts, children below the age of 5 years run the risk of acquiring infection. Rifampicin in a dose of 20 mg/kg daily given orally for 4 days eradicates the carriage of *H. influenzae*.

CHAPTER
39

Salmonella Infections

S Bhasi, KV Krishna Das

Chapter Summary

- General Considerations
- Typhoid Fever
- Pathogenesis
- Pathology
- Clinical Feature
- Diagnosis
- Management
- Antimicrobial Resistance
- Paratyphoid Fever
- Prevention of Salmonella Infections
- Non-typhoid Salmonella Infections

GENERAL CONSIDERATIONS

Salmonella are members of enterobacteriaceae. They are gram-negative motile rods, commonly found in the intestinal tract of humans, several animals and many arthropods. More than 2000 serotypes have been identified. Clinical syndromes caused by *Salmonella* include:

- Typhoid fever and paratyphoid fevers caused by *S. typhi*, *S. paratyphi* A, B and C—collectively known as enteric fevers.
- Gastroenteritis (*Salmonella* food poisoning)
- Bacteremia with or without metastatic infection
- Asymptomatic carrier state.

TYPHOID FEVER

Typhoid fever is an acute systemic infection characterized by sustained fever caused by *Salmonella typhi* with initial lesion in the bowel, bacteremia and subsequent affection of many tissues.

Etiology

Salmonella typhi is an exclusive pathogen of humans. Three antigens have been demonstrated:

1. Somatic antigen (called 'O' antigen)—a lipopolysaccharide cell wall antigen
2. Flagellar antigen (called 'H' antigen)—formed from the structural proteins making up the flagella
3. The polysaccharide envelope VI antigen which confers virulence by masking the 'O' antigen from immunological attack (Fig. 39.1).

Epidemiology

The global incidence is around 15–30 million cases annually with half million deaths. The disease remains a serious public health problem in developing countries. The incidence in India is about 100–1000 cases per 1,00,000 persons per year and enteric fevers continue to be a major infection throughout the country.

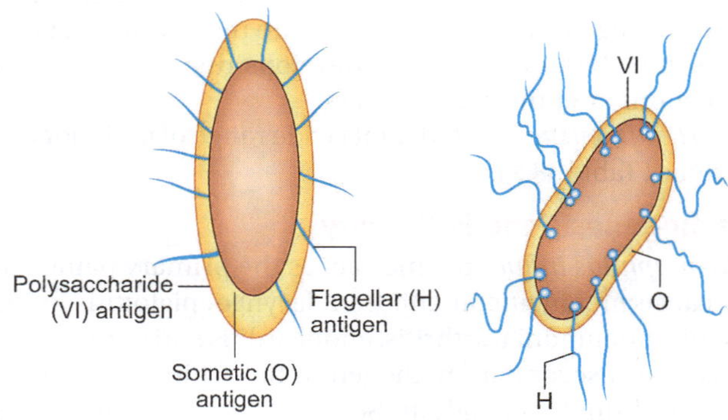

Fig. 39.1: Schematic presentation of the antigens on Salmonella. O-somatic antigen; H-flagellar antigen; VI-virulence antigen

The organisms are excreted in feces and urine of cases of typhoid fever in the acute phase and up to 9 weeks during convalescence. Healthy carriers pass the organism in feces and urine without themselves suffering from the disease for indefinite periods. Disease is spreads from fecal—oral route, infection getting in by contaminated water sources, milk, ice-creams, processed meat, shell fish, food contaminated by infective food handlers and flies. The bacilli remain viable in water or food for considerable periods.

Pathogenesis

Several factors determine the establishment of infection. They are:

- ***Size of the infective dose:*** The average infective dose in immunocompetent subjects is 10^7 organisms. Higher infective doses are required to transmit paratyphoid.
- Normal gastric acid rapidly kills the bacilli. Susceptibility is increased by diluting gastric acid by the ingestion of large quantities of fluids with and before meals, antacids, acid suppressant drugs, vagotomy and prior infection with *H. pylori*.
  - ***Virulence of the infecting strain:*** Multidrug resistant organisms and isolates from fatal cases might vary in their virulence. Highly virulent strains are more invasive.
  - Immune status of the host and the status of bacteria in the upper part of the duodenum and jejunum.

Bacilli enter the epithelial lining of the distal ileum and reach the submucosa where they are phagocytosed by macrophages and polymorphs and reach mesenteric lymph nodes. There, they multiply and enter the blood stream via thoracic duct to produce transient bacteremia. This primary bacteremia results in the organisms reaching the liver, gallbladder, spleen, bone marrow, lymph nodes and other parts of the reticuloendothelial system where further intracellular multiplication occurs inside mononuclear cells throughout the 7 to 14 days incubation period. A second bacteremia follows accompanied by symptoms as the infection spreads throughout liver, gallbladder, spleen, Peyer's patches and bone marrow.

The organism produces endotoxins, which stimulate release of cytokines from macrophages and neutrophils responsible for inflammatory changes in various organs and production of constitutional symptoms including fever.

Pathology

Inflammatory changes mainly occur in the liver, spleen, lymph node, bone marrow and Peyer's patches consisting of mononuclear cell infiltration, hyperplasia and focal necrosis. Focal collections of mononuclear leukocytes are called ***typhoid nodules***. The liver is enlarged and shows cloudy swelling. The Peyer's patches in the terminal ileum becomes swollen and surface undergoes necrosis with formation of ulcers. Blood vessels here may be eroded leading to intestinal hemorrhage. Ulceration may extend to the muscularis mucosa and serosa and may result in intestinal perforation. The rectus abdominis muscle may show ***Zenker's degeneration***.

Clinical Features

The usual incubation period is 7–14 days (range from 3–60 days). Typhoid predominantly affects children and young adults especially in endemic areas. Because of acquired immunity, it is uncommon in elderly. It affects both sexes equally. The clinical manifestations are very variable ranging from fever with little other morbidity to marked toxemia and associated complications involving many systems. In a classical case onset is slow with fever, headache, lethargy, anorexia and malaise. The fever is continuous or remittent; it rises in a step ladder pattern in the first week. Chills and rigor do not occur if antipyretics are not used. Abdominal symptoms such as vague discomfort, pain, constipation in the first week and diarrhea in the second and third weeks occur commonly in the majority of cases. Diarrhea is more common in children. Epistaxis may occur occasionally. Non-productive cough may be prominent in a few and this may be mistaken for a primary respiratory disease.

Physical examination in the ***first week*** reveals relative bradycardia (slow pulse fever) and mild tenderness in the right iliac fossa. Erythematous 2–3 mm diameter maculopapular lesions called ***rose spots*** may appear over the upper abdomen and chest by the 5th or 6th day and fade off in 2–3 days. They are best made out in fair-skinned people. They are rare in Indians. In the ***second week*** temperature reaches around 40°C and remains so for a few days. The tongue is coated in the center. Spleen is palpable 2–4 cm in about 70% of cases and is soft. Abdomen is moderately distended (tumidity) with vague tenderness especially over the right iliac fossa. Palpation may also reveal gurgling due to distended ileal loops. Mild scattered wheeze in the chest is not uncommon. Malena or streaks of blood in feces may be present in a few. This should not be mistaken for typhoid hemorrhage in which bleeding is more pronounced.

Patients with advanced disease and toxemia may show 'typhoid faces' (***typhoid state***)—a thin flushed face with staring apathetic expression. Typhoid encephalopathy may develop in severe cases in the second to fourth week and may present as muttering delirium, tremulousness of the fingers and wrist (***subsultus tendinum***), picking movement of the hands, e.g. picking at the bed clothes (***carphology***) and a staring unarousable stupor—unconscious but eyes open (***coma vigil***). In uncomplicated untreated cases, fever lasts for about 4 weeks and subsides by lysis.

Typhoid in children: Usually a milder illness, diarrhea, vomiting and jaundice are more common. Neonatal typhoid may occur due to vertical transmission from infected mother during late pregnancy. It is rare but could be life-threatening.

Uncommon presentations

- ***Gastroenteritis:*** Acute presentation with vomiting and diarrhea. More common in children especially in paratyphoid.
- ***Acute bronchitis:*** Fever cough and bilateral wheeze.
- ***Acute abdominal pain*** mimicking acute appendicitis.
- ***Jaundice from beginning:*** Seen in about 1–5% cases. This may mimic viral hepatitis, leptospirosis or malaria.

Textbook of Medicine

- *Lobar pneumonia* caused by *S. typhi* (pneumotyphoid) may occur in 1–2%, *S. typhi* may be isolated from sputum culture. The chest lesion may resemble pneumococcal pneumonia.
- *Acute right upper abdominal pain* may be mistaken for acute cholecystitis.
- *Acute glomerulonephritis (nephrotyphoid)* is seen in up to 3% cases—more common in children.
- *Fever with joint pain* may resemble rheumatic fever. This occurs rarely.

Complications: They may develop quite frequently. These may be general or may be confined to specific organ systems. General complications include dehydration, typhoid state, coma vigil, convulsions in children, delirium and septic shock. Systemic complications are listed below:

- *Gastrointestinal (GI) system:* Perforation of ileum with peritonitis, intestinal hemorrhage, paralytic ileus, cholecystitis
- *Respiratory:* Pneumonia
- *Neuropsychiatric:* Typhoid encephalopathy, typhoid meningitis, transverse myelitis, peripheral neuropathy
- *Hematological:* Disseminated intravascular coagulation (DIC), thrombocytopenia
- *Genitourinary:* Glomerulonephritis, pyelonephritis, urinary retention
- *Cardiovascular:* Myocarditis, endocarditis, deep vein thrombosis (DVT), thrombophlebitis
- *Miscellaneous:* Focal sepsis, abscess in liver, spleen, breast, typhoid osteomyelitis, parotitis, arthritis, bone abscess (Brodie's abscess)
- Relapse

Intestinal hemorrhage: Occurs during the second or more commonly, the third week of illness. Mild bleeding manifesting as occult blood or malena is seen in about 20% of cases. Severe bleeding from the ulcerated Peyer's patches occurs in about 2% of cases. Unexplained tachycardia, fall in blood pressure (BP), sudden drop in temperature and pallor indicate the onset of intestinal hemorrhage. Patient passes fresh blood and clotted blood with feces in large quantities. If not treated, hypovolemic shock sets in and death follows.

Intestinal perforation: Occurs usually in third week due to necrosis of Peyer's patches in 1–3% of cases. Terminal 50 cm of the ileum is the site of perforation. The onset of perforation may be heralded by abdominal pain, distension, tenderness and rigidity. The temperature may fall. Severely ill patients may present without classical features and may show only restlessness, tachycardia and hypotension.

Presence of gas under the diaphragm by chest X-ray taken in the erect position is useful for diagnosis. Ultrasonography helps in diagnosis. Secondary infection of the peritoneal cavity with enteric aerobic and anaerobic microorganisms leads to increasing toxemia. In untreated cases mortality exceeds 80%. With prompt treatment mortality can be reduced to less than 10%. In those who survive peritonitis may become localized to form an abscess palpable as a mass in the right iliac fossa.

Relapse: In 2–10% cases 1 to 3 weeks after recovery, fever and other symptoms return. Blood culture often becomes positive again. Relapse rate is lower in those treated with fluoroquinolones or azithromycin, compared to those treated with chloramphenicol or ceftriaxone. Relapses are generally milder than the initial illness. They respond to the same antimicrobials. Usually only one relapse occurs but rarely several relapses may occur in succession, extending the febrile episode to even a few months.

Chronic carriers: There are those who continue to excrete *Salmonella* in feces or urine for more than one year after acute infection, seen in 1–6%. Fecal carriage is more frequent in those with cholelithiasis and other biliary tract abnormalities. They have high levels of systemic immunity and do not develop clinical disease. Urinary carriage may be seen more commonly in people with nephrolithiasis or schistosomiasis. Chronic carriers act as source of infection to others especially if they are working as cooks or food handlers.

Immunity: Infection confers partial immunity, which is unrelated to titer of antibodies against O, H or VI Antigen.

Diagnosis

Clinical: Typhoid fever has to be considered in the differential diagnosis of all prolonged febrile illnesses seen in tropical countries. These include hepatic amebiasis, tuberculosis, infective endocarditis, brucellosis, leptospirosis, typhus, viral hepatitis, malaria, lymphoma, infectious mononucleosis, dengue fever and prolonged viral fever.

Clinical clues to suspect typhoid: Fever more than 5–7 days especially in children and young adults with:

- GI symptoms—vague abdominal pain altered bowel habits ± melena or hematochezia
- Relative bradycardia
- Palpable soft spleen
- Palpable liver ± tenderness
- Central coating of the tongue
- Perforation with peritonitis
- Lower GI bleed
- Severe toxemia.

Laboratory Diagnosis

Isolation of Salmonella typhi

- *Blood culture* is the mainstay of definite diagnosis. Blood is taken directly into 10 times its volume of culture media and incubated. *Blood clot* treated with streptokinase can also be used. Blood culture is usually positive in 72 hours. Sometimes incubation for up to 7 days may be needed. Positivity of blood cultures progressively diminishes from 90 to 75%, 60 and 25% or less respectively from the first week to the fourth week of the illness. Isolates can be tested for drug sensitivity. Culture becomes negative soon after starting specific antibiotics.
- *Bone marrow culture:* This gives the highest positivity. It is especially useful when blood culture is negative. It may remain positive even after starting antimicrobials. 1–2 mL of bone marrow aspirate is sufficient.
- *Bile culture:* Culture of bile aspirated from the duodenum also yields better results.
- *Feces culture:* This gives higher yield in the third week up to 75%. Specificity is limited because of the positive results in carriers.

- ***Skin snip from rose spots:*** This is not commonly done. It is reported to be positive in 75% of cases and it may remain positive even for a few days after starting antibiotics.
- ***Urine culture:*** This is positive in only 25–35% of cases, since bacteriuria may be intermittent. Specificity is limited, since carrier state is known to exist. Positive feces and urine culture results associated with rise in antibody titer is diagnostic.

Widal test: This identifies the agglutinating antibodies against the O and H antigens for *S. typhi* and *S. paratyphi* A and B.

It is a time honored test in vogue for over eight decades introduced by Fernand Widal (French physician, 1862–1929) for the diagnosis of enteric fevers.

Antibody generally appears by the end of first week, steadily increases up to third or fourth week and then gradually declines after varying periods, often months. Patients in endemic areas who are exposed to *Salmonella* antigen earlier (clinical/subclinical infection or TAB vaccination) may give a rapid antibody response.

The O antigen is shared by other *Salmonella* and other members of enterobacteriaceae, this sharing being only partial. Both O and H antibodies increase but the O antibody rises earlier than H antibody. The O antibodies are more specific than H antibody and therefore they are diagnostically more important. A four-fold rise *in antibody titer in paired (acute and convalescent) samples collected 5–7 days apart is a fairly reliable evidence for diagnosis*. The result of a single acute sample should be interpreted taking into account the locally prevalent-Widal titer in the general population. Titers of 1/200 or more are suggestive. In the general population of south India, 10% show H antibody titer up to 1:100 dilution and 2% up to 1:200 dilution. Prevalence of O antibody in the general population is much less.

O antigen of paratyphoid A and B show cross reaction with that of *S. typhi* and hence O antibody titer is not commonly taken into consideration in the diagnosis of paratyphoid fevers. Widal test is simple and cheap compared to blood culture, but lacks specificity. Sensitivity ranges from 47–77% and specificity 50–92%.

The ***Widal test*** has a many disadvantages. These include delay or blunting of the antibody response, rise of only the O or H antibody, pre-existing high titers of antibody, false positive response, false negative and anamnestic reaction.

Anamnestic reaction: This is the rise in antibody levels in patients who have been exposed to antigen by TAB vaccination in the past, when they get any non-specific febrile illness. The rise in titer involves all the antibodies against the *Salmonella* species—*S. typhi* and *S. paratyphi* A and B. Repetition of the test in a week shows that the rise in titer of antibodies does not reach four-fold levels.

Early antibiotic treatment may blunt the antibody response. False positive Widal may occur in malaria, rheumatoid arthritis, chronic liver disease and others.

Other Serological Tests

Many other tests for detection of antibodies, *S. typhi* antigen and *Salmonella* deoxyribonucleic acid (DNA) in the body fluids have been described. These include passive hemagglutination, counter immunoelectrophoresis, latex agglutination and polymerase chain reaction (PCR). An enzyme-linked immunosorbent assay (ELISA) for antibody to the capsular polysaccharide VI antigen is useful for detection of carriers but not for diagnosis of acute illness.

Other laboratory findings: It include mild normocytic-normochromic anemia, mild thrombocytopenia and leukopenia with relative lymphocytosis. Leukocytosis may occur when typhoid is complicated by perforation with peritonitis, secondary sepsis or major bleed. The erythrocyte sedimentation rate (ESR) is generally not elevated in uncomplicated typhoid. Mild to moderate elevation of transaminases—alanine transaminase (ALT) and aspartate aminotransaferase (AST) is common.

Management

- Supportive
- Symptomatic
- Specific—antimicrobial drug
- Prevention.

General Supportive Care

Rest in bed, proper nursing care, measures to avoid bed sores and maintenance of oral hygiene are to be instituted. A nutritious diet helps in recovery. The diet must be easily digestible and of low residue type. At least 1200–1500 calories should be supplied. Fluid and electrolyte balance have to be looked after. Generally 2–3 L of fluid should be given orally if patient tolerates. If not intravenous (IV) fluids are indicated.

Symptomatic Treatment

Paracetamol is useful for treating fever and headache in doses of 500–650 mg 6 hourly. Tepid sponging is also useful to reduce temperature, avoid aspirin, abdominal discomfort and bloated feeling can be reduced by dietary adjustment. Low residue easily digestible articles of food given in small quantities at 2–3 hours intervals.

Specific Antimicrobial Drugs

Typhoid fever is usually treated with a single antibacterial drug. Antibiotic selection depends on local resistance pattern. Effective therapy usually results in clinical improvement within 2–3 days and defervescence in 5–7 days. Treatment of typhoid fever has been complicated by development and rapid dissemination of typhoid organisms resistant to multiple drugs (Table 39.1).

Antimicrobial resistance: This is mediated by plasmids. Chloramphenicol resistance was initially described in 1972 from Kozhikode by Jayaram Panicker, et al. Several reports from Kolkata, Chandigarh and many parts of India and other countries of the world followed soon. The late 1980s witnessed widespread emergence of multidrug resistant *Salmonella*, particularly *S. typhi*, resistant to chloramphenicol, cotrimoxazole and amoxicillin/ampicillin. With the drastic reduction in the usage of chloramphenicol, resistance to this drug fell to less than 20% (re-emergence of sensitivity) by 2000. Resistance to nalidixic acid is a standard criterion used to assess the drug sensitivity of *Salmonella* to fluoroquinolones.

Textbook of Medicine

Table 39.1: Commonly used antimicrobials in typhoid

Antibiotics	Dose mg/kg/day	No. of doses	Route	Duration days
Amoxicillin	75–100	3	Oral/IM/IV	14
Ciprofloxacin	1.5 g/day oral/400 mg IV bd	2/2	Oral/IV	7–14
Ofloxacin	800 mg/day	2	Oral/IV	7–14
Ceftriaxone	60 mg/kg	–2	IV/IM	7–14
Cefotaxime	80 mg/kg	3	IV	7–14
Cefixime	20 mg/kg	2	Oral	7–14
Azithromycin	8–10 mg/kg	1	Oral/IV	7
Chloramphenicol	50–75	4	Oral/IV	14
Cotrimoxazole	6.5–10 trimethoprim	2	Oral/IV	14

Nalidixic acid resistant organisms show decreased susceptibility to clinically important fluoroquinolones, requiring higher dosages and longer duration of therapy or even treatment failure. Resistance to quinolones started appearing in mid 90s at many centers in India and reached up to 50%. Hence, *Salmonella* isolates should be tested directly for ciprofloxacin/ofloxacin. A gradual increase in ceftriaxone minimum inhibitory concentration (MIC) has been observed from 1987–2006 in India, resulting in higher dosage and longer duration. Two isolates of *S. paratyphi* expressing extended spectrum of β-lactamase (ESBL) have been reported from Turkey.

Antimicrobial regimen: With a sensitive agent successful treatment of uncomplicated typhoid usually results in clinical improvement in 2–3 days and defervescence in 5–7 days.

Drug of choice for treatment of typhoid fever in adults:

- Fluoroquinolones such as ciprofloxacin 750 mg BD or ofloxacin 400 mg BD × 7–10 days.
- β-lactam antibiotics such as ceftriaxone 60 mg/kg/day as a single dose or 2 divided doses parenterally for 7–14 days when fluoroquinolones are contraindicated or resistant.
- Azithromycin 1 g on day 1 followed by 500 mg daily orally × 7 days or 1 g daily × 5 days.
- Chloramphenicol 2–3 g/day in divided doses for 14 days.

In situations of drug sensitive typhoid, fluoroquinolones are superior to β-lactam and fluoroquinolones have a low relapse rate of less than 2%. Quinolones are bactericidal and achieve high concentration intracellular and in bile, rapidly eliminating intracellular organisms. Azithromycin in concentrated intracellular at levels 50–100 times greater than serum and is useful for treating typhoid patients including those with resistance. Garenoxacin is a newly developed des-fluoroquinolones with low potential for resistance development showing a wide spectrum of coverage including *Salmonella*. It may be a promising drug for typhoid in the future, though clinical data is now sparse.

The emergence of chloramphenicol sensitive strains have been documented.

Source: Khandeparkar P. Reemergence of chloramphenicol in typhoid fever in the era of antibiotic resistance. J Assoc Physicians India. 2010;58(Suppl):45-6.

Role of Glucocorticoids in Typhoid

There is no consensus regarding the indication, dosage and duration. It may be useful in severe typhoid toxemia manifesting as delirium, obtundation, stupor, coma, shock and others. The dose suggested varies. Usual dose ranges from 2 to 3 mg/kg/bw of dexamethasone IV followed by 1 mg/kg every 6th hourly for 48 hours. Even lower doses may be effective. Short-term uses of corticosteroids along with effective antibiotics and supportive therapy may help to reduce toxemia and favor recovery.

Prognosis: With early diagnosis and proper treatment, prognosis is very good with full recovery in the vast majority. In uncomplicated cases, mortality is less than 1%. Complications such as severe toxemia, hemorrhage, intestinal perforation and meningitis increase the mortality. Septic shock and multiorgan failure are serious complications with high mortality.

Treatment of Complications

Intestinal perforation: If the perforation is recent (within 12 hours) and the general condition satisfactory, emergency surgical closure with broad spectrum antibiotic coverage is indicated. If perforation is more than several hours old and the general condition poor, conservative treatment with IV broad spectrum antimicrobial combinations, IV fluids and other supportive measures should be instituted. With proper care the vast majority of these patients can be saved.

Intestinal hemorrhage: Blood loss has to be corrected with blood transfusion if there are signs of hypovolemia such as increasing pulse rate and fall in blood pressure or active bleeding. In a severe case, rapid replacement of several units of fresh blood may be required.

Treatment of chronic carriers: Most chronic carriers without gallstone disease can be cured by prolonged course of antimicrobials. Fluoroquinolones are most effective with a success rate exceeding 90%. Useful regimens are:

- Ciprofloxacin 750 mg BD or ofloxacin 400 mg BD × 4 weeks.
- Cotrimoxazole 6.5 to 10 mg/kg of trimethoprim in two divided doses × 4 weeks.
- Amoxicillin/ampicillin 100 mg/kg with probenecid in 4 divided doses for 3 months.

For patients with gallstone disease cholecystectomy is indicated in addition.

Treatment of Relapse

Usually relapse also responds to the same antibiotics which are effective for the primary disease. Hence, the same medication should be continued, preferably for a longer period, with bacteriological monitoring.

PARATYPHOID FEVER

These are produced by *Salmonella paratyphi* A, B and C. Incubation period is shorter. The illness generally resembles typhoid in clinical pattern but toxemia and complications are less in the majority of cases. The duration of illness is shorter and mortality is less. At present more severe cases are being reported from south Asian countries. There is also disproportionate increase in paratyphoid fever. Gastroenteritis like presentation is more common, especially in children with paratyphi A infection. In some cases paratyphoid may equal typhoid in severity and complications. Diagnosis is confirmed by isolating the organism and serological tests. Treatment is on lines similar to that of typhoid.

Prevention of Salmonella Infections

Personal hygiene, environmental sanitation and eradication of carriers help to prevent *Salmonella* infection. Washing of hands before eating help to prevent spread of infection and contain the outbreak of typhoid. Disinfection of water sources with bleaching powder, boiling drinking water and anti-housefly measures are helpful. Vaccination is indicated for persons travelling into endemic areas and for contacts and neighbors around index cases. In endemic areas prevention of enteric fever would require implementation of Immunization Programme for young children. Natural infection does not provide complete protection against recurrence.

Vaccines

- **TAB vaccine:** This is the most time-tested vaccine. It is a parenteral, killed, whole cell typhoid-paratyphoid A and B vaccine. It is effective, but largely discontinued in many countries because of side effects. In adults, 2 doses of 0.5 mL given intramuscular (IM) 1–2 weeks apart followed by booster doses every year is the recommended schedule. Adverse side effects include local pain and fever.
- **VI polysaccharide vaccine:** This can be used above the age of 2 years. A single IM or SC injection of 25 µg gives 70–80% protection for 3 years. Re-vaccination is recommended every 3 years.
- **Ty 21a vaccine:** This is a Swiss, live attenuated oral vaccine recommended for persons above 6 years of age. Three doses are to be given on alternate days. Moderate protection occurs for 3 years.

None of the vaccines produces absolute protection and typhoid can occur if the infecting dose is very high.

A new VI-conjugate vaccine has been developed recently and preliminary data shows efficacy. A trial of VI-typhoid vaccine in India (Kolkata) showed that the rate of protection was 61%. Children who were vaccinated between the ages of 2 and 5 years had levels of protection 80%. The overall protection among all VI-vaccine recipients 57%.

Source: Sur D, Ochiai RL, Bhattacharya SK, et al. A cluster-randomized effectiveness trial of Vi typhoid vaccine in India. N Engl J Med. 2009;361(4):335-44.

Non-typhoid Salmonella Infections

These are produced by *Salmonella enteritidis* and *Salmonella typhimurium*. They lead to enterocolitis, bacteremia and localized infections.

Epidemiology: Infection is spread through food and water. Many animals such as chicken, ducks, cattle, sheep, horses, dogs, cats and rodents harbor these organisms as commensals in the intestines. Chicken and duck eggs constitute the largest reservoir of infection. Fish and mussels grown in contaminated water may act as sources for localized outbreaks. Humans develop convalescent or healthy carrier state and excrete the organisms for long time.

Pathogenesis and pathology: After gaining entry through food or drinks the organisms multiply in the small intestine and colon to produce inflammation of the lamina propria of the villi of both the small and large intestines. The lymphoid follicles are enlarged and become swollen. Diarrhea is produced by enterotoxin and direct epithelial invasion. Organisms enter the blood stream to produce bacteremia and metastatic lesions. Conditions like sickle cell anemia and other hemoglobinopathies predispose to the development of recurrent *Salmonella* infections. Osteomyelitis is common in them.

Clinical Features

Enterocolitis: This is also known as *Salmonella* food poisoning. Lesions occur both in the large and small intestines. Incubation period is usually 8–24 hours but can go up to 3 days. Patients present with fever, abdominal pain and diarrhea. The nature of stool varies from profuse watery to frank dysentery. In healthy young adults, *Salmonella* gasetroenteritis is usually a benign self-limiting illness, but in young children and elderly, severe dehydration may develop. Spontaneous resolution usually occurs in three to four days. Bacteremia occurs in 1–2%, more commonly in elderly and immunocompromised subjects. Microscopy of the feces shows cellular exudates and organisms can be cultured from feces.

Treatment: Mainstay is replacement of fluid and electrolytes. Antibiotics do not alter the outcome. Patients who are malnourished, immunocompromised with sickle cell diseases or severely ill should be treated with antimicrobials. Ciprofloxacin, co-trimoxazole, azithromycin or ceftriaxone are effective and to be given for 7–14 days.

Salmonella Bacteremia

This is characterized by prolonged or intermittent fever associated with rigor and chills and positive blood culture. GI symptoms may or may not precede bacteremia. Diagnosis is established by positive blood culture, localized lesions develop in 25% of cases. This includes bronchopneumonia, lung abscess, pleurisy, empyema, pericarditis, endocarditis, nephritis, arthritis, osteomyelitis, bone abscesses and meningitis. Mycotic abdominal aortic aneurysm may occur. Complications tend to occur in the immunocompromised. White blood count (WBC) is usually normal but may be elevated when localized suppuration develops. Treatment is with systemic antibiotics on lines similar to that of typhoid.

Points to Remember
- Typhoid fever is an acute systemic infection with bacteremia caused by *Salmonella typhi* transmitted by fecal oral route.

- Main pathology is inflammation with mononuclear cell infiltration in liver, spleen, lymph node, bone marrow and Peyer's patches in the ileum.
- Prolonged fever, splenomegaly and vague abdominal discomfort—suspect enteric fever.
- Blood culture is the gold standard for diagnosis, maximum positivity exceeding 90% in the first week.
- Most useful antimicrobials are fluoroquinolones, ceftriaxone and azithromycin.

Gram-negative Bacterial Infections
Shigella, Escherichia coli, Klebsiella pneumoniae, Pseudomonas and *Proteus* Infections

S Bhasi

Chapter Summary

- *Shigella* Infections
  - General Considerations
  - Epidemiology
  - Pathogenesis and Pathology
  - Clinical Manifestations
  - Treatment
- *Escherichia coli* Infections
  - General Considerations
  - Clinical Features
  - Treatment
- *Klebsiella pneumoniae* Infections
  - General Considerations
  - Risk Factors
  - Clinical Syndromes
  - Diagnosis
  - Treatment
- *Pseudomonas* Infections
  - General Considerations
  - Conditions Predisposing to Infection
  - Common Lesions
- *Proteus* Infections
  - General Considerations
  - Common Lesions
  - Diagnosis
  - Treatment

SHIGELLA INFECTIONS

General Considerations

Bacillary dysentery is caused by organisms belonging to the genus *Shigellae*. Clinically dysentery is characterized by diarrhea with blood and mucus in the stool. Fever and abdominal pain may be present in the majority. Shigella dysentery is common in the tropics where environmental sanitation is poor and food hygiene is low.

Shigella are gram-negative, non-motile, non-capsulated bacilli belonging to the family enterobacteriaceae. They are classified into 4 species on the basis of antigenic and biochemical features.

1. **Shigella dysenteriae:** Types 1 and 11 (*S. shigae* and *S. schimitzii*). Type 1 is responsible for the most severe form of dysentery. They account for 8–25% of cases in India.
2. **Shigella flexneri:** Most common pathogen responsible for dysentery in developing countries accounts for 50–85% of cases in India.
3. **Shigella sonnei:** Typically causes mild watery diarrhea, most common cause in the west, responsible for 2–24% cases in India.
4. **Shigella boydii:** Least common isolate, usually produces mild disease.

S. shigae is very virulent pathogen, the infective dose can be as low as 10–100 organisms.

Epidemiology

Man is the main host. Infection is transmitted by fecal or oral route. Contaminated water supply, poor personal hygiene, overcrowding, inadequate sewage facilities and proliferation of houseflies contribute to the spread of disease. Apart from contamination of food and water, disease can be acquired through fomites, lavatory seats, door handles and others. During clinical illness and for up to 6 weeks after recovery, organisms are excreted in the feces. These may survive for several months in food and water. Shigellae are relatively resistant to gastric acid.

Pathogenesis and Pathology

Reaching the colon, organisms adhere to the mucosal surface and penetrate the epithelial cell lining where they multiply intracellularly. Maximum involvement is usually in the rectosigmoid region. The entire colon may be affected. Mucosa is inflamed. Shallow ulcers are formed due to necrosis of mucosa. Biopsy specimen shows ulcers and crypt abscess. In severe cases necrosis of the mucosa may occur. The necrosed mucosa may be passed as intestinal casts.

Shigella dysenteriae type 1 produces a powerful exotoxin with enterotoxic and cytotoxic effects which are responsible for the colonic lesions and general toxemia. The toxin may act on the small intestine and lead to secretory diarrhea. Shiga toxin can also cause hemolytic uremic syndrome (HUS) as a complication. *Escherichia*

Textbook of Medicine

coli 0157-H7 can also produce Shiga toxin and lead on to HUS. This toxin is known as **verotoxin**. HUS is more often caused by *E. coli* than *S. shigae*.

Clinical Manifestations

Incubation period varies from 1 to 7 days and in severe cases, it may be as short as few hours. The illness usually starts with fever, colicky abdominal pain and diarrhea with blood and mucus in feces. The stool passed early in the illness contains fecal material, but subsequently it changes into mucus and blood with only small parts of fecal matter. Urgency and tenesmus are marked. Abdominal tenderness is usually prominent in the lower quadrant. The number of stools may exceed 28–30 times per day. In ordinary cases, the symptoms subside within a week. Some cases may be mild and ambulatory.

Fulminant dysentery is characterized by toxemia, electrolyte loss with hyponatremia, prostration and severe bloody diarrhea. In this type mortality may be high especially in children.

Complications

- General—dehydration, electrolyte imbalance and circulatory failure
- Renal failure—either due to hypotension or rarely hemolytic uremic syndrome, especially in children
- Sepsis and septic shock—either primarily due to *Shigella dysenteriae* or due to polymicrobial bacteremia due to other coliforms
- Portal pyemia and multiple abscesses in the liver may occur rarely
- Intestinal perforation, paralytic ileus and intussusception may occur rarely
- Post dysentery complications—1–3 weeks after resolution of the dysentery, arthritis or full-fledged Reiter's syndrome with arthritis, conjunctivitis and urethritis may develop. Presence of human leukocyte antigen (HLA)-B27 predisposes to this complication.

Diagnosis

Clinically the disease should be suspected when dysentery occurs with fever and signs of toxemia. Diagnosis of dysentery is confirmed by observing blood and mucus in feces macroscopically and further by microscopy.

- Microscopic examination of feces reveals large number of erythrocytes, pus cells and macrophages, collectively called **cellular exudates**.
- *Shigella* can be isolated by culture of rectal swab or fresh feces transported to the laboratory in special medium.
- Blood count usually reveals neutrophil leukocytosis.
- Sigmoidoscopy reveals superficial ulcers all along the rectal mucosa with intervening areas also showing hyperemia.

Differential Diagnosis

The common conditions to be differentiated include amoebic dysentery, fulminant ulcerative colitis, staphylococcal food poisoning, salmonellosis, *Campylobacter jejuni* infection and viral enteritis, cholera, necrotizing enterocolitis, antibiotic induced diarrhea, rectal carci-noma and other ulcerating lesions. Sometimes amoebic dysentery and bacillary dysentery may coexist (Table 40.1).

Enteritis caused by *Vitrio cholerae* and other forms of gastroenteritis show watery stools without blood and mucus.

Surgical conditions such as diverticulitis and carcinoma should be excluded if the clinical picture is atypical and response to treatment is unsatisfactory.

Table 40.1: Differentiating features between bacillary and amoebic dysentery

Clinical features	Bacillary dysentery	Amoebic dysentery
Onset	Sudden	Slow
Incubation period	Few days	Weeks to months
Number of stools day	Over 20	Below 15
Nature of feces	Mucus and blood	Mucus, blood + feces
Reaction of feces	Alkaline	Acidic
Clinical course	Acute	Subacute
Microscopy of feces	Cellular exudate	RBCs and *E. histolytica*
Culture of feces	Shigella	Special methods for isolating amoeba

Note: With the improvement in sanitation and the economic progress, amoebic dysentery has become uncommon.

Treatment

- **General and supportive measure:** Correction of fluid and electrolyte losses. Potassium loss may be severe since the mucus is rich in potassium. Majority need oral fluids and electrolytes including potassium. Severe cases should be hospitalized. They may need intravenous (IV) fluids. Diet should be of high calories and low residue, frequently given and in small quantities.
- Antidiarrheal agents that reduce intestinal motility such as diphenoxylate or loperamide should be avoided as they may retard intestinal clearance of the organism. Abdominal pain may require antispasmodics such as hyoscine butylbromide 10 mg oral or 20 mg IM or IV.
- **Antimicrobial therapy:** Mild cases, especially produced by *S. sonnei* are self-limiting and antibiotics are not needed. Severe cases, especially those produced by *S. dysenteriae* benefit from early treatment with 3–5 days course of antimicrobials which decrease the duration of symptoms by 50% and improve the outcome. Ciprofloxacin 500 mg twice daily is the drug of choice in adults. Ampicillin and cotrimoxazole were the preferred agents in the past. Azithromycin is also effective. Multidrug resistant (MDR) strains are now common and hence local sensitivity patterns are also to be considered in selecting the drug.

Prevention

Personal and environmental hygiene is important. Hand washing with soap and water after defecation and before handling food helps to avoid spread of infection. Oral vaccines are in the process of development.

Textbook of Medicine

Points to Remember

- Bacillary dysentery is most commonly produced by *Shigellae*.
- Fever, abdominal pain, loose stool with blood and mucus are important symptoms.
- Feces microscopy showing cellular exudates suggests the diagnosis and can be confirmed by feces culture.
- Severe cases require short course of antimicrobials like ciprofloxacin.
- Correction of fluid and electrolyte balance is the most important.

ESCHERICHIA COLI INFECTIONS

General Considerations

Escherichia coli (E. coli) belongs to the group enterobacteriaceae and is found as a commensal in the intestine of normal man.

E. coli is aerobic gram-negative motile rod. Classification of strains of *E. coli* is based on three antigens—somatic (O) antigen, flagellar (H) antigen and capsular (K) antigen.

Three main types are identified. These are:

1. Commensal strains
2. Intestinal pathogenic strains (enterovirulent *E. coli*)
3. Extraintestinal pathogenic strains.

   Commensal strains are present as normal flora of intestinal tract—they generally lack virulence trait. Occasionally they produce infections in the urinary tract in the presence of urinary catheter, urinary obstruction, immunocompromised situations and the like.

Clinical Features

Intestinal pathogenic strains: These are not commonly present in the fecal flora of healthy humans. They may produce enteritis, enterocolitis or colitis. Five different types are described. These include:

1. ***Enterotoxigenic E. coli (ETEC):*** It is the major cause of endemic diarrhea in tropical and developing countries and also the common cause of traveler's diarrhea. Infections occur by taking contaminated food or fluids. Organism produces a heat labile or heat stable enterotoxin producing secretory diarrhea and vomiting. Incubation period is 1–2 days. Illness is usually mild and self-limiting, improving in 3–4 days. Occasionally life-threatening cholera-like illness may occur. Antibiotics limit the duration of illness.
2. ***Enteroinvasive E. coli (EIEC):*** This may either produce watery diarrhea or an illness similar to *Shigella dysenteriae* due to invasion of colonic mucosa leading to inflammatory colitis. The disease is usually self-limiting.
3. ***Enteropathogenic E. coli (EPEC):*** Most commonly produces acute diarrheal disease in children. Organisms show characteristic affinity to attach to intestinal cell membrane producing effacement of microvilli (attachment and effacement lesion). This interferes with normal intestinal absorption. These cases present with mild or severe diarrhea with or without vomiting. Fever may be present.
4. ***Enteroaggregative E. coli (EAEC):*** This causes prolonged diarrhea in children and is also responsible for traveler's diarrhea. These strains have genetic codes for adhering to small bowel mucosa and produce

a locally active enterotoxin, which causes diarrhea without blood in stools.

5. ***Enterohemorrhagic E. coli (EHEC):*** This strain particularly serotype 0157-H7 produces distinct enterotoxin called ***verocytotoxin*** similar to Shiga toxin produced by Shigella. EHEC produces hemorrhagic colitis. The reservoir of infection is herbivores such as cattle. The source of infection is contaminated meat products, milk, unwashed or uncooked contaminated vegetables and others. Small infective doses are sufficient to produce illness. Incubation period is 1–7 days. Initial watery diarrhea is followed by bloody diarrhea with abdominal pain. Fever and vomiting are not common.

Shiga toxin producing *E. coli* (STEC) produce toxins similar to Shiga toxins 1 and 2. These have genes encoding for 1 or 2 Shiga toxins. They are common causes of HUS. 10–15% of the affected persons may develop HUS, 5–7 days after the onset of symptoms.

E. coli are common to produce traveler's diarrhea in new immigrants and travelers.

Extraintestinal infection by E. coli: *E. coli* producing infection outside the gastrointestinal tract (GIT) are different from commensal and intestinal pathogens. They are more common in hospital settings. The common infections are:

- ***Urinary tract infection (UTI):*** *E. coli* is the single most common pathogen for all UTI syndromes.
- ***Abdominal and pelvic infections,*** e.g. peritonitis due to fecal contamination or spontaneous bacterial peritonitis, appendicitis, diverticulitis, cholangitis and cholecystitis. Rarely septic thrombophlebitis of the portal veins (pylephlebitis) and pyogenic abscess in the liver may occur.
- ***Neonatal infections:*** Bacteremia and meningitis.
- ***Pneumonia:*** *E. coli* is rare to cause community acquired pneumonia. However, *E. coli* and other gram-negative bacilli are common etiological agents for hospital acquired pneumonia, especially in general postoperative and intensive care patients.
- ***Bacteremia and sepsis:*** *E. coli* bacteremia may occur due to:
  - Infections in intravascular devices
  - Primary infections at any other site, most common being UTI followed by intra-abdominal infections
  - Increased permeability of intestines in situations like chemotherapy-associated mucositis, enteritis, colitis and in neonates. Gut flora cross the natural mucosal barrier of the intestines and reach the peritoneum and bloodstream.
- ***Bone and soft tissue infections:*** *E. coli* may cause infections in decubitus ulcers, cellulitis of the leg especially in diabetes, burn site infections and osteomyelitis.

Diagnosis

Culture of *E. coli* from appropriate samples will confirm the diagnosis.

Treatment

In the past, most strains of *E. coli* were sensitive to common antibiotics like ampicillin/amoxicillin, tetracycline, cotrimoxazole and first generation cephalosporins. Now many isolates are resistant to these drugs. Other drugs which are effective include quinolones, third generation cephalosporins, aminoglycosides and extended spectrum pencillins like piperacillin and carbapenems. *E. coli* resistant to multiple drugs especially quinolones and cephalosporins are common in hospital acquired infections [extended spectrum beta-lactamase (ESBL) strains]. Strains resistant to ampicillin/amoxicillin may still respond to ampicillin—sulbactam or amoxicillin—clavulanic acid.

Prevention

Infection rate can be reduced by restricting the use of indwelling catheters and isolation of infected patients. Drug resistance can be reduced by judicious use of antimicrobial agents. *E. coli* transfers its antibiotic resistance to other enteric bacteria like *Salmonella*. Hence, indiscriminate use of antibiotics without proper indication should be avoided.

Points to Remember

- Intestinal pathogenic strains of *E. coli* produces enteritis, enterocolitis or colitis and is a common cause for travelers diarrhea
- EHEC produces an enterotoxin similar to Shiga toxin producing hemorrhagic colitis and is complicated by HUS in 10–15% patients
- Extraintestinal pathogenic strains may produce UTI, abdominal and pelvic infection, neonatal meningitis, bacteremia and sepsis
- Drug resistance is on the increase due to over use and misuse of antimicrobials.

KLEBSIELLA PNEUMONIAE INFECTIONS (ENTEROBACTERIACEAE GROUP)

General Considerations

Klebsiella are capsulated gram-negative bacilli found normally in the throat and intestines in healthy humans. Humans are the primary reservoir. The colonization rate ranges from 5 to 35% in the colon and 1.5% in the oropharynx in the community. Colonization rate increases with wide antibiotic use and hospitalization amounting to > 75% in stool, up to 20% in pharynx and 40% in hand.

Of the pathogenic *Klebsiella*, *Klebsiella pneumoniae* (Friedlander's bacillus) is the most prevalent and clinically important. The bacilli is 1–2 mm long and 0.5–0.8 mm broad. Person to person spread is the predominant mode of transmission.

Risk Factors

Rate of *K. pneumoniae* infection is increased in individuals with impaired host defense mechanisms—diabetes mellitus (DM), alcoholism, malignancy, hepatobiliary disease, chronic obstructive pulmonary disease (COPD), glucocorticoid therapy and renal failure. Most infections are acquired in hospital settings or long-term care facilities. Antibiotic use, indwelling catheters, endotracheal tube and intravascular catheters also increase the risk.

Clinical Syndromes

- ***Pulmonary infections*** occur commonly in diabetics, alcoholics, persons having chronic lung disease and

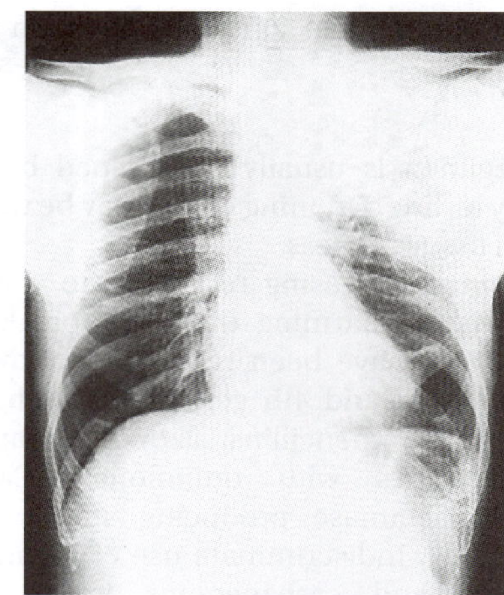

Fig. 40.1: *Klebsiella pneumonia* infection in left upper lobe

hospitalized patients (Fig. 40.1). Lobar pneumonia, bronchopneumonia, bronchitis, lung abscess and empyema may occur. Nosocomial colonization of upper respiratory tract is common in hospitalized patients especially in intensive care unit (ICU) set up. *Klebsiella* from sputum in a hospitalized patient without other signs or symptoms of pneumonia may not be indicative of infection. Pneumonia produced by *Klebsiella* is often associated with marked inflammation and necrosis that can lead to thick mucoid and blood stained sputum—'currant jelly sputum'. There is predilection for involvement of upper lobe with lowering of horizontal fissure downward due to intense consolidation and increase in volume (bulging fissure sign). Mortality rate is higher compared to pneumonia caused by pneumococci.

- ***UTI:*** Cystitis or pyelonephritis may occur. *Klebsiella pneumoniae* is responsible for UTI in 3–4% cases. Rarely prostatitis also may occur. It is seen commonly in complicated UTI including those on indwelling catheters.
- ***Abdominal infections:*** Biliary tract infections, peritonitis and pyogenic liver abscess are usual entities. Pyogenic liver abscess is usually associated with underlying hepatobiliary pathology or cholangitis but may occur as primary pathology also. *K. pneumoniae* is also responsible for spontaneous bacterial peritonitis in about 10–15% cases.
- ***Other infections:*** Usually occur in devitalized tissues or immunocompromised individuals. Examples include, decubitus ulcers, cellulitis in diabetes, burn site infections, nosocomial sinusitis, meningitis associated with neurosurgery, infective endocarditis and others.
- ***Bacteremia:*** Usually spread from primary sites of infection or from intravascular catheters. More common with hospital acquired infections. Biliary tract, genitourinary tract and lung are the usual sites of primary infection.

Diagnosis

Culture of the organism and determination of the antibiotics sensitivity from appropriate material confirms the diagnosis and helps in selecting antimicrobial drug. In

Textbook of Medicine

the setting of pneumonia, sputum Gram stain is useful—sensitivity 50%.

Treatment

Antibiotic regimen is usually determined by results of susceptibility testing. Draining of pus may be warranted in patients with tissue abscess.

Drug resistance: Increasing resistance to a wide range of antibiotic is an alarming trend. Outbreaks of ESBL producing strains have been reported worldwide. They are resistant to 3rd and 4th generation cephalosporins, extended spectrum pencillins, aztreonam and usually to aminoglycosides with quinolones. Carbapenem hydrolysing β-lactamase producing strains have also emerged recently. Indiscriminate use of broad spectrum cephalosporins and carbapenems is an important risk factor for development of resistance. In infections produced by drug sensitive strains, effective antibiotics are 3rd and 4th generation cephalosporins, aminoglycosides, quinolones and carbapenems. Treatment with effective antibiotics has to be continued for 7–10 days.

Points to Remember

- *K. pneumoniae* usually produces infection in hospitalized patients, alcoholics, diabetes and immunocompromised.
- Pneumonia, UTI and intra-abdominal infection are the most common entities.
- Effective antibiotics are 3rd/4th generation cephalosporins, aminoglycosides and quinolones.
- ESBL producing MDR strains are on the increase.

PSEUDOMONAS INFECTIONS

General Considerations

Pseudomonas aeruginosa is the most common human pathogen among the *Pseudomonas* species. They are opportunistic gram-negative bacilli. Most strains of *P. aeruginosa* produce a characteristic bluish-green pigment called pyocyanin which helps in the identification of the organism. The organism has affinity for moist areas and occasionally it colonises the skin, external ear, upper respiratory tract, perineum or colon of healthy human beings. The organism may contaminate medical devices like ventilators, endoscopes or pressure monitors. Health care workers in hospital may transmit the infection from patient to patient.

P. aeruginosa infection is rare in healthy individuals. Infections occur in immunocompromised persons who are predisposed. Most of the infections are acquired in hospitals especially from ICU. Prolonged use of broad spectrum antibiotics favours colonization by the organism and subsequent infection. Severe hospital acquired infection, often MDR, may occur associated with high mortality.

Conditions predisposing to infection are:

- Neutropenia—due to disease, chemotherapy or both
- Mucosal damage—cancer chemotherapy
- Cystic fibrosis with progressive respiratory tract changes
- Respiratory assist devices directly inoculating the organism into the tracheobronchial tree
- Indwelling urinary catheters
- Extensive burns
- Prolonged broad spectrum antibiotic use
- Acquired immunodeficiency syndrome (AIDS).

The organisms enter through the breach in the skin or through urinary, respiratory or GIT. In addition to infection at local site hematogenous spread may also occur.

Common Lesions Produced by *P. aeruginosa*

- Pneumonia commonly occurs in hospitalized patients especially in immunocompromised subjects including AIDS, patient on ventilatory support and those receiving prolonged broad spectrum antibiotics. Organisms reach the lungs via aspirated material from the oropharynx or through the bloodstream. The lungs show microabscesses.
- ***Bacteremia:*** This is common in patients with neutropenia especially those with hematological malignancies. Bacteremia may be primary or it may result from infection elsewhere. Sepsis and septic shock may develop. Mortality is 50–70%. Meningitis may develop.
- ***Endocarditis:*** This may occur in IV drug users, patients after cardiac surgery or those who had suffered from burns.
- UTI caused by *P. aeruginosa* is typically hospital acquired and often it results from urinary tract catheterization, instrumentation or obstruction. It is the third most common pathogen causing hospital acquired UTIs, after *E. coli* and *Enterococci*. Community acquired UTI may occur in patients with urinary tract obstruction, chronic prostatitis and prolonged course of broad-spectrum antibiotic therapy.
- ***Skin infections:*** Wounds, ulcers and burns may be secondarily infected. Bacteremia may lead to ecthyma gangrenosum which appears as indurated purple black areas about 1 cm in diameter with ulcerated centers. Maculopapular and vesiculopustular rashes may occur.
- ***Ear infections:*** *P. aeruginosa* causes four types of ear infections:
  1. Simple otitis externa (swimmer's ear)
  2. Malignant external otitis in elderly diabetes. It is characterized by bacteria penetrating the epithelium invading underlying soft tissues, cartilage and cortical bone
  3. Chronic suppurative otitis media (CSOM)
  4. Perichondritis of the helix or tragus of the ear, usually occurring after trauma or surgery.
- ***CNS infections:*** Meningitis or suppurative brain abscess due to *P. aeruginosa* are rare, but known to occur in patients with serious underlying disease, have recent head trauma or neurosurgical procedures. Mortality is high.
- ***Gastrointestinal infections:*** Uncommon except in selective situations like post endoscopic retrograde cholangiopancreatography (ERCP) cholangitis and enterocolitis of caecum or surrounding gut in patients with chemotherapy induced neutropenia.
- ***Other infections:*** *P. aeruginosa* may also produce osteomyelitis, eye infections like corneal ulcer following trauma, dacryocystitis, blepharoconjunctivitis and orbital cellulitis.

Table 40.2: Antibiotics effective against *P. aeruginosa*

Antibiotic class	Agent
Extended spectrum penicillins	Piperacillin, piperacillin tazobactam
Cephalosporins	Ceftazidime, cefoperazone, cefepime
Carbapenems	Imipenem + cilastatin, meropenem
Monobactams	Aztreonam
Aminoglycosides	Tobramycin, gentamicin, amikacin
Fluoroquinolones	Ciprofloxacin, levofloxacin
Others	Polymyxin B, colistin

Treatment

Antimicrobials used for treating *P. aeruginosa* are shown in Table 40.2. Some experts advocate use of two agents like a beta-lactam plus an aminoglycoside or a beta-lactam plus fluoroquinolones for systemic infection. There is no clear evidence that the combination therapy is superior to monotherapy.

Superficial infections respond to local dressing with polymyxin.

Prophylaxis

Since, pseudomonas is a common cause of nosocomial infections, utmost care should be taken to prevent cross infection by proper hand washing and strict aseptic precautions. Avoid indiscriminate use of prophylactic antibiotics.

Points to Remember
- *P. aeruginosa* are opportunistic pathogens causing infection in hospitalized/immunocompromised patients especially neutropenics.
- Common infections produced include hospital acquired pneumonia, complicated UTI especially associated with indwelling catheter, CSOM, malignant external otitis in elderly diabetics and bacteremia.
- Antimicrobial effective are ceftazidime, cefepime, aminoglycosides, quinolones and carbapenems.

PROTEUS INFECTIONS

General Considerations

The genus *Proteus* includes 3 species pathogenic to man—*Proteus mirabilis, P. vulgaris, P. penneri. P. mirabilis* is part of colonic flora in about 50% of the healthy normal individuals. They are gram-negative rod-shaped bacilli. *P. mirabilis* causes 70–90% of proteus infections.

Common Lesions

- ***UTI:*** *Proteus* causes 1–2% of uncomplicated UTIs and 10–15% of complicated UTIs especially associated with diabetes, urinary tract obstruction or indwelling catheters. In patients with long-term catheterization prevalence rate of infection is as high as 20–45%. *Proteus* infection makes the urine alkaline by producing ammonia from urea. Alkalinization may lead to precipitation of organic and inorganic compounds leading to urinary stone formation.
- ***Other lesions*** are relatively rare. These include pneumonia, sinusitis, biliary tract infections, intra-abdominal abscesses, surgical site infections, decubitus ulcers and diabetic foot infections. In the newborn, the umbilical stump may be colonized by proteus leading to bacteremia and meningitis.
- ***Bacteremia:*** This may result from UTI or occasionally due to infection in intravascular devices.

Diagnosis

Culture of organisms from urine or appropriate specimen confirms the diagnosis.

Treatment

Proteus mirabilis is usually sensitive to most of the antibiotics. Drug of choice in infections caused by sensitive strains is ampicillin. Resistance to ampicillin and first generation cephalosporins are now common. Resistant strains respond to cotrimoxazole, fluoroquinolones, aminoglycosides and third generation cephalosporins in the usual dosage. Fluoroquinolones resistance is also on the increase. *P. vulgaris* and *P. penneri* are more resistant. Third or fourth generation cephalosporins are the drug of choice. Aminoglycosides, cotrimoxazole and carbapenems are alternative agents.

Points to Remember
- Among the pathogenic *Proteus* species, *Proteus mirabilis* is responsible for most infections.
- Most common infection produced is UTI. Other infections are rare.
- Majority of the infections are sensitive to common antibiotics.

CHAPTER
41

Anthrax, Plague, Brucellosis, Melioidosis

S Bhasi, KV Krishna Das, R Sajith Kumar

Chapter Summary

- Anthrax
  - General Considerations
  - Clinical Features
  - Diagnosis
    - Treatment
    - Prevention
- Plague
  - General Considerations
  - Clinical Features

- Diagnosis
- Treatment
- Prevention
- Brucellosis
  - General Considerations
  - Clinical Features
  - Diagnosis
  - Treatment
  - Prevention
- Melioidosis
  - General Considerations
  - Clinical Features
  - Diagnosis
  - Prognosis
  - Treatment

Textbook of Medicine

ANTHRAX

General Considerations

Anthrax is a zoonotic disease, caused by *Bacillus anthracis*. It occurs primarily in herbivorous animals, especially cattle, goats, sheep and horses which form the reservoirs. Recent interest in anthrax has been the fear of using anthrax spores as biological weapons either in battle or by terrorists. In 2001, there were 13 cases of cutaneous anthrax and 11 cases of inhalational anthrax associated with exposure to anthrax spores from contaminated mails.

Etiology

Bacillus anthracis is a large aerobic gram-positive spore forming bacillus. The organism exist as bacillus in the tissues. Spores are produced only outside the body under aerobic conditions and are the infectious form of the organism. They are very resistant, remain viable in soil and animal products for several years (10–71 years on record). Boiling for 10 minutes or treatment with potassium permanganate, formaldehyde, glutaraldehyde and hypochlorite kills the spores. The organism grows well aerobically in ordinary laboratory media.

Epidemiology

Anthrax primarily affects animals. It is prevalent in all countries throughout the world, but only rarely seen in India. Animals get the infection by coming into contact with spores persisting in soil. Most of the human cases are zoonotic in origin. Human to human transmission has not been reported except in the respiratory form. Human infection is mainly caused because of:

- Direct contact with infected animals and consuming contaminated meat—raw or poorly cooked.
- Contact with anthrax spores containing animal products such as wool, hides, hair, skin, bone and inhalation of spore-containing aerosols which may travel long distances in wind. Contaminating the atmosphere with spores may be a method adopted by bioterrorists or for biowarfare.

Pathogenesis

The organisms enter the body:

- Through abrasions in skin
- Gastrointestinal tract (GIT), e.g. eating infected meat
- Inhalation of spores.

The primary foci occur in skin, GIT or lung depending upon the mode of entry. Spores germinate into vegetative bacteria that multiply locally, but may also disseminate to cause systemic infections.

Septicemia and meningitis may occur from any of these primary foci. Changes occur due to tissue invasion by the bacillus, multiplying rapidly extracellularly and the effect of the exotoxin. The main pathological changes in the tissue are edema, necrosis and hemorrhage.

Clinical Features

The disease may present as cutaneous pulmonary, gastrointestinal (GI) and meningeal forms.

Cutaneous Anthrax (Malignant Pustule)

This is the most common manifestation of anthrax. The lesion usually occurs on exposed areas and starts as a small erythematous papule after an incubation period of 1–2 days (usually 2–5 days). It vesiculates and contains serosanguineous fluid which is highly infectious. The vesicle turns into pustule and ulcerate with necrosis; finally progresses to a depressed black eschar. The lesion is usually painless. Lymphangitis and regional lymphadenitis commonly occur. Systemic symptoms are mild. With appropriate antibiotic therapy recovery occurs. Bacteremia can occur with clinical features of systemic infection.

Pulmonary form (Inhalation Anthrax/Woolsorter's Disease)

This occurs as an occupational hazard when spores from wool or hides are inhaled. The spores may also spread from person to person as droplet infection. They reach the mediastinal lymph nodes. The bacilli develop in a few days, but the incubation period can be as long as 60 days.

It is feared that as a part of bioterrorism or biowarfare, dissemination of spores in the environment may lead to a large outbreak of severe and fatal anthrax pneumonia.

Classically a biphasic illness occurs. After an average incubation period of 1–5 days (even up to 6 weeks) symptoms start with malaise, fever, myalgia and non-productive cough mimicking viral respiratory disease. In some, there is transient improvement after 2–4 days followed by second stage with severe dyspnea, fever, cyanosis and hemoptysis. About 50% develop meningitis. Edema of the chest wall and neck may occur. Bacteremia is common. X-ray of the chest may show mediastinal widening due to lymphadenopathy, pulmonary infiltrates and pleural effusion, which is often hemorrhagic. Mortality is high and death usually occurs within 24 hours.

GI Anthrax

This develops 2–5 days following consumption of meat contaminated with spores. Infection of the oropharynx leads to **oropharyngeal anthrax** with ulcers and local lymphadenopathy. Dysphagia and neck edema is common. In the GIT, organisms are deposited in the duodenum, terminal ileum and cecum. The patient presents with fever, abdominal pain, vomiting, bloody diarrhea, hematemesis, hemorrhagic ascites and mesenteric lymphadenitis. Disease may progress to toxemia, shock and death.

Meningeal Anthrax

Any form of primary anthrax may be complicated with meningitis. Cerebrospinal fluid (CSF) is usually hemorrhagic containing bacilli. Mortality is high.

Diagnosis

Clinical suspicion is absolutely necessary for early diagnosis. Occupational history will be helpful.

- Gram staining of the vesicular fluid in cutaneous anthrax, ascitic fluid, oropharyngeal swab, sputum or CSF and demonstration of gram-positive rods arranged in long chains is suggestive.
- Blood culture is positive in cases with bacteremia, if done before starting antibiotics. Culture of fluid expressed from skin lesions, pleural fluids and CSF also useful.
- The capsular and cell wall antigens can be detected by immunohistochemistry.
- Polymerase chain reaction (PCR) useful for detecting genetic material.
- Chest X-ray may show pulmonary infiltrate, pleural effusion and mediastinal adenopathy in pulmonary anthrax.
- Antibodies against anthrax can be demonstrated by enzyme-linked immunosorbent assay (ELISA) test and other methods. Neutrophil leukocytosis is common.

Differential Diagnosis

- Cutaneous anthrax has to be differentiated from tularemia, lymphogranuloma venereum (LGV), cat scratch disease, rat bite fever, bubonic plague, glanders and typhus fever
- Pulmonary anthrax should be differentiated from other forms of pneumonia, especially hemorrhagic pneumonias
- Anthrax meningitis may be mistaken for subarachnoid hemorrhage.

Treatment

Specific: In the past, *Bacillus anthracis* used to be sensitive to most antimicrobials including penicillin, amoxicillin, tetracycline, doxycycline, macrolides, chloramphenicol, rifampicin and quinolones. Recently β-lactamase producing strains are identified conferring resistance to pencillins +/– cephalosporins. Drug of choice is ciprofloxacin 500 mg orally bd or 400 mg intravenous (IV) bd. Levofloxacin and moxifloxacin are equally effective. Doxycycline 100 mg bd oral/IV is an alternative. Combination of 2 drugs is recommended for inhalational anthrax, disseminated disease and cutaneous disease involving face with extensive local edema. The optimal duration of therapy is not known. In naturally occurring disease, 7–10 days for cutaneous disease and 2 weeks after clinical improvement for disseminated, inhalational or GI infection is the current recommendation. Inhalational anthrax resulting from inhalation of aerosol in bioterrorism because of concerns about relapse from latent spores recommendation is to continue drug for 60 days.

Supportive care: Ventilatory support may be required for pneumonia with respiratory distress. Vasopressors and volume repletion are necessary for those in shock.

Prognosis: Self-limiting cutaneous lesions outcome is excellent. Mortality for inhalational anthrax, disseminated disease and intestinal disease is more than 50%.

Prevention

Personal protection for at-risk persons is by using protective clothing and masks and by vaccination.

- Vaccination is available for individuals at high-risk. The vaccine is an inactivated cell free vaccine. Three subcutaneous injections at 2 weeks intervals and additional 3 doses at 6, 12 and 18 months and annual booster doses give adequate protection. An attack of anthrax generally produces permanent immunity.
- GI anthrax can be prevented by public education to avoid consumption of contaminated meat.
- Post-exposure antibiotic prophylaxis should be given for those who are exposed to inhaled spores. Ciprofloxacin 500 mg/day oral is recommened for 60 days.
- Control of anthrax in animals is by immunization.
- Carcasses of animals that have died due to anthrax are to be buried or cremated to avoid sporulation and further contamination.

Procedure to be observed when anthrax spores are used for bioterrorism/warfare:

- Suspect anthrax and alert the public and health personnel
- Early specific therapy
- Burn all infected cattle carcasses
- Disinfection of infective material with 5% formalin
- Vaccination of susceptible population and animals. Protective clothing for those at risk
- Ciprofloxacin prophylaxis for exposed individuals.

> **Points to Remember**
>
> - Anthrax is a zoonotic disease, spores are the infectious forms.
> - Primary focus of infection is either skin (producing cutaneous anthrax), GIT (producing GI anthrax) or lung (pulmonary anthrax).
> - Septicemia and meningitis may occur from any of these primary sites.
> - Diagnosis is by demonstration of organism by Gram staining or culture of the appropriate specimen.
> - Drug of choice is quinolones.

PLAGUE

General Considerations

Plague used to occur in the form of epidemics up to the early part of the 20th century causing more deaths than many other diseases. Now it is a rare disease but still capable of appearing as localized outbreaks. There was an outbreak of plague in Surat in India in 1994. Plague is one of the most virulent and potentially lethal bacterial diseases known.

Etiology

Yersinia pestis, the cause of plague is a gram-negative aerobic coccobacillus. It shows bipolar staining. The organism remains viable for long periods in human sputum and dried flea feces when protected from sunlight and heat.

Epidemiology

Plague is a zoonotic infection. The main animal reservoirs are rats, mongooses and rabbits. Among the rodent

Textbook of Medicine

population plague is spread by transmission from one rodent to another by the bite of the rat flea *Xenopsylla cheopis* (sylvatic plague). The organisms multiply in the alimentary tract of the flea and they regurgitate into the mouth parts. These enter the new host when the flea bites to suck blood. Organisms are also passed in the feces of the flea.

Man is the accidental host. Human epidemics usually arise from infected domestic rodents. Man gets infection:

- When bitten by infected rat flea. Under suitable conditions the flea lives for 1–2 years and remains infective for long periods
- Handling of carcasses/tissues of infected animals. Direct inoculation into the skin predisposes to the development of septicemic plague. Scratches or bites from infected domestic cats may also leads to disease
- Inhalation of respiratory droplets released from infected animals or from dried flea feces
- Man to man transmission in the setting of pneumonic plague by droplet infections. This risk is low and requires close contact
- Laboratory exposure
- Consumption of contaminated food.

Pathogenesis and Pathology

Organisms are transmitted through the skin by the bite of the infected rat flea. At the site of entry a papule or pustule may form. The bacilli reach the local lymph nodes which enlarge and suppurate. This constitutes the bubo. Bacilli proliferate and enter the blood stream to produce metastatic lesions in other lymph nodes, liver, kidneys, spleen, meninges, brain and lungs.

Organisms can directly reach the lung by inhalation of droplets of respiratory secretions of pneumonic cases. Organisms can also remain in the environment by getting released from dried flea feces. The lesion in the lung is pneumonic consolidation. Hemorrhagic manifestations develop due to endothelial damage and disseminated intravascular coagulation (DIC).

Clinical Features

There are three major clinical syndromes associated with plague.

1. **Bubonic plague** is the most common type, accounts for 80–90% cases. The incubation period is 2–6 days. Symptoms start with fever and lymphadenopathy. Buboes are acutely tender and seen most frequently in inguinal or axillary regions depending upon the flea bite. Skin lesion at the site of bite is usually insignificant and may be unnoticed. Buboes may slowly suppurate and discharge their contents. In the absence of treatment initial bubonic stage may be followed by disseminated infection in about 50%. Death may occur due to peripheral circulatory failure.

2. **Septicemic plague:** It accounts for 10–20% of cases. Primary septicemic plague present with sudden onset of chills, fever, tachycardia, headache, vomiting and delirium. Several organs may be affected. Death may occur within a few days before localizing lesions are evident. Hemorrhagic manifestations like petechia, subcutaneous ecchymosis, epistaxis, hematemesis or malena may develop. Meningitis may occur.

3. **Pneumonic plague:** It is rare. Two types of pneumonia occur in plague—primary and secondary. In the **primary** form the organism reaches the lung by inhalation. It can be acquired by inhalation of aerosolized droplets from infected animals, humans or lab exposure. The incubation period is short, ranging from 2 hours to 2 days. **Secondary** form develops via blood-stream spread.

The primary form is more fulminant and rapidly fatal. The onset is abrupt with high fever, tachycardia and dyspnea. In comparison to severity of symptoms and respiratory distress physical signs are less marked. Sputum may be scanty, blood stained or frothy. The term **pestis minor** refers to mild cases seen during epidemics. This presents with only the buboes which suppurate and discharge pus in due course or may resolve without significant systemic manifestations.

Pharyngitis and tonsillitis with cervical lymphadenitis following ingestion may occur rarely.

Diagnosis

High index of suspicion is necessary for early diagnosis. Diagnosis is confirmed by:

- Demonstration of organisms by staining of smear of fluid aspirated from bubo, sputum or buffy coat in blood. In the absence of bubo diagnosis may be missed.
- Culture of blood, sputum or aspirated materials. Yersinia grow well on common laboratory media. Blood culture is positive in 27–96% depending upon the clinical presentation.
- Serological tests—demonstrate rising antibody titer.
- Other tests—neutrophilic leukocytosis with shift to left and thrombocytopenia is common. Radiological appearance of pneumonic plague is not specific to be diagnostic.
- Animal inoculation studies.

Treatment

Therapy should be started immediately when plague is suspected. Streptomycin is the drug of choice. Alternate effective drugs are tetracycline, doxycycline and chloramphenicol. In meningitis, chloramphenicol is preferable. Gentamicin and cotrimoxazole also have been used successfully. Quinolones are also very effective. The duration of treatment is for 10 days (Table 41.1).

Supportive treatment for circulatory failure, DIC, hyperpyrexia, respiratory distress and fluid and electrolyte imbalance has to be instituted early. Buboes may require surgical drainage, at times.

Table 41.1: Antimicrobial regimen for plague

Drug	Daily dose	Doses/day	Route
Streptomycin	2 g (30 mg/kg)	2	IM
Tetracycline	2 g (adult)	4	Oral/IV
Doxycycline	200 mg (adult)	1–2	Oral/IV
Chloramphenicol	50 mg/kg	4	Oral/IV

Abbreviations: IM = Intramuscular; IV = Intravenous

Prognosis

Overall mortality of untreated plague is 50%. Untreated, primary septicemic and pneumonic plague is invariably fatal. Modern antibiotic therapy has improved the outcome considerably.

Prevention

Avoiding exposure to rodents and fleas in endemic areas is the best prevention strategy. Patients with pneumonic plague should be isolated and the attendants must wear masks. Contacts must be given drug prophylaxis. Doxycycline 100 mg bd for 7 days is the ideal. No effective vaccine is available.

> **Points to Remember**
> - Plague is a zoonotic disease, main animal reservoir's are rats. Most common mode of human infection is by bite of infected rat flea producing bubonic plague.
> - Inhalation of respiratory droplets leads to pneumonic plague.
> - Septicemia plague produces multi-organ dysfunction and is often fatal.
> - Diagnosis is by demonstration of organism by staining and culture of appropriate specimen.
> - Drug of choice is streptomycin. Doxycycline and chloramphenicol are also effective.

BRUCELLOSIS

Syn: Undulant fever, Malta fever, Abortus fever

General Considerations

Brucellosis is a zoonotic infection, transmitted to man by contact with fluid from an infected animal or ingestion of contaminated food such as unboiled goat's milk and milk products and meat and also by handling tissues of infected animals.

Etiology

Brucellosis is produced by one of 4 species of *Brucella*.

1. ***Brucella melitensis:*** The most common type spread from goats, sheep and camels.
2. ***Brucella abortus:*** This spreads from dairy cattle. It produces abortion in cattle.
3. ***Brucella suis:*** From pigs.
4. ***Brucella canis:*** From dogs.

Brucella organisms are small, non-capsulated, non-motile, gram-negative aerobic rods or coccobacilli. They are facultative intracellular parasites.

Epidemiology

The disease is worldwide in distribution. The true incidence is not known, but it is definitely many times more than what is reported. Brucellosis is common in the Middle East, USSR, Mexico and South America. It occurs less commonly in India, Europe, USA and other countries. Brucellosis is an occupational disease in veterinarians and farm workers, workers in meat processing industries and slaughter houses, shepherds and laboratory workers. Exposure to the placenta and other products of conception of cattle, swine, sheep, dogs and other animals and contact with sick animals can cause infection.

Mode of Transmission

Infected animals pass the bacillus in their milk for long periods. The placenta, fetus, semen, vaginal discharge and urine of animals are also infective. Human infection occurs by:

- ***Ingestion of untreated milk and its products, raw meat, liver or bone marrow.*** Organisms enter through the mucous membrane of GIT.
- ***Penetration through the abrasion in skin coming in contact with infected material.*** Brucella may also enter through the conjunctiva when infected material gets into the eye accidentally.
- ***Inhalation of aerosol particles:*** Close contact with infected animals can lead to droplet infection.
- Transplacental transmission from mother to fetus may occur. *Brucella* has been isolated from human breast milk. Transmission through sexual contact has been recently reported in humans.

B. melitensis can be used as an agent in biological warfare or bioterrorism.

Pathogenesis and Pathology

After entry the organisms pass through the local lymph nodes to reach bloodstream and localize in reticuloendothelial system. *Brucellae* are unique in that they have no specific virulence factors like exotoxins or endotoxins. Organism which enter the tissue are phagocytosed by reticuloendothelial (RE) cells. 15–30% of the organisms survive in vacuoles within the phagocytes. They are periodically released into the circulation.

In the RE tissues including bone marrow, liver, lymph nodes and spleen, they multiply to produce granulomas made up of epithelioid cells, giant cells, lymphocytes and plasma cells. *Brucella* persists in the tissues through inhibition of apoptosis.

Exposure to infection elicits humoral and cell mediated immunity, which helps to clear the infection.

Clinical Features

The incubation period is 1–4 weeks but may be as long as several months. The clinical syndromes produced by different species are similar but *B. melitensis* produces more aggressive disease often with acute presentation.

B. canis is infrequently associated with human disease and usually present with mild illness.

Brucellosis is a systemic infection with broad clinical spectrum ranging from asymptomatic disease to severe and/or fatal illness. Infection among children is generally more benign than in adults. In pregnant women illness may be complicated with spontaneous abortion, premature delivery, intrauterine infection and fetal death.

The onset is either sudden or gradual with fever, malaise weakness, sweating, chills, arthralgia and backache. The term undulant fever is derived from the characteristic pattern of the temperature. Fever shows wide fluctuation and it persists for long periods, up to several weeks or months.

Bones and joints are commonly affected. Migrating polyarthritis mainly involve major joints like knee, hips, sacroiliac joints shoulder and others. Septic monoarthritis is also known to occur in the knee, hip, shoulder and sacroiliac joints. Spondylitis is more prevalent in older patients and in patients with prolonged illness prior to treatment. Lumbar vertebra more frequently involved than thoracic and cervical vertebrae. Paravertebral, epidural and psoas abscess may complicate brucella spondylitis. This may affect any vertebra, but the fourth lumbar vertebra is the most common site of lesion. Brucella osteomyelitis is rare outside the vertebral column.

Cardiovascular affection is rare but may occur and include myocarditis, endocarditis, pericarditis, endarteritis and thrombophlebitis.

Liver involvement leads to formation of granulomas. Sometimes suppuration may occur. May present like hepatitis with jaundice. Cholecystitis, pancreatitis, hepatic and splenic abscess may occur rarely.

Splenomegaly is common. Cervical, axillary and hilar lymphadenopathy may be seen.

Central nervous system (CNS): Neurobrucellosis may take the form of meningoencephalitis with lymphocytic pleocytosis in the CSF. Other manifestations include myelitis, radiculopathy, cranial or peripheral nerve palsies and vasculitis presenting as stroke.

Genitourinary system: Unilateral or bilateral orchitis/epididymo-orchitis may occur. Acute glomerulonephritis and interstitial nephritis has also been described.

Respiratory system: Lobar pneumonia, interstitial pneumonia and bronchitis are seen in some. Pleural effusion with lymphocytic pleocytosis may occur rarely.

Uveitis may occur as a rare complication.

The term ***chronic brucellosis*** refers to patients with clinical manifestations lasting for more than one year. May present as pyrexia of unknown origin or with chronic spondylitis.

Diagnosis

Prolonged fever with arthritis or spondylitis with risk of exposure should suggest the possibility of brucellosis. Residence in endemic areas should be considered a strong point for making the diagnosis.

Confirmation: By isolation of *Brucella* from blood, bone marrow, liver biopsy specimen or other tissues such as joint fluid, CSF or tissue aspirate. This is positive in about 15–70% cases. The organisms are slow-growing and take about 6 weeks. Culture by BACTEC technique yields positive cultures in 7–10 days. Bone marrow culture is more sensitive.

Serology: The best serological diagnosis of brucellosis is by demonstration of four-fold or greater rise in *Brucella* agglutination titer between acute and convalescence phase serum specimens obtained more than 2 weeks apart and studied in the same laboratory. Positive serology can be present long after recovery in treated individuals. Immunoglobulin M (IgM) antibodies appear early followed by IgG and IgA. A single titer $\geq$ 1:320 is considered highly suggestive. Antibodies can be detected also by alternate methods such as complement fixation test, ELISA and Coomb's antiglobulin test.

PCR: This is more sensitive and quicker than blood culture. It can be performed on blood or any body fluid. Molecular tests are available for identification of genus and species and now used for research purpose only.

Non-specific laboratory findings include anemia and leukopenia. Pancytopenia may be seen in some. Synovial fluid in Brucella arthritis shows lymphocytic dominance in contrast to neutrophilic dominance in septic arthritis. Imaging including magnetic resonance imaging (MRI) may be needed in case of suspected spondylitis.

Treatment

Antimicrobial therapy: For adults with acute brucellosis without localizing lesions elsewhere like bone CNS and others, treatment with a combination of two antimicrobials given for six weeks is ideal. Two major regimens recommended are:

1. Streptomycin 1 g intramuscular (IM) daily for first 14–21 days plus doxycycline 100 mg oral 12 hourly for 6 weeks. Relapse rate with this regimen is about 5%. Aminoglycosides show synergistic activity with tetracycline. This is considered to be the gold standard. Gentamicin 5 mg/kg for 7–14 days may be substituted for streptomycin with equal efficacy.
2. Doxycycline 100 mg oral 12 hourly + rifampicin 600–900 mg oral once daily for 6 weeks. The relapse rate is higher. Monotherapy and duration less than 6 weeks not acceptable.

Treatment of complicated brucellosis:

- ***Spondylitis–streptomycin*** for first 14–21 days plus doxycycline 100 mg bd for 12 weeks. Alternative regimen is doxy plus rifampicin for 12 weeks. Neurobrucellosis, endocarditis and localized suppurative lesions need 12 weeks therapy. A third agent (cotrimoxazole or fluoroquinolones) may be added.
- ***Relapse:*** The following treatment is about 5–10% usually occurring within 6 months after completing treatment. Usual reasons are improper choice of antibiotics, inadequate duration of treatment, lack of adherence to therapy and localized foci of infection.

Prevention

- Control of infection in animals is by active immunization.
- Pasteurization of milk will prevent transmission from milk and milk products.
- Vaccination for prevention of human brucellosis is currently not available in India.

Points to Remember

- It is a zoonotic infection transmitted from animals to man via contamination of milk, meat, handling tissues of infected animal.
- Usually present with prolonged fever—weeks to months.
- Bone and joint involvement especially spondylitis, hepatosplenomegaly and lymphadenopathy are common.
- Diagnosis is confirmed by culture of organism from blood, bone marrow or other appropriate specimens. Detection of antibodies also help.
- Treatment of choice is combination of 2 antimicrobials for 6 weeks. The gold standard is streptomycin 1 g daily for 2–3 weeks + doxycycline 100 mg bd for 6 weeks.

MELIOIDOSIS

General Considerations

Melioidosis (Whitmore's disease) is caused by *Burkholderia pseudomallei* formerly known as *Pseudomonas pseudomallei*. It is a gram-negative motile, aerobic, nonsporeforming bacillus. The organism is widely distributed in soil and most commonly seen in tropical climates of Southeast Asia, Middle East and China. In India it occurs sporadically and is reported from the southern states more. The organism can be employed as a biological warfare weapon, because of the ease with which it can be handled, transmitted and it produces catastrophic results. Biosafety level 3 containment practices are required for laboratory staff when working with cases of glanders and melioidosis. Chlorination of water supplies destroys the organism.

Clinical Features

The organism is found in contaminated environments. It enters the body through abrasions in the skin. This leads to ulceration followed by lymph node enlargement. The incubation period is 4–6 days. When the organisms are inhaled or when they reach the lung through hematogenous route, the incubation period is longer up to 10–14 days. Due to the ability of *B. pseudomallei* to survive in phagocytic cells, many cases of melioidosis result after a long latent period. In this instance, patient develops pneumonia, pulmonary abscess and pleural effusion. In debilitated and immunosuppressed individuals hematogenous dissemination can be followed by septicemia with involvement of the lungs, liver, spleen and other organs. They develop fever, diarrhea, respiratory distress and abscesses on the skin and different parts of the body. Anemia, leukocytosis, hepatic and renal dysfunction and coagulopathy may be observed.

Glanders: It is a similar disease caused by *B. mallei* and more common among animals like horses, mules and donkeys. Occasionally humans are involved and they behave just like melioidosis described above.

Diagnosis

Diagnosis of melioidosis is difficult. It has been called the great imitator because there are no pathognomonic lesions. Any organ can be affected and the lesions have no distinguishing characteristics. The organism can be demonstrated from respiratory secretions or pus from abscesses or ulcers by Gram staining (safety pin morphology with bipolar staining). Blood or pus culture on meat agar helps to isolate the organisms. Serological tests include agglutination tests, indirect hemagglutination, complement fixation, immunofluorescence and enzyme assays. Agglutination tests and IgM ELISA tests are available. Improved methods for rapid diagnosis are being evaluated.

Prognosis

Melioidosis has a high mortality (90%) in the disseminated form and with pulmonary disease. Overall mortality varies from 20 to 50% with relapse rate of about 10%.

Treatment

For localized disease, a 60–150 day course of oral amoxicillin and clavulanate, doxycycline or co-trimoxazole may be used.

For disseminated or pulmonary disease, a parenteral course of ceftazidime or imipenem-cilastatin for two weeks followed by oral co-trimoxazole for 20 weeks is recommended.

Another promising avenue of therapy is inhalational immunotherapy with cationic liposome (deoxyribonucleic acid) DNA complexes (CLDC). These complexes are potent activators of innate immunity within the pulmonary system, thereby making this modality attractive in the event of an inhalational exposure to these bacteria. Abscesses may require surgical drainage.

CHAPTER 42

Diarrheal Diseases of Infective Origin

KV Krishna Das, VP Gopinathan

Chapter Summary

- Cholera
  - General Considerations
  - Etiology and Epidemiology
  - Immunity
  - Pathogenesis
  - Clinical Features
  - Diagnosis
  - Prognosis
  - Complications
  - Treatment
  - Prevention
- Non-Cholera Vibrio
- Acute Diarrheal Diseases of Children
- Rotavirus
  - Clinical Features
  - Diagnosis
  - Vaccination
- Norovirus Infections
  - History
  - Clinical Features
  - Management
  - Vaccination
  - Probiotics
  - Rarer causes of Viral Diarrhea
- Campylobacter Jejuni
  - Epidemiology
  - Pathogenesis

- Clinical Features
- Treatment
- Prevention
- Clostridium Difficile: Pseudomembranous Colitis
  - General Considerations
  - Pathology
  - Clinical Features
  - Diagnosis
  - Treatment
  - Prevention
  - Chronic Life-threatening Clostridium Difficile Infection

Textbook of Medicine

CHOLERA

General Considerations

Word meaning of cholera is ***flow of bile***. Cholera is an acute infectious disease caused by *Vibrio cholerae* occurring in outbreaks, characterized by watery diarrhea and effortless vomiting, often leading to severe dehydration and shock. *Vibrio cholerae* is a comma-shaped, flagellate, motile, gram-negative organism. It was discovered by Robert Koch in 1884. The somatic (O) antigen is of importance in the identification of the organism. Ninety two serogroups are identified based on the O antigen structure. Of these the strain producing epidemic cholera possesses O1 antigen and hence, this vibrio is designated *Vibrio cholerae* O1. *Inaba, Ogawa* and *Hikojima* are the most important pathogenic subtypes. The others are collectively designated non-O1 *V. cholerae*. Among these some have been now identified to be pathogenic. The Eltor biotype is a variant of *V. cholerae* O1 and it is characterized by its hemolytic activity and resistance to polymyxin. Many Eltor vibrios are non-hemolytic at present. Morphologically and antigenically Eltor resembles *V. cholerae*. Differentiation is by phage typing and other tests.

The classic disease is caused by *Vibrio cholerae,* but in the majority of outbreaks occurring in India and neighboring countries in recent times, the main pathogen is the *Eltor* biotype. Eltor biotype was first identified in Eltor village in Egypt in 1905, from Indonesian *Haj* Pilgrims. Cholera has been endemic in the banks of the Ganges and Brahmaputra in India and Bangladesh for several centuries. From these endemic foci the disease used to spread along routes of human communication to other parts during fairs, festivals, floods and famines, causing outbreaks associated with high mortality. Between 1817 and 1923 the disease swept to other parts of the world including Europe and America as pandemics on at least six occasions. *Eltor vibrio* was identified as the cause of the cholera-like disease during 1937–38 in Celebes island of Indonesia. This was identified as a major pathogen causing diarrheal illness in India, Pakistan, Afghanistan, Iran, Iraq and southern parts of Union of Soviet Socialist Republics (USSR) in 1965–66. From this time *Eltor vibrios* are responsible almost exclusively for cases of cholera reported in this subcontinent.

A new strain named *V. cholerae* O139 was found to produce toxin and this was identified as a cause of clinical cholera in 1992. It rapidly spread to several countries in South East Asia and by 1993 it almost replaced the O1 Eltor strain. By 1995–96 Eltor were considerably eliminated even though occasional cases did occur in India and Bangladesh. Recent outbreaks in Ambajogai region of Maharashtra documented the presence of O139 strain in about 25% of cholera like illness.

Etiology and Epidemiology

An estimated 3–5 million cases occur worldwide annually with 1,20,000 deaths (WHO-2003). There is no steady decline in overall incidence in the disease prevalence over the years, even though with socioeconomic development the incidence has come down in such areas. Man and environment form the natural reservoir. Spread occurs through the environment. Organisms are eliminated in feces of acute cases and carriers. Convalescent patients become temporary carriers passing the organisms in feces for 4–7 days after an attack. Rarely chronic carrier state may develop and organisms may be present in feces for years. Unlike the explosive outbreaks of classical cholera, Eltor epidemics follow a protracted pattern with a few cases occurring everyday for several weeks. The pathogenic vibrios can survive outside the human host in the environment for varying periods. Freezing infected water does not kill the vibrios. The medium for infection are water, cooked food kept unhygenically exposed to flies, sea foods, fruits and vegetables. Apart from shell fish and plankton, there are no animal reservoirs. Biofilm, formation and conversion into a visible, but non culturable state due to nutrient deprivation helps the organisms to persist within natural aquatic habitats for long periods. The infective dose is 10^5–10^8 vibrios.

Cholera is predominantly a disease of the lower socio-economic group living in gross insanitary conditions. The organisms are killed in the presence of normal gastric acidity. In different places cholera outbreaks follow seasonal patterns.

Immunity

An attack of classic biotype of *Vibrio cholerae* usually protects against recurrent infection by either type. But, Eltor type cholera does not protect against further attacks. Persons with blood group 'O' are at an increased risk of developing Eltor cholera.

Pathogenesis

Vibrio cholerae are ingested in food or drinks and they multiply in jejunum and small intestine and produce an enterotoxin. This toxin causes the enterocytes (intestinal mucosal cells) to secrete large amount of isotonic fluid. The rate of secretion of the fluid exceeds the rate of absorption which also goes on. The result is watery diarrhea which leads to the loss of isotonic fluid. The fluid loss accounts for all the clinical manifestations. Virulence is determined by genetic factors which favors bacterial colonization and attachment to intestinal epithelium.

Cholera enterotoxin is a protein of molecular weight (mol wt) 84,000 made up of two immunologically distinct regions—A (active) and B (binding). The B region is composed of five subunits of mol wt about 11,500. This region of the cholera toxin is responsible for binding to cell membrane receptors containing GM1 ganglioside. The binding enables the 28,000 MW 'A' region to penetrate the mucosal cells. This toxin leads to the formation of adenylate cyclase which induces excessive production of cyclic-adenosine monophosphate (cAMP), which in turn is responsible for over secretion of electrolytes and water by the enterocytes. The exact mechanism of action of cAMP, however, is not clear. The enterotoxin acts locally and does not invade the intestinal wall, as a result the feces does not show cellular exudates which are characteristic of inflammation. The feces is watery, turbid and often does not contain any visible fecal matter.

The pathophysiological changes result directly from the massive gastrointestinal (GI) loss of fluid isotonic with plasma. The feces are low in proteins and chloride, but relatively rich in sodium, potassium and bicarbonate (sodium 126 ± 9, potassium 19 ± 9, bicarbonate 47 ± 10 and chloride 95 ± 9 mmol/L). Excessive loss of fluid and electrolyte gives rise to hypovolemic shock and metabolic acidosis. Most of the fluid loss is from the small intestine.

Clinical Features

Severity of cholera varies from a completely asymptomatic form to fulminant diarrhea and shock. In Eltor cholera outbreaks, the proportion of asymptomatic and mild cases is higher than the severe cases.

In most cases the incubation period varies from less than a day to 5 days. Mild cases of cholera may be asymptomatic and diagnosis has to be established by stool culture. In some only a mild diarrheal illness may be seen.

In moderate and severe cases the onset is abrupt with uncontrollable painless watery diarrhea and effortless vomiting. The excreta may contain fecal material at the onset but soon it assumes the characteristic 'rice-water' appearance due to the presence of flakes of mucus and large number of vibrios. Rice-water stools contain about 10^{11}–10^{12} vibrios/L. Watery stools are passed in quick succession. In many patients vomiting supervenes either along with the diarrhea or may follow later. Nausea is absent. Vomitus consists of clear, watery fluid. Loss of fluid and electrolytes leads to dehydration, acidosis and shock. Earliest indication of fluid deficit is thirst with dryness of the mouth and tongue. Decreased renal blood flow produces oliguria and renal shutdown. The patient may be unable to talk due to loss of voice. Painful muscular cramps develop due to hyponatremia.

Mental state remains clear. Restlessness is the forerunner of shock. When dehydration is severe, the eyes are sunken, skin is shrivelled, neck veins are collapsed and signs of shock supervene. The rectal temperature is usually normal or raised even though the extremities may be cold. The abdomen is scaphoid and nontender. The illness seldom lasts for more than 3–5 days. Rarely large amounts of fluid may collect in the intestinal lumen and severe dehydration, shock and death may result even before evacuation occurs. The term *cholera sicca* is used to denote such cases.

Diagnosis

Laboratory diagnosis is made by isolating the organisms from proper stool samples collected before the administration of antimicrobial agents. The specimen should be transported to the laboratory without delay. A suitable medium for transporting specimens is Venkatraman and Ramakrishnan (V-R) fluid or Carry and Blair medium. It is very important to make bacteriological diagnosis in all cases of diarrhea since undetected sporadic cases may be starting point of outbreaks. Moreover, cholera being a notifiable disease, should be notified to the Public Health Authorities in order to take preventive measures. Vibrios can be identified in fresh microscopic preparation of feces by their characteristic movement.

Other laboratory findings: These are non-specific, but they help to assess the fluid and electrolyte status and to plan definitive management. These include:

Elevation of PCV	Dehydration
Neutrophil leukocytosis	Lactic acidosis
Fall in serum bicarbonate	Hyponatremia
Increase in anion gap	Electrolytic loss
Hypokalemia	

Differential Diagnosis

A clinically indistinguishable picture can be presented by about 25 intestinal pathogens such as enterotoxigenic *E. coli,* other vibrios, *Campylobacter jejuni,* rotavirus and others. Bacterial and toxin type of food poisoning has to be looked for and excluded. Gastroenteritis may resemble cholera. In gastroenteritis vomiting precedes diarrhea, there is abdominal pain and stools may contain cellular exudates. Fever may be present.

Prognosis

During epidemics mortality may be as high as 30%. Malnutrition, intercurrent illness and need of proper medical attention are adverse factors. Adequate and early replacement of fluid and electrolytes reduces mortality considerably. Introduction of the oral rehydration solution (ORS), recommended widely by the World Health Organization (WHO) and adopted as the first line of treatment in diarrheal diseases, has brought down mortality to a great extent. Many complications can also be prevented by early rehydration.

Complications

Most frequent complication is hypovolemic shock which is fatal if untreated. Hypokalemia may lead to fatal cardiac arrhythmias, abdominal distension and muscle paralysis. Injudicious administration of electrolyte solutions intravenously (IV) without correcting metabolic acidosis may result in acute pulmonary edema. Convulsions may develop in children due to cerebral venous thrombosis. Severe hypoglycemia may also contribute to this symptom. Severe shock leads to renal cortical necrosis and renal failure. Other complications include venous thrombosis, cataract and prolapse of the rectum in children. Florid malnutrition may develop after diarrheal episodes in children from poor communities.

Treatment

All cases with moderate or severe diarrhea should be hospitalized and treated properly. Early replacement of GI fluid and electrolyte losses, maintenance of nutrition

Textbook of Medicine

Table 42.1: Assessment of dehydration and fluid deficit

Signs and symptoms	Mild dehydration	Moderate dehydration	Severe dehydration
General appearance and condition—infants and young children	Thirst, alert, restless	Intense thirst, restless or lethargic but irritable when touched	Drowsy, flaccid, cold sweaty, cyanosis, may be comatose
Older children and adults	Thirst, alert, restless	Intense thirst, giddiness with postural hypotension	Usually conscious, apprehensive, cold, sweaty, cyanotic extremities wrinkled skin of fingers and toes, muscle cramps
Radial pulse	Normal rate and volume	Rapid and weak	Rapid, feeble, thready pulse
Respiration	Normal	Deep, may be rapid	Deep and rapid
Anterior fontanelle	Normal	Sunken	Very sunken
Systolic blood pressure (BP)	Normal	Normal to low	Less than 80 mm Hg, may be unrecordable
Skin elasticity	Pinch retracts immediately	Pinch retracts slowly	Pinch retracts very slowly (> 2 seconds)
Eyes	Normal	Sunken	Deeply sunken
Tears	Present	Absent	Absent
Mucous membrane	Moist	Dry	Very dry
Urine flow	Normal	Reduced amount and dark	Almost stops, empty bladder
Percent body weight loss	4–5%	6–9%	10% or more
Estimated fluid deficit	40–50 mL/kg body weight	60–90 mL/kg body weight	100–110 mL/kg body weight

Note: Material for Tables are taken from the WHO and UNICEF statement 1983.

Table 42.2: Guidelines for rehydration therapy

Severity	Age group	Nature of fluid	Volume of fluid	Duration
Mild	All	ORS solution	50 mL/kg	Within 4 hours
Moderate	All	ORS solution	100 mL/kg	Within 4 hours
		IV Ringer lactate	30 mL/kg	Within 1 hours
Severe	Infants	IV	40 mL/kg	Within next 2 hours
		Ringer lactate		
		Followed by oral	40 mL/kg	Within next 3 hours
		ORS administration		
	Older children and adults	IV Ringer lactate	110 mL/kg	Within 4 hours initially as fast as possible until the radial pulse is palpable

Note: In the management of severe cases all the measures described under mild and moderate dehydration have to be started before hospitalization. Use the largest size needle available for IV drip. A common error is the use small needles for IV drip which will delay fluid administration.

Abbreviations: ORS = Oral rehydration salt; IV = Intravenous

and institution of antimicrobial drugs form the mainstay of treatment. Fluid replacement is done to correct the existing deficit of water and electrolytes (rehydration therapy) and it is continued to replace losses due to continuing diarrhea (maintenance therapy) (Tables 42.1 and 42.2). Fluid replacement therapy should be started as early as possible with ORS, preferably at home itself on the onset of the disease.

Rehydration therapy: In mild and moderate cases, rehydration can be achieved with oral rehydration salt (ORS) solution. The WHO recommended ORS formula contains:

- Sodium (90 mmol/L)
- Potassium (25 mmol/L)
- Chloride (80 mmol/L
- Bicarbonate (30 mmol/L) and
- Glucose (111 mmol/L).

Procedure to prepare ORS at home:

- Sodium chloride 3.5 g
- Sodium bicarbonate 2.5 g
- Potassium chloride 1.5 g
- Glucose 20 g
- Water 1 L.

It can be easily prepared in any household by dissolving sodium chloride 3.5 g, sodium bicarbonate 2.5 g, potassium chloride 1.5 g and glucose 20 g in 1 L of drinking water. Rice-based oral rehydration solutions have been devised. These are made by replacing the glucose with 80 g/L of rice powder and boiling the solution. In addition to the carbohydrate, the glycine liberated by digestion of protein also assists the absorption of sodium and water across the intestinal mucosa.

Mothers are advised to give this fluid at frequent intervals to the children, thirst being the guideline for deciding the quantity and frequency. The efficacy of ORS has been widely tested and accepted. The glucose acts mainly as an agent to favor absorption of sodium. Glucose can be replaced by twice the quantity of sucrose or even other household starches, but they are less efficient. Severe dehydration, with or without hypovolemic shock, should be treated with IV fluids to achieve satisfactory rehydration. Ringer's lactate solution is the best commercially available preparation suitable for all age groups. This contains sodium lactate, sodium chloride, potassium chloride and calcium chloride. If Ringer lactate solution is not available, the next best is a solution containing sodium chloride 4 g potassium chloride 1 g, sodium acetate 6.5 g and glucose 10 g/L. The volume and rate of fluid required depends on the severity.

One of the disturbing aspects which make ORS less acceptable to rural people is the fact that even though it stimulates absorption of electrolytes across the intestinal mucosa, often the stool volume is not reduced abruptly. This disadvantage is partly corrected by rice or cereal-based ORS. Amylase resistant starch obtained from several types of cereals reaches the colon without being digested and absorbed in the small intestine. Bacterial action converts this starch into short chain fatty acids which promote the absorption of fluid and electrolytes from the colon and thereby reduce stool volume. About 10 g of amylase resistant starch added to 200 mL of conventional ORS was found to be beneficial in studies conducted in Vellore South India.

Fluid replacement should cover the losses in stools, vomitus and sweat. In a severe case, fluid balance should be checked hourly. Where facilities permit, replacement of electrolytes should be guided by laboratory estimations. As the dehydration is corrected, the child's mental state improves, the acidosis clears, blood pressure (BP) comes up and urine is passed. It is ideal to achieve a urine flow of 50–60 mL/h. An IV line should be maintained till the child is well on the road to recovery.

Zinc supplemented ORS solutions are available at present. Zinc supplementation has been found to be better among malnourished children and adults who are likely to be zinc deficient. Dose of zinc sulfate for children below 6 months is 10 mg/day and it is 20 mg for children above 6 months.

Maintenance therapy: It is intended to replace continuing losses of fluid and electrolytes and this follows the initial intensive regimen. The principle is to match the input to the output. ORS can be relied upon for maintenance therapy in moderate cases without severe diarrhea. The volume of ORS should be 100 mL/kg bw/day in mild cases. In moderate and severe cases, fluid should be given at the rate of 10–15 mg/kg bw/hour until diarrhea stops. Severe cases should be treated with IV fluids—can deliver only up to 4 mmol of potassium/L whereas ORS contains up to 20 mmol/L. Hence, ORS should be started as soon as the severe phase is tided over.

Antimicrobial drugs: Though cholera is a self-limiting disease, it is customary to use antibiotics when a case is diagnosed. Effective antibiotic therapy reduces purging time by 50%, purging rate by 50% and reduces the period of elimination of vibrios in feces from 5 or more days to 1–2 days. Tetracycline, furazolidone, ciprofloxacin and erythromycin shorten the duration of the illness and stop excretion of vibrios in stools. Recent work has shown that a single dose of azithromycin 1 g given orally at the onset of illness reduces the duration of diarrhea (up to 30 hours) and achieves elimination of bacteria in 78% of cases. These results are much better than those achieved with ciprofloxacin.

Source: Saha D, Karim MM, Khan WA, et al. Single-dose azithromycin for the treatment of cholera in adults. N Engl J Med. 2006;354(23):2452-62.

Dosage of drugs: All given orally.

Tetracycline	2 g od for 3 days or 500 mg 6 h for 3 days
Doxycycline	100 mg bd for 3 days
Ciprofloxacin	500 mg bd for 3 days
Erythromycin	40 mg/kg daily, 6 h for 3 days
Azithromycin	1 g single dose

Dietetic management: Even during the diarrheal phase, food should be given in accordance with the patient's desire and tolerance. Starvation, in addition to the depletion of calories, also reduces the ability of the small intestine to absorb a variety of nutrients. Infants should be breastfed as they demand. Older children and adults should be given easily digestible food with adequate calories depending on customary practices and local availability. Fruit juices, bananas, coconut water and cereals are usually well tolerated. Bananas and apple help to reduce diarrhea and form stools of normal consistency.

Prevention

General Measures

Cholera is a notifiable disease. All suspected cases should be fully investigated bacteriologically and notified to the health authorities to prevent an outbreak. Health education of communities during outbreaks, chlorination of water supplies, control of flies and provision of adequate treatment facilities at the affected areas help to limit the epidemic. Instruction on the use of ORS from the beginning of the diarrheal phase has proved to be of great value in reducing morbidity and mortality.

On a long-term basis, improvement in environmental sanitation, provision of protected water supply, arrangement for proper disposal of excreta and improvement of food hygiene are absolutely essential to wipe out infective diarrhea. Chlorination of water effectively destroys the organism. Spraying the breeding places of flies with deltamethrin will suppress the fly population. Fly-proofing of kitchen and food containers is very effective in arresting the spread of cholera. Vaccination is to be given to special groups such as inmates of refugee camps and following natural disasters such as earthquakes and floods.

Personal prophylaxis: Vaccination is protective against cholera. Many newer vaccines employ equal numbers of classical cholera and Eltor biotypes and the concentration has been raised to 12,000 million organisms per mL. This vaccine is antigenic. The course of immunization consists of 2 subcutaneous injections of 0.5 mL and 1 mL separated by an interval of four weeks. Several well-controlled field trials have shown that conventional cholera vaccines provide only low degree of protection and that too only for 3–6 months. Oral live vaccines are also underway. Shanchol, the Indian made oral vaccine made by Shanta Biolab Hyderabad, India is approved by the WHO for use to prevent cholera. This vaccine is recommended in outbreaks worldwide. It contains killed whole cell organisms and also *V. cholera* serogroup O139. Shanchol is only one-third as costly as vaccine made by other producers. Its storage volume is also smaller. Trial of the modified killed whole cell cholera vaccine along with a placebo vaccine in Calcutta and follow-up for 2 years showed that with 2 doses of oral vaccine, level of protection was 86.6% of more and it persisted for more than 2 years. The vaccine is cheap compared to other makes.

Firdausi Quadri and others working from Bangladesh have reported that 'Shanchol given in doses of 1.5 mL as single dose orally provided 40% protection against cholera for atleast 6 months especially in children above 5 years'.

Source:

1. Sur D, Lopez AL, Kanungo S, et al. Efficacy and safety of a modified killed-whole-cell oral cholera vaccine in India: an interim analysis of a cluster-randomised, double-blind, placebo-controlled trial. Lancet. 2009;374:1694-702.
2. Luquero FJ, Grout L, Ciglenecki I, et al. Use of vibro chlorea vaccine in an outbreak in Guinea. New Eng J Med. 2014;370(22)2111-20.
3. Qadri F, Wierzba TF, Ali M, et al. Efficacy of a Single-Dose, Inactivated Oral Cholera Vaccine in Bangladesh. N Engl J Med. 2016;374(18):1723-32.

An attack of cholera confers temporary immunity for 6–12 months after which the immunity wanes off. Since *V. cholera* forms a part of the normal flora and ecology of the surface water in many places it has not been possible to eradicate the organism in it so far.

NON-CHOLERA VIBRIOS

Other vibrios that are at times pathogenic to humans are *V. parahaemolyticus, V. vulnificus, V. alginolyticus* and a few others.

Infective agent	Pathogenicity
V. parahaemolyticus	Explosive diarrhea
V. vulnificus	• Rapid onset fulminating septicemia • Rapidly spreading cellulitis • Acute diarrhea following consumption of shell fish
V. alginolyticus	Wound infections, mainly opportunis

ACUTE DIARRHEAL DISEASES OF CHILDREN

Acute diarrheal diseases are major killers of infants and young children, accounting for 30–50% of deaths below the age of 5 years. In India about 1.5 million children die annually from diarrheal diseases other than cholera. Disorders in which three or more watery stools are passed daily with or without vomiting are included under this group.

Etiologic agents: The most well-known pathogens are *Shigella, Salmonella,* enteropathogenic *E. coli, Vibrio cholerae, Eltor vibrios, E. histolytica* and *G. lamblia* and these account for only about 20% of the total, the remaining 80% being due to other agents which number about twenty. Diarrhea results either from enterotoxin or through invasive mechanisms. The clinical picture and management are the same as described under cholera.

Viruses account for the majority of diarrheal episodes in infants and young children in both developed and developing countries. These viruses include rotavirus, Norwalk and Norwalk-like agents, coronavirus, adenovirus, caliciviruses and others whose causative role is not yet clearly established. Viral gastroenteritis occurs globally in epidemic or endemic outbreaks.

Epidemic gastroenteritis	Norwalk viruses (present name noroviruses)
Endemic gastroenteritis	Rotavirus, astrovirus and coronavirus

Adenovirus and calcivirus cause both endemic and epidemic outbreaks.

ROTAVIRUS

Rotavirus affects mainly infants and young children aged 6 months to 2 years and above. It is a ribonucleic acid (RNA) virus which is enveloped. In many places rotavirus has emerged as a major pathogen causing wide outbreaks. Forty percent of severe gastroenteritis in children in India is due to rotavirus. Three groups A, B and C are pathogenic to man and produce diarrhea in local or epidemic outbreaks. In developing countries rotavirus accounts for 20–30% of the diarrheal deaths. Most of the rotavirus infections occur in the first year of life.

Infection is by fecal-oral route. Incubation period ranges from 1 to 7 days but usually it is less than 48 hours. The virus affects the enterocytes of the small intestine and the epithelium overlying the Peyer's patches. Destruction of the villi lead to disaccharidase deficiencies and malabsorption of carbohydrates. Recovery of the villi takes 2–3 weeks.

Clinical Features

Vomiting occurs early and it precedes diarrhea. Diarrhea extends over 5–7 days but virus is shed for up to 10 days. The diarrhea may be severe extending 10 stools/day and vomiting may occur in 90%. Asymptomatic infections and mild disease may occur during outbreaks. Breast milk may have a protective role due to the presence of maternal IgA antibodies. Mild forms may also occur.

Diagnosis

It can be established by demonstrating the organism by electron microscopy or rotavirus antigen by enzyme-linked immunosorbent assay (ELISA) test in stool. This is not required in the ordinary case, since, specific antiviral therapy is not widely available. Rotavirus diarrhea responds to standard rehydration therapy as described under cholera. Rare complications include myositis, polio like paralysis and sudden infant death.

Nitazoxanide, in a dose of 7.5 mg/kg bw given orally for 3 days controlled rotavirus diarrhea in hospitalized patients. This drug has been licenced in the United States of America (USA) for treating rotavirus infections.

Vaccination

Three rotavirus vaccines are currently available—Rotarix (GlaxoSmithKline).

1. Monovalent vaccine made from human rotavirus strain and attenuated.
   Dose: 2 oral doses 1st dose 6–14 weeks of age, 2nd dose 4 weeks later.
2. Pentavalent vaccine [RotaTeq (Merck)] made from bovine rotavirus strains and attenuated.

Dose: 3 oral doses 1st dose 6–12 weeks of age, 2nd and 3rd doses 4–10 weeks intervals.

3. A monovalent human bovine (116E) rotavirus vaccine made by Bharat Biotech International, Hyderabad, India was tried in three centres—Delhi, Pune and Vellore between 11th March 2011 and 5th November 2012 on infants aged 6–7 weeks. The vaccine was effective and well tolerated. Incidence of severe rotavirus diarrhea was 1.5/100 person years in the vaccinated group compared to 3.2 in the controls.

Source: Bhandari N, Rongsen-Chandola T, Bavdekar A, et al. Efficacy of a monovalent human-bovine (116E) rotavirus vaccine in Indian infants: a randomised, double-blind, placebo-controlled trial. Lancet. 2014;383(9935):2136-43.

Further studies on oral pentavalent vaccines in infants aged 6–14 weeks showed efficacy in African, Bangladesh and Vietnam studies when given in 3 doses at 6th, 10th and 14th weeks. Studies are in progress.

Several other vaccines are being produced. The Millennium Development Group has suggested the inclusion of rotavirus vaccine in the routine childhood immunization schedule in order to prevent 5% of the deaths occurring in childhood and 4% of deaths due to diarrhea.

Source: Glass RI, Parashar UD, Bresee JS, et al. Rotavirus vaccines: current prospects and future challenges. Lancet. 2006;368(9532):323-32.

NOROVIRUS INFECTIONS

Previously known as (Norwalk and Norwalk-like Agents)

History

Since 1972, these viruses have been identified as the cause of outbreaks, generally mild gastroenteritis occurring in school, community and family settings. The present name is Norovirus which is an enterovirus. It belongs to the group of calicivirus and it is a non-enveloped RNA virus. Several strains are present, the human strains are distinct from those which affect other animals. Infection is by fecal-oral route. Infective dose may be small. Incubation is 1–2 days and the duration of illness is 4–5 days. Outbreaks commonly occur in closed communities such as schools, hospitals and hotels.

Clinical Features

Vomiting, diarrhea and abdominal pain may occur. The diarrhea is generally milder than in rotavirus infections. Vomiting may occur in 50% of cases. Often symptoms are mild and self-limiting. Treatment is supportive. Once an outbreak occurs and subsides, sanitary measures to sterilize the ward are needed to prevent further cases from occurring. The viral antigen can be detected in feces by ELISA test.

Management

General measures such as fluid replacement orally and if needed, parenterally should be instituted without delay. The condition is self-limiting and the child recovers within a few days.

Vaccination

The virus-like particles (VLP) vaccine against norovirus has been developed. It is given intranasally in 2 doses, it provides homologous protection against both norovirus infection and viral gastroenteritis.

Probiotics

At present these are commonly used to restore health in the post diarrheal state. Since diarrheas lead to severe malnutrition, especially in children with subnormal nutritional status, food supplements—calories, proteins, vitamins, minerals and fluids should be started early. Probiotics are live microbes, many of them being normal intestinal flora, e.g. *Lactobacillus, Bifidobacterium,* varieties of *Streptococci, Saccharomyces boulardi* and others. These help to restore normal microbial environment of the gut and inhibit pathogens. They help to restore normal bowel function, provide symptom relief and accelerate recovery. The main probiotic effect is the development, maturation and regulation of mucosa-associated immunological defenses and suppression of atopy and food allergies.

Rarer causes of Viral Diarrhea

Other viral pathogens include adenovirus, astroviruses, other caliciviruses and mini-rotavirus. These produce diarrhea of varying severity.

CAMPYLOBACTER JEJUNI

Epidemiology

Campylobacter jejuni **(previously known as *Vibrio fetus*)** is found in the intestines of birds, particularly in chicken, turkeys, wild birds and also in dogs, cats and calves. *C. jejuni* is a slender spirally shaped gram-negative bacillus, rapidly motile, non-sporing and microaerophilic. The organisms are spread by fecal-oral route. They are acquired from sick puppies, kitten or infected cases. *Campylobacter jejuni* is ubiquitous and has been isolated as the pathogen in several outbreaks. Normal gastric acidity kills the organisms.

Pathogenesis

Campylobacter jejuni invades tissues and produces diffuse bloody exudative enteritis and nonspecific colitis. No enterotoxin has been isolated. Bacteremia and metastatic lesions may complicate the primary lesion.

Clinical Features

Incubation period is 1–7 days. Main symptoms include watery or bloody diarrhea, abdominal pain, malaise, fever, vomiting and constitutional symptoms. The severity may vary. On an average there may be 8–10 bowel movements in a day. Recovery occurs within a week. Campylobacter infection cannot be clinically differentiated from other forms of dysenteries. Rarely a prolonged illness resembling typhoid and meningitis may develop.

Complications include reactive arthritis (1–2%) and possible induction of Guillain-Barré syndrome (GBS). About 14–38% of patients with GBS give a history of recent campylobacter infection. Intestinal hemorrhage, toxic megacolon and hemolytic uremic syndrome may occur rarely. Mortality is low.

Treatment

Since the infection is self-limiting, fluid and electrolyte replacement forms the mainstay of therapy. The organisms

Textbook of Medicine

respond to erythromycin given orally in a dose of 250 mg every 6 hourly. Resistant cases respond to tetracycline in a dose of 250–500 mg every 6 hourly. For bacteremia, gentamicin or chloramphenicol are given systemically.

Prevention

The organisms are destroyed by proper cooking and storage of animal foods, pasteurization of milk and provision of protected water supply. Chlorination of water kills the organisms.

CLOSTRIDIUM DIFFICILE: PSEUDOMEMBRANOUS COLITIS

Syn: Antibiotic associated diarrhea

General Considerations

Clostridium difficile is a gram-positive anaerobic spore-forming bacillus that can cause pseudomembranous colitis and other disease manifestations. It produces two toxins A and B. Generally toxin A is enterotoxin and toxin B is a cytotoxin. In addition, about 6% of organisms produce a third toxin known as binary toxin cytolethal distending toxins (CDT) which is similar to the toxin of *C. perfringens.* The toxins account for its virulence. Transmission occurs primarily in healthcare institutions where exposure to antimicrobial drugs is common. Infected persons with diarrhea spread large number of spores which contaminate their skin, clothing and surrounding surfaces. The presence of spores favor transmission. The predominant infecting strain of *Cl. difficile* is the O27/B1/NAP1 strain. The asymptomatic carriers of the toxic strain of *Cl. difficile* outnumber the cases and they could also be sources of new cases (30% and 29%) respectively. It is proposed that airborne dispersal of spores could also occur. Potential reservoirs also include infants residing in colonies, food materials and animals. 45% of *Cl. difficile* diarrhea are probably acquired from sources other than hospital settings.

Alteration in the intestinal microbial flora contributes to the pathogenicity which is pseudomembranous enterocolitis. With the widespread use of antibiotics, pseudomembranous colitis has come into prominence. Pseudomembranous colitis is a more serious and specific infection caused by *Clostridium difficile* which develops following the use of several antibiotics. Though all antibiotics predispose to infection by *Clostridium difficile,* fluoroquinolones, clindamycin and beta-lactams are more risky. The disease is reported from several institutions in India. The incidences in BYL Nair Charitable Hospital was 2–4% in patients without diarrhea and 7–30% in those with diarrhea as reported in 2012. Asymptomatic carriage was 6%.

Source: Kaneria MV, Paul S. Incidence of Clostridium difficile associated diarrhoea in a tertiary care hospital. J Assoc Physicians India. 2012;60:26-8.

Pathology

The lesions consist of disruption of villous tips, infiltration by neutrophils and the presence of yellow plaque-like lesions on the mucosa, especially in the colon. These are caused by the toxins derived from *Clostridium difficile* which overgrows and become pathogenic.

Clinical Features

A broad spectrum of presentations ranging from mild diarrhea to severe life-threatening illness may occur. The disease is clinically characterized by abdominal pain, fever, leukocytosis, watery diarrhea and rarely toxic megacolon. If not diagnosed and treated early, the mortality may go up to 50–60%.

Diagnosis

Clinical suspicion should lead to the diagnosis. The organism can be isolated from feces. Presence of toxins can be demonstrated in fecal samples by ELISA. It is the most common method of diagnosing *Cl. difficile* associated diarrhea. Sigmoidoscopy reveals erythema with ulceration of the mucosa and patchy adherent membranous plaques.

Treatment

Drug treatment consists of metronidazole in a dose of 400 mg tid for 10 days. An alternative is vancomycin 250 mg qid for 10 days. On stopping therapy recurrence is common. In them addition of rifampicin to vancomycin helps to control the infection. Probiotics like *Saccharomyces boulardii* or *Lactobacillus* help to reconstitute the intestinal flora. In the Indian series the disease is less severe and more amenable to metronidazole unlike as in the West, where the virulent-strain toxin type III is prevalent.

Fidaxomicin, 200 mg twice a day for 10 days is non-inferior to vancomycin in effectiveness. Recurrence of infection is also lower, adverse effects of fidaxomicin and vancomycin are similar.

Prevention

The preventive measures include—isolating the patient with contact precautions and disinfection of surfaces and equipment with sporicidal products such as sodium hypochlorite. Avoidance of overuse of antibiotics help to reduce incidence.

Chronic Life-threatening *Clostridium Difficile* Infection

Recurrent *Cl. difficile* infection is difficult to treat and failure to respond to antibiotics is high. Such cases are treated by fecal reconstitution of the gut microbes. The effect of donor feces infusion into the duodenum by a nasoduodenal tube has been used as a method to reconstitute the microbial flora of the intestines as a form of therapy in such cases. Standard vancomycin treatment 500 mg for 4 days was given followed by bowel lavage with 4/L of macrogol solution. Feces of donors are selected from those who did not have any infections or other diseases of the intestinal tract and are free from hepatitis virus. 141 ± 71 g diluted in 500 mL saline was infused by a nasoduodenal tube at the rate of 50 mL in 2–3 minutes and the tube was withdrawn after 2 hours. The favorable outcome was cure without relapse within 10 weeks of therapy. Side effects include belching, nausea and aversion. Results are better than vancomycin.

Source: Van Nood E, Vrieze A, Nieuwdorp M, et al. Duodenal infusion of donor feces for recurrent *Clostridium difficile.* New Eng J Med. 2013;368(5):407-15.

CHAPTER 43

Bartonellosis, Legionellosis, Listeriosis, Yaws, Pinta, Relapsing Fevers, Lyme Borreliosis

KV Krishna Das

Chapter Summary

- Bartonellosis
  - Carrion's Disease
  - Bacillary Angiomatosis
  - Cat-Scratch Disease
  - Trench Fever
- Legionellosis
  - Legionnaires disease
  - Pontiac Fever
- Listeriosis
  - Gastroenteritis
  - Bacteremia
  - Meningitis
  - Meningoencephalitis
  - Fetal problems
  - Prognosis
  - Treatment
- Yaws
  - General Considerations
  - Clinical Features
  - Diagnosis
  - Treatment
- Pinta
  - Clinical Features
  - Diagnosis
  - Treatment
- Relapsing Fevers
  - Borrelial Infections
  - Louse-Borne Relapsing Fever
  - Tick-Borne Relapsing Fever
- Lyme Borreliosis
  - Clinical Features
  - Lyme Neuroborreliosis
  - Cardiac Manifestations
  - Acrodermatitis Chronica Atrophicans
  - Diagnosis
  - Treatment
  - Prevention

BARTONELLOSIS

Syn: Carrion's Disease, Oroya Fever, Verruga Peruana

The genus *Bartonella* consists of three main pathogens affecting man.

1. *Bartonella bacilliformis*—cause of Carrion's disease
2. *Bartonella henselae*—cause of cat-scratch disease and bacillary angiomatosis in patients with acquired immunodeficiency syndrome (AIDS)
3. *Bartonella quintana*—cause of trench fever, transmitted by body louse.

Carrion's Disease

This name is given in memory of Daniel A Carrion, a Peruvian student who injected infective blood into himself during studies on the infectivity of *Bartonella bacilliformis* and died because of the disease.

Carrion's disease is confined to the valleys of Andes mountains of South America and has not been reported in India. It is caused by *Bartonella bacilliformis,* which is seen inside the erythrocytes. The disease is transmitted by the sandfly *Phlebotomus verrucarum.*

Bartonella bacilliformis is a small gram-negative coccobacillus 0.3–1.5 × 0.2–0.5 μm. It is motile and strictly aerobic.

It presents different clinical pictures at different stages of evolution of the disease. After an incubation period of three weeks, the disease develops. It is characterized by two distinct clinical syndromes. The initial illness is characterized by constitutional symptoms like fever, rigors, nausea, diarrhea and headache. This is called Oroya fever and lasts for 3–4 weeks. Organisms can be demonstrated in blood smears stained by Giemsa's or Wright's stain. Death may occur at this stage due to severe anemia or super infection by *Salmonella.*

The second stage called *Verruga peruana*, is characterized by hemangiomatous tumors of skin and mucous membranes varying in size between 2 and 15 mm, some of which may ulcerate. Mortality is very low at this stage, since immunity develops.

Specific treatment is with chloramphenicol or tetracyclines in addition to supportive measures.

Bacillary Angiomatosis

This is caused by *Bartonella henselae* which is seen in domestic cats. It may produce three clinical syndromes:

1. Chronic bacteremia
2. Bacillary peliosis hepatis
3. Disseminated bacillary angiomatosis.

Skin lesions occur as vascular nodules and may reach large sizes. Such lesions may be seen in internal organ such as liver, spleen, lymph nodes and bone marrow. Prolonged fever is common. Treatment is with antimicrobials such as erythromycin, doxycycline or ciprofloxacin given for 3–8 weeks.

Cat-scratch Disease

This is also caused by *Bartonella henselae*. It is transmitted by bites, licks or scratches by the cat. Local lesion develops as a crusted papule. It is followed by fever and malaise and tender regional lymphadenopathy. The lesion is self-limiting and usually benign. Rarely, complications may occur which include meningitis, myelitis, encephalitis hepatitis and osteomyelitis. Treatment is with erythromycin or doxycycline.

Textbook of Medicine

Trench Fever

This is caused by *Bartonella quintana* which is transmitted from person to person by the body louse. It is seen in persons huddled in trenches, refugee camps and similar situations. Treatment is with erythromycin or doxycycline.

LEGIONELLOSIS

Legionellaceae are gram-negative rods whose natural habitat is water. Man is accidentally infected and human to human transmission is unusual. There are over 36 defined species, among which *L. pneumophila* is the most common human pathogen. Two main clinical syndromes are produced—**Legionnaires disease** and **Pontiac fever**. The former has a low attack rate among those exposed whereas the latter has a high attack rate. Risk factors for infection include cigarette smoking, chronic respiratory diseases, alcoholic liver disease, elderly age and immunocompromised states.

Legionnaires Disease

The first description was given in 1976 following the outbreak of an unusual pneumonic illness among members attending the legion convention at Philadelphia. The organisms have been isolated from air-conditioning systems, water taps, soil and other environment. It is acquired by inhalation, ingestion or through the conjunctiva.

At present legionella has been found to be a common cause of community acquired pneumonia in several countries including India. Infection is by inhalation of aerosols containing the organisms or microaspiration of infected water. *Legionella* exist in water. They can infect and replicate within several protozoa found in the soil, including amoeba. By successive replication its virulence increases.

The incubation period is 2–10 days after which the patient presents with fever, anorexia, weight loss, headache, myalgia and confusion. Severe cases progress to pneumonia and pleurisy.

Pathology

It is mainly confined to the lungs. Reaching the lungs, the organisms are phagocytosed by alveolar macrophages in which they multiply and are released by cell rupture. Successive multiplication takes place in fresh macrophages. Bacterial multiplication and attack of fresh cells are arrested by cytokines produced by macrophages and lymphocytes. The predominant immune mechanism is T-cell mediated. Antibodies of the immunoglobulin M (IgM) and IgG classes are produced. Pathological lesions in the lungs lead to the development of bronchopneumonia with exudates rich in neutrophils and fibrin. Toxins secreted by the organisms lead to encephalopathy.

Lesions: Pneumonia is the most common presentation followed by gastrointestinal (GI) symptoms such as watery diarrhea. Cardiac lesions include myocarditis, pericarditis, post-cardiotomy syndrome and prosthetic valve endocarditis. Neurological manifestation are not common, these include confusion, frank encephalopathy, neuropathy, myositis, cranial nerve palsies and cerebellar disturbances. These have been described in Indian patients.

Source: Kulkarni KH, Thorat SB, Wagle SC, et al. Focal neurological manifestations in Legionellosis. J Assoc Physicians India. 2005;53:731-3.

Pontiac Fever

Pontiac fever also occurs in persons exposed to the infective environment. It is a brief febrile illness resembling influenza, caused by other species of *Legionella*. Mortality is nil. Nosocomial legionella infections may lead to wound infection or prosthetic valve endocarditis, rarely.

Diagnosis

- Culture of the organism from sputum in special media
- Direct fluorescent antibody staining is a quick and ready method, but less sensitive and more non-specific
- Legionella urinary antigen detects legionella in urine.

Radioimmunoassay (RIA) and enzyme-linked immunosorbent assay (ELISA) are available. Rapid serological tests are good for epidemiological investigations, but not for case management. Four-fold rise in antibody titer or an antibody titer of 128 or more is suggestive of infection. Sometimes a few weeks may be required for serology to become positive.

Legionella pneumophila responds to erythromycin and rifampicin if given early in the course of the disease.

Dose of erythromycin is 500 mg 6 h oral.	
Alternate drugs include:	
Roxithromycin	300 mg oral bd
Azithromycin	500 mg oral or intravenous (IV) daily
Ciprofloxacin	500 mg oral—8 h or 750 mg oral bd

In severe cases ciprofloxacin may have to be given IV initially, later to be changed to oral dosage. The total duration of treatment has to be up to 21 days. The disease carries a mortality ranging from 10 to 20%. Immunocompromised subjects suffer more. *Legionella* in water tanks can be sterilized by heating to 70–80°C or chlorination.

LISTERIOSIS

This is a food-borne infection affecting humans, especially dangerous during pregnancy and in immunocompromised hosts. This organism—*Listeria monocytogenes* exists in the environment as a saprophyte which can become invasive and affect many animals including man.

L. monocytogenes is facultative anaerobe, gram-positive, rod-shaped bacteria. Serotypes 1/2a, 1/2b and 4 as pathogenic.

Infection is by ingestion of contaminated food. The organism internalizes into several cells of the host and spreads from cell to cell. The bacterial entry into host's cells is facilitated by the host's surface proteins called internalins. The internalins help the bacteria to cross the natural barriers like intestinal epithelium, blood-brain and maternal-fetoplacental interphases. The β-hemolyins produced by the organism confer pathogenicity. Cellular immunity caused by CD⁺ T-cells is the main protective system of the host against the organism.

Epidemiology: *L. monocytogenes* causes sporadic infection. Mother to fetus transmission may occur if it occurs during pregnancy.

Clinical lesions produced by L. monocytogenes:

- ***Gastroenteritis:*** Incubation period is up to 2 days after ingestion. The symptoms include fever, diarrhea, headache and general symptoms.
- ***Bacteremia:*** Causes fever, chills, arthralgia, mental confusion and meningism. Bacteremia is more common in cancer patients. Rarely endocarditis over diseased or prosthetic valves may occur.
- ***Meningitis:*** In endemic areas this leads to community acquired bacterial meningitis. The clinical picture is one of subacute meningitis. Focal neurological deficits and seizures may develop. The cerebrospinal fluid (CSF) picture is that of aseptic meningitis with moderate pleocytosis with predominant neutrophils. Gram staining of the CSF may reveal the organism.
- ***Meningoencephalitis:*** Direct invasion of brain parenchyma may result in cerebritis, brain abscess, meningoencephalitis and brain stem lesions affecting the medulla and pons.
- ***Listeriosis during pregnancy:*** This is a serious problem starting with subacute fever and general symptoms caused by bacteremia. Blood culture at this stage may reveal the organism.
- ***Fetal problems:*** Include preterm delivery and fetal infection in > 70% of cases. Fetal death occurs in 50%. Generalized infection of the infant leading to military lesions (microabscesses and granulomas) termed ***granulomatosis infantiseptica***. These lesions may be evident at birth. Infants can also develop overt infection postpartum up to 1 month after birth. If the infection is diagnosed early and treatment given to mother—both mother and baby recover.
- ***Prognosis:*** Those receiving treatment before the localization of the disease, recover almost completely. Those who have developed complications may get sequelae like neurological defects, seizures and others. Mortality is around 20–25%. Since, the infection is sporadic in most cases strong clinical suspicion is needed to detect the disease and institute early treatment.
- ***Treatment:*** The drug of choice is ampicillin IV 2 g every 4 h in adults. Penicillin and Trimethoprim (TMP) are both effective alternatives. Dose of TMP is 15–20 mg/kg/bw per day given in divided doses 6 hours.
  An effective regimen in serious cases is to combine ampicillin with gentamicin 1–1.7 mg/kg/bw every 8 h, especially in neonates. Duration of therapy depends upon the lesion—2 weeks for bacteremia, 4–6 weeks for endocarditis and 6–8 weeks for encephalitis/brain abscess. Neonates should receive treatment for > 2 weeks.
- ***Prevention:*** By proper food hygiene, washing hands and vegetables and proper cooking of animal food. Unpasteurized dairy products—especially soft cheese may be avoided, since it is likely to be contaminated.

YAWS

Syn: Framboesia [meaning raspberries (French)]

General Considerations

Yaws and ***Pinta*** are nonvenereal diseases caused by spirochetes which resemble *Treponema pallidum* morphologically and serologically, but differ in pathogenesis and epidemiology. Primary infection is usually acquired in childhood. Transplacental transmission of infection does not occur usually. Pathologic lesions are confined to the skin and bones, the other viscera are not affected as in syphilis.

Yaws is widely prevalent in the tropics and subtropics. It is seen sporadically in all parts of India, though the disease is more prevalent in Africa. The causative organism is *Treponema pallidum pertenue*. The discharges from the primary and early secondary lesions teem with the organisms. *Treponema pallidum pertenue* has corkscrew mobility, dark field microscopy reveals the actively motile spirochete. The pertenue subspecies has been detected in gorilla population in Congo. Serological tests resemble those of syphilis. Several genetic differences between *Treponema pallidum* and *Treponema pallidum pertenue* have been described. Untreated individuals develop strain specific immunity to reinfection. Unless treated, yaws remains an indolent chronic disfiguring disease.

Other treponematosis include Bejel (endemic syphilis) and Pinta which used to be prevalent in South America. Transmission is much more efficient during the wet seasons. Portals of entry are abrasions of the skin. Overcrowding and poor personal hygiene favors the transmission.

Three stages—primary, secondary and tertiary can be identified during the course of the disease. With the improvement in living conditions and advent of penicillin therapy the picture of yaws and its prevalence have changed considerably, though there are some suggestions that the disease is also showing signs of resurgence.

The pathological lesions in the early stages within five years of infection take the form of papillomas. Late yaws develops five or more years after the onset. These take the form of gummatous changes with widespread tissue destruction, mutilation and ulceration (Figs 43.1 to 43.4).

Clinical Features

- ***The primary stage:*** This shows red maculopapular lesions which develop at the site of inoculation of the organism after three to six weeks. These enlarge and become multiple. They are painless but pruritic. Ordinarily they heal without scarring.
- ***The secondary lesions*** develop in crops, weeks to months after the healing of the primary lesions. Though

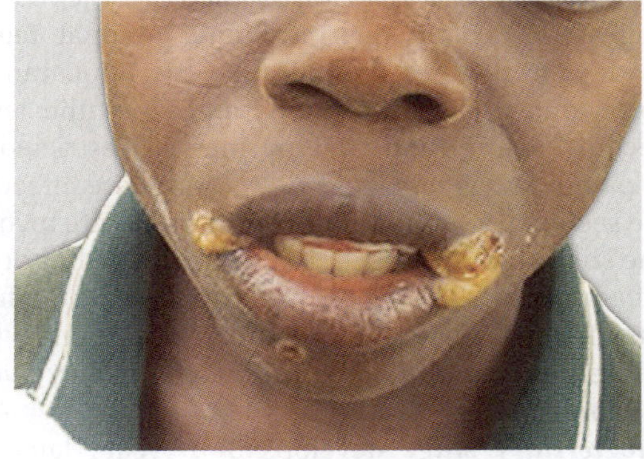

Fig. 43.1: Yaws secondary stage condylomass angles of the mouth

Textbook of Medicine

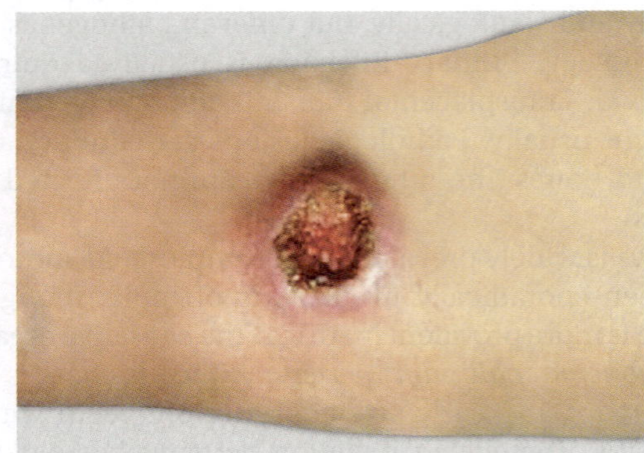

Fig. 43.2: Yaws secondary lesions deep necrotic indolent ulcer leg

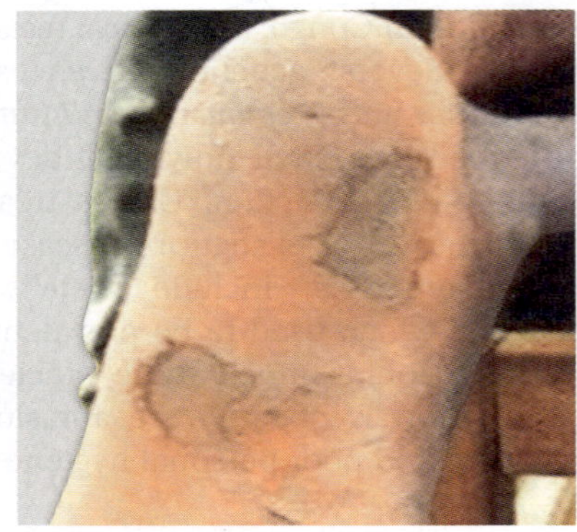

Fig. 43.3: Yaws secondary stage painful superficial and indolent ulcerations of sole of the foot (crab yaws)

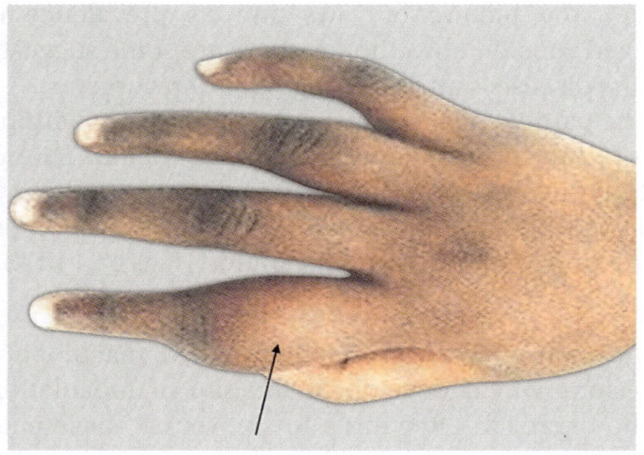

Fig. 43.4: Dactylitis in late stages of yaws. **Note:** Thickening of metacarpophalangeal (MCP) joint right index finger (arrow)

they resemble the primary lesions, they are more numerous and widely distributed over circumoral (Fig. 43.1), axillary, perineal and perianal regions. In the moist areas they assume the appearance of condylomas. Over the palms and soles the lesions become painful and walking may be restricted due to pain *(crab yaws) (Fig. 43.3)*. Bones are affected in the secondary stage. Multiple long bones are involved. The shaft shows cortical rarefaction and subperiosteal inflammation and new bone formation. The affected part is thickened and painful. Nasal bones show thickening *(gondou)* and the tibial lesion may give rise to sabre tibia.

- *The tertiary stage* develops 5–10 years later with gummatous and destructive lesions. The skin and bones are affected. Deep ulcers develop which show overhanging edges. Chronic destructive lesions in the bone may lead to discharging sinuses. Extensive destruction of the facial tissues with gross mutilation of the nose and mouth leads to the formation of a single open cavity *(gangosa)*.

Diagnosis

Clinical suspicion should be strong to diagnose this condition since it occurs sporadically or in families and the condition is likely to be missed by the unwary physician.

Yaws has to be differentiated from other granulomatous lesions involving the skin and bones such as syphilis, tuberculosis, leprosy and mucocutaneous leishmaniasis all of which may cause lesions similar to gondou. The diagnosis is confirmed by demonstrating the treponemes in the discharges from primary and secondary lesions by dark ground illumination. Serological findings resemble those of syphilis.

Treatment

Dramatic improvement occurs with a single dose of 1.2 mega units of benzathine penicillin given intramuscularly (IM). An alternative regimen is to give tetracycline 1–2 g daily for 5 days. Early cases are cured, whereas, in late cases, mutilation may persist.

A single dose of azithromycin in a dose of 30 mg/kg orally gives a 94% clearance of the infection after 6 months. **Source:** Oriol Mitja, et al. Trial in Papua New Guinea. The Lancet. 2012;379:362-67.

PINTA

Pinta, which is also a non-venereal treponemal disease prevalent in South and Central America, is caused by *Treponema carateum.* Transmission occurs by close physical contact and the organism enters through skin abrasions. Exudates from the early skin lesions are highly infective.

Clinical Features

The incubation period is 7–21 days. Three stages are recognizable. The early stage develops in a few months of infection. The primary lesions develop at the site of inoculation as erythematous, pruritic papules, which coalesce to form ulcers, which take a long time to heal. Scarring and depigmentation occur at these sites. The secondary stage develops three to twelve months after the primary stage. This stage is characterized by pruritic and deeply pigmented areas. Morphologically these lesions resemble the primary lesions, but they are smaller and more numerous and widely distributed. Lesions at different stages of development occur simultaneously. Constitutional symptoms may occur at this stage. This stage is infective. When the skin lesions heal, atrophy, scarring and depigmentation result.

Diagnosis

The discharges from early skin lesions reveal spirochetes on dark ground illumination. In late lesions organisms may not be demonstrable. Serological tests for syphilis are positive in such cases.

Treatment

Single dose of 1.2 mega units of benzathine penicillin given IM is curative in most of the cases. The early lesions heal. The serological titers fall but the test may remain positive over low titers over long periods.

RELAPSING FEVERS

KV Krishna Das, K Sreekanthan

Borrelial Infections

Borrelia are helical rods 8–30 μm long and 0.2–0.5 μm in diameter with 3–10 loose spirals, actively motile and stainable by aniline dyes. In man, they cause relapsing fevers and Lyme borreliosis. Relapsing fevers are further classified into louse-borne and tick-borne varieties depending on the vector which transmits the disease viz. body louse or soft tick. Lyme disease is transmitted by hard tick (Figs 43.5A and B).

Louse-borne Relapsing Fever

This disease is caused by *Borrelia recurrentis.* It affects only humans. Epidemics used to follow wars, famines or natural catastrophes such as floods or earthquakes. Overcrowding, malnutrition and unhygienic surroundings start off epidemics in the tropics and temperate zones. Severe epidemics have occurred in north Africa, middle east and Europe following world war II and the mortality was as high as 70%. The vector is the body louse *(Pediculus humanus corporis)* which is infected by blood meal containing the organism from infected persons. The louse becomes infective in 5–15 days and the organisms are found in its body cavity. It remains infective for its whole lifespan (1 month). Lice leave their host when the temperature is high or when the temperature drops due to its death. Pruritus caused by their bites leads to scratching and the lice are crushed. Smearing of their infected body contents and excreta to the bite wound results in infection of the host. Lice do not transmit the infection transovarially to their progeny.

Pathology

In the early phase of infection bacteremia develops and borreliae can be demonstrated in blood films outside the cells. Bacteremia coincides with the change of surface antigens of the borrelia which helps to evade the immune system and cause multiplication and recurrent bacteremia. They invade most of the viscera, especially the spleen, liver, brain, meninges, kidneys and the heart. Skin, mucous membranes and serous surfaces show petechial hemorrhage. Consumption coagulopathy may occur resulting in thrombocytopenia. Renal involvement leads to proteinuria and hematuria. Macrophages in the liver, spleen, lymph nodes and bone marrow may show engulfed borreliae. After an attack of fever the spirochetes disappear from the blood to reappear again during relapse. Probably immunological factors are important in producing clearance of these organisms.

Clinical Features

The clinical features may be varied and affection of different systems may be predominant in different cases. These include neurological features, general febrile illness or GI manifestations. The incubation period varies between 2 and 12 days, but is usually 7–10 days. Onset is abrupt with high fever, rapid pulse, headache, body pains, conjunctival congestion, epistaxis and sometimes a petechial rash. Mild or moderate thrombocytopenia may occur.

Herpes labialis may develop. The liver and spleen enlarge and become palpable. Jaundice, meningism and intestinal hemorrhage may occur. In four to ten days the fever comes down by crisis, but in some cases it returns after 5–7 days. Two or three such relapses may occur in succession. The relapses are generally milder and less prolonged. In epidemics, the mortality used to be as high as 40% especially in children and the elderly. After recovery from the illness immunity lasts for 1–2 years. Louse-borne relapsing fever carries a higher mortality than the tick-borne variety.

Diagnosis

Examination of blood films stained with Giemsa's or Leishman's stain reveal the borreliae. Dark ground or phase contrast microscopy of fresh blood may show the motile organisms.

Polymerase chain reaction (PCR) helps to identify the organisms. Monoclonal antibody tests help to identify the species of Borrelia. Four-fold rise of antibody between acute and convalescent phases strongly supports the diagnosis. ELISA and indirect immunofluorescence. Antibody assay are used for detecting the antibody depending on their availability.

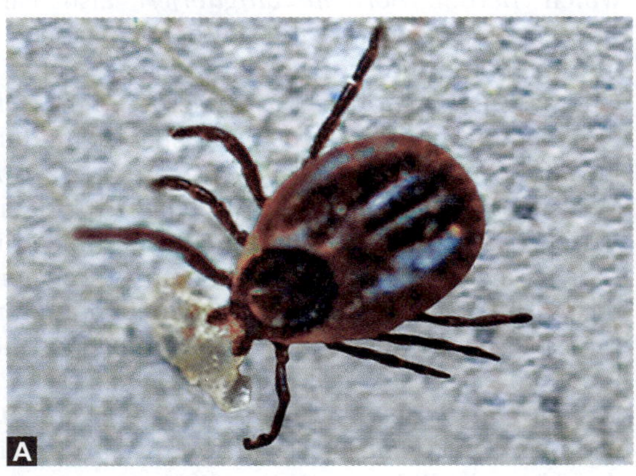

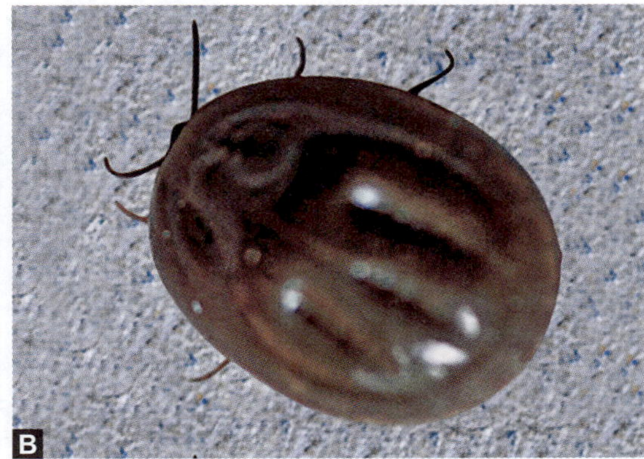

Figs 43.5A and B: **A.** Hard tick; **B.** Soft tick

Textbook of Medicine

Treatment

The disease responds well to penicillin and tetracycline in the usual doses, the former is slower in action. Drug therapy may lead to severe Jarisch-Herxheimer reaction with profound fall in temperature, shock and cardiac failure within a few hours. This potential complication should be expected and supportive measures instituted promptly. Initial administration of procaine penicillin 500,000 units on the first day, followed subsequently by doxycycline 100 mg bd oral/day has been recommended as a safer course. Other antibiotics to which the organism is sensitive include chloramphenicol and erythromycin, both given in doses of 500 mg 6 h for 7–10 days.

In cases with neurological features lumbar puncture (LP) may be done for diagnosis. Antibiotics should be given by the parenteral route in these cases.

Prevention

The disease can be prevented by undertaking delousing measures. Use of 10% dichlorodiphenyltrichloroethane (DDT) powder effectively kills the lice. Boiling the clothes and bed linen for 30 minutes destroys the lice and their eggs.

Tick-borne Relapsing Fever

The causative organism is *Borrelia duttoni* which is transmitted by several species of soft ticks (Argasidae). Several antigenic variants of the same species have been identified in different regions, e.g. *B. novyi, B. carteri,* etc. Endemicity in a region is determined by the vector population. In the middle east, Iran and Afghanistan *Ornithodoros tholozoni* is the main vector. In these regions non-human animal reservoirs like rodents or bats exist. The ticks are infected from them and they transmit the infection to humans accidentally. In north India, relapsing fever is caused by *B. carteri* spread by *O. tholozoni, O. crossi, O. lahorensis* and the fowl tick *Argas persicus.* In central and east Africa, the infection is mainly confined to human and the vector is *O. moubata* which inhabits mud floors, crevices in dwelling places or camp sites. Ticks transmit infection transovarially to the progeny so that a large colony of infected ticks develops which acts as a reservoir of infection. The soft ticks live for 14–21 years and can subsist on blood meals taken at very long intervals. These ticks bite at night and the bite is painless. They attack several animals and man is only incidentally affected. They insert their mouth parts into the skin and remain attached to the body for a few days taking their blood meal, after which they fall off. The site of attachment shows a pruritic erythematous lesion which develops into an eschar. The eschar takes the form of a clean punched-out ulcer commonly seen in the body folds and moist regions. Presence of eschar should be specially looked for and if detected, it is strongly suggestive of the diagnosis. Both the adults and the larval forms suck blood. The saliva, coxal fluid and excreta of ticks contain the organisms. Borrelia enter through the bite wound, abrasions on the skin and also intact mucous membranes. Pathology resembles that of louse-borne relapsing fever, but neurological involvement is more frequent.

Clinical Features

Tick-borne relapsing fever resembles louse-borne relapsing fever, but the febrile bouts may be shorter, lasting only for 3–5 days, so also the apyrexial intervals. Number of relapses are more and may reach up to ten. Neurological complications occur during relapses. These include facial palsy, optic atrophy, spastic paraplegia and other focal paralysis. Mortality is lower than in louse-borne relapsing fever. Though substantial immunity occurs, it is not permanent.

Diagnosis

The clinical diagnosis is supported by the demonstration of the organisms in stained blood smears or by dark ground microscopy. Compared to the louse-borne disease, the organisms are less numerous. Other diagnostic methods such as animal inoculation studies using rats, mice and guinea pigs are available.

Treatment

The disease responds to tetracycline 1 g given daily for seven days and repeated after a week if necessary. Though Jarisch-Herxheimer reaction may develop, it is less pronounced. Doxycycline in a single dose of 200 mg is effective against the borrelia but allergic reactions are more frequent.

Prevention

Ticks can be destroyed by spraying with Lindane 1% (gamma BHC). Visitors to infected areas should be informed of the risk. They should wear protective clothing and use insect repellents. Ticks should be looked for and removed mechanically from the body before going to bed after the day's work.

Note: Relapsing fever are being reported more commonly in several states in India, hence strong clinical suspicion is required to diagnose the condition without missing.

LYME BORRELIOSIS

This is caused by the spirochete *Borrelia burgdorferi,* transmitted by hard ticks *Ixodes ricinus* and *Ixodes persulcatus* in Eurasia and *Ixodes dammini, Ixodes pacificus* and *Ixodes scapularis* in North America. The organisms are present in the saliva of the ticks. Tick bites are generally painless. Ticks inhabit woods. Ticks which harbor *Borrelia burgdorferi* also can harbor *Borrelia miyamotoi*— the latter can affect old and immunocompromised hosts and can cause disease, whereas *B. burgdorferi* (OspA serotype 1) is the main organism in the USA, three other species predominate in Europe. These include *B. afzelii* (serotype 2), *B. garinii* (serotypes 3, 5, 6 and 7) and *B. bavariensis* (serotype 4). Various intermediate and small mammals including rodents act as reservoirs. Birds help to transfer infected ticks over great distances during their migratory flights. Maternal-fetal transmission of infection has been recorded.

Borrelia burgdorferi is 10–30 μ long and 0.2–0.25 μ wide. Unlike *T. pallidum,* it can be grown in artificial media, though with difficulty. Three different genospecies and seven serotypes have been identified. This fact possibly accounts for the different organotropism and virulence exhibited in various geographical areas.

Borrelia miyamotoi was first discovered in Japan in 1995, it may co-exist in Lyme disease vector globally.

Larval and adult ticks may harbor *Anaplasma phagocytophilum*, *Babesia* species and encephalitis virus. These may co-infect patients with *Lyme borreliosis*. Ticks that remain attached to the human host for more than 24 hours transmit the disease more readily.

Pathology

After entry of the organism into the human host they spread locally and produce erythema migrans, in which several rings of erythema can be detected, these are painless. Spread to other organs is through the blood stream or lymph. Both cellular and humoral mechanisms develop to arrest infection.

The disease affects mainly the skin, nervous system, heart and joints. The organisms have been isolated from various specimens such as blood, skin, CSF, eye, joint fluid and myocardium, indicating that the organisms get disseminated widely. The organisms are present in the lesions extracellularly. Histologically the lesions show inflammatory infiltrate consisting mainly of lymphocytes, histiocytes and plasma cells. The total pathogenesis may be the sum total of direct invasion, stimulation of several inflammatory cytokines and autoimmune mechanisms.

Clinical Features

Incubation period ranges from weeks to months. Three clinical stages are seen. The first two stages are early manifestations, the third is late manifestation.

Stage I: Clinical lesion is erythema migrans which is a rash spreading centrifugally.

Stage II: Early disseminated infection.

This develops a few weeks to months after infection. Several organs become affected, probably because of hematogenous spread. Lesions include:

Neurological features (Lyme neuroborreliosis) include meningoradiculitis, meningitis, cranial neuritis involving predominantly facial nerve, plexus neuritis, mononeuritis multiplex and rarely encephalitis, myelitis and cerebral vasculitis.

Meningoradiculitis also known as Bannawarth's syndrome—which is common, is characterized by CSF pleocytosis and severe radicular pain, especially worse at night. Other accompaniments of meningitis such as severe headache and signs of meningeal irritation are not present. Blindness may develop. Neurological sequelae may develop.

Cardiac manifestations include heart block, arrhythmias and heart failure. ***Arthralgias*** and ***myofasciitis*** can develop at this stage. Localized or generalized lymphadenopathy may occur. Ocular involvement presents as conjunctivitis, iridocyclitis, choroiditis and optic neuropathy with papilledema and panophthalmitis. Rarely hepatitis and orchitis may occur.

Stage III: This develops months to years after infection. This is characterized by mono or oligoarticular arthritis affecting the large joints, particularly the knees. Synovial fluid shows neutrophil leukocytosis. In a few cases, complete resolution of arthritis may not occur. Residual disabling arthralgia and arthritis may persist for several months. The joint manifestations and neurological sequelae are due to immune mediated (complement mediated) lysis of the borrelia, recruitment of neutrophils and macrophages to the site of infection and production of proinflammatory cytokines. Histological examination shows infiltration by lymphocytes, macrophages and plasma cells with some degree of vasculitis. All these lead to prolonged disability even after cure of the infection. This stage has been designated as post-Lyme syndrome.

Skin lesions develop in the extremities as bluish-red edematous areas which go on to atrophy and wrinkles. These are called ***acrodermatitis chronica atrophicans (ACA)***.

Rarely progressive Lyme encephalitis and encephalomyelitis characterized by spastic paresis and ataxia may develop. Several other rare manifestations have been described.

Diagnosis

This is based on endemicity, evidence of tick bite and the clinical picture. Only 0.5–1% of tick bites in affected regions transmit the infection. Material removed by biopsy from the margins of the erythema can be used to culture the organism and also demonstrate them by PCR.

Serological tests to demonstrate IgG antibodies by ELISA, indirect immunofluorescence assay (IFA) and western blot are available in specialized laboratories. Both serum and CSF have to be tested to diagnose neuroborreliosis.

The cultivation of the organisms from body fluids is difficult and hence serological tests are used for diagnosis routinely.

Treatment

Stage I: Doxycycline, amoxicillin, cefuroxime and ceftriaxone are the most effective antibiotics.

Stage II: High dose IV crystalline penicillin as is given for meningitis leads to fast resolution of radicular pain. Corticosteroids given concurrently accelerate relief. Other alternatives are ceftriaxone and cefotaxime.

Stage III: Arthritis responds to doxycycline and amoxicillin. Resistant cases respond to ceftriaxone, cefotaxime or high dose IV penicillin (Table 43.1).

Rarely, Jarisch-Herxheimer reaction may develop during treatment.

Prevention

Tick bites can be avoided by wearing protective clothing impregnated with permethrin which is a tick repellent. In endemic areas examination of the body parts after exposure to infective environment and removal of ticks within 36 hours of their bite without breaking their mouth parts and removal of ticks adhering to clothes serve to

Table 43.1: Dose of antimicrobials for Lyme disease	
Doxycycline	2 × 100 mg/day × 14 days
Amoxicillin	3 × 500–1000 mg/day × 14 days
Cefuroxime	2 × 500 mg/day × 14 days
Ceftriaxone	IV 2 g/day × 21 days
Phenoxymethylpenicillin	Oral 3 × 1–1.5 million units/day × 14 days

prevent infection. Chemoprophylaxis consists of giving a single dose of 200 mg doxycycline which is effective if given within 3 days of the tick bite.

Vaccine

Two vaccines were developed against *B. burgdorferi* in 1990, which were highly efficient. Then vaccines were based on the OspA proteins of the bactérie antibodies agent. OspA prevent replication of the organisms in the tick. Studies are going in to prepare vaccines effective against the different strains.

Source: Plotkin SA. Need for a New Lyme Disease Vaccine. N Engl J Med. 2016;375(10):911-3.

Leptospirosis

R Sajith Kumar, KV Krishna Das

Chapter Summary

- General Considerations
- Pathology
- Clinical Features
- Diagnosis
- Treatment
- Prevention

GENERAL CONSIDERATIONS

Leptospirosis is one of the most common zoonotic disease across the world, caused by pathogenic spiral bacteria belonging to the genus *Leptospira*, the family leptospiraceae and the order spirochetales. These are finely coiled, thin, motile, obligate, slow-growing anaerobes. Their flagella allow them to burrow into tissues. The genus *Leptospira* was originally thought to comprise only of 2 species—*L. interrogans*, which is pathogenic and *L. biflexa*, which is saprophytic. Recent work has identified seven distinct species of pathogenic *Leptospira* which appear as more than 250 serologic variants (serovars). The classic *L. interrogans* species, is divided into 7 named and 5 unnamed species as follows.

L. interrogans, L. weilii, L. santarosai, L. noguchi, L. borgpetersenii, L. inadai, L. kirschner and *Leptospira* species 1, 2, 3, 4 and 5. They infect many types of mammals including rats, dogs, cats, cattle, pigs, squirrels, raccoons, mongooses and bandicoots. Leptospires are passed in the urine of infected animals, even though many of them do not suffer from the disease. They remain viable and infective in fresh water for varying periods up to 16 days and in soil for up to 24 days. They infect humans by entering through intact mucosal surfaces of the conjunctiva, oronasal cavity, genitourinary tract and others or disrupted skin, when the person bathes, wades through contaminated puddles and fields or engages in underwater activities. The organisms are killed by even minor changes in the temperature, acidity, salinity, chlorine content and other physical and chemical changes.

Epidemiology

The disease was first recognized as an occupational disease of sewer workers in 1883. In 1886, Adolf Weil described the clinical manifestations in four men who had severe jaundice, fever and hemorrhage with renal involvement. Inada, et al. identified the causal agent in Japan in 1916. Almost all published case series focussed on seasonal outbreaks associated with changes in local water levels, flood conditions and increased risk of exposure of the population to infection. In India most outbreaks follow flooding in monsoon seasons. Andaman, Tamil Nadu and Kerala have been witnessing many epidemics from the middle of the twentieth century. Workers employed in paddy, pineapple and sugarcane cultivation and people engaged in underwater occupations like sand mining, inland water fishing and cleaning of contaminated water logged areas are predisposed to get the infection. The disease is also more common among butchers, veterinary staff and people who handle live cattle, dogs and other pets. Leptospirosis has been encountered in almost all major hospitals all over the country.

Only about 10% of all leptospirosis cases run the classic clinical picture and get diagnosed. The majority may get only a non-specific febrile illness or may be even subclinical. Still all develop antibodies and therefore a large proportion of the population in many endemic regions possess antileptospiral antibodies.

Using microagglutination techniques, the major serogroups prevalent in Kerala were grippotyphosa, australis, autumnalis, icterohemorrhagiae and louisiana. A new serovar Bharathy type Kolenchery has also been identified in Kerala.

PATHOLOGY

Entry of leptospira through the skin or mucous membrane is followed by extensive proliferation of the organism in blood and many tissues. The resulting leptospiremia causes widespread distribution and further damage in many organs. Leptospiremia stage is followed by disappearance of the organisms from blood, but this is followed later by the appearance of leptospira in urine (leptospirosis phase). Most of the pathological manifestations are due to immunologically mediated injury, even though direct invasion by the organism may also cause damage. The true mechanism of injury is not very clear even though

Textbook of Medicine

complex interactions involving endotoxin, hemolysin and lipase are thought to play major roles.

The pathologic findings in many organs include vasculitis of capillaries causing endothelial edema, necrosis and lymphocytic infiltration and hemorrhage. Capillary vasculitis leads to loss of red blood cells (RBC) and fluid through the vascular wall. This causes secondary tissue injury. Platelet count is reduced in a good proportion of patients. Bleeding tendencies such as petechiae and mucosal bleeding (subconjunctival bleeding in particular) occur. Bleeding may not always be directly proportional to thrombocytopenia or alterations in coagulation function since it is multifactorial in origin.

The liver shows vascular congestion and disorganization of the liver cell plates on histology. Hyperbilirubinemia occurs in leptospirosis. This is caused by hepatic injury, also contributed to by muscle damage and release of myoglobin, intra and extravascular hemolysis and hemorrhages.

In kidneys, interstitium, renal tubules and tubular lumen are affected causing interstitial nephritis and tubular necrosis. Renal failure is usually due to tubular damage, but hypovolemia resulting from dehydration and altered capillary permeability are also contributory.

In the lungs either focal or diffuse alveolar capillary injury is common. Interstitial and intra-alveolar edema and bleeding can occur. Fatal adult respiratory distress syndrome (ARDS) may occur without warning.

In the heart, epicardial and endocardial petechiae, interstitial edema and lymphocyte and plasma cell infiltration of the myocardium, myocarditis and coronary arteritis may develop.

CLINICAL FEATURES (FIG. 44.1)

The incubation period is usually 7–12 days, with a range of 2–20 days. Approximately 90% of patients manifest mild anicteric form of the disease. Five to ten percent have the severe form with jaundice, classically known as Weil's disease. The natural course of leptospirosis falls into two distinct phases: leptospiremic and immune phases. During a brief period of 1–3 days between the 2 phases, the patient shows some improvement.

The leptospiremic phase resembles any viral fever with high temperatures, generalized myalgia, sore throat, cough, chest pain, hemoptysis, generalized rash and frontal headache. Conjunctival suffusion and prominent myalgia and tenderness over big muscles are very suggestive of leptospirosis. Many cases recover and the patient may become afebrile within a week.

The next phase, also called immune or leptospirosis phase is associated with the appearance of antibodies in blood and elimination of leptospira in urine. Symptoms may persist for 6 days to more than 4 weeks, with a mean duration of 14 days.

There are two well-defined patterns, icteric and non-icteric. The non-icteric illness is more common.

The Non-icteric Illness

The presenting feature is usually headache, attributable to aseptic meningitis, confusion, irritability and occasionally delirium. Cutaneous manifestations include hemorrhages and maculopapular eruptions on the trunk. ***The involvement of kidneys leads to rapid development of oliguric renal failure, which may necessitate dialysis therapy.*** Hyperkalemia and metabolic acidosis are common.

The Icteric Illness

The icteric illness is usually associated with deep jaundice, acalculous cholecystitis, pancreatitis and gastrointestinal (GI) bleeding. Bilirubin levels may exceed 30 mg/dL. Aspartate aminotransferase (AST) and alanine aminotransferase (ALT) are moderately elevated, the elevation being considerably less compared to the rise in bilirubin. This is in contrast to the picture in viral hepatitis in which the elevation of transaminases is much more prominent.

Cervical, axillary and mediastinal lymph nodes may be enlarged. ***Different types of bleeding*** can occur ranging from epistaxis and gingival oozing to hematuria, hemoptysis and pulmonary hemorrhage. Subconjunctival hemorrhage is common. It is not related to platelet count or coagulation abnormalities. Uveitis and iridocyclitis may occur.

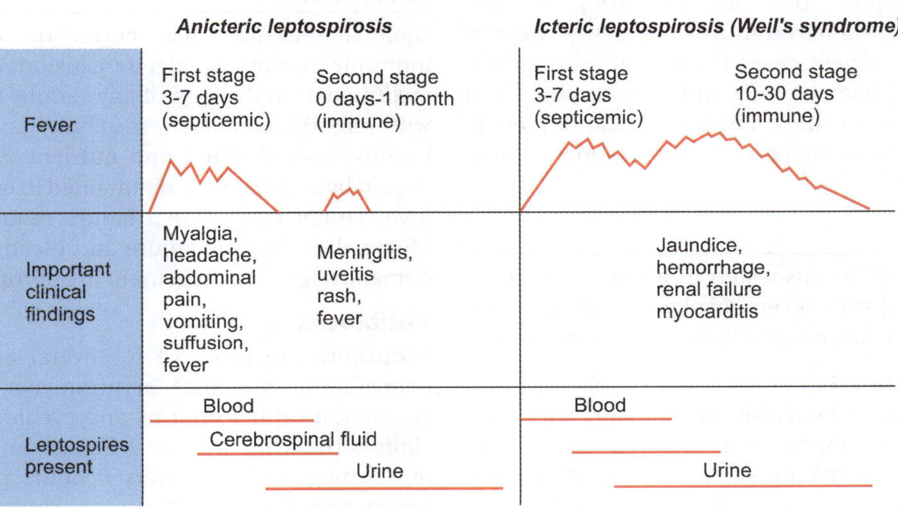

Fig. 44.1: Salient features of anicteric and icteric forms of leptospirosis

Textbook of Medicine

Pulmonary manifestations include cough, hemoptysis and pneumonia. Chest X-ray may show multifocal infiltrates, as well as pleural effusions. ***Respiratory symptoms*** may progress to ARDS, requiring intubation and mechanical ventilation. ***Myocarditis*** and ***coronary arteritis*** may occur. These present as first-degree AV block in 30% of patients early in the disease. It resolves completely with recovery. Atrial fibrillation may occur; this carries a bad prognosis. Electrocardiogram (ECG) changes includes T-wave inversion in 18%, ST-segment elevation in 15% and abnormalities of rhythm in 11%. Renal involvement to produce acute oliguric renal failure is also common.

It is known that clinical features of leptospirosis are not specific to the infecting organism, since considerable overlap may occur in the disease manifestation caused by the different serovars. But some clinical manifestations are more frequently seen by infection by particular serotypes. These include:

Hepatorenal lesions	*L. icterohaemorrhagiae*
Pretibial skin lesion	*L. autumnalis* (Fort Bragg fever)
Meningeal symptoms	*L. canicola*

Weil's Syndrome

- Weil's syndrome is not a specific subgroup of leptospirosis, but indicates severe leptospirosis. It can develop during the second (immune) phase of leptospirosis or as a progressive illness.
- ***Components of Weil's syndrome:*** It is dramatic life-threatening event, characterized by: a) Jaundice, b) acute kidney injury and c) hemorrhage.
  - ***Jaundice:*** The first manifestation of severe leptospirosis is usually jaundice. It develops between 5th and 9th day. Jaundice is deep and is not due to hepatocellular damage, but probably due to cholestasis or sepsis.
  - ***Renal failure:*** Primarily due to impaired renal perfusion and acute tubular necrosis. It presents as oliguria or anuria, with the presence of albumin, blood and casts in the urine.
  - Hemorrhagic manifestations are common and include purpura, petechiae appearing on oral, vaginal or conjunctival mucosa and large areas of bruising. In severe cases there may be epistaxis, hemoptysis, hematemesis and melena (due to GI bleeding), hemorrhage into adrenal glands pleural, pericardial or subarachnoid spaces (subarachnoid hemorrhage).

DIAGNOSIS

Leptospirosis should be suspected in all cases of febrile jaundice associated with severe myalgia, prostration and conjunctival congestion, especially during local outbreaks.

Laboratory Diagnosis

Polymorphonuclear leukocytosis, occasionally with toxic granules and band forms and elevated erythrocyte sedimentation rate (ESR) are seen in about 90% cases. Mild thrombocytopenia may occur in up to 50% cases. Urine examination reveals proteinuria with leukocytes, erythrocytes, hyaline casts and granular casts in the sediment. As noted earlier the gross elevation in serum bilirubin is associated with only a mild or moderate elevation in transaminase values. Creatine phosphokinase (CPK) is markedly elevated, particularly in patients with muscle tenderness. Higher values of serum alkaline phosphatase suggests cholestasis.

Demonstration or culture of leptospira from blood or urine samples demand advanced laboratory facilities. Dark field examination and use of immunofluorescent techniques are helpful in early stages. The serologic tests become positive by the end of the first week. These include macroscopic and microscopic agglutination using antigens for identifying the strains and enzyme-linked immunosorbent assay (ELISA) tests using mono-specific antigens to identify serovars. False positive and false negative results are common. Rising titers are more helpful in diagnosis. More recently, rapid commercial tests such as dipsticks (Dry-dot) which contain antigens and used to detect leptospira antibodies in blood, have been made available. Cerebrospinal fluid (CSF) may show moderate lymphocytic pleocytosis (200–300/mm^3).

Differential Diagnosis

Leptospirosis mimics almost any febrile illness at different stages. These include dengue fever, encephalitis, Hantavirus, hemorrhagic fever with renal syndrome, hepatitis, cholecystitis, yellow fever, rickettsia diseases, falciparum malaria, meningitis, infectious mononucleosis and even enteric fever.

Prognosis

Leptospirosis is a serious illness with mortality ranging from 10 to 30% depending on the stage of disease at which people seek treatment and proper early diagnosis. Serious patients may die within 24 hours of hospitalization. Death is due to renal failure, generalized bleeding, shock, ARDS or myocarditis. Hepatic failure per se is not a common cause of death even in jaundiced patients. Infection acquired in the early months of pregnancy is associated with higher incidence of spontaneous abortion.

TREATMENT

General measures like correction of fluid balance, inotropic support, platelet transfusions and others must be instituted as in the case of any serious illness. All patients with oliguria, confusion, irritability and bleeding should be hospitalized. Fluid and nutrient intake-output chart should be meticulously maintained in order to detect renal involvement early. Renal failure requires early dialysis. Myocarditis, hepatic failure and bleeding manifestations demand special management in appropriate facilities.

Antibiotics

Leptospira are sensitive to several antibiotics such as penicillin, tetracyclines, erythromycin, quinolones, third generation cephalosporins doxycycline and others. Penicillin is the drug of choice. Benzylpenicillin G in a dose of 1.5 mega units IV every 6 hours produces dramatic improvement in 24–72 hours. Penicillin is continued in the same dose till the acute symptoms subside and thereafter in a reduced dose. Rarely ***Jarisch-Herxheimer reaction*** develops at the commencement of bactericidal therapy. This has to be managed with antihistamines, supportive measures and corticosteroids. In those patients who are allergic to penicillin, doxycycline erythromycin, chloramphenicol and quinolones are also effective alternative drugs.

Important points in the management of leptoscpirosis:
- All cases should be hospitalized, since sudden deterioration of apparently mild cases is not uncommon. These require emergency management.
- ***Antibiotic therapy:*** Leptospires are highly susceptible to a broad range of antibiotics. Early antibiotic therapy is indicated to prevent the development of major organ failures and for shortening the illness.
- ***For mild disease:*** Oral administration of antibiotics is sufficient if there is no vomiting. Doxycycline (100 mg orally twice daily) ampicillin (750 mg four times daily), amoxicillin (500 mg four times daily) or azithromycin 500 mg bd may be employed for 4–7 days.
- Severe cases should be treated with intravenous (IV) penicillin started early in a dose of 1.5 million units 6 hourly IV. Alternative drugs include ceftriaxone 1 g twice a day, cefotaxime 1g IV four times a day.
- Complications should be anticipated and treated early. Outcome can be bettered by appropriate intervention.

PREVENTION

Prevention of leptospirosis in animals is difficult. Environmental sanitation to avoid contamination of water sources by animal and rodent urine and care during bathing and wading through contaminated water should reduce infection. Proper washing with soap and water and quick drying of the skin after exposure to contaminated water reduce risk of infection. Treatment with bleaching powder kills the organisms.

Vaccination of domestic cattle and dogs has been tried with success. Dogs are regularly vaccinated in many countries including India.

Chemoprophylaxis

Doxycycline administered orally in a dose of 200 mg once weekly during the period of exposure is protective.

Points to Remember
- Leptospirosis has become a very common infection in many parts of India.
- Several serovars cause the disease.
- Brunt of the disease is borne by the liver and kidney, but several other organs may also be affected.
- Early diagnosis and treatment with penicillin or other antibiotics ensure cure in the vast majority.
- Prompt dialysis therapy saves life in severe renal involvement.

CHAPTER 45

Rickettsial Diseases, Q Fever, Human Ehrlichiosis and Anaplasmosis

KV Krishna Das, VP Gopinathan

Chapter Summary
- Rickettsial Diseases
  - General Considerations
  - Epidemic Typhus
  - Endemic Typhus
  - Scrub Typhus
  - Tick-borne Typhus
- Q Fever
- Human Ehrlichiosis and Anaplasmosis

RICKETTSIAL DISEASES

GENERAL CONSIDERATIONS

Rickettsiae are obligate intracellular gram-negative parasites seen in several parts of the world. These organisms are naturally found in arthropods which act as active vectors without themselves suffering. Rickettsiae are classified into three genera—*Rickettsia*, *Rochalimaea* and *Coxiella*. Tissue culture or the yolk sac of the embryonated egg has to be employed for growing them. Most are zoonoses spread to humans by the bite of arthropods vectors such as body louse, mites, ticks and fleas (except Q fever which is transmitted by ingestion of animal products).

Serological Diagnosis of Rickettsial Diseases

Agglutination of *Proteus vulgaris* (Weil-Felix reaction). Rickettsiae and *Proteus vulgaris* share common antigenic components and therefore infection by some rickettsial strains lead to the development of antibodies that agglutinate some strains of *Proteus vulgaris*. Detection of these antibodies by agglutination forms the basis of the ***Weil-Felix reaction*** which is a commonly used diagnostic test (Table 45.1).

The diagnosis can be confirmed by serologic, molecular, immunohistochemical and/or culture assays. A monoclonal antibody against a lipopolysaccharide has been shown to react with a stable antigen of *R. akari, R. conorii, R. rickettsii* that survive fixation with formaldehyde and embedding in paraffin before immuno-peroxidase staining of tissue. Skin biopsy in relevant cases yields diagnosis even when serology is negative. Table 45.2 summarizes salient features of rickettsia pathogens to humans.

EPIDEMIC TYPHUS

Syn: Louse borne typhus, Typhus exanthematicus, Gaol fever

Epidemic typhus is a severe febrile disease caused by *Rickettsia prowazekii*. Man is the only known host for this

Textbook of Medicine

Table 45.1: Details of rickettsiae pathogenic to man

Group	Agent	Vector and reservoir	Weil-Felix reaction
Typhus group			
• Epidemic typhus	*R. prowazekii*	Body louse (man)	+++ for OX-19
• Endemic typhus	*R. typhi*	Rat flea (rat) (formerly *R. mooseri*)	+++ for OX-19
• Brill-Zinsser disease	*R. prowazekii*	Body louse (man)	Usually negative
Spotted fever group			
• Rocky mountain spotted fever	*R. rickettsii*	Ticks (rabbit, dog and rodents)	++OX-19 and ++OX-2
• Mediterranean fever (fever boutonneuse)	*R. conorii*	Ticks (rodent, dogs)	++OX-19 and ++OX-2
• Rickettsial pox	*R. akari*	Gamasid mite (mouse)	Negative
• North Asian tick borne typhus	*R. siberica*	Tick (wild animals cattle, birds)	+OX-19 and OX-2
• Queensland tick typhus	*R. siberica*	Tick (bush rodents)	+OX-19 and OX-2
• Indian tick typhus	*R. conorii*	Tick (rodents)	+OX-19 and OX-2
• African tick bite fever	*R. africae*	Tick (cattle and goat)	
Scrub typhus (Tsutsugamushi fever)	*R. tsutsugamushi*	Trombiculid mite (small rodent, birds)	+++ OXK
Q fever	*Coxiella burnetii* which is a coccobacillus	Ticks transmit diseases negative in animals, human disease is occupational-cattle, sheep, goat	Negative

Note: Even though Weil-Felix reaction is still employed for diagnosis in many laboratories in India more precise tests are available in many places. These include polymerase chain reaction (PCR) tests, indirect fluorescent antibody (IFA) test (titer ≥ 1:200) and complement fixation test (CFT).

Table 45.2: Salient features of rickettsia pathogens to humans

Diseases	Rickettsial agent	Insect vector	Mammalian reservoir	Clinical features
Typhus group				
Epidemic typhus	*R. prowazekii*	Louse	Human	Fever/chills Myalgia Headache Rash (no eschar) all over body except palm sole and face
Murine typhus (endemic typhus)	*R. typhi*	Flea	Rodents	Fever Myalgia Headache Rash (no eschar) Trunk > extremities Milder form of illness
Scrub typhus	*R. tsutsugamushi*	Mite	Rodents	Fever Headache Rash with eschar Lymphadenopathy
Spotted fever group				
Indian tick typhus	*R. conorii*	Tick	Rodent, dog	Fever Headache Rash with eschar, first appear on wrist and ankle
Rocky mountain spotted fever	*R. rickettsii*	Tick	Rodents, dog	Fever Headache Rash (no eschar) first appear on wrist and ankle Palms and soles involved Systemic complications—R/S, CVS, CNS, renal, hepatic
Rickettsial pox	*R. akari*	Mite	Mice	Mild illness Fever Headache Vesicular rash with eschar Lymphadenopathy Resemblance to chickenpox
Others				
Q fever	*C. burnetii*	Nil	Cattle, sheep, goat	Fever Headache Fatigue Pneumonia, endocarditis No rash
Trench fever	*R. quintana*	Louse	Human	

Abbreviations: RS = Respiratory system; CVS = Cardiovascular system; CNS = Central nervous system

parasite. As age advances the disease assumes more serious proportions. Several epidemics have occurred during famine, war and other natural calamities, when people had to be kept in camps under unhygienic conditions.

Rickettsia prowazekii is transmitted by the body louse (*Pediculus humanus corporis*) and rarely the head louse (*Pediculus humanus capitis*) from man to man. The lice are infected by the blood meal. An infected louse passes the organisms in feces for the rest of its life (4 weeks). When the patient scratches, the lice are crushed and their body contents are smeared on to the bite wound through which organisms enter the host. Inhalation of the dried lice feces is another possible mode of entry. Lice leave dead bodies to seek new hosts and in this process they spread infection. Persons who suffer from typhus acquire lifelong immunity. In some cases, relapse occurs after a long latent period and this is referred to as **Brill-Zinsser disease**. Occasionally epidemics have followed such sporadic cases.

Pathology

Pathologically, the lesions are characterized by angiitis seen in the small blood vessels of various organs including the skin, heart, skeletal muscles and brain. Rickettsiae replicate within the cytoplasm of endothelial cells and smooth muscle cells of capillaries, arterioles and small arteries causing necrotizing vasculitis. The blood vessels are thrombosed or they may rupture. Rickettsiae are seen in the proliferated endothelial cells. Various tissues show infiltration by round cells, macrophages and sometimes lymphocytes and plasma cells. The vascular changes lead to patchy gangrene of the skin, sloughing of skeletal muscles and myocarditis.

Clinical Features

Average incubation period is 7 days (5–21 days). Fever is sudden in onset with malaise and myalgia. Temperature rises to 39–40°C and remains continuous. The face is flushed, conjunctiva are injected and there is severe sore throat. A macular skin rash appears on the fifth day. It is particularly seen in the axilla, abdomen, chest, back and extremities. The rash starts to fade by about the tenth day. Involvement of the central nervous system (CNS) leads to headache, stupor, coma and urinary incontinence. Bleeding from the mucous membranes gives rise to hematemesis, epistaxis, melena and hematuria. Respiratory involvement leads to bronchitis, bronchopneumonia, lung abscess or gangrene of the lung. Myocardial involvement is manifested by tachycardia, hypotension and cardiac failure. In uncomplicated cases the temperature comes down by the twelfth to fourteenth day by lysis.

Complications: It include patchy gangrene of the skin over the extremities, parotitis, cardiac failure and renal failure. Death may occur in the latter part of the second week due to complications. Though the disease used to be associated with high mortality during the epidemics, early diagnosis and specific therapy have considerably lowered the mortality rate.

Diagnosis

The disease has to be diagnosed by the clinical features. Epidemic typhus has to be differentiated from typhoid, malaria, tuberculosis, pneumonia, relapsing fever and other rickettsial diseases. Laboratory diagnosis is by the Weil-Felix reaction and other specific tests including isolation of the organisms. The organisms can be isolated from blood collected during the early phase of the illness. Four-fold rise in titer of Weil-Felix reaction is suggestive. Specific antirickettsial antibodies can be demonstrated.

Polymerase chain reaction (PCR) studies, western blot and microimmunofluorescence can be done in advanced laboratories for specific diagnosis.

Treatment

Chloramphenicol 0.5 g 6 h for 5–7 days and doxycycline 100 mg bd for 5–7 days are specific and highly effective. They have to be continued for a week after the temperature reaches normal in order to avoid relapse.

Prevention

On admission to the wards the clothes of the patient should be disinfested by heat or 10% dichlorodiphenyl-trichloroethane (DDT) or 1% lindane powder. Any ectoparasite remaining on the patient should be removed manually or by use of the pesticides such as benzyl benzoate 20% emulsion, permethrin, synergized pyrethrin or malathion.

Personal prophylaxis may be achieved by vaccination. Vaccines containing either killed rickettsiae (Cox vaccine) or live virulent strains are available.

Doxycycline given in a dose of 100 mg oral daily prevents infection in contacts.

ENDEMIC TYPHUS

Syn: Murine typhus, Flea typhus

This is an acute febrile illness caused by *R. typhi (R. mooseri)* transmitted from rat to man by the rat flea *Xenopsylla cheopis.*

Etiology

The rat flea and the rat louse (*Polyplax spinulosa)* transmit *R. typhi* among rodents. The insect acquires the infection while feeding on an infected rat. The organisms are passed in the feces of the flea after multiplication in the intestinal cells. Man is infected by the flea when it takes a blood meal. The bite wound is contaminated with flea feces and the organisms get in. Infection may also enter through the respiratory tract or the conjunctiva. Since the urine of infected rats contains the organisms, contamination of food with rat's urine is also a possible source of spread. Rats and mice may harbor the organisms in their brain for long periods. Lice have been incriminated as vectors in some areas in Kashmir and China. Compared to epidemic typhus, endemic typhus is milder.

Clinical Features

After the incubation period of 8–16 days, prodromal symptoms like headache, malaise, backache and arthralgia develop, followed soon by the onset of fever. Fever may be associated with frequent chills, rigors, nausea, vomiting, photophobia and congestion of the eyes. The fever persists continuously for 12 days and then comes down by lysis. A morbilliform rash develops in the axillae, arms, abdomen, chest, shoulders and thighs by about the fifth day and it fades away. Bronchitis may develop and this is manifested as cough and the presence of rales on examination. Rare complications include stupor, coma, prostration and renal failure.

Diagnosis

The clinical suspicion should be supported by laboratory investigations.

Treatment

The disease responds to chloramphenicol or doxycycline in usual doses.

SCRUB TYPHUS

Syn: Mite typhus, Mite fever, Tsutsugamushi fever, Japanese river fever

Infection by *Orientia tsutsugamushi* leads to a febrile illness, which lasts for about 2 weeks.

Epidemiology

The disease is being reported from several states in India including Kerala. It is present in South-East Asia, including Japan, Soviet Union, Australia and several other countries. It is transmitted by different species of trombiculid mites. In India scrub typhus is endemic in many regions especially the north and the vector is *Trombicula deliensis*. A recent report from Andhra Pradesh found the vector larval mites as *Leptotrombidium deliense.* Mites are seen in scrub jungles mainly, but they are also seen in sandy beaches, deserts and dense forests. Reservoir of infection is formed by wild rodents and birds. Mites are infected when they take their blood meals during the larval stage (chiggers). Only larval mites suck blood and they transmit the disease. The infected mites transmit the organisms transovarially to the offspring. Thus, a colony of mites which harbor organisms develops which acts as a reservoir of infection for long periods. Immunity to these bacteria is still ill-understood. These bacteria infect dendritic cells and macrophages in the cutaneous sites of the chiggers feeding and from there they spread to infect primarily endothelial cells and secondarily macrophages throughout the body, including lung and brain. Man gets the infection from the bites of mites, which are acquired when engaged in jungle clearing operations, warfare, picnicking and similar activities. Pathologically the lesions resemble those caused by *Rickettsia prowazekii*.

Clinical Features

The incubation period varies from 6 to 18 days. The onset is abrupt with rigor, severe headache, fever and lymphadenopathy. At the site of bite, a necrotic ulcer (eschar) develops with local lymphadenopathy. Fever may go up to 38–39.5°C. It is associated with relative bradycardia. The cutaneous rash appears after the fifth day, first on the trunk and then it spreads to the extremities. It may persist for a few days. Fever lasts for about two weeks and comes down by lysis.

A report of a series from Andhra Pradesh on 176 cases of scrub typhus seen over 18 months, confirmed by Weil-Felix test gives the findings as follows. Symptoms in the order of frequency were cough (15.3%), breathlessness (47.7%), signs of pulmonary consolidation (45.5%), altered sensorium (24.4%), seizures (6.3%), eschar (13%), renal failure (27.8%) and respiratory failure (6.2%). Mortality was 4.2%. Most frequent laboratory findings was elevation of liver enzymes [serum glutamic-pyruvic transaminase (SGPT), serum glutamic oxaloacetic transaminase (SGOT)] seen in 86% cases.

Source: Subbalaxmi MV, Madisetty MK, Prasad AK, et al. Outbreak of scrub typhus in Andhra Pradesh—experience at a tertiary care hospital. J Assoc Physicians India. 2014;62(6):490-6.

Serious complications may occur. These include myocarditis, cardiac failure, renal failure and meningo-encephalitis. The mortality is around 6%. Convalescence tends to be prolonged.

Diagnosis

The diagnosis is made clinically by the presence of eschar rash, high fever, bradycardia, body ache, malaise and/or lymphadenopathy. The disease however is to be differentiated from other febrile conditions relevant to the area/country.

The Weil-Felix reaction is positive for OXK in 50% of cases by two weeks of illness. Rising titers of antibodies demonstrated at the end of three weeks all more suggestive. More sophisticated tests are available. Microimmunofluorescence is the test of choice. Latex agglutination, indirect hemagglutination, immunoperoxidase assay, enzyme-linked immunosorbent assay (ELISA) and PCR are the other tests available. A dipstick test has been developed for rapid diagnosis. Nonspecific, but very suggestive laboratory findings include moderate elevation of liver enzyme such as SGOT and SGPT (100–200 IU/L) and elevation of C-reactive protein (CRP).

Treatment

Doxycycline in the usual dose of 100 mg bd orally for 5–7 days is quite effective and safe. Chloramphenicol and tetracycline are effective against the organisms when given in a dose of 2–4 g/day. Within 24 hours of starting therapy, the temperature falls and recovery starts. Rifampicin in a daily dose of 600 mg given oral is quite effective and clearance of fever and febrile symptoms occurs more rapidly. Azithromycin is also effective in usual doses.

Infection can be avoided in endemic areas by wearing protective clothing and using insect repellents. Hot shower bath with lathering soap will remove most of the mites. Drug prophylaxis consists of chloramphenicol or tetracycline 500 mg given once every five days for 35 days. An alternative is doxycycline 100 mg given once a week for the period of exposure and for 6 weeks after leaving the endemic area. There is a suggestion that rickettsia may develop resistance to doxycycline in endemic areas.

TICK-BORNE TYPHUS

(Spotted Fever Group)

Tick-borne typhus group is characterized by the development of prominent rash. Most of them are transmitted by hard ticks (ixodidae), except *R. akari* which is transmitted by mite. Rickettsiae of this group possess a common antigen and therefore, may show serological overlap. These organisms are found in animals and enzootics occur periodically. They constitute the reservoir for infection. In addition, transovarian transmission of rickettsiae by the female tick to its offspring leads to the formation of an insect reservoir, which tends to persist for long periods on account of the long lifespan of the ticks. Man is affected accidentally. The course of the disease is similar to that of epidemic typhus. Mortality differs from place to place, but is around 15–18%.

The classic disease in this group is *rocky mountain spotted fever*. Hard ticks transmit the diseases. At the site of bite an eschar may develop. Eschar is the necrotic ulcer developing about a week after the bite. The rash occurs around the third day. It is maculopapular and morbilliform. In severe cases petechiae may develop.

In India, spotted fevers are caused by *R. conorii*, which is distributed over extensive areas at the foothills of the Himalayas. The main vector is the dog tick *Rhipicephalus sanguineus,* but other species of ticks like *Hemaphasalis leachi, Amblyomma* and *Hyalomma* may also take part in transmission. ***Rickettsial pox*** is caused by *R. akari*. It is seen in the United States of America (USA).

Q FEVER

It is a zoonosis caused by *Coxiella burnetii*—it is a gram-negative pleomorphic coccobacilli which is having homology with *Legionella pneumophila*. Two forms exist:
1. A small cell variant (SCV)
2. A large cell variant (LCV).

The SCV exists in nature and it is resistant to environmental factors. The LCV develops in the host's monocytes and multiplies. It is the pathogenic form. The disease exists in Australia, India, USA and other areas. In India, the disease has been reported from Delhi, Punjab, South Canara and Rajasthan. Animal reservoirs include cows, goats, sheep, dogs, cats and others. Organisms are shed in milk, feces, urine and products of conception. Humans become infected by ingestion of infective material or droplet infection through the respiratory tract. Incubation period is 12–30 days.

Acute Q Fever

This resembles influenza clinically, with varying degrees of pneumonia and hepatitis. Fever lasts for an average of 10 days (range 10–57 days).

Chronic Q Fever

This occurs in 60–70% of infected persons. It leads to endocarditis which supervenes on pre-existing valvular lesions. Untreated, the condition is fatal. Q fever may recrudesce during pregnancy and lead to abortion. Other manifestations include osteoarticular infections and hepatitis.

Diagnosis

Antibodies can be detected by indirect immunofluorescence.

Treatment

- *Acute Q fever*—doxycycline 100 mg bd po for 14 days
- *Chronic Q fever*—lifelong doxycycline therapy may be necessary.

Addition of hydroxychloroquine 200 mg tds po given for 18 months favors recovery. It acts synergistically with doxycycline.

Prevention

Pasteurization of milk is partly protective. Occupational risk can be reduced by vaccination in persons exposed to the risk.

EHRLICHIOSIS AND ANAPLASMOSIS

Ehrlichiosis and anaplasmosis infections have been occasionally reported in India, especially being transmitted by ticks from the dogs or other animals. Four genera belonging to the family anaplasmataceae (bacterial organism) include *Ehrlichia, Anaplasma, Wolbachia* and *Neorickettsia*.

Human Ehrlichiosis

Ehrlichia are small gram-negative intracellular bacteria that are located in the cytoplasmic vacuoles. They grow in clusters and are termed morulae. They are transmitted by ticks to man from animal vectors. This disease may affect humans and are sporadically seen in many parts in India.

Human Monocytotropic Ehrlichiosis

This is caused by *Ehrlichia chaffeensis* transmitted by the tick *Amblyomma americanum*. Onset is with fever, headache, nausea, body pains, vomiting and diarrhea. Serious complications such as respiratory distress meningoencephalitis, hemorrhagic manifestations and toxic shock syndrome may develop. Caseating granulomas may be seen in bone marrow tissue. At times, peripheral blood smear may reveal morulae in monocytes and macrophages.

Treatment: Doxycycline given in doses of 100 mg bd oral given for 5 days is effective. *Ehrlichia ewingii* is also transmitted by the same tick compared to *Ehrlichia chaffeensis* the disease is milder. Treatment is with doxycycline.

Human Anaplasmosis

The human disease is caused by *Anaplasma phagocytophilum* transmitted readily by the tick. *Ixodes scapularis*. Incubation period is 4–8 days. The disease starts as flu-like illness. Rarely complications such as respiratory lesions (even respiratory distress syndrome in elderly) brachial plexopathy and demyelinating neuropathy have been reported.

Since ticks can habor different pathogens simultaneously, combination of Lyme disease and anaplasmosis or ehrlichiosis have been documented.

Laboratory investigations: It shows thrombocytopenia leukopenia and elevation of hepatic transaminases—SGPT and SGOT. Examination of peripheral blood film may show neutrophil morulae PCR is specific for identifying the organism. Serodiagnosis consists of demonstrating fourfold rise of anti-*Anaplasma* phagocytophilum antibody in paired sera collected at interval of one month.

Treatment: Drug of choice is doxycycline 100 mg given bd orally for 4–7 days. The fever subsides in 2–3 days. Rifampicin 300–400 mg given od is a suitable alternative, especially useful for pregnant women.

Anaerobic Infections: Tetanus and Gas Gangrene

KV Krishna Das

Chapter Summary

- General Considerations
- Diseases caused by Clostridia
- Tetanus
  - Etiology
  - Clinical Features
  - Treatment
    - Tetanus Antitoxin
    - Control of Convulsions
    - Prognostic Factors
    - Working Classification of the Severity
  - Prevention
- Gas Gangrene
  - Pathogenesis
  - Clinical Features
  - Diagnosis
  - Treatment

GENERAL CONSIDERATIONS

Many areas in the body such as mouth, nasopharynx, paranasal sinuses, tonsillar crypts, gastrointestinal tract (GIT) and female genital tract harbor anaerobes as commensals and they far outnumber aerobes. Anaerobes thrive in the anaerobic environment provided by the facultative anaerobes such as *Enterobacteriaceae*, *Staphylococci*, *Streptococci*, *E. coli* and *K. pneumoniae* which use up oxygen. They multiply further and acquire virulence if there is reduction in vascular supply, tissue injury or presence of dead tissue. Most of the anaerobic infections are mixed. These organisms act to facilitate each other to grow, invade tissues and resist the action of drugs. Their multiplication is promptly inhibited even by moderate increase in oxygen tension. For the isolation and identification of anaerobes, special microbiological techniques have to be adopted in collecting specimens and culturing the organisms. Since anaerobic infections produce septic venous thrombosis and embolism, pyemic abscesses are common. The virulence of these organisms depend on their endotoxins, exoprotein, cytokines like interleukin 8 (IL-8) and 17 tumor necrosis factor (TNF) and others. These cytokines facilitate chemotaxis of neutrophils, adhesion to host cells and abscess formation. They liberate endotoxins from their cell walls which lead to endotoxic shock and disseminated intravascular coagulation (DIC). Anaerobes can affect all tissues, especially so, if there is tissue necrosis and presence of foreign material.

Anaerobes which are pathogenic to man:

- **Gram-negative bacilli:**
  - **Bacteroides:** *B. fragilis, B. oralis, B. melaninogenicus, B. corrodens*
  - **Fusobacterium:** *F. nucleatum, F. varium, F. necrophorum*
- **Spore forming gram-positive bacilli:** *Clostridium: C. botulinum, C. tetani, C. perfringens, C. histolyticum, C. septicum, C. novyi, C. bifermentans*
- **Non-spore forming gram-positive bacilli:** *Actinomyces, Subacterium, Bifidobacterium, Propionibacterium, Catenibacterium*
- **Anaerobic cocci:**
  - **Gram-positive:** *Peptococcus, Peptostreptococcus,* microaerophilic streptococci, anaerobic pneumococci.
  - **Gram-negative:** *Veillonella.*

Anaerobic infections should be suspected under following situations:

- Location of lesion, in close proximity to mucosal surfaces
- Foul smelling exudates
- Presence of gas in the tissues
- Black discoloration of exudates, e.g. *B. melaninogenicus*
- Infections associated with gut perforation and ulceration
- Infections after human or other bites
- Aspiration pneumonia and infection associated with the presence of foreign bodies.

Lesions caused by Anaerobes

Central nervous system (CNS): Brain abscess, subdural empyema, septic thrombophlebitis of the cortical veins and venous sinuses.

Head and neck: Chronic sinusitis, mastoiditis, chronic otitis media, dental infection (caries), periodontal disease, Vincent's angina, peritonsillar abscess, cervicofacial actinomycosis and Ludwig's angina.

Female genital tract: Endometritis, myometritis, parametritis, pyometra, pelvic cellulitis, pelvic abscesses, pelvic thrombophlebitis, vulvovaginal abscess, Bartholinitis, Skene's gland infection, salpingitis, tubo-ovarian abscess, vaginal cuff infection, chorioamnionitis, intrauterine or neonatal sepsis and pneumonia, septic abortion and puerperal sepsis.

Respiratory tract: Aspiration pneumonia, necrotizing pneumonia, lung abscess, empyema, mediastinitis, bronchiectasis and pulmonary actinomycosis.

Bloodstream spread: Septicemia and endocarditis.

Abdomen: Peritonitis, appendicitis, diverticulitis, pylephlebitis, intra-abdominal abscess, liver abscess and abdominal actinomycosis.

Soft tissues: Cellulitis, gangrene, infected deep wounds, wound infections after gastrointestinal or gynecologic surgery, infections following human bites, necrotizing fasciitis, decubitus ulcer (perineal or gluteal area), infected sebaceous or pilonidal cysts, diabetic ulcers on the feet.

Textbook of Medicine

Musculoskeletal: Pyogenic arthritis, osteomyelitis and gangrene.

Urinary tract: Renal abscess, perirenal abscess, pyelonephritis, wound infection after nephrectomy, cystitis, chronic prostatitis and abscess and testicular abscess.

Therapeutic Principles

The polymicrobial nature of anaerobic lesions demand the use of antibiotic combinations active against anaerobes and aerobes.

Surgical measures should be employed in time and these are most important. They consist of drainage of abscesses, debridement of necrotic tissue and relief of obstruction to natural passages.

Penicillin is effective against all anaerobes except *Bacteroides fragilis* and it is the drug of choice. It has to be given in very high doses (20–30 mega units in 24 hours). Gentamicin, clindamycin and chloramphenicol act synergistically with penicillin against anaerobes and therefore these antibiotics are combined for therapy. When the organisms are resistant to penicillin, these antibiotics are used as the primary drugs. Beta-lactamase-resistant cephalosporins—cephoxitin and cephamandole—are also effective. Metronidazole, given intravenously (IV) in a dose of 400 mg 8 h as infusion, is a useful drug against many of the anaerobes. It has to be combined with other antibiotics. Oral doses are effective to a lesser degree (Table 46.1).

Other measures include administration of antitoxins, hyperbaric oxygen, local oxygen therapy and use of oxygen-releasing agents locally, e.g. hydrogen peroxide.

Major drawbacks of antibiotics in treating anaerobic infections.

Agent	Major disadvantages
Penicillin G	Ineffective against *B. fragilis*
Chloramphenicol	Hematotoxicity—aplastic anemia
Clindamycin	Poor penetration into CSF, occurrence of pseudomembranous colitis
Carbenicillin	Up to 5–10% of *B. fragilis* strains are resistant, sodium overload, bleeding tendency
Metronidazole	All aerobes are resistant
Cephamandole	Poor penetration to CSF
Cephoxitin	Poor penetration to CSF

Abbreviation: CSF = Cerebrospinal fluid

DISEASES CAUSED BY CLOSTRIDIA

These include tetanus, gas gangrene, food poisoning including botulism and pseudomembranous colitis.

C. tetani	Tetanus
C. perfringens Syn: *C. welchii*	Gas gangrene
C. Septicum	-do-
C. novyi Syn: *C. edematiens*	-do-
C. histolyticum	-do-
C. sordelli	-do-
C. botulinum	Botulism (*See* Section 4, Ch 24)
C. perfringens	Also food poisoning
C. difficile	Pseudomembranous colitis (*See* Section 6, Ch 42)

TETANUS

Syn: Lockjaw

Tetanus has been in existence over several millenniums, as is seen from descriptions from the ancient texts of *Ayurveda* (*Susruta Samhita*) and the writings of *Hippocrates*.

Definition: Tetanus is an acute infectious disease characterized by rigidity, intermittent spasms of the voluntary muscles and convulsions. Trismus, which is a prominent feature, gives it the name 'lockjaw'. The disease is caused by the exotoxin produced by *Clostridium tetani*. *C. tetani* is a gram-positive (also can be gram-negative), obligate anaerobe which is motile and sporing. The spores resist boiling water for three hours and dry heat up to 160°C for one hour.

Etiology

C. tetani is commonly found in the soil and the intestinal tract of animals and man. The organism exists as vegetative forms and spores. They can remain viable *in vitro* for several years. Spores are destroyed by autoclaving at 121°C for 20 minutes. After entry into tissues through wounds they germinate and grow. Rarely, they may remain dormant for considerable periods. *C. tetani* produces exotoxins among which two are most important: (1) A powerful neurotoxin tetanospasmin and (2) a hemolysin-tetanolysin. Tetanospasmin is responsible for the clinical disease.

Table 46.1: Effectiveness of antibiotics against the common anaerobes

Antibiotic	B. fragilis	B. melaninogenicus	Fusobacterium	Clostridia	Propionobacterium	Actinomyces	Peptostreptococcus
Penicillin G	Variable	Variable, but effective	++	+ to ++	+++	+++	+++
Broad spectrum							
Penicillins	++	++	++	++	+++	+++	+++
Cefoxitin second generation	++	+++	++	Variable	+++	+++	+++
Chloramphenicol	+++	+++	+++	++	+++	+++	+++
Metronidazole	+++	+++	+++	+++	–	–	+++
Imipenem with cilastatin	+++	+++	++	+++	+++	+++	+++
Clindamycin	++	+++	+++	+++	+++	+++	+++

Note: + effective, – not effective

Pathology

C. tetani remains strictly localized to the site of multiplication, but the toxin reaches the CNS through the peripheral nerves and bloodstream. Tetanus toxin which is a polypeptide with molecular weight 1,48,000 daltons enters the bloodstream and reaches the nerve endings in the muscles. From here it ascends though the nerves to the CNS. From the motor cells of the brain and spinal cord, the toxin passes retrogradely to bind to the terminals of the inhibitory neurons. Tetanospasmin causes disinhibition of both the alpha and gamma motor systems and thereby leads to generalized muscle rigidity. Spasms occur when external stimuli are applied and also spontaneously. Direct effect of the toxin on the muscle leads to contraction. The toxin acts also on the central sympathetic system and possibly on the cerebral cortex and brainstem. The effects of tetanus toxin are self-limited and they pass off within weeks or months if further absorption of toxin is prevented.

Tetanus is more common after sustaining deep wounds with tissue devitalization and introduction of foreign materials inside. In such sites anaerobic conditions are established and *C. tetani* multiplies. In addition to wounds, chronic otitis media, umbilical sepsis of neonates, parturition, septic abortion, burns, intramuscular (IM) injections and chronic ulcers may be complicated by tetanus. In about a fifth of the cases there may be no obvious focus of entry. This is termed cryptogenic tetanus. Despite all advancements in antimicrobial therapy and effective vaccination, tetanus still occurs frequently in all parts of the country and accounts for considerable mortality.

Clinical Features

Since it is not essential that infection and injury coincide, it is difficult to ascertain the incubation period exactly in all cases. The incubation period is generally less than 2 weeks, although it may range from 2 to 60 days. Cases with shorter incubation periods tend to be more severe and are associated with higher mortality.

The disease starts with premonitory symptoms like vague discomfort, pain around the site of injury and restlessness. The diagnosis becomes evident when lockjaw sets in. It is painless or only mildly painful. Severe pain should suggest a local cause for trismus.

Within hours to days the abdominal and trunk muscles become spastic. Rigidity of the abdominal muscles may simulate peritonitis. Rigidity and spasm of the back muscles result in hyperextension of the spine and neck (opisthotonus). All muscle groups (both the agonists and antagonists) go into spasm at the same time. Risus sardonicus is the characteristic grinning expression brought about by the sustained contraction of facial muscles. Rarely dysphagia can be the first presenting symptom. Spasm of the sphincters leads to retention of urine and feces.

Spasmodic contractions involving different parts of the body develop at variable intervals after the onset of rigidity. The interval between the first symptom and the first convulsion is called the ***onset period***. External stimuli or emotions precipitate these painful spasms which cripple the patient. In severe cases they may develop spontaneously. Asphyxia results from spasm of the laryngeal and respiratory muscles. Regurgitation of gastric contents leads to aspiration into the respiratory tract. With progress of the disease, the spasms become frequent and prolonged and this leads to muscular exhaustion, hyperpyrexia and cardiac failure. Sympathetic over-activity causes hypertension, hyperpyrexia and cardiac arrhythmias. Mind remains alert till the end and in many cases the patient is very anxious. Deep tendon reflexes are generally exaggerated, but the plantar response is flexor.

Course and Prognosis

It takes about three days for the disease to manifest fully. If complications are prevented, the condition remains stable for the next 5–7 days. Thereafter the spasms gradually subside in frequency and intensity to disappear in 2 weeks. Complete recovery may take 4 weeks or more, though in some cases the rigidity may persist even longer.

Local tetanus: In this form, rigidity and other symptoms are confined to a part near the site of injury. This generally runs a mild course and ends in complete recovery.

Cephalic tetanus: This term is used when local tetanus involves the facial muscles only. It is usually unilateral but can be bilateral.

Tetanus neonatorum: This form of tetanus occurs within 10 days of birth. It is usually severe. It manifests as inability to suck the nipple, irritability and excessive crying associated with grimacing movements of the face. The muscles of the back, neck and abdomen may become spastic. In many instances the classical signs may not develop in neonates and premature infants.

Tetanus neonatorum is still an important cause of infant mortality in many developing countries including India. Re-immunization of the pregnant women prevents tetanus in both the mother and the child.

Complications

Respiratory obstruction and aspiration pneumonia are the most frequent complications accounting for death in many cases. Peripheral venous thrombosis may develop and lead to pulmonary embolism. Myocarditis gives rise to cardiac failure and hypotension. Hyperpyrexia is the result of excessive muscular activity and the effect of the toxin on the hypothalamus. Decubitus ulcers and urinary tract infection (UTI) result from prolonged immobility. Fractures of the spine and other bones are seen at times. Sudden death due to laryngeal spasm, cardiac arrhythmias or massive aspiration of gastric contents may occur and these have to be anticipated.

Diagnosis

The disease has to be diagnosed clinically. Repeated observations may be required to make the diagnosis in doubtful cases.

Tetanus has to be differentiated from meningo-encephalitis, strychnine poisoning, local causes of trismus, dystonia due to phenothiazines, tetany and hysteria. Cerebrospinal fluid (CSF) is normal in tetanus.

Treatment

The outcome depends on proper therapy based on the severity of this disease (Tables 46.2 and 46.3).

Table 46.2: Prognostic factors

Age	Neonates and older patients fare badly
Type of injury	Large wounds contaminated with soil, lacerated wounds, compound fractures and septic abortions are associated with severe tetanus. Though rare, tetanus following IM injections tends to be serious
Incubation period	Short incubation periods indicate greater severity. Apparently long incubation period does not necessarily mean that the case is mild
Interval between the onset of trismus and at all the first spasm	Shorter this period, more severe is the disease. In mild cases spasms may not occur
Frequency of spasms	More frequent and more prolonged spasms are poor prognostic signs
Autonomic disturbances	Dysphagia, hypertension, hyperpyrexia and cardiac arrhythmias indicate poor prognosis
Treatment	Early administration of antitoxin, proper surgical toilet, institution of antibiotics, proper anticonvulsive therapy, availability of a team of physicians, surgeons and anesthetists and proper nursing care are the most important factors determining a successful outcome. Inadequacy of treatment is a common cause of death in many cases

Table 46.3: Working classification of the severity of tetanus

	Mild	*Moderately severe*	*Severe*
Incubation period	Above 14 days	7–14 days	Less than 7 days
Onset time	6 days	3–6 days	Less than 3 days
Trismus	Present	Marked	Severe
Dysphagia	Absent	Present	Present
Rigidity	Absent	Mild	Severe
Spasms	Brief and mild	Present, frequent	Frequent, prolonged and generalized convulsions
Ventilation	Not affected	Inadequate ventilation during spasm	Often ventilatory insufficiency
Mortality	Up to 5%	25%	80–90%
Treatment	ATS, oral medications, IM diazepam	ATS, IV drip and medication, Ryle's tube, elective tracheostomy	Early tracheostomy, IV drips and medication, muscle relaxant, artificial ventilation

Abbreviations: ATS = Antitetanus serum; IM = Intramuscular; IV = Intravenous

All cases should be hospitalized. An apparently simple case may rapidly deteriorate and demand specialized care. Best results are obtained if tetanus is managed in institutions where specially trained teams are available. Depending on the severity, treatment has to be planned from the beginning.

General measures: The patient is nursed in an environment where external stimuli such as drafts of air, cold winds, noises and vibrations are minimal. Nutrition is provided by giving adequate calories in the form of glucose and cereals. Fluid and electrolyte balance should be maintained. The main aim of treatment is to arrest the growth of *C. tetani* in the local lesion, prevent further production of toxin, neutralize the toxin already in circulation and to abolish the excitatory effect of the toxin on the muscles. Since the toxin attached to nerve endings cannot be neutralized, antitoxin should be administered without delay to neutralize circulating toxin.

Tetanus Antitoxin/Antitetanus Serum (ATS)

The best available preparation is human tetanus immunoglobulin (TIG) which is to be given in a dose of 2000–5000 units IV or IM. If the wound is heavily contaminated and in severe cases, up to 10000 units may be required. This is more potent and free from risk of anaphylaxis. Human TIG can also be given intrathecally in a dose of 250–1500 units reduces mortality. This measure may help in controlling convulsions more effectively when other measures fail. Protective level of immunoglobulin G

(IgG) antitetanus antiglobulin in blood is > 0.1 IU/mL and above this level tetanus is unlikely. Injections of tetanus toxoid repeatedly for 5 times in addition to primary immunization [Diphtheria, Pertussis, Tetanus (DPT)] gives life-long protection in ordinary cases.

The other preparation is ATS prepared from the horse. It may cause anaphylactic shock in allergic individuals and hence it should be administered only after testing for allergy (skin test and later IV test) and if human immunoglobulin is not available.

All measures to combat anaphylactic shock should be available ready at hand. The dose is 10,000 to 25,000 units given IV or IM. Ordinarily, there is no need to repeat the antiserum.

Surgical Toilet of the Wound

It aims at debridement and removal of necrotic material and foreign bodies, with a view to removing the anaerobic environment. Surgical toilet should be done only after giving the antitoxin.

Antibiotics

C. tetani is sensitive to penicillin and benzylpenicillin in a dose of 0.5 mega unit 6 hourly administered IV helps in preventing the multiplication of the organism and further toxin production. When the infection is controlled, procaine penicillin can be used in a dose of 0.5 mega unit daily. Metronidazole given in doses of 400 mg IV bd has also been found to be effective.

Practical clues to determine immune status and administer TIG		
	Immune if	**Non-immune if**
Injection of tetanus toxoid	Within 6 months of injection 2 doses; for 5–10 years after full course with booster	No vaccination more than 6 months after a course of 2 doses or 10 years after a course of 3 doses without booster
Equine ATS	Within 2 weeks	After 2 weeks
Human TIG	within 6 weeks	After 6 weeks any doubt about vaccination status
Procedure to be followed	Boost up immune status with a shot of tetanus toxoid	Human TIG 250–500 units stat. Start 3 injection tetanus toxoid schedule, the first injection given simultaneously at a different site

Control of Convulsions

Diazepam in adequate doses controls the muscle spasms; 50 mg is added to 600 mL of 5% glucose and it is run as an IV drip, at a rate required to control the spasms. Even up to 200 mg may be required in 24 hours. Paraldehyde 7 mL every 6 h given orally, chlorpromazine 50 mg every 6 h given IM and phenobarbitone 200 mg twice daily given IM are effective in controlling the spasms and producing the required sedation when used in combination with diazepam. A combination of anticonvulsants can be used. Midazolam given IV as a continuous drip in a dose of 5–15 mg/hour is an effective alternative.

In severe tetanus that cannot be controlled effectively by drugs, curarization and assisted ventilation are essential and this regimen has to be undertaken by a team trained for ventilatory assistance (Table 46.4).

Tracheostomy

It maintains patency of the airway and helps in giving effective tracheal toilet. A cuffed endotracheal tube protects against aspiration of gastric contents. In moderate and severe tetanus, tracheostomy is indicated which should be performed without delay.

In severe sympathetic overactivity, beta-adrenergic blockers like propranolol have to be used.

Prevention

Tetanus is an easily preventable disease. Clinical tetanus does not confer immunity and therefore, the patient should be actively immunized when he recovers. Three subcutaneous injections of adsorbed toxoid in a dose of 0.5 mL at monthly intervals produces lasting immunity. As a part of the total immunization program for children the first dose may be given as the DPT vaccine at the fourth month of life and two further doses at monthly intervals. If the full course of DPT vaccine is given, the child gets life-long immunity. Boosters are needed once every 5–10 years. When severe injuries are sustained, one dose of 0.5 mL of toxoid may be given as a precautionary measure. Passive immunization can be achieved in nonimmunized subjects by the administration of 250 IU of TIG or 3000 IU of ATS after test dose. The immunity lasts for about two weeks. Passive immunization is given along with a booster dose of toxoid in separate syringes at different sites to nonimmunized individuals who sustain injury. Active immunization of pregnant women ensures adequate antibodies in the neonate and prevents tetanus neonatorum.

Primary care of the wound like surgical toilet and penicillin therapy considerably reduce the risk of tetanus.

- Effective antibiotics in tetanus are penicillin and metronidazole
- Protective level of IgG antitetanus antiglobulin in blood is > 0.1 IU/mL and above this level tetanus is unlikely to happen
- Injections of tetanus toxoid repeatedly for 5 times in addition to primary immunization (DPT) gives life-long protection in ordinary cases. Intratheral human immunoglobulin given in doses of 1500 IU reduces mortality in tetanus.

Points to Remember
- Tetanus is a life-threatening infection occurring widely in India.
- It is preventable by suitable vaccination starting during pregnancy of the mother.
- Diagnosis is clinical.
- Early treatment using appropriate measures depending on prognostic factors saves lives.

GAS GANGRENE

Syn: Clostridial myonecrosis

Gas gangrene is caused by *Clostridium perfringens (C. welchii), C. septicum, C. novyi (C. oedematiens) C. histolyticum* and *C. sordelli*. These clostridia are commensals in human gut and soil. They produce local necrosis and distant lethal effects.

Table 46.4: Procedure to be followed in the management of severe convulsing tetanus	
Sedation	Diazepam 5 mg IV given at 5 minutes intervals until muscle relaxation is achieved
Airway	Preferably tracheostomy and cuffed tracheostomy tube
Nutrition	Nasogastric tube feeding, 2500 cal with 70 g proteins in 24 hrs. Fluids adequate to maintain urine output of 60 mL/hour
Control of spasms	Diazepam in large doses 10–18 mg or more in 24 hours may be required
Attention to fatal complications such as respiratory arrest, appropriate life-saving measures cardiac arrest and shock	
Antitoxin	Human tetanus immunoglobulin 1500 units IM injection or administration equine ATS 10000 units IV
Wound toilet	Surgical debridement
Immunization	Tetanus toxoid to start early
Severe cases	Management in intensive care room-paralysis by pancuronium 2–6 mg IV and ventilatory support

Textbook of Medicine

Pathogenesis

Necrosis of tissue brought about by anoxia, ischemia or injury is complicated by clostridial infection which may be exogenous (introduced along with the wounds) or endogenous (derived from the intestinal tract). The organisms multiply locally and produce toxins which diffuse out and lead to generalized toxemia. The affected tissues are avascular and appear as if cooked.

Clinical Features

After an incubation period of 1–4 days the wound becomes swollen and tender and exudes brownish foul-smelling fluid. Due to the presence of gas, crepitus may be felt. Blebs filled with purplish foul-smelling fluid develop. These blebs rupture and ulcerate. General symptoms such as restlessness and fever develop and the patient may rapidly go into shock and anuria.

Diagnosis

The condition has to be diagnosed clinically. The organism can be identified by culture. X-ray of the affected part shows gas in the tissues. Gas in the tissues may occur in other conditions such as surgical emphysema and infections by streptococci, staphylococci and *E. coli*.

Treatment

Early institution of therapy is most important for success. Shock is treated on the lines of septic shock. Penicillin which is the drug of choice is given IV in a dose of 2 mega units 2 hourly. Other antibiotics may be tried depending on the sensitivity tests. Metronidazole and gentamicin are effective in most cases. Antitoxin is available for IV use [anti-gas gangrene serum (AGGS)]. It should be given in a dose of 40,000 units initially to be followed by 20,000–40,000 units repeatedly till the condition improves. Keeping the patient under hyperbaric oxygen (3 atmosphere pressure) remarkably improves the result of therapy and this should be instituted wherever it is available. Surgical excision of dead tissue and removal of foreign bodies should be undertaken after administration of AGGS. Gas gangrene can be prevented by taking proper care of the wound and early recognition of the condition.

CHAPTER

47

Sexually Transmitted Diseases

KV Krishna Das, Usha Vaidhyanathan

Chapter Summary

- General Considerations
- Syphilis
  - Classification
  - Pathology
  - Clinical Features—Acquired Syphilis
  - Congenital Syphilis
  - Diagnosis
  - Treatment
  - Prevention
- Gonorrhea
  - Pathology
  - Clinical Features
  - Diagnosis
  - Treatment
- Nongonococcal Urethritis
  - Lifecycle of Chlamydia
  - Epidemiology
  - Clinical Features
  - Diagnosis
  - Treatment
- Lymphogranuloma Venereum
  - Clinical Features
  - Diagnosis
  - Treatment
- Granuloma Inguinale
  - Clinical Features
  - Diagnosis
  - Treatment
- Chancroid
  - Clinical Features
  - Diagnosis
  - Treatment
- Trichomoniasis
  - Pathology
  - Clinical Features
  - Treatment
- Bacterial Vaginosis
  - Diagnosis
  - Treatment

GENERAL CONSIDERATIONS

Infectious diseases which are transmitted by heterosexual or homosexual intercourse and contacts are included under this group. In many developed countries this group constitutes the main bulk of infectious diseases in adults and the incidence is increasing. Increase in promiscuity, change in sex practices, asymptomatic infections, facilities for intercontinental travel, failure to trace sources of infection and lack of awareness of healthy sex practices have contributed to the increase in prevalence.

The present tendency is to include several other diseases like viral hepatitis B which can also be transmitted sexually in the group of sexually transmitted infections (STI).

Common diseases mainly transmitted by sexual contact

Spirochetes	*Treponema pallidum*	Syphilis
Bacteria	*Neisseria gonorrhoeae*	Gonorrhea
	Haemophilus ducreyi	Chancroid
	Donovania granulomatis	Granuloma inguinale
Chlamydia	*Chlamydia trachomatis*	• Urethritis • Cervicitis • Lymphogranuloma venereum
Virus	Herpes simplex virus	Herpes genitalis
	Papillomavirus	Genital warts
	Molluscum contagiosum	Molluscum contagiosum
	Human immunodeficiency virus (HIV)	Acquired immunodeficiency syndrome (AIDS)
Protozoa	*Trichomonas vaginalis*	Trichomonas vaginitis
Fungi	*Candida albicans*	Genital candidiasis
Ectoparasites	*Phthirus pubis*	Pubic lice infestation

SYPHILIS

Syn: Lues venerea

Definition: Syphilis is a chronic infection caused by the spirochete, *Treponema pallidum.* Syphilis is present in all parts of the world. Though the incidence of primary infection continues to be steady, late complications are distinctly rare at present.

T. pallidum is aerobic, very susceptible to antiseptics and is killed by exposure to light in 1–2 hours. It may survive in stored blood for 72 hours. Infection is acquired by the entry of the organism through abrasions in the skin and mucous membranes. In the vast majority of cases, infection is acquired by sexual intercourse. Rarely skin abrasions may be contaminated by infective discharges. The disease can also be transmitted occasionally by needle pricks or by the transplacental route. *T. pallidum* subspecies pallidum (syphilis), *T. pallidum* subspecies pertenue (yaws) and *T. pallidum* subspecies endemicum (endemic syphilis or bejel) and *T. carateum* (pinta) are all morphologically identical. They are tightly coiled helical rods, 5–15 µm long and 0.1–0.5 µm in diameter, motile and demonstrable by dark ground illumination or special staining methods.

Classification

Based on its course, syphilis can be described in 3 stages—primary, secondary and tertiary.

1. **Primary stage:** In the primary stage, local lesions occur at the site of inoculation.
2. **Secondary stage:** The secondary stage is characterized by generalized lesions, most obviously seen in the skin and mucous membranes.
3. **Tertiary stage:** In the tertiary stage, which develops 3–10 years after the initial infection, gummatous and destructive lesions develop in many tissues.

For practical therapeutic purposes, the disease can be conveniently considered in two phases—the early and the late. The early phase extends over the first two years after infection and this includes the primary, secondary, early recurrent and early latent stages. This phase is more contagious. Syphilis of more than 2 years duration is called late phase.

Latent syphilis: It is that stage in which there are no abnormal clinical features. Blood serology is positive, but the cerebrospinal fluid (CSF) does not show any abnormality. History of primary or secondary lesions and abortion during the earlier pregnancies help in identifying this stage.

Clinical Types of Syphilis

- ■ **Congenital syphilis (prenatal infection)**
  - Infantile form—manifests within two years of birth
  - Tardive congenital syphilis (late congenital syphilis)—manifests 2 years or more after birth.
- ■ **Acquired syphilis**
  - Primary
  - Secondary
  - Latent
    - Early phase—within 2 years of infection
    - Late phase—2 years later
  - Late manifestations.

Pathology

The lesions show a chronic granulomatous inflammation and are histologically characterized by epithelioid cells, plasma cells, lymphocytes and giant cells. The small vessels are occluded by obliterating endarteritis. This results in necrosis and scar formation. Inflammation, vascular occlusion and probably immunological factors are contributory to the production of gummata. During the primary and secondary stages, the lesions teem with the organisms. In the late phases, the number of organisms comes down and infectivity diminishes. Syphilitic lesions show a propensity to attract activated CD4+ T lymphocytes. This makes the syphilitic lesions more efficient in disseminating human immunodeficiency virus (HIV) infection as well.

Clinical Features—Acquired Syphilis

Primary stage of syphilis: The incubation period varies from 1 to 3 weeks in most cases, though it may extend up to 90 days. A small macule develops at the site of inoculation which later becomes a papule and ulcerates. This is the primary chancre. It presents a characteristic appearance; a punched out ulcer with a dull red areola and a clear granular base exuding colorless serum which teems with the spirochetes (Fig. 47.1).

The regional lymph nodes enlarge a few days later. They are discrete, rubbery in consistency and are generally

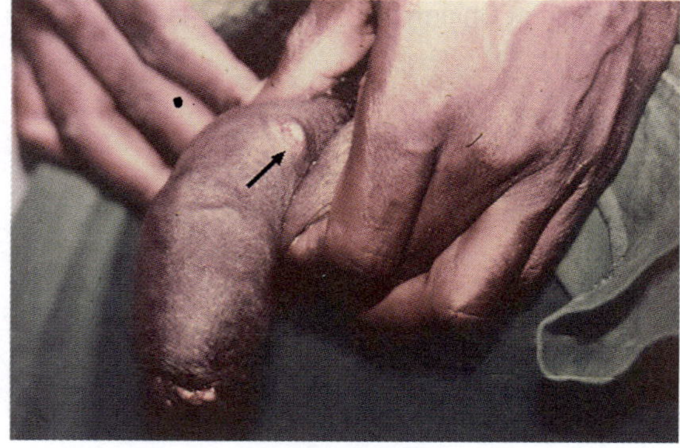

Fig. 47.1: Syphilis primary chancre (arrow)

described as 'shotty'. Even without treatment the chancre heals in 8–10 weeks leaving behind a thin scar. Even after the healing of the chancre the lymph node enlargement persists. Generalized lymphadenopathy may develop at this stage before the secondary stage sets in.

Other ulcers occurring in the genitalia such as herpes genitalis, traumatic ulcers, chancroid, lymphogranuloma venereum (LGV), scabies and carcinoma have to be differentiated from syphilitic chancre.

Secondary stage of syphilis: This stage develops 6–8 weeks after the appearance of the chancre. General symptoms such as malaise, fever, headache, anorexia, hoarseness of voice, arthralgia, nocturnal pains, generalized lymphadenopathy, jaundice and anemia develop.

The ***skin lesions of the second stage*** have certain common characteristics, though some degree of variability is evident. The distinguishing features of secondary syphilitic lesions are:

- Generalized and symmetrical distribution
- Pink, coppery or dusky red color
- Absence of pruritus
- Induration
- Polymorphic (macular, papular or pustular) presentation.

Mucous membrane lesions: Condylomata lata are seen in the mucocutaneous junctions. Basically they are papules which are modified due to the constant moisture and rubbing. They are flat topped, hypertrophic fleshy masses with broad bases. They exude serum rich in treponemes. Mucous patches and snail track ulcers occur in the oral cavity and genitalia. Systemic manifestations of secondary syphilis include acute uveitis which may be unilateral or bilateral, meningitis and hepatitis.

Late syphilis: About 3–12 months after the primary and secondary stages, which are easily distinguishable, the disease enters the latent phase. The first two year period of the latent phase is termed as the ***early latent phase.*** The organisms are located deep in the tissues and the only evidence of infection is the positive serology. Syphilis may remain latent for months or years or even for the whole of the patient's life. In the early part of the latent phase the patient may be infective, but the infectivity diminishes with time.

Tertiary stage: During this stage typical destructive lesions called 'gummata' develops. This is granuloma which may be single or multiple. Histologically the lesions show perivascular infiltration by lymphocytes and plasma cells, followed later by fibrosis. Gummata may occur on the skin, mucous membranes, subcutaneous tissue, bones or viscera. These are asymmetric, small to large in size and indolent with a tendency for healing in the center and spreading at the periphery (Fig. 47.2).

Bone lesions: They occur more commonly in men than in women and the symptoms are very variable and are likely to be missed if clinical suspicion is not strong. The tibia, skull, clavicle and femur are affected most, but any bone may be involved. Two types of lesions may develop— granulomatous periostitis and gummatous osteitis. Periostitis leads to bony proliferation and deposition of new bone beneath the periosteum. Gummatous osteitis

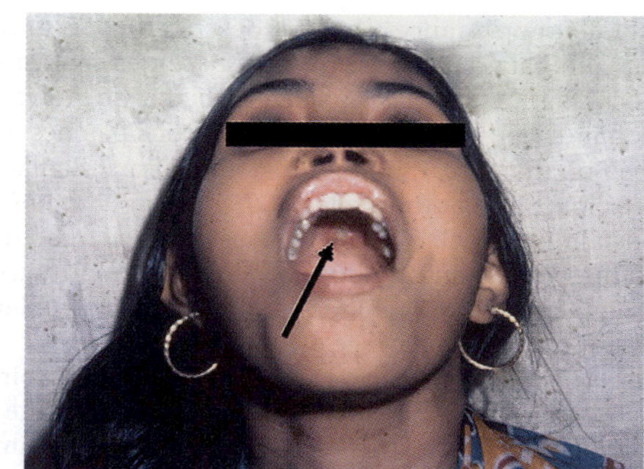

Fig. 47.2: Syphilis tertiary stage gummata tongue (arrow)

produces circumscribed areas of osteolysis surrounded by areas of sclerosis. Syphilitic osteitis and periostitis may occur in the same bone.

Visceral syphilis: Liver is affected most commonly and it is enlarged by multiple gummata. As the lesions heal, sheets of fibrous tissue are formed and the liver is shrunken and distorted. The surface of the liver becomes lobular and this is termed as ***hepar lobatum***. Stomach, intestines, lungs and reproductive organs are affected less commonly.

Cardiovascular and central nervous system (CNS): Lesions occur 10–40 years after the initial infection. Cardiovascular lesions include syphilitic aortitis, aortic regurgitation and aneurysms of the aorta. Neurological involvement is more varied and this may be meningovascular or parenchymal. Meningitis occurs in the secondary stage, but in the tertiary stage meningovascular involvement leads to meningomyelitis, transverse myelitis, syphilitic pachymeningitis, Erb's syphilitic paraplegia and occlusive vascular lesions. Parenchymal lesions are tabes dorsalis, general paralysis of the insane (GPI), taboparesis and optic atrophy.

Congenital Syphilis

T. pallidum can pass from the infected mother to the fetus through the placenta. An infected mother can transmit the disease to her child even in the late stages, but in the late latent phase there is less infectivity to the fetus. Since *T. pallidum* is transmitted only through the fully formed placenta which develops by the fourth month of pregnancy, the fetus is unaffected in the early period. Abortions occurring earlier during pregnancy are not attributable to syphilis. Birth of a syphilitic baby is often preceded by repeated abortions occurring at progressively later months.

The primary stage is not evident in congenital syphilis. The early manifestations are similar to those of secondary acquired syphilis. Sometimes, a syphilitic infant may be clinically normal at birth. The skin lesions consist of dusky red papules with bullae containing serum or pus, most prominent in the palms and soles (syphilitic pemphigus). The discharge contains a large number of *T. pallidum*. Generalized widespread papular skin rashes are seen at times. At the mucocutaneous junctions the papules develop into condylomata. The infant has a wasted and dehydrated appearance which is described as 'old man facies.' The baby fails to thrive and becomes marasmic. Alopecia may occur. Occasionally there may be growth of black hair called the **syphilitic wig**. Mucous patches may be seen on the nose, mouth, throat and larynx. Radiating fissures may form at the angles of the mouth (**rhagades**). Bloodstained, thick, purulent nasal discharge may block the nostrils and produce a bubbling sound during breathing termed as 'syphilitic snuffle.' Feeding problems may develop due to blockage of the nose.

Bony lesions develop within 6 months of birth. The ends of long bones are swollen and tender due to osteochondritis. The restriction of movement is sometimes referred to as **syphilitic pseudoparalysis**. Osteochondritis clears up by six months of age, but syphilitic periostitis persists and tends to become more marked. Subperiosteal new bone is laid down irregularly over the shaft of bones leading to thickening and deformity, e.g. sabre tibia. Due to concentric layering of new bone, the skiagrams may reveal a characteristic onion peel appearance. Painless effusions in one or both knee joints (Clutton's joints) develop between the ages of 10 and 20 years.

Eye lesions include choroiditis and retinitis which develop after the first two years of life. Invasion of the nervous system by *T. pallidum* during intrauterine life may lead to arrest of development of the brain.

Late non-infectious congenital syphilis: This stage sets in after the second year of life. Lesions are more common between 7 and 15 years of age but may occur at any age. Gumma may develop in the skin, mucous membranes or viscera. The lesions resemble those of acquired syphilis.

Interstitial keratitis: It is one of the common lesions occurring in late congenital syphilis. This may develop at any age between 3 and 30 years or even later.

Neurological lesions: Nerve deafness develops due to involvement of the 8th cranial nerve endings and this lesion is suggestive of congenital syphilis. It presents as bilateral progressive loss of hearing which may become total. Congenital neurosyphilis leads either to general paralysis of insane or tabes dorsalis, but these patients develop the disease at a younger age. Meningovascular neurosyphilis is rare. When it occurs it presents as cranial nerve palsies, hemianopia and hemi or monoplegia.

Stigmata of congenital syphilis: Damage to the developing organs *in utero* leads to the permanent stigmata of congenital syphilis. These include localized thickening of the frontal and parietal bones of the skull due to periostitis giving rise to frontal bossing, **hot cross bun skull** and **Parrot's nodes**. **Saddle nose** develops due to the destruction of nasal bones. High arched palate and bulldog facies are all characteristic. The permanent teeth show diagnostic abnormalities. Peg-like incisors (**Hutchinson's teeth**) are diagnostic. Hutchinson's triad is a combination of interstitial keratitis, Hutchinson's teeth (Fig. 47.3) and nerve deafness.

Diagnosis

Serodiagnosis of syphilis: Two types of serological tests have been developed; the nonspecific tests using cardiolipin from beef heart and specific tests using

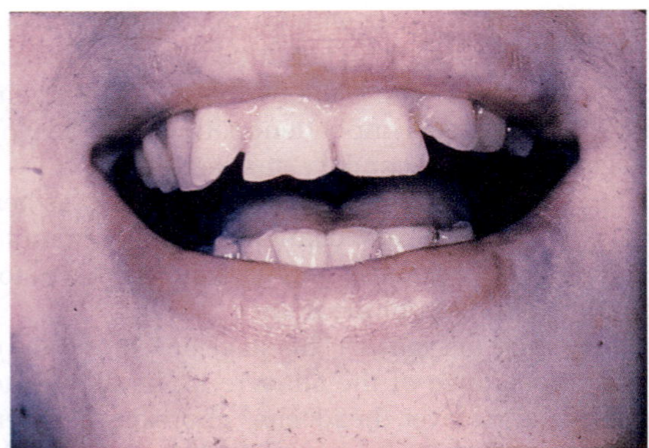

Fig. 47.3: Congenital syphilis—Hutchinson's teeth

live or killed laboratory strains of treponemes or their components. The commonly used nonspecific tests are the rapid plasma reagin (RPR) test and the venereal disease reference laboratory (VDRL) test. Among the specific tests the commonly used one is *Treponema pallidum* hemagglutination (TPHA) test. The fluorescent treponemal antibody-absorption (FTA-ABS) test and the *Treponema pallidum* immobilization (TPI) test are done usually for research purposes. There are several other tests used in different laboratories.

Interpretation of serological tests: The nonspecific serological tests become positive about 4 weeks after infection and the titer progressively increases in the secondary stage. If the disease is treated and cured at this stage the titers fall and the test may become negative in 4–6 months. Treatment instituted late in the disease may not eliminate seropositivity. False positive reactions not due to any technical error are known as biological false positive reactions. This may occur in connective tissue disorders like systemic lupus erythematosus (SLE) and rheumatoid disease, malaria, leprosy, hepatitis, infectious mononucleosis and tuberculosis.

The FTA-ABS test becomes positive early after infection. The TPI test becomes positive only later than the FTA-ABS test. Once positive, they remain so for life. Early treatment in primary stage prevents the development of seropositivity. Nonspecific tests are useful to determine cure, since they decline in titer if the disease is treated sufficiently early.

Frequency of serological tests:

Tests	Primary stage	Secondary stage	Tertiary stage
Nonspecific	50–70%	98–100%	70%
Specific	70–85%	100%	98–100%

In the primary and secondary stages, diagnosis is established by demonstration of the organism by dark ground microscopy and serological tests. All genital ulcers should be investigated for syphilis irrespective of their appearance. Treatment should always be given only after an accurate diagnosis has been made. All suspected cases should be kept underobservation for a minimum period of three months and serological tests for syphilis should be performed at regular intervals. All sexual contacts of the patient during the past six months should be traced and examined. The 2010 Centers for Disease Control and

Prevention (CDC) guidelines recommend that lumbar puncture to assess CNS invasion in early syphilis is needed only if neurologic symptoms are present.

Latent syphilis: It is diagnosed when the standard serological tests for syphilis are positive in the blood without any clinical evidence of the disease.

Late syphilis: It is essential to confirm the diagnosis by serological examination before starting the treatment. The CSF should be examined in all cases of secondary syphilis to exclude meningeal involvement.

Diagnosis of congenital syphilis: The disease should be suspected in children born to mothers who are syphilitic. In the early infectious stage diagnosis can be established by finding *T. pallidum* on dark ground examination of the discharge from the lesions of the skin, mucous membrane and nose. Serological tests have to be interpreted with caution in the early weeks of life. Maternal reaginic antibodies of immunoglobulin G (IgG) class may be passively transferred across the placenta and these may lead to positive serology in the infant even though the baby is not suffering from syphilis. These disappear with time. If the baby is really affected, IgM antibodies develop and the rise in titers can be demonstrated by specific tests (IgM-FTA-ABS). If a non-treponemal test is reactive at 18 months of age, the child should be evaluated and treated for congenital syphilis.

Treatment decisions must be made on the basis of:
- Identification of syphilis in mother
- Adequacy of maternal treatment
- Presence of clinical, laboratory or radiographic evidence of syphilis in the infant
- Comparison of maternal and infant nontreponemal serological titers. Infant's serological titers four-fold higher than maternal titer are significant.

Specific treponemal test on newborn's serum is not necessary. All infants born to women who have reactive serological test for syphilis should be thoroughly examined for evidence of congenital syphilis.

Treatment

The principal aim of therapy is to make the patient non-infectious within the shortest time and to achieve cure. A treponemicidal level of penicillin (0.018 mg/L) has to be maintained in the serum and CSF for 7–10 days or more to achieve cure.

Treatment regimen for syphilis:
- ***Early syphilis*** (primary, secondary and early latent)
  - ***Adults:*** Benzathine benzylpenicillin, 2.4 million IU by intramuscular (IM) injection, given as two injections at separate sites in a single session.
  - ***Children:*** Benzathine penicillin 50000 IU/kg, to a maximum of 2.4 million IU, as a single dose by IM injection.
  - ***Alternative regimen:*** Procaine benzylpenicillin, 1.2 million IU, IM injection for 10 consecutive days.
- ***Late syphilis:*** The dose and choice of the drugs is the same as for early syphilis but the duration is longer. Benzathine penicillin is given once weekly for 3 consecutive weeks, procaine penicillin for 20 days, doxycycline, tetracycline and erythromycin for 30 days.

- ***Neurosyphilis:*** Aqueous benzylpenicillin (crystalline penicillin) 12–24 million IU by intravenous (IV) injection, administered daily in doses of 2–4 million IU every 4 hours for 14 days. Treatment as for late syphilis can be considered after completion of neurosyphilis treatment. Patients with syphilitic eye disease should be treated as neurosyphilis.

Alternative regimen—procaine benzylpenicillin 2.4 million IU IM once daily and probenecid 500 mg qid po, both for 10–14 days.

Congenital syphilis:
- ***Congenital syphilis (up to 2 years of age) and infants with abnormal CSF:*** Aqueous crystalline penicillin 1,00,000–1,5,000 IU/kg/day administered as 50,000 IU/kg/dose IV every 12 hours, during the first 7 days of life and every 8 hours thereafter for a total of 10 days. Alternative regimen is procaine penicillin, 50,000 IU/kg IM, as a single daily dose for 10 days.
- ***Congenital syphilis of 2 or more years:*** Aqueous benzylpenicillin, 2,00,000–3,00,000 IU/kg/day IV or IM, administered as 50,000 IU/kg/dose every 4–6 hours for 10–14 days.

Penicillin allergic children—erythromycin 7.5–12.5 mg/kg qid po for 30 days.

Adverse Effects of Penicillin

In addition to all the adverse side effects of penicillin, syphilitic subjects receiving the drugs may develop ***Jarisch-Herxheimer reaction*** caused by rapid destruction of spirochetes. In addition to the products of spirochete disintegration, cytokines such as tumor necrosis factor (TNF) and others may also play a role. It may develop in up to 50% of cases of secondary syphilis and in a smaller proportion of late syphilis. After 2–3 hours of receiving penicillin, the patient becomes restless and apprehensive and develops severe rigor, fever, tachypnea and rise in blood pressure. In a few hours sweating starts, becomes profuse and the blood pressure (BP) drops. The reaction subsides within a few hours with symptomatic management. However, in patients with general paresis or high CSF cell counts, further neurological damage may develop and lead to extension of paralysis. The lesions of syphilitic aortitis may extend and lead to coronary occlusion which can be fatal. Administration of 20 mg prednisolone starting 24 hours prior to penicillin injections and continued for two days prevents Herxheimer reaction. If Herxheimer reaction occurs, management is the same as for anaphylactic shock. Antibody to TNF which blocks its action has been employed with benefit in severe cases where other routine measures are inadequate.

Treatment of Patients Allergic to Penicillin

Non-pregnant patients: Doxycycline 100 mg orally twice daily for 14 days or tetracycline 500 mg orally 4 times daily for 14 days. A single dose of azithromycin 2 g orally is also effective. There are reports of azithromycin resistant *T. pallidum*. Azithromycin should not be used in men who have sex with men and in pregnant women.

Pregnant patients: They should be desensitized and treated with penicillin.

Textbook of Medicine

Follow-up: Patients should be followed up at the end of 3 months, 6 months and 12 months, clinically and serologically, using a nontreponemal test like VDRL or RPR to assess the results of therapy and to detect possible reinfection.

At all stages of the disease, repeat treatment should be considered when clinical signs or symptoms of active syphilis persist or recur or there is confirmed increase in the titer of a nontreponemal test. Examination of CSF should be undertaken before repeat treatment, unless reinfection and a diagnosis of early syphilis can be established. Retreatment is with schedules as for late syphilis.

When congenital syphilis is detected, the mother also should be investigated serologically. Surveillance plan is the same as for late syphilis. The baby should be followed up late into adult life. ***Interstitial keratitis*** should be treated with local corticosteroids and atropine drops in addition.

Prevention

Congenital syphilis is preventable if the mother is treated before the fourth month of pregnancy. Treatment administered later in pregnancy usually cures both the mother and the fetus, though residual stigmata may be seen in the baby. If syphilis is detected in the pregnant woman, the course of treatment is the same as for primary syphilis. Tetracycline should be avoided in pregnancy. Azithromycin in a dose of 1.8 g orally given on two occasions within six days has been found to prevent the development of syphilis in persons who had infective exposure. This may serve as a short-term measure.

Social measures: When primary or latent syphilis is detected, all sexual contacts should be traced out and examined. Since, a social stigma has been attached to the sexually transmitted diseases (STDs), patients tend to conceal the infection and do not come up for treatment. Hence, great care is required to avoid psychological trauma to the patient and his contacts. High intensity behavioral counseling is recommended, which is counseling and education delivered through multiple sessions, most often in groups with durations from 3 to 9 hours. The doctor should not take an admonishing attitude. Proper instruction on healthy sexual practices, avoidance of direct contact by the use of condoms and periodic examination of commercial sex workers and other personnel engaged in similar practices help to limit to some extent the incidence of STD.

Syphilis and HIV: There is increased interest in syphilis at present, since it often coexists with acquired immunodeficiency syndrome (AIDS) and each aggravates the manifestation of the other. Individuals infected with sexually transmitted infection (STI) are 2–5 times more likely to acquire HIV infection if exposed to the virus. Ulcerative infections provide a portal of entry for HIV. Ulcerative or nonulcerative STIs cause inflammation which increase the concentration of cells in the genital region that serve as targets for HIV. Individuals with HIV infection with another STI are more likely to transmit HIV due to increased concentration of HIV in genital secretions.

All patients with syphilis should be screened for HIV and vice versa. Clinical manifestation of syphilis in HIV may be atypical. A rapid progression from early to late disease is reported. Progression to neurosyphilis occurs more frequently. The diagnosis of syphilis by serologic means become unreliable. Serological tests like VDRL and TPHA may be false negative or quantitatively higher or lower than expected. Dark field microscopy, histology and clinical acumen have to be relied upon. Most HIV co-infected patients respond appropriately to standard treatment of early syphilis. CSF abnormalities are more common. However, unless neurological symptoms are present, CSF examination has not been associated with improved clinical outcomes. Patient should be followed up clinically and serologically at 3, 6, 9, 12 and 24 months after therapy.

Syphilis and pregnancy: All women should be screened serologically for syphilis early in pregnancy, preferably in the first prenatal visit. In populations where prevalence of syphilis is high, a repeat serologic testing should be performed during third trimester, preferably at 28–32 weeks gestation and at delivery. A positive VDRL/RPR test should be confirmed by a specific TPHA.

Pregnant patients should receive the same benzathine penicillin dose appropriate for their stage of infection. In early syphilis, an additional dose one week later can be beneficial.

Patients who are allergic to penicillin should be desensitized and treated with penicillin. Erythromycin and azithromycin should not be used because neither reliably cure maternal infection or treat an infected fetus.

Points to Remember

- The primary chancre on the genitalia appears 3 weeks after the sexual contact.
- The generalized symmetrical, nonpruritic papules of the secondary stage develops 6–8 weeks following the chancre.
- Tertiary stage develops years later.
- Serological diagnosis includes VDRL and TPHA and demonstration of treponema by dark ground microscopy.
- Treatment is with benzathine benzylpenicillin or procaine penicillin.

GONORRHEA

Definition: It is one of the most common STD all over the world. This is caused by *Neisseria gonorrhoeae,* a gram-negative intracellular diplococci, which is present throughout the world. Several strains of *N. gonorrhoeae* produce *beta-lactamase* and this helps them to develop resistance to penicillin to which they were sensitive. At present, occurrence of penicillin-resistant gonorrhea is widespread. The lesions also occur over a wider area, depending on the sexual practices.

Gonococci attach themselves to cells with the help of pili before initiating infection. The organisms are ingested by polymorphs and they survive within the cells for variable periods, being protected from adverse environment. Four types can be distinguished by cultural characteristics. Types T_1 and T_2 are virulent whereas T_3 and T_4 are not. Gonococci are gram-negative diplococci seen intracellularly and also free in the exudate.

Pathology

Gonococci affect columnar and transitional epithelium mainly and infection is initiated in the urethra, anal canal, conjunctiva, pharynx and endocervix. Pus is produced locally. Direct extension from the site of infection leads to complications such as endometritis, salpingitis, peritonitis and bartholinitis in the female and periurethral abscess, epididymo-orchitis and prostatitis in the male. Ocular conjunctiva is affected. Metastatic spread of the organisms leads to arthritis, dermatitis, endocarditis, meningitis, myopericarditis and hepatitis.

Clinical Features

In men the onset of the disease is more acute than in women. Incubation period is usually 3–5 days.

Gonorrhea in the male: In over 90% of cases urethritis presents with a constant burning sensation in the penis and discharge of infective pus which teems with the organisms. Meatal inflammation and penile edema may be obvious. Variable amounts of pus can be milked from the urethra. Micturition is painful and the patient is severely distressed.

Other adnexal structures like epididymis, testes and spermatic cord become inflamed. Rarely the Tyson's glands and the median raphe of the scrotum may be inflamed. Gonococcal prostatitis and seminal vesiculitis are seen but they are rare. If left alone, the acute manifestations subside over a period of weeks or months even-without treatment. Exacerbations occur frequently as a result of sexual indulgence, alcoholism or undue exertion. Ultimately, the anterior and posterior urethra develop stricture. Periurethral abscesses may develop at times. Extension of suppuration into the periurethral tissues and scrotum result in fistulous openings discharging urine from multiple sites ***(watering-can scrotum)***. In 10% of subjects the lesion may be asymptomatic and has to be detected by examination.

The rectum is an important site of ulceration in persons who are habitual catamites in homosexual relationship. The rectum and anal canal are ulcerated and show blood-stained mucopurulent discharge. The condition may present as proctitis and may be mistaken for other ulcerating lesions of this region.

Gonorrhea in the female: In a good number of women gonorrhea may remain asymptomatic. Symptoms include leucorrhea, dysuria, menstrual abnormalities and features of pelvic inflammation. Rectal lesions develop in about 40% of affected women due to contamination by cervical discharges.

The gonococci may pass up from the endocervix leading to acute salpingitis and oophoritis. Chronic salpingo-oophoritis and tubo-ovarian masses may develop. Exacerbations occur during menstrual periods or one or two weeks thereafter. Gonococcal salpingo-oophoritis is a common cause of sterility.

Gonococcal infection in the newborn: Inoculation of gonococci into the baby's eyes from the maternal genital passages leads to ophthalmia neonatorum. This presents with purulent conjunctivitis which may result in blindness. The infection can also disseminate to other tissues and result in arthritis in the newborn.

Disseminated gonococcal infection: This occurs in up to 30% of infected patients, 80% of them being females. Bacteremia spread occurs. Manifestations include cutaneous lesions, septic arthritis, septicemia, endocarditis, myocarditis and rarely, pericarditis and meningitis. Risk of dissemination depends on the type and virulence of the organism. Dissemination is more common from silent foci in the pharynx, rectum or endocervix. The cutaneous lesions take the form of vesicles and pustules which do not usually ulcerate.

Oropharyngeal infections: Pharyngitis and tonsillitis result from oral sex and may affect both sexes. In the majority of cases symptoms are not severe enough to seek medical care. Strong clinical suspicion and microbiological investigations are required to make the diagnosis. Gonococcal pharyngitis may give rise to dissemination.

Diagnosis

Gonorrhea should be suspected in all clinical situations where there is purulent urethral discharge, leucorrhea in women, atypical oropharyngeal ulceration, proctocolitis and ophthalmia neonatorum. Urethritis can be documented on the basis of following signs or tests.

- Mucopurulent or purulent discharge on examination
- Gram stain of urethral secretions demonstrating > 5 white blood cells (WBCs)/oil immersion field. Demonstration of gram-negative intracellular diplococci is diagnostic of gonococcal infection. Similarly, in women, leucorrhea (> 10 WBCs/high power field on examination of vaginal fluid) is associated with cervicitis.
- Positive leukocyte esterase test on first void urine or microscopic examination of first void urine sediment demonstrating >10 WBCs/high power field.

If these criteria are absent, *N. gonorrhoeae* and *C. trachomatis* can be tested using nucleic acid amplification tests.

The organism can be identified by culture and further studies. Culture of cervical discharge is required in women with late manifestations to establish the diagnosis. On rare occasions purulent material may have to be collected by culdocentesis or laparoscopy. Fluorescent antibody techniques help in making quick diagnosis where such facilities exist. Complement fixation test (CFT) is useful in selected cases of chronic gonorrhea with systemic manifestations.

Treatment

The sheet anchor of the treatment of gonorrhea up to the 1970's used to be penicillin to which the organisms were invariably sensitive. A large proportion of gonococcal isolates worldwide are now resistant to penicillin, tetracyclines and other older antimicrobial agents. Therefore, these drugs can no longer be relied upon for the cure of gonorrhea (Table 47.1). Since, dual infections with gonococcus and chlamydia are common, it is recommended that concurrent antichlamydia therapy should be given.

Recommended regimen (CDC guidelines 2010): Ceftriaxone 250 mg IM injection as a single dose + azithromycin 1 g orally single dose/doxycycline 100 mg bd orally for 7 days.

Table 47.1: Clinical type of gonorrhea and the drug of choice

Uncomplicated infections of the cervix, urethra and rectum in adults	Ceftriaxone, cefixime, ciprofloxacin, ofloxacin, levofloxacin
Gonococcal infections in pregnancy	Ceftriaxone, cefixime
Disseminated gonococcal infection in adults (> 45 kg)	Ceftriaxone
Uncomplicated infections of the cervix, urethra and rectum in children (< 45 kg)	Ceftriaxone
Gonococcal conjunctivitis in adults	Ceftriaxone
Ophthalmia neonatorum	Ceftriaxone
Infants born to mothers with gonococcal infection (prophylaxis)	Erythromycin, tetracycline

Alternative regimens

- Ceftizoxime 500 mg IM single dose
- Cefoxitin 2 g IM with probenecid 1 g orally
- Cefotaxime 500 mg IM single dose
- Cefixime 400 mg orally or spectinomycin 2 g by IM injection, as a single dose. These drugs are also effective in adult gonococcal conjunctivitis
- Quinolones are no longer used in the treatment of gonorrhea.

Neonatal gonococcal conjunctivitis: Ceftriaxone 50 mg/kg IM as a single dose to a maximum of 125 mg.

Alternative regimen includes kanamycin or spectinomycin 25 mg/kg IM single dose to a maximum of 75 mg.

Disseminated gonococcal infection: Ceftriaxone 1 g IM or IV injection, once daily for 7 days is the recommended regime. Alternative regimes include cefotaxime 1 g thrice daily or ceftizoxime 1 g IV thrice daily or spectinomycin 2 g IM twice daily for 7 days.

Gonococcal endocarditis—same dosages of ceftriaxone or spectinomycin for 4 weeks.

Prophylactic treatment: Instillation of 1–2% silver nitrate solution or 1% tetracycline ointment or erythromycin ophthalmic ointment 0.5% as a single application into the eyes of newborn babies effectively prevents all forms of ophthalmia neonatorum whether it is of bacterial, viral or chlamydial origin. Use of condoms helps to reduce transmission of STDs.

Follow-up: Patients should be reviewed after 48 hours for subsidence of acute symptoms and at longer intervals for recurrence. Retesting is recommended 3 months post treatment. Sexual partners should be evaluated.

Points to Remember
- Males present with dysuria, frequency and urethral discharge.
- Females complain of vaginal discharge, dysuria and abdominal pain.
- Pelvic inflammatory disease and infertility are late sequelae.
- Treatment is with ciprofloxacin or ceftriaxone.
- Concurrent antichlamydia therapy should be given to all patients with gonorrhea.

NONGONOCOCCAL URETHRITIS

Syn: Nonspecific urethritis

Definition: Urethritis, from which gonococci cannot be isolated, is termed as nongonococcal urethritis (NGU).

While in men the condition is well-defined, in women it is not so. The possible causative organism is *Chlamydia trachomatis* in 60% cases. Other organisms include mycoplasma such as *Ureaplasma urealyticum*, *Mycoplasma hominis*, *M. fermentans* and *M. genitalis*. Other pathogens such as ***herpes simplex virus***, *Trichomonas vaginalis* and *Candida albicans* may rarely produce the picture of NGU. In a proportion of patients organisms may not be identified. Several species of chlamydia cause diseases in humans affecting different organ systems.

C. trachomatis is an obligate aerobic intracellular human pathogen which is a gram-negative bacterium. It can occur in coccoid or rod-shaped forms.

Etiology

- *C. trachomatis* (15–40%)
- *M. genitalium* (15–25%)
- Others (20–50%)
  - *T. vaginalis*
  - *U. urealyticum*
  - Herpes simplex virus (HSV) (in absence of skin lesions)
  - Adenovirus
  - Hemophilus
  - Miscellaneous
    - In association with urinary tract infection (UTI)
    - Bacterial prostatitis,
    - Urethral stricture,
    - Phimosis,
    - Secondary to instrumentation of the urethra,
    - Congenital abnormalities,
    - Chemical irritation
    - Tumors.

Lifecycle of Chlamydia

Chlamydia have a unique lifecycle, it cannot synthesize its own adenosine triphosphate (ATP) supply. So it has to depend on the host cells for metabolism. There are two stages in the lifecycle of *C. tractomatis*—the elemental bodies (EBs) and reticulate bodies (RBs). The bacteria has to replicate within the host cell for survival and the host cell dies in the process. EB is the infective form which attaches and enters host's cells present in the endocervix, urethra, endometrium and fallopian tubes. The organism is phagocytosed by the host's cells. After phagocytosis the EBs prevent the fusion of phagosomes and liposomes and they are protected by host's defense system.

The second phase in the host's cells starts when the EBs secrete glycogen and transform into metabolically active RBs which multiply by binary fission utilizing the ATP of the host's cells. A large cytoplasmic inclusion body consisting of numerous RBs develops. At this stage the RBs revert to the EBs, lyse the cell and escape to infect fresh cells for attack. One complete cycle takes 72 hours.

Epidemiology

NGU occurs worldwide and it is common in India. Infection is initially acquired by sexual intercourse, though relapses may occur without such contact. The chain of transmission is not as clear cut as in gonorrhea. This infection develops only in a few of the sexual partners of patients in both sexes. The reason for this phenomenon is not known. In many centers NGU outnumbers gonorrhea.

Table 47.2: Different chlamydial lesions in humans

Diseases	Organisms
Eyes	
• Trachoma	C. trachomatis A, B, Ba, C
• Inclusion conjunctivitis	C. trachomatis D-K
• Ophthalmia neonatorum	-do-
Genitourinary tract	
Male	
Urethritis, epididymitis, prostatitis	C. trachomatis D-K
Female	
Urethritis, cervicitis, salpingitis, infertility abortion, stillbirth	
Gastrointestinal system	
Proctitis, perihepatitis, periappendicitis	
Respiratory tract	
• Pneumonitis of infants	C. trachomatis D-K
• Pharyngitis, pneumonia	C. pneumoniae
• Psittacosis	C. psittaci (avian strains)
• Pneumonia	C. psittaci (ovine strains)
Sexually transmitted infection	
Lymphogranuloma venereum	C. trachomatis L1-3

Clinical Features (Table 47.2)

NGU in men: The incubation period ranges from a few days to two months. This wide range may suggest the possibility of different pathogens. Clinical features resemble a mild attack of gonorrhea with a subacute onset and a watery, mucoid, mucopurulent or rarely frankly purulent urethral discharge. Gram staining shows the absence of gonococci. Even in untreated cases the urethritis subsides, but mild exacerbations occur from time to time. Treatment with tetracycline, which is the drug of choice, rapidly clears the condition in 90% of cases. Nongonococcal proctitis may occur in homosexual individuals.

Post-gonococcal urethritis (PGU): This term is used for patients with gonococcal urethritis who develop non-gonococcal urethritis after successful treatment with penicillin. It is possible that these patients harbor the organisms of gonorrhea and NGU simultaneously.

Local complications of NGU and PGU: Local abscesses may develop in some cases. Acute unilateral epididymitis develops rarely. ***Chronic prostatitis*** is the most common complication. Identification of this condition may not be easy. The most significant symptom is prostatic pain which is felt in the perineal region as a vague discomfort and this may be referred to the groins, thighs and suprapubic region. Chronic prostatitis can also cause irritative voiding symptoms, pain during or after ejaculation or new onset of premature ejaculation lasting for more than 3 months. Presence of pus cells and numerous prostatic threads in the first sample of urine collected after prostatic massage suggests prostatitis. Around 1–2% of males who develop NGU may suffer from Reiter's syndrome later.

Nongonococcal genital infections in women: This infection is much less clear cut in women than in men. Some women may complain of vaginal discharge. The most important manifestation is salpingitis, which may extend to pelvic tissues to produce pelvic inflammatory

disease. Perihepatitis, bartholinitis, postpartum and post-abortal fever, ascending pyelonephritis, infertility and birth of underweight babies have all been recorded as complications.

Nongonococcal infections in infants and children: Infections may be acquired by the baby during birth, from the maternal genital passages. The newborn may develop nongonococcal ophthalmia neonatorum and infantile pneumonia caused by *C. trachomatis*.

Diagnosis

This is by culture of discharges, cervical swab or urethral discharge, in both sexes. Serological diagnosis is by demonstrating antichlamydia antibodies IgG and IgM. Direct fluorescence antibody test employs immune fluorescence to detect the elementary body by deoxyribonucleic acid (DNA) hybridization in urethral swabs. Other methods include polymerase chain reaction (PCR) for *C. trachomatis*.

Treatment

Recommended regimen: Doxycycline 100 mg orally bd for 7 days or azithromycin 1 g orally in a single dose.

Alternative regimen (7 days treatment): Erythromycin 500 mg qid or ofloxacin 300 mg bd or levofloxacin 500 mg od. Epididymitis responds to ceftriaxone 250 mg IM bd with doxycycline 100 mg bd for 10 days. Azithromycin 1 g single dose is a suitable alternative. Patients with HIV co-infection should receive same treatment. In pregnant women, azithromycin is safe and effective. Repeat testing 3 weeks after completion of therapy is recommended to ensure therapeutic cure.

Recommended regimen: Azithromycin 1 g orally single dose or amoxicillin 500 mg orally tid × 7 days.

Alternative regimen: Erythromycin base 500 mg orally qid × 7 days or 250 mg orally qid × 14 days.

Follow-up: Patients should be reviewed if symptoms persist or recur. Repeat testing is recommended 3–6 months after treatment to detect re-infection. Routine testing 3–4 weeks after treatment is not recommended. If a patient has persistent symptoms, re-treatment is indicated only if objective signs of urethritis are present. Initial regimen can be repeated, if they did not comply with treatment or got re-infected.

Doxycycline resistant *U. urealyticum* or *M. genitalium* can cause persistent urethritis. The following regime is recommended. Metronidazole 2 g orally single dose or tinidazole 2 g orally single dose + azithromycin 1 g orally single dose (if not used for initial episode).

Points to Remember
- NGU presents as urethral discharge which is watery, mucoid or mucopurulent.
- Some patients harbor organisms of gonorrhea and NGU simultaneously and their urethritis persists if gonorrhea alone is treated.
- Treatment is with doxycycline or azithromycin.

LYMPHOGRANULOMA VENEREUM

Syn: Climatic bubo, Lymphogranuloma inguinale

Definition: Lymphogranuloma venereum (LGV) is a common infection of the genitals along with anorectal involvement in the late stages.

Textbook of Medicine

It is sexually transmitted disease caused by *Chlamydia trachomatis* strains L1, L2 and L3, manifesting as inguinal buboes, pseudoelephantiasis. It is present all over the world, more frequently in developing countries. The incubation period ranges from 2 weeks to several weeks.

Clinical Features

The organisms enter by sexual intercourse and a small herpetiform ulcer develops under the prepuce or the labia. This ulcer disappears within 24–48 hours. Rarely may it become secondarily infected and persistent.

The manifestations are different in the two sexes. In *males,* the prominent feature is development of inguinal buboes since lymphatics from the prepuce and penis drain into the inguinal group of lymph nodes. On the other hand, in the females, they drain into the anorectal lymph nodes or directly into the hypogastric lymph nodes. The buboes are usually unilateral, painful, matted, firm or fluctuant and tender. The overlying skin is indurated. If the femoral and inguinal nodes are enlarged, they are separated by Poupart's ligament producing a groove called *groove sign of Greenblatt*, which is pathognomonic. Buboes may be bilateral at times. Sooner or later, the bubo suppurates and multiple sinuses develop and discharge pus. Some buboes may remain indolent for a long time.

In *females,* mild constitutional symptoms like fever, malaise and lower abdominal pain on the side of the bubo, are fairly common. Local peritonitis may develop through peritoneal lymphatics. Other lesions in the female include stricture of the urethra, destruction of the floor of urethra and rectovaginal, urethrovaginal or vesicovaginal fistulae. In debilitated patients extensive tissue damage may develop. Pelvic inflammation may follow.

Esthiomene: This is a pseudoelephantoid condition of the genitalia caused by lymphatic obstruction, due to extensive involvement of deeper pelvic lymph nodes and lymphatics. It is more common in women. Hypertrophy involves the labia, prepuce of the clitoris and sometimes the clitoris. They enlarge to big sizes and the surface is warty, mammilated, verrucous or ulcerated.

Anorectal lesions: These develop late in the disease and are more common in women and in male passive homosexuals. Initial lesion is anoproctitis which may resemble dysentery, but does not respond to usual treatment. Finally it leads to rectal stricture. Rarely, stricture may develop without evidence of preceding anoproctitis. Below the stricture, extensive polyposis and cock's comb like condylomatous masses may develop in the perianal region.

Extragenital manifestations are rare in LGV. These are meningitis, cutaneous eruptions, episcleritis, iridocyclitis and arthritis.

Diagnosis

Diagnosis is clinical. Lesion swab or bubo aspirated can be tested for *C. trachomatis* by culture, direct immunofluorescence or nucleic acid detection tests. The causative organism can be grown in chick embryo or tissue culture, where facilities exist. The LGV CFT becomes positive in 1–3 weeks in 90–95% cases. This test is nonspecific since other chlamydiae may give rise to positive reactions, though not in the same titers as seen in LGV. A four-fold rise in the titer can be taken as diagnostic of LGV.

Treatment

The recommended regimen is doxycycline 100 mg orally bd for 21 days or alternative regime is to treat with erythromycin 500 mg orally qid for 21 days. The suppurating buboes should be aspirated through healthy skin and not incised. Some patients with advanced disease may require prolonged treatment. Surgery is required for excising elephantoid lesions and dilating strictures after treating adequately with tetracycline. Sometimes, even established strictures resolve with simple medical treatment.

Follow-up: Patients should be followed up clinically until signs and symptoms have resolved. Even advanced lesions will resolve with prolonged medical treatment, e.g. rectal stricture and vulvar edema, etc.

- Early treatment is necessary to prevent the chronic phase
- Doxycycline 100 mg orally, twice daily for 14 days
  or
- Erythromycin 500 mg orally, 4 times daily for 14 days
  or
- Tetracycline 500 mg orally, 4 times daily for 14 days
- Fluctuant buboes should be aspirated with a syringe and needle
- Surgical drainage or reconstructive surgery may be sometimes needed.

Points to Remember

- Caused by L1, L2 and L3 strains of *Chlamydia trachomatis*
- Primary asymptomatic ulcer that develops two weeks after the sexual contact is usually unnoticed
- Males present with tender, unilateral inguinal bubo
- Complications are more common in females
- LGV responds to doxycycline or erythromycin.

GRANULOMA INGUINALE

Syn: Granuloma venereum, Donovanosis

Definition: Granuloma inguinale is a specific chronic granulomatous disease affecting primarily the genitalia in both sexes. It is particularly prevalent in the tropical and subtropical regions. It constitutes 1.5–6% of the total number of STD cases seen in clinics in India. There is a higher incidence of this disease in the eastern coastal states, particularly in the states of Orissa, Andhra Pradesh and Tamil Nadu. It has been reported from all regions.

The disease is caused by *Donovania granulomatis* (Syn: *Calymmatobacterium granulomatis, Klebsiella granulomatis*) which is seen either as bacillary forms inside phagocytes in discharges or biopsy specimens. The organism can be cultured *in vitro*.

Clinical Features

The incubation period ranges from a few days to a few months. The disease starts as a subcutaneous papule or vesicle which ulcerates to give rise to a granuloma. The lesion extends by contiguity. Lesions are highly vascular and bleeds easily on touch. Draining lymph glands are not affected and this helps to differentiate the lesion from a primary chancre. Rarely can it present as a subcutaneous swelling in the inguinal region which bursts open to produce a granulomatous ulcer. This is called **pseudo bubo**. The initial lesion may be in the genitalia, groin, thigh, perineum or oral mucosa depending on the sex practices. It may extend to the buttocks or anterior abdominal wall. In most of the cases extragenital lesions on the tongue, cheek or oral cavity are accompanied by a primary lesion in the genitalia. Fusospirochetal infection supervenes as secondary invader and this result in tissue destruction. The ulcers show pouting granulation tissue. Healing leads to scarring and local elephantiasis of the genitalia. Epidermoid carcinoma may develop in 0.5% of cases.

Diagnosis

Granuloma inguinale has to be differentiated from syphilitic chancre and carcinoma. Diagnosis is confirmed by biopsy and demonstration of the organism in tissue spreads obtained from the margins of the ulcer.

Treatment

Treatment halts the progression of disease and healing proceeds inward from the ulcer margins.

Recommended regimen: Doxycycline 100 mg orally bd for at least 3 weeks and until all lesions have completely healed.

Alternative regimens: Azithromycin 1 g orally once a week for at least 3 weeks and till all lesions have completely healed.

Ciprofloxacin 750 mg bd, erythromycin base 500 mg qid or trimethoprim, sulfamethoxazole, double strength (160 mg/800 mg) bd are other alternatives. All should be given for at least 3 weeks and till all lesions have completely healed.

Pregnant and lactating women are treated with azithromycin or erythromycin regimen.

Patients co-infected with HIV, should receive same treatment. Addition of a parenteral aminoglycoside (gentamicin) can be considered.

> **Points to Remember**
> - Granulomatous lesion in the genitalia and neighboring sites
> - Lymph nodes are not affected
> - Treatment is with doxycycline or azithromycin till the lesions heal.

CHANCROID

Syn: Soft chancre, Soft sore, Ulcus molle

Definition: Chancroid is caused by *Haemophilus ducreyi*. The organism is seen in clusters or singly in smears from ulcers and can be grown in special media. The prevalence of chancroid has declined worldwide. Chancroid is a risk factor in the transmission of HIV infection. The disease is seen more in the poor with bad personal hygiene. Incubation period is 5 days.

Clinical Features

Multiple, superficial, non-indurated, painful ulcers which bleed easily develop along the corona glandis or inner aspect of the labia. Inguinal glands may be enlarged and in many cases they suppurate to form inguinal buboes called (inflammatory bubo). Secondary infection with Vincent's spirochetes may develop. In such cases balanoposthitis with offensive discharge may be prominent.

Diagnosis

Diagnosis is confirmed by demonstrating *H. ducreyi* in Gram stained smears from ulcers or by culture. Other ulcerating lesions have to be excluded. Patients should be screened for HIV infection. If initial tests are negative, a serologic test for syphilis and HIV should be performed 3 months after the diagnosis of chancroid.

Treatment

Ciprofloxacin 500 mg bd for 3 days or erythromycin 500 mg qid for 7 days or azithromycin 1 g orally as a single dose is recommended. Alternatively ceftriaxone 250 mg IM as a single dose can be given.

Ciprofloxacin is contraindicated in pregnant and lactating women. No adverse effects of chancroid on pregnancy outcome have been reported. Incision and drainage of fluctuant suppurative bubo may be necessary. Partner should be treated if they had sexual contact with the patient, during the 10 days preceding the patient's onset of symptoms. HIV co-infected patients require repeated or longer courses of therapy.

Follow-up: Patients should be re-examined 3–7 days after initiation of therapy. If no clinical improvement, consider co-infection with another STD, HIV, noncompliance to treatment or treatment resistance.

TRICHOMONIASIS

Definition: Trichomoniasis is infection by the flagellate protozoan, *Trichomonas vaginalis* causing vaginitis in women and rarely urethritis in men. In women the condition is localized to the vagina. In most of the cases infection is acquired by sexual intercourse.

Pathology

The infection is most common in the second and third decade of life and may be associated with gonorrhea. The superficial layers of the vagina are affected. There is marked polymorphonuclear infiltration and changes in the epithelium of the vagina.

Clinical Features

Females: In young women there is a profuse, irritating, offensive, yellow vaginal discharge. Severe cases may show vulval swelling with excoriation of the adjacent skin. The vaginal pH tends to become more alkaline (pH 5–8) than normal (pH 4–5). Symptoms are milder in older women.

Vaginal trichomoniasis has been associated with adverse pregnancy outcomes, particularly premature rupture of membranes, preterm delivery and low birth weight.

Males: Many are asymptomatic carriers. Some may suffer from true trichomonal urethritis or they may harbor *T. vaginalis* in addition to NGU. Occasionally frank purulent urethritis may occur due to this flagellate.

Laboratory diagnosis: It is established by demonstrating the active flagellates in fresh exudates. The sensitivity for microscopic diagnosis is 60–70%. This requires immediate evaluation of wet preparation slide. Food and Drug Administration (FDA) cleared tests include OSOM Trichomonas rapid test, an immunochromatographic capillary flow dipstick technology and a nucleic acid probe test for *T. vaginalis*. Culture is a sensitive and highly specific method of diagnosis. In men, wet preparation is not a sensitive test. Culture of urethral swab, urine or semen is one diagnostic option.

Treatment

Metronidazole or tinidazole, 2 g orally in a single dose is recommended. Alternatively, metronidazole 400 mg or 500 mg orally bd for 7 days or tinidazole 500 mg orally bd for 5 days can be used.

Patient should be followed up after 7 days. If not cured, the treatment is repeated with the 7 day regimen. If there is no response to repeat treatment, metronidazole 2 g orally daily together with 500 mg applied intravaginally at night for 3–7 days is recommended. Vaginal preparations are advised only in refractory infections. Relapse is prevented by treating both sexual partners simultaneously. Relapses of trichomoniasis are unusual. Recurrence of symptoms is usually due to reinfection.

All symptomatic pregnant women should be treated with 2 g metronidazole, single dose. In lactating women, breastfeeding should be withheld during treatment and for 12–24 hours after the last dose. In HIV co-infected women, a 7-day course of metronidazole is preferred over a single dose.

BACTERIAL VAGINOSIS (BV)

It is a polymicrobial clinical syndrome resulting from replacement of the normal vaginal flora with multiple organisms like *Prevotella sp, Mobiluncus sp, Gardnerella vaginalis, U. urealyticum, Mycoplasma hominis* and many other anaerobes. This causes a decrease in the number of hydrogen peroxide producing lactobacilli and a rise in vaginal pH. Most women are asymptomatic.

Diagnosis

At least 3 of the following criteria should be present:
1. Homogenous thin white discharge that smoothly coats the vaginal walls
2. Demonstration of clue cells on microscopic examination
3. Vaginal pH > 4.5
4. Fishy odor of vaginal discharge.

New guidelines for diagnosis expand on the reliable methods. This includes Gram stain, DNA probe test and OSOM BV blue test. Gram stain is considered the gold standard laboratory method for diagnosing BV. If Gram stain is not available, clinical criteria can be used.

Treatment

Relieve the vaginal symptoms and signs of infection.
Recommended regimen
- Metronidazole 500 mg orally bd × 7 days
- Metronidazole gel 0.75%, one full applicator (5 g) intravaginally, od × 5 days
- Clindamycin cream 2%, intravaginally at night for 7 days.

Alternative regimen
- Tinidazole 2 g orally od × 3 days
- Tinidazole 1 g orally od × 5 days
- Clindamycin 300 mg orally bd × 7 days
- Clindamycin ovules 100 mg, intravaginally hs × 3 days.

Follow-up: Women should be advised to return for evaluation if symptoms recur.

Routine treatment of sex partners is not recommended as it does not affect response to treatment or relapse or recurrence in the women. Symptomatic pregnant women are treated with oral metronidazole or clindamycin. HIV co-infected patients have higher recurrences of BV. They should receive the same treatment.

CHAPTER

48

Sexually Transmitted Viral Diseases

KV Krishna Das, Usha Vaidhyanathan, R Sajith Kumar

Chapter Summary

- Herpes Genitalis
  - Clinical Features
  - Herpes Genitalis in the Newborn
  - Diagnosis
  - Treatment and Prophylaxis
- Genital Warts
  - Clinical Features
  - Diagnosis
  - Treatment
  - Prevention
- Molluscum Contagiosum
  - General Considerations and Clinical Features
  - Treatment
- HIV Infection and AIDS
  - Epidemiology
  - Intravenous Drug Users
  - The Present Situation (2014)
  - The Causative Organism
  - Routes of Transmission
  - Use of Drugs to Prevent Transmission
  - Clinical Features
  - Acute Retroviral Syndrome
  - Respiratory System in AIDS
  - Cutaneous Manifestations
    - Kaposi's Sarcoma (KS)
    - Fungal Infections
    - Other Infections

- **Neurological Manifestations**
  - AIDS Encephalopathy
  - Progressive Multifocal Leukoencephalopathy (PML)
  - Cerebral Toxoplasmosis
  - Cryptococcal Meningitis
  - Primary CNS Lymphomas
  - Peripheral Neuropathy
  - Reactivation of CMV Infection
- **Cardiovascular System Involvement**
- **Other Miscellaneous Infections**
  - Esophageal Candidiasis
  - Atypical Mycobacterial Infections
  - Cryptosporidiosis
  - Penicilliosis
  - HBV and HCV Infections

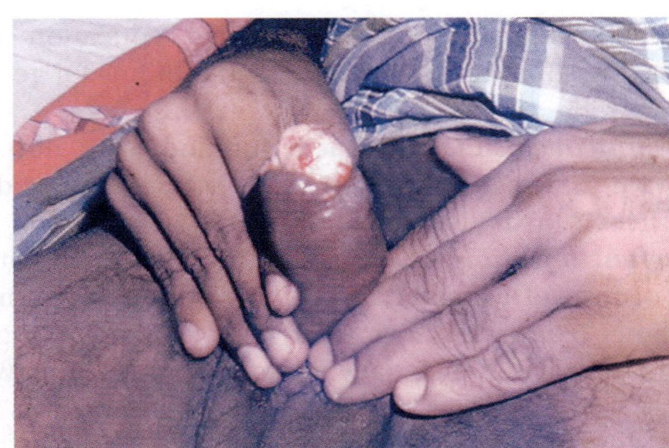

Fig. 48.1: Herpes genitalis male

Several viruses may be transmitted by sexual contact. Important among them are herpes simplex, human papillomavirus (HPV), molluscum contagiosum, hepatitis B virus, cytomegalovirus, Marburg virus and acquired immunodeficiency syndrome (AIDS).

HERPES GENITALIS

Definition: Herpes genitalis is a chronic lifelong infection caused by herpes simplex virus (HSV) type 2 and less frequently by HSV type 1. It is moderately infectious. The virus remains dormant in the presacral sensory ganglion cells. Periodically it moves into the skin through the axons of sensory nerves to produce recurrent attacks of herpes simplex locally. Factors which produce the reappearance of herpes are not clear. In many western countries, herpes genitalis is emerging as the most common among the sexually transmitted disease (STD). The disease is transmitted by sexual intercourse. The virus is shed from the lesions for up to 2 weeks after apparent healing. This asymptomatic viral shedding is more frequent in genital HSV 2 infection than HSV 1 infection, and is an important factor in disease transmission as the patient is unaware of the infection. Infection of the baby during birth leads to neonatal herpes. The misconception that HSV 2 causes cancer should be dispelled.

Clinical Features

The incubation period is 2–4 days or rarely longer. The onset of local lesions may be preceded by burning pain in the S1 to S5 dermatomes.

The lesions occur in the external genitalia of men and in the anal canal of homosexuals. Over the penis, it starts with erythema followed by the appearance of grouped papules or vesicles which soon rupture to form shallow painful ulcers. Ultimately, crusts form which dry up and fall off leaving healed scars which fade. Tender inguinal adenopathy develops in the primary attack but not with recurrences. The lesions are infective throughout. Recurrences are generally much milder. Recurrences are less frequent after initial genital HSV 1 infection (Fig. 48.1).

In women, the primary lesion and recurrent attacks differ from each other considerably. Primary attack is severe, whereas, subsequent attacks are milder. Lesions occur usually in the vulva and adjacent skin areas. Morphology of the lesion is same as in men. During the primary attack retention of urine may develop due to extreme pain on micturition.

Dissemination of the infection is rare in adults, but if it occurs, it can be fatal. The skin, the central nervous system (CNS) and other internal organs may be affected.

Herpes Genitalis in the Newborn

The newborn may acquire herpes during its passage through infected maternal tissues. Lesions develop usually within 2 weeks after birth. These occur more commonly with primary maternal herpes than with recurrent attacks. Both HSV 1 and HSV 2 may be responsible but the latter is more common. The lesions in the newborn include meningoencephalitis or generalized herpetic lesions involving several organs. If not treated, mortality and morbidity are very high.

Diagnosis

Laboratory diagnosis: It is established by isolation of the virus from the lesions. The sensitivity of viral culture is low, especially for recurrent infections. Polymerase chain reaction (PCR) assays for HSV-deoxyribonucleic acid (DNA) are more sensitive. Serological tests using blood include complement fixation test which becomes positive about a week after infection. In primary infection, the first sample is seronegative, the second sample shows a marked rise in titer. In recurrent herpes both samples give the same low titer. Type specific serologic tests are based on HSV specific glycoprotein G2 (HSV 2) and glycoprotein G1 (HSV 1). These tests are sensitive and specific. IgM testing for HSV is not useful because they are not type-specific. Herpes virus can be demonstrated by electron microscopy of vesicle fluid or tissue specimens. In herpes simplex encephalitis, the cerebrospinal fluid (CSF) shows antibodies.

Cytology: Papanicolaou stained smears from vesicles show multinucleated giant cells with eosinophilic inclusions. Cytology for cellular changes are insensitive and nonspecific and should not be relied upon. In meningoencephalitis, CSF shows changes. Computed tomography (CT) scan, magnetic resonance imaging (MRI) and brain biopsy are employed to diagnose herpetic encephalitis.

Treatment and Prophylaxis

Nearly all HSV 2 infections are sexually acquired. The presence of type specific HSV 2 antibodies implies

Textbook of Medicine

anogenital infection and appropriate education and counseling should be done. Treatment options for genital herpes:

First clinical episode: Treatment duration—7–10 days. Acyclovir 200 mg orally 5 times daily or 400 mg tid or valacyclovir 1 g orally bd or famciclovir 250 mg tid.

Recurrent infection: Therapy should be initiated within 1 day of onset of lesions or during the prodrome. Treatment duration—5 days. Acyclovir (oral) 400 mg tid or 800 mg bd or valacyclovir 1 g once daily or famciclovir 125 mg twice daily.

Other dosage options are also available.

Suppressive Therapy

The condition tends to recur often on cessation of treatment. If the recurrence is too frequent (> 6 times a year), suppressive therapy is indicated for prolonged periods. Suppressive therapy decreases the risk of HSV 2 transmission, but does not reduce the risk for human immunodeficiency virus (HIV) acquisition.

Acyclovir 400 mg bd or valacyclovir 500 mg od or famciclovir 250 mg bd continuously.

Recommended regimen for ***severe disease*** is acyclovir 5–10 mg/kg IV every 8 hours for 5–7 days or until clinical resolution is attained, followed by oral antiviral therapy for a total of at least 10 days. Acyclovir resistant severe infections should be treated with foscarnet 40 mg/kg IV every 8 hours till clinical resolution.

Severe herpes with coinfection with HIV: HSV infection might be severe, painful and atypical in HIV coinfected patients. HSV shedding is increased. Suppressive or episodic therapy is effective in reducing the clinical manifestations of HSV. Higher and prolonged doses are required. Acyclovir 400–800 mg orally 2–3 times daily until clinical resolution is attained.

Neonatal infection: Acyclovir 10 mg/kg IV 3 times daily for 10–21 days.

If the mother develops primary attack of herpes genitalis after the 36th week of pregnancy, cesarean section is indicated before the rupture of the membranes to avoid infection of the baby and the baby has to be watched for 2–4 weeks for the development of generalized herpes.

Pregnant women with symptomatic HSV infection should be treated with acyclovir.

> **Points to Remember**
> - This is the most common STD.
> - Primary herpes is severe and is characterized by shallow painful ulcers on the genitalia.
> - Recurrent attacks are milder.
> - Acyclovir is effective.

GENITAL WARTS

Syn: Condyloma acuminata

Definition: Genital warts are benign growths of the skin and adjacent mucous membrane, caused by the human papilloma virus (HPV). More than 100 types exist. They can be broadly classified into: (1) Low-risk non-oncogenic types, e.g. types 6 and 11 which cause benign anogenital warts, condyloma acuminata and (2) high-risk oncogenic

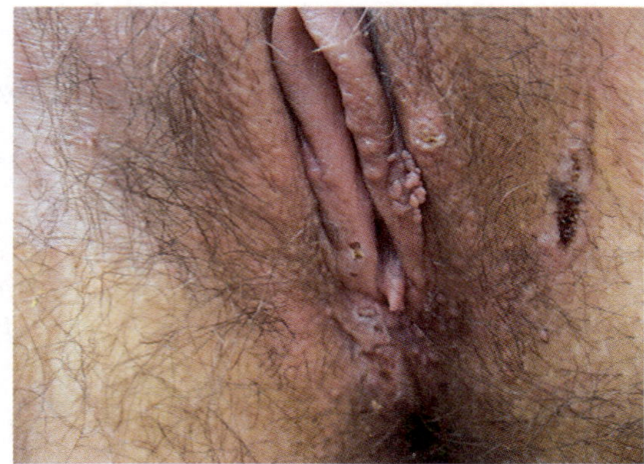

Fig. 48.2: Condyloma acuminata. ***Note:*** Warty growth on the labia minora. Other large lesions on the neighboring skin were removed by electrosurgery

types, e.g. types 16, 18, 31 and 45 which occasionally lead to cancer. Majority of cases of genital warts are sexually transmitted and 90% are caused by HPV 6 or 11. Though usually the incubation period is two to three months, it may be up to a year in some cases.

Clinical Features

Warts are commonly seen on the moist surfaces of the male and female genitalia, especially the coronal sulcus, glans penis, frenum and shaft of the penis in the male and posterior part of the introitus, labia majora, labia minora and clitoris in the female. Warts may develop in the urethral meatus and the cervix uteri. The wart virus is always present in the cervix, even if warts are not seen there. In females, the genital warts enlarge during pregnancy and regress during the puerperium (Fig. 48.2).

Diagnosis

Diagnosis is mainly clinical. The use of HPV DNA testing is not recommended for diagnosis of genital warts because the test results would not alter the clinical management.

Treatment

No specific treatment is effective in eliminating the virus and therefore, recurrences are frequent. If left untreated, warts can resolve on their own, remain unchanged or increase in size or number.

Recommended treatment: Podophyllin resin 10–25% in spirit or tincture of benzoin should be applied carefully to the warts avoiding normal tissue at weekly intervals. It should be washed thoroughly after 1–4 hours of application. Podophyllin is teratogenic and should not be used during pregnancy. Podophyllotoxin 0.5%, one of the active constituents of podophyllin, can be self-applied and it is less toxic. It is used twice daily for 3 days followed by 4 days of no treatment, the cycle repeated up to 4 times. Imiquimod 5% cream applied with a finger at bed time, left on overnight, 3 times a week for as long as 16 weeks can be self-applied by the patient. The treatment area should be washed after 6–10 hours of application.

Sinecatechins 15% ointment, a green-tea extract, applied 3 times daily, 0.5 cm of ointment to each wart, using a finger for not more than 16 weeks is also useful. It should not be washed off after use.

The warts can be cauterized under local anesthesia, using electrocoagulation. Cryotherapy with liquid nitrogen, solid carbon dioxide or a cryoprobe can be used. Large warts are removed surgically.

Prevention

Two HPV vaccines are available. A bivalent vaccine containing HPV types 16 and 18 protects against cervical cancers. A quadrivalent vaccine containing HPV types 6, 11, 16 and 18 protects against genital warts. Vaccines are advised to girls and boys before the onset of sexual activity. Three IM doses over a 6-month period is recommended.

MOLLUSCUM CONTAGIOSUM

(*See* Section 18, Ch 220)

General Considerations and Clinical Features

Molluscum contagiosum is a viral disease which can be transmitted from person to person by sexual or nonsexual contact, the latter is more common. The infective agent is a virus belonging to the pox group. Cellular proliferation occurs in the deeper layers of the skin in the stratum malpighii. Many cells contain ovoid eosinophilic intracytoplasmic inclusions which can be demonstrated by Romanowsky stains. These are called ***molluscum bodies*** and are diagnostic. The cheesy material exuding when the lesion is squeezed is taken up for demonstrating the molluscum bodies. Lesions may develop on any part of the skin. The incubation period varies from 3 weeks to several months. The sexually transmitted lesion develops on the genitalia. The lesions are papular, ranging in size from 2 mm to 1 cm, waxy and pale pink with central depression.

The sexually transmitted variety may be associated with HIV infection in which case even the molluscum lesions tend to proliferate and persist till antiretroviral therapy (ART) is instituted.

Treatment

The lesions can be extracted using a molluscum extractor or by simple needling. Local application of pure phenol or concentrated trichloroacetic acid by a sharpened match stick will destroy the virus. Electrocoagulation is also useful.

HUMAN IMMUNODEFICIENCY VIRUS (HIV) INFECTION AND ACQUIRED IMMUNODEFICIENCY SYNDROME (AIDS)

Definition: AIDS is the name given to a group of disorders related to immunodeficiency produced as a result of the infection by HIV. The syndrome was first described in 1981 in Los Angeles in male homosexuals. In a short span, it has spread all across the globe, affecting various spheres of human life. AIDS is the final consequence of various changes that take place in the immune status of the individual and is characterized by the occurrence of opportunistic infections and specific malignancies.

Epidemiology

It is estimated that more than 35 million people live with HIV infection worldwide as of end of 2013. Since the beginning of the epidemic, more than 75 million people have contracted HIV and nearly 36 million have died of HIV-related causes. In 2012, an estimated 2.3 million people were newly infected with HIV. Of them, 260,000 were under the age of 15. Everyday nearly 6,300 people contract HIV—nearly 262 every hour. In 2012, 1.6 million people died from AIDS; 210,000 of them were under the age of 15. The country of Swaziland has the maximum seropositivity rate of 27% among adults. The current estimates put India as having the second largest load of AIDS patients with 5.3 million infected persons. As per the statistics released by the National AIDS Control Organization (NACO), Government of India, India is estimated to have an adult (15–49 years) HIV prevalence of 0.27%. Children (<15 years) account for 7% of all infections. Thirty-nine per cent (8.16 lakh) of all HIV infections, are among women. In 2011, among the states, Manipur has shown the highest estimated adult HIV prevalence of 1.22%, followed by Andhra Pradesh (0.75%), Mizoram (0.74%), Nagaland (0.73%), Karnataka (0.52%), Goa (0.43%) and Maharashtra (0.42%). Besides these, Odisha, Gujarat, Tamil Nadu and Chandigarh have shown estimated adult HIV prevalence greater than national prevalence (0.27%). Prevalence of the infection among all female sex workers in Mumbai was 44.7%. HIV and AIDS formed 17.6% of all STD clinic attendees in Andhra Pradesh (AP). 22% of intravenous drug users (IVDUs) in Manipur and 2.2% of all expectant mothers in AP were HIV positive. Maharashtra, Tamil Nadu, Manipur, Andhra Pradesh, Karnataka and Nagaland have been identified as high prevalence states with the HIV prevalence exceeding 5% among high-risk groups and 1% among antenatal women. All other Indian States are classified as low prevalence areas.

The adult HIV prevalence at national level has continued its steady decline from estimated level of 0.41% in 2001 through 0.35% in 2006 to 0.27% in 2011. Similar consistent declines are noted among both males and females at national level. Considerable decline in HIV prevalence has been recorded among female sex workers at national level (5.06% in 2007 to 2.67% in 2011) and this has been made possible by constant and long-standing targeted interventions focused on behavior change and increasing condom use. Declines have been achieved among homosexual men (7.41% in 2007 to 4.43% in 2011) also. Stable trends have been recorded among injecting drug users in whom the prevalence of HIV positivity remains stable with only minimal fall at national level from 7.23% in 2007 to 7.14% in 2011. It is estimated that about 1.48 lakh people died in India from AIDS-related causes in 2011. Deaths among HIV infected children account for 7% of all AIDS-related deaths.

Epidemics of AIDS rampaging in several countries in the late 20th century have been responsible for death of millions of adults during their wage-earning period of life, leaving families and several countries economically and socially devastated.

Wider access to anti-retroviral therapy (ART) has led to reduction in estimated annual AIDS-related deaths during National AIDS Control Program (NACP)-III period (2007–2011) by 29%. It is estimated that the scale up of free ART, since 2004 has saved over 1,50,000 lives in India till

2011 by averting deaths due to AIDS-related causes. At the current pace of scale up of ART services, it is estimated to avert around 50,000–60,000 deaths annually in the next five years.

Intravenous Drug Users

They transmit HIV among themselves by needle sharing. The estimated number of injecting drug users (IDU) worldwide is 11–21 million in 2007, among which 3 million were infected with HIV. General prevalence of HIV in IDUs is 20–40%.

Reports from Tamil Nadu show that the commonly injected drugs in the Indian subcontinent include ***cannabis derivatives, pethidine-related drugs, cocaine, amphetamine, opioids, sympathetic and para sympathetic stimulants, hyoscine*** and several others. Addiction to drugs such as amphetamine and related drugs, increase the incidence of HIV, since these drugs promote the sexual urge for heterosexual and homosexual exposure and thus acquire the infection.

Source: Mathers BM, Degenhardt L, Phillips B, et al. Global epidemiology of injecting drug use and HIV among people who inject drug: a systematic review. Lancet. 2008;372:1733-45.

The Present Situation (2014)

As it stands, at present, the results of active interventions such as early detection of HIV infection, mass education campaigns combined with effective ART undertaken free of cost by government sources have all served to convert the deadly disease AIDS into a chronic illness which prolongs life, reduces the transmissibility and enable the patients to follow productive occupations. Due to reduction in mortality, the apparent prevalence of AIDS patients may increase, even though the incidence rates have shown definite decline. In the global scenario, voluntary male circumcision, ART to prevent mother to child transmission, ART to prevent AIDS in HIV infected persons and pre-exposure prophylaxis have all contributed to the reduction. India is estimated to have around 86 (56–129) thousand new HIV infections in 2015, showing 66% decline in new infections from 2000 and 32% decline from 2007, the year set as baseline in the NACP.

The Causative Organism

The disease is caused by infection with HIV which is a retrovirus and belongs to the family of lentiviruses. Infections with lentiviruses typically show a chronic course of disease, a long period of clinical latency, persistent viral replication and involvement of the CNS. There are many viruses which are classified under this name. HIV-1 and HIV-2 are the major ones. Using electron microscopy, HIV-1 and HIV-2 are almost similar. However, they differ with regard to the molecular weight of their proteins, as well as having differences in their accessory genes. Both HIV-1 and HIV-2 replicate in CD4+ T-cells and are regarded as pathogenic, HIV-2 being less pathogenic. HIV-1 is subdivided into groups: M (for main) and O (for outlier), antigenically. Within group M are the vast majority of HIV-1 strains subdivided into subtypes (currently 10: A–J) based on genetic variation. HIV-1 subtype B is more prevalent in homosexuals and IV drug users. However, most of the ongoing HIV-1 epidemic around the world is due to non-B subtypes, especially subtype C in Sub-Saharan Africa and India. But almost all subtypes have been identified in all parts of the world.

HIV viruses are ribonucleic acid (RNA) viruses. HIV-1 viral particles have a diameter of 100 nm and are surrounded by a lipoprotein membrane. After entry, HIV starts replication in the mucosa, sub-mucosa and draining lymphoreticular tissues. For 7–21 days, virus cannot be detected in plasma (eclipse phase). CD4+ cells and Langerhan's cells are the first targets of the virus regardless of the route of infection and the first cells affected. Within a few days viral replication the virus converges in the lymphoreticular system of the gastrointestinal tract (GIT). The CD4+ cells lacking activation markers and expressing low levels of the C-C chemokine receptor type 5 (CCR5) are the most infected cells.

The virus is present in blood, body fluids, tissue fluids semen, placenta and breast milk and entry of the organism is through abrasions in the skin, mucus membranes or through active procedures like sexual intercourse, needle pricks or introduction of infective material including blood and blood products and during unprotected deliveries.

During the process of budding, the virus may incorporate, different host proteins, such as HLA class I and II proteins or adhesion proteins from the membrane of the host cell into its lipoprotein layer.

HIV has greatest affinity towards CD4 receptor bearing T helper lymphocyte group. Two proteins found on immune cells, CCR5 and fusin (also known as CXCR4) are considered as coreceptors. Certain chemokines are also considered important in modulating the entry of virus into the CD4 cell. After HIV successfully attaches and fuses with the cell, the RNA strands are transcribed to DNA by the timely activation of reverse transcriptase, a viral enzyme. The DNA strands thus formed in the cytoplasm migrate to the nucleus and integrate with the human DNA (with the help of enzyme integrase). This is an irreversible bonding and leads to the beginning of a permanent HIV infection.

The integrated human CD4 cell may take various routes. Some of them are detected by the person's immune system and are eliminated promptly. Some of them get activated against other antigens or allergens and start producing chemical mediators. When parts of the DNA correspond to that of the virus, the proteins so produced will contain the amino acid sequences needed for the virus replication too. These 'viral' proteins are cleaved into correct sequence by the enzyme protease. The newly synthesized viral proteins acquire their coating from the CD4 cell surface and 'bud out' damaging the cell membrane. This leads to significant damage to the cells and they are destroyed in large numbers. Some of the cells undergo fusion and form syncytia. Some may be destroyed by cell mediated, complement mediated or antibody dependent cytotoxic mechanisms. Some CD4 cells undergo apoptosis (programed and premature cell death). Thus the virus infection over a period of years leads to fall in the number of CD4 cells. The virus can also produce direct effects on cells in the brain, heart and bowel and reticuloendothelial system. HIV can replicate aggressively and up to 10 billion virus particles may be produced in a day with an average half-life of 6 days.

The CD4 count in a normal person is between 800 and 1200 cells per mm³ in peripheral blood. The CD4 cell is responsible for the smooth and coordinated function of all arms of the immune system. Once the CD4 function is compromised, various abnormalities occur. Both physiologic and deregulated activation contribute to the profound immune activation and accelerated cell death that characterizes HIV infection. In early HIV infection, CD8+ T-cell numbers tend to increase, reflecting expansion of memory CD8+ T-cells, particularly HIV-reactive cells. CD8+ cell expansion persists until far advanced stages of HIV disease, when all T-cell numbers tend to fall. A number of immunological abnormalities have been described including:

- Leukopenia and lymphopenia
- Loss of T4 lymphocytes from the peripheral blood
- Hypergammaglobulinemia
- Skin test anergy
- Decrease in lymphocyte proliferation, cytotoxic T-cell response and antibody production to new antigens
- Elevated levels of immune complexes, interferon and β_2-microgobulin.

Immunodeficiency manifest in three different patterns:

1. Reactivation of dormant infections like tuberculosis and herpes infections
2. Infections by opportunistic pathogens
3. Atypical manifestations of common infections.

The immune dysregulation also leads to development of specific malignancies such as Kaposi's sarcoma related to human herpesvirus 8 (HHV-8) infection.

Routes of Transmission

HIV is susceptible to destruction by many physical and chemical agents. Close contact and exchange of blood or body fluids is necessary for transmission. The most rampant route is sexual intercourse. Male homosexuals practicing anal sex have the highest risk. Heterosexual anal sex, heterosexual vaginal sex, oral sex and sex using condoms have been stratified in the decreasing order of risk involved. The infection is common amongst IV drug users in whom sharing of contaminated needles, syringes and drugs is the risky factor. The infection can also be transmitted from the mother to the child during pregnancy, at the time of labor or during breastfeeding. The transmission is most effective following transfusion of infected blood. Occasionally needles and sharps used in hospitals can act as sources of infection to healthcare professionals if proper precautions are not taken. HIV does not spread through casual contact, furniture, touching, sharing the food, utensils, toilet or through air or water. Person to person transmissibility of infection is closely correlated with the viral burden in blood. Each time the viral burden in blood increases 10 times, the transmissibility increases 2.5 times. Transmissibility in chronically infected person is less, probably due to presence of neutralizing antibodies. The penile foreskin and urethra of men harbor critical viral receptor cells; removal of penile foreskin by circumcision can prevent at least 60% of HIV infections in men. Introduction of male circumcision as an important preventive strategy in African countries have served to reduce transmission rates considerably.

Source: Newell ML, Iwuji C. HIV treatment as prevention: applicable in Sub-Saharan Africa? Lancet Infect Dis. 2016;16(7):754-5.

Transmission by sexual intercourse is increased in the presence of other sexually transmitted diseases leading to ulcerative or inflammatory lesions in the genitalia. HIV infected mothers transmit the disease to their babies during labor and also through breast milk. Efficiency of transmission depends upon the viral load and clinical stage of the mother, the nature of delivery and time spent in labor. It can vary from 14 to 40%.

The risk of transmission by accidental needle pricks in hospitals is calculated to be less than 0.3%.

Use of Drugs to Prevent Transmission

The antiretroviral (ARV) drug tenofovir when used as a topical application in vagina before sexual exposure reduces HIV infection rate by 39% and this effect is dependent on the vaginal concentration of the drug. Use of pill once a day containing tenofovir plus emtricitabine gives a 44% protection in addition to other methods of prevention.

Route of infection in India	Percentage	Efficiency (%)
Sexual (mainly heterosexual)	85.96	0.1–1
Perinatal transmission	3.64	14–45
Blood and blood products	2.00	~100
Injecting drug users	2.39	0.5
Others (not specified)	6.01	

Risk of AIDS defining infections in relation to CD4+ counts

Mild immunodeficiency 200–500 cells/mm³	Encapsulated bacteria, *Mycobacterium tuberculosis* (MTB)
Moderate immunodeficiency < 200 cells/mm³	Bacteria, MTB, *Pneumocystis jiroveci*
Severe immunodeficiency < 100 cells/mm³	Bacteria, MTB, *Pneumocystis jiroveci*, nontuberculous mycobacteria, fungi, CMV

Clinical Features

The spectrum of diseases caused by HIV is quite wide. The clinical patterns are grouped into four stages.

1. Acute retroviral syndrome
2. Asymptomatic stage
3. Early symptomatic stage
4. Advanced immunodeficiency.

The possibility of AIDS should be suspected in the following situations:

- Sexual history—unprotected sex with multiple partners, especially homosexuals, ano-oral sex, needle sharing population
- Occurrence of any of the AIDS—indicating conditions
- Clinical syndromes attributable to AIDS
- In many cases routine testing for AIDS during investigations for other diseases may reveal evidence of HIV infection.

Textbook of Medicine

AIDS indicator conditions

- Candidiasis of esophagus, trachea, bronchi or lungs
- Cervical cancer, invasive*
- Coccidioidomycosis, extrapulmonary*
- Cryptococcosis, extrapulmonary
- Cryptosporidiosis with diarrhea longer than 1 month
- Cytomegalovirus of any organ other than liver, spleen or lymph nodes
- Herpes simplex with mucocutaneous ulcer for more than 1 month duration or bronchitis, pneumonitis, esophagitis
- Histoplasmosis, extrapulmonary*
- HIV-associated dementia—disabling cognitive and/or motor dysfunction interfering with activities of daily living*
- HIV-associated wasting—involuntary weight loss >10% of baseline plus chronic diarrhea (2 loose stools/day 30 days) or chronic weakness and documented enigmatic fever 30 days*
- Isosporiasis with diarrhea greater than 1 month*
- Kaposi's sarcoma in patient under 60 years (or over 60 years*)
- Lymphoma of brain in patient under 60 years (or over 60 years*)
- Lymphoma, non-Hodgkin's of B-cell or unknown immunologic phenotype and histology showing small, noncleaved lymphoma or immunoblastic sarcoma
- *Mycobacterium avium* complex or *M. kansasii* disseminated tuberculosis*
- Nocardiosis*
- *Pneumocystis jiroveci* pneumonia
- Pneumonia, recurrent-bacterial (2 episodes in 12 months)*
- Progressive multifocal leukoencephalopathy
- *Salmonella septicemia* (nontyphoid), recurrent*
- Strongyloidiasis, extraintestinal
- Toxoplasmosis of internal organs.

* Requires positive HIV serology

Note: Criteria of Center for Disease Control and Prevention (CDC), Atlanta.

Acute Retroviral Syndrome

Also called primary HIV infection or seroconversion illness, occurs 2–6 weeks after the entry of HIV into human body. The illness is associated with fever, papular eruptions, arthralgia, lymph node swelling and oral ulcers (Figs 48.3A to C).

The CD4 count falls and viral load increases during this period. The symptomatic phase of acute HIV-1 infection lasts between 7 and 10 days, and rarely longer than 14 days. The severity and duration of symptoms have prognostic implications. Severe and prolonged symptoms are associated with more rapid disease progression, which may be unnoticed in the majority of cases. The infected person recovers completely to an asymptomatic stage with the return of CD4 count to normal but becomes HIV antibody positive thereafter.

In the next few years many changes take place in the immune system even though the person is grossly asymptomatic. Immune mediated events like lymph node enlargement, thrombocytopenia, demyelinative disorders of CNS, occur with increasing frequency. Most of these are because of misdirected immunologic activity. The occurrence of persistent generalized lymphadenopathy (defined as enlargement of two or more extrainguinal lymph nodes of size 2–3 cm persisting for more than a month) is common at some time in this stage.

As the CD4 count drops to below 500 cells/mm^3, the person experiences reactivation of dormant organisms like tuberculosis (pulmonary and extrapulmonary), herpes zoster, disseminated herpes, *M. contagiosum*, etc. Fungal infections of the genital tract, extensive non genital warts, exaggerated insect bite reactions on the exposed skin, etc. are seen in this stage (Fig. 48.4).

As the CD4 count drops below 200 cells/mm^3, the opportunistic infections appear. This is also the time when neoplasms like high-grade B cell lymphoma, Kaposi's sarcoma, cervical intraepithelial neoplasia and primary CNS lymphoma appear. Many infections which remain localized in immunocompetent subjects tend to become disseminated (e.g. *M. tuberculosis, Toxoplasma gondii, Cytomegalovirus, Cryptococcus neoformans* and *Histoplasma capsulatum*).

Respiratory System in AIDS

Respiratory system gets involved in almost all patients at some stage (Box 48.1).

The most important among these are *Pneumocystis carinii pneumonia* (now re-named as *P. jiroveci*) and tuberculosis.

Pneumocystis jiroveci pneumonia (PCP) (*See* also Ch 62): The organism is an unusual type of fungus. PCP gives rise to interstitial pneumonia with the classic symptoms of

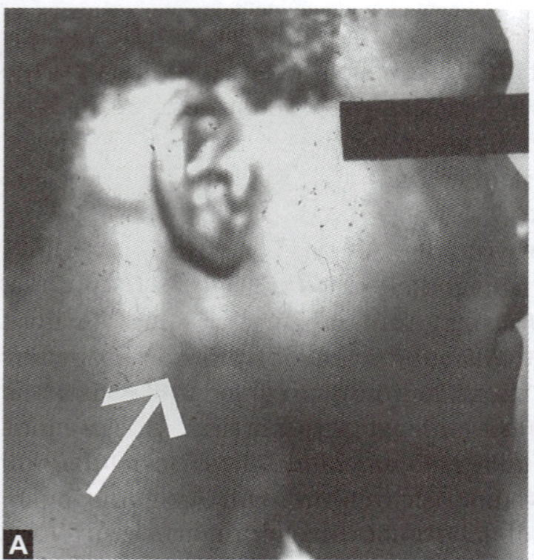
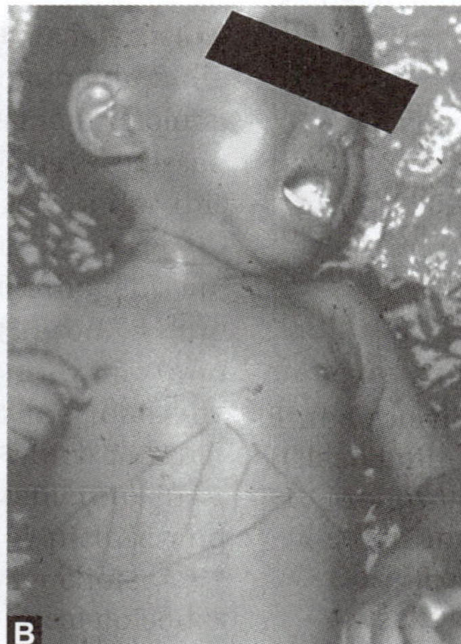
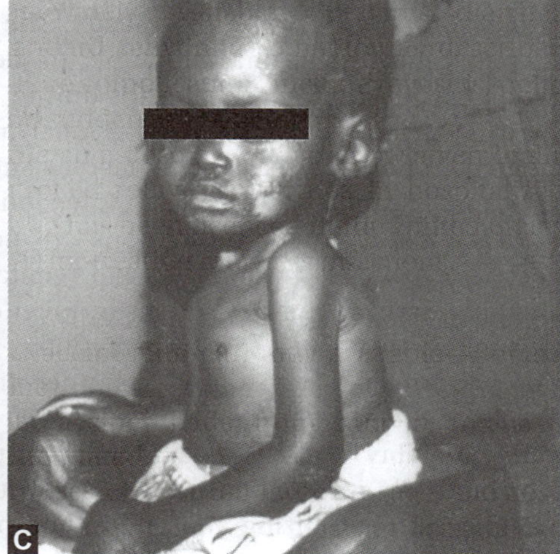

Figs 48.3A to C: *AIDS:* **A.** Persistent lymphadenopathy neck (arrow); **B.** Oral candidiasis; **C.** Cachexia diarrhea

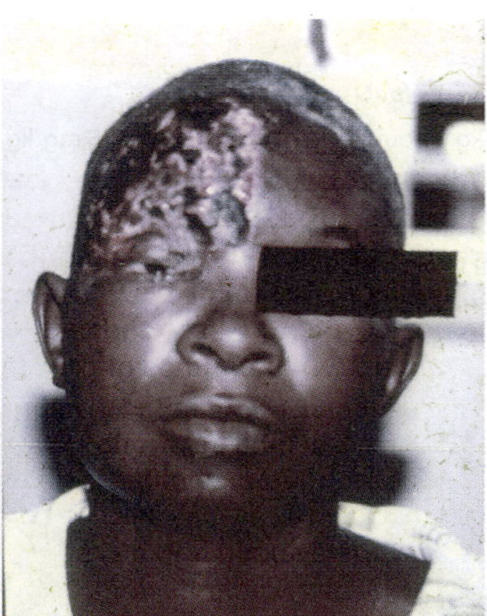

Fig. 48.4: Severe herpes zoster

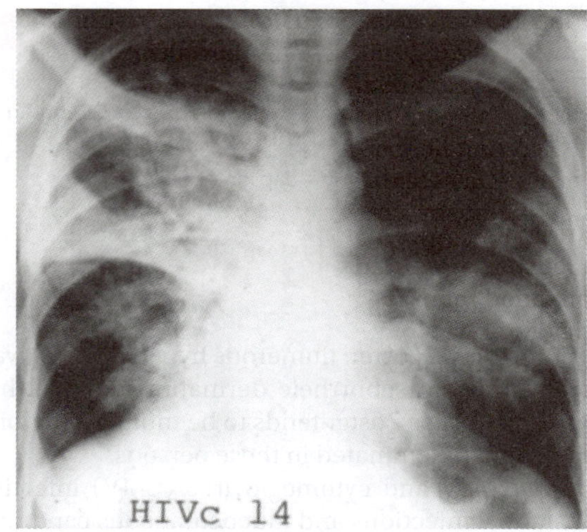

Fig. 48.5: Chest X-ray showing pneumocystis pneumonia

Sexually Transmitted Viral Diseases

Box 48.1: Pulmonary complications in patients with HIV infection

Infections	Neoplasia	Others
• **Pneumocystis jiroveci**	• Kaposi's sarcoma	• Lymphocytic interstitial pneumonia
• **Bacterial pneumonia**		
• S. pneumoniae		
• S. aureus		
• H. influenzae		• Non-specific interstitial pneumonia
• B. catarrhalis	• Non-Hodgkin's lymphoma	
• P. aeruginosa		• Pulmonary hypertension
• Rhodococcus equi	• Hodgkin's lymphoma	
• Nocardia asteroides		
• **Mycobacteria**		• Chronic obstructive pulmonary disease (COPD)
• M. tuberculosis	• Bronchial carcinoma	
• Atypical mycobacteria		
• **Other**		• Bronchial hyper reactivity
• Cytomegalovirus		
• Aspergillus spp.		
• Cryptococcus neoformans		
• Histoplasma capsulatum		
• Toxoplasma gondii		

dry cough, with or without fever and very gradual onset of dyspnea on exertion. The patient may be cyanosed, by the time he reaches a physician. The diagnosis may be delayed weeks or months. Diagnosis is clinched by a chest X-ray and if possible, high resolution computed tomography (HRCT) of the lungs. The chest X-ray often shows relatively characteristic findings with a butterfly-shaped (perihilar) interstitial infiltrate. In the early stages, the focus is on the mid and lower fields (Fig. 48.5). Cystic changes may also occur. Indistinct, diffuse changes are more easily visible on HRCT than on chest X-ray. There is almost always partial respiratory insufficiency, which should be confirmed by arterial blood gas analysis. Lactate dehydrogenase (LDH) is often elevated. High levels of LDH reflect the severity of the PCP. Sputum specimens are generally not useful for identification of the organism. Bronchoalveolar lavage (BAL) aspirate is usually necessary.

Methenamine silver staining and PCR demonstrate the fungus. The organism may be demonstrable for a few days more after starting treatment.

Treatment should be initiated immediately if there is clinical suspicion. In cases of mild PCP with arterial pO_2 > 70–80 mm Hg, ambulatory treatment can be attempted, oral medication is effective. Respiratory insufficiency is an indication for hospitalization. Therapy with cotrimoxazole (2 DS tablet three times daily for adults) should be given for 21 days. Patients with documented or suspected PCP and moderate-to-severe disease, defined by room air pO_2 < 70 mm Hg or Alveolar-arterial O_2 gradient $\geq$ 35 mm Hg, should receive adjunctive corticosteroids as early as possible and certainly within 72 hours after starting specific PCP therapy. In patients who cannot tolerate cotrimoxazole, intravenous pentamidine is the drug of second choice. Induction therapy consists of 200–300 mg pentamidine in 500 mL 5% glucose or normal saline, as IV trip. Half this dose is given from days 6 to 21. Dapsone, a combination of clindamycin and primaquine, atovaquone are other drugs proved to be useful. ART should be initiated as soon as possible (Table 48.1).

Prevention: Patients with CD4 T-cell count less than 200/mm³ are at risk and should therefore receive prophylaxis, ideally with cotrimoxazole daily or three times weekly. Monthly inhalation of pentamidine is a well-tolerated alternative. PCP prophylaxis regimens can be discontinued safely when the CD4 T-cell count rises above 200/mm³ and remain so at least for three months.

Tuberculosis and HIV disease are closely linked. This is described in Ch 49.

Cutaneous Manifestations

Cutaneous manifestations are quite common in AIDS. A broad spectrum of cutaneous infections caused by viruses, bacteria, fungi, protozoa and parasites as well as many unusual manifestations of common dermatoses is seen.

Acute primary HIV infection may lead to a transient, generalized, morbilliform eruption on the trunk and the arms. With the person developing immunosuppression, nonspecific skin changes occur. These include common disorders with atypical clinical features, including

Table 48.1: Summary of indication for treatment of PCP based on severity

Mild cases	Moderate to severe cases (paO$_2$ < 70 mm Hg)
Trimethoprim 5 mg/kg 6 hourly + sulfamethoxazole 25 mg/kg 6 hourly orally	Trimethoprim 5 mg/kg 6 hourly + sulfamethoxazole 25 mg/kg 6 hourly IV
Trimethoprim 5 mg/kg 6 hourly + dapsone 2 mg/day	Pentamidine 4 mg/kg/day IV
Pentamidine 4 mg/kg/day IV	Clindamycin (600 mg qid) + primaquine (30 mg od)
Atovaquone 750 mg tid	In all cases, add prednisolone 40 mg bd for 5 days, then 40 mg/day for 5 days and then 20 mg/day for 11 days

recurrent varicella zoster, numerous hyperkeratotic warts, treatment-resistant seborrheic dermatitis and oral hairy leukoplakia. Herpes Zoster tends to be multi dermatomal, recurrent and disseminated in these persons.

Chronic HSV and cytomeglovirus (CMV) infections, mycobacterial infections and mucocutaneous candidiasis occur in late stages.

Kaposi's Sarcoma (KS)

This was the first malignancy detected to be associated with HIV infection. In the mid-1990s, approximately 1 in 4 homosexual men contracted the disease. This number has decreased precipitously with the advent of safer sexual practices in the early 1990s and accelerated with the introduction of highly active antiretroviral therapy (HAART) in the mid-1990s due to improved immune reconstitution. Presently the rate is around 1.6 per 100,000 in this group. The incidence in other HIV risk groups initially was 10% in IV drug abusers, 4% in hemophiliacs and 3% in children with AIDS. It has decreased in these groups as well to a relatively steady rate of 2%, which is now the same rate for homosexual men. Most of the patients are homosexual men. KS is due to proliferation of endothelial cells induced by **HHV-8 (also referred to as KS herpes virus-KSHV)**. KS begins as pink macules that become disseminated and palpable. Purplish or brown macules and plaques may become nodular. Mucosal and visceral involvement is common. The size varies from a few millimeters to many centimeters and can have different shapes. AIDS-related KS, unlike other forms of KS, tends to have an aggressive clinical course. Morbidity may occur from extensive cutaneous, mucosal or visceral involvement. In patients receiving HAART, the disease often has a more indolent clinical course or may regress spontaneously. The most common causes of morbidity include cosmetically disfiguring cutaneous lesions, lymphedema, gastrointestinal involvement or pulmonary involvement. Being a highly vascular tumor, hemorrhage can occur from any of the lesions (Fig. 48.6).

Other malignancies can also occur more commonly with HIV infection. AIDS-related B-cell non-Hodgkin's lymphomas may lead to skin nodules. Anal carcinoma and cervical intraepithelial neoplasia are papillomavirus-associated tumors. These tumors tend to be more progressive and aggressive. An increase in squamous cell carcinoma of the anal mucosa has been reported, especially in young homosexual men. Intraoral or multiple squamous cell carcinoma, Bowen's disease and metastatic basal cell carcinoma have occasionally been reported. Malignant melanoma occurring in patients

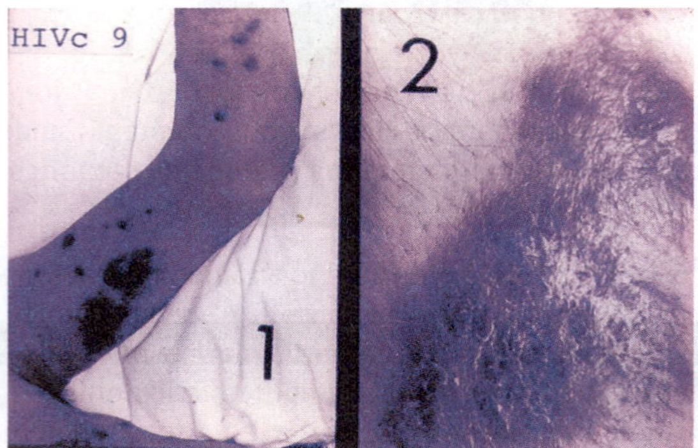

Fig. 48.6: Kaposi's sarcoma. **Note:** (1) General appearance—pigmented lesions, (2) enlarged view × 100

with HIV is more aggressive than in individuals without HIV. Children with AIDS have a higher risk of developing leiomyosarcoma, although the incidence is still low in this population. Primary CNS lymphoma is a disease almost exclusively seen in HIV infected persons and manifests as a space occupying lesion.

Fungal Infections

It occur extensively on the skin and mucus membranes. Recurrent and persistent mucocutaneous candidiasis is common. Recurrent vaginal candidiasis can occur in any stage of the disease. In adults, generalized dermatophytosis or tinea capitis, which is typically caused by *Trichophyton rubrum* is common. Onychomycosis in HIV infected may continue for many years.

Deep fungal infections like cryptococcosis, histoplasmosis and coccidioidomycosis may disseminate to the skin, usually as hemorrhagic papules or nodules.

Other Infections

Mycobacterium tuberculosis; Mycobacterium aviumintracellulare complex, rarely *Mycobacterium kansasii* may present as acneiform papules and indurated crusted plaques. Impetigo and folliculitis may be recurrent and persistent in HIV disease, particularly in children. Disseminated furunculosis, gingivitis, gangrenous stomatitis and abscess formation can occur. Bacillary angiomatosis, which is caused by *Bartonella henselae* and rarely by *Bartonella quintana,* usually manifests as red papules and nodules. This is usually considered in the differential diagnosis of KS, but can be managed with antimicrobials like doxycycline, clarithromycin or rifampicin. Atypical or Norwegian scabies, which is characterized by widespread hyperkeratosis, scaly maculopapular eruptions or crusted plaques, can occur. Seborrheic dermatitis like eruptions are observed in 83% of patients with AIDS. Seborrheic dermatitis may be the initial cutaneous manifestation of HIV disease. The eruption, which is characterized by widespread inflammatory and hyperkeratotic lesions, may progress to erythroderma in some patients.

Pruritic papular eruption and eosinophilic folliculitis also presents with papular eruptions.

Nail and hair changes (graying and other pigmentary changes), photosensitive eruptions and diffuse alopecia are noticed.

Among sexually transmitted diseases, chancroid, syphilis in homosexual men and lymphogranuloma venereum are more commonly associated with AIDS. Syphilis coexisting with HIV creates special problems (*See* Ch 47).

Treatment: Almost all cutaneous manifestations in HIV can be managed by the same modalities as in seronegative persons.

Neurological Manifestations
(*See* also Section 17, Ch 199)

- *AIDS encephalopathy:* Infection of the CNS by HIV leads to encephalopathy (HIVE) which is also known by terms such as *AIDS dementia complex, AIDS dementia* and *HIV associated cognitive motor complex.* HIVE is a late manifestation when there is a profound immune suppression with CD4 counts below 200/mm^3. HIVE is a subcortical dementia, caused by leukoencephalopathy typically emerging over the course of weeks and months. Typical complaints are slowing of reasoning, forgetfulness, difficulties concentrating, lack of energy and drive, mild depressive symptoms and emotional blunting. MRI often shows patchy, diffuse, hyperintense and relatively symmetrical lesions in the white matter. These changes indicate leukoencephalopathy. HIV-associated myelopathy whose histopathological hallmarks are vacuoles, most prominent in the cervical and thoracic parts of the spinal cord, hence called *vacuolar myelopathy.*

- *Progressive multifocal leukoencephalopathy (PML)* is a severe demyelinating disease of the CNS predisposed to AIDS. It is caused by John Cunningham virus (JCV), which is a polyoma virus found worldwide. The main focus of disease is the white matter of the cerebral hemispheres, but the cerebellum and in some cases the grey matter may also be affected. The median interval between the onset of the first symptoms and death was between 3 and 6 months. Patients usually die of secondary complications after being bedridden for many weeks. In addition to cognitive disorders, which may range from mild impairment of concentration to dementia, focal neurological deficits are very typical of PML. Mono and hemiparesis are observed most frequently, as well as defects of speech and vision. MRI usually shows asymmetrical high signal intensity lesions in T2-weighted imaging, hypointense in T1-weighted images. Usually they do not show gadolinium enhancement or mass effect. Non-involvement of the grey matter is characteristic. The lesions are almost always asymmetrical.

- *Cerebral toxoplasmosis* almost always results from the reactivation of a latent infection with *Toxoplasma gondii*, Patients may present with seizure, headache or focal neurological deficits. Cerebral toxoplasmosis is extremely rare above a CD4 T-cell count of 100/mm^3. It should always be expected when the CD4 T-cell counts fall below 100/mm^3. CT or MRI scan of the head should be performed promptly in all cases of focal neurological deficit. Ring enhancing lesions and solitary or multiple abscesses should suggest the infection. Up to 97% of patients with cerebral toxoplasmosis have IgG antibodies and therefore absence of these antibodies help to rule out toxoplasmosis. Treatment is described in (*See* Ch 65, pp 466).

- *Cryptococcal meningitis* is more common in advanced immunodeficiency when the CD4 count is less than 200 cells/mm^3. *C. neoformans* is transmitted by droplet infection. This should be suspected when the HIV infected patient presents with indolent headache lasting for many weeks. Early CSF study is recommended. The non-staining capsulated organisms are identified in India by ink stained smear. *Treatment:* Drug of choice is amphotericin B along with flucytosine or fluconazole. The recommended schedule for adults is amphotericin B deoxycholate (0.7–1.0 mg/kg/day IV) plus flucytosine (100 mg/kg/day orally in 4 divided doses) for at least 2 weeks. This is followed by fluconazole 6 mg/kg (400 mg per day orally) for a minimum of 8 weeks. The response is good even though the disease carries a mortality of around 10%. Patients are put on lifelong prophylaxis with fluconazole. Relapses are common and must be managed with the same induction regime.

- *Primary CNS lymphomas* are late complications of HIV infection, occurring in up to 10% of AIDS patients. Almost all cases are EBV-associated. Neurological deficits occur depending on their location.

- *Peripheral neuropathy* may complicate all stages of HIV infection. Acute inflammatory demyelinating polyneuropathy (AIDP) and Guillain-Barré syndrome (GBS) usually occur during seroconversion or during the latent stages of HIV infection. Chronic inflammatory demyelinating neuropathy, vasculitic neuropathy, distal symmetrical sensory polyneuropathy and drug induced neuropathies are all reported. Many ARV drugs also frequently cause peripheral neuropathy.

- *Reactivation of CMV infection:* When the CD4 count falls below 50/mm^3 reactivation of CMV infection can lead to retinitis. Any visual impairment occurring subacutely or acutely, such as blurred vision or floaters especially unilaterally should prompt immediate ophthalmological examination. Oral and/or intravitreal ganciclovir or valacyclovir will be useful if started early. Primary prophylaxis is not effective against CMV retinitis.

Cardiovascular System Involvement
Cardiovascular involvement is common in HIV-infected patients.

Textbook of Medicine

Pericardial diseases: Pericardial effusion (usually tuberculous), pericarditis (viral, bacterial, fungal), neoplasms (KS, lymphoma).

Myocardial involvement: HIV-associated dilated cardiomyopathy, acute or chronic myocarditis, KS or lymphoma and adverse effects of ARV drugs.

Endocardial involvement: Infective endocarditis—bacterial or fungal and nonbacterial thrombotic endocarditis.

Vascular diseases: Arteriosclerosis, vasculitis, perivasculitis, pulmonary artery hypertension.

Other Miscellaneous Infections

Esophageal candidiasis: Candidiasis takes the form of extensive and persistent superficial lesions over the oropharynx, the buccal mucosa, tonsillar ring, tongue and the esophagus. Candida esophagitis usually occurs with oropharyngeal involvement, but in about one third of the cases there may not be oral lesions. Esophagitis presents with odynophagia (painful dysphagia) and retrosternal pain. Fluconazole therapy rapidly clears the infection.

Atypical mycobacterial infections: *M. avium* complex (MAC) infection supervenes when the CD4 cell count falls below 50/mm³. The symptoms of disseminated MAC infection are usually nonspecific. Fever, weight loss and diarrhea in a patient with CD4 count less than 100/mm³ should always raise the possibility of atypical mycobacteriosis. Elevation of serum alkaline phosphatase is a strong evidence for the diagnosis of MAC infection. Similarly development of anemia with constitutional symptoms may be due to bone marrow involvement by MAC. Hepatosplenomegaly and lymphadenopathy may occur. Atypical mycobacteria grow more readily in blood culture compared to *M. tuberculosis*. MAC infection responds to treatment with a macrolide, clarithromycin or azithromycin with ethambutol and rifabutin given for a period of six months or more.

Cryptosporidiosis: It caused by *Cryptosporidium parvum* may occur as a complication in AIDS. It presents as severe diarrhea (*See* Ch 65).

Penicilliosis: Most fungi belonging to the Penicillium species are not pathogenic. One exception is *Penicillium marneffei*, which seems to be a problem mainly for HIV patients in South East Asia including parts of Manipur state in India. The clinical symptoms consist of prolonged high fever, lymphadenopathy, hepatosplenomegaly, weight loss, malaise, cough and hemoptysis, diverse cutaneous and mucocutaneous lesions resembling molluscum and abnormal increase in liver enzymes. Amphotericin B and itraconazole are effective in control in the infection.

HBV and HCV infections: Coinfection of hepatitis B and/or C viruses with HIV occurs frequently, since they share the same modes of transmission. Parenteral drug users and recipients of blood products are particularly susceptible. Primary HBV infection leads to chronic hepatitis in 2–5% of immunocompetent adults, whereas in HIV-infected patients the chance for the disease to become chronic is five times more. Viral replication of HBV is more active in AIDS patients. In general, patients with chronic hepatitis B should be screened for hepatocellular carcinoma (HCC) every 6–12 months.

The progress of hepatitis C is also more rapid, particularly in patients with CD4 counts below 100/mm³. The unfavorable course of hepatitis C in HIV infection can be improved by treatment of HIV infection by HAART. In addition, the development of liver failure can also be delayed. Hepatitis C infection can aggravate the potential hepatotoxicity of several drugs used in HAART regimens, especially nevirapine. Up to 10% of patients have to discontinue HAART due to severe hepatotoxicity. The response to treatment of HCV infection is less satisfactory due to lower clearance rates and adverse side effects of drugs which prevent continuation of therapy. Results are better if HCV RNA is < 2 million copies/mL, HCV genotype is 2 or 3 and the age of the patient is < 50 years. Histologically low grade fibrosis of the liver, normal γ-glutamyl transferase and stable HIV infection are good prognostic factors. Since the advent of more effective drugs which are directly viricidal to HCV genotype 1 and which can be given orally (with a clearance rate of 91–98%) future results are bound to be better. For treatment of HCV (*See* Ch 55).

All infections, irrespective of their nature can affect immunosuppressed persons in general and produce more serious outcome. This should be borne in mind when infections are encountered with unusual severity in patients, out of proportion to the usual picture.

Diagnosis

HIV infection is a laboratory diagnosis and is made by demonstration of:

- HIV antibodies by enzyme linked immunosorbent assay (ELISA) or solid state card/spot tests
- Circulating antigens (p24)
- The viral RNA itself by PCR–qualitative and quantitative—in peripheral blood.

Since false positive tests are not uncommon, it is advisable to repeat the tests using different types of ELISAs or different antigens before labeling an asymptomatic person as positive. If classical clinical symptoms have manifested, two positive tests are considered enough.

Laboratory Diagnosis of HIV Infection

- ***Diagnosis can be established by:*** Detection of antibodies in blood and body fluids by ELISA which detects antibody and also p24 antigen simultaneously.
- ***Other tests:***
  - Rapid immunoassays such as HIV spot test, immuno Combi test, dot-blot immunoassay and agglutination assay
  - Presence of viral antigen in blood and body fluid by p24 antigen assay which detects the viral capsid (core) p24 protein by basic antibody sandwich ELISA test
  - Detection of viral nucleic acid by PCR or nucleic acid sequence based amplification (NASBA).
- HIV DNA PCR can be done on dried blood spots specimens which are done for diagnosis for HIV infection in newborns and children.
- ***Take away HIV test:*** A saliva-bound antibody test for HIV has been approved by the FDA (US) which can be offered across the counter. The sensitivity and specificity are comparable to other saliva based tests.

Fallacies of the Tests

- The test become positive only after the 'window' period, i.e. 4–6 weeks or more after infection, by which time only the antibodies appear.
- In the late stage when antibodies are too low, the tests may be only weakly positive or even negative.

Note: Testing for HIV should be done along with pre- and post-test counseling. Integrated testing and counseling centers attached to major government institutions provide free counseling, testing and follow-up guidance. A minimum of three tests is done in these centers on every positive sample, as per World Health Organization (WHO) testing guidelines.

AIDS is defined as the presence of one of the AIDS defining conditions or a decline of CD4 cells to less than 200/mm³ in an HIV infected person.

Management of HIV Infection

The first contact physician has to suspect HIV infection in all probable cases, make the diagnosis by serology and molecular techniques and refer the case to the center where there are facilities provided by the government or non-governmental agencies to undertake full investigations and supply drugs (if needed free of cost) regularly and monitor the progress.

In a situation where specialist help is not available and drugs cannot be supplied free of cost in an uninterrupted manner, the primary care physician will not be able to undertake complete treatment in an individual capacity. The following description gives only the principles of treatment due to space constraint. Grass root details available in monographs on the subject are not given.

General measures: HIV infection should be confirmed beyond doubt by appropriate investigations. The immunological status is assessed by CD4 estimation. Severity of infection can be assessed by estimating the viral load using PCR test or other methods. The coexistence of other sexually transmitted infections and opportunistic infections should be confirmed by investigations. Regular repetition of CD4 T-cell count and RNA viral load helps to assess the progress of the disease.

The interventions in HIV disease can be grouped into three major headings.

- Nonpharmacologic modifications
- Prophylaxis and treatment of opportunistic infections
- Antiretroviral therapy (ART).

Source: Guidelines for the use of antiretroviral agents in HIV-1-infected adults and adolescents. Panel on Antiretroviral Guideline for Adults and Adolescents. Department of Health and Human Services. Available at http://aidsinfo.nih.gov/contentfiles/lvguidelines/AdultandAdolescentGL.pdf

Antiretroviral Therapy

It aims at bringing down the virus levels to undetectable levels, i.e. below 20 copies per mL with the presently available tests. This will ensure immune reconstitution with the return of CD4 counts above 200/mm³. Symptom free survival is also prolonged. Different groups of drugs are used. These include ***reverse transcriptase inhibitors (RTIs), protease inhibitors (PIs), entry inhibitors and integrase inhibitors (Table 48.2).*** The RTIs belong to two

Table 48.2: List of currently available ARV drugs. Several new drugs are in the process of development

Nucleoside reverse transcriptase inhibitors (NRTIs)
Zidovudine (AZT, ZDV)
Didanosine (DDI)
Stavudine (D4T)
Lamivudine (3TC)
Abacavir (ABC)
Emtricitabine
Non-nucleoside RTIs (NNRTI)
Nevirapine
Efavirenz
Nucleotide reverse transcriptase inhibitors (NtRTI)
Tenofovir
Protease inhibitors (PIs) and Boosted protease inhibitors (PIs)
Ritonavir
Indinavir
Nelfinavir
Amprenavir
Lopinavir
Atazanavir
Fosamprenavir
Entry (fusion) inhibitors
Enfuvirtide (T-20)
Integrase inhibitors
Raltegravir
Dolutegravir
CCR5 (coreceptor) antagonist
Maraviroc

Note: More than 25 ARV drugs are available for treating AIDS.

groups, nucleoside reverse transcriptase inhibitors (NRTIs) and nucleotide reverse transcriptase inhibitors nucleotide analog reverse transcriptnase inhibitors (NARTIs) and non-nucleoside RTIs (NNRTIs). The reverse transcriptase inhibitors block the transcription of DNA from viral RNA, without which the genetic material cannot be incorporated into the human DNA. The protease inhibitors block the protease enzyme, effectively preventing the formation and release of new virions. The fusion inhibitors block the virus fusion with the CD4 and other receptors on the cell membrane, thus preventing the entry of the virus into a new cell. The integrase inhibitors prevent the integration of the freshly transcribed DNA with host cell DNA.

The principle of treatment is to use a combination of three or more drugs belonging to the different groups. Several protocols are under trial. Different protocols are used in many countries. India follows the National AIDS Control Organization (NACO) guidelines. The first line therapy is using a combination of two RTIs with one NNRTI or a combination of one NtARTIs (tenofovir) with one NRTI and one NNRTI. The most favored regimen uses a combination of tenofovir, emtricitabine and lamivudine or efavirenz. Protease inhibitors based regimes and integrase inhibitor based regimes are also recommended as initial therapy in certain situations. Treatment is also recommended as prevention in cases of discordant couples. Monotherapy should be avoided due to the risk of developing resistance by HIV. The importance of adherence with regard to dosage and relationship with food must be stress in a therapeutic counseling setting. Patient should be willing and able to commit to treatment and should understand the possible risks and benefits of treatment and importance of adherence. More than 95% adherence to the schedule is needed for the desirable result. There is no consensus at present about the duration of therapy. Therefore, once started, the drugs have to be continued lifelong. When the first line drugs fail due to resistance or become intolerable due to toxicity, second or third line drugs are begun. The second line and third line drugs are more expensive and require closer monitoring. Recent studies has shown that treatment started even in asymptomatic patients before the CD4+ counts fall below 500/mm³ gives better results in terms of mortality and morbidity.

Source: Kitahata MM, Gange SJ, Abraham AG, et al. Effect of early versus deferred antiretroviral therapy for HIV on survival. N Engl J Med. 2009;360(18):1815-26.

Several treatment schedules have been advocated from time to time and all of them are in vogue. A standard regimen recommended by WHO is a combination of lamivudine 150 mg bd and efavirenz 400–600 mg od. More than 25 ARV drugs are available to treat AIDS. Further drugs are also being actively produced even now. The choice of drug therapy is determined by the effectiveness, availability, cost, adverse effects and comorbid conditions. For mass therapy, drugs supplied by the Indian pharmaceutical producers have been preferred due to their lower cost.

Single tablet treatment of HIV undergoing review: A single tablet containing, elvitegravir (ENG), cobicistat (COB1), emtricitabine (ATCC) and tenofovir disoproxil fumarate (TDF) given as a single dose on diagnosis helps to prevent the development of AIDS. Studies are progressing.

Source: The Lancet, 30th June, 2012, pp – 2429-2465.

Effective ART improves immune function and functions of cardiovascular system and liver. The increased risk of development of malignancy continues to persist.

Indications for Starting Therapy

Over the years and across countries there have been wide fluctuations in selecting the criteria for starting therapy in treatment naïve HIV infected persons. WHO consensus recommendations are summarized below.

- As a priority, ART should be initiated in all individuals with severe or advanced HIV clinical disease (WHO clinical stage 3 or 4) and individuals with CD4 count ≤ 350 cells/mm³.
- ART should be initiated in all individuals with HIV with a CD4 count >350 cells and ≤ 500/mm³ regardless of WHO clinical stage. This recommendation is not included in NACO guidelines.
- ART should be initiated in all individuals with HIV regardless of WHO clinical stage or CD4 cell count in the following situations:
  - Individuals with HIV and active TB disease
  - Individuals coinfected with HIV and HBV with evidence of severe chronic liver disease
  - Partners with HIV in serodiscordant couples should be offered ART to reduce HIV transmission to uninfected partners
  - Pregnant and breastfeeding women with HIV.

Outcome of therapy: The desired outcome of therapy will be a rise in CD4 count in 6-8 weeks and a fall in viral load to 'undetectable' range in 3–6 months. Following initiation of therapy, viral load should fall below 5,000 copies/mL within one month. Fall in viral load is measured in logs and one log reduction (ten times fall) is to be expected in 6–8 weeks. At present it is possible to arrest the multiplication of HIV and reduce the chances for opportunistic infections by judicious drug combinations. This highly active antiretroviral therapy (HAART) is the goal initiated by the WHO and accepted by several countries.

Adverse side effects: All ARV drugs are associated with adverse side effects.

Drug	Major side effects
Zidovudine	Bone marrow suppression
Nevirapine	Skin rash, hepatotoxicity, lactic acidosis
Stavudine	Peripheral neuropathy, lactic acidosis, lipodystrophy
Protease inhibitors	Mitochondrial toxicity, lipodystrophy

Severe toxic effects warrant change of drug schedule. Failure of response can also happen when the virus acquires resistance. This is due to the changes in the nucleoside sequence of the new viruses occurring during reverse transcription and other stages of viral multiplication. Many developed nations are performing drug resistance studies before start of therapy and for monitoring. Two types of tests—genotyping and phenotypic; both are available in many Indian laboratories as well. Genotypic resistance testing is detection of the occurrence of alterations in the nucleotide chains. This gives an indirect clue to resistance of the virus. Phenotypic resistance studies look for the survival patterns of growth of the virus in a cell culture medium in the presence of ARV drugs. These tests are now available in India too.

With the introduction of HAART death rates have come down and the quality of life of AIDS patients has improved considerably. Review of the therapy in developing and developed countries has shown very encouraging results in preventing transmission, reducing fresh infections and reducing non AIDS related deaths also.

Pregnancy complicating AIDS: The fetus may be infected by the virus. Infection rate is higher in mothers who have HIV RNA levels exceeding 1000 copies/mL. At higher viral loads the baby is infected earlier in pregnancy. HIV infection during pregnancy does not produce congenital birth defects in the baby.

Prevention of parent to child transmission (PPTCT) protocols (e.g. ACTG 076, Thai Harward, HIVNET012, PeTRa) are available, which includes use of zidovudine and nevirapine in the expectant mother, during labor and to the newborn child after delivery. PPTCT guidelines are being followed after regular testing of all antenatal women. Most of the ARV drugs cross the placenta if administered during pregnancy. Treatment reduces the transmission rate to ± 2% if started early. Administration of single drugs to the mother for preventing transmission to the child should be avoided due to the risk of developing drug resistance in the child later. Women with HIV RNA loads above 1000 copies/mL may be offered cesarean delivery. Cesarean delivery without trial of labor reduces the risk of transmission to the baby from 10.5 to 1.8%.

Prevention

Present role of ART is to reduce viral RNA to less than 50 copies/mL and maintain it. At this level, viral RNA is not detectable by commercial kits, but detectable only by highly sensitive microarrays. HIV infection leads to increased aging of the immune system with reduction in the number of memory T-cells (immunosenescence). HIV infection is a risk factor for end organ diseases involving the CVS, CNS and others.

A single-tablet treatment for preventing AIDS is undergoing review. A tablet containing elvitegravir (EVG)/cobicistat (COBI)/emtricitabine (FTC)/tenofovir disoproxil fumarate (TDF) given soon as diagnosis helps to prevent the development of AIDS. Studies are in progress.

Source: DeJesus E, Rockstroh JK, Henry K, et al. Co-formulated elvitegravir, cobicistat, emtricitabine, and tenofovir disoproxil fumarate versus ritonavir-boosted atazanavir plus co-formulated emtricitabine and tenofovir disoproxil fumarate for initial treatment of HIV-1 infection: a randomised, double-blind, phase 3, non-inferiority trial. Lancet. 2012;379(9835):2429-38.

AIDS, though a dreaded disease, is preventable too. Sex with a regular uninfected partner is the safest way to prevent HIV infection through sex. However, condoms if properly used offer almost complete protection against acquiring infection during natural sexual intercourse. Strict screening of blood products for transfusion reduces the risk considerably. Transmission in parenteral drug abuse groups is tackled by supply of sterile syringes by governmental and other agencies. Other measures to reduce illicit use of habituating drugs include counseling, group therapy and legal measures to prevent drug trafficking. Transmission in hospital settings can be reduced by proper practice of universal (standard) precautions.

Postexposure Prophylaxis Protocols in Healthcare Personnel are Mandatory

These consist of administration of basic ARV regimen as early as possible after exposure to the risk, ideally within 2 hours. The standard regimen is to give zidovudine 300 mg and lamivudine 150 mg twice daily for a period of 4 weeks. In the expanded regimen, a PI is also added. Many newer regimes are also advocated depending on the therapy used in source patient and based on the availability of drugs. There are recommendations for post sexual exposure and pre-exposure prophylaxis (based on several guidelines) as well.

Vaccines

Several attempts to produce anti-HIV vaccines for prevention and therapy are taking place under the International AIDS Vaccine Initiative (IAVI). National AIDS Research Institute (NARI) Pune also has developed a vaccine which is undergoing field trials. The need for proper health education and awareness are promoted as the major preventive strategy.

Global Measures and Future Prospects

Provision of regular supply of ARV drug to patients in developing countries has been taken up by the WHO aided agencies and several philanthropic non-governmental funding sources. At present the government of India and State Governments have made primary anti-HIV drugs available free of cost in major government hospitals. Several international governmental and non-governmental organizations have come forward to help needy nations with funds, manpower and drugs. Several Indian drug manufacturers have contributed to this global venture. With proper treatment, AIDS is converted into a chronic illness with considerable increase in life span. The mortality has dropped from 175/1000 person years in 1999–2000 to 9.1 deaths in 2009–2011. Present aim of therapy is to reduce viral RNA below 50 copies/mL (not detectable by the usual commercial tests). The treatment has to be continued indefinitely, since complete elimination of the virus has not been achieved even though tell-tale cases of total cure are on record. Widespread use of ART has given rise to drug resistance, but this is not considered to be a contraindication to pursue ART with alternate drugs.

Challenges in the elimination of pediatric HIV infection

The baby may be infected during pregnancy, delivery or breastfeeding. Relative proportion of HIV-1 transmission from an untreated mother to her infant according to gestational period and mode of infant feeding.

Antenatal period and intrapartum period early < 28 weeks and late > 28 weeks.

- Formula fed infants: 20–25%; 75–80%
  During pregnancy: 25–30%
  Labor and delivery: 65–75%
- Breastfed infants
  During pregnancy: 20–25%
  Labor and delivery: 35–50%
  Postpartum period breastfeeding: 25–35%

Treatment of lactating women with ARV drugs effectively reduces transmission through breast milk to less than 2%. It has now become the standard care to initiate treatment of pregnant women as soon as HIV-1 is diagnosed irrespective of CD4+ counts. With this new strategy, the number of newly infected infants has come down by 58% worldwide (520,000 in 2000 to 220,000 in 2014). Despite enormous benefits by treating the pregnant women with anti-HIV drugs, minor adverse effects like preterm delivery and pregnancy loss may rarely occur.

Early combination therapy to reduce infant mortality

Untreated children have more rapid progression of HIV-1 than untreated adults. 53% of untreated children die within 2 years and 75% die before the age of 3 years. Infants affected *in utero* or intrapartum 60% have higher risk of death than those infected through breastfeeding (60% versus 36%). Since maternal HIV-1 antibodies passively pass to the baby in the third trimester of pregnancy all children born at term to HIV positive mothers will be seropositive. Babies in whom treatment has been started

Textbook of Medicine

before 3 months of life have lower DNA levels and virus load than those treated after 3 months. Virus replication rebounds after weeks of discontinuing ART.

Source: Luzuriaga K, Mofenson LM. Challenges in the Elimination of Pediatric HIV-1 Infection. N Engl J Med. 2016 Feb;374(8):761-70.

Children Growing up with HIV Infection

An estimated 3.4 million children and adolescents are growing up with HIV infection receiving ART. Consequences of HIV infection in the crucial period of growth and development are being realized at present. Long standing HIV infection leads to growth failure and damage to heart, lung, brain and probably other organs which may not be correctable later. Disabilities like impairment of vision, hearing and learning abilities are common, so also sexual problems crop-up during the period of sexual maturation. Social problems such as loss of affected parents, lack of financial support and others add to the dimension of disabilities. These problems are also beginning to be felt, most intensively in sub Saharan African countries. Comprehensive management programs have to consider this aspect as well.

Source: Bernays S, Jarrett P, Kranzer K, et al. Children growing up with HIV infection: the responsibility of success. Lancet. 2014;383(9925):1355-7.

Points to Remember

- India has the potential to become one of the most heavily affected countries by AIDS if the medical fraternity, government and non-governmental organizations do not take steps to arrest the spread of infection.
- AIDS affects directly or indirectly almost all systems in the body.
- Morbidity caused by AIDS and the heavy cost of treatment and rehabilitation of bereaved families cause heavy financial burden to the country.
- Several drugs have been introduced to arrest progress of the disease, if started early.
- Primary treatment for AIDS patients is available in several centers in the country free of charge.
- This devastating illness is preventable by adopting safe sex habits, especially meticulous use of the condom.
- It is the duty of all medical men to procure the best available treatment offered by governmental agencies to the patents for continued medication and follow-up.

CHAPTER

49

Mycobacterial Infections
Tuberculosis, Nontuberculous Mycobacteria and Leprosy

KV Krishna Das, Usha Vaidhyanathan

Chapter Summary

- Tuberculosis (TB)
  - General Considerations
  - Epidemiology
  - Pathogenesis and Pathology
  - Immunity against TB
  - Pulmonary TB
  - Primary Pulmonary TB
  - Postprimary TB
  - Complications of Pulmonary TB
  - Diagnosis
  - Investigations
  - Sputum Examination
  - Radiology
  - Other Tests
  - Treatment
  - Drugs used in the Treatment of TB
  - Directly Observed Treatment Shortcourse (DOTS)
  - Drug Resistance and Reserve Drugs
  - Treatment of MDR-TB and XDR-TB
  - Special Points in Anti-TB Treatment
  - Treatment of TB in HIV Positive Patients
  - Immune Reconstitution Inflammatory Syndrome
  - Prevention of TB
  - Miliary TB
  - Tuberculous Meningitis
- Nontuberculous Mycobacteria
  - Lesions caused by Nontuberculous Mycobacteria
  - Choice of Drugs for Atypical Mycobacteria

- Leprosy
  - General Considerations
  - Pathology
  - Clinical Features
  - Indeterminate Leprosy
  - Tuberculoid Leprosy
  - Lepromatous Leprosy
  - Lucio Leprosy
  - Borderline Leprosy
  - Pure Neuritic Leprosy
  - Leprosy and HIV Infection
  - Reactions in Leprosy
  - Diagnosis
  - Management
  - Prevention and Control

TUBERCULOSIS (TB)

GENERAL CONSIDERATIONS

Even now TB remains a top infectious disease affecting humans and several animals globally. It is one of the most widely prevalent chronic infectious diseases affecting mankind. TB is caused by *Mycobacterium tuberculosis* (MTB) which may involve all organs in the body, but lungs are the most common sites. Robert Koch discovered the organism in 1882. Man is affected most commonly by the human strain and less commonly by the bovine strain. With the availability of pasteurized milk and improved animal husbandry practices, the frequency of the bovine tubercle bacillus infection has fallen considerably. Phage typing helps to subclassify the strains further. MTB can survive in dark moist environment for very long periods (up to years). In sputum, it remains viable for 20–30 hours. In droplet nuclei and dust, the viability is much longer.

TB is a major and still neglected cause of death and disability. The number of TB cases in the world is still very high. TB eradication is included in the Millennium Development Goals (MDGs). TB has a very complex relationship to poverty and immunosuppression especially human immunodeficiency virus (HIV). More than 9 million new cases of TB occur globally every year. The incidence rate is falling at less than 1% annually. MDGs aims at reducing incidence of TB to < 1% by 2050 and halt and begin to reverse the incidence of TB by 2015. Globally, multidrug-resistant TB (MDR-TB) were 4,40,000 new cases in 2008. In India, drug resistance surveillance in 2006 shows MDR prevalence at 2.8%. The estimated incidence of all forms of TB in India (2006) was 170/1,00,000 population, MDR-TB notified in 2008 was 0.3% [World Health Organization (WHO)].

A third of affected patients are not diagnosed and treated. Latent TB affects two billion people globally and this reservoir sustains the global burden of the disease. India contains a large proportion of the total global burden of TB including MDR-TB.

Tubercle bacilli are non-motile, non-sporing non-capsulate straight or curved rods about 3 × 0.3 μm in size. They grow only in special enriched media. They are obligate aerobes. Ultraviolet (UV) light and pasteurization of milk destroy the bacillus. Genotyping of *M. tuberculosis* has been completed and the fingerprint is available. Genetic studies employing **restriction fragments length polymorphism (RFLP)** help to make accurate epidemiological observations. Genetic studies also help to distinguish relapse from reinfection. In many countries, shelters, workplaces, healthcare facilities and bars are common sites for transmitting the disease. Infection in teachers spreads readily to the children at school. About 4.5% of households contacts of a newly detected case of TB have active TB at the time of diagnosis, additional cases developed as the contacts continued.

EPIDEMIOLOGY

All over the world, TB was in the forefront as a major cause of morbidity and mortality before the middle of this century. The present estimate of WHO is that there are about 15–20 million infectious cases in the world at any one time and that three million deaths occur annually. The three major killers in the developing world are HIV disease, TB and malaria. In India, TB still remains as a major cause of death from a curable infection. In the study launched by Indian Council of Medical Research (ICMR) in 1955–8, the prevalence of sputum positive pulmonary TB was 4/1000. Such nationwide surveys have not been performed subsequently. Only limited data is available.

Tuberculin surveys are employed to detect infection in the community. A limited study conducted in Trivandrum (South India) in 1980 showed that by the age of 14 years, 7.4% of school children were tuberculin positive. The WHO has suggested that the tuberculin positivity rates in children below 14 years has to be brought down below 1% to achieve control of this disease. It is evident that India has still a long way to go in achieving this goal. Despite the vigorous measures to control the disease undertaken by the **National Tuberculosis Control Programmes (NTCP),** the disease tends to persist because of the poor socioeconomic and educational levels of the population, reluctance to accept treatment and non-compliance with the prolonged drug regimen. HIV increases the risk of getting TB 20-fold. Undernutrition, smoking, diabetes, alcohol misuse, indoor air pollution and immunosuppressive treatment all increase risk of TB.

Immunodeficiency states—both iatrogenic and acquired immunodeficiency syndrome (AIDS) led to a resurgence of the disease in several parts of India. Vitamin D deficiency impairs the ability of monocytes to inhibit growth of *M. tuberculosis.* HIV predisposes to TB infection because of the reduction of Th1 lymphocytes which produce gamma interferon. TB accelerates the progression of AIDS and thereby hasten death. Both pulmonary and extrapulmonary lesions are more frequent.

Latent TB: In the majority of individuals infected by *Mycobacterium tuberculosis*, the immune system suppresses the infection and the patient harbors the dormant bacteria. The person develops cell mediated immune memory to the organism (Mantoux test). This state is termed as latent TB. Individuals with latent TB are at risk of progression to active TB; about 5–10% being the lifetime risk of progression. This risk of progression from latent to active TB is more during the first two years after infection. Several occupations and habitual exposures increase the risk of TB activation.

Susceptibility to TB conferred by other disease state: The lifetime risk of developing overt TB in an infected child is 10%. Among such children, 50% develop TB within 2 years of infection. There is a genetic predisposition to develop TB in some individuals.

In HIV negative individuals who develop TB, over 80% manifest as pulmonary TB. In HIV positive individuals, the occurrence of nonpulmonary manifestations is relatively higher. In India, co-infection of HIV and TB is seen in 10–11% of TB cases. Co-infection by the two diseases decreases the cure rate with treatment and also increases mortality. Susceptibility to develop TB is increased 2.4 times in patients with chronic renal failure. In persons receiving corticosteroid therapy for immunosuppression, the risk is twice the normal. TB remains predominantly a disease of the poor. Twenty-two countries where the per capita income is < $760 contain more than 80% of the total global burden of TB patients.

PATHOGENESIS AND PATHOLOGY

The portal of entry of the organisms is inhalation, ingestion or inoculation. Inhalation is the most common route. Droplets containing MTB are released when a patient coughs. Larger droplets fall to the ground. Medium-sized droplets are trapped in the mucosa of the upper respiratory tract from where they are cleared without causing infection. Tiny droplets (< 25 mm in diameter) evaporate immediately leaving particulate organisms to float in the air. These particles escape the trapping mechanisms and reach the lungs, where even a single bacterium can initiate infection. Given adequate exposure, TB is highly contagious. About 45–60% of children of parents with sputum positive patient gets the infection. One open case may infect at least 20 persons of whom 10%, i.e. 2 persons develop overt disease-one will be infectious and the other non-infectious. Smoking increases the incidence of TB.

Source: Gajalakshmi V, Peto R, Kanaka TS, et al. Smoking and mortality from tuberculosis and other diseases in India: retrospective study of 43000 adult male deaths and 35000 controls. Lancet. 2003;362(9383):507-15.

The primary site of infection depends on the mode of entry. It may be in the lungs, tonsils, mucous membranes, intestines or skin. The development of hypersensitivity plays a major role in determining further events. The pathological process occurring in an individual who has not been sensitized to the organisms, i.e. occurring for the first time, is known as *primary TB.* Subsequent infection occurring in the sensitized individual who possesses immunity gives rise to a different course of events. This is known as *postprimary TB*. T-lymphocytes play a major role in conferring immunity against *M. tuberculosis.* Tuberculosis bacillus circulates in blood and the number of circulating bacteria may reach high counts in immunocompromised hosts. They can be detected by polymerase chain reaction (PCR).

The host's reaction to the bacilli which enter is initially exudative and later proliferative. Initially, the exudate is composed mainly of neutrophils. Later, lymphokine activated macrophages accumulate and these engulf the organisms. These phagocytes are derived from the fixed tissue macrophages, the alveolar macrophages of the lungs and the monocytes from blood. Macrophages with engulfed organisms get transformed into epithelioid cells. Multinucleated foreign body type of giant cells *(Langhans giant cells)* are formed by the fusion of epithelioid cells. These are surrounded by lymphocytes and fibroblasts. At the center of the lesion caseation necrosis occurs. The secret of the organism's success is its ability to evade the immune system by penetrating into macrophages without being destroyed by them. Activated macrophages prevent replication of the tubercle bacillus, but may not kill them altogether. The pathological hallmark of TB is the tubercle which consists of an area of central caseation, around which there is infiltration by epithelioid cells, giant cells, round cells and peripherally by fibroblasts. Several such microscopic tubercles form the macroscopic tubercles which are seen in affected tissues.

Granuloma formation is usually adequate to limit the infection. The lesion becomes quiescent and surrounding fibroblasts produce scar tissue which may become calcified. Some bacilli remain in this tissue as *persisters* which, when reactivated produce postprimary disease.

In a minority of cases the infection progresses without being localized and gives rise to serious manifestations of the primary infection such as progressive primary lesion in infants, pleurisy, renal lesion, bone TB, meningitis and so on. If a primary focus ruptures into a blood vessel, miliary TB develops, with affection of all organs, particularly the meninges and brain.

Immunity against TB: Organisms possess nonspecific and specific immunity against TB. Nonspecific immunity is present in people living in areas of high prevalence. Depression of the general immune mechanism in diseases such as diabetes, malnutrition, immunosuppressed states and therapy with corticosteroids predispose fresh infection by *M. tuberculosis* and reactivation of quiescent lesions.

Specific immunity in TB is T-lymphocyte mediated. Though humoral antibodies are demonstrable, they do not play any protective role. *M. tuberculosis* can survive and replicate within macrophages thereby evading the immune defenses of the host. The infection also suppresses the reaction of macrophages to activating cytokines. One attack of TB does not confer solid immunity so that both reactivation of a quiescent focus and reinfection are possible. Abdominal TB occurring in HIV +ve subjects is characterized by visceral involvement with necrosis, best made out on computed tomography (CT) scans. Abdominal TB in HIV –ve subjects leads to omental thickening, ascites and peritonitis more often. Though the T-lymphocyte function is demonstrable as tuberculin sensitivity (Mantoux testing), sensitivity and immunity are not identical. Tuberculin sensitive individuals possess a degree of resistance to further infection by TB, but this immunity is not absolute.

PULMONARY TUBERCULOSIS

In man, lungs are the most frequently affected organs. All those who develop the disease for the first time manifest primary TB irrespective of their age. The pathological lesions in primary TB show prominent lymph nodular enlargement (usually hilar) with only minimal parenchymal lesions. Postprimary TB presents mainly as parenchymal disease with only minimal lymph node enlargement.

In primary TB, the bacilli multiply rapidly in the lesions and dissemination by lymphatics and blood-stream is frequent. Extensive tissue necrosis is rare.

Primary Pulmonary Tuberculosis

Lung is the most common site for primary TB. Children are affected most, though no age is immune. The initial lesion is a subpleural tubercle located in the lower part of the upper lobe, upper part of the lower lobe or middle lobe. This parenchymal lesion *(Ghon's lesion)* with its enlarged regional lymph nodes and interconnecting lymphangitis is known as the primary complex *(Ghon's complex)*. More than 80% of cases of primary TB do not produce systemic disturbances and the lesions heal spontaneously. These remain undetected. The tuberculin test becomes positive within 4 to 6 weeks of infection. Once it becomes positive, it usually remains so for life.

In 10–15% of children the primary lesion goes on to progressive disease. This may be due to poor general resistance, immunosuppression, high infective dose or virulent strains of bacilli. AIDS, measles and whooping cough lower the resistance and favor progression. The hilar

Textbook of Medicine

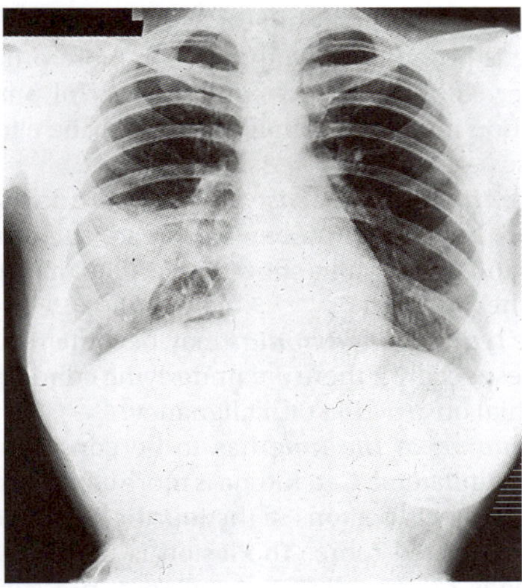

Fig. 49.1: Chest X-ray tuberculosis—middle lobe consolidation right lung

lymph nodes enlarge progressively and undergo caseation. Compression of the neighboring bronchi, especially of the middle lobe, leads to collapse-consolidation and bronchiectatic changes. This may present later as the 'middle lobe syndrome' (Fig. 49.1).

When a caseated node ruptures into a bronchus, spread occurs to other parts of the lungs and tuberculous bronchopneumonia develops. Erosion of a vessel and discharge of the caseous material into the bloodstream leads to wide dissemination and the development of miliary TB. Rarely the pulmonary lesion may increase in size to produce cavitation. It may also spread to the other regions of the lung parenchyma. Spread to the pleura results in pleurisy with effusion.

Clinical Features

Progressive primary TB is invariably symptomatic. Onset may be acute or insidious. Fever, loss of appetite, loss of weight and cough are early symptoms. Lethargy, vague ill-health, failure to thrive and delay in the milestones may be the presenting features in children. At this stage, the disease can be diagnosed only if the clinical suspicion is strong. Allergic manifestations like **phlyctenular conjunctivitis** or **erythema nodosum** may herald primary TB in some cases. Erythema nodosum manifests as reddish, indurated, painful, swellings usually seen in front of the tibia. These persist for varying periods. Occasionally the disease predisposes to recurrent respiratory infection. Acute pleural effusion may develop in some. Other presentations in children include tuberculous pneumonia, hemoptysis or asthma. Miliary TB may manifest as meningitis in many.

Physical examination may not give any positive finding in many patients and the diagnosis has to be based on investigations. In some, the signs of pulmonary consolidation, collapse or pleural effusion may be present. Tuberculin skin test is positive in the vast majority. Blood examination shows raised erythrocyte sedimentation rate (ESR) and lymphocytosis.

If the parenchymal lesion is small, expectoration may not be present. Chest X-ray reveals hilar lymphade-nopathy and on careful examination the pulmonary lesion may be detectable. The diagnosis of primary TB is based on the history of tuberculous contact, clinical symptomatology, X-ray findings and recent tuberculin positivity. Bacteriological confirmation is usually difficult to get.

Postprimary Tuberculosis

Pathogenesis and Pathology

Postprimary TB occurs in one of four ways:
1. Direct progression of primary lesion
2. Reactivation of a quiescent primary focus
3. Hematogenous infection of lung from lymph nodes, tonsils, etc.
4. Reinfection or superinfection.

Postprimary pulmonary TB is characterized by tendency for early cavitation, limitation of the disease process and healing. The upper lobes are more commonly affected, unlike as in primary TB. Depending upon the resistance, two pathological forms are seen.
1. Slowly progressive nodular form in individuals who possess resistance
2. Fibrocaseous form with tendency for cavitation if the resistance is low.

In the nodular form, the sputum shows only less number of tubercle bacilli, whereas the reverse is true in the latter.

Mainly the lung parenchyma shows lesions, the lymph node changes are minimal. The initial lesion is an exudative pneumonia. Subsequently tubercles form. They coalesce to give rise to large macroscopic lesions. The caseous material is discharged into a bronchus and coughed out, leaving behind a cavity. The wall of the cavity teems with the bacilli and its surroundings show many tubercles. Blood vessels in the cavity become unsupported. Many of them are occluded by thrombosis, but those that remain patent become aneurysmal (**Rasmussen's aneurysms**). They may rupture and give rise to massive hemoptysis. Healing, occurs with replacement fibrosis.

Clinical Features

Adolescents and young adults are more frequently affected, though no age group is spared. The disease manifests insidiously with respiratory symptoms such as mild and persistent cough, low-grade evening fever, anorexia, loss of weight and general weakness. The fever is moderate and comes on in the evening to subside with sweating by midnight. In a few cases the onset may be acute with high fever, cough and hemoptysis and the lesion may resemble lobar pneumonia. The nodular type is generally silent and in many cases it is detected radiologically. Sputum is mucoid or mucopurulent, initially scanty, later it is more copious. Mild streaky hemoptysis may occur initially, but later, profuse hemoptysis occurs due to erosion of blood vessels. The larynx is affected and laryngitis results in hoarseness of voice. In some cases, pleural effusion, empyema or pneumothorax may be the initial presentation.

Physical examination of the chest may reveal signs of consolidation, cavitation, collapse, fibrosis, pleural effusion or pneumothorax. As the condition proceeds, the

Textbook of Medicine

patient becomes emaciated. Cough with expectoration is pronounced and extreme cachexia develops (phthisis). If left untreated, death occurs due to extensive disease, cachexia, intercurrent infection or any of the complications. The classic picture of well-established lesion is rarely only encountered at present. Due to the free availability of chest X-ray and strong clinical suspicion, cases are diagnosed at earlier stages.

Complications of Pulmonary Tuberculosis

Several complications may develop during different stages of the disease. These may occur in the early part of the disease or much later. Some may be delayed by several years.

These are listed below:

Early: Occurring within months

- Mild hemoptysis
- Pneumothorax
- Pleural effusion
- Poncet's syndrome.

Intermediate: Occurring within several months or a few years

- Massive hemoptysis
- Secondary infection of cavities
- Pneumothorax, pleural effusion, empyema
- Progressive fibrosis with dyspnea
- Spread to other organs such as larynx, pericardium and others
- Nonhealing of lesion due to drug resistance of organisms.

Late: Occurring after several years

- Pulmonary fibrosis with compensatory emphysema, cor pulmonale, pleuropulmonary fibrosis
- Bronchiectasis
- Persistence of open cavities without healing
- Aspergilloma, i.e. growth of *Aspergillus fumigatus* in the cavities in the form of a fungus ball
- Coexistence of apical TB with carcinoma
- Secondary amyloidosis.

Diagnosis

TB should be suspected in all patients suffering from chronic respiratory disease, especially if associated with night sweats, fever, emaciation and hemoptysis. Other conditions which should be differentiated are bronchiectasis, lung abscess, cystic disease of the lung, chronic pneumonias, malignancy and tropical eosinophilia. Cough persisting for more than two weeks without other obvious causes should alert the physician to investigate for pulmonary TB.

Differential Diagnosis

In bronchiectasis, the lesions are often bilateral, involving usually the lower lobes. The condition is more chronic extending over several years. Finger clubbing and history of postural cough with copious sputum may be present. In majority of cases of pulmonary TB, finger clubbing does not occur, except in the bronchiectatic form and in the chronic fibrotic stage. Tuberculous bronchiectasis is usually confined to the affected part, unlike as in primary bronchiectasis.

Lung abscess usually affects the lower lobes. Postural coughing is prominent, symptoms are more pronounced and finger clubbing occurs early. History of pneumonia or aspiration into the respiratory tract may be elicitable in some cases.

Congenital cystic disease manifests in adolescence or adulthood. Lesions are more widespread, clubbing is only minimal and radiographs show thin-walled multiple cysts, more in the lower zones.

Some types of pneumonias may become recurrent or chronic, especially if there are underlying conditions such as bronchial obstruction or malignancy.

Carcinoma of the lung has to be considered when lesions are unilateral. Carcinoma is more common in heavy smokers. It affects persons in the fourth and fifth decades. Males are affected more. The lesion is more around the hilum. Signs of consolidation, collapse, pressure effects like Horner's syndrome or diaphragmatic paralysis should suggest this possibility. Clubbing of fingers occurs early and supraclavicular or pretracheal lymph nodes are palpably enlarged in most cases.

Tropical eosinophilia may present with cough, fever and loss of weight, especially in adolescents and young adults. Physical examination may reveal signs of bronchospasm and scattered rales. There may not be evidence of any localized lesions. Blood eosinophil count is high (often above 3000/mm^3). The sputum shows numerous eosinophils.

TB should be considered as a probable underlying cause in all cases presenting with asthma of recent onset, prolonged fever and pneumonias which tend to persist even after administering a standard therapy. Onset of TB in otherwise apparently healthy persons should raise the possibility of diabetes mellitus (DM) or AIDS as possible predisposing factors.

Poncet's syndrome is a hypersensitivity reaction to the infection, manifesting as arthritis, which may resemble rheumatoid or other forms of arthritis.

Investigations

Sputum examination: The most important diagnostic investigations are the demonstration of acid-fast organisms in sputum by Ziehl-Neelsen method and radiology. Positivity of smears and cultures depends on the bacterial count in the sputum. While examining a sputum smear, at least 100 fields should be seen for 10 minutes before declaring it as negative. At least 3 bacilli should be seen before the smear is declared positive (Fig. 49.2).

Concentration methods are available using 24-hour collection of sputum to detect acid-fast bacilli (AFB) when direct smears are negative. Sputum microscopy and culture detect only 70% v/v of the active cases, therefore a negative test does not totally exclude the diagnosis of TB. A common cause for sputum-negativity in India is partial treatment with anti-TB drugs.

Fluorescence microscopy is being employed to identify tubercle bacilli. It is more rapid and this method has the advantage of better coverage of the smear. Modern techniques using PCR have been found to be very useful in making early specific diagnosis.

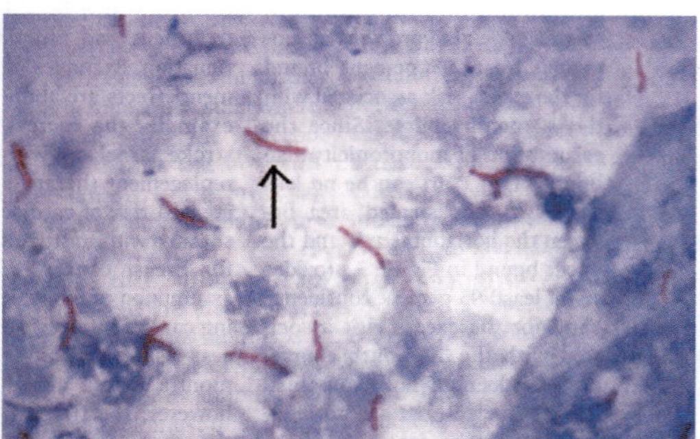

Fig. 49.2: Sputum: Zeihl-Neelsen stain. Acid-fast bacillus (arrow)

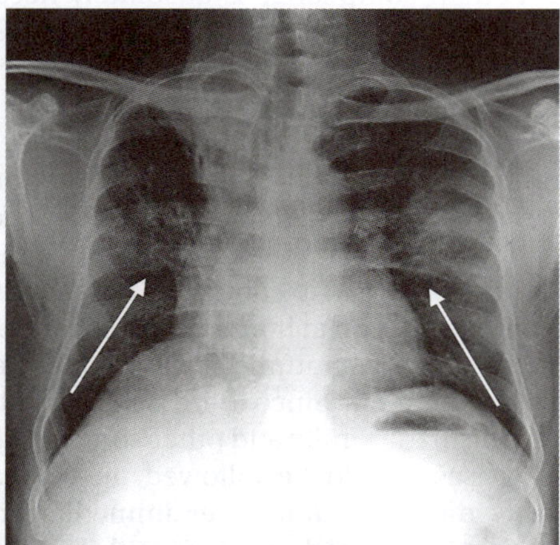

Fig. 49.3: Chest X-ray tuberculosis. Bilateral infiltrations (arrows)

Further confirmation is obtained by identification of *M. tuberculosis* in sputum culture. In high prevalence areas, it may not be practicable to do culture in all cases. For all practical purposes, two consecutive morning sputum examinations can be accepted as confirmatory of the diagnosis. When the sputum is difficult to get, as in children and psychiatric patients, laryngeal swab or material collected by gastric aspiration may be used. Laryngeal swab is 25% and gastric aspirate about 50% as efficient as sputum examination in identifying the organism. Sputum may be collected by transtracheal aspiration in comatose patients. Bronchoscopic aspiration is resorted to in exceptional cases. In high prevalence areas, sputum culture and animal inoculation studies should be reserved for cases with negative sputum smears, but with suggestive radiological features and in whom drug resistance is suspected.

Radiology: In day-to-day practice, radiology is the easiest and most readily available investigation to visualize the pulmonary lesion. Early cases show infiltration in the upper zones (Fig. 49.3).

Later the lesions coalesce to produce consolidation. When cavitation occurs, thin-walled cavities are seen, often multiple, with intervening fibrosis. As the lesion becomes fibrotic, the opacities become dense, with reduction in pulmonary volume and shifting of the trachea and mediastinum towards the side of lesion. Such lesions occupying the upper zones, especially if bilateral, should raise the strong suspicion of TB and the diagnosis has to be confirmed or excluded by appropriate tests.

With treatment, infiltration, consolidation and even early cavitation may heal completely leading to full resolution of the radiological abnormality. Once cavitation is chronic and fibrosis has set in, the radiological abnormalities do not clear up with further treatment even though the disease becomes arrested. In such cases, it is essential to distinguish residual radiological abnormalities from active disease.

Blood examination: It shows mild lymphocytosis and raised ESR in most cases. Since these findings are non-specific, they have only a limited diagnostic value. Progressive fall of ESR and clearance of radiological abnormalities are fairly reliable and simple practical methods to follow-up the progress of the disease with treatment.

OTHER TESTS

Presence of organisms in blood can be detected by PCR. PCR is a highly sensitive and specific test taking only a few hours for diagnosis. Sputum, blood, cerebrospinal fluid (CSF), pleural fluid and other tissues may be subjected to PCR. Different kits containing appropriate probes are available. Deoxyribonucleic acid (DNA) detected by PCR may remain so for long periods even after the infection is cured or suppressed.

Amplified mycobacterium TB detection (AMTD): This test uses the principles of transcription mediated amplification of ribosomal ribonucleic acid (RNA) of MTB. The detection of t-RNA indicates the presence of actively multiplying MTB. RNA is a much more short-lived molecule compared to DNA which persists for long periods. Specimens such as sputum, aspirated fluids, CSF, bone marrow and fine-needle aspiration cytology (FNAC) tissue can be used for the test. It takes 24 hours to get the result and costs approximately ₹ 1,000/-.

Interferon gamma release assays (IGRAs): These tests are useful to detect latent infection. Indications for these tests are situations where there is chance of exacerbation such as recent infection from active cases, HIV infection, injection drug use, homeless persons and immunosuppression. These tests tend to be positive in recent infections. They do not cross react with Bacillus Calmette-Guérin (BCG) vaccine immunity.

Enzyme-linked immunospot (ELISPOT) assay technique: They have been developed and different commercial kits are available. These are based on detection of interferon-γ produced by T-cells in response to antigens specific to *M. tuberculosis* (T-SPOT.TB, QuantiFERON-TB Gold) which have been tested in children and approved by the Food and Drug Administration (FDA). It has sensitivity of 83% to detect TB in children, whereas Mantoux test has sensitivity of only 63%.

Moreover, unlike Mantoux test which may be influenced by immunosuppressed conditions, the ELLISPOT test is unaffected. Nontuberculous mycobacteria (NTM) and BCG vaccination does not interfere with the ELLISPOT test.

Source: Liebeschuetz S, Bamber S, Ewer K, et al. Diagnosis of tuberculosis in South African children with a T-cell-based assay: a prospective cohort study. Lancet. 2004;364(9452):2196-203.

Textbook of Medicine

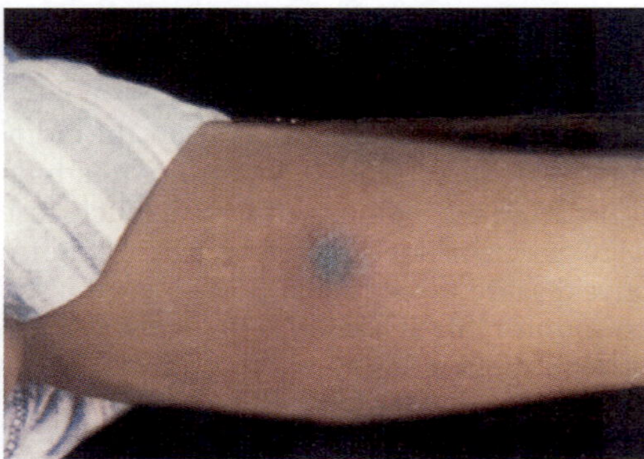

Fig. 49.4: Forearm showing accelerated reaction to Mantoux test in a male having active tuberculous lymphadenopathy

Proteomic finger printing methods: They are being developed to detect TB early, by identifying serum markers.
Tuberculin skin test (Mantoux test): This test is usually done by injecting one unit of purified protein derivative (PPD) in the volar surface of the forearm intradermally. The formation of induration depends on the presence of long standing cellular immune responses especially central memory T-cells. The result is read after 48 hours and the area of induration is recorded. In a positive test, the diameter of the induration exceeds 12 mm. Negative results do not always rule out tuberculous infection, since conditions like malnutrition, immunosuppression therapy and Hodgkin's disease, suppress the test. Patients suffering from active TB show an accelerated Arthus reaction with necrosis. Though the occurrence of ***accelerated reaction*** is not a wholly reliable parameter, invariably it points to active TB (Fig. 49.4).

The diagnostic value of tuberculin test is in those individuals who are ***recent converters***. This should suggest the occurrence of infection by mycobacteria. In infants below the age of one year, tuberculin positivity should be taken as recent infection and therefore it is an indication for starting anti-TB treatment.

Tuberculin testing is widely employed to assess the prevalence of the disease in the community. Prevalence of tuberculin positivity in the young subjects is related to the number of infective cases. This is of help in planning TB control programs. BCG vaccination if successful, gives rise to tuberculin-positivity.

Other methods to test tuberculin-sensitivity include Heaf multiple puncture test and tuberculin Tine test. Infection by NTM may give rise to positive tuberculin test. Differential tuberculin testing using PPD prepared from these mycobacteria helps to identify such infections.

TREATMENT

The goals of treatment are:
- To ensure cure without relapse
- To prevent death
- To prevent spread
- Prevent the development of resistance. Since MTB can remain dormant for long periods, all anti-TB treatment programs have two phases.
  - i. An ***active phase*** intended to kill actively growing and a proportion of the dormant organisms

ii. The ***second phase*** intended to eliminate the persisting bacilli.

Modern therapy is mainly dependent on the powerful anti-TB drugs currently available. With judicious combinations, virtually all lesions can be rendered bacteria-free and allowed to heal. Early lesions heal without any residual damage, whereas late lesions heal with fibrosis and calcification in some cases. It is important to institute treatment without delay after establishing the diagnosis. The drugs are always given in combination to avoid the development of resistance and for synergistic effect. A strict schedule should be instituted. Patient compliance is absolutely necessary to ensure cure and prevent the development of resistance. Lack of motivation of the patient and the long course of treatment are the most important factors which account for many dropouts after receiving incomplete therapy. Since most of the cases can be treated at home with excellent results, domiciliary treatment is preferable. Moreover, it is now well understood that once the case is notified, the risk of spread to contacts is only slight. Simple precautions like isolation at home, use of separate utensils and disinfection of the sputum are advised to the patient and his family members. Since there is likelihood of other cases occurring in the family and other contacts, detection of all fresh cases should be followed up with a survey of the family members and other immediate contacts. Hospitalization is required for cases with high fever and toxemia, hemoptysis, pleural effusion, pneumothorax, extreme cachexia and coexistence of other diseases like uncontrolled DM. Rendering the patient sputum-negative is the most effective method to control spread to others.
Drug schedules: Adequate chemotherapy administered without interruption for the optimal duration is the cornerstone of success. The available drugs are classified into standard or first line drugs and reserve or second line drugs based on their efficacy, cost, availability and toxicity (Table 49.1).

Short Course Chemotherapy

At present short course chemotherapy using isonico-tinylhydrazide isoniazid known as (INH), rifampicin, ethambutol and pyrazinamide is the preferred method, on account of its efficacy, ease for supervision and better patient compliance. Though the drugs are expensive, the government supplies the drugs free of cost from the TB control centers. Short course chemotherapy extending over 6–9 months is adequate to cure 95–98% of all forms of TB and in all age groups. Alternate drugs or longer period of treatment are indicated when drug resistance or intolerance of the primary drugs exists. Among the anti-TB drugs INH, rifampicin, pyrazinamide and streptomycin are bacteridal; the other drugs are bacteriostatic. Rifampicin absorption is better when taken with fatty food. Absorption of fluoroquinolones is inhibited by concurrent administration of antacids. INH, rifampicin and pyrazinamide blood levels are lower when taken with food.

Response to therapy occurs in three stages:
1. Within the first two weeks of starting therapy the majority of actively replicating bacteria in cavity

Table 49.1: Drugs used in the treatment of tuberculosis, dosage, route or administration and toxicity

Name of drug	Daily dose for adults	Children	Route of administration	Diffusion in CSF	Main toxic effects
First line drugs					
Isoniazid (INH)	5 mg/kg bw for ordinary cases 12 mg/kg bw in miliary TB and meningitis	10 mg/kg bw	Oral	Good	Hypersensitivity,* hepatitis, peripheral neuropathy
Rifampicin	Persons weighing below 50 kg:450 mg, above 50 kg:600 mg	10–20 mg/kg	Oral	Good	Gastrointestinal toxicity, hepatitis, enzymes, hypersensitivity, flu-like syndrome, blood dyscrasia especially thrombocytopenia
Pyrazinamide	Persons weighing up to 50 kg:1.5 g, 51–74 kg:2 g, above 75 kg:2.5 g (i.e.) 20–35 mg/kg bw	40 mg/kg maximum 2 g	Oral	Good	Arthralgia, hepatitis, hyperuricemia
Ethambutol	800 mg/day (24 mg/kg bw) for 2 months thereafter 15 mg/kg bw		Oral	Good	Retrobulbar neuritis, rare if dose is kept below 15 mg/kg
Streptomycin	Below 30 kg bw or above the age of 60 years:0.75 g, above 30 kg bw:1 g (20 mg/kg bw)	20 mg/kg bw	IM inj	Fair	Deafness, nephrotoxicity, vestibular dysfunction
Second line drugs					
Thiacetazone	150 mg	4 mg/kg bw	Oral	±	Gastrointestinal, hepatitis, exfoliate dermatitis
Ethionamide	500–750 mg	–	Oral	±	Gastrointestinal, metallic taste in the mouth, hepatitis
Cycloserine	0.5–1.0 g	–	Oral	Good	Confusion, slurring of speech, convulsions, psychosis
Kanamycin	15 mg/kg bw	–	IM inj		Ototoxicity and nephrotoxicity
Capreomycin	30 mg/kg bw:up to 1 g/daily for 4 months, followed by 1 g, 2–3 times a week	–	IM inj		Nephrotoxicity, vestibulotoxicity
Viomycin	3–4 g weekly	–	IM inj		Nephrotoxic and vestibulotoxic
Amikacin	15 mg/kg bw	–	IM inj		Ototoxicity, nephrotoxicity
Rifabutin is an analogue of rifampicin—used for treatment of rifampicin resistant mycobacteria.					
Rifapentine	600 mg once a week		Oral		Serum half-life 10–15 hours suitable for once-a-week schedules
Reserve drugs					
Ofloxacin	400 mg bd		Oral		Abdominal distress
Ciprofloxacin	750 mg bd or tid		Oral		Headache, anxiety, tremor, thrush, drug interaction
Clarithromycin	500 mg bd		Oral		Allergy

Note:

1. *Acute INH toxicity—acute overdose of INH 35–40 mg/kg/bw (8 tablet of 300 mg) causes seizures which tend to be recurrent and not responding to ordinary anticonvulsants. Ingestion of 6–10 g (20–30 tablets) is fatal, if untreated. Toxicity appears as soon as 30 minutes with nausea, vomiting, metabolic acidosis, seizures or coma. Treatment consists of removal of unabsorbed drug and administration of IV pyridoxine equal to the weight of INH ingested. If the dose of ingested INH is not known 5 g pyridoxine HCl can be given IV safely repeatedly. If IV preparation is not available, repeated oral doses of 5 g may be given but the effect is less. Morinamide is a derivative of pyrazinamide given orally in a dose of 40 mg/kg bw which is less toxic.
2. Prothionamide is a derivative of ethionamide, given in the same dosage. Its toxicity is possibly less. Both these drugs are only seldom used.
3. Para-aminosalicylic acid (PAS) is not used in regular therapy, but at times it is used as a second line drug.

walls are killed, mainly by INH, but also by rifampicin and pyrazinamide. The slow reactors may be even replicating or may be dormant. The latter is called the persistent group.

2. In the succeeding few weeks, rifampicin and pyrazinamide kill the less active bacteria lurking within macrophages, caseous material and exudates.
3. With maintenance therapy, the dormant bacilli are killed by rifampicin during their short bursts of activity. Emergence of drug resistant bacilli is uncommon if the shortcourse therapy is given properly under supervision.

Relapses, if they occur, are still caused by drug-sensitive bacilli, though rarely it may be by drug-resistant strains. Several regimens for short course chemotherapy are recommended.

Domiciliary Treatment

Success of domiciliary treatment has been established by several studies. Contacts of a notified case naturally maintain isolation and therefore spread from such cases is less common. Open cases of TB should maintain restricted isolation so that they do not transmit the disease to others.

Textbook of Medicine

They may be advised to confine to home till the sputum becomes AFB-negative. Separate utensils for eating and drinking are preferable. Infective materials like sputum should be disinfected by burning or burying deep in soil. All contacts with an infective case of TB should be followed up with a view to detect infection early.

DIRECTLY OBSERVED TREATMENT SHORTCOURSE (DOTS)

Standard therapy		
Drugs		
Initial phase first 2 months		
Rifampicin	450 mg	
INH	600 mg	Given under observation thrice a week
Ethambutol	1200 mg	
Pyrazinamide	1500 mg	
Maintenance treatment 4 months		
Rifampicin	450 mg	Given under observation thrice a week
INH	600 mg	

Modifications are done under special circumstances:
Category I: Severe forms of pulmonary TB with sputum positivity.
Category II: Defaulters of past treatment and failed cases from category I.

To the standard regimen add streptomycin 0.75 g IM thrice a week for 3 months. This period is extended to 4 months if clearance of lesion is not satisfactory.

Maintenance with three drugs INH 600 mg, rifampicin 450 mg and ethambutol 1200 mg thrice a week for 4 months. Total 8 months.

Category III: Extrapulmonary TB and sputum negative cases—regimen is the same as for standard therapy.

Note: Some regimen do not include ethambutol in the initial phase. Only three drugs are used.

India has launched the ***Revised National Tuberculosis Control Programme (RNTCP)*** in 1993 based on DOTS. This has been very successful. RNTCP has achieved cure rates of 80%.

All the anti-TB drugs are given together in full dosage on an empty stomach in the morning, since absorption is best at this time. Any food is allowed only at least 30 minutes later.

Since *M. tuberculosis* develops drug resistance rapidly when exposed to a single drug, combination therapy should always be insisted upon. Late relapses are more likely to occur if the full duration of treatment is not completed. INH which is still the most popular anti-TB drug behaves differently in slow and fast acetylators. Fast acetylators are persons who have high levels of acetyltransferase activity in the liver. This enzyme metabolizes INH much faster and so fast acetylators require higher doses. In slow acetylators, the half-life of INH is over 2 hours, whereas in fast acetylators, it is 0.5–1.5 hours. Above 70% of Indian subjects are slow acetylators.

The standard regimen is adequate for all forms of TB, both for human and bovine strains of mycobacteria.

Patients with uncomplicated TB, receiving uninterrupted treatment for the entire period, should be considered cured, unless proved otherwise. Up to 2% cases relapse after successful chemotherapy. The risk of relapse is more in the first three years after completing treatment. The DOTS program launched in 1993 has achieved the following results in India. More than 200,000 health workers have been trained. Forty percent of the population has access to DOTS regimen; 800,000 received treatment. The World Bank, Danish and UK National Agencies and the Government of India have funded the program.

Course and prognosis: With successful regimen the lesions become sterile and the vast majority heal by fibrosis. Surgery is indicated only under exceptional situations. These include open healed cavities with aspergilloma, grossly destroyed lung with secondary infection, bronchiectasis and persistence of tubercle bacilli resistant to all drugs, especially in cavitary lesions.

Common causes for failure of therapy are:
- Inadequate drug dosage
- Noncompliance with the schedule
- Early stopping of therapy
- Drug toxicity
- Initial drug resistance.

DRUG RESISTANCE AND RESERVE DRUGS

Resistance to drugs may be of different types:
- Some strains of *M. tuberculosis* are naturally resistant to drugs. This is rare.
- ***Primary drug resistance:*** Bacilli which are initially resistant to drugs may be the infecting organism.
- ***Secondary drug resistance:*** This is drug resistance acquired by initially sensitive bacilli, due to irregular and inadequate chemotherapy.
- In some cases, initial resistance may be either primary or secondary, especially when a patient conceals the history of earlier chemotherapy.
- ***Transient resistance:*** This is a bacteriological phenomenon which occurs sometimes during successful chemotherapy. One or two cultures may be reported as resistant but later these cases may also become sensitive. This is not an indication to change the drugs.

Patients with cavitary lesion in which the bacterial population is very high, are more likely to develop drug resistance. Resistance should be suspected when a lesion fails to become sputum negative and heal, despite adequate chemotherapy.

MDR-TB: WHO estimates that 4,40,000 cases of MDR-TB occurred in 2008 contributing 3.6% of estimated total incident TB. Resistance to drugs arise as a result of spontaneous mutations in the genome of MTB. Thus in the patients with active TB subpopulation of MTB spontaneously arise and multiply. Once created, drug resistant strains can infect fresh patients. The total problem of MDR-TB is due to a combination of acquired resistance and primary transmission. Use of second line drugs such as fluoroquinolones for other diseases also contribute to silent development of resistance in MTB as well. Lab testing for INH and rifampicin sensitivity can detect MDR-TB and this is needed for all fresh cases.

Alternate drugs: These are used when the organisms are resistant to one or more of the standard drugs or toxicity is severe. The regimen consists of 3–4 drugs administered for a period of 2 years or more. The drugs include rifampicin, ethambutol, pyrazinamide or morinamide, ethionamide or prothionamide, cycloserine, kanamycin, viomycin and capreomycin. There should be at least two bactericidal drugs. Lifelong follow-up is necessary in cases where reserve drugs have been used.

MDR-TB is increasing due to noncompliance and poorly supervised treatment programs. Resistance to INH and rifampicin in MDR-TB is highly dangerous. In HIV –ve individuals, it causes 22% mortality. In HIV +ve case, it is about 50%. Concurrent MDR-TB and HIV infection carries a high mortality. Early detection and treatment of this combination is needed for successful outcome. Prevalence of MDR-TB in some surveys in India give the following figures:

Mahajan, et al. Delhi 1996	Tiwari, et al. Pune 1994
• Resistance against INH 26–48% • Resistance to Streptomycin (SM) 18–63%	• Resistance to 1 drug—38% • Resistance to 2 drugs—28% • Resistance to 3 drugs—13%

MDR-TB may be classified as ***basic MDR-TB*** in which the resistance is only to INH and rifampicin and ***MDR-TB plus*** in which there is resistance to several other drugs as well. The molecular basis for resistance has been elucidated. Even with combination drug regimen the cure rates for MDR-TB is only 50–60%.

Whenever drug resistance is suspected, preferably in all cases it is better to do culture and sensitivity of the organism before administrating the appropriate anti-TB regimen. At present drug resistance of the organism can be detected by molecular studies.

Example: Rapid molecular detection of TB and rifampicin resistance—a multicentric trial including 310 patients from Hinduja National Hospital, Mumbai, reported a fully automated Xpert MTB/RIF test performed on sputum. In smear positive cases: 98% and in smear negative case: 72.5% were positive for rifampicin resistance. This test is a rapid method to detect TB and rifampicin resistance.

Source: Boehme CC, Nabeta P, Hillemann D, et al. Rapid molecular detection of tuberculosis and rifampin resistance. N Engl J Med. 2010;363(11):1005-15.

Treatment of MDR-TB

- Start treatment with at least three drugs to which the organisms is sensitive *in vitro*
- Use bactericidal drugs as far as possible
- Avoid drugs that impair absorption of anti-TB drugs, e.g. antacids
- Never add a single agent to a failing regimen
- Malabsorption is common in AIDS and therefore check the serum levels
- Always use directly observed therapy
- Surgical measures should be considered early so as to eradicate infection
- Consider treatment as successful only if two sputum cultures done at least two weeks apart are negative

- Continue treatment for at least 18–24 months after bacteriological clearance
- Strict isolation of the patients.

Extensively drug-resistant (XDR) TB: This newly coined term denotes extensive resistance to drugs in the first and second line also. XDR-TB is classified as cases resistant to three or more of the second line drugs. The reason for developing. XDR-TB is misuse and mismanagement of second line drugs. This problem is widespread in many countries. In India also this is cropping up. The mortality is $\pm$ 80%.

Treatment of MDR-TB and XDR-TB RNTCP PMDT (programmatic management of drug-resistant TB) guidelines: The diagnosis of MDR-TB must be confirmed wherever possible. This can be done either by culture and conventional drug susceptibility testing on solid or liquid media or by molecular methods. There are two WHO endorsed rapid molecular methods available in the RNTCP for diagnosis of drug resistance: Xpert MTB/RIF (Gene Xpert) and line probe assay (LPA). While Xpert provides only information on rifampicin resistance, LPA detects both isoniazid and rifampicin resistance. All patients at high-risk for MDR-TB, i.e. those with previous anti-TB treatment or who have failed treatment, patients in contact with a known MDR-TB patient and all HIV+ patients can be referred for free drug-resistance testing to the program. Only in life-threatening situations like meningitis or in children where bacteriologic confirmation may not always be possible, should MDR-TB treatment be started empirically. The tables below provide the drug regimen and dosages to be used for treatment of MDR and XDR-TB (Tables 49.2 to 49.4). Close follow-up and monitoring are required for early detection and management of adverse reactions.

RNTCP regimen for MDR-TB: 6 (9) km Lvx Eto Cs Z E/18 Lvx E to Cs E (Reserve/substitute drugs: PAS, Mfx, Cm).

The dosages for higher weight patients include use additional dosages of same 2nd line drugs for MDR-TB cases in patients weighing > 70 kg taking the dosage to kanamycin/capreomycin (1 g), ethionamide (1 g), cycloserine (1 g), ethambutol (1.6 g) and pyrazinamide (2 g). Other drugs dosages would remain the same. All these are well within the maximum permissible dosage for each drug as per the WHO guidelines.

RNTCP regimen for XDR-TB: 6–12 cm, PAS, Mfx, high dose-H, Cfz, Lzd, Amx/Clv/18 PAS, Mfx, high dose-H, Cfz, Lzd, Amx/Clv (Reserve/substitute drugs: Clarithromycin, Thiacetazone).

Recently, two new drugs, with novel mechanism of action, have been developed for use in MDR-TB. Bedaquiline is manufactured by Janssen and has been approved by FDA for use in M/XDR-TB while Delamanid is manufactured by Otsuka and is approved by European Medicines Agency (EMA). Neither drug is approved by Central Drugs Standard Control Organization (CDSCO) or available in India. However, they can be imported for compassionate use in exceptional circumstances. Another novel compound, pretomanid (PA-824) is beginning phase II trial in MDR-TB in India.

Table 49.2: Regimen for MDR-TB dosage and weight band recommendations

S. no.	Drugs	16–25 kg	26–45 kg	46–70 kg
1	Kanamycin	500 mg	500 mg	750 mg
2	Levofloxacin	250 mg	750 mg	1000 mg
3	Ethionamide	375 mg	500 mg	750 mg
4	Ethambutol	400 mg	800 mg	1200 mg
5	Pyrazinamide	500 mg	1250 mg	1500 mg
6	Cycloserine	250 mg	500 mg	750 mg
7	Pyridoxine	50 mg	100 mg	100 mg
8	Na-PAS (80% weight/vol)	5 g	10 g	12 g
	Moxifloxacin (Mfx)	200 mg	400 mg	400 mg
	Capreomycin	500 mg	750 mg	1000 mg

Table 49.3: Dosage of regimen for MDR-TB for pediatric age group <16 kg

Drug	Daily dose (mg/kg body weight)
Kanamycin/capreomycin	15–20 mg/kg
Levofloxacin/moxifloxacin	7.5–10 mg/kg
Ethionamide	15–20 mg/kg
Cycloserine	15–20 mg/kg
Ethambutol	25 mg/kg
Pyrazinamide	30–40 mg/kg
Na-PAS	150 mg/kg

Table 49.4: Regimen for XDR-TB dosage and weight band recommendations

Drug	Dosage/day	
	≤ 45 kg	> 45 kg
Inj capreomycin (Cm)	750 mg	1000 mg
PAS	10 g	12 g
Moxifloxacin (Mfx)	400 mg	400 mg
High dose INH (high dose-H)	600 mg	900 mg
Clofazimine	200 mg	200 mg
Linezolid (Lzd)	600 mg	600 mg
Amoxyclav (AMx/Clv)	875/125 mg bd	875/125 mg bd
Pyridoxine	100 mg	100 mg
Reserve/substitute drugs		
Clarithromycin (Clr)	800 mg bd	500 mg bd
Thiacetazone (Thz)*	150 mg	150 mg

* Depending on availability, not to be given to HIV positive cases.

Source: Soumya Swaminathan, Director, ICMR, Tuberculosis Research Center, Chennai.

Special Points in Anti-TB Treatment

- Pregnancy and lactation are not contraindications to standard anti-TB treatment. The drugs are not embryotoxic. If a sputum-positive mother gives birth, the baby should be removed, given BCG and preferably brought back to the mother only after it becomes Mantoux-positive. The baby should be observed for the development of primary TB. INH therapy is advocated as prophylaxis after BCG vaccination has taken effect.
- *Hepatic disease:* It is better to avoid rifampicin, INH and thiacetazone since these drugs are metabolized in the liver.
- *Renal failure:* Streptomycin and ethambutol are to be avoided. Rifampicin, INH and pyrazinamide are well tolerated.

TREATMENT OF TUBERCULOSIS IN HIV POSITIVE PATIENTS

Co-infection with the two diseases presents special problems. Primarily the resistance against TB is considerably reduced. So also the progression of AIDS is also accelerated. The special problems include drug-drug interactions, overlapping toxicities, additional pill burden, problems of compliance and development of immune reconstitution inflammatory syndrome (IRIS). All HIV-TB patients should be treated with standard four-drug anti-TB therapy. Intermittent (once a week or twice a week) therapies should be avoided. The exact duration of treatment is not well-defined, but drug susceptible TB should be treated for 6 months. Those with slow response, i.e. sputum cultures positive even at 2 months should receive treatment at least for 9 months. TB involving the central nervous system (CNS) should receive treatment at least for one year.

In those with HIV and TB, the treatment has to be instituted against both diseases simultaneously as early as possible taking precautions against the risk of immune reconstitution inflammatory syndrome. Despite starting treatment for TB, the death in the subsequent one month may still be mostly attributable to TB, whereas deaths occurring later may be due to other causes as well.

What drug regimen should be given to treat HIV in the presence of TB? Rifampicin causes enzyme induction in the liver and this may lead to reduction in the blood level of nevirapine and other antiretroviral (ARV) drugs. It also predisposes to nevirapine induced hepatitis, especially in women with CD4 T-cell counts > 250/mm^3. Therefore, the treatment of HIV should consist of two non-nucleoside reverse-transcriptase inhibitors (NNRTI) with efavirenz in a daily dose of 600–800 mg. After completion anti-TB therapy, a cheaper NNRTI drug like nevirapine can be substituted.

IMMUNE RECONSTITUTION INFLAMMATORY SYNDROME (IRIS)

This phenomenon is not uncommon. This condition arises when antiretroviral therapy (ART) partially restores the immunosuppression in AIDS. This manifest

Textbook of Medicine

as exacerbation of tuberculous lesion such as lymphadenopathy, hepatosplenomegaly, fever, aches and pains, granulomas, suppuration, necrosis of tissues, rise in intracranial tension, flare up of pulmonary lesions and several others. Similar exacerbation may occur in other AIDS-related infections as well. This may mimic drug reactions and it may even be life-threatening. IRIS is more likely to occur in patients where CD4 T-cell counts are <100/mm³ and in whom highly active antiretroviral therapy (HAART) is started within the first 2 months of starting anti-TB therapy. The usual time for manifestation is 3 months after starting the therapy.

Treatment

Some cases clear up spontaneously on continuing the combination therapy. At times if IRIS is life-threatening, such as worsening of lesions, the HAART has to be temporally withdrawn. Nonsteroidal anti-inflammatory drugs (NSAIDs) and prednisolone in adequate doses may have to be used. In any case development of IRIS is not a reason for abandoning specific treatment for both conditions.

PREVENTION OF TUBERCULOSIS

Elimination of TB strategy—this involves three pillars.
1. Integrated patient care and prevention
2. Bold policies and supporting systems
3. Intensified research and innovations.

Source: Uplekar M, Weil D, Lonnroth K, et al. WHO's new end TB strategy. Lancet. 2015;385(9979):1799-801.

Improvement in economic and social factors and education of the community are associated with reduction in incidence of TB. Specific immunization is by BCG vaccination. BCG mounts up CD4 T-cell mediated immunity. Recent trials conducted in south India have thrown doubts on the full efficacy of BCG vaccination. However, the WHO still recommends BCG vaccination as a protective measure against TB especially in children. BCG vaccination prevents severe disease and reduces the mortality in children, but protection against the development of pulmonary TB in children and adults is doubtful. As at present it is included in the primary vaccination program of infants. There are attempts to modify BCG vaccine to improve its immunogenicity.

The vaccination is given intradermally over the left shoulder just below the insertion of the deltoid with 0.1 mL of the liquid or reconstituted dry vaccine. For infants below 4 weeks 0.05 mL is the recommended dose. Ideal time is to give BCG at the third month of life but in practice the vaccine is given in the neonatal period in many centers, for administrative convenience. A nodule develops which ulcerates and heals in 8–12 weeks, leaving a scar. Though BCG was given only to tuberculin negative subjects previously, it is now given routinely even without routine tuberculin testing. Relative immunity starts to appear in 4–6 weeks which wears off with the passage of time and disappears in 5–7 years. In some countries revaccination is done at 7 years intervals in high-risk groups till the age of 21 years. Rare complications include non-healing of the ulcer, abscess formation in the axillary lymph node and keloid formation. Dissemination may occur in immunosuppressed individuals. Nonhealing ulcers or troublesome lymphadenopathy responds promptly to local or systemic INH therapy, but chemotherapy also eliminates the protective role of the vaccine.

Chemoprophylaxis: INH has been found to offer effective prophylaxis against TB in high-risk groups. Chemoprophylaxis may either be primary or secondary depending on whether prophylaxis is given to a person who is tuberculin negative or tuberculin positive respectively. Primary prophylaxis is given to the contacts of sputum-positive TB patients before they develop the disease, e.g. newborns of infective parents.

Secondary chemoprophylaxis is employed only rarely. When corticosteroids or immunosuppressants have to be administered, INH may be given to prevent exacerbation of healed tuberculous lesion.

INH plus ART to prevent TB: In a randomized double blind placebo controlled trial, 12 months isoniazid preventive therapy reduced the incidence of TB in individuals infected with HIV-1, established on ART or newly starting ART. INH was given in dose of 200 mg/day for those with body weight below 50 kg and 300 mg/kg for those with more than 50 kg body weight, along with 25 mg pyridoxine for 12 months. The INH is well tolerated in patients with negative tuberculin skin test or interferon gamma release assays. This therapy did not increase the resistance to INH.

Source: Rangaka MX, Wilkinson RJ, Boulle A, et al. Isoniazid plus antiretroviral therapy to prevent tuberculosis: a randomised double-blind, placebo-controlled trial. Lancet. 2014;384(9944):682-90.

Surveillance: Persons who are at high-risk of developing TB occupationally (danger group) such as hospital staff, school teachers, bus conductors, barbers, hotel employees and others should have periodic medical examination.

The 'End-TB strategy' of WHO launched in 2015 aims are at reducing the incidence of TB to below 10 cases/10,00,000 population which will result in 90% reduction in TB incidence and 90% reduction in deaths due to TB. This is to be achieved by:
- Increase in global investment to improve rapid diagnosis by molecular methods
- Treatment and prevention of TB, all forms of TB including MDR-TB and HIV associated TB
- Development of a new molecular test to detect TB and resistance to rifampicin which is expected to be available shortly.

The present treatment of TB is not considered ideal since it is prolonged, expensive, management intensive and likely to be defaulted. Several different regimens are being tried in order to improve efficacy, reduce duration, avoid non-compliance and reduce the development of drug-resistance.

One regimen which has been introduced is a short course of INH and rifapentine given as single oral weekly dose for 12 weeks. The authors' claim that this course will eradicate latent TB. Similar other studies are also in progress.

Source: Sterling TR, Villarino ME, Borisov AS, et al. Three months of rifapentine and isoniazid for latent tuberculosis infection. N Engl J Med. 2011;365(23):2155-66.

WHO has developed the 'stop-TB strategy' with the following targets: Year 2015—reduce prevalence of TB and deaths due to TB by 50% relative to the levels that existed in 1990.

Year 2050—eliminate TB as a public health problem that is < 1 case per million population.

24th March of every year is designated the ***World TB day*** by the WHO. TB is included along with malaria and AIDS in the MDGs for urgent implementation.

MILIARY TUBERCULOSIS

Syn: Acute hematogenous tuberculosis

Tubercle bacilli entering the bloodstream are diffusely disseminated and results in miliary TB. This is more common in young children in whom it is seen as a complication of primary TB. Postprimary TB may also lead to hematogenous spread when the general resistance is low.

Pathogenesis and Pathology

Entry of the bacilli into the bloodstream is through lymphatics or by erosion of blood vessels by caseating lesions. Areas of caseous vasculitis (***Weigert's foci***) occurring in veins or arteries may result in the discharge of bacilli into the circulation. Numerous tubercles develop in the affected tissues. These coalesce to form multiple lesions of the size of millet seeds. All organs are affected, especially the lungs, liver, spleen, kidneys, meninges, brain, bones and joints, intestines, skin, choroid of the eye and serous membranes. The lesions may become confluent with the progress of the disease.

Clinical Features and Diagnosis

Majority of cases present varying grades of pyrexia. Localizing signs may not be evident in the beginning. In some cases, meningitis and in a few others, pneumothorax or pneumomediastinum may be the presenting manifestation. About one-third of the cases show enlargement of the liver and spleen. Generalized lymphadenopathy may occur. The lymph nodes are small or moderately enlarged in size and discrete. Choroid tubercles may occur rarely. Evidence of an underlying tuberculous lesion may be present in a few cases, but this is more an exception than the rule.

Diagnosis

Clinically the diagnosis of miliary TB should be considered in the differential diagnosis of fevers, especially so in children. Skiagrams of the chest are most helpful. This shows numerous, small rounded shadows—the miliary mottling. The upper lobes are more affected and this helps to distinguish miliary TB from other conditions such as pulmonary hemosiderosis, eosinophilia, disseminated carcinoma, pneumoconiosis, sarcoidosis and histoplasmosis in which mottling of the lungs is more prominent in the lower zones. Since the radiological findings of typical military opacities take time to develop, repetition of X-ray will be needed if clinical suspicion is strong. There is no characteristic abnormality on blood examination. Sputum examination is often unrewarding. Tuberculin test may be positive only in some cases. Histologically, the diagnosis may be made through biopsy of tissues like the liver, lungs or bone marrow (trephine biopsy). Choroid tubercles are diagnostic if they occur, but in Indian subjects they are only rarely found.

Treatment

Standard chemotherapy has to be started early and in most cases the condition dramatically improves within weeks. Corticosteroids may be given along with full anti-TB treatment to reduce toxemia in severe cases. Results of treatment, if started early, are excellent and complete resolution is the rule.

TUBERCULOUS MENINGITIS

About 25–30% of the total number of cases of meningitis seen in many hospitals in India were presumed to be due to TB. Children suffer from this disease most, but all age-groups can be affected. The proportion of tuberculous meningitis is coming down (*See* also Ch 199).

Pathogenesis and Pathology

Tuberculous meningitis develops commonly as a complication of miliary TB. The organisms reach the CNS in the bloodstream. The other source of infection is rupture of a subcortical caseous focus. Small granulomas are formed in the superficial layers of the brain ***(Rich foci)***. Bacilli reach the subarachnoid space from these lesions and set up leptomeningitis. Tubercles are formed most commonly at the base of the brain and along the cerebral vessels. There is increased production of CSF. Adhesions develop in the base of the brain and these block the foramina. The CSF pressure is increased. Autopsy reveals thickening and cloudiness of the pia and arachnoid. The surface shows a creamy white exudate. In advanced disease, the whole of the base of the brain may be covered by thick granulation tissue, which envelops the cranial nerves and the major arteries. The cerebral vessels may develop endarteritis obliterans and thrombosis. This may lead to cerebral infarcts. Surfaces of the cerebral hemispheres and the choroid plexuses may show tubercles. The inflammation spreads to the inner lining of the cerebral ventricles as well.

Clinical Features

The onset is generally insidious with vague ill-health. The child may show nonspecific symptoms like fever, restlessness, irritability, vomiting and loss of appetite. In others, the onset may be acute with convulsions, high fever and signs of intracranial tension. A few cases develop abnormality of behavior which may progress to stupor and coma. Death occurs in 4–8 weeks in untreated cases.

Physical findings depend on the stage at which the patient is first seen. Signs of meningeal irritation may not be evident in very early stages, but soon these become obvious. Neck stiffness is less prominent in younger children. Complications such as cranial nerve palsies, hemiplegia or monoplegia may be evident. Papilledema may be present in some. An acute presentation resembling purulent or aseptic meningitis is not rare. In a few cases the onset may be with brainstem involvement and acute pulmonary edema. Other features of miliary TB may be evident, especially in children.

Textbook of Medicine

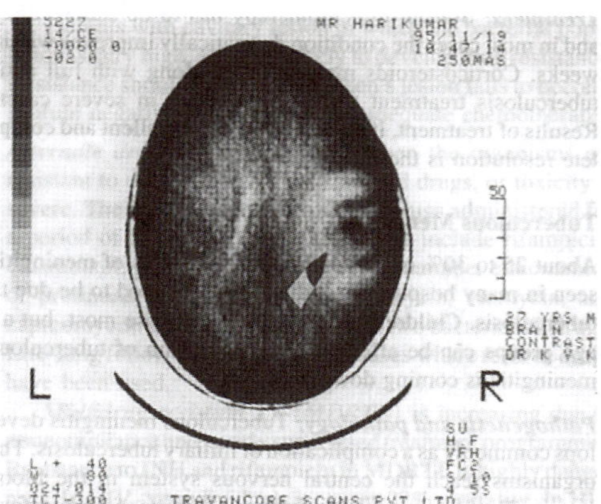

Fig 49.5: *CT scan:* Tuberculoma right parietal lobe (see arrowhead). Male aged 26 with epilepsy. Completely cleared with therapy

Complications

Complications are invariably present in those cases which are seen late in the disease. Acute complications include internal hydrocephalus, cerebral infarction, cranial nerve palsies, convulsions, fluid and electrolyte disturbances and bed sores. The chronic complications are obstructive hydrocephalus, optic atrophy, subdural effusions, diffuse or localized spinal arachnoiditis, spinal cord compression and the development of tuberculoma in the brain and spinal cord (Fig. 49.5). In cases where treatment is delayed for four weeks or more, focal paralysis, intellectual impairment, epilepsy, hypothalamic disturbances and intracranial calcification may persist as sequelae. The overall mortality in large series varies from 10 to 15%.

Diagnosis

Early diagnosis is possible only if the clinical suspicion is strong. History of contact with tuberculous cases, evidence of miliary TB and the presence of choroidal tubercles should suggest the underlying cause. The clinical picture of advanced disease is that of a child, dehydrated, lying in opisthotonus with the typical meningitic cry. This picture is rarely seen now. Differential diagnosis includes other forms of meningitis, encephalitis, acute or subacute demyelinating lesions, cerebral space occupying lesions such as brain abscess, subdural hematoma or tumors, leukemic and carcinomatous meningitis and all other conditions causing coma.

Meningitis is diagnosed by examination of the CSF. *Lumbar puncture* should be done as early as possible on suspecting the diagnosis. If lumbar puncture fails due to spinal block, CSF should be obtained by cisternal puncture or ventricular puncture. Examination of the CSF shows rise in pressure, turbidity and a rise in lymphocytes up to 500–1000 cells/mm³. A mixed pleocytosis may occur in some rare cases. A fine coagulum *(cobweb)* forms in the CSF when kept at room temperature for 6-24 hours. Though this is highly suggestive of tuberculous meningitis, it may rarely be seen in other types of meningitis as well. Proteins are moderately increased up to 200–300 mg/dL. Sugar is reduced to less than 50% of the blood sugar. In severe cases, depression of CSF sugar is even more marked. The chlorides are diminished as a part of generalized hypochloremia due to electrolyte

losses. With meticulous care, *M. tuberculosis* may be demonstrable by culture and animal inoculation in up to 50% of cases. AFB may be demonstrable in the cobweb in about 15–20% of cases.

Tuberculous meningitis has to be distinguished from other forms of meningitis. In purulent meningitis, the CSF shows neutrophil predominance and the organism may be demonstrable by Gram stain. Cryptococcal meningitis may closely resemble tuberculous meningitis. The fungus is demonstrable in CSF by India ink staining.

In partially-treated purulent meningitis the CSF picture shows mainly lymphocytes. This should not be mistaken for tuberculous meningitis. Leptospira, viruses, leukemic infiltration and carcinomatosis may all give rise to CSF pleocytosis and biochemical abnormalities. These should be kept in mind.

Treatment

The most important factor deciding a favorable outcome is early institution of chemotherapy. General treatment includes correction of dehydration and electrolyte imbalance, maintenance of nutrition, good nursing care with special attention to the skin, bladder and bowels, analgesics to relieve headache and anticonvulsants to stop convulsions.

Standard anti-TB chemotherapy is instituted as early as possible. INH is administered at a higher dose of 12–15 mg per kg (600 mg for an average adult). *Systemic corticosteroids* help to reduce morbidity, especially those due to adhesions and fibrosis and speed up recovery. They are employed after establishing specific chemotherapy. Prednisolone is started at a dose of 0.5–1 mg/kg and is tapered off in 4–8 weeks. In severe cases dexamethasone in doses of 4–8 mg should be given twice or thrice daily IM or IV till the patient can tolerate oral medication for children the dose is 200–500 mcg/kg bw daily.

The progress is monitored by clinical assessment and also repetition of CSF studies at weekly intervals. When the cell count reaches normal levels, dosage of INH is reduced to 6 mg/kg bw. Thereafter, standard chemotherapy is continued as for pulmonary TB. The sugar content of CSF is the last to return to normal. Ambulation should be permitted only after the CSF sugar returns to normal.

CT scanning is an excellent method to demonstrate meningitis, obstructive hydrocephalus, presence of tuberculoma and for excluding conditions such as subarachnoid or subdural hemorrhage and primary space occupying lesions. Wherever possible, this facility should be employed for diagnosis, as well as follow-up (Fig. 49.5).

Prognosis

Specific therapy given within two weeks of onset of symptoms gives complete recovery. If treatment is delayed for 4-6 weeks, complications and sequelae may develop. Treatment started beyond six weeks is unrewarding in many cases.

Points to Remember

- Despite prolonged efforts over half century, TB still continues as a major cause of death in India and several other developing countries.

- The main reasons are the high infectivity of the organism, its capacity to remain dormant, need for prolonged multi-drug therapy and the development of drug-resistance.
- The HIV epidemic has caused a boost to study the incidence and complications of TB all over the world.
- Development of drug-resistance is a serious problem which has to be avoided at all costs.
- The government of India has accepted the RNTCP with collaboration from international agencies. The DOTS program which was developed by WHO with active participation of Indian scientists is the mainstay of TB control.

Source: API Consensus Expert Committee. API TB Consensus Guidelines 2006: Management of pulmonary tuberculosis, extra-pulmonary tuberculosis and tuberculosis in special situations. J Assoc Physicians India. 2006;54:219-34.

NON-TUBERCULOUS MYCOBACTERIA (NTM)

Several mycobacteria other than *M. tuberculosis* affect man as opportunistic invaders. These are known by several names such as opportunist mycobacteria, atypical mycobacteria, anonymous mycobacteria and unclassified mycobacteria. Some of these cause pulmonary lesions indistinguishable from TB, while others involve the lymph nodes, skin or subcutaneous tissues. Superinfection in cystic fibrosis cases is more common NTM are free living organisms that are widespread in nature (Table 49.6).

Based on their rate of growth and pigment production they are divided into four groups.

1. ***Group I—photochromogenic:*** The colonies produce yellow or orange pigment on exposure to light, e.g. *M. kansasii, M. marinum.* These have been described from the USA and European countries.
2. ***Group II—scotochromogenic:*** This group produces yellow orange or reddish pigment in the dark, e.g. *M. scrofulaceum.* It may give rise to cervical lymphadenitis in children.
3. ***Group III—nonchromogenic:*** This group does not produce pigment on exposure to light, e.g. *M. avium-intracellulare, M. ulcerans.*
4. ***Group IV—rapidly growing mycobacteria:*** These organisms grow rapidly at 25°C, e.g. *M. fortuitum, M. chelonae.*

Mycobacterium avium-intracellulare complex consists of two distinct, but closely related mycobacteria.

Mycobacterium avium was described in chickens in 1890 referred to as avium tubercle bacillus. *M. intracellulare* was first cultured in 1969 from the

Table 49.6: Lesions caused by nontuberculous mycobacteria (NTM)

M. marinum (swimming pool bacillus, fish tank bacillus)	Ulceration of skin
M. ulcerans	Extensive ulceration of skin and subcutaneous tissue (Buruli ulcer)
M. kansasii	Pulmonary disease, local abscesses
M. scrofulaceum	Bone and joint lesions, lymphadenopathy
M. chelonae	Pulmonary disease, local abscesses
M. fortuitum	Furunculosis
M. avium	Lymphadenopathy, pulmonary intracellulare lesions, AIDS related and non-AIDS related disseminated lesions

Table 49.7: Choice of drugs for atypical mycobacteria

Name	Drug of choice
Mycobacterium marinum	Trimethoprim sulfamethoxazole, minocycline
M. ulcerans	Rifampicin, clofazimine and others
M. kansasi	Anti-TB drugs such as SM, rifampicin, INH and ethambutol for 3 months. Nonhealing lesions may require surgical excision
M. scrofulaceum	Same as for *M. avium* or rifampicin, clarithromycin and ethambutol
M. cheloni	Four drug regimen including gentamicin, amikacin, erythromycin, SM and ethionamide
M. fortuitum	Treatment as for TB. In resistant cases 3–4 drug combination from clarithromycin, amikacin, doxycycline, imipenem, quinolones or the fourth generation cephalosporins
M. avium intracellulare	Four drug combination as for TB or rifabutin, SM, clarithromycin and ethambutol for 2 years

sputum of TB patients at the Battey state hospital in Rome, Georgia, USA. *M. avium-intracellulare* complex is ubiquitous, isolated from all parts of the world from soil, house dust, fresh water plants, animal foods, bedding, chickens and other birds. *M. avium* complex grows slowly. They are nonphotochromogenic, smooth, cream colored colonies unlike *M. tuberculosis* which produces rough flat dry colonies. In AIDS patients, *M. avium* complex organisms may show plasmid induced virulence and the colonies may be rough.

Treatment

Mycobacterium avium complex are very common pathogens in advanced AIDS and they produce infection and bacteremia. Clarithromycin 500 mg bd oral is an excellent drug to treat *M. avium* complex (Table 49.7).

A three drug combination using rifabutin 600 mg/day, ethambutol 15 mg/kg/bw/day and clarithromycin 1000 mg has been found to be effective in producing resolution of lesions in 70% of cases. Rifabutin produces uveitis in high doses. Adverse effects of clarithromycin include taste perversion and rectal problems. Clarithromycin is effective as prophylactic in AIDS patients with CD4+ below 50/mm^3.

Infection by these bacteria also leads to tuberculin sensitivity. Person-to-person spread of organisms does not generally occur.

In immunocompromised subjects, these mycobacteria cause extensive disseminated lesions. Various regimens based on one or more of the following drugs have given fully or partly successful results. Treatment consists of a combination of a macrolide such as clarithromycin or azithromycin with ethambutol and rifabutin given for six months or longer.

LEPROSY

Syn: Hansen's disease

GENERAL CONSIDERATIONS

Leprosy is a chronic communicable disease caused by *Mycobacterium leprae.* Mainly the nerves and skin are affected but it may also involve mucous membranes and other internal organs. Gerhard Armauer Hansen identified the organism in 1873 and so the disease is named after him. *M. leprae* though considered to be an exclusive human pathogen, has been described as a natural parasite of the ring-banded armadillo in the Unites States from which human infection has occurred.

Source: Truman RW, Singh P, Sharma R, et al. Probable zoonotic leprosy in the southern United States. N Engl J Med. 2011;364(17):1626-33.

Leprosy has been known to affect mankind from biblical times. At present it is common in tropical regions of Asia, Africa, Central and South America. Low standards of living, poverty and overcrowding favor its transmission and prevalence. But the disease is not confined to this group. Persons belonging to all socioeconomic groups may be affected.

By global efforts initiated by WHO, the prevalence and incidence of leprosy has been brought down considerably. Whereas the WHO figures for prevalence of leprosy worldwide was 10–12 million in 1985, it came down to 1.15 million in 1997 with an annual incidence of 5.6 lakhs. During 2009, 2,44,796 new cases were detected globally and 1,33,717 new cases from India. At the beginning of 2010, the global registered and reported point prevalence was 2,11,903 cases. Leprosy has been included under the group of **neglected tropical diseases** and the WHO has taken up reduction of the prevalence of the disease to low levels and eradicate transmission to the extent possible.

The Organism

Mycobacterium leprae is a rod-shaped, gram-positive, AFB varying in size from 1.8 to 2.5 μm in length. It is less acid fast than *M. tuberculosis.* 5% sulfuric acid is used for decolorization and staining by Zeihl-Neelsen method. The bacterial morphology helps in assessing the viability and the effects of drug therapy. Viable bacilli appear as regular rods. Bacilli which appear irregular and granular are probably dead. *M. leprae* is grown experimentally in the foot pads of mice and in the nine-banded armadillo. *M. leprae* multiplies maximally at a temperature of 27–30°C. Consequently, the infection is maximum in the cooler parts of the body, i.e. 34–35°C. The organisms infect the skin, cutaneous nerves, peripheral and autonomic nerves.

Transmission

Portal of entry is through abrasions in the skin or mucous membranes of the upper respiratory tract. Untreated subjects with lepromatous leprosy shed numerous bacilli in nasal discharges and minor abrasions in the skin even before they are clinically detectable. Other possible sources of spread such as insect vectors have also been incriminated but not proved.

The incubation period is ordinarily 2–7 years, but this may vary from a few months to 30 years. The incubation period for paucibacillary leprosy is 2–5 years and for multibacillary is about 5–10 years. Since man has natural immunity against lepra bacilli, lesions do not develop in the majority of cases or they remain subclinical. The clinical disease manifests in 1/350 of those infected with the organisms in endemic areas. Adults are more resistant, but 30% of children living in intimate contact with infective cases develop early lesions. In most of them the lesions heal spontaneously. Chronic progressive disease develops only in about 8% cases. Majority of the patients initially present with the disease within the first three decades of life. In lepromatous leprosy, males are twice more commonly affected than women, but in tuberculoid leprosy such a predilection is not noted.

Irrespective of the virulence of the infecting organism, the clinical outcome is so varied, depending on the immune status of the individual which is the deciding factor in pathogenesis. Both cellular and humoral immune mechanisms operate. The cellular immunity is protective, whereas the humoral antibodies are not. Cell-mediated immunity (CMI) which develops against the lipid components of *M. leprae* determines the progress of the disease. Based on the immune response, a wide clinical spectrum varying from the well-localized tuberculoid leprosy to the generalized lepromatous leprosy may be encountered.

The two polar forms are the lepromatous and tuberculoid types. Borderline leprosy denotes the variable clinical patterns seen in between the two polar forms.

PATHOLOGY

During the early stages of infection, the clinical and histological changes are non-specific. The dermal nerve twigs show infiltration with round cells and histiocytes. *M. leprae* has tropism for laminin 2, a component of Schwann's cells, which are present in peripheral nerves. Mycobacteria may be seen in nerves and muscles of the skin and this is diagnostic. This stage is known as the **indeterminate stage**, since it is not possible to predict the clinical outcome at this stage. The lesion heals due to natural resistance in 75% of cases. In those with progression of lesions tuberculoid lesions develop in the presence of good immunity whereas lepromatous lesions develop in its absence.

Tuberculoid Leprosy

This type is characterized by well-localized granulomatous lesions in and around the nerves. The cells are derived by the mobilization of phagocytic macrophages which are transformed into epithelioid and giant cells. These are surrounded by lymphocytic infiltration. This granuloma extends into the epidermis. The dermal nerves are destroyed by the cellular infiltration. Caseation is rarely seen in the nerves. The bacilli are very few and are not generally demonstrable in these lesions. Such patients are noninfective.

Lepromatous Leprosy

In contrast to tuberculoid leprosy, lepromatous lesions teem with organisms. Mononuclear phagocytes ingest the organisms which multiply within and fill them completely. These bacterial masses are called **globi** and such cells are called **lepra cells**. Their cytoplasm is foamy. Lymphocytes are only a few or absent. There is no attempt at tubercle formation. The dermis is infiltrated throughout its entire thickness. The nerves, arrector pili muscles and endothelial lining of blood vessels also show similar changes. The epidermis is spared and a clear cell-free zone exists below the epidermis. The organisms are disseminated through the bloodstream to other parts of the skin and organs such as eyes, respiratory mucosa, testes, liver, kidneys and muscles of the hands, feet and face. As a late complication, amyloidosis may develop.

Borderline Leprosy

When the immunity is variable, borderline leprosy develops in which the histological picture tends to vary. With good cell-mediated immunity, the picture resembles tuberculoid leprosy and this is called **borderline tuberculoid (BT)**. There is differentiation of mononuclear phagocytes into epithelioid cells, but giant cells are not common. Lymphocytes are usually present but do not show tubercle formation. The subepidermal zone is clear and nerves are infiltrated but are still recognizable. In peripheral neuropathy occurring in leprosy, the nerves are damaged mainly by the cellular reaction to the components of dead bacilli. When the immunity wanes the picture resembles that of lepromatous leprosy and this is called **borderline lepromatous (BL)**.

> **Points to Remember**
> - Infection is spread by nasal droplets.
> - Manifestation depends upon the degree of cell-mediated immunity (CMI). Those with strong CMI develop tuberculoid type and those with poor immunity develop lepromatous type. Borderline lesions develop in those whose immune status is in between.
> - *M. leprae* have a predilection for nerves and dermis.

The lepromin test: The lepromin skin test detects delayed hypersensitivity. It is indicative of the immune status of the individual. It is positive in tuberculoid and negative in lepromatous type. This test was in vogue for diagnosis and prognosis. This is seldom used now.

CLINICAL FEATURES (TABLE 49.8)

Indeterminate Leprosy

The disease starts with a single lesion or a few multiple lesions which appear as small hypopigmented or erythematous macules. Careful testing may reveal hyperesthesia, paresthesia, hypoesthesia or hypoalgesia. At this stage nerve trunks are not thickened. Slit skin smears are usually negative for AFB. Lepromin reaction may be negative or doubtfully positive. Evolution into the polar forms takes a long-time after infection. In the early stage, which is known as indeterminate leprosy, the distinctive features are absent. Though diagnosis is possible, it is difficult to predict the clinical outcome and the type.

Tuberculoid Leprosy (TL)

In this form the skin lesions are only a few (3 or less) and they vary in size. They are hypopigmented or erythematous and the margins are well-defined. The lesions may be flat or raised. Either the entire lesion or only the margins may be elevated. The surface is dry, rough and anhidrotic. By this time the temperature and pain sensations are impaired. Nerve trunks, especially in the vicinity of the raised lesions, are palpably thickened. Supraorbital and great auricular nerves in the head and neck, ulnar, cutaneous branch of radial, the main radial and median nerve in the upper limb and lateral popliteal (common peroneal), posterior tibial, musculocutaneous and sural nerve in the lower limbs are the common nerves palpated. Facial palsy manifesting over parts of the face either on one or both sides may develop. Slit skin smear does not show AFB and lepromin test is positive. Early lesions may heal spontaneously without complications. More advanced lesions also heal ultimately, but residual damage to nerves may occur due to reactions, which complicate the illness (Figs 49.6 to 49.9).

Lepromatous Leprosy (LL)

In this form the bacilli spread rapidly from the skin, both by local extension and through the bloodstream, to other parts of the body. Extensive involvement of nerves, mucosa of the upper respiratory tract and the internal organs occurs. Eyes, testes, lymph nodes, marrow of the phalanges, superficially placed muscles, liver, spleen and kidney may all be affected in varying degrees.

The morphology of the skin lesions depends upon the stage of the disease. Early lesions are flat, smooth, shiny, hypopigmented or coppery red, with ill-defined margins (Fig. 49.10). Numerous small lesions are distributed symmetrically. The entire body surface may be involved except certain areas like the axilla, groin and the flexor aspects of the limbs. In dark subjects they may be inconspicuous and can be made out only by careful search. Early lesions do not show sensory loss. As the disease progresses, papules and nodules appear especially on the ears and face (Fig. 49.11). The eyebrows are lost. The face is described as leonine and this is caused by infiltration and thickening of skin of the face. The mucosal lesion leads to ulceration of the nose, mouth, trachea

Table 49.8: Salient features of the major clinical types of leprosy			
	Tuberculoid leprosy	*Borderline leprosy*	*Lepromatous leprosy*
Number of lesions	Few (<5)	Some	Many
Lesions borders	Well-defined	Less well-defined	Rough and elevated
Sensory impairment	Marked	Moderate	Variable
Distribution of skin lesions	Asymmetrical	Asymmetrical	Generally symmetrical
Peripheral nerves	Thickened	Normal/just thickened	Normal
Type of leprosy	Paucibacillary	Intermediate multibacillary	Multibacillary
Slit skin smear for acid-fast bacilli	–/1+	2+/3+	4+ and above

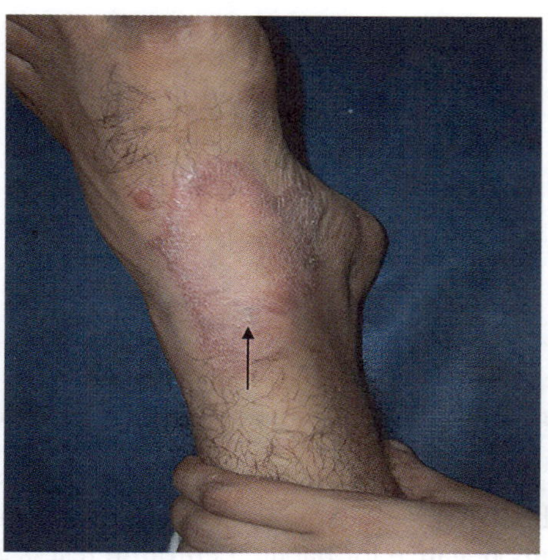

Fig. 49.6: Hansen's disease—borderline tuberculoid. ***Note:*** The raised plaque (arrow)

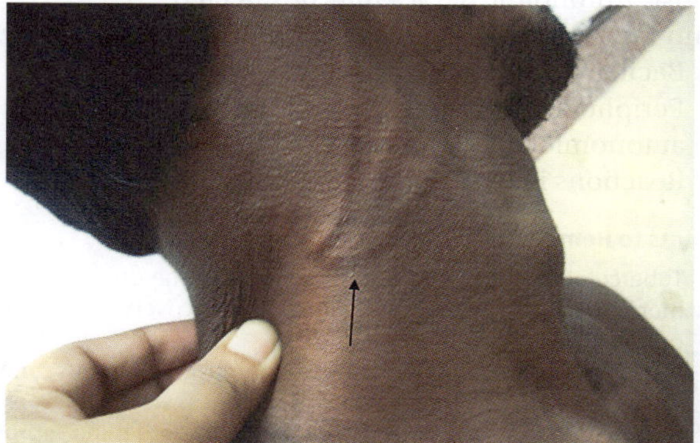

Fig. 49.7: Nerve thickening in tuberculoid leprosy great auricular nerves (arrow)

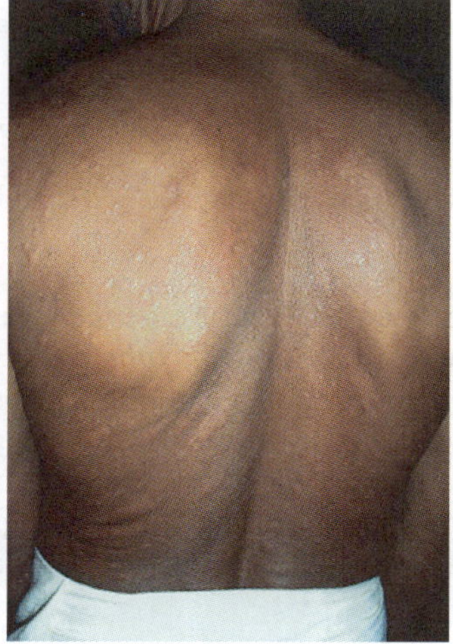

Fig. 49.10: Hansen's disease—lepromatous leprosy

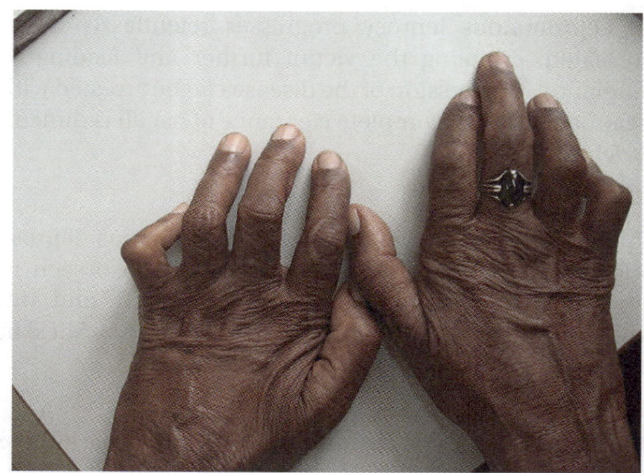

Fig. 49.8: Ulnar palsy and muscle wasting in late stages of Hansen's disease (neurotic type)

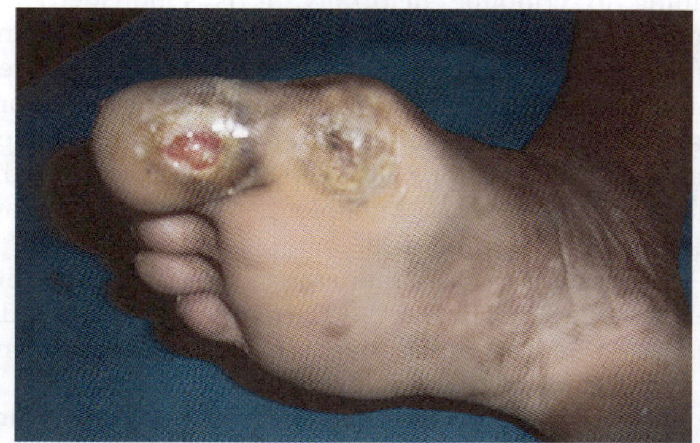

Fig. 49.9: Plantar ulcer in Hansen's disease late stages of peripheral neuropathy

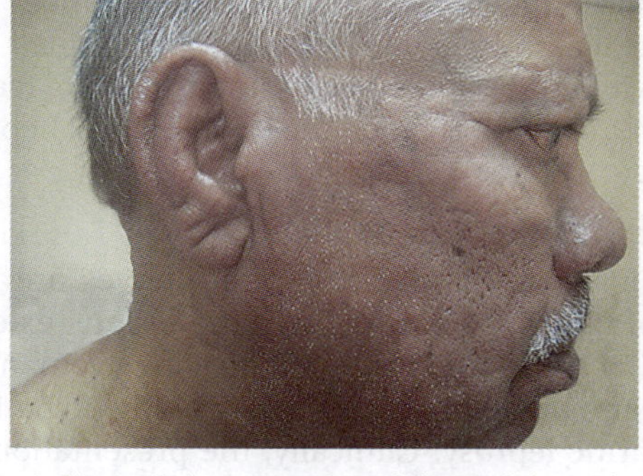

Fig. 49.11: Infiltrated plaques and ear lobe nodules in lepromatous leprosy

and larynx. Nasal discharge teems with the bacilli. Nasal bones may be destroyed resulting in deformity of the nose. Involvement of the premaxilla leads to loss of the upper incisors.

Clinical evidence of nerve damage occurs late in lepromatous leprosy. The nerve trunks are symmetrically enlarged and soft to feel. Dorsal aspects of the forearms and legs show anesthesia and anhidrosis. Gradually anesthesia spreads over the whole body except the palms, soles, axillae and groins. Motor weakness follows further nerve damage. Tendon reflexes are preserved till late stages. Paradoxically, the wasted muscles may be hyper-reflexic. In addition to neural damage, muscular dysfunction may result from direct invasion of the muscles by the bacilli. Affection of the testes gives rise to impotence and enlargement of the breasts.

Ocular involvement may occur by extension from the skin or by hematogenous spread. Common lesions include miliary lepromata on the iris and superficial punctate keratitis. All parts of the eye except the retina may be affected.

Lepromatous leprosy progresses relentlessly if left untreated, crippling the victim further and leading to mutilation. Progression of the disease can be arrested with treatment, though complete clearance of bacilli is difficult to achieve.

Lucio Leprosy

This is a special type of diffuse lepromatous leprosy originally described from Mexico, but it is also seen in other areas. The whole skin becomes smooth and stiff with loss of body hair, especially on the eyebrows. Slit skin smears are always positive for the organisms.

Borderline Leprosy

Borderline leprosy is immunologically unstable. There is a tendency to move towards tuberculoid spectrum if the immunity improves or may downgrade to lepromatous spectrum. Nerve damage is more common leading to crippling deformity. It is subdivided into borderline tuberculoid (BT), mid borderline (BB) and borderline lepromatous (BL), based on clinical features, bacteriological index and lepromin test. Skin lesions are usually hypopigmented or erythematous. Macules, plaques, annular lesions and punched out lesions are the characteristic features. Multiple peripheral nerves are thickened but asymmetrical.

Skin lesions are less numerous, dry with partly well-defined edges in BT (Fig. 49.12). Hair growth is markedly decreased. Sensory impairment is more marked. AFB is nil or scanty in lesions. Lepromin is weakly positive.

In BL, the lesions are smaller, more numerous, shiny and smooth with ill-defined edges. Sensory impairment is slight. Hair growth in lesions is slightly diminished. Many AFB are detected in lesions. AFB in nasal scrapings are not seen in borderline leprosy. Lepromin is negative.

Large bizarre geographic lesions and small satellite lesions with moderate sensory impairment are features of BB (Fig. 49.13). AFB is moderate in BB lesions. Lepromin is negative.

Pure Neuritic Leprosy

Though in all forms of leprosy the nerves are the first targets of attack, sooner or later the lesions extend into the skin. In some patients only nerve involvement is seen without any perceptible skin lesions. This form is called pure neuritic leprosy. Clinically, the presentation is with the affection of single or multiple large nerve trunks. The

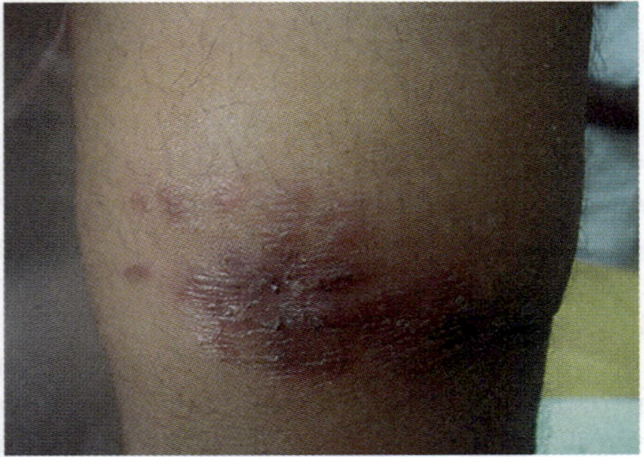

Fig. 49.12: Hansen's disease BT—partly well-defined plaques on upper limb

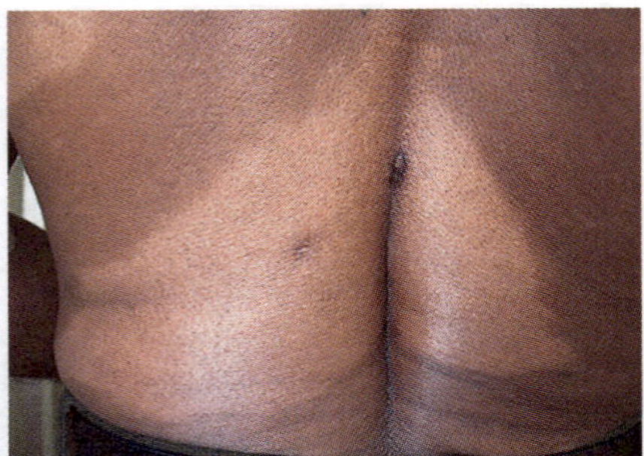

Fig. 49.13: Hansen's disease-mid borderline. ***Note:*** Bizarre lesions

nerves are enlarged, firm and tender. Both sensory and motor abnormalities are demonstrable. The affected parts are usually negative for bacilli. Lepromin test is generally positive but it may be doubtful or negative in some. Definite diagnosis of this stage can be made only by nerve biopsy. Autonomic nerves may be affected.

Main causes of tissue damage in leprosy:

- Bacillary infiltration—lepromatous leprosy
- Peripheral neuritis—loss of sensory, motor and autonomic functions
- Reactions in leprosy.

> **Points to Remember**
>
> - Tuberculoid spectrum—lesions are less numerous, drier and more anesthetic with well-defined borders. Nerve thickening occurs in early stages.
> - Lepromatous spectrum—lesions are more numerous, more shiny and less anesthetic and vague edges. Nerve thickening occurs in late stages. If downgraded from borderline leprosy, nerve thickening may be present earlier.
> - Indeterminate type—the CMI is not determined and the patient can go to any spectrum. Lesion is always macular.
> - Nasal symptoms (stuffiness, crusting, blood-stained discharge) and edema of legs are the earliest manifestations of LL.
> - Skin, nerves, mucous membranes, bones, testes, eyes, kidneys, muscles and lymph nodes can be involved in LL.
> - Diagnosis is clinical and by demonstration of *M. leprae* by slit skin smears.
> - Treatment is with rifampicin, dapsone and clofazimine.

Leprosy and HIV Infection

Interaction between HIV and *M. leprae* is far more subtle than that between HIV and *M. tuberculosis*. There is no increase in HIV prevalence among leprosy cases and no alteration in clinical spectrum of leprosy among co-infected patients. Type 1 reactions occur more often in co-infected patients. They respond equally well to multidrug therapy (MDT) and have similar side effect profiles.

REACTIONS IN LEPROSY (LEPRA REACTION)

Episodes of acute inflammation called 'reactions' occur during the course of leprosy. In some patients occurrence of a reaction may be the precipitating event to seek medical help. Immune reactions may be caused either by delayed hypersensitivity (***Jopling type 1 reactions***) or to the formation of antigen antibody complexes (***Jopling type 2 reactions, erythema nodosum leprosum***).

Type 1 reaction occurs in patients with borderline leprosy cases. There is a sudden change in cellular hypersensitivity. These reactions may be spontaneous or precipitated by therapy occurring within six months.

Existing lesions increase in size and severity and may become erythematous, edematous and tender. New lesions may develop. The nerves become swollen, painful and tender and nerve abscesses may form. The neurological deficit may increase. Edema of feet, hands and face may occur. Constitutional symptoms like fever are rare.

Type 2 reaction is caused by vasculitis resulting from the deposition of immune complexes, without a shift along the immunological spectrum. This type of reaction is seen in about one-half of the patients with lepromatous leprosy and one-fourth with borderline leprosy. Commonly this reaction occurs during the second year of treatment. These reactions may be associated with the appearance of tender erythematous nodules, which are called ***erythema nodosum leprosum (ENL)***. Type 2 reactions are characterized by general inflammatory phenomena such as fever, rigor, pain and tenderness in the skin and nerves, arthritis, lymphadenopathy, iritis and keratitis. Further damage to nerves and eyes may develop and repeated reactions aggravate the disability.

Lucio Phenomenon

This is a severe form of type 2 reaction occurring in lucio leprosy. It is characterized by the formation of erythematous macules which become purpuric or ulcerated. Later they heal with atrophic scarring.

DIAGNOSIS

The diagnosis of leprosy is based on clinical signs and symptoms. A case of leprosy is defined as a person having one or more of the following features and who has yet to complete a full course of treatment.

- Hypopigmented or reddish skin lesion(s) with definite loss of sensation.
- Involvement of the peripheral nerves, as demonstrated by definite thickening with loss of sensation and/or weakness of the muscles supplied by that nerve.
- Demonstration of AFB in skin lesions by standard slit skin smears or histological diagnosis of granuloma affecting the nerves.

Demonstration of M. leprae in the skin is by preparing a slit skin smear from the ear lobe or other areas by scraping the subepidermal tissue through a small incision. The material is stained by modified Zeihl-Neelsen method. The disease should not be diagnosed if only nerve thickening is present, without any other accompanying symptoms or signs.

Quantitative estimation of the bacterial count is obtained by noting the density of the bacilli in the smear which is recorded as the ***bacterial index***. Presence of many clumps of bacilli in an average field is recorded as 6+ whereas presence of 1 to 10 bacilli in hundred fields is recorded as 1+. In addition, the morphology of the bacilli enables the observer to assess their viability. This ***morphological index*** is used for recording progress with treatment. Nasal mucosa shows organisms and nasal smears give an idea of the infectivity of the patient. In borderline leprosy, *M. leprae* are scanty and in tuberculoid leprosy, they are not present in skin smears.

None of the cardinal diagnostic criteria like sensory changes, thickened nerves or organisms may be present in indeterminate leprosy. A high index of suspicion and familiarity with the early signs and symptoms are the only factors which help to diagnose this stage. Diagnosis has to be confirmed by the demonstration of *M. leprae* inside nerves or erector pili muscle.

Differential Diagnosis of Skin Lesions

Many other common skin conditions give rise to macular lesions. These are pityriasis alba, tinea versicolor, nutritional dyschromias, birth marks and early vitiligo. Raised lesions or plaques have to be differentiated from fungus infections, cutaneous TB, lupus erythematosus and lichen simplex. Psoriasis and lichen planus do not give rise to problems in diagnosis due to their distinctive features. Post kala-azar dermal leishmaniasis has to be distinguished from lepromatous leprosy. Reaction in leprosy may be mistaken for other forms of vasculitis as in systemic lupus erythematosus (SLE) or polyarteritis nodosa. Other conditions that produce localized sensory loss are entrapment neuropathies and injury to peripheral nerves. Rarely nerves may be thickened, in hypertrophic polyneuritis, Refsum's disease, amyloidosis and traumatic neuromas.

MANAGEMENT

The clinical diagnosis of leprosy should always be confirmed by the laboratory tests, before starting treatment, in view of the socioeconomic and psychological implications. The lepromin test is seldom done for clinical purposes because clinical differentiation along with bacteriological and histological diagnosis is quite satisfactory for management. Education of the patient on the nature of the disease, outcome of treatment and measures to avoid spread is absolutely essential for success.

General Treatment

This includes measures to improve general health and treatment of intercurrent illness.

Chemotherapy

At present, six effective antileprosy drugs are available. Among these, dapsone, rifampicin and clofazimine are used in standard regimens. The others which are used in special situations include minocycline, ofloxacin and clarithromycin. Newer drugs include moxifloxacin, a fluoroquinolone and rifapentine. Moxifloxacin 400 mg once daily is found to be more potent than these drugs. Rifapentine, a semisynthetic derivative of rifamycin is more bactericidal than rifampicin. None of these should be used as monotherapy.

Dapsone: The time honored and basic drug for the treatment is dapsone. The drug is inexpensive and relatively nontoxic in the doses used. Delayed hypersensitivity reactions and less commonly agranulocytosis have been reported. Mild hemolytic anemia is common, but severe anemia is rare except in glucose 6 phosphate dehydrogenase (G6PD) deficiency. This suggests that the rifampicin-resistant mutants in an untreated patient with LL are likely to be eliminated by 3–6 months of treatment with dapsone-clofazimine component of

Textbook of Medicine

the standard. ***Dapsone syndrome*** is a rare but severe form of hypersensitivity reaction to dapsone. It usually manifests within 4–6 weeks after initiation of therapy and is characterized by fever, generalized exanthematous rash, lymphadenopathy, hepatitis, jaundice, leukopenia, eosinophilia and mononucleosis. Genetic factors play an important role in drug induced hypersensitivity reactions. Recent studies have shown that carriers of the HLA-B 13:01 allele are at high risk of developing dapsone syndrome.

The drug is cumulative in the system. Dapsone is weakly bactericidal in a dose of 100 mg daily. Dapsone combined with clofazimine kills more than 99.999% of *M. leprae* within 3 MDT regimen.

Rifampicin: Rifampicin is the most powerful bactericidal drug against *M. leprae* and three monthly doses of 600 mg kills 99.999% of viable *M. leprae*. It is relatively nontoxic, although occasional cases of renal failure, thrombocytopenia, influenza-like syndrome and hepatitis have been reported.

Clofazimine: It is bacteriostatic when given in a dose of 50 mg a day. It has also got anti-inflammatory properties in high doses. Pigmentation of the skin is common but it clears completely after treatment is discontinued. Higher doses may cause gastrointestinal symptoms.

Though most of the patients are rendered non-infectious within a few weeks, clinical improvement may not be apparent for several months. Complete resolution may take a few years.

> **Clinical Classification for Control Programs**
>
> The eighth report of WHO expert committee concluded that patients could be classified into two groups, if skin smears are not available.
> 1. Paucibacillary (PB) leprosy (1–5 skin lesions)
> 2. Multibacillary (MB) leprosy (6 or more skin lesions)
>
> When classification is in doubt, the patient should be treated as having MB leprosy. All smear positive cases should be treated as MB leprosy.

Standard MDT Regimens (eighth report of the WHO expert committee on leprosy-2010)

PB cases (for adults)
Rifampicin 600 mg once a month (supervised)
Dapsone 100 mg daily (self-administered)
Duration—6 months

MB cases (for adults)
Rifampicin 600 mg once a month (supervised)
Dapsone 100 mg daily (self-administered)
Clofazimine 300 mg once a month (supervised and 50 mg daily self-administered)
Duration—12 months

PB cases (for children)
Rifampicin 450 mg once a month (supervised)
Dapsone 50 mg daily
Duration—6 months

MB cases (for children)
Rifampicin 450 mg once a month (supervised)
Dapsone 50 daily
Clofazimine 150 mg once a month (supervised and 50 mg on alternate days)
Duration—12 months.

Children below 10 years of age
Rifampicin 10 mg/kg monthly
Dapsone 2 mg/kg/day
Clofazimine 1 mg/kg (alternate days).

MB patients should complete 12 months doses within a period of 18 months and PB patients, 6 monthly doses within 9 months period. Patients should receive their drugs in monthly, calendar blister packs. WHO operational guidelines recommend to continue treatment for more than 12 months in MB patients with a high bacteriological index.

A patient who relapses should be treated with a further course of MDT. A defaulter is a patient who started MDT but who has not received treatment for 12 months. If such a patient returns to the health center for treatment and shows signs of active disease, he should be given a new course of MDT. In the absence of activity, there is no need to restart MDT and the patient should be educated to report promptly on the appearance of any of these signs. Patients should be actively followed for a minimum period of 8 years after completion of treatment.

Alternative MDT Regimens

- For patients who do not tolerate clofazimine, ofloxacin 400 mg (O) or minocycline 100 mg (M) could be used as substitutes for clofazimine for 12 months. An alternative regimen is to give monthly doses of ROM for 24 months.
- No modification of regimen is required for MB leprosy. For PB leprosy, clofazimine is substituted for dapsone in the standard PB regimen for 6 months.

Treatment of Reactions

Reactions with neuritis should be treated with prednisolone, 1 mg/kg bw for 12 weeks. The patients harboring rifampicin resistant *M. leprae* are very often resistant to dapsone and their treatment depends on clofazimine. The recommended regimen for adults (MB cases) is daily administration of 50 mg of clofazimine together with ofloxacin 400 mg and minocycline 100 mg for 6 months. For at least an additional 18 months, clofazimine with either minocycline or ofloxacin should be administered. Moxifloxacin can be used instead of ofloxacin, if available.

Because of the high risk of permanent damage to the peripheral nerve trunks, ***Type 1 reaction*** (reversal reaction) needs to be diagnosed as soon as possible and treated adequately. Prednisolone is the drug of choice. To begin with, 40–60 mg of prednisolone is given daily and gradually tapered (over 12 weeks) weekly or fortnightly and eventually stopped.

Type 2 reactions vary in severity, duration and organ involvement. Mild erythema nodosum leprosum (ENL) can be treated with analgesic or antipyretic drugs such as aspirin, while severe lenalidomide, 100 mg three to four times daily is also effective for the treatment of severe ENL. It should be used only in male or postmenopausal female patients who have become dependent on corticosteroids and must be given only under close medical supervision.

Clofazimine in a dose of 300 mg daily in divided doses is also effective for ENL but is less potent than corticosteroids and often takes 4–6 weeks to develop its full effects. So it should never be started as the sole agent for the treatment of severe ENL. Clofazimine is started at a dose of 100 mg tid for 12 weeks, then tapered to 100 mg bd for 12 weeks and then 100 mg od for 12–24 weeks. The total duration of high dose clofazimine therapy should not exceed 12 months. If a patient develops type 2 reaction while on treatment, the standard treatment should be continued. If type 2 reaction occurs after MDT is completed, should not restart MDT.

Other Measures

Splinting and physiotherapy help to prevent nerve damage and its sequelae. Care of hands and feet, protective footwear, physiotherapy and rehabilitation are integral parts of patient care in subjects with sensory loss.

PREVENTION AND CONTROL

All studies have shown protection against MB and PB disease with primary BCG vaccination, which can last for decades. BCG is very widely used around the world and has contributed substantially to global leprosy reduction. Some countries recommend a repeat BCG vaccination. The reliable way to control the spread of leprosy in contacts is regular 6 monthly examinations. Close contacts with high risk of transmission can be given chemoprophylaxis with 15 mg/kg rifampicin once a month for 6 months.

Early diagnosis and treatment are the sure ways to arrest the disease, prevent spread and avoid disability. Educating the public, increasing the awareness of the problem and eliminating the social stigma through propaganda have helped to implement mass programs and prevent spread.

The global target for elimination of leprosy as a public health problem, set by world health assembly resolution in 1991 was defined as reducing the prevalence to below 1 per 10,000 population at the global level by the year 2000. Diagnosis and treatment was simplified using MDT blister packs, made available to all new patients free of cost. The result was a dramatic reduction in the prevalence of > 90% and the global target was reached by the end of the year 2000.

Rehabilitation of the disabled patient is to be undertaken along with curative measures. This includes surgical correction of deformities, plastic surgery especially of the hand to make the hands more functional, avoidance of burn injuries to hands and feet, protection of the eyes from exposure keratitis and other community measures needed to ensure social rehabilitation.

The National Leprosy Control Program: This was launched in India in 1955. This program emphasized the need for health education. Centers were established for survey, education and training (SET centers) in areas of high endemicity for early detection and mass treatment. In addition, training and research centers for leprosy were established at different parts of the country. This program was redesignated ***National Leprosy Eradication Program (NLEP)*** in 1982. More than 250 nongovernmental organizations are active in India working for prevention of leprosy and offering other services to the victims.

CHAPTER
50

Chlamydial Respiratory Infections: Psittacosis and Primary Atypical Pneumonia

KV Krishna Das

Chapter Summary

- Spectrum of Human Diseases caused by Chlamydiae
- Psittacosis
  - Epidemiology
  - Pathology
  - Clinical Features
  - Diagnosis
  - Treatment
  - Control
- Primary Atypical Pneumonia (Community Acquired Pneumonia)
  - Clinical Picture
  - Diagnosis
  - Treatment

SPECTRUM OF HUMAN DISEASES CAUSED BY CHLAMYDIA

	Acute lesions	*Chronic lesions*
Chlamydia trachomatis		
Serovar A to C	Conjunctivitis	Trachoma
Serovar D to K	Urethritis	Proctitis, pelvic inflammatory disease, urethritis, Reiter's syndrome, tubal obstruction epididymo-orchitis
LGV serovars	Lymphogranuloma venereum	Multiple sinuses esthiomene

Textbook of Medicine

C. pneumoniae	Pharyngitis, sinusitis, bronchitis, community acquired pneumonia	Atherosclerosis asthma
C. psittaci derived from parrots, canaries, pigeons, turkeys, ducks, chickens, cats, ewes	Atypical pneumonia, hepatic and renal dysfunction, endocarditis, conjunctivitis abortion	

PSITTACOSIS

Syn: Parrot fever

Definition: Psittacosis is an infectious disease caused by the organism *Chlamydia psittaci* which is a primary pathogen of birds. *Chlamydia psittaci* is a gram-negative obligate intracellular parasite.

Epidemiology

The disease is present all over the world. Psittacine birds (parrots, parakeets and cockattoos) are commonly affected, but all types of birds may suffer. Infection in man results from close contact with birds. The organism is present in the feces of infected birds. Humans acquire the infection by inhalation of bird's feces or handling the tissues of infected birds.

Pathology

Chlamydia psittaci reaches the pulmonary alveoli and the reticuloendothelial cells of the spleen and the liver. In the lung, patchy consolidation develops. Liver and spleen are enlarged due to congestion. The heart, meninges and the brain also show congestion. The alveolar exudate is mainly mononuclear.

Clinical Features

The average incubation period is about ten days. The onset is sudden with fever, malaise, sore throat and intense photophobia. Temperature ranges from 37 to 39°C. There is relative bradycardia. Tachypnea may occur. There may be cough with scanty mucopurulent sputum. Signs of pulmonary consolidation may be evident. After about 10 days of fever the temperature comes down by lysis. Mortality may reach 20%. Respiratory failure and toxemia are the usual causes of death.

Diagnosis

Psittacosis has to be differentiated from viral pneumonia, typhoid fever, influenza and Q fever. History of contact with birds is the most helpful clue to diagnosis.

In the first few days of the illness the organisms can be isolated from the sputum and blood by inoculation into mice or into the yolk sac of embryonated eggs or into irradiated cell cultures. Diagnosis can be established by demonstrating antibodies by enzyme linked immunosorbent assay (ELISA) or microimmunofluorescence.

Treatment

Doxycycline 100 po bd up to 3 weeks is effective in most cases. Erythromycin given 500 mg qid oral for 1–2 weeks is a suitable alternative.

Control

Quarantine of birds imported from other countries should be insisted upon and the infected birds should be killed. Carrier state among the birds is reduced by incorporating tetracycline in bird feeds.

PRIMARY ATYPICAL PNEUMONIA (COMMUNITY ACQUIRED PNEUMONIA)

Clinical Picture

In addition to sexually transmitted diseases (STD), psittacosis and trachoma, the role of chlamydia in community acquired pneumonia has come to the forefront. In many areas, 10–20% of community acquired pneumonias are due to *Chlamidophile pneumoniae*. The widespread prevalence of this organism in nature is evident from the presence of the antibody in 50–75% of the population. In women, 5–20% may be harboring chlamydia in the uterine cervix and this may pass on to the neonate during birth. Neonates may develop conjunctivitis, upper respiratory lesions such as naso-pharyngitis or even pneumonia.

Pneumonia caused by chlamydia is the cause of atypical pneumonia similar to mycoplasma pneumoniae or legionella. The infection is by inhalation. Incubation period is 3–4 weeks, upper respiratory symptoms, fever, cough, with expectoration and skin rashes may develop. In patients with chronic obstructive lung disease chlamydial infection leads to exacerbation.

The **clinical picture** is mild to moderate pulmonary symptoms, if untreated, resolution occurs only slowly taking 2–3 months.

Diagnosis

It can be established by demonstrating specific DNA in nasorespiratory secretions or sputum by polymerase chain reaction (PCR) techniques. Antibodies are produced slowly over 4–6 weeks, immunoglobulin M (IgM) during acute phase and IgG in the later phase.

Treatment

Doxycycline 100 mg bd oral for 10–14 days is effective. Macrolides like azithromycin are also effective.

Viral Infections

KV Krishna Das, R Sajith Kumar

Chapter Summary

- General Considerations
  - Viral Multiplication
  - Viral Spread
  - Interferons
- Laboratory Diagnosis
- Prevention of Viral Diseases

GENERAL CONSIDERATIONS

Most of the viruses are not visible under light microscope. They vary in size from 300 to 20 nm. Each virus contains a nucleic acid molecule with either ribonucleic acid (RNA) or deoxyribonucleic acid (DNA) as its genome. A complete viral particle which contains the genetic material (genome) and the surrounding protective coat which serves as vehicle for its transmission from one cell to another is called *virion*. Viruses lack enzymes required for the synthesis of their components and for energy metabolism. They are therefore, dependent on the metabolic pathways and components of their host cells. They are obligate intracellular parasites. They cause lesions in several living organism such as animals, insects, plants and bacteria. Many viruses may live in their host cells without producing disease but some are pathogenic.

Of late many viruses which have not been commonly affecting humans have come into the picture of severe infective agents with high mortality. Among these important ones are: Non-polio enteroviruses, variants of influenza virus which cause severe acute respiratory syndrome such as influenza group A, H_5N_1 virus, H_1N_1 influenza virus, coronaviruses, Nipah virus, human metapneumovirus, betacoronavirus of Middle East respiratory syndrome (MERS), outbreaks of Ebola virus and several others. As it stands at present viral diseases seem to overtake the incidence of bacterial diseases numerically and in severity. For many of them specific treatment or vaccination are still not available.

Viral Multiplication

Multiplication of viruses is controlled by the genetic information contained in the viral nucleic acid. Viral multiplication involves six sequential steps. These are: (1) adsorption to the host cell, (2) entry to the cell, (3) release of viral nucleic acid into the cell contents, (4) biosynthesis of viral components, (5) maturation of the virus particles and (6) release of numerous virus particles from the host cell.

Viral infection causes demonstrable changes in the host cell such as cytolysis and destruction of the cell. Sometimes the virus may become latent and persist within the cell to be reactivated later. Incorporation of viral nucleic acid into the genome of the host cell may result in malignant transformation. Several cells may fuse together to form giant cells. In the central nervous system (CNS) demyelination may occur. Many tissues infected by virus show inclusion bodies within the cytoplasm or the nucleus. These are made up of aggregates of virion at the site of synthesis or these may merely represent products of degeneration caused by virus infection.

Viral Spread

The mechanism of transmission and portal of entry of viruses vary.

Common Routes of Entry

- Respiratory tract, e.g. coryza, influenza, measles and smallpox
- Alimentary tract, e.g. enteroviruses and hepatitis A and E
- Abrasions or wounds on the skin which may be due to animal bites (rabies), arthropod vectors (arboviruses), injection (virus B hepatitis) or abrasions of skin (papillomavirus)
- Intact conjunctiva (adenovirus and measles)
- From mother to fetus through the placenta [rubella cytomegalovirus, human immunodeficiency virus (HIV)]
- From the genital tract, during birth (herpes simplex virus type II, HIV)
- Sexual transmission, e.g. HIV, hepatitis B virus (HBV) and hepatitis C virus (HCV), hepatitis D virus (HDV), human papillomavirus (HPV), Epstein–Barr virus (EBV) and herpes viruses.

The outcome of infection by a virus depends on its virulence and the resistance of the host. The effects on the host may be divided into specific and nonspecific. *Specific* response is the production of immunity, while the *nonspecific* response includes fever and production of interferons. Both humoural and cellular immune responses play their roles in viral infections.

Proteins of the viral capsid stimulate the formation of humoral antibodies which neutralize the virus. They also cause complement mediated lysis of the infected host cells. Although in many cases the antibodies are protective, sometimes these are harmful, causing immune complex type of tissue injury to the renal glomeruli, synovia of joints or the skin. Immunoglobulin A (IgA) antibodies secreted into the respiratory tract protect against infection by other respiratory viruses. Humoral immunity is vital for recovery from many viral infections, e.g. enterovirus infections. Some viruses like herpes, rubeola and proline oxidase (POX) stimulate cell-mediated immunity which plays the major role in defense. Post infective autoimmune

Textbook of Medicine

phenomenon can occur following many viral infections and immunizations.

Some viral infections can be associated with chronic infections characterized by varying asymptomatic periods which may continue indefinitely or be followed by clinical manifestations, e.g. hepatitis B and C, HIV. Some viruses can remain dormant, usually in the nuclei and become reactivated in between when immunity is compromised transiently, e.g. varicella-zoster, herpes simplex, cytomegalovirus (CMV).

Interferons

Interferons are protein substances produced by the host cells in the early phase of infection. Other stimuli also may stimulate the production of interferons and hence, this response is not strictly specific. Interferon protects the cell against the virus by interfering with the translation of viral messenger and thereby inhibiting viral multiplication. The interferons are not virus specific, but they show species specificity. Only interferons produced in human or primate cells have protective effect against human infections. Viruses show variation in their susceptibility to interferons. Interferons exert their protective role even before humoral antibodies develop. At present interferons are produced commercially by DNA technology.

LABORATORY DIAGNOSIS

- *Isolation of the organism:* Viruses can be isolated by inoculating material removed from the subject at the optimum time, into suitable cell systems like tissue culture media, chick embryos or experimental animals. Specimens include throat swabs, sputum, rectal swabs, blood, urine, cerebrospinal fluid (CSF) or vesicle fluid. Since the virus is present in the host in the early part of illness, specimens have to be collected early to isolate the organism. They have to be transported in sterile screw-capped bottles containing Hank's balanced salt solution. Such specimens can be stored at –70°C without affecting the viability of the virus. These methods are mainly used for research purposes at present.
- *Demonstration of viral inclusions, viruses and viral antigens:* Viral infection used to be diagnosed by the demonstration of inclusion bodies under light microscopy, e.g. rabies and smallpox. Some viruses can be identified by electron microscopy, e.g. rotavirus in feces. The presence of viruses or viral antigens in tissues can be demonstrated by immunofluorescence, immunodiffusion, immuno-electron microscopy, radioimmunoassay, counter current immunoelectrophoresis and enzyme-linked immunosorbent assay (ELISA) techniques. These methods are being employed increasingly when viral isolation is difficult or impossible.

- *Polymerase chain reaction (PCR) and other techniques* employed in molecular biology are widely employed to make specific diagnosis. Apart from identifying the virus, these methods also help to quantitate the viral load.
- *Antibodies against viruses:* These can be demonstrated in the serum of the patient. Paired samples of sera are collected, the first sample in the acute phase and the second sample after an interval of 12–14 days. Humoral antibodies can be demonstrated by techniques such as virus neutralization, complement fixation, hemagglutination inhibition, indirect hemagglutination, immunofluorescence, radioimmunoassay and ELISA. In the acute phase, IgM antibodies are formed, which give place to IgG antibodies as the infection becomes chronic or with the passage of time.

The diagnosis of the viral infection can be confirmed by isolating the virus and demonstrating a four-fold increase in the specific antibody titers in paired samples of serum. However, a negative serology does not exclude the diagnosis of a viral infection. In the epidemic periods, specific diagnosis need not be insisted on every case. Cross reacting antibodies can produce false positive results also.

PREVENTION OF VIRAL DISEASES

Active Immunization

At present, protection against many viral infections is possible by specific immunization. Live vaccines or inactivated vaccines are used for this purpose. Live vaccines are used in the cases of poliomyelitis (Sabin's oral vaccine), yellow fever, varicella, rotavirus, measles, mumps and rubella. Killed virus vaccines are used for prevention of rabies (human diploid cell vaccine and duck embryo vaccine), poliomyelitis (Salk vaccine), Japanese encephalitis and several others. Recombinant antigens are used in viral hepatitis B. The vaccines may be related to different changing strains like influenza vaccine, whose composition is changed every year depending on the prevalent strain. In virus infections where multiple subtypes are involved, as in Dengue fever, polyvalent vaccines are used.

Passive immunization against diseases such as varicella, measles, mumps, rabies and infective hepatitis can be conferred by the use of human disease specific gammaglobulin or convalescent sera, early during the incubation period. In many such instances, combined active and passive immunization is also advised, e.g. rabies. Hyperimmune serum, which gives better protection, is used for the prevention of rabies.

Specific identification of the viral infection is important since specific methods for prevention and specific antiviral drugs are available against many viruses.

CHAPTER 52

Viral Infections of the Respiratory Tract
Coryza, Influenza, Parainfluenza, RSV, SARS, Nipah Virus, Human Metapneumovirus

R Sajith Kumar, KV Krishna Das

Chapter Summary

- Coryza
- Influenza
- Avian Flu
- Parainfluenza
- Respiratory Syncytial Virus (RSV) Infection
- Severe Acute Respiratory Syndrome (SARS)
- Other Paramyxoviruses
  - Nipah Virus
  - Human Metapneumovirus
- Middle East Respiratory Syndrome (MERS)

CORYZA

Several viruses cause the clinical picture of coryza. Of these, rhinoviruses are the most important and common. The disease spreads by droplet infection and the portal of entry is the upper respiratory tract. Epidemics occur in early autumn, mid-winter and spring. Incubation period varies from a few hours to 3–4 days. Hyperemia and edema of the mucosa of the nose and rhinopharynx are the early lesions. Copious amounts of watery fluid rich in glycoproteins exude. After a short course, the disease spontaneously subsides completely without any residual damage.

Clinical Features

Onset is abrupt with headache, nasal congestion and obstruction. It is followed by sneezing and watery discharge from the nose, which becomes mucopurulent and tenacious later on. Mild fever (37.5–38°C) and muscle pains set in within a few hours. The whole course lasts for 2–3 days. Coryza predisposes to the development of secondary bacterial infection. Physical examination is negative except for nasal congestion, conjunctival injection and pharyngitis. Complications are sinusitis, infection of the lower respiratory tract and otitis media.

Diagnosis

Clinical diagnosis is easy. Secondary bacterial infection should be looked for. Coryza has to be distinguished from allergic rhinitis in which nasal congestion may be prominent. In this, there may be other signs of allergy like pruritus and asthma extending for long periods. The causative organism of coryza can be cultured from throat washings or nasal swabs.

Treatment

Treatment is symptomatic. Confinement to home and avoidance of contact with others help to shorten the course of the illness and limit its spread. Paracetamol 0.5 g given thrice daily provides symptomatic relief of aches and pains. Medicated inhalations, throat lozenges and decongestant nasal drops are all helpful. Specific protection using vaccines which contain a few strains of rhinoviruses has been attempted on a limited scale.

INFLUENZA

Influenza is a common viral disease which presents as an acute febrile illness. It is caused by three groups of *myxoviruses,* important among them being ***influenza virus A, B and C*** which are antigenically different. Influenza A has occurred in pandemics on several occasions. India experienced influenza pandemics in 1781, 1889, 1918, 1957, 1968 and 1977. The pandemic that took place in 1977 was due to hemagglutinin type 1 and neuraminidase type 1 (H_1N_1). During these pandemics the antigenicity of the causative organisms has changed due to the development of new mutants. Influenza A, B and C consist of at least four subgroups each. The virus is spherical (80–120 nm in diameter) or filamentous in shape. The virus has a glycoprotein coat possessing hemagglutinin (H) and neuraminidase (N) activity. The subtypes of influenza viruses differ in their surface proteins-hemagglutinins (H) and neuraminidase (N). The usual human subtypes are H_1N_1, H_1N_2 and H_3N_2. Influenza viruses undergo reassortment of their genetic material between different influenza viruses and new strains emerge, so that existing vaccines may be ineffective to protect against newer strains.

During epidemics, children and the elderly suffer more. Dissemination of the virus occurs more readily when people are crowded together. Infection is through the respiratory tract. Influenza can also occur as inter-pandemic illness. This takes the form of sporadic illness or local outbreaks.

Influenza B causes localized outbreaks in closed communities such as schools, military camps and dormitories. Influenza C leads to human disease only rarely.

Pathology

Virus spreads by the respiratory route. Viral multiplication reaches its peak in 24–72 hours after the onset of the clinical illness. The virus multiplies in cells lining the respiratory tract including the ciliated epithelium, alveolar cells, mucous gland cells and macrophages. The infected cells show degenerative changes like cytoplasmic granulation, vacuolation and swelling. Ultimately the cells undergo necrosis and they slough away. The mucosa is hyperemic and edematous. Focal hemorrhages are common in these sites. Pneumonia may occur primarily due to viral infection, though it is more common to get secondary bacterial pneumonia. In viral pneumonia intra-alveolar hemorrhage may occur. Secondary bacterial infection occurs in about 25% of cases and it gives rise to suppurative inflammation.

Textbook of Medicine

Clinical Manifestations

The incubation period ranges from a few to 48 hours. Onset is sudden with fever, severe generalized myalgia and prostration. There is spasmodic non-productive cough. Conjunctiva is injected. Temperature varies from 38 to 40°C and may last for 3–4 days. In an uncomplicated case, there is relative bradycardia. Severe complications may occur in a few, especially at the extremes of age and in debilitated subjects. Mortality is higher in the age groups below 2 and above 65 years.

Complications

Pulmonary Complications

These include primary influenza virus pneumonia, influenzal pneumonia with secondary bacterial infections and bacterial pneumonia with multiple organisms.

- *Primary influenza virus pneumonia:* This is a serious condition associated with high mortality. These subjects present with high fever, cough with blood stained expectoration, dyspnea and cyanosis. Examination of the chest may reveal bilateral rhonchi and crepitations. Pulmonary involvement is diffuse. Fever and respiratory signs persist despite antibiotic therapy and other symptomatic measures. The course is more acute and serious in those cases with rheumatic heart disease, myocardial infarction (MI) or chronic obstructive airway disease.
- *Influenzal pneumonia with secondary bacterial infection:* In addition to viral pneumonia, localized consolidation may also develop.
- *Bacterial pneumonia:* Condition is caused by multiple organisms such as *Staphylococci, H. influenzae,* group A *Streptococci* and *Pneumococci.* This type of pneumonia carries a grave prognosis.

Cardiac Complications

Toxic myocarditis may occur. This gives rise to tachycardia and cardiac failure. The electrocardiogram (ECG) may be abnormal.

Neurological Complications

These include febrile convulsions, meningitis, meningo-encephalitis and encephalitis. A rare complication is the development of Reye's syndrome, which is more frequently seen in children. It presents as hepatic failure with encephalopathy and rise in intracranial tension. Reye's syndrome is associated with ingestion of aspirin. Apart from influenza A and B other viruses may also lead to this syndrome, e.g. varicella. Reye's syndrome develops as a result of serious derangement of mitochondrial function.

Diagnosis

The diagnosis is not difficult during an epidemic. Coryza may be mistaken for a mild attack of influenza. Nasal symptoms predominate in coryza but are less marked in influenza.

A *confirmed case* of novel influenza A (H_1N_1) virus infection is defined as a person with an influenza-like illness with laboratory confirmed novel influenza A (H_1N_1) virus infection by one or more of the following tests:

- Real-time reverse transcription polymerase chain reaction (RT-PCR)
- Viral culture.

Swabs (nasal, oral, secretions-respiratory) can be used for virus isolation.

Adenovirus infection, which may resemble influenza, can be diagnosed by the prominence of sore throat and pharyngitis. Primary atypical pneumonia has to be differentiated from influenza virus pneumonia. In primary atypical pneumonia the sputum is more purulent. It is of gradual onset and the clinical course is milder.

Streptococcal pharyngitis may present as a short duration fever with sore throat. Its incidence is higher in children. Cervical adenitis is present and blood shows neutrophil leukocytosis. The severe pain and body ache of influenza may be mistaken for dengue fever and sand-fly fever.

Specific diagnosis can be made by isolating the virus from throat washings or sputum and by demonstration of four-fold rise in titer of antibodies in paired sera by hemagglutination inhibition test.

Prognosis

The disease runs a benign course without complications in majority of cases. Uncomplicated cases recover within a week or two. Complications increase the mortality. In many cases convalescence may be prolonged. Generalized vague ill-health may persist for several weeks.

Influenza occurring during pregnancy is a serious complication since both maternal and fetal health are affected and mortality is increased. Primigravida suffer more than multigravida.

Treatment

Bed rest is essential during the period of illness and during convalescence. If there is secondary bacterial infection, a course of appropriate antibiotics should be given.

Specific drugs include **amantadine, rimantadine, zanamivir** and **oseltamivir**. These drugs act on the virus in different ways.

Amantadine in a dose of 100 mg given twice daily for 10–14 days offers chemoprophylaxis against influenza A virus, but not B. It protects the host cell from virus invasion. These drugs interfere with viral uncoating within the cell. Amantadine and rimantadine reduce the duration of fever by 1–2 days. These are ineffective against avian influenza. Prolonged administration during outbreaks reduces the incidence of fresh infections by 50% and ameliorates the disease in 70–100% of clinical cases. Side effects of amantadine include nausea, headache and neurological features. **Rimantadine** which is an analogue of amantadine is also effective.

Neuraminidase Inhibitors

Neuraminidase promotes influenza virus release from infected cells and facilitates viral spread within the respiratory tract, two neuraminidase inhibitors have been licenced for human use—zanamivir and oseltamivir. Unlike amantadine and rimantadine that target M2 protein of influenza A virus, these inhibit the replication of both of influenza A and B viruses. Zanamivir is given by inhalation due to its low availability when given orally. Oseltamivir is active when given orally. Both the drugs are good for chemoprophylaxis. When given early during the disease they reduce the severity, complications and duration. Compared to amantadine and rimantadine, development of resistance is also less.

Dose: Zanamivir (manufacturers BioTE/Glaxo)

Inhalation: 5 mg zanamivir + (20 mg lactose). After a single inhalation drug is detectable in sputum for 2–7 days.

Oseltamivir (Tamiflu) given in dose of 75–150 mg bd orally early in the disease probably controls the infection. Success is directly correlated with earlier administration of the drug. In children the dose is 30 mg bd oral for 5 days. Resistance of the virus to oseltamivir is being reported.

Oseltamivir and zanamivir help to reduce the symptom duration of influenza by 16.8 hours. These drugs reduce mortality by 50% if started within 2 hours of onset of symptoms. With each day's delay in starting treatment mortality rates increase.

Specific Prevention

Vaccines containing inactivated viruses are available for use during pandemics or epidemics and these offer 90% protection. Since the viral characteristics change from time to time, the composition of the vaccine has also to be different at times.

The general direction for the vaccine is given by the World Health Organization (WHO), taking into consideration the most prevalent viral strains. Usually the vaccine contains A and B strains. One dose in previously exposed individuals and two doses in unprimed subjects give a 90% protection rate. Mild local and general side effects may occur in a few. Sensitivity to egg protein is a contraindication for the vaccine. Pregnancy is not a contraindication.

Vaccination against influenza is a priority during pregnancy, since it reduces maternal illness and improves fetal outcomes such as prematurity and also protects the new born for six months. Repeated pregnancies should be protected with repeated vaccinations which are safe during pregnancy for both mother and fetus.

Emergent influenza A viruses infections such as A (H_7N_9) and A (H_5N_1) circulate in the community and produce outbreaks, they lack person to person transmissibility, still they can produce outbreaks.

AVIAN FLU

(Influenza group A H_5N_1 virus)

The Threat of a Pandemic by the Avian Influenza Virus

The subtype H_5N_1 influenza virus is a natural pathogen of chicken, ducks, turkeys and others. Though it was thought to be pathogenic only to them, the subtype H_5N_1 has crossed over to infect humans and caused small outbreaks. Hong Kong (1977) Thailand, Cambodia, Indonesia and several other Asian countries have reported outbreaks in poultry by H_5N_1 virus. In India, H_5N_1 virus has been identified in Nawapur and Jalagon in Maharashtra State. As on 26th April 2006, the WHO cases has reported the occurrence of 205 confirmed cases in humans with 113 deaths (55%). If human to human transmission of the virus becomes efficient, devastating pandemic more severe than the previous ones is likely to breakout. **Hence this matter is of great concern to all nations.**

Pathologically the lesions resemble those of classic influenza, but hemophagocytic histiocytosis may also be seen.

Clinical Features

The incubation period for human influenza viruses is short 2–3 days (range 1–7 days). However with influenza A (H_5N_1), the median time between exposure and onset of illness is 3 days (range 2–4 days). Most cases have occurred in previously healthy children and young adults. Symptoms of bird flu in humans include fever, cough and sore throat, pneumonia, acute respiratory distress and life-threatening complications. The symptoms of bird flu may vary depending on the type of virus. Primary viral pneumonia and multi-organ failure are common. In the present outbreak, more than half of those infected with the virus have died. Death is due to respiratory failure and multi-organ failure especially respiratory, renal and cardiac failure.

Case Definitions

Criteria for suspecting avian flu: Persons with illness characterized by fever (temperature > 38°C), cough and/or sore throat, severe respiratory symptoms and one or more of the following:

- Contact with a confirmed case of influenza A H_5N_1 during the infectious period
- Recent (less than 1 week) visit to a poultry farm in an area known to have outbreaks of HPAI (highly pathogenic avian influenza)
- Worked in a laboratory that is processing samples from persons or animals suspected to be having HPAI infection.

Procedure to Establish the Diagnosis

- Suspect the disease and start investigations. Virus can be isolated from pharyngeal secretions 2–15 days after the onset of illness. Nasal secretions, blood, cerebrospinal fluid (CSF) and feces also contain the virus. Children may continue to shed the virus in nasal discharges for over 2 weeks after recovering from the acute attack.
- Positive immunofluorescence antibody (IFA) using H_5N_1 monoclonal antibodies can be demonstrated in serum.

Diagnosis is confirmed by the following tests:

- Positive viral culture for influenza A H_5N_1
- Positive real time PCR for influenza A H_5N_1
- Four-fold rise in H_5N_1-specific antibody titer.

Management

Avian influenza virus is resistant to amantadine and rimantadine. Oseltamivir 75 mg orally twice daily for 5 days and zanamivir would probably be useful if started as early as possible. No vaccine is available now to protect against H_5N_1 virus for general use.

Two dose regimen of 90 µg of subvirion influenza A (H_5N_1) given IM over deltoid muscle at 28 days interval generates neutralizing antibody. This vaccine is under trial.

Infection Control Precautions for Hospital Staff

Patients who have visited endemic regions within 10 days and who present with severe febrile illness and respiratory symptoms should be observed for avian influenza, with isolation, barrier nursing and other precautions.

- Proper hand washing before and after contact with the patient
- Use gloves and gowns for all patient contacts. Use separate equipment for individual patients
- Protection of the eyes with goggles or face shields
- Precautions against droplet infection. Patients should be isolated in monitored negative air pressure ventilation systems. Healthcare staff should use a fit-tested respirator or approved N-95 filtering mask when entering the room
- Suspected poultry meat and eggs should be properly cooked so that the whole item reaches a minimum temperature 70°C which is needed to destroy the virus.

PARAINFLUENZA

This is caused by parainfluenza viruses which belong to the group of paramyxoviruses. Other members of the group include mumps measles respiratory syncytial virus and human metapneumovirus. These viruses are 80–120 nm in size. They cause respiratory infection. Based on antigenic differences, parainfluenza viruses are divided into four types. Parainfluenza has nothing in common with influenza virus. Parainfluenza viruses affect mostly children. Mainly the respiratory tract is involved.

Clinical Manifestations

After an incubation period of 5–6 days, it starts with fever which is a constant feature. Type I infection causes laryngotracheobronchitis or croup. Type II infection causes tracheobronchitis, bronchiolitis and bronchopneumonia in infants and children. Submandibular lymph nodes may become enlarged and tender. *Complications* include secondary bacterial infection leading to otitis media, sinusitis and bronchiectasis.

Treatment

There is no specific drug against this virus. Secondary bacterial infection has to be treated with antibiotics.

RESPIRATORY SYNCYTIAL VIRUS (RSV) INFECTION

It is a major pathogen of the lower respiratory tract in infants and elderly persons, especially immunocompromised. It belongs to the family Paramyxoviruses and the genus *Pneumovirus*. According to WHO data a third of the deaths in children below 5 years of age is due to respiratory tract infections caused mainly by *S. pneumoniae, H. influenzae* and RSV. There is no clear data of the epidemiology of RSV infection in India. Still it is most likely that the infection is quite prevalent. Route of infection is the upper respiratory tract, especially the nasopharynx and the eyes. Incubation period is 3–5 days. Main pathological lesions are in the bronchiolar epithelial cells leading to inflammation and edema of the peribronchial region. Plugs containing mucus and epithelial debris lead to ball-valve obstruction of distal airways with air trapping. Cellular immunity plays a major role in the recovery from infection.

Clinical Features

Most common manifestations are rhinitis, cough and fever at times. Otitis media, bronchiolitis, pneumonia and croup are common in children. Severe bronchiolitis may lead to respiratory failure.

In adults, RSV infection leads to exacerbation of chronic bronchitis and emphysema. Diagnosis is established by demonstration of RSV antigens in nasopharyngeal washings by enzyme-linked immunosorbent assay (ELISA).

Prophylaxis

Vaccines are under trial. In immunocompromised infants a humanized monoclonal antibody may be tried with benefit during epidemics. While attending to cases, hand washing and avoiding contamination by oronasal discharges are important.

Management

In many cases the disease is self-limiting and only supportive measures are needed. Ribavirin is probably effective as an antiviral agent and this should be employed in severe cases.

SEVERE ACUTE RESPIRATORY SYNDROME (SARS)

General Considerations

SARS is an emerging infectious disease caused by a novel coronavirus first described from China and Hong Kong and was reported in 2003, which threatened to assume pandemic dimensions. The disease spreads widely, probably by the respiratory route by droplet infection even by very short periods of exposure. Possibly the secretions from other sites and excreta are also infectious. Direct exposure, closed environment in aircrafts and air travel contributed to the dissemination of the virus in many parts of the world. The disease was effectively contained from spreading, by prompt action directed by the WHO and taken up internationally. India did not have proved cases of SARS during this period.

Clinical Features

The cases presented with fever initially with or without chills or rigor, influenza-like symptoms and radiological signs compatible with pneumonia. History of contact with established cases was present. The mean age of the patients were 35–40 years. Presenting symptoms include pyrexia (90%), chills or rigor (71%), cough (52%), vague symptoms (50–60%), dyspnea (30%) and diarrhea (25%).
Common laboratory findings include lymphopenia in 58%, thrombocytopenia in 40% and raised lactate dehydrogenase (LDH) in 70%. Viral ribonucleic acid (RNA) can be identified by RT-PCR from nasopharyngeal aspirate, stool and urine. Seroconversion occurs slowly and immunoglobulin G (IgG) might be detected by 8–10 weeks.

Radiological abnormalities were present in all cases on admission or follow-up. In 70% they were bilateral. The abnormalities include subtle haziness (36%), mild infiltrates and ground-glass appearance (57%), denser infiltrates and dense confluent opacities (7%).

The *differential diagnosis* includes atypical pneumonia, influenza, parainfluenza, respiratory syncytial virus and adenovirus infections and pneumocystis pneumonia. The disease carries a high mortality exceeding 50%, if unrecognized.

Textbook of Medicine

Management

SARS should be suspected in acute febrile illnesses with moderate or severe respiratory embarrassment. Isolation of the patient and protection of healthcare staff should be instituted as described for avian flu (*See* previous page).

Environment and contaminated materials are disinfected by domestic bleach (1,000 ppm hypochlorite solution) for non-metallic articles and 70% alcohol for metallic objects.

Specific Therapy

- ■ *Antibacterial drugs:* Treatment with levofloxacin 500 mg once a day IV or oral should be started without delay in patients above 18 years of age. In patients younger than 18 years, pregnant women and patients suspected to have tuberculosis clarithromycin 500 mg orally bd with co-amoxiclav (amoxicillin and clavulanic acid) 375 mg tds is the combination of choice.
- ■ If chest radiograph shows extensive lesions or clinical features are worsening the antiviral drug ribavirin should be started in doses of 400 mg 8 h (1200 mg/day) IV for 3 days or till the condition becomes stable and thereafter 1200 mg oral bd (total 2400 mg/day) for 10–14 days.
- ■ Corticosteroids should be started along with ribavirin. The standard protocol consist of a 21 day regimen as follows:
  - Methylprednisolone 1 mg/kg bw 8 h IV (total 3 mg/kg bw/day) for 5 days
  - Methylprednisolone 1 mg/kg bw/day IV for 5 days
  - Prednisolone oral 0.5 mg/kg bw/bd daily for 5 days
  - Prednisolone oral 0.5 mg/kg bw od daily for 3 days
  - Prednisolone oral 0.25 mg/kg bw od for 3 days.

Ventilation should be assisted in those having ventilatory problems. Success rate of treatment is high, if instituted early.

> **Points to Remember**
> - SARS is an emerging, serious life-threatening infection by a coronavirus which ushered in several parts of the world in 2003.
> - Prompt recognition of the mode of spread and international action helped to prevent the spread of the disease.
> - All healthcare professionals should be aware of such infections and early reporting to public health authorities is vital, to prevent devastating outbreaks.

Source: So LK, Lau AC, Yam LY, et al. Development of a standard treatment protocol for severe acute respiratory syndrome. Lancet. 2003;361:1615-7.

OTHER PARAMYXOVIRUSES

Nipah Virus

Other paramyxoviruses infections are being reported in recent times. Nipah virus is a member of this group which was identified to produce local outbreaks of encephalitis-like illness in persons working in pig farms and abattoir workers handling pigs in Singapore. Further reports are likely to follow.

Human Metapneumovirus

Human metapneumovirus is a common respiratory pathogen especially in children. It is a RNA virus. It causes bronchitis in 59%, pneumonia in 8%, croup in 18% and exacerbation of asthma in 14%. Nasal wash specimen is used to isolate virus.

MIDDLE EAST RESPIRATORY SYNDROME (MERS)

General Considerations

MERS is a newly identified cause of acute respiratory distress syndrome (ARDS) caused by a virus belonging to the coronavirus family. The virus is technically referred to as EMC/2012 (HCoV-EMC/2012), which is a positive-sense, single-stranded RNA virus of the genus β-coronavirus. Cases have been reported from Saudi Arabia, Malaysia, Jordan, Qatar, Egypt, the United Arab Emirates, Tunisia, the Philippines and the United States. There is a potential for spread to various countries. As of April 2014, there are 339 confirmed cases in Saudi Arabia, with 102 deaths. The mortality rate as per this data is 30%. There are so many epidemiologic similarities with SARS, which is also caused by a coronavirus. The first few cases were reported from Amman, Jordan in 2012. An Egyptian virologist Dr Ali Mohamed Zaki isolated and identified a previously unknown coronavirus from the lungs of a man who died from a pneumonia with renal involvement. The virus has a peculiar tropism for non-ciliated respiratory epithelium and suppresses interferon response. Cd26 receptors are thought to be important in attachment. Related virus and antibodies have been demonstrated in bats and camels. Isolation of the causative coronavirus from respiratory secretions showed exactly similar genetic pattern with the oronasal secretions of his patient's sick camel. Serological studies revealed evidence for circulating virus in the camel, but not in the patient. This gives strong clue to the source of infection.

Source: Azhar EI, El-Kafrawy SA, Farraj SA, et al. Evidence for camel-to-human transmission of MERS coronavirus. N Eng J Med. 2014;370(26):2499-505.

Clinical Features

Fever, cough with expectoration, breathlessness occur after a usual incubation period of 12 days. Severe acute pneumonia and renal failure was present in almost all fatal cases. Though immunofluorescence detection is available, cross reactivity with other coronaviruses is common. The virus can be detected in the sputum or bronchial fluids by PCR, which is confirmatory. No specific treatment is available as of now.

The disease may spread by eating infected material or by close contact with cases. Healthcare personnel may be particularly at risk.

Treatment

No specific treatment is available as yet. Management consists of isolation supportive measures and barrier nursing to prevent spread to contacts.

Prevention and Surveillance

General measures to prevent viral spread should be undertaken.

Appropriate vaccines should be administered.

CHAPTER
53

Exanthems and Enanthems

KV Krishna Das

Chapter Summary

- Measles
  - Pathogenesis and Pathology
  - Clinical Features
  - Complications
  - Laboratory Diagnosis
  - Differential Diagnosis
  - Treatment
  - Prevention
- Smallpox
  - General Considerations
  - Pathology
  - Clinical Manifestations
  - Complications
  - Course and Prognosis
  - Diagnosis
  - Treatment
  - Prevention
- Chickenpox
  - General Considerations
  - Pathogenesis and Pathology
  - Epidemiology
  - Clinical Features
  - Complications
  - Diagnosis
  - Laboratory Diagnosis
  - Treatment
  - Prophylaxis
- Herpes Zoster
  - General Considerations
  - Clinical Features
  - Complications
  - Diagnosis and Differential Diagnosis
  - Specific Treatment
- Herpes Simplex
  - General Considerations
  - Clinical Features
  - Diagnosis
  - Treatment
- Rubella
  - Epidemiology
  - Pathogenesis
  - Clinical Features
  - Diagnosis
  - Treatment
  - Prevention

MEASLES

Syn: Rubeola

Measles or rubeola (red spots-Arabic) is an acute exanthematous febrile illness caused by a specific virus of the paramyxoviruses group affecting children primarily. It is a ribonucleic acid (RNA) virus varying in size from 150 to 300 nm.

The present day major killers of children globally are measles, diphtheria, whooping cough, tetanus, tuberculosis, polio-like paralysis and to some extent poliomyelitis.

In developing countries, 10% of all deaths in children below 5 years of age are measles related.

Pathogenesis and Pathology

Man is the only natural host. The disease may occur in localized or wider outbreaks once in 2–3 years, especially during spring. The virus is present in the nasopharyngeal secretions and infection is by droplets. Portals of entry are the respiratory mucous membrane and the conjunctiva. The period of infectivity starts 5 days after the exposure to the virus and lasts until 5 days after skin eruptions have appeared. Infants do not generally suffer, presumably because of the persistence of maternal antibodies in them.

The virus multiplies in the epithelium of the respiratory tract and then causes viremia. Hematogenous spread occurs to various tissues. The virus can be isolated from blood, conjunctiva, lymphoid tissues and secretions of the respiratory tract for a few days before and for 1 or 2 days after the appearance of rashes and from the urine as long as 4 days after the rash. Following the viremic phase the virus localizes in the skin and respiratory tract in addition to several tissues. There is interaction between the virus and the T-cells. ***Koplik's spots*** are pathognomonic.

The mucous membrane lesions (enanthem) known as Koplik's spots seen in the cheeks, consist of vesicles and necrotic epithelium. Microscopically the lesions show cytoplasmic and intranuclear inclusions, giant cells and intercellular edema. Aggregates of virion in the affected cells can be demonstrated by electron microscopy.

Multinucleated giant cells with acidophilic nuclear and cytoplasmic inclusions ***(Warthin Finkeldey cells)*** may be found in the hyperplastic lymphoid tissues of lymph nodes, tonsils, spleen and thymus. Chromosomal breaks may be seen in leukocytes. Epithelium of the respiratory tract is disrupted and this favors secondary bacterial infection. Lungs show interstitial pneumonia with giant cell infiltration. In patients, who develop encephalomyelitis, the brain shows focal hemorrhage, congestion and perivenous demyelination.

Clinical Features

Incubation period is 9–11 days. The initial manifestations are malaise, irritability, high fever and conjunctivitis with excessive lacrimation, edema of the eyelids, photophobia, hacking cough and nasal discharge. These symptoms last for 3–4 days (up to 8 days) and then the rashes start. Koplik's spots appear as small, red irregular lesions with bluish-white center on the mucous membrane of mouth 1–2 days before the skin rash. They are best seen in the buccal mucosa opposite the upper molar teeth. Lesions similar to them may occur in the conjunctiva and intestinal mucosa. The rashes are red and maculopapular, first appearing on the forehead and behind the pinna, later on spreading down to the face, neck, trunk and limbs. Maximum affection is on the face and shoulders. These rashes persist for about 3 days and disappear in the order in which they appeared. In partially immune persons, the rash and symptoms may be less severe. The disease becomes more severe in adults in whom complications are likely to be more. The general symptoms disappear 1–2 days after the appearance of skin rash. Cough may persist throughout the illness.

The term ***atypical measles*** is used to denote a paradoxical reaction in children who have received formalin–inactivated measles vaccine and who have partial immunity who develops high fever with rashes on the periphery of the extremities which may become even petechial. Toxemia in high. Respiratory complications such as pneumonia and/or plural effusion may occur. The possible reason for this phenomenon may be abnormal immune response to vaccination resulting in formation of immune complexes and abnormal clinical responses.

Complications

These are common, though in the majority, the disease is self-limiting. Respiratory complications include croup, bronchitis, bronchiolitis and rarely interstitial giant cell pneumonia. These are more common in immuno-compromised persons and malnourished children. The eye lesion may progress to corneal ulceration, keratitis and blindness. Myocarditis develops in 20% of cases and this causes transient electrocardiographic (ECG) changes, but clinically this may remain silent. Acute abdominal pain may occur due to mesenteric lymphadenitis. In pregnant women, fetal loss may occur in 20% of cases. Measles occurring in adults is more serious. Primary viral pneumonia with bronchospasm, more severe and con-fluent rashes and bacterial superinfection may develop.

Secondary bacterial pneumonia by *Staphylococcus, Streptococcus, Pneumococcus* and *H. influenzae* is common and may progress to lung abscess and empyema. Otitis media may develop commonly. Stomatitis may develop and progress to cancrum oris, especially in malnourished children. Quiescent tuberculous lesions may flare up or fresh tuberculous infection may develop. Diarrhea may occur as a complication and may prove troublesome. Mortality is high in children below 2 years of age.

Neurological Complications of Measles

Acute postinfectious measles encephalitis caused by cell mediated autoimmune response to measles virus-frequency 1/1000 cases. ***Encephalomyelitis***, another serious complication, occurs in 1/1000 patients, usually occurring 4–7 days after the appearance of the eruption. It is characterized by high fever, headache, drowsiness and coma ending fatally in 10% of cases.

Progressive encephalitis may develop in 1–6 months after measles in immunosuppressed children. ***Measles***

inclusion body encephalitis (MIBE) occurs only in immunocompromised subjects.

It is a subacute infection occurring 1–7 years after infection. Measles virus persists in the brain. It presents as alterations in cognition, convulsions and coma. This disease is invariably fatal.

Subacute sclerosing panencephalitis (SSPE) is a late complication of measles developing 5–15 years after the acute disease. In SSPE the virus persists in the brain, possibly with alteration of matrix proteins. It is characterized by progressive dementia and motor weakness and movement disorders. In this disorder the measles virus tends to persist for long in neural tissue and bring about slow degenerative lesions and a clinical picture similar to slow virus infections result. SSPE is estimated to occur with a frequency of 1/8000 in children infected with measles (*See* Section 17, Ch 199).

Laboratory Diagnosis

Laboratory investigations are essential to diagnose atypical cases and also for differentiating measles from rubella. Leukopenia is frequent in the early stages. Leukocytosis occurs with secondary bacterial infection. Cerebrospinal fluid (CSF) shows raised protein and lymphocytosis in encephalomyelitis.

Demonstration of multinucleated giant cells in Giemsa stained smears of nasal secretions is a simple side room laboratory test. Virus antigen can be detected in the cells by immunofluorescence. Virus can be isolated in human embryonic kidney and amnion cells.

Demonstration of rising antibody levels by complement fixation test, hemagglutination inhibition test and neutralization test in paired sera help to make serological diagnosis. Rise in immunoglobulin M (IgM) measles specific antibody in acute phase and four-fold rise in IgG antibody in convalescent phase are diagnostic. IgM antibodies appear within 3–4 days of onset of the illness and may be detectable up to 4–8 weeks.

Reverse transcriptase polymerase chain reaction (RT-PCR) amplification of RNA can detect the virus in nasal, oral and conjunctival secretions. This also helps to confirm the infection and characterize the genotypes of the viruses.

Laboratory diagnosis of SSPE: The diagnostic investi-gation is the presence of anti-measles antibody in serum above 1/256 and in CSF above 1/4 dilution.

Electroencephalogram (EEG) shows bilateral poly-phasic intermittent synchronous high voltage (200–500 mV) bursts of stereotyped delta waves repeating at regular intervals of 4–10 seconds. This typical EEG is seen during the myoclonic phase. Magnetic resonance imaging (MRI) with gadolinium contrast enhancement reveals patchy areas of white matter involvement, particularly in the temporal and parietal lobes. Brain biopsy shows panencephalitis.

Differential Diagnosis

Rubella has to be differentiated from measles. Rubella is a milder illness of short duration without significant respiratory complaints. Infectious mononucleosis, toxo-plasmosis, secondary syphilis, adenovirus and entero-

Textbook of Medicine

viruses infections, scarlet fever and drug rashes have to be differentiated.

Treatment

There is no specific drug against the virus and therefore, management is symptomatic. Bacterial infection has to be treated with antibiotics based on clinical and bacteriological findings. Supplementation of vitamin A 200,000 units/day for 2–3 days is beneficial. Children who continue to be ill after an attack of measles should be investigated for the presence of tuberculosis.

Prevention

Administration of gamma globulin 0.25 mL/kg given intramuscular (IM) up to a maximum of 15 mL within 5 days of exposure effectively prevents or attenuates the attack. Children below 3 years, pregnant women, immunocompromised persons and those who suffer from tuberculosis should be given gamma globulin for passive immunization which persists for 3–4 weeks.

Live attenuated measles vaccine, prepared from *Edmonston B strains of measles virus* is used for active immunization. Immunity lasts for a period of over 10 years. Vaccination after 12 months of age is more effective, though earlier vaccination can be done in measles prevalent areas. In those vaccinated before 12 months, a second dose should be given at the age of 15–18 months. The vaccine may be given alone or in combination with rubella and mumps vaccines. Vaccination is contraindicated in pregnancy, tuberculosis, leukemia, lymphoma and immunocompromised patients. Combined vaccines for measles, mumps and rubella (MMR vaccine) are available. Adverse effects include fever in 5–15% and rashes. MMR vaccination 2 doses give seroconversion in 98% for measles and only 88% for mumps. So the vaccinated persons are more susceptible to mumps than measles.

Measles vaccine is supplied free of cost along with the general immunization schedule. MMR vaccine is available at cost for those who prefer to take it (*See* Section 1, Ch 3).

Though the World Health Organization (WHO) recommended vaccination coverage of 90% of the children by 2000 AD, this target has not been achieved. Vaccination is very effective in preventing measles and SSPE.

Aerosol vaccines using Schwartz or Edmonston-Zagreb strains of the virus have been compared with the standard subcutaneous injection. The antibody response at one month and one year are reported to be comparable.

Measles eradication is feasible since, there are no non-human hosts for the virus and immunization is effective.

SMALLPOX

Syn: Variola

General Considerations

Smallpox is a natural infection in man caused by variola virus and the virus affects only humans. The virus is 200–250 nm in size and belongs to the group of poxviruses which are double-stranded deoxyribonucleic acid (DNA) viruses. The variants of variola virus—*variola major* and *variola minor* can be distinguished in the laboratory. Studies to sequence the genome of the virus are in progress. Variola minor causes milder disease compared to variola major.

The virus is transmitted from man-to-man by the respiratory route. There are no animal reservoirs or insect vectors in the transmission of this disease. The transmission may be direct from patient-to-patient or through fomites and other contaminated articles. Nasopharyngeal secretions, vesicle fluid and dried scabs contain the virus. The virus can remain viable in dried scab for over one year. The patient is infective from the onset of early symptoms till the last scab has fallen off.

Though smallpox was one of the most dreaded diseases and outbreaks occurred in the tropics regularly, at present, the disease has been eradicated by worldwide efforts undertaken by the WHO from 1967 to 1977. The world was declared free of natural infection in October 1977. In India, the last case was reported in 1976. Except for the stock cultures of the virus maintained in a few laboratories, the virus is believed to have disappeared. This achievement was made possible by an intensive program of mass vaccination and early case reporting. Absence of any non-human reservoir and vector and the solid immunity produced by vaccination have contributed to this achievement. Variola virus proteins modulate the immune system. Since the virus can be grown easily and modified genetically to evade the vaccination induced immunity, it is a good candidate for bioterrorism and warfare.

Pathology

After entry, the virus reaches the lymph nodes, where it multiplies and then enters the circulation. Viremia disseminates the virus to lymphoid tissues from which the skin and mucous membranes are affected thereafter. Cellular, humoral and innate immunity influence the course of smallpox. The affected epithelial cells show acidophilic cytoplasmic inclusion bodies called *Guarnieri bodies*. These are aggregates of the virus particles which are called *Paschen bodies.*

Clinical Manifestations

The incubation period is 12 days (8–16 days). Prodromal symptoms occur 2–4 days before the eruption starts. These consist of high fever, myalgia, headache, backache, delirium and abdominal pain. The rash starts on the third day and the fever subsides when the rash appears. Fever reappears after varying intervals, when the rash becomes pustular. The temperature comes down with scabbing. The rashes are characteristic. They are distributed in a centrifugal pattern. The face, arms and legs are more often and more heavily affected. Presence of vesicles in the palms and soles is characteristic. Initial lesions are erythematous macules, which progress successively into papules, vesicles, pustules and scabs at 48-hour intervals. The vesicles and pustules are deep-set in the skin, multiloculated and the center is umbilicated (Figs 53.1A and B). Unlike as in chickenpox, all the vesicles are at the same stage of development. When the scab separates, pitted scars are left behind, which tend to remain permanent.

In vaccinated individuals who possess residual immunity, the clinical picture is modified and this is

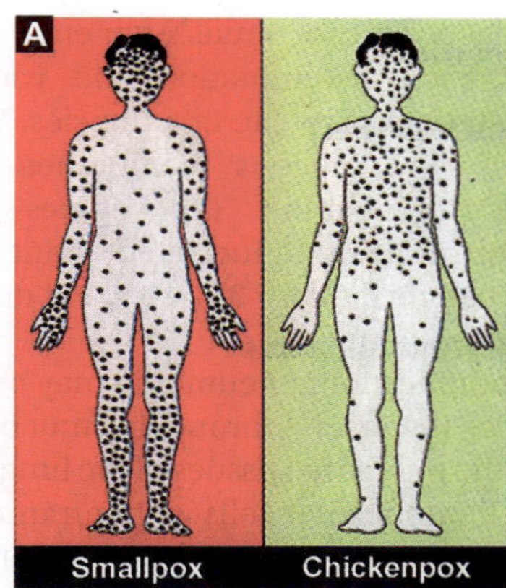
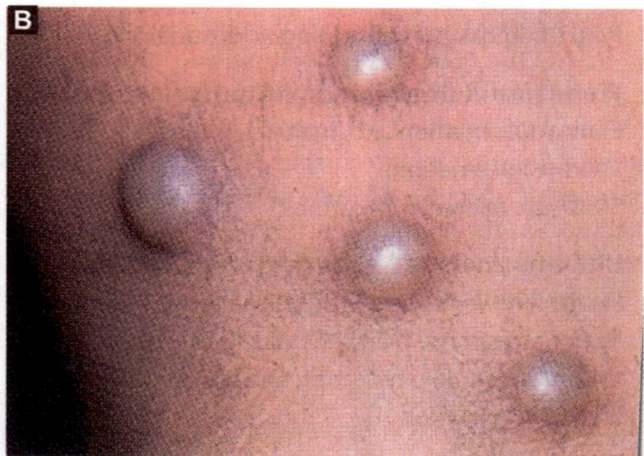

Figs 53.1A and B: Smallpox **A.** Distribution of rash; **B.** Deep seated vessels, all at the same stage of development

termed as varioloid. This is abrupt in onset with the development of only a few rashes. The course is benign. Smallpox may occur without the characteristic rash, *variola sine eruption*. A less virulent form of the virus capable of producing milder manifestations, *variola minor (alastrim),* has also been recognized.

Other serious clinical types may occur less commonly. These are hemorrhagic smallpox which is highly fatal and the flat form (malignant form) in which the papules are velvety, may become vesicular and lead to peeling off of the whole epidermis. Both these severe forms are uniformly fatal.

Complications

Secondary infection by staphylococci occurs during the stage of postulation. This may lead to septicemia, pneumonia, osteomyelitis, septic arthritis, otitis media and pyelonephritis. Death is due to coagulopathy, hypotension and multi-organ failure. In the eye, vesicles in the cornea may suppurate and lead to panophthalmitis and blindness. Smallpox was a common cause of blindness in India till six decades ago. Neurological complications include demyelinating lesions such as encephalitis, encephalomyelitis and peripheral neuritis. Laryngeal edema may occur, leading to respiratory obstruction.

Osteomyelitis Variolosa

In this form of destructive osteomyelitis, the metaphysis are infected with the virus during the phase of viremia, but symptoms are late to develop. Destruction and detachment of the epiphyses lead to permanent bone and joint deformities which persist in later life (Fig. 53.2).

Course and Prognosis

Till the middle of this century smallpox used to be a major killer among children with a mortality of 20–80% among unvaccinated subjects. Death is due to severe toxemia or secondary infection.

Diagnosis

Clinically, smallpox should be suspected when an unvaccinated person gets high fever with prodroma and rash occurring on the third day. The distribution and progress of the rash strengthens the diagnosis. Since the world has been declared free of smallpox, physicians have to be alert to detect initial cases and

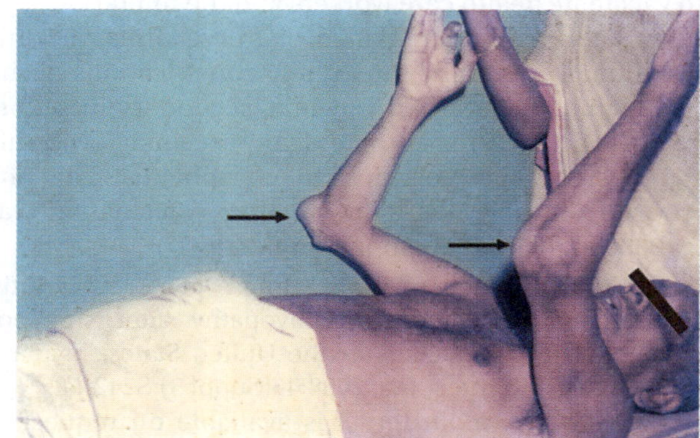

Fig. 53.2: Osteomyelitis variolosa (arrows)

subject them to through laboratory investigations. By international agreement, reporting of fresh cases to the health authorities carries a cash award. Chickenpox, drug rashes and erythema multiforme are to be differentiated from smallpox. Rickettsial pox and pustular syphilis may resemble mild cases of smallpox.

Laboratory Diagnosis

- Demonstration of the virus in material from vesicles or crusts by electron microscopy. Characteristic brick-shaped virus can be identified. PCR assays confirm the presence of virus
- Identification of Guarnieri bodies from the vesicular material
- Isolation of the virus.

Treatment

The treatment is mainly supportive. Antibiotics are used when secondary bacterial infection occurs. After exposure, the attack can be prevented by administering methisazone in a dose of 1.5–3 g twice daily for four days. Methisazone offers protection in unvaccinated individuals but it has no curative effect when the disease is manifest. Vaccinia immunoglobulin can be administered and it has a protective role. Early notification of cases, strict barrier nursing and large scale immunization of the surrounding population should be undertaken to prevent the spread of the disease. Since the vaccine is not at present available for regular use, vaccination programs have to be undertaken by the appropriate health authorities.

Textbook of Medicine

Prevention

Vaccination used to be the most effective method to prevent smallpox. It was introduced by Edward Jenner on May 14, 1796. Since the world is declared free of smallpox, regular vaccination of infants is not insisted upon at present. Several strains of vaccinia of low pathogenicity are used for the vaccine. Single clones are used for vaccine production. Attenuation is achieved by serial passage in non-human tissue. Third generation vaccines are available. The immunity is solid; the exact duration is not clear. There is evidence that the conventional vaccine diluted ten times still maintains its immunogenicity. Vaccination done within 3–4 days of exposure will prevent or allay the disease manifestations. Due to the fear of bioterrorism, many countries have produced smallpox vaccine. Priority is to vaccinate health care workers and the military.

The vaccine contains killed or freeze dried vaccinia virus. Though generally safe, rarely complications occur. These include generalized vaccinia, secondary infection, eczema vaccinatum, progressive vaccinia (vaccinia gangrenosum) and postvaccinal encephalitis. The rate of possible myocarditis after smallpox vaccination was 5.5/10000 in the civilian population in the US.

Source: Morgan J, Roper MH, Sperling L, et al. Myocarditis, pericarditis, and dilated cardiomyopathy after smallpox vaccination among civilians in the United States, January-October 2003. Clin Infect Dis. 2008;46(Suppl 3):S242-50.

Vaccine immune globulin: It is available on request to treat severe vaccination reaction.

The doctors working in India have to keep smallpox in mind and report the first suspicious case to prevent the occurrence of a devastating epidemic in a non-immune population.

WHO website on additional information on smallpox are available at http://www.who.int/topics/smallpox.

CHICKENPOX

Syn: Varicella

General Considerations

Chickenpox is a common viral infection occurring frequently in children. The disease is highly contagious. It is characterized by fever and disseminated vesicular eruptions. Though in children the disease is benign and self-limiting, as age advances the disease becomes more serious and produces grave complications.

The etiological agents of varicella and herpes zoster are identical in all respects. The varicella-zoster (V-Z) virus is a double-stranded DNA virus measuring 100–150 nm in diameter belonging to the family Herpesviridae. It multiplies in the nuclei of infected cells and produces intranuclear inclusions.

It is an exclusively human herpesvirus that causes chickenpox (varicella), become latent in cranial nerves and dorsal root ganglia, to be reactivated later to produce shingles (zoster) and postherpetic neuralgia.

Pathogenesis and Pathology

Cases of chickenpox are most infective in the early stages of illness and virus is present in the lesions and the respiratory discharges. Infection occurs by respiratory route, contacts or nosocomial. After entry there is a period of bloodstream dissemination and widespread organ involvement demonstrable in autopsies. Vesicles develop in the skin and mucous membranes. The epidermis undergoes degeneration. The vesicles contain serum, polymorphs and multinucleated giant cells. Virus is present in vesicle fluid for 3–4 days, but not after the onset of crusting.

As a complication, pneumonia may occur. In varicella pneumonia, the tracheobronchial mucosa, the alveolar septa and the interstitial tissues of the lungs are edematous and show mononuclear cells with intranuclear inclusions and giant cells. Pneumonia develops as nodular areas of consolidation in the lungs. Ultimately these lesions may become calcified. Encephalomyelitis which resembles that seen in measles may occur as a complication. During the acute phase of the disease infants and children may develop acute encephalopathy with fatty infiltration of the viscera ***(Reye's syndrome).***

Epidemiology

The infectious period extends from a day or two before the onset of the rash to six days after the appearance of new skin lesions or until all vesicles have started crusting. Chickenpox develops commonly due to exposure to other cases of chickenpox and rarely in contacts of herpes zoster. Herpes zoster is mainly a disease of adults who have partial immunity to the virus. Though chickenpox produces good immunity, it wanes off after 10 years and second attacks may develop.

Clinical Features

The rashes appear 14–16 days after exposure (range 10–23 days). Prodromal symptoms are mild in children, the first manifestation in whom is the appearance of vesicles. Early symptoms in adults include fever, headache, backache, sore throat and malaise which last for 2 or 3 days. Enanthem occurs over the palatal and pharyngeal mucosa even before the skin rash appears. The skin rashes ***(exanthem)*** come up in crops starting from the first day of fever and these continue for 3–4 days so that lesions at different stages—macule, papule, vesicle, pustule and scab—may be present simultaneously ***(polymorphism).*** The rashes are centripetal, maximally affecting the trunk and sparing the distal parts of the limbs. Face may be affected variably (Fig. 53.3). The axillae are almost invariably affected. The vesicles are unilocular, superficial, elliptical in shape and contain clear fluid in the beginning (tear drop vesicles). These become pustular in 24 hours. Intense pruritus may develop and scratching disrupts these vesicles. The pustules dry up to form scabs in a few days. When the scabs fall off, superficial scars are left behind which clear up in due course. Recovery is the rule in vast majority of healthy subjects. Complications and death may occur in immunosuppressed persons and children receiving glucocorticoids. In them progressive varicella develops and organ involvement is more common.

Complications

- Thrombocytopenia may develop leading to hemorrhage into the vesicles, conjunctiva and intestines.

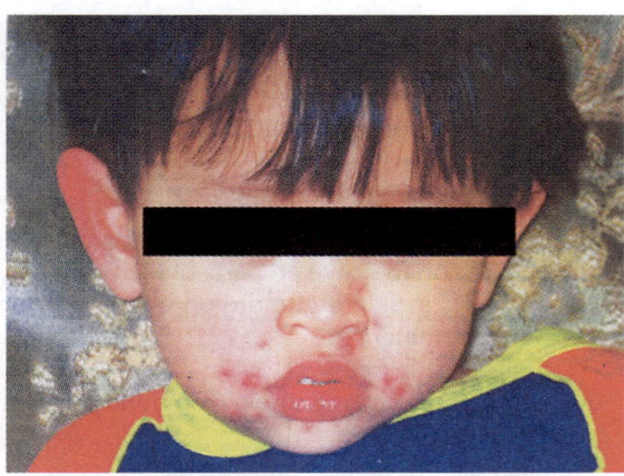

Fig. 53.3: Chickenpox. ***Note:*** Superficial vesicles in different stages of development the face is invariably affected

- Staphylococcal infection may supervene leading to bacteremia and delayed healing.
- Children with impetigo may develop bullous lesions.
- Superinfection by hemolytic streptococci causes varicella gangrenosa.
- Around 15% of adults with chickenpox may develop primary varicella pneumonia. This is manifested 1–6 days after the onset of the rash. This may be asymptomatic or it may present with high fever, tachypnea, cough, pleuritic chest pain, cyanosis and hemoptysis. Physical examination may not give evidence of extensive consolidation. It may show only a few rhonchi, scattered rales or rarely pleural effusion. Radiologically extensive nodular lesions are seen in both lungs. As the rashes subside and general condition improves the pulmonary lesions clear up.
- Neurological complications develop more in immuno-compromised individuals at all ages. In elderly persons these may occur in immunocompetent individuals as well. The central nervous system (CNS) lesions include myelitis, encephalitis, encephalomyelitis ventriculitis and meningitis. The major pathological change in varicella-zoster encephalopathy is a vasculitis affecting the small and large vessels. Clinically, presentations include transient cerebellar ataxia, encephalomyelitis, polyneuritis cranialis, ascending paralysis, transverse myelitis and optic neuritis.
- Other systemic complications that may develop rarely are myocarditis, keratitis, iritis, nephritis, arthritis, purpura, orchitis and appendicitis. Quiescent tuberculosis may be reactivated. Chickenpox occurring in the first two trimesters of pregnancy may give rise to congenital malformations in 9%.
- ***Varicella during pregnancy:*** Congenital varicella syndrome in the fetus occurs in the third trimester of pregnancy especially between 8 and 20 weeks. Clinical features include skin lesions, neurological and eye defects, limb hypoplasia, intrauterine growth retardation (IUGR) and other manifestations due to direct viral invasion. Risk of developing this syndrome is 0.7% in first trimester and 2% in the second trimester. Detailed ultrasound examination is diagnostic. Abnormalities include limb deformities microcephaly, hydrocephalus, polyhydramnios and soft tissue calcification. These are detectable at least

5 weeks after maternal varicella. If the mother develops the rash between four days prior to delivery and two days thereafter, it is highly probable that the newborn is infected. The disease is associated with high mortality in the neonate.

Complications in varicella	

• Secondary bacterial infection of skin lesions
• CNS (rare)
  ▪ Cerebellar ataxia
  ▪ Encephalitis
  ▪ Aseptic meningitis
  ▪ Transverse myelitis
  ▪ Guillain-Barré syndrome
• Varicella pneumonia (interstitial)
	• Myocarditis
	• Acute glomerulonephritis
	• Corneal lesions
	• Arthritis, osteomyelitis
	• Bleeding diatheses
	• Hepatitis
	• Reye's syndrome with aspirin use
	• Perinatal varicella
	• Congenital varicella (extremely uncommon)

Diagnosis

Clinical diagnosis is not difficult in typical cases. Fever with vesicular rash occurring on the trunk and milder prodromata is suggestive of chickenpox. Smallpox used to be an important differential diagnosis. Though smallpox has been eradicated, it is extremely important to identify any similar illness and subject the patient to full investigation. The clinical differentiation between chickenpox and smallpox is given in Table 53.1. When the disease is modified by immunization or immunosuppression, laboratory confirmation becomes necessary.

Laboratory Diagnosis

Examination of material scraped from the vesicles (Tzanck smear) reveal eosinophilic intranuclear inclusion bodies within epithelial cells and multinucleated giant cells. Virus can be isolated from vesicular fluid. Serological diagnosis can be made by complement fixation, immunoadherence, hemagglutination, indirect immunofluorescent antibody detection tests or enzyme-linked immunosorbent assay (ELISA). Presence of IgM antibodies or four-fold rise of IgG antibodies in paired sera are diagnostic. Presence of the virus in blood vessels can be detected by PCR.

Treatment

In the majority of cases only symptomatic treatment is required, when the illness is mild. Paracetamol in a dose of 0.5 g given thrice daily serves to relieve pain. To prevent secondary infection, local antiseptics like chlorhexidine can be used. Pruritus can be reduced by local application of peanut oil containing 1% phenol. Antiviral drugs such as acyclovir have to be given parenterally in complicated cases.

For normal hosts acyclovir 20 mg/kg bw orally as tablets up to a maximum of 800 mg 4–5 times a day for 5 days is effective. Valacyclovir in a dose of 1 g orally tid for 5–7 days is also quite effective. The other alternative is famciclovir given orally in a dose of 500 mg tid for 5–7 days.

In immunocompromised hosts and in normal hosts with pneumonia or meningoencephalitis the dose is 10 mg/kg intravenous (IV) 8 hourly for 7–10 days or more. If started early the results are excellent. Painful neuritis may require judicious use of analgesics drugs like

Textbook of Medicine

Table 53.1: Clinical differentiation between chickenpox and smallpox

Signs and symptoms	Chickenpox	Smallpox
• Prodromal symptoms	Absent or mild	Prodromal symptoms more

• Rash
  ▪ Appearance of vesicles
  ▪ Distribution
 	
  ▪ Nature of eruption
	• Within 24 hours of onset of fever
	• Centripetal rash, i.e. more on the body and less on the face and limbs
	• Superficial and more on flexor regions
	
	• Axilla involved
	• Rash appears in crops for 3–4 days
	• Vesicles are oval or elliptical
	• Rash in different stages occur simultaneously
	• Unilocular vesicles without umbilication, which collapse on puncture
	• Superficial scars which fade off
		• 3rd or 4th day of illness
		• Centrifugal, i.e. rash more on the face and extremities and less on the covered parts of the body
		• Deep-set in skin and more on extensor regions and bony prominences
		• Axilla usually free
		• Rash comes out as a single crop during 1–2 days
		• Vesicles are round
		• Rash is in the same stage all over
		• Multilocular and umbilicated vesicles, do not collapse on puncture
		• Deep permanent scarring

gabapentin intense antiviral therapy parenterally and glucocorticoids along with antiviral therapy.

Patients with pneumonia may require ventilatory support and intensive care. Neurological complications of chickenpox may be associated with worse prognosis in terms of mortality and morbidity.

Prophylaxis

Spread of infection can be prevented by isolation of the patient and heat sterilization of contaminated articles. Immunosuppressed children who are exposed to chickenpox should be given protective immunoglobulin. Varicella-zoster immune globulin (VariZIG) prepared from pooled human plasma contains antibodies against varicella and when given in a dose of 12.5 units/kg body weight within 72 hours of exposure it gives passive immunity. Secondary bacterial infection should be treated with antibacterial agents.

Live attenuated varicella zoster virus (VZV) vaccines are available for use in special situations. The vaccine is prepared by growing the attenuated virus in human diploid cells. It may be given to children after the age of 1 year.

Age	Dose
1 year to 12 years	0.5 mL subcutaneous injection
Above 12 years	0.5 mL two doses at an interval of 6–10 weeks in between vaccination is indicated for children who are likely to undergo immunosuppressive therapy

It is available commercially as Varilrix (SmithKline and Beecham). Vaccination should be avoided during pregnancy and within one month of measles vaccination. Pregnancy has to be avoided for three months after chickenpox vaccination. Immunity persists for two decades or more. A second dose of vaccine boosts up immunity.

Vaccination protects against incidence of varicella and also reduces the occurrence of severe cases. Efficacy of one dose vaccination is only 65.41%. Two doses of varicella vaccine are recommended for protection (94.9–99.5%).

Varicella vaccine can be given separately or combined with MMR vaccine. Such vaccines have been licensed in European countries. Adverse effects of vaccination include injection site redness and fever.

Source: Prymula R, Bergsaker MR, Esposito S, et al. Protection against varicella with two doses of combined measles-mumps-rubella-varicella vaccine versus one dose of monovalent varicella vaccine: a multicentre, observer-blind, randomised, controlled trial. Lancet. 2014;383(9925):1313-24.

HERPES ZOSTER

Syn: Shingles

General Considerations

Herpes zoster is an acute eruptive disorder characterized by painful radiculitis and vesicular eruptions in the corresponding dermatomes. It is seen more commonly seen in subjects above the age of 40 years. Chickenpox and herpes zoster are caused by the same virus, the latter occurs in persons who have acquired partial immunity. Following the episode of chickenpox, the VZV becomes latent in ganglia along the entire neuraxis, particularly the trigeminal ganglia and the dorsal root ganglia, remaining mainly in the cytoplasm of the neurons. Later the perineural cells of the ganglia are also involved. The virus persists in non-infectious form with intermittent periods of reactivation and shedding. The exact factors leading to reactivation are not fully known. The virus can be isolated from these tissues by appropriate methods. Attacks of herpes zoster are often precipitated by immunodeficiency states, hematological or neurological malignancies or trauma. Involvement of the cerebral arteries by VZV produces unifocal or multifocal vasculopathy, i.e. granulomatous arteritis. The localized form occurs in immunocompetent and the multifocal form occurs in immunocompromised subjects. This usually occurs after reactivation from the ganglia. This virus travels transaxonally to involve the cerebral arteries. This leads to vascular occlusion and stroke. Intensive IV administration of acyclovir helps to resolve the lesion when used along with other supportive measures.

Clinical Features

The eruption has an abrupt onset after a prodromal illness characterized by malaise, fever and severe pain in the corresponding dermatomes lasting for 3–4 days. The pain may be lancinating, deep-boring, burning or vague and in many cases it is unbearable. The common sites for the eruptions are the ophthalmic and maxillary divisions of the trigeminal nerve, geniculate ganglion of the facial nerve and thoracic and abdominal nerve roots.

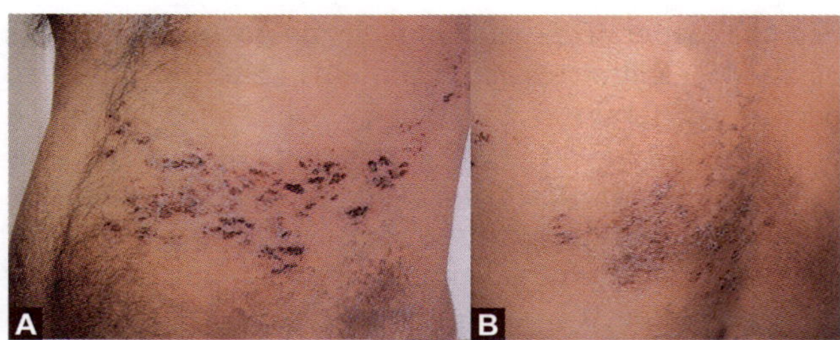

Figs 53.4A and B: Herpes vesicles. ***Note:*** The dermatomal pattern (A) front and (B) back

After a variable period of pre-eruptive neuralgia, the rash begins as reddish papules which soon develop central vesiculation. The vesicular fluid becomes turbid in three days and crust formation occurs after a week. The rash may involve a whole dermatome or only parts of it. The eruptions seldom cross the midline (Figs 53.4A and B).

With the formation of pustules the initial pain may subside, but in many elderly patients it may persist in the same form or in an altered form for months or even years. This is referred to as ***postherpetic neuralgia.*** Vague paresthesia, varying degrees of sensory loss and even lesser degree of motor loss may persist over the affected segments for considerable periods. In general the condition is benign, but the development of neuralgia may lead to severe distress and even suicidal tendencies in susceptible subjects. Incidence of postherpetic neuralgia is more in elderly subjects (9–34%) with severe prodromal symptoms and painful confluent lesions. VZV involvement of CNS is accompanied by high leukocyte count in the CSF. Presence of virus in CSF detectable by PCR.

Complications

- ***Secondary infection:*** The vesicles may be infected by bacteria, giving rise to fever. Deep scarring may occur.
- ***Ophthalmic herpes:*** In herpes involving ophthalmic division of the trigeminal nerve, keratitis may develop. Optic neuritis and oculomotor palsy may occur less commonly.
- Herpes of the geniculate ganglion presents as facial nerve palsy and vesicles over the ipsilateral external auditory meatus (Ramsay Hunt syndrome). Generally the facial nerve palsy tends to persist. Zoster occurring in the distribution of the maxillary and mandibular divisions of the trigeminal nerve may lead to osteo-necrosis and spontaneous less of the teeth.
- Paralysis of muscles corresponding to the involved spinal segment is a rare sequel. Cervical herpes zoster may give rise to weakness of the arm. Encephalitis and myelitis have been reported rarely.
- In leukemic subjects and those on immunosup-pressant therapy extensive vesiculation may develop (generalized herpes).
- ***Pregnancy:*** The fetus may be infected and this may lead to congenital malformations.
- Postherpetic neuralgia.
- VZV vasculopathy and strokes.

Diagnosis and Differential Diagnosis

Once the eruption has occurred over the sensory root distribution, diagnosis becomes easy. Before the onset of the eruption, the preherpetic neuralgia may be mistaken for other serious conditions depending on its location. These include trigeminal neuralgia, vascular headache, painful ophthalmic problems, MI, pleurisy, cholecystitis, appendicitis or any surgical abdominal emergency. Careful examination of the part in bright light may show at least erythematous rashes in many cases and this should suggest the diagnosis. Examination of the serum and CSF may reveal anti-VZV IgG in serum and CSF, the levels being relatively higher in CSF. Even in cases with clear-cut diagnosis, an attempt should be made to bring out an underlying malignancy like lymphoma or carcinoma, especially in the elderly subjects.

Specific Treatment

Immunocompetent individuals: Acyclovir 800 mg orally five times a day for 7–10 days. A new drug famciclovir is a more effective analogue given in a dose of 250 mg tid orally for 5–7 days. If started early, it may even prevent the occurrence of postherpetic neuralgia.

Immunocompromised individuals: Acyclovir 500 mg/m^2 IV eighth hourly for 7 days. Steroid should be given only under cover of acyclovir.

Local treatment consists of keeping the area dry and clean. Analgesics like aspirin and dextropropoxyphene are required in the eruptive stage. A short course of adrenocorticotropic hormone (ACTH) or prednisolone has been recommended in the elderly patients with a view to prevent postherpetic neuralgia. Opinions are divided on this issue. The risk of dissemination of infection is a real danger.

Preherpetic neuralgia: This develops in herpes zoster before the appearance of the rash. This is due to ganglionitis. The area of pain and site of rash usually coincide in most of the cases, but not always so. Aseptic meningitis and acute meningoencephalitis may occur with the occurrence of the rash.

Postherpetic neuralgia: The most troublesome comp-lication of herpes zoster is postherpetic neuralgia. Age is the most important single factor to predict its occurrence. There is no reliable method to prevent the neuralgia.

Treatment: It consists of administration of analgesics, tricyclic antidepressants and anticonvulsants. The pain is often refractory to analgesics. Diphenylhydantoin (300–400 mg/day), carbamazepine (200–1000 mg/day) and tricyclic compounds (amitriptyline, imipramine and doxepin) have been used with some benefit. Other therapeutic modalities like transcutaneous nerve stimulation (TNS) have benefitted some patients. Aspirin dissolved in chloroform and allowed to evaporate topically reduces pain. Capscicine applied as ointment over the affected segment may bring about relief. Early specific treatment of herpes zoster reduces the chance for neuralgia.

Zoster sine herpete

- This condition is characterized by recurrent severe shooting pains, but no vesicular eruptions. The diagnosis can only be made based on rising titers of antibody to VZV.
- Characteristic localization of pain to a dermatome with serologic evidence of herpes zoster, in the absence of skin lesion is diagnostic.

Prevention

Efficacy of adjuvanted herpes zoster subunit vaccine in older adults.

A varicella-zoster recombinant subunit vaccine containing varicella zoster glycoprotein E and the AS01$_\beta$ adjuvant system (called Hz/su) is being put to phase 3 trails. The vaccine reduces the risk of herpes zoster in adults above 50 years. It is given as IM injection 2 doses at an interval of two months, over the deltoid muscle. Efficacy is 96–98%, the duration of immunity is being observed.

Source: Lal H, Cunningham AL, Godeaux O, et al. Efficacy of an adjuvanted herpes zoster subunit vaccine in older adults. N Engl J Med. 2015;372(22):2087-96.

Live attenuated vaccine against herpes zoster (Zostavax-Merck) containing the Oka strain VZV is licensed for use in adults. It reduces the risk of herpes zoster in adults above 50 years. With advancing age, the efficacy is less (only 38% above 70 years). The vaccine also reduces the incidence of postherpetic neuralgia by 66%. Duration of protection is 8–10 years. Live attenuated vaccine is contraindicated in immunocompromised individuals.

HERPES SIMPLEX VIRUS (HSV)

Syn: Herpes febrilis, Fever blister, Cold sore

General Considerations

Infection by **HSV**, also known as **Herpesvirus hominis (HVH)**, produces recurrent crops of vesicles over the mucocutaneous regions. The virus remains in the skin and nerve ganglia in the dormant form to be activated periodically to give rise to recurrent eruptions. Herpes viruses are DNA viruses and the pathogenic types are two different antigenic variants herpes simplex virus type 1 (HSV 1) and herpes simplex virus type 2 (HSV 2). The former causes lesions around the mouth, noses, cornea and conjunctiva and around the nails—herpetic whitlows. This is a non-venereal infection. HSV 2 (herpes genitalis) is a sexually transmitted disease (STD) described in Chapter 48.

Clinical Features

Fever, exposure to sunlight, physical or emotional stress, malignancy and immunosuppressant drugs lead to exacerbation. Fevers, especially pneumonia, malaria and meningitis are commonly associated with herpes labialis. HSV is rare in enteric fevers. A crop of vesicles develop following a short period of tingling pain and paresthesia over the affected region. The vesicles remain for 7–10 days after which they start to heal with the formation of crusts. Healing is complete in 21 days. When the crusts fall off, thin scars persist for some time. Common sites of eruption are around the mouth and external nares. Less commonly HSV keratitis, recurrent gingivostomatitis and vulvovaginitis may occur. HSV can cause mild fever.

Serious complications may occur in susceptible persons and in immunosuppressed subjects. These include HSV encephalitis and **Kaposi's varicelliform eruptions (KVE) (eczema herpeticum)**. HSV encephalitis may lead to necrosis of the temporal lobe and rise in intracranial tension. KVE develops in infants and adults with eczema. In such subjects the eruptions become generalized and this leads to excessive loss of fluid, electrolytes and proteins. Herpes tends to become generalized in subjects who have sustained burns. Generalized HSV occurring in wrestlers is called **herpes gladiatorum**. HSV pneumonia occurs in immunocompromised hosts.

HSV infection is more serious in pregnancy especially after 31 weeks of gestation. HSV hepatitis and dissemination of infection occurs. Case fatality rate is about 39% for the mother and the neonate.

Diagnosis

HSV has to be differentiated from pustular or vesicular rashes and herpes zoster; the latter is nonrecurrent. HSV can be isolated from the vesicle fluid. Serological diagnosis is by demonstrating complement fixing antibodies. In HSV encephalitis the virus can be demonstrated in CSF by PCR.

Treatment

Local lesions which are benign may be left alone with simple cleaning and application of gentian violet. Topical idoxuridine (0.1% hourly as drops or 0.5% ointment) is effective in herpetic keratitis. Acyclovir ointment is available for local use over the vesicles. This gives relief of pain and prevents recurrence. In severe cases and complicated cases systemic therapy with acyclovir has to be given. Dose is 800 mg orally 5 times a day for 5 days. In case of HSV encephalitis, acyclovir should be given in a dose of 10 mg/kg bw IV 8 hour for 10–14 days. Forneonatal HSV infections the dose is 10 mg/kg bw IV for 10–14 days. Famciclovir 500 mg oral tds for 5 days is a suitable alternative.

Note: HSV2 infection (genital herpes) is described along with STDs in Chapter 48.

RUBELLA

Syn: German measles (three days measles)

Rubella is an exanthem caused by a RNA virus (50–85 nm in size) belonging to the family of togaviruses. The disease is characterized by mild constitutional symptoms and rash. Its importance is due to the risk of producing serious fetal abnormalities and abortion if it occurs in women during the early months of pregnancy, even though the illness it produces in adults is only mild.

Epidemiology

The infection spreads through droplets and entry is through the nasopharynx. Infective period starts one week before the onset of the rash and it lasts for one week after the rash fades. Virus is present in the nasopharyngeal secretion one week before the onset of the illness. In the early stage, viremia occurs. The virus reaches the fetus through the placenta and causes lesions in the fetus. The baby sheds the virus at birth and continues to be infective for 6–31 months. The disease is prevalent in the community and small epidemics may occur from time-to-time. Many cases may be subclinical. An attack confers lifelong immunity. In western countries it is estimated that 10–15% of adult women are susceptible to infection. In India the disease is not infrequent, though reliable statistical figures are not available.

Textbook of Medicine

Pathogenesis

The virus is present in blood up to two days before the onset of the rash. Lymph nodes are moderately enlarged, showing edema and hyperplasia. When the fetus is affected, the virus multiplies in the liver, spleen, bone marrow and all other tissues and leads to various structural malformations in the heart, nervous system, eyes and the limbs.

Once the fetus is infected, the infection persists throughout the pregnancy and up to the 12 months after birth. Such babies will be shedding the virus in oropharyngeal and nasal secretions, urine and body fluids. Such infants may form the starting point for small outbreaks of rubella.

Clinical Features

Rubella in Adults

The incubation period is usually 2–3 weeks. The onset is sudden with malaise, fever, rashes and characteristic enlargement of the occipital, posterior auricular and posterior cervical lymph nodes.

The rash which resembles that of measles begins on the face and neck and spreads to the trunk and limbs, but the rash is less extensive. Enanthem may occur consisting of discrete rose colored spots on the palate and fauces. The rash becomes discrete by the second day and it disappears in 3–4 days.

Compared to measles, constitutional symptoms are mild in children. In addition to fever and malaise, arthralgia, joint stiffness and headache may occur. Rarely serious neurological complications like encephalitis, encephalomyelopathy or polyneuropathy develop 5–10 days after the onset. Thrombocytopenia may develop in a few (Table 53.2).

Diagnosis

Clinically the disease should be suspected when fever, posterior cervical lymphadenopathy and rash occur in a young subject. Rubella has to be distinguished from measles, secondary stage of syphilis, drug rashes, infectious mononucleosis and echovirus, coxsackievirus and adenovirus infections. The leukocyte count is normal in rubella. Specific diagnosis is established by finding a four-fold increase in hemagglutination inhibition antibodies in paired sera or by isolating the virus from nasopharyngeal secretions and blood.

Table 53.2: Differential diagnosis between measles and rubella		
Symptoms	**Measles**	**Rubella**
Prodrome	Nasal congestion and cough more severe	Mild
Rash	Confluent reddish and pinkish maculopapular rash—slower progress and clearance	Discrete maculopapular—rapidly progressing and clearing
Temperature	Rises abruptly with rash	Does not rise abruptly with rash
Lymph nodes	Not characteristic	Retroauricular, posterior cervical or posterior occipital are characteristic
Koplik's spots	Pathognomonic	Nil

Congenital Rubella Syndrome

Rubella embryopathy results either from inhibition of cell growth or cellular necrosis. Fetal defects include retardation of growth, eye defects like cataract, glaucoma or retinopathy, congenital heart defects, nerve deafness, mental retardation, hepatosplenomegaly and skeletal abnormalities. Rubella occurring in women in the first 16 weeks of pregnancy leads to fetal malformation in up to 50–80% of cases. Miscarriages, premature delivery and fetal death may occur. In those who do not have the rubella embryopathy, the infant may show purpuric rash thrombocytopenia and extramedullary erythropoiesis particularly in the dermis without any congenital organ defect. Risk of fetal affection reduces if the infection is acquired later in pregnancy.

Active Rubella in Pregnant Women

Presence of IgG antibodies persisting throughout pregnancy indicates immunity in the mother. Rising titers of IgM and/or IgG antibodies (four-fold) during pregnancy indicates that the infection is acquired during pregnancy and the risk of fetal infection is high.

Congenital Rubella in the Baby

Presence of congenital defects such as cataracts, hearing defects and heart lesions should point to congenital rubella syndrome (CRS). Lab diagnosis is the same as for adults, several other intrauterine infections can lead to congenital defects in the baby and they should be considered before confirming rubella embryopathy.

The rubella antibody may persist for up to 1 year after birth without diminution. In affected children the IgG antibody persists for 1 year and beyond whereas in passive transfer of material antibody it fades off within 4–6 months. Rubella virus can be identified in infected babies by RT-PCR.

Treatment

As the disease is generally benign, it is desirable to acquire rubella before the child-bearing age. No specific treatment is indicated. Medical termination of pregnancy (MTP) has to be considered if there is proof of rubella infection in early pregnancy.

Prevention

Vaccination using live attenuated virus confers immunity. Live attenuated rubella virus RA 27/3 grown in human diploid fibroblast cells is effective, when given in a dose of 0.5 mL as a single injection. Vaccination confers solid immunity over 10 years. If facilities are available, vaccination should be considered for girls in the age group of 11–13 years and women in the child-bearing age who are antibody-negative and are desirous of child-bearing. The vaccine virus passes into the fetus and so pregnancy should be avoided for eight weeks following vaccination. Gamma globulin administered to the mother after exposure aborts an overt-attack, but safety of the fetus cannot be guaranteed. Ideal time for vaccination is after 12 months of age. The combined MMR vaccine takes care of rubella as well. In women while planning pregnancy, it is safe to give vaccination 2 months prior to the pregnancy.

CHAPTER
54

Mumps

KV Krishna Das

Chapter Summary

- General Considerations
- Pathology
- Clinical Features
  - Complications
  - Diagnosis
- Treatment
- Prevention

GENERAL CONSIDERATIONS

This common childhood infection is caused by mumps virus, which belongs to the group of paramyxoviruses. It is a ribonucleic acid (RNA) virus. The infection is worldwide in distribution and spreads through droplets. The disease runs a subclinical course in 30–40% of cases. Man is the only known host and the infection spreads directly from man-to-man. Infectivity rate among contacts is not high. Second attacks do not occur since mumps produces solid lifelong immunity.

PATHOLOGY

Organisms enter through the respiratory tract. The virus is present in the saliva from 7 days before to 8 days after the onset of parotitis. In susceptible hosts viral multiplication leads to viremia. Thereafter the virus localizes in several organs such as the salivary glands, pancreas, central nervous system (CNS), testes, ovaries, thyroid gland and others. The salivary glands are enlarged and histology shows mononuclear infiltration. Neurological lesions take the form of meningoencephalitis or encephalomyelitis. Testicular lesions include intense interstitial edema, perivascular lymphocytic exudate, focal hemorrhages and destruction of germinal epithelium, which may be patchy or generalized.

CLINICAL FEATURES

Incubation period is 18 days (range 12–21 days). Initial symptoms are fever, pain over the region of the parotid gland, especially on opening the jaw, trismus, dryness of the mouth and headache. Soon the parotids and less commonly the other salivary glands become tender and enlarged. Unlike suppurative parotitis, redness and edema are absent. Sialadenitis is usually bilateral, but rarely it may be unilateral (Fig. 54.1).

After 5–7 days the fever and glandular enlargement subside. In the uncomplicated case, there is leukopenia with relative lymphocytosis. A few atypical lymphocytes may be present. When complications occur, neutrophil leukocytosis may develop. Around 50% of cases show cerebrospinal fluid (CSF) pleocytosis.

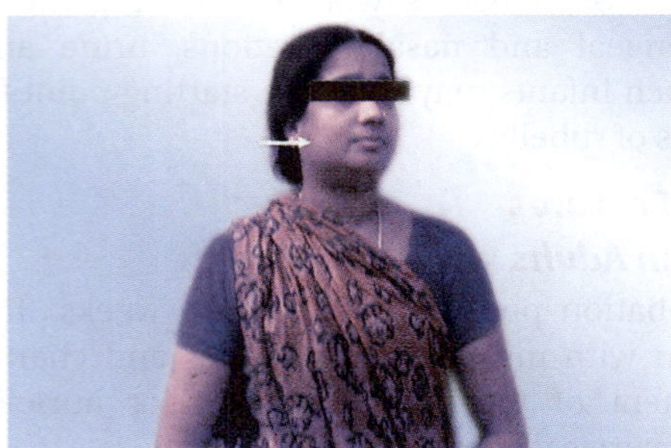

Fig. 54.1: Female mumps (arrow)

Complications

In the vast majority, the course is benign and uncomplicated. If the disease occurs in adult males, 25% develop unilateral or bilateral **orchitis**. The affected testes are red, swollen, tender and painful. Reactive hydrocele may develop. Sterility may follow bilateral involvement. **Oophoritis** may develop in women. Though parotitis is present in most of such cases, rarely gonadal lesions occur without obvious parotitis.

Pancreatitis should be suspected when patients with mumps complain of upper abdominal pain. In a few cases, serum amylase level may be increased. Pancreatitis usually subsides without sequel. Thyroiditis develops in some cases. The occurrence of *meningitis* is heralded by intense headache and signs of meningeal irritation. CSF shows lymphocytic pleocytosis. Encephalomyelitis is a rare complication. Arthritis follows the acute illness after 2–3 weeks. Mumps occurring in pregnancy is not associated with fetal or maternal complications.

Diagnosis

Bilateral enlargement of the parotid and other salivary glands with mild constitutional disturbances should suggest possibility of mumps. Diagnosis is easy during outbreaks, but it may be difficult when the presentation is atypical such as unilateral parotitis/meningitis. Mumps virus can be isolated from throat washings obtained 48 hours before 7 days after parotid swellings develop. Rise in antibody titers can be demonstrated in paired sera by complement fixation, hemagglutination inhibition/ELISA. Polymerase chain reaction (PCR) helps to identify the viral antigens.

TREATMENT

Symptomatic treatment consists of analgesics and antipyretics in addition to bed rest. This is all that is required in most of the cases. Troublesome dryness of the mouth can be relieved by frequent sips of water.

When orchitis is present, local dressing with ichthammol glycerin and supportive bandage give

Textbook of Medicine

relief. Prednisolone 40 mg daily for 4–7 days may help in reducing the inflammation. The meningitis also subsides with symptomatic measures. Corticosteroids produce early clinical improvement though there is no objective benefit demonstrated by controlled studies.

PREVENTION

Specific prophylactic measures are not generally required, since the infection runs a benign course and produces lasting immunity. A live attenuated vaccine (*Jeryl-Lynn strain*) is available for administration along with measles, mumps and rubella (MMR) vaccines. This produces a noncommunicable subclinical infection. The vaccine is administered to children above the age of 13 months. MMR vaccines can be given together as a single injection safely between the ages of 13–15 months. Booster doses are not required. Rarely fever, rashes and seizures may occur as adverse reactions.

CHAPTER

55

Viral Hepatitis

KV Krishna Das, KR Vinaya Kumar

Chapter Summary

- General Considerations
- Hepatitis A Virus (HAV)
- Hepatitis B Virus (HBV)
- Hepatitis C Virus (HCV)
- Pathogenesis and Pathology
- General Clinical Features
  - Special Characteristics of HCV
- Hepatitis Delta Virus (HDV)
- Hepatitis E Virus (HEV)
- Hepatitis G Virus (HGV)
- Investigations Common to all the Hepatitis Viruses
- Complications and Sequelae
- Diagnosis of Viral Hepatitis
  - Salient Features of Different Hepatic Lesions resembling Viral Hepatitis
- Prognosis
- Management
  - Treatment of HBV
  - Treatment of HCV
  - Prophylaxis

GENERAL CONSIDERATIONS

Several viruses can cause the syndrome of acute viral hepatitis. This is characterized by diffuse inflammation of the liver as the predominant feature. Five viruses are mainly responsible for the vast majority of cases—hepatitis A virus (HAV), hepatitis B virus (HBV), hepatitis C virus (HCV), hepatitis delta virus (HDV) and hepatitis E virus (HEV).

HAV and HEV are transmitted predominantly through fecal-oral (enteric) route. The others are transmitted parenterally. Viruses A and E produce acute hepatitis. Chronicity and delayed damage to the liver are very rare. On the other hand HBV causes both acute and chronic hepatitis, the latter develops in 5% of cases. In the case of Hepatitis C, 80% of patients develop chronic infection and 3–11% of them with chronic HCV infection will develop liver cirrhosis within 20 years with associated risks of liver failure and hepatocellular carcinoma. HDV is exceptional in that it can exist only in the presence of HBV infection. It acts as a co-infecting agent and modifies the clinical picture and outcome in HBV hepatitis. The problems of hepatitis viruses in terms of infectivity, morbidity, mortality and economic loss and loss of quality of life have been recognized by the World Health Organization (WHO) and 28th of July every year has been designated as *World Hepatitis Day.*

Several other viruses cause hepatic lesions in addition to lesions in other parts of the body. These include cytomegalovirus, *Epstein-Barr virus*, herpes simplex, varicella zoster, dengue, yellow fever, rubella, hemorrhagic fever viruses, human immunodeficiency virus (HIV) and others (Table 55.1).

HEPATITIS A VIRUS (HAV)

It is a single stranded ribonucleic acid (RNA) virus belonging to the genus *Hepatovirus*. There are four genotypes of the virus showing antigenic cross reactivity.

It is present in feces of cases from 2 weeks before the onset of the symptoms. Infection is by the fecal-oral route. In tropical countries and in communities where food hygiene is low, this infection is prevalent and vast majority of sufferers are children. Contamination of drinking water supply with sewage is responsible for several outbreaks from time-to-time. Most of the adults acquire immunity due to subclinical infection or overt disease. They show the presence of specific antibody which is protective. With improvement in hygiene, the disease becomes less common in children and older age groups are affected more. Other methods of transmission include oral-anal sexual contact in homosexual men and rarely the parenteral route if the blood donor incubates the infection. The incubation period varies from 2–6 weeks. This virus has been grown in tissue culture. This infection does not become chronic. HAV used to be known as short-incubation hepatitis. HAV is relatively acid stable, it resists drying and can remain for at least a month under room temperature. The virus multiplies in the liver and is passed

Table 55.1: Important features of the viruses primarily causing hepatitis

	HAV	HBV	HCV	HDV	HEV	HGV
Type of virus	RNA	DNA	RNA	RNA	RNA	RNA
Source of infection	Fecal-oral, rarely parenteral	Parenteral, sexual and mother to baby	Parenteral, rarely sexual and mother to baby	Parenteral	Fecal-oral, rarely parenteral	Parenteral
Incubation period (weeks)	2–6	8–48	2–22	4–8	2–9	–
Onset of clinical illness	Acute	Insidious	Insidious	Acute	Acute	Possibly a passenger virus
Presence of jaundice	50%	33%	25%		20%	
Diagnostic markers	IgM HAV	HBsAg	Anti-HCV IgM	Anti-HDV IgM	Anti-HEV	HGV RNA
Establishment of chronic carrier state	Nil	5–10%	Up to 60%	Vast majority	Nil	–
Vertical transmission	–	+	+	+	–	–
Chronic hepatitis	Very rare	5%	30–50%	70%	Rare	–
Fulminant hepatitis	0.1%	Up to 1%	Not known	Up to 17%	Up to 10% in pregnant women	
Vaccination	Available	Available	No	–	No	No

Abbreviations: HAV = Hepatitis A virus; HBV = Hepatitis B virus; HCV = Hepatitis C virus; HDV = Hepatitis delta virus; HEV = Hepatitis E virus; HGV = Hepatitis G virus; RNA = Ribonucleic acid; DNA = Deoxyribonuleic acid; IgM = Imunoglobulin M; HBsAG = Hepatitis B surface antigen

into bile 2–3 weeks before the onset of jaundice and the feces contains the virus. Maximal infectivity is during the later part of the incubation period. Once jaundice occurs infectivity comes down even though the virus is present in feces. The initial antibody response is immunoglobulin M (IgM) anti-HAV. This runs parallel to serum transaminase levels. After the eighth week, the levels come down. Immunoglobulin G (IgG) anti-HAV rises during recovery and this confers life-long immunity. Radioimmunoassay (RIA) and enzyme linked immunosorbent assay (ELISA) tests are available for detecting these antibodies. Polymerase chain reaction (PCR) test can identify the virus specifically and distinguish between the different hepatotropic viruses.

HEPATITIS B VIRUS (HBV)

HBV is the prototype member of the Hepadnaviridae [hepatotropic deoxyribonucleic acid (DNA) virus]. It is 42 nm in diameter. Chronic hepatitis B affects 350 million people, approximately 5% of the world population. Carrier state of the virus ranges from 0.1 to 20% in different parts of the world. Prevalence has been classified as high (> 8% of population affected), intermediate (2–7%) and low (< 2%). Prenatal transmission is high in prevalence areas.

In India, the prevalence ranges from 1.2 to 12.2%, the average carrier rate is 3.34%. Eight genotypes A–H have been identified and the prevalence in different geographical areas varies. In India, A and D genotypes are more prevalent. The different genotypes vary in their pathogenicity, especially in severity, chronicity and oncogenic potential. Mothers who are chronic carries of infection and those who develop acute hepatitis B in the last trimester transmit the disease to their babies in the perinatal period. If the hepatitis B surface antigen (HBsAg) and hepatitis Be antigen (HBeAg) are positive, the chances for transmission exceeds 90%. Infection is acquired by the infant during its passage through the vagina and inoculation of mother's blood and liquor amnii. Infection acquired during the neonatal period leads to chronicity in > 90% of cases, whereas infection acquired during adult life leads to chronicity only in 5–10% of cases. HBV transmission to fetus can also occur transplacentally. The viral load in the mother correlates with the frequency of transmission. HBe positive mothers transmit the disease more readily to their infants than HBe negative women.

HBV spreads by parenteral introduction of the infective agent along with blood or blood products or through needle pricks. In communities where the carrier rate is low (1 in 1000 or less), HBV infection is seen in special population groups such as newborns of carrier mothers, homosexuals, drug addicts and personnel working in dialysis units and laboratories. Since the virus is present in semen, it can also spread by hetero- or homosexual intercourse. In homosexuals, the transmission rate is high. Risk factors include multiple casual sexual partners, anal intercourse and a high carrier rate among these subjects. Oral-to-oral spread occurs by kissing, since the virus is present in saliva. Accidental contamination by infected blood can transmit the disease. In India, the main mode of transmission is horizontal—from child to child or adult to adult. Other than the liver and plasma, the virus may be present in saliva, tears, vaginal secretions, semen, breast milk, sweat and urine. It is highly infectious. Infection is by parenteral route or contact with abraded skin or mucosal surfaces. Risk of infection from needle stick injures in healthcare workers is as high as 30%. HBsAg was positive in 5–10% in drug addicts in 29 countries and >10% in 10 countries. Worldwide 6.4 million injecting drug users (IDUs) are anti-HBV core antigen positive (CI 2.3–9.7 millions) and 1.2 million (0.3–2.7 millions) are HBsAg positive.

This risk of transmission can be prevented by immunization. Gastric acid and pancreatic enzymes destroy the virus. It is demonstrable in sera of patients many weeks before the acute illness and it may be demonstrable for 3 months or more after clinical recovery.

Viral Morphology

The virus consists of a central core consisting of hepatitis B core antigen (HBcAg), HBeAg, a specific DNA polymerase and a circular DNA (HBV DNA). Under electron microscope the virus is seen as spherical particles called ***Dane particles***. The virus consists of a lipoprotein outer coat which is secreted in excess by hepatocytes and released into serum. Presence of excess of envelope antigen HBsAg is a special feature of HBV. This surface antigen circulates in the plasma in the form of rods or spheres with a diameter of 22 nm. This is detectable as HBsAg 1–10 weeks after infection and 2–8 weeks before onset of symptoms. This is diagnostic of the presence of infection. Some cases of HBV hepatitis do not show HBsAg in blood, even though the viral genome may be demonstrable. HBsAg is itself not infective to others. HBsAg was described in 1965 first by Blumberg in the blood of an Australian aboriginal and was hence termed as Australian antigen. HBsAg can be detected by RIA or ELISA tests. Its presence is pathognomonic of recent or chronic HBV infection. With the onset of clinically detectable hepatitis and jaundice, the level of HBsAg falls. Clearance of HBsAg indicates resolution of infection.

Immune Markers of HBV Infection

Antibodies to HBsAg develop (anti-HBs) and these may be IgM and IgG in serum and IgA in secretions. These antibodies provide immunity to future infection by HBV. IgM is short lived, whereas IgG antibody persists. Anti-HBs antibody (anti-HBsAb) can be estimated to detect protective immunity. These are detectable in patients who recover from the disease and in these who are successfully vaccinated. Antibody levels above 10 μIU/mL are protective.

Antibodies to other HBV components develop in due course. HBcAg is not detectable in serum, but with the onset of clinical illness anti-HBc IgM (IgM antibody to core antigen) appears and remains elevated throughout the course of the disease. Detection of anti-HBc IgM is diagnostic of HBV hepatitis. This also helps to rule out superinfection in an HBV carrier by other hepatitis viruses. Anti-HBc IgM is the only serological marker of HBV infection when HBsAg has disappeared and anti-HBsAg has not reached detectable levels. Anti-HBcAb is not a neutralizing antibody and therefore it is not protective. Initial antibody is IgM type later it is replaced by IgG

type. Persistence of anti-HBc IgG in high titer indicates continuing infection.

HBeAg is a circulating peptide derived from the core genome and transported from liver cells. HBe positive mothers transmit the disease more readily to their infants (73%) than HBe negative mothers (13%).

Detection of HBeAg indicates active replication of the virus and presence of infective agent in the liver. HBeAg appears within 1 week of appearance of HBsAg and disappears within 4 weeks of onset of symptoms. Persistence of HBeAg beyond 10 weeks should suggest progression to a carrier state and it may also portend the development of chronic hepatitis. In those who overcome the infection, antibody to HBe (anti-HBe) appears within 4 weeks of onset of symptoms. Presence of anti-HBe suggests good immunological response and chance of recovery.

Presence of virus in blood is demonstrable directly by the presence of circulating viral DNA (HBV DNA). In India, about 25% of HBsAg + subjects show also HCV positivity. Coexistent hepatitis C infection suppresses markers of HBV replication.

HBV DNA and DNA polymerase appear in the serum at the same time as HBeAg. These also are markers of HBV replication and potential infectivity. HBV DNA is detected by PCR. Levels of HBV DNA correlate with transaminase levels and HBsAg in the serum.

HBV infection is tolerated by the body and once infection occurs, 5–10% become chronic carriers. ***Younger the age of getting the infection, greater is the chance of developing carrier state. In vertical transmission from mother to newborn, the carrier state may develop in 80–90%, whereas in transmission in adult life the chances are less.*** Most of the carriers tolerate the virus which replicates in the liver. They show HBsAg positivity and viremia, but at the same time do not suffer from the disease. They are the main source of spread to others. This state may persist lifelong. Risk of primary carcinoma of the liver is high in them and many of the cases of liver cell cancer occurring in young adults, especially in India and other neighboring countries are attributable to HBV.

The lifecycle of HBV can be divided into four stages (Table 55.2):

1. ***Stage 1:*** Immune tolerance occurs. Viral replication occurs even without elevation of hepatic serum

Table 55.2: Four stages of hepatitis B infections

Disease marker	Replicative phase		Integrative phase	
	Stage 1	Stage 2	Stage 3	Stage 4
HBsAg	Positive	Positive	Positive	Negative
Antibody to HBsAg	Negative	Negative	Negative	Positive
HBV DNA	Strongly positive	Positive	Negative	Negative
Antibody HBcAg	Positive	Positive	Positive	Positive
HBeAg	Positive	Positive	Negative	Negative
Antibody to HBeAg	Negative	Negative	Positive	Positive
Aspartate and alanine aminotransferase levels	Normal	Elevated	Normal	Normal

Abbreviations: HBsAG = Hepatitis B surface antigen; HBV = Hepatitis B virus; DNA = Deoxyribonuleic acid; HBcAg = hepatitis B core antigen; HBeAg = Hepatitis Be antigen

Textbook of Medicine

glutamic-pyruvic transaminase (SGPT). This is the incubation period. HBeAg and HBV DNA levels in serum are high.

2. **Stage 2:** Immunological response develops leading to production of cytokines, direct cell lysis and the inflammatory process. Secretion of HBsAg continues. This is the stage of active symptomatic hepatitis. This may last for 2–4 weeks. In those with chronic hepatitis, this stage may extend to several years, leading to cirrhosis and its complications. If the host is able to mount an immune response that eliminates the infected hepatocytes, active viral replication ends and this marks the onset of the third stage.

3. **Stage 3:** This is the stage at which the bulk of the virus infected cells have been cleared. At this stage HBeAg is no longer detectable but anti-HBeAb becomes demonstrable. Viral DNA levels drop even through PCR may still be able to detect it. In most cases the infection is cleared and the SGPT levels become normal. However HBs positivity may still persist, presumably because of the integration of the viral genome with that of the hepatocyte.

4. **Stage 4:** At this stage the virus is cleared and protective antibody is abundant. Most patients eventually become negative for HBsAg and positive for anti-HBsAg (HBsAb). HBV DNA is no longer detectable and the patient is immune to further infection.

The factors affecting the stage wise progression of the infection and the ultimate outcome include:

- Genetic predisposition of the host
- Co-infection with other virus (hepatitis C and D)
- Treatment with immunosuppressant drugs
- The appearance of HBV mutants.

HEPATITIS C VIRUS (HCV)

This was first identified in 1989. It is an RNA virus belonging to the family flaviviridae. At least six genotypes, HCV 1 to HCV 6 are identified and subtypes are denoted by letters A, B, etc. In India, HCV 3 is more prevalent. In voluntary blood donors in West Bengal, the prevalence rate was 1.8%, in Chandigarh it was 2.8% and in Delhi it was 1.85%. The genotypes determine the response to treatment. Types 2 and 3 are more responsive to pegylated interferon (PEG-IFN) and ribavirin (85%) whereas the others are less so (48%). Genotype 1b is most aggressive in course and least amenable to drugs.

The virus is present in blood, tissue fluids, saliva, vaginal secretions and semen of infected persons. Infection is acquired mainly by parenteral route. Transfusion of blood and blood products and sharing of contaminated needles for injection account for more than 85% of cases. Sexual transmission occurs from unprotected sexual intercourse. Male to female transmission by the sexual route is more efficient and infection rate is 1.6% among sexual partners. As in the case of hepatitis B, chronic IDU form a major reservoir of hepatitis C virus. Sixty to eighty percent of IDUs have anti-HCV in 25 countries and greater than 80% in 12 countries. About 10 million IDUs (range 6–15 million) worldwide may be anti-HCV positive. China (1.6 million), USA (1.5 million) and Russia (1.3 million) have the largest number. IDUs have anti-HCV more frequently than HIV infection. Co-infection with HIV enhances the rate of sexual transmission. Healthcare staff gets infection by entry of the virus through contamination by blood and body fluids coming into contact with cuts and wounds or needle stick injuries. Infection rates among healthcare workers are 0.6 to 4.5%. Hemodialysis patients have infection rates ranging from 0.6 to 4.5%. Perinatal transmission rate is 2–3%. In general HCV is less infectious compared to HBV.

The course of HCV is progressive if untreated. Unlike HBV, more than 80% of cases develop chronic hepatitis. Of these 20–50% develops cirrhosis over a period of 10–20 years. Twenty-five percent among these cirrhotic patients may develop hepatocellular carcinoma. In contrast to HBV, HCV infection acquired during childhood runs a more benign course than that in adults. Older age, alcoholism and co-infection with HBV and HIV increase the risk of diseases progression and chance of developing decompensated cirrhosis. In thalassemic children with iron overload, HCV runs a more aggressive course.

After infection by HCV, the viral RNA becomes detectable in serum within 1–2 weeks. Thirty percent of cases are anicteric, 85% go into chronicity. The natural history of HCV infection is variable. In more than 60%, the infection persists and the virus is demonstrable in blood for over 5 years; 10% may recover completely.

PATHOGENESIS AND PATHOLOGY

The hepatitis viruses cause injury to liver cells by direct invasion and immunological processes. Under most circumstances, HBV and other viruses by themselves do not kill the hepatocytes. An intact immune system is necessary to cause cell injury as well as ultimate clearance of the virus. Immune complexes appear in blood prior to the onset of liver injury. They may account for the serum sickness like syndrome observed in the early phase. Cellular immunity also plays a role in altering the host's response to the virus and the progression to the chronic carrier state. For practical purposes, the severity of hepatocyte injury also reflects the vigor of the immune response. The most complete immune response is also associated with the chance of viral clearance and full recovery.

The lesions caused by viruses A, B and others are all similar. In uncomplicated hepatitis, the essential lesions are ballooning of hepatocytes, acidophilic degeneration leading to the presence of **Councilman bodies** and focal necrosis or cell dropouts. Changes are more pronounced in the centrizonal regions. There is infiltration by small lymphocytes, plasma cells and eosinophils, most marked in the portal regions. Kupffer cells undergo hyperplasia. Many large multinucleated hepatocytes are formed. There is also a variable degree of cholestasis. The pathological changes are seen diffusely involving all the lobules.

Necrosis of liver cells is a prominent feature in severe cases. Necrosis involving many adjacent hepatocytes is described as **confluent necrosis**. The term **submassive necrosis** is used to denote necrosis involving several adjacent lobules. The necrosis may extend between adjacent central zones, portal zones or between adjacent central and portal zones. If the reticulum is intact, full regeneration is possible and recovery is complete. If the reticulum collapses, collagenous tissue is laid down and this leads to fibrosis, which bridges adjacent zones. These cases have a more unfavorable prognosis and many of them progress to subacute necrosis or to chronic hepatitis and cirrhosis. When necrosis is submassive or massive and fulminant, the liver shrinks in size and this carries a grave prognosis. With the onset of recovery, regenerative changes and Kupffer cell activity become evident.

HBV and HCV predispose to cirrhosis and carcinoma. In India, posthepatitic cirrhosis is caused mainly by HBV and also by HCV. In endemic areas with a high carrier rate, chance for vertical transmission of the virus from mother to child, primary carcinoma of the liver occurring in young adults may be a late sequel to these infections (*See* Section 9, Ch 88, 'Chronic HBV Hepatitis').

GENERAL CLINICAL FEATURES

Hepatitis presents a clinical spectrum ranging from mild and inapparent infection to the most serious, fulminant and rarely fatal acute hepatic failure. Subclinical infection is recognized by the rise in antibody titer during epidemics. In many others, clinical illness without jaundice may develop. In these cases of anicteric hepatitis, prodromal symptoms and biochemical abnormalities may develop but jaundice may not occur. Such anicteric cases far outnumber the icteric cases during epidemics. As a general rule the onset of HAV hepatitis is more acute than that of HBV. The onset of the other viral infections is generally similar, but variable in intensity. The clinical picture is similar, but HBV and HDV hepatitis tends to be more severe.

Prodromal Symptoms

The classic attack of viral hepatitis is heralded by a prodromal phase which lasts for three to five days or longer, before the onset of jaundice.

The prodrome consists of general malaise, headache, fatigue, nausea, vomiting and mild pyrexia. Severe anorexia and aversion for smoking and alcohol are characteristic. Symmetrical non-migrating polyarthritis with or without effusions may occur in 15% of cases. Features like anosmia, dysosmia, hypogeusia or dysgeusia, urticaria, maculopapular rashes, polyarteritis and thrombophlebitis may occur less commonly.

The Icteric Phase

The prodromal phase is followed by the icteric phase (Fig. 55.1). Urine becomes deep yellow and the stools pale in color with the appearance of jaundice. Nausea and vomiting subside and appetite returns. The patient becomes afebrile and feels better. Transient pruritus might appear. Discomfort in the right hypochondrium may be felt. Liver may be moderately enlarged and mildly tender. Spleen is enlarged in 20% of cases. The jaundice deepens over the first 1 or 2 weeks, after which it gradually subsides to clear up in 3–4 weeks. Initially the jaundice is hepatocellular in type, later it becomes obstructive. Convalescence may be prolonged in many cases. HBV and HCV may produce symptoms related to other systems

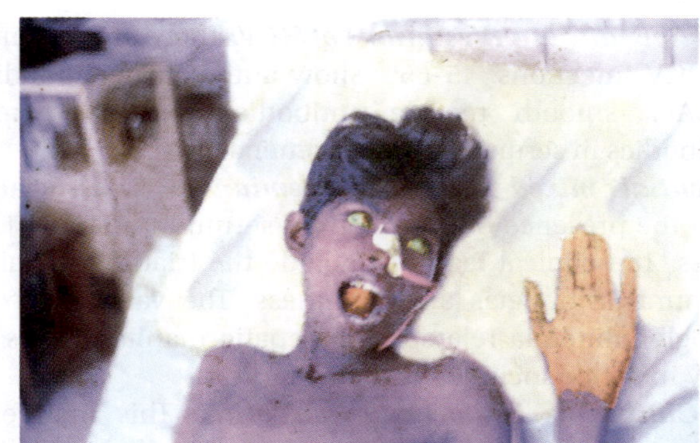

Fig. 55.1: Obstructive jaundice in viral hepatitis

such as arthralgia and arthritis, lymph node enlargement and skin rashes, glomerulonephritis, keratoconjunctivitis and others.

Stage of Recovery

In most of the cases clinical and biochemical recovery is complete within 4 to 6 months of the onset of jaundice. Loss of weight, general weakness and vague ill health may persist for varying periods in many.

Special Characteristics of HCV

The three types of clinical presentation are:

1. Florid stage with high viremia
2. Symptomless carriage with low viremia
3. Recovery without viremia—this occurs only in a few.

In contrast to HBV—there is no state of immune tolerance. Liver shows subacute or chronic lesions varying in severity. Hepatitis C is a very common cause for hepatic transplantation in many areas. Often the graft also gets infected by hepatitis C.

Acute HCV infection: It is asymptomatic in many, except for the presence of elevated transaminase levels in serum (15 times the normal levels). Within 2–26 weeks, 30% have symptoms such as anorexia, weight loss abdominal pain, myalgia and mild jaundice. These resolve in 1–3 months— PCR detects the virus in serum within a week of exposure. Antibody response occurs in 4–8 weeks and this can be demonstrated by ELISA tests.

Chronic HCV Infection: 60–70% of cases go into chronicity, among which a third are symptomatic. Clinical features include fatigue, right hypochondrial pain, hepatomegaly in 30–70%, splenomegaly in 15% and cirrhosis in a few. Carrier state with normal transaminase levels occur in 70% and with elevated transaminase levels in 30%. Those with elevated transaminase levels follow an unpredictable course. Transition from hepatitis to cirrhosis may take 3–30 years. Hepatocellular carcinoma develops in 20–30 years, the annual risk being 1.4%. Male gender, alcoholism, age above 45 years, host immune factors, viral genotype 1b and co-infection with HIV are adverse prognostic factors. Several markers has been employed to detect and follow-up hepatic fibrosis. These include simple tests such as aspartate and amino transaminases ratio index (APRI), other biomarkers such as alpha 2, macro globulin, alpha 2 globulin, gamma globulin, apolipoprotein-A1 and several others.

Extrahepatic manifestations of HCV: These are common in HCV infections. 45–65% show antinuclear antibodies (ANAs), smooth muscle antibodies and antithyroid antibodies in serum as epiphenomena.

Essential mixed cryoglobulinemia: It is associated with the presence of HCV RNA in serum in up to 84% of cases. The clinical features include the triad of palpable purpura, arthralgias and weakness. The various mixed cryoglobulinemia-related extrahepatic manifestations of HCV infection include the following:

- ***Cutaneous leukoclastic vasculitis:*** This manifests as palpable purpura in the lower limbs, which ulcerate due to plugging of the dermal capillaries by precipitated cryoglobulins containing the virus. Severity of manifestations directly correlates with the viral load. Interferon treatment allays the lesions.
- ***Renal disease:*** Membranoproliferative glomerulone-phritis (MPGN) is associated with cryoglobulinemia in 20% of cases. The renal lesions confer poorer prognosis.
- ***Locomotor system:*** Fifty percent have one or other musculoskeletal manifestations. These include arthralgia, myalgia, polymyositis, dermatomyositis, Behcet's syndrome, antiphospholipid antibody syndrome, fibromyalgia and others. Joints affected include ankles, wrists, elbows, hands and toes. Response to antiviral therapy is good.
- ***Nervous system:*** Neuropathies occur in 10–20% of cases. Lesions include cerebral infarction, stupor, mononeuritis multiplex and cranial nerve palsies.
- ***Miscellaneous conditions***
  - Pulmonary vasculitis and respiratory distress syndrome
  - Sjogren's syndrome
  - Porphyria cutanea tarda (PCT) (20–50% of cases)
  - Lichen planus, polyarteritis nodosa, prurigo, erythema nodosum and immune thrombocytopenic purpura.

HEPATITIS DELTA VIRUS (HDV)

Syn: Delta agent

This is an RNA virus which is incomplete and therefore requires prior infection by HBV for establishing and replicating in the host. This virus was discovered by Rizetto, et al. in 1977 in long-term carriers of HBV. Fourteen percent of HBV infected persons show antibodies to HDV also. HDV is a single stranded circular RNA genome complexed with the viral protein—delta antigen. The HDV genome is encapsulated by hepatitis B surface antigen which forms the viral envelope. HDV suppresses HBV replication. Transmission is by parenteral inoculation, sexual contact and intravenous drug users (IVDUs). Co-infection with HBV occurs in 10–75%. HBV and HDV may enter together or separately and cause co-infection of the recipient or HDV may cause superinfection on a person already suffering from HBV. Receptor for HDV and HBV on liver cell is the same. Vertical transmission from mother to offspring is rare. Eight HDV genotypes have been known. HDV genotype 1 is more serious than HDV genotypes 2–8.

Co-infection is more serious. Superinfection rapidly leads to cirrhosis. In pregnancy, mortality may go up to 4–59% with fetal mortality up to 69%.

HDV can lead to acute or chronic liver disease when co-infecting with HBV. This combination is more severe than simple HBV. Clinical presentation of HDV ranges from asymptomatic carrier state, acute and chronic hepatitis, cirrhosis and liver failure.

Diagnosis is by detecting anti-HDV DNA IgG antibody, real time PCR and HDV genotyping. Liver biopsy reveals the tissue pathology. Non-invasive method of staging liver fibrosis is by transient elastography. Follow-up of the progress is by real time PCR.

Treatment of HDV is by using peginterferon alfa 2b 1.5 mg/kg/bw weekly + adefovir dipivoxil 10 mg oral. Viral clearance occurs in 25% of cases over 48 weeks. Direct response to interferon, ribavirin and lamivudine is minimal if any. Control of HBV indirectly controls HDV as well.

HEPATITIS E VIRUS (HEV)

This is a single stranded RNA virus transmitted mainly by the enteral route (fecal-oral) and is associated with poor sanitation. Four genotypes occur and they fall into 2 major groups. Genotypes 1 and 2 are human pathogens, occurring as water and food borne infections—often in epidemics. Genotypes 3 and 4 are common in swine domestic animals and wild pigs. The virus is shed in feces and so fecal-oral route of infection accounts for most of the cases. HEV antigen has been identified in the cytoplasm of hepatocytes in patients suffering from the disease.

HEV can give rise to small or large outbreaks. Waterborne outbreaks of HEV hepatitis have been described from several parts of India (Ahmedabad, Kolhapur, Srinagar and others). HEV RNA or anti-HEV antibodies have been reported from swine, cows, goats and rodents. Infection by consuming uncooked deer meat has been recorded.

Epidemic HEV infections occurs more in developing countries, genotypes 3 and 4 occur in all countries and occur as autochthonous infection (originating from that land itself). Infections may be sporadic or in limited epidemics. Differences between epidemic and autochthonous types are given in Table 55.3.

Volunteer self-inoculation study published from postgraduate institute (PGI), Chandigarh revealed the following:

- Incubation period was 15–20 days. Initial symptoms include anorexia, epigastric pain and high colored urine. All these were well-established by 30 days post-inoculation. Icteric phase started from day 38 and lasted till day 120 associated with rise in serum bilirubin and transaminases.
- HEV was first identified in blood on day 22 and could be detected till day 46. HEV antibodies appeared on day 41 and persisted beyond 2 years. Recovery was complete and follow-up for 2 years did not reveal any sequel. Since HAV and HEV appear in blood before the onset of jaundice, there is risk of transmission by blood transfusion during the window period.
- Clinical features are similar to those of HAV—jaundice, anorexia, hepatomegaly abdominal pain, nausea,

Textbook of Medicine

Table 55.3: Difference between epidemic and autochthonous HEV infection

	Epidemic	Autochthonous
Geographic distribution	More in developing countries	All countries
Genotypes	1 and 2	3 and 4
Pattern of spread	Epidemic	Autochthonous
Species specificity	Human	Swine, human
Major route of spread	Fecal-oral, waterborne	Food borne
Secondary spread	Uncommon	Rare
Rate of icteric illness	High	Low
Age distribution	Adolescents and young adults	Older age groups
Sex distribution	Both	More in men
Mortality	High in pregnancy	More in old
Extrahepatic features	A few	Neurologic complications
Chronic infection	None	Common in immunosuppression
Therapy	None	Ribavirin and Peginterferon
Prevention	Vaccine available	Vaccine available

vomiting and fever. Mortality in the general population is 0.5–4%, but in pregnant women the disease is more serious and mortality may go up to 20%. HEV is being reported from developed countries as well.

- In general, hepatitis E infection does not go to chronicity and continuing liver damage, but chronic HEV infection may persist in old and immunocompromised persons and progress to chronic liver disease. Chronic HEV infection have been described in patients recovering from liver, kidney, pancreas and heart disease, hematological stem cell transplantation, cancer chemotherapy, HIV patients and those on steroid therapy.

Diagnosis

Tests for anti-HEV antibodies IgM and IgG are available commercially. Tests for HEV RNA in serum and stool are confirmatory. Serological tests for anti-HEV antibodies are less sensitive and therefore hepatitis E nucleic acid testing is preferable.

Treatment

Drugs: Ribavirin—600–800 mg daily for 12 weeks and peginterferon is also beneficial.

HEV vaccination is available for genotype 1 (cross immunity occurs). Hepatitis E vaccine against HEV genotypes prepared and tested in China offered protection for up to 4.5 years after 3 injections given at 0, 1 and 6 months. Work is in progress.

Source:

1. Zhang J, Zhang XF, Huang SJ, et al. Long-term efficacy of a hepatitis E vaccine. N Engl J Med. 2015;372(10):914-22.

2. Hoofnagle JH, Nelson KE, Purcell RH. Hepatitis E. N Engl J Med. 2012;367(13):1237-44.

HEPATITIS G VIRUS (HGV)

As early as 2000 AD, many workers have described two viral agents belonging to the flavivirus family, HGV and GV virus type C (GBV-C) in humans. Probably, they are the same and are commonly referred to as HGV. These could infect the South American monkeys (tamarins). These agents can spread by parenteral exchange of body fluids and sexual contacts in humans. Distribution of GBV-C is global. Possibly this is only a passenger virus without being a pathogenic in humans. The exact pathogenesis role of HGV is yet to be established. HGV is not further discussed in this chapter.

INVESTIGATIONS COMMON TO ALL THE HEPATITIS VIRUSES

Urine

Bilirubin is present early in the disease. This is followed by the appearance of urobilinogen. With the onset of the obstructive phase, urobilinogen temporarily disappears from the urine to reappear during recovery. The feces is clay-colored during the obstructive phase.

Blood

Initially there is leukopenia with relative lymphocytosis which reverts to normal with the onset of jaundice. Atypical lymphocytes may be present in small numbers. The erythrocyte sedimentation rate is mildly elevated in the pre-icteric phase returning to normal as jaundice appears.

Biochemical Tests

These depend upon the severity of hepatic functional impairment. The prothrombin time may be prolonged. Serum bilirubin increases in the first two weeks to reach levels of 10–15 mg/dL or more. This is a mixture of conjugated and unconjugated pigment, the former predominating. Serum bilirubin levels return to normal in 3 to 4 weeks. Serum transaminase values-alanine and aspartate transaminases (SGPT and SGOT) increase considerably to reach peak levels just before or after the onset of jaundice. In majority of cases, the enzyme levels are in the range of 200–600 IU/L. Raised levels may persist even for a few months after apparent clinical recovery. In some cases, the enzyme levels reach much higher values. Apart from the transaminases, alkaline phosphatase, 5-nucleotidase, gamma glutamyl transpeptidase and serum lactate dehydrogenase (LDH) are moderately elevated. Serum alkaline phosphatase level rarely goes above twice the normal value and this helps in differentiating viral hepatitis from extrahepatic obstructive jaundice. Persistent elevation of the enzymes beyond six months would point to the development of chronic liver disease.

Serological Markers for Diagnosis

Serological markers are diagnostic of different viruses. Second and third generation ELISA helps to demonstrate viral antibodies. Recombinant immunoblot assay detects antibody to HCV and qualitative PCR measures the viral RNA.

Hepatitis B virus: Acute hepatitis due to HBV may be associated with HBsAg and IgM HBc. If IgM HBc is negative, the hepatitis may be due to other causes as well.

Presence of HBsAg alone indicates the carrier state. Modern tests can detect HBsAg levels as low as 1 ng/mL. The usual values in acute hepatitis vary from 10,000 to 100,000 ng/mL.

Presence of HBeAg indicates infectivity. Generally HBsAg and HBeAg are positive in most cases. Routine testing of HBeAg is not indicated. In chronic cases presence of HBeAg is an indication for starting treatment. Favorable response results in the production of antibody to HBeAg. Anti-HBe antibody (anti-HBeAb) appears in the serum and this indicates resolution and success of therapy.

Anti-HBe is found in both acute and resolved cases of HBV hepatitis. In acute hepatitis, IgM anti-HBe is elevated in all cases and its presence is diagnostic. In chronic infections it is the IgG antibody.

Anti-HBs antibody is not a reliable test to determine the prevalence of HBV infection in the population, but it is a good test to determine the success of vaccination against HBV.

Hepatitis C: It is diagnosed by demonstrating anti HCV antibodies and PCR tests to detect the viral RNA. Genotyping helps to characterize the virus, assess the prognosis and plan treatment.

Liver biopsy: Liver biopsy is not indicated in ordinary case. Biopsy is indicated to differentiate viral hepatitis from extra hepatic obstruction and confirm the presence of chronic hepatitis if the condition does not resolve and diagnostic parameters are not clear-cut. It is advisable to have biopsy confirmation of the persistent hepatic lesion before starting on interferon therapy.

COMPLICATIONS AND SEQUELAE

Complications occur in a small proportion of cases whereas vast majority of cases recover uneventfully.

- ***Relapse:*** About 15% of patients may get relapse after initial clearance of jaundice. Premature resumption of physical activity favors relapse. With proper management this also subsides completely.
- ***Prolonged cholestasis:*** Cholestasis may persist due to the development of intrahepatic obstruction. This is more frequently seen with acute HAV and HEV infections. With rest and supportive measures these patients usually recover completely within weeks or months.
- ***Fulminant hepatitis:*** This is a serious complication occurring in 1–2% of patients, more so in type B hepatitis. Hepatic function deteriorates rapidly with the onset of hepatocellular failure. When hepatic encephalopathy occurs within 8 weeks of onset of jaundice, it is called fulminant hepatic failure. If this occurs between 8 and 28 weeks, it is called subacute hepatic failure. Hepatitis B is responsible for 30–60% of cases of acute hepatic failure. The liver shrinks progressively. The condition is fatal in 80% of patients, irrespective of the treatment. Death is due to cerebral edema, brainstem damage, gastrointestinal (GI) hemorrhage, infections or renal failure. The overall mortality is 2% in HBV infections, but 10% or more in post-transfusion hepatitis, since the infecting dose is high in the latter.

- ***Chronic hepatitis:*** This is defined as continuing inflammation of the liver persisting for more than 6 months. HBV is responsible for chronic hepatitis in 30–50%. Chronic hepatitis may take the form of chronic persistent hepatitis which is benign and self-limiting or chronic active hepatitis which is more sinister and often ends up in hepatic failure or cirrhosis.
- ***Cirrhosis:*** HBV and HCV can progress to cirrhosis directly or passing through a stage of chronic active hepatitis. HCV relentlessly progresses to chronic liver failure and it is a frequent cause for hepatic transplantation. Median time from infection to cirrhosis is ± 30 years.
- ***Hepatocellular carcinoma:*** Both HBV and HCV are oncogenic. Persistence of the virus in the system for 25 years or more predisposes to carcinoma. The risk of developing hepatocellular carcinoma is high in HBV carriers. The incidence of cancer in a community correlates directly with the HBV carrier rate. In areas where HBV carrier rate is very high (15%), the mean age for carcinoma is 25 years, since a good number of subjects get infected perinatally. In areas where the HBV carrier rate is low (1% or less), the mean age for cancer is 50 years or more, since the main source of infection is parenteral or sexual route. Malignancy may follow hepatitis directly or through a phase of cirrhosis. HCV is also carcinogenic.
- ***Posthepatitis syndrome:*** Sometimes symptoms of ill-health persist for many months after apparent recovery. The liver may remain slightly enlarged with evidence of mild or moderate dysfunction. Such persons generally show anxiety and loss of morale which aggravate the disability. If followed-up, many recover. Only reassurance is needed.
- ***Extrahepatic manifestations:*** Patients with HBV or HCV infection have circulating immune complexes, which lead to the development of serum sickness-like picture early in the disease. These are more prominent in the case of HCV.
- ***Aplastic anemia:*** Aplastic anemia may follow HAV and HCV infection rarely. This is an immune mediated process.

DIAGNOSIS OF VIRAL HEPATITIS

Viral hepatitis is diagnosed by its clinical features, epidemiology, clinical circumstances like injection, illicit drug use and others and the presence of jaundice, mild to moderate hepatosplenomegaly, absence of severe tenderness over the liver, leukopenia, biluria (presence of bile in urine), marked rise in hepatic transaminases (600–2000 units/dL or more) and a subacute course except in the fulminant type.

Drug-induced hepatitis, intrahepatic cholestasis due to other causes and cholangitis present with jaundice and these have to be differentiated. Though hepatic amebiasis is not generally associated with jaundice, in a few cases it may create problems when mild or moderate jaundice occurs. Hepatic amebiasis presents with tender hepatomegaly, moderate leukocytosis, no impairment of hepatocellular function and recovery with antiamebic drugs. Outbreaks of liver damage resulting from toxic products (e.g. veno-occlusive disease and aflatoxicosis) may be initially mistaken for viral hepatitis. Falciparum malaria should be excluded in all cases. Leptospirosis is a common cause for acute hepatitis at present.

Salient Features of Different Hepatic Lesions Resembling Viral Hepatitis

- ***Drug induced hepatitis:*** Rise of alanine transaminase (ALT) is only moderate—compared to the rise in bilirubin, toxic substances reduce diagnostic clues. Their presence may be demonstrated by chemical analysis.
- ***Alcoholic hepatitis:*** History of acute or chronic alcoholism and changes in the liver depending upon the stage of the disease are diagnostic. Jaundice is rare and elevation of transaminases is not high.
- ***Falciparum malaria:*** This should be considered in all cases and excluded by repeated examination of blood smear.
- ***Gallstone disease with acute biliary obstruction:*** The transaminases may rise moderately or abruptly to high levels which come down rapidly. Serum bilirubin and alkaline phosphatase may rise later. Ultrasonography is most often diagnostic.
- ***Acute anoxic damage to liver:*** This occurs in passive venous congestion occurring abruptly. This may lead to abrupt rise of SGPT to very high levels even 10000 IU/L, but unlike as in viral hepatitis where LDH level is only moderately increased, here LDH is also very much raised.
- ***Leptospirosis:*** This presents with acute hepatitis and jaundice, proteinuria, hemorrhagic manifestations and neutrophil leucocytosis. Leptospira antibodies are demonstrable. Rarely leptospira can be demonstrated in blood and urine.

In the common clinical setting in India, almost in all places acute leptospirosis by different strains of leptospira (Weil's disease) poses diagnostic difficulties before full investigations are available (Table 55.4).

PROGNOSIS

Virus A hepatitis is a benign disorder which recovers uneventfully in most of the cases with mortality below 2%. In children, the disease runs a milder course whereas in the elderly patients, complications occur. Fulminant hepatitis carries a grave prognosis. During pregnancy, viral hepatitis carries a higher risk of mortality and morbidity, especially in the malnourished subjects. The prognosis of HBV is more serious, mortality and morbidity being higher. Though vast majority recover, 1–2% go on to chronic hepatitis and carcinoma. In 5–10% of cases, the carrier state persists and such people can be infective to others.

HBV and HCV

HCV follows the same long-term behavior as HBV. Unlike HBV which can exist in a carrier state with no lesion in the liver, HCV tends to produce chronic lesions in the liver in most cases. At present, HCV and HBV induced chronic liver disease and carcinomas are the major indications for hepatic transplantation. Till recently, drug treatment for HCV and HBV were at best only partially successful (viral clearance rate 25–50% or less). Recently, powerful orally administrable anti-viral drugs have been introduced, but they are very expensive (1000–2000 $/day or 8–12 weeks therapy). In a high proportion of cases, HCV produces chronic liver disease and mortality.

HDV aggravates the clinical picture of HBV and leads to greater incidence of acute hepatic failure. HDV gets eradicated when HBV disappears.

HEV is more benign, except when it occurs in pregnant women in whom the mortality may reach up to 40%. Recently, chronic hepatitis E progressing to cirrhosis has been documented in immunocompromised individuals.

MANAGEMENT

General Management

Adequate bed rest is recommended if symptoms are pronounced. Strenuous exercise should be avoided. Inadequate oral intake and dehydration due to persistent nausea and vomiting may require hospital admission for intravenous 10% glucose administration.

There are no specific dietary recommendations for acute viral hepatitis, however alcohol and hepatotoxic drugs should be avoided. Normal diet can be resumed once appetite returns.

Patients are managed as outpatients with symptomatic treatment. Assurance should be given to the patient that uncomplicated recovery is the norm in most cases. Inpatient care is recommended when patient has either hepatic encephalopathy, International Normalized Ratios (INR) prolongation (>1.5) indicating hepatic parenchymal failure, signs of sepsis or patient is unable to maintain hydration and nutrition.

Treatment of HBV

The currently approved drugs for hepatitis B fall into the broad categories of nucleoside and nucleotide analogs (NUCs or NAs) and interferons.

Nucleoside analogs have good safety profile and excellent antiviral efficacy and are the drug of choice in patients with decompensated cirrhosis. The NUCs act as competitive inhibitors of the viral reverse transcriptase and DNA polymerase by replacing natural nucleosides

Table 55.4: Difference between Weil's disease and viral hepatitis

	Weil's disease	Viral hepatitis
Onset	Sudden	Gradual
Headache	Constant	Occasional
Muscle pains	Severe	Mild
Conjunctival injection	Present	Absent
Prostration	Great	Mild
Disorientation	Common	Rare
Hemorrhagic diathesis	Common	Rare
Nausea and vomiting	Present	Present
Abdominal discomfort	Common	Common
Bronchitis	Common	Rare
Albuminuria	Present	Absent
Leukocyte count	Polymorph leukocytosis	Leukopenia with lymphocytosis

during the synthesis of the first or second strand or both of HBV DNA.

Lamivudine (Zeffex Glaxo Smith Kline)

Lamivudine was the first nucleoside analog approved for the treatment of hepatitis B in 1998. The drug has been shown to be a relatively potent inhibitor of viral replication, convenient to administer and free of severe adverse effects. The recommended dose of lamivudine for adults with normal renal function (creatinine clearance more than 50 mL/min) is 100 mg orally daily. The recommended dose for children is 3 mg/kg/day with a maximum dose of 100 mg/day. Emergence of viral resistance has been the major setback with lamivudine and viral resistance of 38% at two years and 65% at year five years have been reported. Patients in whom lamivudine resistance has developed, hepatitis flares. For this reasons, the drug is no longer recommended as first-line therapy.

Adefovir Dipivoxil (Hepsera Gilead)

Adefovir dipivoxil was approved for HBV treatment in 2002. Adefovir has been shown to be effective in suppressing wild-type as well as lamivudine-resistant HBV in *in vitro* and clinical studies. The recommended dose of adefovir for adults with normal renal function (creatinine clearance more than 50 mL/min) is 10 mg orally daily.

Adefovir and lamivudine differ greatly in their resistance profiles and as a result, adefovir is effective in patients with lamivudine-resistant HBV. Therefore, most clinicians continue to use lamivudine when starting adefovir therapy in patients who have become resistant to lamivudine. However, adefovir is being replaced as first-line therapy with more potent drugs such as entecavir and tenofovir.

Telbivudine

Telbivudine is an L-nucleoside analog of thymidine that has been shown to be more potent than lamivudine in patients with HBeAg-positive and HBeAg-negative hepatitis B. The approved dose of telbivudine is 600 mg daily if the creatinine clearance is more than 50 mL/minute. Unfortunately, after 1 and 2 years of treatment, genotypic resistance was found in 5% and 25% of HBeAg-positive patients respectively. Telbivudine has a higher rate of resistance than entecavir and tenofovir and has fallen out of favor as a treatment for HBV infection.

Entecavir

Entecavir was approved by the United States Food and Drug Administration (USFDA) in 2005. Entecavir blocks HBV replication by inhibiting the priming of HBV DNA polymerase and the synthesis of the first and second strands of HBV DNA. Entecavir is effective against both wild-type and lamivudine-resistant HBV. Entecavir is used in a dose of 0.5 mg in previously untreated patients, whereas 1 mg was used in patients who were resistant to or exposed to lamivudine. Entecavir resistance is rare (approximately 1% at five years) in treatment-naive patients but is common in patients with prior lamivudine resistance.

Tenofovir Disoproxil Fumarate-Viread (Gilead)

Tenofovir was approved in 2008 for the treatment of HBV infection. The approved dose of tenofovir is 300 mg orally once daily with dose adjusted for patients with creatinine clearance less than 50 mL/min. Resistance to tenofovir has not occurred after 2 years of treatment in either HBeAg-positive or HBeAg-negative patients. Tenofovir has been reported to cause Fanconi syndrome, renal insufficiency as well as osteomalacia. Serum creatinine levels should be monitored regularly during prolonged use of tenofovir and if the serum creatinine level rises, the dose may need to be modified or the drug discontinued to reduce the risk of further nephrotoxicity.

Interferon Alfa (IFN-α)

Interferon is an immune modulator and it works by improving immune defense of the cells which eliminates the virus in the presence of anti-viral drug administered simultaneously.

This is used for hepatitis B, hepatitis C and also hepatitis D infections. This treatment is effective.

Interferon therapy is started when there is no further chance of natural cure and if the abnormal liver functions and liver biopsy findings persist after 6 months of clinical remission.

Combination of ribavarin 1000 mg oral bd and interferon 2–3 million units IM daily gives better results than either drug given alone. With higher doses of interferon, the cure rate may go up to 60%.

Side effects of interferon include malaise, fever, shivering and 'flu' like symptoms within a few hours of injection. With successive injections, the side effects came down. These side effects can be controlled by paracetamol 500 mg given orally. Other side effects include anorexia, hair loss, depression weight loss, marrow suppression, seizures and susceptibility to bacterial infection. Beneficial effects are monitored by the level of transaminases and clinical improvement. Majority of the cases that improve do so within 2 months. Maintenance of normal transaminase levels for 6 months or more after cessation of therapy indicates cure.

- Cure rates in HBV on interferon are 25–40%
- In HCV, 6–12 months therapy gives cure rates of up to 40%
- In HDV, the remission rate is up to 25%.

Earlier the treatment is started, better is the response. Absence of cirrhosis, absence of high levels of hepatic iron in biopsy before therapy and HCV genotypes 2 and 3 indicate favorable prognosis.

IFN-α is available as standard or conventional interferon and PEG-IFN and had been licensed for the treatment of chronic hepatitis B since 1992. The major advantage of interferon is its finite duration of treatment and unlike the nucleoside analogs, has not been associated with drug resistance.

Interferon has direct immunomodulatory properties, it enhances human leukocyte antigen (HLA) class I antigen expression on the surface of infected hepatocytes and augments CD8+ cytotoxic T lymphocytes (CTL) activity. Interferon reduces the amount of the HBV cccDNA thereby leading to the loss of HBsAg that occurs in interferon-treated patients.

Pegylated IFN-α

Pegylated interferon (PEG-IFN) (interferon attached to polyethylene glycol) which has longer duration of action gives better cure rates with less of side effect. The drug is more expensive. Two forms of PEG-IFN are available with similar efficacy and safety profile. PEG-IFN-α 2a has been used as a dose of 180 µg subcutaneously per week and α 2b at a dose of 1.5 µg per kg subcutaneously per week.

Response of hepatitis B virus to interferon appears to depend on the viral genotype. Studies have shown that HBV genotype A demonstrated HBeAg loss and HBsAg clearance more frequently than those with genotypes B, C and D (47% vs 44%, 28% and 25%, respectively).

Response-guided Therapy with PEG-IFN

The principle of response-guided PEG-IFN therapy is that on treatment HBsAg levels could be used to identify either early responders for whom prolongation of treatment to week 48 could be beneficial or non-responders who should be withdrawn from PEG-IFN treatment and 'rescued' with alternative therapy.

Indications for Stopping PEG-IFN Therapy

HBeAg-positive patients: Two stopping rules at week 12 have been advocated.

1. For HBeAg-positive patients:
   - No HBsAg decline
   - HBsAg levels >20000 IU/mL.
2. For HBeAg-negative genotype D patients
   - No HBsAg decline and <2 log copies/mL decline in HBV DNA at 12 weeks
   - HBsAg levels >7500 IU/mL at 24 weeks.

Indications for Specific Therapy in HBV Infections

Chronic Hepatitis B

Two different types of drugs can be used in chronic HBV infection: Conventional and PEG-IFN and nucleoside/nucleotide analogues (NAs) are lamivudine, adefovir, entecavir, tenofovir and telbivudine. PEG-IFN, tenofovir or entecavir is preferred for first line monotherapy due to high resistance barrier in long-term treatment duration (for NAs) and finite duration of therapy (for PEG-IFN).

The indications for treatment are generally the same for both HBeAg-positive and HBeAg-negative chronic hepatitis B (CHB). This is based mainly on the combination of three criteria:

1. Serum HBV DNA levels
2. Serum ALT levels
3. Severity of liver disease.

Patients should be considered for treatment when they have HBV DNA levels above 2000 IU/mL, serum ALT levels above the upper limit of normal (ULN) and severity of liver disease assessed by liver biopsy showing moderate to severe active necroinflammation and/or at least moderate fibrosis. In patients who fulfill the above criteria for HBV DNA and histological severity of liver disease, treatment may be initiated even if ALT levels are normal.

Patients with HBeAg-positive or negative chronic hepatitis B with ALT greater than 2 times normal and HBV DNA >20,000 IU/mL should be considered for treatment without liver biopsy.

Duration of treatment: PEG-IFN has finite duration of therapy and is given as weekly subcutaneous injection for 48 weeks. NAs are given for long-term with end points being disappearance of HBV DNA from serum with HbsAg seroconversion to Anti-HBs (ideal) or undetectable HBV DNA with HBeAg seroconversion to Anti-HBe when there is no HBsAg loss. At least 6 months of additional consolidation therapy is recommended after achieving the end points.

Cirrhosis Patients

In well compensated cirrhosis, treatment is same as that for chronic HBV. However they require long-term therapy with careful monitoring for resistance and flares.

In decompensated cirrhosis, treatment should be started with any detectable HBV DNA irrespective of titer and continued lifelong.

Antiviral Therapy in Special Population

Acute Viral Hepatitis B

Complete immunological recovery occurs in >95% from acute viral hepatitis B. Patients with protracted, severe acute hepatitis (increase in INR > 1.5 and deep jaundice persisting for more than 4 weeks) and acute liver failure must be evaluated for liver transplantation. Antiviral treatment is recommended in these group of patients. Entecavir or Tenofovir should be started and continued for at least 3 months after Anti-HBs seroconversion or at least 12 months after Anti-HBe seroconversion without HbsAg loss.

Viral Hepatitis B in Pregnancy

If a patient on anti-HBV therapy becomes pregnant, treatment indications should be re-evaluated. The indications are same as that for chronic hepatitis B but treatment agents should be reconsidered. PEG-IFN must be stopped and patient should be continued on FDA **category B** NAs, preferably tenofovir. For prevention of perinatal HBV transmission, traditionally active and passive immunization with HBV immunoglobulin (HBIG) and HBV vaccination of the newborn is recommended. In mothers with high viremia (HBV DNA >$10^{6\text{-}7}$ IU/mL) >10% chance exist for perinatal transmission despite immunization strategy. Thus, telbivudine, lamivudine or tenofovir (as a potent FDA category B agent) may be used for the prevention of perinatal and intrauterine HBV transmission in the last trimester of pregnancy in HbsAg positive mothers with high viral load. Antiviral drugs can be discontinued within 3 months of delivery.

Treatment of HCV

Acute HCV infection: IFN-α 2b, 5 million units/day IM injection for 4 weeks and thereafter 3 times a week for 20 weeks. In chronic hepatitis C, the pattern is different. Hepatitis C is more susceptible to interferon and smaller doses (3 million units given thrice a week for 6 months) are sufficient. Patients without cirrhosis do better than those with cirrhosis. In 50% of cases, the transaminases fall to normal level and HCV RNA disappears from serum by the end of therapy. Relapses are more common and only 20–25% get permanent cure.

Chronic Hepatitis C: PEG-IFN with ribavirin has been the standard of care for chronic hepatitis C infection. The

Textbook of Medicine

treatment duration is 48 weeks for genotypes 1, 4, 5, 6 and 24 weeks for genotype 2 and 3. The dose of PEG-IFN α-2a is 180 µg subcutaneously per week together with ribavirin using doses of 1,000 mg for those <75 kg in weight and 1,200 mg for those >75 kg.

The dose of PEG-IFN α-2b is 1.5 µg/kg subcutaneously per week together with ribavirin using doses of 800 mg for those weighing <65 kg, 1,000 mg for those weighing >65 kg to 85 kg, 1,200 mg for >85 kg to 105 kg and 1,400 mg for >105 kg.

PEG-IFN + ribavirin has a clearance rate of only <14%. For patients with cirrhosis and platelet count <100,000/cm³ or serum albumin <35 g/dL. PEG-IFN, ribavirin and boceprevir are contraindicated.

Newer Treatment Modalities in Hepatitis C

Directly acting antivirals (DAAs)

The major drugs in this group fall under the categories of protease inhibitors and polymerase inhibitors. Boceprevir and telaprevir were the first protease inhibitors approved for HCV genotype-1 treatment along with PEG-IFN and ribavirin. Sofosbuvir is the first polymerase inhibitor in HCV treatment and has shown pan genotypic effect and efficacy both in treatment naive and interferon resistant cases. Both these drugs are inhibitors of HCV/NS3/4A serine protease. Better response rates (66–75%) were obtained by treatment for 24–48 weeks. This combination is more toxic than PEG-IFN and ribavirin medication.

Further developments of direct acting anti-HCV drugs include simeprevir which is also a HCV/NS3/4A serine protease inhibitor with the advantage of a once-a-day dosage.

Simeprevir was better tolerated. Simeprevir can be used with sobosfuvir or ribavirin for 12–24 weeks.

Follow-up: Prolonged follow-up is necessary in cases which have developed complications.

Newer drugs in the pipeline

Several newer directly acting anti-HCV drug are being introduced as single oral drug therapy for chronic HCV. These include ledipasvir, sofosbuvir, ombitasvir, dasabuvir, ABT-450/r ritonavir and probably others.

Action of these drugs:

ABT	Inhibitor of HCV non-structural 3/4 A (N53/4A) protease
Ritonavir	No action on HCV but inhibits ABT450 metabolism increasing its blood levels and prolongs its action to overdose dosage
Ombitasvir	(ABT267) HCV NS5A inhibitor
Dasabuvir	(ABT333) A non-nucleotide HCV NS5A RNA polymerase inhibitor
Boceprevir and telaprevir	Protease inhibitors
Sofosbuvir	Polymerase inhibitor

Treatment with once daily single tablet regimen of ledipasvir and sofosbuvir in a fixed dose tablet resulted in a high rate of virological response in 94–95% (CI 87–97%) in those receiving the drug for 12 weeks and 99% (CI 95–100%) in those receiving the drug for 24 weeks.

Ledipasvir + Sofosbuvir + Ribavirin
Dose: Ledipasvir—90 mg; sofosbuvir—400 mg (given once a day). Ribavirin 1000 mg daily given oral as 2 doses for patients <75/kg and 1200 mg for those >75 kg.

Oral drugs: HCV are highly effective even without concurrent use of interferons. Some newer regimens are given below:

- 150 mg of ABT 450
- 100 mg ritonavir
- 25 mg ombitasvir + 250 mg bd dasabuvir
- Ribavirin as per body weight { 1000 mg as 2 doses daily for persons <75 kg/bw; 1200 mg as 2 doses for persons >75 kg/bw

These have been tried for 12 and 24 weeks. On 12th week post treatment, virological clearance occurred in 91.8% (CI 87.6–96.1). For those on 24 weeks treatment, clearance rate was 95.9% (CI 92.6–99.3). Adverse effects include fatigue, headache and nausea. At present the new oral drugs are prohibitively costly ($1000/tablet) and are unavailable in India at moderate cost. But in course of time the prices may come down a little.

Source:

1. Afdhal N, Reddy KR, Nelson DR, et al. Ledipasvir and sofosbuvir for previously treated HCV genotype 1 infection. N Engl J Med. 2014;370(16):1483-93.

2. Poordad F, Hezode C, Trinh R, et al. ABT-450/r-ombitasvir and dasabuvir with ribavirin for hepatitis C with cirrhosis. N Engl J Med. 2014;370(21):1973-82.

3. Ghany MG, Gara N. QUEST for a cure for hepatitis C virus: the end is in sight. Lancet. 2014;384(9941):381-3.

Prophylaxis

HAV and HEV

HAV and HEV infections can be prevented by boiling drinking water for 10 minutes during the epidemics. General precautions to prevent fecal-oral spread should be instituted. These include personal hygiene, disposal of excreta and control of flies.

Passive immunization: Immune serum globulin (ISG or pooled human gamma globulin) prevents or modifies virus A infection. The dose is 0.02–0.12 mL/kg given IM within 14 days of exposure. Passive immunization is indicated in contacts of HAV hepatitis, pregnant women at risk, travellers to endemic areas and those who have received probably infected blood. The protection lasts for 4–5 months, therefore, the dose has to be repeated at 5 months intervals. Sexual and familial contacts of cases of HAV hepatitis during the incubation period should be given gamma globulin.

Active immunization: Hepatitis A can be prevented by vaccination. The vaccine is effective in 94–100% of the cases. Formalized inactivated HAV vaccine is available.

- Dose 2–18 years of age—2 doses of 0.5 mL at intervals 6–18 months.
- Above 18 years of age—2 doses of 1 mL at an interval of 6–18 months apart.

HAV vaccine is indicated for children in endemic areas, high-risk groups such as hospital staff and travellers into endemic areas. Immunity against HAV lasts for several years (>6). Further prolonged follow-up is needed to assess the exact period of immunity. The vaccines costs about INR 700/dose. Adverse effects include local pain and mild general symptoms.

Combined HBV and HAV vaccines (TWINRIX) is available. Schedule is the same as for HBV (i.e.) 1 mL each at 0, 1 and 6 months. The immunity agent HBV is strong for 10 years after which it may wane.

Vaccine Against Hepatitis E Virus

At present, vaccines against HEV are not commercially freely available, but several vaccines are being developed and tried. A recombinant anti-HEV vaccine has been tried in Nepal. Three doses were given IM at 0, 1 and 6 months. Compared to placebo, it gave 95.5% protection. Further trials are in progress. In 2011, a vaccine against HEV 239 has been registered in China, but it is not available globally. **Source:** Shrestha MP1, Scott RM, Joshi DM, et al. Safety and efficacy of a recombinant hepatitis E vaccine. N Engl J Med. 2007;356(9):895-903.

Hepatitis B

Avoidance of professional blood donors, avoidance of pooled blood products and screening of all blood donors for HBV and HCV help to minimize the risk of transmission. Boiling all equipment for ten minutes or autoclaving will destroy the virus. Those who have had jaundice during the past 6 months and those who are known to have caused post-transfusion hepatitis should be rejected as blood donors. Use of disposable needles and syringes for injections helps to safeguard against hepatitis.

Active Immunization

Effective vaccines are available widely for immunization. Commercial vaccines are prepared from two sources mainly.

1. Vaccine prepared by HBsAg of carriers—this plasma vaccine is cheaper and still used widely in many countries (Heptavac). Cost/dose around ₹ 50. Side effects include local soreness and mild febrile reactions.
2. Vaccine produced by recombinant DNA technology in yeast. This vaccine is more expensive costing about ₹ 400/- per mL. Each mL contains 20 mg of the material.

Vaccination is given to children after the first year of life by which time the maternal antibodies would have disappeared.

Children age	Dose
2–18 years	0.5 mL (720 ELISA units) at 0, 6 and 12 months by IM injection

Adults age	Dose
Above 18 years	1 mL (1440 ELISA units) at 0, 6 and 12 months.
	Antibodies start appearing by 3 weeks after vaccination. Immunity lasts for 10 years. The vaccine should not be frozen.

Side effects are few and it is one of the safe vaccines.

Passive Immunization

It is required for those who have no demonstrable antibody against HBsAg. HBIG contains a high titer of anti-HBs and affords passive protection for three months if given within two days of exposure. The initial dose is 0.05–0.07 mL/kg body weight intramuscularly. A second dose is given 25–30 days later. The immunity lasts for a period of 6 months.

Indications for HBIG

- Needle prick injury
- Spouses and sexual partners of acute HBV hepatitis patients
- Accidental transfusion of HBsAg positive blood or blood product
- Mucosal contact with HBsAg positive blood or other infective material in laboratory workers
- Babies born to HBsAg positive mothers.

Babies born to mothers who develop hepatitis B during the third trimester or who are positive for HBsAg at the time of delivery should be given 5 mL HBIG on the day of birth and then every 5 weeks for 6 months till the baby is actively immunized. HBIG is available in India, but the cost is high. Immunization against HBV also protects against HDV.

Indications for Vaccination

- **High-risk groups:** Medical students, medical and paramedical personnel. Those receiving hemodialysis, peritoneal dialysis, repeated doses of blood and blood products, babies born to HBsAg positive mothers, spouses and sexual contacts of HBsAg positive subjects.
- **Elective:** Since the best method to reduce carrier state is to prevent the spread of infection, vaccination is indicated to all persons (irrespective of the age at onset of vaccinating schedule), if facilities permit.

In many countries, hepatitis vaccine has been included in the schedule for vaccination of infants, along with the DPT, polio and measles vaccines.

Schedule for vaccination

	1st dose	2nd dose after 1 month	3rd dose after 6 months
Adults Infants and newborns	1 mL	1 mL	1 mL
Booster at 5 years	0.5 mL	0.5 mL	0.5 mL

For infants of HBsAg positive mothers, HBIG and vaccine are given within 12 hours of birth and thereafter at 1 and 6 months. Protective titer of antibodies are not impaired by concurrent administration of HBIG and vaccine. The protective antibody level is 10 μIU/mL.

Immunity starts in about 1 month of first dose and is strong by the 3rd month. By 6 months, more than 90% are immune. When the protection is desired early, accelerated course of vaccination can be given. This consists of 3 doses given at 1 month intervals and a booster at 12 months. Immunogenicity is more if IM injections are given over the deltoid region than over the gluteal region and therefore the former site should be chosen.

Intradermal injection of 0.1 mL of vaccine is also effective, but the immunization rates are lower.

Procedure to be followed if healthcare personnel get needle stick injuries with HBsAg positive blood con-

tamination: Passive immunization should be given with 3 mL HBIG (1 mL = 200 units) as early as possible and active immunization should be started simultaneously. Extensive vaccine coverage over the previous three decades have significantly reduced the incidence of hepatic cirrhosis and carcinoma in young adults in several countries.

Points to Remember
- Hepatitis viruses belong to six different families
- Infection is very common
- Viruses A and E are feco-oral transmitted
- Virus B, C and D are transmitted by parenteral inoculation
- Viruses B and C lead to cirrhosis and carcinoma of the liver
- Effective preventive measures are available for HAV and HBV.

Enteroviruses

KV Krishna Das

Chapter Summary

- Poliomyelitis
- Echoviruses
  - Aseptic Meningitis
  - Acute Hemorrhagic Conjunctivitis
- Coxsackieviruses
- Enteroviruses caused Diseases

These are viruses which are found in the alimentary tract of man. These include poliomyelitis, coxsackie, echo and several other viruses. They are isolated from the feces of healthy and sick individuals. Most of them are host specific and antigenically distinct. They are single-stranded ribonucleic acid (RNA) viruses.

POLIOMYELITIS

Syn: Heine-Medin disease, Infantile paralysis

Poliomyelitis is an acute contagious disease producing a wide clinical spectrum ranging from a non-paralytic illness in which the patient develops symptoms and signs of meningeal involvement without paralysis to a severe paralytic form in which flaccid paralysis results from affliction of spinal motor neurons and brainstem nuclei. Poliomyelitis viruses belong to the group of *picornaviruses*. Three types are pathogenic—types 1, 2 and 3. Type 1 is most common and is responsible for the majority of paralytic cases. Types 1, 2 and 3 do not show cross-immunity.

Epidemiology

The disease is worldwide in distribution, spreads by the feco-oral route. The virus is eliminated in feces by cases and carriers. The virus sheds from the oropharyngeal secretions for up to 3 weeks after infection and in feces for up to 3 months. The disease may occur sporadically or in outbreaks. Majority of cases of infection are inapparent with only transient nonspecific symptoms and a rise in antibody levels. Classic paralytic polio develops only rarely. Poliomyelitis used to be common in India with an incidence of 20–30/100,000 of the population. About 90% of children aged 5 years and above showed the presence of neutralizing antibodies to all the three types of polio viruses acquired naturally during the 1980s. Worldwide efforts to contain poliomyelitis started in 1988 with the aim of eradicating poliomyelitis from the world. Only humans act as reservoir of the virus and therefore it may lend itself to eradication by eliminating the human reservoir by vaccination coverage. By intensive and extensive mass vaccination programs conducted nationwide, the incidence of poliomyelitis has been considerably reduced, though India is still not polio-free. With the decrease in incidence of paralytic poliomyelitis, the relative frequency of non-polio paralytic lesions caused by other enteroviruses have increased. In the gastrointestinal tract (GIT) virulent poliovirus can mutate and become invasive at times.

Pathogenesis and Pathology

The virus enters the system by ingestion. It proliferates in the cervical and mesenteric lymph nodes and Peyer's patches. At this stage the virus may be present in the oropharyngeal secretions and feces. The next stage is of viremia. The virulence of the virus and immune status of the host determine the localization of the virus to the central nervous system (CNS). Even a genetic predisposition to paralytic polio has been postulated. Physical exhaustion, intramuscular injections, tonsillectomy and local injury have all been known to be associated with paralysis localized to the affected part. Immunity to poliomyelitis is mainly humoral, immunoglobulin G (IgG) antibodies being protective. IgA antibodies in the GIT inhibit viral replication and viral shedding.

The virus reaches the CNS through the neural pathways. In the paralytic cases, the anterior horn cells of the spinal cord and the medullary nuclei are swollen and congested. As the condition proceeds, chromatolysis and pericellular infiltration occurs. The neurons are totally destroyed. Occasionally other parts of the CNS such as roof of the fourth ventricle and vermis, midbrain, substantia nigra, thalamus, globus pallidus and hypothalamus may be involved. In the early stages, the cerebrospinal fluid (CSF) shows increase in cells, mainly polymorphs, but this gives way to lymphocytic increase with the passage of time. Protein level may be moderately increased (up to 150 mg/dL) and the sugar level is normal.

Clinical Features

The incubation period is 7–14 days. The disease manifests a bimodal pattern, the initial features are due to viremia and the second one is due to neurological damage. Initial symptoms are nonspecific such as fever, headache, muscle pain and diarrhea. The second phase, which sets in after a period of 3 to 4 days, is characterized by paralysis. In many of the patients infection may be subclinical.

Nonparalytic polio: Features of meningitis develop in nonparalytic polio. These include fever, headache, neck rigidity and muscle pains. Physical examination may reveal signs of meningeal irritation. The condition subsides without further events within a week.

Paralytic polio: In paralytic polio, paralysis may involve the spinal group of muscles, bulbar muscles or a combination of both.

Spinal form: The initial manifestations in this form are followed by diffuse muscle twitching and cramps. The muscles may be tender. Transient fasciculations may be noted. Paralysis of muscles sets in rapidly by the third or fourth day of illness. The spectrum ranges from mild weakness of a limb or a part thereof to extensive flaccid quadriplegia. Paralysis usually takes place within hours in the majority of cases, rarely it may take 4 to 5 days or more. There seems to be a predilection for the cervical and lumbar segments of the spinal cord. The tendon jerks are abolished. Objective sensory changes do not occur. The paralysis is asymmetrical, maximal in the beginning and tends to recover with time. Total destruction of neurons leaves behind complete paralysis, partially affected groups recover to varying degrees. The final picture is one of different combinations of muscle paralysis. Often part of a muscle is affected, leaving the remaining part unaffected. Ventilatory insufficiency may develop if the diaphragm and intercostal are paralyzed. Respiratory failure manifests as restlessness and tachypnea, with shallow irregular respiration.

Bulbar form: Affection of the lower cranial nerves occurs early in this form. It may precede or follow the spinal involvement. Dysphagia, dysarthria and dysphonia occur commonly. Facial palsy may develop less commonly.

Involvement of the nuclei of the medullary reticular formation results in dysfunction of the vital areas such as the respiratory and vasomotor centers. These manifest as irregularity of respiration with apneic spells, vasomotor collapse, transient hypertension and acute pulmonary edema.

Polioencephalitis: This form is unusual and is characterized by alteration in the level of consciousness, convulsions, signs of brainstem involvement and varying combinations of spastic or flaccid paralysis. This condition may mimic other forms of encephalitis.

Diagnosis

Poliomyelitis should be diagnosed clinically in any unimmunized child who develops an initial febrile illness and proceeds to acute paralysis within a few days. The clinical features and the CSF findings help to make a bedside diagnosis in almost all cases. Rarely coxsackie and echoviruses are also capable of producing paralytic disease. There are reports of increasing incidence of Japanese encephalitis virus causing polio like presentation with asymmetric flaccid paralysis of limbs, meningism and lymphocyte pleocytosis in the CSF.

Laboratory Investigations

The virus can be grown in tissue culture from specimens such as feces, rectal swab and CSF. Polymerase chain reaction (PCR) studies help to identify the virus and distinguish it from other wild polio viruses. CSF shows moderate lymphocytic pleocytosis (100–200 cells/mm³) and mild elevation of proteins (40–50 mg/dL). These changes occur in several other conditions and therefore may not help in specific diagnosis. Serological diagnosis is established by demonstrating rising titers of neutralizing and complement fixing antibodies in the serum.

Differential Diagnosis

Nonparalytic poliomyelitis has to be differentiated from other conditions causing aseptic meningitis. ***Acute motor polyneuropathy*** occurring in nutritional and toxic neuropathies, viral encephalitis and Guillain-Barré syndrome (GBS) may cause difficulty in diagnosis. In ***GBS***, there is a considerable rise in CSF proteins without rise in cells (albuminocytological dissociation), whereas in polio, the cellular response occurring before the rise in proteins is marked. Nerve conduction studies also help in diagnosis. Slowing of the velocity of nerve conduction in the peripheral nerves and nerve roots is suggestive of GBS. ***Acute intermittent porphyria*** may present rarely with motor paralysis. Other features of the disease such as psychiatric disturbances, abdominal pain and hypertension may be evident. Demonstration of excess of porphobilinogen in the urine supports the diagnosis. Sometimes painful conditions near the joints result in restriction of movement of the part. Such ***pseudoparalysis*** may occur in osteomyelitis, periosteitis, arthritis, hemophilia, scurvy with subperiosteal bleeding, syphilitic epiphysitis, etc. These have to be carefully looked for and excluded by local examination. Rarely hysterical paralysis may be mistaken for poliomyelitis. This has to be borne in mind when other features of hysteria are suggestive.

Prognosis

In the spinal form of paralytic poliomyelitis in children, mortality is 2–5%. Morbidity is variable. In adults mortality may go up to 15–30%, reaching 75% in bulbar polio. Death is due to respiratory paralysis, autonomic disturbances and encephalitis syndrome. With passage of time considerable return of power occurs in many muscle groups and varying degrees of activity may return.

Treatment

Complete bed rest, analgesics and local heat to sore muscles give symptomatic relief. Since there is no specific treatment, supportive measures are all important. The tendency to tire out muscles which are in a state of partial paresis should be avoided. The respiratory rate, deglutition and blood pressure should be closely monitored to detect complications early. In cases with bulbar polio, feeding by nasogastric tube and parenteral administration of nutrients and fluids may be required. Cases showing signs of respiratory embarrassment should be nursed in a respiratory intensive care unit (ICU). When the vital capacity drops to 25–30% of normal, endotracheal intubation and artificial respiration are called for. Normal vital capacity (VC) for adults = 25 × height in cm; VC for children is 200 × age in years. If ventilatory failure tends to persist, tracheostomy is indicated.

Once the acute phase is over, the muscle strength returns to varying degrees. This improvement is brought about by the recovery of partially damaged neurons, compensatory hypertrophy of the remaining motor units and sprouting of the peripheral nerve endings. In most cases considerable improvement in function is evident in 3–4 months. Further improvement is facilitated by active physiotherapy which is intended to prevent wasting and contractures and stimulate and restore function in partially paralyzed muscles.

Deformities of the axial skeleton develop in severely paralyzed patients. The affected limb fails to grow whereas the normal one undergoes compensatory hypertrophy. Contractures may result in further loss of function of the limbs. Planned orthopedic surgery and rehabilitation help to relieve functional and cosmetic disability in such cases.

Postpolio syndrome (PPS): This is progressive muscular atrophy and muscle weakness occurring several years after apparent recovery from poliomyelitis with residual paralysis. The distinctive features include weakness, pain, fasciculations and atrophy of muscles. Muscles supplied by bulbar nuclei and diaphragm may be affected. Sleep apnea may develop. The exact pathogenesis is not clear. The severity of PPS bear some relation to the severity of the original attack of polio.

The possibilities include:

- Progressive attrition of surviving motor neurons and eventual loss of the axonal terminals.
- Following paralytic polio some of the surviving neurons sprout new endings in an attempt to restore muscle function. This may account for partial recovery of strength for several years following the acute attack. It is likely that the metabolic function of these neurons deteriorate and this leads to PPS.

The CSF shows elevation of immunoglobulin M (IgM) and interleukin-2 which point to an immunological basis for this syndrome.

Prevention

By and large poliomyelitis is a preventable disease. Prophylactic vaccination has significantly reduced the occurrence of polio epidemics. Two types of vaccines are available—live vaccine (Sabin) which is given orally and the killed vaccine (Salk) which is given subcutaneously. The live vaccine is more widely used. The vaccines contain all the three viruses. The trivalent vaccine is given in three doses in the second, fourth and sixth months of age. The immediate response is the formation of IgM antibodies, to be followed later by the appearance of IgG antibodies in 90–99% of cases. In addition, the

live attenuated vaccine also stimulates the formation of local immunoglobulin A (IgA) which gives immunity in the gut also. Booster doses are given at the age of 1.5 and 5 years. Clinical trials conducted in several parts of India have suggested that the standard course of oral vaccination gives protective levels of antibody only in 60–70% cases. Therefore, five doses are recommended at monthly intervals (2, 3, 4, 5 and 6 months) for better protective levels.

The vaccines are generally safe. Oral vaccine has produced limited outbreaks of minor paralytic disease, but with the present vaccines this risk is very low. While immunizing children in closed community like a slum or a hostel, it is advisable to cover all the eligible children (up to the age of ten years if they have not been previously vaccinated). The killed vaccine may produce trivial adverse effects like pain at the site of injection and fever.

Rarely the viral capsid protein may get altered and give rise to wild type sequence giving rise to invasive polio virus especially in those with common variable immune deficiency in whom, polio infection may remain chronic. The risk of vaccine associated paralytic polio in persons with primary B cell immune deficiency is increased 3000 times than that of normal. Such persons will also shed polio viruses for much longer periods. Many countries including United States of America (USA) have discontinued oral polio vaccine and use only killed vaccine despite its higher cost and need for injection.

Eradication of poliomyelitis can be achieved by full coverage of the population by vaccination, provision of protected water supply and general improvement in hygiene. Continued surveillance is absolutely essential to prevent outbreaks. In several countries, occurrence of fresh cases has been arrested. India is near to the goal of eradication.

As part of a strategy to eradicate the major infectious diseases of childhood, especially poliomyelitis, the Indian Medical Association (IMA) has recommended the regime in Table 56.1 for immunization.

At present, IMA is the main agency working with governmental institutions in giving effect to the Pulse Polio Programme.

Recent studies from India show that injectable polio vaccine given to children who have received oral polio vaccine (OPV) previously, boosts up both humoral

Table 56.1: Regime recommended as per Indian Medical Association			
S. No.	**Age of child**	**Vaccine**	**Other care**
1	At birth	BCG, OPV	
2	6 weeks	DPT, OPV	
3	10 weeks	DPT, OPV	
4	14 weeks	DPT, OPV	
5	9 months	Measles	Vitamin A
6	16 months (Booster)	DPT, OPV	Vitamin A

Abbreviations: DPT = Diphtheria, Pertussis and Tetanus; BCG = Bacillus Calmette–Guérin; OPV = Oral polio vaccine

neutralizing antibody levels and also intestinal mucosal immunity.

Source: Jafari H, Deshpande JM, Sutter RW, et al. Polio eradication. Efficacy of inactivated poliovirus vaccine in India. Science. 2014;345(6199):922-5.

OTHER ENTEROVIRUSES

These include coxsackie virus, echovirus and enterovirus which have several serotypes each and cause pathological lesions in humans. There is considerable overlap in pathogenicity and clinical features (Table 56.2).

ECHOVIRUSES

Syn: Enteric cytopathogenic human orphan viruses

These are RNA viruses ranging in size from 20 to 30 nm which produce a spectrum of diseases ranging from mild upper respiratory infection, fever with rash and aseptic meningitis to acute hemorrhagic conjunctivitis. Over 30 serotypes have been identified by using virus neutralization tests.

Pathogenesis

The virus gets in by ingestion and the mode of spread is feco-oral. After an initial period of viral multiplication in the epithelium of the intestines and respiratory tract, they enter the bloodstream to produce viremia. The organisms reach the various target organs from the bloodstream.

Clinical Features

The incubation period is generally 2–5 days but for hemorrhagic conjunctivitis, it is shorter (12–72 hours).

The clinical manifestations include nonspecific fever, upper respiratory tract infections, exanthems, diarrhea, pneumonia, myopericarditis and serious neurological involvement.

Aseptic Meningitis

Aseptic meningitis may occur as a result of infection by several strains of echoviruses. Signs of meningeal irritation or rise in intracranial tension may be evident. The acute phase may last for 4–7 days.

Table 56.2: Different lesions caused by enterovirus serotypes

Lesions	Virus types
Exanthems	Coxsackie (Cox), Echovirus (Ech) and Enterovirus (Ent)
Encephalitis	Cox, Ech
Aseptic meningitis	Cox, Ech
Hand, foot and mouth disease	Cox, Ent
Myocarditis and pericarditis	Cox, Ech, Ent
Pleurodynia	Cox, Ech
Pneumonia	Cox, Ech, Ent
Acute hemorrhagic conjunctivitis	Cox, Ech
Paralytic lesions	Cox, Ech, Ent
Herpangina	Cox, Ech, Ent
Infantile infections	Cox, Ech

The CSF shows lymphocytic pleocytosis usually less than 500/mm³. Mixed pleocytosis may occur in some cases. Complete recovery is the rule, but rarely complications such as transverse myelitis, bulbar paralysis, GBS, cerebellar lesions and coma may develop.

Treatment

There is no specific treatment and therefore, treatment is symptomatic and supportive. Prophylactic measures include improvement of environmental sanitation, provision of protected water supply and elimination of flies. Vaccines are not available for general use.

Acute Hemorrhagic Conjunctivitis (AHC)

This disease occurs in pandemics from time to time (1971, 1981). Most of the cases are caused by the ***enterovirus type 70 (EV70)***. All age groups are affected, children being more. The age group of 21–40 are more prone to develop neurologic complications. Infection is acquired by direct spread to the eyes from contaminated fingers or by fomites. Incubation period is 12–72 hours. Initial symptoms are bilateral conjunctivitis with irritation of the eyes and watery discharge. The conjunctiva may show blotchy hemorrhage. In vast majority of cases, the symptoms subside without other local complications within 7–10 days. Secondary bacterial infection and keratitis may develop. The virus can be isolated from the conjunctival secretions. In a small proportion, constitutional symptoms such as fever, malaise and limb pains may occur.

Neurological complications may develop in a few, usually within 2–3 weeks (even up to 4 months). Adult males are affected more. These may take one of three forms—spinal, cranial or combined.

Spinal form: Asymmetric flaccid paralysis of the proximal muscles of the lower limbs, associated with backache and followed by muscular wasting.

Cranial form: Isolated or combined cranial nerve palsies.

Combined form: A variable combination of both. Sensory symptoms are absent or minimal. Examination of the CSF during the early stages may reveal mild lymphocytosis and moderate rise in proteins. Neutralizing antibodies against EV70 can be demonstrated in the majority of cases, in the serum as well as CSF. Treatment is symptomatic.

COXSACKIEVIRUSES INFECTIONS

Coxsackieviruses are picornaviruses which can be grouped into A and B. They were first isolated from the village of Coxsackie in New York by Dalldorf in 1948 and the name is derived therefrom. About 30 immunological types have been isolated. Many strains are commensals in the alimentary and respiratory tract of man. Spread is by the feco-oral route and small outbreaks occur especially in summer. The causative role of these viruses in any specific illness can be established only by isolating it from specific lesions in the affected organs or tissue fluids.

Pathogenicity

Several lesions are produced by these viruses group A and B. These include: (1) Neurological lesions, (2) respiratory disorders, (3) carditis and (4) hand-foot and mouth disease and others. The incubation period is 2–14 days.

Clinical Features

Neurological lesions: The clinical syndromes include polio-like paralysis, meningoencephalitis and aseptic meningitis. The pathological lesions are:

- Neuronophagia of the anterior horn cells of the spinal cord and perivascular infiltration by lymphocytes
- Meningoencephalitis
- Scattered foci of degeneration in the spinal cord, cerebral hemispheres, pons and cerebellum.

Respiratory lesions: Pleura is most characteristically involved. The syndrome of pleurodynia (***devil's grip, Bornholm's disease, epidemic myalgia***) is caused by Coxsackie B group viruses.

Severe pain develops in the chest and upper abdomen, after a prodromal febrile illness. Breathing becomes painful, short, shallow and rapid. Physical examination may reveal pleural rub, pleural effusion, pneumonia, myocarditis, pericarditis, hepatitis or orchitis. The acute phase subsides in 2–3 days but mild fever and pain may persist for a longer period. Pleurodynia has to be distinguished from acute myocardial infarction, other forms of pleurisy and surgical abdominal emergencies. Symptomatic treatment with rest and analgesics gives relief. Enteroviruses are etiological agents for childhood pneumonias.

Cardiovascular lesions: The heart is affected by both groups of Coxsackie viruses, but group B is more common to produce acute myocarditis and pericarditis. Infection acquired congenitally or neonatally tends to be serious and rapidly fatal. This may be associated with encephalitis or adrenal necrosis. Pericarditis is more common in older children and adults. Myocarditis may lead to cardiac failure, arrhythmias or the late development of chronic cardiomyopathy and calcific or constrictive pericarditis. Electrocardiographic (ECG) changes may occur. Congenital heart disease is associated with Coxsackie B types 3 and 4 infection acquired *in utero.*

ENTEROVIRUSES CAUSED DISEASES

Hand, Foot and Mouth Disease

It is a not a rare childhood exanthem caused by human enterovirus, species of the family Picornaviridae—most commonly by EV71 and coxsackievirus A16. Children below 5 years are most affected and they are liable to develop neurological complications. With the elimination of poliomyelitis, the neurological lesions caused by these viruses are coming to the forefront. EV71 virus was identified in 1961 in the USA, subsequently several epidemics of hand, foot and mouth disease have been described in Malaysia, Taiwan, far Eastern countries, China, France and others.

Based on the variable VP1 structural gene, EV71 has been classified into four genetic lineages A, B, C and D. Newer strains with different genetic lineages B3, B4, B5, C3, C4 and C5 have been detected. Recombination of different strains of EV71 have been described, adding to the genetic diversity. Spread is by feco-oral transmission comparable to that of poliomyelitis.

Clinical Features

The clinical presentation and severity varies between epidemics. Majority of infections are asymptomatic. Mild cases manifest as upper respiratory infections, herpangina and hand, foot and mouth disease.

The vesicular lesions occur on the palms of hands, soles of the feet, mouth and buttocks where they may ulcerate. This disease is self-limiting.

Neurological lesions which may occur include brain stem encephalitis [demonstrable by magnetic resonance imaging (MRI) scan], acute flaccid paralysis and aseptic meningitis which are serious and may lead to mortality and permanent morbidity. Brainstem encephalitis affects the hypothalamus, brain stem, spinal cord and cerebellar dentate nucleus and the lesions are caused by direct affection by EV71 viruses. These lesions are more likely to result in permanent sequelae. The flaccid paralysis is caused by lytic lesions in the anterior horn motor neurons of the spinal cord.

Neurogenic pulmonary edema may occur progressing rapidly over a period of 24–36 hours and is associated with high mortality. Serious complications are more common in children below 2 years of age.

Diagnosis

Hand, foot and mouth disease may be mistaken for chickenpox, aphthous stomatitis or herpangina. In chickenpox the vesicles are more widely distributed, multiple crops occur and pustulation and scab formation are seen. These are absent in hand, foot and mouth disease. The virus can be isolated from the vesicle fluid. Neutralizing and complement fixing antibodies are also demonstrable. Treatment is essentially symptomatic.

Management

There is no specific antiviral drug; treatment is symptomatic and supportive. In many countries, attempts to make suitable vaccines are actively pursued. Phase 3 clinical trial of inactivated EV71 vaccine were completed in 2013. Further trails on EV71 vaccines manufactured in China report effectiveness of protection against EV71 associated hand, foot and mouth disease and herpangina in children. Neutralizing antibody titers above 1:16 were found to be protective. Two intramuscular doses given 28 days apart gave suitable protection. Present day vaccines protect against the specific strains, but not against EV71 viruses and coxsackieviruses of other lineages. Multivalent vaccines are being formulated.

Source: McMinn PC. Enterovirus vaccines for an emerging cause of brain-stem encephalitis. N Engl J Med. 2014;370(9):792-4.

Other Manifestations

Herpangina

Coxsackieviruses have been implicated in the production of herpangina (painful vesicles in the throat and pharynx), lymphonodular pharyngitis, hepatitis, exanthematous fevers and pancreatitis.

Laboratory Diagnosis of Enteroviruses

Enteroviruses can be isolated by appropriate methods from feces and upper respiratory and pharyngeal secretions. Since these viruses may exist in body cavities without causing disease, isolation of the virus may not be conclusive evidence of pathogenicity.

Serological tests are often nonspecific, since the serotypes of these viruses which can be pathogenic are large in number and varied. Isolation of virus from body fluids is more reliable to judge pathogenicity.

Treatment of Enterovirus

This infection is mainly supportive. There is no specific therapy. Majority of cases recover completely in 1–6 weeks. Absolute bed rest and symptomatic treatment should be continued till the ECG becomes normal. Immunoglobulin containing high titers against the infecting virus has been used in serious situations with possible success.

CHAPTER
57

Adenovirus Infections

KV Krishna Das

Chapter Summary

- General Considerations
- Clinical Features
  - Acute Febrile Respiratory Illness
  - Acute Pharyngoconjunctival Fever
  - Epidemic Keratoconjunctivitis
  - Pneumonia and Diarrheal Disease
- Diagnosis
- Treatment
- Prevention

GENERAL CONSIDERATIONS

Adenoviruses are a group of double-stranded deoxyribonucleic acid (DNA) viruses which cause a range of febrile disorders characterized by inflammation of the respiratory tract and conjunctiva and accompanied by submucosa and regional lymphadenopathy. The name is derived from the fact that these viruses were first isolated from adenoid tissue removed surgically. More than 50 serotypes of human adenoviruses have been identified.

The virus is 60–90 nm in size. Several serotypes are known. Adenoviruses are implicated in the production of acute respiratory disease, intestinal infections and mesenteric adenitis. Adenovirus is a common cause of respiratory disease especially in children below 15 years of age. The disease spreads by droplet infection. Oronasal secretions of infected persons contain about 10^6–10^7 virus particles/mL. Even as low as 5 viral particles can result in infection and therefore the infection spreads fast. The incubation period varies between 3 and 14 days. A good proportion of adults show antibodies against adenoviruses indicating the prevalence of this infection in the community acquired during childhood.

CLINICAL FEATURES

Several clinical disorders are caused by these viruses.

- ***Acute febrile respiratory illness*** occurs more frequently in children. Paroxysms of cough may occur. X-ray shows patchy lobular pneumonia. Encephalitis may develop as a complication.
- ***Acute pharyngoconjunctival fever*** produces the classical triad of fever, pharyngitis and conjunctivitis. The disease subsides in 1–2 weeks. Unilateral or bilateral simple conjunctivitis may develop in some.
- ***Epidemic keratoconjunctivitis*** may occur in outbreaks, affecting particularly shipyard workers and in harbor personnel. The onset is sudden with unilateral edema, conjunctivitis, superficial corneal opacities and lymphadenopathy. Later the other eye is also involved. The course is for 3–4 weeks. The majority recover completely, though in a small proportion blindness may result from corneal lesions.
- ***Pneumonia and diarrheal disease:*** Small outbreaks of adenovirus pneumonia and diarrheal disease have been reported military personnel especially in the United States of America (USA).

DIAGNOSIS

Specific diagnosis is established by isolation of the virus or demonstration of viral DNA by polymerase chain reaction (PCR).

TREATMENT

It is symptomatic and supportive. Severe pneumonia in infants and epidemic keratoconjunctivitis require special management. The antiviral ribavirin and cidofovir are active against adenoviruses *in vitro*. Empirical treatment with these drugs in severe systemic disease may give benefit.

PREVENTION

Vaccines against adenovirus types 4 and 7 have been developed for the use of military recruits in the USA. This consists of live unattenuated virus held in oral capsules, they cause local immunity against infection and systemic humoral immunity against respiratory lesions. This vaccine is not available in India.

KV Krishna Das, Sajith Kumar

CHAPTER 58

Arenavirus Infections, Filovirus Infections and Hemorrhagic Fevers

Chapter Summary

- General Considerations
- Arenaviruses
- Lymphocytic Choriomeningitis
- Lassa Fever
- South American Hemorrhagic Fevers
- Hantavirus Infections
- Marburg Virus and Ebola Virus Infections
- Crimean-Congo Hemorrhagic Fever
- Omsk hemorrhagic Fever
- Chandipura Virus Encephalitis

GENERAL CONSIDERATIONS

Since 1930, several viruses especially arenaviruses are known to produce hemorrhagic manifestations, though other groups of viruses can also cause the same. The hemorrhagic fevers can be grouped under three headings depending upon the virus and the vector. Localized or generalized hemorrhage may occur as alarming symptoms in infections by dengue, yellow fever, chikungunya, Kyasanur forest disease (KFD) and arenavirus infections.

- ■ *Mosquito-borne hemorrhagic fevers,* e.g. dengue types 1, 2, 3 and 4, chikungunya, yellow fever virus.
- ■ *Zoonotic viruses which may be transmitted to man,* e.g. Korean hemorrhagic fever, Argentine hemorrhagic fever and Lassa fever (Lassa virus) (Table 58.1).
- ■ *Tick-borne hemorrhagic fevers,* e.g. KFD. Omsk hemorrhagic fever and Crimean-Congo hemorrhagic fever (CCHF) group. The vectors in some hemorrhagic fevers have not been identified yet.

Newer and newer viruses capable of producing this syndrome are being added to the list even now.

Hemorrhagic fever of South Asia: Viral hemorrhagic fevers occurring in Philippines, Malaysia, Vietnam and eastern parts of India are collectively referred to as 'hemorrhagic fevers of South East Asia'. These are all transmitted by *Aedes aegypti* mosquitoes.

Outbreaks of dengue hemorrhagic fever have occurred in all parts of India in the recent past and are being reported frequently even now despite several precautionary measures undertaken to limit the infection. All types of dengue viruses (especially type 2) are responsible for most of the cases.

ARENAVIRUSES

They are ribonucleic acid (RNA) viruses belonging to three families. They may be spherical, oval or pleomorphic, ranging in size from 110 to 130 nm. Under the election microscope they resemble grains of sand and hence the name arenaviruses (Latin: arenosos) means sandy.

They belong to two genetic branches:

1. Lassa virus and lymphocytic choriomeningitis (old world)
2. South American hemorrhagic fevers (new world viruses).

They all occur as natural inhabitants in rodents.

Except Machupo virus, the others exists without producing diseases in them. The infection is transmitted from parent to offspring *in utero* and thus a reservoir of infection is maintained among the rodents. Man may get the infection directly through cuts and wounds or by inhalation of infective aerosols and close contact with rodents and their excreta.

A groups of viruses which are zoonotic can be transmitted to man. Those produce sporadic infection

Table 58.1: Zoonotic viruses transmitted to humans		
Genus/groups	*Viruses*	*Natural hosts*
Arenaviridae	Lymphocytic choriomeningitis, Lassa fever	Rodents
Arenaviridae	South American hemorrhagic virus, Machupo, Junin viruses	Rodents
Bunyaviridae–Bunyavirus	Bunyamwera virus	Mosquito vector and vertebrate host
Phlebovirus	Sandfly virus	Sandfly vector man
Nairovirus	Hantavirus, Crimean-Congo hemorrhagic fever	Rodent, ticks and man
Flaviviridae	Ebola and Marburg viruses	Not known? Bats and other animals
Flaviviridae (mosquito borne)	Yellow fever, dengue fever	Mosquito vector human reservoir
Flaviviridae (tick borne)	Russian spring-summer encephalitis (Omsk hemorrhagic fever)	Ticks and humans
Rhabdoviridae	Vasculo virus, Chandipura virus	Sandfly vector, vertebrate host transovarial passage
Togaviridae	Alphavirus, chikungunya virus	Mosquito, vertebrate host

Textbook of Medicine

leading to clinical features of varying severity, many with hemorrhagic complications during their clinical course.

LYMPHOCYTIC CHORIOMENINGITIS

Lymphocytic choriomeningitis virus (LCMV) was one of the earliest viruses to be isolated in the mid-1930s. It belongs to the family arenaviridae which contains about 20 known viruses affecting different rodents which shed the virus without themselves suffering from disease.

LCMV has assumed importance with the infection occurring more commonly in transplant recipients. Most of the cases are subclinical with < 1% developing meningitis and with mortality < 1%. LCMV infection may be transmitted by donors who themselves do not show signs of overt disease.

Incubation is one week. Disease starts with prodrome and fever. Meningitis occurs by about 15–20 days. Cerebrospinal fluid (CSF) shows moderate lymphocytosis, up to 700/mm^3. LCM occurring in transplant recipients is generally obscure and fatal if, on detected.

Another pattern of LCMV infection is that of a fatal hemorrhagic fever typical of that of Lassa fever which is also an arenavirus.

Ribavirin is effective against the virus. LCMV infection occurring in pregnant women may lead to hydrocephalus, mental retardation and chrioretinitis in the newborns.

LASSA FEVER

This occurs mainly in Africa. Majority of infections are subclinical. Symptomatic cases may present with chest pain, sore throat, cough, abdominal pain, vomiting, diarrhea, facial puffiness, myocarditis and conjunctivitis. Minor hemorrhagic manifestations may develop due to increase in capillary leak. Nerve deafness may occur as a complication.

Treatment is symptomatic. Ribavirin given orally in dose of 1000–1200 mg/day may be beneficial.

SOUTH AMERICAN HEMORRHAGIC FEVERS

Important in this group are **Argentine** and **Bolivian hemorrhagic fevers** and **Venezuelan hemorrhagic fever.** The general symptoms include fever, malaise, myalgia, hypotension, petechiae, capillary leak syndrome and neurological complications including convulsions and coma.

Serological tests may show antibody by enzyme linked immune sorbent assay (ELISA). Virus can be isolated from blood and other tissues by cell-culture. Mortality ranges from 10 to 20%. Mainstay of treatment is intensive care with correction of fluid and electrolytes and symptomatic management of hemorrhagic manifestations. Vaccines against Argentine hemorrhagic fever and Lassa fever are under trial in endemic areas.

HANTAVIRUS INFECTIONS

Hantavirus is a natural inhabitant of rodents and the virus is shed in their urine, feces and saliva. Infection is by inhalation of rodent excreta particles. Urine and feces of rodent contain the virus and they become aerosolized and inhaled. The virus remains in the environment for 9–15 days. This virus affects the vascular endothelium and causes two major syndromes:

1. Hemorrhagic fever with renal syndrome (HFRS)
2. Hantavirus cardiopulmonary syndrome (HCPS).

Antibodies to these virus has been reported in 15% of febrile patients in Vellore (India). Infection is by aerosol inhalation of infective material. Incubation period is about 3 weeks.

The virus affecting the endothelium leads to immune response against viral antigens expressed on the endothelial cells of the heart, lungs, kidney and lymphoid organs. The immune reactions are mediated by T-lymphocytes and macrophages. Tumor necrosis factor (TNF)-α and interleukin (IL)-1β increase capillary permeability. Nitric oxide released by TNF leads to vasodilation and shock.

HFRS: Nonspecific constitutional symptoms occur followed by hemorrhagic manifestations along with renal lesions.

Shock, oliguria and disseminated intravascular coagulation (DIC) follow. Survivors enter a diuretic phase by day 10–14. **Blood findings** include thrombocytopenia, left-sided shift of granulocytes, atypical lymphocytosis and hemoconcentration. Increase in the number of circulating immunoblasts (up to 10% of circulating lymphocytes) and increase in serum levels or lactate dehydrogenase (LDH) should suggest the diagnosis. Specific tests include the demonstration of immunoglubulin M (IgM) and IgG antibodies by ELISA.

HCPS: Pulmonary syndrome is described in North America and Europe. Constitutional symptoms lasting for 3–7 days are followed by hypotension and shock. Noncardiogenic-bilateral-interstial pulmonary edema, cardiac arrhythmias and cardiac arrest may occur. Pulmonary edema is presumably caused by T-cell response to viral infection of the microvascular pulmonary endothelial cells. Cause of death is cardiogenic shock and hence the name 'Hantavirus cardiopulmonary syndrome' is used.

Renal lesions may develop leading to oliguria lasting for 3–8 days and later followed by polyuria.

Treatment

It is supportive with intravenous (IV) fluids, inotropes, mechanical ventilation and blood products. Hantavirus pulmonary syndrome causes hypoxemia and bilateral intestinal noncardiac pulmonary edema. The disease should be suspected in conditions of exposure to mouse and rodent excreta. Diagnosis is by demonstration of IgM and IgG antibodies to the virus. Extracorporeal membrane oxygenation may be lifesaving. Ribavirin has been used in usual doses with variable results. Mortality may be as high as 36%.

Source: Chandy S, Mitra S, Sathish N, et al. A pilot study for serological evidence of hantavirus infection in human population in south India. Indian J Med Res. 2005;122(3):211-5.

MARBURG VIRUS AND EBOLA VIRUS INFECTIONS

These are single-stranded RNA viruses belonging to the family of Filoviridae both the types being native to African countries. The two types Ebola and Marburg can be

Textbook of Medicine

distinguished serologically, biochemically and genetically, though they are morphologically similar and their pathogenicity also is similar. The term Ebolavirus is derived from the name of a river in Congo. Marburg is a town in Germany where early descriptions of the virus occurred. These viruses cause immune dysfunction in humans and endothelial damage leading to the fatal hemorrhagic complications and multi-organ failure. Viral replication occurs in the cytoplasm of cells, main involvement is in the liver, kidney and lymph nodes.

Epidemiology

In 2004–2005, an outbreak occurred in Angola with a case fatality of about 90%. Apes, man and fruit bats and other mammals were the reservoir. Ebolavirus is transmitted by eating infected animals, contact with cases and handling infected bats. Transmission is also by close contact with body secretions and tissue fluids of cases. Incubation is from 4 to 10 days. Though the infections were considered to be rare, recent outbreaks (March to October, 2014) in the East and Central African States with the possibility of spread globally has brought these diseases into prominence and global preventive measures have been geared up under control of World Health Organization (WHO). The number of cases infected in the recent epidemic has exceeded 2500 with deaths exceeding 1500 (60% mortality or higher); 80% deaths occurring in the healthcare personnel. The fact that there is no specific antiviral agent currently available and that the mortality may go up to 90% make these infections as top priority. There are no authentic reports about the presence of these diseases in India. The Indian government is seized of the situation and has given directions to contain the disease from spreading. Marburg virus infection leads to 25% mortality.

Ebola Virus Disease (EVD) in West Africa

Clinical Features

Early symptoms include high fever, temperature above 40°C, malaise, fatigue and body aches.

Fever persists and by the 3rd to 5th day of illness, gastrointestinal (GI) symptoms start with epigastric pain, nausea, vomiting and diarrhea. At this stage, testing for Ebola virus is invariably positive by polymerase chain reaction (PCR) test. In many cases there was no history of contact to get the disease. Large volume diarrhea (more than 5 L/day or more–like that of cholera) starts suddenly and persists for 7 days and tapers off. Associated signs included symptoms of asthenia, headache, conjunctival injection, chest pain, abdominal pain, arthralgias, myalgia and hiccups delirium and less commonly, RH.

In the absence of fluid replacement, severe lethargy and prostration develop. Shock was associated with confusion or coma with peripheral thready pulses, severe metabolic acidosis. Clinically significant hemorrhage from upper or lower GIT occurred in less than 5% of cases often before death. Sudden death occurred between 7 and 12 days of illness. Those who survived 10 days started improving, those who survived 13 days, ultimately recovered. Children below 5 years, pregnant women and elderly were particularly vulnerable. Patients were discharged if they were afebrile for 3 days and PCR was negative.

Treatment should consist of fluid replacement and treatment of shock from the beginning. IV fluids and electrolytes may help. Aggressive antiemetic therapy may help to reduce morality.

Analysis of the results of management of confirmed Ebola virus disease in the United States and Europe has been published. Twenty-seven patients (median age 25–75) were treated, out of which 70% were males, 9 patients had comorbidities, 24 patients were evacuated from west Africa with the disease. Main symptoms included fatigue, fever or feverishness and weakness, myalgia headache, decreased appetite, lethargy arthralgia, sore throat, rhinorrhea, diarrhea, nausea, abdomen pain, cough and vomiting. Predominant laboratory findings were hypoalbuminemia, hyponatremia, hypokalemia and hypocalcemia and hypomagnesemia. Nine patients had oliguria of whom 5 had anuria.

Ebola virus DNA levels in blood peaked at a median of 7 days after onset of illness. Aminotransferase levels peaked at a median of 9 days after onset. All patients were treated with IV fluids and electrolytes supplementation. 9 received assisted ventilation, 5 received continuous renal replacement therapy and 21 received empirical antibiotics. Aggressive support, IV fluid and electrolyte substitution, nutritional support and critical care for respiratory and renal failure were needed. 81.5% of those who received this care survived. The median time to clearance of viremia was 17.5 days. 5 patients (18.5%) died, 3 of them had respiratory and renal failure.

Source: Uyeki TM, Mehta AK, Davey RJ Jr, et al. Clinical management of Ebola Virus Disease in the United States and Europe. N Eng J Med. 2016;374(7):636-46.

Vaccination: Development of vaccine against Ebola virus is being pursued by several countries. A monovalent chimpanzee adenovirus. Ebola vaccine boosted with modified vaccinia virus Ankara (MVA) strain encoding the same Ebola virus glycoprotein has been tried at Oxford United Kingdom. This vaccine produced B and T cells immune response better than previously tried vaccines.

Phase 1 Trial of rVSV Ebola Vaccine in Africa and Europe

Replication competent recombinant vesicular stomatis virus based vaccine expressing a Zaire Ebola virus glycoprotein was tried in Europe and Africa. This vaccine is reactogenic, but immunogenic after a single dose and warrants further evaluation for safety and efficacy.

Source: Agnandji ST, Huttner A, Zinser ME, et al. Phase 1 Trials of rVSV Ebola Vaccine in Africa and Europe. N Engl J Med. 2016;374(17):1647-60.

CRIMEAN-CONGO HEMORRHAGIC FEVER (CCHF)

Originally discussed as early as 12th century from Tajikistan, the name CCHF was coined in 1967.

Virus: A member of genus norovirus, family Bunyaviridae (Hantavirus also belongs to same family). It is an RNA virus. Thirty-four strains have been identified.

Vector: Ixodid (hard ticks) and argasid (soft ticks) transmit the disease. Ticks can maintain the reservoir. Human contamination is caused by blood and body fluids. Tick bites and contact with infected animals and animal products helps to spread infection.

Recently this infection broke out in Kolat Village, 30 km southwest of Ahmedabad in Gujarat State—it was well controlled and studied reported by Times of India 19th January, 2011.

Pathology and pathogenesis include: Endothelial damage, procoagulant activity and DIC like manifestations:

Clinical features: Incubation period is 3–8 days.

Prehemorrhagic phase: Fever, chills, temperature ranging from 39 to 41°C, fatigue and vague symptoms. Hemorrhagic phase ushers with bleeding from mucus membranes and skin. Convalescence lasts for 2–3 weeks.

Diagnosis: Blood shows neutropenia and thrombocytopenia. Antibodies are demonstrable by ELISA (IgG and IgM) by 6–7 days. Virus culture may be positive if done early. PCR detects the viral genome. Only laboratories with biosafety level 4 should undertake the tests since risk of nosocomial spread is high.

Prognosis: Case fatality 15–70%.

Treatment: Specific treatment includes ribavirin 30 mg/kg as initial dose, thereafter 15 mg/kg 6 h for 4 days and then 75 mg/kg 8 h for 6 days. Ribavirin is available in the Indian market as 200 mg tablets (cost of 10 day treatment is ₹ 6000).

Prevention: Postexposure prophylaxis with ribavirin 200 mg twice a day for 5 days is effective. Long-term measures include control of ticks, protective clothing and acaricides.

Source:

1. Bajpai S, Nadkar MY. Crimean Congo hemorrhagic fever: requires vigilance and not panic. J Assoc Physicians India. 2011;59:164-7.

2. Patel AK, Patel KK, Mehta M, et al. First Crimean-Congo hemorrhagic fever outbreak in India. J Assoc Physicians India. 2011;59:585-9.

OMSK HEMORRHAGIC FEVER

Omsk hemorrhagic fever was first detected in Osmk region of Siberia of Russia, the animal hosts being the musk rat and others. Vectors are ticks—*Dermacentor reticulatus* and *Dermacentor marginatus*. Other vectors may also be important. The virus belongs to Flavivirus family, infection is acquired from ticks and oral or respiratory routes. Incubation period is 3–7 days. Symptoms include fever, headache, cough, GI symptoms, hemorrhages from nose, mouth and uterus. Blood shows neutrophilia, monocytosis and thrombocytopenia. Mortality is up to 2.5%. Specific treatment is by the antiviral drug ribavirin. Larifan and rivastin which are interferon inducers are tried in doses of 0.5–1.5 mg given parenterally. Vaccine is also available in endemic places.

CHANDIPURA VIRUS ENCEPHALITIS

This is a rapidly developing encephalitis which has occurred in several parts of India from time to time. The virus belongs to the genus of Vesiculovirus and family Rhabdoviridae. An outbreak was documented in Jamshedpur in 1954. An outbreak was described in 2003 in Andhra Pradesh and adjoining areas of Maharashtra. In 1980, the virus was isolated from a case in Madhya Pradesh. It has also been reported from Senegal and Nigeria. The virus was originally discovered in 1965 at the National Institute of Virology, Pune. Vectors are most probably female sandflies—phlebotomus.

The onset is with sudden fever, rigor, drowsiness leading to unconsciousness and death in 6–48 hours. The age group ranged from 2.5 to 15 years. The case fatality was 52.3%.

Soucre: Rao BL, Basu A, Wairagkar NS, et al. A large outbreak of acute encephalitis with high fatality rate in children in Andhra Pradesh, India, in 2003, associated with Chandipura virus. Lancet. 2004;364(9437):869-74.

CHAPTER

59

Rabies

KV Krishna Das, K Sreekanthan, Aswini Kumar

Chapter Summary

- General Considerations
- Clinical Features and Complications
- Diagnosis
- Treatment
- Prophylaxis

GENERAL CONSIDERATIONS

Syn: Hydrophobia, Lyssa

Rabies is an acute viral disease, primarily of animals, clinically characterized by rapidly progressive and fatal encephalitis, acquired by man through the bites or licks of infected animals.

Etiology

The etiological agent is a ribonucleic acid (RNA) virus belonging to the group of rhabdoviruses. The rhabdoviridae consists of five genera, each of which has several species. Rabies virus is a species of (serotype1) of the genus Lyssa virus of the family rhabdoviridae. It is a rod-shaped virus approximately 180 by 75 nm. When isolated first from animals, it was called ***street virus***. This has a long incubation period and the virus multiplies in the salivary glands and

Textbook of Medicine

the central nervous system (CNS). By repeated intracerebral passage in laboratory animals, it adapts to them. At this stage, it is called *fixed virus*. It has a uniformly shortened incubation period (4 to 6 days) and it loses its ability to multiply in the salivary glands. It has reduced pathogenicity and is used in vaccine production. Rabies virus is rapidly inactivated by heat. At 56°C, the virus dies in less than a minute, whereas at 37°C, it survives for several hours under moist environment. The virus is also inactivated by ultraviolet light, detergents and soap solution, ethanol, iodine and quaternary ammonium compounds.

Distribution and Incidence

Rabies is enzootic worldwide except in a few countries. Rabies is widely prevalent in India, but human rabies is generally under reported. In India, 30,000 deaths were reported to the World Health Organization (WHO) in 1998. Other countries reporting high incidence of human rabies are Bangladesh, Nepal, Sri Lanka, Pakistan, Vietnam, Philippines, Indonesia, Mexico and Ethiopia.

All warm-blooded animals are susceptible to rabies. Dogs are most important in transmitting the disease to man. Among mammals, different animals differ in their susceptibility to infection. Very highly susceptible animals include wolves, foxes, jackals, kangaroo rats and cotton rats. Highly susceptible animals include hamsters, skunks, raccoons, domestic cats, rabbits, bats and cattle. Dogs and primates are moderately susceptible. Opossums have low susceptibility. *Dogs and other animals may or may not succumb to the infection.*

Transmission and Epidemiology

Virus enters through cuts or wounds caused by bites, scratches or licks of rabid animals, which contain virus in their saliva. Rare modes of transmission include inhalation of virus aerosols. When dogs bark, the saliva may be sprayed to a distance of up to 2 meters. Inhalations of aerosols created in caves inhabited by vampire bats, which suck blood from animals and man, have also resulted in rabies. Laboratory accidents of rabies following inhaled aerosols of fixed virus also been reported. Less commonly injury from cats, jackals, mongoose, wolves and other canines may transmit the disease. Rabies following accidental injection of vaccines containing live rabies virus are also reported.

Human-to-Human Transmission

Man-to-man transmission from contact with human saliva is extremely rare, though theoretically possible. Transmission has occurred through grafting of infected corneas and organ transplantation.

Pathogenesis

After entering a susceptible host, the rabies surface glycoprotein attaches to a cell and enters it by endocytosis. The surface envelope of the virus fuses with the vesicle membrane and the ribonucleoprotein enters the cytoplasm. Local replication may occur in striated muscle near the site of the bite, but there may also be direct invasion of nerve cells. Postsynaptic nicotinic acetylcholine receptors at neuromuscular junctions are important binding sites. Once inside the peripheral nerves, the virus is carried in the flow of axoplasm at the rate of about 3 mm/hour to the dorsal root ganglia where replication occurs. This may give rise to prodromal paresthesia at the site of the bite. In the CNS, there is massive replication with viral budding from intracellular membranes of neurons and trans-synaptic transmission of virus from cell to cell. Passive centrifugal spread of virus from the CNS in the axoplasm of many efferent nerves including those of the autonomic nervous system occurs. By this route the virus spreads to the salivary glands and to lacrimal glands and several other tissues.

Pathology

The white and the gray matter of the cerebrum show severe congestion. Perivascular and perineuronal infiltration with mononuclear cells occur. Intracytoplasmic inclusion bodies (Negri bodies) are formed and these are demonstrable in 80% of the cases. Negri bodies are seen in large numbers in the hippocampal gyrus, Purkinje cells of the cerebellum and the pyramidal cells. They are also seen in the basal ganglia and the cranial nerve nuclei and spinal cord. While their presence is diagnostic of rabies, their absence does not exclude the diagnosis. Extra neural changes include focal degeneration of salivary and lacrimal glands, pancreas, adrenal medulla and lymph nodes. Interstitial myocarditis with round cell infiltration may occur.

Immune Responses

The immune response to natural rabies infection is insufficient to prevent rabies. Rabies can produce immunosuppression and only a minority of unvaccinated patients develop a measurable antibody response. Patients developing a cellular immune response tend to have the furious form rather than the paralytic form and die faster than those who do not mount such a response. The virus may persist in macrophages and may later emerge to produce disease. This may explain some cases with very long incubation periods.

CLINICAL FEATURES AND COMPLICATIONS

Animal Rabies

In dogs, the incubation period is usually between 2 weeks and 4 months (extreme range, 5 days to 14 months). The illness may start with 2 to 3 days of prodromal symptoms, e.g. a change in behavior, fever and intense irritation. Dogs with the less common but more familiar, furious form of the disease become aggressive, wander away from home and may develop convulsion, dysphagia, pharyngeal paralysis causing an altered bark and hyper salivation. Those with paralytic or dumb rabies hide themselves and develop paralysis of the jaw, neck and hind limbs. Dysphagia and drooling of saliva may raise the suspicion of a foreign body stuck in the throat. Virus may be excreted in the saliva for 2–3 days before there are signs of rabies and the animal usually dies within the next 7 days. A small proportion of infected animals recover and may continue to excrete virus for long periods. Horses and cats usually exhibit furious symptoms whereas paralytic disease is the rule in foxes and bovines. Hydrophobia is not seen in animals but inability to drink is a common symptom of rabies.

Human Rabies—Clinical Features

Incubation period is usually between 20 and 90 days (extreme range, 4 days to more than 19 years). Relatively short incubation periods are observed after facial and severe multiple bites. Bites from stray wild animals are more risky and dangerous. The disease manifests with prodromal symptoms like excitement, fever, malaise, anorexia, nausea and headache and nonspecific upper respiratory tract symptoms. Attention to the site of bite may be drawn by tingling pain and paresthesia especially itching, which develops before the appearance of spasms. Psychotic behavior with irrational and violent spells with intervening periods of calm may develop.

Neurological involvement may present as: (1) The spastic (furious) form and (2) the paralytic form. In the former, the lesions are more marked in the brainstem, cranial nerves, limbic system and higher centers. In the paralytic form, the lesions are mostly in the medulla, spinal cord and the spinal nerves.

The spastic form: Sets in at various intervals (hours to a day or so) after the prodromal symptoms. Sensory stimuli, which may be tactile, auditory or photic, provoke painful spasms. These are most marked and characteristic in the oropharynx. Swallowing liquid and later on a spray of water, its sight or even thought of it produces painful oropharyngeal spasms with respiratory distress. This symptom is called **hydrophobia**. Though not pathognomonic, this is almost confirmatory of the diagnosis. Aerophobic spasms caused by a draught of air on the face or switching on the fan are also diagnostic. The whole course extends to less than 5 days in almost all cases. The patient becomes comatose and death is due to respiratory paralysis resulting from bulbar involvement.

Paralytic form: This is characterized by ascending paralysis. It may start as monoplegia or paraplegia. Spasms are not prominent. Paralytic form is known to occur more often after vampire bat bites. Hydrophobia is rare. Patients may survive for a month even without intensive care. In India, the primary paralytic form occurs only in less than 20% of cases.

Complications

Neurologic, cardiac and pulmonary complications may develop.

- ***Neurological:*** Cerebral edema, generalized convulsions, polyneuropathy, severe autonomic dysfunction and inappropriate secretion of antidiuretic hormone.
- ***Cardiac:*** Tachy or bradyarrhythmias, hypotension, myocarditis with congestive cardiac failure.
- ***Pulmonary:*** Hyperventilation, respiratory alkalosis, hypoxia, aspiration pneumonia, pneumothorax, pulmonary edema, respiratory failure and respiratory arrest.
- ***Gastrointestinal tract (GIT):*** Hematemesis due to ulceration or tears in the mucosa of the upper GIT.

DIAGNOSIS

Development of mental excitement, hydrophobia and spasm or paralysis in persons who have sustained bites or licks from any warm-blooded animal within 6 months should suggest the possibility of rabies. A bite by an unusually excitable or partially paralyzed mammal indicates high-risk of exposure to rabies. However, in up to 16% of cases, no history of exposure can be elicited. In the initial stages the diagnosis of rabies may be difficult.

Differential Diagnosis

Rabies has to be differentiated from encephalitis and other neurological disorders leading to paralysis. Paralytic rabies may be mistaken for adverse reaction to vaccination in persons receiving anti-rabies vaccination. The spasms of tetanus may resemble hydrophobia especially if they involve the pharyngeal muscles (hydrophobic tetanus). Psychiatric conditions, such as maniac excitement and hysteria and drug reactions such as akathisia have to be differentiated at times. Hysterical subjects adopt hydrophobic manifestations, but absence of aerophobia excludes this condition.

Laboratory Diagnosis

In practice, diagnosis of rabies is primarily clinical where laboratory facilities exist, tests are available for confirmation of diagnosis. The virus can be isolated in saliva or cerebrospinal fluid (CSF) for the initial 2 weeks of the illness, but this takes about 3 weeks and hence is not a practicable method for day-to-day use.

Neutralizing antibodies against rabies virus can be demonstrated after the initial 10 days of onset. Levels of antibody are much higher in CSF, compared to serum. Vaccinated individuals develop antibodies by 8 days after vaccination, but the titers are much higher in the patients who develop clinical rabies.

Antigen Detection

Rapid rabies diagnosis by polymerase chain reaction (PCR) tests on saliva—CSF and skin biopsy are available in a few reference laboratories. A ***direct immunofluorescent antibody*** (IFA) test also rapidly identifies antigen in frozen sections of the skin biopsies taken from a hairy area, usually nape of the neck. Rabies-specific immunofluorescence appears in nerve twigs around the base of hair follicles. This test is 60–100% sensitive. False positives have not been reported.

Prognosis

In the ordinary settings, rabies is invariably fatal. This underscores the need for preventing the development of rabies in persons exposed to the risk either by animal bites or by occupation. Recent reports of stray survivors by intensive and continuous prolonged life support measures are available.

TREATMENT

Once the disease is manifested, treatment is only symptomatic. There is no specific treatment. Treatment aims at controlling spasms with muscle relaxants, maintenance of hydration by intravenous (IV) fluids and assistance to ventilation. Those who attend on the patients should use gloves, masks and protective goggles. Though the virus eliminated in human saliva is not very virulent, as a matter of abundant caution, attendants who have been inadvertently exposed to very close contact with rabies may be advised to take a course of prophylactic inoculation.

Local treatment of bites, scratches and licks: Thorough cleaning of the wound by washing with soap and water repeatedly and then by 40–70% alcohol or 0.1% quaternary ammonium compounds *(Cetavlon)* eliminates the virus present superficially. Bite wounds should not be sutured straight away. In severe bites local injection of anti-rabies serum or hyperimmune globulin helps in reducing the risk further.

Assessment of the risk (Table 59.1): Animals incubating the disease may be apparently normal for five days before becoming symptomatic. Once they develop the disease, majority of them die within 5 days. Therefore, the animal should be observed for 10 days, to decide on the need for vaccination. If the animal is obviously rabid or it is not traceable, vaccination is started straightaway without any delay. If the risk is only class I or II, vaccination can be undertaken after observing the animal. In class III risk, vaccination is started, but if the animal is normal, it can be stopped. A rabid dog shows features like recent change in behavior, aggressiveness, characteristic howl, tendency to bite objects indiscriminately, ataxia, paralysis and excessive salivation. Paralysis of bulbar muscles may be mistaken for impaction of foreign bodies in the throat.

Post-exposure Prophylaxis (PEP)

Active immunization: This is achieved by anti-rabies vaccination. Vaccination affords considerable degree of protection, though this is not absolute. Immunity is established after 10–14 days of starting the course and it lasts up to 1 year. Anti-rabies vaccine was originally introduced by Louis Pasteur in 1885. ***All the vaccines used for anti-rabies prophylaxis are killed vaccines.*** The original vaccines were nerve tissue vaccines in which the fixed virus grown in the nervous tissue of sheep was killed by phenol or beta-propiolactone. The course of injections used to be long, injections were painful and about 6 to 10% of patients used to get minor or moderate complications. A smaller number used to get serious neuroparalytic and encephalitic complications. These vaccines are practically

Table 59.1:	Assessment of risk

Class I (light risk)

- Licks except on face and fingers
- Licks on intact mucous membranes
- Light bites and scratches over parts of the body except head, neck, face and fingers
- Consumption of unboiled milk or handling raw flesh of rabid animal

Class II (moderate risk)

- Licks on fresh wounds and cuts and abrasions on fingers
- Scratches on fingers

Class III (great risk)

- Licks on fresh cuts, scratches and bites on head, neck or face
- Bites on fingers and all lacerated wounds
- Jackal and wolf bites
- Any class II patient who has not received anti-rabies vaccination within 2 weeks

never given now due to this risk and the availability of safer and more effective cell culture vaccines.

Avian embryo vaccines: These are produced in chick (Flury) or duck embryos. Though allergic reactions may occur, neuroparalytic accidents are much less common with this vaccine. The vaccines are used mainly for active immunization of dogs and other pets.

Cell Culture Vaccines

The available popular vaccines are:

- Monkey kidney cell vaccine marketed as Verorab
- Purified chick embryo cell vaccine marketed as Rabipur
- Human diploid cell vaccine (HDCV)—the human cell derived vaccine costs about ₹750/dose, whereas the other two cost about ₹250.

All are equally antigenic. Dose of monkey kidney cell vaccine is 0.5 mL that of HDCV is 1 mL each time. All these vaccines are safe, painless and free from permanent neuroparalytic accidents. At present, all these vaccines are imported. Immunity starts by the seventh day after the first dose. It lasts for 3 years.

Five injections of the vaccine on day 0, 3, 7, 14 and 28 given intramuscular (IM) give rise to sufficient protection. A booster dose of 1 mL is given on day 90, if antibody level is not adequate. Injections over the deltoid are more immunogenic than gluteal injections.

The course of cell culture vaccine is the same for all classes of bites and the classification of the risk is only to decide the need and timing of vaccination. Being a killed vaccine, there is no contraindication for antirabic vaccination during pregnancy.

Passive immunization: If the risk is class III or even II, passive immunization should be given as early as possible, since active immunization will not be completed within the incubation period. Antirabic serum prepared in ***human rabies immunoglobulin (HRIG)*** should be given in a dose of 20 units/kg IM at a site away from the vaccine dose. If there is a lacerated wound, 50% of the dose should be infiltrated around it and the remainder should be given IM. The half-life of HRIG is for 21 days and this is probably the duration of passive immunity.

Antirabic serum (ARS): Produced in horses is also used in a dose 40 u/kg bw IM. If horse serum is used the risk of anaphylaxis is higher. The equine antiserum is much cheaper than the human immunoglobulin. Both are effective. When the former is used, prior skin testing should be done to avoid anaphylactic reactions.

Pre-exposure immunization: Personnel who have occupational risk of rabies, e.g. veterinary surgeons and kennel trainers can be actively immunized with HDCV. When an immunized person is exposed to the risk of rabies, he should receive booster doses of the vaccine.

Three doses of cell culture vaccines given as IM injections on day 0, 7, 21 or 28 give adequate antibody levels for up to 2 years. If facilities permit, antibody levels should be estimated and if the titer is inadequate, a booster dose of 1 mL should be given. It is better to administer booster doses only when indicated, since over-immunization can be associated with serum sickness-like reaction in up to 6% of cases.

Textbook of Medicine

An alternate method is to give HDCV in a dose of 0.1 mL intradermally on days 1, 7, 21 or 28. Protection starts after four weeks. The intradermal route is inadequate for post-exposure prophylaxis. In persons who have received pre-exposure prophylaxis, if risk of infection occurs two booster doses of the vaccine should be given on days 0 and 3. Local washing of the wound and wound toilet are absolutely necessary to reduce the risk.

Total dose—0.8 mL in 4 sessions given intradermally (Table 59.2). Government of India approved Intra-Dermal Rabies Vaccination (IDRV) in 2006. In Kerala, this was approved in 2008.

Post Script

Several countries have reduced frequency of infection in wild life by mass vaccination programs of terrestrial carnivores. Newer Lassa viruses causing clinically indistinguishable diseases have been detected in several species of bats in different countries, especially in the

Table 59.2: Thai Red Cross Regimen for immunization

Day of bite	Dose	Total Volume
0	0.1 mL each arm	0.2 mL
3	0.1 mL each arm	0.2 mL
7	0.1 mL each arm	0.2 mL
28	0.1 mL each arm	0.2 mL

New World (America). These viruses are antigenically distinct from the presently available vaccine strains. Bats may be blood sucking types (vampire bats) or fruit bats. Bat population is more in caves and instances of infection by the virus acquired by the respiratory route has been on record.

Source: Fooks AR, Banyard AC, Horton DL, et al. Current status of rabies and prospects for elimination. Lancet. 2014;384(9951):1389-99.

CHAPTER
60

Arboviruses

K Sreekanthan, KV Krishna Das, R Sajith Kumar

Chapter Summary

- General Considerations
- Dengue Fever
  - Clinical Features
  - Dengue Hemorrhagic Fever
  - Dengue Shock Syndrome
  - Treatment
- Sandfly Fever
- Yellow Fever
- Kyasanur Forest Disease
- Chikungunya
- Japanese Encephalitis
- Zika Virus Infections

GENERAL CONSIDERATIONS

Arthropod borne (ARBO) viruses are a group of viruses with complex transmission cycles involving arthropods. These viruses have diverse physical and chemical properties and are classified into several virus families.

The arboviruses are transmitted by blood sucking arthropods from one vertebrate host to another. The vector acquires a lifelong infection through the ingestion of blood from a viremic vertebrate. The viruses multiply in the tissues of the vector without evidence of disease or damage. Some arboviruses are maintained in nature by transovarian transmission in the vector. The main pathogenic arboviruses include members of the flavivirus, togavirus and bunyavirus families. The main vectors include mosquitos and pigs.

The major arbovirus diseases worldwide are dengue fever (DF), yellow fever, sandfly fever, Kyasanur Forest disease, chikungunya fever, West Nile fever and various forms of encephalitis like Japanese encephalitis, St. Louis encephalitis, Western equine encephalitis, Eastern equine encephalitis, Russian spring-summer encephalitis and others. A new entrant in this class is the Zika virus, included in 2015.

The diseases with public health importance in India are DF, chikungunya fever, sandfly fever, West Nile fever, Kyasanur Forest disease, yellow fever and Japanese encephalitis.

DENGUE FEVER (DF)

Syn: Break bone fever, Dandy fever

Dengue is an acute febrile illness, characterized by high fever, severe pain of bones and joints, lymphadenopathy and a characteristic rash.

History

Benjamin Rush in Philadelphia first described the clinical syndrome in 1789. Viral etiology and mode of transmission by mosquitoes were established in early 20th century. DF is found mostly during and shortly after the rainy season in tropical and subtropical areas of India, Africa, Southeast Asia, China, Middle East, Caribbean islands and Central and South America. In 1954, dengue became epidemic in many areas of tropical Asia. Large outbreaks of DF have occurred in many areas of India after 2000 and in Kerala particularly during July–August 2003. At present, sporadic

Textbook of Medicine

cases occur all over the country throughout the year. In Kerala, cases are reported mostly in summer months following intermittent rains.

Etiology

Dengue is caused by four distinct serotypes of dengue viruses (Type DEN-1 to DEN-4) within the *Flavivirus* genus of the family flaviviridae. Dengue viruses are small 40–50 nm spherical particles composed of a lipoprotein envelope and nucleocapsid of single strand ribonucleic acid (RNA) genome. The major envelope glycoprotein E which is exposed on the virion surface contains type-specific and group specific antigens. There are genetic variations within serotypes. They share limited identity (around 60–75%) at the amino acid level. Viruses within the same serotypes have a 3% difference in the amino acid level and 6% difference in the nucleotide level. These viruses are phylogenetically divided into genotypes and clades. Particular serotypes and clades have been associated with differential clinical manifestation and disease. Some genetic variants within each serotype appear to be more virulent or have more epidemic potential. After primary infection, each serotype provides specific lifetime immunity and short term cross-immunity.

New Dengue Classification

A revised World Health Organization (WHO) case classification was introduced in 2009, replacing the classic classification into DF, dengue shock syndrome (DSS) and dengue hemorrhagic fever (DHF). Present classification is 'dengue with and without warning signs' and 'severe dengue.'

This classification helps to plan treatment early. Severe dengue can present with hepatitis, neurologic abnormalities, myocarditis or severe bleeding with plasma leakage or shock. Bronchial asthma, diabetes, sickle disease and ethnic susceptibility worsens the outcome.

Source: WHO/TDR. Dengue guidelines for diagnosis, treatment, prevention and control. New edition. Geneva-World Health Organization, 2009.

Transmission

Man is the usual reservoir of infection. The main vectors are *Aedes aegypti, Aedes albopictus* and to a lesser extent *Aedes polynesiensis.* These are fresh water breeders existing in domestic surroundings and which bite frequently several persons during all times of the day. They also have a tendency to bite the lower ankles and feet more mostly around dawn and dusk. They do not fly long distances and remain inside the rooms during most of the day-time. The extrinsic incubation period in the mosquito is 8–14 days by which time the mosquito becomes infective and it remains so for the rest of its life (15–65 days). There is transovarial transmission of the dengue virus with the *A. albopictus* mosquito. The virus is reported to survive in eggs and get reactivated in mosquitoes even after one year (Fig. 60.1).

Pathogenesis and Pathology

First attack of dengue: After the bite of an infected mosquito, the virus replicates in regional lymph nodes and is disseminated via the lymphatics and the blood to other

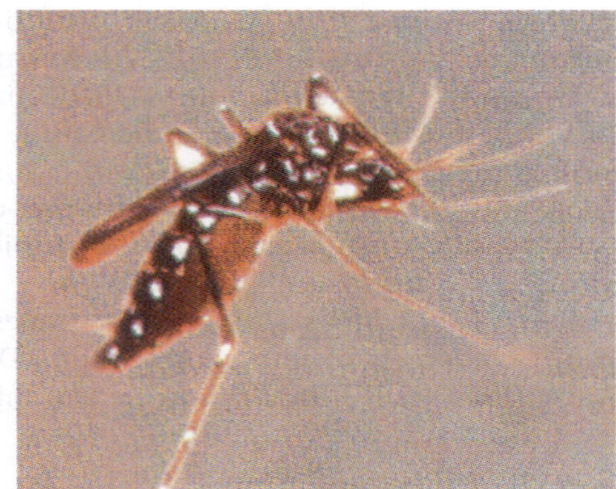

Fig. 60.1: Aedes mosquito vector which transmits dengue, yellow fever and Zika virus

tissues. Replication in the reticuloendothelial system and skin produces viremia, which begins 3–7 days after infection. Viremia is present for the first 3 days early in the illness. After the clearance of viremia, the virus persists in the infected mononuclear cells. In majority of dengue infections, the disease is self-limited.

Subsequent attacks of dengue: First infection produces long-term type specific immunity and short-term cross immunity. This cross immunity fades after a few months. Therefore, reinfection with remaining serotypes can occur. The speed and extent of viral spread is much higher in subsequent infections by different serotypes of dengue viruses compared to the first attack. In this group, some develop severe complications such as DHF and DSS. Infection by DEN-2 following DEN-1 infection is likely to be more serious in this regard.

The hallmarks of DHF–DSS are increase in the permeability and fragility of the capillaries and abnormalities of hemostasis. Ninety percent of cases of DHF-DSS occur during subsequent infections. Less commonly, infants born to mothers who transmit dengue antibodies transplacentally are sensitized to the dengue virus may develop DHF-DSS in the first attack itself.

The immune status of the host plays an important role in determining the course of dengue infection and subsequent complications. The presence of non-neutralizing antibodies to a heterologous dengue virus may form virus-antibody complexes and facilitate the entry of dengue virus into the mononuclear cells and viral multiplication (antibody-dependent enhancement). The increased numbers of infected cells (monocytes and lymphocytes) with the release of cytokines like tumor necrosis factor (TNF)-α and complement activation leads to endothelial swelling of small blood vessels, perivascular edema and mononuclear cell infiltration. The pathologic changes in complicated cases and DHF include arrest of megakaryocyte multiplication in the bone marrow and thrombocytopenia. Hemorrhages occur due to thrombocytopenia, platelet dysfunction and coagulopathy. There is also generalized abnormality of the vascular endothelium resulting in extensive leakage of fluid from the intravascular compartment.

In DHF, there is widespread dissemination of the virus into several organs including liver, spleen, heart, bone marrow and rarely the brain. Liver shows focal midzonal necrosis, fatty changes and hyaline necrosis of hepatocytes.

Clinical Features

DF is an acute febrile disease with headache, musculo-skeletal pain and rash, but the severity of illness and clinical manifestations vary with age. All age groups are affected. Dengue can present in the following clinical syndromes.

- Undifferentiated fever, particularly in children
- Classic DF
- Dengue hemorrhagic fever
- Dengue shock syndrome.

Undifferentiated fever: Infection is asymptomatic in 80% of infants and children. In the ordinary case, the illness presents as fever, malaise or irritability, pharyngeal injection, upper respiratory symptoms and rash. This resembles other common childhood infections.

Classic DF: This is most common in adults and older children. The incubation period is 3–8 days. It starts abruptly with fever, headache, pain in the muscle, bone and joints, retro-orbital region and lumbosacral ache. A transient generalized macular rash may be present during the first 24–48 hours. Generalized myalgia increase in severity. Other symptoms such as anorexia, nausea, vomiting, marked lassitude, cutaneous hyperesthesia and dysgeusia appear on the second to the fourth day. Orbital pain may develop and movements of the eyeball may be painful. The temperature rises up to 40–41.5°C with relative bradycardia. Conjunctival congestion is common. Posterior cervical, epitrochlear and inguinal lymph nodes are enlarged, but nontender.

The fever usually subsides after three days. A second bout of fever may occur after two days. This is milder than the first and lasting for 2–3 days (saddle back pattern). The second episode of fever comes down by lysis.

A maculopapular rash occurs with the second bout of fever on the trunk, limbs and face. It disappears as the temperature falls. Mild hemorrhagic phenomena such as petechial hemorrhages, ecchymosis at injection sites, epistaxis and menorrhagia may occur during the course of the illness, even in uncomplicated cases.

Ogilvies syndrome: It has been reported in dengue. This is a clinical condition in which symptoms, signs and radiological features of large bowel obstruction without mechanical obstruction develop due to colonic atony (autonomic disturbance) and pseudo-obstruction, more severe complication is colon perforation.

The Stage of Complications

Transition from the febrile to the critical phases, occurs between days 4 and 7 of the illness. Impending signs of deterioration usher in with persistent vomiting, severe abdominal pain, tender hepatomegaly, increasing hematocrit values and development of thrombocytopenia. Typically shock and rapid deterioration, occurs on the second to fifth day of illness. Hemorrhagic manifestations are most common during this critical period with nadir platelet counts below 20,000/mm³. Apart from hemorrhage and shock, other life threatening complication such as liver failure, myocarditis and encephalopathy may develop.

Dengue Hemorrhagic Fever

This syndrome, characterized by increased capillary permeability and hemostatic derangements, occur more frequently in children. Based on the severity, cases of DHF can be categorized into four grades (WHO guidelines).

Grading Severity of Dengue Hemorrhagic Fever (DHF)

DHF is classified into four grades of severity, where grades III and IV are considered to be DSS. The presence of thrombocytopenia with concurrent hemoconcentration differentiates grade I and II DHF from DF.

Grade I: Fever accompanied by nonspecific constitutional symptoms; the only hemorrhagic manifestation is a positive tourniquet test and/or easy bruising.

Grade II: Spontaneous bleeding, in addition to the manifestations of grade I patients, usually in the form of skin or other hemorrhages.

Grade III: Circulatory failure manifested by a rapid, weak pulse and narrowing of pulse pressure or hypotension, with the presence of cold, clammy skin and restlessness.

Grade IV: Profound shock with undetectable blood pressure or pulse.

The minimum diagnostic criteria for DHF are a positive tourniquet test or spontaneous hemorrhages from multiple sites, thrombocytopenia (<100,000 /mm³) and evidence of plasma leakage as shown by increase in hematocrit by 20% or more from baseline, ascites or pleural effusion.

Early in the illness, these children are clinically identical to those with classical dengue. But around the time of defervescence, a second phase of illness develops. This is characterized by petechiae, ecchymoses, epistaxis and other spontaneous hemorrhages including gastrointestinal hemorrhage and menorrhagia. Variable ascites or pleural effusion, more common on the right side may develop. Liver may be enlarged and tender.

Dengue Shock Syndrome (DSS)

It is the most serious complication of dengue hemorrhagic fever, seen widely in Asia and South America. It is seen in all hospitals in India, though infrequently. Some patients manifest signs of restlessness, abdominal pain and shock with cold and clammy extremities, diaphoresis, circumoral cyanosis, irritability or change in mental status. Hypotension with narrowing of pulse pressure below 20 mm Hg, severe shock and rapid deterioration, typically occurs on the second to fifth day of illness. Untreated, 50% of such patients may die. Patients with less severe illness or those successfully treated recover rapidly after a 1–2 day period of acute illness.

Other manifestations: Less commonly dengue may present with encephalopathy, intracranial bleed, renal failure, fulminant hepatitis and acute respiratory distress syndrome (ARDS).

Diagnosis

Dengue should be suspected when fever with severe body pain and rash occurs. In the initial stage, it should be differentiated from influenza, leptospirosis, malaria

Arboviruses

and typhoid fever. In endemic areas sandfly fever and chikungunya have to be kept in mind.

Investigations

Usually there is leukopenia, mainly neutropenia and mild thrombocytopenia. Severe thrombocytopenia may occur in DHF. *S. bilirubin* is usually normal unless there is hepatic involvement; serum transaminases show mild elevation even in uncomplicated cases.

Blood urea and creatinine are elevated in complicated cases. Chest X-ray may show pleural effusion. Ultra-sonogram of abdomen may reveal serous effusions.

Virological Diagnosis

Virus isolation is by cell cultures, done with blood culture within the first week of illness in specialized laboratories for special purposes. Viral RNA can be identified by reverse transcriptase polymerase chain reaction (RT-PCR). Subtyping of the virus is also possible by PCR.

Detection of the virus-expressed soluble non-structural protein 1 (NS1) is by enzyme linked immunosorbent assay (ELISA) test. Even though false negatives do occur. For primary infections in persons who have not been infected previously, NS1 antigen can be detected as early as the first day of illness and the diagnostic sensitivity of NS1 detection in the febrile phase will be above 90%. Even after the resolution of fever, antigenemia may persist for several days. Compared to the primary infection, in those with repeated infections by other dengue subtypes, the sensitivity of NS1 detection is only (60–80%).

Serology

Complement fixation and neutralizing antibody titers can be demonstrated in paired sera drawn at intervals of 7–14 days.

The IgM antibody capture ELISA has improved the serodiagnosis of dengue. By the end of first week, IgM antibodies are detectable. They rise rapidly and by 2–3 months they become undetectable. A very high rise of IgG antibodies early in the disease indicates a second dengue infection. IgM antibodies are relatively specific for dengue without cross-reaction with other heterologous flaviviruses, but IgM antibodies do not distinguish individual dengue serotypes.

Treatment

Vast majority of patients can be managed as outpatients with paracetamol for fever, antiemetics, oral fluids, reassurance and rest. Indications for inpatient treatment are fever above 40.5°C, prostration, severe vomiting requiring intravenous (IV) fluids and other complications. It should be remembered that an apparently mild case of dengue may turn to be severe with complications and high mortality, therefore close watch and monitoring of laboratory parameters such as platelet count should be done repeatedly till resolution is complete.

Treatment of Complicated DF, DHF and DSS

The treatment is mainly supportive. Patient has to be treated in an intensive care facility with proper monitoring of vital parameters, attention to nutrition and fluid and electrolyte balance. The blood pressure (BP), hematocrit, platelet count, bleeding manifestations, urinary output and level of consciousness should be monitored systematically to identify complications.

Hypotension, signs of increased capillary fragility and toxemia are indications for IV fluids. Normal saline, 5% dextrose saline, Ringer lactate, colloid plasma expanders and plasma have to be given with proper monitoring to maintain the BP and vital functions. It is important to correct fluid and electrolyte balance early in the disease in order to prevent irreversible changes.

Indications for Blood Components/Transfusion

Thrombocytopenia in DF is multifactorial and hence transfusion of platelets based on platelet count alone is discouraged. Many studies have negated the need for platelet replacement in most of the cases. One unit of platelet supplementation will raise the count by 5,000–10,000 only. Platelet transfusions should ideally be restricted to those situations where an invasive procedure (like dialysis, aspirations/biopsy, etc.) is planned.

The treatment of massive bleeding is by packed red cell transfusion.

Great emphasis has to be paid to the components of hemoconcentration and hypoperfusion. Oral fluid and electrolyte replacement works in the majority of persons. IV fluid therapy should be properly monitored and stopped at the appropriate time so as to avoid fluid overload.

There is no specific antiviral therapy. Secondary bacterial infections and concurrent infections like malaria should be looked for and treated appropriately.

Prevention

General measures include anti-mosquito operations and personal protection using nets or mosquito repellents. As the mosquito is peridomestic, clearance of water holding containers (indoor like flower vases, air coolers and outdoor like tyres, glass pieces, plastic covers) plays a major role in vector control and should be repeated at least once weekly. Live attenuated vaccines (quadrivalent) acting against all 4 serotypes are currently under development.

A phase 3 vaccine trail against dengue is reported. An observer masked randomized controlled multicenter phase 3 trial in five countries in Asia Pacific region between June 3 and December 1st 2011 done on 10,275 children aged 2–14 years is reported.

Three injections of a recombinant live attenuated dengue vaccine (CYD-TDV) or placebo were given by injection at 0, 6 and 12 months and patients were followed up for 25 months. There was 56.5% efficacy in the vaccine group against the development of dengue. The vaccine gave 80% protection against dengue hemorrhagic fever after 1 injection and 88.5% after 3 injections.

Source:

1. Wilder-Smith A. Dengue vaccines: dawning at last? Lancet. 2014;384(9951):1327-9.

2. Capeding MR, Tran NH, Hadinegoro SRS, et al. Clinical efficacy and safety of a novel tetravalent dengue vaccine in healthy children in Asia: a phase 3 randomised, observer-marked, placebo-controlled trial. Lancet. 2014; 384(9951):1358-65.

Points to Remember

- Dengue, which was considered to be a mild infection is emerging as a serious problem.
- Four distinct viruses can cause the disease. No cross protection is present. But may produce DHF and DSS in subsequent attacks.
- Main cause of death—DHF and DSS—increased capillary permeability.
- Early fluid replacement and supportive measures save life.

SANDFLY FEVER

Syn: Phlebotomus fever, Pappataci fever, 3 days fever

It is a short, self-limited, undifferentiated febrile illness caused by sandfly-borne viruses.

Etiology

The disease is caused by members of phlebovirus subgroup of the family Bunynaviridae.

The disease is present in India, mainly in northern states and Himalayan areas. It is prevalent in other tropical countries, Middle East and Mediterranean countries.

It is transmitted by the sandfly *Phlebotomus papatasi*. Female phlebotomus sucks blood. It becomes infective 6–7 days after an infective feed and remains infective for the rest of its life. Sandfly fever viruses are transovarially transmitted in their vector species. In the tropical environment, sand flies are active throughout the year. In temperate climates, they are seen only in summer. They are small (2–3 mm) and readily pass through bed nets and screens. They are nocturnal biters.

Clinical Features

Incubation period is 2–6 days. The illness starts abruptly with fever and rigor. The temperature rises rapidly to 40°C with headache, malaise, retro-orbital pain, photophobia, myalgia, nausea and vomiting. The absence of rash, lymphadenopathy, and respiratory symptoms may help in differentiating the illness from other viral syndromes. The acute febrile illness lasts approximately 3 days. This may be followed by a period of weakness, fatigue and depression lasting 1–2 weeks. Aseptic meningitis can occur in 12% of cases. There is associated neck rigidity, changes in mental status and sometimes convulsions. There is cerebrospinal fluid (CSF) pleocytosis with predominant mononuclear cells. The disease resolves without sequel.

Diagnosis

The diagnosis is mainly clinical. There is leukopenia. The diagnosis is established by culture of the virus, PCR test or serological assays. The most commonly used test is IgM capture ELISA. This is to be done 4–5 days after onset of symptoms. It gives only a probable diagnosis. By 7–10 days IgG antibodies develop in the majority.

Prognosis and Treatment

The disease is self-limiting, benign and nonfatal. Treatment is symptomatic with analgesics and supportive measures.

Prevention and Control

No vaccine has been developed. Spraying residual insecticides can control sandflies. Personal protection is achieved by using insect repellents. A new strategy tried in Vietnam against *Aedes aegypti* is to grow predator copepods in domestic water collecting vessels and tanks.

YELLOW FEVER

Yellow fever is an acute mosquito-borne infection of varying severity characterized by the triad of hepatitis, hemorrhagic diathesis and proteinuria.

Etiology

The causative virus is an arbovirus belonging to the genus *Flavivirus*, in the family Flaviviridae.

Epidemiology

Yellow fever is prevalent in many parts of Africa, tropical parts of South America and Panama. The disease has not been reported in India. The presence of the efficient vector *Aedes aegypti* mosquitoes and the nonimmune population pose a threat of the disease spreading in India, if the virus is introduced. Hence, this disease is of importance to India.

Yellow fever is notifiable under the International Health Regulations.

Transmission

Epidemic (urban) yellow fever is transmitted from human to human by *Aedes aegypti* mosquitoes. Infected monkeys and the vector mosquitoes maintain the reservoir of infection in the jungle. These act as a source of infection when the humans intrude into endemic areas.

Pathology and Pathogenesis

The incubation period after an infectious mosquito bite is 3–6 days.

Liver and kidneys show maximal lesions but hemorrhage may occur in all organs. Hepatic changes include widespread necrosis and degeneration of liver cells. Renal changes include acute tubular necrosis and subcapsular hemorrhages.

Bleeding diathesis is due to depletion of hepatic clotting factors, intravascular coagulation, and platelet abnormalities. Direct damage to the myocardium, kidneys and other organs and the effects of vasoactive cytokines, lead to fatal complications such as multi-organ failure and shock.

Clinical Features

In the majority of cases the disease is self-limited with fever and myalgia. Twenty-five to fifty percent of cases may develop the full syndrome with complications such as hemorrhages, jaundice, renal involvement and shock.

The first stage (i.e. period of infection) is due to the direct effect of the virus. It starts abruptly with fever, headache and myalgia. In severe illness there is nausea, vomiting, abdominal pain and distressing pain in the back and limbs. There is relative bradycardia. This stage lasts about 3 days and by 4th day the temperature comes down and ***the second stage (period of remission)*** starts. Many cases recover without going to the third stage. Some progress to ***the third stage (period of intoxication)***. It starts after a day or a few days, with resumption of high fever, body pains, nausea, vomiting, abdominal pain and changes in the level of consciousness. Bradycardia, jaundice, widespread hemorrhages and renal failure may supervene. Death is due to hepatic or renal failure and shock.

Textbook of Medicine

Diagnosis

In endemic areas, fever, leukopenia and proteinuria with or without jaundice should suggest the possibility of yellow fever. Specific diagnosis is established by the isolation of the virus from the blood in the first few days of fever or demonstration of rising titer of antibodies in serum.

Treatment

There is no specific antiviral treatment. Symptomatic and supportive measures should be instituted. Hepatic and renal failure have to be anticipated and managed accordingly.

Prevention

Vaccination using live attenuated vaccine (17D strain) is very effective. Vaccination gives immunity starting from ten days and full protection for 10 years. Though side effects are generally negligible, children below 9 months may develop encephalitis. Pregnancy is not a contraindication for vaccination.

India and many other countries insist on yellow fever vaccination for persons entering the country or remaining during transit, if they come from endemic areas. Persons travelling to endemic areas have to take vaccination. Yellow fever vaccination is available at recognized centers in India.

KYASANUR FOREST DISEASE (KFD)

KFD is an acute febrile illness caused by a **group B arbovirus,** clinically characterized by sudden onset of fever with rigor, severe body pains, headache, meningism, delirium, mental confusion and dehydration. The original description was from Shimoga district of Karnataka State in South India in 1956. There have been a few reports from various parts of South India and even from the hilly forest areas close to the Western Ghats in Kerala.

The disease was prevalent among people living in the villages around the forest area. The infection developed in persons who had gone into the forest (usually to fetch wood) and who had come into contact with dead monkeys. The ticks *Hemaphysalis spinigera* and *Ixodes* act as vectors to transmit the disease from animals to man. Monkeys (black faced langur and macaques), shrews and rats are known to harbor the virus. Man gets infection by the bite of the nymph of *H. spinigera.* Infected ticks carry the virus for long periods. Personnel working in laboratories handling the virus or investigators working in the affected areas are susceptible to infection. In addition to vector transmission, infection can also be spread by inhalation of infected material.

Clinical Features

After the incubation period lasting for 2–7 days, sudden fever sets in with chills and rigor. Fever is associated with headache and severe myalgia in the nape of the neck, back and calf. These may be mistaken for DF. Abdominal pain, diarrhea and vomiting may occur between the third and the seventh day. Uncommonly, bleeding tendencies such as epistaxis, bleeding gums and melena may develop around third day. Lymphadenopathy of the neck and axilla and conjunctival injection may also be seen. Bradycardia

and hypotension may develop. Hepatosplenomegaly may occur in some cases. Alteration in mental state, neck rigidity, giddiness, tremors, listlessness and dyspnea have all been reported.

In uncomplicated cases, the fever lasts for about 10–12 days and temperature comes down. A second febrile phase may follow 2–12 days after the temperature has touched normal and this may continue so for 9–21 days. The mortality rate is around 5%. Death is usually caused by pulmonary edema.

Laboratory Diagnosis

Leukocyte count is low (about 3000/mm^3). The virus can be isolated from blood during the course of the fever. Paired sera show rise in antibody titers. During the second febrile phase, CSF may show features of aseptic meningitis.

Treatment

In the absence of specific treatment only supportive therapy is to be given.

Prevention

Anti-tick measures have to be instituted during jungle clearing operations. Persons at risk should use protective clothing and insect repellents. Though a vaccine was developed against KFD, it was not found to be very effective.

CHIKUNGUNYA (CHIK)

This fever is an acute infective disease, characterized by symmetrical polyarthropathy, fever, rash and rarely, generalized hemorrhages and central nervous system (CNS) symptoms. The disease derives its name from the sudden onset of severe joint pain, which cripples the victim. The disease was first described in 1955 following an outbreak in Africa in 1952.

Etiology

CHIK virus is an *Alphavirus* in the Semliki Forest complex (Togaviridae) and most closely related to **O'Nyong Nyong (ONN)** virus.

Distribution and Incidence

CHIK is widely distributed in Africa, the Middle East and Asia. The disease has now become endemic in several parts of India. Epidemics have been reported from southern and eastern parts of India including Tamil Nadu and Kerala. In 1964, an epidemic occurred in Tamil Nadu and surveys showed 38% of the population had antiviral antibodies. It is possible that sporadic or small outbreaks may occur from time to time. A localized outbreak is reported from Tamil Nadu during June–July 2006. Thiruvengadam, et al. studied epidemic of CHIK which occurred in the Madras Metropolitan Area in 1964. The virus was isolated and rise in antibody titer was confirmed at the Indian Council of Medical Research (ICMR) Virus Research Laboratory Pune in a third of the patients studied. Many parts of India including Kerala experienced a serious epidemic in 2004–10 when millions were affected and many districts continued to report sporadic cases throughout the year. It is possible that the original virus has undergone genetic mutation. At present, the disease has spread to several countries reducing major outbreaks and disabling outcomes.

Transmission and Epidemiology

In India, *Aedes aegypti* mosquito is the main vector. *Aedes albopictus* is also implicated. In Africa, there is a sylvian cycle involving forest mosquitoes, humans and possibly other mammals. In Asia, sylvatic viral reservoirs have not been defined. Vertical transmission from mother to baby has been reported. In such cases encephalitis may occur. Hemorrhagic manifestations are rare and this contrasts with dengue.

Clinical Features

The incubation period varies from 2–10 days, usually 3–7 days. The onset is sudden with abrupt fever (above 40°C), chills and rigor, headache, body pains and joint pains. There may be mild conjunctivitis, pharyngitis an erythematous rash over the body and face. The joints may be so inflamed that normal activities, standing and walking become painful. Arthropathy is symmetric, affecting the extremities and less often the shoulders and hips. Definite joint effusion is seen in 10% of cases. Small joints of the hands and feet and major joints of the lower limbs are affected most. The joint involvement usually selects those joints which had more wear and tear from occupations. Pain may be excruciating, crippling the patient quite out of proportion to the general disability. Fever and joint pains persist for up to six days after which they subside. Residual arthropathy lasting for months may occur in up to 30% of adults, especially in elderly patients. Morning stiffness and pain may persist for even a few months. Pre-existing joint problems like rheumatoid arthritis (RA) and neurological disorders may be aggravated and considerably worsen the disability and delay recovery. Joint pains are milder and may be even entirely absent in children. Migratory polyarthritis with synovitis have been reported in 70% of cases. Unlike as in RA, distal interphalangeal (DIP) joints were also affected. Various cutaneous manifestations have been noted ranging from transient erythematous eruptions to bullous lesions and ulcerations in the face, axilla, back, groin, scrotum and aphthous like ulcers in mucous membranes. Persisting hyperpigmentation of nose, cheeks and malar areas have been observed. Complications such as hyperpyrexia, hemorrhagic manifestations, encephalitis, polyneuropathy of the Guillain-Barré type and electrocardiogram (ECG) changes suggestive of myocarditis were recorded in the Madras outbreak. Behavioral abnormalities and depression have been reported to be aggravated or precipitated in a few during the epidemic. Among asymptomatic subjects 38.4% showed hemagglutination inhibition (HI) antibodies to chikungunya virus (CHIKV), confirming the presence of the virus in the community.

Hemorrhagic manifestations occur occasionally. CNS manifestations like meningism, convulsions and acute polyneuropathy has been reported in a minority of patients, especially children and infants.

Course and Prognosis

The disease may run a benign course with slow recovery even if untreated. Arthropathy may persist for varying periods and can be disabling. Worsening of joint symptoms during subsequent febrile illnesses has been a common observation. The acute illness in children and infants and elderly persons can rarely be fatal. The primary role of uncomplicated CHIK as a cause of death is not established. It produces considerable morbidity and impairment of the quality of life for prolonged periods.

Diagnosis

Routine laboratory investigations are not specific. The erythrocyte sedimentation rate (ESR) may be elevated to 20–50 mm/hour and C-reactive protein (CRP) may also be elevated. Isolating the virus or identifying genomic products by PCR in acute phase blood specimens can confirm the diagnosis. Serologically specific IgM or other antibodies can be demonstrated by IgM capture ELISA test. The test may become positive after a few weeks also. The test continues to be positive in those with residual activity. This test will distinguish the condition from dengue which is also transmitted by the same vector. During the prevailing epidemic in south Kerala, a few cases of co-infection by CHIK and dengue have been observed. Chronic CHIK arthritis may mimic rheumatoid and other poly or monoarthritis. At present there are no classic defining features for chronic CHIK arthritis. Diagnosis is clinical and by exclusion.

Treatment

Rest and symptomatic treatment with nonsteroidal anti-inflammatory drugs (NSAIDs) give relief. Powerful NSAIDs and steroids may be required in a few cases. Prolonged arthropathy demands symptomatic treatment. Chloroquine given in a dose of 250 mg od or bd (or hydroxychloroquine) has been reported to be useful. Steroids produce a transient relief but have been observed to produce a relapse like picture almost always. In any case, results are not impressive. There are a few reports of improvement with ribavirin treatment. Chronic cases in the quiescent phase may require drugs such as salazopyrin, methotrexate and others as for rheumatoid arthritis.

Prevention and Control

An experimental live attenuated vaccine has been shown to produce high levels of neutralizing antibody in human volunteers but efficacy has not been tested. A virus like particle (VLP) based vaccine was found to be immunogenic, has a proved safety record and elicits the production of neutralizing antibodies. This vaccine has been found to protect nonhuman primates from viral infection. Protection is afforded by the neutralizing antibody. Further studies are necessary to assess the vaccine effect completely in humans.

Antimosquito measures and personal protection with mosquito repellents will reduce the spread.

Source:

1. Thiruvengadam KV, Kalyanasundaram V, Rajgopal J. Clinical and pathological studies on chikungunya fever in Madras city. Indian J Med Res. 1965;53:729-44.

2. Charrel RN, de Lamballerie X, Raoult D. Chikungunya outbreaks—the globalization of vector-borne diseases. N Engl J Med. 2007;356(8):769-71.

3. Ganu MA, Ganu AS. Post-chikungunya chronic arthritis—our experience with DMARDs over two year follow up. J Assoc Physicians India. 2011;59:83-6.

4. Chang LJ, Dowd KA, Mendoza FH, et al. Safety and tolerability of chikungunya virus-like particle vaccine in healthy adults: a phase 1 dose-escalation trial. Lancet. 2014;384(9959):2046-52.

JAPANESE ENCEPHALITIS (JE)

It is a severe mosquito-borne infection of the CNS, is a leading cause of childhood encephalitis in Asia.

Etiology and History

The causative *Flavivirus* is related antigenically to West Nile virus (WNV). The virus was first isolated from human brain of an epidemic case in Japan in 1924 and its transmission by mosquito was proved in 1936. It is an RNA virus. This disease has been reported from several countries in both tropical and temperate zones.

Distribution and Incidence

The disease is widespread in India and south-east Asian countries. Surveys done by National Institute of Virology, Pune, suggest that the flaviviruses are widely distributed in India. Neutralizing antibodies to JE virus were demonstrated in all regions, which had epidemics. In north and north-east India, the disease occurs more during the summer monsoon, whereas the maximum incidence in the south is from September to January. Epidemics occur in several parts of India from time to time. About 30,000 cases occur annually. The outbreaks coincide with the density of mosquito population.

Transmission and Epidemiology

The virus exists in reservoir hosts and man is affected from them. Pigs, birds such as pond herons, cattle-egrets, bats, buffaloes and cattle harbor the virus. In India, pigs constitute the major reservoir in which the virus multiples. Migration of birds account for the regional spread of infection. Though the virus is seen in several animals, it is pathogenic only to man and a few other mammals like horses. Poverty, unsatisfactory dwelling conditions and co-existance with cattle, birds and pigs facilitate transmission.

The vector Culicine mosquitoes act as the main vectors. Important among them are *Culex tritaeniorhynchus*, *Culex pseudovishnui* and *C. vishnui*. *Anopheles barbirostris* can also transmit this virus.

The natural transmission cycle of the virus is birds → mosquito → bird and pig → mosquito → pig. Human infection occurs only when the mosquito population increases and man—mosquito contact is established. Risk for infection is highest in rural locations where rice fields, pigs and humans coexist.

In the vast majority, the infection remains subclinical. The ratio of overt to inapparent infection varies from 1:300 to 1:1000. Children below 15 years suffer more. The peak incidence is between 2 and 10 years and males suffer more.

Pathogenesis and Pathology

After an infective bite by the mosquito, the virus propagates locally and in the regional lymph nodes. Viremia leads to affection of several organs mainly the brain unless the infection is modulated by prompt immune response. Neuroinvasion probably occurs as the virus grows through vascular endothelial cells to the parenchymal side. The virus enters the neurons and leads to widespread degenerative and necrotic changes. Most marked lesions occur in the cerebral cortex, thalamic nuclei, corpus striatum and brainstem with relative sparing of the white matter. Cerebellar cortex and spinal motor neurons may also be affected, but less marked. There is occlusion of the smaller arterioles leading to extensive focal ischemia and necrosis. Perivascular hemorrhages and mononuclear infiltration are seen.

Clinical Features

The incubation period ranges from 5 to 15 days. Three stages are recognizable-prodrome, acute encephalitis and convalescence.

Prodromal stage: The onset may be gradual (4–5 days) or acute (12–24 hours) or abrupt (1–6 hours). The disease starts as fever with chills, headache, meningism, convulsions, psychotic behavior and coma. Majority of cases recover in 4–5 days and clinical diagnosis can be made initially, only during epidemics.

Acute encephalitic stage: The fever persists at 40–41°C, the pulse is rapid and neurological manifestations predominate. Symptoms such as convulsions (70%), altered sensorium (90%), focal neurological deficits, signs of meningeal irritation (30%) and coma supervene. Supra-nuclear ocular palsies are common. Cranial nerve palsies and papilledema are uncommon. These features help to identify JE from tuberculous meningitis. Rapid onset of paralysis such as hemiplegia or monoplegia is characteristic. Plantar responses are bilaterally extensor. Other manifestations of brain involvement include cerebellar signs, extrapyramidal signs and dystonic postures. The syndrome of inappropriate secretion of antidiuretic hormone (SIADH) occurs in about 30% of cases reported from Kerala.

Convalescence: Neurological function is regained gradually over several weeks, most of them by 6–12 weeks. For the rest further recovery occurs after discharge over intervals of months to years.

Laboratory Findings and Diagnosis

Leukocytosis may be present and liver enzymes may be mildly elevated. CSF shows lymphocytic pleocytosis. The cell count varies from 10 to 1000 cells/mm^3, with an average of 100–200 cells. CSF protein may be raised to 50–250 mg/dL; sugar is usually normal. Electroencephalogram (EEG) abnormalities are present in the acute phase. These include a pattern of diffuse delta wave activity and rarely, spike and wave discharges. EEG findings are not helpful in predicting the outcome. ECG may show nonspecific ST-T changes indicating myocarditis.

Magnetic resonance imaging (MRI) reveals diffuse white matter edema and abnormal signals mainly in the thalamus, often with evidence of hemorrhage in the basal ganglia, cerebellum, midbrain, pons and spinal cord. The clinical diagnosis is easy during epidemics. Since this disease often occurs sporadically, JE should always be considered in cases of encephalitis.

Textbook of Medicine

Laboratory diagnosis in most cases depends principally on the serologic testing of the serum and also CSF by antibody capture enzyme linked immunosorbent assay (ELISA).

IgM and IgG antibodies can also be detected by indirect immunofluorescence assay. The assay is more than 95% sensitive when serum specimens are tested 7–10 days after the onset.

HI or complement fixing antibodies can be demonstrated in paired sera and these give evidence of infection in retrospect. Neutralizing antibody titer of 80 in the serum is suggestive. Four-fold rise in titer is confirmatory. CSF neutralizing antibody titer of 10 is confirmatory.

The virus can be isolated from blood only during the first few days of illness, usually preceding the onset of neurologic symptoms. Isolation of the virus from the CSF indicates the absence of protective antibodies and therefore, poor prognosis.

Differential Diagnosis

Features of JE have to be distinguished from various types of meningitis and encephalitis, cerebral malaria, toxic encephalopathies, cerebral tumors and Reye's syndrome.

Prognosis

Complete recovery occurs in one-third of cases, neurological sequelae occur in another one-third and mortality in the rest. In India, mortality rate is 25–45%. Death is usually due to neuronal damage, cerebral edema, pulmonary edema or intercurrent complications like infections from stasis ulcers, urinary tract infection (UTI), pneumonia and bacteremia. Prognosis has to be guarded since it is not always possible to predict the outcome from the clinical features. Neurologic sequelae such as intellectual impairment, motor deficits, extrapyramidal features and cerebellar disturbances are common. Polio like flaccid paralysis may occur rarely. Parkinsonism is uncommon and this stands in contrast to encephalitis lethargica. The first attack of JE produces immunity, but second attacks do occur since immunity is not lifelong. JE occurring in the first or second trimester of pregnancy may lead to fetal infection and fetal death. Cases acquired in the third trimester have not been reported to interrupt pregnancy.

Treatment and Prevention

Treatment

There is no specific treatment. Supportive treatment includes correction of fluid and electrolyte abnormalities, measures to control cerebral edema, anticonvulsants and maintenance of nutrition. Use of human immunoglobulin in a dose of 150–200 mg/kg bw early in the disease has been claimed to reduce the severity and mortality of the disease. There is preliminary data on the possible effectiveness of alpha-interferon for treatment of JE. Further studies are required to confirm the effect.

Prevention

Killed vaccine using Nakayama Yoken strain of the virus is available for prophylaxis. Indian vaccine is available, originally prepared from Nakayama JE virus at Central Research Institute, Kasauli, Himachal Pradesh. It is a formalin-inactivated vaccine. It is supplied as freeze dried vaccine, which has to be stored below 10°C. The reconstituted vaccine should be used within eight hours if kept cold. It should not be frozen. The recommended schedule for adults in JE endemic areas is two doses of 1 mL each given SC at an interval of 1–2 weeks. Protection starts one month after second dose. A booster dose should be given after one month but within one year. One more booster should be given after three years for full protection. In non-endemic areas repeated booster doses should be given every three years.

For children below three years the dose of vaccine is 0.5 mL, other conditions remaining the same. The vaccine is immunogenic and safe with only rare side effects.

A live attenuated cell culture derived vaccine (SA14-14-2 strain) has been used safely and with high effectiveness in China and parts of India.

Note: Zydus Biogen manufactures this vaccine in India.

Antimosquito measures help to limit the spread. Travellers to endemic areas should protect themselves against mosquito bite.

Points to Remember

- JE is endemic in several parts of India occurring sporadically and as small outbreaks
- Co-existence of birds, cattle and humans and proliferation of culex mosquitoes provide the ideal environment
- Once the disease occurs, treatment is only symptomatic
- Effective vaccination is available for producing solid immunity.

ZIKA VIRUS INFECTIONS

Zika virus infection has been known for over six decades as a mild inapparent dengue like illness with fever, myalgia, eye pain, prostration and maculopapular rash. Hemorrhagic tendency or mortality has not been recorded.

This virus was discovered in Uganda in 1967 in the course of regular vector surveillance. The main reservoir of virus has been wild primates in Africa and mosquitoes such as *Aedes africanus*. Human infection was rare.

Zika virus is a member of the *Flavivirus* genus in the family Flaviviridae. This has shot up into prominence due to the explosive pandemic of Zika virus infection which occurred in South American countries, Central America and the Caribbean in the later part of 2015. In 2013, the epidemic of chikungunya was followed by Zika infection in many countries due to the presence of the vectors *Aedes aegypti* and susceptible population. Thirty-three countries in the Americas reported the infection.

In India, due to the presence of the vector and susceptible population, outbreaks can develop if careful preventive measures are not undertaken. It is also likely that Zika virus may adapt to other mosquitoe vectors such as *Aedes albopictus*. The virus may be transmitted to sexual partners during sexual intercourse by infected persons. Breast milk may contain the virus. Incubation period is unknown but it is likely to be less than one week.

Clinical Features

Initial symptoms include fever, maculopapular rash, arthralgia or arthritis nonpurulent conjunctivitis, myalgia, retro-orbital pain and vomiting. The pattern of the present epidemic is that of a milder asymptomatic dengue like disease. Recent observations have brought out neurological complications like Guillain–Barré syndrome and other neurological complication like meningoencephalitis in Polynesians. The Zika virus epidemic occurred in Brazil in March 2015 affecting 1.3 million Brazilians. In Brazil, an epidemic of microcephaly has been recorded following Zika infection in pregnant women in 2014–2015. Though the association of Zika virus with microcephaly in the newborn has not been proved, this possibility is still strong and Zika virus may prove to be more harmful in pregnant women and their babies. Maximum risk is in the first trimester, most often between 7–13 weeks of gestation. Ocular abnormalities in the fetus such as focal pigment mottling, choroidal-retinal atrophy optical nerve abnormalities, neuroretinal atrophy, lens subluxation and coloboma have been recorded.

Diagnosis

During the times of epidemics, clinical diagnosis may be easy. Both dengue and chikungunya may present with similar clinical pattern. Commercial test for Zika has not been developed. Detection viral nuclei by RT–PCR and the detection of specific IgM, 5 days after the conjunctivitis suggests the diagnosis. Cross relation between IgM produced by other flaviviruses may occur. Zika virus RNA can be detected in urine for longer periods.

Management

Mainstay of management include bed rest and supportive care. Broad-spectrum antivirals, if available are to be employed since the occurrence of arboviruses infection may overlap and also reliable testing methods to pinpoint the infections are not yet available.

The microcephaly can be detected as early as 15–20 weeks of gestation in some cases, though in many cases the abnormality can be detected only in late pregnancy. Recent reports of CNS lesions occurring in adults are being reported. A case of 81-year-old male developing meningoencephalitis as the primary clinical picture has been reported.

Source: Carteaux G, Maquart M, Bedet A, et al. Zika Virus Associated with Meningoencephalitis. N Engl J Med. 2016;374(16):1595-6.

Prevention

Zika virus vaccines are not yet available. Best preventive methods to follow antimosquito measures at homes as well as the environment.

Source:

1. Fauci AS, Morens DM. Zika Virus in the Americas—Yet Another Arbovirus Threat. N Engl J Med. 2016;374(7): 601-4.
2. Bajpai S, Nadkar MY. Zika Virus Infection, the Recent Menace of the Aedes Mosquito. J Assoc Physicians India. 2016;64(3):42-45.

CHAPTER

61

Other Viral Infections
Epstein-Barr Virus, Cytomegalovirus, Parvovirus

KV Krishna Das

Chapter Summary

- Epstein-Barr Virus—Infectious Mononucleosis
  - Introduction
  - Pathogenesis
  - Clinical Features
  - Diagnosis
  - Treatment
- Cytomegalovirus (CMV) Infection
  - Clinical Features
  - Treatment
- Parvovirus Infections
  - Clinical Features
  - Treatment

EPSTEIN-BARR VIRUS—INFECTIOUS MONONUCLEOSIS

Introduction

This is worldwide in distribution, occurring in young individuals more frequently and caused by Epstein-Barr virus (EBV). EBV has been associated with several diseases both benign and malignant. These include infectious mononucleosis, Burkitt's lymphoma, oral hairy leukoplakia seen in relation to acquired immune deficiency syndrome (AIDS), nasopharyngeal carcinoma prevalent in China and postorgan transplantation lymphomas.

EBV is a member of the herpesvirus family. It infects B-lymphocytes. Major histocompatibility complex (MHC) class II molecules act as cofactors for infection. The virus infects epithelial cells primarily and replicates in them, leading to lysis of the cells. In EBV induced pharyngitis, the saliva contains infective virus. Other sites of invasion are the cervical epithelium and B-lymphocytes. Immunosuppressant therapy predisposes to, and augments the development of EBV induced lymphoproliferative syndromes. One of the modes of spread of infection is through saliva and kissing is attributed to play a role. In some, saliva may contain the virus even lifelong.

Pathogenesis

Only B-lymphocytes have receptors for EBV and therefore, EBV attacks B-lymphocytes initially. These cells begin to proliferate and are altered antigenically. Though T-lymphocytes are not affected by EBV, they also proliferate enormously. Around 90% of the atypical lymphocytes which are characteristic of the disease have T-lymphocyte markers, whereas only 10% have B-lymphocyte markers. The T-cells destroy EBV infected B-cells resulting in the liberation of antigenic materials which stimulate the formation of autoantibodies. The antigenic stimulus to heterophilic antibody is not known. Both cellular and humoral responses occur, the former is more effective in conferring immunity. The virus develops strategies to elude the immune system and the infection tends to persist. EBV may persist in B-lymphocytes lifelong. Initially antibodies of immunoglobulin M (IgM) types are formed, later they are immunoglobulin G (IgG). Since, cytomegalovirus (CMV) and human immunodeficiency virus (HIV) occurring in pregnancy are much more serious, they should be excluded by appropriate tests in women developing infectious mononucleosis during pregnancy.

Clinical picture resembling infectious mononucleosis can be evoked by *Toxoplasma gondii*, **primary HIV infection** and **CMV**, but in these the heterophile antibody response is not seen.

Clinical Features

The incubation period may range from 1 to 10 weeks, usually 2 weeks. The clinical spectrum may vary from that of a mild benign illness to that of a more severe and prolonged one. In children, the infection is less severe whereas in adolescents and adults, it produces the syndrome of infectious mononucleosis. The onset is usually insidious with general malaise, headache, diffuse myalgia, variable grades of fever and other constitutional symptoms. A petechial rash occurring at the junction of the soft and hard palate associated with sore throat may herald the onset. The sore throat may persist for days and this may be mistaken for follicular tonsillitis. The posterior cervical lymph nodes enlarge initially, later generalized lymphadenopathy may occur. Spleen is moderately enlarged to 2–3 cm below the costal margin, is soft and nontender. If gross splenomegaly occurs, the organ tends to rupture even with slight trauma. The period of risk of splenic rupture is 3–7 weeks of diagnosis, therefore convalescence is required during this period, rarely jaundice and neurological manifestations may develop.

Complications may occur. These include hemolytic anemia, thrombocytopenia, aplastic anemia, myocarditis, hepatitis, genital ulcers, splenic rupture and Guillain-Barré syndrome (GBS). Some cases go into chronicity.

Diagnosis

Clinically the disease should be suspected when small outbreaks occur in closed communities like hostels and dormitories or when there is close personal contact with cases. The presence of oral lesions, posterior cervical lymphadenopathy, splenomegaly and erythematous rashes are suggestive. Diagnosis should be strongly suspected if the proportion of atypical lymphocytes exceeds 20%.

Blood: Initially there is leukopenia due to decrease in neutrophils, but this is followed by leukocytosis in

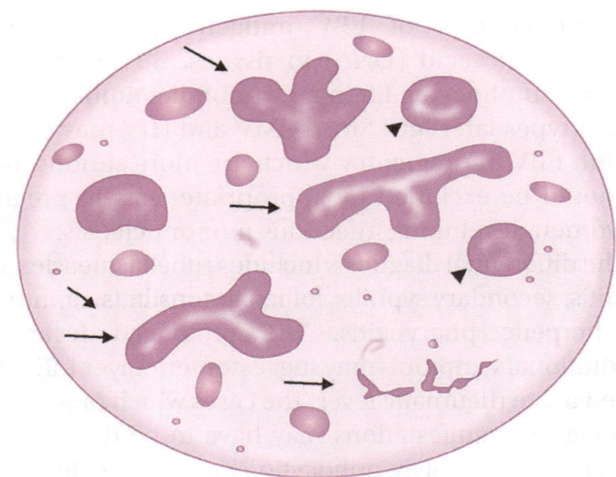

Fig. 61.1: Blood film showing atypical lymphocytes—line drawing, arrows—amoeboid shapes, arrowheads—neutrophils

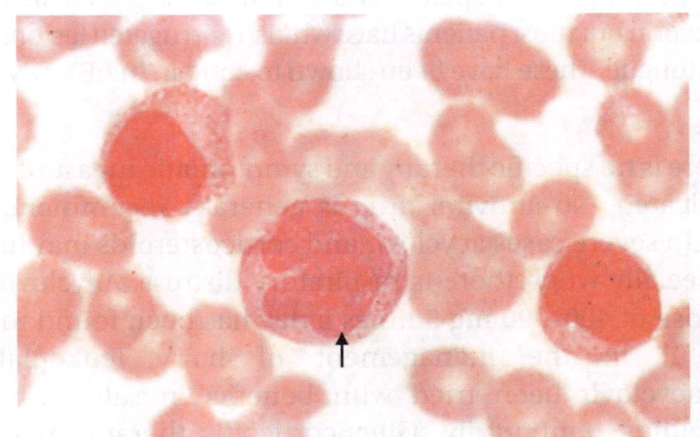

Fig. 61.2: Infectious mononucleosis—blood film; arrow points to atypical lymphocyte

which the leukocyte count may go up to 15–20,000/mm³. The characteristic finding is the presence of atypical lymphocytes which may form 60–80% of the total. The nuclei of the atypical lymphocytes do not have a regular shape but may be kidney shaped, oval, lobulated or polymorphic. Nucleoli are not seen. The cytoplasm is non-granular, foamy, vacuolated and appears amoeboid. The rest of the cells are mononuclear cells. In uncomplicated cases platelet count is normal (Figs 61.1 and 61.2).

Presence of heterophile antibodies demonstrable by the ***Paul-Bunnell test (sheep-cell agglutination)*** strongly suggests the diagnosis of infectious mononucleosis. The titer of antibodies increases with the passage of time. They are detectable for 4–6 weeks. Since, similar antibodies develop in serum sickness as well, differential absorption techniques are employed to differentiate infectious mononucleosis antibodies from those due to serum sickness.

Recently, a rapid slide test called ***monotest*** has become available for quick diagnosis. Specific antibody to EBV can be demonstrated by enzyme linked immunosorbent assay (ELISA), immunofluorescence, complement fixation and gel diffusion wherever facilities exist.

Chronic active EBV infection is diagnosed by the following features:

- Severe illness more than six months duration
- Histological evidence of organ involvement such as pneumonitis, hepatitis, bone marrow hypoplasia and uveitis

Textbook of Medicine

- Demonstration of EBV antigens or EBV deoxyribonucleic acid (DNA) in tissues. EBV may persist in B-lymphocytes lifelong. Antibodies initially are of IgM types later IgG. Since CMV and HIV may coexists with EBV in pregnancy which are more serious, these should be excluded by appropriate tests in pregnant women developing infectious mononucleosis.

The differential diagnosis includes rubella, measles, viral hepatitis, secondary syphilis, follicular tonsillitis, diphtheria, and herpetic pharyngitis. The prolonged fever and constitutional symptoms may suggest enteric fever, influenza, or even acute rheumatic fever. The cases which present with neurological manifestations may have to be distinguished from encephalitis or lymphocytic choriomeningitis. Other hematological disorders like acute leukemia and lymphoma have to be distinguished by suitable tests.

Oral hairy leukoplakia is a lesion usually seen in HIV infection but most patients have whitish corrugated lesions on the tongue. These have been shown to contain in EBV DNA.

Treatment

There is no specific therapy and symptomatic measures are indicated. No antiviral drug is generally recommended, but in severe cases acyclovir and corticosteroids may help, especially when there is respiratory distress. Acyclovir in a dose of 400–800 mg 5 times a day has been found to be useful in the management of hairy leukoplakia. Valacyclovir been tried with benefits in salivary viral shielding temporarily. Glucocorticoids therapy may be required for preventing and controlling complications like tonsillar hypertrophy, autoimmune hemolytic anemia, hemophogocytic syndrome and severe thrombocytopenia. It is seen that ampicillin aggravates the lymphadenopathy, skin rash and laryngeal edema in many cases and hence this drug should not be employed. Other antibiotics may be used only if there is evidence of secondary infection.

In the vast majority, recovery is usually complete in 3–4 weeks without any sequelae. Recent epidemiological evidence suggest that in some cases, due to continued antigenic stimulation, a lymphomatous process may be triggered off. Attempts to produce a vaccine are going on.

CYTOMEGALOVIRUS (CMV) INFECTION

This virus which belongs to the family herpesviridae commonly affects humans and 40–90% of adults may show antibodies to the virus. The virus is shed in saliva and urine and from the genital tract. Infection is acquired by contact with saliva or urine or by sexual contact. Uncomplicated CMV infection in immunocompetent subjects may be asymptomatic in vast majority.

Clinical Features

CMV infection of child may occur through breastfeeding. Feces of infants and children commonly contains CMV. Clinical illness resembles infectious mononucleosis caused by EBV with rash. Hepatitis, retinitis and neuropathy resembling GBS may occur rarely.

In immunocompromised states, the virus produces more severe illness leading to retinitis, pneumonitis, enteritis and generalized infection. It may occur as a co-infection in AIDS when the CD4 counts falls below 50/mm³. Patients receiving immunosuppressive therapy after organ transplantations may get CMV superinfection. CMV superinfection may complicate ulcerative colitis patients who are on glucocorticoids. CMV colitis shows erythema, granularity of mucosa and deep ulceration with surrounding edema on colonoscopy. Pregnant women who develop CMV infection may transmit the same to the fetus in up to 40%. Congenital infection may lead to hepatosplenomegaly, purpura, encephalitis, deafness and mental retardation in a small proportion.

Treatment

The drug of choice is ganciclovir 5 mg/kg bw given intravenous (IV) as infusion slowly over 1 hour, bd for 2 to 3 weeks. Maintenance dose is 5 mg/kg/day for long periods. An oral preparation of ganciclovir is available for prophylaxis in immunocompromised persons. Valacyclovir, an analogue of ganciclovir has been tried with benefit in patients with temporary salivary viral shedding.

Another effective drug is foscarnet given IV in a dose of 90 mg/kg bd for 14 to 21 days. Alternate drugs include valganciclovir and cidofovir. Neutropenia and thrombocytopenia may occur with ganciclovir and the other drugs. Renal toxicity may occur with foscarnet and cidofovir. A new drug letermovir is a potent anti-CMV drug with a novel mechanism of action targeting the viral terminase subunit pUL56. The dose varies from 60 to 240 mg/day. The drug was tried in hematopoietic cell transplant cases with good results and without hepato and nephrotoxicity. This drug is not yet available in India.

IV administration of hyperimmune anti-CMV globulin given during pregnancy protects the fetus. Vaccines against CMV infection are being developed.

Source: Chemaly RF, Ullmann AJ, Stoelben S, et al. Letermovir for cytomegalovirus prophylaxis in hematopoietic-cell transplantation. N Engl J Med. 2014;370(19):1781-9.

PARVOVIRUS INFECTIONS

Parvoviridae is a large family containing several members pathogenic to vertebrates. Of particular importance is parvovirus B19 (PVB19) belonging to the genus erythroparvovirus and it propagates best in erythyroid progenitor cells. Spread is by respiratory droplets and through transfusion of blood and blood products. The virus does not have a lipid envelope and therefore it is resistant to heat-inactivation and solvent detergents. Infection is very common and more than 50% of people acquire antibodies to the virus by 15 years of age. The natural host for PVB19 is the human erythyroid precursor cells which contain globoside, a neutral glycolipid which acts as a cellular receptor (also known as group P antigen) on the red blood cell (RBC). Antibodies develop against the virus. These help to limit and eliminate the infection. Failure to produce antibodies results in persistence of the infection. Most of PVB19 infections go without consequence. Active infection can lead to significant pathology especially in those with impaired red cell production, accelerated destruction or immunosuppression. PVB19 directly infects erythroid progenitor cells leading to their lysis. The impaired erythropoiesis lasts for 7–10 days, with a drop of hemoglobin of up to 2g/dL in otherwise normal people. Markers of infection include B19 IgM and/or B19 DNA.

Clinical Features

Several syndromes are caused by PVB19.

- ***Fifth disease in children:*** This manifests as fever with rash on the cheek-called erythema infectious. This rash is due to the deposition of immune complexes in the skin. The rash may tend to recur.
- ***Arthralgia and even arthritis*** in older age groups.
- ***Pure red cell aplasia:*** This may lead to insidious onset of anemia in normal people. Generally the infection is short lived and spontaneous recovery is the rule. In hemolytic anemias where erythrocyte life span is reduced such as sickle cell disease, hereditary spherocytosis, thalassemia, congenital aplastic anemia and even iron-deficiency anemia, the virus causes aplastic crises.

- ***Persistence of parvovirus infection:*** This leads to severe pure red cell aplasia of prolonged duration.
- In pregnant women the virus may infect the fetus and produce fetal loss or hydrops fetalis. Twenty percent of non-immune mediated hydrops fetalis is due to parvovirus infection.
- Edema may occur due to change in capillary permeability and development of capillaritis.

Treatment

Diagnosis can be established by demonstrating the antibodies. ***Treatment*** is symptomatic.

Systemic Fungal Infections

CHAPTER

62

Systemic Fungal Infections

KV Krishna Das, R Sajith Kumar

> **Chapter Summary**
>
> - General Considerations
> - Candidiasis
> - Aspergillosis
> - Histoplasmosis
> - Cryptococcosis
> - Rhinosporidiosis
> - Pneumocystis jirovecii Infection
> - Other Fungal Infections

GENERAL CONSIDERATIONS

Fungi are present in abundance in the soil as saprophytes and they generally invade immunologically compromised hosts. In the human body, they are present as commensals abundantly in the mucosal regions, skin and alimentary tract. The normal flora keep the fungi under check. With the widespread use of antibacterial drugs and immunosuppressive therapy, fungal infections have assumed greater importance. Advances in surgery, organ transplantation, widespread use of prosthetic materials inside tissues, extensive use of broad-spectrum antibacterial agents and long-term use of immunosuppressant drugs have paved the way for the emergence of life-threatening fungal infections. Prophylactic drugs against such infections are sometimes effective. Vigorous curative therapy has to be undertaken to achieve the desired benefits in such patients.

Fungi may be unicellular such as *Cryptococcus* or multicellular such as dermatophytes and they show varying degrees of differentiation. Hyphae are elongated tubular structures formed by the cells. Hyphae may be septate or nonseptate. A tangled mass of hyphae is called mycelium.

Pathogenic fungi may be classified into four groups morphologically.

1. ***Yeasts:*** These are unicellular fungi, spherical or ellipsoidal in shape, which reproduce by simple budding, e.g. *Cryptococcus neoformans.*
2. ***Yeast-like fungi:*** These show spherical and hyphal forms, e.g. *Candida albicans.*
3. ***Moulds:*** These are filamentous fungi which are capable of spore formation, e.g. dermatophytes.
4. ***Dimorphic fungi:*** These may grow as yeasts in tissues and moulds in the soil. Most of the systemic mycoses are due to such organisms.

Another basis for classification takes into account sexual spore formation. According to this classification, fungi may be divided into phycomycetes, ascomycetes, basidiomycetes and fungi imperfecti. Most of the human fungal pathogens belong to the class of fungi imperfecti.

Diagnosis of fungal diseases is established by demonstration of the organism in tissue specimens, body fluids or discharges. Fungi can be easily cultured in prepared media such as Sabouraud's glucose agar at pH 5.4.

Fungal lesions occurring in man can be broadly classified into superficial and deep mycoses. Superficial mycoses are more common and include the various types affecting the skin, nails, hair and mucous membranes. They are more common in those parts which are prone to be moist, such as intertriginous areas of skin, e.g. groin, gluteal folds and webs of fingers. They occur in individuals who are otherwise healthy (*See* Section 18, Ch 220).

Primary systemic fungal infections are caused by organisms that are mostly soil saprophytes and the infection is accidental. Immunocompromised individuals run the risk of opportunistic infections by fungi that are usually avirulent such as *Mucor, Cryptococcus, Candida* and *Aspergillus*, but which become invasive when body resistance goes down.

Textbook of Medicine

A range of antifungal drugs are available at present for topical and systemic use. Early detection of fungal infection and appropriate therapy are essential for successful result.

CANDIDIASIS

Candida albicans is a common inhabitant of the oropharyngeal, genital and intestinal cavities of man. Candidiasis is infection by *Candida albicans*. In most of the cases it remains as a local infection affecting the skin or mucous membranes of the mouth or genitalia. In the mouth it presents as oral thrush which is seen at the extremes of ages, those on antibiotic therapy or in immunosuppressed individuals.

Clinical Features

Oral candidiasis especially in severe immunosuppression is usually associated with esophageal candidiasis and patients present with painful dysphagia (odynophagia). The oral and esophageal mucosa may show whitish coatings or eroded bleeding mucous membrane, when the patches are shred or removed. In the genitalia it usually presents as vulvovaginitis in diabetic women whose diabetic status is not well-controlled. Cutaneous candidiasis usually affects the intertriginous areas.

Systemic candidiasis occurs in immunocompromized individuals and in drug addicts who share needles. The fungus becomes invasive and spreads through the blood stream to produce several lesions.

- **Localized lesions:** Urinary tract, liver, catheter and cannulae, heart valves, meninges and peritoneal cavity.
- **Widely disseminated:** Associated with septicemia (candidemia).

In disseminated candidiasis, the main targets of attack are kidneys, brain, liver, gastrointestinal tract (GIT), eye (endophthalmitis) and heart valves. Mortality in disseminated candidiasis is around 40%, even with many new therapies.

Diagnosis

The organism can be demonstrated microscopically by examining samples from local lesion. A potassium hydroxide smear, Gram stain or methylene blue is useful for direct demonstration of fungal cells. In tissues, periodic acid-Schiff (PAS) staining or methenamine silver staining reveals the organism. It should be borne in mind that the respiratory, GI and genitourinary tract can harbor these organisms without being the cause of infection.

The fungus can be grown in Sabouraud's medium. Antibodies to *Candida* can be detected by enzyme linked immunosorbent assay (ELISA) or immunodiffusion. The *Candida* antigen can be demonstrated by ELISA or radioimmunoassay. A new polymerase chain reaction (PCR) based detection is also available.

Treatment

Fluconazole, ketoconazole, itraconazole and amphotericin B are all effective in appropriate dosage to control the systemic infection. Most of the cases will respond to fluconazole, oral and/or parenteral.

Doses

- Fluconazole 150–400 mg/day for 14–21 days.
- Ketoconazole 400 mg/day for several weeks.
- Itraconazole 200–400 mg/day.
- Amphotericin B up to 50 mg/day IV for 1–2 weeks and more.

Ketoconazole tablets should no longer be prescribed as a first-line therapy for any fungal infection, including *Candida* and dermatophyte infections, because of the risk for severe liver injury, adrenal insufficiency and adverse drug interactions. Superficial skin and mucous membrane lesions respond well to nystatin ointment or nystatin mouthwashes.

Fluconazole given orally is very effective to cure vaginal candidiasis and esophageal candidiasis. Infections in human immunodeficiency virus (HIV) infected persons tend to recur even after an apparent cure. With extensive use of fluconazole in HIV infected persons, candida is developing resistance to the drug. Doubling the daily dose may be tried in these cases.

Voriconazole has also been approved for use in candidemia in patients who are not neutropenic. Voriconazole can be used at 6 mg/kg intravenous (IV) bd initially. The drug can also be given orally twice a day, in mild cases. Maintenance dose is 3 mg/kg bw (or 200 mg orally bd).

The echinocandins have become first-line therapy in many situations because of their efficacy and low incidence of adverse events and drug interactions. Caspofungin is a broad-spectrum semisynthetic echinocandins. It is an effective alternative for severe mucosal infections and systemic infections due to candida, other than *Candida albicans*. Caspofungin can be initiated as a 70 mg loading dose. This is followed by 50 mg/day IV to a total duration of a minimum of 2 weeks. Local surgical therapy should be aimed at removal of the source of infection, e.g. splenectomy for splenic abscess, surgical debridement for osteo vertebral lesions, vitrectomy for ophthalmitis and removal and replacement of prostheses or cannulae.

ASPERGILLOSIS

The species of *Aspergillus* pathogenic to man are *Aspergillus fumigatus, Aspergillus niger, Aspergillus flavus, Aspergillus terrens* and *Aspergillus nidulans*. Of these, *Aspergillus fumigatus* is most common. Infection occurs when general resistance is lowered or local disease favors superinfection. *Aspergillus* is very widespread in nature and their spores are found in dust. Both superficial and systemic lesions may develop. The most common superficial lesion is otomycosis. Systemic infection may be pulmonary or disseminated. Major portal of entry is the respiratory tract.

Clinical Features

Pulmonary form: There are four types of pulmonary aspergillosis: (1) Allergic bronchopulmonary aspergillosis (ABPA), (2) Invasive aspergillosis, (3) Chronic necrotizing aspergillosis and (4) Aspergilloma.

Allergic alveolitis may develop due to inhalation of fungal spores in sensitized individuals. *Aspergillus* may grow in the bronchi to produce invasive bronchopulmonary

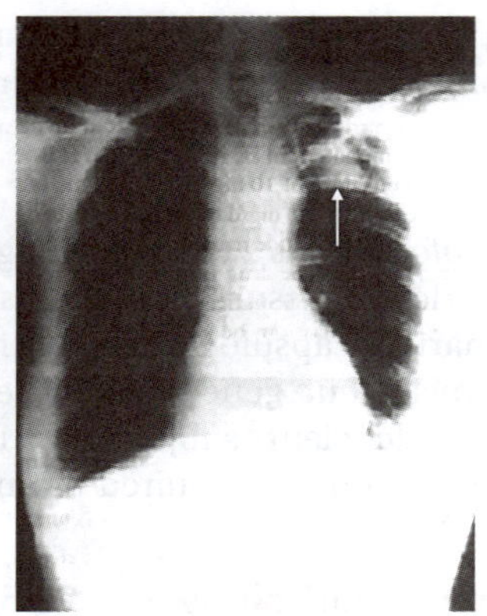

Fig. 62.1: Skiagram: Aspergilloma in cavity, left lung and upper zone (arrow) fungal ball

disease. The hyphae may obstruct the lumen. Healed tuberculous cavities or other types of cavities may be the seat of colonization by the fungus. The mycelia grow to form a tangled fungal ball which is recognizable in X-rays (aspergilloma).

It may remain asymptomatic or may cause massive hemoptysis with pleuritic chest pain. Invasive aspergillosis occurring in immunosuppressed individuals leads to widespread pulmonary necrosis with marked systemic symptoms. It presents as pneumonia with large nodular shadows in the lungs. Halo sign on chest X-rays and air crescent sign on computed tomography (CT) scans is supportive for a diagnosis of aspergilloma (fungal ball) (Fig. 62.1). Invasive aspergillosis is associated with very high mortality (80–90%). *Aspergillus* infection can occur in intensive care unit (ICU) patients with intravascular access lines and if not detected and treated promptly fatal results may occur.

Other Sites of Lesions

Other sites of lesion are the central nervous system (CNS) and naso-orbital cavities. Diagnosis can be made by histological demonstration of the fungus and isolation of the organism from the exudates. Since *Aspergillus* is a common contaminant in respiratory secretions, mere isolation does not prove its pathogenic role. Galactomannan (cell wall polysaccharide) assays may help before clinical features become typical. ELISA tests are also available. The samples used are serum, bronchoalveolar lavage (BAL) fluid, urine or cerebrospinal fluid (CSF) depending on the organ involvement. Precipitating antibodies can be demonstrated by gel diffusion test and this test is of great value in diagnosis.

Treatment

Amphotericin B in a dose of 1 mg/kg/day is effective in systemic aspergilloma. Amphotericin B and 5-fluocytosine are effective in CNS disease. Steroids are recommended to suppress the hypersensitive phenomenon with ABPA. The underlying predisposing factor should be attended to cavities containing aspergilloma producing intractable hemoptysis have to be removed surgically. Otherwise they are closely monitored and kept undisturbed. Other drugs like clotrimazole which is also effective *in vitro* is being evaluated. Other drugs effective against aspergillus include oral fluconazole itraconazole, voriconazole and posaconazole. Dose of voriconazole is 200–300 mg 12 hour given orally for long periods. Parenteral preparation (200 mg vial) is also available. Posaconazole can be given pro-phylactically against *Aspergillus* and other fungal infec-tions in neutrophilic patients. The dose is 200 mg tds oral. Caspofungin is a new antifungal drug effective against *Aspergillus* and other yeast species.

HISTOPLASMOSIS

Syn: Darling's disease, Cave disease

Etiology

This infection is worldwide in distribution but maximum number of cases has been reported from the West, especially the United States of America (USA). Histoplasmosis is an under-recognized disease in India and should be considered in the differential diagnosis of patients with prolonged fever, adrenal enlargement, hepatosplenomegaly, oral ulcers and granulomatous disease on histopathology. Occasional cases have been reported from Kerala too. *Histoplasma capsulatum* is seen in soil enriched by the droppings of birds, especially fowls. When the spores are inhaled, yeast-like forms develop in tissues. It grows as a mould in its natural habitat and *in vitro*.

Pathology

The lesions are granulomas produced in several organs. Reticuloendothelial organs, lungs, adrenals, brain and other tissues may be affected. Lesions may resemble tuberculosis. Healing occurs with calcification. Cerebral lesions can be mistaken for those of cerebral thrombosis or hemorrhage.

Clinical Features

The majority of cases are asymptomatic. Approximately 10% of patients with histoplasma infection can develop progressive disseminated histoplasmosis. They present with any of the following manifestations such as fever, malaise, hepatosplenomegaly, lymphadenopathy, pancy-topenia, renal failure, disseminated intravascular coagula-tion, skin lesions, GI manifestations like diarrhea and vomiting, neurologic manifestations like encephalo-pathy, focal parenchymal lesions and some-times adrenal insufficiency. Pulmonary lesions may resemble different types of tuberculosis (Fig. 62.2). Common manifestations include fever, cough, hilar adenopathy, pneumonitis, apical infiltrates, fibrocavitary lesions and subpleural solitary pulmonary nodules. Scattered miliary calcification may develop in disseminated histoplasmosis (Fig. 62.3). Other manifestations include mediastinal syndrome, uveitis and adrenal insufficiency. GI involvement (of the intestines) is rare—both immunocompromised and immunocompetent persons may be affected. It presents with diarrhea, weight loss, fever and emaciation and may be mistaken for tuberculosis. Endoscopic biopsy helps in diagnosis. Skin and mucus membrane ulcers may develop.

Diagnosis

Chest X-ray shows the pulmonary lesions. Delayed hypersensitivity test using histoplasmin is helpful in diagnosing past infection. The test shows cross-sensitivity with other fungi. It is more useful for epidemiological

Textbook of Medicine

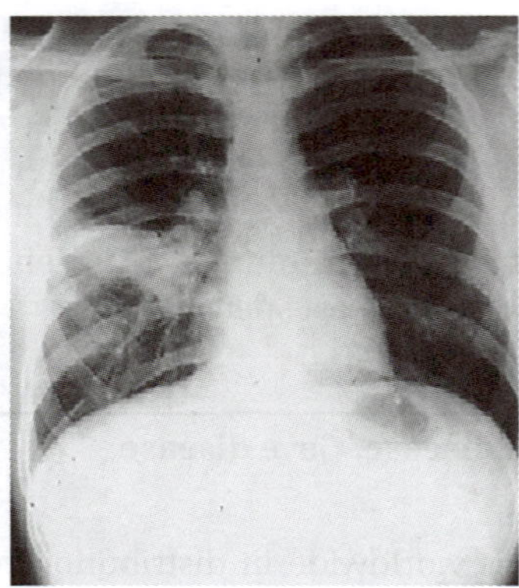

Fig. 62.2: Chest X-ray histoplasmosis—lesion resembling tuberculosis

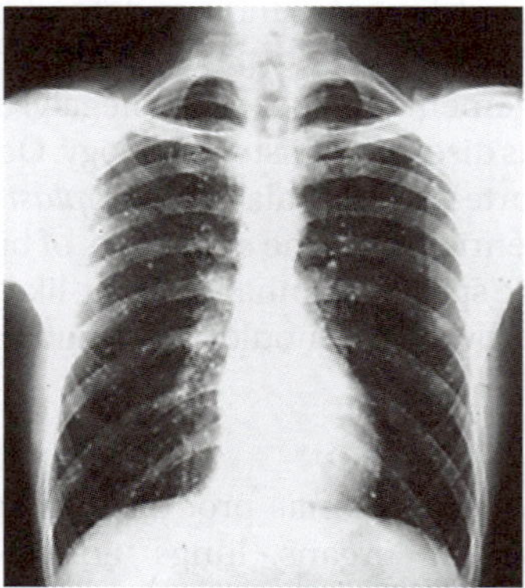

Fig. 62.3: Chest X-ray histoplasmosis—miliary calcification

studies to determine the prevalence of histoplasmosis in the community. Its use in the diagnosis of individual cases is limited. Complement fixing antibodies are detectable in the serum and these, being more specific, are useful in diagnosis. Diagnosis can be confirmed by demonstrating the fungus in tissue biopsies or other suitable material.

Prognosis

Histoplasmosis is generally benign. The mortality in disseminated histoplasmosis can be as high as 80%, even though with the right treatment this can be reduced to around 20%.

Treatment

Specific treatment is not indicated in asymptomatic cases. In disseminated disease and chronic pulmonary lesions, IV liposomal amphotericin B is given for 10–12 weeks is curative.

The dose is 0.5–0.6 mg/kg bw daily or 1.0–1.2 mg/kg bw on alternate days. Immunocompromised subjects should receive amphotericin as the drug of choice. Oral fluconazole and oral itraconazole 200 mg bd for 6 months is curative, but relapse rate is more (20–30%). Persistent cavities and mediastinal fibrosis may demand surgical management.

CRYPTOCOCCOSIS

Syn: Torulosis, European Blastomycosis, Busse-Buschke's disease

Infection by *Cryptococcus neoformans* leads to a clinical picture of subacute or chronic meningoencephalitis commonly. Sometimes the infection becomes generali-

zed and lungs, skin, bones and viscera may be involved. The fungus is present in nature especially in soil contaminated by the droppings of birds like fowls and pigeons.

Etiology

Cryptococcus neoformans is a yeast like fungus, distributed all over the world. In tissues, it remains encapsulated in a polysaccharide capsule. Infection in majority of cases is subclinical, but generalized disease occurs in immunologically deficient subjects. It is a common opportunistic infection in acquired immunodeficiency syndrome (AIDS).

Pathogenesis and Pathology

It is probable that the fungus reaches the lungs by inhalation. The pulmonary lesions tend to heal spontaneously without becoming symptomatic. Histologically, the lesions range from mild inflammatory reaction to definite granulomas. Intracranial infection leads to basal meningitis. The organism reaches the meninges by the bloodstream.

Clinical Features

The pulmonary involvement may be subclinical. It may be detected during routine investigation or accidentally, as inflammatory or tumor-like lesions. Often these, lesions are mistaken for tuberculosis. Meningoencephalitis closely resembles tuberculous meningitis. The patient presents with persistent progressively severe headache. CSF study is mandatory for the diagnosis (*See* Ch on AIDS). Papilledema and cranial nerve palsies occur in some cases. The course is prolonged with remissions and exacerbations.

Papular or suppurative lesions occur in the skin in 10% cases. These ulcerate and discharge hairy material containing the fungus. Other viscera such as liver, pericardium and endocardium may be affected.

Diagnosis

Diagnosis is confirmed by finding the encapsulated fungus in the sputum, urine, tissues and CSF. The fungus can be cultured and identified. The encapsulated organism can be demonstrated in the CSF by microscopic examination after mixing with a drop of India ink (Fig. 62.4). Histology of the lesions may reveal the fungus. Serological tests like complement fixation and latex agglutination are available, but being nonspecific, they are

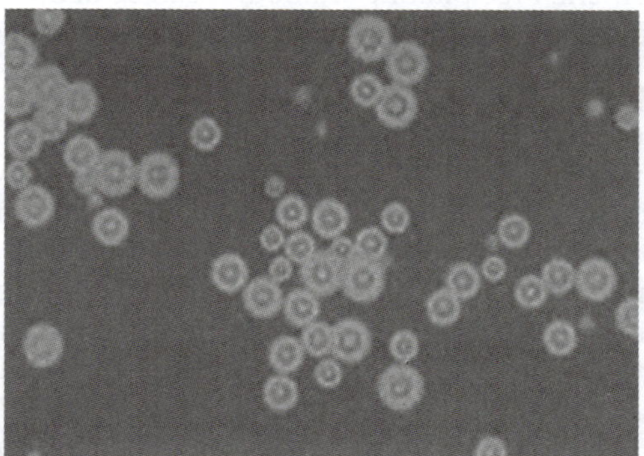

Fig. 62.4: Cryptococcus in wet preparations with Indian ink in CSF in cryptococcal meningitis. ***Note:*** Encapsulated organisms

not of great help. Cryptococcal antigen can be detected in CSF or blood by enzyme immunoassay.

Treatment

Cryptococcosis of the CNS is treated with flucytosine, given 150 mg daily orally in four divided doses or IV amphotericin B. Amphotericin B is started in a daily IV dose of 10 mg in a drip as the initial dose and it is increased to 50 mg/day to reach a total dose of 2 g or more. Mild toxic effects include nausea, vomiting, chills, fever, headache and malaise. The drug is nephrotoxic and increase in blood urea is a contraindication for further therapy. Fluconazole 400 mg/day can be given IV daily for 14 days of more.

Combination of amphotericin B 0.7 mg/kg bw and fluconazole 200–400 mg IV daily along with other drugs results in earlier resolution of both meningitis and pneumonia. In cases where cryptococcosis complicates AIDS treatment has to be continued till the CD4+ count rises about 200/mm^3 with ART. Oral Fluconazole is recommended for secondary prophylaxis.

RHINOSPORIDIOSIS

It is a chronic localized proliferative lesion caused by *Rhinosporidium seeberi* which affects the mucous membranes of the nose, larynx, eyes, ears, mouth, genitalia, rectum and skin. A case of disseminated cutaneous rhinosporidiosis is reported from Kottayam Medical College in 2008.

Source: Anoop TM, Rajany A, Deepa PS, et al. Disseminated cutaneous rhinosporidiosis. J R Coll Physicians Edinb. 2008;38:123-5.

Etiology

The etiological agent which is most probably a fungus was included under the class phycomycetes. The source of infection is stagnant water or aquatic life. The disease is endemic in Sri Lanka and India, but only rarely seen in other parts of world. Mode of infection is not clearly known.

Pathology

Typical lesions are soft, nodular and polypoid with grayish-white areas over the surface. Chronic inflammatory cell infiltration may be demonstrable. Histology shows a large number of fungal spherules containing endospores, embedded in a stroma of vascular connective tissue.

Clinical Features

The incubation period is not clearly known. The patients often seek medical help only when polypoid masses have developed. The symptoms depend on the site of affection. Nasal cavity is affected most commonly (Fig. 62.5). Symptoms include local pruritus, presence of mass, nasal block and epistaxis. The polyps are soft, pink, friable and easily bleed on touch. Their sizes vary and they show small yellowish dots on the surface. Cutaneous lesions resemble warts and are initially painless but become painful and nodulo-ulcerative later, varying in size from 0.5 to 2 cm.

Diagnosis can be made clinically in endemic areas. Nasal discharge may show free spores demonstrable microscopically. Histology is confirmatory. The organism

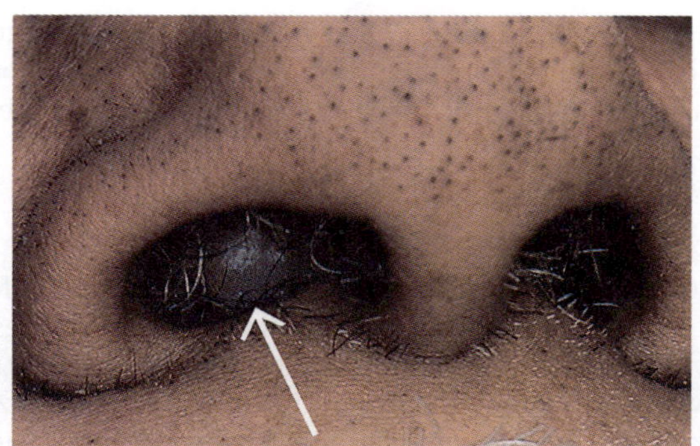

Fig. 62.5: Rhinosporidiosis—polypoid lesions (arrow)

can be observed with typical fungal stains like Gomori methenamine silver (GMS), PAS and hematoxylin and eosin (H&E).

Treatment consists of surgical removal. Some success with oral dapsone has been reported but the cutaneous lesions may be resistant.

PNEUMOCYSTIS JIROVECII INFECTION

General Considerations

This organism, previously known as *Pneumocystis carinii,* is considered to be more similar to fungi, though for several decades it was included among the protozoa. The parasite that is specific to man has been redesignated as *Pneumocystis jirovecii*. It is a pathogen of low virulence. It measures 1–8μ and is round or elongated. It is seen widely in nature in man and several animals. Air borne transmission has been proved. It may spread from the environment or from person to person. In those with suppression of immunological function, it becomes invasive and causes pneumonia. This parasite has unique tropism for the lungs if it remains as an alveolar pathogen without invading deeper tissues. Tissue reaction to infection leads to inflammation and diffuse alveolar damage. Immunity is CD4 T-cell mediated.

Clinical Features

Pneumocystis jirovecii infection complicates hemato-logical malignancies, immunosuppressant therapy and organ transplantation.

Homosexual men and subjects with AIDS show predilection. In children, pneumocystosis may supervene on congenital immunodeficiency states and protein-calorie malnutrition.

Immunodeficiency also predisposes to infection by cytomegalovirus, candida and mycobacteria which may coexist with pneumocystosis. In many patients with AIDS, the presentation is pneumocystis pneumonia. Impaired diffusing capacity, decrease in lung volumes and hypoxemia with an increased alveolar arterial oxygen gradient occur. Infection is heralded by fever, non-productive cough and progressive dyspnea. The condition generally deteriorates within weeks to months. Acute respiratory distress syndrome (ARDS) like presentation is reported in advanced immunosuppression. Physical examination may show nil or only minimal signs. Lactate dehydrogenase (LDH) levels are elevated and come down

Textbook of Medicine

with successful treatment. X-ray shows infiltration, going on to extensive consolidation. Less commonly, other organs such as lymph nodes, spleen, liver, bone, bone marrow, meninges, pancreas and endocrine glands may show lesions (*See* also Ch 48).

Diagnosis

Pneumocystis pneumonia should be suspected when fever and respiratory symptoms occur in immunosuppressed individuals. Chest skiagram may be normal or may show diffuse interstitial infiltrates mostly in mid zone (sparing the apical regions in most cases) with occasional pneumatoceles. Pleural effusion can occur rarely. High resolution computed tomography (HRCT) will show patchy areas of ground-glass attenuation with a background of interlobular septal thickening. Normal CT does not exclude the diagnosis. The organisms can be demonstrated in Bronchoalvelar lavage (BAL) or lung biopsy specimens taken at bronchoscopy or by needle biospy. Though positive results confirm the diagnosis, negative results do not exclude the condition. Detection by PCR can also be tried. Arterial blood gas (ABG) will show hypoxia with metabolic alkalosis.

Treatment

Cotrimoxazole in doses up to 6–7 g/day, in divided doses, for 2 weeks is beneficial. Pentamidine isothionate given intramuscularly in a dose of 2–4 mg/kg body weight daily for 10–14 days is also effective as a curative drug. If the drug is started early, results are good. Improvement starts in 5–7 days. Other drugs which are also beneficial include dapsone and pyrimethamine.

Table 62.1: Other fungal infections

Disease	Organism	Geographical distribution
Coccidioidomycosis	*Coccidioides immitis*	Worldwide
Paracoccidioidomycosis	*Paracoccidioides brasiliensis*	South America
Blastomycosis	*Blastomyces dermatitidis*	Worldwide
Sporotrichosis	*Sporothrix schenckii*	Worldwide
Chromoblastomycosis and mycetoma	*Fonsecaea* and *Cladosporium*	Tropics
Zygomycosis	*Absidia, Mucor, Rhizopus*	Worldwide

If the results are not good with the specific drugs alone, addition of prednisolone in a dose of 1 mg/kg bw brings about rapid relief. This has to be tapered off with improvement. The underlying condition should also receive attention.

Prophylaxis against pneumocystis pneumonia should be instituted in patients infected with HIV when the CD4 lymphocyte count falls below 200/mm^3. Cotrimoxazole is very effective in preventing infection, if given in a dose of one double strength tablet daily for prolonged periods. Secondary prophylaxis is mandatory, but can be stopped when CD4 counts go above 300 cells/mm^3.

OTHER FUNGAL INFECTIONS

With the advent of numerous antimicrobial drugs and immunosuppressant drugs, the number of immuno-compromised subjects has increased. The epidemic of HIV has rendered many patients immunosuppressed. Due to all these factors the number and variety of fungal infection have also increased. Some of the less common fungal infections are given in Table 62.1.

Actinomyces and Nocardia

KV Krishna Das, R Sajith Kumar

Chapter Summary

- Actinomycosis
- Nocardiosis
- Mycetoma

These are gram-positive bacteria with branching filaments sometimes forming a mycelium. These are included under the order Actinomycetales. Mostly they are soil saprophytes. Two genera—*Actinomyces* and *Nocardia* are pathogenic to man.

ACTINOMYCOSIS

Syn: Ray-fungus disease

Actinomycosis is a chronic, slow-growing, progressive, granulomatous lesion caused by *Actinomyces israelii*. *Actinomyces* are bacteria. They form mycelia like fungi.

They are susceptible to antibiotics and in this regard behave more akin to bacteria. They are gram-positive. The two genera of medical importance are *Actinomyces* and *Nocardia*. *Actinomyces* are anaerobic or microaerophilic whereas *Nocardia* are aerobic. *Actinomyces israelii* is present in the mouth as a commensal and tissue invasion occurs due to minor trauma.

Pathology

The lesions are granulomas with added suppuration. The pus shows microcolonies of the organisms as yellowish granules (sulfur granules). These granules become more distinct when the pus is shaken vigorously with water.

Clinical Features

The disease presents as the cervicofacial form, thoracic form, abdominal form and bony lesions. Symptoms depend on the anatomic location.

- ***Cervicofacial form:*** Fourty to sixty percent of the total. This form starts as painless, slow growing lump near the jaw or a painful lesion resembling an abscess. The lesion progresses to involve deeper tissues and bone and sinuses develop. Trismus may occur. Lymph nodes are generally spared. Systemic symptoms are few or absent. The lesion progresses slowly to destroy all tissues and discharge the characteristic pus. Presence of extensive destructive lesions in the presence of minimal general symptoms should suggest the possibility of actinomycosis.
- ***Thoracic form:*** This form results from aspiration of the organism from the mouth. Manifestations include pulmonary infiltration and cavitation, pleurisy, empyema and pericarditis. Pulmonary lesions may be unilateral or bilateral and may closely resemble tuberculosis. The lesion may spread to the pleura and chest wall leading to periostitis of the ribs and formation of discharging sinuses.
- ***Abdominal form:*** This form results from ingestion of the organisms. Lesions occur in the cecum and appendix. The disease may present as acute appendicitis or a slow growing lump in the right iliac fossa. This may resemble ileocaecal tuberculosis, Crohn's disease or malignancy. The lesion may become adherent to the anterior abdominal wall and form sinuses. Rarely the liver and genitals may be involved.
- ***Bony lesions:*** These include osteomyelitis of the mandible, ribs and lumbar vertebrae.

Diagnosis

Strong clinical suspicion is necessary to make the diagnosis. Microscopy of the discharges reveals the mycelia. Histopathological examination confirms the diagnosis. The organism can be grown in culture anaerobically.

Prognosis

Early diagnosis and proper treatment result in resolution of the lesions.

Treatment

Penicillin is the drug of choice giving cure rates over 80% in 6–8 weeks. Tetracycline and stilbamidine have to be given when penicillin is contraindicated. Erythromycin, fusidic acid, lincomycin and rifampicin are all effective. Surgery may be necessary in advanced cases if drug treatment fails.

NOCARDIOSIS

General Considerations

This is infection by gram-positive bacteria of the type aerobic actinomycosis of in the genus *Nocardia*. The organisms are branching beaded filaments that are gram-positive and weakly acid fast. These organisms are found in the soil, decaying vegetable matter and contaminated water sources. They may become air borne when they can reach the lungs and cause pulmonary lesions. There are more than nine pathogenic species.

Clinical Features

Nocardia brasiliensis causes skin infections leading to mycetoma. Primary cutaneous nocardiosis manifests as cellulitis or abscess and as lymphocutaneous infection like sporotrichoid nocardiosis.

Systemic nocardiosis can lead to acute, subacute or chronic infectious disease that occurs as cutaneous, pulmonary and disseminated forms. Pleuropulmonary nocardiosis manifests as an acute, subacute or chronic pneumonitis and cavity formation. Local spread to another intrathoracic organs has been reported.

Disseminated nocardiosis may involve any organ. Brain and meningeal lesions are more common particularly in immunocompromised persons.

Diagnosis

Respiratory samples, aspirates or pus and affected tissue can be subjected to culture, even though growth rates are slow. Cerebrospinal fluid (CSF) in meningitis due to *Nocardia* has features of bacterial meningitis only.

Treatment

Surgical drainage may be required in localized abscesses. Drugs recommended in treatment of nocardiosis include sulfonamides (cotrimoxazole), third generation cephalosporins, carbapenems, tigecycline, linezolid, oral amoxicillin-clavulanic acid and minocycline. Six to twelve months of therapy may be needed.

MYCETOMA

Syn: Madura foot, Maduramycosis

Definition

This is a chronic granulomatous inflammation caused by several species of *Nocardia*, *Actinomycosis* and fungi. *Nocardia* are normally present in soil and infection may be exogenous.

The classic lesions are Madura foot and other mycetomas. The organisms causing Madura foot are *Nocardia madurae*, *N. asteroides* and *N. brasiliensis*. In addition to *Nocardia actinomycosis* and fungi can also lead to mycetoma.

The lesion starts in the subcutaneous tissues and later on involves deeper structures, including the bones, to form sinuses leading to the eventual destruction of the part. This condition was described in Madurai in 1842 by Gill. This disease is confined to the tropics and is particularly endemic in India, Africa and South America. Most of the cases in India have been reported from Tamil Nadu, Andhra Pradesh and Maharashtra.

Pathogenesis and Pathology

The organisms enter through abrasions on the skin. The lesions manifest after a long incubation period. A granuloma develops. The organisms are seen to lie in abscesses, surrounded by a zone of chronic inflammatory cells. The organism can be easily identified on microscopic examination. The inflammation spreads along fascial planes by contiguity. Nerves and tendons are highly resistant to invasion. Regional lymph nodes are not generally affected.

Clinical Features

A small painless firm subcutaneous tumor develops in both the nocardial and actinomycosis types. The lesions slowly progress to destroy the part. Sinuses develop which discharge pus containing the organisms. The progress of an actinomycosis granuloma is more rapid than that of a nocardial lesion.

The most common site is the dorsum of the foot, but other regions like the hands, buttocks, back, scalp and orbits may be affected. Systemic symptoms do not occur.

Radiological Features

Bone destruction and endosteal or periosteal new bone formation may be demonstrable in localized areas or more diffusely.

Progressive painless destructive lesions of the extremities occurring in endemic areas should raise the possibility of mycetoma. The differential diagnosis includes chronic osteomyelitis, tuberculosis, syphilis, elephantiasis and neoplasms. Histology of the lesion and isolation of the organism from the lesion help to establish the diagnosis. Antibodies to the organism can be demonstrated by agar-gel precipitation tests.

Treatment

Drug treatment is effective for actinomycosis lesions, but not so readily for nocardial lesions. Actinomycetoma respond well to prolonged treatment (6–12 months) with dapsone (200 mg/day), cotrimoxazole, nalidixic acid or rifampicin. Therapy of choice for nocardia is cotrimoxazole.

Surgery

In addition to drug therapy, surgery may be needed to excise early lesions or to amputate grossly damaged limbs. The lesion may recur after surgery. Mycetomas can be prevented by regular use of footwear and proper foot hygiene.

CHAPTER 64

Disease caused by Protozoa
Malaria, Leishmaniasis, Trypanosomiasis

PK Sasidharan, KV Krishna Das, VP Gopinathan

Chapter Summary

- Protozoal Diseases
  - General Considerations
- Malaria
  - General Considerations
  - Epidemiology
  - Lifecycle of the Parasite
  - Pathogenesis
  - Immunity against Malaria
  - Clinical Features
  - Complications
  - Tropical Splenomegaly Syndrome
  - Laboratory Findings
  - Diagnosis
  - Treatment
  - Prevention
  - Malaria Vaccines
  - Other Community Measures
- Leishmaniasis
  - Visceral Leishmaniasis
  - Post-Kala-azar Dermal Leishmaniasis
  - Cutaneous Leishmaniasis
  - American Cutaneous and Mucocutaneous Leishmaniasis
- African Trypanosomiasis
- American Trypanosomiasis

PROTOZOAL DISEASES

General Considerations

Protozoa are unicellular organisms containing cytoplasm, nuclei and other organelles. Based on the mode of locomotion, protozoa have been classified into flagellates, ciliates, amebae and sporozoa. Even though differences occur between different classes, basic similarities exist. The cytoplasm is divided into an outer ectoplasm and inner endoplasm. Both layers contain several organelles, the ectoplasm performs the functions of protection, locomotion, respiration, nutrition and excretion.

The nucleus is made up of fine delicate filaments studded with masses of chromatin granules and is enclosed by the nuclear membrane. The karyosome lies in the center of the nucleus. It may be minute or large and conspicuous. Under adverse conditions, free-living protozoa change from the vegetative to the cystic form by encasing themselves in a tough membranous wall.

Protozoa are found extensively in the environment. Many, such as *Entamoeba coli* and *Trichomonas hominis* are free living commensals, while others become invasive and pathogenic when circumstances are favorable, e.g. *Entamoeba histolytica* and *Giardia lamblia*. Some are obligate parasites of man or other vetebrate hosts, e.g. malarial parasites, trypanosomes and leishmania. These have a developmental cycle in arthropod vectors. Distribution of the vector determines the endemicity to particular geographical regions. Rise in vector population leads to outbreaks of epidemics from time to time. Since tropical climate offers the ideal situation for breeding and proliferation of the vector arthropods, such vector-borne diseases are most prevalent in the tropical belt. High density of population, low socioeconomic conditions and poor hygienic environment favor the persistence and spread of many of the diseases—both feco-orally transmitted and vector-transmitted.

MALARIA

General Considerations

Malaria is characterized by high fever, occurring in paroxysms with chills and rigor or as continuous fever

Textbook of Medicine

or remittent fever with or without chills and rigor, splenomegaly, sometimes hemolysis and is capable of running a recurrent and chronic course. It is one of the most common serious infections affecting mankind in the tropical countries and is caused by the protozoan parasite *Plasmodium*. Alphonse Charles Laveran, a French military surgeon, detected moving protozoal parasites in fresh blood studies and described it in 1880. He won the Nobel Prize in 1907 for this. It was Ronald Ross, an English doctor in Indian Medical Service, who, while working in Hyderabad, demonstrated transmission of malarial parasite to human beings by anopheline mosquitoes and got Nobel Prize for this discovery. Among the 10 species which can cause malaria in humans, five species account for almost all the human infections. They are *Plasmodium vivax, Plasmodium falciparum, Plasmodium ovale, Plasmodium malariae* and *Plasmodium knowlesi*.

Epidemiology

It is mainly a disease of the tropics. In South East Asia itself, there are 10 endemic countries. Malaria is endemic in countries like India, Bangladesh, Myanmar, Middle East, Sri Lanka and several African nations. Eighty percent of malaria is occurring in Africa and South East Asia. More than 3 billion people are exposed in 109 countries and is a major public health problem. It leads to 1–2 million deaths every year. It has now been eliminated from several countries like USA, Canada, Europe and Russia and the heavy burden in the endemic countries pose a threat to them. In epidemics, children suffer more and mortality is higher in them. In recent years, there is resurgence in incidence of malaria, as a consequence of environmental, socioeconomic and public health changes related to industrialization and globalization. Vivax malaria is more infective and spreading due to earlier development of gametocytes compared to *Plasmodium falciparum* and it tends to be persistent. Malaria is transmitted by some species of anopheline mosquitoes and transmission does not occur at temperatures below 16°C and at altitudes >2,000 meters. The optimum conditions for transmission are high humidity and an ambient temperature between 20 and 30°C. In the places where the disease occurs, the most important issue is accumulation of all kinds of wastes, especially the plastic bags and containers, bottles, coconut shells, tumblers and tyres thrown around carelessly which can hold water, creating a stagnant water-body or can cause stagnation of water in the drainages—all facilitating mosquito breeding. Although rainfall provides breeding sites for mosquitoes, excessive rainfall can destroy the larvae. In India, around one million cases are reported annually among which majority is due to *P. vivax* and *P. falciparum*. Sixty-seven percent of India's population live in low transmission areas, 22% in high transmission and 11% only in malaria free areas (Fig. 64.1). Malaria, like all other killer diseases, is linked to marginalization, lack of social security and human development and the consequent issues like poor waste disposal habits, poor waste management facilities and malnutrition which need to be tackled on a priority basis for efficient control and eradication.

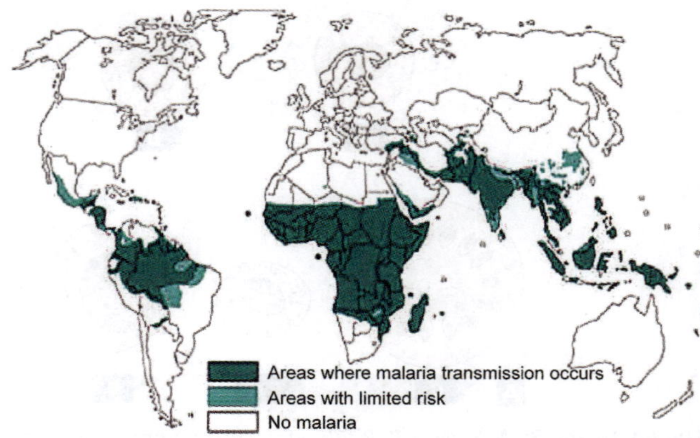

Fig. 64.1: Epidemiology of malaria

The prevalence of malaria in endemic areas is indicated by spleen rate, parasite rate and infant parasite rate. Spleen rate is the percentage of children aged 2–9 years showing palpable spleen in an endemic area. Parasite rate is the percentage of positive cases of malaria detected by examination of thick and thin blood smear in the community. Infant parasite rate is the percentage of positive smears among infants of 0–11 months. Any region is hypoendemic when spleen rate and parasite rate are 0–10%, mesoendemic when these are 11–50%, hyperendemic when it is above 50%. A place is holoendemic when the spleen rate and parasite rate are more than 75%. The common species of mosquitoes transmitting malaria are *Anopheles culicifacies, A. stephensi, A. fluviatilis, A. dirus, A. sundaicus* and others.

Lifecycle of the Parasite

Malaria is transmitted by female anopheline mosquitoes which inoculate plasmodial sporozoites from the salivary gland along with saliva during the bite. They are carried rapidly to the liver, where they invade hepatocytes and multiply inside them. This form of asexual cycle is called intrahepatic or pre-erythrocytic schizogony or merogony. The fully developed pre-erythrocytic schizont in a hepatocyte contains as many as 12,000–30,000 merozoites. The swollen infected hepatocyte eventually bursts and releases the motile merozoites into the bloodstream. These merozoites may enter into red cells to start their erythrocytic schizogony or re-enter the hepatocytes to continue the exo-eryhtrocytic schizogony. In *P. vivax* and *P. ovale* infections, a proportion of the intrahepatic forms may remain dormant for several weeks to a year or longer before reproduction begins. These dormant forms or hypnozoites, are the cause of the relapses that characterize infection with these two species.

Incubation period	
P. falciparum	12 days (8–15 days)
P. vivax	14 days (12–30 days)
P. ovale	15 days (12–20 days)
P. malariae	18 days (15–35 days)

Finally, merozoites are released into blood by rupture of hepatocytes. These merozoites rapidly invade the red blood cells (RBCs) and become trophozoites. During erythrocytic schizogony, the parasite passes through the

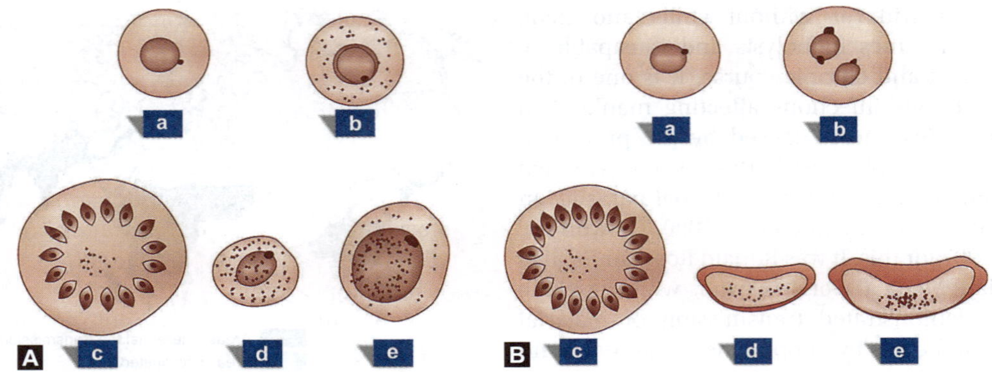

Figs 64.2A and B: A. *P. vivax;* **B.** *P. falciparum* (diagrammatic presentation)
Keys: a. Ring form, b. Trophozoite, c. Schizont with merozoites (rosette), d and e. Male-female gametocytes

following stages: Trophozoite, schizonts and merozoites (Figs 64.2A and B). They multiply six- to twenty-folds every 48–72 hours and consume all the hemoglobin and grow in size to occupy most of the RBC and are now fully mature schizonts. When the maturation is completed, the RBC enlarges and is unable to hold the parasite any longer and bursts to release the merozoites. The febrile paroxysm coincides with this process. The free merozoites released from RBCs attack new RBC and continue the erythrocytic schizogony. The maturation of red cell schizont happen over varying periods for each species— 48 hours for *P. vivax, P. ovale* and *P. falciparum* or 72 hours for *P. malariae*. Sometimes the parasite lifecycle in the erythrocyte takes shorter than 48 hours for *P. falciparum,* especially in fulminant infection with complications. The RBC ruptures to release 6–30 daughter merozoites, each potentially capable of invading a new RBC and repeating the cycle. After a series of asexual cycles (*P. falciparum*) or immediately after release from the liver (*P. vivax, P. ovale, P. malariae*), some of the parasites develop into longer-lived sexual forms (female and male gametocytes) which are morphologically distinct circulating in the bloodstream. These are taken up by the mosquitoes during a blood meal.

When the biting female anopheline mosquito takes up these gametocytes during a blood meal, the male and female gametocytes unite to form a zygote in its midgut. This zygote matures into an ookinite which penetrates and encysts in the insect's gut wall. The resulting oocyst expands by asexual division until it bursts to release the motile sporozoites which migrate to several organs including salivary glands of the mosquito and await inoculation into another human being during the next blood meal. Once infected, the mosquito is infective for its lifespan of approximately one month. Parasite multiplication in humans is by mitosis, whereas it is by meiosis in the mosquito.

Pathogenesis

The clinical manifestations of malaria are due to effects of parasites on RBCs as well as due to the host response. Inside the RBC, the growing parasites consume and degrade the intracellular proteins including hemoglobin which is degraded to hemozoin (malaria pigment). The paroxysms of fever are caused by rupture of RBC and release of parasite debris including malarial pigment,

hemozoin and glycosylphosphatidylinositol (GPI). Parasitized RBCs are also destroyed in spleen giving rise to a state of hemolysis. In addition, in falciparum malaria, membrane protuberances, which are parasite-derived adhesive proteins, appear on the surface which mediate attachment to receptors on the endothelium in capillaries and venules. The cytoadherence and the sequestration of RBC in falciparum malaria is caused by the interaction between parasite derived molecules on the surface of RBC and the receptors on vascular endothelium. Intercellular adhesion molecule-1 (ICAM-1) is probably most important receptor in the brain vascular endothelium. Upregulation of ICAM-1 and other endothelial receptors by tumor necrosis factor TNF-α leads to adherence of erythrocytes, platelet and thrombi to cerebral microvasculature. RBCs containing the falciparum malarial parasite are very sticky because of this phenomenon of cytoadherence and they stick to endothelium or between themselves by rosetting or agglutination and eventually block capillaries and venules. Rosetting occurs when infected and sticky RBCs adhere to normal RBCs and agglutination occurs by sticking together of infected RBCs. All these can lead on to 'sequestration' of parasites with vascular occlusion in vital organs causing organ ischemia and dysfunction. This phenomenon causes reduction of the number of parasites in the peripheral blood despite high parasite load and severe disease. Only the younger ring forms of the asexual parasites are sometimes seen in the peripheral blood in falciparum malaria and the level of peripheral parasitemia underestimates parasite load.

Plasmodium falciparum releases large number of pro-inflammatory cytokines like interleukin 1 beta (IL1β), IL6, IL8 and TNF. Severe malaria has several features in common with severe sepsis syndrome with all its consequences including disseminated intravascular coagulation (DIC) and acute respiratory distress syndrome (ARDS).

Coagulation system is deranged leading to DIC and its consequences and coexisting deep vein thrombosis or cerebral vein thrombosis (CVT) with or without hemorrhage, which can complicate the clinical picture. Vascular occlusion in liver can sometimes lead to severe ischemic necrosis of the liver presenting even with hepatic encephalopathy mistaken for fulminant hepatitis. This process is often compounded by nonsteroidal anti-inflammatory drugs (NSAIDs) intake which adds to liver and kidney injury.

In the other three forms of malaria which are less severe, cytoadherence and sequestration does not occur and all the stages of parasite's development are demonstrable in peripheral blood. Co-morbidities including bacterial infections, human immunodeficiency virus (HIV) and the coexisting malnutrition worsen the outcome. Due to severe life-threatening complication caused by *P. falciparum,* it used to be referred to as malignant tertian malaria whereas the *P. vivax* used to be referred to as benign tertian malaria. At present reports of more severe form of *P. vivax* malaria are appearing in the literature.

Immunity against Malaria

Clinically obvious or subclinical malnutrition and the consequent poor cell mediated immunity is one of the major causes permitting the parasite to multiply in the body and for the poorer outcome in some individuals. Nonspecific and specific immune responses to infection also help to control the infection to some extent, but adequate immunity exists only in the presence of normal nutrition. Both humoral immunity and cellular immunity are involved in this protection against malaria but the mechanisms involved are poorly understood. Immune individuals have elevated levels of antibodies [immunoglobulin (Ig) IgM, IgG or IgA] to a variety of parasite antigens limiting replication of the parasite. Repeated exposures confer protection against severe disease but do not prevent infection. As a result of this, a state of infection without illness is possible and they remain asymptomatic with parasites in peripheral blood and are capable of transmitting the disease. This phenomenon is very common in holo or hyperendemic areas. Passively transferred maternal antibodies (IgG) from an immune mother can protect the infant from severe malaria in the first month of life. The complex immunity which confers protection against the disease declines when the person leaves the endemic area. The complexity of the immune responses in malaria and the complex antigenic structure of the parasite and the ability of the parasite to evade the defense mechanisms all are the reasons for the inability to develop an effective vaccine against malaria.

Red cell disorders like sickle cell disease, thalessemia, hemoglobin C, glucose-6-phosphate dehydrogenase (G6PD) deficiency and pyruvate kinase deficiency and probably other intrinsic defects confer some protection against death from falciparum malaria. A person with sickle cell trait has six-fold reduction in the risk of dying from falciparum malaria. This could be due to reduced parasite growth in low oxygen levels inside the RBC containing sickle hemoglobin (HbS). Sickle cell Hb disease is more frequent in areas endemic for *P. falciparum*. It is hypothesised that the heterozygote forms of these disorders develop as a result of mutations arising under the high pressure of malaria in the community and are supposed to have evolved as a natural protective mechanism against malaria. After severe infection, patients without the mutations die and those with mutations would survive. Thus over several decades of presence of malaria in a society, large number of heterozygous (HbAS) individuals for these defects survive as a natural selection process and consequently when two heterozygotes mate, a homozygous progeny is born (HbSS). Thus, sickle cell disease (HbSS) or the homozygous state is a natural consequence of large number of HbAS in a community. This phenomenon is termed balanced polymorphism.

Clinical Features

Fever is the most classical symptom which is usually high grade with or without chills and rigor. The classic triad of fever, rigor and sweating paroxysms is established especially in *P. vivax, P. ovale* and *P. malariae*, after a few weeks of onset of the disease. In the early phase, the fever may resemble any other febrile illness. In the case of *P. falciparum*, even after considerable periods, the typical paroxysms may be absent, adding problem for clinical diagnosis.

The classic malarial paroxysm has three stages—cold stage, hot stage and sweating. During the cold stage the skin is cold, goose pimples appear on skin, patient uses a blanket and has visibly shaking movements which is followed by the hot stage and has high fever. After that the sweating stage occurs with profuse sweating and the fever subsides with or without the use of paracetamol. The classic picture of malaria occurs in the non-immune individuals having uncomplicated malaria. Traditional description of febrile paroxysms with chills and rigor (every other day for *P. vivax, P. ovale* and *P. falciparum* and every third day for *P. malariae*) is rarely observed nowadays, when it is seen it is more common in vivax malaria. Therefore, in any febrile patient residing in an endemic area or those with history of travel to endemic areas, malaria should be considered in the differential diagnosis of all types of fevers especially when there are no clinical features of other febrile illness. The common conditions to be differentiated in early phase are acute pyelonephritis, enteric fever, scrub typhus, common viral fevers, dengue fever and leptospirosis. After five days of fever the differential diagnosis is usually between enteric fever, scrub typhus and malaria. Unlike viral fevers, there are usually no respiratory symptoms, rhinitis, sore throat or severe myalgia. Presence of arthralgia, myalgia or diarrhea often suggests another diagnosis. Sometimes there may be associated nonspecific headache, myalgia and malaise mimicking viral infections like dengue fever, but in malaria the fever persists even after five days. High index of suspicion and awareness of the clinical features and epidemiological settings help to arrive at the diagnosis in the majority.

Physical examination is basically to look for clinical features of other common febrile illness, the absence of which favor malaria in the appropriate epidemiological setting. There may be mild anemia, jaundice or splenomegaly which favors the diagnosis. Spleen may not be palpable in the first or second week and when it is palpable it is often firm unlike in enteric fever which is almost always a soft spleen. In nonimmune individuals, it takes several days for the spleen to become palpable. But splenic enlargement is seen in otherwise healthy individuals in malaria endemic areas, which suggests repeated infections. The spleen enlarges with every paroxysm and therefore repeated abdominal examinations are necessary. Rash of any kind is uncommon and the presence of rash or lymphadenopathy should suggest alternative diagnosis.

Simple investigations like hemogram, erythrocyte sedimentation rate (ESR) and urine routine, help almost always to differentiate between the major possibilities in a febrile patient—in other words after a good clinical evaluation, often the investigations done are to exclude other causes rather than confirming malaria. The specific tests which are considered as the gold standard for diagnosis for malaria are demonstration of the parasite in the blood smear or bone marrow and indirect methods to demonstrate the organisms such as fluorescence microscopy. Parasites are detectable in blood when the parasite density is 50/μL of blood or when the total number of parasites is 100 million and above. This occurs in 6–8 days after the release of the hepatic merozoites from the liver.

A competent laboratory technician should be able to detect the parasites and identify the species and stages in almost all cases in fresh blood smears stained with Romanowsky stains (Leishman's, Giemsa, Wright or May-Grünwald–Giemsa). Smear positivity is increased by repeating examination during subsequent paroxysms and examining thick blood smears. Early diagnosis depends on the epidemiological setting and clinical features supported by simple laboratory tests.

Complications

Life-threatening complications are due to falciparum malaria and they are listed below:

- Impaired consciousness/coma—cerebral malaria
- Repeated generalized convulsions
- Hypoglycemia (plasma glucose < 50 mg/dL)
- Metabolic acidosis
- Renal failure (serum creatinine > 3 mg/dL)
- Hepatocellular damage [very high serum glutamate-pyruvate transaminase (SGPT), serum bilirubin > 3 mg/dL]
- Pulmonary edema/ARDS
- Severe anemia (Hb < 5 g/dL)
- Circulatory collapse/shock [systolic blood pressure (BP) < 80 mm Hg, < 50 mm Hg in children]
- Bleeding tendency and DIC
- Hemoglobinuria
- Hyperpyrexia (temperature > 42°C or > 106°F)
- Hyperparasitemia (> 5% RBCs contain the parasite and > 10% parasitized RBCs contain > 1 parasite)
- Mixed infections
- Malaria in pregnancy.

Coma and Cerebral Malaria

Cerebral malaria can be defined as unarousable coma in a patient with definite or probable *Plasmodium falciparum* infection, in whom other causes of encephalopathy have been excluded. Coma of varying grade is the hallmark of cerebral malaria and the onset may be gradual or sometime sudden when it occurs following a convulsion. The manifestations in cerebral malaria are often due to multiple factors. It is always due to severe falciparum malaria producing diffuse ischemia in the brain due to clogging of the microcirculation. Studies from east Lansing and Malawi shows that brain swelling occurring in cerebral malaria predisposing to death. Among fatal cases, 84% had brain swelling whereas only 27% had this feature among the survivors. There is diffuse cerebral dysfunction with impaired consciousness, coma, delirium or seizures. Except for the presence of fever, cerebral malaria looks like a metabolic encephalopathy and sometimes hypoglycemia or hyponatremia could be contributing to the encephalopathy. Coexisting hepatic encephalopathy or uremia also can compound the clinical picture. Metabolic acidosis is common. Cytokine induced metabolic encephalopathy also occurs. Seizures are relatively common and are due to multiple factors like CVT and metabolic problems including hypoglycemia and hyponatremia. Convulsions occur in 10% of adults and 50% of children with cerebral malaria. Rarely, fever may be even absent at the time of presentation leading to a wrong diagnosis of encephalitis or metabolic encephalopathy. The plantar responses may be flexor or extensor. Signs of meningeal irritation like neck stiffness are often absent. Focal signs are rare but both are possible due to CVT and its complications. Retinal hemorrhage and other retinal abnormalities can be seen in a significant number of patients. Malarial retinopathy is due to sequestration in the retinal vasculature demonstrable by fluorescence angiography. It correlates with the severity of cerebral malaria. Even with treatment, cerebral malaria carries a mortality rate of 15–20%, especially if specific treatment is delayed. Around 10% of the children can have residual neurological deficit in the form of cognitive dysfunction, language abnormalities, cerebral palsy, cortical blindness, hemiplegia and others.

Hypoglycemia

Hypoglycemia is a very common complication of severe malaria which can be the cause for encephalopathy and would coexist with other manifestations. It is likely to be missed, unless looked for. Usual physical signs of hypoglycemia may be absent and the neurological manifestations due to the disease cannot be distinguished from that of hypoglycemia. Hypoglycemia in malaria is an ominous sign; it should be prevented during treatment especially while giving quinine. Quinine and quinidine are powerful stimulants for pancreatic insulin secretion. Diminished hepatic gluconeogenesis (due to ischemic damage to liver is common) and increased consumption of glucose by the host and the parasite, with reduced intake, aggravate the picture further. Prevention of hypoglycemia, early identification and its correction are extremely important for recovery, especially so, in children and pregnant women.

Metabolic Acidosis

Metabolic acidosis is very common and is multifactorial in origin. This has been considered to be mainly lactic acidosis, although ketoacidosis (and sometimes salicylate intoxication) may predominate in children. Lactic acidosis can occur due to the following reasons:

- Anaerobic glycolysis in host tissues due to the ischemia resulting from cytoadherence and sequestration
- Lactate production by the parasite
- Hypovolemia or septic shock resulting in hypoperfusion
- Defective hepatic and renal lactate clearance.

In severe malaria, the arterial, capillary, venous and cerebrospinal fluid (CSF) concentrations of lactate rise in direct proportion to disease severity.

Metabolic acidosis of renal failure is common in adults. It is an important cause of death in severe falciparum malaria, both in adults and children.

Renal Failure

Renal failure is a complication of falciparum malaria, found more commonly among adults and usually manifests as acute tubular necrosis. Apart from ischemia due to sequestration, hypovolemia and hemolysis, nephrotoxic drugs including NSAIDs taken during fever may contribute to renal impairment.

Jaundice and Malarial Hepatopathy

Mild to severe jaundice due to hemolysis is common in malaria. Severe hepatic dysfunction with moderate to very high levels of transaminases mimicking severe acute hepatitis can be seen in falciparum malaria. This is due to erythrocyte sequestration and ischemic damage to liver. To differentiate this condition from acute viral hepatitis, the presence of high grade fever with chills and rigor or persistence of fever even after five days helps. It could also be associated with multiorgan dysfunction, hypoglycemia and thrombocytopenia. Sometimes severe hepatocellular dysfunction could be due to coexisting acute viral hepatitis or other causes of acute or chronic hepatocellular damage due to alcohol, NSAID intake or coexisting non-alcoholic fatty liver disease (NAFLD) which is also common. Some patients can have deep jaundice due to a combination of hepatocellular damage, hemolysis and cholesatsis. Severe hepatocellular damage can contribute to hypoglycemia and lactic acidosis.

Noncardiogenic Pulmonary Edema

Noncardiogenic pulmonary edema or ARDS can occur in severe falciparum malaria. Falciparum malaria should be considered as an important cause of septicemia with ARDS in tropics. It can be worsened by overhydration with intravenous (IV) fluid. It is like any other systemic inflammatory response syndrome (SIRS) causing ARDS. But in falciparum malaria, erythrocyte sequestration in the capillaries and venules in the lung may contribute to the pathogenesis of ARDS.

Severe Anemia and other Hematological Abnormalities

Malaria can be associated with various hematological abnormalities. Anemia is the most important problem which can complicate the clinical course especially in children. Anemia in the setting of malaria occurs due to:

- Hemolysis of parasitized red cells
- Increased splenic clearance of parasitized erythrocytes which have diminished deformability
- Cytokine induced suppression of hematopoiesis or dyserythropoiesis
- Shortened erythrocyte survival
- Intravascular hemolysis with hemoglobinuria.

Anemia in malaria can be worsened by concurrent helminthic infections and malnutrition. Rarely, there can be rapid fall in hemoglobin with hemoglobinuria necessitating blood transfusion. ***Black water fever*** is intravascular hemolysis with hemoglobinuria in malaria and is characterized by cola-colored urine which was considered as an ominous sign. It can follow primaquine administration; it can be transient and can occur without renal dysfunction. G6PD deficiency should be ruled out in such patients. Thrombocytopenia is also common in malaria and is related to the severity of the disease but can be multifactorial including DIC and underlying folic acid deficiency or liver disease.

Mixed Infections

Mixed infections with *Plasmodium vivax* and *Plasmodium falciparum* are common in endemic areas (up to 20%). Complicated or severe malaria is almost always caused by *P. falciparum* and is associated with grave prognosis, and is a medical emergency. Vivax malaria also can sometimes present with severe manifestations but this could be a mixed infection as falciparum malaria may not be sometimes picked up by peripheral blood examinations. Bone marrow examination may reveal the falciparum infection in such cases, but this may not be possible at all times. Repeated attempts to document falciparum has sometimes failed and finally autopsy only shows falciparum malaria in brain, liver and other visceral organs; not an uncommon situation in the endemic areas. Some studies have described pernicious complications in *Plasmodium vivax* as thrombocytopenia, leucopenia, ARDS, severe jaundice, acute renal failure, cerebral malaria, anemia, metabolic acidosis and death. But these patients were all treated with artemesin based combination therapy and primaquine along with supportive measures. It is likely these were mixed infections. The role of pure *P. vivax* malaria in producing life-threatening complications is still under study. Several reports from India highlighting the more serious consequences of *P. vivax* infection point to the more dangerous complications in vivax malaria too. The mortality due to vivax malaria is increasing in many places in India. Morality increases with age, thrombocytopenia and renal, hepatic, pulmonary and cerebral involvement. In a retrospective study of 680 cases of malaria in TYL Nair hospital, 336 were *P. vivax*, 206 were *P. falciparum* and 136 were mixed infection. One hundred sixty two had severe malaria of which 31% were *P. vivax*, 39% were *P. falciparum* and 30% had mixed infection.

Other common infections can also coexist and complicate the clinical course and outcome. Malaria with acute viral hepatitis or typhoid is a relatively common situation. Salmonella septicemia may coexist and complicate the clinical picture and course of falciparum malaria especially in children.

Source:

1. Nadkar MY, Huchche AM, Singh R, et al. Clinical profile of severe Plasmodium vivax malaria in a tertiary care centre in Mumbai from June 2010-January 2011. J Assoc Physicians India. 2012;60:11-3.

2. Limaye CS, Londhey VA, Nabar ST. The study of complications of vivax malaria in comparison with falciparum malaria in Mumbai. J Assoc Physicians India. 2012;60:15-8.

Malaria in Pregnancy

Malaria poses a very severe risk in pregnancy especially in primipara and in all the trimesters. In plasmodium falciparum malaria, the parasite localizes in the placenta and produces severe complications in both the mother and the fetus. In malaria endemic areas, more than 45 million pregnancies occur annually. In hyperendemic and holoendemic areas, pregnant women with heavy parasite load in placental microcirculation can remain asymptomatic and can lead on to low birth weight (LBW) infants or congenital malaria. In areas of unstable transmission, pregnant women with malaria can have severe infections, fetal distress, premature labor, stillbirth or fetal death. The common problems encountered by pregnant women with malaria are: (1) Maternal anemia, (2) stillbirths, (3) premature delivery, (4) intrauterine growth retardation (IUGR) and (5) LBW infants. Special precautions are to be taken to select the appropriate safe antimalarial in them (see treatment).

Tropical Splenomegaly Syndrome

In malaria endemic areas, some individuals have an abnormal immunological response to repeated infections which manifests as massive splenomegaly and hepatomegaly. They present with problems due to splenomegaly like vague abdominal discomfort in the left upper quadrant and early satiety. Constitutional symptoms may be mild or absent at times. Some degree of pancytopenia due to hypersplenism can develop. Malarial parasites are not found in peripheral blood. High titers of IgM malarial antibody may be demonstrable. Some may evolve into clonal malignant lymphoproliferative disorder. If other causes of splenomegaly are excluded, this may be considered in differential diagnosis. Some of them respond often to prolonged chloroquine administration for three weeks to six months.

Laboratory Findings

Usually there is normocytic normochromic anemia but it is also decided by baseline nutritional status and other comorbidities. White cell count is normal to high with slight monocytosis, lymphopenia and eosinopenia. Reactive lymphocytosis and eosinophilia could be observed in the weeks following the acute infection. Acute phase reactants like ESR and C-reactive protein (CRP) are moderately high. Thrombocytopenia is a common finding (median count-100,000/mm^3). Abnormal coagulation profile is seen when there is DIC or liver dysfunction. Hypoglycemia, hyponatremia, metabolic acidosis, abnormal liver and renal function are seen in severe falciparum malaria. These are not specifically diagnostic.

Diagnosis

The most important prerequisite for diagnosis is good clinical skill, high index of suspicion and familiarity or awareness of the varied clinical presentations, which would enable prompt diagnosis. Demonstration of the parasite

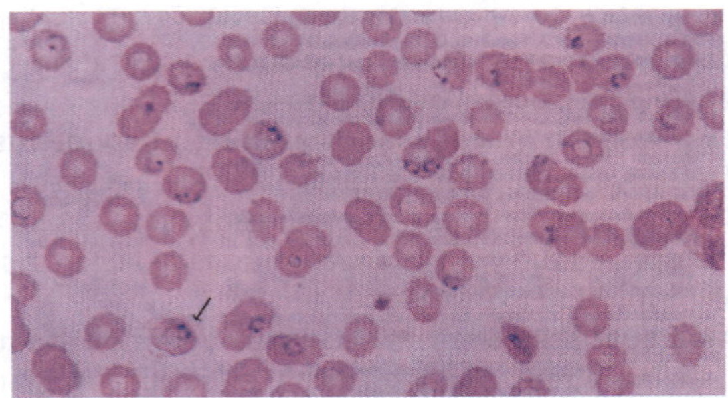

Fig. 64.3: Peripheral blood slide *Plasmodium falciparum* malaria. Arrow points to parasite in RBC

by microscopy is the confirmatory test in the appropriate epidemiological and clinical setting. Identification of the parasite may not be possible always in falciparum malaria and hence if other diseases are unlikely, empirical treatment and prompt response could suggest diagnosis of malaria. Since in hyperendemic areas, asymptomatic individuals also may have parasites in peripheral blood, detection of the parasite does not necessarily mean that the fever is due to malaria. It is possible that the febrile illness may be due to other conditions in the carrier of malaria.

Light Microscopy

Demonstration of the parasite in peripheral smear is the most important diagnostic test (Fig. 64.3), but negative smear does not rule out the diagnosis; repeat smears are essential. Both thick smears and thin smears are important in patients with suspected malaria. Thick smears should be dried thoroughly and stained without fixing. Thick smears are useful for diagnosis and for measuring parasite density, especially at low levels of parasitemia. Thin smears are used for the identification of the species and stage of circulating parasite, as well as measurement of parasite density. Thin smears should be air dried and fixed in anhydrous methanol and stained. Giemsa stain at a pH 7.2 is the preferred stain. Level of parasitemia is expressed as number of parasitized RBCs/1000.

Morphological Differentiation (Table 64.1)

P. falciparum: Usually RBCs are of normal size. Trophozoites and schizonts are seldom seen in peripheral blood. Gametocytes only are often seen in peripheral blood and they are crescent-shaped with chromatin as a single mass in the female gametocyte (macrogametocyte) or is diffuse in the male gametocyte (microgametocyte). Their number may vary. The malarial parasite is identified by the cardinal features: (1) It is intra-erythrocytic, (2) cytoplasm is blue and (3) the chromatin is red. Shape of the parasite depends up the stage of development.

P. vivax: In *P. vivax* infections erythrocyte will be enlarged in size with fine Schuffner's dots.

P. ovale: Normal to slightly enlarged RBCs with occasional fimbriation and Schuffner's dots can be seen.

Parasitemia of $>10^5$ parasites/μL is associated with high mortality, but nonimmune individuals can have complications even with lower levels of parasitemia. In severe malaria, predominance of more mature *P. falciparum* parasites (i.e. >20% of parasites with visible pigment) in the peripheral blood film or by the

Textbook of Medicine

Table 64.1: Morphological features of the different species of *Plasmodium*

Features	P. vivax	P. falciparum	P. malariae	P. ovale
Size of parasitized erythrocyte	Larger	Not larger	Normal size	Variable, the erythrocyte is often oval
Common stages present in peripheral blood	All stages	Only rings and gametocytes	All stages	All stages
Pigmentary change in erythrocyte	Schuffner's dots seen in the erythrocyte outside the parasite	Maurer's clefts	Nil	Schuffner's dots
Number of merozoites in the schizont	8–16	12–24	6–12	8–12
Morphology of the rings	Thick and large	Fine rings-marginal forms (applique)*	Large coarse ring	Large ring
Multiple infection in erythrocyte	Nil	Present	Nil	Nil
Number of chromatin in the rings	One	One or two	One	One
Gametocyte	Oval or circular	Crescentic	Oval or circular	Oval or circular

* Applique forms of *P. falciparum* are the ring stages of the parasite attached along the margin of the erythrocyte.

presence of phagocytosed malarial pigment in >5% of neutrophils indicates poor prognosis. According to World Health Organization (WHO), hyperparasitemia of >5% parasi-tized RBCs qualifies for severe malaria. It should be noted that a negative smear will not rule out malaria and they should be repeated every 12–24 hours; repeat smears with repeating paroxysms of fever increases the chance of detection. When peripheral blood is negative for falciparum malaria, bone marrow can be used for demonstration. Intradermal smears are shown to be more sensitive than routine smears and may be as sensitive as bone marrow smears.

Rapid diagnostic test (RDT): They are important in areas lacking facilities for microscopic examination. These are simple, rapid, sensitive and relatively specific dipstick or card tests for the diagnosis of malaria based on antibody detection of malaria specific antigens. Currently used antigens are *Plasmodium falciparum* histidine-rich protein 2 (PfHRP2), parasite lactate dehydrogenase and aldolase. Antibodies capturing the parasite antigen are read out as colored bands. In lactate dehydrogenase (LDH) based assays one band will be genus specific (all malarial parasites) and the other is specific for *P. falciparum.* RDT can have sensitivity almost equivalent to that of thick smears. PfHRP2 based kits may show false positive result up to 3 weeks after successful treatment.

Treatment

Various antimalaria drugs are listed in Table 64.2.

Trial of artemisinin combination reports of the study conducted in sub-Saharan Africa.

Table 64.2: Available antimalarial drugs and their effects

Drugs	Mechanism effects	Adverse effects
Chloroquine	Activity against the blood stages of susceptible strains of *P. vivax* and *P. falciparum*, *P. ovale* and *P. malariae*	Vomiting, headache, pruritus, retinopathy and myopathy (only on chronic use), hypotension and cardiac arrhythmias if drug is given parenterally
Quinine	Mainly on trophozoites, kills gametocytes of all except falciparum	Bitter taste, cinchonism (tinnitus, nausea, headaches, dizziness and disturbed vision), hypoglycemia and cardiac arrhythmias
Amodiaquine	Same as cholorquine	Agranulocytosis and hepatitis, increased toxicity if HIV infected. This drug is not commonly used in India
Mefloquine	Same as above	Seizures, psychosis, encephalopathy, nausea conduction defects, pneumonitis
Primaquine	Prevents relapse of *P. vivax* and *P. ovale* malaria by eliminating dormant hypnozoites, active against the pre-erythrocytic stage and gametocytes of *P. falciparum*	Gastrointestinal upset, hemolytic anemia in G6PD deficiency
Lumefantrine	As for quinine	Well tolerated
Halofantrine	As for quinine	Prolonged QT interval and PR interval
Sulfadoxine/pyrimethamine	Dihydrofolate reductase (DHFR) inhibition and dihydropteroate synthase (DHPS) inhibition respectively. Available as fixed combination	Mild gastrointestinal symptoms, hemolysis in G6PD deficiency, allergy to sulfa moiety
Artemisinin derivatives	Rapid clearance of blood stages, active against gametocytes, not against liver stages	Rare type 1 hypersensitivity, neurotoxicity reported in animal studies
Proguanil	Active form is cycloguanil, acts on tissue stages	Safest antimalarial, may cause oral ulcers and abdominal discomfort
Atovaquone	Combined with proguanil due to resistance	Usually well tolerated

Textbook of Medicine

- ***Artemether/lumefantrine:*** Fewer side effects with acceptable cure rates but the post-treatment prophylactic period is short.
- ***Dihydroartemisinin/piperaquine:*** This has the best efficacy and safety profile. This combination is safe in pregnancy.

Source: Kakuru A, Jagannathan P, Muhindo MK, et al. Dihydroartemisinin-Piperaquine for the Prevention of Malaria in Pregnancy. N Engl J Med. 2016;374(10):928-39.

It is desirable that all malaria cases be confirmed with microscopy or rapid diagnostic test before initiation of treatment. If the infecting species is not definitely established or when mixed infection is suspected, the treatment should be as if it is for falciparum malaria with quinine or artemisinin derivatives.

Uncomplicated Vivax Malaria

Chloroquine is the preferred drug in uncomplicated vivax malaria. Confirmed *P. vivax* cases should be treated with chloroquine at a dose of 25 mg/kg divided over three days. It is given initially as 1 g (4 tablets) and 500 mg after six hours and then 500 mg daily for another three days. For prevention of relapse, primaquine should be given at a dose of 0.25 mg/kg bw daily (15 mg in adults) for 14 days under supervision. Primaquine is contraindicated in known severe G6PD deficient patients, infants and pregnant women. In mild G6PD deficiency, 0.75 mg of base/kg should be given once week for 6–8 weeks. At present *P. vivax* is showing chloroquine resistance and the resistant strains are rapidly spreading (Table 64.3).

Newer Drugs

Tafenoquine which is a new 8-aminoquinoline (8AQ) has anti-hypnozoite action on the liver stages of the parasite. Given in a single dose of 300 mg, coadministered with the standard dose of chloroquine, it eradicates the infection. Side effects are similar to those of primaquine–hemolysis in G6PD deficient persons and QT prolongation in 30% of patients.

Source: Llanos-Cuentas A, Lacerda MV, Rueangweerayut R, et al. Tafenoquine plus chloroquine for the treatment and relapse prevention of Plasmodium vivax malaria (DETECTIVE): a multicentre, double-blind, randomised, phase 2b dose-selection study. Lancet. 2014;383(9922):1049-58.

Treatment of Falciparum Malaria

Chloroquine resistance is high in falciparum malaria and therefore this drug is not used as the first line management.

Genetic markers for resistance have identified. Mutation of the 'propeller' domain of ketch protein gene is responsible for the development of resistance.

WHO and National guidelines recommend artemisinin combination therapy (ACT) for all *P. falciparum* cases. ACT consists of an artemisinin derivative combined with sulfadoxine-pyrimethamine or a long-acting antimalarial like mefloquine, amodiaquine or lumefantrine. This is to be accompanied by single dose primaquine (0.75 mg/kg bw) on day 2 of treatment. But in practice, it is probably better to give primaquine as in the case of vivax malaria (15 mg/day for 14 days) for the reason that up to 20% of cases are mixed infections, which may not be readily picked up.

The ACT recommended in the national program in India is artesunate + sulfadoxine-pyrimethamine. It is given as artesunate (4 mg/kg qid for 3 days) plus sulfadoxine (25 mg/kg)/pyrimethamine (1.25 mg/kg) as a single dose. Other fixed dose combinations available are artesunate + mefloquine, artemether + lumefantrine, artesunate + amodiaquine. Monotherapy with artimesinin derivatives are banned in India due to the probability of developing resistance.

In severe cases of malaria, parenteral antimalarials have to be given. These include artemisinin derivatives or quinine. Both drugs are effective against *P. falciparum* and *P. vivax* but artemisinin derivatives are more effective than quinine (Table 64.4).

Artemisinin derivatives clear infection and also arrest transmission. Resistance to artemisinin derivatives is being reported in Thai-Cambodia border area. This phenomena is seen in the neighborhood countries as well. Artemisinin resistance of *P. falciparum* malaria.

Resistance is associated with a single point mutation in the 'propeller' region of the *P. falciparum* kelch protein gene on chromosome 13 (kelch13)—detected in South East Asia.

Source: Ashley EA, Dhorda M, Fairhurst RM, et al. Spread of artemisinin resistance in Plasmodium falciparum malaria. N Engl J Med. 2014;371(5):411-23.

In severe cases, administration of artesunate rectally at home before reaching a hospital may be lifesaving. Capsule containing 100 mg artesunate may be used for this purpose. Parenteral artesunate is equal to or better than IV quinine in severe falcipram malaria.

Quinine at a dose of 10 mg/kg salt tid for 7 days (approximately 600 mg 8th hourly) can be equally effective in treating falciparum malaria. It should be combined with another drug like doxycycline (3 mg/kg qd for 7 days) or tetracycline (4 mg/kg qid for 7 days) or clindamycin (10 mg/kg bd for 7 days).

Parenteral Quinine

Quinine hydrochloride is available for IV use in vials containing 600 mg/mL. This is given in doses of 10 mg/kg bw as IV injection diluted in 5% glucose given slowly or as IV infusion over 20 minutes. This dose is repeated 8 hourly till the patient can accept oral medication. In severe falciparum infections a loading dose of 20 mg/kg bw may be given initially.

Table 64.3: Grading of chloroquine resistance of *P. falciparum* (WHO 1973)		
	Recommended symbol	**Response**
Sensitive	S	Clearance of asexual parasitemia within 7 days of treatment without any recrudescence
Resistance (mild)	R1	Clearance of asexual parasites within 1 week but reappear within 28 days (7-28)
Resistance (moderate)	R2	Significant regression but no clearance
Resistance (severe)	R3	No marked reduction or increase, with persistent symptoms

Table 64.4: Preparations of qinghaosu derivatives

Drugs	Dose	Route	Effect
Artemisinin	80 mg day 1, 40 mg on days 2–4	IM injection, oral or rectal	Schizonticidal on all species including *P. falciparum*
Artesunate, an ester of artemisinin	120 mg day 1, 60 mg for 4 days	Oral, IM and rectal	Effective particularly used for cerebral malaria
Artemether methyl ether derivative of artemisinin	80 mg bd 3.2 mg/kg/bw for 3 days	IV/IM and oral	Same as above
Arteether	150 mg/day for 3 days	IM	Same as above + gametocidal

Note: Chinese researcher Tu Youyou identified the artemisinin and demonstrated its effect. Tu Youyou received the Lasker award of $250,000 in 2011 at the age of 81 years.

Adverse side effects include anaphylactic shock, severe hypoglycemia, reactions at site of injection.

Mixed Infection (PF + PV)

Artemisinin combination therapy is to be given as described earlier for treatment of falciparum malaria. But primaquine should be given for 14 days.

Malaria in Pregnancy

In uncomplicated *P. vivax* infection, chloroquine is the drug of choice in all trimesters.

Treatment of uncomplicated falciparum malaria in pregnancy: In unconfirmed but suspected falciparum malaria, if not severe, chloroquine is the best drug if the parasite is sensitive. If the parasite is likely to be resistant to chloroquine, quinine is the drug of choice in the first trimester, in a dose of 10 mg/kg 8 hourly IV or orally for 7 days. In pregnant women and children under 8 years of age; instead of doxycycline, clindamycin 10 mg/kg bw 12 hourly for 7 days should be used. During second and third trimesters, ACT is the treatment of choice.

- ***First trimester:*** Quinine + clindamycin (7 days), ACT should be used if it is the only effective treatment even though it is contraindicated in first trimester.
- ***Second and third trimesters:*** ACT given as artesunate + clindamycin (7 days) or quinine + clindamycin (7 days).
- Lactating women should receive standard antimalarial treatment (including ACTs).

Treatment of Severe Malaria

Severe malaria is an emergency and treatment should include intensive supportive measures as well as specific antimalarials. The fact that the risk of death due to malaria is highest in the first 24 hours underscores the importance of early diagnosis and prompt treatment. Parenteral artemisinin derivatives or quinine should be used irrespective of chloroquine sensitivity in severe malaria. Studies comparing artemesinin derivatives and quinine suggest IV artesunate as the preferred treatment in areas where it is available. It is found that water soluble derivative like artesunate which can be given IV clears parasitemia more rapidly than quinine.

Artesunate: 2.4 mg/kg bw IV or IM given on admission (time = 0), then at 12 hours and 24 hours, then once a day for 4–5 days (care should be taken to dilute artesunate powder in 5% sodium bicarbonate provided in the pack). Patients receiving artemisinin derivatives should get full course of oral ACT. However, ACT containing mefloquine should be avoided in cerebral malaria due to neuropsychiatric complications.

Quinine: Quinine hydrochloride is available as vials containing 600 mg/mL; 20 mg quinine salt/kg bw on admission (IV infusion in 5% dextrose/dextrose saline over a period of 4 hours) followed by maintenance dose of 10 mg/kg bw 8 hourly. Infusion rate should not exceed 5 mg/kg bw per hour. Loading dose of 20 mg/kg bw is not required if the patient has already received quinine. Parenteral quinine may be given for 7 days or switched over to oral quinine 10 mg/kg bw three times a day to complete a course of 7 days, along with doxycycline 3 mg/kg bw per day for 7 days. In pregnant women and children under 8 years of age, instead of doxycycline, clindamycin 10 mg/kg bw 12 hourly for 7 days should be used.

New Drug for Resistant Malaria

Resistant malarial parasites which are resistant to *artemisinin* drugs contain molecular markers can be demonstrated in P. falciparum and P. vivax. Mutations of Pf CRT and Pf MDR genes are associated with resistance to *aminoquinolines*. Never antimalarial drugs are being developed.

Drugs are being developed against resistant strains. Spiroindolone is a new drug developed by Novartis against both *P. vivax and P. falciparum.* The drug is effective both against the sexual and asexual forms. The drug acts on the plasma membrane of the parasite on the Na$^+$ATPase. Dose is 30 mg/day orally for 3 days. Rapid clearance of parasites occurs.

Prevention

Chemoprophylaxis

It is important in travelers to highly endemic areas. Chemoprophylactic agents are of two types. The dihydrofolate reductase (DHFR) inhibitors (pyrimethamine, proguanil, chlorproguanil) and atovaquone inhibit parasite development in the liver (pre-erythrocytic activity) and in the erythrocyte and are called causal prophylactics. These drugs also inhibit development in the mosquito. Chloroquine and mefloquine acts on the blood stages which are described as suppressive prophylactics. These drugs also have gametocytocidal activity against *P. vivax, P. malariae* and *P. ovale*, but not *P. falciparum.* Other prophylactic agents are atovaquone, proguanil, doxycycline and primaquine. More important is to avoid

Textbook of Medicine

exposure to mosquito bite and improving nutrition and lifestyle; but if mosquito bites are unavoidable in a highly endemic area, chemoprophylaxis may be considered in a person visiting that area. Choice of prophylactic agent depends on resistance pattern and host factors. National guidelines recommend: Mefloquine—5 mg/kg bw (up to 250 mg) weekly and should be administered two weeks before, during and four weeks after leaving the area (for long-term prophylaxis >6 weeks).

Most important step in prevention of malaria, undoubtedly is vector control and improving nutrition and lifestyle of the people to reduce the impact of infection. Both are social issues which are not tackled appropriately in malaria endemic regions and are largely neglected. Again vector control is primarily an issue of proper environmental hygiene including empowering the people to adopt proper waste disposal habits and the society organizing the most appropriate waste management techniques to prevent unwanted water stagnation and the consequent mosquito breeding. This kind of primary prevention should get priority over all the other measures adopted now to stop malaria in the society.

Personal Protection

At individual level, it is by using insecticide-treated bed nets (ITNs) and indoor spraying of insecticides. Regarding ITNs, commonly used insecticides are pyrethroids.

Indoor spraying with residual insecticides serves as a potential vector control measure in many areas with its effect lasting for about 3–6 months. The nets have an effective life for about six months after which they have to be re-impregnated with the insecticide.

Other measures include protective clothing avoiding exposure of parts of the body. Insect repellents applied over bare areas of the skin and over light clothing have their role in individual cases. Diethylbenzamide 12% w/w cream is effective for 3–4 hours after applications.

Malaria Vaccines

Although research towards the development of malaria vaccines has been pursued since 1960s, as yet there are no licensed malaria vaccines. However, a number of candidate vaccines are being evaluated in clinical trials, with one candidate vaccine currently being assessed in phase 3 clinical trials (RTS, S/AS01) and about 20 others in Phase 1 or Phase 2 clinical trials. Though no effective vaccine is so far developed against malaria, it is an area where a lot of research is going on. Of them, the vaccine against *P. falciparum* known as RTS, S/ASO1 is a promising step.

Vaccine Candidate RTS, S/AS01

The RTS, S/AS01 vaccine targets *P. falciparum*. Now in Phase 3 clinical trials, the vaccine is being developed in a partnership between Glaxo-Smith Kline (GSK) and PATH malaria vaccine initiative (MVI), with MVI receiving funds from the Bill & Melinda Gates Foundation. The vaccine comprises a fusion protein of a malaria antigen—the carboxy terminus of the *P. falciparum* circumsporozoite (CS) antigen—with hepatitis B surface antigen and includes a new and potent adjuvant. The manufacturer's clinical development plan for the vaccine focuses on

infants and young children living in malaria-endemic African countries. In October 2013, a third set of results on the efficacy of the RTS, S/AS01 vaccine were reported for 6–14 weeks and 5–17 months age groups. In the 5–17 months age groups, efficacy estimates, pooled across all trial sites, remained statistically significant against clinical malaria (46%) and severe malaria (35.5%). Reductions in both malaria hospitalizations (41.5%) and all-cause hospitalizations (19%) were noted over 18 months. By contrast, the 6–14 weeks age groups, the efficacy estimate for severe malaria was not statistically significant.

Other Community Measures

Several trials using intermittent administration of sulfadoxine-pyrimethamine universally to all persons in endemic areas have been used. Results are varying. Salt has been fortified with sulfadoxine-pyrimethamine in a few countries.

Newer methods such as mobile phone alerts to health workers in Kenya to adhere to malaria treatment guidelines have yielded beneficial results in treatment efficacy and reduction in transmission. The effect of mobile phone text reminders on Kenyan health workers adherence to malaria treatment guidelines; a cluster randomized trial.

Source: Zurovac D, Sudoi RK, Akhwale WS, et al. The effect of mobile phone text-message reminders on Kenyan health workers' adherence to malaria treatment guidelines: a cluster randomised trial. Lancet. 2011;378(9793):795-803.

The WHO, United Nations International Children's Emergency Fund (UNICEF), United Nations Development Programme (UNDP), World Bank and other national organization and other charities such as Melinda & Bill Gates Foundation are pursuing commendable global efforts to control the major infectious diseases such as malaria, tuberculosis and acquired immune deficiency syndrome (AIDS) in several countries. India is a beneficiary in this venture.

WHO has defined the 25th of April every year as the World Malaria Day.

References

World Health Organization

- Guidelines for the treatment of malaria, 2nd edn. Geneva, World Health Organization, 2010. (who.int/malaria/publications/atoz/9789241547925/en/).
- Guidelines for Diagnosis and Treatment of Malaria in India 2011 (2nd edition) Government of India, National Institute of Malaria Research, New Delhi. World Malaria Report 2013 of WHO.
- Harrison's Textbook of Medicine, 17th Edition, Volume 1.

LEISHMANIASIS

General Considerations

Leishmaniasis is a group of infectious diseases caused by various species of the protozoan parasites of the genus *Leishmania*. The major clinical presentations that are prevalent in India are: (1) Fatal visceral leishmaniasis (VL) which is also known as kala-azar and post kala-azar dermal leishmaniasis, (2) cutaneous

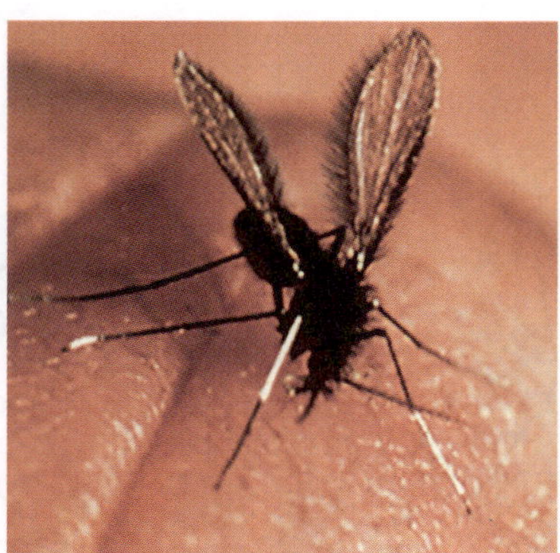

Fig. 64.4: The sandfly

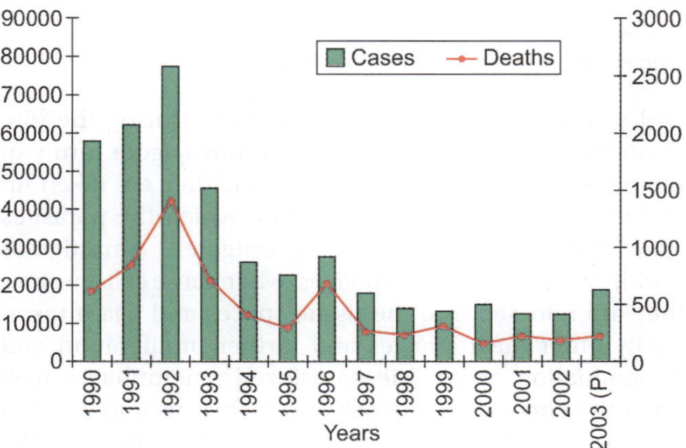

Fig. 64.5: Kala-azar situation in India

leishmaniasis (CL), which may present as chronic and indolent, but spontaneously healing skin ulcers and (3) as more serious mucocutaneous leishmaniasis (MCL).

Epidemiology

The disease remains as a major public health problem, being currently prevalent in 98 countries. About 2 million cases occur annually, about 12 million individuals are affected and another 350 million people are at risk of developing it. The geographical distribution of leishmaniasis is restricted to tropical and temperate regions where the vector sandflies (Fig. 64.4) are seen but the disease is seen in the developing and less developed countries of the world. More than 90% of cases of VL occur in six countries: Bangladesh, India, Nepal, Sudan, Ethiopia and Brazil. India, Nepal and Bangladesh harbor 70% of the global burden. In India, it is endemic in the States of Bihar, West Bengal, parts of Uttar Pradesh and the North Eastern States and the adjoining areas, but is seen in almost all states sporadically (Fig. 64.5). Like all other parasitic diseases, leishmaniasis also affects poor communities, generally in remote rural areas. Migration of population, malnutrition, lack of control measures and HIV co-infection are the main factors driving the increased incidence of visceral leishmaniasis. Conditions that favor the multiplication of the sandflies and the presence of susceptible populations determine the endemicity of the disease. Human leishmaniasis is on the increase worldwide with outbreaks in previously unreported areas. There is a small pocket now in Kerala in Palakkad district. The first case from this region was seen by the author in 1987 in a 26-year-old tribal from Nilambur with typical features of VL. Subsequently 5 cases of VL were diagnosed from the same area.

VL has been listed among the neglected tropical diseases (NTDs) included for elimination by 2020. Partnership between governments, public and private partners including drug companies have decided by London Declaration of 2012 to eliminate as far as possible the NTDs. Other diseases in this category include soil transmitted helminths, lymphatic filariasis. Onchocerciasis, schistosomiasis, trachoma, guinea worm, Chagas disease and human African trypanosomiasis.

Leishman working in England and Donovan working in Madras (present Chennai) discovered the parasite simultaneously in 1903. Leishmaniasis is spread by the bite of a female sandfly. Sandflies bite the victims during sleep; dogs, foxes and rodents serve as the animal reservoir for most *Leishmania* species. However, in India and Bangladesh, animal reservoirs are not reported and humans serve as both the natural reservoir and the host for infection. Sandflies have only a short flying range and therefore, they must live close to the mammalian reservoirs for perpetuation of transmission.

Cutaneous and visceral disease can both have epidemic or endemic transmission patterns. Outbreaks tend to occur when susceptible hosts move into an area of endemic transmission or when a sandfly habitat is disturbed, such as with encroachment or settlements into forest areas. Both visceral and CL are increasing in prevalence globally because of rapid urbanization, increase in rodent population, ecological changes resulting from war and increase in the number of immunosuppressed and susceptible hosts due to multiple reasons such as malnutrition, HIV and unhealthy lifestyle habits.

Lifecycle of the Parasite and Pathology (Fig. 64.6)

VL in India is caused by *Leishmania donovani* which is most prevalent. Leishmania exist in nature in two morphologic states: (1) As intracellular amastigotes within macrophages of mammalian hosts and (2) As extracellular promastigotes within the gut of their sandfly vectors (Figs 64.7 and 64.8). Amastigotes are nonmotile, they are seen within macrophages in tissues particularly in the spleen, bone marrow, lymph nodes and others. In the circulation they are seen in the monocytes. The amastigotes in cells are identified by the presence of nucleus and the kinetoplast.

In the sandfly and in *in vitro* cultures (Fig. 64.9), the parasites develop flagella and become the motile leptomonad form (promastigotes). In the leptomonad form the flagella arises from the kinetoplast.

Over 20 species of sandflies transmit leishmaniasis. In India, the main sandfly vector is *Phlebotomus argentipes*. Only female sandflies transmit the disease. In India, VL is a disease of humans with possibly no animal reservoirs. In other endemic regions of the world, dogs, raposa (a fox-like animal) and rodents also harbor the parasite.

Transmission

Sandflies ingest the amastigote parasites from the circulation and cutaneous macrophages. These develop

Textbook of Medicine

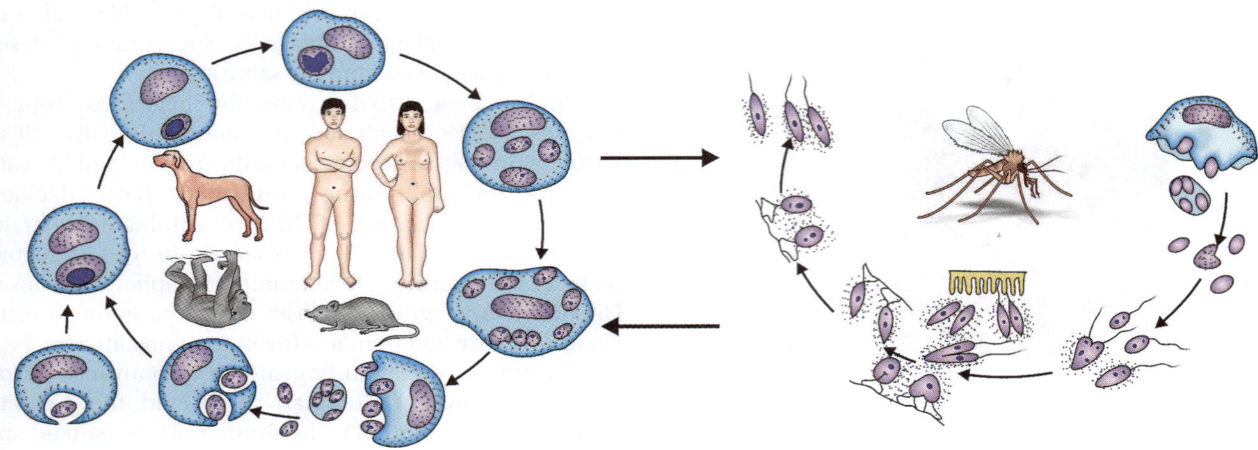

Fig. 64.6: Leishmanial form multiplying taken the vector roundfly. Leptomonad form in the roundfly and *in vitro* culture

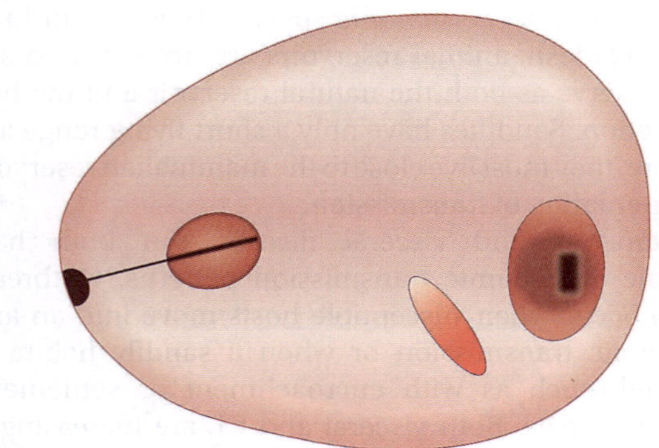

Fig. 64.7: *Leishmania donovani*—leishmanial form (LD body) seen *in vivo* in man—general morphology (diagrammatic presentation)

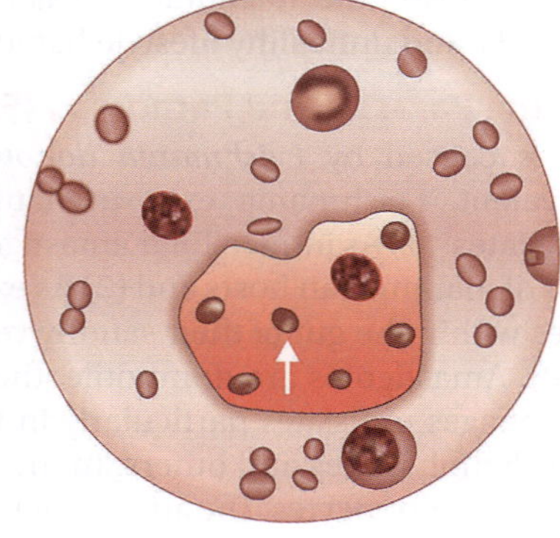

Fig. 64.8: *Leishmania donovani* in macrophages and outside cells (diagrammatic presentation)

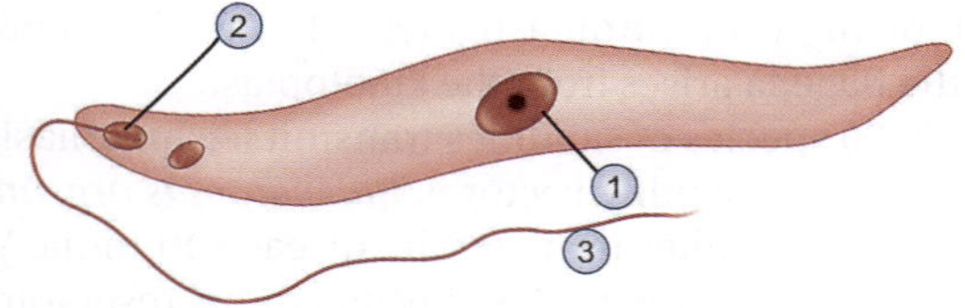

Fig. 64.9: Leishmaniasis-leptomonad form seen *in vitro* cultures and in the vector (diagrammatic presentation).
Keys: (1) Nucleus, (2) kinetoplast, (3) flagellum

into promastigotes in the mid gut of the sandfly within 4–14 days depending on the climatic conditions; they multiply

and extend anteriorly to the proboscis. During the bite of an infected sandfly, flagellated promastigote forms of the parasite are injected into the skin. They are taken up by local tissue macrophages, within which the parasites transform into intracellular amastigotes. Amastigotes multiply within the macrophages; when these cells rupture they are released into the tissue spaces and again taken up by other macrophages and further proliferation and dissemination occur. The parasitized macrophages may enter the circulation to reach several organs and develop further. Infected macrophages may either remain in the skin or disseminate throughout the reticuloendothelial system producing disseminated disease depending on the immune status of the infected person. The site of inoculation is often inapparent, but a small papule may form. By contrast, a local ulcer may rarely be seen in those who develop visceral syndromes.

VL is caused by two leishmanial species, *L. donovani* or *L. infantum*, depending on the geographical area. *Leishmania donovani* is seen in Indian subcontinent and Africa. *Leishmania infantum* is seen in Europe and New World. *L. infantum* infects mostly children, whereas *L. donovani* infects all age groups. There are an estimated 500,000 new cases of VL and more than 50,000 deaths from the disease each year, a death toll that is surpassed, among the parasitic diseases, only by malaria.

In the infected human beings, the parasites reside in macrophages in tissues and monocytes in circulation. In VL, the organs which are maximally affected are spleen, liver, bone marrow and lymph nodes. The spleen can be enlarged to moderate or massive size. Macrophages with LD bodies are seen in large numbers in the splenic pulp. Liver is enlarged with Kupfer cells distended with LD bodies. Bone marrow also becomes hypercellular with parasitized macrophages in the reticuloendothelial cells. Lymph nodes also may contain macrophages with LD bodies. In general all the patients with kala-azar are malnourished with impaired cell mediated immunity. Specific IgM and IgG antibodies are produced, which are not protective. Even in clinically cured cases the parasite may persist in vacuoles in the cytoplasm of the macrophages. HIV co-infection further lowers the cell mediated immunity but can return to normal with successful therapy.

Visceral Leishmaniasis (VL)—Clinical Features

VL was described at the end of 19th century in India as kala-azar (black fever). The incubation period is difficult to evaluate precisely. It is generally 2–6 months, but can range from 10 days to many years. Long incubation periods, up to 10 years, have been occasionally reported. Majority of patients remain asymptomatic with subclinical infection even while harboring the parasites if the cell mediated immunity is relatively better. When symptomatic, fever is the major symptom in acute presentations as well as in the chronic forms. Fever can be intermittent and irregular or remittent or low grade with a double or triple rise per day. All types of fever have been described—continuous, undulant or remittent with rigor and chills. The febrile illness in the early stages of VL can be mistaken for typhoid or malaria and later for tuberculosis or lymphoma. Later stages the fever may be mild or insignificant and the patients feel apparently alright without even recognizing the presence of fever till they come to clinical attention due to the anemia, splenomegaly or weight loss.

Massive splenomegaly and mild hepatomegaly are characteristic of the disease in late stages (Fig. 64.10). Splenomegaly appears early and is almost invariably present when the patients present. It is firm, smooth and painless and the size increases steadily, in relation to the duration of the disease. Hepatomegaly is less frequent and occurs later than splenomegaly. When hepatomegaly is present, it is generally mild and is painless. Rarely jaundice appears in late stages and is considered to indicate poor prognosis. Discrete superficial lymph node enlargement can appear during evolution. The nodes are small, firm painless and mobile. In some patients despite the low grade fever they remain apparently well till they have advanced disease with severe pallor and massive splenomegaly.

In India, patient's skin has a grayish pigmentation, which gives rise to the local name of the disease as kala-azar. Progressive pallor is the most frequent hematological manifestation. Anemia is generally of normochromic and normocytic type, it progressively and steadily worsens until it is very severe with hemoglobin levels are around 7–10 g/dL and can decrease down to even

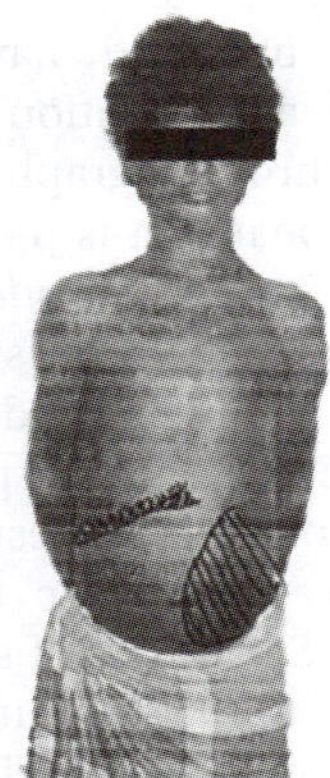

Fig. 64.10: Patients with advance kala-azar. **Note:** The gross spleno-hepatomegaly and emaciation—adult 26-year-old

4 g/dL or less. Leukopenia with neutropenia is frequently reported and when it is severe can be responsible for numerous associated infections. Platelet numbers are low normal or decreased. Severe thrombocytopenia (below 40000/mm^3) can sometimes occur and when it is associated with alterations of coagulation factors due to liver involvement, is responsible for bleeding manifestations, which can be quite dramatic. Very often in later stages of the disease, they present with the classical picture of pancytopenia, which is commonly associated with visceral leishmaniasis.

Ascites is considered as a late sign and is of bad prognosis, sometimes associated with edema and pleural effusion. These unusual signs are more common in Indian kala-azar. As a result of immune complex deposition, renal involvement with albuminuria may occur as a late complication. They may also present with various other infections which these people are even otherwise predisposed to develop; the infections which can coexist with leishmaniasis and bring them to clinical attention include tuberculosis, pneumonia, herpes zoster, scabies and gastrointestinal (GI) infections like amoebic or bacillary dysentery or because of the additional problems they develop due to co-infection with HIV. If untreated, the patients with severe disease invariably die.

HIV Co-infection in VL

Immunocompetent individuals may harbor the infection and remain asymptomatic for considerable periods. Intact cell mediated immunity is required to control leishmaniasis; individuals with malnutrition and those infected with HIV are prone to more severe clinical manifestations. HIV infected people are more vulnerable to VL. HIV infection increases the risk of developing active VL by several hundred times, especially when they have very low CD4 counts. VL is more common in patients with CD4 counts less than 300/μL. Disseminated disease occurs when the CD4 count is less than 50/μL. Similar situation is possible in those taking immunosuppressive drugs for organ transplants, hematological malignancy or autoimmune diseases. In HIV infected persons, atypical presentations are common, serological diagnosis is not reliable and relapse is more frequent. The HIV-VL co-infection would change the clinical picture of both diseases and both are mutually reinforcing. VL would accelerate the progression of HIV infection to AIDS. VL is an AIDS defining illness in an endemic region. Immunosuppressed individuals with VL, when they have HIV co-infection, have clinical features similar to classic disease but can also have involvement of other organs and can present with unusual features. Fever, hepatosplenomegaly, lymphadenopathy and pancytopenia are found in the majority of patients with HIV-VL co-infection. In addition, extensive GI involvement with mucositis and ulcers with presence of the amastigote forms of the parasites in the rectal, jejunal, duodenal, gastric and esophageal mucosa can occur. The amastigotes can be recovered from mucosa of any of these areas. The GI involvement can lead to symptoms such as dysphagia, odynophagia, epigastric pain, severe watery diarrhea,

Textbook of Medicine

intestinal hemorrhage and rectal pain. Splenomegaly may be absent sometimes. They may also develop diffuse papular skin lesions and involvement of the central nervous system (CNS), larynx and lungs. Pulmonary involvement may lead to pleural effusions and pulmonary nodules. Aplastic anemia has also been described. One must remember that malnutrition is the most common cause for poor cell mediated immunity and low CD4 count and it is only natural that they harbor several infections simultaneously especially when they have co-infection with HIV also.

Treatment failure for VL is high in the presence of HIV co-infection and they eventually relapse and die unless they are given antiretroviral treatment and proper nutrition as well. Because of higher prevalence of HIV in urban settings, outbreaks of severe VL might occur in these regions if the sandflies reach the urban settlements—with changing epidemiology and potential threat for epidemics in urban areas too.

Diagnosis

Clinical

The disease should be suspected based on epidemiologic setting and clinical features. Since sporadic incidence of leishmaniasis is being reported from several parts of India, VL should be kept in mind in the differential diagnosis of prolonged febrile diseases with splenohepatomegaly. Several conditions need to be differentiated based on the stage of the clinical presentation. These include enteric fever, malaria, miliary tuberculosis, brucellosis, lymphoma and leukemia besides differentiation from other causes of moderate to massive splenomegaly.

Laboratory

Nonspecific laboratory findings: Laboratory findings in VL include anemia or pancytopenia, hypergamma-globulinemia with albumin globulin reversal and elevated alkaline phosphatase. The anemia seems to develop from a combination of factors including nutritional deficiencies, hypersplenism, blood loss, hemolysis and bone marrow suppression. Hypergammaglobulinemia results from polyclonal B-cell activation. In addition to nonspecific antibodies, specific antibodies to leishmania are common.

Parasite Detection

The gold standard for diagnosis is demonstration of the amastigote form of the parasite (LD bodies) by microscopic examination of aspirates from spleen, bone marrow or lymph node (Fig. 64.11). Although the specificity is high, the sensitivity of microscopy varies, being higher for aspirates from spleen (93–99%) than for bone marrow (53–86%) or lymph node (53–65%) aspirates. The peripheral smear or buffy coat preparation may demonstrate LD bodies in monocytes especially in HIV co-infection. But the accuracy of microscopic examination is influenced by the experience and competence of the laboratory personnel and the quality of the reagents used. Leishmania in sections of tissue biopsies appear as round or oval intracellular parasites that are 2–3 μm in diameter. They can be stained with Giemsa, Wright's or hematoxylin and eosin stain. In addition to visualization

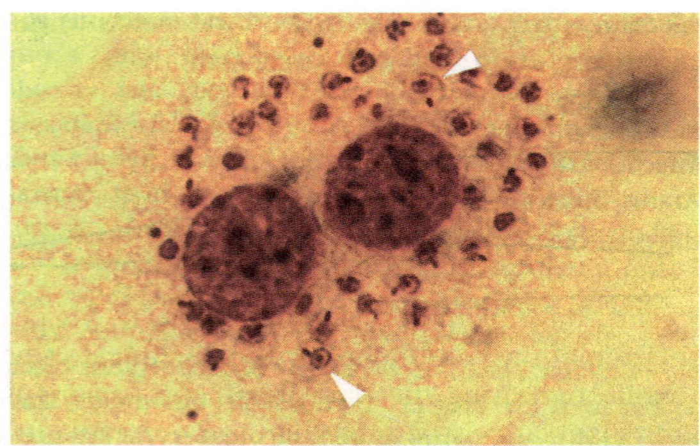

Fig. 64.11: Bone marrow smear LD bodies (Giemsa stain × 1000)

of the organisms, granulomas are often detected at sites of infection, particularly when there is better cell mediated immune response.

Leishmania can be grown in culture in NNN (Novy-MacNeal-Nicolle) medium or a liquid medium containing calf serum such as Schneider's medium, using splenic or bone marrow aspirate. Leishmania grow at 26–28°C and the promastigotes forms can usually be identified within a few days in heavy infections but may take several weeks if there is only low parasite load. Thus, cultures should be maintained and examined for a minimum of 4 weeks. The detection of parasites in the blood or organs by molecular techniques for parasite DNA by PCR is more sensitive than microscopic examination but these techniques remain restricted to referral hospitals and research centers.

Antibody-Detection Tests

Serologic tests alone are neither sufficiently sensitive nor specific to definitively confirm or exclude leishmaniasis. Serology may be positive in individuals from endemic areas because of past exposure and may not be indicative of current active disease. But it becomes useful with appropriate and adequate clinical data. While immuno-competent patients with VL usually have a high titer of antibodies, immunocompromised patients often do not have detectable parasite-specific antibodies; thus, serology may not be a sensitive test in these hosts.

Serological tests based on indirect fluorescence antibody (IFA), enzyme-linked immunosorbent assay (ELISA) or Western blot have shown high diagnostic accuracy in most studies but are poorly adapted to field-settings. Two serological tests have been specifically developed for field use and have been sufficiently validated—the direct agglutination test (DAT) and the rK39-based immunochromatographic test (ICT). The rK39 is a 39-amino acid repeat that is part of a kinesin-region of amastigotes (LD) in *Leishmania chagasi*. An rK39-based ELISA showed excellent sensitivity (93–100%) and specificity (97–98%) in many VL-endemic countries.

The rK39 based ICTs are easy to perform, rapid (10–20 minutes) and give reproducible results. Of the currently available non-invasive diagnostic tests, rk39 strip test seems to be the best. Sensitivity of strip test is very good with blood and sera (~100%). But in HIV co-infected patients, the sensitivity of serological tests is low and hence not reliable. They are currently the best available diagnostic tool for VL for use in remote areas.

Montenegro Skin Test

The Montenegro skin test (or leishmanin skin test) is performed by injecting the antigen of leshmania promastigotes intradermally to induce a cutaneous delayed-type hypersensitivity reaction. The injection site is examined 48 hours later; an induration of 5 mm or more is considered a positive test. It is negative in active VL cases but is positive in primary cutaneous forms. After recovery from VL, the test can become positive indicating improvement in the immune status. Even though this test is often referred to, in order to establish the immune competence of CL, it is not clinically used routinely.

Management of VL

Treatment of leishmaniasis remains difficult due to multiplicity of the existing co-morbidities and their often variable susceptibility to available drugs, which are toxic and expensive. Since the 1920s, treatment has been based on pentavalent antimonial compounds. Following the increasing incidence of VL cases in immunocompromised patients and the rise of acquired resistance to antimonials, amphotericin B has joined the antimonials as a first-line drug for leishmaniasis. Miltefosine, a new oral compound has shown promising results and appears to be an efficient alternative for the treatment of Indian kala-azar (VL).

Pentavalent Antimonials

Two closely related pentavalent antimonials are currently used—sodium stibogluconate 100 mg/mL and meglumine antimoniate 85 mg/mL have been the mainstay of the treatment of all forms of leishmaniasis all over the world for more than seven decades. However, the mechanism of action of antileishmanial agents remains unclear. It may involve inhibition of ATP synthesis. It might be possible that antimonial salts have to be concentrated within the macrophage or parasite and transformed into active trivalent metabolites to be efficient. Antimonials have poor oral absorption and therefore are administered by the parenteral route. They are rapidly excreted by the kidneys. Various treatment regimens are used and the exact duration and efficacy vary depending upon the type of leishmaniasis, the severity of the lesion and the endemic area concerned.

IM injections at a dose of 20 mg/kg per day for 28–30 days were the usual regime. Minor adverse effects from the pentavalent antimonials are common and include nausea, vomiting, myalgias, arthralgias, headache and malaise. More severe dose-dependent reactions can also occur, such as leukopenia, agranulocytosis, thrombocytopenia, behavioral changes and cardiac arrhythmias. Electrocardiographic (ECG) changes include: T wave flattening, nonspecific ST segment changes, prolongation of the QT interval and ventricular arrhythmias. Renal insufficiency, proteinuria and elevation of hepatic and pancreatic enzymes have also been described. Over the years reports of unresponsiveness appeared and up to 30% of VL cases are resistant at present. Increasing the dosage and duration have been of no avail and therefore other drugs have become the mainstay of treatment.

Amphotericin B

During the last 15 years it has become an alternative first-line drug. The use of amphotericin B for treatment of leishmaniasis is biochemically rational because its target is ergosterol-like sterols, which are the major membrane sterols of leishmania as well as fungi. High cure rates (> 96%) are reported with amphotericin treatment. Amphotericin B is administered as a slow (6–8 h) IV infusion (0.5–1 mg/kg) dissolved in 500 mL of 5% dextrose daily or on alternate days. The common regimens range from 14 to 20 infusions, for a total dose of 1.5–2 g.

Liposomal Amphotericin B

It has been used in several countries for VL treatment. It is less toxic than conventional amphotericin B. It can be given in higher doses, more rapidly, IV in shorter duration with low toxicity and improved efficacy, but the cost is considerably higher. Short-course treatment consists of IV infusions given as 3–4 mg/kg/day for five days followed by one more injection of the same dose on the 10th day (total dose 10–15 mg/kg). This regimen is effective even in refractory kala-azar. Single dose liposomal amphotericin at a dose of 10–15 mg/kg is also found to be equally effective.

Side-effects of amphotericin B during infusion include chills, headache, cramps, hypotension, vertigo, paresthesias, vomiting and exceptionally, anaphylactic shock or cardiogenic shock. These manifestations are usually controlled by addition of corticosteroids within the liquid suspension or by slowing down the infusion rate.

Paromomycin

It is a wide-spectrum antibiotic of the aminoglycoside family with minimal reversible ototoxicity and no nephrotoxicity. It is a safe, affordable and effective drug for the treatment of visceral leishmaniasis. An injectable formulation of paromomycin was registered in India in 2006. The recommended dose for administration by IM injection or IV infusion is 15 mg/kg per day, given for 20 days. It gives cure rates as high as 95% and is effective in antimony and miltefosine therapy failed patients. Paromomycin appears to be an excellent substitute for antimony and amphotericin B and can be considered as a first line antileishmanial drug.

Miltefosine (Hexadecylphosphocholine)

Miltefosine is a phosphocholine analogue that can be given orally. It has antileishmanial activity *in vitro* and *in vivo*, probably via effects on cell-signaling pathways and membrane synthesis. A number of studies on treatment of VL in India have demonstrated benefit from miltefosine. The recommended dose is 50 mg daily for patients weighing < 25 kg and 50 mg twice daily for patients weighing > 25 kg. For children it is 2.5 mg/kg. Duration of treatment is four weeks. Cure rate is around 94%. GI side-effects are frequent with mild vomiting (40%) or diarrhea (20%) in most patients. Sometimes transient elevation of liver enzymes may develop. This drug is teratogenic and therefore should not be used in pregnancy and in those refusing contraception during the treatment period and for two months more.

Combination Therapy

Combination therapy is the suggested way forward to increase treatment efficacy, prevent the development of drug resistance, reduce treatment duration and perhaps to decrease cost of treatment. The combination of sodium stibogluconate and paromomycin was found to be safe and effective in early trials conducted in India and East Africa. Drug combinations including liposomal amphotericin and miltefosine are currently being studied in India.

Treatment of HIV-VL Co-infection with Lieshmaniasis

Treatment is essentially similar to treatment of other patients. Liposomal amphotericin B is the drug of choice for HIV/VL co-infection—both for primary treatment and for treatment of relapses. A total dose of 40 mg/kg, administered as 4 mg/kg on days 1–5, 10, 17, 24, 31 and 38, is considered optimal but most patients relapse within one year. Pentavalent antimonials and amphotericin B deoxycholate can also be used where liposomal amphotericin B is not available. Active antiretroviral treatment effective for AIDS has to be initiated early and continued.

Post Kala-Azar Dermal Leishmaniasis (PKDL)

Syn: Post Kala-Azar Dermal Leishmaniasis of Brahmachari

PKDL is a chronic granulomatous lesion of the skin containing parasitized macrophages, lymphocytes and plasma cells. It develops as a sequel to VL occurring 6 months to five years after treatment in 5–15% of cases. This could be due to breakdown of cell mediated immunity. Therefore it is important to improve the nutrition of the patients to avoid this complication. The disease develops in a variety of clinical forms from hypopigmented macules to infiltrated papules or nodules of pinhead size to large patches. PKDL persists as a chronic dermatosis without complication in most cases. The other unusual variants of PKDL include the annular, warty, papillomatous growths, fibroid with erythematous plaques and xanthomatous growth. The lesions may be seen on any part of the body; occasionally large tumor like lesions appear on face, limbs and trunk. Complications can occur depending on the site, the most serious being blindness due to corneal ulceration. The incidence of PKDL may have important implications in transmission of leishmaniasis, as PKDL provides the only known reservoir of the parasite in India. The hypopigmented form of PKDL has been often misdiagnosed as vitiligo but the parasite load is scanty in them; the nodular form may be easily confused with a number of dermatological conditions among which leprosy is the most important. Most patients have more than one type of lesions and constitutional symptoms are absent. When the parasite is not demonstrated in skin biopsies, the diagnosis of the PKDL hinges on the endemicity of VL in the area and previous history of infection. 15–20% of PKDL patients come without a past history of VL suggesting subclinical infection followed by spontaneous recovery probably due to incidental improvement in immunity and later breakdown of immunity and it poses difficulty for diagnosis. The lesions have to be differentiated from all granulomatous lesions of the skin like lepromatous leprosy, skin tuberculosis, fungal granulomas and lupus erythematosus. The diagnosis is based on history and clinical findings, but rK39 and other serologic tests are positive in most cases. Indian PKDL is treated with pentavalent antimonials for 60–120 days. This prolonged course frequently leads to noncompliance. The alternative is several courses of amphotericin B spread over several months—but is expensive and unavailable for many patients.

Cutaneous Leishmaniasis

It is primary infection of the skin by direct inoculation and localization of the lesion confined to the skin without any visceral involvement because of better cell mediated immunity in the affected person or low virulence of the parasite. In India, it is caused by *L. tropica* and *L. major*. In other places, *L. aethiopica*, *L. mexicana* and *L. braziliensis* complexes are responsible. The typical incubation period between the time of the sandfly bite and clinical manifestations is one week to several months. The lesions are granulomatous ulcers which are indolent and chronic, persisting for several months to years; the lesions contain promastigotes in macrophages. ***Oriental sore, Delhi boil, Baghdad boil*** and ***Aleppo boil (Syria)*** were some of the synonyms used for the skin lesions. Cutaneous lesions tend to occur on exposed areas of skin, beginning as a red papule that enlarges to form an ulcer with granulomatous tissue at the base and raised, heaped up margins. There is usually no surrounding induration. The ulcers are characteristically painless unless secondarily infected. Localized adenopathy may develop, especially in the early stages of the infection. Some individuals have multiple lesions and lesions may occur in the distribution of lymphatic drainage. Nodular, psoriasiform and verrucous forms arise less commonly. The lesions typically undergo spontaneous resolution. The pace of this resolution varies according to the infecting *Leishmania* species and the immune reaction of the host. A residual hypopigmented, depressed scar at the site is common following cure. Generally CL gives rise to permanent immunity from the same species.

L. major tends to cause an exudative, 'pizza-like' or 'wet ulcer'. The ulcer usually has a raised outer border, a granulating base and an overlying white purulent exudate. After a typically short incubation period of one week to two months, the ulcer frequently grows to a size up to 6 cm in diameter over a short time period. Spontaneous healing also occurs quickly, usually within six months. Multiple lesions are common.

L. tropica tends to evolve more slowly. It has a typical incubation period of two months to two years and the ulcer does not usually grow larger than 1 to 2 cm. This ulcer is characterized as a 'dry ulcer' because it usually has a central crust and no exudates.

Diagnosis

In an endemic area or after visiting an endemic area, development of any isolated skin lesion of undetermined etiology or non-healing ulcer should suggest the diagnosis. Other diseases like cutaneous tuberculosis, fungal infections, leprosy, sarcoidosis and malignant ulcers are sometimes mistaken for CL. A skin aspirate or scraping or biopsy is optimal for demonstrating the organisms. The organism can be cultured in NNN medium also. PCR is more sensitive than microscopy and culture and allows identification of the *Leishmania* species responsible.

Treatment

CL does not always need therapy because of their tendency to resolve spontaneously. However, lesions that are large, multiple, progressing or in cosmetically important areas such as the face, are usually treated. A pentavalent antimonial is the first-line drug for all forms of CL and it is used in a dose of 20 mg/kg for 20 days as for VL. The exceptions to this rule are CL caused by *L. guyanensis*, for which pentamidine isethionate is the drug of choice (two injections of 4 mg of salt/kg separated by a 48-h interval) and CL due to *L. aethiopica*, which responds to paromomycin (16 mg/kg daily) but not to antimonials. Relapses are common and treated with the same drug. Ketoconazole 200–400 mg daily or itraconazole 100–200 mg daily have been used with mixed responses but have not been adequately assessed for this indication in clinical trials. Small lesions (< 3 cm in diameter) may conveniently be treated with intralesional injections of a pentavalent antimonial at a dose adequate to blanch the lesion, 0.2–2.0 mL weekly until cured. An ointment containing 15% paromomycin sulfate plus 12% methylbenzonium chloride cures 70% of lesions due to *L. major* in 20 days and may be suitable for lesions caused by other species as well.

Diffuse Cutaneous Leishmaniasis (DCL)

It is a rare syndrome that occurs mainly with *L. aethiopica*, *L. mexicana* and *L. amazonensis*. The primary lesion does not ulcerate; rather amastigotes progressively disseminate to macrophages in other areas of skin. Patients with DCL usually have a defect in the cell mediated immune response and are anergic. Nodules or plaques typically occur on the face and the cooler extensor surfaces of the limbs. DCL characteristically follows a relapsing or chronically progressive course. Generalized skin nodules can develop over months to years, leading to marked deformity. These lesions may be mistaken for lepromatous leprosy. DCL does not heal spontaneously and is difficult to treat. If relapse and drug resistance are to be prevented, treatment should be continued for some time after lesions have healed and parasites can no longer be isolated. Repeated 20-day courses of pentavalent antimonials are given, with an intervening drug-free period of 10 days. Miltefosine has been used for several months with a good initial response. Combinations should be tried. In *L. aethiopica* infection, a combination of paromomycin (14 mg/kg per day) and sodium stibogluconate (10 mg/kg per day) is effective.

American Cutaneous and Mucocutaneous Leishmaniasis

Mucosal leishmaniasis (ML) occurs only in the New World and is mainly associated with *L. braziliensis* infection. Months or years after resolution of the primary cutaneous lesion, recurrence at a distal mucosal site can follow due to hematogenous or lymphatic dissemination. This is also known as *espundia*. It has been estimated that the lifetime risk of developing a mucosal lesion is 1 to 5% after a primary *L. braziliensis* lesion. ML is associated with erosive disease of mucosal surfaces, most commonly of the nose, nasal septum or mouth. Ulceration of the nasal septum can lead to septal perforation. The palate can also be destroyed. Patients may present with bleeding of mucosal surfaces. Primary lesions of *L. braziliensis* tend to be large, frequently associated with regional lymphadenopathy. *L. braziliensis* can be associated with mucocutaneous leishmaniasis. *L. mexicana* generally produces small chronic ulcers, usually with only one or a few lesions. These tend to heal rapidly and spontaneously, often within three to four months. Lesions frequently occur on the ear, which relates to the biting habit of the vector. These lesions are referred to as **Chiclero's ulcers**. Tissue biopsy is essential for identification of parasites, but the rate of detection is poor unless PCR techniques are used.

Treatment

The regimen of choice is a pentavalent antimonial drug administered at a dose of 20 mg/kg for 30 days. With failure of therapy or relapse, patients may be given another course of an antimonial but then become unresponsive, presumably because of resistance in the parasite. In this situation, amphotericin B should be used. Amphotericin B dose totaling 25–45 mg/kg is appropriate. The more extensive the disease, the worse is the prognosis; thereby emphasising the role of prompt and effective treatment and regular follow-up.

Prevention of Leishmaniasis

The aim of prevention is avoiding host infection (human or canine) and its subsequent disease. It includes means to prevent intrusion of people into natural zoonotic foci and ways to protect against infective bites of sandflies. Prevention can be at an individual or collective level. Control programs are intended to interrupt the lifecycle of the parasite, to limit or ideally, to eradicate, the disease. The two main targets in control programs are the vector and the reservoir, which are not mutually exclusive. As the majority of the leishmaniases are zoonoses, control programs are generally limited and rarely pass beyond the experimental stage. Whatever type of intervention strategy is selected, an active participation of the population is essential to succeed. Public information on the natural history of the parasite, transmission and the disease is a prerequisite for any preventive measure or development of a control program. A simple preventive measure is to avoid the vicinity of sandfly development or resting sites in endemic areas during critical periods (seasons and activity cycles of the vector).

Mechanical means include wearing clothes that cover as much skin as possible and using bed nets. Sandflies bite uncovered skin and do not have the ability to bite through clothes, even when it is made of thin material like cotton. Wearing full clothes during the hours of sandfly activity is a good preventive measure. Sandflies can generally pass through the mesh of mosquito bed nets and therefore insecticides impregnated bed nets should be used. Neither chemoprophylaxis nor vaccines are available against leishmaniasis.

Source: Sundar S, Sinha PK, Rai M, et al. Comparison of short-course multidrug treatment with standard therapy for visceral leishmaniasis in India: an open-label, non-inferiority, randomised controlled trial. Lancet. 2011;377(9764):477-86.

AFRICAN TRYPANOSOMIASIS

Syn: Sleeping sickness

African trypanosomiasis or sleeping sickness is caused by two subspecies of *Trypanosoma brucei, T. gambiense* and *T. rhodesiense.* These hemoprotozoa are transmitted by the bite of infected tsetse flies (Glossina).

Geographic Distribution

Trypanosoma brucei gambiense is found in West Africa, Congo, Southern Sudan and Uganda. *Trypanosoma brucei rhodesiense* is found in Central and Eastern Africa. Endemicity is closely related to the distribution of the vector tsetse flies and the reservoir hosts. The disease is not present in India.

Trypanosomes are hemoflagellates seen as actively motile spindle-shaped organisms in periphersal blood. In Leishman stained preparations, trypanosomes measure 14–33 × 1.5–3.5 microns. They possess a central nucleus and a kinetoplast situated near the posterior end. A flagellum arises from the blepharoplast situated close to the kinetoplast and passes forwards along the free margin of the undulating membrane and becomes a free flagellum protruding forward from the anterior end (Fig. 64.12). Trypanosomes are seen actively moving in the plasma in fresh preparations. *Trypanosoma gambiense* and *Trypanosoma rhodesiense* are morphologically similar, but the latter is more virulent in laboratory animals.

Incidence

20,000 to 30,000 people are infected by trypanosomes each year.

Transmission

The vectors are mainly *Glossina palpalis (G. fuscipes)* and *G. tachinoides* for *Trypanosoma gambiense* and *G. morsitans, G. pallidipes* and *G. swynnertoni* for *Trypanosoma rhodesiense.* Both sexes of tsetse flies suck blood and transmit the disease. They live for 2–5 months.

T. gambiense and *T. rhodesiense* are widespread parasites of several herbivorous animals in endemic areas and these form the reservoir. Humans form the major reservoir for *T. gambiense* and animals form the major reservoir for *T. rhodesiense.*

Tsetse flies get infected by feeding on infected animals or man. The parasites multiply in the gut of the fly and pass anteriorly to the proventriculus and the salivary glands. The infective metacyclic forms develop and multiply there further and pass into the proboscis after 3–7 weeks.

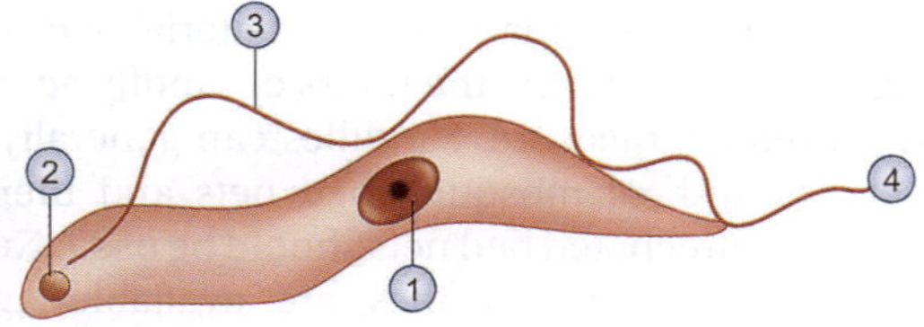

Fig. 64.12: Trypanosomes—general morphology

Keys: (1) The nucleus, (2) kinetoplast, (3) undulating membrane and (4) the flagellum

The fly remains infective for its life. The metacyclic forms are introduced into the host during the next bite. The metacyclic forms transform into trypanosomes within 48 hours and multiply in the tissue space. Ultimately, they pass to lymph nodes and the bloodstream and then reach several organs.

Indian Scene

Sporadic cases of trypanosomiasis by various *Trypanosomes (T. evansi*—cattle, *T. lewisi*—rodents and rats and others) have been reported in India from the northern regions and Pune. Cattle trypanosomiasis is common. People in cattle rearing areas show antitrypanosomal antibodies.

Pathology

Lymph nodes and the CNS show maximal lesions. There is localized or generalized lymph node enlargement. The nodes are congested and show hemorrhagic areas which contain trypanosomes. Later, these undergo fibrosis. In liver, Kupffer cell hyperplasia occurs with portal infiltration, but clinical hepatosplenomegaly is rare. Pancarditis occurs because of extensive cellular infiltration and fibrosis.

Affected organs show infiltration of the blood vessels by monocytes, macrophages and plasma cells causing endarteritis. This increases vascular permeability.

In CNS, main lesion is leptomeningitis seen over the brain and spinal cord. Histologically there is perivascular cuffing with lymphocytes and plasma cells. Later, trypanosomes invade the brain tissue, particularly the frontal lobe, pons and medulla. Parasites are seen in the CSF during the meningitic stage. Other changes include rise in pressure, moderate rise in protein and lymphocytosis. Complement-mediated hemolytic anemia may develop in some. IgM class antibodies are demonstrable in the serum and CSF.

Clinical Features

The incubation period varies from one to three weeks. Though the symptoms of *T. gambiense* and *T. rhodesiense* infections are broadly similar, the rhodesian type is usually more severe and runs a more acute course with a higher mortality. The initial lesion is the formation of a painless nodule at the site of bite **(tryponosomal chancre or trypanids)**. This nodule occurs 5–15 days after the bite. *Trypanosomes* are seen in this lesion. Irregular fever and parasitemia occur within 1–2 weeks. Lymphadenopathy occurs usually after 3 weeks of the bite. Cervical, femoral and axillary groups of lymph nodes enlarge. Lymph nodes are more pronounced in the posterior triangle of the neck in *T. gambiense* infection. Enlargement of these groups of lymph nodes is called **Winterbottom's sign**. The spleen is often enlarged. Anemia develops in due course due to slow inanition and hemolysis. Fever, lymphadenitis, anemia and debility continue for several months.

The CNS involvement is late in the gambian type while symptoms of CNS involvement develop within a few months in the Rhodesian type. The whole course runs over 2–3 years, but the course is shorter in the Rhodesian type and death may occur in 6–9 months.

Several unusual manifestations may develop. These include circinate erythematous skin rashes, localized edema over the face, eyelids and neck, ulnar hyperesthesia (Kerandel's sign) neuralgic pains, formication, myocarditis, pericardial effusion and jaundice. The sleeping sickness stage sets in when the parasites enter the CNS. The debility and languor increase, the gait becomes slow, shuffling and swaying, the speech becomes slurred and tremors of the tongue and lips develop. The patient may become demented. Mask-like vacant expression, drooping of eyelids, tendency to fall asleep during daytime and restlessness at night are all seen in endemic areas. The patient becomes severely emaciated and serious complications like pneumonia, dysentery, hyperpyrexia, convulsions and coma may supervene and prove fatal. Though untreated cases of sleeping sickness are generally fatal, the gambian type may recover spontaneously at times (Table 64.5).

Diagnosis

History of residence in an endemic area, irregular fever, enlargement of cervical lymph nodes and hepatosplenomegaly should point to this diagnosis. Trypanosomes are demonstrable in peripheral blood (Figs 64.13A and B), lymph node aspirate and CSF. Serological tests such as indirect fluorescent antibody test and ELISA are helpful. Newer tests based on proteomics signature analysis are available. These are more specific and reliable for diagnosis and follow-up.

Card agglutination test for *T. gambiense* can be done with serum, capillary blood or from impregnated filter papers. It is a rapid screening test with 87–98% sensitivity and 93–95% specifity.

CNS disease is diagnosed by the CNS findings. More than 5 WBC/mm³ of CSF, presence of trypanosomes or increased protein contents of more than 300 mg/L are diagnostic.

Drug Treatment

Early cases limited to blood and lymph nodies respond to suramin which is a derivative of urea. Dose is 20 mg/kg bw given IV as a 10% solution on days—1, 3, 7, 14 and 21. The drug is nephrotoxic. Anaphylactic reaction may develop.

Late cases with neurological involvement respond to melarsoprol (Mel-B) which is a trivalent arsenical, combined with BAL (British anti-Lewisite). The drug has to be administrated under supervision due to adverse side effects. The drug is quite effective in curing even late cases with neurological involvement. Resistance of the parasite to arsenicals may develop. Other drugs which are also effective include difluoromethylornithine (eflornithine) given in a dose of 200–400 mg/kg bw daily IV for 4 weeks and nitrofurazone given in a dose of 10 mg/kg given 8 h orally for 10 days. With treatment, clinical and parasitological clearance occurs even in late cases. Patients should be watched for 2 years to ensure cure.

Pentadimine is the drug of choice for first stage of *T. gambiense*, dose – 4 mg/kg/bw IV at 24 hours interval for 7 days.

Source: Brun R, Blum J, Chappuis F, et al. Human African trypanosomiasis. Lancet. 2010;375(9709):148-59.

Prevention

Anti-tsetse fly measures including proper clothing and insect repellent creams (Di-meepol) or diethylbenzamide and elimination of the reservoir hosts are effective. Drug prophylaxis with suramin or pentamidine are also available.

AMERICAN TRYPANOSOMIASIS

Syn: Chagas disease

General Considerations

It is one of WHO's 13 neglected tropical diseases. The Brazilian physician—Carlos RJ Chagas discovered *Trypanosoma cruzi* in 1909. Chagas disease is caused by *Trypanosoma cruzi* (schizotrypanum) which is transmitted by species of reduvid bugs to man (Fig. 64.14). It is seen in all countries of Central and South America. Main vector is *Triatoma infestans* in Brazil.

Other means of transmissions include the oral route by ingestion of contaminated food such as meat, sugarcane or Euterpe oleracea fruit juice, organ transplant, needle sharing and laboratory contamination.

Source: Prata A. Clinical and epidemiological aspects of Chagas disease. Lancet Infect Dis. 2001;1(2):92-100.

Due to frequent and increasing inter country migration of population, Chagas' disease is being reported in non-endemic countries as well. Chronic disease may develop in up to 30% of cases 10–30 years after acute infection.

Trypanosoma cruzi is a broad trypanosome, about 20 μ in length and is C-shaped. The motile stage of the parasite

Table 64.5: Comparison of disease caused by *T. brucei gambiense* and *T. brucei rhodesiense*

	T. b. gambiense	*T. b. rhodesiense*
Disease produced	Gambian sleeping sickness	Rhodesian sleeping sickness
Distribution	West and central Africa	East Africa
Vector	Glossina palpalis or tachinoides (riverine tsetse)	Glossina morsitans (savanna tsetse)
Reservoir	Humans and domestic animals	Wild animals
Course	Slow—months to years. Less acute course	More rapid—up to one year. More acute course
CNS symptoms	More characteristic	Less marked
Results with treatment	Good	Not satisfactory
Chemoprophylaxis	Useful	Not reliable

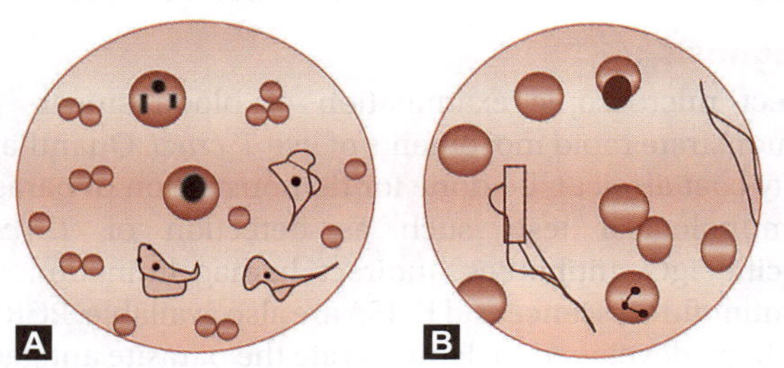

Figs 64.13A and B: Trypanosomes in peripheral blood. **A.** *T. cruzi*, **B.** *T. gambiense*

Disease caused by Protozoa

Textbook of Medicine

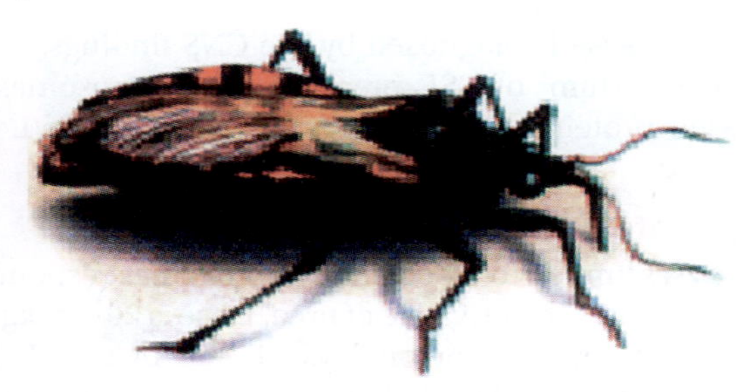

Fig. 64.14: Reduvid bug

is found only for a short period after infection. It soon develops into the leishmanial form that multiplies in the cells of mesenchymal origin. Reduvid bugs of the genera *Triatoma, Rhodnius* and *Eratyrus* are the principal vectors. ***Triatoma magista:*** These bugs inhabit the floor and walls of rural houses. These come out at night and suck blood from the sleeping inhabitants. During the blood meal they defecate. Reservoir hosts are formed by dogs, cats, opossums and armadillos. Reduvid bugs are infected by taking blood meal and in 6–15 days infective metacyclic forms are passed in feces. Organisms enter the body when the feces is smeared on to the bite wound. Other methods of transmission also exist. Infected mothers can transmit the disease to the fetus, giving rise to congenital Chagas disease. Spontaneous abortion may occur in many, but 2–5% of babies may manifest infection at birth.

Other vehicles for transmission of infection are blood or donated organs from infected individuals. Migration of population has led to introduction of this disease into several parts of the world which were free. When the reduvid bug sucks blood, motile trypomastigotes enter the bloodstream and invade many nucleated cells. In these cells the motile trypomastigotes transform into non-motile amastigotes and replicate over 4 days. By this time they become trypomastigotes, rupture the parent cell and enter the bloodstream to be ingested by the vector.

Incidence

An estimated 16–18 million people are infected in 18 Latin American countries. Chagas disease results in 45,000–50,000 deaths per year. Major cause of death is cardiac involvement. This disease is not reported from India.

Pathology

At the site of inoculation, the organisms multiply and produce a local lesion—chagoma. They are seen in the bloodstream for a short period. They are taken up by macrophages later. *Trypanosoma cruzi* multiplies and produces focal lesions in the cardiac and skeletal muscles and neuroglia. Cardiomyopathy develops as a result of cardiac involvement. From the foci of multiplication, active trypanosomes enter the bloodstream and are demonstrable.

Granulomatous lesions occur in the spleen, liver and lymph nodes. CNS involvement in children leads to meningoencephalomyelitis. Chronic Chagas disease manifests several years or decades later in 10–30% of cases. The direct effect of the parasite as well as immunological processes account for the late results. Common presentation is cardiomyopathy. Pathological changes include biventricular enlargement, thinning of ventricular walls, apical aneurysm, mural thrombi and varying degrees of heart block. Parts of the alimentary tract are also affected.

In the esophagus and colon, dilatation occurs giving a picture of acquired achalasia cardia and megacolon seen. The alimentary lesions are due to destruction of the Auerbach's plexus.

Clinical Features

In children Chagas disease occurs in an acute form, presenting with fever, rash. Without itching and the rash clears in several days. Symptoms of the acute phase may also include malaise, myalgia, headache, asthenia and anorexia. Mortality in the acute phase, is low (<5%) and it is due to acute myocarditis and/or meningoencephalitis, Children younger than 2 years suffer more.

Chagoma (furunculoid and peeling cutaneous lesion) which is nodular occurs at sites of entry of the parasite through the skin, generalized lymphadenopathy, myocarditis and rarely meningoencephalitis develop. The ***Romaña sign*** develops in 20–50% of cases in which the route of entry is through the conjunctiva. It is a painless, periophthalmic, unilateral edema of both palpebral conjunctiva, frequently accompanied by conjunctivitis and local lymph node enlargement. It persists for 30–60 days. The manifestations of the acute disease resolve spontaneously within 3–8 weeks in approximately 90% of individuals who are infected.

They enter the chronic, latent or indeterminate asymptomatic phase of the disease. A direct progression from the acute phase to the symptomatic chronic form of Chagas disease occurs in fewer than 5% of patients. In the chronic type, cardiomyopathy and achalasia cardia and atonic dilation of the colon and the small intestine are seen. Approximately two-thirds of cases develop cardiac manifestations leading to arrhythmias, cardiac failure, thromboembolic phenomena and sudden death. In the endemic areas of South and Central America, cardiomyopathy due to Chagas' disease used to be a common cause of cardiovascular death among patients aged 30–50 years.

Involvement of the GIT leads to megaesophagus and/or megacolon in approximately one-third of chronic cases; these chronic lesions do not resolve spontaneously.

Diagnosis

Direct microscopic examination of blood smears will demonstrate rapid movements of live *T. cruzi*. Quantitative buffy coat also can be done for demonstration of parasite. Immunological tests such as detection of *T. cruzi* specific IgG antibodies, indirect hemagglutination test, immunofluorescence and ELISA are also available. PCR test has been developed to demonstrate the parasite antigen.

ECG may show arrhythmias, heart block especially right bundle branch (RBB) and block of the anterior branch of the bundle of His. This combination is typical of Chagas' cardiomyopathy. Cardiac involvement determines the prognosis.

Xeno Diagnosis

Feeding laboratory reared triatoma vector as the patient and examining the gait contents of the vector for *T. cruzi* after 30–60 days; only 30–60% of cases of chronic chagas disease are positive. Affection of the other systems can be demonstrated by appropriate tests.

Treatment

In acute phase, benznidazole is the drug of choice. Benznidazole (Rochagan) is given as an oral dose of 6 mg/kg for 30–60 days. This has to be given under supervision. Primaquine has been found useful in a dose of 15 mg daily for about 6 months in acute Chagas disease. At present Nifurtimox (Lampit) a nitrofurantoin, is available for oral use. The dosage is 8–10 mg/kg/day for adults and 15–20 mg/kg/day for children and the drug has to be administered for 120 days. Cure rates of 80% in acute and 90% in chronic cases have been claimed. The drug is toxic and hence has to be given under supervision. Permanent lesions occurring in others organ systems demand management on their own merits.

Posaconazole which is a systemic antifungal agent shows promise as an anti *T. cruzi* drug. Fatal arrhythmias have to be treated with pacemakers or defibrillator. In an intractable case, cardiac transplantation may be necessary.

Control

Improvement in housing and sanitation and use of insecticides limit the spread of the reduvid bugs. Treatment of active cases and attention to the animal reservoir reduce the reservoir pool.

Amebiasis, Giardiasis, Balantidiasis, Toxoplasmosis and Cryptosporidiosis

CHAPTER 65

Amebiasis, Giardiasis, Balantidiasis, Toxoplasmosis and Cryptosporidiosis

KV Krishna Das, VP Gopinathan

Chapter Summary

- Amebiasis
  - General Considerations
  - Pathology
  - Clinical Manifestations
  - Acute Amebic Dysentery
  - Hepatic Amebiasis
  - Treatment of Amebiasis
- Primary Amebic Meningoencephalitis
- Giardiasis
- Balantidiasis
- Toxoplasmosis
- Cryptosporidiosis

AMEBIASIS

General Considerations

Fedor Aleksandrovich Losch in Russia first described amebiasis in 1875. The term amebiasis includes all lesions caused by infection by the protozoan parasite *Entameba histolytica*. These amebae cause ulcerative lesions in the large intestine causing dysentery and from there they spread to several organs to produce necrotic lesions. There is a great tendency for the intestinal infection to become chronic and persistent for long periods. *E. dispar* is morphologically identical to *E. histolytica*, but nonpathogenic. It is genetically different. It is a commensal. However, *E. histolytica* can also remain in the bowel for many years without causing major symptoms.

Amebiasis is worldwide in distribution, but it is very prevalent in tropical climates. In many parts of India, the infection rate used to be as high as 40–50%. Chronic carrier state, poverty, insanitary disposal of excreta, unhygienic food handling and proliferation of flies are responsible for this high prevalence. Though all age groups are susceptible, adults suffer more often.

Due to the wide prevalence of intestinal parasitism and want of full information on the prevalence of other chronic gastrointestinal disorders, such as irritable bowel syndrome and motility disorders, there was a general tendency to overestimate the prevalence of intestinal amebiasis. In areas where the environmental sanitation has improved and the use latrines is popular, the prevalence of amebiasis has considerably fallen. Intestinal endoscopic studies done in many institutions reveal that at present amebic lesions are relatively less common.

Parasitology

Amebae are widely distributed in nature. The common pathogen is *E. histolytica*. It exists in two forms—**the cyst** and **the trophozoite**. The cysts are round or oval in shape and measure 10–15 μ in diameter. In iodine-stained preparations, the cysts show one, two or four nuclei depending on their maturity. Cysts resist adverse environment. In addition to the nucleus, one or more rod-like structures called chromidial bars and a glycogen mass are also seen. Cysts are formed in the bowel when the environment becomes unfavorable for the trophozoite and are then passed out in feces. Cysts are responsible for transmission of the disease from person to person. The vegetative form (trophozoite) is actively motile by the aid of pseudopodia. It measures 20–50 μ in diameter. Invasive trophozoites are identified by the hematophagous nature

Textbook of Medicine

(presence of ingested erythrocytes within them). Amebae multiply by binary fission. The trophozoite is the invasive form and is responsible for all lesions. A large number of trophozoitesis are seen in the feces of dysenteric patients. Trophozoites and cysts occur in the feces of carriers. Outside the body, the trophozoites survive only for an hour or so. Normal gastric juice destroys them in the stomach. Cysts survive external environment for long periods.

Transmission

Humans are the only reservoir for *E. histolytica*. Cysts are passed in the feces of cases and carriers. These are ingested along with food or water. Cysts resist acid digestion in the stomach. Excystation occurs in the intestines, trophozoites develop from cysts and they establish themselves in the colon, feeding on the bacteria and desquamated epithelial cells. They multiply by binary fission. These noninvasive forms may persist for long periods without producing any symptoms. Under favorable conditions these become invasive.

Pathology

Intestinal amebiasis: The invasive trophozoites adhere to colonic mucosa with the help of specific lectins and ulcerate the mucous membrane and penetrate deep into the submucosal layers of the colon. The basic pathological process is a lytic necrosis of tissue. This is due to an extra-cellular cysteine kinase enzyme causing proteolytic destruction of the tissue, producing flask shaped ulcers. *E. histolytica* which produce lytic enzymes kills host cells which come into contact with them. The host cells become immobile on contact with *E. histolytica* and the cells die. *E. histolytica* can also induce apoptosis in host cells. The cellular response consists of mononuclears and a few polymorphs. Amebae are seen in the invading margins of the lesions. Cecum, ascending and descending colon and rectum are the sites of predilection. The appendix may be involved. The terminal ileum may be affected rarely. The ulcers have undermined edges and are covered by dense yellow or brown slough. The mucous membrane between ulcers is healthy. Ulceration may extend to blood vessels causing severe hemorrhage at times. Perforation of the bowel may occur, but it is rare. Sometimes ameboma or amebic granuloma develop due to repeated infection by ameba and bacterial pathogens. The acute inflammatory process has a tendency to subside spontaneously. In many patients, chronic infection persists with microscopic lesions which harbour *E. histolytica* for many years. The lesions may heal in a few cases. Persistence of the chronic lesions accounts for the carrier state.

E. histolytica infection is associated with transient immunosuppression. Activated macrophages form the major defense against invasive amebae. Tumor necrosis factor (TNF) which is a cytokine derived from macrophages has parasticidal properties. The resistance against invasive amebiasis is mainly cell mediated immunity.

Extra-intestinal Lesions

Amebic liver abscess: Invasive amebae reach the liver through the portal blood stream from the colon which is the primary seat of infection. In the liver they multiply and cause colliquative necrosis of liver cells to produce abscess.

Possibly, malnutrition, alcoholism and consequent immunosuppression favor the development of liver abscess. Unlike pyogenic abscess, the wall of the amebic abscess is made up of necrotic and compressed liver tissue and it is devoid of granulation tissue. Active amebae are found near the expanding margins. The pus is made up of necrotic tissue which shows amorphous material and erythrocytes. It is sterile on culture. In most cases, the color of the pus is reddish brown or chocolate. This pus is classically described as anchovy sauce pus because of its appearance. Amebae are seen only rarely in the pus aspirated from the center of the abscess, they are more often demonstrable in the pus aspirated from near the walls on subsequent occasions. The site of the abscess is more commonly the right lobe. It is usually single and may attain very large size. The abscess may enlarge progressively and spread by contiguity to the chest wall, colon, diaphragm, pleura and pericardial cavities. Amebic abscess does not impair hepatic function significantly. Jaundice is generally mild or absent, but pressure over a major hepatic duct can give rise to obstructive jaundice. On aspirating the pus, the liver tissue comes into apposition and complete healing occurs without structural damage or fibrosis.

During acute amebic dysentery, the liver may enlarge as a result of diffuse inflammation caused by the products of inflammation of the colonic tissue and bacteria reaching the liver in the bloodstream. The hepatic lesion clears up with cure of the dysentery. This lesion should not be mistaken for liver abscess.

Other foci for embolic lesions include the lungs, brain, spleen and other tissues. Direct invasion of the skin by active vegetative amebae leads to extensive spreading necrotic ulceration-cutaneous amebiasis.

Clinical Manifestations

The incubation period varies from a few weeks to months.
Spectrum of illnesses caused by E. histolytica:
Intestinal amebiasis
- Asymptomatic infection
- Symptomatic noninvasive infection
- Acute proctocolitis (dysentery)
- Toxic megacolon
- Chronic nondysenteric colitis
- Ameboma
- Perianal ulcers

Extraintestinal amebiasis
- Liver abscess
- Pleuropulmonary involvement
- Pericarditis
- Peritonitis
- Brain abscess
- Genitourinary disease.

Acute Amebic Dysentery

This presents with sudden or subacute onset of lower abdominal pain and diarrhea with blood and mucus in stools. The frequency ranges from 3 to 10 in a day. At times, watery diarrhea with large amounts of blood and mucus may occur. Constitutional symptoms are mild and these include low grade fever and vague discomfort. Palpation of the abdomen reveals colonic tenderness and mild hepatomegaly. The feces is semisolid or liquid, showing fecal matter mixed with blood and mucus. Microscopic examination shows erythrocytes, a smaller number of leukocytes and trophozoites of *E. histolytica*. In majority of cases, the condition subsides after several weeks even without treatment, to exacerbate again with dietary irregularity, psychological stress or other factors. Complications are rare but in a few cases extensive destruction of mucosa and submucosa may lead to severe hemorrhage and occasionally perforation. Rectal prolapse, intussusception and colonic stricture may develop in some. ***Amebomas*** may develop in the cecum or other parts of the colon and these may be mistaken for tumors. These resolve completely with specific treatment.

Nondysenteric Amebiasis

This is a common mode of presentation in endemic areas. The condition starts insidiously with abdominal discomfort, flatulence, intermittent diarrhea with constipation and presence of mucus in stools. Asymptomatic intervals and periods of dyspepsia alternate for many months or years. Vague general symptoms like feverishness, mild depression, fear and anxiety may be prominent. Physical examination may reveal palpable tender cecum and sigmoid and sometimes tender hepatomegaly. An amebic granuloma (ameboma) may be felt as a sausage-shaped mass in the right iliac fossa and this may be mistaken for malignancy or tuberculosis. Mucosal ulcers may be seen on sigmoidoscopy. Examination of the mucus collected by sigmoidoscopy may show active trophozoites. Repeated examination of fresh stool or sigmoidoscopic specimen may be necessary to establish the diagnosis. Sigmoidoscopic biopsy reveals ulceration and parasite in the mucosa.

Hepatic Amebiasis

Hepatic involvement used to be very common, almost all patients give a history of alcoholism. Around 50% of patients suffering from hepatic amebiasis gives history of dysentery. Liver involvement manifests as insidious onset of pain in the right hypochondrium or right lower chest with high fever, chills and sweating. Loss of weight and anemia may be pronounced. In the early stage, the liver is enlarged as a whole. The pathological process is not inflammatory, but it consists of multiple necrotic lesions caused by amebae diffusely distributed in the liver. In this stage, the organ is enlarged as a whole and it is acutely tender. This stage may persist for varying periods and may resolve either spontaneously or with treatment, without proceeding to abscess formation. At present, the occurrence of liver complications has come down.

In those in whom abscess develops, the liver is considerably enlarged and tender. When the abscess spreads to the abdominal wall, there is superficial edema and severe local tenderness. The majority of liver abscesses are in the right lobe. Left lobe lesions are palpable over the epigastrium. Diaphragmatic involvement causes pleuritic pain in the right lower chest. Physical examination reveals diminished air entry, impaired percussion note and crepitations over the lower part of the right chest. Jaundice is rare. Blood shows high leukocytosis (about 12,000–14,000/mm^3) with polymorphonuclear cells dominating the field. The erythrocyte sedimentation rate (ESR) is usually high. Fluoroscopy reveals elevation of the right dome of the diaphragm and diminished movement. Ultrasonography is the standard method by which liver abscess is diagnosed with certainty. Computed tomography (CT) scan and isotopic scanning also help to locate the site of the abscess.

Complications of liver abscess include rupture into neighboring organs or cavities leading to peritonitis, right sided empyema, bronchohepatic fistula and pericarditis. Untreated, the mortality may go up to 10%.

Cutaneous amebiasis occurs over the genitalia, perianal region, opening of sinuses and around colostomy wounds. Rarely, metastatic lesions from the liver develop in the lungs and brain. Rupture of a liver abscess into the peritoneum causes the clinical picture of an acute abdominal emergency with shock.

Differential Diagnosis

Amebic dysentery has to be differentiated from bacillary dysentery, ulcerative colitis and tuberculous enterocolitis. Ameboma may closely resemble carcinoma. Hyperplastic ileocecal tuberculosis is another possibility to be thought of. Chronic intestinal amebiasis may be mistaken for irritable bowel syndrome, diverticulitis and neurasthenia or malabsorption state. Hepatic amebiasis is a common cause of prolonged fever in the tropics and when liver enlargement and tenderness are not marked, it resembles enteric fever, brucellosis or tuberculosis.

In an endemic area, enlargement and tenderness of the liver should suggest the diagnosis of amebic liver abscess. Other conditions such as alcoholic liver disease, primary and secondary tumors of the liver, subdiaphragmatic abscess and pyogenic liver abscess have to be differentiated. In case of doubt, the diagnosis is confirmed by ultrasonography and later, aspiration. Prompt response to antiamebic drugs is a point suggesting a diagnosis of hepatic amebiasis.

Laboratory Diagnosis

Examination of the feces: Fresh stool examination by light microscopy invariably reveals *E. histolytica* in dysentery. Active *E. histolytica* shows characteristic ameboid movement and ingested erythrocytes. In chronic amebic colitis, cysts are present in feces in varying numbers. These can be identified in saline preparations but cellular details are better demonstrable in iodine stained specimen. Unlike bacterial dysentery, the feces does not contain innumerable leukocytes. Plenty of erythrocytes are present. Stool occult blood may be present in invasive intestinal disease. Stool enzyme immunoassay also will be useful (Figs 65.1A to D and 65.2A to E).

E. histolytica has to be distinguished from the non-pathogenic *Entameba coli* by the following features.

Features	E. histolytica	E. coli
Saline wet smear		
Movement	Progressive	Non-progressive
Ingested RBC	Present	Nil

Textbook of Medicine

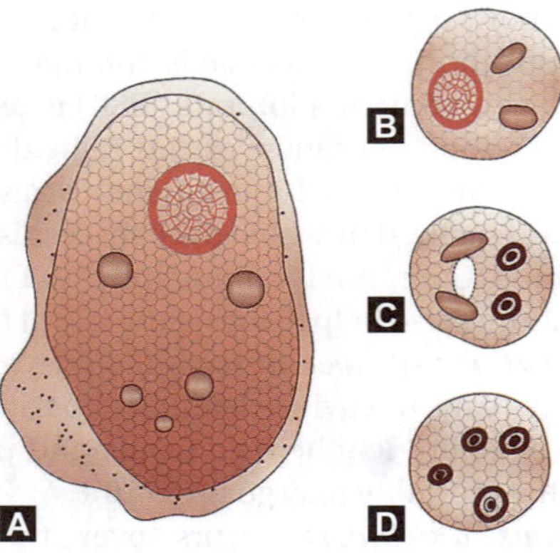

Figs 65.1A to D: *Entameba histolytica* in stools. **A.** Trophozoite (vegetative motile form) with ingested erythrocytes; **B.** Uni- and bi-nucleated cysts; **C.** Chromatoid bars and glycogen vacuole; **D.** Mature cyst with four nuclei

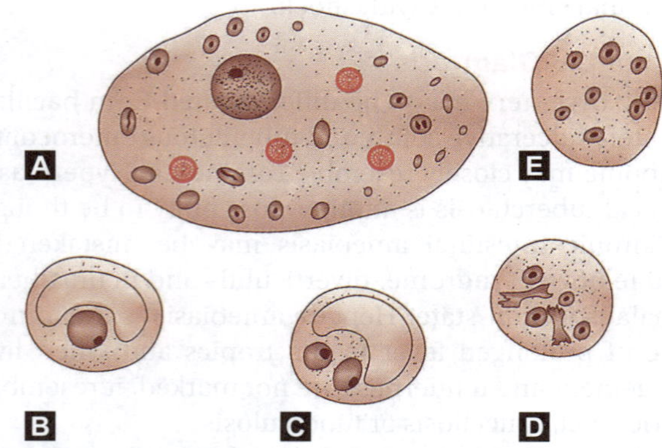

Figs 65.2A to E: *Entameba coli* in stools. **A.** Trophozoite; **B, C and D.** Uni-, bi- and quadrinucleated cysts with glycogen vacuole and chromidial bars; **E.** Mature cyst with eight nuclei

Iodine stained preparation		
Nuclear chromatin	Central	Eccentric
Number of nuclei in the cyst	1 or 4	1, 2 up to 8
Chromidial bars	Short and thick	Filamentous

Apart from feces, vegetative *E. histolytica* can be demonstrated in the following specimen.

- Liver abscess pus
- Sputum in pulmonary amebiasis
- Discharge from cutaneous amebiasis.

Serological tests: These tests are mainly used in extraintestinal disease. Indirect hemagglutination antibody test is positive in 95% of extraintestinal and 70% of intestinal amebiasis. Other tests also have been developed. Indirect immunofluorescence is positive in more than 60% of cases. Countercurrent electrophoresis and agar gel diffusion are other methods employed.

Imaging studies:

- ***Ultrasonography:*** A single lesion in the postero-superior aspect of the right lobe of the liver is commonly seen. However, multiple abscesses may also occur in some patients. Deep seated abscess may be missed on clinical evaluation. Multiple abscesses should suggest the possibility of pyemic etiology.
- ***CT scan:*** In cerebral amebiasis, CT may show irregular lesions without surrounding capsule or enhancement.

Other investigations: Blood counts may show mild anemia, leucocytosis, elevated ESR and elevated alkaline phosphatase.

Endoscopy: Rectosigmoidoscopy and colonoscopy may reveal small mucosal ulcers covered with yellowish exudates and the intervening mucosa appears normal. For demonstrating vegetative amebae, the fresh mucus exudates should be examined as a saline preparation, microscopically.

In chronic intestinal amebiasis, feces show amoebic cysts, when the disease is quiescent. With acute exacerbation, trophozoites appear from time to time. Charcot-Leyden crystals may be seen as a result of chronic bleeding foci. These crystals are needle shaped, refractile and are made up of lysophopholipase.

Treatment of Amebiasis

Drug treatment consists of amebicidal drugs. These may act on the parasites found in the lumen of the gut or on the invasive forms seen in the tissues. They are grouped as luminal amebicides and tissue amebicides. Some drugs, however, have action on both sites.

The most effective amebicides in current use are given in the following box.

Metronidazole	400 mg 3 times/day orally for 10 days (or) 800 mg tds for 5 days
Tinidazole	600 mg 2 times daily for 5 days orally
Diloxanide furoate	500 mg 3 times daily for 10 days
Chloroquine	500 mg 2 times daily for 2 days 250 mg bd for 2–3 weeks

- ***Metronidazole:*** This drug has effect on both tropho-zoites and cysts. It is well-absorbed after an oral dose to produce adequate tissue levels. It is effective for the treatment of acute and chronic intestinal amebiasis and in hepatic amebiasis. In severe cases, the drug can be used intravenously in a dose of 500 mg twice a day as an infusion. Though side effects are not serious, they are common. These include distaste in the mouth, anorexia, nausea, abdominal discomfort, vertigo, dizziness and ataxia. Peripheral neuropathy may develop rarely. The drug is generally avoided during pregnancy on account of its possible teratogenic effects in laboratory animals.
- ***Tinidazole:*** This drug belongs to the group of nitroimidazole derivatives, structurally related to metronidazole. The therapeutic spectrum is similar to metronidazole, but the drug is more potent and is also better tolerated. Newer drugs in this group with more prolonged action are being introduced, e.g. secnidazol 2 g single dose for intestinal amebiasis and 1.5 g as a single daily dose for five days for hepatic amebiasis.
- ***Diloxanidefuroate:*** It is a safe drug effective only on the intestinal forms of the parasite. It is used in the treatment of acute and chronic intestinal lesions in doses of 500 mg tds oral for 10 days. In amebic dysentery, the symptoms subside in 5–7 days. In chronic intestinal amebiasis, clearance rates approximate 80–90%. This drug is rarely used now.
- ***Chloroquine:*** It has amebicidal properties in hepatic lesions. This is brought about by the high tissue concentration of the drug obtained in the liver. It is

effective in the treatment of hepatic amebiasis along with metronidazole or tinidazole. It has no action on the trophozoites or cysts in the intestine.

Acute amebic dysentery: Metronidazole, which produces symptomatic relief in 3–5 days, is the drug of choice. General management consists of treatment of fluid and electrolyte imbalance, especially potassium loss. The diet should be soft, low residue type with high caloric value. After the full course of treatment, stool examination should be done to ensure parasitological cure.

Chronic intestinal amebiasis: When symptoms are mild and chronic, metronidazole or diloxanide furoate are the drugs of choice. A single course may bring about parasitological cure in 80–90% cases. Repeated courses are required to completely eliminate the infection in most cases. Even with repeated courses some cases may prove to be resistant.

Hepatic amebiasis: Metronidazole and chloroquine are administered in full doses. During the acute phase, metronidazole 500 mg infused intravenous (IV) twice a day till the pain and tenderness subside and then followed up by oral dosage is ideal. Addition of chloroquine is optional, but it probably acts together to bring about better results. Small abscesses may even resolve completely with medical treatment. Large abscesses should be aspirated 2–3 days after starting drug therapy by which time the surrounding edema would have partly cleared.

Aspiration used to be done at the site of maximal tenderness and edema of the chest wall. The site of the abscess can be accurately determined by ultrasonography and in most cases aspiration under ultrasonographic guidance is done in order to safely locate the pus and also to confirm the aspiration of all lesions. Since, there is no granulation tissue to wall off the cavity in amebic liver abscess, needle aspiration is adequate to remove the pus and favor healing. Most of the cases clear up with two to three aspirations. Emergency aspiration has to be done if the abscess threatens to rupture or has just ruptured. In case of left lobe abscesses, it is preferable to do aspiration under ultrasonographic guidance in order to ensure full drainage and avoid injury to neighboring structures.

The main complications of aspiration are hemorrhage, vasomotor collapse and introduction of infection into the cavity. Secondary infection should be treated with full doses of broad spectrum antibiotics. In uncomplicated liver abscess, the pus is chocolate colored or yellow, odorless, sterile and does not show predominance of pus cells on microscopy. When the abscess is infected, the pus is yellow or greenish, foul smelling and microscopic examination shows predominance of pus cells. Gram staining and culture help in demonstrating the organisms. Small liver abscesses may resolve with medical treatment even without aspiration.

When infection supervenes on amebic liver abscess, the patient shows more serious symptoms such as high fever, chills and rigor and toxemia. Systemic antibiotic therapy should be instituted along with antiamebic drugs. Surgical drainage may be needed if the abscess cannot be cleared by aspiration and drug therapy.

In all cases of hepatic amebiasis, a course of intestinal amebicides should be given to prevent relapse of the hepatic lesions and to clear the carrier state.

Other lesions caused by E. histolytica: Amebic lesions of the brain, lung and skin respond to a course of metronidazole or tinidazole.

Dehydroemetine is indicated if the response is unsatisfactory. The dose in 60 mg/day by intramuscular (IM) injection. The drug is toxic particularly causing myocarditis. A course should not exceed a cumulative dose of 600–900 mg. The drug is seldom used now.

Resumption of alcohol intake predisposes to relapse of liver abscess.

Asymptomatic cyst passers: It is advisable to treat them with metronidazole to avoid the risk of future hepatic amebiasis and to eradicate the carrier state. A full course of metronidazole or tinidazole given for 5–10 days clears 80% of cases. Repeated courses are needed for better results. Diloxanide furoate, either singly or in combination with metronidazole can also be employed with success.

Results of treatment: Both acute and chronic intestinal amebiasis respond satisfactorily to drug therapy. In endemic regions, reinfection is quite common unless proper hygienic measures are instituted. Complications like gut perforation and amebic peritonitis carry a high mortality if treatment is delayed. Prompt supportive measures and therapy with antiamebic drugs and antibiotics considerably improve the outlook. Mortality due to liver abscess is about 10% if the condition is not diagnosed and treated in time. Prompt treatment gives very satisfactory results. The liver recovers completely without residual damage. Amebic abscess of the brain clears up with specific therapy and other symptomatic measures, but it is fatal if missed.

Prevention: The most important steps are to observe food hygiene, provide safe drinking water and arrange for sanitary disposal of human excreta. Ordinary chlorination of drinking water does not kill the cysts. Cooks and food handlers should be periodically examined and the infection eradicated. Fruits and vegetables can be rendered safe by washing with soap and peeling off the skin wherever possible.

PRIMARY AMOEBIC MENINGOENCEPHALITIS

***(See* Section 17, Ch 199)**

General Considerations

Some species of free-living soil amebae of the genus *Naegleria* may produce primary amebic meningoencephalitis, which is a rapidly fatal disease. The organisms are carried in the nose and throat of asymptomatic carriers. It is seen worldwide, occurring sporadically. The disease is present in India.

Naegleria gruberi is the common pathogen. The genus *Hartmannella* (syn: Acanthamoeba) can also affect man. In most of the cases, a history of swimming or bathing in contaminated water may be obtained. The organisms enter through the roof of the nose and spread up the cribriform plate to reach the subarachnoid space. The brain is edematous and covered by a blood stained

Textbook of Medicine

purulent exudate, especially in the basal cisterns. Amebae are also seen invading the gray matter.

Clinical Features

The incubation period is 2–14 days after a possible exposure. The clinical picture resembles acute meningitis. The cerebrospinal fluid (CSF) is under tension and it is turbid or blood stained. Microscopy shows erythrocytes, numerous polymorphs and motile amebae containing ingested erythrocytes, which may be mistaken for macrophages. The species of ameba can be identified by suitable staining. CT scan shows generalized cerebral edema with increased vascularity in postcontrast study suggestive of meningitis. Azithromycin in the dose of 7.5 mg/kg/day for 5 days has been tried with partial success. Amebic meningoencephalitis is associated with high mortality within 2–5 days. Present treatment is not fully satisfactory. In addition to meningoencephalitis, occasionally granulomatous amebic encephalitis may develop. This is caused by *Acanthamoeba* species and *Balamuthia mandrillaris*, particularly in immunocompromised subjects.

Treatment

Amphotericin B given intravenously in a dose of 0.25 mg/kg daily for 8 days is partially effective against *Naegleria*. The drug can also be given intrathecally in a dose of 0.5 mg diluted in 5 mL of CSF, thrice a week. Rifampicin, doxycycline and sulfisoxazole are beneficial if given as adjunct therapy.

Acanthameobae (Hartmannella) are free-living amebae seen in soil and water. These become pathogenic to immunocompromised hosts. They gain entry through the nasal mucosa, abrasions on the skin or eyes. Pathogenicity is similar to that of *Naegleria*.

Source: Tungikar SL, Kulkarni AG, Deshpande, Gosavi VS. Primary Amebic meningoencephalitis. J Assoc Physicians India 2006;54:327-9.

GIARDIASIS

Giardiasis is infection of the small intestine by the flagellate protozoon—*Giardia intestinalis (G. lamblia)*. In the tropics and subtropics, this parasite is very widely prevalent, particularly in children.

Giardia lamblia is a flat pear-shaped organism, 12–18 μ in diameter with eight flagella, two nuclei and a large ventral sucker placed anteriorly. These flagellates are found in large numbers in the duodenum and jejunum in between the villi and attached to them by their suckers. Occasionally, biopsy specimens may show giardia between villi. With the aid of the flagella, giardia moves actively and this helps to identify the organisms in fresh stools or duodenal aspirates. Cysts are formed which are passed in feces (Figs 65.3A and B).

Transmission occurs by ingesting the cysts along with food and water. Infection rates are high in closed communities. New immigrants and travelers may get the infection from endemic areas. Hypochlorhydria and hypogammaglobulinemia predispose to heavy infection.

Pathogenesis

Though the exact mechanism is not known, it is possible that a large number of flagellates adhering to the mucosal

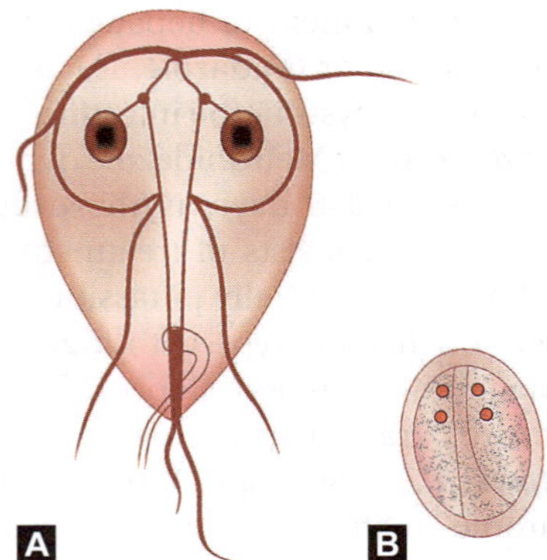

Figs 65.3A and B: *Giardia lamblia* seen in stools. **A.** Actively motile form; **B.** Cyst

surface may reduce the area for absorption. In addition, irritation of the brush border of the villi, alteration in bacterial flora in the small intestine and invasion of the submucosa have been suggested as contributing factors. Many cases show increased intestinal motility.

Clinical Features

Presenting symptoms range from mild abdominal discomfort to explosive diarrhea. Some infections may be asymptomatic but the majority are subacute or chronic. Nonspecific symptoms include failure to thrive, abdominal pain, epigastric distress, intermittent diarrhea and general ill-health. Features of malabsorption may occur, especially in children and this should suggest the possibility of giardiasis.

In some outbreaks, explosive diarrhea with watery foul smelling stool may be the presenting symptom. Giardiasis is a frequent cause for traveler's diarrhea in endemic regions. The acute attack lasts for 3–4 days but in children, the course may be prolonged for weeks or months and it results in malabsorption state. Many cases go into spontaneous remission and carrier state develops in them.

Diagnosis

Giardiasis is a common cause of diarrhea in children and vague abdominal discomfort in adults. Fresh feces should be examined for identifying the motile flagellate. Presence of the active flagellate in fresh stool or in the duodenal aspirate confirms the diagnosis. In many cases, mixed infection with *Giardia* and other intestinal pathogens like *E. histolytica* or helminths is common. Clinical severity does not always correlate with the number of parasites seen in feces. In mild infections, repeated examination and concentration methods (formol-ether concentration method or zinc sulfate floatation) may be required to establish the diagnosis. In some cases, when feces do not show the parasites, duodenal aspiration has to be done for recovering them. Presence of cysts indicates the carrier state. These can be identified by examining iodine-stained preparations of feces.

Treatment

The drug of choice is metronidazole in a dose of 15 mg/kg/day given for 7 days. In 80–90% of cases, infection is eliminated. In resistant cases, this course can be repeated. Single administration of metronidazole in a dose of

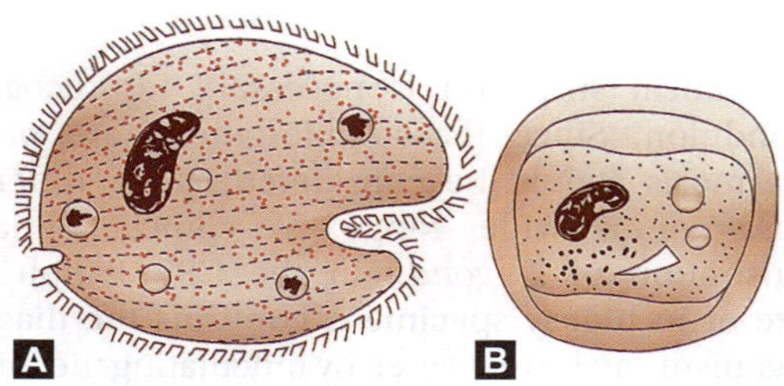

Figs 65.4A and B: *Balantidium coli* in stools. **A.** Trophozoite—motile ciliate; **B.** Cyst

30 mg/kg repeated after a week is also effective and it may be more suited for mass treatment on account of better patient compliance. Chloroquine 250 mg thrice a day for 5 days and tinidazole are also effective.

Giardiasis can be prevented by improving food hygiene and environmental sanitation. Heavy chlorination of water supply is required for killing giardia cysts.

BALANTIDIASIS

Balantidiasis is infection by *Balantidium coli* which affects the large intestine of man. *Balantidium coli* is a large ciliate (200 × 80 μ), actively motile with the help of numerous cilia in fresh specimens of stools. The cysts are rounded and smaller (Figs 65.4A and B). These are seen in carriers. Infection occurs when cysts are ingested. It is primarily a pathogen of pigs. Malnourished persons with low gastric acidity are more commonly infected. Compared to giardiasis and amebiasis, incidence of balantidiasis is very rare in India, but it is encountered from time to time.

Pathology

Balantidium coli primarily invades the colonic mucosa and produces flask-shaped ulcers which resemble amebic ulcers. Proteolytic enzymes and hyaluronidase are secreted by the organism. The mucosa shows infiltration by lymphocytes and polymorphs around the ulcers. Secondary infection and hemorrhage may occur as complications. In fulminant cases necrosis of the colon and perforation may result rarely. In addition to the colonic lesions, uterine, vaginal and vesical lesions may also develop at times.

Clinical Features

These resemble cases of mild to moderately severe amebic dysentery. Mild infections may be asymptomatic.

Diagnosis

It is established by demonstrating the active parasite in feces or sigmoidoscopic aspirate material. Presence of cysts indicates the carrier state.

Treatment

Tetracycline given in divided doses of 10 mg/kg daily for 10 days eliminates the infection. Many cases show a tendency towards spontaneous remission and development of carrier state. Metronidazole is also effective but the results are not consistent. Recently nitazoxanide has been recommended in a dose of 500 mg twice daily for 3 days.

TOXOPLASMOSIS

Infection by *Toxoplasma gondii* causes toxoplasmosis. This parasite undergoes its full life cycle only in cats and other canine hosts but it affects many mammals, birds and reptiles. Chickens lambs and pigs may be affected. The parasite was first discovered in 1908 in a North African rodent—the gondii. *Toxoplasma gondii* is a crescent shaped organism 4.6 × 2 μ size demonstrable by Giemsa or Wright stain. It is seen intracellularly in endothelial cells, monocytes or tissue cells. It may be seen free in tissues and tissue fluids.

T. gondii is a sporozoan parasite which is intracellular. In its life cycle, there is a sexual cycle in the intestinal epithelium of cats and other feline hosts. Immature oocysts develop into mature infective sporozoites in the enviornment within 2–3 days. When humans and other intermediate hosts ingest them, trophozoites (also known as tachyzoites) are released. They invade the cells of the gastrointestinal mucosa and then disseminate through the circulation to most of the organs. In the nucleated cells, the parasite proliferates. This leads to death of the host cell. If the host develops immunity, the trophozoites encyst. Each cyst contains about 3000 organisms. Encystment protects the organisms. They persist thought the lifespan of the host. The dormant organism within in the cysts are called bradyzoites. They are morphologically identical to tachyzoites, but they multiply slowly and are functionally different.

Human infection is acquired by ingesting the oocysts passed in cat's feces or contaminated meat of animals and birds. *Toxoplasma gondii* may be found in the milk of infected animals. Transplacental transmission to the fetus from the mother occurs if she gets infection during early pregnancy. At times, the maternal infection may be silent. Other rarer modes of transmission include inoculation of infected material into skin, blood transfusion, organ transplantation and entry through the respiratory tract. The disease is worldwide in distribution and limited serological surveys reveal that it is prevalent in India.

Pathology

The congenital form occurs in 3–5% of babies of infected mothers. If the fetus is affected heavily transplacentally during early pregnancy, abortion or stillbirth may result. If the fetus is affected in late pregnancy, the baby is normal at birth but symptoms develop after a few months. Lesions are seen widespread in the central nervous system (CNS), eyes, heart, lungs and adrenals. The parasite disappears from all tissues except the CNS and retina. Brain and spinal cord show extensive areas of necrosis, cyst formation and patchy calcification. Retina shows choroidoretinitis (Fig. 65.5).

In the acquired form, the parasite gets disseminated through the blood and lymphatics from the intestinal epithelium. Lymph nodes and spleen are commonly affected. Other tissues such as the liver, lungs, skeletal muscles, myocardium, meninges and brain may also be involved.

Clinical Features

Congenital toxoplasmosis presents predominantly with neurological involvement. The child develops chronic encephalomeningomyelitis which results in hydrocephalus, microcephaly, convulsions, tremors, focal paralysis and contractures (*See* Section 17, Ch 199). Eye lesions include

Textbook of Medicine

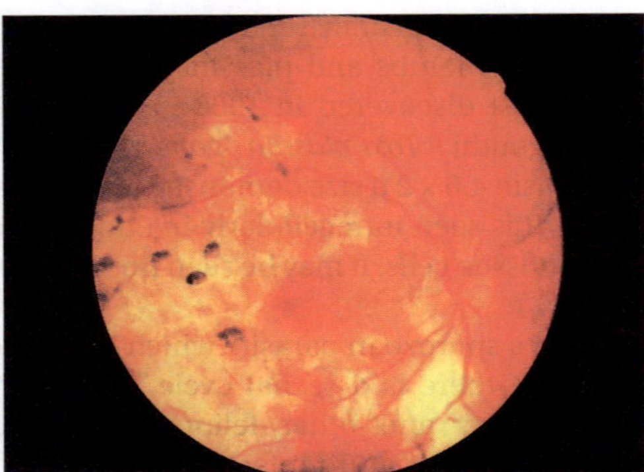

Fig. 65.5: Chronic burnt out choroidoretinitis probably *Toxoplasma*

Table 65.1: Lesions in the different forms of toxoplasmosis

Congenital	Acquired
	Often asymptomatic, detected by serological survey
• Hydro- or microcephaly	• Maculopapular rash
• Convulsions	• Fever
• Ocular palsies	• Hepatomegaly
• Bilateral choroidoretinitis	• Lymphadenopathy-tender non-suppurative, anterior and posterior cervical groups
• Hepatosplenomegaly	• Encephalitis
• Jaundice	• Myocarditis
• Maculopapular rash	• Choroidoretinitis rare, unilateral
• Cerebral calcification	• Pneumonia

microphthalmia, nystagmus, blindness and bilateral choroidoretinitis. In cases with meningoencephalitis, CSF is xanthochromic with rise in protein and mononuclear cells but with normal sugar. *Toxoplasma gondii* may be demonstrable. Other manifestations such as hepatosplenomegaly with jaundice, thrombocytopenic purpura, lymphadenopathy and rashes have been described.

Unlike congenital toxoplasmosis, acquired toxoplasmosis may be symptomless in the vast majority, detectable only by serological tests (Table 65.1).

Symptomatic cases may occur in two forms—acute and chronic. The acute form presents frequently with fever, aches and pains, cough, pneumonitis, profound malaise and maculopapular rash. Rarely jaundice, myocarditis and meningoencephalitis may develop. In the chronic form, there is generalized painful lymphadenopathy which is more marked in the cervical region, lymphocytosis with atypical lymphocytes in peripheral blood, hepatomegaly and rarely unilateral choroidoretinitis. In persons with latent infection or those who have undergone remission, depression of immune status of the individual results in recrudescence.

TOXOPLASMOSIS IN AIDS

Toxoplasmosis is one of the frequent opportunistic infection in human immunodeficiency virus (HIV) positive individuals. It mainly affects CNS. Toxoplasmosis occurs when CD4 count falls below 100 cells/mm³. It presents with fever, headache, focal neurological deficits like hemiparesis, aphasia and seizures. It also presents with pneumonia, pericarditis and choroidoretinitis. For further details (*See* Section 6, Ch 48).

Diagnosis

Strong clinical suspicion is necessary for recognizing the condition. Since the manifestations are protean, toxoplasmosis should be considered in the differential diagnosis of a wide range of clinical situations. Demonstration of *T. gondii* in the CSF, lymph gland aspirate or in biopsy specimens confirms the diagnosis. The organism can be recovered by inoculating the infective material into laboratory animals like mice, hamsters and guinea pigs. Isolation of the organism points to acute lesion. Polymerase chain reaction (PCR) done on CSF in meningoencephalitis cases may reveal the organism.

When acute *T. gondii* infection is suspected in a pregnant woman, the diagnosis should be pursued. Toxoplasmosis usually is diagnosed on the basis of antibody detection. In acute infection, immunoglobulin M (IgM) and later immunoglobulin G (IgG) antibody levels generally rise within one to two week. IgM antibodies indicate the occurrence of recent infection. IgG antibodies develop later and persist for considerable periods.

Toxoplasmosis in Pregnancy

When a pregnant woman is found to be infected with *T. gondii*, the next step is to determine whether the fetus is infected. It is done by demonstrating PCR testing of amniotic fluid to diagnose congenital toxoplasmosis. PCR testing of amniotic fluid is safer and more sensitive than fetal blood sampling and it allows earlier confirmation of fetal infection. However, false-positive and false-negative tests may occur with PCR tests.

Other investigations like complement fixation test, neutralizing antibody test, indirect hemagglutination test and enzyme-linked immunosorbent assay (ELISA) test are also available. The IgM-immunofluorescent antibody (IgM-IFA) test is particularly useful to detect recent infection. Immunocompromised subjects may not show rise in antibody titer. Ocular toxoplasmosis can be diagnosed by funduscopy on seeing typical lesion, associated with the positive serological tests.

The cerebral lesions can be visualized by contrast enhanced CT scan and magnetic resonance imaging (MRI) which show single or multiple ring-enhancing lesions near the basal ganglia, brainstem and subcortical region with space occupying effect and surrounding edema. In the investigation of pregnant women and neonates for infection, toxoplasmosis is always looked for.

Course and Prognosis

The lymphatic form tends to be mild and chronic which runs over several months, but is ultimately self-limiting. Congenital toxoplasmosis and acquired neurological lesions are associated with high mortality and morbidity. Congenital toxoplasmosis is a major cause of developmental anomalies.

Treatment

The organism is susceptible to a combination of pyrimethamine (daraprim) 25 mg/day and sulfadiazine 1 g every 6 hours for 14 days. Pyrimethamine is a folate-antagonist and therefore, megaloblastic anemia may develop during prolonged therapy. In children, the dose of pyrimethamine is 2 mg/kg. In acute cases, large doses of pyrimethamine, i.e. a loading dose of 200 mg, followed by a maintenance dose of 25–75 mg/day and sulfadiazine 100 mg/kg daily in three divided doses may be needed. At this dose, folinic acid 10 mg should be given daily to prevent the development of megaloblastic anemia. The course of treatment has to extend for 4–6 weeks.

Clindamycin is also effective and this can be combined with the standard drugs in resistant cases. The dose is 1200 mg/day in divided doses. Other drugs effective against *T. gondii* include azithromycin (250 mg bd) given with pyrimethamine (25 mg) or atovaquone monotherapy. In ocular toxoplasmosis, oral corticosteroid therapy given in addition to pyrimethamine—sulfadiazine is beneficial.

Treatment of Toxoplasmosis in Pregnancy

Women who are seropositive should be advised to take spiramycin 1 g qid for 4–6 weeks before undertaking pregnancy. This drug is safe for use during pregnancy. If the clinical features and laboratory investigations confirm that a pregnant woman has an active infection, the next step is to determine whether the fetus is infected. Prenatal tests including amniocentesis and ultrasound may help to determine whether the fetus is infected. If the fetus is infected, the mother is given pyrimethamine and sulfadiazine after the first trimester along with folinic acid in doses of 20 mg/day. Pyrimethamine is teratogenic and hence contraindicated in the first trimester of pregnancy. Other effective drug schedules include azithromycin + pyrimethamine or atovaquone monotherapy.

CRYPTOSPORIDIOSIS

This is caused by infection by *Cryptosporidium parvum*. *Cryptosporidium* is coccoid protozoa. Distribution is worldwide. Domestic animals such as cattle, sheep, pigs and horses act as reservoir hosts. Infection occurs by ingesting the oocysts. This infection has been reported in Kerala. In a study of stools in 148 diarrheal patients, *C. parvum* was seen in 1.5% of cases. Maximum prevalence was in children below 2 years of age and in immunocompromised patients.

On reaching the small intestine, infective sporozoites are released from the oocysts. They undergo asexual development in the apical enterocytes of the small intestine. After two cycles of development, sexual stages develop with the formation of zygotes and more oocysts. The oocysts sporulate, mature fully in the gut and are passed in feces, ready to infect other hosts. Incubation period after ingestion ranges from 3 to 11 days.

Clinical Features

Onset is with acute watery diarrhea associated with fever and general malaise. In healthy individuals, the disease runs a benign course and is self-limiting.

Cryptosporidiosis is a common opportunistic infection in acquired immune deficiency syndrome (AIDS). In such patients, the disease runs a more aggressive down-hill course, leading to severe weight loss and general debility. Toxic dilation of the colon may occur in a few.

Diagnosis

Demonstration of oocysts using concentration techniques and modified Ziehl-Neelsen staining help to establish the diagnosis.

Treatment

No specific drug was available. Clindamycin, erythromycin and spiramycin may reduce the severity of diarrhea.

In AIDS patients, zidovudine clears the infection temporarily. Nitazoxanide in a dose of 7.5 mg/kg bw controls the disease when given for 5–7 days. This is a thiazolide drug, the active metabolite being tizoxanide. Adverse side effects are minimal.

CHAPTER
66

Helminthiasis: General Considerations

RK Shenoy, KV Krishna Das

Chapter Summary

- General Biology
- Pathogenesis
- Diagnosis
- Treatment
- Prevention

GENERAL BIOLOGY

Helminths constitute the most widespread parasites affecting humans all over the world. In India, the problems of helminths is a serious one leading to considerable morbidity, mortality and economic retardation. *Ascariasis,* *ancylostomiasis, schistosomiasis* and *filariasis* are the most widespread helminthic parasites affecting extensive geographical belts and millions of people. The three main soil transmitted helminths—*Ascaris lumbricoides, Trichuris trichura* and the hookworms—*Necator americanus* and *Ancylostoma duodenale* are common in most parts of India, where the soil is contaminated by human feces.

In many poor communities, helminthiasis may be evident even at the age of 1 year, it reaches its maximum by the age of 10–12 years and then its severity declines. Helminths affecting man can be divided into three groups—*roundworms (nematodes), tapeworms (cestodes)* and *flukes (trematodes).* Helminths have well-developed

Textbook of Medicine

reproductive, excretory and nervous systems and may also possess alimentary tracts. They have complex life cycles and for majority of parasitic helminths, the reproductive and transmission cycles require presence of two or more hosts. Both adults the larvae are capable of producing disease depending on the parasite. Several mechanisms operate to produce lesions in different helminthic infections, examples of which are mentioned under pathogenesis. Allergy plays a part in producing symptoms during the stages of larval development. In many infections, mild to moderate, eosinophilia may develop. This reflects the immunological reaction of the host. Eosinophils have a protective role. They are seen to accumulate around helminthic larvae and destroy them, e.g. filaria.

World Health Organization (WHO) goal about soil transmitted helminths is to reduce illness from moderate or heavy infestation in school age children to below <1%. Soil transmitted helminths, lymphatic filariasis, onchocerciasis, guinea worm, schistosomiasis have all being included under the general term ***neglected tropical diseases*** by international committee consisting of heads of states, public and private charities and major pharmaceutical companies which held their deliberations in London in the later part of the previous decade and resolved to eliminate these infections or contain them by 2020.

PATHOGENESIS

Pathogenetic mechanisms in helminthiasis:

- Competition for nutrients in small intestine, e.g. *Ascaris lumbricoides* adults, *Diphyllobothrium latum.* They derive their nutrition by absorbing nutrients that pass through the intestines. Hookworms and whipworms get their nutrition and oxygen from the blood that traverses their intestinal tracts.
- Ingestion of host's blood and causing blood loss from the intestine, e.g. hookworms, *Trichuris trichiura.*
- Adults undergoing development in host's tissues and giving rise to tissue lesions, e.g. *Strongyloides stercoralis* and *Trichinella spiralis* in submucosa of small intestine, schistosomes in blood vessels, *Fasciola hepatica* in biliary passages, *Paragonimus westermani* in lungs.
- Dilation of lymph vessels caused by adult parasites, which later becomes prone to secondary bacterial infection resulting in clinical disease, e.g. *Wuchereria bancrofti* and *Brugia malayi* filariasis.
- Larval forms producing tissue lesions, e.g. migrating phase of roundworms, hookworms and strongyloides producing pulmonary and other tissue lesions; larval forms of *Echinococcus granulosus* (hydatid cysts), *Taenia solium* in cysticercosis, *Trichinella spiralis* in muscles and *Onchocerca volvulus* in skin and eyes.
- Tissue irritation by eggs, e.g. schistosomes.
- Irritation by the presence of adults, e.g. *Enterobius vermicularis* over the perianal region, *Ascaris lumbricoides* in the intestinal tract, biliary passages and respiratory tract.
- Allergic manifestations—both local and systemic, e.g. Loeffler's syndrome caused by larval forms of nematodes, larva migrans caused by *Ancylostoma braziliense* and *Strongyloides*, tropical pulmonary eosinophilia caused by filariasis.

- Give rise to severe functional damage to intestines to produce malabsorption state, especially in immunocompromised hosts, e.g. strongyloidiasis, trichuriasis and ascariasis. Ascariasis may lead to lactose intolerance and malabsorption of vitamin A.
- Toxic effects due to absorption of the metabolites or products of dead worms, e.g. roundworms, microfilaria.
- ***Risk of malignancy:*** Constant irritation by the adults or the ova in the tissues or natural passages has been associated with higher incidence of cancers in these sites, e.g. *Opisthorchis viverrini* in Thailand, Laos and Malaysia and *Clonorchis sinensis* in Japan increase the risk of cholangiocarcinoma 25–50 times. *Schistosoma haematobium* is associated with the increased incidence of cancer of urinary bladder.

With the introduction of sanitary latrines and potable water supply, the prevalence of intestinal helminths has come down considerably in several communities especially in Kerala but in many parts of India, the soil transmitted helminths infection is very rampant. The problem with regard to tissue helminthiasis, especially lymphatic filariasis remains the same and larger areas of India are now identified to be endemic for the disease.

Host parasite interaction: Several factors contribute to the survival and persistence of these worms in human host. The worms produce antiproteolytic substances, which help them to escape the digestive enzymes. They modify the immune mechanisms of the host so as to avoid acute and formidable reactions in the host, thereby, enabling them to complete their life span in the human host including residence, feeding and reproduction. Except *Enterobius vermicularis* and *Strongyloid stercoralis,* the others do not multiply in the same host. Increase in number is mainly due to continuous infection.

Helminths secrete substances which make them refractory to host immunity. Whip worms produce anti-inflammatory cytokines. They induce production of cyto-kines [interleukins (IL) 4, 5, 10 and 11], parasite specific immunoglobulin (Ig) and nonspecific IgE and also expansion and mobilization of mast cells, eosinophils and basophils [T Helper 2 (Th2) immune response].

DIAGNOSIS

Helminthiasis is diagnosed in the vast majority of instances by the demonstration of the adults, larvae or eggs in appropriate specimens. Indirect methods include immunological tests like immunoelectrophoresis and enzyme-linked immunosorbent assay (ELISA).

TREATMENT

Many subjects harboring worms acquire heavy worm loads due to the long lifespan of the parasites and repeated infection. Effective anthelmintics can produce temporary reduction or elimination of the worm-load, but reinfection occurs if the subject continues to live in the same environment (Table 66.1). Even regular periodic deworming fails to eradicate intestinal helminths from communities, unless simultaneous steps are taken to improve environmental sanitation.

Table 66.1: Choice of drugs for helminthiasis

Worms	First choice of drugs	Alternatives
Roundworm	Albendazole, mebendazole, pyrantel pamoate	Levamisole, ivermectin
Hookworm	Albendazole, mebendazole, pyrantel pamoate	Levamisole
Threadworm	Albendazole, mebendazole, pyrantel pamoate	Ivermectin
Strongyloides stercoralis	Ivermectin, thiabendazole	Albendazole, mebendazole
Whipworm	Albendazole, mebendazole	Ivermectin
Trichinella spiralis	Thiabendazole, albendazole	Mebendazole
Filariasis	Diethylcarbamazine	Ivermectin, albendazole, doxycycline
Tapeworm	Praziquantel, albendazole	Niclosamide, mebendazole
Hydatid disease	Albendazole, mebendazole	–
Guineaworm	Metronidazole	–
Flukes	Praziquantel	Albendazole

Cure rates with the common anthelmintic drugs single dose

Drugs	Cure rate
Albendazole	
Hookworms	59.8%
Roundworms	92%
Mebendazole	
Hookworms	17.4%
Roundworms	91.2%
Oxantel pamoate	
Roundworms	94.4%

PREVENTION

Strict personal hygiene, proper disposal of excreta and provision of potable water supplies are most important to ensure freedom from intestinal helminthic infestations. Vector control assumes importance in infections caused by tissue nematodes. More recently, mass drug administration to 'at risk' population in endemic countries is adopted as a measure to prevent transmission of filarial infection and schistosomiasis.

Points to Remember

- Helminths infecting man belong to the class nematodes, cestodes and trematodes.
- Pathogenesis ranges from simple competition for nutrients to risk of malignancy.
- Availability of broad-spectrum anthelmintics like albendazole and praziquantel has improved the ease and efficacy of treatment.
- Good personal hygiene, vector control and mass drug administration are important to prevent different types of helminthic infections.

CHAPTER
67

Intestinal Nematodes

RK Shenoy, KV Krishna Das

Chapter Summary

- Ascariasis
- Hookworm Infection
- Trichuriasis
- Strongyloidiasis
- Enterobiasis
- Trichinosis
- Larva Migrans

ASCARIASIS

Ascariasis is worldwide in distribution and is caused by the nematode *Ascaris lumbricoides.* In India, it is the most widely distributed intestinal parasite.

Morphology and Habitat

The worm measures 20–35 cm in length. The female is larger than the male. The females lay several thousand eggs every day. The eggs are elliptical, 30–40 μ × 50–60 μ in size with an outer dense mammillated shell and a smooth translucent inner shell. They are passed in feces. They become embryonated and infective in the soil in 2–3 weeks and they can remain viable under optimum conditions for years.

Life Cycle

Embryonated eggs are ingested with food or water and the larvae hatch out in the small intestine (Figs 67.1A and B). They penetrate the intestinal mucosa to enter the venules or lymphatics and travel to the lungs, where they develop for about 10 days. They then enter the alveoli to be coughed up and swallowed. During the pulmonary phase, the larvae undergo four moultings and become resistant to gastric acid. The larvae grow and mature in 2–3 months. Lifespan of this worm is 6–15 months.

Pathogenesis

During the stage of larval migration, pulmonary symptoms like cough, wheezing and hemoptysis may occur (Loeffler's syndrome) and used to be a common cause of respiratory symptoms in children.

The adult worms ingest nutrients from the small intestine and lead to nutritional deprivation. Large number of adults may form tangled masses and obstruct

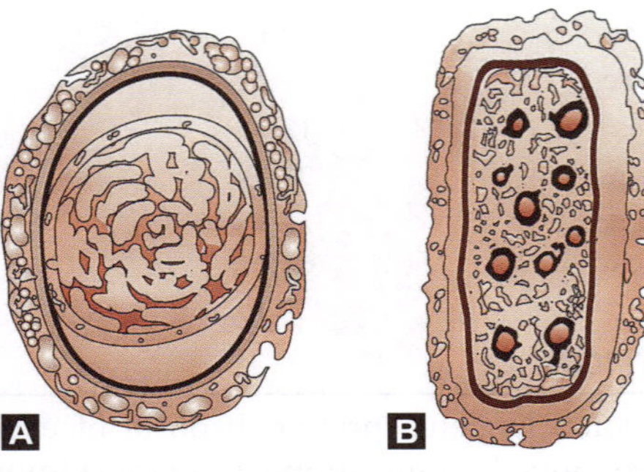

Figs 67.1A and B: Ova of *Ascaris lumbricoides.* **A.** Embryonated; **B.** Non-embryonated

the small intestines. The worm may migrate to ectopic sites like the stomach, nasal cavity, biliary tree, pancreatic ducts, respiratory passages, female genital tract or others.

Absorption of the products of living and dead worms leads to the development of allergy and toxic symptoms.

Clinical Features

Those due to larvae: Respiratory symptoms such as cough, hemoptysis or wheezing may develop 1–5 days after swallowing the eggs. Eosinophilia may be present. Clinical severity depends upon the worm load and reactivity of the host.

The liver may be enlarged and histology may show centrilobular necrosis. Rarely larvae may reach the brain, giving rise to convulsions. Other organs may also be affected.

Those due to adult worms: Light infestations are asymptomatic. Moderate worm loads produce abdominal pain, pica, diarrhea, abdominal distention and grinding of the teeth (bruxism). Infected children have voracious appetite but they remain malnourished despite adequate intake of food. Migration of worms to biliary ducts or pancreatic ducts lead to obstruction. In heavy infection, the masses of worms may lead to intestinal obstruction and they may be palpable (Fig. 67.2).

Diagnosis

It is made from the history of passing roundworms in the stool or the children may vomit roundworms. Diagnosis is confirmed by demonstrating the characteristic ova in feces. In the rare event of infection by male worms alone, ova may not be present in feces. During the stage of larval migration, the diagnosis has to be presumptive.

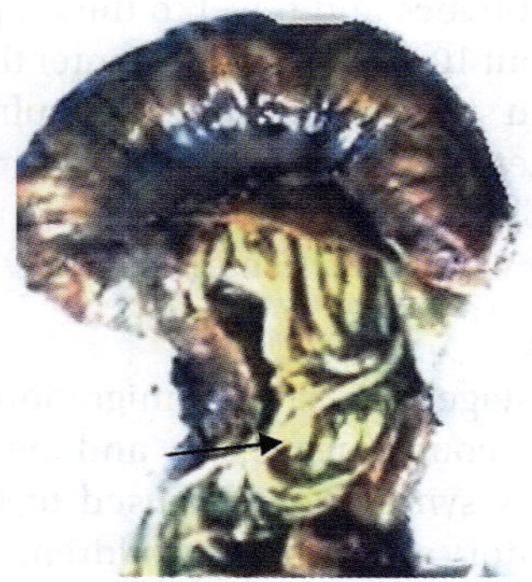

Fig. 67.2: Surgical resected specimen of partially devitalized ileum in *Ascaris lumbricoides* infection. ***Note:*** The large bunch of worms (several hundreds) (arrow)

Treatment

The adult worms respond to a variety of anthelmintics.

Effective, safe and polyvalent anthelmintics are preferred at present. In more than 30% of patients, multiple helminths occur, common combination being roundworm, whipworm and hookworm and broad-spectrum anthelmintics are more advantageous in them. Benzimidazole drugs, which include albendazole and mebendazole bind to nematode b tubulin and inhibit parasite microtubule polymerization which causes death of adult worms. This may take a few days to complete.

Albendazole in single dose of 400 mg for adults and 200 mg for children is the drug of choice due to its safety, ease of administration and easy availability. ***Mebendazole*** in a dose of 100 mg twice a day for three days is another equally effective alternative. The worms are killed and are eliminated in a partly digested manner. There is no danger of irritation of worms, exacerbation of symptoms or other untoward effects. The eradication rate of roundworms after single dose reaches 80–90% and above 95% after two doses given at weekly interval. Albendazole is ideal for mass therapy in community practice on the merit of its effectiveness, ease of administration and safety. Adverse side effects include gastrointestinal upsets, nausea, vomiting, abdominal pain, dizziness and rarely granulocytopenia. Albendazole is contraindicated during pregnancy.

Pyrantel pamoate, in a dose of 11 mg/kg given as a single dose at bedtime is a limited broad-spectrum anthelmintic active against roundworm, hookworm and pinworm. The drug eliminates the worms in up to 50% of subjects. It is safe in children.

Ivermectin 200 µg/kg in single oral doses is also effective against roundworms.

Children with intestinal obstruction are managed conservatively with intravenous (IV) fluids, gastric suction and antibiotics for 24 hours. If the mass of worms remains in the same position in the presence of severe abdominal colic and tenderness or if the general condition deteriorates as indicated by rising pulse rate and toxemia, etc. surgery is indicated. The worms are manipulated to break the mass without opening the intestine. Delayed surgery carries a high mortality.

Prevention

Improvement in nutritional status of children, health education, especially pertaining to personal hygiene and environmental sanitation reduce the infection rates. Mass deworming campaigns are helpful in endemic areas to reduce worm loads temporarily but reinfection within months is the rule.

Points to Remember

- No direct human-to-human transmission since *Ascaris* ova have to develop in the soil before they become infective.
- There is a pulmonary phase in the developmental cycle.
- No multiplication of roundworm in humans and the worm load depends on the number of eggs ingested.
- Clinical symptoms could either be due to the larvae or the adult worm.
- After administration of albendazole, usually intact worms are not seen in the stools, as the dead worms are partly digested.

Textbook of Medicine

HOOKWORM INFECTION

Syn: Ancylostomiasis

Hookworm infection is prevalent in hot damp areas throughout the tropics and subtropics. Two species of hookworms—*Ancylostoma duodenale* and *Necator americanus* are seen to parasitize the small intestine of man. *Ancylostoma* is more harmful than *Necator* because it is more persistent in the environment and causes heavier blood loss. *Ancylostoma* is seen in the tropical and temperate zones whereas *Necator* is more widespread in the tropics.

In the rural communities in India, the prevalence for hookworm in adults ranges from 10 to 35%. In children with increasing age, the prevalence rates also increase, being 0.5% at 1 year of age to 10% in the 12th year. In 60–70% of affected persons, *Ascaris lumbricoides* and *Trichuris trichiura* may also be present. In almost all parts of India, Far East, Africa and South America both types of hookworms are seen. In South India, *N. americanus* predominates. Some persons show a special predilection to acquire and sustain different intestinal nematodes.

Morphology and Habitat

Man is the natural host. The adults remain in the small intestine. Eggs are passed in feces.

Adult worm of *Ancylostoma duodenale* is 8–13 mm long and is thread-like in thickness. The buccal cavity has four pointed hook-like teeth. *Necator americanus* is smaller than *A. duodenale*. The buccal cavity contains two chitinous cutting plates (Figs 67.3 and 67.4).

The worms attach to the intestinal villi of the jejunum and duodenum by their mouthparts. They produce

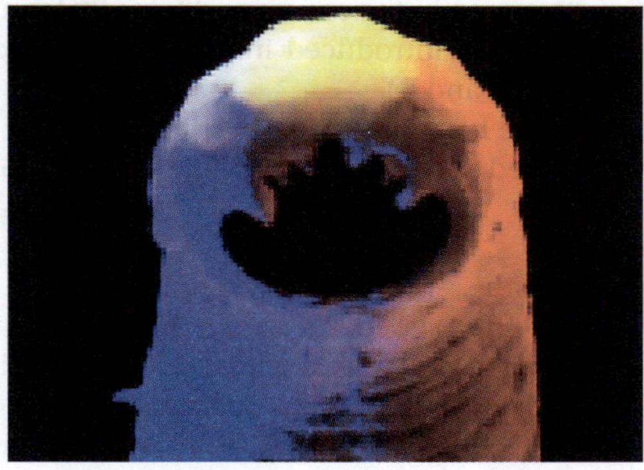

Fig. 67.3: Adult worm mouth parts *Ancylostoma duodenale*

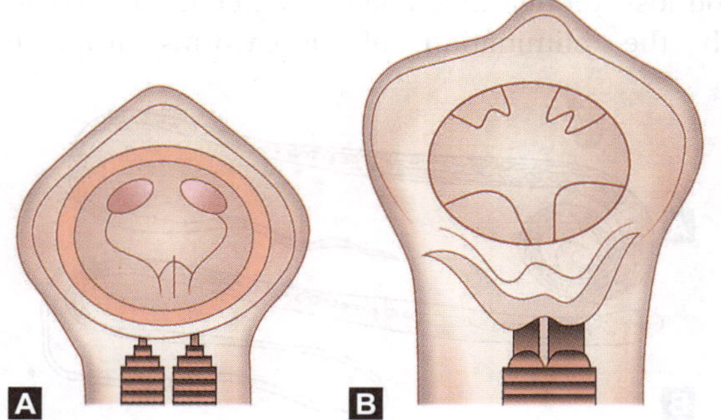

Figs 67.4A to B: Hookworms—buccal capsules. **A.** *Necator americanus*; **B.** *Ancylostoma duodenale*

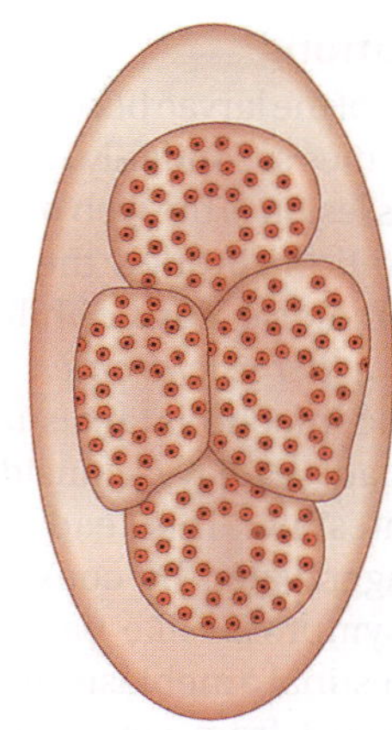

Fig 67.5: Hookworm eggs—the segmented embryo

bleeding points from which the blood passes through the alimentary canal of the worm continuously. This blood is required for the nutritive and respiratory functions of the worm. Hookworms produce pathogenesis-related proteins which prevent clotting by combining with platelets and inactivating them. In addition, factors that inhibit factor Xa, VIIa and tissue factor are also secreted. Thus, the worms ensure a continuous flow of blood through their intestinal tract. The loss of blood caused by a single ancylostoma is estimated to be 0.1–0.2 mL per day. Necator causes a blood loss of 0.01–0.03 mL. Worm loads above 40 can give rise to significant iron deficiency anemia over a period of time if there is added malnutrition as well.

The fertilized female can lay up to 20,000 eggs a day. The eggs measure 40–60 μm and are embryonated when passed. *Necator americanus* lays fewer eggs than *A. duodenale*, but the eggs are larger (60–70 μm) (Fig. 67.5).

Rarely two other species of hookworms—*Ancylostoma cyclonicum* and *Ancylostoma braziliense* may infect man. *A. cyclonicum* is a hookworm of cat found in the far East, which occasionally reaches maturity in humans. *A. braziliense* is a hookworm of dogs and cats, which may also infect man but does not reach maturity.

Life Cycle

Eggs are passed in feces and within 5 days they hatch in warm moist soil. The rhabditiform larvae come out and they moult twice on the third and fifth days and develop into filariform larvae, which develop a sheath. These are infective to man. The larvae can persist in the soil for two months, feeding on bacteria and other organic matter. On coming into contact with the skin of man, the sheath is shed and the larvae penetrate into the subcutaneous tissues and enter the lymphatics and venules.

Within three days of entry into the skin, the larvae pass through the right side of the heart and the pulmonary capillaries to enter alveolar spaces. Foci of inflammation develop in the lungs. Then they enter the bronchi and pass up the trachea, larynx and back of the pharynx to be swallowed. In the esophagus, a third molting occurs and a terminal buccal capsule is formed. In the small intestine, they attach to the villi and grow into adults in 3–5 weeks. Average lifespan of the worm is 2 years, but sometimes it may exceed 10 years.

Textbook of Medicine

Clinical Manifestations

Skin: The site of entry of the larvae becomes itchy and sodden. It ulcerates and becomes secondarily infected (ground itch). Common site for this lesion is the web of the toes.

Lungs: Larval migration through the lungs may lead to allergic symptoms, malaise, eosinophilia, dyspnea, cough and hemoptysis—*Loeffler's syndrome.*

Intestinal tract: Mild infections are usually asymptomatic. When the worm load is heavy, considerable blood loss occurs from the intestine. This leads to iron deficiency anemia, which is aggravated by coexistent malnutrition. Vague abdominal symptoms like pain resembling peptic ulcer or chronic intestinal amebiasis may develop.

Heavy infection: Apart from severe anemia, it leads to stunted growth, apathy, reduction of learning abilities in children, frequent absence from work and school, diminished productivity, impairment of immune responses, frequent respiratory infections and increased susceptibility to tuberculosis.

Diagnosis

The diagnosis is established by demonstrating the ova in feces. Ova of *A. duodenale* and *N. americanus* are indistinguishable. The feces gives positive reaction for occult blood. The worm load can be quantitated by egg counting using Kato-Katz cellophane thick smear technique or by Stoll's method when there is heavy infection. Each worm produces 30 eggs per gram of feces per day. Identification of species is carried out by examining the adult worms passed after a vermifuge.

Treatment

Specific treatment can be administered directly if the hemoglobin is above 7 g/dL. In severely anemic patients, proper diet and iron supplements are given to raise the hemoglobin to 5 g/dL or more before administering the anthelmintic. Though this is a golden rule to be followed in outpatient practice, specific anthelmintic treatment can be started much earlier using **albendazole** or **mebendazole**, which are considerably less toxic. Elimination of the worms leads to quicker recovery of the nutritional status as well.

Albendazole 400 mg single dose causes partial elimination of the worms along with other nematodes. Repeated doses may be required for complete elimination. The drug is best absorbed when given along with a fatty meal. It is available as 400 mg tablets and 200 mg suspension. Children above 2 years can be given the full doses. Younger children should be given 200 mg. Since the drug reaches several tissues, it may act on tissue forms of helminths as well. Albendazole has become more acceptable for mass therapy on account of its effectiveness, safety and convenience of dosage. The side effects are mild including gastrointestinal upset, allergy, headache, alopecia and rarely convulsions. Albendazole is contraindicated in pregnancy due to risk of teratogenicity.

Mebendazole is given in the dose of 100 mg twice daily for three consecutive days after food (for adults). It is poorly absorbed from the intestine and therefore its effect is mainly on the adult worms. This drug produces clearance of 80% of worms in a single course and almost complete clearance if two courses are administered at an interval of 2 weeks. Due to risk of teratogenicity, the drug is contraindicated during pregnancy and infancy.

Pyrantel pamoate, which is also a broadspectrum anthelmintic, given in a single dose of 11 mg/kg body weight is very effective in clearing the infection.

Prophylaxis

Personal measures include the use of proper footwear and sanitary disposal of excreta.

> **Points to Remember**
> - Ancylostomiasis is a geohelminth infection where skin lesions may be present at the site of larval entry.
> - There is a pulmonary phase during larval migration.
> - Clinical manifestations are mainly due to blood loss.
> - Occult blood may be present in stools in heavy infection.
> - Protective footwear, completely covering the feet, is important in preventing transmission.

TRICHURIASIS

Syn: Whipworm infection

Trichuris trichiura is worldwide in distribution. It is especially prevalent in the tropics. The prevalence rate in India varies from 6 to 25% in different communities. There is considerable geographical variation. Coinfection with roundworm and hookworm is very common.

Morphology and Habitat

The adult worm measures 30–50 mm in length, the females being larger than males. The anterior three-fifths is slender and filiform and the posterior two-fifths is bulky and fleshy. The worms are seen in the cecum and large intestine with their anterior ends introduced into the mucosa to suck blood (Figs 67.6A and B).

The eggs are barrel-shaped, translucent, 20–50 μm in size, thick-walled and possess knob-like ends (Fig. 67.7).

Life Cycle

The eggs become embryonated and infective in three weeks after being passed. They are ingested. Hatching occurs in the small intestine. The larvae get attached to the intestinal villi and after variable periods migrate to the large intestine where they mature in about 3 months. Though not exactly known, the lifespan of the worm is probably several years. The adults suck blood and lead to blood loss, though in a smaller degree than hookworms. With the elimination of hookworms from many

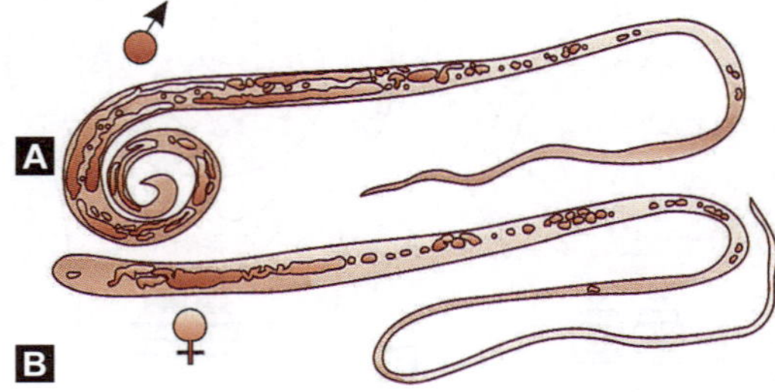

Figs 67.6A and B: *Trichuris trichiura*—adult. **A.** The slender anterior end; **B.** The thick posterior end

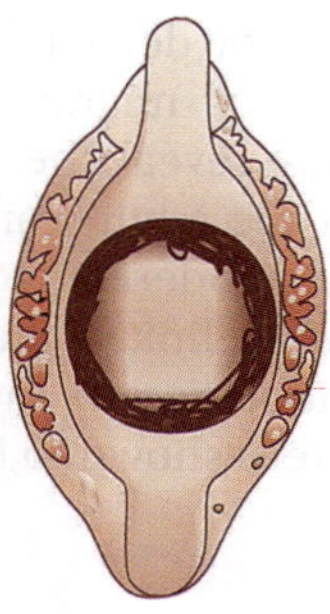

Fig. 67.7: *Trichuris trichiura—ovum*

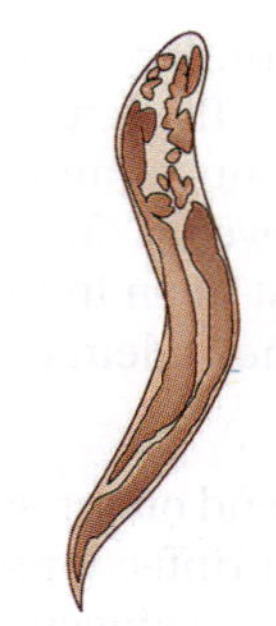

Fig. 67.8: Larva of *Strongyloides stercoralis*

communities, whipworms have emerged as a major cause of intestinal blood loss.

Clinical Manifestations

Mild infections pass unnoticed and the diagnosis is made by routine examination of feces. Heavy infection, which is common in children and certain susceptible subjects, is accompanied by nausea, vomiting, diarrhea and dysenteric symptoms. Diarrhea with mucus and even blood-streaking may occur. Rectal prolapse may develop. Malabsorption leads to wasting and stunting of growth in children. Iron deficiency anemia may develop.

Diagnosis

Demonstration of the eggs in feces establishes the diagnosis. Adult worms may be seen hanging from the walls of the colon on sigmoidoscopy.

Treatment

Albendazole, the drug of choice, given in a single dose of 400 mg gives a clearance rate of 30–90%. Administration for 2 to 3 days continuously increases the clearance rate and this may be required in heavy infection.

Mebendazole 100 mg tablets twice daily for three consecutive days produces a cure rate of 50–80%. Repeated courses improve the clearance rate. This drug should be used with caution in children and pregnant women.

Ivermectin, a newly introduced anthelmintic, is also effective against trichuriasis.

Oxantel pamoate 20 mg/kg/bw given on one or two days with albendazole 400 mg/day cured 31.2% of *T. trichiura* infection compared to 11.8% with mebendazole 500 mg given as single dose oral. Combination of oxantel pamoate and albendazole was more effective in *T. trichiura* infection. Side effects of oxantel pamoate were mild—such as abdominal cramps and headache.

Source: Speich B, Ame SM, Ali SM, et al. Oxantel pamoate-albendazole for Trichuris trichiura infection. N Engl J Med. 2014;370(7):610-20.

> **Points to Remember**
> - Trichuriasis is a geohelminth infection.
> - There is no phase of larval migration.
> - Like hookworm infection, trichuriasis can cause blood loss and anemia.
> - Severe infections may be associated with symptoms of dysentery.

STRONGYLOIDIASIS

Strongyloidiasis is infection of the small intestine by *Strongyloides stercoralis*. Adult females are small

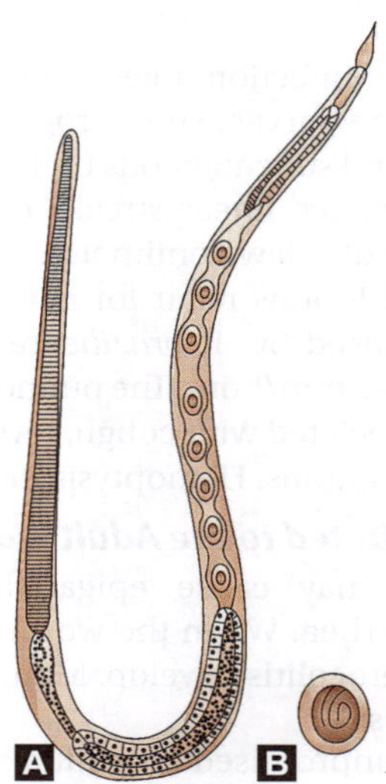

Figs 67.9A and B: *Strongyloides stercoralis.* **A.** Gravid female; **B.** Egg containing larva

measuring 2 mm in length. They live in the mucosa of the duodenum and lay eggs.

Life Cycle

The eggs are laid inside the mucous membrane. Soon the eggs hatch and the rhabditiform larvae enter the intestinal lumen by breaking the mucosa. These larvae are seen in fresh stools and their spring-like movement is diagnostic. *Strongyloides stercoralis* is known to take one of three life cycles (Figs 67.8 and 67.9).

1. ***In the soil:*** They develop into the infective filariform stage within three to four days. The larvae penetrate human skin to enter the blood vessels. An alternate mode of infection is accidental ingestion of infective larvae. They pass through the lungs and after a period of development, they are coughed up and swallowed. In the small intestine they mature and copulate. The fertilized female burrows into the mucosa of the jejunum while the males are passed in feces. Lifespan of the worm is not clearly known.

2. ***Free living cycle:*** *Strongyloides stercoralis* can develop as free-living worms in the soil. The rhabditiform larvae in soil may develop into free-living adults, which reproduce in the soil independent of the human host. Under favorable conditions, the free-living larvae can change into filariform larvae, which can enter the human skin and initiate a new cycle.

3. ***Autoinfection:*** By this life cycle, the worm perpetuates itself without leaving the host. The rhabditiform larvae

Textbook of Medicine

change into filariform larvae in the large intestine or in the perianal skin. The latter penetrate the mucosa or skin to enter venules and reach the pulmonary circulation and develop further. In this way, the infection can persist in an individual for long periods even after leaving the endemic area.

Clinical Features

Clinical symptoms depend on the severity of infection and reactivity of the host. Mild infections may be asymptomatic. In immunocompromised subjects hyperinfection occurs which may be fatal.

Larval Migration

Local allergy and infection may appear at the site of penetration by the larvae. The progress of the larvae through the skin and subcutaneous tissue (cutaneous larva migrans) may produce linear streaks of urticaria, which progress at a rate of a few centimeters every hour. Crops of these urticarial lesions recur for considerable periods. Larva migrans caused by *A. braziliense* and *A. caninum* move at a rate of 1–2 mm/hour. The pulmonary phase of the larvae may be associated with cough, fever, breathlessness and asthmatic symptoms. Hemoptysis may occur rarely.

Symptoms Attributed to the Adult Worm

Heavy infection may cause epigastric pain, nausea, vomiting and diarrhea. When the worm load is very high symptoms of enterocolitis develop. Meningeal irritation is seen in a few cases.

In immunocompromised individuals, strongyloidiasis may take a severe and fatal form of hyperinfection; may present as malabsorption syndrome or chronic diarrhea resembling Crohn's disease. Elimination of larvae in feces may be episodic and therefore the diagnosis may be missed by single examination of feces. Diagnosis can be confirmed by biopsy of small intestine. Extensive dissemination of the larvae can present with respiratory, cardiovascular, hepatic and central nervous manifestation rarely. Immunosuppressive interventions in persons harboring chronic strongyloides infection may lead to strongyloides hyperinfection syndrome. Glucocorticoid therapy, human immunodeficiency virus (HIV) infection, human T-cell lymphotropic virus (HTLV) infection, use of monoclonal antibodies and immunosuppressants may precipitate this syndrome. Rapid proliferation of the larvae and worms occur with accelerated autoinfection and bloodstream invasion. Organ involvement includes invasion of the liver, brain, kidneys, meninges and skin by filariform larvae. Penetration of the intestinal wall leads to transfer of intestinal bacteria to the peritoneum. The bacteria include Gram-negative *Enterobacteriaceae* species and *Streptococcus bovis* (present name *Strep. gallolyticus-subspecies pasteuriansis*). This can lead to meningitis. Treatment consists in management of meningitis and use of ivermectin.

Source: Keiser PB, Nutman TB. Strongyloides stercoralis in the Immunocompromised Population. Clin Microbiol Rev. 2004;17(1):208-17.

Diagnosis

It is established by demonstrating the larvae or adult worms. Larvae can be demonstrated in fresh fecal samples. The larvae may be detected in the sputum during the pulmonary phase of migration. Accidentally, the duodenal aspirate may reveal the larvae and intestinal biopsy may bring out the adult worm. During the phase of larval migration, moderate to high eosinophilia may be seen. Enzyme linked immunosorbent assay (ELISA) detecting antibodies to the excretory-secretory antigens of the parasite is shown to be highly specific and sensitive.

Treatment

Once the infection is diagnosed, treatment must be given, irrespective of the symptoms. Ivermectin is the drug of choice. It is given in doses of 200 µg/kg orally for 1–2 days. Cure rates reported range from 82 to 98%.

Thiabendazole, which is available as tablets or suspension, is the alternative drug. This is given in a dose of 25 mg/kg twice a day for 3 days. Thiabendazole is generally safe, but vomiting and vertigo may occur at times, which are self-limiting. Clearance of the worms occurs in over 80% of cases. Repetition of the drug after 3 months may be necessary if the larvae are demonstrable in feces or allergic manifestations persist.

Albendazole in a dose of 400 mg orally once a day is also effective. Repetition of 3 doses at weekly intervals gives higher clearance rates.

Ivermectin in doses of 200–400 µg/kg bw depending on the response, is highly effective and lifesaving.

Prevention

The general principles mentioned in the case of hookworms are applicable in the case of *Strongyloides*, but treatment has to be repeated to eradicate the infection due to the phenomenon of autoinfection.

Points to Remember

- *Strongyloides stercoralis* is known to have three different life cycles.
- Infection tends to be severe and fatal in immunocompromised host.
- Apart from lungs, larval migration can occur through the skin.
- Only larvae (not ova) are seen in the stools.
- Ivermectin is the drug of choice.

ENTEROBIASIS

Syn: Oxyuriasis, Threadworm, Pinworm, Seat worm

Enterobiasis is caused by *Enterobius vermicularis* (also known as *Oxyuris vermicularis),* the adults of which inhabit the large intestine, especially the cecum, rectum and anal canal. The infection occurs worldwide and is seen more in children.

The female is 8–13 mm long and has the thickness of a thread. The male is 2–5 mm long. The egg, which contains a well-formed larva when passed, is plano-convex, 20 × 50 µm in size and is infective when laid (Figs 67.10 and 67.11).

Life Cycle

The gravid female comes out of the anus to lay eggs in the perianal and perineal skin, usually during sleep. Intense itching results in scratching and the ova contaminate fingers of the host. These are swallowed accidentally by the same host or may be spread to others. The ova hatch in the intestine and the larvae migrate to the colon to mature.

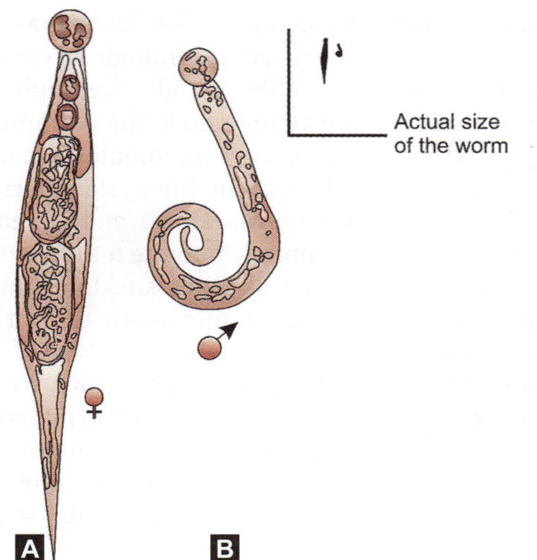

Figs 67.10A and B: *Enterobius vermicularis*—adult. **A.** Male; **B.** Female

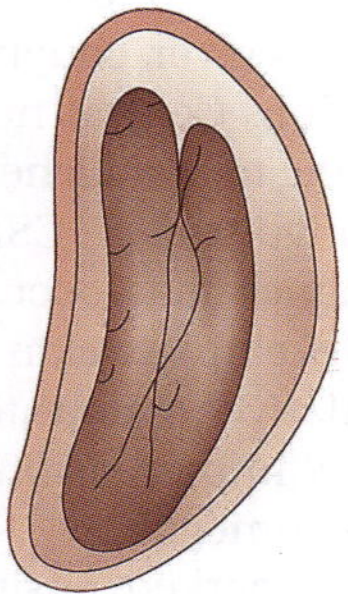

Fig. 67.11: Ovum of *E. vermicularis*. **Note:** Larva inside

Lifespan is 4–6 weeks. This infection can perpetuate itself in the same host for long periods.

Clinical Features

The patient may complain of passing pinworms in stools. Symptoms are produced by the adult female, which migrates to lay eggs. It results in perianal pruritus and excoriation due to scratching. In females, severe pruritus vulvae and mild vulvitis may develop. Children may suffer from nocturnal enuresis, insomnia and allergic manifestations.

Diagnosis

The condition can be diagnosed by observing the worms in the perianal region while the child is asleep or on the surface of the feces. Ova can be demonstrated by examining a scotch-tape swab prepared from the perianal skin. A cellophane tape is applied to the uncleansed perianal region in the morning, with the sticky side up, to collect the ova. After removal it is placed on a clean glass slide, sticky side down with a drop of toluene over the slide and examined under the low power of the microscope to detect the eggs.

In heavy infections, material collected by digital examination of the rectum shows the ova.

Course

The infection is self-limiting if autoinfection is prevented, otherwise it persists for long periods due to reinfection. Members of the same household get cross infection.

Treatment

Single dose oral treatment with mebendazole 200 mg, albendazole 400 mg or pyrantel pamoate 10 mg/kg are all effective. The parasite can be eradicated from the household only if all affected persons are treated simultaneously. Some persons have a particular predilection to get the infection repeatedly. In them repeated deworming may be required. Ivermectin 200 µg/kg in single oral doses is also effective against threadworms.

> **Points to Remember**
> - Threadworm infection presents with nocturnal, perianal pruritus and in females pruritus vulvae.
> - Ova are not seen in stools and are demonstrated only by scotch tape technique.
> - Because of direct human infection, members of whole household need to be treated.
> - Repeated courses of treatment necessary due to high incidence of reinfection.

TRICHINOSIS

Syn: Trichinosis, Trichinellosis

This is only rarely seen in India. Trichinellosis is caused by *Trichinella spiralis*, a nematode parasite of several animals such as the rat, pig, polar bear, etc. Infection in humans occurs when meat containing infective larvae is ingested without proper cooking. The disease has been reported from many parts of Europe, North and West USA, African countries and China.

Common mode of infection is through partially cooked pork sausages. The pig acquires infection by eating infected rats or the offal of infected pigs. Both adults and larvae are seen in the same hosts, but two hosts are required to complete the life cycle.

Morphology and Life Cycle

The adult female varies in size from 3–4 mm × 40–60 µm. The male is only half this length. When meat containing viable larvae is ingested, the larvae escape in the intestinal lumen, penetrate the mucosal cells of the duodenum and grow into adults in 5–7 days. After fertilization, the female discharges larvae, which embolize to many tissues. Those reaching the muscles encyst themselves in an oval capsule measuring 0.8 mm, grow, mature and become infective after 16 days. They remain viable for 6 months and thereafter die and become calcified. Each female may liberate 1000–1500 larvae during its lifespan. The male lives for about a week, while the female lives for 3–16 weeks. Intercostal muscles, pectoral muscles, diaphragm and shoulder girdle muscles are heavily affected.

Clinical Features

Symptoms depend upon the heaviness of infection. Mild infection may be asymptomatic. Within the first 1–2 days after ingestion, fever, abdominal pain, nausea, vomiting and diarrhea may develop. Larval dissemination starts around the seventh day and is marked by urticarial rash, remittent fever, edema of the eyelids, conjunctivitis and subungual splinter hemorrhages. Neurological manifestations include polyneuritis, polio-like paralysis, myasthenia, meningoencephalitis and psychosis. The cerebrospinal fluid (CSF) does not show any abnormality. Myocarditis may occur. This is characterized by persistent tachycardia

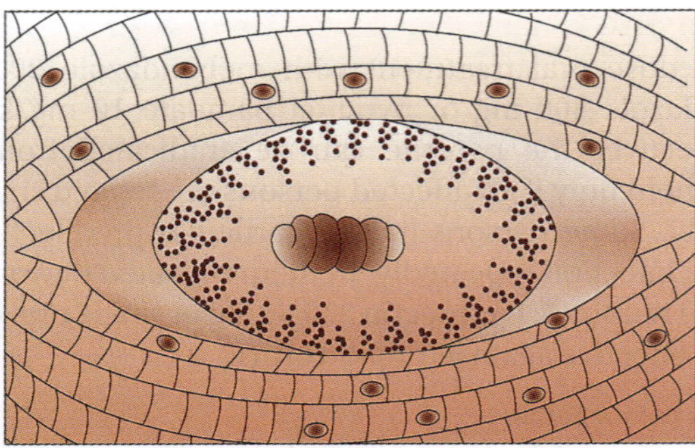

Fig. 67.12: *Trichinella spiralis* larva in striated muscle biopsy

and congestive failure. In 20% of cases, electrocardiography (ECG) shows ST-T wave changes and conduction defects.

Diagnosis

Eosinophilia is a constant finding in the early stages. Erythrocyte sedimentation rate (ESR) is invariably normal. Serum muscle enzymes are elevated. Skin test using the larval antigen is not useful to diagnose active infection since it remains positive for even up to 20 years after infection. Useful serological tests are ELISA, immunofluorescent test and bentonite flocculation test. Muscle biopsy from the deltoid or gastrocnemius shows encysted or calcified larvae and evidence of myositis (Fig. 67.12).

The acute stage of larval migration has to be differentiated from other conditions characterized by allergic manifestations and muscular pains such as dermatomyositis, other forms of polymyositis, polyarthritis nodosa, serum sickness and food poisoning.

Treatment

Available anthelmintic drugs are not proved to be effective once the parasite invades the muscles. They may be useful during the intestinal phase of infection. Thus albendazole 400 mg twice a day for 10 days; mebendazole 200–400 mg thrice a day for 10 days or thiabendazole 25 mg/kg given twice daily for 5-7 days all are effective. During the phase of muscle invasion, antihistamines, corticosteroids and analgesics may be required for obtaining symptomatic relief. The overall mortality is around 2%.

Prevention

The larvae in meat can be destroyed by proper cooking or deep-freezing at –18°C for 24 hours.

Points to Remember
- Trichinellosis is rare in India.
- This parasitic infection has to be differentiated from common collagen vascular diseases.
- Eosinophilia associated with normal ESR is suggestive of *Trichinella spiralis* infection.
- Anthelmintics are not proved to be of use in the muscle invasion phase.

LARVA MIGRANS

Visceral Larva Migrans

The term ***visceral larva migrans*** is used to denote the manifestations produced by larvae of nonhuman ascarids, when they migrate through human tissues. Most often the ascarids of dogs and cats—*Toxocara canis* and *Toxocara*

catis—are the common offenders. Possibly larvae of other helminths also may be causative. Though larvae migrate in human tissues for variable periods, the adults do not develop in man. The larvae migrate in the pulmonary and visceral capillaries evoking a granulomatous reaction in various organs. They die and the life cycle is terminated at this stage in noncanine hosts. However, in female dogs the larvae pass transplacentally into the fetus *in utero* and into the puppies through milk while suckling. The adults develop in the puppies. They eliminate the eggs in feces in the first few months.

Children between the age of one and four, who are in close contact with puppies, are at high risk of infection. The infection is acquired by ingesting dirt containing the ova. The larvae are liberated in the jejunum and they migrate into tissues like liver, lungs, heart, brain, ocular structures, kidneys and muscles.

Clinical Features

In the majority of cases the condition is asymptomatic. In a few, symptoms such as fever, cough, wheeze, abdominal pain and pallor develop. Central nervous system (CNS) may be involved leading to headache, visual disturbances, strabismus and convulsions. CSF pleocytosis with eosinophil predominance may occur. Nodular eruptions and urticaria may develop as skin manifestations. Eye lesions include exudative endophthalmitis and retinal granuloma. These may impair vision considerably. Some children develop hepatomegaly.

Leukocytosis with marked eosinophilia is common during acute phase of infection. ELISA detecting larval antibodies is highly specific and sensitive.

Treatment

Visceral larva migrans is self-limiting, since the encysted larvae die out after varying periods. Involvement of liver, lung, brain or eyes calls for treatment.

Available anthelmintics have not proved to be effective in ***visceral larva migrans***. Albendazole, mebendazole, thiabendazole and ivermectin are tried empirically. Albendazole 400 mg twice daily or mebendazole 200–400 mg twice daily are given for 21 days. Thiabendazole is given in a dose of 50 mg/kg bw in divided doses daily for 2–3 days.

Antihistamines and corticosteroids are required to suppress the allergic response. Pulmonary lesion, chorioretinitis and neurological involvement are indications for corticosteroids. Ocular lesions may progress further even after specific anthelmintic therapy and, therefore, prolonged follow-up is necessary in such cases.

Larva migrans can be prevented by proper deworming of newborn pets and avoiding contamination of children's playground with the excreta of these animals.

Cutaneous Larva Migrans

The larvae of *A. braziliense* and *A. caninum* (dog's and cat's hookworms) and *Strongyloides stercoralis* cause creeping eruption. The larvae, which are present in soil penetrate the intact skin and enter the tissues. In the subcutaneous tissues, they cause multiple, intensely pruritic serpiginous tracts. While the larvae of *A. braziliense* and *A. caninum* progress forwards at a rate of 2–3 mm per hour, those of *S. stercoralis* progress a few cm at a time. At the anterior end of the eruption the larva is present and a bleb may form. Since the larvae ultimately die, the lesions are self-limiting. The eruptions due to strongyloides tend to persist for several years, if left untreated.

Treatment

Albendazole 400mg given orally for 5 days or ivermectin 200 µg/kg single dose are the treatment of choice on account of their safety. Antihistamines help to suppress the pruritus.

Points to Remember

- Larva migrans in humans is mostly caused from accidental infection by helminths from animals.
- Marked eosinophilia is common during active infection.
- Anthelmintics are generally not proved to be effective.
- *S. stercoralis* can cause rapidly progressing cutaneous larva migrans.

68

Cestodiasis

RK Shenoy, KV Krishna Das

Chapter Summary

- General Considerations
- *Taeniasis saginata*
- *Taeniasis solium* and Cysticercosis
- Echinococciasis
- *Diphyllobothriasis latum*
- *Hymenolepis nana*
- *Hymenolepis diminuta*
- *Dipylidium caninum*

GENERAL CONSIDERATIONS

Cestodes or tapeworms are segmented flat ribbon-like hermaphrodite worms that inhabit the small intestines of men or animals. The head (scolex) is at the anterior end and the body (strobila) is made up of segments. The head is small in size and it is provided with suckers, which help the worm to attach to the intestinal mucosa. The scolex contains hooklets in some species. The body consists of a short neck and a chain of successive segments (proglottids). Every proglottid is a complete hermaphrodite unit. The proglottids are formed near the head as the worm grows. The segments near the head are immature, the intermediate ones are mature with fully developed gonads and the distal ones are gravid, filled by the uterus containing numerous eggs. Cross-fertilization occurs between adjacent segments. Tapeworms have no body cavity or digestive tract. Nutrients are absorbed by the surface. They require 2 or 3 hosts for completion of their life cycle. More than 30 species have been found to infect man but only six of them are common. These are *Taenia solium, T. saginata, T. echinococcus, Diphyllobothrium latum, Hymenolepis nana* and *H. diminuta*.

TAENIASIS SAGINATA

Syn: Beef tapeworm, Unarmed tapeworm

Taeniasis saginata is infection caused by *Taenia saginata*. This is the most common among the large tapeworms found in man and is distributed worldwide. Prevalence is highest in areas where beef is a major source of meat. The adult worm grows to a length of 10 meters and may consist of over 2000 segments. It lies free in the jejunum and ileum, the head being attached to the mucosa. The scolex is 2 mm in diameter and bears no hooklets, but has four suckers. The gravid segments are actively motile and they come out in chains along with feces or wriggle out singly due to their intrinsic muscular action. The uterus has about 20 lateral branches.

The eggs are spherical measuring 30–45 µ in diameter and the eggshell is thick, striated and bile-stained. The embryo or oncosphere bears six hooklets and it remains viable for 4–8 weeks. The adult worm may live for 10–25 years.

Life Cycle

Man is the definitive host and cattle and llamas form the intermediate hosts. Eggs passed in feces contaminate soil. These are ingested by grazing cattle. The oncospheres are liberated in the intestine and they penetrate the mucosa, enter the blood stream and reach various muscles, mainly those of the heart, tongue, shoulder, neck and loins. On reaching these sites, the oncospheres lose their hooks and grow into the cystic stage known as ***cysticercus bovis*** in 60–70 days. The cysticercus is ovoid, measures 8 × 5 mm and contains a single sprouting scolex. Cysticercus remains viable for 1–3 years within the muscles. Heavily infected meat is easy to distinguish by the presence of numerous cysts.

On ingesting undercooked meat, the cyst wall is digested and the head attaches itself to the intestinal mucosa and rapidly grows to reach the adult size in 6–8 weeks. A host usually harbors only one or two worms.

Clinical Features

Majority is asymptomatic, though vague symptoms such as abdominal pain, diarrhea and increased appetite may occur in a few. The motile segments emerging out of the anus may cause pruritus and anxiety to the host. Appendicitis and biliary obstruction have been reported rarely.

Diagnosis

History of passing segments and seeing the segments in feces confirm the diagnosis. The species can be identified by observing the number of lateral branches of the uterus. An easy method is to press the segment between two glass slides and to hold it against light. *Taenia saginata* segment has more than 15 lateral branches, whereas *Taenia solium* has only less than 13.

Eggs can be demonstrated by microscopic examination of the feces or by examining perianal scotch tape swab. The eggs of *T. saginata*, *T. solium* and *T. echinococcus* cannot be differentiated from each other.

Treatment

Both niclosamide (Yomesan) and praziquantel are effective against *T. saginata*. Niclosamide kills the scolex and segments on contact. Four tablets, each of 0.5 g, are given as a single dose to be thoroughly chewed in the morning with a gulp of water. The worm is passed partially digested 24–36 hour later. If the whole worm including the scolex is not passed, the worm regrows and segments reappear in stools within 3 months. In this case the drug is repeated in the same dose.

Praziquantel in a dose of 10–15 mg/kg bw given as a single dose orally is adequate to dislodge the intestinal adult worm in almost all cases. The drug is generally safe. Side effects include dizziness, headache, vomiting and allergy. It is available as tablets of 500 mg and 600 mg.

Prevention

Taenia saginata infection can be prevented by avoiding infected beef, inspection of slaughterhouses and proper disposal of excreta.

> **Points to Remember**
> - *T. saginata* is the longest tapeworm infecting humans.
> - Passing motile segments in stools is diagnostic.
> - Morphology of ova does not help to differentiate the different tapeworms.
> - There is no tissue invasion in humans.

TAENIASIS SOLIUM AND CYSTICERCOSIS

Syn: Pork tapeworm, Armed tapeworm

The adult of *Taenia solium* inhabits the small intestine of man. The larval stage of *T. solium* may remain encysted in several tissues. This condition is called cysticercosis. *Taenia solium* is seen all over the world, especially in those countries where pork is a major source of meat. With the availability of computed tomography (CT) and magnetic resonance imaging (MRI) of brain, more and more cases of cysticercosis are being diagnosed in many parts of India. *T. solium* is present in all areas, though it is less common than *T. saginata* (Figs 68.1A and C).

Morphology

The adult worm is 3 meters in length and the proglottids are less than a thousand in number. The scolex is globular and 1 mm in diameter. It bears a rostellum with a row of hooklets and four suckers. The name solium is derived from the shape of the rostellum, which resembles the conventional figure of the sun.

The gravid uterus has a main stem with 8–10 compound lateral branches on either side. The worm has a long life span anecdotally stated as extending up to 25 years but, actually may be only up to 5 years. Eggs are

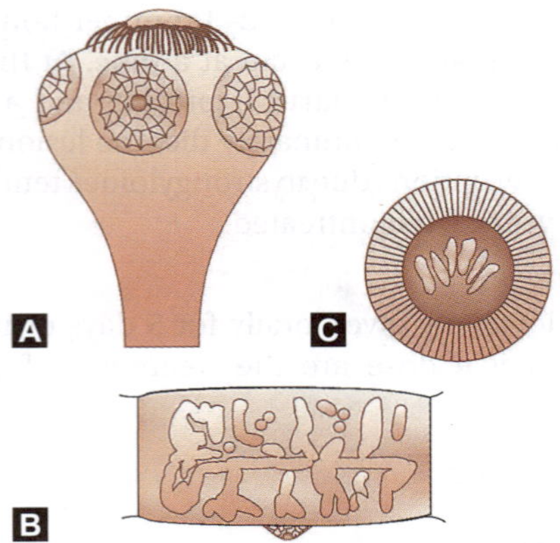

Figs 68.1A and C: *Taenia solium*. **A.** Scolex; **B.** Gravid proglottids; **C.** Ovum

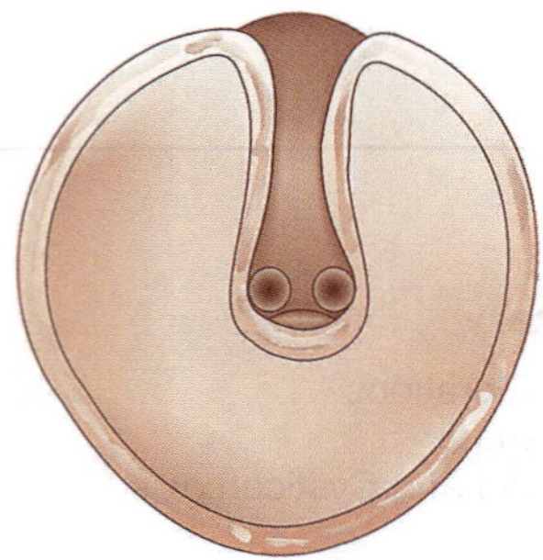

Fig. 68.2: *Taenia solium*—cysticercus cellulosae

indistinguishable from those of *T. saginata*. Larvae are found encysted in tissues. The cyst is oval in shape (5 × 20 mm) and contains an invaginated scolex (Fig. 68.2).

Life Cycle

Man is the definitive host. Pigs and occasionally man form the intermediate hosts. Segments containing eggs passed in the feces are eaten up by pigs. The hexacanth embryos liberated in the intestine of the pig penetrate the gut wall and reach several tissues through the blood stream. Muscles of limbs, tongue and neck are affected more. Within 60–70 days, the embryos develop into cysts called ***cysticercus cellulosae*** (bladder worm). The cysticerci live up to 8 months after which they die. Heavily infected pork is known as ***measly pork***. Man gets the infection by eating undercooked infected pork. The larvae are liberated in the intestines. They attach to the jejunal mucosa and grow into adult worms in 2–3 months after which segments are passed in stools.

Clinical Manifestations

Intestinal infection leads to minimal symptoms or none at all. The patient may complain of passing segments in strips and this may lead to anxiety.

Cysticercosis

When man ingests the eggs or when the gravid segments with ova reach the stomach by reverse peristalsis, the eggshell is digested and larvae escape. The liberated embryo penetrates the mucosa. The larvae are disseminated to various tissues in the circulation and they develop into cysticerci. Cysticercosis is the result of the complex encounter between a highly sophisticated

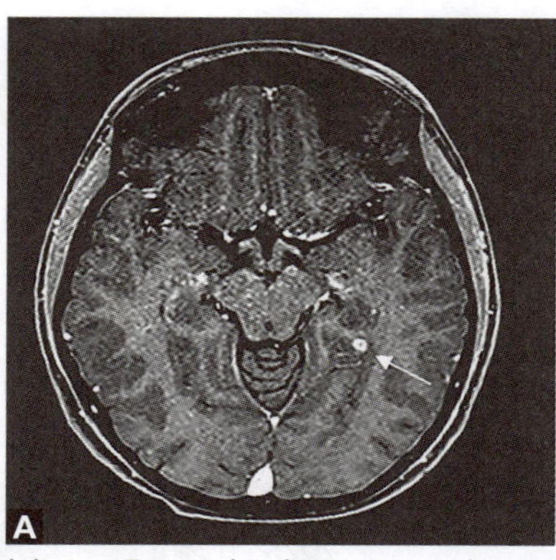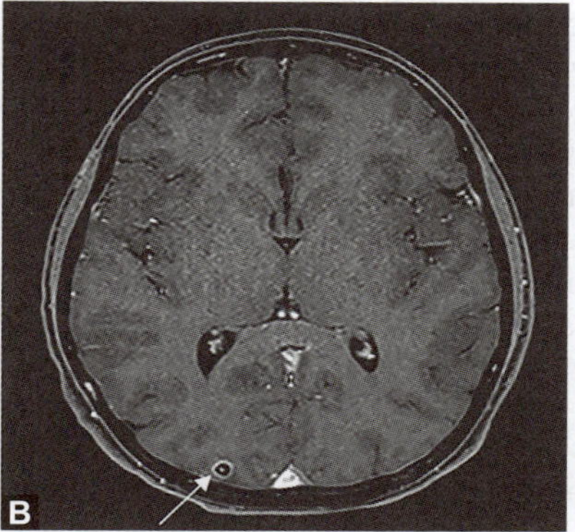

Figs 68.3A and B: Post gadolinium T1 weighted MRI: Ring enhancing lesions in medial. **A.** Left temporal lobe; **B.** Right occipital lobe. Arrow showing cysticercosis

parasite and an elaborate immune response. This can lead to rapid elimination of the parasite in some cases. In others the parasites persist and grow. The cysts are found mostly in the subcutaneous tissues, eyes, brain and bones and they remain viable for three years. Viable cysts do not cause any tissue reaction. When they die, the cysts swell up and provoke foreign body reaction in the tissues and general symptoms in the form of fever, eosinophilia, arthralgia and muscular pain. Ultimately, the cysts get calcified and can be seen in X-rays. The disease may be seen in strict vegetarians as well.

Neurocysticercosis

This has emerged as a common cause of seizures and intracranial space occupying lesion in many parts of India. The cysts developing in the nervous system may be situated in the parenchyma of the brain, subarachnoid space, meninges and ventricles or rarely in the spinal cord. They may present with focal or general neurological manifestations such as epilepsy, focal neurological deficits referable to brain or spinal cord, rise in intracranial tension and progressive or intermittent hydrocephalus. The commonest presentation is late onset epilepsy. The cysts in the brain do not calcify readily as in other tissues. In the eyes, the cysts provoke uveitis and retinal hemorrhage and they can be seen by ophthalmoscope. In the skin and muscles, they are palpable as small nodules. Sometimes affected muscles undergo pseudohypertrophy.

The advent of CT has revealed that cysticercosis exists in all communities irrespective of their dietary habits.

Diagnosis

T. solium is diagnosed by observing the gravid segments or eggs in feces. The gravid segments show distinctive features. The ova of all the Taeniae are identical morphologically. Examination of feces is quite adequate to diagnose the infection in almost all cases. Sophisticated tests to detect specific coproantigen by enzyme-linked immunosorbent assay (ELISA) are available. So also specific deoxyribonucleic acid (DNA) based studies are available to detect carrier state.

Cysticercosis is suspected by history and clinical examination. Calcified cysts may be seen by radiological examination of soft tissues. Occasionally, ocular cysticerci can be seen at funduscopy. CT scan and MRI scan are excellent methods to visualize cysticerci, which give diagnostic patterns. Both CT and MRI are reliable methods to dia-

gnose neurocysticercosis and follow-up treatment results (Figs 68.3A and B). Parenchymal cysticerci appear as multiple cortical and subcortical circumscribed lesions about 1 cm in diameter with perilesional edema appearing as a ring lesion. Contrast enhancement suggests active inflammation. The differential diagnosis includes tuberculosis and fungal infections. ELISA to detect antibodies to cysticercal antigens is helpful in diagnosis. Enzyme-linked immunoelectrotransfer blot (EITB) is shown to be more specific and sensitive.

Treatment

Niclosamide is effective in killing the adult worms in a dose of 2 g, but the worm is disintegrated and this may liberate the ova. Due to the risk of cysticercosis, this drug is better avoided. Praziquantel in a single dose of 15–20 mg/kg is effective against the adult. It is preferable since it has action against cysticerci too.

Treatment of Neurocysticercosis

The drug of choice is **albendazole** given orally in a dose of 15 mg/kg/day for 8 days**.** It is a benzimidazole compound, which is readily absorbed from the gut. Albendazole prevents glucose uptake by the parasite membrane, thereby leading to energy depletion. It reaches high concentration in most of the tissues and so it exerts wormicidal effects in tissue forms of helminths. The success rate is 80%. Albendazole can be safely administered with anticonvulsant drugs without affecting their efficacy.

Being embryotoxic and teratogenic, albendazole is contraindicated in pregnancy. Toxic effects include abdominal pain, nausea, vomiting, dizziness, headache, rashes, pruritus, leukopenia, alopecia, eosinophilia, jaundice and nonspecific rise of hepatic transaminases.

Praziquantel which is also a broad-spectrum anthelmintic is effective against cysticerci when given in a dose of 50 mg/kg/day for 15 days. The success rate is 60–70%. It exerts its action by producing muscular paralysis and destroying the scolices.

Treatment using albendazole or praziquantel should be started only after hospitalizing the patient. This is necessary since the dying parasites induce inflammatory reactions in the surrounding tissue resulting in features of meningism or signs of raised intracranial tension. These reactions require measures to reduce the inflammation and raised tension, along with antiepileptic drugs.

In late cases, where arachnoiditis and hydrocephalus have set in, results may not be fully satisfactory even after eradicating the cysticerci.

Symptomatic measures include the control of seizures by antiepileptic drugs, control of cerebral edema and anti-inflammatory drugs. Rarely surgery may be required to relieve obstructive hydrocephalus. Corticosteroids are indicated when there is raised intracranial tension, signs of meningoencephalitis or ocular cysticercosis.

Prevention

The infection can be prevented by cooking pork thoroughly and by proper disposal of human excreta.

Eradication of cysticercosis:

- Avoid open defecation which contaminates pig's environment.
- Treating pigs and humans who harbor *T. solium* with niclosamide.
- A vaccine has been developed at the University of Melbourne, Australia which clears the pigs of the infection. It is still used only in veterinary medicine.
- The drug oxfendazole clears the pigs of the infection.
- Diagnosis of cysticercosis by detecting parasite antigens in infected humans is possible which is a more sensitive method of diagnosis.
- World Health Organization (WHO) is starting programs for control of human and pig cysticercosis with a view to eradication of the disease.

Source: Maurice J. Of pigs and people—WHO prepares to battle cysticercosis. Lancet. 2014;384(9943):571-2.

> **Points to Remember**
> - Cysticercosis can occur both in vegetarians and nonvegetarians.
> - Neurocysticercosis is a common cause of epilepsy and focal neurological deficits in endemic areas.
> - A high index of suspicion is required to make a clinical diagnosis of neurocysticercosis.
> - Treatment with albendazole or praziquantel should be given after hospitalization due to risk of inflammation induced by the dying parasites.

ECHINOCOCCOSIS

Syn: Dog tapeworm or Hydatid worm

Definition

Infection of human tissues by larval form of *Echinococcus granulosus* and less commonly *E. multilocularis* is termed echinococcosis. The disease is worldwide in distribution. It is more common in sheep-rearing countries, both in the tropic and temperate zones. Close contact between man, dog and sheep favors this infection. *E. granulosus* is widely distributed in India and the disease is seen endemically or sporadically.

Morphology

The adult worm is small, measuring only 3–6 mm in length. The scolex bears four suckers and rostellum with two rows of hooklets. There are only three segments. The last segment is mature and gravid. Dogs pass the ova in their feces. The ova resemble those of *T. saginata* and contain the infective embryo. Larval forms occur within hydatid cysts. A single metastasized larva settles in tissues and grows to form a hydatid cyst. The germinal layer of the hydatid cyst gives rise to successive generations of embryos, ultimately

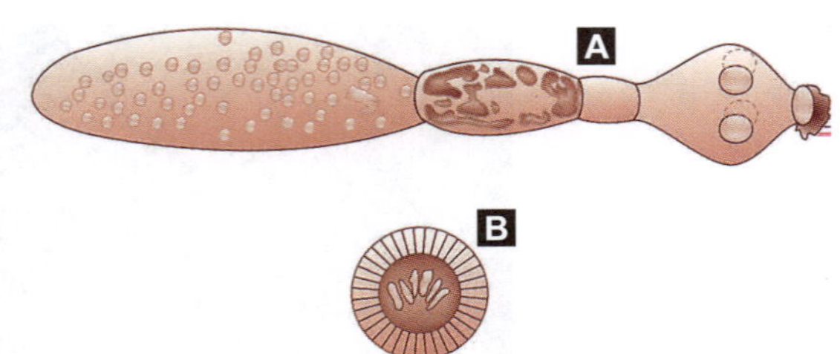

Fig. 68.4: *Echinococcus granulosus.* **A.** Adult; **B.** Ovum

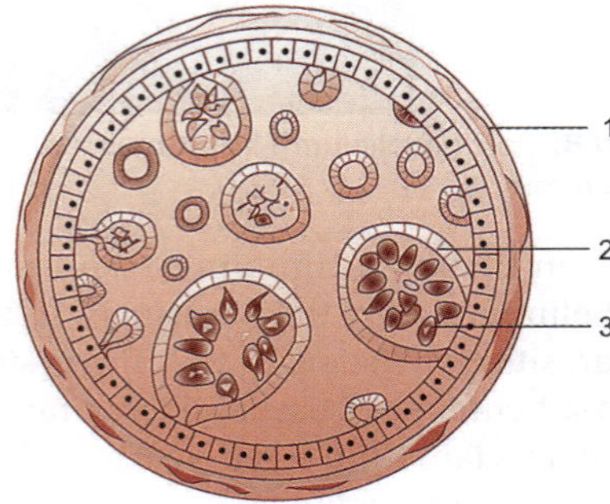

Fig. 68.5: Hydatid cyst (diagram): 1. Outer wall, 2. Brood capsules and 3. Scolices

leading to the development of several thousand infective larvae from a single egg (Figs 68.4 and 68.5).

Life Cycle

Definitive hosts are the dogs, wolves, jackals and other canines. Intermediate hosts are sheep, pigs, goats and humans. Sheep are the optimum intermediate hosts and they serve to perpetuate the natural life cycle of the parasite. The eggs passed in dog feces are ingested by the intermediate hosts. The embryos are liberated in the intestines. They penetrate the mucosa and enter the portal radicles to reach the liver. The larvae are arrested mainly in the liver and lungs but some may escape into the systemic circulation to reach other viscera like the brain, bones and kidneys. Within 3–6 weeks they grow into vesicles 5–10 mm in diameter and these are known as hydatid cysts (hydatids = drops of water). They grow to reach large sizes and the parasite multiplies in number.

The hydatid cyst has a thick fibrous outer wall and an internal germinal layer, from which brood capsules containing budding scolices arise. These may separate from the capsule and float inside as daughter cysts. The hydatid fluid is a clear colorless fluid, which is highly antigenic. On keeping it, a granular deposit forms at the bottom (hydatid sand), which contains free scolices and brood capsules.

When the hydatid cyst or scolices are ingested by the definitive hosts, they attach to the intestinal mucosa and grow into adults. Each animal may harbor many worms.

Clinical Features

Infected dogs are asymptomatic. In human hydatid disease, symptoms are due to allergic reactions and mechanical compression of the surrounding tissues. Local symptoms depend on the site and size of the cyst. Clinical features are those of an enlarging mass. Common presentation is with hepatomegaly, hemoptysis or neurological symptoms. In about 75% cases, the right lobe

Textbook of Medicine

of the liver is the seat of large cysts. Lungs, brain orbits and bones are affected not uncommonly. An interesting physical finding is the hydatid thrill, which is elicitable by percussion over large hydatid cysts, particularly over the liver region. Place three fingers of the left hand firmly over the enlarged liver and percuss on the middle finger with the right hand and feel the sensation over the other two fingers, produced by the movement of the free floating daughter cysts in the cyst cavity. This is called hydatid thrill.

Allergic manifestations occur either as nonspecific allergy such as urticaria, eosinophilia or rashes. Sometimes rupture of a cyst and entry of the fluid into tissues evoke anaphylactic reactions.

Diagnosis

Strong clinical suspicion is necessary to suggest the diagnosis of hydatid disease.

- *Blood:* Mild eosinophilia is invariably present.
- *Casoni's reaction:* This intradermal test using sterile hydatid fluid used to be an important diagnostic test which was in vogue till three decades ago and it is no longer used because of poor specificity and cross reaction with other helminths.
- *Immunological tests* such as hemagglutination test using sensitized sheep red cells and immuno-fluorescence are useful for screening.
- *Immunoelectrophoresis* and *ELISA techniques* are specific, though technical difficulties restrict their wide use.
- *X-rays:* The cysts are radio-opaque and are seen as sharply outlined masses in the lungs (Fig. 68.6).
- *Imaging:* Ultrasonography gives the most valuable information about the nature of the mass and its contents. CT and MRI are also useful imaging techniques. Calcification of the cyst wall on CT is suggestive of hydatid cyst. Isotope scans of the liver bring out cold areas.

Closed aspiration as a diagnostic procedure is generally contraindicated since escape of the contents may result in anaphylactic shock and secondary infection.

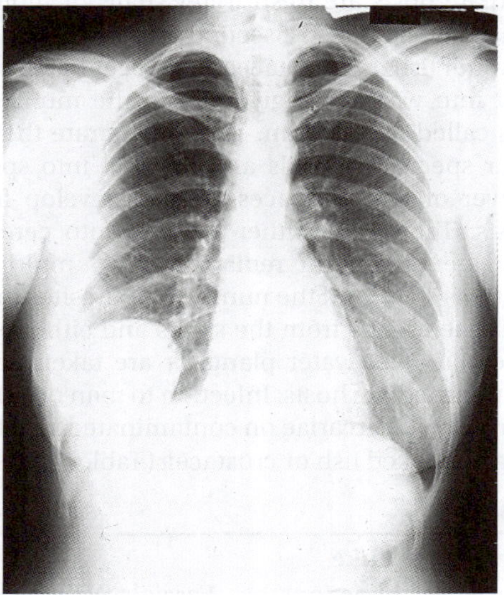

Fig. 68.6: Chest X-ray, hydatid disease left lower zone

Treatment

Planned surgery offers the best chance of cure for symptomatic cysts as drug therapy fails to clear the mass fully. Due to problems associated with surgery, presently ultrasound guided percutaneous aspiration and infusion of scolicidal agents like ethanol or hypertonic saline followed by reaspiration of the contents is recommended for uncomplicated cysts.

Albendazole, which is the drug of choice, is effective in sterilizing the scolices and reducing the size of the cysts. This drug is given pre- and post-operatively to sterilize the cysts and to prevent recurrence due to spillage during surgery. The dose is 800 mg given orally as two doses for 30 days. Pregnancy is a contraindication for this drug. Concurrent administration of corticosteroids help to reduce systemic reactions.

Praziquantel 50 mg/kg/day for 2 weeks is shown to destroy the protoscolices within the cysts but has no action on the germinal layer.

Prophylaxis

Care should be taken in handling dogs. Domestic dogs should be regularly dewormed. Monthly treatment with praziquantel 5 mg/kg eliminates *T. echinococcus* and *Hymenolepis nana* in dogs. Oxibendazole which is a veterinary drug given a dose of 30 mg/kg bw given orally, eradicates the inflectional animals in > 95%.

Contamination of children's playgrounds with dog's feces should be avoided.

Points to Remember

- Hydatid cyst should be considered in the diagnosis of an otherwise asymptomatic space occupying lesion in the liver and lungs.
- Ultrasound and CT findings are diagnostic, especially calcification in the cyst wall.
- Aspiration of the cyst is associated with risk of spillage of the contents and anaphylactic shock.
- Planned surgery is the definitive treatment since albendazole alone does not clear the cyst completely.

DIPHYLLOBOTHRIASIS LATUM

Syn: Diphyllobothrium latum, Fish tapeworm

Infection by *Diphyllobothrium latum* is extremely rare in India. It is more common in the Union of Soviet Socialist Republics (USSR), Baltic regions, Switzerland and Japan. The adults are seen in human small intestine and may range in length from 3 to 10 meters. The eggs are operculated. Two intermediate hosts are required for completing the life cycle, the fresh water cyclops and fresh water fish. Man gets infected by eating uncooked fish. The parasite may compete for vitamin B_{12} in the intestine, leading to vitamin B_{12} deficiency in the host.

Both niclosamide and praziquantel are effective vermicides.

HYMENOLEPIS NANA

Syn: Dwarf tapeworm

This is the smallest tapeworm found in man, measuring 1–4 cm in length. Children acquire infection by swallowing eggs. The larvae hatch out and grow in the small intestine.

Niclosamide and praziquantel are very effective in clearing the infection.

Tissue Invasion and Possible Malignancy of the Parasite

Instances of *H. nana* invading host tissues and proliferating into malignant tissue have been reported previously. These have been described as aberrant or anomalous developments. These include malignant transformation as well. More recent descriptions of aberrant intraepilthelial and epithelial mesenchymal involvement leading to neoplastic proliferation have been recorded.

Source: Muehlenbachs A, Bhatnagar J, Agudelo CA, et al. Malignant Transformation of Hymenolepis nana in a Human Host. N Engl J Med. 2015;373(19):1845-52.

HYMENOLEPIS DIMINUTA

This tapeworm is a parasite primarily affecting rats and mice. Man is accidentally infected by consuming the infective larva present in fleas, along with cereal grains. Both niclosamide and praziquantel are curative.

DIPYLIDIUM CANINUM

This is a tapeworm seen in cats and dogs. Many get infected accidentally by consuming the infective larvae present in fleas. Niclosamide and praziquantel are effective drugs.

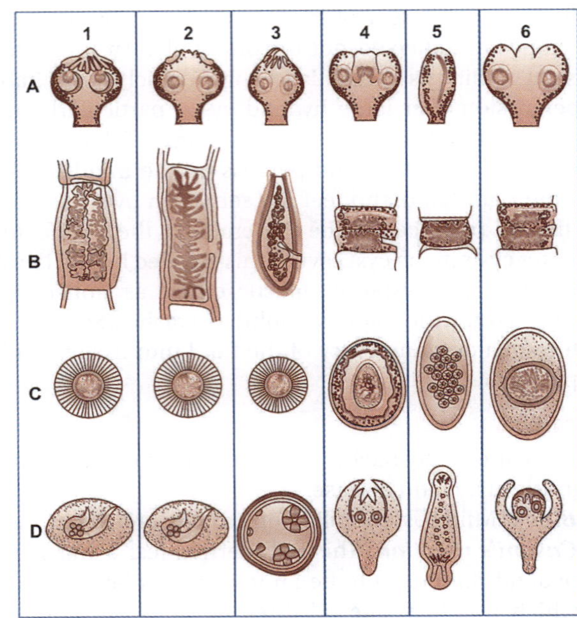

Fig. 68.7: Comparative diagram of tapeworms: **1.** *T. solium*, **2.** *T. saginata*, **3.** *T. ecchynococcus*, **4.** *H. nana*, **5** *D. latum* and **6.** *H. diminutum*. **A.** Scolices, **B.** Proglottides, **C.** Eggs and **D.** Larvae

Comparative morphology of the pathogenic tapeworms is given in Fig. 68.7.

69

Trematode (Fluke) Infections

RK Shenoy, KV Krishna Das

Chapter Summary

- General Considerations
- Fascioliasis
  - Morphology, Life Cycle and Pathogenesis
- Heterophyiasis
- Chlonorchiasis
- Schistosomiasis

GENERAL CONSIDERATIONS

Trematodes (flukes) are flat leaf-shaped unsegmented worms, which have a long lifespan. Except schistosomes, all are hermaphrodites. Compared to the other worms, human fluke infection is rare in India.

The common features are:

- Majority of them gain entry through the digestive tract except schistosomes
- Intermediate host is a snail and the infective metacercaria encyst on vegetables or develop in some aquatic animals which are ingested
- The eggs are operculate except in the case of schistosomes.

General Life Cycle

Man and other mammals form the definitive hosts. Intermediate hosts are fresh water snails or molluscs. In addition, some have also a second intermediate host such as fresh water fish or a crustacean. The eggs hatch out when liberated into water and give rise to the motile ciliated embryos called miracidium. These penetrate the body of particular species of snails and develop into sporocysts in the liver or lymph spaces. Rediae develop from the sporocysts. The rediae either develop into cercariae or a second generation of rediae. Asexual multiplication occurs at this stage and the number of parasites increases. The cercariae escape from the snails and either encyst as metacercariae over water plants or are taken up by the second intermediate hosts. Infection to man occurs due to ingestion of metacercariae on contaminated vegetables or by eating uncooked fish or crustacea (Table 69.1).

FASCIOLIASIS

Syn: Sheep liver fluke

Fascioliasis is infection by *Fasciola hepatica*. It is essentially a parasite of cattle and sheep and is worldwide

Table 69.1: General characteristics of some of the common pathogenic trematodes

Species of Flukes	Hosts	Habitat of adult
Intestinal flukes		
Fasciolopsis buski	Pig, occasionally dog, man	Duodenum and jejunum
Heterophyes heterophyes	Cat, dog, fox, man	Small intestine
Metagonimus yokogawai	Fish eating mammals, pelican, man	Small intestine
Gastrodiscoides hominis	Pig, man	Cecum and colon
Liver flukes		
Clonorchis sinensis	Dog, pig, cat, man	Biliary passages
Opisthorchis felineus	Dog, cat, fox, several other animals, man	Biliary and pancreatic passages
Fasciola hepatica	Sheep, cattle, rabbit, man	Liver and biliary passages
Lung flukes		
Paragonimus westermani	Tiger and other crab eating animals, man	Lungs
Schistosoma		
S. haematobium	Man	Urinary tract
S. mansoni	Man	Intestines and liver
S. japonicum	Man and other animals	Intestines, liver, lungs and brain

in distribution. Infection among cattle is not uncommon in India but human infection is less common.

Morphology, Life Cycle and Pathogenesis

This fluke measures 3.5 × 1.5 cm. The eggs measure 140 × 80 μm. They are operculate and are passed in feces. The snail vector is *Limnaea truncatula*. The cercariae encyst on aquatic vegetation. Man gets the infection by eating contaminated watercress. When ingested, the parasites excyst in the intestine and penetrate the wall to enter peritoneal cavity. They enter the liver by piercing the capsule. In the liver, they mature into adults in the bile ducts. Ova appear in feces 3–4 months later.

Clinical features: During parasitic invasion prolonged fever, abdominal pain, tender enlargement of the liver, urticaria and eosinophilia develop. Thereafter, the disease remains latent for months to years. The third stage is one of obstruction of the bile duct leading to jaundice and biliary cirrhosis.

Treatment: Triclabendazole given orally in a dose of 10 mg/kg bw in 2 single doses, 2 days apart is the drug of choice.

Bithional in a dose of 30–50 mg/kg given orally on alternate days for 10–15 days or praziquantel in a dose of 75 mg/kg daily in three divided doses for 5 days is also effective.

> **Points to Remember**
> - Infection by *Fasciola hepatica* is one of the causes of obstructive jaundice and biliary cirrhosis.
> - Triclabendazole is the drug of choice.
> - In endemic regions, watercress should not be eaten raw.
> - Cooking destroys the parasite.

HETEROPHYIASIS

Heterophyes heterophyes is a small fluke found in large numbers in the small intestine of man, dog, cat and wolf. It is distributed widely in the far East and Egypt. In India, it is occasionally seen in visitors or immigrants. The operculated eggs measure 13–16 μm in size and are passed in feces. They resemble those of *Clonorchis sinensis*. The snail vector is *Pironella conica*. The second intermediate hosts are the mullets and other types of fish, which are infective when eaten raw or improperly cooked. Inflammatory reactions occur at the point of attachment to the intestinal mucosa. Heavy infections lead to diarrhea and abdominal pain. Ectopic worms and ova in the heart had been reported. These unusual sites are reached through the bloodstream.

Treatment: Praziquantel given in a single oral doses of 20 mg/kg body weight clears the infection.

CLONORCHIASIS

Syn: Chinese liver fluke

Infection of the biliary passages by *Clonorchis sinensis* causes clonorchiasis. This disease is prevalent in the far East among fish eating mammals such as dogs, cats, pigs and man. In India, it has been reported among the Chinese immigrants.

Morphology, Life Cycle and Pathogenesis

This fluke is 11–20 × 3–4 mm in size. Eggs measure 30–16 μm and are passed in stools. The snail vectors belong to the *Bythinia* species. The cercaria are ingested by fresh water fishes (more than 40 species), which form the second intermediate hosts. Metacercariae develop in their muscles. When such fishes are ingested uncooked, the cyst wall is digested and the larvae are set free in the duodenum. They pass up through the ampulla of Vater to the smaller biliary passages and sometimes the pancreatic ducts. In course of time the biliary epithelium proliferates and the ducts dilate to form cystic cavities. The liver is enlarged and biliary cirrhosis, suppurative cholangitis and rarely malignancy may occur as complications.

Clinical features: Include diarrhea, hepatomegaly, recurrent jaundice and eosinophilia.

Diagnosis: The eggs can be demonstrated in the feces or duodenal aspirate.

Treatment: Praziquantel in a dose of 75 mg/kg given in three divided doses for 1–2 days is curative. Bithionol given orally in doses of 50 mg/kg on alternate days for 2–3 weeks is also effective.

> **Points to Remember**
> - There are two intermediate hosts in the life cycle of *Clonorchis sinensis*.
> - Clonorchiasis clinically presents with obstructive jaundice from cholangitis, biliary cirrhosis.
> - This is one of the causes for cholangiocarcinoma.
> - Proper cooking of fish prevents infection.

SCHISTOSOMIASIS

Syn: Bilharziasis

Infection by *Schistosoma haematobium, S. mansoni* or *S. japonicum* constitute schistosomiasis. *Schistosoma haematobium* affects the urinary tract. *S. mansoni* affects the large intestine, liver, lungs and also spinal cord. *S. japonicum* affects mainly the small intestine and upper part of large intestine, but the liver, lungs and the central nervous system (CNS) are also affected frequently. *S. hematobium* and *S. mansoni* parasitize only man whereas *S. japonicum* may also affect other animals such as the dog, cat, rat, field mouse and cattle. More than 200 million people are affected by the worm, worldwide.

Schistosomiasis in India: Gadgil and Shah reported a few cases of *S. haematobium* from Ratnagiri in Maharashtra.

Source: Theodor Bilharz (1825-1862). Pai-Dhungat JV. J Assoc Physicians India. 2015;63(3):62.

Morphology and Life Cycle

The life cycle of all the species is similar. Definitive host is man. Eggs are discharged in urine or feces. The eggs hatch out immediately in water and liberate free-swimming miracidia, which penetrate specific snail hosts within 24-hour (genus *Bulinus* for *S. hematobium, Biomphalaria* for *S. mansoni* and *Oncomelania* for *S. japonicum*). Two sporocyst generations develop within the snail. Cercariae are formed within 4–6 weeks. These escape from the snail into water and remain infective for 2–3 days. A snail infected by one miracidium can shed thousands of cercariae daily for months. The cercariae penetrate intact human skin and the oral mucous membrane when there is a thin film of water. Infection is acquired by contact with fresh water containing the cercariae. After entry, the cercariae lose their tails and they reach the peripheral venules and lymphatics. Within 24 hours, they pass through the lungs, diaphragm and liver. Then they enter the systemic circulation. The parasites finally reach the portal venous system and develop into adult worms. The adult worms measure 1–2 cm in length and have a lifespan of 4–30 years. The male is broader and holds the female within its fold. The female is longer and more slender and cylindrical than the male (Fig. 69.1).

Within 4–6 weeks of infection, they reach their destination through the venules draining the pelvic viscera and start laying eggs. *S. japonicum* passes through the superior mesenteric vein and *S. mansoni* passes through the inferior mesenteric veins. Finally, they both reach the submucosal vessels of the intestine. *S. japonicum* affects the small intestine and the ascending colon, while *S. mansoni* lodges in the descending colon and rectum. *S. haematobium* reaches the bladder and other pelvic organs. They feed on blood and globulins by anaerobic glycolysis.

The females lay about 3,000 eggs daily in the terminal blood vessels. The eggs contain ciliated miracidium larvae which secrete proteolytic enzymes that help them to migrate into the lumen of the bladder or the intestine. The worms slowly retreat as the terminal vessels get progressively blocked. The eggs remain viable for 1 week.

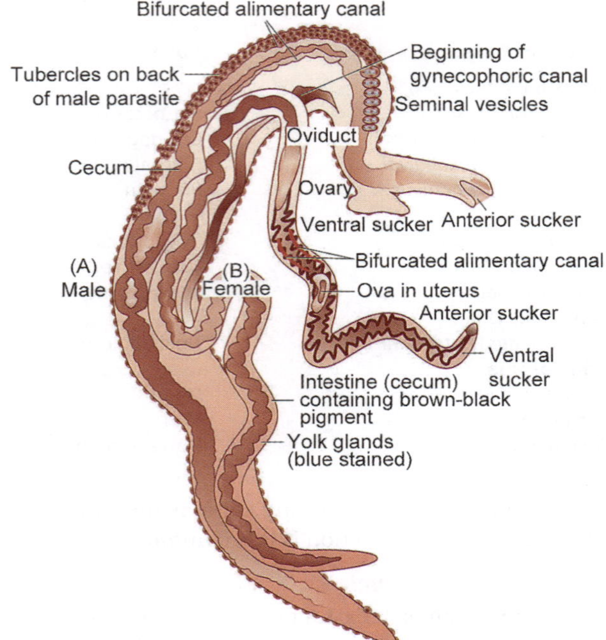

Fig. 69.1: Adult schistosome—(A) Male and (B) Female

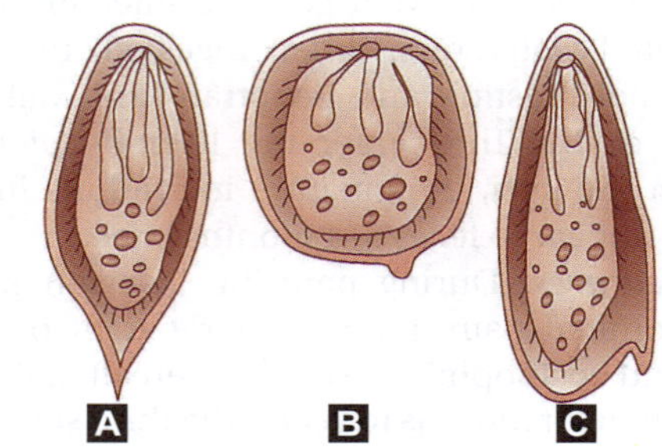

Figs 69.2A to C: Ova of schistosoma. **A.** *S. hematobium;* **B.** *S. japonicum;* **C.** *S. mansoni*

The eggs of *S. haematobium* containing miracidia appear in urine. The eggs of *S. mansoni* and *S. japonicum* are passed in feces (Figs 69.2A to C).

Epidemiology

Though schistosomiasis is one of the more widespread helminthic infections affecting about 200 million people in 71 countries, it is only rarely reported from India. There is a pocket of infection by *S. haematobium* in Maharashtra state. Highest prevalence is in Africa and the Middle East. *S. haematobium* and *S. mansoni* occur in Africa, Middle East and South America. *S. japonicum* is prevalent among the field workers in China, Japan, Philippines, Celebes, Lagos, Thailand, Vietnam and Myanmar. Newer areas have become endemic with the construction of dams and irrigation projects.

Pathology and Pathogenesis

Eggs are laid in the tissues, but many are discharged into the lumen and are passed in urine or feces. About 50% of the eggs are retained in the tissues. The eggs produce proteolytic enzymes which lead to typical eosinophilic inflammatory and granulomatous reactions, leading to fibrosis. Granulomatous lesions occur especially in liver, intestines, urinary bladder, uterus and lungs, resulting in complications. The tissue reaction is determined by the intensity of infection and the reactivity of the host. Ultimately further reinfection is limited by immunity developed by the host in endemic areas.

Clinical Features and Complications

Three phases are recognizable:

1. *Earliest lesion* is caused by penetration of the skin by cercariae. It results in itching and papular rashes at the sites of penetration *(swimmer's itch, cercarial dermatitis)*. This phase is more common in infections caused by non-human schistosomes.
2. In about 4–6 weeks, the *second stage* starts with fever, severe toxemia and allergic reactions. Marked eosinophilia develops in about 4–6 weeks. This stage is called *Katayama syndrome*. This serum sickness like reaction is seen during oviposition and it is most severe in *S. japonicum* infection.
3. *Late complications* are seen three months to several years after the initial infection. These are due to granulomatous lesions and fibrosis occurring in various organs. The manifestations of this stage differ in the three species.

S. haematobium (genitourinary schistosomiasis): It affects the urinary bladder, ureters and the prostate in males, whereas vagina, cervix and uterus are also involved in females. Urinary symptoms predominate depending on the stage of the disease. *S. haematobium* infection predisposes to vesical carcinoma.

S. mansoni infection (intestinal schistosomiasis): The early stage is characterized by abdominal pain and dysenteric symptoms. The lesion extends to the liver due to retrograde passage of eggs into the portal system and the liver. Periportal fibrosis resulting in presinusoidal portal hypertension develops in the liver. Massive splenomegaly may occur. The ova may reach all organs through the portal-systemic collaterals. The ova in the brain lead to neurological symptoms. *S. mansoni* infection favors the development of carrier state for *Salmonella typhi*. There is no rise in the risk of cancer.

S. japonicum infection (Katayama disease, Asiatic schistosomiasis): Since this worm produces more eggs than the others, its pathogenicity is greater. Major pathological lesions are seen in the small intestine, mesentery and ascending colon. This leads to ulcerations, fibrous thickening and polyp formation. Early symptoms are abdominal pain and bloody mucoid stools. Cirrhosis of liver develops with all its attendant complications. Five percent of cases develop ectopic foci of infection, especially in the lungs and CNS. Symptoms include Jacksonian epilepsy, focal paralysis, paraplegia and coma. Embolization of eggs in the pulmonary circulation leads to obstruction of small arterioles resulting in pulmonary hypertension. Granulomas develop in the lungs, which result in fibrosis. Such patients present with asthma, bronchitis or pulmonary emphysema.

Diagnosis

Schistosomiasis is diagnosed by demonstrating the eggs in appropriate specimens or in tissue biopsy. Concentration technique like Kato-Katz quantitative method is useful to enhance the egg count results. Investigation for *S. haematobium* includes plain X-ray abdomen for bladder calcification, excretory urograms and cystoscopy with biopsy, especially when there are no eggs or miracidia in urine. Rectal biopsy, sigmoidoscopy, barium enema and colonoscopy with biopsy are necessary to diagnose *S. mansoni* and *S. japonicum*. Serological tests like enzyme linked immunosorbent assay (ELISA) and immunoblot are available for diagnosis.

Modern investigations such as ultrasonography, computed tomography (CT) and magnetic resonance imaging (MRI) help to assess lesions in the liver, portal venous system, kidneys, bladder, brain and spinal cord. With the availability of these facilities, structural lesions can be diagnosed and appropriate corrective treatment instituted.

Treatment

It should be the aim to start treatment early since at this stage lesions are reversible. *S. haematobium* is most susceptible and *S. japonicum* is more resistant to drug therapy.

Praziquantel

This is an acylated quinoline-pyrazine derivative. It is given as a single oral dose of 30–45 mg/kg and the drug is effective in all types of infections. Cure rates of 72–95% have been reported and side effects are few, spasmodic abdominal pain being the most common. Being effective in a single dose, it can be utilized for mass therapy. Therefore at present it is the drug of choice. *S. haematobium* responds to 30 mg/kg bw, whereas *S. mansoni* and *S. japonicum* require above 40 mg/kg for proper response. The drug is available as 600 mg tablets. After a single dose 70–100% of patient cease to discharge eggs. A follow-up dose repeated 6–12 week later ensures killing of developing prepatent worms as well. Katayama fever is primarily treated with corticosteroids and praziquantel.

Oxamniquine: It is a quinoline derivative specific for *S. mansoni* infection. It is given orally in a dose of 20–30 mg/kg/day for 3 days. Fever and eosinophilia may develop 2–3 days after completing treatment.

Metrifonate: This is an organophosphorous compound specific for only *S. haematobium*. It is given orally in a dose of 10 mg/kg every 2 weeks for a total of 3 doses.

Preventive measures

- Proper environmental sanitation and health education.
- Mass therapy with oral drugs to reduce the worm load.
- Destruction of snails by proper control of water and use of molluscides.
- Avoidance of infection by wearing protective clothing.

CHAPTER
70

Tissue Nematodes

RK Shenoy, KV Krishna Das

Chapter Summary

- Filariasis
  - General considerations
- Lymphatic filariasis
- Loiasis
- Onchocerciasis
- Other filarial infections
  - *M. perstans*
  - *M. streptocerca*
  - *M. ozzardi*
- Dracontiasis

FILARIASIS

General Considerations

Infection by nematodes belonging to the superfamily Filarioidea constitutes filariasis. *Wuchereria bancrofti, Brugia malayi, Brugia timori, Loa loa, Onchocerca volvulus, Dipetalonema perstans, Dipetalonema streptocerca* and *Mansonella ozzardi* parasitize man. The distribution of these parasites depends upon the geographical and climatic conditions and the prevalence of the appropriate vector. In India, the two species prevalent are *W. bancrofti* and *B. malayi*. The parasites are distributed in different parts of Africa, South America and possibly other areas. The morbidity burden caused by filariasis in India is considerable. Extensive areas are endemic for this disease.

LYMPHATIC FILARIASIS

This is caused by *W. bancrofti, B. malayi* and *B. timori*. The first two infections are considered in this chapter since, *B.timori* is rare and is confined to a few islands in Indonesia. The adult worms living in the lymphatic vessels are responsible for the lesions and hence the name.

Epidemiology

Eighty one countries have lymphatic filariasis. It is estimated that 120 million people throughout the world are infected with *W. bancrofti* or *B. malayi*. Out of this disease burden, India and Sub-Saharan Africa account for about 40% and 38% respectively. Infection by *W. bancrofti* is endemic between latitudes 41° north and 30° south, involving most parts of India, Myanmar, Africa, South-East Asia, West Indies, Central America, the Pacific Islands and eastern coastal plains of South America. Infection due to *B. malayi* is restricted to South-East Asian countries and several pockets in India particularly along the coastal and backwater regions of Kerala, Andhra Pradesh and Odisha. It is now becoming clear that many areas hitherto unsuspected, coastal, midland and even mountainous are

endemic for bancroftian filariasis. During the early phase of infection, the person remains apparently healthy, but serves as a source of transmission. About 5–7 years after infection symptoms start. By itself lymphatic filariasis is nonfatal but infective complications can be fatal. *W. bancrofti* infection constitutes ~90% of the incidence of lymphatic filariasis (LF) world over, while *B. malayi* is responsible for only 10% of the remaining.

Morphology

The adults of *W. bancrofti* are 4–10 cm long, whereas those of *B. malayi* are only 3–5 cm. The males are smaller than females. The adults are seen coiled in clusters in the lymphatic vessels and their lifespan ranges probably from 7 to 15 years. Periodically, the female worm discharges numerous embryonated eggs [microfilaria (Mf)] into the lymphatics. These circulate in blood. In India, the Mf are most numerous in the peripheral blood at night, whereas in other geographical areas like the Pacific Islands, they are present during daytime as well. This phenomenon probably corresponds with the biting habits of the vector mosquitoes and the sleep rhythm of the patients.

When they are not present in peripheral blood, the Mf remain in the central parts of circulation in the lungs, liver and spleen. The Mf are sheathed, vary in length from 200 to 300 μ, and are actively motile. The Mf of *B. malayi* differ from those of *W. bancrofti* by certain characteristics like increased length of the cephalic space, secondary kinks in the curvature and presence of terminal nuclei in the tail (Figs 70.1 and 70.2). These help to identify them morphologically. Man is the only known definitive host for *W. bancrofti*, but animals like monkeys, dogs, cats and wild carnivores also harbor *B. malayi*.

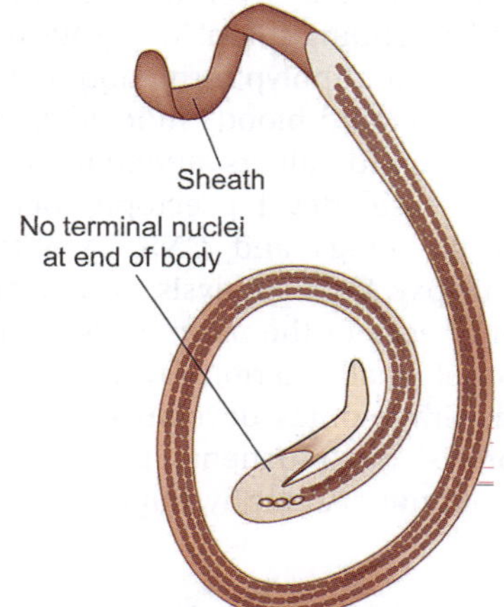

Fig. 70.1: Microfilaria *W. bancrofti*

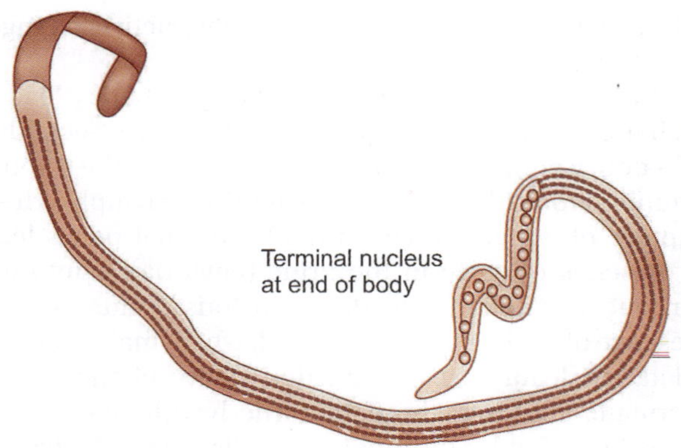

Fig. 70.2: Microfilaria *B. malayi*

Life Cycle

The Mf are ingested by the vector mosquitoes during blood meals. For *W. bancrofti*, many species of *Culex* and some species of *Anopheles* mosquitoes act as vectors. *B. malayi* is transmitted by *Mansonia* and *Anopheles* mosquitoes, the former being more important. The adult worms do not multiply in the host, nor do the larvae multiply in mosquitoes, so that the extent and severity of infection ultimately depend on the number of bites by the infective vector. Further development occurs when the Mf are ingested by the appropriate mosquito vectors. In the mosquito, the Mf shed their sheath, reach the wing muscles, become shorter and thicker, moult twice, and develop further to become the infective form. Depending on the temperature and humidity of the environment and species of the mosquitoes, this takes 10–14 days. The infective L3 larvae, which measure 1.4–2 mm × 18–23 μ migrate to the proboscis-sheath to be deposited at the bite wound caused by the mosquito. The larvae enter the skin at puncture sites and reach the lymphatics to grow, mature and mate. Microfilariae appear in circulation 6–12 months after entry of the larva. The severity of infection is determined by the number of adult worms harbored by the host. The Mf remain viable for 2–3 months after which they die and are removed by the macrophages of the liver and the lungs.

Pathology

The adult worms living in the lymph vessels are responsible for the early changes in these vessels. The severity of the pathology depends on the number of adult worms, their location and the host immune response. At one end of the disease spectrum, there are many, who in spite of repeated exposure, do neither have microfilaremia nor any lesions. The largest group of affected individuals are asymptomatic who harbor the adult worms and show Mf in their peripheral blood, but without clinical disease. The commonest clinical presentation is lymphedema involving the extremities or occasionally the genitalia in both sexes and rarely breasts in the females. In bancroftian filariasis in adult males, hydrocele is the more common manifestation. At the other end of the clinical spectrum is tropical pulmonary eosinophilia syndrome, which results from an exaggerated immune response of the host. It is classified under occult filariasis.

Spectrum of disease in lymphatic filariasis
- Endemic normals
- Asymptomatic microfilaraemia
- Clinical disease
- Tropical pulmonary eosinophilia syndrome.

Recent studies have revealed that the earliest lesion in lymphatic filariasis is dilatation of the lymph vessels harboring live adult worms. This is demonstrable by ultrasound scan and lymphoscintigraphy, in even asymptomatic microfilaremics. Dilation is responsible for the later lymphatic dysfunction and lymph stasis. It predisposes to secondary bacterial infections and development of lymphedema in the affected regions. The alterations in the immune response of the host and the parasite products probably contribute to the lymphatic dilatation (Figs 70.3 to 70.6).

Infection by *Str. haemolyticus* and occasionally other bacteria produces recurrent episodes of acute adenolymphangitis (ADL), also termed acute dermato-lymphangioadenitis (ADLA) because of the sequence of events, i.e. inflammation of the skin, lymph vessels and then lymph nodes. These involve the limbs or sometimes genitalia, where there is underlying lymphatic damage. ADL presents as acute febrile episodes. In most patients with acute ADL attacks, sites of entry for the bacteria are demonstrable in the limb involved. These include fungal infections of the interdigital spaces (Fig. 70.7), minor injuries or other lesions that disrupt the skin barrier allowing entry of bacteria. Moisture and damp environment favor the development of the skin lesions. This accounts for their greater frequency during rainy season. Repeated ADL attacks lead to progression of the lymphedema and

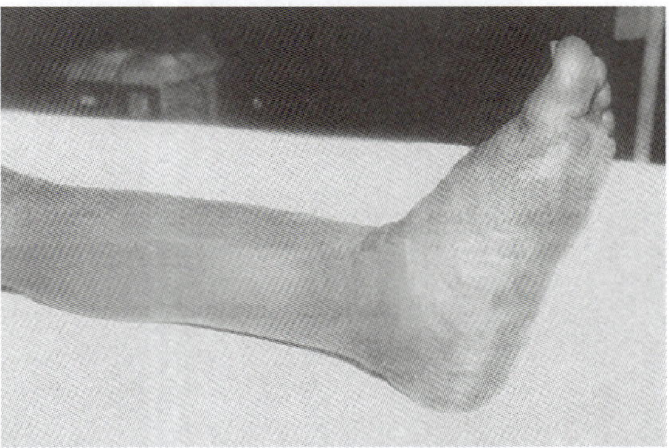

Fig. 70.3: Filarial lymphedema with acute adenolymphangitis

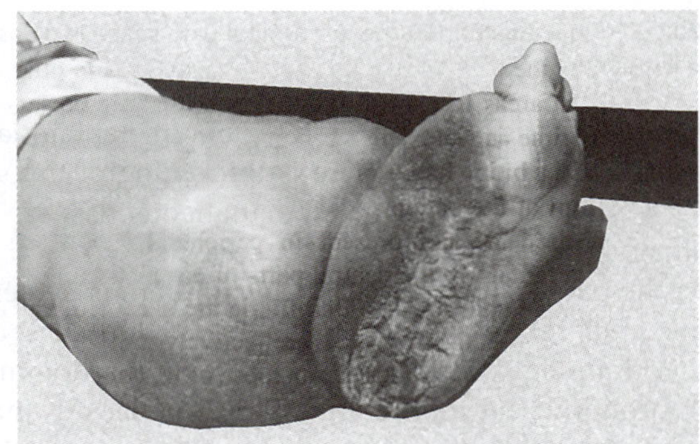

Fig. 70.4: Late stage of filarial lymphedema of leg

Textbook of Medicine

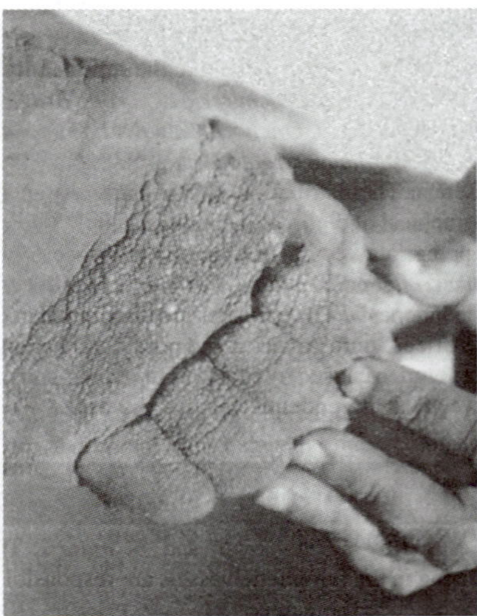

Fig. 70.5: Warty excrescences in a filarial foot

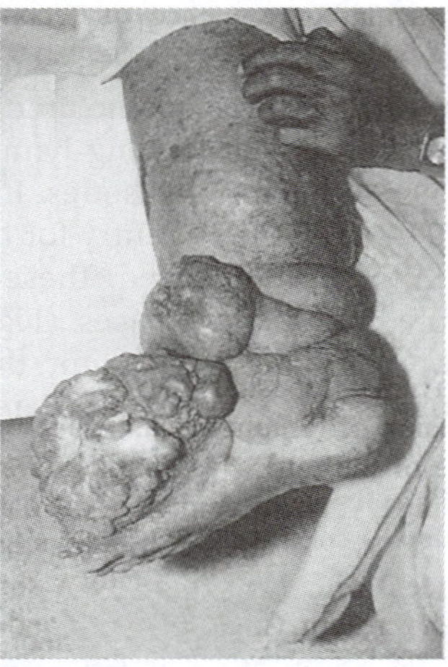

Fig. 70.6: Large nodular excrescences in a filarial leg

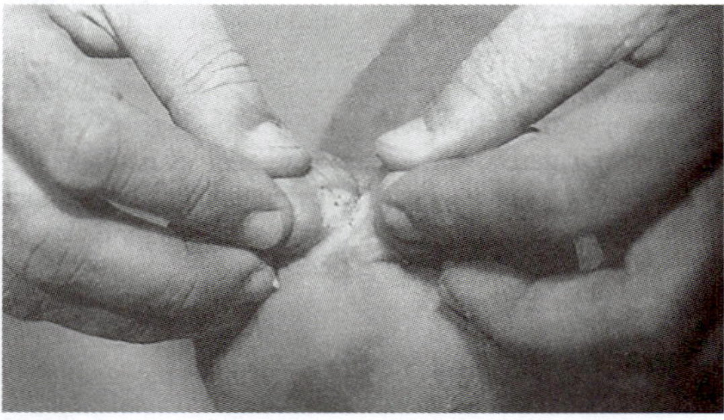

Fig. 70.7: Fungal infection in the interdigital web space in a case of filarial lymphedema

later elephantiasis of the affected region. In elephantiasis, the edema is nonpitting. There is thickening of the skin and gross hypertrophy of the subcutaneous tissues. The skin may show warty or nodular excrescences.

In the early stages of lymphedema, there is evidence of subacute inflammation in the affected tissues and in the draining lymph nodes. There is predominant polymorphonuclear infiltration. As the disease advances, there is further dilatation of lymphatics, proliferation of the lymphatic endothelium and new lymph vessel formation.

Late stages of lymphedema show obstructive changes, gross thickening and fibrosis.

The dilation and rupture of the lymphatics lead to oozing of lymph—***lymphorrhage***. This favors secondary infection. Common sites of lymphorrhage are the scrotum (lymph scrotum) and lower extremities (lymphorrhea). Rupture of lymph varices around the renal pelvis leads to presence of chyle in the urine (chyluria). Rupture of peritoneal lymphatics leads to chylous ascites, i.e. the presence of chyle in the ascitic fluid, which makes it milky. Dilatation leading to dysfunction of lymphatics of the spermatic cord and the para-aortic lymphatics leads to collection of fluid in the tunica vaginalis testes—***hydrocele***. Similarly chylocele may occur due to the rupture of these lymphatics.

When the adult worms die, this leads to granulomatous changes with predominant eosinophilic infiltration. The dead worms may get calcified.

Immunology

Immune mechanisms play a major role in the pathogenesis and clinical manifestations of filariasis. The adult worms remain in the host for long periods without evoking host defense response by producing anti-inflammatory substances. The T lymphocyte responses lead to production of interleukins 4 and 5 (IL4 and IL5). B lymphocytes are stimulated to produce immunoglobulin E (IgE) and immunoglobulin G4 (IgG4) which are associated with eosinophilia. IgG4 blocks the action of IgE, thereby reducing the host immune response. In the tropical pulmonary eosinophilia (TPF) syndrome, the hyperimmune response with high levels of IgE is characterized by increase in eosinophils in the absence of Mf in peripheral blood.

Role of Wolbachia in Lymphatic Filariasis

Recent studies have shown the presence of endosymbiotic bacteria of the genus *Wolbachia* in the adult filarial worms and Mf. *Wolbachia* are required for the homeostasis of their hosts. Destruction of these bacteria by drug intervention results in profound effects on the development, viability and fertility of the adult parasite. The role of these bacteria in the pathogenesis of filariasis and the inflammatory episodes is currently under investigation.

Clinical Features

The incubation period is from 5 to 12 months. There are acute and chronic clinical manifestations.

Acute Manifestations

Attacks of ADL are the most common acute clinical manifestations, which may occur both in the early and late stages of the disease. These are characterized by fever, lymphangitis, lymphadenitis or epididymo-orchitis. Fever is usually moderate and intermittent but sometimes it may be high, associated with severe rigor, sweating and delirium. The affected area is painful, tender, warm, red and swollen. Inguinal, axillary and epitrochlear lymph nodes, lower and upper limbs or genitalia are frequently affected. In *B. malayi* infection genital involvement is rare, and lower limbs below the knee and upper limbs below the elbow alone are involved. These acute ADL attacks recur many times a year in patients with lymphedema. Common sites for lymphangitis are the inner aspects of the thighs, legs, and arms. Repeated episodes of lymphangitis lead to distal edema, which resolves initially but later on tends to persist. Other acute manifestations are funiculitis, orchitis and epididymitis. Rarely scrotal pain, abscess formation in the breast in females or lymphadenitis in the abdomen resembling a picture of acute appendicitis or psoas abscess may occur. Hematuria, usually microscopic is seen sometimes in patients with microfilaremia.

Acute manifestations directly caused by adult worm death are usually rare and they occur when the adult worms are destroyed in the body either spontaneously or by drugs like diethylcarbamazine (DEC) or albendazole. These true attacks of acute filarial lymphangitis (AFL) are characterized by formation of small tender nodules at the location of adult worms either in the scrotum or along the lymphatics in the limbs. Lymph nodes may become tender. Inflamed large lymphatics may stand out as long tender cords underneath the skin, usually along the lateral aspect of chest or upper arm and axilla associated with painful restriction of movement of affected limb. Unlike ADL, these episodes are not associated with fever, toxemia or evidence of secondary bacterial infection.

Manifestations of lymphatic filariasis	
Early silent phase	• Clinically asymptomatic • Mf present in peripheral blood • Dilatation of lymphatics demonstrated by ultrasonography and lymphoscintigraphy
Acute manifestations	• Acute adenolymphangitis • Acute epididymo-orchitis, funiculitis • Acute onset hydrocele due to inflammation • Abscess formation • Acute abdominal lymphadenitis • Hematuria
Chronic manifestations	• Lymphedema/elephantiasis of extremities, genitalia and breasts • Hydrocele • Lymph scrotum • Chyluria, chylocele, chylous ascites • Lymph node enlargement • Lymphadenovarix

Chronic Manifestations

The commonest permanent sequel of the disease is lymphedema, which may be pitting on pressure in the early stages. But in later stages, it is nonpitting, leading on to elephantiasis, which may attain enormous sizes. Lower limbs, external genitalia in males and upper limbs are affected in the order of frequency. In females, the breast and the genitalia may develop elephantiasis at times. This feature is rare in India. Repeated ADL episodes are responsible for the progression of lymphedema.

Hydrocele of the tunica vaginalis is a common manifestation resulting from involvement of the para-aortic group of lymphatics. The skin of the scrotum may be covered with vesicles distended with lymph giving a soft velvety feel known as lymph scrotum. Chylous ascites and chyluria, often associated with hematuria may result from rupture of dilated peritoneal or perirenal lymphatics. Spongy lymphadenovarix is another chronic manifestation. In this condition, the lymph nodes, usually in the groin are enlarged, soft and spongy, the swelling becoming prominent in erect posture. Usually there is associated lymph scrotum, chylocele or chyluria.

Lymphatic Filariasis in Children

Infection acquired in childhood: It is now known that filarial infection is first acquired mostly in childhood. Lymphedema of the limbs, hydrocoele and ADL attacks are known to occur in children and young adults in endemic areas. Recent studies have indicated the extent of microfilaremia and circulating filarial antigens in children aged 3 years and above. Lymphoscintigraphy has demonstrated lymph vessel dilatation and ultrasound has shown presence of adult worms in lymph nodes and lymph vessels in children. The current understanding is that lymphatic dilatation once established is irreversible and promotes future progression of the disease. Most children with microfilaremia or lymph vessel dilatation are asymptomatic. Acute ADL attacks and lymphedema are later manifestations, which may be the first clinical presentation (Fig. 70.8).

Diagnosis

The diagnosis is evident when a patient presents with unilateral or asymmetrical bilateral edema of the limbs of long duration associated with recurrent febrile episodes of lymphangitis in an endemic area or if there is history of residence in an endemic area. But diagnosis of filarial infection is not possible clinically in the early asymptomatic phase. The following tests help in the diagnosis of lymphatic filariasis in its various stages.

Microfilaria (Mf) Detection Tests

Due to the periodicity of the parasite, Mf are detected usually by examination of peripheral blood at night. They are detectable in the early stages of the disease even before clinical manifestations develop. Once lymphedema develops Mf are rarely seen in the peripheral blood. But hydrocele may be associated with microfilaremia.

Examination of a blood smear obtained by finger prick method from the patients between 10 PM and 2 AM and stained with Leishman or Giemsa stain helps in the identification of the parasite and species. Motile Mf are generally seen in fresh thick wet films and this helps in rapid diagnosis. Concentration methods and techniques to filter the Mf through nuclepore membrane filters are

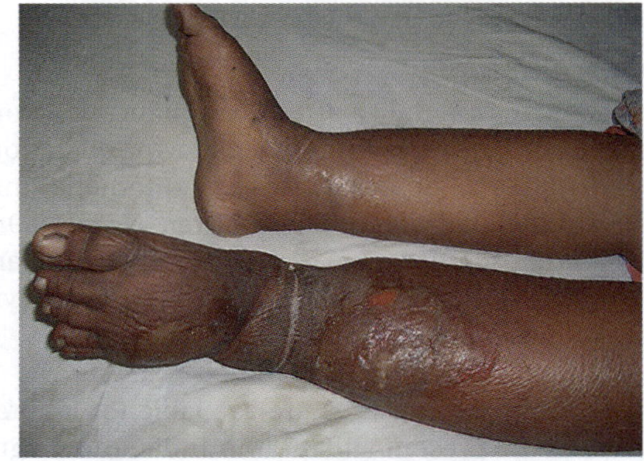

Fig. 70.8: Filarial lymphedema with acute adenolymphangitis

Tissue Nematodes

Textbook of Medicine

Table 70.1: Differences between chylous and pseudochylous urine

Characteristics	Chylous urine	Pseudochylous urine
Appearance	Milky	Cloudy
On keeping for hours	Fat containing high triglycerides float on top	Pus and debris settle in the bottom
Triglyceride content	>110 mg/dL	<110 mg/dL
Mixing with ether, other fat solvents	Fat dissolves, urine becomes relatively clear	No change
Microscopy	Red blood cells (RBCs), lymphocytes, fat, microfilariae	Cellular debris, pus cells or malignant cells

available to enable easy detection even when Mf counts are low and also to quantify the load of infection.

A moderate rise in eosinophils (up to 20%) is usually present, though this is not invariable. Chylous urine and hydrocele fluid may show Mf.

Sometimes pyuria with disintegration of the cells may superficially appear milky. This is termed pseudochylous urine (Table 70.1). Histological examination of lymph nodes or swellings may reveal the adult worms.

Immunochromatographic Test (ICT)

Both card and ELISA based ICT are highly specific and sensitive for the diagnosis of *W. bancrofti* infection. This is a filarial antigen detection test, which can be done on blood collected even during daytime. This test is positive in early stages of the disease when the adult worms are alive and becomes negative once the worms are dead. This test is not currently available commercially.

For *B. malayi* infection, a recombinant antigen-based ELISA and its modification, the 'Brugia Rapid' dipstick test, are currently available in cassette form. This test detects filariasis specific IgG4 antibody in *B. malayi* infection. Both these tests are highly sensitive and specific.

Ultrasonography

Live *W. bancrofti* adult worms can be visualized in the scrotal lymphatics of microfilaremic post pubertal males by ultrasonography using special techniques. Filarial dance sign (FDS) is the demonstration of the wriggling movements of the live adult worms on ultrasonography. Recent studies have demon-strated FDS in the inguinal and axillary lymphatics in children and adult females, in the latter the adult worms are located in the breast tissue as well.

Lymphoscintigraphy

Another imaging modality of the lymphatics is lympho-scintigraphy. This procedure has shown dilatation of lymph vessels in the limbs of asymptomatic micro-filaremic individuals including children (Figs 70.9 and 70.10). Lymphoscintigraphy is also useful in advanced lymphedema to delineate the pathology in the lymph channels and to determine their patency to plan lymphovenous shunt procedures.

Even though several tests are available for laboratory diagnosis, in the present situation in India, the diagnosis has to be arrived at by clinical findings, geographical

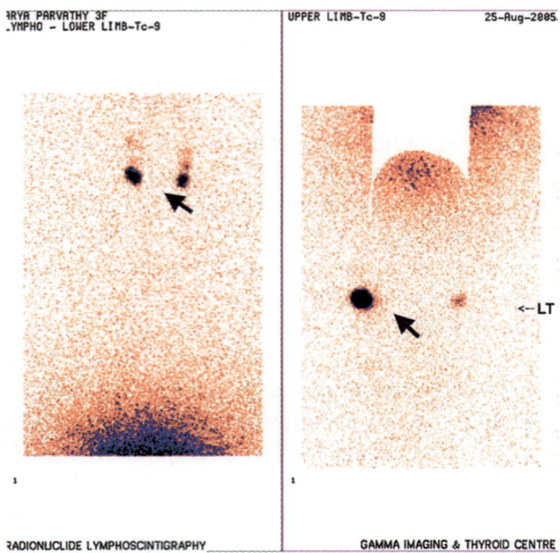

Fig. 70.9: A normal lymphoscintigram of the lower and upper limbs after injecting Tc99m tagged sulfur colloid in the interdigital spaces. The inguinal and axillary lymph nodes are imaged. Normal lymph vessels are not visualized

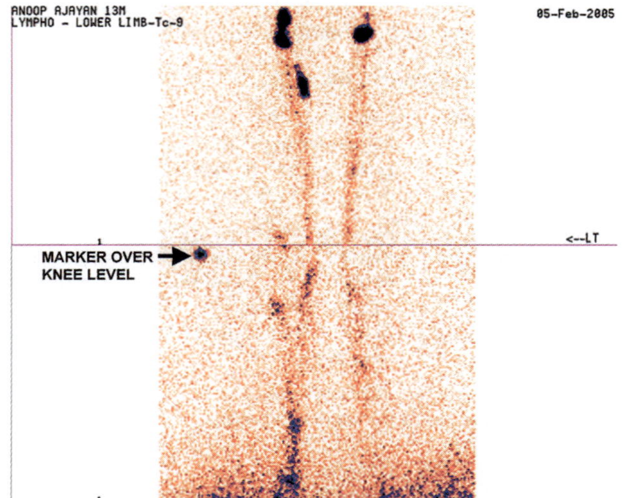

Fig. 70.10: Lymphoscintigram showing dilated lymph vessels in both legs of a child with asymptomatic microfilaremia. Dilation of the lymph vessels is caused by the adult worms

considerations and probability. The fact that Mf are seen in the night blood only in the asymptomatic phase and that too in around 30% of the cases, makes early diagnosis difficult.

Definite differentiation between filariasis due to *W. bancrofti* and *B. malayi* is possible only during the early asymptomatic microfilaremic phase, by examining the morphological characteristics of the Mf. The ICT helps in the diagnosis *of W. bancrofti* infection when the adult worms are alive. Table 70.2 lists some of the differences between the diseases produced by these two species.

Mixed infections by both the parasites are encountered occasionally in some endemic regions where both are known to co-exist, while blood is examined for microfilariae. The diagnosis of mixed infection is possible only at this stage since Mf are not generally seen once symptoms appear.

Table 70.2: Differences between *W. bancrofti* and *B. malayi* infection

Characteristics	*W. bancrofti*	*B. malayi*
Global prevalence	106.2 million	12.9 million
Global distribution	Tropical regions of Asia, Africa, China, Pacific and America	China, India and other South-East Asian countries
Distribution in India	12 States and Union Territories	7 states only
Incubation period	5–12 months	2–12 months
Sites of involvement	Extremities, genitalia and breasts	Only extremities: • Lower limbs below knee • Upper limbs below elbow
Immunology tests	ICT and ELISA for circulating filarial antigen	Brugia Rapid and ELISA for filariasis specific IgG4
Sensitivity to drugs	Less sensitive to DEC	More sensitive to DEC

Abbreviations: ICT = Immunochromatographic card test; ELISA = Enzyme-linked immunosorbent assay; DEC = Diethylcarbamazine; IgG4 = Immuno-globulin G4

Differential Diagnosis

Filarial etiology should be considered in the differential diagnosis of the following clinical situations:

- Repeated or single attacks of lymphangitis, lymphadenitis or cellulitis in the limbs
- Unilateral or asymmetrical bilateral swelling of limbs
- Swelling of the scrotum, funiculitis, epididymo-orchitis
- Fever with chills, rigor and delirium
- Persistent eosinophilia.

Lymphedema and elephantiasis are also known to occur in other conditions where there are congenital anomalies of the lymphatics, following irradiation to the lymph nodes for treatment of malignancies or following surgical excision of the lymph nodes. Lymphedema of the legs simulating filariasis may also be seen in late stages of carcinoma cervix or carcinoma of the prostate with pelvic floor secondaries. Rarely still, damage to the lymphatics following absorption of ultrafine silica particles from the soil in certain geographic areas also result in lymphedema.

Podoconiosis is a tropical lymphedema of lower limbs occurring in persons walking bare footed in places where exposure occurs to red clay soil derived from volcanic rock. It occurs in 10 countries—including Africa, Central and South America and pockets of North India. Familial and human leukocyte antigen (HLA) associations have been described. The final picture of the limb resembles elephantiasis. Papillomatosis cutis lymphostatica is rare disease characterized by long-term lymphatic obstruction, chronic lymphedema and partly hyperkeratotic verrucose papules and lymphedema associated damage to lymphatic vessels. This may superficially resemble elephantiasis. ***It should be remembered that more than 95% of chronic unilateral non-dependent lymphedema is due to lymphatic filariasis in endemic areas.***

In all the above situations where there are abnormalities in the lymphatics, recurrent ADL episodes are known to occur in the affected limbs due to secondary bacterial infections, thus worsening the edema leading on to elephantiasis, indistinguishable from that of filarial etiology.

Management

Treatment of lymphatic filariasis is described under following heads:

- Use of drugs acting against the parasite
- Treatment and prevention of acute ADL attacks
- Treatment of lymphedema, elephantiasis and hydrocele
- Control and prevention of filariasis.

Drugs acting Against the Filarial Parasite

There are three drugs now available in this group:

1. ***Diethylcarbamazine (DEC)*** is the drug of choice, which is effective in destroying Mf even in single annual doses of 6 mg/kg. It is easily available, effective, cheap and has a high safety profile. DEC is shown to kill only over 50% of the adult worms in those who harbor them. By ultrasonography it is shown that even single doses of DEC kill the adult worms when they are sensitive to the drug. If insensitive, even repeated doses do not produce any effect on the adult parasite. This drug does not act directly on the parasite and its action is mediated through the host immune system.

   The earlier recommended dose of this drug was 6 mg/kg given daily for 12 days. The rationale of this dosage is under scrutiny in the light of above recent observations. The sustained microfilaricidal effect of this drug even in annual single doses makes it a good tool to prevent the transmission of this disease. The adverse effects produced by the drug in patients with microfilaremia are due to the rapid destruction of the Mf and are associated with fever, headache, myalgia, sore throat or cough lasting for 24–48 hours. They are usually mild and self-limiting, requiring only symptomatic treatment with analgesic and antipyretic drugs. Direct adverse effects related to the drug are very rare. DEC is known to produce unpleasant side effects in microfilaremia of *O. volvulus* and *Loa loa* infections.

   DEC is indicated when there is active filarial infection as evidenced by presence of Mf in blood or in hydrocele fluid, demonstration of adult worms by ultrasonography or positive antigen/antibody tests. Single dose of 6 mg/kg is as effective as the 12 days dose both against Mf and adult worms. In cases of established lymphedema and ADL, usually there are no adult worms or Mf. Recent studies have clearly shown that the ADL attacks respond promptly to antimicrobials and local treatment and that the role of specific antifilarial drugs is not substantiated.

   DEC is also the drug of choice in the treatment of tropical eosinophilia syndrome where the drug is to be given for longer periods of 3–4 weeks.

2. ***Ivermectin:*** This drug acts directly on the microfilariae and in single oral doses of 200–400 µg/kg keeps the blood Mf counts at very low levels even at the end of one year. The adverse effects noticed in microfilaremic

patients are similar to those produced by DEC but milder due to the slower clearance of the parasitemia. Ivermectin is not effective against the adult parasite, during ADL attacks or in tropical eosinophilia. So this drug has no role in the treatment of clinical manifestations of lymphatic filariasis. Other benefits of ivermectin are clearance of lice infestation, scabies and some of the intestinal helminths.

3. ***Albendazole:*** When given in doses of 400 mg bd for 2 weeks, this drug is shown to destroy the adult filarial worms, inducing severe scrotal reactions, which is the common site in adult males where the adult worms are killed.

Albendazole has no direct action against the Mf. But when given in single dose of 400 mg in combination with DEC or ivermectin, the microfilaricidal action of the these drugs becomes more pronounced and sustained. Because of this effect and its action against many intestinal nematodes, albendazole combination with DEC or ivermectin is currently recommended for the ***Global Programme to Eliminate Lymphatic Filariasis (GPELF).***
Use of antibiotics against Wolbachia: Studies in animals and recent trials in humans indicate that treatment targeted at *Wolbachia*, which are intracellular symbionts in the filarial worms may be useful to destroy the adult parasites. Treatment with tetracycline and doxycycline daily for 4–6 weeks results in elimination of the bacteria with profound effects on the adult worms like dysembryogenesis and death.

The utility of this form of treatment in lymphatic filariasis is still under trial.

Treatment and Prevention of Acute ADL Attacks

Systemic antibiotics, particularly ampicillin-cloxacillin combination should be instituted. Microbiological examination of the local infective sites help to select the suitable antibiotic. Attention to local site of entry of the organisms is important. Bed rest, analgesics and nonsteroidal anti-inflammatory drugs (NSAIDs) give symptom relief.

Prevention of further attacks is crucial to reduce the morbidity and economic loss from this disease. Proper foot-care has to be instructed to all patients. We have found the following regimen to be very effective, giving statistical significant results.

- The feet should be washed with soap and water daily and wiped dry before going to bed, with special attention to the interdigital folds, cracks and abrasions. Presence of moisture in inter digital spaces promotes fungus infections and excoriation of skin inducing ADL.
- Keep the nails short, clean and promptly clipped.
- Antiseptics such as povidone iodine or chlorhexidine ointment should be applied over cuts and wounds. Antifungal drugs like Whitfield's ointment or clotrimazole cream should be applied over sites predisposed to fungal infection.
- Proper footwear should be worn.
- Edematous limb should be kept elevated during sleep.
- Light exercise of the affected limb promotes lymph drainage.

Local care will not be prefect when there is gross elephantiasis with excrescences, warty growths and so on. Such cases may benefit from short- or long-term systemic antimicrobial therapy.

Treatment of Lymphedema, Elephantiasis and Hydrocele

Use elastocrepe bandage or tailor made stockings while ambulant. The patient should be instructed to apply the bandage effectively. ADL should be prevented by proper foot hygiene measures.

There are various surgical options like lymph nodovenous shunts, omentoplasty and excisional surgery available for established cases of elephantiasis. In elephantoid scrotum and breasts, the thickened skin and subcutaneous tissue can be surgically excised and reconstructed.

Surgery for hydrocele: Surgery is the treatment of choice for patients with persistent hydrocele due to filariasis.

Control and Prevention of Filariasis

Once the clinical disease is established, lymphatic filariasis cannot be cured. This is due to the irreversible damage to the lymph vessels caused by the adult worms. So prevention assumes great importance. *GPELF* has been started in filariasis endemic countries from the year 2000 consist of two arms.

1. Mass chemotherapy using combinations of either DEC or ivermectin with albendazole in single annual doses for 4–6 years or regular use of DEC medicated cooking salt.
2. Alleviation of disability in those who have the disease.

Annual mass treatment with above drug regimens for prolonged periods reduces the Mf counts to very low levels. This brings down the disease transmission rate in the community. Mosquito control measures have to be instituted on a long-term basis. Personal protection against mosquito bites can be achieved by the use of bed nets and insect repellents.

Points to Remember
- Adult worms are responsible for the basic pathology. Mf do not cause any symptoms.
- Acute ADL attacks are caused by secondary bacterial infection and not by the adult worms.
- AFL due to adult worm death is very rare.
- In chronic disease neither the adult worms nor Mf are usually present.
- Once established, the pathology cannot be reversed by treatment with antifilarial drugs.
- Mass drug administration is a feasible way to control transmission of lymphatic filariasis.

LOIASIS

Loa loa is prevalent in West and Central Africa and this is commonly known as the African eye worm. The adult worms migrate in the subcutaneous tissues of several parts of the body including the eyes. Adult female measures 70 mm in length whereas the male measures only 30 mm. The thickness ranges from 0.3–0.4 mm. They live for 10–15 years. Sheathed Mf are produced and these appear in the blood during day time. This infection is transmitted by *Chrysops* (*C. silacea* and *C. dimidiata*), which act as vectors. In many endemic areas, monkeys form the reservoir.

The disease manifests as Calabar swellings, which are recurrent localized allergic inflammatory swellings. The swellings may overlie the adult worms at times. They commonly appear over the limbs or trunk. When the eyes are affected, intense lacrimation and pain may result. The adult worm may be seen in the eye during its subconjunctival migration. Rarely the microfilariae invading the nervous system may result in encephalitis, myelitis or focal seizures. The examination of cerebrospinal fluid (CSF) may show the larvae. Diagnosis usually clinical, is confirmed by demonstrating the characteristic microfilariae in the blood during daytime. Eosinophilia is invariably present.

Treatment consists of the administration of diethyl-carbamazine, which kills both adults and Mf. The dose is 6 mg/kg given for 14 days. Treatment with this drug may produce severe reactions, including encephalitis, in people with heavy microfilaremia. So, ivermectin or albendazole are suggested for initial treatment of patients with high Mf counts.

ONCHOCERCIASIS

Syn: African river blindness

This is a cutaneous form of filariasis caused by *Onchocerca volvulus* prevalent throughout tropical Africa, Mexico, Guatemala, Eastern Venezuela and Northern Brazil. This disease has not been identified in India.

The female worm measures 35–70 cm and the male 2–3 cm in length. The adult worms lie tangled together in the subcutaneous nodules and they live for 7–15 years. The microfilariae, which are unsheathed, are widely distributed in the adjacent skin. The vectors are female black flies belonging to the genus *Simulium*.

Pathology

The lesions are caused by the Mf. Inflammatory and allergic processes play their roles in pathogenesis. The adults form local granulomas, which appear as subcutaneous nodules. The microfilariae are distributed around these nodules. Their extent and density vary. Dead or dying microfilariae are responsible for the pathological changes occurring in both anterior and posterior chambers of the eye leading to permanent blindness. The role of *Wolbachia*, obligate intracellular bacteria of filarial parasites, in the causation of ocular pathology is under investigation.

Clinical Features

The adult worms give rise to subcutaneous nodules, which are 0.5–5 cm in diameter. These are firm, nontender, freely movable and are most commonly seen around the head and shoulders or the pelvic girdle. The skin manifestations are intensely itchy lesions, which in the early stages are seen as papular-erythematous rashes. Later, the skin becomes thickened, hyperkeratotic (crocodile skin) and depigmented. The penis and scrotum may show elephantoid changes.

Ocular lesions develop especially if the adults are numerous over the head and neck. These are punctate

keratitis, iridocyclitis and rarely choroidoretinitis, all of which ultimately lead to blindness.

Diagnosis

Demonstration of Mf in the skin shavings or skin snips taken from the affected area or the adults in biopsy of the nodules, establishes the diagnosis. Antifilarial antibodies may be detected in 95% of cases.

Treatment

The Mf are rapidly destroyed by diethylcarbamazine but the drug is ineffective on adult worms. The drug is started in a low dose and gradually worked up to 100 mg given thrice daily for 7–10 days. Severe allergic reactions may complicate the initial phase of therapy. Diethylcarbamazine is no more used in the treatment of onchocerciasis due to the severe systemic and ocular reactions induced by rapid destruction of Mf.

Presently **ivermectin** is the drug of choice for the treatment of onchocerciasis. Ivermectin given in a single dose of 150–200 μg/kg bw orally is very effective in destroying Mf and clearing the systemic and ocular lesions. Thereafter, the drug dose is repeated every 6 months or yearly intervals. In the vast majority, lesions clear up within six months. This drug is safe and side effects due to destruction of microfilariae are mild and do not adversely affect the eyes.

The drug **suramin**, a complex urea derivative, is effective against the adult worms. It is given intravenously in doses of 1 g weekly for five to six weeks. Due to complexities of dosage and toxic effects like renal damage this drug is not routinely used.

Recent animal and human studies have indicated that tetracycline or doxycycline given for 6 weeks has macrofilaricidal effect. This is due to the action of these drugs in clearing *Wolbachia* bacteria, endosymbionts of *O. volvulus*.

Ocular lesions have to be treated with mydriatics and topical steroid applications. The adult worms are removed by excision of nodules wherever they are accessible.

Control of infection in endemic areas is achieved by antivector measures, personal prophylaxis and recently, mass therapy for endemic population. Regular administration of ivermectin 150–200 μg/kg repeated every 6 months or yearly intervals helps to reduce Mf rates and transmission from person to person.

OTHER FILARIAL INFECTIONS

Mansonella Perstans

This parasite is prevalent in central Africa, South America and the Caribbean. Adults are seen in the subserosal layer of viscera. The pleura, pericardium and peritoneum are involved. In many cases the mesentery is a frequent site. The Mf are unsheathed, nonperiodic and are demonstrable in blood. The vectors are the blood sucking midges—*Culicoides*. Though in the majority of cases infection is asymptomatic, some cases may develop fever, pruritus, skin rashes and abdominal pain. Demonstration of the microfilariae in peripheral blood confirms the diagnosis. *Mansonella ozzardi*, Mf are unsheathed. This parasite does not respond to the standard antifilarial

Textbook of Medicine

drugs. Endosymbionts such as *Wolbachia* perpetuates the infection. Often it exists along with *W. bancrofti*.

Treatment

Diethylcarbamazine is generally ineffective. Repeated doses of ivermectin effectively reduce the blood Mf levels. Success has been reported with mebendazole given in a dose 100 mg twice daily for 30 days and albendazole 400 mg twice daily for 10 days. Doxycycline in a dose of 200 mg/day for long periods reduces the microfilaia in blood.

Mansonella Streptocerca

It is prevalent in parts of Africa. It is transmitted by *Culicoides.* Adult worms are seen in the dermis and subcutaneous tissues. The Mf are nonperiodic and they are seen surrounding the adult worms and are demonstrable in skin snips taken from the lesions. Clinical features consist of pruritic papular rashes, edema and hypopigmentation. This worm responds to diethylcarbamazine in the usual doses. Ivermectin 150 µg/kg single dose causes sustained suppression of microfilaremia.

Mansonella Ozzardi

This infection has been reported from the tropical regions of South America. Adult worms are found in the visceral adipose tissue. Mf are nonperiodic and are seen in peripheral blood. Vectors include *Simulium* and *Culicoides.* In majority of cases, this infection is nonpathogenic, though fever, lymphadenopathy and erythematous skin rashes may occur at times. Treatment with diethylcarbamazine is generally ineffective. Single dose of ivermectin is shown to be effective in the treatment of this infection.

DRACONTIASIS

Syn: Guinea worm, Serpent worm, Dragon worm

Infection by *Dracunculus medinensis* used to be seen in several endemic pockets in India, Pakistan, Iran, Middle East, West Indies, South America and East, West and Central Africa. In India the disease was common in Punjab, Madhya Pradesh, Gujarat, Maharashtra, Andhra Pradesh and Tamil Nadu. At present India has been declared disease-free by the World Health Organization (WHO). Endemic pockets are present in some African countries.

Morphology and Habitat

Adult male is 2.5 cm long and is short lived. The female worm is 60–100 cm long and 1.5–1.7 mm in diameter, cylindrical, white and is viviparous. The posterior end is tapering and hook-shaped. Opening of the uterus is at the anterior end. Adult females may live up to one year. Larvae are discharged in batches when the anterior end of the worm comes in contact with water.

Life Cycle

The larvae are taken up by fresh-water cyclops, belonging to the family Crustacea and these form the intermediate hosts. The larvae become infective to man in 10 days. Man gets infected by ingesting the cyclops in water. The larvae are liberated in the intestine and these migrate to the subcutaneous connective tissues to grow into adults in 9-18 months. After fertilization, the females come to lie subcutaneously under those parts of the body, which come in contact with water. A blister develops in the skin where the anterior end of the worm lies, which breaks down to form an ulcer. When the part comes in contact with water, the worm protrudes its anterior end through the ulcer and discharges a milky fluid containing a large number of larvae. Over a period of 3 weeks the worm is extruded and the ulcer heals. Infection is generally acquired when the drinking water source is infested with cyclops and people with open lesions contaminate it.

Clinical Features

Initial symptoms include urticaria, eosinophilia, wheezing, nausea, vomiting and diarrhea. Formation of the blister is accompanied by local pain, itching and inflammation. The tissue around the blister may become red, tender, and edematous. Secondary infection of the ulcer is common. Periarthritis and pyarthrosis may occur if the worms are in the neighborhood of joints. The ulcer may even act as a portal of entry for *Clostridium tetani.* Sometimes, the female worm may be palpable in the subcutaneous tissue. Worms that fail to reach the surface die and get calcified. Aseptic abscesses may develop around the worms.

Diagnosis

It is easy to diagnose if the worm is seen in the centre of the ulcer, which is characteristic. The worm can be induced to discharge the larvae by applying water over its anterior end. Under the microscope the motile larvae are demonstrable in the discharge from the ulcer. X-ray may demonstrate calcified worms. Blood shows eosinophilia.

Treatment

Local dressing and administration of antibiotics serve to minimize local infection. Removal of the worm is achieved mechanically. The worm is induced to discharge its larvae in water for a few days by which process it protrudes more and more. As the anterior end comes out progressively it is tied with a fine silk thread and rolled up over a matchstick till it is extracted fully over a course of 15–20 days. Live worms are easier to extract. If the worm breaks and its anterior end retracts, the track is likely to be infected. Surgical measures are indicated when conservative treatment fails.

Drug Therapy

Thiabendazole given in a dose 25 mg/kg for 3 days or metronidazole 400 mg daily for 10–20 days offer relief of symptoms, but do not kill the adult worms.

Prevention

The transmission of *D. medinensis* can be interrupted by public education; avoidance of contamination of drinking water source by persons with infective lesions; vector control by chemical treatment of water source and boiling or proper filtration of drinking water. India launched the National guinea worm eradication programme in 1984 with technical assistance from WHO. Since 1996 no fresh case has been reported. Eradication of this parasite is in the agenda of WHO.

CHAPTER
71

Rare Helminthic Infestations

KV Krishna Das, RK Shenoy

Chapter Summary

- Multiceps Multiceps
- Intestinal Capillariasis
- Anisakiasis
- Angiostrongyliasis
- Gnathostoma Spinigerum
- Sparganosis

Sporadic cases of exotic helminthic infections are reported from time to time, man being accidentally infected by helminths parasitizing animals. These include ***multiceps, intestinal capillariasis, anisakiasis, angiostrongyliasis, gnathostomiasis and sparganosis***.

MULTICEPS MULTICEPS

This is a tapeworm, the adults of which live in the intestines of dog. The larvae (bladder worm) are seen in the brain of sheep and other herbivores—*Coenurus cerebralis.* Accidentally man may be infected when the brain or eye harbor the larvae.

INTESTINAL CAPILLARIASIS

This has been described from Thailand and Philippines. The adults (*Capillaria philippinensis)* parasitize birds. Fish and crustaceans are the possible intermediate hosts. Infection is acquired by eating raw or partially cooked intermediate hosts. The larvae mature and live in the crypts of the small intestines. They multiply in large numbers and lead to malabsorption state or protein losing enteropathy. Eggs are passed in feces and their identification helps to establish the diagnosis. Prolonged treatment using ***mebendazole*** and ***albendazole*** is effective.

ANISAKIASIS

This is caused by *Anisakis* species, which are intestinal nematodes of marine animals. Several species of fish act as intermediate hosts and infection occurs by eating raw or partially cooked fish. Cases have been reported more often from Japan, Netherlands and Scandinavia. The larvae penetrate the stomach wall or intestinal wall, giving rise to pain and symptoms, sometimes simulating acute abdomen. No drug is effective against this parasite. Albendazole is reported to be useful.

ANGIOSTRONGYLIASIS

Man may become infected by *Angiostrongylus costaricensis* or *Angiostrongylus cantonensis*. Adults parasitize several species of rats. *A. costaricensis* is described from Central and South America. Man acquires the infection by eating molluscs, which act as the intermediate hosts. Symptoms include abdominal pain, which may even resemble acute abdomen.

A. cantonensis is described from far East and also from India. Man gets infected by eating molluscs, prawns or crabs, which harbor the larvae. The larvae migrate in tissues. Some reach the brain to give rise to meningitic symptoms. Spinal fluid may show lymphocytes and eosinophils. In the vast majority, the disease is self-limiting.

There is no specific treatment available. Angio-strongyliasis can be prevented by proper cooking of crabs, prawns and molluscs before consumption.

GNATHOSTOMA SPINIGERUM

This is an intestinal nematode affecting dogs and cats. The intermediate hosts are fish, which when consumed uncooked leads to human infection. Infection is reported from far East, especially Thailand. The larvae do not develop into adults in man, but migrate and lead to the development of eosinophilic granulomas, mostly seen in subcutaneous tissue and brain. Eosinophilia may develop. Central nervous system (CNS) involvement leads to neurological features. Biopsy of subcutaneous nodules may help to give a histological diagnosis. Serological diagnosis can be made by enzyme-linked immunosorbent assay (ELISA) testing. Treatment with ivermectin 200 µg/kg for 2 days and albendazole 400 mg twice a day for 21 days is effective.

SPARGANOSIS

Sparganum is the second larval stage of tapeworms of the genera *Spirometra* and *Diphyllobothrium* that are common in various canines and felines. The ova are ingested by cyclops and the first stage larvae (procercoids) develop in them. The ***Sparganum***, which is the second stage larva, develops in frogs, crustacea and fishes that ingest cyclops. Man may acquire sparganosis by ingesting infected cyclops or by the application of infected frogs or fish as poultices over wounds or inflamed eyes. The condition is seen in far East. The larva (*Sparganum mansoni*) grows and forms a cyst, which appears as nodular lesion. ***Treatment*** is to remove the nodules surgically.

CHAPTER
72

Abnormalities of Water and Electrolyte Balance

R Kasi Visweswaran

Chapter Summary

- General Considerations
- Disorders of Sodium and Water Balance
  - Hyponatremia
  - Hypernatremia
- Disorders of Potassium Homeostasis
  - Hypokalemia
  - Hyperkalemia
- Disorders of Calcium Homeostasis
  - Hypercalcemia
  - Hypocalcemia
- Disorders of Phosphate Homeostasis
  - Hyperphosphatemia
  - Hypophosphatemia
- Disorders of Magnesium Homeostasis
  - Hypermagnesemia
  - Hypomagnesemia

GENERAL CONSIDERATIONS

Water constitutes approximately 60% of body weight. As fat contains less water, obese persons have proportionately less body water compared to lean individuals. Thus, the proportion of body water may vary from 80% in the newborn baby to 60% in lean and young males and 40% in obese and elderly women. The water in the body is distributed in two major compartments—intracellular fluid (ICF) and extracellular fluid (ECF) in a ratio of 66–34%. The ECF compartment is further subdivided into interstitial fluid (65%), intravascular fluid (25%) and transcellular fluid (10%). In the intravascular compartment, only 10% is in the arterial system. Majority of the fluid is distributed in the capillary system (55%) and venous system (35%). The transcellular fluid which is about 10% of ECF is distributed as cerebrospinal fluid (CSF), gastrointestinal (GI) fluid, serosal fluid, fluids in the eye and others. The remaining part of the body water is constituted by ICF. The composition of the fluid in the intra- and extracellular compartment are markedly different.

The total number of anions and cations are equal in all these compartments. Sodium (Na^+) is the predominant extracellular cation and potassium (K^+) is the most abundant intracellular cation. The intracellular concentration of magnesium (cation) is also high. Chloride and bicarbonate are the major anions in the extracellular compartment. Phosphates, sulfates and

Table 72.1: Composition of intra- and extracellular fluid compartments

Substance	ICF	ECF
Sodium (Na^+)	10 mmol/L	140 mmol/L
Potassium (K^+)	150 mmol/L	4 mmol/L
Chloride (Cl^-)	2 mmol/L	104 mmol/L
Bicarbonate (HCO_3)	6 mmol/L	24 mmol/L
Calcium (Ca^{++})	50–100 nanomoles/L	2.25–2.65 mmol/L
Magnesium (Mg^{++})	0.5 mmol/L	0.75–1 mmol/L
Phosphates	1.4 mmol/L	0.8–1.5 mmol/L

Note: For univalent ions, the mEq and mmol are the same.

protein contributes to the anions of the ICF compartment (Table 72.1).

Water Homeostasis

Under normal circumstances, water intake and water elimination are equal and the osmolality of the body fluids is maintained. Water balance is regulated by formation of concentrated or dilute urine. The diluting mechanisms permit the excretion of up to 12–15 L of urine daily, whereas the urinary concentrating ability can achieve full elimination of the daily metabolic waste in as little as 500 mL urine. In health, the urine osmolality could vary from 50 to 1200 mOsm/kg. The water intake is mainly regulated by the thirst mechanism. When the plasma osmolality increases by 3–5 mOsm/kg, the osmoreceptors in the medulla oblongata are stimulated resulting in thirst. Hypovolemia, hypotension and angiotensin II are also stimuli for thirst. The antidiuretic hormone (ADH) or vasopressin regulates the concentration of urine. In the presence of ADH, the collecting tubule becomes more permeable to water and more of water is reabsorbed leading to formation of concentrated urine. When the fluid in the collecting tubule traverses the renal medulla, water is reabsorbed into the hypertonic medullary area through these permeable tubules. The increased permeability is achieved by insertion of water channels called aquaporin channels into the luminal side of tubule cell membrane. In addition to the renal losses which can be regulated to some extent, water loss also occurs through the skin, lungs and gastrointestinal tract (GIT). The loss through the skin and lungs depends upon the climate, exercise and body temperature. Under normal circumstances, the GI loss is approximately 120–160 mL per day. If the daily water loss in a person remaining indoors with outside temperature of 32°C is 200 mL, the loss during heavy exertion outside at temperature over 40°C may be even 5–6 L.

When there is excess water in the body, the volume expansion results in stretching of the atria, release of atrial natriuretic peptide and promotion of natriuresis and diuresis. The ADH secretion decreases. The collecting tubules become less permeable to water (the aquaporin channels are delinked from the cell membrane) and the dilute tubular fluid is passed out as urine. Thus, the excess water in the body is eliminated.

Sodium (Na$^+$) Homeostasis

In a healthy adult, the total body Na$^+$ is approximately 5,000 mEq. About 90% is in the extracellular compartment. The main function is to maintain the ECF volume, osmolality and BP. Under normal circumstances, the salt intake and excretion are equal. The salt intake of individuals or communities is highly variable. The daily salt requirement is about 6 g or 100 mmol (one level teaspoon = 6 g). In addition to the diet, Na$^+$ intake could occur through parenteral fluids or Na$^+$ containing drugs. Significant Na$^+$ loss could occur in those with excessive sweating and in diarrhea. In health, the kidney is the main route for elimination of ingested Na$^+$. In diseases, Na$^+$ loss could occur through other sources also.

Na$^+$ is freely filtered by the glomerulus. The concentration of Na$^+$ in the glomerular filtrate is the same as in blood. As the filtrate traverses the proximal tubule, 60–65% of Na$^+$ and water are reabsorbed. Thus, the glomerular filtrate remains iso-osmotic at the end of proximal tubule. The next segment contributing to Na$^+$ reabsorption is the thick ascending limb of the loop of Henle where Na$^+$-K$^+$-2 chloride co-transport pump reabsorbs chloride, Na$^+$ and K$^+$. About 25–30% of Na$^+$ is reabsorbed here. This segment of the tubule is impermeable to water and is involved in reabsorbing only solutes, the fluid leaving the loop of Henle is hypo-osmolar (osmolality <100). The remaining 10% of the Na$^+$ reabsorption occurs in the distal tubule and collecting duct. The reabsorption here is mediated through Na$^+$ and chloride co-transporter and Na$^+$/K$^+$ ATPase. This reabsorption is regulated by aldosterone which causes reabsorption of Na$^+$ in exchange for K$^+$. The fine tuning of the Na$^+$ excretion occurs in these segments. Thus, the urine may contain only < 1% of the filtered Na$^+$. In those with high salt intake and normal renal Na$^+$ regulation, the urinary Na$^+$ excretion will be higher.

The controlling mechanism for renal Na$^+$ excretion is mediated through afferent and efferent limb. The afferent impulses are from the receptors in atria and pulmonary vascular bed. Activation of these receptors by distension, stretching or pulmonary congestion cause decrease in sympathetic outflow, decreased renal sympathetic tone and natriuresis. Conversely, low central venous pressure (CVP) leads to sympathetic stimulation and Na$^+$ reabsorption. The efferent limb consists of the sympathetic system, hormones and the forces acting on the Starling equilibrium. The **Starling forces**—the capillary hydrostatic pressure, tissue oncotic pressure, capillary oncotic pressure and tissue hydrostatic pressure play a significant role in the reabsorption of Na$^+$ in the proximal tubule. The sympathetic stimulation causes increased cardiac output, BP, activation of renin angiotensin system and these enhance Na$^+$ reabsorption. The hormonal factors regulating Na$^+$ handling are angiotensin II, atrial natriuretic peptide, prostaglandins and arginine vasopressin (AVP).

DISORDERS OF SODIUM AND WATER BALANCE

The ECF fluid volume and osmolality are maintained in a narrow range despite wide variations in the intake of salt and water. Disorders in water balance result from abnormalities of concentrating or diluting capacity of the kidney. The major causes include renal disease, abnormalities in vasopressin release or action and defective thirst mechanism. Urinary concentrating ability is diminished both in central and nephrogenic diabetes insipidus (DI). Both present with polyuria and dilute urine. The other disorders of urinary concentration include renal insufficiency, solute diuresis, water diuresis, use of osmotic diuretics, loop diuretics and severe protein malnutrition.

Urinary diluting capacity is diminished in conditions like renal failure, cirrhosis liver, nephrotic syndrome, capillary leak syndrome, congestive cardiac failure (CCF) and conditions associated with decreased arterial blood volume. Severe chronic hypokalemia, hypothyroidism and syndrome of inappropriate ADH (SIADH) secretion are other important causes. SIADH release is a common cause of hyponatremia in hospitalized patients. Disorders of urinary dilution often manifest as hyponatremia.

The new term SIAD (syndrome of inappropriate anti diuresis) is gradually replacing the term SIADH.

Hyponatremia

Contrary to common belief, hypo- and hypernatremia are primarily disorders of water metabolism. Hyponatremia is a common problem in hospitalized patients and is defined as plasma Na$^+$ of less than 135 mmol/L.

Before confirming the diagnosis of hyponatremia based on low plasma Na$^+$ level, **pseudohyponatremia** and **translocational hyponatremia** must be excluded. **Pseudohyponatremia** is a condition characterized by low serum Na$^+$ readings when plasma is tested in patients with hyperlipidemia and hyperproteinemia. This occurs because the 'solid phase' of plasma is increased and the Na$^+$ is low when the plasma is assayed. The osmolality is often normal. This fallacy can be overcome by using potentiometry which measures the true liquid based Na$^+$. Substances like glucose, mannitol or glycine increase serum osmolality while decreasing serum Na$^+$. For every 100 mg increase in blood glucose level, the serum Na$^+$ decreases by 1.6 mmols and is due to movement of water from the ICF to ECF compartment due to high sugar. This is an example of **translocational hyponatremia**. Although, there may be no symptoms

Box 72.1: Classification of hyponatremia based on ECF volume status

- Hyponatremia with decreased ECF volume and low total body sodium (hypovolemic hyponatremia)
  - Due to renal losses
    - Diuretic use
    - Salt losing nephropathy
    - Osmotic diuresis
    - Cerebral salt wasting.
  - Due to extrarenal losses
    - Vomiting
    - Diarrhea
    - Burns
    - Pancreatitis—third space loss
    - Trauma.
- Hyponatremia with increased ECF and high total body sodium (hypervolemic hyponatremia)
  - Cirrhosis liver
  - CCF
  - Nephrotic syndrome
  - Advanced CRF.
- Hyponatremia with normal ECF and normal total body sodium (euvolemic hyponatremia)
  - Glucocorticoid deficiency
  - Hypothyroidism
  - Severe K^+ depletion
  - Postoperative administration of salt free fluids
  - Drugs such as antipsychotics, nicotine, tolbutamide, chlorpropamide, chlorpromazine, carbamazepine and others
  - SIADH.

Abbreviations: ECF = Extracellular fluid; SIADH = Syndrome of inappropriate antidiuretic hormone secretion; CCF= Congestive cardiac failure; CRF = Chronic renal failure

till the level of Na^+ falls < 120, proper identification and appropriate treatment are necessary. The treatment is to control blood sugar and not give Na^+. Hyponatremia could occur acutely (within 48 hours) or may be chronic (over 48 hours). It is classified depending on the ECF status (Box 72.1).

Hyponatremia with decreased ECF volume and decreased total body Na^+ occurs due to selective loss of intravascular fluid and ECF.

Hyponatremia with increased ECF volume and increased total body Na^+ occurs in conditions associated with fluid retention and edema. In these conditions, there may be Na^+ retention and increase in total body water. Na^+ and the disproportionately high water retention causes the hyponatremia. This is predominantly a 'dilutional' hyponatremia.

Hyponatremia associated with normal ECF volume and normal total body Na^+ is a common disorder. Although the ECF volume may be slightly higher, there is no edema and the water is distributed throughout ICF and ECF compartments.

Clinical Features

Most patients are asymptomatic and the diagnosis is based on low Na^+ levels detected by biochemical tests. The signs and symptoms depend on the rate of onset and severity of hyponatremia. Mild and moderate cases are generally asymptomatic. Symptoms of acute hyponatremia are due to cerebral edema. Cellular edema occurs because the intracellular compartment is hypertonic compared to ECF. Therefore, water moves into the cells by osmosis causing cellular edema. Although intracellular swelling occurs in most cells, it manifests as neurological symptoms because the brain is encased in the bony calvarium and edematous brain tissue is compressed by the rigid skull. The symptoms are often vague and nonspecific. Anorexia, lethargy, nausea and headache followed by muscle cramps, drowsiness, coma and convulsions.

The early clinical signs of hypovolemic hyponatremia include postural tachycardia and postural hypotension, dryness of the mouth, lack of sweating in axilla and poor skin turgor. The urine volume may be reduced and there may be elevation of urea and uric acid. Urinary Na^+ is more than 20 mmol/L in renal causes and less than 10 mmol/L in extrarenal causes of hypovolemic hyponatremia. Clinical edema occurs when more than 5 L of fluid accumulates in the interstitial fluid compartment.

Management of Hyponatremia

If acute hyponatremia has developed in less than 48 hours and is symptomatic, aggressive correction is warranted, since complications due to cerebral edema may occur. Correction should be done with normal saline or 3% (hypertonic) Na^+ chloride. Total correction of Na^+ to 'normal blood level' of around 140 mmol/L should not be attempted. Initially, hyponatremia may be corrected to achieve blood level of 120 mmol/L or till symptoms improve. The rate of correction should not be over 1.5–2.0 mmol/L/hr and should not exceed 8 mmol/L in 24 hours. The amount of Na^+ required in mmols can be calculated. *See* below box for formula and example.

For example: A person weighing 54 kg has serum sodium 110 mmol/L and is symptomatic. The aim is to correct at 1.5 mmol/L/hr initially up to a maximum of 6–8 mmol/L per day.
Amount of sodium in mmols required = (120-present serum Na^+ level) × 0.6 × body weight in kg.
Amount of sodium in mmols = (120 − 110) × 0.6 × 54 = 324 mmols.
1 L of 3% sodium chloride = 512 mmol Na^+ and 1 L of 0.9% NaCl (normal saline) = 154 mmol of Na^+.
The required sodium will be provided in this case by > 2 L normal saline or about 600 mL of 3% NaCl to be given over 24 hours. Depending on the fluid status, the clinician could decide the replacement fluid. Not more than 400 mL of 3% NaCl over 16 hours and 1 L normal saline over 8 hours.

In chronic and asymptomatic hyponatremia, aggressive correction is not required. In chronic hyponatremia, the low ECF osmolality causes movement of osmotically active substance K^+ and osmotically active intracellular substance called 'idiogenic osmoles' or 'osmolytes' (inositol, taurine, sorbitol, glutamate and glutamine) to move from neurons to CSF and removed. Thus, the intracellular osmolality also decreases and a new osmotic equilibrium is established between ICF and ECF and the patient is asymptomatic. If any aggressive correction is undertaken at this stage, it may lead to higher osmolality of ECF compared to ICF. This osmotic difference results in movement of water from intracellular to extracellular space leading to cellular dehydration and damage. Damaged neuronal cells undergo demyelination. The neurons in the area of central pons are most susceptible to such damage but other parts of the nervous system like basal ganglia can also be affected. This syndrome of osmotic demyelination, also called ***central pontine myelinolysis*** may manifest as extrapyramidal syndromes. Irreversible brain damage may also occur in severe cases. Chronic symptomatic hyponatremia evolves in more than 48 hours. Correction must not be aggressive. Initial correction of 10% (approximately 10 mmol/L) is achieved over 24–48 hours. This is followed by correction at the rate of 1–1.5 mmols/L/day. Hypertonic saline should be avoided after initial correction. Fluid restriction is the mainstay in chronic asymptomatic hyponatremia. Now, AVP receptor antagonists belonging to the class known as vaptens (e.g. tolvaptan) are available for reversing hyponatremia. Vaptens are particularly useful in hypervolemic hyponatremia and in the long-term management of SIADH. Other underlying problems like hypothyroidism, adrenal insufficiency and conditions causing SIADH or intake of drugs like lithium should be looked for and corrected.

Hypernatremia

It is a disorder of water homeostasis associated with serum Na^+ level of more than 145 mmol/L. It may be symptomatic or asymptomatic. Hypernatremia may occur when there is more loss of water compared to Na^+ or more gain of Na^+ compared to water gain in the body. It is common in elderly and in hospitalized patients. If free access to water is denied, hypernatremia may result. As in hyponatremia, it can be associated with ECF volume contraction, ECF volume expansion or normal ECF volume (Box 72.2).

Risk Factors for Hypernatremia

Hypernatremia is common in extremes of age. The physiological responses may not have developed in infancy or they would have been blunt in old age. Inability to maximally concentrate the urine results in polyuria which, when combined with denial of access to free water intake may lead to hypernatremia. This occurs more often in hospital settings where the patient is in the intensive care unit (ICU) or has impaired cognitive function, fever, stroke and impaired thirst mechanism, associated with decreased water intake.

Intravenous (IV) normal saline or Ryle's tube feeding with hyperosmolar enteral feeds aggravate hypernatremia. Diseases like uncontrolled diabetes mellitus (DM) (causing solute diuresis), DI (causing excessive loss of hypotonic fluid as urine), postobstructive diuresis or diuretic phase of acute tubular necrosis (causing free water loss) lead to development of hypernatremia. Water deficiency results in dehydration which in turn causes avid Na^+ reabsorption from the nephron and this combination results in hypernatremia. The resultant increase in ECF osmolality causes movement of water from ICF to ECF with a view to establish an osmotic equilibrium and cell shrinkage occurs. Shrinkage of neurons may cause intracerebral or subarachnoid bleed due to traction on the capillaries. When water content decreases, presence of K^+, Na^+, chloride and idiogenic osmoles in the ICF help to equilibrate the osmolality of ICF and ECF. Aggressive correction of ECF osmolality may lead to movement of excessive fluid into the ICF causing cerebral edema and seizures.

Clinical Features

Infants, elderly patients, those with underlying polyuria, hypertonic fluid infusions, osmotic diuretics, ICU patients with stroke or low Glasgow coma scale (GCS) score, those on mechanical ventilation, or uncontrolled diabetes are at increased risk for hypernatremia. Since hypernatremia represents a hyperosmolar state, the signs and symptoms are related mainly to the central nervous system (CNS).

Since hypernatremia often occurs in hospitalized sick patients and in predictable clinical settings, careful monitoring and prevention is very important. The mortality in children due to acute hypernatremia varies (50 ± 20%). Many of the survivors may have long-term neurological squeal. The mortality in chronic hypernatremia is about 10%.

Management of Hypernatremia

The primary aim of therapy is to restore the serum tonicity. If hypovolemic hypernatremia is associated with hypotension or orthostatic hypotension, initially these patients are given IV normal saline till the systemic hemodynamic and hypotension are corrected. Subsequently, administration of plain water by mouth or 5% dextrose can be used to replace water alone.

In hypervolemic hypernatremia, the aim is to eliminate the excess Na^+ but at the same time administering water. Use of diuretics combined with 5% dextrose IV can achieve this. Those with renal impairment may need dialysis because the response to diuretic may not be prompt. In euvolemic hypernatremia, the water loss from the body is in excess of salt loss. These patients can be managed by 5% dextrose infusion or encouraging oral intake of plain water approximately 2–3 L per day. The dietary Na^+ and protein are restricted. Thiazide diuretics cause more natriuresis than water diuresis. The correction or hypernatremia should be gradual and not at a rate

Box 72.2: Causes of hypernatremia

- Hypernatremia associated with low ECF volume (more water loss compared to sodium loss)
  - Hyperosmolar nonketotic diabetic coma
  - Use of osmotic diuretic—mannitol
  - Tube feeding with high osmolar fluid
  - Hot humid weather, febrile convulsion, excessive sweating
  - Postobstructive diuresis and recovering stage of ATN
  - Gastroenteritis
  - Peritoneal dialysis with high concentration dextrose solutions.
- Hypernatremia with hypervolemia (higher salt intake compared to water)
  - Excessive intake of $NaHCO_3$
  - Excessive infusion of normal/hypertonic saline
  - Drinking excessive quantities of salt water or near-drowning in salt water.
- Hypernatremia with normal ECF volume (mainly due to loss of free water and defective thirst mechanism)
  - Central DI
  - Nephrogenic DI
  - Psychogenic/polydipsia.

Abbreviations: ECF = Extracellular fluid; ATN = Acute tubular necrosis; DI = Diabetes insipidus

greater than 1.0 mEq/L/hr and the total correction can be achieved over 48–72 hours. Serum K^+ and magnesium should be monitored and appropriate corrections given. Aqueous vasopressin, 5 units subcutaneously or desmopressin (DDAVP) by subcutaneous or intranasal route helps the kidneys to retain water.

DISORDERS OF POTASSIUM (K^+) HOMEOSTASIS

Potassium (K^+) is the major intracellular cation. The body contains approximately 3,500 mmol of K^+ (roughly 50 mmol/kg) and is distributed as 90% intracellular, 8% in bone and 2% is in the ECF and serum. The presence of K^+ in the ECF is critical for cellular depolarization and the serum K^+ is maintained between 3.5 and 5.5 mmol/L. The level of serum K^+ does not reflect the total body K^+. The average normal intake of K^+ is 60–80 mmol/day. This is eliminated mainly through urine (80%), GIT (15%) and sweat (5%). Fruits, fruit juices, dry fruits, tender coconut water, beans, chocolates and vegetables are rich in K^+. Dietary K^+ is absorbed and it is driven into the cells by insulin. The Na^+–K^+ ATPase pump in the cell wall constantly shifts the K^+ to the inside and Na^+ out of the cell. In the kidneys, the K^+ is completely filtered by the glomerulus. The K^+ in glomerular filtrate is conserved or eliminated depending on the needs of the body. About 65–70% of K^+ is reabsorbed in the proximal tubule. About 25% reabsorption that occurs is in the thick ascending limb of the loop of Henle and is mediated by the Na^+ K^+ Cl^- co-transport system on the luminal side of the tubular cells. The fine control of renal K^+ elimination occurs in the collecting duct. There are two types of cells in cortical collecting ducts—*the principal cells and the intercalated cells*. Principal cells are concerned with K^+ secretion. This is enhanced by increased luminal flow rate, Na^+ concentration, aldosterone and pH. In the intercalated cells, K^+ reabsorption occurs in exchange for H^+ ions through the K^+-H^+ ATPase. Thus, the normal kidney regulates the serum K^+ level. Aldosterone controls K^+ excretion by its action on the principal cells in the collecting tubule. It also acts through the distal colon and increase fecal elimination. When serum K level is low, suppression of aldosterone and feedback redistribution of K from intracellular compartment occurs. In addition, three important factors regulate the serum K^+ level.

1. Insulin stimulates intracellular K^+ uptake and can reduce extracellular and serum K levels.
2. Catecholamines like epinephrine increases intracellular influx of K.
3. The third and most important factor is the acid base status. Acidemia produces hyperkalemia due to shift of K from ICF to ECF and the opposite occurs when there is alkalemia. However, metabolic alkalosis may be associated with significant urinary K^+ loss.

In hypokalemia, urinary loss of > 30 mmol/day reflects renal K^+ wasting and in hyperkalemia urinary loss of < 30 mmol/day suggests primary renal disease. Trans-tubular K^+ gradient (TTKG) provides an indirect measurement of the net K^+ secretion in the distal nephron. It is calculated as follows:

$$TTKG = \frac{Urinary\ K^+}{Serum\ K^+} \times \frac{Serum\ osmolality}{Urinary\ osmolality}$$

Note: Normal TTKG is 5–10. TTKG is not generally used at present.

In hypokalemia, if the kidney is functioning normally, the TTKG will be less than 5. If the TTKG is > 10, it suggests inability of kidney to reabsorb K^+ and hypokalemia is due to primary renal disease, e.g. renal tubular acidosis (RTA) (types I and II) and Bartter syndrome.

In hyperkalemia, if the kidneys are functioning normally, TTKG will be more than 10. If the TTKG is < 5, it suggests inability of the kidneys to excrete K^+ ions and hyperkalemia is due to renal failure, aldosterone deficiency or resistance to aldosterone.

Hypokalemia

In hypokalemia, the serum K^+ level is less than 3.5 mmol/L. In early stages, it is asymptomatic and may be detected incidentally during investigations. Many conditions are associated with development of hypokalemia. Common causes includes:

- *Diuretic therapy:* Most diuretics except the K^+ sparing diuretics can lead to hypokalemia.
- *Pyloric stenosis and continuous gastric drainage:* Loss of gastric hydrochloric acid (HCl) and volume contraction will lead respectively to alkalosis and activation of renin angiotensin—aldosterone axis. Aldosterone causes Na^+ reabsorption and K^+ excretion and leads to hypokalemia.
- *Alcoholism:* Combination of poor intake, gastric loss due to vomiting and urinary loss of K^+ leads to hypokalemia.
- *Renal tubular acidosis (RTA):* Urinary K^+ loss which occurs in both distal (type I) and proximal (type II) RTA leads to hypokalemia.
- *Antibiotic induced hypokalemia:* Antibiotics like penicillin, carbenicillin and gentamicin cause hypokalemia due to excessive secretion of K^+ by renal tubules.
- Amphotericin B produces type I (distal) RTA and hypokalemia.
- *Hyperaldosteronism:* Any condition causing primary and secondary hyperaldosteronism causes hypokalemia.
- *Bartter syndrome:* It is a syndrome characterized by hyperreninemia, hyperaldosteronism, metabolic alkalosis and hypokalemia and is associated with hyperplasia of juxtaglomerular apparatus. Severe form of Bartter's syndrome is associated with failure to thrive, polyuria and muscle cramps.

Other conditions causing hypokalemia are acute leukemia, magnesium deficiency, chronic diuretic or laxative use, salt losing nephropathies, familial hypokalemic periodic paralysis, Cushing's syndrome, steroid therapy, ectopic adrenocorticotropic hormone (ACTH) secretion, insulin administration, use of β2-adrenergic agonists (salbutamol) and metabolic alkalosis.

Clinical Manifestations

Even though the laboratory report may show low levels of K^+, most patients are asymptomatic till serum K^+ levels are below 3 mmol/L. In hypokalemia, major manifestations

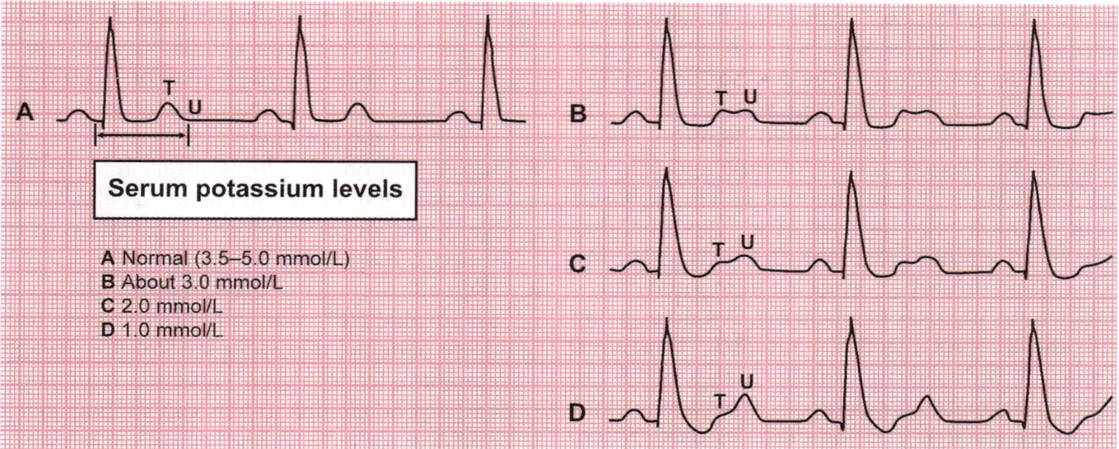

Fig. 72.1: Hypokalemia—ECG. **Note:** (1) Flat/inverted T waves, (2) Prominent U waves (3) Prolonged QT interval

are due to functional cellular abnormalities in skeletal muscle, smooth muscle, cardiac muscle and renal cells. Initially, the motor power is diminished particularly in the lower limbs. This is followed by weakness or paralysis. The deep tendon reflexes may remain normal initially. The severe myopathy may progress to rhabdomyolysis, myoglobinuria and acute kidney injury. Paralysis of respiratory muscles may also occur. The manifestations relating to cardiac muscle involvement is more common in digitalized patients or those with ischemic heart disease (IHD). The electrocardiographic (ECG) changes are non-specific ST-T changes and more specific U wave changes (Fig. 72.1). In the kidney, hypokalemia manifests as polyuria, polydipsia, metabolic alkalosis with increased ammonia synthesis and increased acid excretion in urine. There is vacuolation of renal tubular cells, leading to the presence of acid urine in the setting of metabolic alkalosis, and is called ***paradoxical aciduria.*** It is a common feature in hypokalemic states. The other renal manifestations include reversible renal failure due to the changes in the renal tubule, phosphaturia, hypophosphatemia, hypocalcemia and water retention. In hypokalemic states, the release of insulin from pancreas is blunted resulting in hyperglycemia. In the gastrointestinal system, severe hypokalemia, often associated with hypomagnesemia below 1 mg/dL, results in paralytic ileus.

Management of Hypokalemia

While attempting to correct hypokalemia, certain important guidelines are followed. The normal intake of about 60 mmol/day of K^+ often prevents the development of hypokalemia. However, cardia patients on long-term diuretics, digitalis therapy, those on large doses of steroids, IHD and postoperative patients may need higher K^+ intake. Since K^+ is an intracellular ion, serum K^+ level does not truly reflect the total body K^+. One mmol/L fall in serum K^+ level represents approximately a total body deficit of 200–400 mmol. If the serum K^+ is < 2 mmol/L, the deficit may be >600 mmol of K^+. Administration of K^+ should be carefully monitored in those receiving K^+ sparing diuretics, angiotensin converting inhibitors or angiotensin II receptor blockers (ARBs) and patients with renal failure or oliguria and anuria since this can precipitate hyperkalemia. Oral route is sufficient in most situations. In severe hypokalemia, with paralysis, K^+ is given as IV infusion. K^+ should never be given as a bolus injection or rapid IV infusion since it may cause cardiac arrest and instantaneous death. IV K^+ infusions are given only in intensive care units (ICUs) where monitoring facilities are available. The rate of infusion should not exceed 10 mmol/hour and the administration and response should be continuously monitored.

If IV K^+ administration is needed for severe hypokalemia and in those with symptoms or signs like cardiac arrhythmia, paralytic ileus, respiratory muscle paralysis, severe myopathy or familial periodic paralysis, 100 mmol of K^+ chloride in 1,000 mL normal saline is given over 10–12 hours. The subsequent dose is decided based on response and blood level. Appropriate supportive measures including ventilatory/respiratory assistance should be available. The correction must be steady and gradual. If the response is not adequate in 48 hours, concomitant hypomagnesemia must be looked for and corrected with oral or IV magnesium. The two important causes for nonresponsive nature of hypokalemia are ongoing K^+ loss and associated hypomagnesemia. K^+ supplements are continued as a long-term treatment for those with constant urinary K^+ loss.

Once the acute stage is corrected and the renal functions are normal, K^+ sparing drugs can be used as adjuvant therapy. Often, it is not necessary to give K^+ supplements along with K^+ sparing diuretics like spironolactone, amiloride and triamterene.

If the serum K^+ is between 3 and 4 mmol/L and the patient is asymptomatic, no aggressive treatment is necessary. However, if the patient is receiving diuretic, or laxative or has chronic diarrhea, appropriate K^+ supplements in the form of fruits and vegetables or oral K^+ chloride supplements may be given. In patients with IHD or on digitalis, K^+ level should not be allowed to drop below 3.5 mmol/L as it may induce life-threatening arrhythmias. Serum K^+ level of <3 mmol/L requires treatment. Oral K^+ replacement is adequate in most patients. Administration of oral K^+ chloride alone is

Textbook of Medicine

sufficient for correction of hypokalemia associated with alkalosis because, it dissociates into K^+ and Cl^- and is absorbed in the gut in exchange for Na^+ and HCO_3^- respectively. Thus, the hypokalemia and alkalosis are corrected simultaneously. The dose is 20–40 mmol orally, 2–4 times a day. In those with hypokalemia and acidosis (RTA types I and II), K^+ bicarbonate or K^+ citrate-based replacement solution may be used. The recommended oral dose is 20–40 mmol of KCl four times a day. During therapy, serum and urinary K^+ levels are monitored daily.

Spironolactone, in doses of 25–50 mg, 3–4 times a day is given till the K^+ level reaches 4 mmol/L. Thereafter, the dose may be reduced and smaller doses of 25 mg daily are given as maintenance dose. Triamterene and amiloride are the other K^+ sparing diuretics used. Since, hypomagnesemia, hypophosphatemia and alcoholism are associated with chronic hypokalemia, correction of the primary conditions is necessary on long-term management. In rare situations of acidosis with hypokalemia, K^+ supplements are administered initially to correct hypokalemia before attempting to correct acidosis with IV bicarbonate. For diluting K^+ chloride, normal saline is preferred to 5% dextrose. Ringer lactate contains K^+. Most oral rehydration fluids also contain K^+.

Hyperkalemia

In hyperkalemia, serum K^+ is greater than 5 mmol/L. It is considered moderate if K^+ level is between 5.5 and 6.5 mmol/L and severe if > 6.5 mmol/L. Severe hyperkalemia may cause cardiac arrest. A functioning kidney is able to eliminate the K^+ from the body efficiently and so most cases of hyperkalemia are due to renal failure. Pseudohyperkalemia may be due to errors in blood collection, hemolysis of the sample, leukocytosis or thrombocytosis. In such cases, plasma K^+ is rechecked using a properly collected specimen. Though K^+ is excreted mainly by the kidney, when the kidney function deteriorates gradually as in chronic renal failure (CRF), the gastrointestinal excretion increases and K^+ homeostasis is maintained. The risk of hyperkalemia increases when such patients develop oliguria, infection, sepsis or they consume K^+ rich diets or use K^+ retaining drugs. Stored blood, fruit juice, angiotensin converting enzyme (ACE) inhibitors, spironolactone or K^+ containing drugs may precipitate hyperkalemia in patients with milder degrees of renal failure.

Causes

- Hyperkalemia in these situations may be due to following mechanisms:
  - *Kidney diseases:* Failure of excretion of K^+ could occur either due to decreased glomerular filtration or due to defective tubular secretion of K^+. Both acute and CRF can cause hyperkalemia. Defective K^+ secretion is due to either deficiency or cellular unresponsiveness to aldosterone. Since the kidney cannot eliminate the K^+ rapidly, any rapid increase in exogenous K^+ intake invariably causes hyperkalemia.
  - Rapid release of K^+ from the intracellular compartment may occur with rhabdomyolysis, tumor lysis syndrome, intravascular hemolysis, trauma causing crush injury, infection and transfusion of stored blood. In most patients with normal renal function and normal urine output, the excess K^+ is eliminated gradually.
- Redistribution of K^+ from intracellular to extracellular compartment as in diabetic ketoacidosis, use of drugs like β-adrenergic blockers and digitalis overdose can cause hyperkalemia.
- Hypoaldosteronism may be primary or secondary as in diabetes with tubulointerstitial disease. In these patients, the hypoplasia of the juxtaglomerular apparatus leads to hyporeninemia, hypoaldosteronism and hyperkalemia. When the tubular cell is unresponsive to aldosterone as in sickle cell anemia, systemic lupus erythematosus (SLE), amyloidosis or following renal transplantation, hyperkalemia occurs.

Clinical Manifestations and Diagnosis

Hyperkalemia is very often asymptomatic and the diagnosis is made by investigation. Muscular weakness and paresthesias may be the only initial symptoms. Rarely hyperkalemic periodic paralysis may occur. Mild to severe chest discomfort resembling cardiac pain may be the only symptom when the patient presents with ventricular fibrillation or cardiac arrest.

The diagnosis is confirmed by demonstrating serum $K^+ > 5.5$ mmol/L.

ECG changes of hyperkalemia evolve through the following stages as the serum K^+ level increases from 5.5 to more than 9 mmol/L. The relationship between the ECG changes and blood levels is quite variable. The ECG changes are (Figs 72.2A and B):
- Tall peaked T waves (serum K^+ 6–7 mmol/L)
- Prolongation of PR and absent P wave (serum K^+ 7–8 mmol/L)
- Widening of QRS (serum K^+ 7–8 mmol/L)
- Sine wave, ventricular tachycardia, ventricular fibrillation (serum K^+ 8–9 mmol/L)
- Cardiac arrest (serum K^+ more than 9 mmol/L).

In patients with recurrent chronic hyperkalemia, the following points should be particularly looked for:
- History of intake of K^+ in diet or as K^+ supplements.
- Drugs causing hyperkalemia such as K^+ sparing diuretic, β-blockers, ACE inhibitor, H_2 receptor blockers and nonsteroidal anti-inflammatory drugs (NSAIDs).
- The combination of hyperkalemia with hyponatremia should suggest Addison's disease.

Management of Hyperkalemia

In mild and moderate hyperkalemia, attention to potassium intake, avoidance of drugs causing hyperkalemia and correction of acidosis are often sufficient. Cation exchange resins such as Na^+ or calcium polystyrene sulfonate given orally or as retention enema exchanges Na^+/calcium for K^+ and helps to eliminate K^+ from the body. Two gram of resin exchanges 2 mmol Na^+ or 1 mmol of calcium for 2 mmol K^+. For oral administration, the resin is given in

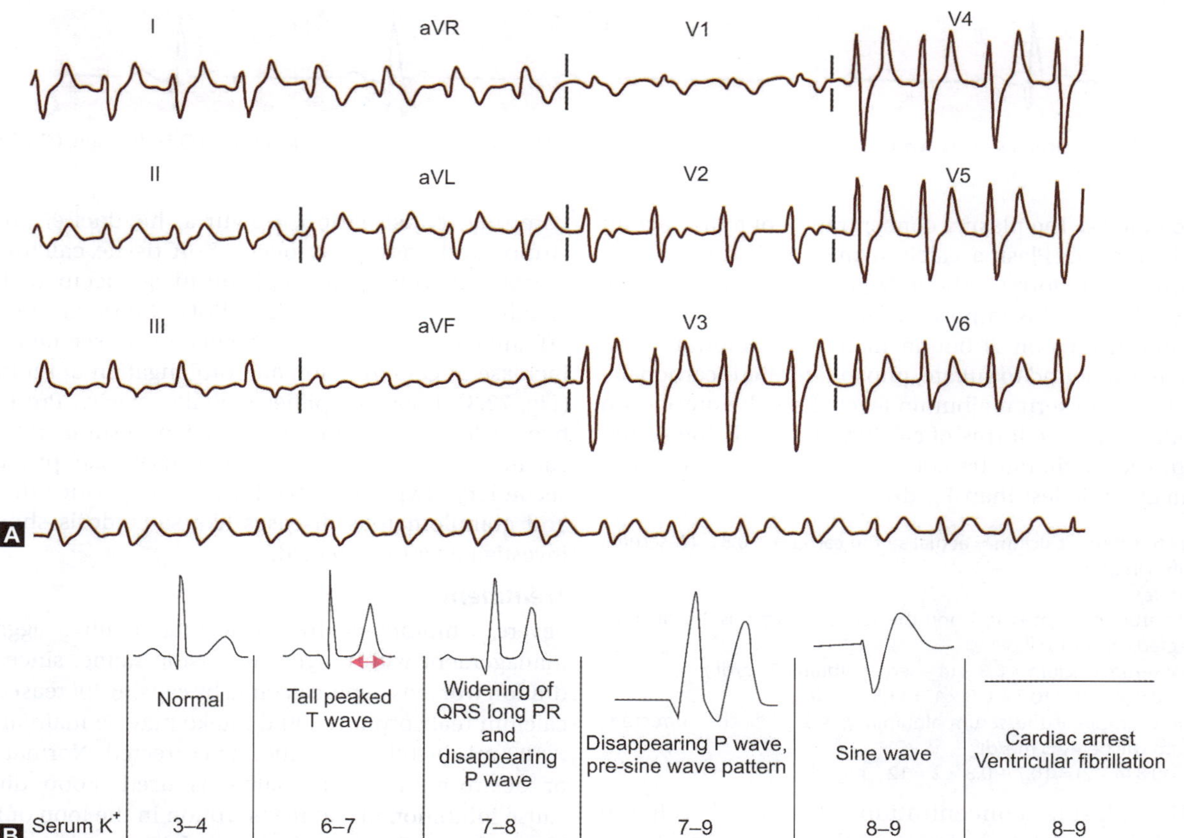

Figs 72.2A and B: Hyperkalemia—ECG. **A.** 12-lead ECG characteristic features of hyperkalemia; **B.** Diagram showing progressive changes in ECG pattern with raising serum potassium levels

20% sorbitol. For retention enema—10% dextrose is used as the vehicle.

Severe hyperkalemia is a medical emergency and is managed as follows:

Step 1A: 20 mL of 10% calcium gluconate is given as a steady slow IV injection over 5–10 minutes and repeated once if necessary. The solution should not be injected rapidly as a bolus. Calcium stabilizes the myocardial membrane against the arrhythmias caused by K^+ but the effect is very transient and lasts for the period of infusion only.

Step 1B: If the patient is acidotic, 100 mL of 7.5% Na^+ bicarbonate is given IV. 10 mL normal saline should be given through the needle or cannula after the calcium injection before giving IV bicarbonate. Use of same syringe for loading calcium and bicarbonate must be avoided since calcium salts and $NaHCO_3$ are physically incompatible. White precipitation of calcium carbonate occurs when they come into contact with each other. $NaHCO_3$ causes temporary reversal of acidosis and reduces serum K^+ level by causing movement of K^+ into the intracellular compartment. If the patient is acidotic, we may proceed to Step 2 after Step 1A.

Step 2: 100 mL of 25% glucose along with 5 units of regular (crystalline) insulin is infused in 2 hours. Insulin also promotes entry of K^+ into the cells and controls hyperkalemia. Thus, it helps to gain time for initiation of dialysis.

Step 3: High doses of adrenergic agonists such as albuterol or salbutamol (5 mg/mL) when given as nebulization in doses of 10–20 mg over approximately 10 minutes also shifts the K^+ to the intracellular compartment, thereby reducing serum K^+ level.

Step 4: Both hemodialysis (HD) and peritoneal dialysis (PD) help to remove K^+ rapidly from the body. HD does it faster and more efficiently. The K^+ concentration of the HD concentrate or PD fluid can be altered depending on the clinical circumstances.

Step 5: If dialysis facility is not available, removal of K^+ from the body can be achieved by the regular use of Na^+/calcium polystyrene sulfonate. The recommended dose is 15 g 6 hourly orally and it is continued till the serum K^+ falls below 5.5 mmol/L. Thereafter, smaller doses are given to prevent rise in K^+ levels. In all patients with renal failure, low K^+ diet and avoidance of offending drugs are necessary.

Hyperkalemia suggests mainly impaired K^+ elimination by the kidney and is an asymptomatic 'silent killer'. So, early diagnosis and prompt treatment are life-saving.

DISORDERS OF CALCIUM HOMEOSTASIS

Calcium plays a crucial role in cellular functions and is an important ingredient of the bone. Calcium exists in 2 forms, bound and free forms. The bound calcium which constitutes more than 99% of the body's calcium is in bones. In the intracellular compartment, calcium concentration in cytoplasm is low but it is very high in the

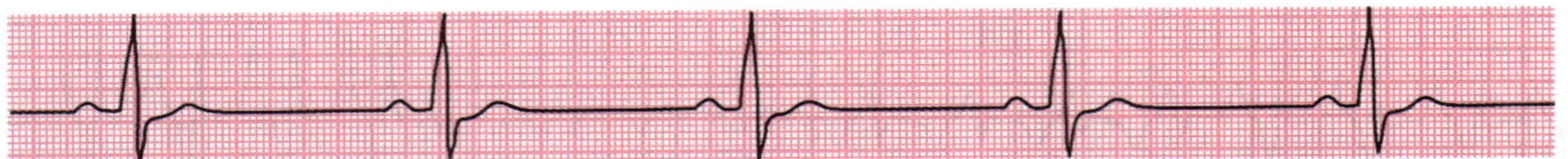

Fig. 72.3: Hypercalcemia—ECG. *Note:* (1) ST segment short or absent, (2) Short QT interval, (3) Slight increase in QRS duration, (4) PR interval may be prolonged

mitochondria. The plasma concentration of total calcium is 9–11 mg/dL. Plasma calcium may be in the ionized or nonionized forms. About 50% of calcium is in the ionized form and is important for cellular functions. The nonionized fraction is bound mainly to albumin (40%) and the rest bound to sulfate, phosphate and bicarbonate. Any change in serum albumin level alters the proportion of bound and free forms of calcium in blood. The serum calcium level should be corrected for any reduction in serum albumin less than 4 g/dL.

> Corrected serum calcium = actual serum calcium + 0.8 × (4–serum albumin in g/dL).
>
> **Example:**
> If the serum calcium is 10.7 and the serum albumin is 3 g/dL, the corrected calcium will be:
> Actual serum calcium + 0.8 × (4 – serum albumin in g/dL)
> 10.7 + 0.8 (4 – 3) = 10.7 + 0.8 × 1 = 11.5 mg/dL
> In the example, if the serum albumin was 2 g/dL, the corrected calcium will be: 12.3 mg/dL
> 10.7 + 0.8 (4 – 2) = 10.7 + 0.8 × 2 = 12.3 mg/dL

The plasma concentration of ionized calcium is tightly regulated by parathormone, calcitriol 1,25-dihydroxyvitamin D_3 [1,25$(OH)_2D_3$] and calcitonin. The ionic calcium is influenced by the acid-base status, estrogen and prolactin. Alkalosis causes fall in ionized calcium. The dietary calcium, approximately 800–1100 mg/day, is absorbed from the intestine and transported to the ECF compartment. In the extracellular space, it is deposited in the bone or eliminated via the kidney. The entry and exit between the skeletal and nonskeletal compartments are equal under steady-state conditions. The kidneys, intestine and skeleton are important in the short, mid and long-term homeostasis respectively.

Parathormone facilitates reabsorption of calcium from bone. In the kidney, it increases reabsorption of filtered calcium from renal tubules and aids in 1α-hydroxylation of vitamin D. Thus, the serum calcium increases. The high level of calcium and active vitamin D in plasma suppresses parathyroid hormone (PTH). Calcitonin on the other hand decreases the plasma calcium level by inhibiting bone reabsorption and increasing urinary excretion. Other factors like hyperphosphatemia decreases calcium levels. Metabolic alkalosis is often associated with hypocalcemia because of decreased release of calcium from bone.

Hypercalcemia

It is defined as total serum calcium more than 11 mg/dL. Hypercalcemia results from increased intestinal calcium absorption, stimulation of bone resorption or decrease in urinary calcium excretion (*See* Section 11, Ch 100).

The clinical manifestations of hypercalcemia depends on the degree and rate of its development. Symptoms like fatigue, muscle weakness, nausea, vomiting, constipation, polyuria, headache, amnesia stupor and coma may occur. Soft tissue calcification, nephrocalcinosis and nephrolithiasis occur with long standing hypercalcemia. The ECG shows shortening of QT interval, reduction or absence of ST segment, slight increase in QRS duration and prolongation of PR interval (Fig. 72.3). It also amplifies digitalis toxicity. Presence of hypercalcemia can be confirmed by estimating serum calcium level. The underlying causes like primary or secondary hyperparathyroidism, neoplastic disorders and granulomatous diseases like sarcoidosis should be investigated and corrected.

Treatment

Severe symptomatic hypercalcemia requires aggressive management with rehydration using saline, since dehydration worsens hypercalcemia by causing increased renal calcium reabsorption. Fluid intake may be maintained at > 100 mL/hr till dehydration is corrected. Normal saline or dextrose in normal saline is used. Loop diuretics cause inhibition of Na^+ reabsorption in the loop of Henle. Na^+ reabsorption is linked to calcium and so calcium excretion in the urine increases. Use of calcitonin 4 IU/kg IV is used in emergencies to reduce calcium levels rapidly. Bisphosphonates (etidronate and pamidronate) inhibit bone reabsorption and help to normalize high plasma calcium levels. Other drugs which can be used are glucocorticoids which inhibit calcitriol production. Steroids may be used in hypervitaminosis D, sarcoidosis and hematopoietic tumors such as myeloma, lymphoma and solid tumors like breast cancer. Gallium nitrate which is used in hypercalcemia of malignancy. Correction of acid base imbalance, also improves calcium level. The use of calcitonin and mithramycin (tumoricidal antibiotic causing hypocalcemia) are reserved for malignant hypercalcemia with serum calcium above 15 mg/dL. A new class of *calcium receptor (CaR) agonists or calcimimetics* which increase the sensitivity of calcium sensing receptors are used in primary and secondary hyperparathyroidism. In severe and symptomatic hypercalcemia, dialysis with low calcium dialysate can be undertaken.

Hypocalcemia

It is defined as serum calcium below 8.5 mg/dL. Calcium level should be corrected for albumin concentration before confirming hypocalcemia. Symptoms of hypocalcemia occur only when ionized calcium level decreases below 4.5 mg/dL. Acute hypocalcemia may occur following hyperventilation and respiratory alkalosis. Alkalemia decreases ionized calcium level. Chronic hypocalcemia is caused by hypoparathyroidism, pseudohypoparathyroidism, vitamin D deficiency states, CRF and magnesium deficiency (*See* Section 11, Ch 100).

Textbook of Medicine

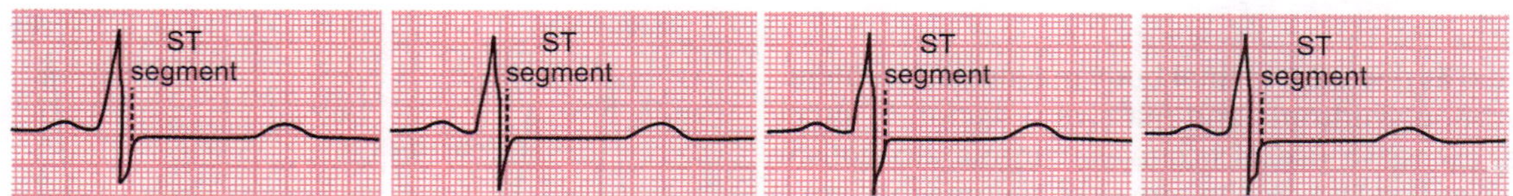

Fig. 72.4: Hypocalcemia—ECG. ***Note:*** (1) Prolongation of the QT interval, (2) Flat or inverted T waves in severe hypocalcemia, (3) Slight decrease in QRS duration, (4) ST segment lengthening

The diagnosis is confirmed by corrected serum calcium level of < 8.5 mg/dL. If hypocalcemia is associated with high plasma phosphorus, conditions like hypoparathyroidism, pseudohypoparathyroidism and advanced renal failure are the possibilities. In steatorrhea, vitamin D deficiency, acute pancreatitis and recovering acute renal failure (ARF), combination of hypocalcemia and hypophosphatemia is seen.

The ECG signs of hypocalcemia include prolongation of the QT interval, flat or inverted T waves in severe hypocalcemia, slight decrease in QRS duration and ST segment lengthening (Fig. 72.4).

DISORDERS OF PHOSPHATE HOMEOSTASIS

Phosphorus is present in the ICF and ECF. It participates in most metabolic processes including the release of energy from adenosine triphosphate (ATP). Apart from being an abundant component of skeleton along with calcium, it is also present in various tissues and cell structures. The plasma phosphorus level is controlled by hormones like PTH and calcitriol. Long-term maintenance of phosphate homeostasis is regulated by renal tubular reabsorption. About 60% of dietary phosphate is absorbed by the intestine. There is a constant turnover daily between blood and bone phosphorus. The daily renal phosphate excretion equals the intestinal absorption.

Hyperphosphatemia

It is defined as serum phosphorus > 5 mg/dL. The most common cause is reduced renal excretion as seen in renal failure. Normally, 85–90% of filtered phosphorus is reabsorbed. When the glomerular fitration rate (GFR) is declining, even though the remaining nephrons eliminate 90% of phosphorus, the serum phosphorus increases because of decrease in the number of functioning nephrons. Other causes of hyperphosphatemia include, hypoparathyroidism, chronic hypocalcemia, acromegaly, hypercatabolic states (tumor lysis and crush injury) and vitamin D intoxication.

Severe hyperphosphatemia decreases serum calcium level which in turn stimulates PTH. This causes increased phosphate excretion and normalization of hyperphosphatemia. The occurrence of severe hypocalcemia with tetany and ectopic calcification is the most severe manifestation of hyperphosphatemia.

Treatment of the underlying cause of hyperphosphatemia is most important. Low phosphate diet, low protein diet, oral phosphate binders like calcium acetate and magnesium salts may be used. Aluminium containing phosphate binders should be used cautiously in CRF because of toxicity due to aluminium accumulation. A new nonabsorbable aluminium and calcium free phosphate binding resin—***sevelamer*** is now available and can be used in doses of 800 mg in 3 divided doses.

Hypophosphatemia

It is defined as plasma phosphate level of less than 2.5 mg/dL. It may be caused by genetic diseases or acquired conditions. Inherited hypophosphatemia include Fanconi's syndrome, X-linked hypophosphatemic rickets and distal RTA.

Acquired conditions include malnutrition, alcoholism, diabetic ketoacidosis, acute respiratory alkalosis, oncogenic osteomalacia and total parenteral nutrition. The clinical manifestations depend on the severity of hypophosphatemia. Metabolic encephalopathy, muscle weakness, rhabdomyolysis, hemolysis, thrombocytopenia and leukocyte dysfunction may occur. The cause of hypophosphatemia is identified and treated appropriately. Oral phosphate supplementation is achieved by increasing intake of milk products. Joule's solution containing disodium hydrogen phosphate buffered in phosphoric acid may be used orally for long-term treatment. In severe symptomatic deficiency, parenteral K^+ phosphate infusions may be given.

DISORDERS OF MAGNESIUM HOMEOSTASIS

Magnesium is predominantly an intracellular cation. It is involved in metabolic processes like protein synthesis, regulation of mitochondrial function and immune and inflammatory processes. It is also involved in the maintenance of vasomotor tone, neuronal activity, cardiac excitability and neuromuscular transmission. The dietary magnesium averages about 12 mmols/day. Only about 50% is absorbed. The plasma magnesium concentration is maintained between 0.75 and 1.0 mmols/L (1.8–2.4 mg/dL). The absorbed magnesium reaches the ICF and is either deposited in the bone or soft tissue. The renal elimination approximately equals the intestinal absorption and the magnesium homeostasis is maintained.

Hypermagnesemia

It is defined as serum magnesium level more than 1.9 mg/dL (or 1 mmol/L). The common cause are renal failure and use of magnesium containing drugs. The signs and symptoms are due to the effect of magnesium on the CNS and cardiovascular system (CVS). Mild cases are asymptomatic. When the serum level increases to 7–9 mg/dL (3 mmols/L), deep tendon reflexes are lost. When the level is more 12 mg/dL (5 mmols/L), respiratory paralysis, hypotension, cardiac conduction abnormalities and loss of consciousness occur. The initial step in the emergency management of symptomatic hypermagnesemia is administration of IV calcium.

Hypomagnesemia

It is defined as decrease in total body magnesium content. Malabsorption syndrome and massive resection of small intestine, excessive use of laxatives, chronic alcoholism and uncontrolled DM are the causes of hypomagnesemia. Use of drugs like gentamicin, cisplatin, cyclosporin and overuse of diuretics may also lead to hypomagnesemia. Moderate to severe magnesium depletion may result in general weakness, neuromuscular hyperexcitability with hyper-reflexia, carpopedal spasm, tremor and rarely, tetany. The ECG changes include widening of QRS, prolongation of QT interval, ST depression, low or inverted T wave and occasional U waves (Figs 72.5A and B). Treatment is by using oral magnesium salts. In emergency, parenteral magnesium sulfate may be used. 1.5–3.0 g of magnesium sulfate is given by deep intramuscular route. It provides 150–300 mg of elemental magnesium.

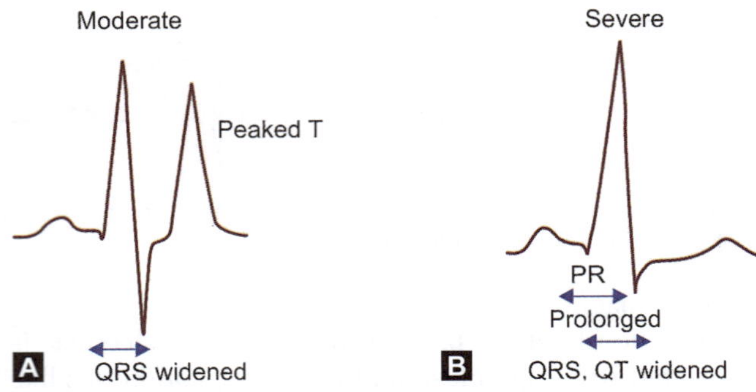

Figs 72.5A and B: ECG changes in hypomagnesemia (1) Peaked T waves, T wave amplitude falling progressively in severe deficiency (2) QRS widened, QT widened (3) PR interval prolonged (4) 'U' waves may develop (5) ST segment depressed

Hypermagnesemia: It is uncertain whether hypermagnesemia per se leads to any pathognomonic ECG changes.

Abnormalities of Acid-base Balance

R Kasi Visweswaran

Chapter Summary

- General Considerations
- Body Buffers and Buffering Systems
- Primary Disturbances in Acid-base Balance
- Interpretation of Arterial Blood Gases (ABG) and Biochemical Reports
- Practical Clinical Situation Examples
- Serum and Urinary Anion Gap
  - Urinary Anion Gap
- Compensatory Response to Acid-base Disturbance and their Limits of Compensation
- Respiratory Acidosis
- Respiratory Alkalosis
- Metabolic Alkalosis
- Metabolic Acidosis
  - Uremic Acidosis
  - Lactic Acidosis
  - Ketoacidosis
  - Drugs and Toxins
- Mixed Acid-base Disorders
- Case Studies

GENERAL CONSIDERATIONS

In the body, acid-base homeostasis is maintained by the kidneys, lungs, liver and buffering mechanisms. The pH of the blood represents the concentration of free H^+ ions. When the pH is 7.0, the H^+ concentration is greater than 80 nmol/L and can be potentially lethal. The normal pH is 7.40 and represents H^+ ion concentration of 40 mmol/L. Within the ranges of body pH in health and disease, the H^+ ion concentration in nmol/L can be calculated by taking away (subtracting) the numbers in the decimal part of the pH, from the number 80.

Examples:

pH 7.40 = (80 – 40) = 40 nmol/L
pH 7.35 = (80 – 35) = 45 nmol/L
pH 7.45 = (80 – 45) = 35 nmol/L
pH 7.25 = (80 – 25) = 55 nmol/L
pH 7.55 = (80 – 55) = 25 nmol/L

Free H^+ ions bind avidly to proteins, increase the net positive charge and alter their structure and function. The pH of extracellular fluid (ECF) must be maintained constantly between 7.35 and 7.45 for viability, normal metabolism and enzyme functions of the cells in the body. Although the daily acid load to the body varies from time to time even in a healthy person, the pH of blood is avidly maintained in above range. Diet contributes to the production of acids and alkali. Metabolism of amino acids like lysine, arginine, methionine, cysteine or organophosphates yield acid. Some amino acids like glutamate and aspartate or substances like acetate and citrate yield alkali on metabolism. Generally, nonvegetarian diet gives rise to more acid production. In addition, the body produces small quantities of organic acids like acetic acid, lactic acid and pyruvic acid. The endogenous H^+ (acid) production is approximately 1 mEq/kg/day. The acids are added to the body as volatile and nonvolatile acids (phosphoric and sulphuric). They are immediately buffered and transported to the lungs and kidneys for elimination. Carbonic acid (H_2CO_3) is volatile since, it dissociates into carbon dioxide and water ($H_2CO_3 \rightarrow H_2O + CO_2$).

The lungs help to eliminate approximately 15,000 millimoles of CO_2 daily and regulate the CO_2 concentration. This capacity is much more than the CO_2 produced in health.

For each H^+ ion excreted by the kidney, the body gains one mmol of bicarbonate. Thus, the kidneys regulates the bicarbonate concentration. Kidneys help to excrete the H^+ ion as titratable acid and ammonia, e.g. disodium hydrogen phosphate in the tubular fluid is converted into sodium dihydrogen phosphate and is excreted ($Na_2HPO_4 + H^+ \rightarrow NaH_2PO_4 + Na^+$), thus eliminating one atom of hydrogen.

BODY BUFFERS AND BUFFERING SYSTEMS

Buffers are the immediate defense mechanisms against challenges with acids. They consist of chemical substances which can bind acid or alkaline ions rapidly. The buffers may be intracellular or extracellular. Buffering takes place by many mechanisms:

- Intracellular organelles have endomembrane acid-base transporters which respond appropriately to acute changes in intracellular acid or base in such a way that the pH in the cytoplasm is maintained. The intracellular pH of cells is variable and is often lower than the blood pH. The intracellular pH of some important cells is given below:
  Skeletal muscle $\rightarrow$ pH = 6.9–7.2
  Hepatocyte $\rightarrow$ pH = 7.2
  Neuronal cell $\rightarrow$ pH = 7.1
  Cardiac muscle $\rightarrow$ pH = 7.0–7.4
- Hemoglobin/inorganic and organic acid, ammonia and phosphates serve as buffers in blood and body fluids.
- Biochemical buffer systems may generate or consume H^+ ions [e.g. adenosine triphosphate (ATP) hydrolysis, phosphorylation of adenosine diphosphate (ADP) and glycolysis].
- Basic physiochemical buffer systems.
  Buffers are solutions which can resist changes in the pH caused by the addition of acid or alkali. Physicochemical buffers are of two types:
  1. Mixture of weak acids with their salt with a strong base.
  2. Mixture of weak base with their salt with a strong acid.
  For examples:
  - Bicarbonate buffer—carbonic acid (weak acid) H_2CO_3/sodium bicarbonate (salt of strong base) $NaHCO_3$.
  - Acetate buffer—acetic acid (CH_3COOH)/sodium acetate (CH_3COONa)
  - Phosphate buffer $\rightarrow$ disodium hydrogen phosphate (Na_2HPO_4)/sodium dihydrogen phosphate (NaH_2PO_4). This is the most effective buffer system in the body. The phosphate buffer system is effective in a wide range of pH.

The action of acetate buffer is explained to highlight how the buffer behaves on addition of acid or alkali to it.

When hydrochloric acid (HCl), a strong acid, is added to the acetate buffer, the salt sodium acetate reacts with HCl forming acetic acid (weak acid) and sodium chloride.

$$HCl + CH_3COONa \rightarrow NaCl + CH_3COOH$$

When sodium hydroxide (NaOH), a strong base, is added to the acetate buffer, the acetic acid reacts with NaOH and forms salt, sodium acetate (weak base) and water.

$$NaOH + CH_3COOH \rightarrow CH_3COONa + H_2O$$

The buffer systems in the body are very important in preventing the shift of pH of the ECF. The bicarbonate-carbonic acid buffer system is the most important buffer system in the ECF. The other buffer systems include hemoglobin, plasma proteins, phosphate ions and the bone. Bone is a huge alkali reserve in the body. Dissolution of the bones provides alkaline calcium salts and adds bicarbonate to the ECF. The bone buffers are utilized in conditions associated with chronic metabolic acidosis. In the initial stages, there are no symptoms and the bone damage may go unnoticed. Patients may become symptomatic only when advanced stage is reached.

PRIMARY DISTURBANCES IN ACID-BASE BALANCE

When the pH of blood falls less than 7.35, the condition is called acidemia and when it rises more than 7.45, it is called alkalemia. The term acidosis and alkalosis are used to denote the pathophysiological process causing the shift in the pH. Hypercarbia is carbon dioxide retention (high $PaCO_2$) and hypocarbia is carbon dioxide washout (low $PaCO_2$). Hypoxemia is low PaO_2 levels in blood.

Thus, we can visualize four primary disturbances in the acid-base equilibrium.
1. Fall in bicarbonate $\rightarrow$ metabolic acidosis
2. Rise in bicarbonate $\rightarrow$ metabolic alkalosis
3. Rise in PCO_2 $\rightarrow$ respiratory acidosis
4. Fall in PCO_2 $\rightarrow$ respiratory alkalosis

The body has built in mechanisms to combat the primary disturbances of acid-base to some extent. It can be understood well by the simple equation derived from the Henderson-Hasselbalch equation for pH.

Henderson-Hasselbalch's equation for pH $\rightarrow$ $pH = pKa + \log \dfrac{HCO_3}{H_2CO_3}$

The simplified formula derived from the above is $\rightarrow \dfrac{HCO_3}{PCO_2}$

If the primary change is an increase in the numerator (HCO_3) of the above simplified equation, i.e. metabolic alkalosis, the pH would also increase. In order to minimize the increase in pH, the value of the denominator (PCO_2) should also increase. In other words, the 'compensation' by the body for the primary event of metabolic alkalosis ($\uparrow HCO_3$) is respiratory acidosis ($\uparrow PCO_2$). Similarly, any upward or downward change in numerator should be associated with similar change in the denominator and vice versa. Thus, the compensatory mechanisms of the body follow the 'same direction rule' for the numerator and denominator of the modified equation above. The primary event and compensatory mechanisms follow the *same direction rule* for each primary acid-base disorder as shown in Table 73.1.

Table 73.1: Primary acid-base abnormality, compensatory event and the direction of shift in the equation

Primary event	Compensatory event	Directional change in equation
Metabolic acidosis	Respiratory alkalosis	↓HCO_3/⇓PCO_2
Metabolic alkalosis	Respiratory acidosis	↑HCO_3/⇑PCO_2
Respiratory acidosis	Metabolic alkalosis	⇑HCO_3/↑PCO_2
Respiratory alkalosis	Metabolic acidosis	⇓HCO_3/↓PCO_2

Note: ↓↑ arrows represent primary event. ⇓⇑ arrows represent compensatory event.

INTERPRETATION OF ARTERIAL BLOOD GASES (ABG) AND BIOCHEMICAL REPORTS

Recently, a new concept of 'strong anion' approach has been developed but it has not gained wide acceptance for clinical use now and the conventional method is explained in this section.

A proper history and clinical examination will help to suspect the acid-base disorder even before the results are available and the clinical scenario help to suspect and diagnose the acid-base disorders. Coexistence of multiple disorders may yield normal arterial blood gases (ABG) reports.

In order to recognize and interpret the acid-base disorder, four parameters are used:

1. $PaCO_2$ is measured by ABG analysis machine using 'anaerobically' collected heparinized arterial blood sample. The test is performed immediately in the ABG machine which is usually available in most well-equipped intensive care units (ICUs).
2. pH can be observed from the printout/monitor of the ABG machine or it can be measured using a pH meter.
3. HCO_3 is assayed in a biochemistry laboratory and used to cross check the values obtained from the ABG machine.
4. Anion gap (AG) is the difference between the measured cations (Na^+) and anions (HCO_3^-, Cl^-) in blood.

The normal values for arterial blood obtained from ABG machine (at sea level) are:

pH (measure of acidity)	7.4 ± 0.05 (*7.36 ± 0.05)
PCO_2 (partial pressure of CO_2 in blood)	40 ± 4 mm Hg (*46 ± 5)
HCO_3 (calculated bicarbonate)	24 ± 2 mmol/L
PaO_2 (partial pressure of oxygen in blood)	>80 mm Hg (*35 ± 5)
CO_2 (carbon dioxide content)	23–30 mmol/L (*variable)
Na^+	140 ± 5 mmol/L
Cl^-	99 ± 3 mmol/L
AG	10 ± 2 mmol/L
Base excess/deficit (loss of buffer base to neutralize acid)	± 3 mmol/L
SO_2 (oxygen saturation)	>94% (75% for venous blood)

Note: The values marked * are for venous blood.

The ABG machine measures mainly pH and PCO_2. It calculates HCO_3 from pH and PCO_2 and also calculates the excess or deficit of base (HCO_3) from normal. It will be necessary to cross check the result obtained from ABG by biochemical estimation of HCO_3. The report often contains another calculated parameter 'base excess' or 'base deficit'. 'Base deficit' means that 10 mmols of bicarbonate has been used up to neutralize metabolic acids. The same thing can be expressed as 'base excess'—minus 10.

The following steps if followed systematically will help in identification of the acid-base disorder:

Step 1: Obtain ABG and serum electrolytes simultaneously. There are many methods of interpretation. It is necessary that one familiarizes oneself with one of these methods:

- Look at pH first and correlate with PCO_2 and HCO_3
- Look at PCO_2 first and correlate with pH and HCO_3
- Look at HCO_3 first and correlate with pH and PCO_2.

In this chapter, the method of approach (b) starting from pH is followed.

Step 2: Look at pH whether it is high (> 7.45), low (< 7.35) or normal (7.35–7.45 range).

Step 3: Look at PCO_2 and HCO_3 and decide if the change in pH co-relates with the change in PCO_2 and HCO_3.

If the abnormal value of PCO_2 or HCO_3 correlates with abnormal pH, it is often the primary disorder. When PCO_2 decreases, pH should increase and vice versa. Similarly, when the HCO_3 decreases, the pH should decrease and vice versa.

Step 4: Confirm the primary acid-base disorder. PCO_2 is high or HCO_3 is low in acidosis and PCO_2 is low and HCO_3 high in alkalosis.

From the initial change, four primary acid-base disorders can be identified (Table 73.1).

Step 5: *See* if the compensatory change is appropriate. The body tries to normalize the abnormality caused by the primary event by a compensatory change. The direction of the compensatory change will be the same as that of the primary change (Table 73.1).

Step 6: If the compensatory change is less or more than expected or totally variable suspect mixed acid-base disorder.

PRACTICAL CLINICAL SITUATION EXAMPLES

Example–1

pH—7.21	PCO_2—51 mm Hg	HCO_3—27mmol/L

First, look at the pH. It is 7.21. It is 'abnormal and low'. There is acidemia. Look at PCO_2, 51 mm Hg—abnormal and high; HCO_3, 27 mmol/L—abnormal and high. If change in HCO_3 was the primary event, the pH should have increased. So, high HCO_3 is unlikely to be the primary event whereas, high PCO_2 is associated with acidosis. Since, the pH is towards the acidic side (7.21), we may conclude that the patient has primary respiratory acidosis. Both PCO_2 and HCO_3 are high suggesting that the 'same direction rule' is followed in this case.

Example–2

pH—7.55	PCO_2—25 mm Hg	HCO_3—20 mmol/L

First, look at the pH. It is 7.55—abnormal and high; PCO_2, 25 mm Hg—abnormal and low. Now look at the HCO_3, 20 mmol/L—abnormal and low. If change in HCO_3 was the primary event, the pH should have decreased. So, low HCO_3 is unlikely to be the primary event whereas low PCO_2 is associated with alkalosis. Since, the pH is towards the alkaline side (7.55), we may conclude that the patient has primary respiratory alkalosis. Both PCO_2 and HCO_3 are low suggesting that the 'same direction rule' is followed in this case.

Textbook of Medicine

Example–3

pH—7.57	PCO₂ —50 mm Hg	HCO₃—40 mmol/L

Again, look at pH, it is 'abnormal and high'. There is alkalemia; PCO_2, 50 mm Hg—abnormal and high; HCO_3, 40 mmol/L—abnormal and high. If high PCO_2 was the primary event, the pH should have decreased. So, high PCO_2 is unlikely to be the primary event whereas high HCO_3 is associated with alkalosis. Since, the pH is towards the alkaline side (7.57), we may conclude that the patient has primary metabolic alkalosis. Both PCO_2 and HCO_3 are higher than normal suggesting that the 'same direction rule' is followed in this case.

Example–4

pH—7.15	PCO₂—20 mm Hg	HCO₃—8 mmol/L

First, look at pH, it is 7.15—abnormal and low. There is acidemia. Look at PCO_2, 20 mm Hg—abnormal and low; HCO_3, 8 mmol/L—abnormal and low. If change in PCO_2 was the primary event, the pH should have increased. So, low PCO_2 is unlikely to be the primary event whereas, low is HCO_3 associated with acidosis. Since the pH is towards the acidic side (7.15), we may conclude that the patient has primary metabolic acidosis. Both PCO_2 and HCO_3 are high suggesting that the 'same direction rule' is followed in this case also. In a case of metabolic acidosis, assessment of serum AG helps to establish whether it is a high or normal AG metabolic acidosis (*See* AG later in this chapter).

Example–5

pH—7.32	PCO₂—40 mm Hg	HCO₃—18 mmol/L

The pH is 7.32 suggesting acidemia. Here, the PCO_2 is 'normal'. Therefore, it is not a primary respiratory disorder. However, the HCO_3 is reduced suggesting metabolic cause and the pH is towards acidic side. Therefore, metabolic acidosis, however there is no 'compensation' by respiratory alkalosis and the 'same direction rule' is not followed in this example.

SERUM AND URINARY ANION GAP

Cations are positively charged ions, e.g. sodium, potassium, calcium, magnesium and globulins. Anions are negatively charged ions, e.g. bicarbonate, chloride, sulfate, phosphate, organic acid and albumin. The number of cations and anions in the body fluids should be equal so as to maintain electrical neutrality (Fig. 73.1).

There is therefore no actual 'gap' in the serum between anions and cations. Only sodium, bicarbonate and chloride are taken into consideration for the calculation of serum AG. So, the cationic compartment will consist of sodium and all other cations on one side and the anionic compartment will have sum of chloride and bicarbonate with all other unmeasured anions (UA) on the other side.

$$\text{Serum anion gap} = Na^+ - [HCO_3^- + Cl^-]$$

This 'gap' represents the difference between the unmeasured anions and cations which is calculated from the measured parameters as mentioned above. The normal value for AG is approximately 12 + 6 mmol/L. For the purpose of calculation of serum AG, UA as well as unmeasured cations (UC) including potassium are discarded. Since, albumin is negatively charged, it contributes to the AG significantly. The normal AG is approximately three times the serum albumin level. Therefore, if the patient has hypoalbuminemia, the interpretation of AG has to be modified as AG is decreased.

Increased AG occurs when anions other than HCO_3 and chloride accumulate (Table 73.2). Increased levels of albumin, accumulation of substances like sulfates, phosphates, lactic acid, ketoacids or uremic anions lead to increased AG. There is no change in chloride but the bicarbonate is reduced. Normal AG metabolic acidosis may occur when there is loss of both anions and cations. Loss of alkali rich intestinal secretions is associated with sodium loss resulting in normal AG metabolic acidosis. Here, the acidosis is due to alkali loss and the AG is not altered because sodium (cation) is also reduced. In conditions like renal tubular acidosis or acetazolamide therapy, there is failure to excrete acid or reabsorb bicarbonate in the renal tubule and the body loses bicarbonate and there is no accumulation of anions. The chlorides are increased in order to maintain electrical neutrality. Hyperchloremic metabolic acidosis with normal AG is encountered in such conditions.

In acidosis, if the bicarbonate is used up by other anions like ketoacid, lactic acid or uremic anions, AG will be increased. If there is simultaneous reduction in sodium level or when the low bicarbonate is offset by increase in chloride, normal AG acidosis develops (Fig. 73.2).

Delta ratio, in other words, $\Delta AG/\Delta HCO_3$ ratio is a useful parameter for assessment of elevated AG metabolic acidosis. It helps to determine if a mixed acid-base disorder is present. This ratio can be calculated by dividing the number by which AG has increased and by the number by which the HCO_3 has decreased. Example, if measured AG is 25 and measured bicarbonate is 10, $\Delta AG = (25 - 12) = 13$ and ΔHCO_3 is $(24 - 10) = 14$. The delta ratio is 13/14 = nearly 1:1.

Each molecule of metabolic acid added to ECF consumes one molecule of bicarbonate and the ratio will be 1:1. When (fall) ΔHCO_3 is greater than (rise) ΔAG, (delta value below 1:1), say 1:2, it suggests that fall in HCO_3 is more than the rise in AG. This suggests that more HCO_3 is used up that can be explained by the increase in AG. This situation occurs when mixed metabolic acidosis, i.e. combined elevated AG acidosis and a normal AG acidosis occurs. For example, lactic acidosis superimposed

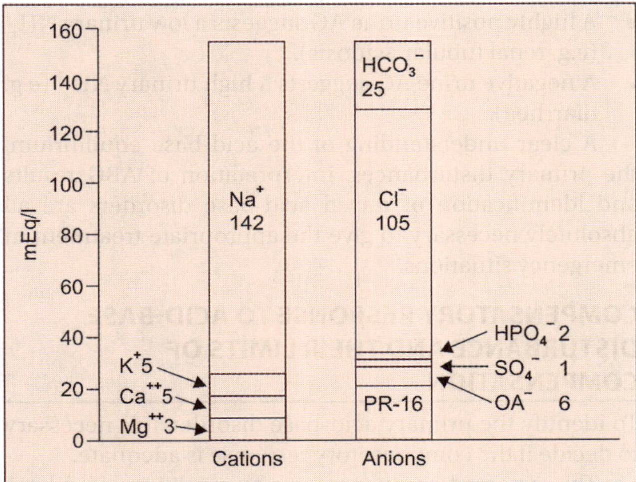

Fig. 73.1: Cations and anions in serum—equal

Table 73.2: Abnormalities in anion gap and their features

High anion gap	Normal anion gap	Decreased anion gap
Increased anions (not Cl⁻ and HCO₃⁻)	*Hyperchloremic metabolic acidosis*	*Increased cations* (not Na⁺)
Increased albumin	Renal tubular acidosis	Increased calcium/magnesium/lithium/immunoglobulins/bromium
Increased inorganic anions (phosphate/sulfate)		
Increased organic anions (lactate/ketones/uremia)		*Decreased anions* (not HCO₃⁻ and Cl⁻)
Exogenous anions (salicylates/ethylene glycol/methanol/paraldehyde)		Hypoalbuminemia/acidosis (for every 1 g decrease of serum albumin from 4.5, anion gap decreases by 2.5)
Increased unidentified anions (Myoglobinuric renal failure/hyperosmolar nonketotic coma/other toxins)		
Decreased cation (not Na⁺) calcium/magnesium		

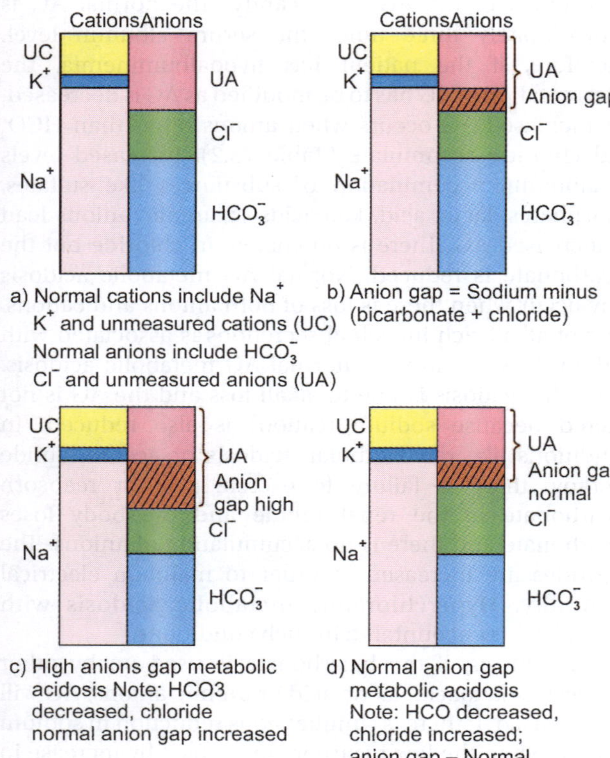

a) Normal cations include Na⁺ K⁺ and unmeasured cations (UC) Normal anions include HCO₃⁻ Cl⁻ and unmeasured anions (UA)

b) Anion gap = Sodium minus (bicarbonate + chloride)

c) High anions gap metabolic acidosis Note: HCO3 decreased, chloride normal anion gap increased

d) Normal anion gap metabolic acidosis Note: HCO decreased, chloride increased; anion gap – Normal

Fig. 73.2: Anions, cations, anion gap and types of metabolic acidosis

on severe diarrhea. Delta value above 2:1 indicates a lesser fall in (HCO₃⁻) compared to the (increase) change in the AG. Thus, a delta ratio more than 2:1 suggests concurrent metabolic alkalosis or a pre-existing high HCO₃⁻ level due to conditions like chronic respiratory acidosis.

Urinary Anion Gap (UAG)

Glutamine is hydrolyzed to ammonia (NH₃) by the enzyme glutaminase in the renal tubular cells. NH₃ diffuses into tubular lumen, where it combines with H⁺ ion and forms ammonium (NH₄) and later combines with Cl to form NH₄Cl (ammonium chloride). Since this cannot diffuse back, it is excreted in urine. For every H⁺ ion thus excreted, the body gains 1 mmol bicarbonate. Estimation of urinary ammonia helps to assess if the kidneys are capable of appropriately acidifying urine and to differentiate between renal to

extrarenal causes of normal AG metabolic acidosis. Renal causes are defective net acid excretion by the kidney as in renal tubular acidosis. Nonrenal causes are increased exogenous acid load, endogenous acid production or bicarbonate loss that overwhelms renal ability to excrete acid. If the cause of normal AG metabolic acidosis is renal, urinary ammonia is low whereas in extrarenal causes, urinary ammonia is increased. Urinary AG helps to indirectly assess urinary ammonia excretion. The main cations in the urine are Na⁺, K⁺ and NH₄⁺. Since, there is no significant bicarbonate in urine, only chloride is taken into consideration in the calculation of urinary AG. UAG is calculated by:

$$UAG = (U_{Na^+} + U_{K^+}) - (U_{Cl^-})$$

Normally, UAG is positive–range from +30 to +50. If UAG is negative, it suggests that UC (NH₄⁺) is higher. Since, urinary pH does not help to differentiate between metabolic acidosis due to renal or extrarenal causes, we have to rely on net acid excretion in urine which can be assessed by urinary NH₄ levels.

Extrarenal causes of metabolic acidosis are associated with high urinary ammonium exertion and negative urinary AG. If it is due to primary renal disease, it will remain positive. UAG may not be reliable if there is increased Na⁺ excretion due to diuretic or factors like diabetic ketoacidosis.

- A highly positive urine AG suggests a low urinary NH₄⁺ (e.g. renal tubular acidosis).
- A negative urine AG suggests a high urinary NH₄⁺ (e.g. diarrhea).

A clear understanding of the acid-base equilibrium, the primary disturbances, interpretation of ABG results and identification of mixed acid-base disorders are all absolutely necessary to give the appropriate treatment in emergency situations.

COMPENSATORY RESPONSE TO ACID-BASE DISTURBANCE AND THEIR LIMITS OF COMPENSATION

To identify the primary acid-base disorder, it is necessary to decide if the compensatory response is adequate.

The expected compensations to a primary acid-base disorder are as follows:

- In metabolic acidosis, for every mmol fall in HCO_3, PCO_2 will fall by about 1.25 mm Hg.
- In metabolic alkalosis, for every mmol rise in HCO_3, the PCO_2 will rise by about 0.75 mm Hg.

The extent of compensatory response in primary respiratory disorders may differ in acute and chronic situations. In acute respiratory acidosis, the pH may not usually decrease to less than 7.15 and PCO_2 does not increase to > 90 mm Hg. In chronic respiratory acidosis, the PCO_2 level may be higher (up to 110 mm Hg) and also the HCO_3 (up to 50 mmol/L) but the pH change will be limited to 7.25–7.35.

- In acute respiratory acidosis, for every 10 mm Hg increase in PCO_2, the HCO_3 will increase by about 1 mmol/L.
- In chronic respiratory acidosis, for every 10 mm Hg increase in PCO_2, the HCO_3 will increase by about 4 mmol/L.
- In acute respiratory alkalosis, for every 10 mm Hg fall in PCO_2, the HCO_3 will fall by approximately 2 mmol/L.
- In chronic respiratory alkalosis, for every 10 mm Hg fall in PCO_2, the HCO_3 will fall by approximately 4 mmol/L.

If the compensatory response is inadequate or excessive or if the 'same direction rule' is not followed, more than one acid-base disorder may coexist.

ILLUSTRATION OF CLINICAL EXAMPLES

Example–6

pH—7.30	PCO_2—41 mm Hg	HCO_3—16 mmol/L
Na—140	Cl—100	AG—24

First look at pH, it is 7.30—abnormal and low. There is acidemia. PCO_2 is 41, nearly normal. HCO_3 is low. AG is 140–(100 + 16) = 24. So, it is high-AG metabolic acidosis. In metabolic acidosis, for every mmol reduction of HCO_3, the PCO_2 should decrease by about 1.25 mm Hg. In this example, the expected PCO_2 should have been around 28–32 mm Hg. Since, it is 41 mm Hg, hyperventilation and CO_2 washout have not occurred, suggesting associated respiratory acidosis.

Note: Same direction rule is not truly followed here. HCO_3 is low and PCO_2 is tending to higher than normal. This is a combination of high AG metabolic acidosis with respiratory acidosis.

For example, severe pneumonia with shock and pulmonary edema.

Example–7

pH—7.55	PCO_2—25 mm Hg	HCO_3—30 mmol/L

First, look at the pH—7.55; it is case of alkalemia. PCO_2 is 25 that means it is 'abnormal and low'. Low PCO_2 associated with high pH suggests respiratory disorder (respiratory alkalosis). The compensation is by metabolic acidosis. The fall in HCO_3 is expected to be (considering both acute and chronic) 2–4 mmol for every 10 mm Hg of fall in PCO_2. Difference in PCO_2 (ΔPCO_2) is 40 – 25 = 15. So, difference in bicarbonate (ΔHCO_3) should be between 3 and 6 mmol/L. That is, the bicarbonate values should be between 18 and 21 mmol/L. Here, it is 30 mmols suggesting a combination of respiratory and metabolic alkalosis. It may be noted that the numerator (HCO_3) and denominator (PCO_2) of the pH equation mentioned earlier in this section have not observed the 'same direction rule' and

moved in opposite directions. Whenever the PCO_2 and HCO_3 are abnormal and in opposite directions, i.e. one above normal while the other is reduced, a mixed respiratory and metabolic acid-base disorder exists. As a rule of the thumb, we should always remember that:

- When the PCO_2 is elevated and the HCO_3^- reduced, respiratory acidosis and metabolic acidosis coexist.
- When the PCO_2 is reduced and the HCO_3^- elevated, respiratory alkalosis and metabolic alkalosis coexist.

RESPIRATORY ACIDOSIS (BOX 73.1)

It occurs as a result of alveolar hypoventilation and is characterized by rise in PCO_2. When there is diminished central respiratory drive, neuromuscular diseases airway obstruction or restriction of lung expansion due to any factor could lead to development of respiratory acidosis (Box 73.1). Hypoxemia invariably occurs and is often the cause of death. The body tries to compensate by trying to maintain the pH in normal range. In acute respiratory acidosis, buffering mechanisms come into play immediately and the bicarbonate will increase by 1 mmol/L for every 10 mm Hg increase in PCO_2. In chronic respiratory acidosis, the renal mechanisms take over by 24 hours and cause elevation of HCO_3 by up to 4 mmol/L for every 10 mm Hg rise in PCO_2.

Clinical Features

The clinical features vary depending on the rapidity of onset, severity, duration of illness and presence of

Box 73.1: Causes of respiratory acidosis

- ***Neurologic causes***
  - Inhibition of respiratory center (central)
  - General anesthesia
  - Sedative overdose
  - Head injury/cerebrovascular accident/tumors
  - Encephalitis/brainstem lesions
- ***Neuromuscular causes***
  - Spinal cord injury
  - Poliomyelitis
  - Multiple sclerosis
  - Muscular dystrophy
  - Guillain-Barré syndrome
  - Status epilepticus (SE)
  - Amyotrophic lateral sclerosis
- ***Respiratory muscle paralysis***
  - Tetanus, botulism
  - Myasthenic crisis
  - Periodic paralysis
  - Diaphragmatic paralysis
  - Myopathies
  - Succinylcholine administration
  - Organophosphorus poisoning
- ***Upper and lower airway obstruction***
  - Sleep apnea
  - Aspiration
  - Laryngeal edema/vocal cord palsy
  - Bronchoconstriction
  - Emphysema
  - Chronic interstitial lung disease
  - Thymoma/aortic aneurysm
- ***Restriction of expansion of lung***
  - Obesity
  - Bilateral pleural effusion/pneumothorax
  - Pleural fibrosis
  - Pleural thickening/lung stiffening.

hypoxemia. The usual symptoms include severe breathlessness, anxiety, disorientation, confusion, hallucinations, tremor, myoclonus, headache, asterixis, incoherence and drowsiness. Blurring of optic disc, papilledema and symptoms of increased intracranial pressure are due to vasodilatory effects of CO_2. Sometimes, injudicious administration of high flow O_2 may precipitate coma. The vascular manifestations are due to vasodilatation. Congestive cardiac failure (CCF) and cardiac arrhythmias may occur. These patients may also develop salt and fluid retention. Investigations reveal coexisting hypercarbia (CO_2 retention) and hypoxemia (low PaO_2).

Treatment

Treatment of respiratory acidosis depends on its severity and rate of onset. Measures to reverse the underlying cause is together with providing adequate alveolar ventilation—the mainstay. This will help to relieve hypoxemia, hypercarbia and acidosis. Since hypoxemia is mainly responsible for the mortality, careful O_2 administration is the mainstay in the treatment. Injudicious O_2 administration may lead to suppression of respiratory drive particularly in patients with chronic obstructive pulmonary disease (COPD). In acute respiratory acidosis, the treatment principles include maintenance of airway, administration of oxygen and judicious use of antibiotics, bronchodilators and corticosteroids. Noninvasive ventilation or intubation and mechanical ventilation may be used for more severe cases with pH < 7.15 and PCO_2 > 80. Bicarbonate administration may be necessary to bring the pH to 7.20 in severe acute cases.

Chronic respiratory acidosis is difficult to treat. When correcting chronic respiratory acidosis, adequate urine flow should be maintained and K^+ and Cl^- must be administered with a view to eliminate the accumulated bicarbonate by the kidney. Measures to treat chronic respiratory acidosis include:

- Maximize lung function
- Stop smoking
- Judicious use of oxygen
- Bronchodilators
- Corticosteroids
- Diuretics
- Physiotherapy.

RESPIRATORY ALKALOSIS

It is characterized by hypocapnia (fall in PCO_2). The rate of production of CO_2 in the body is relatively constant. Therefore, any fall in PCO_2 can only be due to alveolar hyperventilation. It is a common acid-base disorder and occurs in normal pregnancy and at high altitude. It also occurs in critically ill patients as a simple disorder or as a part of mixed disorder (Box 73.2). The primary fall in PCO_2 does not increase pH to levels above 7.55 and severe alkalemia is unlikely. Acute respiratory alkalosis is associated with immediate lowering of HCO_3 by non-bicarbonate buffers. After a few hours, the renal buffering takes over and reduces titratable acid and ammonium excretion. This helps to maintain the HCO_3 low.

Box 73.2: Causes of respiratory alkalosis

- **Hyperventilation**
  - Voluntary
  - Psychogenic
  - Anxiety
  - Pain
  - Pregnancy (high progesterone)
- **Central nervous system (CNS) stimulation**
  - Brainstem lesions
  - Encephalitis
  - Salicylates intoxication (direct stimulation of medullary chemoreceptors)
  - Fever/sepsis
- **Stimulation of intrathoracic receptors**
  - Pneumothorax
  - Hemothorax
  - Flail chest
  - Pneumonia
  - Asthma
  - Pulmonary edema
  - Pulmonary embolism
  - Pulmonary fibrosis
  - Acute respiratory distress syndrome
- **Stimulation of peripheral chemoreceptor**
  - High altitude—hypoxemia
  - Hypotension
  - Severe anemia
  - Drowning—aspiration
- **Drugs**
  - Respiratory stimulants (doxapram, nikethamide)
  - Salicylates
  - Nicotine
  - Epinephrine/norepinephrine
- **Miscellaneous**
  - Mechanical hyperventilation
  - Hepatic failure
  - Recovery from metabolic acidosis

Clinical Features

The clinical features are variable and depend on the primary disorder, rate of onset and severity of respiratory alkalosis. The symptoms are usually due to the causative disorder. The usual initial symptoms attributable to respiratory alkalosis include tingling sensation in the extremities and circumoral region, light headedness and confusion. Later, muscle cramps, carpopedal spasm and brisk deep tendon reflexes may be noted. Cardiac arrhythmias and seizures may also occur in severe cases. The occurrence of symptomatic respiratory alkalosis or PCO_2 less than 20–25 mm Hg in critically ill-patients suggests a grave prognosis.

Diagnosis and Treatment

The diagnosis can be established by the history, physical examination and laboratory data including ABG. The treatment is directed towards the underlying cause. Often, no treatment is required for mild respiratory alkalosis if it is not associated with symptoms. In psychogenic hyperventilation, rebreathing into a closed bag can be tried. Acute mountain sickness can be prevented by slow ascent, pretreatment with acetazolamide and oxygen therapy. In case of salicylate intoxication, first step is to remove unabsorbed salicylate from the gut. This is achieved by inducing emesis or gastric lavage.

Textbook of Medicine

Absorption of salicylates may be prevented by administration of activated charcoal with sorbitol. The absorbed salicylates can be removed from blood by alkaline diuresis or hemodialysis. In patients on assisted ventilation with respiratory alkalosis, appropriate adjustments in the mode of ventilation may have to be undertaken. In hypoxemia, oxygen therapy is useful.

If the pH is more than 7.55 and patient has hemodynamic instability or altered mental status, more aggressive measures are warranted. Attempts must be made to bring the pH to less than 7.5. This can be achieved by either reducing HCO_3 or increasing PCO_2. The bicarbonate can be reduced by the use of acetazolamide, ultrafiltration or hemodialysis using low bicarbonate dialysate or by isotonic saline replacement. The PCO_2 can be increased by rebreathing into a closed system or by giving controlled hypoventilation using a ventilator.

METABOLIC ALKALOSIS

It is characterized by increased pH primarily due to increased HCO_3. The compensatory mechanism to combat the acid-base abnormality is increase in PCO_2 level. Metabolic alkalosis is a common disorder in hospitalized patients and in ICUs. Many cases go unrecognized because it is not looked for. It occurs more often as a part of mixed acid-base disorder than a single entity. Two important factors operate in the metabolic alkalosis—the initiating factor and main-taining factor. Unless both are present, metabolic alkalosis is not sustained. Metabolic alkalosis may be initiated by loss of acids from the body or gain of alkali. Normally, such events are effectively handled by the kidney by removing the excess bicarbonate from blood. Therefore, certain additional factors are required for maintaining metabolic alkalosis. The chief maintaining factors are chloride and potassium deficiency causing low ECF volume and low glomerular filtration rate (GFR), increasing renal H^+ ion secretion, increased ammonium production and action through renin and aldosterone.

If metabolic alkalosis is associated with low ECF volume as in vomiting or diuretic use, there is prompt correction of alkalosis with administration of chloride. This is called ***chloride responsive metabolic alkalosis***. Metabolic alkalosis is associated with normal or increased ECF in hyperaldosteronism and Cushing's syndrome, respectively. In these conditions, alkalosis will be sustained only if renal functions are markedly reduced or if alkali loading is very high. Such alkalosis persists despite chloride administration and it is called ***chloride resistant alkalosis***. The urinary chloride helps to distinguish between these two types of metabolic alkalosis. In chloride responsive type, the urinary chloride is less than 10 mmol/L and in chloride resistant alkalosis, the urinary chloride is more than 10 mmol/L. The body tries to minimize the degree of metabolic alkalosis by reducing ventilation and increasing $PaCO_2$.

Classification

The metabolic alkalosis is classified as chloride respon-sive, chloride resistant and miscellaneous.

■ ***Chloride responsive metabolic alkalosis***
- Gastric acid loss
  - Vomiting
  - Gastric drainage
  - Pyloric stenosis
- Urinary loss—diuretic therapy (thiazides, metola-zone, furosemide, torsemide, bumetanide and ethacrynic acid)
- Fecal loss—congenital chloride diarrhea, villous adenoma of colon
- Recovery from chronic hypercapnia.

■ ***Chloride resistant metabolic alkalosis***
- Hyperaldosteronism
  - Conn's syndrome
  - Cushing's syndrome
  - Bartter's syndrome
  - Liddle's syndrome
  - Liquorice ingestion

■ ***Miscellaneous***
- Alkali administration
  - Milk-alkali syndrome
  - Massive blood transfusion, due to excess of citrate
  - Alkali supplements
- Hypercalcemia
- Poorly absorbable anion administration (e.g. anti-biotic like carbenicillin).

Clinical Features

Metabolic alkalosis is generally, well-tolerated and patients are not symptomatic. The symptoms are generally related to hypoxemia, hypokalemia, hypocalcemia and alkalemia. Symptoms like lethargy, confusion or stupor are often related to hypoxia and hypoventilation and are particularly worse in those with COPD. The clinical manifestations related to hypokalemia are weakness, ECG changes or even flaccid paralysis. Tetany may occur due to fall in ionic calcium level.

Diagnosis

The finding of serum bicarbonate of >30 mmol/L associated with hypokalemia is pathognomonic of meta-bolic alkalosis. Although, HCO_3 may be high in chronic respiratory acidosis, it is not associated with hypokalemia. Since metabolic alkalosis may co-exist with other acid-base disturbances, mixed acid-base disorders should be looked for. Mixed metabolic alkalosis and metabolic acidosis can be diagnosed only if the metabolic acidosis is high AG acidosis. A single measurement of urinary chloride in a spot sample of urine is sufficient to classify if it is chloride responsive or chloride resistant metabolic alkalosis. Urine chloride of < 10 mEq/L suggests chloride responsive metabolic alkalosis. If the urinary chloride is >15–20 mEq/L, it suggests chloride resistant metabolic alkalosis.

Management

The primary disorder is identified and treated accordingly. In chloride responsive metabolic alkalosis, the aim is to replace the chloride deficit and normalize the ECF

Textbook of Medicine

volume and sodium and potassium concentrations. Thus, the mainstay of treatment is sodium chloride (NaCl) infusion with additional potassium orally or intravenously (IV). The amount of NaCl required depends on volume contraction and is guided by central venous pressure (CVP) monitoring. Usually, with the correction of chloride, the kidneys effectively eliminate the excess bicarbonate. In patients with cirrhosis liver, digoxin therapy or respiratory failure, the alkalosis may have to be corrected by exogenous administration of acids or acid precursors. Treatment includes administration of dilute IV 0.1 N hydrochloric acid, ammonium chloride or arginine hydrochloride. Dialysis with low bicarbonate dialysate is the treatment modality of choice in severe cases associated with renal failure.

METABOLIC ACIDOSIS

Metabolic acidosis occurs when acid is added to the body from exogenous sources or when alkali is lost from the body. Endogenous acid production and accumulation of lactic acid and ketoacids often occur in sepsis or diabetic ketoacidosis (DKA). Failure to excrete endogenous acids occur in uremia. Diarrhea and drainage of alkali rich intestinal fluids like bile or pancreatic juice lead to acidosis due to loss of alkali. Consumption of external acid or highly acidic substances may occur in poisoning and is a rare cause of metabolic acidosis. Metabolic acidosis is broadly classified as high AG metabolic acidosis and normal AG 'hyperchloremic' metabolic acidosis. Both may occur due to renal or extrarenal causes. When metabolic acidosis occurs, the body tries to compensate for the metabolic shift causing reduction of pH by hyperventilation leading to CO_2 wash out resulting in reduction of PCO_2. The deep sighing respiration also known as ***Kussmaul breathing*** occurs in metabolic acidosis. If the renal functions are normal, kidneys respond to metabolic acidosis by increasing urinary production and excretion. Severe acidosis occurs in renal diseases because this compensation fails to occur in uremia and renal tubular acidosis.

Classification

- ***Metabolic acidosis with high AG***
  - Renal causes: Uremic acidosis due to accumulation of uremic anions in acute and chronic renal failure when the GFR is < 20 mL/min.
  - Extrarenal causes:
    - Accumulation of lactic acid—(due to incomplete carbohydrate oxidation) lactic acidosis, e.g. shock, sepsis, cirrhosis, malignancies, phenformin and very rarely metformin.
    - Accumulation of ketoacids due to incomplete oxidation of fat, e.g. diabetic ketoacidosis, starvation ketoacidosis, alcoholic ketoacidosis.
    - Poisoning, e.g. ethylene glycol, methanol, ethanol, isopropyl alcohol, salicylate.
    - Gain of exogenous acid, e.g. hydrochloric acid, ammonium chloride, methionine and IV hyperalimentation.

- ***Metabolic acidosis with normal AG***
  - Renal bicarbonate loss:
    - Proximal renal tubular acidosis (type II RTA)
    - Distal renal tubular acidosis (type I RTA)
    - Hyperkalemic distal RTA (type IV RTA)
    - Acetazolamide
    - Chronic kidney disease with mild renal insufficiency.
  - Gastrointestinal (GI) bicarbonate loss:
    - Diarrhea
    - Pancreatic/biliary fistula
    - Ureterosigmoidostomy (reabsorption of H^+ ions and ammonia in urine in exchange for bicarbonate in the gut). Use of cholestyramine is also preferred.

Since AG is an important factor in classifying metabolic acidosis, its interpretation should be made very carefully. If serum albumin is lower than 4.5 g/dL, the normal AG should be calculated as lower by 2.5 for every 1 g reduction in serum albumin. For example, if the serum albumin of a patient is 2.5, the normal AG for the patient should be calculated as (12 – 5) = 7 ± 2. In normal AG metabolic acidosis, the reduction of HCO_3 is associated with a reciprocal increase in chloride so that the AG remains unaltered. This is also called hyperchloremic metabolic acidosis. There is no accumulation of anions to account for the enlargement of the 'unmeasured anion pool'. The ΔCl^- equals ΔHCO_3^-. In high AG metabolic acidosis, also called AG metabolic acidosis, the accumulated anions use up the available HCO_3 to the same extent as the excess of anions. Therefore, in simple AG metabolic acidosis, the $\Delta AG = \Delta HCO_3$.

Clinical Features and Diagnosis

The clinical features due to metabolic acidosis are similar irrespective of the etiology. In mild degrees of acidosis, increase in respiratory rate and in severe acidosis, deep sighing respiration (Kussmaul breathing) occurs. A careful history of recurrent stone disease, diabetes, alcoholism, drug therapy, poisoning or overdose should be elicited. Physical examination, investigations including urinalysis for sugar, ketones, blood sugar, blood ketones, lactate, renal function, electrolytes, osmolality and ABG help to differentiate the four common causes of high AG metabolic acidosis.

- ***Uremic acidosis:*** In early renal failure, there may be normal AG metabolic acidosis. Later, the retention of phosphorus, sulfate and other acidic ions accumulate resulting in AG metabolic acidosis. Since the bone buffers are used up, hypercalciuria, nephrocalcinosis, and nephrolithiasis may be seen in chronic acidosis. As acidosis accelerates protein and amino acid breakdown, the patient may go into negative nitrogen balance.

- ***Lactic acidosis:*** Metabolism of glucose yields lactic acid in the tissues. Some lactate is buffered by sodium bicarbonate, converted to sodium lactate which is again converted in the liver to bicarbonate. However, if the production of L-lactic acid is greater than the ability to convert it back to HCO_3, accumulation of lactic acid may occur. Type A lactic acidosis results from tissue hypoxia whereas type B lactic acidosis occurs from overproduction of lactic acid from leukocytes or tumors. Enzyme deficiencies like glycogen storage disease, drugs like metformin and liver disease may cause type B lactic acidosis. A condition called D lactic acidosis occurs due to bacterial overgrowth in the gut. The excessive D lactate may be produced and absorbed through the gut in conditions like short bowel syndrome, paralytic ileus, and intestinal obstruction or after prolonged use of oral antibiotics. The toxic products from the gut rather than the D lactate that cause the toxicity.

- ***Ketoacidosis:*** Diabetic ketoacidosis occurs in patients with uncontrolled diabetes who develop complications like intercurrent infection. Insulin deficiency and other factors increase fatty acid metabolism and results in accumulation of acetoacetic acid and beta-hydroxybutyric acid. The usual presentation is with nausea, vomiting, weakness and symptoms of uncontrolled diabetes. Nausea, vomiting, hyperglycemia and polyuria causing severe dehydration combined with accumulation of ketone bodies in the body leas to AG metabolic acidosis.

  In alcoholic ketoacidosis, starvation and accumulation of beta-hydroxybutyric acid accumulation occurs. Since vomiting is a predominant feature, loss of acid and metabolic alkalosis is seen associated with AG metabolic acidosis. In this case, the ΔAG to ΔHCO_3 will help in suspecting this mixed acid-base disorder.

- ***Drugs and toxins:*** Drugs like mannitol, radiocontrast agents or substances like alcohol or toxins like ethylene glycol or acetone can cause high AG metabolic acidosis. These substances also contribute to 'osmolar gap' (*See* the following section on osmolar disorders). Osmolar gap is the difference between the measured osmolality and the 'calculated' osmolality. The osmolality can be calculated from serum sodium, urea and blood sugar. Patients with ethylene glycol poisoning present with cardiac failure, pulmonary edema or seizures and coma. Ethylene glycol is converted to glycolic acid and oxalic acid. Lactic acid accumulation also occurs. Thus, high AG metabolic acidosis, with increased osmolar gap, acute kidney injury due to tissue deposition of oxalate occur. Methyl alcohol (methanol) consumption is a medical emergency and the accumulation of formaldehyde causes damage to nervous system, particularly optic nerve. It also produces high AG metabolic acidosis with high osmolar gap. Most laboratories do not have the osmometer to measure osmolality. It is important to remember that the calculated osmolality is 'normal' in these cases.

Salicylate intoxication is a cause of a characteristic mixed acid-base disorder characterized by high AG metabolic acidosis and respiratory alkalosis. Acetyl salicylic acid is converted to salicylic acid which interferes with mitochondrial metabolism resulting in accumulation of lactic acid and ketoacids which contribute to high AG metabolic acidosis. The salicylates directly stimulate the respiratory center causing hyperventilation and respiratory alkalosis.

Management

Management depends on the correction of the underlying disorder. Correction with IV sodium bicarbonate is indicated if acidosis is symptomatic and severe (pH <7.2 and HCO_3 <12). The dose of bicarbonate is calculated by the formula: Bicarbonate required = 0.3 × bw in kg × deficit. The deficit is calculated by noting the difference between required HCO_3 (usually 12–16) and observed bicarbonate (available lab value). The correction is achieved within 2–4 hours and ABG is repeated. In high AG metabolic acidosis due to intoxications, removal of the toxins by appropriate measures may be undertaken.

In advanced renal failure—stage IV and V of chronic kidney disease, oral bicarbonate supplementation to maintain serum HCO_3 level more than 20 mmol/L is advised. Once this level is achieved, the HCO_3 level can be maintained by supplementing 0.5–1 mmol/kg bw per day. Regular use of sodium bicarbonate tablets may be associated with gaseous distension of the stomach due to liberation of CO_2 ($NaHCO_3$ + HCl → NaCl + H_2O + CO_2). As long as aluminium containing antacids are not coadministered, ***Shohl's solution*** which is a buffered solution of sodium citrate with citric acid can be used. One mL of Shohl's solution gives 1 mmol of HCO_3 to the body. It can be given diluted with water, buttermilk of added to the prepared salt free food.

In L-lactic acidosis, attempts to improve tissue perfusion should be undertaken first. In severe cases with pH < 7.1, bicarbonate infusions may be given temporarily. 40 mL of 7.5% $NaHCO_3$ added to 500 mL or half normal saline or 5% dextrose can be given as infusion to bring the pH to around 7.25.

In diabetic ketoacidosis, the main treatment is with normal saline to control dehydration, insulin to correct hyperkalemia and hypophosphatemia with appropriate potassium and phosphate supplements, once ketosis is controlled. Bicarbonate supplementation is often not necessary because of the chances of developing overshoot alkalosis in the recovery stage. In alcoholic ketoacidosis, administration of glucose and careful refeeding with supplementation of phosphates, potassium and magnesium are necessary. Bicarbonate supplements are not needed.

For methanol poisoning, administration of ethanol oral or IV drip combined with early hemodialysis will help to remove methanol and formic acid from the body. Once the formic acid is fixed to the tissue, its removal by dialysis is impossible.

For other substances consumed, gastric lavage, use of activated charcoal, IV bicarbonate infusion and early dialysis may be considered.

Prevention or relief of stasis and eradication of bacterial overgrowth in the intestine is the first step in the treatment of D-lactic acidosis. Use of drugs to increase bowel motility, avoiding oral feed for a few days and use of oral metronidazole are the other measures.

MIXED ACID-BASE DISORDERS

When two or more acid-base disorders occur simultaneously, the condition is called ***mixed acid-base disorder***. This could be two or three disorders combined. The usual compensation of the body to a primary acid-base disorder is not considered as a mixed disorder. Mixed acid-base disorders are commonly observed in hospitalized patients particularly in the ICUs. The clinical settings in which they occur include cardiorespiratory arrest, sepsis, drug intoxication, complications of diabetes mellitus (DM), renal, hepatic, pulmonary or cardiac failure and those on artificial life support. A few examples are enumerated and explained below. The acid-base disorders and clinical conditions are enumerated below causative mechanisms within brackets.

- ***Respiratory alkalosis and metabolic alkalosis***
  - Hyperemesis gravidarum (hyperventilation in pregnancy and acid loss due to vomiting).
  - Congestive heart failure (CHF) on diuretic therapy (tachypnea and diuretic therapy).
- ***Respiratory acidosis and metabolic alkalosis***
  - Pulmonary insufficiency/COPD with diuretics/volume depletion (vomiting/hypokalemia/steroids/post-hypercapnic alkalosis).
- ***Acute respiratory acidosis with chronic respiratory acidosis***
  - Acute pneumonia causing exacerbation of COPD
  - Sedative administration/improper oxygen therapy in COPD patient.
- ***Respiratory alkalosis with metabolic acidosis***
  - Salicylate intoxication [stimulation of respiratory center (hyperventilation) with accumulation of salicylate and lactic acid]
  - Gram negative sepsis (hyperventilation leads to respiratory alkalosis and shock causes lactic acidosis).
- ***AG metabolic acidosis and metabolic alkalosis***
  - Lactic acidosis, uremia or DKA with vomiting or nasogastric suction
  - Lactic acidosis/DKA given sodium bicarbonate therapy.

Note: In single disorders like high AG metabolic acidosis, the reduction of bicarbonate and increase in AG will be identical. So, difference in HCO_3 (ΔHCO_3) and difference in AG (ΔAG) will be equal. The mixed acid-base disorder as shown above can be identified if the ΔHCO_3 is less than ΔAG. The difference signifies presence of another process like bicarbonate therapy or loss of acid increasing HCO_3 without affecting AG.

- ***High AG metabolic acidosis and respiratory acidosis:*** Cardiopulmonary arrest—cardiac arrest (lactic acidosis) and respiratory acidosis.
- ***AG metabolic acidosis and normal AG metabolic acidosis***
  - Lactic acidosis superimposed on severe diarrhea (loss of alkali)
  - DKA with type IV RTA.
- ***Two types of AG metabolic acidosis***
  - Uremia and DKA
  - Ketoacidosis and sepsis (lactic acidosis).
- ***Two types of metabolic alkalosis***
  - Vomiting and diuretic therapy
  - Potassium deficiency and mineralocorticoid excess.

Note: Respiratory alkalosis and respiratory acidosis cannot occur concurrently in a patient.

CASE STUDIES

Case 1: A 22-year-old lady, a known case of type 1 diabetes for 5 years is brought to emergency with polyuria, polydipsia, nausea, vomiting and abdominal pain of two days duration. She had dehydration, tachycardia, postural hypotension and Kussmaul's breathing. The urine examination showed glycosuria but no ketonuria. The blood sugar was 720 mg/dL, urea: 64 mg/dL, creatinine: 2.8 mg/dL, Na: 132, K: 6.0, Cl: 93, HCO_3: 11 and serum albumin: 4.5 g/dL. The ABG showed pH: 7.27, PCO_2: 23, calculated HCO_3: 10, base deficit: 14.

Approach:

- From the history, it can be suspected that she is in ketoacidosis, metabolic acidosis with dehydration and metabolic alkalosis due to vomiting.
- pH is 7.27 suggesting acidemia. PCO_2 is 23 cannot explain acidemia but low HCO_3 can account for acidemia. Hence, she has metabolic acidosis. Since, the AG is [132 – (93 + 11)] = 28, its AG metabolic acidosis. The compensatory response in PCO_2 is following the same direction rule.
- Next step is to decide if the 'compensatory response is adequate or not. We will apply the correlation in metabolic acidosis, for every mmol fall in HCO_3, PCO_2 will fall by about 1.25 mm Hg.
- The expected PCO_2 should have been lower by (base deficit × 1.25) = 17.5. The PCO_2 should have been 40–18 = 22. The actual PCO_2 was 23, falls within the estimated range suggesting that the response is adequate.
- Next calculate ΔAG and ΔHCO_3. Here, ΔAG is 28 – 12 = 16 and ΔHCO_3 is 24–11 = 13. Since, ΔAG to ΔHCO_3 ratio is not high, it is a case of compensated AG metabolic acidosis.

Case 2: A 70-year-old man who has previous admissions for CCF is admitted with history of shortness of breath, orthopnea and leg swelling. On examination, there was bilateral, symmetrical, pitting, non-tender edema up to knees. Lungs showed bilateral coarse basal crepitation. The ABG reports showed that, pH: 7.24, PCO_2: 60 mm Hg, PO_2: 52, HCO_3: 27.

Approach:

- From the history, we can suspect cardiac failure with acute pulmonary edema with acute respiratory acidosis.
- Since, the pH is 7.24, there is academia. Elevation of PCO_2 is consistent with acidosis and the HCO_3 is also elevated follows the 'same direction rule'. So, the primary disorder is acute respiratory acidosis.
- The expected HCO_3 for the given rise in PCO_2 will be guided by the following. 'In acute respiratory acidosis, for every 10 mm Hg increase in PCO_2, the HCO_3 will increase by about 1 mmol/L'.

- The expected ΔHCO_3 in this case should be equal to $\Delta PCO_2/10 = (60 - 40)/10 = 2$.
- Since, the actual bicarbonate is 27 and the expected bicarbonate is very close to it, the disorder is acute respiratory acidosis with adequate 'compensation' due to acute pulmonary edema.
- In acute respiratory acidosis, the ΔpH will be equal to $\Delta PCO_2 \times 0.008$. In this case, ΔPCO_2 is $(60 - 40) = 20$ and the ΔpH should be $(20 \times 0.008) = 0.16$, i.e. pH should be $7.40 - 0.16 = 7.24$. Since, the pH is as expected, it suggests a simple disorder. By this method also, we can rule out mixed acid-base disorders with acute respiratory acidosis.

Case 3: A 30-year-old lady who had been diagnosed as Sjogren's syndrome attends the clinic with two day history of diarrhea. Although, she was relatively asymptomatic except for tachypnea, the emergency room resident ordered ABG and other biochemical tests. Subsequently, the consultant asked for urine chemistry also. The relevant results are ABG—pH: 7.30, PCO_2: 28, HCO_3: 14 mmol/L, Na: 138, K: 4, Cl: 110, base excess: minus 10. The urinary electrolytes were Na: 100, K: 31 and Cl: 105.

Approach:
- This young lady with Sjogren's syndrome coming with short diarrhea and tachypnea, it may be having acidosis whether due to alkali loss or due to Sjogren's syndrome which could be associated with renal tubular function defects.
- The pH is towards academia and the low bicarbonate suggests metabolic acidosis. The AG is $138 - (110 + 14) = 14$. So, this is a normal AG metabolic acidosis.
- The base excess is minus 10 (the base deficit is 10). The expected compensation for metabolic acidosis is in metabolic acidosis, for every mmol fall in HCO_3, PCO_2 will fall by about 1.25 mm Hg.
- For ΔHCO_3 of 10, the expected ΔPCO_2 will be 12.5, i.e. PCO_2 should be $40 - 12.5 = 27.5$. The observed PCO_2 is 28 suggesting normal compensation.
- To find out if the renal ability to excrete ammonia is preserved or not, we need to check the urinary AG. $UAG = (Na + K)-Cl = (100 + 31) - 105 = 26$.
- ***Remember*** extrarenal causes of metabolic acidosis are associated with high urinary ammonium exertion and negative urinary AG. If metabolic acidosis is due to renal cause, the urinary AG remains positive. Extrarenal causes of metabolic acidosis are associated with high urinary ammonium exertion and negative urinary AG.
- Diagnosis of normal AG metabolic acidosis due to renal tubular acidosis possibly following Sjogren's syndrome.

Case 4: A 40-year-old man was admitted in a dehydrated condition following acute severe diarrhea of three days duration. Physical examination showed signs of mild dehydration, tachycardia and postural fall in blood pressure (BP) of 10–20 mm Hg. The relevant blood results are ABG—pH: 7.31, PCO_2: 30 mm Hg, HCO_3: 16, PO_2: 93 mm Hg, Na^+: 134, K^+: 2.9, Cl^-: 108, HCO_3^-: 16, blood urea nitrogen (BUN): 31, Cr: 1.5.

Approach:
- Based on the clinical presentation, the patient could have normal AG acidosis from diarrhea and/or elevated AG acidosis secondary to lactic acidosis as a result of hypovolemia and poor perfusion.
- The pH is low—academia.
- PCO_2 is 30 and low PCO_2 occurs in alkalosis. The HCO_3 is 16—suggesting low metabolic acidosis.
- The HCO_3 and PCO_2 have moved in the same direction (downwards). Therefore, unlikely to be mixed acid-base disorder.
- Low PCO_2 is a compensatory response. If we apply the rule in metabolic acidosis, for every mmol fall in HCO_3, PCO_2 will fall by about 1.25 mm Hg, the expected PCO_2 will be $40 - (8 \times 1.25) = 30$ (within the estimated range). Hence, the compensation is adequate and there is no separate respiratory disorder present.
- Since, it is metabolic acidosis, calculate AG $[Na-(Cl + HCO_3^-)] = 134-(108 + 16) = 10$ (normal range).

We can conclude that the patient has normal AG acidosis with adequate compensation secondary to severe diarrhea.

Case 5: A 72-year-old man with history of chronic obstructive pulmonary disease (COPD) presents to the hospital with alcoholic ketoacidosis. If it is known that his AG was 12 earlier and the present serum chemistry is as follows, Na: 136, K: 5.1, Cl: 85, HCO_3^-: 25, Urea: 54, Cr: 1.4 and ABG—pH: 7.20, PCO_2: 60, HCO_3: 25, PO_2: 75. Urine showed ketones 3+, we will approach the acid-base abnormality.

Approach:
- From the history, it is clear that he had COPD which may have contributed to respiratory acidosis with high PCO_2 and corresponding increase in HCO_3. At this time, his AG was 12 (normal). When he developed alcoholic ketoacidosis, it is likely that he developed severe AG metabolic acidosis.
- The present ABG values show the pH is 7.2—academia is present. The PCO_2 is high—possibly chronic respiratory acidosis. He must have had elevated HCO_3 as a compensation for high PCO_2.
- However, the present HCO_3 is within 'normal' range and patient is in alcoholic ketoacidosis.
- How is this possible? If the initial HCO_3 was very high and the recent metabolic acidosis has brought it down, normal HCO_3 may occur.
- The AG is $136 - (85 + 25) = 26$. In any condition where the AG is more than 24, there must have been pre-existing metabolic alkalosis with higher values of HCO_3.
- In this case, the previous AG was 12 and is now 26. The ΔAG is 14. The present HCO_3 is 25. So, before the starting of the acute event, in this case, alcoholic ketoacidosis, ΔAG and ΔHCO_3 should be equal. So, the patient must have had serum bicarbonate level = present $HCO_3 + \Delta AG - 25 + 14 = 39$ mmol/L.

We can conclude that in this patient, chronic respiratory acidosis well-compensated by metabolic alkalosis with HCO_3 level –39 mmol/L. When he developed alcoholic ketoacidosis, the ketoacids neutralized HCO_3 to the extent of ΔAG and the patient has chronic respiratory acidosis complicated by AG metabolic acidosis—even though the HCO_3 level is 'normal.'

Case 6: A 50-year-old lady was brought in a semiconscious state. She was a diabetic with cardiac failure who had been ill for several days. She had been using digoxin and diuretics for the cardiac failure. The relevant biochemical reports and ABG were urine ketones: 3+, serum chemistry—Na: 132, K: 2.7, Cl: 79, HCO_3^-: 19 mmol/L, glucose: 815 mg/dL, lactate: 0.9, ABG—pH: 7.41, PCO_2: 32, HCO_3^-: 19 and PO_2: 82.

Approach:

- Based on the history and clinical features, she is likely to have elevated AG acidosis secondary to DKA and metabolic alkalosis in view of the thiazide diuretic use.
- Since, the pH is within the normal range, it may suggest a normal acid-base status or a mixed acid-base disorder.
- PCO_2 is low suggesting respiratory alkalosis and HCO_3 ($\Delta HCO_3 = 24 - 19 = 5$) are low suggesting metabolic acidosis.
- It is difficult to decide the primary event since, the pH is normal.
- Since, she has hyperglycemia with ketonuria, we assume that she has DKA with high AG metabolic acidosis.
- The AG here is $132 - (79 + 19) = 34 \rightarrow$ (high) $\rightarrow \Delta AG$ is $34 - 12 = 22$.
- This confirms high AG metabolic acidosis.
- Why is the pH normal then? Possibly, there is associated disorder increasing the HCO_3. Diuretic therapy, vomiting due to DKA or associated chronic respiratory acidosis could be the cause of the initial high HCO_3.
- In this case, concurrent use of thiazide diuretic could be responsible for the pre-existing metabolic alkalosis on top of which, the patient has developed high AG metabolic acidosis due to DKA.
- The delta ratio ($\Delta AG/\Delta HCO_3$) in this case is $22/5 = 4.4$. When delta ratio is over 2:1, it suggests concurrent metabolic alkalosis.

Table 73.3: Quantitative and molar composition of different solutions used for infusion

Solution	Chemical composition
2, 5, 10, 40% dextrose	Corresponding number of g% of dextrose
0.85% NaCl (normal saline)	145 mmol/L of Na and Cl
0.45% NaCl	77 mmol/L of Na and Cl
3.0% NaCl	513 mmol/L of Na and Cl
15% potassium chloride (10 mL ampoules)	2,000 mmol/L of K and Cl or 2 mmol/mL of K and Cl
1.5% $NaHCO_3$	178 mmol/L of Na and HCO_3
7.5% $NaHCO_3$ (10 mL ampoules)	890 mmol/L of Na and HCO_3 (roughly 1 mmol/mL)
1/6 molar lactate or (1.87% $NaC_3H_5O_3$)	167 mmol/L of Na and HCO_3
Composition of Ringer's lactate:	
NaCl	130 mmol/L
Sodium lactate	27 mmol/L
KCl	4 mmol/L
$CaCl_2$	4 mmol/L

Table 73.4: Equivalent of 1 g of solute

Solute	mmol
NaCl	17.24
KCl	13.3
CaCl	9.0
$CaCO_3$	10.0
$MgSO_4$	8.3
$NaHCO_3$	11.9
Na_2HPO_4	7.0
NaH_2PO_4	8.2

We may conclude that this is a case of mixed elevated AG metabolic acidosis and metabolic alkalosis due to DKA and thiazide diuretics.

The composition and availability of commonly used IV fluids is summarized in Tables 73.3 and 73.4.

CHAPTER
74

Disturbances of Osmotic Equilibrium

KV Krishna Das, R Kasi Visweswaran

Chapter Summary

- Concept of Osmolality
- Regulation of Plasma Osmolality
- Measurement of Osmolality and Osmolar Gap
- Disorders of Osmolality
  - Hyperosmolar States
  - Hypo-osmolar Disorders
    - Evaluation and Causes of Hyponatremia
- Central Pontine Myelinolysis (Osmotic Demyelination)

Clear understanding of the concepts of osmolality will enable easier comprehension of disorders of water and electrolyte balance, particularly water and sodium homeostasis. This will also help in the diagnosis of certain poisonings and prevent complications like osmotic demyelination syndrome (ODS).

CONCEPT OF OSMOLALITY

If two solutions of varying solute concentration are separated by a semipermeable membrane that does not

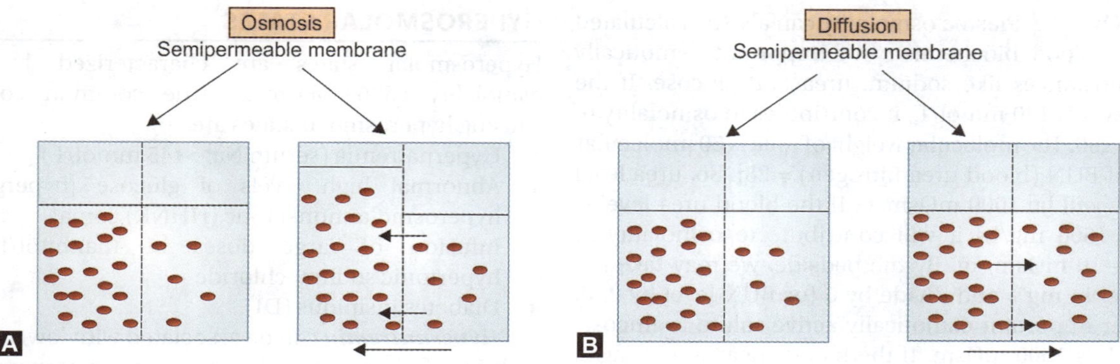

Figs 74.1A and B: Difference between osmosis and diffusion. **A. *Osmosis:*** Movement of water (solvent) from a region of lower solute concentration to a region of higher solute concentration across a semipermeable membrane; **B. *Diffusion:*** Movement of solute from a region of higher solute concentration to a region of lower solute concentration across a semipermeable membrane.

allow solutes to pass through, but it permits only solvent, the solvent (often water) will move from the solution of lower solute concentration to the solution with higher solute concentration. This movement of the solvent (water) is called ***osmosis*** (Fig. 74.1A). The driving force for osmosis is determined by the number of osmotically active solutes in the solution.

If two solutions of varying solute concentrations are separated by a semipermeable membrane that permits solutes to move, the movement of solutes from higher solute concentration to that of lower solute concentration occurs and this process is called ***diffusion*** (Fig. 74.1B).

There is difference between osmolality and osmolarity. ***Osmolality*** is defined as the amount of osmotically active solutes in one kilogram of solvent (water). ***Osmolarity*** is the amount of osmotically active solutes in 1 L of the solution. In the case of water, since 1 kg equivalent to 1 L, osmolality and osmolarity are the same. The unit for measuring osmotic pressure is the ***osmole (Osm or osmol)***, which is defined as the amount of solute that dissolves in solution to form 1 mole of particles. One mole of any substance is equal to the atomic/molecular weight of the substance in gram. Therefore, a solution with osmolality of 1 means 'one gram molecular weight' of the solute is dissolved in 1 kg of solvent. Atomic weight of sodium is 23 g/mol and the molecular weight of glucose is 180 g/mol. If 23 g/mol of sodium is dissolved in 1 kg water, the osmolality is 1 osmol/kg or 1000 milliosmoles (mOsm)/kg. Similarly, 180 g/mol of glucose is dissolved in 1 L of water, the osmolality is 1 osmol/kg or 1000 mOsm/kg. The sodium (cation) in serum is accompanied by an equivalent quantity of anion. So, if the serum sodium is 140 mmol/L, the osmolality contributed by sodium and accompanying anion will be 280 mOsm/kg.

REGULATION OF PLASMA OSMOLALITY

Plasma osmolality varies from 285 to 290 mOsm/kg. The major contributor to the plasma osmolality is the sodium. In order to increase the osmolality of a fluid compartment, the solute must remain confined to that compartment. Those solutes which remain confined to a particular compartment, e.g. sodium or administered mannitol, remains in extracellular fluid (ECF) and increase osmolality thereby, causing significant osmotic gradient between ECF and intracellular fluid (ICF). Since they facilitate net movement of water, they are 'effective' osmole. Urea can freely diffuse between the compartments and is distributed in both the ICF and ECF almost equally. When the blood urea increases, there is parallel increase in the osmolality of both ICF and ECF. Thus, there is effectively no gradient between these two compartments. Thus, it is an 'ineffective' osmole.

In health, plasma osmolality is maintained within 1–2% of the normal range. The osmoreceptors located close to supraoptic nucleus of hypothalamus respond by increase in osmolality and these osmoreceptors cause release of vasopressin from the posterior pituitary gland. Vasopressin acts on vasopressin 2 (V2) receptors on collecting duct in the kidney which regulate the expression of water channels known as ***aquaporin channels***. Normally, some aquaporin channels remain dormant inside the cell. Under the influence of vasopressin, they move to the luminal membrane and are inserted on to the cell membrane. Since, these are free water channels, more water is reabsorbed from the lumen of the collecting tubule as it travels through the hypertonic renal medullary interstitium. This increases body water content and helps to normalize plasma osmolality. Hyperosmolality also stimulates the thirst center resulting in sense of thirst and if the subject is conscious and has access to water, he/she consumes water so that the osmolality is normalized. Any decrease in osmolality causes the opposite effect wherein the water intake is reduced because of reduced thirst and the urine output is increased by reduced release of vasopressin (antidiuretic hormone). The aquaporin channels are delinked from the luminal membrane of the collecting tubule cells and go into dormant state inside the cell. Nonosmotic stimuli including hypovolemia, pain, nausea and pregnancy which may also stimulate vasopressin release.

MEASUREMENT OF OSMOLALITY AND OSMOLAR GAP

Osmolality of plasma can be measured using an ***osmometer***, which measures the osmolality from the freezing point. A solution with osmolality 1 (1000 milliosmoles) freezes at the temperature of 1.86°C. So, if a solution freezes at –0.93°C, we can say that the osmolality is 500 mOsm/kg. Plasma osmolality can also be calculated from the blood biochemistry of important osmotically active substances like sodium, urea and glucose. If the serum level is 140 mmol/L, it contributes to osmolality of $140 \times 2 = 280$. The molecular weight of urea is 60 [molecular weight of BUN (blood urea nitrogen) = 28]. So, urea level of 60 g/L will be 1000 mOsm/L. If the blood urea level is 60 mg% (600 mg/L) it will contribute to osmolality of $600/60 + 10$ mOsm/kg. By the bedside, we may take the urea level in mg% and divide by 6 (or BUN level by 2.8). The other important osmotically active solute is glucose, 180 mg/L is 1000 mOsm. If the blood sugar is 180 mg%, (1800 mg/L) it will contribute to $1800/180 = 10$ mOsm/L. We may take the blood sugar in mg%/18 or if the result of glucose in mmols as obtained from some labs. Thus, the osmolality can be calculated using the following formula:

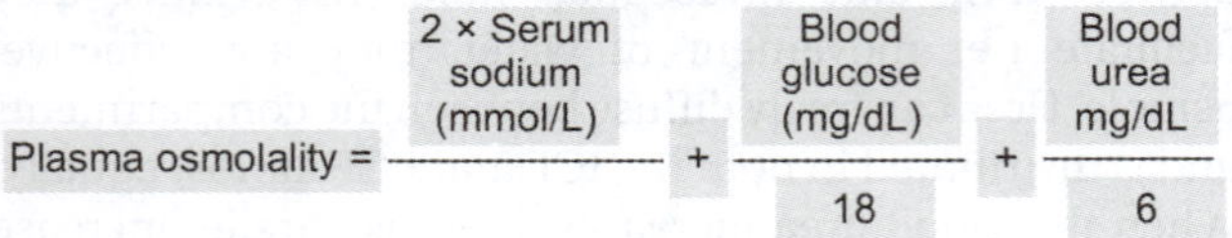

Note: If BUN is provided instead of blood urea, BUN must be divided by 2.8 in place of 6. If values of urea and glucose is given as mmols, it is used directly.

If serum sodium is 140, blood glucose is 145 and blood urea is 36, the calculated plasma osmolality will be $2 \times 140 + (145/18) + (36/6) = 280 + 15 + 6 = 301$ mOsm/kg water. If serum sodium is 140, blood glucose 900 and blood urea 180, the plasma osmolality will be $2 \times 140 + (900/18) + (180/6) = 280 + 50 + 30 = 360$ mOsm/kg water.

Such values are seen in patients with hyperosmolar nonketotic diabetic coma.

Osmolar gap is the difference between measured osmolality and the calculated osmolality. Presence of osmolar gap of more than 10, suggests the presence of osmotically active unmeasured exogenous substances/toxins in plasma.

Osmolar gap = Measured osmolality – calculated osmolality

Osmolar gap can be observed when serum sodium is spuriously low as in pseudohyponatremia (hyperlipidemia or hyperproteinemia) or due to accumulation of osmolytes, other than sodium, urea and glucose in the blood. Substances like acetone, mannitol, radiocontrast agents, methyl alcohol, ethyl alcohol, isopropyl alcohol, acetone, ethylene glycol and propylene glycol are the common causes of toxin associated with high osmolar gap metabolic acidosis.

DISORDERS OF OSMOLALITY

Hypo-osmolar and hyperosmolar disorders are disorders of osmolality characterized by either a decrease or an increase in the plasma osmolality. Since plasma sodium is the main determinant of plasma osmolality, true hypo-osmolar states are reflected by hyponatremia and hyperosmolar states are manifested by hypernatremia. Although plasma sodium level may indicate the total body sodium concentration, most often hypo/hypernatremia are in fact a reflection of abnormal water balance.

HYPEROSMOLAR STATES

Hyperosmolar states are characterized by serum osmolality >320 mOsm/kg. The common conditions causing hyperosmolar states are:

- Hypernatremia (serum Na^+ >145 mmol/L)
- Abnormal high levels of glucose [hyperglycemic hyperosmolar nonketotic (HHNK) coma]
- Infusion of large doses of mannitol/fructose/hypertonic sodium chloride
- Diabetes insipidus (DI).

Hypernatremia can be associated with low, normal or high ECF fluid volume (*See* section on hypernatremia for more details).

Hyperglycemic hyperosmolar nonketotic diabetic coma is a complication of type 2 diabetes mellitus (DM) and often occurs in the elderly people. Severe hyperglycemia with polyuria leading to severe dehydration occurs without development of ketosis. It is often precipitated by myocardial infarction, stroke, infection or other illnesses. If the person is deprived of water intake in spite of excessive urine output, severe dehydration occurs and oliguria develops. Since, there is no insulin deficiency, ketosis does not develop and the symptoms are mild. The patient visits the hospital often late in the course of the disease with severe dehydration and complications. The patient may have vague neurological symptoms like disorientation or may be in coma. Physical examination would show evidence of severe dehydration with poor skin turgor, sunken eyeballs, tachycardia and hypotension. Patient will have high blood sugar levels often >600 mg% with no ketonuria. The plasma osmolality will be high and is due to high sodium and glucose. It is managed by appropriate fluid administration to correct the fluid and electrolyte deficit and insulin infusions for bringing down the blood glucose level. Both are performed simultaneously under close monitoring. Potassium supplements are often needed early in the treatment (even before starting insulin). If the serum potassium is less than 3.5 mmol/L, administration of insulin without potassium supplementation may even lead to fatal hypokalemia. Initial correction is with isotonic saline, followed by half normal saline. The initial replacement could be about 1 L/hour and the total requirement may go up to 8–12 L over 24–36 hours. If facilities are available or if cardiac illness is suspected, fluid should be administered with central venous pressure (CVP) monitoring. With good supportive treatment, the outlook and prognosis have improved.

Administration of high osmolar solutions as intravenous infusions, total parenteral nutrition, and radiocontrast agents should be closely monitored so as to prevent the development of hyperosmolar state. Since, dehydration is an adverse prognostic factor, adequate hydration and urine flow rate should be maintained for preventing development of complications related to hyperosmolality.

In DI, there is either a decreased production of antidiuretic hormone (ADH) (central DI) or the collecting tubules are resistant to the action of ADH (nephrogenic

DI). These two conditions are clinically distinguished by the *water deprivation test*.

Water deprivation test is the scenario in which the patient is deprived of water till he loses 3–5% of body weight, develops tachycardia, postural hypotension or till three consecutive urine samples have an osmolality of within 10% of each other. In normal individuals, water deprivation results in increase in urine osmolality >500 mOsmol/kg and the plasma vasopressin level increases to more than 2 pg/mL. If the osmolality remains low, exogenous vasopressin is administered. If the patient has central DI (vasopressin deficiency), the urine volume decreases and the osmolality increases within the next hour. If no response occurs, it suggests the vasopressin is not acting. Since, the renal tubules do not respond appropriately and the diagnosis is nephrogenic DI. Administration of exogenous vasopressin does not increase the urine osmolality.

Central DI may be congenital and inherited as autosomal dominant or autosomal recessive disorder. It can follow head injury, encephalitis and meningitis, granulomatous diseases like tuberculosis or sarcoidosis, tumors, infiltrative disorders like histiocytosis or may be without a known cause (idiopathic). The urine osmolality is < 150 osmol/kg, with no increase in plasma ADH even after water deprivation. On administration of exogenous vasopressin, urine osmolality increases promptly to >800 mOsm/kg water.

Nephrogenic DI on the other hand could occur following hypokalemia, hypercalcemia, sickle cell disease, use of lithium or during pregnancy. The urine osmolality is often over 300 but does not exceed 500 mOsm/kg in spite of water deprivation, vasopressin level increases to > 5 pg/mL after water deprivation. Since, vasopressin is ineffective, there is no increase in urine osmolality even after administration of exogenous vasopressin.

HYPO-OSMOLAR DISORDERS

Plasma contains 93% fluid and 7% solid components. The sodium, distributed in the aqueous phase is the major contributor of plasma osmolality. Any true reduction in sodium will be associated with hypo-osmolality. When there is paraproteinemia or hyperlipidemia, the solid phase in the plasma increases. Therefore, there is an apparent reduction in serum sodium level. This causes pseudohyponatremia and is associated with normal plasma osmolality. Accurate liquid based sodium in plasma can be measured by using potentiometer which measures the sodium in plasma and overcomes the fallacy of pseudohyponatremia. Another type of apparent hyponatremia occurs in patients with hyperglycemia and increased serum osmolality. It causes movement of water from ICF to ECF resulting in low levels of sodium, even though there is no deficiency of sodium. For every 100 mg increase in blood glucose level, the serum sodium decreases by 1.6 mmols and is due to movement of water as explained above. This is an example of *translocational hyponatremia*. Other substances like mannitol or glycine also increases serum osmolality while decreasing serum sodium. Once the above two conditions are ruled out, true hyponatremia can be diagnosed. It is a hypo-osmolar disorder often due to a disturbance in urinary dilution leading to water retention.

Evaluation and Causes of Hyponatremia

The initial evaluation in case of true hyponatremia is to determine the volume status of the patient (hypovolemic, euvolemic or hypervolemic) and to determine the urinary spot sodium concentration Flowchart 74.1.

The most common causes of hyponatremia are diuretic use, hypervolemic states like congestive cardiac failure (CCF), nephrotic syndrome, cirrhosis liver and syndrome of inappropriate antidiuretic hormone secretion (SIADH).

Flowchart 74.1: Algorithm for diagnosis of true hyponatremia

Abbreviations: SIADH = Syndrome of inappropriate antidiuretic hormone; CCF = Congestive cardiac failure

Hypovolemic Hyponatremia

Diuretics are among the most common cause of hyponatremia. Thiazide diuretics saluretic (causing more salt loss) compared to loop diuretics which are aquaretics (causing more water loss). Hence, use of thiazides is more commonly associated with hyponatremia especially in elderly women compared to loop diuretics. In cases of extrarenal fluid loss, there is loss of total body sodium and water leading to hypovolemia. However, the body tries to maintain effective arterial volume at the expense of osmolality with resultant increase in ADH level. Since, there is loss of sodium and water, replacement fluid is normal saline. Inappropriate choice of hypotonic fluids like 5% dextrose will lead to worsening of hyponatremia in such situations. Cerebral salt wasting is another cause of hypovolemic hyponatremia seen in neurological diseases like in cerebral trauma, infection or following neurosurgical procedures. It is often not suspected and the diagnosis may be missed. Although, the exact mechanism is unclear, it is thought to be due to increased release of brain natriuretic peptide leading to natriuresis and volume contraction. This in turn stimulates ADH release and the syndrome closely mimics SIADH. The difference is that SIADH is normovolemic, whereas cerebral salt wasting is hypovolemic. These two can be differentiated by checking serum uric acid level. Since, cerebral salt wasting is a hypovolemic state, uric acid level is increased whereas, in SIADH, the patient is euvolemic and the serum uric acid is normal.

Euvolemic Hyponatremia

Hypothyroidism is a common cause of euvolemic hyponatremia. The exact reason is unclear; it is also thought to be closely related to ADH action. Drugs are an important cause of hyponatremia. They act by different mechanisms such as:

- ***Vasopressin analogue:*** DDAVP (desmopressin)
- ***Enhanced vasopressin release:*** Chlorpropamide, clofibrate, carbamazepine, vincristine
- ***Enhanced renal action of vasopressin:*** Chlorpropamide, cyclophosphamide
- ***Unknown mechanisms:*** Haloperidol.

A diagnosis of SIADH is made after the exclusion of thyroid, pituitary and renal diseases and absence of diuretic intake. The cause for SIADH must be sought and corrected.

- Fluid restriction—to prevent excess water reabsorption due to increased activity of vasopressin
- Pharmacological inhibition of vasopressin

Vaptans: These are drugs which act on the V2 receptors in the collecting duct and block the action of ADH. Three oral agents (tolvaptan, lixivaptan and satavaptan) and one parenteral preparation (conivaptan) are available. Tolvaptan is used in a dose of 15–60 mg/day.

Demeclocycline: Blocks the action of ADH on the collecting duct and can be used as an alternative. Usual dose is 600–1200 mg/day. It can cause photosensitive reactions and should be used with caution in patients with liver disease. Before the availability of the vaptans, this drug is employed more frequently.

Syndrome of inappropriate ADH secretion (SIADH) (Refer to Section 1, Ch 7)

This is one of the common cause of hyponatremia in hospitalized patients. It is diagnosed by excluding other potential causes of hyponatremia. Normally, the 'appropriate stimuli' for the release of ADH are hyperosmolality and hypovolemia. However, when there is ADH release in the absence of these appropriate physiological stimuli, the clinical condition is called SIADH. It is most commonly associated with central nervous system (CNS) and pulmonary diseases. Some of the causes of SIADH are explained in Box 74.1.

Diagnosis of SIADH

SIADH is a diagnosis of exclusion. There are essential and supplemental criteria for diagnosing SIADH that are explained in Box 74.2.

Hypervolemic Hyponatremia

Hypervolemic hyponatremia is seen in conditions like nephritic syndrome, CCF and cirrhosis liver. The fluid accumulation is mainly in the ECF compartment. The reduction in effective arterial volume results in an appropriate ADH release. This ADH action enables more water reabsorption and this coupled with ingestion of hypotonic fluids results in hypervolemia and hyponatremia. The development of hyponatremia in CCF is an independent predictor of mortality.

Clinical Features

The clinical features depend on:

- The rapidity of development of hyponatremia
- The primary cause of hyponatremia
- The osmotic adaptation of the patient to hyponatremia.

In general, plasma sodium levels more than 125 mEq/L are well-tolerated and the patients are often asymptomatic or may have anorexia and headache.

Box 74.1: Causes of SIADH

Central nervous system (CNS) disorders	Encephalitis/meningitis/trauma/tumor/cerebrovascular accident/subarachnoid hemorrhage/Guillain-Barre syndrome/acute intermittent porphyria
Pulmonary disorders	Pneumonia/tuberculosis/abscess/mesothelioma
Malignancy	Carcinoma of bronchus/stomach/pancreas lymphoma, thymoma
Miscellaneous	Human immunodeficiency virus (HIV) or acquired immune deficiency syndrome (AIDS)

Box 74.2: Supplemental criteria for diagnosing SIADH

Essential criteria	Supplemental criteria
• Low serum osmolality (<270 mOsmol/kg) • Raised urine osmolality (>100 mOsmol/kg) • Clinical euvolemia • Urine Na >30 mEq/L with normal salt and water intake • Absence of pituitary, thyroid or adrenal insufficiency • No history of diuretic intake	• Abnormal water load test (inability to excrete at least 90% of 20 mL/kg water administered in 4 hours inability to lower urine osmolality < 100 mOsmol/kg) • Inappropriately raised plasma vasopressin level with respect to plasma osmolality • Correction of plasma sodium with water restriction

Textbook of Medicine

Rapid fall in plasma sodium level to less than 125 mEq/L is associated with lethargy, personality changes, muscle weakness, confusion and alteration in mental status. Levels below 115 may be associated with drowsiness, hyporeflexia and even seizures. Untreated hyponatremia carries high mortality. Symptomatic acute hyponatremia (occurring within 48 hours in patient who had normal serum sodium and osmolality earlier) is a medical emergency. The sudden fall in plasma osmolality alters the osmotic equilibrium between the ECF and ICF and results in osmotically mediated movement of water from ECF to ICF compartment. Intracellular edema manifests in the neurons in the form of cerebral edema. The neurological symptoms in acute hyponatremia signify cerebral edema.

Treatment

The mainstay of treatment is to restrict salt and water along with administration of furosemide which promotes the renal clearance of solute free water. Treatment depends on the cause, rapidity of onset and whether the patient is symptomatic. The cause must be identified and corrected. In most cases, the cause of hyponatremia is retention of water and not deficiency of salt. The following principles are applied in the treatment of all types of hyponatremia:

Guidelines and Principles for Correcting Acute Symptomatic Hyponatremia

- Even severe and symptomatic hyponatremia should not be corrected faster than 2 mmols/L/hour.
- Maximum permissible correction during 24 hours is 10 mmols/L.
- A target should be set every day for correction based on the above guidelines.
- Full correction should never be attempted overnight.
- The initial target should be set around 120–125 mEq/L to avoid over-correction.
- In most situations, water restriction is the mainstay in treatment.
- For hypovolemic hyponatremia, oral replacements are sufficient unless there are contraindications.
- Saline infusions are necessary only for correction of hypovolemic hyponatremia.

Steps for Correction with Saline

Calculate the required sodium to be corrected to achieve the target set from the following formula:

(Desired sodium – Actual sodium) × Total body water
(Total body water is approximately 0.6 × bw in males and 0.55 × bw in females). If it is desired to raise sodium from 110 to 118 mmol/L in 24 hours in a 60 kg male, the required sodium is calculated as follows:
Required sodium = (118 – 110) × (60 × 0.6) = 8 × 36 = 288 mmols
(1 L of normal saline contains 154 mEq of Na and 1 L of 3% saline contains 514 mEq of Na).

If the patient is clinically dehydrated, approximately 2L isotonic sodium chloride (NaCl) (normal saline) nearly 310 mEq Na may be given over 24 hours. If the patient does not need such fluid intake, 300 mL of 3% NaCl (153 mEq) and 1 L normal saline (154 mEq) may be administered slowly and uniformly over 24 hours. Hypertonic sodium chloride (3% NaCl) should be given only in the ICUs with close monitoring. This is expected to raise the sodium by 8–10 mmols. Reassessment and planning for the next day will depend on the reports of serum biochemistry the next day.

CENTRAL PONTINE MYELINOLYSIS (CENTRAL OSMOTIC DEMYELINATION)

This is a dreaded complication resulting from the rapid correction of chronic hyponatremia. In chronic hyponatremia, the brain undergoes osmotic adaptation by losing osmotically active chemicals (osmolytes) from the neurons so that a new osmotic equilibrium is established in the brain and restores the brain osmolality to that of the plasma. In such a patient, with well-adapted hyponatremia who is asymptomatic, if hyponatremia is corrected rapidly, the serum osmolality rises fast. The high osmolality in the ECF will cause movement of water from ICF to ECF resulting in cellular dehydration. Since, the neurons lose water into the plasma, cerebral dehydration and cell shrinkage occurs. The response of damaged neurons is to undergo demyelination. The neurons in the central area of the pons are highly vulnerable to such damage. Other parts of the nervous system can also be affected. Clinically, this is manifested as cranial nerve palsy, behavioral changes and ends up locked-in state. This condition is more common in alcoholics, malnourished elderly women on thiazides and in liver transplant recipients. This is called *ODS or central pontine myelinolysis*.

CHAPTER 75

Digestive Organs: General Considerations

KR Vinaya Kumar, KV Krishna Das

Chapter Summary

- Applied Anatomy and Physiology
- Symptoms in Alimentary Disorders
- Investigations in Alimentary Disorders

APPLIED ANATOMY AND PHYSIOLOGY

ESOPHAGUS

Esophagus is a muscular tube ranging in length from 25 to 30 cm extending from the cricopharyngeal sphincter to the lower esophageal sphincter (LES) above the cardia of the stomach. Its immediate relations are the trachea, left main bronchus, the aortic arch and the left atrium. The blood supply is derived from the small branches of the descending thoracic aorta. The inferior thyroid artery supplies the upper most part and the left gastric artery supplies the lower end. Veins from the upper part drain into the superior vena cava (SVC), those from the middle third drain into the azygos system and the veins of the lower third drain into the portal system through the gastric veins. These veins are interconnected. The vagus nerve, fibers of which anastomose with the Auerbach's plexus, acts as the chief motor nerve. The cervical sympathetic ganglia and the fibers from the thoracic sympathetic ganglia provide sympathetic innervation. The cervical lymph nodes receive lymphatics from the upper third, mediastinal nodes from the middle third and the celiac and gastric lymph nodes from the lower third. The lymphatics anastomose freely. The upper one-third of the esophagus contains striated muscle and the lower two-third contains smooth muscle. The esophagus has no serosa. It is lined by stratified squamous epithelium. Under abnormal conditions when gastric acid regurgitates into the esophagus, the lining of the lower end undergoes metaplasia, to resemble columnar epithelium resembling the gastric mucosa.

Physiology

The cricopharyngeal sphincter remains tonically closed except during swallowing. On swallowing, a wave of peristalsis (called primary peristalsis) sweeps down. Secondary peristalsis is set up when gastric contents regurgitate into the esophagus. On swallowing, the LES relaxes and the food bolus passes into the stomach. Reflux of gastric contents into the esophagus is prevented by the LES. The LES involves the distal 3–4 cm of esophagus and at rest is tonically contracted. The proximal part of LES is normally 1.5–2 cm above squamocolumnar junction and the distal segment is about 2 cm in length which lies with in the abdominal cavity, thus maintaining gastroesophageal competence during intra-abdominal pressure excursions. This sphincter is controlled by inhibitory and excitatory neural influences. Several other factors also influence the LES tone.

Below box shows factors about increasing and decreasing LES tone.

Factors increase LES tone:	*Factors decreases LES tone:*
Prostaglandins, cholinergic agents, cisapride, metoclopramide, alkalies, high protein meal, gastrin, motilin	Secretin, cholecystokinins, somatostatin, alcohol, chocolate, smoking, gastric acidity, obesity, pregnancy, hiatal hernia, tricyclic antidepressants

STOMACH

The stomach is the most distensible part of the gastrointestinal tract (GIT). Capacity of the adult stomach is 1–1.5 L. Stomach wall is made up of mucosa, submucosa, muscle coat and serosa. Thickness of stomach is about 5 mm. The stomach volume reaches from about 30 mL in the neonate to 1.5–2 L in adulthood. Branches of the celiac axis and to a lesser extent branches of superior mesenteric artery provide arterial blood. Veins accompany the arteries and drain into the portal circulation. Lymphatic drainage is into four main groups of lymph nodes, left gastric, pancreaticosplenic, right gastroepiploic and pyloric. From these primary nodes, further drainage occurs into the celiac group of preaortic nodes and then into cisterna chyli. The stomach receives sympathetic and parasympathetic nerves. The two vagus nerves which are parasympathetic, reach the stomach through the esophageal hiatus and anastomose with the ganglion cells in the layers of the organ. Parasympathetic stimulation leads to gastric secretion, contraction of the stomach and relaxation of the pylorus. The sympathetic fibers derived from T6 to T10 segments reach the stomach through the celiac ganglia and celiac plexus. Sympathetic stimulation constricts blood vessels, contracts the pylorus and inhibits secretion and motor activity.

Structure

The gastric glands differ in the three regions of the stomach and are called the cardiac glands, oxyntic glands and the pyloric glands. The oxyntic glands have cell types—the chief cells, oxyntic or parietal cells, mucous neck cells and enterochromaffin (EC) cells and D cells. The chief cells produce pepsinogen, the parietal cells produce hydrochloric acid and intrinsic factor and the mucous neck cells produce mucus and D cells producing stomatostatin. The pyloric glands have G cells producing gastrin, mucus secreting cells, D cells and EC cells.

Structure of glands		
Cardiac glands	Oxyntic glands	Pyloric glands
Mucus secreting cells	• Chief cells—pepsinogen • Parietal cell—hydrochloric acid, intrinsic factor • Mucus secreting cells • D cells—stomatostatin • Ghrelin (Gr) cells • EC cells—atrial natriuretic peptide (ANP), serotonin, histamine	• Mucus secreting cells • G cell–gastrin • EC cell • Gr cells • D cells

Physiology

The proximal part of the stomach acts as a reservoir to receive ingested food and the distal portion (antral mill) churns the food and converts it into chyme. Gastric emptying is controlled by the antral contractions. Liquids leave the stomach faster than solids. The antrum contracts at a rate of 3/min. Gastric emptying depends on factors such as volume and composition of the meal and by the activity of the duodenum and small bowel which is mediated through neurohumoral mechanisms. Gastric emptying is slowed by *glucagon, gastrin, secretin, cholecystokinin, vasoactive intestinal polypeptide (VIP), gastric inhibitory polypeptide (GIP)* and *increased acidity.* Hyperglycemia causes delay in gastric emptying while hypoglycemia accelerates it.

The *gastric juice* contains hydrochloric acid, pepsinogens, intrinsic factor and mucus. The endogenous stimulants of gastric acid secretion are gastrin, histamine and acetylcholine. Food is the most important physiologic stimulus for gastric acid secretion. Distension of the stomach enhances acid secretion through cholinergic reflexes. Amino acids and peptides in the stomach induce acid secretion through the release of gastrin. Pepsins, which are the proteolytic enzymes in the gastric juice, are stored as inactive precursors; the pepsinogens, which are converted to pepsin in the presence of acid. Cholinergic reflexes, gastrin and histamine stimulate secretion of pepsin. Intrinsic factor is produced by the parietal cells and normally the quantity of intrinsic factor far exceeds the amount required for vitamin B_{12} absorption. Intrinsic factor secretion is stimulated by vagal stimulation, cholinergic agents, histamine and gastrin.

SMALL INTESTINE

The small intestine is 6–7 meters long (range 300–850 cm). If the length is reduced below 200 cm, it leads to 'short bowel syndrome'. The widest part is the duodenum and it is fixed. The rest of the small intestine is arbitrarily divided into jejunum and ileum without any sharp demarcation. Thickness of small intestine is around 3 mm.

The duodenum is the first 20 cm of the small intestine and is the thickest section. The jejunum is 1.5–2.5 m (5–8 feet) long and forms two-fifths of the length of the small intestine. The other three-fifths is the ileum which is 2.5–3.5 m. The small intestine derives its arterial supply from the celiac and superior mesenteric arteries. Its veins drain into the portal system. The vagus provides parasympathetic innervation. Sympathetic fibers originate from T9 and T10 segments. The wall of the small intestine has four layers. They are *mucosa, submucosa, muscular layer* and *serosa*. The small intestine is the main site of digestion and absorption. The mucosa is thrown into convoluted folds, the *valvulae conneventes*, which are more numerous in the jejunum. The luminal surface is covered by villi which are taller in the jejunum than in the ileum. The villi are lined by a single layer of tall columnar epithelial cells. The area between the villi is occupied by the crypts. The crypt epithelial cells are the precursors of the villous epithelial cells. In addition, the crypt contains *Paneth cells, goblet cells* and *endocrine cells.* The crypt epithelial cells migrate towards the villi where they mature and are finally shed off from the tip. The villus epithelium is constantly being replaced and the migration time from crypt to villus is 2–6 days. In addition to the tall columnar cells, the mucosa contains goblet cells which secrete mucus and EC cells with endocrine function. The luminal end of the epithelial cells has the brush border, composed of tall closely packed microvilli. This region contains the enzymes for digestion of carbohydrates and proteins. The Paneth cells are trapezoid cells with basophilic cytoplasm seen at the base of the crypts. They secrete growth factors, antimicrobial peptides and digestive enzymes.

The Brunner's glands are seen in the submucosa of the duodenum. They secrete alkaline mucus, epidermal growth factor and pepsinogen II.

The *lamina propria* contains blood vessels, lymphatics, nerve fibers, lymphocytes, plasma cells, eosinophils, macrophages and mast cells. The lymphocytes and plasma cells of the lamina propria and the epithelium form part of the immune system. *Peyer's patches* are aggregations of lymphoid tissue seen in the submucosa of the ileum.

Motility of the GIT

The stomach and intestines undergo regular co-ordinated peristaltic movements. Motility and intraluminal pressures can be recorded by manometry at different levels.
Movement occurs in three phases:
Phase 1: Quiescent phase.
Phase 2: Occurs after eating in which the fasting pattern gives place to the fed pattern in the stomach and small intestine. At this stage, the migratory pattern stops and bursts of contractions occur which help to mix the contents and enhance digestion and absorption.
Phase 3: This occurs during fasting. The movements are known as *migrating motor complex (MMC).* Regular motility occurs at a rate of 3 cycles per minute in the duodenum and passes down the intestine.

The peristaltic activity is controlled by mechanical and neurohumoral factors. Chyme is mixed up by segmenting movements and propelled forwards by peristaltic movements. Movement of chyme is faster in the jejunum than in the ileum.

Two major functions of the small intestine are: (i) digestion and absorption of food and (ii) barrier function against luminal micro-organisms and toxins. Intestinal failure leads to three major problems:

1. Malnutrition
2. Sepsis
3. Symptoms which impair the quality of life—diarrhea, vomiting and abdominal pain.

Lesions and resection of the distal parts of the small intestine produce greater abnormalities of digestion and absorption. Removal of long segments of the small intestine also leads to secondary hypersecretion in the stomach as a result of decrease in the production of the inhibitory hormones.

LARGE INTESTINE

Syn: Colon

The large intestine, which begins at the ileocecal junction and ends at the anal canal, is 90–125 cm long. The caliber of the colon diminishes progressively from cecum to the sigmoid. The portion proximal to the midtransverse colon is derived from the midgut and it derives its blood supply from the superior mesenteric artery. It is absorptive in function. The distal half is derived from the hindgut and it derives its blood supply from the inferior mesenteric artery and its main function is storage. The lower end of the rectum and anal canal is supplied by paired middle and inferior rectal arteries which arise from the internal iliac artery. The veins accompany the arteries and ultimately reach the portal system through the superior and inferior mesenteric veins. The rectum provides a site for portal-systemic anastomosis. The lymphatics of the colon and rectum accompany the superior and inferior mesenteric vessels. Lymphatics from the anus drain into the superficial inguinal nodes. Sympathetic and parasympathetic nerves supply the colon. Sympathetic fibers arise from T11 to L2 through the sympathetic ganglia and splanchnic nerves and finally reach the colon along with the blood vessels. Parasympathetic fibers arise from the vagus and the sacral outflow.

Colonic mucosa is lined by a single layer of columnar epithelial cells which are flat. The surface of the mucosa shows the *crypts of Lieberkühn*. There are numerous goblet cells in the mucosa. The crypts show argentaffin cells also. The luminal surface of the epithelial cells shows villi. The lamina propria contains blood vessels, lymphatics, nerve fibers, lymphocytes, plasma cells and histiocytes.

Physiology

The essential function of the large intestine is to process the intestinal wastes, to store them and to discharge them at periodic intervals. In addition, it plays an important role in the maintenance of fluid and electrolyte balance. The colon absorbs water, sodium and chloride and nutrients and secretes potassium and bicarbonate. The motor activity of the colon consists of segmenting and propulsive movements. The segmenting movements facilitate the absorption of water and electrolytes. Due to the absorption

of water, the liquid contents are transformed into solid material as the contents pass down. Distension of the rectum initiates the defecatory reflex. The goblet cells of the mucosal surface secrete mucus, which lubricates the feces and facilitates propulsion.

The amounts of water and the major electrolytes entering and leaving the colon in 24 hours are as follows.

	Entering	Leaving
Water	1500–1800 mL	100–150 mL
Sodium	180–220 mmol/L	5 mmol/L
Potassium	5 mmol/L	9–13 mmol/L
Chloride	117–157 mmol/L	2 mmol/L

Upto 400 calories can be provided through the colon by intracolonic infusion. Colonic function supplements function of the small intestine. If the colon is normally functioning, a patient can be maintained even with only 50 cm length of small intestine. At least 100 cm of small intestine is absolutely necessary to manage a patient whose colon is nonfunctional.

Digestion and Absorption

Digestive processes start in the mouth and proceed as the food passes down. The ultimate function of the GIT is the assimilation of ingested nutrients. The food materials which are in macromolecular form have to be broken down to smaller molecules before they can be absorbed. This process is called digestion. Absorption is the process of transfer of digested nutrient molecules across the mucosal epithelium from the intestinal lumen into the tissues. Digestion and absorption are closely interrelated. A part of the digestion occurs in the stomach. Exocrine pancreatic secretion and the bile salts aid in the process of digestion. The digestive processes of some of the nutrients continue in the brush border of the small intestinal epithelium. Small intestine is the major site of absorption of nutrients and most of the water and electrolytes. Calcium and iron are preferentially absorbed in the duodenum. Vitamin B_{12} and bile salts are absorbed mainly from the ileum. The rest of vitamins, minerals and nutrients in the diet are absorbed from the jejunum. The large intestine absorbs mainly water and electrolytes.

Digestion and Absorption of Fat

The pancreatic lipase splits the triglycerides into monoglycerides and fatty acids. The bile acids help to bring these insoluble products into soluble form which is absorbed. The products of digestion of fat are incorporated into the center of the micelles formed by bile salts to form mixed micelles. The brush border of the intestinal epithelium absorbs monoglycerides and fatty acids from the mixed micelles. The fatty acids are again converted to triglycerides in the epithelial cells and covered with a lipoprotein coat to form chylomicrons. The chylomicrons are discharged into the lacteals from where they reach the systemic circulation. Medium chain triglycerides are those composed of short chain fatty acids. They are more readily absorbed and they enter the portal vein directly instead of the lacteals. The salivary (lingual) and gastric lipase also contribute to fat digestion; however in a minor way.

Textbook of Medicine

Digestion and Absorption of Carbohydrates

Starch, sucrose and lactose constitute the important carbohydrates in the diet. Salivary amylase initiates digestion of carbohydrates in the mouth, but dietary carbohydrates are mainly digested in the upper small intestine with the help of pancreatic amylase. Starch is broken down to **maltose, maltotriose** and **alpha–limit dextrins.** These products and other disaccharides like sucrose and lactose are broken down further into monosaccharides by the **disaccharidase enzymes** located at the brush border of the intestinal epithelium. On further breakdown, glucose is formed from maltose, maltotriose and alpha-limit dextrins; glucose and fructose are formed from sucrose and glucose and galactose are formed from lactose. Glucose and galactose are actively absorbed. Fructose is absorbed by facilitated diffusion.

Digestion and Absorption of Proteins

Digestion of proteins starts in the stomach where pepsin is present. However, the major site of digestion of dietary protein is the upper small intestine. This is effected by the pancreatic enzymes.

The **proteolytic enzymes** are secreted as inactive precursors and are activated by the duodenal mucosal enzyme—**enterokinase** and by **trypsin.** Trypsin, chymotrypsin and elastase are endopeptidase that cleave specific peptide bonds adjacent to specific amino acids.The proteolytic enzymes breakdown the proteins to produce small peptides of 2–6 amino acids. These small peptides are further broken down by the **oligo peptidases** in the brush border of intestinal epithelium. Dipeptides and tripeptides may be actively taken up as such into the epithelial cell. They are hydrolyzed to free amino acids in the cell before they pass into the portal circulation.

Vitamins: Jejunum is the main site of absorption of all the vitamins except vitamin B_{12}, which is absorbed in the ileum.

Water and electrolytes: About 9L of fluid [2 L intake plus 7 L of gastrointestinal (GI) secretions] pass through the alimentary tract daily. Only 100–200 mL is excreted in the stools. Water is transported in the alimentary tract passively by the osmotic or hydrostatic pressure gradient generated by active solute transfer.

Sodium is absorbed mainly in the small intestine and its active transport is linked with the absorption of glucose.

ENDOCRINE FUNCTIONS OF THE GUT AND THE REGULATORY PEPTIDES

General Considerations

The term hormones (derived from the Greek word for 'I arouse to activity') is used to describe the chemical messengers acting at a distance. The other mechanism of control of bodily functions is neural. These two apparently different mechanisms of control of bodily functions act in an integrated manner. The same active principles (regulatory peptides) can be produced and released by endocrine and neural tissues and these may act as circulating hormones, local regulators, neurotransmitters or all these. The term **regulatory peptides** has been coined to describe active peptides capable of exerting their effects in one way or the other. Though these regulatory peptides were originally identified in the gut, brain or both, it is now realized that their distribution is much wider and that they are present practically in all the tissues.

Gastrointestinal Hormones

The regulatory peptide system of the GIT has received particular attention in recent times. Some of the regulatory peptides are secreted either by the endocrine cells interspersed among the mucosal cells or the enteric nerves, while others are present in both sites.

The peptidenergic nervous system is a complex system composed of different types of peptidenergic neurons. The cell bodies of the neurons lie either in the submucosal plexus or the mesenteric plexus. These neurons can cause gut movements independently and these belong to the noncholinergic, nonaderenergic class of autonomic nerves. Several peptides including VIP, substance P, somatostatin, enkephalin and others have been identified in these nerves. Table 75.1 gives the regulatory peptides.

Enteroinsular Axis

Gut hormones play an important role in the regulation of insulin secretion and glucose homeostasis. They control postprandial glucose levels by stimulation of insulin secretion from pancreatic beta cells and inhibition of hepatic gluconeogenesis by suppression of glucagon secretion. Approximately 50% of insulin released after a meal is due to GI hormones that potentiate insulin secretion. This interaction is called enteroinsular axis. These gut peptides are called incretins. The major incretins are glucagon like polypeptide-1 (GLP-1) and GIP.

Gut Flora in Health and Disease

Human alimentary tract normally contains about 100 trillion micro-organisms. It is sterile at birth; but soon after delivery, it gets inhabited by the microbial flora mainly from the fecal organisms of the mother and those from the surroundings. There are over 400 different species of microbes in the normal gut flora and they may reach a few hundred grams. The microbial density is less in the stomach and upper small intestine due to the presence of gastric acid and intestinal peristalsis. Anaerobes far outnumber aerobes.

In addition, *Peptococcus, Peptostreptococcus, Klebsiella, Proteus* and others may also occur (Table 75.2).

Physiological Role of Gut Flora

Gut flora are metabolically very active. They synthesize vitamin K and B-complex vitamins. They metabolize unabsorbed lipids to short chain fatty acids (SCFA) which are the main energy source for colonocytes. They ferment nondigestible dietary residues and endogenous mucus. They help absorption of calcium, magnesium and iron. In the proximal colon, the pH is 5–6 (acid). The microbial growth is maximum and saccharolytic is predominant. In the rectum and distal colon, the pH is neutral, bacterial growth is slow and proteolysis is predominant.

Textbook of Medicine

Table 75.1: Regulatory peptides

Peptide	Main distribution	Established actions
Gastrin	Stomach, duodenum	Stimulate gastric acid secretion
Cholecystokinin	Duodenum, jejunum and brain	Stimulate contraction of gallbladder and secretion of pancreatic enzymes
Secretin	Duodenum and jejunum	Stimulates secretion of pancreatic bicarbonate
Vasoactive intestinal polypeptide (VIP)	Central and peripheral nervous system and gut	Stimulates muscle relaxation, vasodilatation, secretion
Gastric inhibitory polypeptide (GIP)	Small intestine (duodenum and jejunum)	Stimulates secretion of insulin, inhibits secretion of gastric acid
Glucagon, enteroglucagon	Pancreas, gut, brain, ileum and colon	Regulates carbohydrate metabolism (pancreatic glucagon), trophic to gut (enteroglucagon)
Motilin	Small intestine	Stimulates gut motility
Pancreatic polypeptide	Pancreas	Inhibits pancreatic enzyme secretion and gallbladder contraction
Substance P	Centeral and peripheral nervous system	Sensory and vasodilatory role, stimulates muscle contraction
Neurotensin	Ileum, adrenal, brain	Vasodilatory, inhibits gastric acid secretion
Bombesin	Gut, brain, lung	Stimulates release of peptides (? antagonistic to somatostain)
Somatostatin	Gut, pancreas, thyroid, brain	Inhibits release and action of many peptides
Enkephalins and endorphins	Gut, brain, sympathetic nervous system, carotid body, adrenal	Opiate effects
Thyrotropin releasing hormone (TRH)	Brain and gut	Endocrine action and bioactivity on the brain
Insulin	Pancreas, gut	Carbohydrate, lipid and other metabolic functions
Miscellaneous: Adrenocorticotropic hormone, growth hormone, angiotensin II	Mainly endocrine tissue	Probable activity on the gut and brain
Amylin	Pancreas	Suppresses glucagon secretion, delay gastric emptying, induces satiety
Glucagon like polypeptide-1 (GLP-1)	Small intestine	Stimulates insulin secretion

Table 75.2: Bacterial contents in the normal gastrointestinal tract (GIT)

Parameter	Stomach	Jejunum	Ileum	Colon
Bacteria	Streptococci Staphylococci Fungi	Streptococci Staphylococci Lactobacilli	Coliforms Bacteriodes Bifidobacterium Clostridium	Bacteriodes Bifidobacterium Clostridium Enterococci
Bacterial density (per mL of contents)	10^{0-3}	10^{0-4}	10^{5-9}	10^{10-12}
pH	2–4	6–7	7.5	6.8–7.3

They also reduce cholesterol to coprostanol which is unabsorbable and thus they play an important role in cholesterol balance. They are also responsible for deconjugating conjugated bile salts, converting unabsorbed protein and urea to ammonia and fermentation of dietary fibers. The gut flora stimulate and favor the spread of MMC of the gut. Trophic functions include the control of epithelial cell proliferation and differentiation and homeostasis of the immune system. They play a role in the maintenance of normal gut endocrine function and detoxification of dietary carcinogens.

Protective function against pathogenic bacteria is achieved by preventing their growth and colonization. Adherent nonpathogenic bacteria prevent the attachment and subsequent entry of pathogens into the epithelial cells.

Protective function	Structural function	Metabolic function
• Pathogen displacement • Nutrient competition • Receptor competition • Production of antimicrobial factors like bacteriocins and lactic acid	• Barrier fortification • Induction of IgA • Apical tightening of tight junctions • Immune system development	• Synthesize vitamins, e.g. biotin and folate • Iron absorption • Metabolism of dietary carcinogens • Ferment nondigestable dietary residue and endogenous epithelial derived mucus

Gut Flora in Disease

Excessive proliferation leads to malabsorption, bloated feeling due to fermentation and nutritional deficiencies (bacterial overgrowth syndrome). It may play an important role in the pathogenesis of inflammatory bowel diseases (IBD), especially Crohn's disease and irritable bowel syndrome (IBS). Bacterial translocation is an important factor in the pathogenesis of spontaneous bacterial peritonitis (SBP), necrotizing pancreatitis and systemic sepsis following surgery, shocked states, major injuries and burns.

Probiotics and Prebiotics

Probiotics are live micro-organisms which, when administered, confer a health benefit to the host. They are approved by World Health Organization (WHO) for clinical use. *Saccharomyces boulardii* and *Lactobacillus delbrueckii* are the main probiotics in clinical use. Prebiotics are non-living nutrient elements which are not broken down by the intestinal enzymes. They nourish the probiotic flora to enhance their function.

- Adhere to colonic mucosa, there by reducing sites at which pathologic bacteria attach
- Probiotics release bacteriocins that are detrimental to pathologic bacteria
- Enhances intestinal barrier function
- Decrease the production of inflammatory cytokines.

Disorders where probiotics may be beneficial include:

- Ulcerative colitis
- Pouchitis
- Irritable bowel syndrome
- Antibiotic associated diarrhea
- Acute pancreatitis.

SYMPTOMS IN ALIMENTARY DISORDERS

Ptyalism: There is excessive salivation in this condition. This is a frequent complaint and it develops due to local causes in the mouth such as dentures, dental fillings, gingivitis or other painful lesions. Excessive salivation may occur reflexly in peptic ulcer, esophagitis and other lesions of the upper GIT. Ptyalism may be troublesome in parkinsonism. Excessive salivation in association with distaste is a common side effect of drugs like parasympathomimetic agents, antibiotics and iron salts.

Dryness of the mouth (xerostomia): This may be a prominent accompaniment of dehydration, diabetes mellitus (DM) or drugs like atropine. Mouth breathing, chronic sialadenitis and Sjögren's syndrome are local conditions which make the mouth dry. Mouth and conjunctiva are dry in sicca syndrome. Dryness of the mouth predisposes to infection and interferes with speech and deglutition.

Halitosis: Bad odor of the mouth is commonly caused by poor oral hygiene, periodontal sepsis or infections in the paranasal sinuses. Deep seated lesions like lung abscess, bronchiectasis or achalasia cardia may also give rise to halitosis. The bad smell is produced by anerobic organisms multiplying in these areas.

Bleeding from the gums: Bleeding on brushing the teeth is usually caused by gingivitis and periodontal infections like pyorrhea alveolaris. Spontaneous bleeding occurs in hemorrhagic disorders and scurvy.

Bruxism: It is grinding of the teeth, especially during sleep. This is more common in children. Reflex irritation from the digestive organs may give rise to this symptom, though in many cases no cause is detectable.

Dysphagia: It is difficult in swallowing which may be due to mechanical or neurogenic causes. ***Odynophagia*** is painful swallowing.

Mechanical causes are due to surgical conditions like carcinoma, stricture, diverticula and foreign bodies in the esophagus or pressure from without as in mediastinal tumors, enlarged left atrium, retrosternal goiter or mediastinitis. The obstruction is gradual in onset and difficulty is more during the swallowing of solids than liquids.

The swallowing mechanism is deranged in paralysis of the lower cranial nerves or affection of the muscles. Neurological causes of dysphagia are paralysis of 9th, 10th or 12th cranial nerves, myasthenia gravis, motor neuron disease and cranial myopathies.

Hunger: It is an unpleasant awareness of the desire to eat when the stomach is empty. It is accompanied by irritability and a sensation of abdominal discomfort.

Appetite: It is a pleasurable desire to eat food and it may not bear any direct relationship to hunger. Many factors like emotions, social customs and training modify appetite. Satiety is the feeling of fullness after the ingestion of food.

Anorexia: It is a morbid loss of desire to eat. Unlike satiety, which occurs only on taking food, anorexia may be present even when the person is hungry. Anorexia may accompany GI and liver diseases, infections like tuberculosis or psychological disturbances like depression.

Nausea and vomiting: Nausea is the feeling of impending desire to vomit. It is usually associated with salivation, inhibition of gastric peristalsis and rise in tone of the duodenum and proximal jejunum. Duodenogastric reflux occurs. The spasmodic and abortive respiratory movements in the presence of a closed glottis cause retching. During retching, the distal part of the stomach contracts and the proximal part relaxes. The gastric contents are forcibly ejected through the mouth. Vomiting is controlled by the two medullary centers—the vomiting center and the chemoreceptor trigger zone.

Weight loss: This is not a phenomenon specific to GI diseases, but in many alimentary disorders, considerable weight loss occurs. Diminution of food intake, malabsorption, loss of nutrients, accelerated metabolism and parasitism may contribute to the weight loss. Diseases like GI and hepatic malignancy and liver cirrhosis may present with considerable weight loss before the local symptoms develop.

Abdominal pain: It may be classified into: (i) Visceral pain, (ii) parietal pain and (iii) referred pain. Pain arising from the abdominal organs is visceral pain.

- ***Visceral pain:*** It is carried by the C fibers and therefore, it is poorly localized. Visceral pain is evoked by stretching, rise in tension in the wall of hollow organs due to spasm and dilatation or traction on the mesentery or the blood vessels.

  Pain from solid organs is caused by stretching of the capsule, inflammation, ischemia or neoplastic infiltration of the free nerve endings. Pain from solid organs tends to be of constant dragging, lancinating or throbbing nature, aggravated by movements and respiration. Pain arising from hollow viscera such as the esophagus, intestines, biliary tract and urogenital

Textbook of Medicine

tract tend to be intermittent, often associated with contraction of the viscus against resistance or hyperperistalsis. The nature is colicky, in which the pain starts, works upto a maximum and passes off after varying periods, with relief. These episodes tend to recur at intervals. The pain is described as gripping, twisting or squeezing. The site of pain may correspond to the dermatomal distribution of the organ or may be over its surface marking.

Biliary colic arising from the gallbladder tends to be a steady pain despite its name. It is severe and intermittent. It starts abruptly and lasts up to five hours in uncomplicated cases. It may be felt over the right hypochondrium and epigastrium or may radiate to the right scapula or shoulder.

- ***Parietal pain:*** Pain arising from the parietal peritoneum is generally more intense and more precisely localized because it is transmitted by overlying somatic nerves.
- ***Referred pain:*** Sometimes pain felt in the abdomen may be referred from other sites such as the pleura, lungs or heart or it may result from spinal root irritation (T7–T11).

Diarrhea: Diarrhea is defined as the passage of stools of fluid consistency more frequently than is usual (usually more than 3 times per day). The wet weight of the stool is increased. Diarrhea results from several factors like intestinal hypermotility, malabsorption of water and electrolytes, inflammation of the GIT or use of laxatives. In addition to the development of dehydration and malabsorption state, diarrhea and vomiting along with abdominal pain impair the quality of life. Acute diarrhea clears up within 2 weeks. Chronic diarrhea exceeds 2 weeks in duration. The presence of fresh blood in stools is called ***hematochezia***.

Infections or irritants cause acute diarrhea whereas chronic diarrhea may result from many causes.

Constipation: It is a condition of infrequent evacuation with harder consistency of feces. Any reduction in frequency of normal bowel movement in an individual should be considered as constipation. There is no single definition for the term constipation. Different attributes include one or more of the following—hard stools, infrequency (less than thrice a week), excessive straining, sense of incomplete evacuation, excessive time taken for defecation and unsuccessful defecation. Common causes are reduction of dietary bulk, dehydration, lack of exercise, recumbency, social factors like change of place and travel, drugs reducing intestinal motility, increased intracranial tension in children, myxedema, megacolon, intestinal obstruction and psychiatric disorders. Both diarrhea and constipation should receive more attention when they are of recent onset since they may the warning signals of serious underlying diseases such as malabsorption or cancer.

INVESTIGATIONS IN ALIMENTARY DISORDERS

EXAMINATION OF FECES

Wherever possible, examination of the total quantity of feces passed at a time should be done. This helps in assessing the volume, color, consistency and abnormal constituents of feces. On an average Indian diet, the weight of feces ranges from 250 to 500 g/day. The consistency may vary from semisolid to hard even among normal individuals. The color is derived from products of bile pigments. Clay colored stools are seen in obstructive jaundice. Presence of altered blood makes the feces black and tarry (melena). Black color may be due to ingestion of heavy metals or other dietary articles.

Microscopic examination: The microscopic examination of fresh feces helps in identifying protozoa such as *E. histolytica* and *G. lamblia*. Other abnormalities commonly seen are helminthic ova and larvae, cellular exudates, fat globules and muscle fibers. Protozoal cysts and helminthic eggs are better detected by concentration techniques and staining with aqueous iodine.

Microbiological investigations: These are done for the identification of pathogenic bacteria, fungi or viruses. Fresh fecal specimens, rectal swabs or material obtained during proctoscopic examination are used for this purpose.

Biochemical tests: Occult blood may be present in stools and is detected by the ***o-toluidine blue*** or ***guaiac test***. As a rule, it is better to avoid iron containing drugs and consumption of meat for 3–5 days before collecting feces for occult blood test. Two mL of blood in the stool is necessary to produce a positive result. Two samples of each of three consecutive (daily) stools should be tested. Avoid red meat, peroxidise containing vegetables and foods like cauliflower, raddish and medications like nonsteroidal anti-inflammatory drug (NSAID), vitamin C and iron tablets. The sensitivity of a single stool guaiac test to pick up bleeding has been quoted as 10–30%, but if a standard three tests are done as recommended, the sensitivity rises to 92%.

Fecal Immunochemical Testing (FIT)

This test utilizes specific antibodies to detect globin and picks up as little as 0.3 mL of blood in the stool. Presence of occult blood points to a bleeding source in the GIT such as benign ulceration or malignancy. Absence of occult blood in feces on repeated testing is a strong point against such lesions.

Quantitative estimation of the fat content of the stool helps to establish steatorrhea. More than 7g/day is abnormal. Other biochemical tests such as estimation of the electrolytes, pH value, nitrogen content, stercobilinogen, porphyrins, etc. are done at times in special situations.

DIGITAL EXAMINATION OF THE ANAL CANAL AND RECTUM

This is a very valuable method which gives information on the pathology in the anal canal, rectum and even the lower parts of the sigmoid colon. Digital examination is done with the gloved index finger, properly lubricated with vaseline, keeping the patient in the left lateral decubitus or in the knee chest position. Proper explanation to the patient is necessary to ensure his co-operation. The external parts of the anus, tone of the anal sphincter and mucosal surface of the anal canal and rectum are systematically palpated. Fissure-in-ano, hemorrhoids, carcinoma, other growths, abnormalities of the prostate and other pelvic organs can all be diagnosed with reasonable certainty. Fecal masses and foreign bodies can be identified. Examination of the material on the finger helps to diagnose bleeding from upper or lower GIT. Microscopy of the material and further studies help to diagnose dysentery and other ulcerative lesions.

The findings on digital examination can be further clarified by proctoscopy, anorectal manometry and further imaging procedures.

GASTRIC ACID ANALYSIS

The time honored method of fractional test meal has been replaced by measurement of basal and maximal acid output. Maximal acid secretion is obtained by stimulating with histamine (0.04 mg/kg), histalog (1.5 mg/kg) or pentagastrin (6 µg/kg) given parenterally. Acid output values are expressed as mmol/h—*maximal histamine test.*

Anticholinergic drugs should be avoided at least for 48-hour before the test. After fasting overnight, a tube is passed through the mouth and its tip is positioned at the junction of the lower and the middle-third of the stomach under fluoroscopic control. Basal secretion is collected by continuous suction and histamine is given subcutaneously. The gastric juice is collected by continuous suction and four 15-minute samples are collected separately. Volume of each specimen and the amount of hydrochloric acid are determined. For Indians, basal acid output (BAO) varies from 1 to 4 mmol/h and maximal acid output (MAO) from 6 to 30 mmol/h. By using insulin as the stimulant, the test can be employed to assess the completeness of vagotomy *(Hollander test).* With the advent of endoscopic studies, the value of gastric secretory studies in the diagnosis of gastric and duodenal ulcer and gastric carcinoma has come down. In these conditions, the acid levels show considerable overlap and, therefore, may be misleading. However, very high gastric acid values are valuable clues in the diagnosis of *Zollinger-Ellison syndrome* and complete absence of gastric acid (achlorhydria) is suggestive of pernicious anemia. The patients with gastrinoma demonstrate hypergastrinemia with elevated basal acid output.

SAMPLING OF INTESTINAL CONTENTS

Sampling of intestinal contents from various levels has been employed for chemical and microbiological studies in conditions such as malabsorption states and hepatic and pancreatic diseases. Contents of the GIT can be aspirated by using special tubes, the tip of which can be accurately positioned at a particular site under fluoroscopic control. Endoscopy has revolutionized the procedure for aspiration. Conventional methods using tubes or biopsy capsule blindly have been totally replaced by aspiration or biopsy from specific areas, under vision.

RADIOLOGICAL EXAMINATION OF THE DIGESTIVE SYSTEM

These time-honored studies are of considerable help in diagnosis. Diagnostic accuracy has been considerably improved by several technical refinements. Endoscopy is more reliable to visualize mucosal lesions and to take biopsies. But to demonstrate other structural lesions, displacements, fistulae, etc. and for studying the progress of the contrast medium, radiological studies are regularly undertaken.

Plain X-ray of the abdomen: Liver, spleen, kidneys and tumors can be identified in a plain X-ray and their size determined. Calculi in the gallbladder, bile duct, urinary tract or pancreas, calcification of organs such as the pancreas and adrenals and radiopaque foreign bodies and fetal parts are all classically demonstrable in a plain radiograph.

A plain X-ray of the abdomen taken in the erect posture after proper bowel preparation may show presence of gas under the diaphragm, gas in organs such as gallbladder, biliary tree and liver that normally do not contain gas. Presence of gas under the diaphragm indicates perforation of a hollow air-containing viscus such as the stomach or intestine. Gas in the biliary tree and gallbladder should suggest fistula formation with the gallbladder, perforation or infection by gas-forming organisms. Intestinal obstruction gives rise to the presence of multiple dilated loops with fluid levels.

Contrast studies of the GIT: Several contrast materials have been employed to visualize different organs.

Barium swallow: It is done to visualize the esophagus. After overnight fast, the patient is made to swallow a thick freshly prepared paste of barium sulfate as rapidly as possible. Since most patients swallow considerable amounts of air also simultaneously, the air distended esophagus is well visualized. Barium swallow brings out lesions such as strictures, neoplasms, diverticula, esophagitis, ulcers, tears, esophageal varices and external compression. The function of the esophagus and the lower sphincter can be assessed from the passage of the barium downwards and the pattern of peristaltic waves.

Barium meal: For barium meal studies, a large quantity (250–500 mL) of freshly suspended emulsion of barium sulfate is swallowed rapidly. The rate of transit of the barium and the contours of the stomach and intestines can be assessed by fluoroscopy or television. Pictures are taken at regular intervals to delineate the different parts. Double contrast technique using air and barium helps to bring out even minute mucosal abnormalities. Barium meal studies for stomach and duodenum are indicated in suspected peptic ulcer, neoplasms of the stomach, mucosal erosions, obstructions, persistent vomiting and vague upper abdominal symptoms.

The intestines are visualized by taking pictures in the intestinal phase of the meal. The time taken for the passage of barium, pattern of distribution in the intestinal lumen and morphological abnormalities can be assessed. Several newer techniques have helped in increasing the diagnostic efficiency and minimizing the discomfort to the patient.

ENTEROCLYSIS (SMALL BOWEL ENEMA)

Barium contrast is administered directly into jejunum through a tube introduced through the nose or mouth and positioned under fluoroscopy across the duodenum. In conventional barium study, adequate quantity of barium may not enter the jejunum freely due to the action of the pyloric sphincter. Better delineation of the small intestine can be obtained by enteroclysis.

Hypotonic duodenography: The medial wall of the duodenum, which is closely apposed to the pancreas, can be better visualized by instilling barium after using a relaxant drug such as propantheline bromide (probanthine) 30–60 mg intramuscularly (IM) or 15 mg intravenously (IV).

Barium enema: The large intestine up to the ileocecal junction can be visualized by barium enema. Meticulous preparation of the large bowel before examination is absolutely essential to ensure accuracy. The patient should be on a low residue diet for 2 days prior to the examination. Evacuation is achieved by a purgative and if needed, a thorough bowel wash. Barium sulfate suspension is given as an enema to fill the whole large intestine and the progress of barium is watched under the fluorescent screen. Pictures of the barium-filled colon are taken. After evacuation of the barium, air is pumped through the anal canal to fill the colon and further pictures are taken. This double contrast study helps to demonstrate mucosal lesions clearly. Barium enema is indicated in lesions of the colon and rectum such as carcinomas, ulcerative colitis, diverticulitis, polyposis, strictures and megacolon.

GASTROINTESTINAL ENDOSCOPY

The advent of flexible fiberoptic endoscope has revolutionized endoscopy. Incorporation of video screens in which magnified images can be seen simultaneously has made the procedure much more efficient. Almost all parts of the stomach, many parts of the duodenum and small intestine and almost the whole of the colon can be visualized using endoscopes which are capable of manipulation to bring to focus several areas such as the fundus of the stomach, cecum, ileocecal region and others which could not be fully visualized by the earlier endoscopes. At present the procedure is very reliable, freely available in many centers and almost noninvasive. Endoscopy enables direct examination of the lesions, biopsy, cytology of suspicious areas and documentation by photography. Therapeutically, endoscopes are used to remove polyps and foreign bodies, dilate strictures and cauterize ulcers and bleeding points. At present all parts of the alimentary tract are accessible to endoscopy.

SPECIAL TYPES OF ENDOSCOPES

Upper alimentary endoscopy: Examination of the esophagus, stomach and duodenum is done by a panendoscope. Upper alimentary endoscopy is indicated in patients with upper GI bleeding, all types of chronic dyspepsia and when lesions are demonstrable by X-ray but their pathological nature is not clear. Whenever facilities are available, endoscopic examination should be undertaken to confirm the nature of mucosal lesions. Endoscopic esophageal variceal injection, variceal ligation, percutaneous feeding gastrostomy and similar procedures are commonly undertaken in gastroenterology departments at present. Endoscopic ultrasonography is a technique which gives more precise data from locations usually inaccessible to conventional ultrasound. It gives better imaging of the pancreas and even tumors less than 3 cm in diameter can be detected. Endocrine adenomata and cancer with vascular invasion arising from pancreas and small lesions arising from other parts of the GIT are particularly well seen by endoscopic ultrasonography.

- ***Capsule endoscope:*** A battery powered computer chip camera is assembled inside a capsule. Patient swallows it orally and the signals are recorded, which can be viewed in the monitor screen. The cost of an endoscopic capsule may come to ₹ 30,000.
- ***Zoom endoscopes:*** The lesions can be zoomed to 50–150 times magnification.
- ***Laparoscopy-assisted panendoscopy (LAPE):*** Endoscope is introduced per orally and the small intestine is sleeved on to the endoscope with the help of the laparoscope. The entire small intestine can be visualized. It is very useful in obscure GI bleeding.

Proctoscopy: Anal canal and rectum are visually examined with the proctoscope. Digital examination of the rectum is mandatory before introducing the proctoscope. Proctoscopy is contraindicated in severely painful lesions and strictures of the anal canal. Digital examination and proctoscopy help to diagnose vast majority of lesions in the rectum and anal canal. These procedures should be done as part of the clinical examination in all patients presenting with symptoms pertaining to the lower alimentary tract.

Digital examination is contraindicated in the first 3–4 days following myocardial infarction (MI), since there is the risk of triggering off serious arrhythmias.

Further refinements in the study of the anal sphincter mechanism especially in the investigation of fecal incontinence, are ultrasonography to detect tears of the external sphincter muscle, pudendal nerve latency to assess nerve conduction and anal canal manometry.

Proctosigmoidoscopy: The anal canal, rectum and distal sigmoid colon can be visualized through a sigmoidoscope. Rigid and flexible sigmoidoscopes are available. The simplicity of the procedure and availability of the instrument in all hospitals have contributed to widespread use of this procedure. Hemorrhoids, polyps, acute and chronic inflammatory bowel disease, neoplasms, ulcerating lesions and sources of bleeding can be diagnosed by sigmoidoscopy and biopsy.

Colonoscopy: Flexible fiberoptic colonoscopes are available and the whole of the large intestine can be examined with them. Proper bowel preparation using an osmotically active cathartic is mandatory to clear the colon of fecal matter and enable full visualization. Indications for colonoscopy are:

- In lower GI bleeding not accessible to the sigmoidoscope.
- In inflammatory bowel disease, to assess the extent.
- In the evaluation of radiologically demonstrable abnormalities in the large bowel situated beyond the reach of the sigmoidoscope.
- Therapeutically, these instruments are used to remove polyps and foreign bodies and to arrest bleeding points.

Textbook of Medicine

- ***Peritoneoscopy (laparoscopy):*** Examination of the peritoneal cavity is safely carried out using a peritoneoscope (laparoscope). Under aseptic precautions, air is introduced into the peritoneum and the laparoscope is introduced through a small incision on the anterior abdominal wall. Liver, spleen, gallbladder, omentum, loops of intestines, pelvic organs and peritoneum can be seen directly. Localized lesions can be biopsied under vision through the peritoneoscope. Laparoscopy is indicated for detecting the cause of ascites, diagnosing liver diseases and in detecting metastatic carcinoma. Surgical procedures can also be undertaken through the laparoscope. Heart disease, acute infections, hemorrhagic diathesis and peritoneal adhesions are contraindications for laparoscopy. Rarely, complications such as hemorrhage, peritonitis and perforation of organs may occur.

- ***Choledochoscopy:*** In this procedure, an endoscope is passed into the biliary tree, usually during surgery. It helps to visualize the major biliary passages, remove stones and release obstructions.

- ***Endoscopic retrograde cholangiopancreatography (ERCP):*** This is a procedure undertaken to delineate the common bile duct and pancreatic duct. After fixing the endoscope at the ampulla of Vater, the ampulla is cannulated using special catheters and several procedures can be performed. These include collection of the respective digestive juices, contrast injection and visualization of the duct pattern, removal of stones and growths, sphincterotomy and others.

- ***Angiography:*** Abdominal angiography may be required for investigation of several GI diseases. With the help of suitable catheters, celiac, superior and inferior mesenteric arteries and their branches can be selectively cannulated and contrast injected. Angiography is indicated to detect the site of acute and chronic GI bleeding, determine the cause of ischemic bowel disease and in other vascular disorders of the GIT. Therapeutic indications include the administration of vasoconstrictor drugs (e.g. pitressin), clotting factors or microemboli to arrest bleeding and local cytotoxic drugs for neoplasms.

ULTRASOUND IMAGING

Ultrasound scanning is a safe, noninvasive, simple and relatively inexpensive examination. It is useful in imaging solid, cystic or air-containing tissues and organs. Ultrasound examination is indicated in hepatobiliary diseases like primary or secondary tumors, liver abscess and differentiation of medical from surgical jaundice, cholelithiasis and various lesions of the pancreas. In skilled hands, ultrasound examination is a very reliable procedure. This has become a primary investigation to establish hepatobiliary diseases, organomegaly, ascites, pregnancy and others. Ultrasound-directed percutaneous biopsies from lesions and aspiration of pus from abscess cavities are undertaken regularly at present. The average cost for ultrasonography of the abdomen is around ₹ 400–600.

Esophageal manometry: This test is done in specialized laboratories where GI mortality studies are undertaken.

The test is done after fasting for 8 hours, using a thin, pressure-sensitive tube passed through the nose, down the esophagus and into the stomach. Pressure at various levels of esophagus are recorded and analyzed. The function of the lower esophageal sphincter and the muscles of the esophagus can be assessed.

COMPUTED TOMOGRAPHY (CT) SCAN

This technique is widely employed in the investigation of diseases of abdominal organs. Solid tissues like liver, pancreas, kidneys, adrenals and tumors of lymph nodes and fluid-containing masses like cysts and abscesses produce diagnostic images. It is also useful in the investigation of biliary tract disease and in the differentiation of medical from surgical jaundice. With the help of CT scan, percutaneous biopsy needles can be accurately positioned to get biopsies. This investigation has the advantage of being noninvasive, but its high cost and nonavailability in smaller cities and towns are disadvantages. The cost of CT scanning of the abdomen is around ₹ 3000–5000. Several newer techniques using CT scanning have been introduced.

Virtual colonoscopy is a CT technique which generates high resolution two-dimensional axial images from which three-dimensional images of the colon resembling those seen on colonoscopy are reconstituted.

The reliability of this imaging procedure in detecting colonic lesions including cancer is being investigated.

MAGNETIC RESONANCE IMAGING (MRI)

MRI scans are increasingly used in complicated abdominal conditions. MRI is more useful than CT scan in defining soft tissue lesions and is especially useful in conditions like internal intestinal fistulae.

ISOTOPIC INVESTIGATIONS

These are of great value in diagnosis. Absorption and fecal elimination of many substances such as cyanocobalamin and fats can be studied by using suitable isotopes. Functions of several organs can be assessed.

BIOPSY

Histology is a valuable aid in confirming the diagnosis. The advent of flexible endoscopes have made all parts of the alimentary tract accessible for biopsy.

At present endoscopic biopsy is preferred for all the tubular organs. For solid organs such as the liver, pancreas, lymph nodes and solid tumors ultrasound directed or CT directed biopsy is done on account of its reliability and safety.

Laparoscopy: This is a procedure to visualize intra-abdominal and pelvic structures *in vivo* using appropriate laparoscopes. Several refinements and modifications have resulted in the manufacture of sophisticated instrument and development of techniques which make it possible to inspect almost all organs in the peritoneal cavity. Laparoscopy is safe and minimally invasive. In experienced hands, the findings are quite reliable. Biopsy procedures and surgical interventions can be undertaken at the same time.

However, when the other non-invasive tests are not conclusive and particularly so when malignancy is suspected, early laparotomy has to be undertaken. In some centers, minilaparotomy is used as a diagnostic tool in the investigation of jaundice and other hepatobiliary problems. By this procedure, after exposing the left lobe of the liver, liver biopsy, transhepatic cholangiography, portal manometry and collection of bile for cytology can be carried out.

Investigative techniques have reached a high level of perfection. With the availability of modern facilities, it is possible to arrive at a proper diagnosis in almost all cases, without resorting to surgery. These investigations also help the physician in assessing the functions of organs accurately, so as to plan the therapy more objectively. The proper selection and interpretation of the tests demands diagnostic skills of the physician and a very meticulous clinical examination.

CHAPTER
76

Diseases of the Mouth and Tongue

KR Vinaya Kumar, KV Krishna Das

Chapter Summary

- Inflammation of the Salivary Glands
- Recurrent Aphthous Ulcer
- Oral Submucous Fibrosis
- Orofacial Granulomatosis
- Nonspecific Inflammatory Diseases of Periodontium
- Dental Caries
- Vincent's Infection
- Diseases of the Tongue
- Oral Cancer

INFLAMMATION OF THE SALIVARY GLANDS

Syn: Sialadenitis

Causes of Generalized Sialadenitis

- **Bacterial infections:** *Staphylococcus aureus, Pseudomonas aeruginosa, Streptococcus viridans* and rarely *Streptococcus pneumococci* and *Escherichia coli.*
- **Viral infections:** Mumps.
- **Other conditions:** Sjögren's syndrome, leukemia, lymphoma, sarcoidosis *(Heerfordt's syndrome),* lupus erythematosus, tuberculosis, other mycobacteria, actinomycosis, obstruction of the ducts, salivary calculi and rarely Reiter's syndrome.

Causes of Parotid Enlargement

- **Reaction to drugs** such as iodides, guanethidine, chronic toxicity by copper, lead or mercury.
- **Alcoholism, Laennec's cirrhosis** and **calcific pancreatitis**.
- **Suppurative parotitis:** This may complicate prolonged fevers like typhoid. Infection reaches the gland from the mouth through the duct. Dehydration and poor oral hygiene predispose to infection. An abscess develops in the parotid gland. Once the abscess forms, pus has to be drained by incision. Suppurative parotitis is prevented by proper care of the mouth in predisposed individuals.

Causes of Bilateral Parotid Enlargement Include

- **Local disease**
  - Mumps—more commonly in children than adults
  - Parotitis
  - Uveoparotid fever
  - Sjögren's syndrome
  - Tumor infiltration.
- **Systemic disease**
  - Sarcoidosis
  - Tuberculosis
  - Alcoholism
  - Myxoedema
  - Cushing's disease
  - Diabetes/insulin resistance—about 25% of patients with overt or latent diabetes have bilateral asymptomatic enlargement of the parotid glands
  - Liver cirrhosis
  - Gout
  - Bulimia nervosa
  - Human immunodeficiency virus (HIV) in children may cause bilateral parotid enlargement.
- **Drugs**
  - Thiouracil
  - Isoprenaline
  - Phenylbutazone
  - High estrogen contraceptive pills.

Bilateral parotid enlargement may also be seen in:
- Severe dehydration
- Malnutrition.

RECURRENT APHTHOUS ULCER

Syn: Cancer sore, Mikulicz aphthae, Aphthous stomatitis

Aphthous ulcers are the most common lesions affecting the oral mucous membrane. The exact etiology is unknown. Recent observations suggest an autoimmune etiology. Microscopically, the lesion shows a nonspecific ulcer with necrosis of subepithelial small blood vessels.

Textbook of Medicine

Clinical Features

Crops of painful ulcers occur periodically at intervals of weeks to months. The ulcers can be divided into minor (60–70%) and major aphthae (30–40%).

Minor Aphthous Ulcers

These occur mainly on the labial, buccal and tongue mucosa. They are shallow, measuring 2–4 mm in diameter. The floor is covered with fibrin and the periphery is erythematous. Rarely, the ulcers may become secondarily infected, but they heal without scarring.

Major Aphthous Ulcers

These appear commonly in the soft palate and lower labial mucosa. They are larger, measuring over 1 cm in diameter and are deep and indurated. They persist for more than 4 weeks and heal with scar formation. Other clinical features are similar to those of minor aphthae.

Diagnosis is clinical. Minor aphthae have to be differentiated from the oral manifestations of herpes simplex, agranulocytosis, infectious mononucleosis and cyclic neutropenia. Major aphthae showing induration should be differentiated from malignancy.

Treatment

There is no specific treatment. Topical application of steroids in the initial phase may abort an attack. Pellets of glucocorticoids or 0.1% triamcinolone in orabase applied locally four times daily are effective in 2–3 days. Rarely systemic corticosteroids may be required.

Other modalities of treatment include tetracycline mouth wash and 2% anesthetic ointment or jelly. Castor oil 5–10 mL administered at bed time in milk for 3–4 days helps in shortening the duration and aborting an attack (personal observation-KVK).

ORAL SUBMUCOUS FIBROSIS

Submucous fibrosis is commonly seen among all races inhabiting South-East Asia. It is common in South India. There may be an increase in incidence in those who chew betel nut continuously for several months. Recent studies have shown a high content of copper in some of the nut preparation available commercially. The significance of this finding needs further study.

Pathology

Pathological changes include ribbon-like atrophy of subepithelial collagen and moderate infiltration by chronic inflammatory cells. There may be dysplastic changes in the epithelium and many cases develop squamous cell carcinoma on follow-up.

The disease starts insidiously and runs a chronic course. Early symptoms include burning sensation of the mouth and difficulty to tolerate spicy foods. Gradually, fibrosis sets in and this may interfere with opening of the mouth. In advanced cases the uvula becomes fibrotic and small. The fibrotic process may rarely extend to the pharynx and esophagus in advanced cases. Later on, recurrent erosions and ulcers develop which heal slowly. Carcinoma develops from these erosive or ulcerated areas and not uncommonly it is multicentric.

Clinical diagnosis is based on the symptoms and the leathery inelastic feel of the oral mucosa. Diagnosis is confirmed by biopsy.

Management

There is no specific treatment. Smoking and chewing of tobacco and betel nut should be stopped. Repeated submucous infiltration of 25 mg of hydrocortisone hemisuccinate into the fibrous areas may help in resolving early lesions and improving the mobility of the lower jaw and tongue. All patients have to be followed-up and suspicious lesions biopsied. If malignancy is detected, it is treated by irradiation.

OROFACIAL GRANULOMATOSIS

Oral lesions are common in patients suffering from Crohn's disease of the intestines. These include aphthae, diffuse swelling of lips and cheeks, chronic inflammatory hyperplasia with fissuring of the mucosa, mucosal tags, vertical fissuring of lips and hyperplastic gingivitis. Sometimes similar lesions may occur even in the absence of the intestinal lesions.

Outlook for orofacial granulomatosis is variable. Some cases are self-limiting. Drugs which are found to be partially effective include danazol and clofazimine.

NONSPECIFIC INFLAMMATORY DISEASES OF PERIODONTIUM

Limited surveys reveal that periodontal disease occurs in up to 90% of several communities in India. Periodontium comprises gingiva, periodontal membrane and the alveolar bone which support the teeth. All the nonspecific infections together are called as ***pyorrhea***. Pyorrhea is common in persons past middle age. Dental infection is the most common focus of sepsis in any individual. The infection takes the form of gingivitis in the beginning and then it progresses to periodontitis and finally the teeth fall off. Many local and systemic factors influence the course of the disease. Local factors that aggravate the progress of periodontal disease are traumatic occlusion, malalignment of teeth, mouth breathing, calculus, ill fitting appliances and xerostomia. Systemic conditions include protein malnutrition, puberty, pregnancy, menopause, diabetes, anemia, scurvy, granulocytopenia, drugs like phenytoin and immunodeficiency states.

The earliest change is the formation of a bacterial plaque in the cervical margin of the tooth. The plaque contains *Streptococcus viridans, Staphylococcus albus, Staphylococcus aureus,* lactobacilli, *Helicobacter pylori* and actinomycetes. The toxins produced by the bacteria evoke an inflammatory response in the gingival crevice. The gingiva and interdental papilla become edematous and bleed on palpation. Further bacterial proliferation and toxin formation occur and inflammation progresses.

The gum attachment migrates apically. The periodontal fibers undergo degeneration and the alveolar cristal bone also undergoes resorption. This stage is called periodontitis. At this stage an acute periodontal abscess may form, continued inflammation and resorption of alveolar bone leads to loosening and loss of teeth.

Clinical Features

Gingivitis may be symptomless except for halitosis and painless bleeding from gums on brushing. The gingiva are red and the normal stippling is absent. Periodontitis is characterized by dull pain. Periodontal abscess causes throbbing pain which increases when the patient is recumbent. Pus can be expressed from the gingival crevice.

Diagnosis

The diagnosis of nonspecific periodontal disease is made by clinical examination. Depth of the gingival pocket can be measured by a periodontal probe.

Intraoral bite wing X-rays are useful in assessing the pattern and extent of bone loss. In all cases of severe periodontal disease full clinical examination and investigation should be done to exclude the underlying systemic disorders.

Management

The disease can be prevented by avoiding the formation of dental plaques. Plaques can be removed by regular brushing and flossing. The calculus formed should be removed by scaling. Analgesics and antibiotics are required to control pain and infection respectively. Acute gingival or periodontal abscess has to be drained. If there are deep pockets, gingivectomy has to be done. Loose teeth have to be extracted if they cannot be refixed by appropriate dental management.

Causes of gum hypertrophy drugs	
• Gingivitis	• Sarcoidosis
• Pregnancy	• Wegener's granulomatosis
• Puberty	• Nifedipine, cyclosporine, phenytoin
• Leukemia	

DENTAL CARIES

Dental caries is defined as the local destruction of susceptible hard tissues by acidic byproducts formed by bacterial fermentation of dietary carbohydrates. Caries may affect the crown or the root of the tooth.

Dental caries is one of the most widespread diseases present all over the globe, but shows wide variation in prevalence among different communities. In several parts of India, the prevalence is 65–70% among the general population. It results from demineralization and dissolution of the enamel and dentine. The etiology of dental caries is complex and several factors serve to start off the process. Factors which affect the extent and progress of the disease are the composition of the enamel, food habits, content of carbohydrates in the food, oral hygiene, heredity and fluoride intake in food and water. Food debris and bacteria accumulate on the pit and fissure surface of the teeth to form a plaque consisting of bacteria, mucus and desquamated epithelial cells. Refined carbohydrates like sugars adhere to the plaque and help in liberating acid products by action of the mixed bacterial flora, the most important among them being *Streptococcus mutans.* The infant acquires *Streptococcus mutans* from the mother or other primary care givers. Under the plaque, the pH is lowered below 5.3 and this causes demineralization of the enamel. The calcium salts are removed, leaving the tooth surface rough and chalky white. At this stage, the proteolytic organisms destroy the protein matrix of enamel rods. This process proceeds towards the dentine and a cavity is formed. In the dentine, the progress is faster and the pulp is reached. The response of the pulp depends upon the age and general resistance of the individual and virulence of the organism. Either an acute pulpitis with necrosis may develop or the inflammation may become chronic. Secondary dentine may be formed from the pulp in an attempt to limit the infection. At times the pulp may undergo hyaline degeneration and calcification.

Finally, the bacteria and their toxins reach the periapical tissues and produce acute periapical periodontitis and progress to acute periapical abscess. If the host resistance is poor, the infection can spread to adjacent tissues, maxillary sinuses, base of the skull and through the bloodstream. More often the inflammation becomes chronic leading to the formation of a granuloma which acts as a chronic focus of sepsis. An inflammatory cyst may be formed (Fig. 76.1).

Clinical Features

In children, caries is usually seen in the pit and fissures of the occlusal surfaces whereas in elderly persons it is noticed more in the cervical margins of the teeth, though any surface may be affected. The whole process may proceed slowly over the years or can be rapid to develop within months. Widespread acute caries involving all surfaces of several teeth is referred to as ***rampant caries.***

The condition remains asymptomatic till the lesion reaches the dentinoenamel junctions, since there are no nerve endings in the enamel. Early lesions appear as chalky white areas on the enamel surface which can be detected by a probe. These are translucent on X-ray examination. Later, the chalky areas become brown or black. Initial symptom is sensitivity to sweet, cold or hot drinks produced by stimulation of nerve endings in the dentine. Pain develops when the pulp becomes hyperemic. Acute pulpitis causes unbearable pain, often described as toothache, on the affected side. The pain is only poorly localized and the patient may not be able to pinpoint

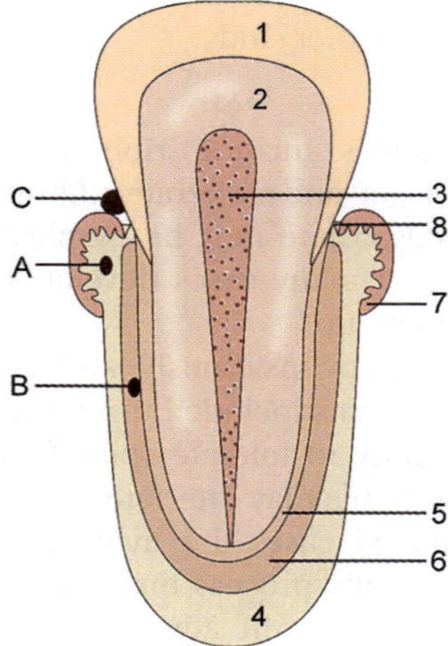

Fig. 76.1: Tooth and gum. 1. Enamel; 2. Dentine; 3. Pulp; 4. Soft tissues; 5. Cementum; 6. Alveolar bone; 7. Gingiva; 8. Gingival crevice; A and B. Site for periodontal abscess; C. Site of accumulation of plaque

the affected tooth. As the acute condition subsides, pain becomes dull. If the pulp undergoes necrosis, pain is abolished and the condition remains symptomless for a while. As the inflammation extends outside the tooth, pain returns. Exacerbations and remissions alternate for considerable periods of time.

Treatment

Powerful analgesics give moderate relief of pain in the acute stage. Prompt relief is obtained by injection of a local anesthetic. A broad spectrum antibiotic like ampicillin 250 mg 6 hour or ciprofloxacin 500 mg bd is required for 3–5 days to control infection. Abscesses have to be drained surgically. Since appropriate dental care is to be instituted, the case should be immediately referred to a dental surgeon.

Caries is incurable once it is established, since the dentine is not capable of undergoing repair. Early lesions are treated by removal of the affected parts and filling up the defect with suitable materials. Technical advances in dentistry have been remarkable and even grossly affected teeth can be restored to functional stage, without recurrence of pain. If the tooth is grossly damaged beyond repair, it has to be extracted. At present, the policy is to restore the tooth to normal functions and preserve it as far as possible.

Prevention

Dental caries is an easily preventable disease. Prevention should start during pregnancy, when the teeth of the fetus are getting mineralized. Adequate supplements of calcium, vitamin D and other nutrients to mothers during pregnancy and later to the child, ensure proper teeth formation. Inclusion of fresh vegetables and fruits which require proper mastication helps to keep the teeth and gums healthy. The habit of allowing the baby to sleep with the milk feeding nipple in the mouth helps to promote caries. Soft drinks which contain sugar favor the growth of organisms and promote the development of caries. Proper brushing of the teeth and massage of the gums before the child goes to bed is an effective preventive measure against caries.

Fluoridation of community water supplied at 1 ppm reduces the incidence of caries. Fluoride applied topically either directly or by using fluoridated toothpastes or chewing gums improves local resistance of the teeth. Fluoride tablets containing 2.2 mg of sodium fluoride (equivalent to 1 mg fluorine) have been used to supplement the intake in babies. One tablet is dissolved in 1.25 L water and this water is used for making up milk formula and cooking for children below the age of 3 years. Above the age of 3 years, 1 tablet may be administered daily. Periodic dental check-up of preschool and school children and education of the mothers are absolutely essential to lower incidence of caries in the community. In many parts of India where the fluoride content of drinking water is high, additional supply of fluoride through toothpastes has been incriminated as a factor aggravating fluorosis. This has to be borne in mind while making recommendations for fluoride supplementation.

VINCENT'S INFECTION

Syn: Vincent's angina, Acute necrotizing ulcerative gingivitis

It occurs as a painful condition caused by a mixed bacterial flora consisting of *fusiform bacilli* and *Vincent's spirochetes.* It may be associated with extensive necrotizing ulcerative mucositis or acute pseudomembranous lesions of the pharynx or tonsils. The condition is predisposed to by poor oral hygiene, food impaction, excessive smoking and local trauma.

The gums are painful, swollen, hemorrhagic and foul smelling. A serious complication is noma which begins at the corners of the mouth and proceeds to rapid necrosis of the entire thickness of the cheeks. Rarely septicemia and meningitis may occur.

Treatment

The organisms respond dramatically to penicillin in the usual dosage. Metronidazole 200 mg given orally thrice daily for 7 days gives good relief and is a satisfactory alternative.

DISEASES OF THE TONGUE

Glossitis: It is inflammation of the tongue and in general denotes soreness and redness of the tongue. The tongue appears beefy red and the papillae are prominent. In some cases, the papillae may be ironed out. Glossitis may result from deficiency of B complex vitamins, megaloblastic anemia, cirrhosis of liver, irritants like alcohol, excessively spicy foods and all causes of stomatitis. Specific lesions of syphilis, gonorrhea, tuberculosis, actinomycosis and acquired immunodeficiency syndrome (AIDS) may start in the oral cavity.

Leukoplakia: This is a chronic lesion characterized by the presence of white, firm, smooth patches over the tongue present over a variable extent. Though painless at first, it may become fissured and painful later. Being a precancerous condition, persons who develop leukoplakia have to be regularly followed-up. The chance of transformation into oral squamous cell carcinoma varies from 0% to about 20% and this may occur over 1–30 years.

Oral Hairy Leukoplakia

Oral hairy leukoplakia (OHL) is a (hairy) white lesion found on the sides of the tongue caused by opportunistic infection with Epstein-Barr virus on severely immuno-deficient subjects, almost always due to HIV infection. It is one of the most common oral lesions seen in patients with HIV infection. Development of OHL often heralds the transition from HIV to AIDS.

Erythroplakia

Is a flat red patch or lesion in the mouth. The most common areas in the mouth where erythroplakia is found are the floor of the mouth, the tongue and the soft palate. It appears as a red macule or plaque with well-demarcated borders. The texture is characteristically soft and velvety. An adjacent area of leukoplakia may be found along with the erythroplakia.

Microscopically, the tissue exhibits severe epithelial dysplasia, carcinoma-*in-situ* or invasive squamous cell

Textbook of Medicine

carcinoma in 90% of cases. There is an absence of keratin production and a reduced number of epithelial cells. Since the underlying vascular structures are less hidden by tissue, erythroplakia appears red when viewed in a clinical setting.

Geographical tongue: It is the name given to chronic migrating superficial glossitis. Though, it appears fierce, it is not clinically significant. The cause is not clear.

Glossodynia: It is pain arising from the tongue, which is apparently normal.

Atrophy of the tongue (bald tongue): Mucosal atrophy occurs in iron-deficiency anemia, pellagra, vitamin B_{12} deficiency or syphilis. The tongue may be sore. Lesions of the hypoglossal nerves or their nuclei cause atrophy of the muscles. In this condition, the tongue shows longitudinal furrows.

Pigmentation of the tongue and oral mucosa: Main causes of this condition are given below:

- Poor oral hygiene
- Irritation due to dentures or extensive metal fillings
- Addison's disease
- Side effects of drugs like phenothiazines and oral contraceptives
- Peutz-Jeghers syndrome
- Accumulation of heavy metals like lead, mercury and bismuth
- Malignant melanoma.

Fissured tongue (scrotal tongue): The dorsal and lateral surfaces of the tongue are covered by deep fissures which are soft, painless and often asymptomatic except for the appearance. This may cause anxiety to the patient.

Hairy tongue: This abnormality develops due to elongation of the filiform papillae at the dorsum of the tongue, as a result of failure of the keratin layer to desquamate normally. Staining by food, tobacco, *pan* or chromogenic microbes gives this a black or brown color.

ORAL CANCER

This is the most frequent form of cancer in Indian subjects, especially males. More than 95% cases have squamous cell carcinoma. The sites of predilection are the lips, posterior two-third of the tongue, inner aspects of the cheek and gingival margins. The growth is single in the majority of cases but cancer arising from submucous fibrosis may be multiple.

Etiology

Excessive chewing of tobacco in the form of *pan* (betel leaf, lime and tobacco) and retention of the cud in the mouth are closely associated with oral cancer in India. Other associations are cigar or pipe smoking, smoking with the lighted end of the cigar or *beedi* inside the mouth (as in Andhra Pradesh) and keeping snuff in the mouth.

Conditions like submucous fibrosis, alcoholism, syphilitic glossitis, chronic irritation by misaligned teeth and **Plummer-Vinson syndrome** are associated with higher risk of cancer. Leukoplakia is a common precancerous lesion.

Since, the early lesions are painless, there may be considerable delay in seeking medical aid. Presence of induration of the ulcer or growth should draw attention to the possibility of cancer. All chronic ulcerating or indurated lesions in the mouth should be examined carefully by palpation and biopsied without delay to detect carcinoma and the case may be referred to the appropriate speciality services.

Treatment

Mainly local irradiation is advised. Surgical measures are employed in special circumstances.

Regular attempts to educate the public and training of volunteers to detect oral cancer in the community by the Regional Cancer Center, Thiruvanthapuram has served to bring oral cancer cases at a much earlier stage for therapy.

CHAPTER
77

Diseases of the Esophagus

KR Vinaya Kumar, KV Krishna Das

Chapter Summary

- Symptoms in Esophageal Disease
  - Esophageal Pain
  - Dysphagia
- Vomiting
- Esophagitis
  - Eosinophilic Esophagitis
- Achalasia Cardia
- Diffuse Esophageal Spasm
- Esophageal Hiatus Hernia and Peptic Esophagitis
- Gastroesophageal Reflux Disease (GERD)
- Carcinoma of Esophagus

SYMPTOMS IN ESOPHAGEAL DISEASE

Diseases of the esophagus manifest as esophageal pain and/or dysphagia. The esophagus is not readily accessible to physical examination and the examiner has to interrogate regarding these symptoms. Investigations include contrast radiography using barium swallow, esophagoscopy and biopsy from different regions under vision.

Esophageal Pain

It may be of three types:

1. Heartburn—burning sensation produced by reflux of acid gastric contents into the esophagus.

2. Odynophagia—pain during deglutition which is due to inflammation of the esophagus.
3. Colicky pain—caused by vigorous contraction or distension of the esophagus. Esophageal pain may arise either because of obstruction by food or diffuse esophageal spasm. Esophageal pain may be mistaken for angina pectoris. Presence of dysphagia suggests that the pain arises from the esophagus. Autonomic disturbances like sweating may accompany these attacks. Nitrates may relieve the pain of esophageal spasm.

Causes of odynophagia

Caustic ingestion
- Acid
- Alkali
- Pill-induced injury
- Alendronate and other bisphosphonates
- Aspirin and other nonsteroidal anti-inflammatory drugs (NSAIDs)
- Iron preparations
- Potassium chloride (especially slow-release form)
- Quinidine
- Tetracycline and its derivatives
- Zidovudine

Infectious esophagitis
- Cytomegalovirus (CMV)
- Herpes simplex virus (HSV)
- Human immunodeficiency virus (HIV)

Severe reflux esophagitis

Esophageal carcinoma

Dysphagia

It may be oropharyngeal or esophageal.

Causes of dysphagia

- Neuromuscular causes
  - Parkinson's disease
  - Polymyositis or dermatomyositis
  - Stroke
  - Thyroid dysfunction

Oropharyngeal Dysphagia

- Processes that affect the mouth, hypopharynx and upper esophagus.
- The patient is often unable to initiate a swallow and repeatedly has to attempt to swallow. Patients frequently describe coughing or choking when they attempt to swallow.

The answers to four questions are crucial:

1. What type of food or liquid causes symptoms?
2. Is the dysphagia intermittent or progressive?
3. Is there any weight loss?
4. Does the patient have heartburn?

Causes of oropharyngeal dysphagia

- Neuromuscular disorders
  - Lower cranial nerve paralysis
  - Myasthenia gravis
  - Oropharyngeal myopathies
  - Motor neuron disease
  - Hydrophobia
  - Iron deficiency states.
- Mechanical obstruction
  - Tumors
  - Stricture
  - Diverticula or webs as in iron deficiency anemia (IDA).

Esophageal Dysphagia

This can be distinguished by the onset of dysphagia when the patient initiates swallowing. The passage of food is delayed. Though some degree of localization of the pain is possible, on many occasions, it is referred to other regions like the suprasternal notch. Mechanical causes lead to obstruction to solids whereas neuromuscular causes lead to difficulty in swallowing solids and fluids.

Neuromuscular causes: These include achalasia cardia, diffuse esophageal spasm, vagal paralysis, progressive systemic sclerosis and Chagas' disease.
Mechanical causes: These may be intrinsic or extrinsic.
Intrinsic causes: These include:
- Carcinoma
- Strictures
- Diverticula
- Esophageal rings and webs, e.g. the mucosal or muscular ring at the junction of the squamous and columnar epithelium (Schatzki ring).

Extrinsic causes: These include compression by mediastinal masses like lymph nodes, tumors, enlarged left atrium, aortic aneurysm, mediastinitis or infiltration by bronchogenic carcinoma.

Dysphagia should be fully investigated to find out the cause. If none is detected, the investigations should be repeated after a suitable interval. Carcinoma of the esophagus may present with bizarre symptoms for long periods of time and a high index of suspicion is necessary to make an early diagnosis.

Note: *Dysphagia lusoria:* Symptoms arising from vascular compression of esophagus by an aberrant right subclavian artery.

VOMITING

Vomiting is a forceful expulsion of the gastric contents through an open mouth. This has to be distinguished from regurgitation which is the effortless entry of the gastric or esophageal contents into a closed mouth. This may be spat out or swallowed.

Vomiting may be caused by different mechanisms. The common causes of vomiting are given as follow:

Gastric causes: Irritant foods, drugs or other chemicals, bleeding into the stomach, gastritis and pyloric obstruction.
Neurological causes: Rise of intracranial tension, intracranial bleeding, inflammation of brain or meninges, vertebrobasilar ischemia and migraine.
Metabolic causes: Uremia, hepatic failure, diabetic ketoacidosis (DKA), lactic acidosis, acute intermittent porphyria and poisoning.
Endocrine causes: Hypoadrenal crisis, hyperparathyroidism, hyperthyroidism and pheochromocytoma.
Reflex causes: Labyrinthine stimulation occurring in motion sickness, ocular causes.
Psychogenic vomiting: Anxiety state, hysteria, depression.
Pregnancy: Hyperemesis gravidarum.

Drugs

Several drugs lead to nausea and vomiting as prominent side effects. This may be due to local irritation as in the case of antirheumatic drugs, antibiotics and iron salts or vomiting may be caused by stimulation of the medullary centers. Anticancer drugs, oral contraceptives and estrogenic steroids come under this group.

Vomiting is a very unpleasant symptom due to the associated autonomic phenomena such as sweating, salivation, palpitation and tachypnea. Severe vomiting leads to dehydration, hyponatremic hypokalemic hypochloremic alkalosis and ketosis. Repeated vomiting may also lead to gastroesophageal tears (Mallory-Weiss syndrome), esophageal rupture, subconjunctival hemorrhage or even intraocular and intracranial hemorrhage.

Management

Precise diagnosis of the underlying condition and specific treatment is required in all cases. Correction of the metabolic derangement should be instituted in severe vomiting as in hyperemesis gravidarum. In severe cases, infusion of intravenous (IV) normal saline should be started without delay. Further management depends upon the degree of electrolyte and acid base disturbances. Infusion of fluid should be started as soon as the patient is first seen. Even in the presence of moderately severe vomiting, frequent small sips of fluids (30 mL given every 10 minutes) help to retain some fluid and in many cases this is very beneficial.

Fluid can be administered rectally. Up to 1.5 L of normal saline can be given in 24 hours by this route. Fluid is given through a narrow bore urinary catheter introduced high up in the rectum and given at the rate of 75–100 mL/hour. The infusion bottle should be suspended 30–50 cm above the bed. If fluid is given at greater pressure into the rectum, the fluid may be ejected. Prokinetic agents such as metoclopramide, domperidone and cisapride can restore normal gastric motility and give good symptomatic relief. Antihistamines, such as pheniramine 25–50 mg oral are useful to prevent vomiting in motion sickness. Phenothiazines, such as trifluoperazine hydrochloride 5–10 mg oral are effective in mild forms of vomiting due to neurological causes. In more severe forms, injection of prochloperazine maleate 12.5–25 mg intramuscular (IM) may be required. Vomiting can be very disturbing in cancer chemotherapy. Selective 5-hydroxytryptamine receptor antagonists such as ondansetron 4–8 mg given slowly IV before starting chemotherapy prevents this complication.

ESOPHAGITIS

Inflammation of the esophagus may occur in several diseases, some of which are listed below:

Irritants	Corrosive, alcohol, spicy foods and drugs
Infections	HSV, CMV, *Candida albicans*, *Mycobacterium tuberculosis*, HPV, *Trypanosoma cruzi*
Peptic esophagitis	Associated with GERD
Postradiation	
Drugs	Doxycycline, bisphosphonates, ferrous sulfate, doxorubicin, potassium chloride
Eosinophilic esophagitis	Autoimmune mediated (TH2) mechanism

Abbreviations: HSV = Herpes simplex virus; CMV = Cytomegalovirus; HPV = Human papillomavirus; GERD = Gastrointestinal reflux disease; TH2 = T helper2

Management: When a specific cause is identified, it should be removed. Small feeds given frequently and administration of demulcents and antacids gives symptomatic relief. Omeprazole, 20 mg oral bd given for 3–4 days may help. If swallowing is difficult, ranitidine injection, 50 mg IM 8 hour will be beneficial.

In the case of infections, specific anti-infective agents are indicated. Management of corrosive poisoning is given in Section 4.

Eosinophilic Esophagitis

This condition, previously thought to be rare, is reported more frequently at present and it affects all populations. The condition is encountered when investigating dysphagia and food impaction in children and adults. This is distinct from Gastroesophageal Reflux Disease (GERD). It is a distinct entity which does not completely respond to acid suppression. All age groups may be affected.

Definition

Eosinophilic esophagitis is a chronic autoimmune mediated or antigen mediated lesion characterized by symptoms related to esophageal dysfunction and eosinophil prominent inflammation. The antigens seems to be food related. Histology shows eosinophils in the exudates at least 15/high power field. The mechanisms is T helper 2 (TH2) related activity.

Symptoms include feeding problems, vomiting and abdominal pain in children. In adolescents and adults, food impaction may occur. Differential diagnosis includes other forms of esophagitis, allergic vasculitis, Crohn's disease and others.

Contrast esophagoscopy reveals abnormalities of the esophageal wall. Routine esophagoscopy reveals exudates, mucosal edema, linear furrows, esophageal rings and strictures which are long, unlike those seen in GERD. The condition is not precancerous. Associated diseases include, connective tissue diseases, celiac disease and Crohn's.

The antigens can be identified by prick tests, patch tests or specific serum immunoglobulin E (IgE) testing. The six common foods causing allergy include wheat, milk, soya bean, nuts, eggs and sea food.

Treatment

Special diet consisting of exclusive amino acid formula, excluding antigens is initiated.

The mainstay of treatment is to give glucocorticoids as throat spray or as viscous preparation (fluticasone). Up to 90% cases improve within two weeks; systemic steroids may be required at times. Proton pump inhibitors (PPIs) are generally ineffective or less effective. Those with esophageal eosinophilia may respond to PPIs at times.

Repeated esophageal dilatation may be required to maintain relief.

Source: Furuta GT, Katzka DA. Eosinophilic Esophagitis. N Engl J Med. 2015;373(17):1640-8.

ACHALASIA CARDIA

Syn: Cardiospasm

In this disorder, there is abnormality of lower part of the esophagus which results in failure of relaxation of the sphincter when food reaches the lower end. The esophagus

Textbook of Medicine

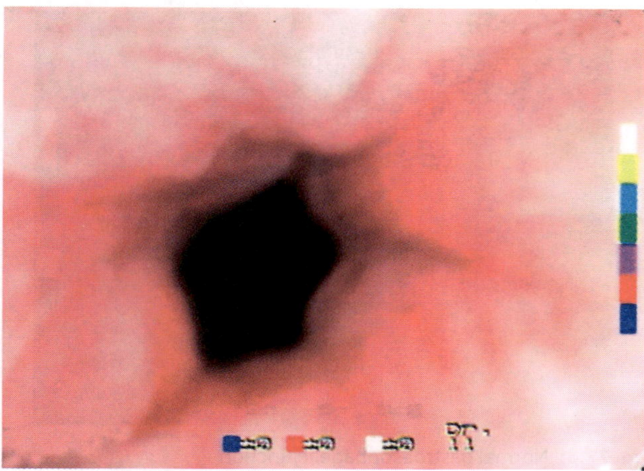

Fig. 77.1: Achalasia cardia: Dilated esophagus above the stricture

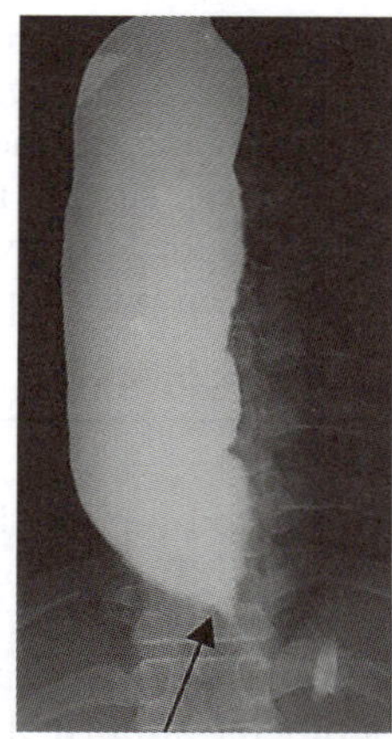

Fig. 77.2: Achalasia cardia: Barium swallow (arrow). **Note:** The grossly detailed esophagus with sharply tapering lower end (arrow)

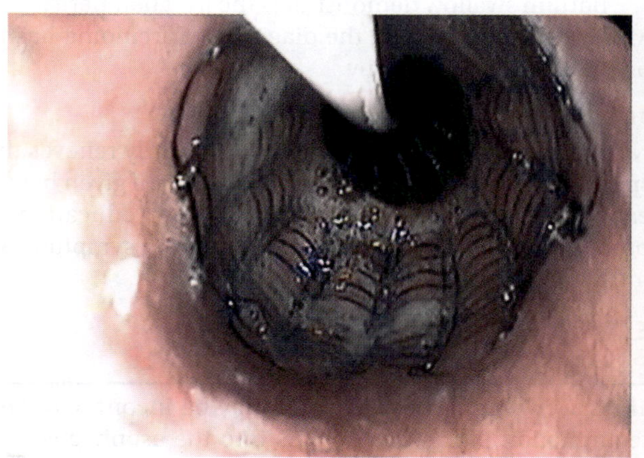

Fig. 77.3: Esophageal stent in stricture esophagus

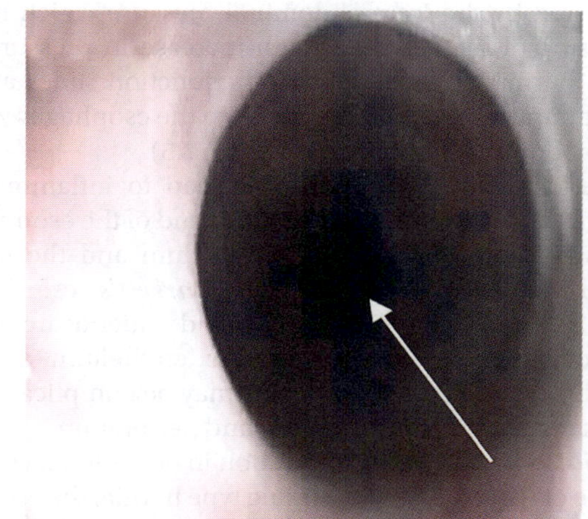

Fig. 77.4: Stricture esophagus endoscopy (arrow). **Note:** The irregular narrowing

progressively dilates and becomes atonic. The dysfunction is due to degeneration in the Auerbach's plexus and vagal fibers (Fig. 77.1).

Note: Cause of ganglion cell degeneration—there is increasing evidence of autoimmune process due to latent infection with herpes simplex virus1 (HSV-1).

Clinical Features

The presentation may be varied. There may be dysphagia, recurrent respiratory infections or vague upper abdominal symptoms. Even with dysphagia, the general health is preserved. At the end of the meal, the patient exerts pressure which opens the sphincter and the food material passes down to the stomach with a gurgle. Food collected in the dilated esophagus undergoes fermentation. Repeated aspiration of this material into the respiratory tract results in recurrent bouts of respiratory infection. Carcinoma *(squamous cell carcinoma)* may supervene on achalasia cardia.

In some cases of achalasia, there may be vigorous contractions of the esophageal muscles causing chest pain *(vigorous achalasia)*.

Diagnosis

Clinically, the condition should be diagnosed when long-standing dysphagia is accompanied by good general health. Some cases may be identified for the first time from chest radiographs. The presence of a mediastinal shadow with a horizontal fluid level produced by the dilated fluid-filled esophagus should draw attention to this condition. Barium swallow confirms the diagnosis (Fig. 77.2). In all cases, esophagoscopy and biopsy should be done to exclude stricture and carcinoma.

Other conditions which produce esophageal lesions similar to achalasia are gastric carcinoma infiltrating into the lower end of the esophagus, amyloidosis and Chagas' disease.

Treatment

Conservative management consists of dietary adjustment such as frequent small feeds, anticholinergic drugs like probanthine, 15–30 mg thrice a day 15 minutes before meals and attention to general health. Calcium channel blockers such as nifedipine have been tried with limited success. Stenting the esophagus is possible in suitable cases, especially associated with structure (Figs 77.3 and 77.4).

Pharmacotherapy is often unsatisfactory and unpredictable. All symptomatic patients require a definitive therapy such as balloon dilatation, injection of botulinum toxin or surgical cardiomyotomy *(Heller's operation)*. Balloon

Textbook of Medicine

dilatation under endoscopic or fluoroscopic control is a quick and safe procedure which gives lasting relief. It is the first choice in many centers. Endoscopic injection of botulinum toxin also gives similar results for varying periods. It has to be repeated. Surgery gives permanent relief but regurgitation is a complication.

DIFFUSE ESOPHAGEAL SPASM

Syn: Corkscrew Esophagus

This is caused by disordered peristalsis. Multiple contractions occur simultaneously in addition to normal contractions induced by deglutition. The disorder may be primary or secondary to esophagitis and carcinoma. The lower esophageal sphincter is normal. Emotional stress and hurried eating precipitate symptoms. These patients complain of retrosternal pain induced by swallowing.

Barium swallow demonstrates the irregular peristalsis. Motility studies confirm the diagnosis. Carcinoma has to be ruled out by endoscopy.

Treatment

Nitroglycerin in a dose of 0.5 mg sublingually relieves the spasm and it also helps in relieving the pain if given before eating. General measures to allay anxiety, education in proper eating habits and reassurance clears symptoms in most cases.

ESOPHAGEAL HIATUS HERNIA AND PEPTIC ESOPHAGITIS

The lower esophageal sphincter may be incontinent and regurgitation of gastric contents into the esophagus may occur in a variable proportion of normal subjects, but in a few cases it causes symptoms. The sphincteric action is assisted by the intra-abdominal pressure which helps in closing of the sphincter with increase in pressure. In hiatus hernia, the esophagogastric junction slides above the diaphragm and reflux occurs into the esophagus when intra-abdominal pressure rises (Fig. 77.5).

Gastric acid, pepsin and bile lead to inflammatory changes in the esophagus. The lower end of the esophagus may show metaplasia of the epithelium and the lining may resemble gastric mucosa (***Barrett's esophagus Fig. 77.5).*** Peptic ulceration and adenocarcinoma may develop in such metaplastic epithelium as late complications. Peptic esophagitis may be complicated by hemorrhage, stricture formation and perforation.

Hiatus hernia is more common in obese females. This may be of two types. In the sliding type hernia, the esophagogastric junction slides through the diaphragmatic hiatus. In the paraesophageal type of hernia, a knuckle of the fundus of the stomach passes up to the thorax alongside the esophagus. These hernias as such may be symptomless but symptoms start appearing when peptic ulceration develops.

Clinical Features

The common symptoms is heartburn felt at the lower part of the sternum, when the patient lies down flat, stoops forward as in tying the shoe lace or lifts heavy objects. The pain is relieved by adopting the erect posture. Certain

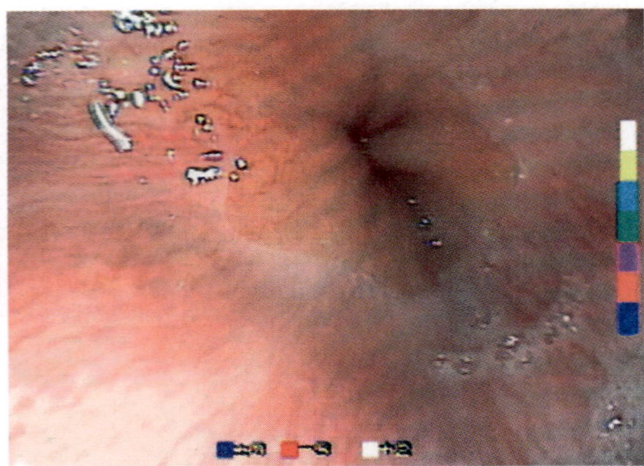

Fig. 77.5: Normal gastroesophageal junction

foods aggravate this pain. Rarely gastric contents may regurgitate into the mouth or may be aspirated into the respiratory tract.

Diagnosis

It is confirmed by radiology and esophagoscopy. The lesion is demonstrable by barium meal taken in the ***Trendelenburg position.***

GASTROESOPHAGEAL REFLUX DISEASE (GERD)

This term denotes reflux of the acidic gastric contents into the esophagus. It is not a disease. It is seen in many subjects, especially children. Normally, the lower esophageal sphincter maintains a pressure 15 mm Hg above the gastric pressure and so, there is no regurgitation of gastric contents into the esophagus.

GERD becomes a disease when it is causing symptoms such as heartburn or when it is associated with endoscopic changes or histopathological changes in the esophageal mucosa. It is a common disease and about one third of the adult population have symptoms at some point in their lifetime. Obesity and smoking are weakly associated with GERD. Males suffer more.

Heartburn and regurgitation are common symptoms of GERD. Dysphagia chest pain, dysphonia and globus are also seen in severe cases. Laryngitis, reflux bronchospasm, precipitation or aggravation of asthma and strictures and ulcerations of the lower end of esophagus are seen as complications. Severe disease may be associated with Barret's esophagus. Ambulatory pH monitoring done with a pH probe positioned 5 cms above the gastroesophageal sphincter records the GERD throughout the day.

Endoscopy and pH-metry are the diagnostic investigations. Endoscopy can assess the severity of the illness and can also detect complications such as strictures, Barret's lesions, ulceration and esophageal adenocarcinoma (Fig. 77.6).

Los Angeles classification of GERD	
Grade A	One or mucosal breaks confined to folds ≤ 5 mm
Grade B	One or more mucosal breaks >5 mm confined to folds but not continous between tops of mucosal folds
Grade C	Mucosal breaks continuous between tops of two or more mucosal folds but not circumferential
Grade D	Circumferential mucosal break

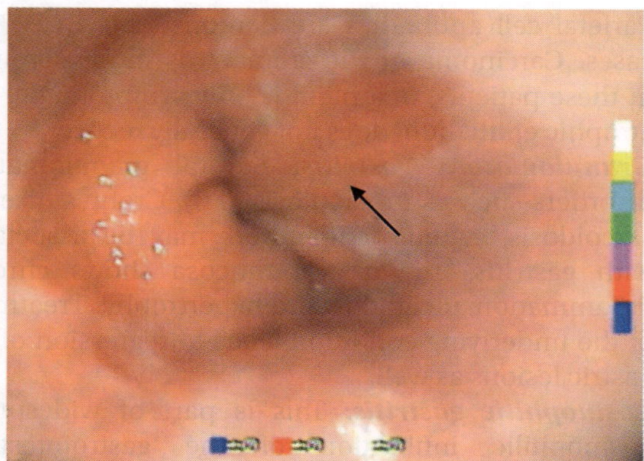

Fig. 77.6: Barrett's esophagus. **Note:** Gastric metaplasia in the esophagus (arrow)

Treatment

The medical treatment of GERD and esophageal hiatus hernia is similar in the early stages and hence, they are described together. Mild cases require only dietary regulation, elevated position of head during sleep and antacids. Weight reduction and short causes of treatment with prokinetic drugs such as metoclopramide 10–15 mg bd or mosapride 10 mg bd help to relieve symptoms. H_2 receptor blockers such as ranitidine or famotidine are useful, but PPIs such as omeprazole 40 mg bd or pantoprazole 40 mg bd are more effective. Severe cases require high doses of PPI for long duration (several years). Cases resistant to medical therapy may be benefited with surgical interventions such as laparoscopic fundoplication. Complications such as esophageal strictures are managed with endoscopic balloon dilation.

Source: Moayyedi P, Talley NJ. Gastro-oesophageal reflux disease. Lancet. 2006;36(9528):2086-100.

Paraesophageal hernias: These may not be symptomatic in many cases since the lower esophageal sphincter is intact but sometimes large hernias may produce symptoms like cardiac arrhythmias, dyspnea and dysphagia. Gangrene or perforation may present as surgical emergencies at times.

CARCINOMA OF ESOPHAGUS

This is common in India, especially in the southern states. Thirty to forty percent of all esophageal carcinomas occur at the lower end of the esophagus—95% is squamous cell carcinoma and 5% is adenocarcinoma. In many countries, the proportion of adenocarcinoma is increasing. Etiological factors include smoking, alcoholism, Barret's esophagus, obesity, poverty, burns of the esophagus and Plummer-Vinson syndrome.

Due to the absence of serous coat, esophageal cancer disseminates early. The growth may be ulcerating, polypoid or annular.

Progressive dysphagia, initially to solids and later to fluids as well, is the time honored description, but in a minority of cases, symptom may be vague and atypical. Loss of weight is an early symptom. Barium swallow, esophagoscopy and biopsy confirm the diagnosis. These investigations must be undertaken in all patients with symptoms referable to the esophagus.

Treatment

Lesions in the distal third are more amenable to therapy. Surgical resection and irradiation are beneficial in early cases. In advanced cases, irradiation may give symptomatic relief. A feeding gastrostomy may prolong life, but the miserable condition of the patient after the surgery is a strong point against palliative surgery. Self-exapandable metallic stents are available which can be introduced endoscopically. Radiation can be applied over the stent.

Early esophageal carcinoma	Endoscopic therapy (endoscopic resection,endoscopic submucosal dissection)
Locally advanced resectable	Surgery, neoadjuvant chemoradiotherapy followed by surgery
Locally advanced unresectable	Chemoradiation (in patients without metastatses), chemotherapy (in patient with metastatses), endoscopic palliation (laser tissue ablation therapy, dilatation and stent placement).

CHAPTER

78

Diseases of the Stomach

KR Vinaya Kumar, KV Krishna Das

Chapter Summary

- Gastritis
- Ulcers
  - Peptic Ulcer
  - Duodenal Ulcer
  - Gastric Ulcer
- Zollinger-Ellison Syndrome
- Carcinoma of the Stomach
- Gastric Outlet Obstruction
- Hematemesis
- Melena
- Fresh Blood in Stools

GASTRITIS

Gastritis denotes an inflammatory process involving the wall of the stomach, particularly the mucosa due to various etiological factors.

Classifications

There are two types of gastritis—(i) acute gastritis and (ii) chronic gastritis. Chronic gastritis is further classified into: (a) chronic superficial gastritis, (b) atrophic gastritis, (c) granulomatous gastritis, (d) eosinophilic gastritis and (e) hyperplastic gastritis.

Acute Gastritis

Chemicals like strong acids or alkalies, drugs such as salicylates and indomethacin, ethanol, ionizing radiations, acute mental and physical stress, shock, hypoxia and renal failure may cause acute gastritis. The pathological change leads to breakdown of gastric mucosal barrier. The hydrogen ions (H^+) diffuse into the mucosa from the lumen. Vascular damage occurs. Acute hemorrhagic gastritis may be localized or diffuse. Superficial erosions may develop due to necrosis of the epithelium and extravasation of blood from the damaged vessels in the lamina propria.

Symptoms include upper abdominal pain, nausea, vomiting, hematemesis and melena. Endoscopy reveals edema of the mucosa, hyperemia, surface erosions and hemorrhages. Proper treatment results in complete recovery within a few days.

Treatment

Removal of the cause, bland frequent diet, antacids and correction of fluid and electrolyte levels give relief. Hematemesis may develop which demands emergency management. H_2 receptor blockers such as ranitidine 150 mg oral bd or famotidine 40 mg oral bd help to bring early relief. Proton pump inhibitors (PPIs) such as omeprazole 40 mg bd are very effective.

Chronic Gastritis

Chronic gastritis can be subdivided into types A and B. Type A gastritis is probably an immune-mediated disorder. Some of these cases develop pernicious anemia. *Helicobacter pylori* is causally associated with type B or chronic bacterial gastritis. Many drugs such as nonsteroidal anti-inflammatory drugs (NSAIDs) and others may produce chronic chemical gastritis. Attention to these factors helps to relieve the condition in many cases.

- *Chronic superficial gastritis:* In this form, the gastric glands are normal but cellular infiltration consisting of lymphocytes and plasma cells occur in the lamina propria adjacent to the surface and the gastric pits. The body and fundus of the stomach are affected leaving the antrum free.
- *Chronic atrophic gastritis:* This is more common as age advances. It is associated with pernicious anemia, diabetes mellitus (DM), thyroid disorders, Addison's disease and iron deficiency anemia (IDA). Mucosa over the body and fundus is diffusely affected. Mucosal cells atrophy partially or completely resulting in variable thinning of the mucosa. Gastric epithelium may undergo metaplasia and be transformed into intestinal type of epithelium. There is also infiltration by lymphocytes and plasma cells. Acid secretion falls. Majority of cases are symptomless, but pernicious anemia or gastric bleeding may develop in some.

Parietal cell antibodies are demonstrable in 60% of cases. Carcinoma of the stomach is more common in these patients, treatment is only symptomatic. The atrophic epithelium does not generally recover.

- *Granulomatous gastritis:* Several granulomatous disorders such as tuberculosis (TB), Crohn's disease, sarcoidosis, syphilis and others may be associated with gastritis. The gastric mucosa shows chronic inflammation, ulceration and hypertrophy. Treatment of the underlying condition leads to regression of the gastric lesions as well.
- *Eosinophilic gastritis:* This is part of widespread eosinophilic infiltration of the gastrointestinal tract (GIT), the cause is not evident in many cases. Peripheral blood may show increase in eosinophils. Treatment with corticosteroids and antihistamines is often successful.

  At times, larval forms of nematodes such as *Anisakis marina* may cause infestation of the gastric mucosa. This is associated with secondary eosinophilic infiltration.
- *Hypertrophic gastritis:* This is characterized by large hypertrophic folds of gastric mucosa. There are two varieties:
  1. This causes hypersecretion of gastric juice poor in acid and rich in protein. This is called *Ménétrier's disease.* The excessive protein loss may lead to hypoproteinemia and edema. Treatment consists of high protein diet and symptomatic measures.
  2. In the other variety, gastric juice is rich in acid and low in protein. This hyperacidity responds to H_2 blocker drugs or omeprazole.

Other rarer causes of gastritis include infections caused by pyogenic bacteria or anaerobes and *Candida albicans.* External irradiation leads to both acute and chronic gastritis.

ULCERS

PEPTIC ULCER

Erosions: Break in the mucosa without perceptible depth.
Ulcers: Break in the mucosa with appreciable depth (involvement of submucosa).

This term refers to nonmalignant ulceration of gastric or duodenal mucosa as a result of acid-peptic influences. These are seen in the stomach, duodenum or other sites where gastric type mucosa may be present, e.g. lower end of esophagus or Meckel's diverticulum. Peptic ulceration may be acute or chronic.

- *Acute peptic ulceration* may result from ingestion of corticosteroids, NSAIDs, corrosive agents and unwholesome food. Severe stressful conditions such as mental stress, burns, shock and others may lead to acute mucosal ulceration and these present as hematemesis and melena complicating the primary disease.
- *Chronic peptic ulceration* generally affects the stomach or duodenum and less commonly other ectopic sites of gastric mucosa. Normally, the ulcerogenic effect of acid and pepsin is counteracted by the mucosal resistance of the gastroduodenum. Ulceration results when this equilibrium is upset.

This is 10–20 times more common in males than in females and it is 12–30 times more common than gastric ulcer. Chronic duodenal ulcers occur in the first part of the duodenum just distal to the pyloroduodenal junction. Fifty percent are on the anterior wall. Multiple ulcers occur in 10–15%. In 10%, duodenal and gastric ulcers coexist. The pathogenesis of duodenal ulcer is not completely understood. It is more common in the rice-eating population of India.

Hereditary factors, dietary habits, heavy smoking and chronic use of drugs like aspirin, antirheumatic drugs and corticosteroids may predispose to this disorder. Psychological stress aggravates ulceration and precipitates bleeding. Duodenal ulcer is associated with serotype HLA-B$_5$ as reported from the West. It is also more common in blood group O nonsecretor subjects. The ulcer is sharply demarcated and the site of predilection is the first part of the duodenum. The role of *Helicobacter pylori* in the pathogenesis of ulceration has been established.

Helicobacter Pylori

It is a gram-negative spiral organism which is now accepted as the major causative factor in chronic duodenal ulcer, gastric ulcer and chronic gastritis. It plays a role in the pathogenesis of gastric carcinoma and mucosa associated lymphoid tissue (MALT) lymphoma of the stomach. It is demonstrable in almost all cases of duodenal ulcer and over 80% of cases of gastric ulcer. About 50% of the adult population is infected with *H. pylori* and this is possibly one of the most common bacterial organisms colonising humans. Some cases of pernicious anemia are also closely associated with the presence of *H. pylori. H. Pylori* infection is more prevalent in the low socioeconomic groups. Spread of infection is by the oral route, ingestion. Family contacts, especially children are affected more. Once infection occurs, spontaneous elimination of the organism is rare.

H. pylori moves under the mucus layer in the stomach by its flagella and thrives in this location. Presence of urease helps the organism to produce carbon dioxide and ammonia from urea and this mechanism protects it from gastric acid. *H. pylori* produces a vacuolating cytotoxin (VacA) which enters the epithelial cells. Its pathogenic role is not fully known. *H. pylori* causes inflammation of duodenal mucosa, hyperacidity and duodenal ulcers. Genotypes of *H. pylori,* Cytotoxin Associated Gene A (CagA) and VacA differ in their predisposition to cause gastric cancer. *H. pylori* infection raises the risk of gastric cancer 6-folds, compared to those not infected. It leads to atrophic gastritis and intestinal metaplasia both of which predispose to cancer. Inflammation of the stomach may lead to hypochlorhydria and predispose to gastric carcinoma.

The organism is demonstrable beneath the mucus layer adjacent to the cells, mainly in the mucosa of the gastric antrum and duodenum, especially if there is gastric metaplasia of the mucosa. Only some types of *H. pylori* are pathogenic. It is also known that *H. pylori* which can cause gastric adenocarcinoma can protect against esophageal adenocarcinoma. There are reports that *H. pylori* may even protect against reflux esophagitis. So, eradication is indicated only under appropriate situations. The indications for investigation to demonstrate *H. pylori* as follows:

- All patients with peptic symptoms <45 years of age.
- Patients <45 years with alarm symptoms. Endoscopy is also indicated.
- Patients <45 years with recent onset of symptom. They also require endoscopy.

Indications for testing and treatment of H. pylori infection:

- Active peptic ulcer disease (gastric or duodenal ulcer)
- Confirmed history of peptic ulcer (not previously treated for *H. pylori* infection)
- Gastric MALT-lymphoma (low grade)
- Following endoscopic resection of early gastric cancer
- Uninvestigated dyspepsia (if the *H. pylori* prevalence is high in the population).

H. pylori has been implicated (either beneficial or detrimental) in diseases like Raynaud's disease, idiopathic urticaria, acne rosacea, migraine, thyroiditis, Guillain-Barre syndrome, coronary artery disease and immune thrombocytopenic purpura.

In NSAID induced ulcers and Zollinger-Ellison syndrome, *H. pylori* has no major pathogenic role. *Helicobacter heilmannii* is a native organism in animals. Rarely, it may infect humans. It may cause mild gastritis. This infection is more associated with MALT lymphoma.

Diagnosis of H. pylori

- ***Noninvasive tests:*** These include serology (IgG, *H. pylori*), urea breath test and stool antigen test.
- ***Invasive tests:*** Includes histology which is the gold standard, rapid urease test, culture and polymerase chain reaction (PCR) study.

Biopsy of the ulcers can be done for demonstrating the organism.

Clinical Features of Peptic Ulcer

The classical feature is the hunger pain felt in the epigastrium, relieved by food. Pain starts within three hours of eating food and it may be described as burning, aching, pressure, fullness or as a sensation of hunger. The pain comes on everyday for a few weeks and then subsides for considerable periods. Pain may be more prominent at night. The pain is usually relieved by food, antacids or even by vomiting. A small proportion of ulcer subjects may be asymptomatic. Occurrence of complications may be the first sign of disease in them. Compared to the disabling symptoms, physical signs are only minimal. Physical examination may reveal tenderness in the epigastrium or to the right of the midline. Ulcer patients are able to localize the pain and this feature helps to distinguish them from cases of functional dyspepsia.

Differential Diagnosis

Epigastric pain is a common symptom in several alimentary disorders such as gastric carcinoma, pancreatic carcinoma, pancreatitis, biliary tract disease, peptic ulceration of the esophagus, duodenitis and ancylostomiasis. The pain of irritable bowel syndrome may mimic peptic ulcer. At times, pain of ischemic heart disease (IHD) may resemble heart burn.

Diagnosis

The history of pain coming on with hunger and relieved by hot fluids or antacids is suggestive, but final diagnosis depends on the demonstration of the ulcer by gastro-duodenoscopy. Endoscopy confirms the presence of ulcers and also confirms the absence of ulceration. Since, the clinical features of benign ulcers show considerable overlap with those of malignancy, upper GI endoscopy should be done to see the lesion and confirm it histologically in all cases, where the clinical presentation is not straightforward. Duodenal ulcer is seen as an ulcer crater in the proximal part of the duodenal bulb in the barium meal. The duodenal bulb may show marked deformity (trifoliate appearance). Indirect demonstration of the lesion is by barium meal examination. In all cases, where symptoms persist for more than a few weeks in spite of dietary and pharmacological therapy, upper gastroduodenal endoscopy should be done to exclude malignancy and other more serious conditions. In the hands of a trained endoscopists, endoscopy and biopsy are very reliable and safe.

Alarm symptoms indicating urgent need for endoscopy include the following:

- Unintentional weight loss
- Dysphagia
- Odynophagia
- Persistent vomiting
- Hematemesis, melena
- Recent onset iron deficiency state
- Epigastric mass
- Previous gastric surgery
- NSAIDs use
- Family history of upper gastrointestinal cancer
- Jaundice
- Left supraclavicular lymphadenopathy.

There is a great tendency to recur after initial healing. It is seen even after surgery. The persistence of *H. pylori* infection is the most common cause for recurrence.

Course and Complications

Acute ulcers and those caused by stress or offending drugs such as corticosteroids and NSAIDs may heal with dietary regime and short course drug therapy. Acute complications include severe ulceration with intractable hematemesis and perforation.

Chronic duodenal ulcer persists with exacerbations and remissions over several years. Precipitating factors are change in diet and lifestyle, drugs and mental stress. If left untreated, complications occur in chronic peptic ulcer. Major chronic complication is the development of cicatricial stenosis of the pylorus resulting in pyloric obstruction, penetration of the ulcer outside the peritoneum leads to development of adhesions with the omentum and neighboring viscera and ulceration of the structures adjacent to the posterior wall of the stomach and duodenum, especially the pancreas. Pyloric obstruction develops 10–20 years after onset of duodenal ulcer. When this develops, the clinical picture changes. Once pyloric obstruction is established, surgical treatment becomes inevitable.

Hematemesis presents as an acute medical emergency. It is often precipitated by the use of non-steroidal antirheumatic drugs, corticosteroids or aspirin. Perforation presents with sudden onset of severe pain, tenderness over the epigastrium, rigidity of the abdominal wall, signs of peritonitis and presence of gas under the diaphragm, demonstrable by X-ray taken in the erect posture. If this emergency is not recognized, the condition rapidly proceeds to local and general peritonitis with its associated high mortality. Ideal treatment is to close the perforation surgically at the earliest opportunity.

Management

Aims of Therapy

- Relief of pain as early as possible
- Favor healing of ulcer
- Prevent complications
- Avoid recurrence.

General measures: The patient should be advised to take food regularly at 2.5–3 hour intervals to avoid pain. A cup of milk taken at bedtime often helps to abolish nocturnal pain in many cases. Sometimes patients report that milk leads to worsening of acidity. Excepting highly spiced food, there is no choice between the various foods to be avoided. Till the advent of H_2 receptor blocking drugs, one of the mainstay of management was strict dietary therapy. In some cases, dietary adjustment itself may give considerable relief and even help in gradual healing of the ulcer. It is important that persons who are predisposed to develop peptic ulcer should maintain this dietary discipline for life, to avoid relapse.

Tobacco smoking should be stopped forthwith, since it favors ulcerogenesis and hinders ulcer healing. Resumption of smoking is a common cause for relapse of ulcer-symptoms. Alcohol should be avoided, especially the spirits. It is advisable to restrict coffee to two cups daily or less.

Drug Therapy

Several drugs are available for treating peptic ulcers. Table 78.1 shows the available groups of drugs, their main actions and major side effects. Anti-ulcer drugs are among the most widely used drugs in modern medical practice.

Specific drugs should be started along with the general measures. Choice of drugs depends on the individual case. Though antacids are effective in relieving pain and are cheap, they achieve ulcer-healing only in a smaller proportion of cases. Therefore, it is better to add a ***H_2 receptor blocker*** or ***PPIs*** concurrently. These drugs are available as tablets for oral use. They are very powerful inhibitors of gastric acid, giving pain-relief within a few days of administration. Cimetidine 300 mg and ranitidine 50 mg are also available as IM or IV injections and they are indicated when oral medication is not possible or when more urgent relief is needed as in hematemesis or melena.

Table 78.1: Drugs used for peptic ulcer

Drugs	Action	Dose for oral administration	Major side effects
Antacids			
Aluminium hydroxide Magnesium hydroxide Magnesium trisilicate Magnesium carbonate	Neutralizes gastric acid	15–30 mL of suspension one and three hours after each meal and at bedtime for 6 weeks	Diarrhea or constipation, inhibition of absorption of iron, calcium and phosphates and milk-alkali syndrome
Mucosal protecting agents			
Sodium alginate	Coats the mucosa	0.5–1 g after food and at bedtime	Nil
Carbenoxolone sodium		100 mg tid for 4–8 weeks	Retention of sodium and loss of potassium
Sucralfate (aluminium salt of sucrose-octasulfate)		1 g four times a day	Nil
Anti-helicobacter pylori			
Colloidal bismuth: Tripotassium dicitrato bismuthate (De-nol) Omeprazole, amoxycillin, Clarithromycin	Eliminates *H. pylori*, thereby hastening ulcer-healing and preventing relapse	20 mL three or four times a day for 30 days	Unpleasant taste, staining of mouth and teeth
H_2 receptor blocking agent			
Cimetidine	Suppression of acid secretion and favor ulcer-healing	200 mg 6 hrs and 400 mg bedtime oral	Drowsiness, allergy, gynecomastia, impotence and inhibition of gastric intrinsic factor
Ranitidine		150 mg BD or 300 mg bedtime oral	Reduction of gastric acidity may predispose to
Famotidine		20 mg BD or 40 mg bedtime 50 mg IV or IM in emergencies	Salmonella infection
Mizatidine		150 mg oral hs	
Roxatidine		150 mg oral hs	
Proton-pump inhibitors			
Omeprazole lansoprazole, pantoprazole, esmoprazole and rabeprazole	Inhibits H^+K^+ ATPase and suppresses acid secretion,	10–20 mg twice a day and 20 mg bedtime favors ulcer-healing	Very few, diarrhea, skin rashes headache, impotence and gynecomastia 30 mg od
Prostaglandins			
Misoprostol	Cytoprotection and reduces acid production	200 mg four times a day	Diarrhea

Note: Antacids and acid inhibiting drugs are continued for 4–8 weeks in full doses and then maintenance treatment is given depending on the individual response.

Abbreviations: H. pylori = Helicobacter pylori; IV = Intravenous; IM = Intramuscular; H+K+ ATPase = Hydrogen potassium ATPase

Both H_2 receptor blockers and PPIs favor ulcer-healing when given for 3–6 weeks. Their role in preventing relapse of ulcer is less definite. Still, long-term continuation of treatment may help to reduce relapse rate in those who are otherwise prone to relapse. In the vast majority, these drugs can be stopped after 6–12 weeks of therapy. Newer H_2 receptor blockers are nizatidine 300 mg hs oral for 4–5 weeks and ranitidine 150 mg hs for 4–6 weeks.

PPIs in common use are omeprazole 20–40 mg oral daily, lansoprazole 15–30 mg oral daily, and pantoprazole 20–40 mg daily, esmoprazole 20 mg bd and rabeprazole 20 mg bd. Adverse effects of PPIs include GI upsets, allergy and susceptibility to food and water borne infections. Rarely inhibition of absorption of vitamin B_{12} may occur, if treatment is prolonged.

Eradication of H. pylori

Though *H. pylori* is very sensitive to many antibiotics *in vitro,* it is difficult to eradicate it due to its location in the mucus layer of stomach where antibiotics do not reach readily. Multiple drugs are required for prolonged duration. Present day triple therapy given for 10–15 days gives an eradication rate of 95%.

A common regimen effective in the vast majority of cases is listed below:

Omeprazole	20 mg bd or 40 mg od
Amoxicillin	1g bd
Clarithromycin	500 mg bd, all given for 10 days consecutively

Elimination rate is about 95%. Repeated courses and quadruple therapy including metronidazole or tinidazole to the triple drug regimen may be slightly more effective. Colloidal bismuth augments the efficacy of this regimen.

Metronidazole resistance is widespread in India. In resistant cases and in relapses, quadruple therapy including tetracycline 500 mg 6 hour and tinidazole 300 mg tid are effective.

Note:

1. Sequential therapy: PPI+amoxicillin for 5 days followed by PPI + clarithromycin + tinidazole for 5 days.
2. Rescue therapy (when primary treatment fails): PPI + amoxicillin + either levofloxacin (250 mg bd) or rifabutin (150 mg bd).

It is ideal to assess the success of treatment by endoscopy which will reveal healing of the ulcer. Apart from specific treatment aimed at the local problem in the stomach, other drugs including analgesics such as dextropropoxyphene 65 mg, parasympatholytic drugs such as propantheline bromide 10–20 mg and anxiolytic drugs such as chlordiazepoxide 10 mg, may be required to control symptoms.

Surgical Measures

At present, treatment of peptic ulcer is by and large a medical problem. More than 90% of ulcers heal with proper treatment. Surgery is indicated in a small proportion of cases which fail to heal or where there is suspicion of malignancy. The usual procedure is highly selective vagotomy in which the vagal fibers supplying the parietal cell bearing area of the stomach are interrupted, leaving the rest of the nerve intact. This operation serves to reduce the acid secretion and thereby favor ulcer-healing.

Indications for Emergency Surgery

- Bleeding of the ulcer, not responding to conservative management.
- Perforation of the ulcer. This is an urgent indication.
- Pyloric stenosis and gastric outlet obstruction.
- Frank carcinoma or atypical features on histology of the ulcer.

GASTRIC ULCER

Gastric ulcers occur in the mucosa of the stomach, 90% being located along the lesser curvature. Gastric ulcers are seen more frequently in males, in the sixth decade of life. Chronic analgesic users are affected more. Most of the benign ulcers are single and 90% are located in the antrum immediately distal to the junction of the antrum with the acid secreting mucosa of the body of the stomach.

The exact mechanism of ulcerogenesis is not known. Unlike as in duodenal ulcer, gastric ulcer patients have only normal or low acid levels. NSAIDs and *H. pylori* are the two most common causes. Corticosteroids and acute stress may cause acute ulceration manifesting frequently as hematemesis.

Clinical Features

Gastric ulcer patients present with epigastric pain of long duration. The pain is generally precipitated by intake of food but in many cases, it is indistinguishable from that of duodenal ulcer. Nausea, vomiting and significant weight loss may be present. Physical examination is unrewarding in the majority of cases.

Diagnosis

It is confirmed by endoscopy which should not be delayed if symptoms persist for a few weeks or more. Endoscopy and biopsy should be performed in all cases. Not

Table 78.2: Radiological differences between benign and malignant ulcers	
Benign	**Malignant**
Flat, broad or conical crater with smooth margins	Irregular crater with fissure-like expansions and a nodular contour of its base
Radiating gastric folds converge on the ulcer and they arise from the margins of the ulcer crater.	Radiating folds are absent due to tumor infiltration of gastric wall.

Note: Even in the presence of slightest double proceed to endoscopy.

infrequently, gastric ulcers are malignant. It is, therefore, important to establish the exact nature of the ulcer before starting therapy. Carcinoma of the stomach may start as ulcer or very rarely malignant change may supervene on a benign ulcer. Gastric ulcer in association with achlorhydria is almost always suggestive of malignancy.

Indirect demonstration of the ulcer is by barium meal imaging, by which the ulcer crater and abnormal patterns in the gastric mucosa can be demonstrated. With the advent of gastroduodenoscopy and biopsy, barium imaging in gastric lesions has lost its prime importance. But, in the diagnosis of motility abnormalities, gastroesophageal reflux and stasis, barium studies are still extremely helpful. Size of the ulcer as revealed by X-rays is not a reliable guide to the nature of the lesion. Table 78.2 gives the radiological differences between benign and malignant ulcers.

Management

Dietary regimen is similar to that for duodenal ulcer. Antacids, ranitidine and omeprazole constitute the sheet anchor of treatment. Over 90% of ulcers generally heal in about six weeks. Drugs which encourage healing of duodenal ulcer are very effective in benign gastric ulcers as well. Repeat endoscopy is essential to confirm ulcer healing. If the ulcer has not healed by three months or if the ulcer size has increased at the end of four weeks, surgery may be considered. The recommended surgical procedure is antrectomy with Billroth I anastomosis. General management, indications for surgery and complications are similar to those described under duodenal ulcer. If there is evidence of *H. pylori* infection, it should be eradicated.

Long-term management: In all cases of peptic ulcers, recurrence of the condition can be prevented by strict avoidance of tobacco smoking and alcohol, adherence to timely diet, measures to lessen the effects of mental stress and avoidance of ulcerogenic drugs such as corticosteroids, aspirin, NSAIDs, anticoagulants, antifibrinolytic drugs and the like.

ZOLLINGER-ELLISON SYNDROME

Compared to peptic ulcer, this syndrome is rare. This syndrome consists of recurrent ulceration of the stomach, duodenum and jejunum and marked increase in gastric acid secretion caused by a gastrin-secreting tumor, commonly arising from the non-β cells of the islets of Langerhans. Most common site is the duodenum (70%). Others include the pancreas (25%) and extraintestinal areas (5%).

Textbook of Medicine

About 60% of gastrinomas are malignant, the rest are benign. Around 90–95% of patients with gastrinomas show marked hyperacidity and ulceration of the GIT. Majority of the ulcers occur in the first part of duodenum or the stomach. Multiple ulcers are common. The ulcers are generally fulminant, progressive and resistant to medical therapy. Symptoms include abdominal pain, features of recurrent gastric ulceration, diarrhea and evidence of malabsorption. Due to the very high gastric acid, the intestinal pH remains low and therefore several nutrients do not undergo proper digestion and absorption.

Diagnosis

In suspected cases, the maximal histamine test is done. By maximal histamine test, the basal acid output exceeds 10 mmols/hour and this should suggest the diagnosis. Increased levels of serum gastrin can be demonstrated by radioimmunoassay. Normally, fasting serum gastrin level is below 160 pg/mL. Values above 1000 pg/mL are diagnostic of gastrinoma. Injection of secretin in normal individuals results in the fall of serum gastrin levels, but in gastrinomas, there is a paradoxical rise, which is specific. Location of the tumor can be made in some of the cases by computed tomography (CT) scan or magnetic resonance imaging (MRI). Endosonography, selective angiography, MR angiography and operative sonography are useful for precise localization. Selective catheterization of portal venous blood enables to identify the source of gastrin production.

Management

Medical treatment consists of large doses of antisecretory drugs. Large doses of H_2 receptor antagonist drugs or PPIs help to give symptomatic relief and ulcer healing in some cases. Surgical treatment of choice is total gastrectomy or excision of the gastrinoma if it can be identified.

CARCINOMA OF THE STOMACH

Gastric carcinoma is common in Indians. Men are affected more than women. Atrophic gastritis and gastric polyps predispose to gastric carcinoma. It is more common in persons with blood group A. The growth may be polypoid, ulcerative, diffuse or infiltrative and superficially spreading. Gastric carcinomas are mostly adenocarcinomas (Fig. 78.1). Proximal cancers are related to gastroeso-

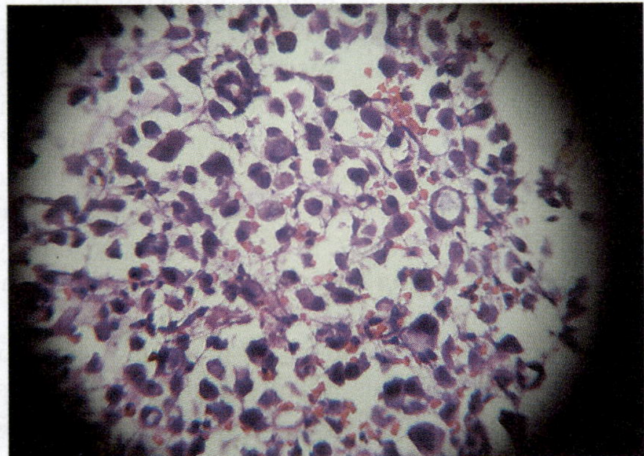

Fig. 78.1: Adenocarcinoma of stomach

phageal reflux. Male:female ratio is 2:1. Familial cancer may occur as diffuse gastric cancer.

Risk Factors

H. pylori infection, cigarette smoking, high intake of salt, bilroth II Surgery, family history of GI cancers, genetic factors, hereditary nonpolyposis colorectal cancer (HNPCC).

- ■ **Genetic factors** have been studied in detail. Germline mutation in one allele of the E-cadherin gene (CDH1) leads to diffuse familial gastric cancer, lifetime risk being 67% in men and 83% in women. Other hereditary syndromes leading to gastric cancer are Lynch syndrome (mutation in one of the mismatch repair genes 1) and Peutz Jeghers syndrome (STK11 mutation).
- ■ **Protective factors:** High intake of fresh fruits, high ascorbate intake, regular use of aspirin.

The antrum or body of the stomach may be equally affected. Around 10–20% involve the cardiac. Extension of the tumor may occur by direct spread in the gastric wall and to the perigastric tissues. Lymphatic metastases develop in the perigastric, para-aortic, portal and splenic nodes. Spread through the thoracic duct leads to enlargement of the left supraclavicular lymph nodes *(Virchow's sign)*. Distant metastases, especially to the liver, occur through the bloodstream.

Clinical Features

Upper abdominal discomfort or pain, anorexia and weight loss are the prominent features. When antral tumors produce pyloric obstruction, they lead to vomiting of stale food. Affection of the cardia around the esophageal opening causes dysphagia. Late features include anemia and widespread metastasis.

Physical Examination

Physical examination may reveal tenderness in the epigastric region or a mass in advanced cases. A gastric mass has to be distinguished from hepatic enlargement and other organs in the epigastrium. Barium meal examination helps to demonstrate the tumor. Final diagnosis can be made by endoscopy and biopsy or exfoliative cytology. Routine upper GI endoscopy and cytology helps in diagnosing the lesion before the tumor is demonstrable radiologically. Treatment of the tumor at this stage gives considerably better results. Gastroscopy, therefore, should be performed without delay in all cases of persistent upper abdominal symptoms. When endoscopy is available, this is the investigation of choice for early and definitive diagnosis (Figs 78.2A and B). Time should not be lost for radiological diagnosis since the false-negative rate is quite high and only moderately advanced lesions can be demonstrated by barium meal examination.

Prompt surgical removal of the tumor early in the course of the disease offers the only chance of cure. Metastases have to be excluded by detailed investigation. If the lesion is resected at a very early stage, the 5-year survival exceeds 90%. If the lesion does not involve the serosa or lymph nodes, the 5-year survival rate is around

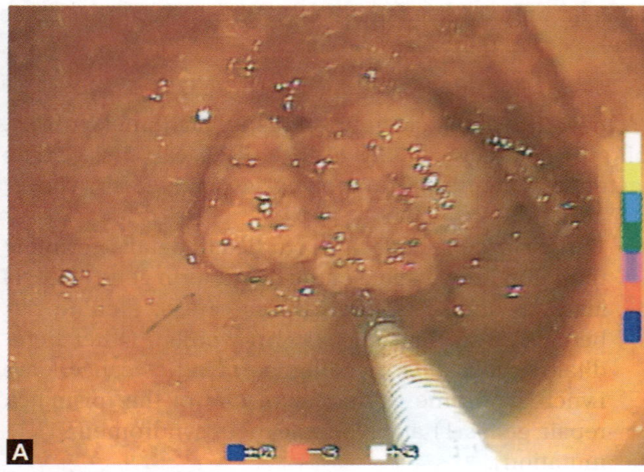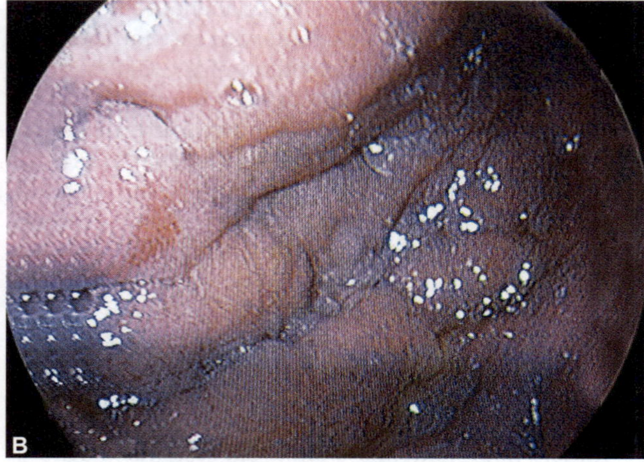

Figs 78.2A and B: Carcinoma stomach (gastroscopy). **Note:** The cauliflower growth (arrow)

Table 78.3: Methods of treatment in various stages of gastric cancer

Early gastric cancer	Endoscopic mucosal resection and dissection
Resectable cancer • Proximal and diffuse gastric cancer • Distal gastric cancer • With metastases	• Total gastrectomy • Distal gastrectomy • Neoadjuvant chemotherapy (5-fluorouracil epirubicin, cisplatin) followed by surgery
Unresectable cancer	• Chemotherapy (epirubicin, oxaliplatin, capecitabine) • Palliation (endoscopic stenting, gastrojejunostomy).

Note: Primary prevention includes avoidance of smoking, avoidance of toxic food preservatives, high intake of fresh fruits and environmental sanitation.

50%. If the nodes are affected, survival falls to 10% or less. In advanced cases, chemotherapy using 5-fluorouracil in combination with methyl-CCNU and adriamycin may induce temporary remission. Chemotherapy is generally used as an adjunct to surgery in such cases (Table 78.3).

GASTRIC OUTLET OBSTRUCTION

Syn: Pyloric obstruction

This is a common condition seen in clinical practice. Cicatrization due to peptic ulcers, antral carcinoma, pancreatic carcinoma, foreign bodies and lymphomas may lead to pyloric obstruction. Rare causes are postsurgical stenosis, pyloric and duodenal diaphragm, adult hypertrophic pyloric stenosis, annular pancreas and acute pancreatitis.

Gastric outlet obstruction produces colicky pain, visible peristalsis and vomiting of stale food. The general condition of the patient rapidly deteriorates. Gastric peristalsis has to be distinguished from small-intestinal peristalsis. Gastric peristalsis is always from left to right, while intestinal peristalsis follows a stepladder pattern without any fixed direction. Another physical sign is succussion splash which is elicitable from the stomach even after several hours of ingesting food or fluids. Normally, the stomach is emptied within three hours after food. On gastric aspiration, a residue is greater than 300 mL four hours after a meal or overnight fasting gastric residue greater than 200 mL is suggestive of gastric outlet obstruction. Barium meal studies and endoscopy with biopsy or cytology can confirm the diagnosis.

Conservative treatment consists of fluid and electrolyte replacement, gastric aspiration, stomach wash, antacids and anticholinergics. The definitive treatment is surgical.

A common cause of gastric outlet obstruction in babies is ***congenital pyloric stenosis*** which is a familial disorder affecting more often males. In them, the circular muscle coat of the pylorus is hypertrophied and this may become palpable. Pyloromyotomy relieves the obstruction.

HEMATEMESIS

Hematemesis or vomiting of blood occurs when bleeding arises from the GIT proximal to the duodenojejunal flexure (ligament of Treitz). The concentration of hydrochloric acid (HCl) in the stomach and the amount of food present, determine the color of the vomited blood. Action of the acid makes the blood brownish so that if vomiting occurs briskly after extravasation, the vomitus is bright blood, otherwise it is dark brown. A bout of hematemesis is often followed by melena which may last for up to 5 days. The common causes of hematemesis are peptic ulcer, erosive gastritis, rupture of esophageal varices and carcinoma. Drugs such as aspirin, corticosteroids, antirheumatics especially NSAIDs and anticoagulants may produce hematemesis in susceptible subjects. Gastric erosions may complicate cerebral and subarachnoid hemorrhage, burns, renal failure, hepatic failure, viper bites and shock and hematemesis may develop in them. Rare causes include ***Mallory-Weiss syndrome*** (mucosal laceration of the cardia due to vomiting), gastric polyps, leiomyomas, lymphoma and blood dyscrasias such as purpuras and coagulopathies.

If bleeding from the upper GIT is small, it leads only to melena. Hematemesis results from more massive bleeding. Hemorrhage leads to hypovolemic shock which depends on the extent and rate of hemorrhage and presence of other diseases. Loss of 20% of the blood

Textbook of Medicine

volume results in postural hypotension and tachycardia. Shock supervenes if the bleeding continues or recurs.

Risk stratification of nonvariceal bleed	
Pre-endoscopic scoring systems	• Blatchford score • Clinical Rockall score • Artificial neural network
Postendoscopic scoring systems	• Complete Rockall score • Baylor scoring system • Cedars-Sinai bleeding index

Of these scores, Rockall and Blatchford scores are used commonly.

Blatchford Scores

Admission risk marker	Value	Score component value
Blood urea	≥6.5 < 8.0 ≥8.0 < 10.0 ≥10.0 < 25.0 ≥25	2 3 4 6
Hemoglobin (g/L) for men	≥12.0 < 13.0 ≥10.0 < 12.0 <10.0	1 3 6
Hemoglobin (g/L) for women	≥10.0 <12.0 <10.0	1 6
Systolic blood pressure (mm Hg)	100–109 90–99 < 90	1 2 3
Other markers	Pulse ≥100 (per min) Presentation with melena Presentation with Syncope Hepatic disease Cardiac failure	1 2 2

Blatchford score of 6 or more are associated with a greater than 50% risk of needing an intervention.

Rockall Scoring System

Variable	Score 0	Score 1	Score 2	Score 3
Age	<60	60–79	>80	
Pulse rate (beats/minute)	<100	>100		
Systolic blood pressure (mm Hg)	Normal	>100	<100	
Co-morbidity	Nil major		CHF, IHD, major morbidity	Renal failure, liver failure, metastatic cancer
Diagnosis	Mallory–Weiss or no lesion observed	All other diagnoses	GI malignancy	
Evidence of bleeding	No stigmata or dark spot in ulcer base		Blood, adherent clot, visible vessel, active bleeding	

Rockall scores 0–2 are associated with low risk and good outcome. Score of 8 or more is associated with rebleeding rate and mortality of 41%. Endoscopic evaluation of bleeding peptic ulcer.

Abbreviations: CHF = Congestive heart failure; IHD = Ischemic heart disease; GI = Gastrointestinal

Forrest Classification

Grade forrest	Endoscopic picture
Ia	Active spurting
Ib	Oozing
IIa	Nonbleeding visible vessel (NBVV)
IIb	Adherent clot
IIc	Flat pigmented spot
III	Clean based ulcer

Management

Emergency management consists of proper assessment, general measures to combat shock and replacement of lost blood.

In many cases, the initial bout of bleeding may subside but soon fierce bleeding recurs and leads to hypovolemic shock. Due to this possibility, it is essential to hospitalize all patients with genuine hematemesis, even though the initial episode may be apparently mild. The patient should be monitored in an acute care ward.

- The patient is sedated with IV diazepam in doses of 5–10 mg given slowly over a period of 3–5 minutes.
- The pulse, respiration and blood pressure are charted at 5 minutes intervals to assess the condition and detect internal bleeding. The amount of blood lost from the stomach and in feces should be recorded.
- An IV line using a wide-bore needle is established. Central venous pressure (CVP) recording is also established for monitoring proper volume replacement.
- Present management of hematemesis has changed due to comorbidities, use of drugs such as NSAIDs, antiplatelet drugs, anticoagulant and other risk factors. Endoscopic treatment and acid suppression by PPIs form the corner stone of management. Radiological interventions and treatment of patients who are on anticoagulant medication, with high cardiovascular risk are difficult problems. Risk scores such as Rockall scores and Blatchford scores assess the risk of severe bleeding.
- ***Blood transfusion:*** Previously compatible fresh blood used to be administered at the same rate as the blood is lost till the bleeding stopped. In an ordinary case, several units of blood used to be given. At present, the policy on blood transfusion has changed. The policy is to give restricted transfusion is to raise hemoglobin above 7 g/dL. Liberal transfusion is to give blood components to raise hemoglobin above 9 g/dL. Several studies have shown that the oxygen carrying capacity is adequate at this level of hemoglobin and that mortality is not adversely influenced. If blood is not readily available, normal saline or a plasma volume expander like 6% W/V dextran can be started as IV drip till blood is procured. Mortality of severe bleeding exceeds 10%. IV erythromycin acts as a prokinetic agent which helps to clear the stomach of blood for endoscopy.
- The stomach contents are aspirated at regular intervals through a nasogastric tube which is kept in position. This helps to detect intragastric bleeding promptly and also to administer foods and medications. Through the nasogastric tube ice-cold saline lavage can be instituted. It is beneficial in some cases. Iced milk can be introduced in small quantities at regular intervals when brisk hemorrhage subsides.

Textbook of Medicine

- ***Drug therapy:*** PPIs—omeprazole and pantoprazole are highly effective in controlling bleeding and reducing rebleeding rates. Dose of omeprazole is 80 mg IV bolus followed by 8 mg/hour infusion.

Elective Endoscopic Management

Attempts must be made to establish the diagnosis. Emergency gastroduodenal endoscopy is indicated if the bleeding does not stop or recurs frequently. The bleeding spot can be visualized and cauterized by modern techniques. These include the use of bipolar electrodes, heater probes, neodymium:yttrium-aluminum-garnet (Nd:YAG) lasers and local injection of vasoconstrictor agents like adrenaline. Esophageal varices can be occluded by injecting sclerosing solutions or banding. In the case of esophageal varices, compression with Sengstaken–Blakemore tube is an effective temporary measure in trained hands.

Indications for Emergency Surgery

- Recurrent and profuse bleeding not amenable to conservative measures even after 12 hours of admission. This period may be extended if modern facilities for intervention and adequate supply of blood are available.
- In elderly subjects due to arteriosclerosis and hypertension, the bleeding tends to persist. Moreover, bleeding is poorly tolerated by such subjects. They go into metabolic complications like uremia and vascular complications like shock and disseminated intravascular coagulation (DIC). Hence, surgery should be considered early. Large ulcers and posterior ulcers in the duodenum may require early surgery.
- Presence of other medical conditions which are aggravated by blood loss.

Surgical techniques consist of ligation of bleeding vessels, undersewing the ulcer bed or excision of the bleeding area in intractable cases.

MELENA

This term denotes visible presence of altered blood in feces. Bleeding from any part of the GIT proximal to the middle of the colon can give rise to melena, if the bleeding is gradual and the blood gets partially digested during its downward passage. After a single isolated episode of bleeding, the blood may be detectable in feces for up to five days. At least 60 mL of blood should be present to produce this symptom. The black color and tarry consistency are caused by partial digestion of the blood. When bleeding in the upper GIT is brisk, the blood may pass down rapidly without allowing time for digestion and in this condition the stools may contain fresh blood. Melena occurring in a patient with obstructive jaundice imparts a silvery color to the feces.

FRESH BLOOD IN STOOLS

Syn: Hematochezia

Bleeding lesions of the large intestine or rectum generally give rise to fresh blood in stools. Conditions which produce serious bleeding per rectum are ulcerative colitis, diverticulitis, typhoid ulceration, carcinomas, polyps, Henoch-Schonlein purpura (HSP), fulminant bacterial dysentery and ischemic colitis. Bleeding from diverticulitis, ulcerative colitis, typhoid ulceration, fulminant bacterial dysentery, HSP and ischemic colitis can be massive. Polyps, carcinomas and other lesions such as angiodysplasia give rise to bleeding of variable severity. They are usually recurrent.

Hemorrhoids is probably the most frequent cause for the presence of fresh blood in stools, in all parts of the world. The blood is passed either along with the passage of stools or in drops after defecation. When the whole stool is collected in a pan, the blood will be seen on the surface of the stool or apart from the main stool mass. Proctoscopy reveals the lesion.

Presence of fresh blood in stools is an urgent indication for full investigation. The investigation should include the following.

- Examination of the whole stools passed at one time, collected in a bed pan, while defecating. This will help to settle whether the bleeding is from hemorrhoids or from higher up in the colon
- Digital examination of the rectum, proctoscopy and sigmoidoscopy
- Colonoscopy, if the lesions are beyond the reach of the sigmoidoscope
- Contrast studies—barium enema
- Isotope studies and selective angiography
- Investigations to diagnose hemorrhagic disorders.

Management of Lower GIT Bleeding

This depends upon the cause. General measures include blood transfusion and attention to the primary cause.

If the lesions can be visualized by endoscopy, procedures to arrest bleeding such as cauterization or ligation may be undertaken. Systemic diseases such as typhoid and HSP have to be managed on their own merits.

Diseases of the Small Intestine

KR Vinaya Kumar, KV Krishna Das

Chapter Summary

- Malabsorption States
  - General Considerations
  - Celiac Disease
  - Tropical Sprue
  - Carbohydrate Intolerance
  - Intraluminal Bacterial Proliferation in the Intestines
  - Parenteral Nutrition
- Irritable Bowel Syndrome (IBS)
  - General Consideration
  - Rome Diagnoistic Criteria
  - Red Flag Signs
- Crohn's Disease
- Abdominal Tuberculosis
- Intestinal Polyposis
- Vascular Disorders Affecting the Small Intestine
- Carcinoid Tumors Syndrome

MALABSORPTION STATES

General Considerations

This term includes several conditions where intraluminal defective of food and/or its subsequent absorption are defective. The processes that are impaired may be: (i) Intraluminal digestion, (ii) transfer across the mucosal lining and (iii) transport from the mucosa to the circulation and to the target organs. In some cases, the pathological mechanism is well-defined and evident, e.g. lactase deficiency. In others, several mechanisms may be involved, e.g. blind loop syndrome in which there is bacterial overgrowth, short circuiting of intestinal contents and also mucosal abnormality.

Malabsorption state is quite common in India and this may result from a number of different conditions. The clinical picture is the total outcome of: (i) nonabsorption of ingested materials resulting in steatorrhea and creatorrhea, (ii) malnutrition manifesting as loss of weight and specific deficiencies and (iii) symptoms of the underlying disease such as tropical sprue, tuberculous enterocolitis or chronic pancreatitis.

Causes of Malabsorption

- ***Abnormalities of the stomach:*** These are (i) partial or total gastrectomy, (ii) gastrocolic fistula, (iii) hypertrophic gastritis (this leads to excessive protein loss in feces) and (iv) Zollinger-Ellison syndrome.
- ***Pancreatic disorders:*** These include chronic pancreatitis, cystic fibrosis and carcinoma.
- ***Biliary disorders***
  - Long-standing obstructive jaundice leads to defective digestion and absorption of fat and fat-soluble vitamins.

- Deficiency of bile acids which may occur in two groups of conditions.

- ***Interruption of the enterohepatic circulation of bile acids:*** Bile acids, which are normally absorbed from the distal ileum, cannot be absorbed if the distal ileum is diseased or removed. Bile acids pass into the colon and are lost in the feces. They stimulate secretion of water and electrolytes in the colon. Since, the bile salts are not secreted in the bile through the enterohepatic circulation, they are not available in the proximal jejunum and therefore, fat digestion and absorption become defective, leading to diarrhea which is known as ***bile acid diarrhea***.

  When the upper small intestine is colonized by bacteria, the bile salts are deconjugated, micelle formation is inadequate, fat absorption is impaired and steatorrhea results, known as ***fatty acid diarrhea***

- ***Intestinal diseases:*** These lead to defective transport across the gut mucosa. The mucosa may show gross pathological lesions or may be histologically normal. Mucosal damage occurs in intestinal tuberculosis, tropical sprue, celiac disease, Crohn's disease, Whipple's disease and intestinal lymphoma.

  Parasitic infections like giardiasis, strongyloidiasis, schistosomiasis, trichuriasis, ascariasis, coccidiosis and cryptosporidiosis and intestinal capillariasis may interfere with absorption. The tapeworm, *Diphyllobothrium latum* uses up vitamin B_{12} from the small intestine and deprives its host of this nutrient. Soil-transmitted helminths such as *Ascaris lumbricoides* may lead to lactose intolerance in some cases. Heavy infestation by *Trichuris trichiura* can lead on to inflammatory and motility changes and result in malabsorption.

  The mucosa is histologically normal in specific enzyme defects like lactase deficiency. In pernicious anemia where absence of intrinsic factor results in the malabsorption of vitamin B_{12}, the intestine is normal histologically.

- ***Impairment of transport from the small intestine:*** Blockage of lymphatics draining the small intestine prevents the discharge of absorbed chylomicrons into the systemic circulation. This occurs in intestinal lymphomas, intestinal and mesenteric tuberculosis and primary lymphangiectasia of the mesenteric lymphatics.

  Though diarrhea is the prominent symptom in the vast majority of cases, rarely selective malabsorption (e.g. vitamin B_{12}) may be encountered even in the presence of constipation. Since different nutrients are processed at different regions of the gastrointestinal tract (GIT), the severity and type of malabsorption vary with the site of lesion. Absorption of fat and fat soluble vitamins is affected much earlier than that of the water-soluble vitamins. Loss of blood and exudates from the ulcerated mucosa further aggravates the condition in disorders like tuberculous enterocolitis and Crohn's disease. The onset may be insidious as in sprue and intestinal tuberculosis and many patients seek medical help only several months after the onset. The onset can be explosive in conditions like giardiasis.

Classification and Etiology

Disorders of intraluminal digestion	
Defect in substrate hydrolysis	
• Enzyme deficiency • Enzyme inactivation • Rapid transit of food through gut • Chronic pancreatitis	• Cystic fibrosis • Pancreatic carcinoma • Zollinger-Ellison syndrome • Gastroenterostomy • Partial gastrectomy
Defect in fat solubilization	
• Reduced transit of food through gut • Reduced bile secretion • Bile salt deconjugation and precipitation in gut • Increased bile salt loss in feces • Parenchymal liver diseases • Cholestatic jaundice	• Zollinger-Ellison syndrome • Stagnant loop syndrome or blind loop syndrome • (Colonization of small bowel by bacteria) • Terminal ileal disease (e.g. Crohn's disease, tuberculosis) • Terminal ileal resection
Defect in luminal availability of factors	
• Lack of intrinsic factor • Increased vitamin B_{12} consumption in gut	• Pernicious anemia • Stagnant loop or blind loop syndrome
Disorders of transport in the intestinal mucosal cell	
Defect in brush-border hydrolysis (mucosa normal histologically)	
Defect in epithelial transport (mucosa often abnormal histologically)	
• Lactase deficiency • Celiac disease • Tropical sprue • Lymphoma • Whipple's disease	• Giardiasis • Radiation enteritis • AIDS (acquired immuno-deficiency syndrome)
Disorders of transport from mucosal cell	
• Lymphatic obstruction • Defect in epithelial processing • Abdominal lymphoma	• Tuberculosis • Lymphangiectasia • Abetalipoproteinemia

Drugs Causing Malabsorption

Drug	**Mechanisms**
• Colchicine	• Inhibits crypt cell division and lactase
• Neomycin	• Precipitation of bile salts in gut; inhibition of lactase
• Methotrexate	• Folic acid antagonist causing inhibition of crypt cell division
• Cholestyramine	• Multiple mechanisms
• Laxatives	• Vitamin B_{12} malabsorption
• Proton pump inhibitor—on long- term therapy	

Clinical Features

Gastrointestinal (GI)

In most of the cases, GI symptoms predominate. Common presentations are diarrhea, especially steatorrhea, distension of the abdomen, abdominal discomfort and increased amounts of flatus which may be very foul-smelling, especially when digestion is impaired.

Diarrhea is more prominent during the early part of the day, with relief in the later part. Nutritional inadequacy results from general malabsorption. It manifests as weight loss, fatigue, lethargy and failure of growth and development in children. Anemia occurs due to deficiency of iron, folate and/or B_{12}. Rickets, osteomalacia and tetany may develop due to defective absorption of vitamin D and calcium. Nutritional edema develops due to impairment of protein absorption. Glossitis, angular stomatitis, peripheral neuropathy and pellagra develop due to malabsorption of B complex factors (Fig. 79.1). Bleeding tendency results from vitamin K deficiency. Vitamin A deficiency leads to night blindness and other ocular manifestations.

Psychiatric symptoms such as anxiety, loss of confidence, irritability and depression are very common, especially when diarrhea is the prominent symptom.

Symptoms

Symptoms and signs of malabsorption and relevant pathophysiology are listed in Table 79.1.

Investigations

Examination of feces: The stools are large, bulky, greasy and pale. There is a tendency to froth and stick to the toilet. In normal persons, the stool fat is below 6–7 g per day on a diet which contains up to 100 g of fat. In malabsorption states, the fat content is increased and this is referred to as ***steatorrhea***. If the pancreatic digestion is unaffected, the fat is present as fatty acids. If the pancreatic function is defective, the fat is present as neutral fat. Microscopic examination reveals fat globules.

Fecal nitrogen should be less than 2.5 g per day in normal subjects. Values above this level suggest malabsorption. Presence of intact muscle fibers in stools, demonstrable microscopically is called ***creatorrhea***.

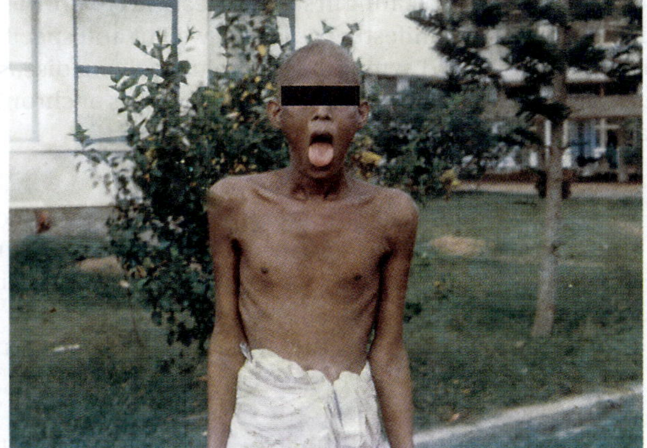

Fig. 79.1: Malabsorption state (male; 40) intestinal resection. ***Note:*** Loss of weight and glossitis

Textbook of Medicine

Table 79.1: Symptoms and signs of malabsorption and relevant pathophysiology

Symptom or sign	Pathophysiologic explanation
Gastrointestinal (GI)	
Diarrhea	Osmotic activity of carbohydrates or short-chain fatty acids Secretory effect of bile acids and fatty acids Decreased absorptive surface Intestinal loss of conjugated bile acids
Abdominal distension, flatulence	Bacterial gas production from carbohydrates in colon, small intestinal bacterial overgrowth
Foul-smelling flatulence or stool	Malabsorption of proteins or intestinal protein loss
Pain	Gaseous distention of intestine
Ascites	Protein loss or malabsorption
Musculoskeletal	
Tetany, muscle weakness, paresthesias	Malabsorption of vitamin D, calcium, magnesium and phosphate
Bone pain, osteomalacia, fractures	Protein, calcium or vitamin D deficiency; secondary hyperparathyroidism
Cutaneous and mucosal	
Easy bruisability, ecchymoses, petechiae	Vitamin K and C deficiency
Glossitis, cheilosis, stomatitis	Vitamin B complex, vitamin B_{12}, folate or iron deficiency
Edema	Protein loss or malabsorption
Ichthyosis, Acrodermatitis, scaly dermatitis	Zinc and essential fatty acid deficiency
Follicular hyperkeratosis	Vitamin A deficiency
Hyperpigmented dermatitis	Niacin deficiency (pellagra)
Koilonychia	Iron deficiency
Perifollicular hemorrhage	Malabsorption of vitamin C
Others	
Weight loss, hyperphagia	Nutrient malabsorption
Growth and weight retardation, infantilism	Nutrient malabsorption in childhood and adolescence
Anemia	Iron, folate or vitamin B_{12} deficiency
Kidney stones	Increased colonic oxalate absorption
Amenorrhea, impotence, infertility	Multifactorial (including protein malabsorption, secondary hypopituitarism, anemia)
Night blindness, xerophthalmia	Vitamin A deficiency
Peripheral neuropathy	Vitamin B_{12} or thiamine deficiency
Fatigue, weakness	Calorie depletion, iron and folate deficiency, anemia
Neurologic symptoms, ataxia	Vitamin B_{12}, vitamin E or folate deficiency

Blood examination: Serum albumin may be reduced in severe cases and they may show dependent edema. Serum iron, folate, vitamin B_{12}, carotene and cholesterol are lowered depending on the severity and duration of the malabsorption state. Vitamin K-dependent coagulation factors are deficient and this results in prolongation of prothrombin time. Blood picture may be microcytic or macrocytic depending on the predominant deficiency.

Studies of Intestinal Absorption

- ***Xylose absorption test:*** In this study, 5 g of xylose is given orally and the urinary excretion over the next 5 hours and the serum levels are determined. Normal persons excrete at least 1 g in urine in 5 hours and the blood levels reach 25 mg/dL 2 hours after the oral dose. In malabsorption due to mucosal disease affecting the upper small intestine, urinary elimination is lowered. This test is not foolproof since delayed gastric emptying, renal disease and sequestration of D-xylose in muscles and edema fluid reduce the urinary excretion.

- ***Lactose absorption:*** This will be defective in lactase deficiency. Normal subjects absorb lactose and the blood level of glucose should increase 20–30 mg/dL 2 hours after oral administration of 50–100 g of lactose. The blood levels will be deficient in subjects with lactase deficiency. The specific test for lactase deficiency is demonstration of diminished amount of the enzyme by biochemical estimation in biopsy specimens of intestinal mucosa.

- ***Vitamin B_{12} absorption (Schilling test):*** Radioactive vitamin B_{12} is administered orally and the fecal loss and urinary elimination are estimated. Normally, more than 7% of administered vitamin B_{12} is eliminated in urine in 12 hours. Vitamin B_{12} absorption is impaired in lesions affecting the distal ileum.

- ***Fecal fat estimation:*** Generally, feces is collected for three days for the estimation of fat. Absorption studies employing radiolabeled fat (***^{14}C-triolein test***) reveals excessive loss of ingested fat which appears in feces.

- ***Fecal protein loss:*** Fecal nitrogen is grossly increased in protein-losing enteropathy. This is diagnosed by

Textbook of Medicine

labeling serum protein with radioactive chromium and detecting its appearance in feces.

- **Radiology:** Radiological study of the GIT after ingestion of barium-meal reveals reduction in transit time of the intestinal contents and segmentation and flocculation of barium in the small intestine. Anatomical abnormalities such as ulceration, strictures, tumors, fistulae and blind loops are demonstrated.

- **Sampling of the intestinal contents:** Using special tubes which can be passed under fluoroscopic control, the intestinal contents can be sampled from different levels. Endoscopic aspiration can be performed from sites accessible to the endoscope. Aliquots obtained by aspiration are examined for enzyme content and nutrients and also microbiologically. The effect of secretory stimulants like secretin and pancreozymin can also be studied.

- **Biopsy studies:** Using the Crosby capsule, peroral biopsies used to be obtained from various sites. This is seldom used at present. Endoscopic biopsies can be obtained where facilities are available. The mucosa can be examined under the dissecting microscope to assess the villus pattern. Further histopathological and histochemical studies can be undertaken. In malabsorption, intestinal villi show blunting, confluence, atrophy and varying degrees of round cell infiltration.

  Since minor degrees of villus atrophy and cellular infiltration may be found in normal individuals, mucosal biopsy alone cannot be considered pathognomonic, especially if the abnormalities are mild. It gives valuable information when considered in the light of other investigations. Biopsy is the mainstay of diagnosis in conditions like tuberculosis, Crohn's disease and Whipple's disease.

- **Breath tests:** They are useful in the diagnosis of steatorrhea, bacterial overgrowth of the intestines, lactase deficiency and ileal disease. ^{14}C-labeled triolein is given with a lipid meal and breath $^{14}CO_2$ is estimated. Level of $^{14}CO_2$ in breath correlates with the capacity for fat absorption. ^{14}C-cholylglycine breath test is a screening test for bacterial overgrowth in the intestine and impaired ileal absorption of conjugated bile salts. Estimation of breath hydrogen levels after an oral dose of 12.5–25 g of lactose gives an indication of the capacity to absorb lactose. In malabsorption states, the unabsorbed lactose is acted upon by bacteria in the colon to produce excess hydrogen which appears in blood and is eliminated in the breath. Increased levels of breath hydrogen indicate bacterial overgrowth in the intestine. Lactulose can be given instead of lactose for the same purpose.

Treatment

- **Dietary management:** The diet has to be modified depending upon the type and severity of malabsorption. Since fats and to a lesser extent carbohydrates cause diarrhea, these have to be restricted. Proteins do not cause diarrhea and they should be given in the usual form or as predigested proteins to avoid negative nitrogen balance. All vitamins have to be supplemented. Parenteral supplementation of nutrients has to be resorted to if oral feeding is not tolerated or is ineffective. Vitamins and minerals have to be given parenterally regularly.

- **Specific management:** This depends upon the cause. Several diseases leading to malabsorption are curable, e.g. giardiasis, lactase deficiency, tuberculous enteritis. Many conditions which may not be curable ultimately, can be treated symptomatically and normal health restored, e.g. pernicious anemia. Such conditions should be looked for and treated appropriately.

Celiac Disease

Syn: Gluten-induced enteropathy

This disease is produced by immunologically mediated or direct inflammatory response initiated by gliadin which is present in gluten, which is a component of wheat, rye, barley and oats. Pathological changes are seen in the mucosa from the duodenojejunal junction to variable lengths distally. Circulating antibodies to gluten are demonstrable in many cases. The disease is less common in India compared to the West. In the West, the prevalence of celiac disease in the general population is 1/266. Human leukocyte antigen (HLA) associations include HLA-DQ2 (DOA1-*05/DOB1/*02) or HLA-D08 (DOA1* 0301/DQBI*0302).

Gluten triggers the production of certain immunoglobulin A (IgA) class antibodies called R1 type reticulin and endomysial antibodies (EMA). These include IgA anti-endomysial antibodies, anti-tissue transglutaminase antibodies (anti-tTG) and IgA-anti-gliadin antibodies (IgA-AGA). Their presence is pathognomonic. The reticulin and EMA are directed against fibroblast derived extracellular matrix-proteins known as *celiac disease* autoantigen proteins. The disease is self-perpetuating unless the trigger gliadin is removed.

Clinical Features

The disease is more prevalent in young persons. Symptoms start between the ages of 1 and 3 when cereals are introduced into the diet. The child fails to thrive, becomes irritable and develops characteristic steatorrhea. The symptoms show periodic remissions and exacerbations over the years. There is increased incidence of intestinal lymphoma in these subjects.

Adult celiac disease may occur at any age. It is characterized by anemia, loss of weight, diarrhea and varying degrees of malabsorption of iron, folic acid, vitamin D and vitamin B_{12}.

Dermatitis herpetiformis: This is a frequent association of celiac disease. Skin shows blistering subepidermal eruptions. This is a classic non-GI manifestation of celiac disease. Histology shows granular IgA deposit in the affected sites. Withdrawal of gliadin clears the skin lesion also.

Avoidance of gluten in the diet relieves the skin lesions as well. In intractable cases, dapsone given orally in a dose of 50–200 mg/day helps to clear the lesions.

Diagnosis

It is made from the history, demonstration of malabsorption and characteristic histology. Improvement on withdrawal of wheat or rye and aggravation on reintroduction suggest the diagnosis. Histologically, the mucosal atrophy increased intraepithelial lymphocytes, crypt hyperplasia and villous atrophy during the active stages of the disease and its clearance during abstinence from gluten containing diet can be demonstrated.

Serologic diagnosis

The serologic tests available are IgA, EMA, IgA-tTG, IgA-AGA and IgG-AGA, IgG-deamidated glycopeptides (DGP). AGA has lower sensitivity. EMA are directed against the connective tissue surrounding the smooth muscles. It is sensitive and specific, but expensive. The epitope against which EMA is directed is identified as tTG. IgA-tTG is more specific and sensitive. It is also cheaper. In low-prevalence areas, a negative tTG test virtually rules out celiac disease. IgA-anti-tTG antibody is the preferred single test for detection of celiac disease in individuals over the age of 2 years. In patients in whom low IgA or selective IgA deficiency is identified, IgG-based testing (IgG-DGP and IgG-tTG) should be performed.

Complications:
- **GI malignancies:** An increased incidence of both GI (e.g. **Carcinoma of the esophagus**) and non-GI neoplasms as well as enteropathy-associated T cell lymphoma (EATCL) is observed in celiac disease
- Development of intestinal ulceration independent of lymphoma **(ulcerative jejunitis),** refractory sprue and collagenous sprue
- **Nonresponsive celiac disease:** Few patients do not improve on a strict diet
- Refractory celiac disease
- Pneumococcal infections
- Dermatitis herpetiformis
- Osteomalacia.

Treatment

Avoidance of wheat, barley, rye and oats in all forms brings about dramatic relief within weeks. Full recovery takes a few months to years. Apparent failure of therapy is due to inadvertent inclusion of the offending cereals in the diet. In addition to the gluten-free diet, patient with newly diagnosed celiac disease should receive nutritional supplementation of calcium, iron, vitamin D, vitamin B_{12}, folic acid and other trace elements. Glucocorticoids are reserved for severly ill patients with acute celiac crisis manifested by severe diarrhea, dehydration, weight loss, acidosis, hypocalcemia, hypoproteinemia.

Tropical Sprue

This is a syndrome which occurs exclusively in the tropics. It is characterized by morphological abnormalities of the small intestine associated with malabsorption of two or more unrelated substances without any detectable cause. This disease has been reported from various parts of Asia, Africa and South America. In India, the disease is present sporadically in all regions, but maximum number of cases have been reported from Vellore, Tamil Nadu. Foreigners who have resided for varying periods in India and other neighboring countries may be affected. In the indigenous population, sprue is more common among poor malnourished young adults. Folate deficiency precipitated by pregnancy and severe malnutrition can aggravate the disease. More cases are seen during the hot humid months. The disease occurs sporadically though several small outbreaks have also been recorded.

In celiac disease, involvement of proximal small intestine predominates whereas tropical sprue affects the distal small intestine and terminal ileum.

The etiology of tropical sprue is not clearly understood. The prevalence of the disease in residents of certain localities, occurrence of several cases in the same household (sprue houses), seasonal prevalence and the favorable response to antibiotics suggest an infective etiology. The onset is insidious. The clinical features are mainly steatorrhea and the sequelae of generalized malabsorption.

The jejunal histology is variable. The changes seen are epithelial cell damage, lengthening of the crypts, broadening and shortening of the villi and varying degrees of chronic inflammatory cell infiltration. Complete villous atrophy seen in some patients with celiac disease is not seen in tropical sprue. A normal jejunal mucosal biopsy rules out tropical sprue.

Treatment

Many patients improve with hospitalization and correction of malnutrition. In addition to general treatment, administration of tetracycline 1 g daily in divided doses for 6 months results in clinical improvement, reduction of jejunal bacterial counts and correction of the histological abnormality. Folic acid 10 mg orally four times daily is given for 6 months. In cases of severe malabsorption, folic acid in intramuscular (IM) dose of 10 mg may have to be given for the initial few days. The condition is likely to recur in many cases if proper dietary care is not followed.

Whipple's Disease

Whipple's disease is a chronic systemic infection caused by Gram–positive actinomycete *Tropheryma whipplei*. The bacteria has high infectivity, but low virulence. Almost any organ can be affected characterized by diarrhea, steatorrhea, abdominal pain, weight loss, migratory large-joint arthropathy and fever, ophthalmologic and central nervous system (CNS) symptoms. It is a sporadic disorder with a predilection for middle-aged white men. The steatorrhea in these patients is generally believed to be secondary to both small-intestinal mucosal injury and lymphatic obstruction secondary to the increased number of periodic acid-schiff (PAS)-positive macrophages in the lamina propria of the small intestine.

The diagnosis of clinically suspected Whipple's disease is by endoscopy with mucosal biopsy. Obtaining tissue biopsies from the small intestine or other organs that may be involved (e.g. liver, lymph nodes, heart, eyes, CNS or synovial membranes), based on the patient's symptoms, and is the primary approach to establish the diagnosis of Whipple's disease. The presence of PAS-positive macrophages containing the characteristic small bacilli is suggestive of this diagnosis. The swollen cytoplasm of macrophages appear foamy when stained with hematoxylin-eosin (H&E). PAS stain shows numerous granular particles due to glycoprotein content of bacterial cell wall. Electron microscopy shows uniformity in size and shape of bacteria with an external diameter of 0.2–0.25 µm and a length up to 2.5 µm. Now, polymerase chain reaction (PCR) analysis is a preferred confirmatory test.

Treatment

Induction phase treatment with either penicillin G plus streptomycin or a third generation cephalosporin for two weeks followed by treatment with trimethoprim-sulfamethoxazole for atleast one year. Rifampin, chloramphenicol, erythromycin, doxycycline are alternative drugs.

Carbohydrate Intolerance

Disaccharidase Deficiency

This is a common condition which is often missed. Carbohydrate intolerance may result from:

- Deficiency of specific disaccharidase
- Impairment of transport of monosaccharides in the intestine
- Diffuse mucosal disease resulting in deficiency of disaccharidases and impairment of monosaccharide transport.

Symptoms are vague and they consist of bloated feeling, gaseous distension, belching, colicky pain, borborygmi and diarrhea following ingestion of lactose or other carbohydrates. Diarrhea results from the osmotic effect caused by unabsorbed low molecular weight carbohydrates. Flatulence is produced by fermentation of carbohydrate in the intestines.

Most widespread enzyme deficiency is that of lactase. This may be acquired or congenital. The former manifests in later years whereas the latter is present from birth. Causes of acquired deficiency include diarrheal states, intestinal parasitism and primary intestinal diseases. These tend to be transient and are relieved when the underlying condition is corrected.

Diagnosis is suggested by lactose absorption tests and breath tests showing excessive hydrogen after oral lactose challenge.

Treatment

Many patients learn to avoid symptoms by omitting the offending articles of diet. Exclusion of lactose (milk and dairy products and baked foods containing dairy products) from the diet gives relief.

Intraluminal Bacterial Proliferation in the Intestines

Normally, the jejunal contents show only less than 10^5 bacteria/mL. Most of these are derived from swallowed bacteria. Gastric acidity and intestinal motility help to keep down the bacterial counts. Impairment of these functions results in bacterial overgrowth. The bacteria hydrolyze conjugated bile salts in the jejunum and this leads to defective micelle formation and absorption of fat. Deconjugated bile salts also damage the mucosa directly. In addition, proliferating bacteria use up essential vitamins like vitamin B_{12} from the proximal small intestine before they reach the ileum and thus deprive the host of these vitamins. Paradoxically, folate levels may be high since the bacteria produce folate.

Causes

- **Structural lesions:** Diverticula, blind loops, fistulae, strictures occurring in intestinal tuberculosis, vascular lesions, radiation enteritis and Crohn's disease, postoperative or traumatic adhesions and afferent loop stasis after gastric operations.
- **Fistulae:** Gastrocolic, jejunocolic, jejunoileal and others.
- **Hypochlorhydria and achlorhydria:** Postgastric surgery, mucosal atrophy, total gastrectomy, vagotomy, atrophic gastritis, pernicious anemia and severe malnutrition including iron deficiency anemia (IDA).
- **Abnormalities of intestinal motility:** Systemic sclerosis, amyloidosis, diabetic and other autonomic neuropathies, paralytic ileus, pseudo-obstruction and postvagotomy ileus.
- **Hypo- or agammaglobulinemia.**

Symptoms of the primary disease may be present. In addition, those due to malabsorption may also be present.

The condition is diagnosed by quantitative culture of the intestinal contents. Breath tests using lactulose or ^{14}C-labelled cholylglycine are helpful. Appropriate investigations are indicated to detect the underlying cause and plan definitive therapy.

Treatment

Rifaximin eradicates bowel overgrowth syndrome in as many as 80% of patients. The standard dose is 600 or 800 mg/day oral. Higher doses (1200 or 1600 mg/day) are more effective. Administration of tetracycline in a dose of 1 g/day in divided dosage for 3–4 weeks relieves the symptoms temporarily. Since tetracycline is not freely available at present, other antibacterial agents such as metronidazole, amoxicillin-clavulanate, ciprofloxacin and co-trimoxazole have been tried with benefit. Surgical treatment for anatomical abnormality should be advised if the lesion is correctable.

Parenteral Nutrition

See also Section 5 Nutrition

General Considerations

Parenteral alimentation is necessary when ingestion and absorption of nutrients are inadequate, impossible over long periods of time or contraindicated. In several situations such as organ transplantation, postoperative states, post-traumatic states, burns and others where ingestion of food is not possible or excess have to be given to overcome hypercatabolic states, parenteral alimentation becomes mandatory. If excess of calories are administered, this is called **hyperalimentation**. When the process has to be continued over several days or weeks, a central venous line is necessary. Proprietary preparations are available. These are highly expensive. It is preferable to use an infusion pump and monitor the rate of nutrient delivery.

Nutrient Solutions

Carbohydrates and fats form the two main sources of calories. Supply of 200–250 g of glucose daily is adequate to prevent starvation ketosis. Adequate calorie supply can be achieved by administration of 600–700 g glucose given as a 20–30% solution through a central venous catheter.

Textbook of Medicine

Administration of glucose in this concentration into peripheral veins causes damage to the venous walls and leads to thrombophlebitis.

Lipids can be given as a 10% emulsion intravenous (IV). Fat emulsions being isotonic, can be infused into peripheral veins. Addition of amino acids and glucose to the fat emulsion provides all the proximate principles. The source of fat is soybean or cottonseed oil and the fatty acid is oleic or linoleic acid. The common source of nitrogen is crystalline amino acids and the equivalent of 8–16 g is to be supplied daily. Amino acids are supplied as mixture of essential and nonessential amino acids in a ratio of 1:1.5. Amino acids will be used for anabolic activity only if 150–250 carbohydrate calories are also supplied simultaneously for each gram of nitrogen.

Vitamins, minerals and other electrolytes have to be supplied; their quantity is to be determined by biochemical estimations. Optimal quantities of electrolytes have to be supplied to ensure complete metabolic utilization of the nutrients in solution.

In general, for every 1000 calories, NaCl–10 mmol, K^+–20 mmol, PO_4–30 mmol, Mg^{2+}–8 mmol and Ca^{2+}–5 mmol are to be supplied in addition to daily losses. Several solutions are available commercially for parenteral nutrition (PN).

When nutrients are administered into a peripheral vein without recourse to a central venous catheter, it is referred to as ***peripheral PN***.

In the commercially available parenteral solutions, energy is provided by glucose and long chain triglycerides in almost equal proportions. 150–250 calories should be provided with 1 g of nitrogen which is provided mainly as amino acids. For providing nutritional balance, energy supply should be 25–40 cal/kg bw/hour. Nitrogen should be provided at the rate of 0.2–0.3 g/kg bw/hour.

Complications include sepsis, blockage of the catheter and other mechanical problems. The metabolic complications associated with PN include hyperglycemia, hypoglycemia, hyperlipidemia, hypercapnia, refeeding syndrome, acid-base disturbances, liver complications, manganese toxicity and metabolic bone disease. After initial hospitalization to set up PN, subsequent treatment can be continued at home. The solutions are prohibitively expensive for routine use.

IRRITABLE BOWEL SYNDROME (IBS)

General Considerations

This condition has been known by several synonyms such as mucous colitis, spastic colon, irritable colon and colonic neurosis. In the West, 20–30% of GI disorders are constituted by IBS. In India, this is very common and many cases used to be diagnosed as chronic amebiasis in the past. It is a functional disorder to the intestine characterized by alteration of the bowel habits and abdominal pain in the absence of any detectable organic pathology.

There is no morphologic, histologic, microbiologic or biochemical abnormality in IBS. Changes in gut motility are observed in several studies though they poorly correlate with the symptoms. In the constipated variety, the frequency of high altitude peristaltic contractions is less whereas nonpropulsive segmentation contractions are more. Moreover, food induced hypermotility of the colon occurring normally about one hour after the meal is reduced in many patients. This may account for their postprandial symptoms. Emotional stress is seen to aggravate the motility disorder.

Normally, gut has two types of myoelectrical activity— the basic electric rhythm (BER) and spike activity (SA). The BER is in the continuous wave form at a rate of 6 cycles per minute. The SA is the form of electrical bursts superimposed on BER and this is responsible for the mechanical contraction of the gut. IBS patients have a slow BER at a rate of 3 cycles per minute. In normal people, feeding induces SA immediately which peaks in 30 minutes and lasts for about 50 minutes. But in IBS patients, the feeding induced SA is dampened in the first 50 minutes, but it becomes stronger later on.

Clinical Features

In India, the female to male ratio is 1:3, though in the West, females suffer more. The clinical spectrum is wide.

Types of IBS

- IBS with constipation (hard or lumpy stools ≥25%/ loose or watery stools <25% of bowel movements)
- IBS with diarrhea (loose or water stools ≥25 %/ hard or lumpy stools <5% of bowel movements)
- Mixed IBS (hard or lumpy stools ≥25%/ loose or watery stools ≥25% of bowel movements)
- Unsubtyped IBS (insufficient abnormality of stool consistency to meet the above subtypes).

The common age group is 20–40 years. Symptoms are vague and these include abnormal bowel habits ranging from constipation to diarrhea (often alternating irregularly), pellet like stools, increased gastrocolic reflex, vague abdominal pain ranging from dull ache to severe colic, flatulence relieved by belching, capricious appetite and insomnia. Around 20% of subjects complain of weight loss. All patients are emotionally tense and they tend to exaggerate the disability.

Examination does not reveal any abnormality except for vague tenderness over the abdomen, palpable cecum and sigmoid, increased bowel sounds and signs of anxiety. Majority of these patients go from doctor to doctor getting repeated prescriptions such as amebicides, antibiotics, sedatives, tranquilizers and massive doses of vitamins. Most of them are wrongly diagnosed as amebiasis, neurosis or other colonic disorders.

Clinical examination should always be followed by macroscopic examination of a total stool, passed in a clean container. The feces is large in volume, the consistency may vary from hard to semisolid, it may froth and mucus may be present, but, there is no blood. Microscopy helps to exclude dysentery, amebiasis and other intestinal parasites. IBS seriously reduces the quality of life of the affected individuals and is an important medical cause of reduced work output. Investigations such as colonoscopy and tests for malabsorption need be done only in those patients with alarm symptoms.

Diagnosis

This condition (IBS) should be diagnosed clinically and other similar conditions should be excluded by investigations. Amebiasis, giardiasis, malabsorption states, tuberculous enterocolitis, ulcerative colitis, diverticulitis, purgative abuse and heavy helminthic infestations should be excluded. Till recently, IBS remained a diagnosis arrived at by exclusion of similar conditions. At present, diagnostic criteria have been laid down. These include:

Rome III diagnostic criteria for IBS
Recurrent abdominal pain or discomfort at least 3 days per month in the last 3 months associated with 2 or more of the following:
- Improvement with defecation
- Onset associated with a change in frequency of stool
- Onset associated with a change in form (appearance) of stool.

Investigations

The blood picture in IBS is usually normal. Stool examination repeated thrice including one concentration smear helps to exclude amebiasis and other intestinal parasites. All IBS patients do not require extensive investigation. Routine investigations may be done in all patients. Investigations such as colonoscopy, small bowel barium studies and tests for malabsorption are required only in a limited number in whom the diagnosis is not clear.

Sigmoidoscopy and colonoscopy reveal only hyperemia and normal nonfriable mucosa with excess of mucus. This helps to differentiate IBS from ulcerative colitis and amebiasis. Intestinal biopsy is normal. Barium enema is not diagnostic and may show only nonspecific changes. It is ideal to reassure the patient only after excluding more serious underlying disease.

Red flag signs of IBS:
- More than minimal rectal bleeding
- Weight loss
- Unexplained IDA
- Nocturnal symptoms
- Family history of selected organic diseases including colorectal cancer, IBS or celiac sprue
- Fever.

Management

Reassurance and psychological support is most important in allaying anxiety and this is very effective in majority of cases. Even if the diagnosis of IBS seems to be the most likely one, it is advisable to follow-up the patient at frequent intervals for at least one year to detect weight loss, development of anemia, presence of blood in stools and other systemic disturbances, which all should raise the possibility of more serious colonic diseases.

Diet

All offending articles of diet which aggravate symptoms should be avoided. In general, a moderate-roughage diet is advisable. The use of high-fiber diets has been advocated in spastic colon but the results are not uniformly encouraging.

Substances that increase stool bulk like methylcellulose (*Isogel, ispaghula husk*) or bran generally improve stool consistency and give relief. Several drugs are in vogue for management of IBS. In practice, the ideal drug regimen has to be determined by trial and error since no drug may act predictably. As a rule of the thumb, the following drugs may be tried first depending on the symptoms.

- ***Diarrhea predominant:*** Loperamide 4 mg, diphenoxylate 5 mg, anticholinergics, codeine phosphate 30 mg.

  The 5-hydroxytryptamine ($5HT_3$) antagonists such as alosetron have proved effective in preventing urgency for defecation. Alosetron taken prophylactically helps to avoid embarrassment during travel and social functions.
- ***Constipation predominant:*** Dietary fiber, osmotic laxatives, stool softeners like liquid paraffin, cisapride and enemata. Tegaserod which is a $5HT_4$ antagonist helps to relieve constipation.
- Pain, gas, bloating, etc. Anticholinergics, anti-gas preparations such as methyl siloxane or activated charcoal and antidepressant drugs.

Tranquilizers are indicated if there is severe anxiety. Psychiatric counseling helps in the majority of cases. Amitriptyline 10–25 mg given at night may benefit a few who have depression and despair.

Long-term favorable clinical results have been achieved with rifaximin in patients with IBS.

Advances in treatment of IBS: A new drug ***eluxadoline*** which is a new class of drug with opioid receptor effect (μ and κ-opioid receptor agonist and δ-opioid receptor antagonist); given in doses of 100 mg orally twice daily, reduces diarrhea in both cases, the drug was found to be effective over a 6 month period. Abdominal pain also reduced.

Source: Lembo AJ, Lacy BE, Zuckerman MJ, et al. Eluxadoline for Irritable Bowel Syndrome with Diarrhea. N Engl J Med. 2016;374(3):242-53.

CROHN'S DISEASE

Syn: Regional enteritis, Granulomatous colitis

This rare disorder is mainly characterized by localized areas of granulomatous inflammation of the small intestine. Rarely, all other parts of the GIT may be affected. The etiology is unknown. It is more common in West especially among Jews and it is rare in India. There is evidence that the incidence is increasing in India.

Etiology

Though the exact cause is not known, factors such as genetic predisposition, infective agents and autoimmune phenomena have been implicated.

Pathology

The role of disturbances in gut flora is being investigated. Viable ***Mycobacterium avium paratuberculosis*** has been detected in a substantial proportion of cases. Specific genes related to the development of Crohn's disease include NOD2 (also called CARD15). This gene is expressed in monocytes, macrophages, dendrite cells and also intestinal epithelial cells including Paneth cells. Lesions are maximal in the terminal ileum. The bowel is edematous, swollen and narrowed. Later the mucosa appears nodular and ulcerated. Classically normal and abnormal segments alternate and this is referred to as ***skip lesions***. The mesentery and lymph nodes are involved. Histologically, lesions are characterized by chronic granulo-

Textbook of Medicine

matous inflammation containing lymphocytes and plasma cells extending through all the layers of the intestinal wall. In 50% cases, there are well-defined non-caseating granulomas containing multinucleate giant cells.

Clinical Features

The disease affects persons aged 15–35 years more and it is characterized by remissions and relapses. Presenting symptoms include fatigue, weight loss, right lower quadrant pain and diarrhea. The pain is continuous and localized but may be colicky. Moderate diarrhea follows; the feces is not visibly mixed with blood.

Physical Examination

Physical examination reveals a tender mass in the right lower quadrant made up of inflamed loops of bowel. Acute ileitis may resemble acute appendicitis and sometimes the diagnosis is made on laparotomy. Rarely, the disease may present as prolonged pyrexia, intestinal obstruction, fistulization and malabsorption syndrome. Enteropathic arthritis is a frequent complication.

Diagnosis

Diagnosis should be suspected clinically. Laboratory investigations are nonspecific and are of little value. The erythrocyte sedimentation rate (ESR) may be moderately raised. There may be leukocytosis, anemia and presence of occult blood in stools. Antineutrophil cytoplasmic antibodies (ANCA) and anti-saccharomyces cerevisiae antibodies (ASCA)—ANCA and ASCA have been proposed as a means for diagnosing ischemic bowel disease (IBD) and distinguishing Crohn's disease (CD) from ulcerative colitis.

A barium examination of the small bowel reveals loss of mucosal pattern, rigidity and narrowing of the affected segments and a *cobble stone* appearance. The characteristic radiological feature is the *string sign* which is produced by the narrowing of the diseased segment with dilatation of the normal intestine on either side. Fistulous tracts, strictures and fibrosis may be demonstrable in advanced cases (Fig. 79.2). Stomach and duodenum may be involved and the picture may resemble an infiltrative tumor. Barium enema reveals colonic lesions. Endoscopy reveals the lesions, strictures, fistulae and other complications. Endoscopic biopsy is also confirmatory.

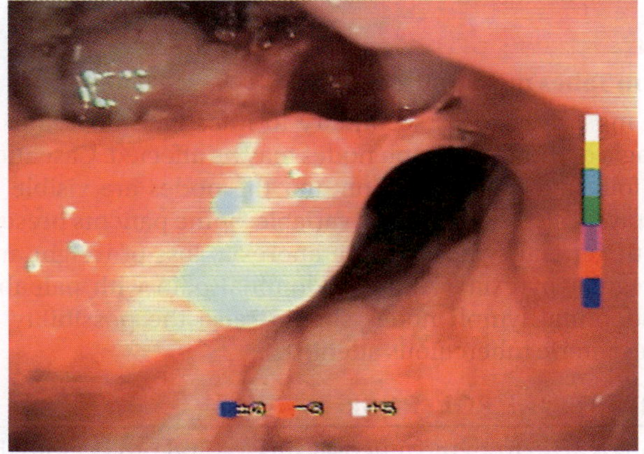

Fig. 79.2: Crohn's disease: Fistulous tract—endoscopic view

Differential Diagnosis

Crohn's disease may be mistaken for tuberculosis of the ileocecal region, lymphoma, appendicular abscess, amebiasis, carcinoma cecum and ulcerative colitis.

Prognosis

In acute regional enteritis, the prognosis is good since in two-third of the cases, the condition subsides without recurrence. In chronic regional enteritis, the disease tends to be recurrent and chronic.

Principles of Treatment

Low residue diet containing adequate calories and protein should be instituted. Diarrhea is relieved by drugs like diphenoxylate (lomotil) 2–5 mg/day or codeine 30–60 mg orally 2–3 times a day.

Sulfasalazine 2–6 g/day is moderately effective. This drug is less effective in this condition than in ulcerative colitis. Corticosteroids are given if active disease persists. Prednisolone 40–60 mg/day is started and reduced over a few months. Budesonide which is a topically active glucocorticoid is effective in relieving symptoms, when given orally in a dose of 8 mg/day. Methotrexate, azathioprine, ciprofloxacin in combination with metronidazole have all been used.

Newer drugs: Mongersen given orally in dose of 10, 40 or 160 mg daily for 2 weeks was tried in recurrent Crohn's disease. Fifty five percent as 40 mg and 65% of those on 160 mg reached remission compared to 12% on placebo, as Mongersen is prepared as a modified release tablet designed to deliver the active ingredients primarily into the lumen of the terminal ileum and right sidede colon.

Source: Monteleone G, Neurath MF, Ardizzone S, et al. Mongersen, an oral SMAD7 antisense oligonucleotide, and Crohn's disease. N Engl J Med, 2015; 372(12):1104–13.

Acute exacerbation of Crohn's disease is difficult to treat. Remission can be induced with parenteral steroids, parenteral alimentation and IV antibiotics such as metronidazole and ciprofloxacin. *Infliximab* which is a monoclonal antibody to tumor necrosis factor-alpha (TNF-α) may be useful in resistant cases and in complications such as fistulae. It can also be used as a primary modality in severe and complicated cases. *Sargramostim* which is a recombinant human granulo-cyte macrophage colony–stimulating factor (GM-CSF) has been found to be beneficial in reducing inflammation and improving the quality of life. Natalizumab is a humanized monoclonal antibody against α4-integrin that inhibits leukocyte adhesion and migration into inflamed tissue. It is administered intravenously at a dose of 300 mg every four weeks. It is the first new class of drugs approved for the treatment of Crohn's disease since infliximab's approval in 1998.

Surgery is reserved for complications like obstruction, fistulae or abscesses.

ABDOMINAL TUBERCULOSIS

Abdominal tuberculosis may be divided into:

- Intestinal tuberculosis
- Tuberculosis of mesenteric lymph nodes
- Tuberculous peritonitis.

Intestinal Tuberculosis

This is the most common granulomatous disease of the bowel in India. The lesions may be secondary to a focus in the lung or they may develop primarily within the intestinal tract. The latter is fairly common. Highest incidence is in young adults in their second and third decades and women are more affected than men.

Pathogenesis and Pathology

Human and bovine strains of *Mycobacterium tuberculosis* produce intestinal lesions but human strain is more common. The infection may reach the intestine by four different routes—enterogenous, hematogenous, through the lymph channels and by direct extension from tuberculous lesions in the female genital tract.

The most common site is the ileocecal region (85% cases). Stasis of the intestinal contents and the close contact of tubercle bacilli with the mucosal surface in this region make this part vulnerable. Ileum, cecum, colon, jejunum and duodenum may be involved in that order of frequency. The lesion may be ulcerative, hypertrophic or ulcerohypertrophic. Pathological picture depends on the reaction of the host and virulence of the invading bacilli.

The bacilli infiltrate through the lymphatics into the submucosa. Tubercles are formed and intense inflammation with caseous necrosis occurs around the lymphatic channels. Endarteritis and lymphangitis lead to the formation of shallow mucosal ulceration. The ulcers are typically triangular running circumferentially (napkin ulcers). They heal by fibrosis leading to short segment strictures. Mesenteric lymph nodes are enlarged initially, later they may caseate and calcify.

Recurrent localized infection leads to the hypertrophic form. In this form, there is increased fibrosis and fat. Ulcerohypertrophic type shows large stellate ulcers with necrosis. The abdominal mass is made up of adherent mesenteric lymph nodes, fat and fibrous tissue.

Clinical Features

The clinical manifestation may be classified into five following groups.

1. **Constitutional symptoms:** For example, fever, weakness, anorexia, night sweats and weight loss.
2. **Ulceration of the intestine:** Leading to abdominal discomfort, diarrhea, malabsorption, perforation and rarely hemorrhage.
3. **Hypertrophic and ulcerohypertrophic forms:** Present with features of subacute intestinal obstruction, e.g. postprandial distress and distension, nausea, vomiting, constipation, colicky pain, borborygmi and visible peristalsis. A tender lump may be palpable in the right iliac fossa.
4. **Involvement of adjacent tissues like peritoneum and lymph nodes:** Lead to the formation of localized or free ascites. Single or multiple masses in the abdomen, enlarged lymph nodes and matted intestinal loops may be present. Extension of the disease to the pelvic adnexa gives rise to the formation of tubo-ovarian masses.
5. **Symptoms produced by tuberculosis in other parts of the body.**

Complications

Intestinal tuberculosis leads to complications such as intestinal obstruction, perforation, malabsorption state and rarely massive hemorrhage. Malabsorption is the result of reduction in the absorptive surface, blind loop syndrome and obstruction to lymphatics. Abdominal pain, weight loss and diarrhea form the symptom-triad of intestinal tuberculosis.

Diagnosis

Clinically, abdominal tuberculosis should be suspected in all cases of vague dyspepsia associated with malabsorption. Presence of obstructive symptoms, ascites and palpable masses strengthen the clinical suspicion. Evidence of tuberculosis elsewhere in the body strengthens the possibility further. Increased ESR and anemia occur in the majority.

A plain film of the abdomen may reveal dilated small bowel loops with fluid levels. Calcified lymph nodes may be seen. In the barium meal study, small-intestinal loops show irregular widening of mucosal folds, irregularity and upward displacement of the cecum. Constricted segments with proximal dilatation may give rise to the 'string sign' as in the case of Crohn's disease. The ascending colon may be shortened.

Other investigations like ascitic fluid analysis, peritoneal biopsy and peritoneoscopy may be helpful in arriving at a diagnosis. Endoscopic biopsy of the lesion is confirmatory. Adenosine diaminase (ADA) test in ascitic fluid is specific for tuberculosis and it is a useful and reliable test. PCR is useful to detect tubercle bacilli in peritoneal fluid and in endoscopic biopsy materials. The test is very sensitive, but too expensive for routine clinical use at present.

Treatment

General chemotherapy is given on the same lines as for the pulmonary tuberculosis. A low-residue diet is advocated when there are obstructive symptoms. Most of the cases respond fully to antituberculosis treatment.

Surgery may be very rarely required under the following conditions:
- Intestinal obstruction
- Perforation and hemorrhage
- If there is doubt of malignancy
- When the diagnosis is uncertain, laparoscopy or laparotomy may be required.

Tuberculosis of the Mesenteric Lymph Nodes

Syn: Tabes mesenterica

In most cases, it is secondary to intestinal tuberculosis, single or multiple lymph nodes may be affected. Caseation is followed by calcification and the nodes are visible in X-rays. The presentation is variable. Some patients present with general symptoms like anorexia, loss of weight and irregular pyrexia. Central abdominal pain with palpable abdominal lymph nodes should raise the possibility of mesenteric tuberculous adenitis.

INTESTINAL POLYPOSIS

Polyps arise from the mucosal surface and project into the lumen. They may be benign or malignant.

Textbook of Medicine

Adenomatous Polyps

These are the most common. They may be sessile or pedunculated, solitary or multiple. The rectum and sigmoid colon are the most common sites accounting for more than 80% of the total. Majority of polyps are silent, but at times they produce bleeding and intermittent obstruction due to intussusception. Some polyps become malignant, especially if the diameter exceeds 1 cm, the smaller ones are benign. Polyps can be visualized by barium studies and endoscopy. Endoscopic removal of polyps within reach is feasible. Since recurrence occurs in 50% cases, all subjects must be followed up regularly.

Villus Adenoma

This occurs usually in the rectum or sigmoid. This is sessile, soft and friable and it tends to bleed on mild trauma. Around 40–60% turn malignant in due course. Watery diarrhea and hypokalemia may develop rarely. Management consists of surgical excision and prolonged follow-up. Risk factors for malignant change in colonic polyps:

- Large size (> 2 cm)
- Multiple polyps
- Villous architecture
- Dysplasia.

Familial Colonic Polyposis (*See* Fig. 80.5)

This is a rare, autosomal dominant disorder characterized by the presence of numerous adenomatous polyps in the entire colon, especially the rectum and sigmoid, starting to appear from childhood and adolescence. These patients may present with lower abdominal pain, weight loss, diarrhea, tenesmus and presence of blood and mucus in stools. There is almost a complete tendency to develop malignancy and hence prophylactic colectomy is indicated (Fig. 79.3 and *See* Fig. 80.5). Systematic follow-up of the patient and his or her family members is necessary.

Juvenile Polyposis

This condition occurs in infants and children and is familial. Polyps are seen mainly in the colon and only sometimes in the small bowel. It presents with rectal bleeding and growth retardation. Histologically, inflammatory changes are seen in addition to columnar epithelium and mucus cysts. Therefore, these are also known as inflammatory polyps. There is no risk of malignancy and only symptomatic polyps should be removed. Prophylactic colectomy is not advised.

Peutz-Jeghers' Syndrome

In this condition, multiple hamartomatous polyps occur in the small intestine and colon along with spotted melanin pigmentation in the buccal mucosa, lips and skin around the mouth, palms and soles. Malignant change is less common. Treatment is required only if the polyps become symptomatic.

VASCULAR DISORDERS AFFECTING THE SMALL INTESTINE

Arterial supply to the small intestine is derived from the celiac and superior mesenteric which are extensively connected to provide adequate collateral circulation. The distal transverse colon, the splenic flexure and the junction of the superior and middle portions of the rectum are vulnerable to ischemia. The causes of ischemic bowel disease are given in Box 79.1.

The clinical features of arterial insufficiency depend on the site and degree of obstruction and the rapidity of onset. Clinical presentation ranges from transient malabsorption to frank infarction of extensive areas of the gut (Box 79.2).

Infarction of the Bowel

This may occur acutely or subacutely. It presents with severe colicky pain around the umbilicus which later leads to peritonitis, GI bleeding, toxemia and hypovolemic

Box 79.1: Causes of ischemic bowel disease

- ***Arterial occlusion***
  - Atherosclerosis
  - Thrombosis
  - Embolism
  - Aorto-arteritis
  - External compression (e.g. median arcuate ligament of the diaphragm)
  - Trauma
- ***Small vessel disease***
  - Vasculitis
  - Connective tissue disorders
  - Anaphylactoid purpura
  - Radiation enteritis
- ***Venous occlusion***
  - Primary
  - Secondary
  - Thrombophilic states
- ***Nonocclusive mesenteric infarction***
- ***Steal syndromes.***

Box 79.2: Clinical manifestations of ischemic bowel disease

- ***Acute intestinal ischemic syndromes***
  - Infarction of the bowel
  - Ischemic colitis and enteritis
- ***Chronic intestinal ischemic syndromes***
  - Intestinal angina
  - Stricture
  - Local ulcer
  - Celiac axis obstruction (median arcuate ligament syndrome)
  - Intramucosal or intramural bleeding ('thumb printing' on X-ray)
  - Malabsorption syndrome

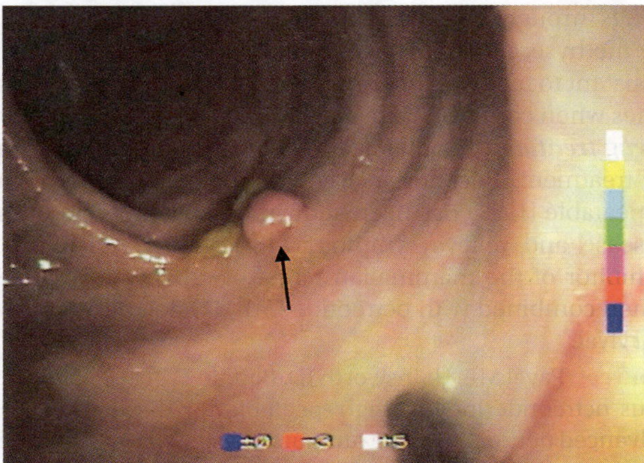

Fig. 79.3: Polyp colon: Endoscopic view, often polyps are precancerous

Textbook of Medicine

shock. Fever indicates definite infarction. Stools contain frank or altered blood. Management is surgical if infarction has occurred. Gangrenous bowel is resected and vascular reconstruction is attempted.

Intestinal angina occurs in partial obstruction of the superior mesenteric artery, especially when the other blood vessels are also diseased. The blood supply is inadequate to meet the demands of intestinal muscles after intake of food.

Twenty to thirty minutes after a heavy meal the patient develops severe crampy or colicky abdominal pain around the umbilicus lasting for 2–4 hours. The patient is afraid of taking food and therefore, he or she loses weight (sitophobia). Often intestinal angina is a forerunner to intestinal infarction. Auscultation may reveal arterial bruit in the abdomen. Abdominal aortography or selective mesenteric angiography helps in locating the obstruction.

Treatment

The diet should consist of small quantities of easily digestible or predigested food given at short intervals. Surgical measures to revascularize the ischemic segments should be considered. Thrombophiliac states should be excluded by investigations and managed appropriately.

CARCINOID TUMORS SYNDROME

General Considerations

Carcinoids are neuroendocrine tumors. Carcinoid tumors arise from the endocrine argentaffin cells in the small intestinal mucosa. Argentaffin cells are most abundant in the cecum and appendix and these are the most common sites for carcinoid tumors. Carcinoid tumors may be associated with multiple endocrine adenomas. The tumors may arise singly or multifocally in 20% of cases. They vary in size from a few millimeters to a few centimeters. Those larger than 2 cm in diameter are malignant and they may spread to the liver, lungs, bones and local lymph nodes. The degree of malignancy is low and even with metastases, about one-third of cases survive for more than 5 years. Atypical sites for carcinoids are stomach and bronchi. Extensive lesions produce metabolic abnormalities due to the production of large amounts of serotonin, 5-hydroxytryptamine, (5-HT) by the tumors and their secondaries. Several other substances like kallikrein, bradykinin, other kinin peptides, prostaglandins and histamine have also been identified. The substrate for production of 5-HT is tryptophan; 5-HT is deaminated by amine oxidase to 5-hydroxyindoleacetic acid (5-HIAA) which is excreted in urine in excess, i.e. more than 30 mg in 24 hour.

Carcinoid Syndrome

This is produced by excessive production of 5-HT.

Clinical Features

Carcinoid syndrome is characterized by frequent episodes of flushing and watery diarrhea. Repeated flushing may give rise to facial edema and development of telangiectasia. Asthmatic symptoms are prominent due to bronchospasm. Severe abdominal colic associated with borborygmi may occur. These attacks are precipitated by emotional upset, alcohol and excessive foods. Right-sided heart lesions like pulmonary and tricuspid stenosis, tricuspid incompetence and right-sided heart failure may develop in long-standing cases. Death is due to intractable right-sided cardiac failure. Since tryptophan, which is the precursor of niacin, is used up for formation of 5-HT, conditioned deficiency of niacin (pellagra) may develop. Carcinoid tumors arising from the intestines are late to produce symptoms. In gut carcinoid tumors, 5-HT and other vasoactive molecules are released into portal system. They are metabolized in the liver first pass and hence, such tumors will have no systemic symptoms early in the diseases. Later, when hepatic metastases develop the vasoactive substance are released into systemic circulation.

Thus, typical carcinoid symptoms are late and often indicate hepatic metastases.

Diagnosis

Clinically, carcinoid syndrome should be suspected in all cases of severe abdominal colic associated with hyper-motility of the bowel, flushing and palpable mass in the ileocecal region. Demonstration of excessive urinary 5-HIAA and raised serum levels of 5-HT will confirm the diagnosis. Foods like pineapples, bananas and walnuts and drugs like phenothiazines, mandelamine and glyceryl guaiacolate which increase urinary levels of 5-HIAA should be avoided for 3 days before undertaking the tests. Two endocrine markers of carcinoids are circulating chromogranin A and 5-HIAA.

Cardinal features of carcinoid syndrome
- Skin
  - Telangiectasia cyanosis
  - Flushing
  - Pellagra
- GIT
  - Diarrhea and cramping
- Heart
  - Valvular lesion
- Respiratory tract
  - Bronchoconstriction.

Treatment

Surgical excision of the primary tumor and the metastases, is undertaken. The results are dramatic in most cases. Another method is to perfuse the tumor with cytotoxic drugs through the hepatic artery. The diarrhea is controlled by methysergide 4 mg given four times daily. The flush is resistant to medical treatment. Treatment is given on usual lines when cardiac failure occurs.

Drug treatment: Somatostatin analogues are the first line of treatment. Recently, octreotide analogues, long-acting repeatable (LAR) has been shown to delay progress of the disease and relieve symptoms. Everolimus which is an inhibitor of the mammalian target of rapamycin (mTOR) when combined with octreotide LAR, is shown to improve survival.

Source: Pavel ME, Hainsworth JD, Baudin E, et al. Everolimus plus octreotide long-acting repeatable for the treatment of advanced neuroendocrine tumours associated with carcinoid syndrome (RADIANT-2): a randomised, placebo-controlled, phase 3 study. Lancet 2011;378:2005-12..

Diseases of the Colon

KR Vinaya Kumar, KV Krishna Das

Chapter Summary

- Idiopathic Ulcerative Colitis
- Cancer Prophylaxis
- Genetics of Colon Cancer
- Diverticulitis
- Carcinoma of Colon
- Prophylaxis

IDIOPATHIC ULCERATIVE COLITIS

The term *inflammatory bowel disease* (IBD) encompasses immune-mediated chronic intestinal inflammation. The major members in this group are idiopathic ulcerative colitis and Crohn's disease.

Ulcerative colitis (UC) is the idiopathic inflammation affecting the mucosa of the large intestine. Some patients have extraintestinal manifestations also.

This disease is present in all parts of the world and it is not uncommon in India. It is characterized by repeated bouts of diarrhea with blood and mucus, produced by inflammation and ulceration of the colon.

Many authors consider UC and Crohn's disease together under the term IBD. The former affects only the large intestine, whereas the latter can affect all parts of the alimentary tract, though the predominant and most frequent involvement is in the distal part of the small intestine. Clinically and histologically, the two conditions show overlap (Box 80.1).

UC results from environmental factors triggering loss of tolerance for normal intestinal flora in genetically susceptible individuals. Cigarette smoking confers a protective effect against this disease. The role of alteration in the normal protective gut flora in the causation of IBD is established.

Protective factors in UC include:

- Tobacco smoking
- Appendectomy.

Etiology

The etiology is unknown. Psychological factors such as emotional stress, anxiety or bereavement are evident in many cases. Since UC may be associated with diseases like arthritis, uveitis, erythema nodosum, hepatitis and autoimmune hemolytic anemia, an autoimmune basis has been suggested. Other postulations include transmissible viruses, bacteria, allergy to milk proteins and genetic factors.

Pathogenesis

The disease usually starts from the rectum which is involved in 95% of cases. Whole of the colon up to the cecum may be affected with extension to the terminal ileum. In the ordinary case, the inflammation is confined to the mucosa and submucosa. Initially, the mucosa is hyperemic, swollen, roughened and easily bleeding on contact. Superficial ulcers are seen which show diffuse infiltration of lamina propria and submucosa by chronic inflammatory cells. Crypt abscesses (cryptitis) may develop in 40% of the cases. The damage to mucosal epithelium is compensated by hyperplasia of regenerating mucosa which appears as pseudopolyps.

Clinical Features

Moderately Severe Form

Majority of cases occur between 20 and 40 years. In the west, males and females are equally affected, but in India, the male to female ratio is 2:1. The disease starts with looseness of the bowel with blood and mucus, abdominal pain, weight loss and fever. The severity varies. The condition tends to be prolonged, unlike bacterial dysentery. In majority of cases, the condition is mild with less than four stools per day and the patient is afebrile. In the moderately severe form, there are disabling constitutional symptoms and the number of stools varies from 6 to 12 day (Table 80.1).

In a few cases, the disease takes a fulminant form and may be mistaken for severe bacterial dysentery. It is characterized by fever, bloody diarrhea, dehydration and electrolyte disturbances. Toxic megacolon occurs in a few cases in whom the inflammatory process affects all the layers of the bowel and mortality is high in such cases.

Box 80.1: Difference between Crohn's disease and ulcerative colitis (UC)

	Crohn's	UC
Macroscopy		
Thickened bowel wall	Typical	Uncommon
Luminal narrowing	Typical	Uncommon
Skip lesion	Common	Absent
Fissures and fistulas	Common	Uncommon
Confluent linear ulcers	Common	Uncommon
Circumscribed ulcers	Common	Absent
Pseudopolyp	Absent	Common
Microscopic		
Transmural inflammation	Typical	Mucosal
Submucosal fibrosis	Typical	Absent
Fissures	Typical	Rare
Granuloma	Common	Absent
Crypt abscesses	Uncommon	Typical
Immunological marker	ASCA+	p-ANCA+

Abbreviations: ASCA = Antisaccharomyces cerevisiae antibodies; UC = Ulcerative colitis; p-ANCA+ = Perinuclear antineutrophil cytoplasmic antibodies

Textbook of Medicine

Table 80.1: Features characteristics of severity of the disease

Feature	Mild	Moderate (in between mild and severe)	Severe
Bloody stools/day	<4	4 or more	≥6
Pulse	<90/min	≤90/min	>90/min
Temperature	<37.5°C	≤37.8°C	>37.8°C
Hemoglobin	>11.5 g/dL	≥10.5 g/dL	<10.5 g/dL
ESR	<20 mm/hr	≤30 mm/hr	>30 mm/hr
CRP	Normal	≤30 mg/dL	30 g/dL

Abbreviations: CRP = C-reactive protein; ESR = Erythrocyte sedimentation rate

Diagnosis

The diagnosis should be suspected in all patients with a history suggestive of dysentery, but not relieved by the usual antiamebic and antibacterial drugs. Examination of the feces, colonoscopy and barium enema help in establishing the diagnosis. The feces is mixed with blood and mucus. Microscopy shows erythrocytes, neutrophils and macrophages. These findings are similar to those found in bacillary dysentery.

Sigmoidoscopy/Colonoscopy

The mucosa is friable, granular and it is covered with a thick inflammatory exudate consisting of pus, mucus and blood. Frank ulcerations, pseudopolyps and strictures may be seen in advanced cases. A rectal biopsy confirms the diagnosis. Microscopic examination of the fresh exudate helps in excluding amebiasis.

Colonoscopic grading of severity

- Normal mucosa
- Loss of vascular pattern
- Granular nonfriable mucosa
- Friability of mucosa
- Spontaneous bleeding with ulceration.

Barium Enema

This investigation helps to assess the extent and severity of the disease and its complications. Barium enema should not be done during the acute phase. In early cases, no abnormality may be detectable or may show only loss of haustrations. Later, the mucosal surface is serrated or spiculated due to shallow ulceration. The picture reveals pseudopolyps and strictures in advanced stages of the disease. The presacral space is widened in the lateral view.

Colonoscopy

This should be done to assess the state of the disease and its extent. During follow-up, repetition of colonoscopy at every 2 years interval helps to detect the development of cancer early, in cases with duration above 10 years (Fig. 80.1).

Differential Diagnosis

Acute bacillary dysentery: This forms the most important differential diagnosis. The diagnosis is made on stool culture, since microscopic examination of the feces and sigmoidoscopic appearance are indistinguishable.

Amebiasis is to be differentiated by examination of the feces, sigmoidoscopy and biopsy. Other conditions

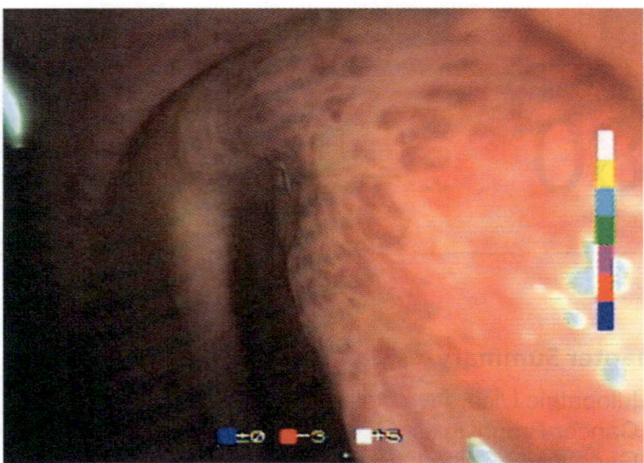

Fig. 80.1: Ulcerative colitis—endoscopy at early stage. ***Note:*** Hyperemia and bleeding tendency

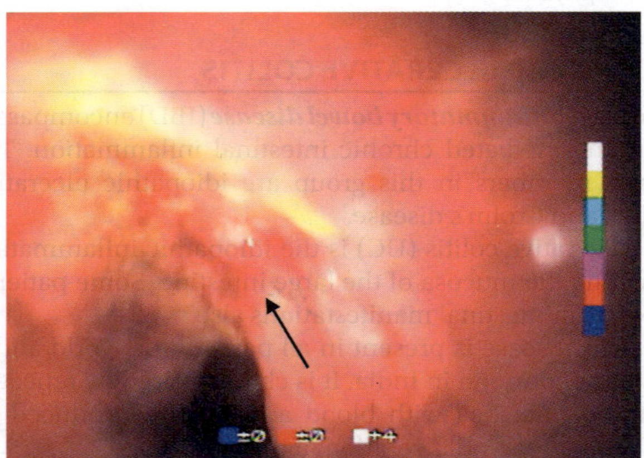

Fig. 80.2: Ischemic colitis—endoscopy. ***Note:*** Mucosal ulceration and bleeding (arrow)

such as inflamed hemorrhoids, ulcerating growths of the colon, tuberculosis of the colon, ischemic colitis (Fig. 80.2), irritable bowel syndrome (IBS) and Crohn's disease have to be differentiated by appropriate investigations. Gonococcal proctitis and acquired immunodeficiency syndrome (AIDS)-related bowel disease have to be excluded in susceptible individuals.

Complications

These may be local or systemic. The local complications are:

- ***Toxic megacolon:*** It is seen in 1–1.5 % of cases, especially in fulminant colitis. This is characterized by acute dilatation of the whole or part of the colon to a diameter greater than 6 cm, usually measured at the mid transverse level. The symptoms include fever, tachycardia, prostration and abdominal distension with diminished or absent bowel sounds. Plain X-ray of abdomen reveals dilated transverse colon. Perforation is identified by the presence of air under the diaphragm. In toxic megacolon, the mortality is 12–30%.
- ***Colonic stricture***
- ***Carcinoma of the colon*** is 7–11 times more frequent if subjects with UC than in controls and more so in the chronic continuous form with extensive involvement. Risk of cancer is associated with the extent and duration of the disease. It is 1.7% for those with disease

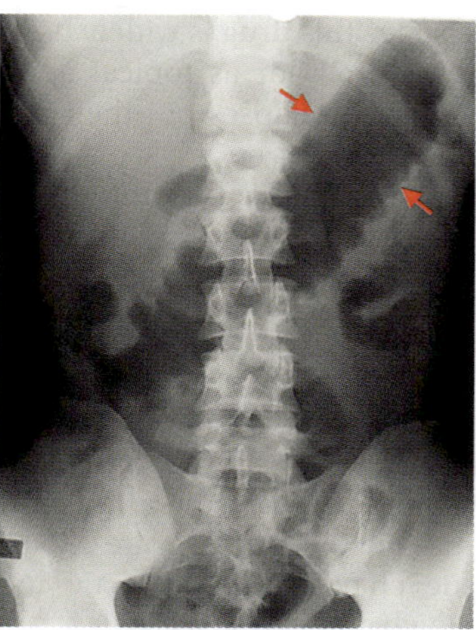

Fig. 80.3: Complication of ulcerative colitis toxic megacolon. **Note:** The grossly dilated transverse colon (arrows)

localized to the rectum, 2.8% for those with disease extending beyond the rectum to the hepatic flexure and 14.8% for those with disease extending proximal to the hepatic flexure.

- ***Venous thromboembolism*** is more frequent in IBD compared to controls especially during active exacerbations. During exacerbation, the risk is 8.4 times and during remission it is 2.6 times than in controls. Non-hospitalized patients have greater risk. Low molecular weight heparin (LMWH) and oral anticoagulants may be used when venous thrombosis develops.
- ***Toxic megacolon:*** Occurs in association with inflammation of the colon (Fig. 80.3).
- ***Ogilvie's disease:*** This is megacolon occurring without colonic inflammation, acute megacolon develops due to disruption of intestinal motility.

Extraintestinal Manifestations of IBD

- Musculoskeletal
- Arthritis—colitic type, ankylosing spondylitis, isolated joint involvement such as sacroiliitis
- Hypertrophic osteoarthropathy—clubbing, periostitis, metastatic
- Miscellaneous—osteoporosis, aseptic necrosis, polymyositis, osteomalacia.

Skin and Mouth

- Reactive lesions—erythema nodosum, pyoderma gangrenosum, aphthous ulcers, vesiculopustular eruption, necrotizing vasculitis, Sweet's syndrome.
- Specific lesions—fissures and fistulas oral Crohn's disease, drug rashes.
- Nutritional deficiency—acrodermatitis enteropathica (zinc), purpura (vitamins C and K), glossitis (vitamin B), hair loss and brittle nail (protein).
- Associated diseases—vitiligo, psoriasis, amyloidosis, epidermolysis bullosa acquisita.

Hepatobiliary

- Specific complications—primary sclerosing cholangitis (PSC) and bile duct carcinoma, small duct PSC, cholelithiasis.

- Associated inflammation—autoimmune chronic active hepatitis, pericholangitis, portal fibrosis and cirrhosis, granuloma in Crohn's disease.

Ocular

Uveitis iritis, episcleritis, scleromalacia, corneal ulcers, retinal vascular disease, Crohn's keratopathy.

Course and Prognosis

The course and severity of UC is variable. In the majority of cases, symptoms are recurrent with complete symptomatic remission between attacks. In 5–10% of cases, there are no recurrences after the initial attack; 5–15% follow a chronic continuous course without any remission.

Factors that determine the prognosis are: (i) severity of initial attack, (ii) extent of colitis, (iii) duration of illness prior to hospitalization and (iv) age of the patient at the onset. Total involvement of the colon, severe disease, short fulminant course and elderly age are adverse prognostic factors. About 4–6% of patients will be dead within one year of the onset of illness and 13–20% within 5 years. Complications like toxic megacolon, associated liver disease, hypokalemia and hypoalbuminemia also worsen the prognosis.

Management

Management of UC depends upon its severity and extent of the involvement. Patients with mild disease confined to the rectum and sigmoid respond to treatment satisfactorily. In moderate and extensive disease, relapses occur in 75% of cases.

Treatment of Moderately Severe Patients

The diet should be bland, low-residue type and with a high protein content. In patients with mild or moderately severe disease, initial therapy consists of sulfasalazine or analgesics. Salazopyrin has a sulfa moiety and an aminosalicylate moiety. The colonic bacteria split it into 5-amino salicylate (5-ASA) which enters the mucosa to exert its anti-inflammatory action. The beneficial action is due to the amino salicylate whereas the side effects are mainly due to sulfa moiety. The newer drugs which also deliver 5-ASA are mesalamine and olsalazine. They do not contain the sulfa moiety and hence, side effects are considerably less. Sulfasalazine (salazopyrin) is started in a dose of 500 mg thrice daily after food and then increased to 1 g three to four times daily, depending on the tolerance. Side effects include headache, malaise, skin rashes, hemolytic anemia and very rarely, agranulocytosis. Mesalamine is effective in doses of 400–1200 mg thrice a day. Olsalazine is another drug with similar action. It is not freely available in India.

Corticosteroids form the mainstay of therapy in acute exacerbations of severeUC. They may be given intravenous (IV), orally or as retention enemas depending on the condition. Prednisolone is given in the dose of 1–1.5 mg/kg body weight daily (40–60 mg) for a week and then tapered off in 4–8 weeks. Steroids can be administered through rectal route as retention enema containing hydrocortisone 100 mg in 200 mL normal saline or as rectal suppositories which produce a foam inside. Beclomethasone, budesonide and prednisolone, metasulfobenzoate are topical steroids which produce good results. They are especially useful for severe ulcerative proctitis.

In some patients, prednisolone may be ineffective and corticotropin gel given in a single daily intramuscular (IM) dose of 60–120 units is effective.

Antibiotics are not normally indicated for the colonic lesions, unless systemic symptoms like fever or toxemia develop. Diarrhea may be partially allayed by drugs like codeine phosphate. General management includes reassurance by the physician, anxiolytic drugs such as chlordiazepoxide 10 mg, attention to nutrition especially supplements of proteins, iron and vitamins and regular follow-up.

Treatment of Seriously Ill Patients

Features which indicate severity include:
- Bowel movement   > 9/day
- Pulse   > 100 minute
- Body temperature   > 38 °C
- Serum albumin   < 3 g/dL
- Plain X-ray abdomen showing intestinal dilation.

Note: These patients may require surgery.

Such cases should be managed by the physician and surgeon jointly. At the outset, an intensive regimen is started and continued for five days.

Only sips of water should be allowed by mouth. Hydrocortisone hemisuccinate is given IV in a dose of 300 mg in 24 hour. As an alternative, corticotropin gel is given in a dose of 60–120 units administered IM or IV. Hydrocortisone retention enemas are given twice a day. Proper maintenance of fluid and electrolyte balance and replacement of blood form the essential supportive measures. In successful cases, the temperature falls rapidly with return of the appetite and feeling of well-being. It takes a few days for the bowel frequency to return to normal. Surgical treatment has to be considered if the condition of the patient does not improve with conservative treatment in 3–4 days.

The onset of toxic megacolon is indicated by the presence of air-filled colon with abnormal haustral pattern and irregular margins in plain X-ray of the abdomen. Since late surgery is associated with high mortality and morbidity, decision for undertaking surgery should not be unduly delayed.

Indications for Surgery in UC
- Colonic dysplasia or carcinoma
- Colonic hemorrhage and uncontrollable
- Colonic perforation
- Growth retardation
- Intolerable or unacceptable side effects of medical therapy
- Medically refractory disease
- Systemic complications that are recurrent or unmanageable
- Toxic megacolon.

Long-term Management
Once the acute attack is controlled, the next step is to prevent relapses. Sulfasalazine given orally in doses of 2–4 g daily, continuously over a prolonged period exerts a suppressive effect to prevent relapse and maintain a symptom-free state. This drug is widely used. Small doses of corticosteroids orally or as topical applications have been used to prevent relapses but their value is still not firmly established.

Immunosuppressants like azathioprine can be used singly or together with corticosteroids for maintenance treatment in severe cases.

Cancer Prophylaxis
Since the risk of colon cancer is high in UC of long duration, there should be periodic evaluation for cancer detection. This is best achieved by colonoscopy every 1–3 years, starting 10 years after the initial diagnosis, suspicious areas in the mucosa are biopsied to detect even dysplastic changes. Prophylactic total colectomy is indicated in high grade dysplasias.

DIVERTICULITIS

The colonic mucosa may herniate through the muscularis mucosa to form diverticula. These small hernia sacs follow the course of the blood vessels on the mesenteric side and their wall consists of only mucosa and serosa. Many asymptomatic persons have colonic diverticula demonstrable by barium enema. This condition is referred to as diverticulosis. The most common site is the sigmoid colon. Only rarely is the proximal colon affected. Inflammation of these diverticula leads to diverticulitis. Diverticula are reported in 20–50 % of the western population over the age of 50. In India, though large population surveys are not available, the condition seems to be distinctly less common.

Pathogenesis
Diverticula are more common in people consuming low-residue diets, which tend to lower the bulk of feces. Rise in intraluminal pressure required to move the colonic contents is probably responsible for diverticula formation in such persons. Inflammation sets in when fecaliths get impacted in the diverticula and cause reduction in blood supply and secondary infection. Intramural or pericolic abscesses may develop. It is, however, rare to produce generalized peritonitis. Sometimes the inflamed mucosa may bleed.

Clinical Features
The disease may present in several ways and clinical severity varies widely. The pain of acute diverticulitis may resemble that of acute appendicitis, but it is left-sided and worsened by defecation. Signs of peritoneal inflammation may be present. The subacute form presents with alteration in bowel habits or as discomfort and tenderness in the left iliac fossa. Though in 25% of cases occult blood can be detected in feces, gross bleeding is rare. Rarely dysenteric symptoms may occur. In chronic cases, narrowing of the colon may lead to subacute obstruction. Physical examination may reveal palpable and tender sigmoid colon.

Diagnosis
Diverticulitis should be considered when an elderly person presents with subacute or chronic colonic pain associated with alteration in bowel habits. Diagnosis is confirmed by barium enema examination. The diverticula

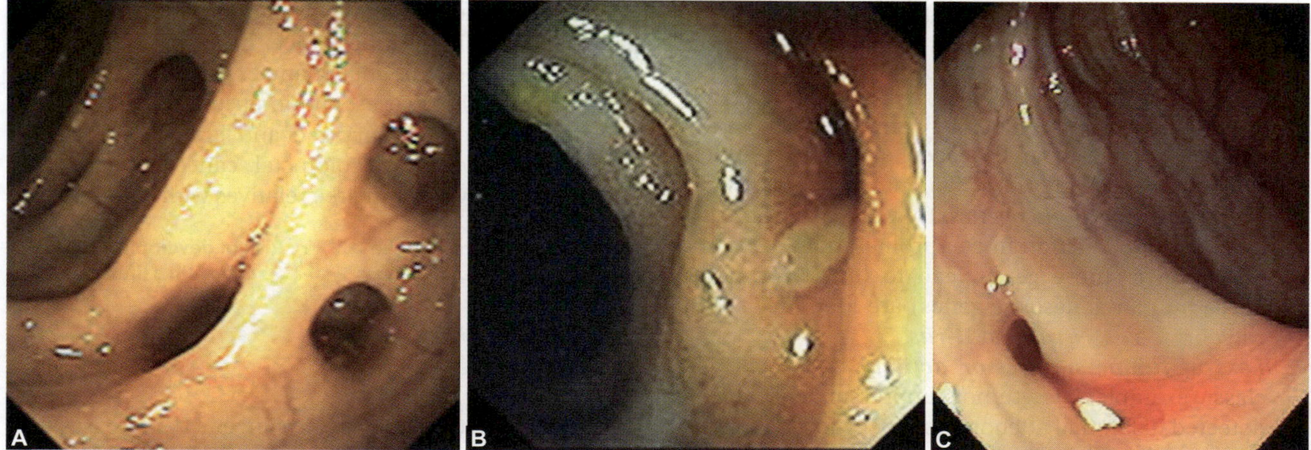

Figs 80.4A to C: Various types of colonic diverticula—sigmoidoscopy

are seen as outpouchings of the colon. They are brought out better in films made with air insufflation into the rectum after voiding the barium. Rigidity, narrowing and loss of haustrations of the affected segment should suggest the presence of inflammation. Sometimes differentiation from carcinoma is difficult. Contrast radiography should not be undertaken in the acute stage since it may lead to rupture of an inflamed sac (Figs 80.4A to C).

Differential Diagnosis

Diarrhea and pain have to be differentiated from other forms of colitis. Severe hemorrhage may resemble that occurring in carcinoma, polyps, angiodysplasia or hemorrhoids. The subacute form with obstruction may resemble carcinoma.

Complications

These include free perforation, fistula formation, fibrosis, strictures and massive hemorrhage.

Treatment

An acute attack of diverticulitis requires seven days of metronidazole (400 mg 8 hourly orally), along with either a cephalosporin or ampicillin (500 mg 6 hourly orally). Severe cases require IV fluids, antibiotics, analgesia and nasogastric suction. In mild cases, conservative management consisting of bed rest, stool softeners and broad-spectrum oral antibiotics like tetracycline or ampicillin serve to tide over the acute phase. Introduction of high residue diet helps to regularize the bowel movements. Antispasmodics have to be given to relieve pain. Administration of isabgol husk in a dose of 5–10 g after the evening meal helps to produce satisfactory bowel movement and relieve symptoms.

Complications like intestinal obstruction, perforation, abscess formation or massive hemorrhage are indications for surgical intervention. Surgery consists of a diverting colostomy and resection of the involved colon with subsequent reanastomosis.

CARCINOMA OF COLON

Carcinoma of the colon is common in India. The etiology is unknown. Villous adenoma, familial polyposis of the colon (Fig. 80.5), chronic UC and rarely adenomatous polyps (Fig. 80.6) may develop into malignant lesions. The peak incidence is between the fifth and the seventh decades.

Colorectal cancer is the third leading cause of death among malignancies all over the world. The incidence begins to increase after the age of 50 years and it

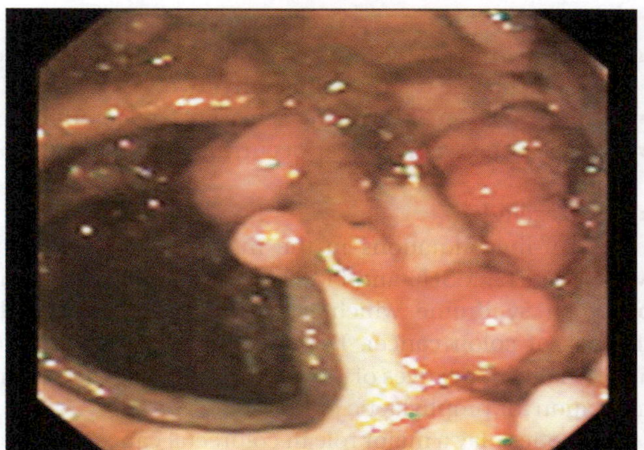

Fig. 80.5: Familial polyposis. **Note:** The multiple polyps which are often premalignant

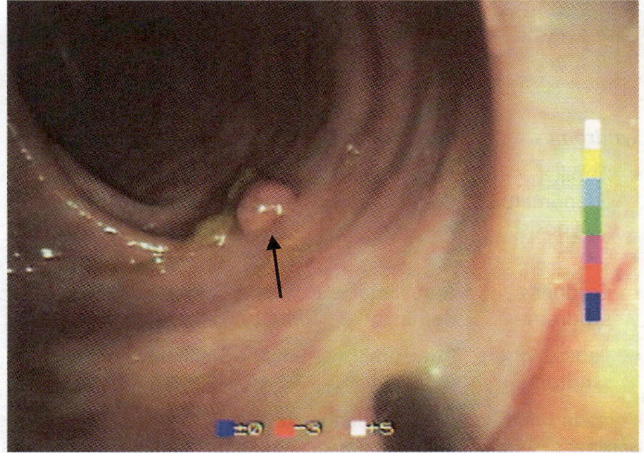

Fig. 80.6: Polyp colon—endoscopic view (arrow), often polyps are precancerous

Textbook of Medicine

doubles with each decade. Incidence is higher in the western world. In India, this form of malignancy is quite common.

Genetics of Colon Cancer

Genetics of colon cancer has been extensively studied. Changes can be generally classified into three classes.

1. ***Changes in proto-oncogenes:*** They play a role normally in signal transduction in cell proliferation. Abnormal activation of these genes lead to tumor formation. Three human genes (ras genes) are identified in this category ***K-ras, N-ras*** and ***H-ras***.
2. ***Loss of tumor suppressor activity:*** APC gene is a classic example. It is a tumor suppressor gene which is detected in familial adenomatous polyposis (FAP).
3. ***Abnormalities in genes involved in deoxyribonucleic acid (DNA) mismatch repair:*** Classic example is gene mutation in hereditary nonpolyposis colon cancer (HNPCC).

Risk factors include increasing age, male sex, previous colonic polyps, previous colorectal cancer, and environmental factors such as excess red meat in diet, high-fat diet, inadequate intake of fiber, obesity, sedentary lifestyle, smoking and high intake of alcohol.

Modified Amsterdam Criteria for Diagnosis of HNPCC

- At least, three relations with colon cancer, one must be the first degree relative of the other two
- Colorectal cancer involving at least two generations
- At least one colon cancer occurring before the age of 50 years
- FAP excluded.

Germ-line mutations in the mismatch repair genes MLH1, MSH2, MSH6 and PMS2 lead to the development of Lynch syndrome which is strongly associated with the risk of colon cancer. Demonstration of this genetic abnormality in relatives of patients with colon cancer is an indication for prophylactic measures.

Genetics play a major role in colorectal cancer. Several forms of intestinal polyposis lead to cancer (Table 80.2). HNPCC syndromes are also described. These include site specific colorectal cancer (Lynch syndrome I) and cancer

Table 80.2: Common inherited polyposis syndromes and the risk of developing cancer

Syndromes	Inheritance	Cancer risk	Distribution of polyps
• Familial adenomatous polyposis	Autosomal dominant	Near 100%	Colon 100%, Stomach 30–50%, Duodenum over 90%, Small bowel about 50%
• Gardner's syndrome	Autosomal dominant	Near 100%	Colon 100%
• Peutz-Jeghers syndrome	Autosomal dominant	About 50%	Small bowel > 90%

Note: In 1 and 2, polyps are adenomatous. In 3, they are hamartomas. Gardner's syndrome is also associated with other abnormalities such as osteomas, epidermoid cysts, fibromas, dental abnormalities, desmoid tumors and retinal lesions.

family syndrome (Lynch syndrome II). Both these show autosomal dominant inheritance. In the later condition, other extraintestinal malignancies are also present, particularly in the ovaries, endometrium, stomach, small intestine, pancreas, urinary tract and larynx.

Risk of developing colorectal cancer is higher in persons who have first-degree relatives with colon cancer.

Number of first-degree relative with colon cancer	Risk of developing colon cancer in a lifetime
1	18%
2	33%
3	50%

In adenomatous polyps, the cancer risk increases with the size of the polyp. Histological pattern also influences the cancer risk.

Pathology

These tumors grow from the epithelial cells of crypts of Lieberkühn. The lesion may be annular, tubular, ulcerative or papilliferous. The annular type produces obstructive symptoms early. About 75% of tumors are seen in the descending colon, rectosigmoid and rectum. Cecum and ascending colon are affected in 15% and the transverse colon is affected in 10% cases. Rectal examination and sigmoidoscopy are able to detect 50% of colonic cancers. Metastases occur initially by lymphatic spread to the lymph nodes and later through the bloodstream to the liver.

Clinical Features

Symptoms vary depending on the site of the growth. Growths in the cecum or ascending colon are usually flat or polypoid and they remain silent for long periods. Nonspecific symptoms like anemia, weight loss, anorexia or malaise may be the presenting features in some cases. Blood stained stool is the presenting complaint in 25% of right-sided lesions.

Left-sided lesions cause obstruction early since the contents are solid. Common symptoms are recent changes in the bowel habits and diarrhea alternating with constipation. Growths of the sigmoid colon may present with tenesmus. Colicky pain is often present. Rectal bleeding occurs in 70% of left-sided growths.

Diagnosis

The diagnosis is difficult when the symptoms are nonspecific. Digital examination of the rectum and sigmoidoscopy can pick up more than 50% of cases. Presence of occult blood in feces is suggestive of ulcerated growths.

Barium enema brings out the lesions in many cases. A growth may be seen as a filling defect or distortion of the colonic mucosa or as an ulcer. Postevacuation air insufflated film is very useful for outlining colonic mucosal lesions.

In lesions beyond the reach of the sigmoidoscope, colonoscopy is diagnostic. Even when barium enema is not definite, colonoscopic examination and biopsy serve to establish the diagnosis (Figs 80.7A to C). Wherever possible, histological diagnosis by endoscopic biopsy

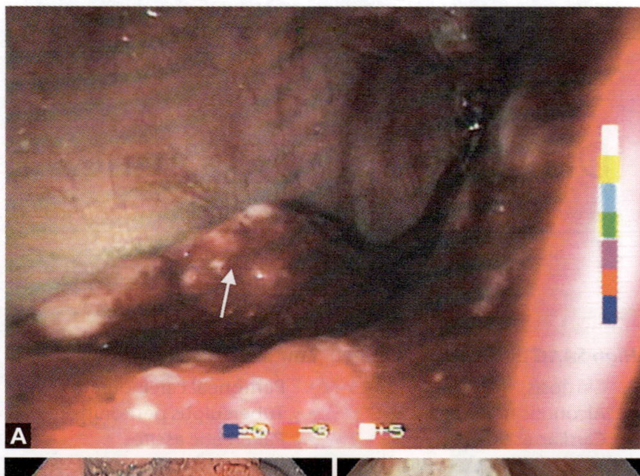

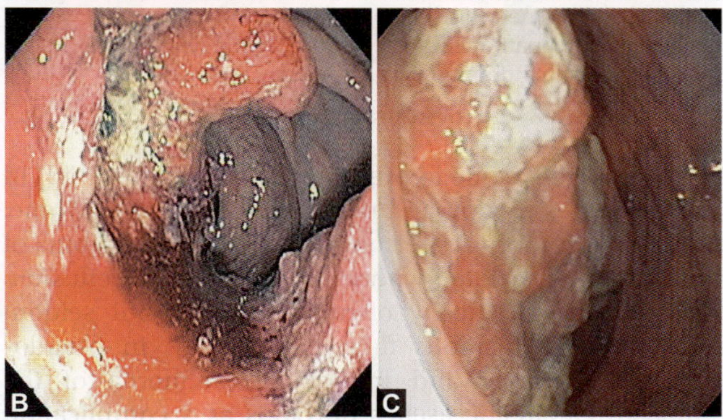

Figs 80.7A to C: Carcinoma colon advanced—endoscopy. **Note:** Cauliflower growth (arrow)

should be made before radical surgery since granulomas and ameboma may clinically resemble neoplasm.

Use of aspirin 600 mg/day in carriers of lineage syndromes and hereditary colorectal cancer syndrome for 25 months, reduced incidence of cancer when followed up for 55.7 months. Further studies for duration of treatment and dose are proceeding.

When secondaries occur in the liver, serum alkaline phosphatase and 5-nucleotidase are elevated. Carcino-embryonic antigen (CEA) is elevated in colonic cancer. Though this is not specific for colonic carcinoma, its use is mainly in following up patients who have undergone surgery. Rise in the level of CEA indicates recurrence of the growth or development of metastases. Computed tomography (CT) colonoscopy, pelvic magnetic resonance imaging (MRI) and enhanced hepatic ultrasound studies are all newer diagnostic methods with high efficacy.

Differential Diagnosis

Carcinoma of the colon should be differentiated from all other conditions which cause dysenteric symptoms and recent change in bowel habits, such as UC, polyps, diverticulitis and intestinal tuberculosis. In chronic amebiasis, granulomatous masses (ameboma) may develop and these have to be differentiated. Lymphoma, lymphogranuloma venereum and endometriosis may also cause difficulty in diagnosis. It should be remembered that carcinoma may coexist with other lesions.

Complications

These include metastases, obstruction, intussusception, volvulus, bowel perforation, local peritonitis, massive hemorrhage and spread to neighboring organs like ureters, bladder and uterus.

Treatment

In early cases, colonic resection with colostomy is the treatment of choice. Preoperative radiation is advocated in rectal cancer. Even when the tumor is not removable, palliative surgery to overcome the obstruction may be required. Adjuvant chemotherapy with 5-fluorouracil (5-FU) and levamisole has good survival advantage. Even a few metastases in the liver is not a contraindication for surgery, since the liver metastases can also be removed.

Prognosis

Surgery offers almost cure, if colon cancer is detected early. Since most cases are detected late, either when the growth is fixed or has metastasized, the prognosis is poor. In large series, overall five-year survival for patients undergoing radical surgery is about 50%. When the tumor is confined to the bowel wall, the five-year survival is 75–80%, whereas in those with lymph node metastases, the survival is only 25%.

Prophylaxis

Carcinoma of the colon is largely preventable if premalignant conditions such as UC and colonic polyposis are regularly followed up with annual endoscopic examination. Colectomy should be undertaken early if malignancy supervenes.

It has been observed that regular use of statins have shown reduction of colon cancer. Regular use of nonsteroidal anti-inflammatory drugs (NSAIDs) such as sulindac and celecoxib has been shown to be associated with suppression of adenomatous polyps and regression of familial adenomatous polyposis and reduction of colon cancers. The therapeutic role of these observations is not fully evaluated. Regular use of aspirin 150 mg/day for 5–6 years reduces the risk of cancer in carriers of gene for colon cancer after 55.7 months of treatment.

People with genetic risk should have guaiac test for occult blood in stools every 2 yearly and screening by flexible sigmoidoscopy every 5 years.

Diseases of the Peritoneum

KR Vinaya Kumar, KV Krishna Das

Textbook of Medicine

Chapter Summary

- Ascites
- Peritonitis
- Malignant Lesions of the Peritoneum
- Retroperitoneal Fibrosis
- Pseudomyxoma Peritonei
- Abdominal Compartment Syndrome

ASCITES

Collection of excess of free fluid in the peritoneal cavity is called **ascites**. A small quantity of fluid resembling lymph is normally present in the peritoneum. Increase in the hydrostatic pressure in the portal capillaries and the colloid osmotic pressure of the ascitic fluid favor further transudation into the peritoneum. Return of the ascitic fluid into the capillaries is brought about by the osmotic pressure of the plasma and the hydrostatic pressure in the peritoneum. The rate of formation and amount of fluid collecting in the peritoneum are determined by these two opposing forces. The peritoneal fluid is in dynamic equilibrium with blood and about 50% of the fluid enters and leaves the peritoneal cavity every hour. The extensive visceral peritoneum and its subjacent capillaries account for this free exchange. In all conditions where the ascitic fluid is a transudate, several factors operate simultaneously.

Cirrhosis of the liver accounts for the majority of cases of ascites in India. In cirrhosis of liver, in addition to rise of portal venous pressure, other factors also operate which help the accumulation of fluid in the peritoneum. These are hypoalbuminemia, secondary hyperaldosteronism which results in the retention of sodium and increased secretion of antidiuretic hormone (ADH) which favors the retention of water. Splanchnic arterial vasodilation caused by nitric oxide (NO) produced locally acts as a major factor in the development of ascites. Portal hypertension leads to the production of NO locally. Combination of portal hypertension and splanchnic arterial vasodilation increases intestinal capillary pressure and permeability resulting in the accumulation of fluid within the peritoneal cavity. As the disease progresses, marked impairment of renal excretion of free water and renal vasoconstriction develop. The former leads to dilutional hyponatremia and the latter to hepatorenal syndrome (HRS) respectively.

On the other hand, ascites in peritonitis is mainly the result of local inflammation and exudation. Table 81.1 lists the main causes of ascites.

Hemorrhagic fluid occurs in malignancy, acute pancreatitis or infarction of organs like the spleen or gut.

Table 81.1: Main causes of ascites

High SAAG ≥ 1.1 g/dL	Low SAAG < 1.1 g/dL
Cirrhosis	Peritoneal carcinomatosis
Alcoholic hepatitis	Tuberculous peritonitis
Cardiac ascites	Pancreatic ascites
Massive liver metastasis	Bowel infraction
Fulminant hepatic failure	Nephrotic syndrome
Budd-Chiari syndrome	Biliary ascites

Abbreviation: SAAG = Serum ascites albumin gradient

The fluid is milky due to presence of fat (chylous fluid) in lymphatic obstruction and rarely in nephrotic syndrome. Meig's syndrome is a rare condition in which a fibroma of the ovary is associated with ascites and pleural effusion. It is a clinical curiosity often mentioned, but seldom encountered. Mucinous fluid accumulates in pseudomyxoma peritonei and in colloid carcinoma of the stomach. Pancreatic ascites develops as a complication of pancreatitis when a fistulous communication develops between the pancreatic duct and the peritoneal cavity. In this condition, the ascitic fluid shows high levels of amylase and proteins.

Clinical Features

The onset may be acute as in the case of inflammatory exudates or insidious as in cirrhosis liver. The common symptom is progressive distension of the abdomen. The abdomen is uniformly distended and the flanks are full. In the early stages, fluid may be detectable only in the flanks, later as accumulation proceeds the whole of the abdomen is filled. Due to rise in intra-abdominal pressure (IAP), the umbilicus becomes everted as a result of the development of an umbilical hernia. Inguinal, femoral or incisional hernias may develop. Striae develop due to stretching of the abdominal wall. Free fluid in the peritoneum can be demonstrated by eliciting shifting dullness on percussion with changing positions of the patient. For this sign to manifest, the fluid should be free so as to shift in the peritoneal cavity and the mesentery should be free so as to allow the intestines to float up and give the hyper-resonant note. When the fluid is very tense or when the intestines are fixed due to involvement of the mesentery, shifting dullness may not be elicitable.

When the quantity of fluid is less than 200 mL, it can be detected only by eliciting dullness to percussion around the umbilicus, the patient being examined in the knee elbow position—'puddle sign'. Fluid thrill can be elicited over the abdomen when the fluid is large in amount and under tension. In obese individuals, the abdominal fat transmits **thrill** in the transverse direction and this should not be mistaken for fluid thrill.

Associated Findings

Ascites and pleural effusion may coexist. Fluid from the peritoneum may pass into the pleural cavities through defects in the diaphragm or lymphatic channels. The raised IAP pushes up the diaphragm, resulting in the diminution of the respiratory excursions of the lower portion of the chest. The cardiac apex may be displaced upwards. Elevation of the diaphragm also leads to secondary rise in intrapleural and right atrial pressure (RAP). The jugular vein may be full due to this reason.

Differential Diagnosis

Free fluid in the peritoneum has to be differentiated from localized fluid collections such as abscesses, cysts, hydramnios and large hydronephrosis. Rarely, a very much distended bladder may give rise to doubt. Localized fluid does not give rise to shifting dullness. Solid organs like enlarged uterus and ovarian tumors do not produce fullness of the flanks.

Diagnosis

Presence of fluid is readily detectable by ultrasonography and this is the investigation of choice. In addition to fluid, solid masses and metastases can also be detected. The diagnosis should be confirmed by paracentesis, which is necessary to determine the etiology. Even when a major cause such as cirrhosis liver is evident, it is still advisable to do a diagnostic paracentesis to exclude other coexisting lesions like tuberculous peritonitis or hepatoma. The ascitic fluid is examined microscopically, biochemically and microbiologically.

Microscopic Examination

A fresh specimen of uncentrifuged fluid should be examined after adding one drop of methylene blue. This brings out the cells clearly. Further identification of cells can be done by examining the stained deposit or by Papanicolaou's technique. When parasites such as microfilaria are suspected, the deposit should be examined after centrifugation. Presence of inflammatory cells is characteristic of exudates. Lymphocytes predominate in tuberculosis, malignancy and pancreatic ascites. In pyogenic infections like acute peritonitis, neutrophils predominate. Malignant cells are identifiable in wet-stained preparations but they are better identified by Papanicolaou's technique. Bacterial organisms can be identified by Gram stain and Ziehl-Neelsen's stain.

Biochemical Tests

Protein content of the ascitic fluid is high in exudates. In transudates, the protein level seldom exceeds 2.5 g/dL. Higher values suggest infection, malignancy or infarction. Determination of serum-albumin ascitic fluid gradient (SAAG) is helpful in deciding upon the cause of ascites. Increase in alpha-fetoprotein (AFP) suggests the presence of hepatoma. Rise in amylase levels above 100 units/L together with higher protein content suggests pancreatic ascites.

Laparoscopy

It helps to visualize the peritoneum and abdominal organs and also aids in the selection of suitable sites for biopsy.

Closed biopsy of the peritoneum can be performed using special **(Cope's or Abrams)** needles if facilities for laparoscopy are not available. This is helpful in the diagnosis of extensive diseases such as tuberculous peritonitis and disseminated malignancy.

Course and Prognosis of Ascites

These depend upon the cause. In hepatic cirrhosis, the ultimate prognosis depends upon the state of liver function. If the liver function is considerably reduced, 40% cases die within 2 years of onset of ascites.

In peritonitis, the outcome depends on early diagnosis and prompt treatment. Ascites occurring in malignancy generally denotes advanced disease and this has a poor prognosis. Ascites secondary to hypoproteinemia, nephrotic syndrome and cardiac failure clears up with improvement of the underlying condition.

Treatment

In all cases where the ascites is secondary to a treatable disease, cure of the primary disorder relieves the ascites as well. When the underlying cause is irreversible such as cirrhosis of liver, measures to relieve the ascites are undertaken.

PERITONITIS

The peritoneum is an extensive serous cavity lined by flattened epithelium. It is generally resistant to infection and in healthy subjects infection is promptly localized.

Peritonitis is inflammation of the peritoneum. It may be acute or chronic and localized or generalized. Acute peritonitis presents as a surgical emergency with severe pain, toxemia and shock. Physical examination reveals extreme tenderness, board-like rigidity and absence of peristaltic sounds because of intestinal paresis. If exudation develops into the peritoneal cavity, signs of ascites become evident. Chronic peritonitis presents with ascites.

Acute Peritonitis

Common causes of this condition include appendicitis, perforation of viscera occurring in peptic ulcer, typhoid fever, cholecystitis, Crohn's disease, ulcerative colitis, dysentery, diverticulitis, gangrene, strangulated internal hernias and injury by foreign bodies. *Gonococci* and *Pneumococci* may cause localized or generalized peritonitis as a primary infection or by spread from other foci.

Diagnosis

Examination of the ascitic fluid shows the presence of intestinal contents organisms and large number of neutrophils. Plain X-ray of the abdomen may reveal dilated loops of intestines and subdiaphragmatic gas in the case of perforation. Ultrasonography (USG) is very helpful.

Acute peritonitis is a surgical emergency. Principles of management consist of correction of fluid and electrolytes, antibiotic therapy, measures to combat shock and surgical measures. All cases should be managed under the combined care of the surgeon and physician without delay.

Chronic Peritonitis

This condition is commonly caused by tuberculosis, malignancy or chemical causes, e.g. peritoneal dialysis. It presents as progressive ascites or peritoneal adhesions with intermittent subacute intestinal obstruction. Diagnosis is established by examining the ascitic fluid which shows increase in protein and chronic inflammatory cells. Treatment for the underlying causes relieves the condition.

MALIGNANT LESIONS OF THE PERITONEUM

Many neoplasms metastasize into the peritoneum early and therefore, secondary tumors are much more common. The primary may be abdominal neoplasms from the stomach, liver or ovaries or extra-abdominal sites like carcinoma of the breast and lungs. These patients present with rapidly developing ascites and cachexia and they run a downhill course. Examination may reveal nodular masses in the abdomen, presence of **Virchow's glands** and periumbilical subcutaneous tumor deposits **(Sister-Joseph's nodules)**.

Sister Mary Joseph (1856–1939) surgical assistant to Dr William Mayo, noted the association between para-umbilical nodules and metastatic intra-abdominal cancer. Ascitic fluid may be hemorrhagic in many cases and microscopy reveals tumor cells. Chemotherapy may be palliative in some cases.

Primary tumors are rare. Histologically, these are mesotheliomas. In many cases, there is association with exposure to asbestos.

RETROPERITONEAL FIBROSIS

Retroperitoneal fibrosis may develop as an adverse side effect of therapy with drugs like methysergide. Other recognized causes are retroperitoneal lymphoma, carcinomatous secondaries and postirradiation fibrosis.

The etiology is unknown in many cases. The disease is more common in middle-aged males. Progressive fibrosis of the peritoneum on the posterior abdominal wall leads to constriction of the ureters and bilateral obstructive uropathy. Surgical measures are required to relieve ureteric obstruction. Clinical features include malaise, back pain, normochromic anemia and raised erythrocyte sedimentation rate (ESR). Contrast urogram shows the obstruction at the level of the pelvic brim with distension proximally, often the distension is asymmetrical. Computed tomography (CT) scan may show the fibrosis as a para-aortic mass.

Treatment: To relieve the obstruction surgically. Withdrawal of methysergide early during the course of the illness arrests further progress and the fibrosis may even regress.

PSEUDOMYXOMA PERITONEI

It is a rare metastatic peritoneal disease, the primary being in the ovary or the appendix. This is characterized by the accumulation of a jelly-like material in the peritoneal cavity. The condition is very indolent and many patients survive more than five years after diagnosis. Surgical debulking of the tumor and local drugs administered intraperitoneally may be beneficial.

ABDOMINAL COMPARTMENT SYNDROME

Sustained elevation of IAP above 20 mm Hg with or without abdominal perfusion pressure below 60 mm Hg that is associated with organ dysfunction and failure is termed **abdominal compartment syndrome**.

This condition is being increasingly recognized in septic shock. It is an independent predictor of death. The lethal triad in trauma includes coagulopathy, acidosis and hypothermia. Severity of the coagulopathy is directly related to the severity of injury.

Damage control laparotomy is an emergency procedure to control hemorrhage and remove contamination-elective surgery is undertaken later.

CHAPTER 82

Hepatobiliary System: General Considerations

KR Vinaya Kumar, KV Krishna Das

Chapter Summary

- Anatomy
- Physiological Considerations

ANATOMY

The liver weighs 1.2–1.5 kg in the adult. It is comparatively bigger in infants, weighing around 6% of the birth weight. It is held in its place by the general intra-abdominal pressure and also by its peritoneal and vascular attachments.

Anatomically, falciform ligament divides the liver into a large right lobe, which is six times the size of the left lobe. The right lobe has two other lesser segments—the quadrate lobe in its inferior aspect and the caudate lobe located posteriorly. A portion of the left lobe is felt in the epigastrium in normal subjects. Based on its vascular supply and biliary drainage, the liver can be divided into physiological right and left lobes. The line of functional division lies to the right of the falciform ligament (Figs 82.1A and B). Liver is the second largest organ in human body and the largest endocrine organ.

Structure of Liver

The basic architecture of the liver is formed by the hepatic lobules which measure about 1 mm in diameter and are polyhedral in shape. Clear cut demarcation between the lobules is not present in the human liver as is seen in the pig. Traditionally, the central hepatic vein was thought to be at the center of the lobule and portal triad at its periphery. The portal triad contains the radicles of the portal vein, hepatic artery and the bile duct, a few round cells and some connective tissue. A limiting plate of hepatic cells surrounds the portal tract.

Rappaport gave the acinar concept with the central vein at the periphery and the portal tracts at the center. An acinus is made up of a group of liver cells which is supplied by the terminal branches of the hepatic artery, portal vein and bile duct. The acinus is the functional unit of the liver. A group of acini forms a complex acinus. The hepatocytes near the central vein are having the least oxygen supply and are more vulnerable to hypoxic injury.

The liver cells are arranged in the form of sheets (hepatic laminae) which are connected by interlaminar bridges. In between the sheets of liver cells are vascular spaces—the sinusoids. The liver tissue is pervaded by two systems of tunnels formed by the portal tract and by the hepatic venous radicles. These two systems interlace in such a way so that, they do not come in contact. They are separated in the terminal portions only by a few liver cells that extend from the central vein to the portal triad.

The sinusoids are lined by a layer of endothelial cells. In between the hepatocyte and the endothelial cells is a narrow space—*the space of Disse*, which contains lymph. The hepatocytes account for 60% of the weight of the organ. They are polygonal, 30 μ in size and show a central nucleus 8–10 μ in diameter. Life span of the hepatocyte is

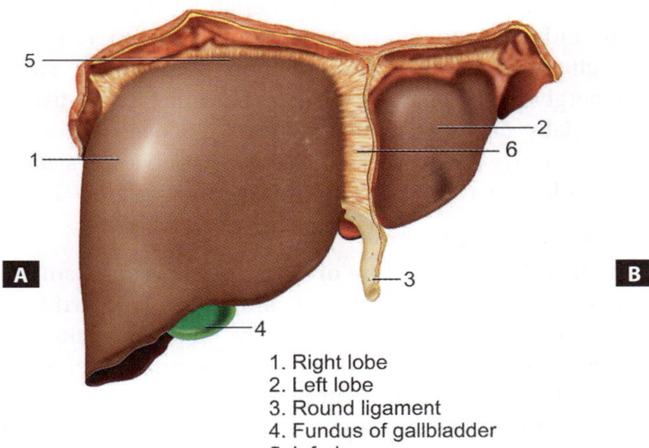

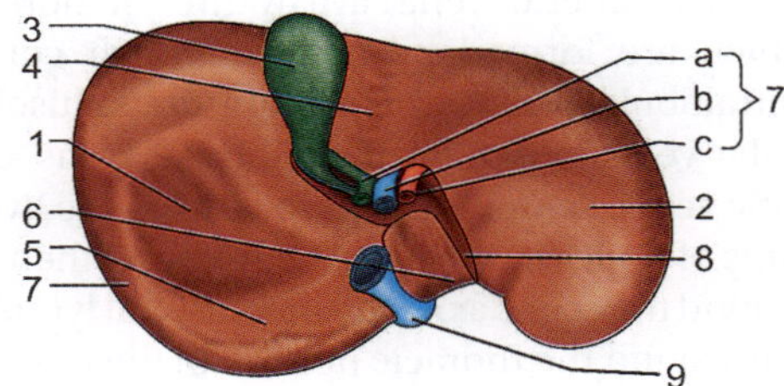

Figs 82.1A and B: **A.** Dorsal and anterior aspect of the liver; **B.** Ventral surface of the liver

Textbook of Medicine

150 days. The bile canaliculi are found between adjoining liver cells. The hepatocyte has several complex metabolic functions to perform.

The phagocytic cells in the liver are the **Kupffer's cells** which belong to the reticuloendothelial system. They are situated in the walls of the sinusoids. In addition to Kupffer's cells, the sinusoidal walls contain endothelial cells, fat storing cells known as lipocytes or **Ito cells** and **pit cells** which have probably an endocrine function.

Under the electron microscope, hepatocytes reveal desmosomes which are anchoring pegs on the sides of contact of the cells. Microvilli project into the bile canaliculi. In the sinusoidal border, microvilli project into the perisinusoidal tissue **space of Disse**. The mitochondria contain several enzymes concerned with various metabolic activities including β-oxidation of fatty acids. The rough endoplasmic reticulum (RER) synthesizes several proteins, including albumin, clotting factors and enzymes and the smooth endoplasmic reticulum (SER) is the site of bilirubin conjugation, detoxification of many drugs and steroid synthesis. Adjacent to the bile canaliculi, dense pericanalicular bodies are seen and these lysosomes contain many hydrolytic enzymes. Some of the pericanalicular dense bodies are termed as microbodies. Golgi apparatus lies near the bile canaliculi. Lysosomes, microbodies and Golgi apparatus are concerned with the sequestration and elimination of ingested materials and this system is deranged in cholestasis. The hyaloplasm contains granules of glycogen, lipids and fine fibrils. The cytoskeleton is formed by microtubules and microfilaments.

Blood Supply

The liver receives a dual blood supply; 1500 mL of blood perfuses the liver every minute. The arterial blood supply is from hepatic artery which supplies 20% of blood. The remaining 70–80% of blood (1000–1200 mL) come from the portal vein. More than 70% of the oxygen supply to the liver is derived from the portal vein. When the portal venous oxygen tension is low during digestion, the major source of oxygen supply is the hepatic artery. The portal blood also contains some hepatotropic factors which are essential for hepatic regeneration. The normal portal pressure is 7 mm Hg (90–120 mm water). The blood is drained into the inferior vena cava by three or more hepatic veins which are formed by radicles which commence in the intralobular veins which drain the sinusoids. The interlobular veins join to form sublobular veins and then the hepatic veins. Lymphatic channels from the liver drain into groups of nodes in the porta hepatis and then into the nodes around the celiac axis. The mediastinal lymph nodes and those around the thoracic portion of the inferior vena cava also receive some lymphatics from the liver.

Secretion of Bile

Bile secreted into the bile canaliculi by the hepatocytes drains into the intrerlobular cholangioles which join to form the larger interlobular bile ducts in the portal tracts. From each physiological lobe, the interlobular bile ducts join to form the right and left hepatic ducts which join to form the common hepatic duct. The common bile duct is formed by the union of the cystic duct from the gallbladder

Table 82.1: Normal composition of bile	
Water	97.62%
Total solids	2.38%
Bile salts	0.90%
Mucin and pigments	0.50%
Lipids	0.25%
Inorganic salts	0.73%

with the common hepatic duct. It travels behind the head of the pancreas to open into the second part of the duodenum at the ampulla of Vater. Bile is secreted continuously and stored in the gallbladder which is a pear-shaped sac with a capacity of 50 mL. Normally, this organ is not palpable, but when it enlarges it becomes palpable under the edge of the liver. The neck of the gallbladder shows a sacculation **(Hartmann's pouch)** which is a common site for lodgement of gallstones. The gallbladder contracts to release bile into the duodenum and this is related to the passage of food. The bile contains secretory and excretory products. The normal composition of bile is given in Table 82.1.

PHYSIOLOGICAL CONSIDERATIONS

The liver plays a key role in the metabolism of carbohydrates, proteins, lipids, hormones, bilirubin, porphyrin, bile salts and many drugs. It is only natural, therefore, that liver diseases may lead to a wide variety of systemic manifestations as the liver has a tremendous reserve capacity, the manifestations of disease occur only when the liver disease is advanced. Regardless of the etiology, the systemic features of liver disease are fairly similar.

Glucose Metabolism

One of the major functions of the liver is to maintain normal blood glucose level. Even though man is an intermittent feeder, the liver acts to dampen the effects of absorption and prevents surges in the blood glucose level and maintains blood glucose levels in the normal range. A fairly steady blood sugar level is to be maintained by the processes of glycolysis, glycogenolysis, glycogenesis and gluconeogenesis. Liver disease can lead to hypoglycemia or hyperglycemia. Fulminant hepatitis and hepatomas can induce even fatal hypoglycemia due to reduction of gluconeogenesis and reduction of glycogen stores. Hyperglycemia may occur in chronic liver disease, especially cirrhosis, which reduces glucose uptake and glycogenesis by the liver, coupled with hepatic resistance to insulin, are responsible for this feature.

Protein Metabolism

The liver is the major site of amino acid metabolism. The enzymes responsible for transamination and oxidative deamination are found in very high quantities in hepatocytes except for branched chain amino acids. The majority of amino acids entering the liver are catabolized. Levels of aromatic amino acids normally metabolized in the liver are increased and branched chain amino acids metabolized by the skeletal muscle which are depressed in liver disease. The alteration of the ratio between the two types of amino acids has been incriminated in the pathogenesis of hepatic encephalopathy.

The liver synthesizes not only the protein but it also need many export proteins (all plasma proteins except immunoglobulins), the most important of which is albumin. Albumin contributes significantly to the plasma oncotic pressure.

Coagulation Factors

Many of the blood clotting factors such as I, II, V, VII, VIII, IX and X are synthesized in the liver. The vitamin K dependent factors (II, VII, IX and X) are synthesized in the liver and are made functionally active by vitamin K (*See* also Ch 30). In addition to coagulation factors, intrinsic antithrombotic proteins such as protein C and protein S which are also vitamin K dependent are synthesized in the liver. The capacity of the liver to produce coagulation factors is limited. Therefore, in hepatic failure, coagulation function is deranged early.

Lipid Metabolism

Fatty acids produced by lipolysis in adipose tissue and those absorbed from the intestine may reach the liver. Some fatty acids may be esterified with cholesterol, conjugated to phospholipids or converted to triglycerides. The triglycerides are cleared from the liver as lipoproteins by combination with apoproteins. Disturbances in these—either increased entry of fatty acids into the liver or decreased clearance—can lead to fatty liver. It is now realized that obesity and the development of metabolic syndrome (syndrome X) are predisposing factors for pathological fatty change in the liver.

Alterations in cholesterol and lipoprotein metabolism are seen in patients with cholestatic liver disease. The liver contains an enzyme lecithin-cholesterol acyltransferase (LCAT). A decrease in the production of LCAT is responsible for the increase in free cholesterol in serum. The reduced level of LCAT is also correlated with the appearance of lipoprotein-X (LP-X) in patients with cholestasis. LP-X has a high concentration of free cholesterol and triglycerides.

Hormonal Metabolism

The metabolism of various hormones is affected in liver disease, e.g. insulin, glucagon, thyroxine, steroids and sex hormones. Abnormalities of sex hormone metabolism account for spider angioma, loss of axillary and pubic hair, testicular atrophy and gynecomastia seen in patients with chronic liver disease. In addition to the hepatic dysfunction, the factors which lead to liver injury also directly impair gonadal function, e.g. alcohol and hemochromatosis.

Physiological Functions of Liver

Glucose metabolism	Gluconeogenesis, glycogenesis, glycolysis
Protein metabolism	Synthesis of albumin and other plasma proteins except immunoglobulin
Lipid metabolism	Synthesis of lipoproteins
Hormone metabolism	Insulin, glucagon, thyroxine, steroids and sex hormones
Coagulation factor synthesis	Factors I, II, V, VII, VIII, IX, X
Inhibitors of coagulation	Protein C, S

Various Zones in Liver and Metabolic Functions

Zone 1 Periportal	Zone 3 Perivenular
• Gluconeogenesis • Glycogen synthesis from lactate • β-oxidation of fatty acids • Amino acid catabolism • Urea synthesis • Cholesterol synthesis • Bile acid secretion	• Glycolysis • Glycogen synthesis from glucose • Lipogenesis • Removal of ammonia from blood by glutamine • Detoxification, biotransformation of the majority of drugs and toxins, glucuronidation • Ketogenesis • Bile acid synthesis • Increase in Kupffer cell phagocytic activity

CHAPTER
83

Jaundice

KR Vinaya Kumar, KV Krishna Das

Chapter Summary

- Biochemical Abnormalities in Jaundice and Classification
- Diagnosis
- Complications due to Jaundice
- Management of Jaundice

DEFINITION

Jaundice is yellow discoloration of skin, sclera, mucous membranes and other tissues due to excess of bilirubin in the blood. The normal level is 0.5–1.0 mg/dL. Clinically, jaundice is to be manifested when serum bilirubin rises above 3 mg/dL (50 μmol/L). The term 'latent jaundice' is used when the level is between 1 and 2 mg/dL. Examination in bright daylight is absolutely essential to detect mild jaundice (Fig. 83.1).

BIOCHEMICAL ABNORMALITIES IN JAUNDICE AND CLASSIFICATION

Approximately 30 mg of bilirubin is formed in the body every day of which 80% is derived from senescent erythrocytes and 20% from other sources. Bilirubin combines

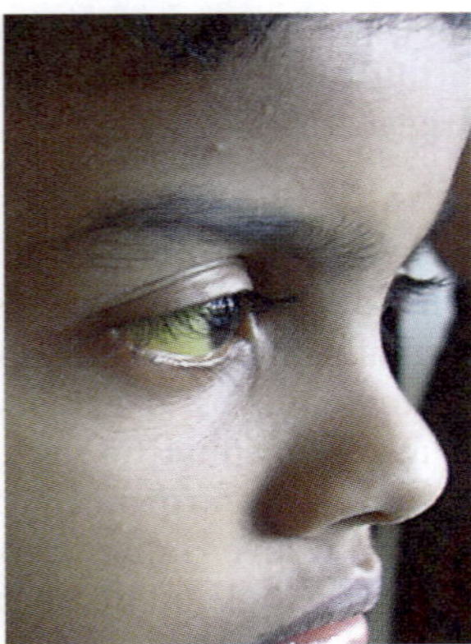

Fig. 83.1: Ten-year-old girl with mild jaundice due to hereditary spherocytosis

with albumin and this product is being insoluble in water does not appear in urine. In hemolytic jaundice in which most of the bilirubin is unconjugated, urine does not contain bilirubin. Three main phases are recognized in the metabolism of bilirubin. These are: (i) Entry into the liver cell, (ii) conjugation and (iii) excretion into the bile. After uptake, bilirubin is conjugate with glucuronic acid in the endoplasmic reticulum of hepatocytes with the help of glucuronyl transferase and it reduces the level of enzyme that are responsible for certain forms of congenital hyperbilirubinemias like *Crigler-Najjar syndrome*. Conjugated bilirubin is water-soluble and it freely passes into urine. *Bilirubin* diglucuronide in the gut is acted upon by bacteria present in the distal small intestine and the colon and is converted into urobilinogen. Urobilinogen is reabsorbed mainly from the small intestine and to a small extent from the large intestine into the portal blood. It is subjected to enterohepatic circulation. The portion that is present in stool without being absorbed is called *stercobilinogen*.

Both unconjugated and conjugated bilirubin stain tissues. Collagenous and elastic tissues have the maximum affinity for bilirubin and therefore, tissues rich in these are stained early and most deeply.

In adults, bilirubin does not cross the blood-brain barrier and the brain is not stained. In neonates, the blood-brain barrier is not well-developed and it is disturbed in inflammations (e.g. Weil's disease). In such situations, the brain and cerebrospinal fluid (CSF) are also stained. Presence of bilirubin in ocular fluids may lead to yellow vision-xanthopsia which is extremely rare. Sweat, milk, semen and synovial fluid may contain bilirubin in most cases, but tears, saliva and pancreatic juice are discolored only if, the jaundice is severe. In long-standing jaundice, the skin shows a greenish tinge due to the formation of biliverdin, an oxidation product of bilirubin.

Jaundice can be classified in different ways (Table 83.1).

A clinically useful classification of jaundice with indication of etiology which used to be in vogue is given below:
- Overproduction of bilirubin—hemolytic
- Decreased hepatic uptake—hepatocellular dysfunction
- Decreased hepatic conjugation and release into biliary canaliculi—hepatocellular dysfunction

Table 83.1: Classification of jaundice based on the types of pigment

Predominantly unconjugated hyperbilirubinemia
- ***Overproduction of bilirubin***
  - Hemolysis—intra- or extracorpuscular causes
  - Ineffective erythropoiesis
- ***Impaired hepatic uptake***
  - Drugs—rifampicin, cholecystography dye
  - Familial—Gilbert's syndrome
- ***Impaired bilirubin conjugation (decreased glycoronyl transferase activity)***
  - Hereditary absence or deficiency of transferase—Crigler-Najjar syndrome—types 1 and 2
  - Immaturity of transferase (neonatal jaundice)
  - Acquired transferase deficiency
    - Drug effect—chloramphenicol, novobiocin
    - Hepatocellular disease—hepatitis and cirrhosis

Predominantly conjugated hyperbilirubinemia
- ***Impaired hepatic excretion (intrahepatic defects)***
  - Acquired disorders of the liver cells—viral hepatitis, leprospirosis, drug-induced hepatitis, e. g. isoniazid, methyldopa, alcohol
  - Hereditary disorders—Dubin-Johnson syndrome, Rotor's syndrome
- ***Intrahepatic cholestasis***
  - Viral hepatitis
  - Drug induced cholestasis, e.g. oral contraceptives, anabolic steroids methyltestosterone, sulfadiazine, chlorpromazine, thiouracil, p-aminosalicylic acid (PAS)
  - Primary biliary cirrhosis
  - Extensive involvement of liver by malignant secondaries, Hodgkin's diseases, etc.
  - Intrahepatic biliary atresia
- ***Extrahepatic causes for cholestasis (surgical jaundice):*** Gallstones, carcinoma head of the pancreas, biliary stricture, carcinoma of the ampulla of Vater, obstruction of masses in the porta hepatis

- Obstruction to the biliary passages—cholestasis with regurgitation of bile into the blood.

Though, in majority of cases, jaundice runs true to type. In many instances more than one factor may be operative and this tends to make the biochemical picture more complex. For example, in long-standing hemolytic jaundice, biliary calculi may develop and produce obstructive jaundice as well. In the setting of isolated hyperbilirubinemia, presence of more than 15% direct fraction indicates direct hyperbilirubinemia and less than 15% direct fraction indicates indirect hyperbilirubinemia.

Differentiation of the types of jaundice: Differentiation between ***medical, i.e. prehepatic and hepatic types*** or ***surgical, i.e. posthepatic and extrahepatic cholestasis,*** is crucial in deciding upon the management. The investigations have to be planned suitably. Medical jaundice is to be treated mainly with drugs whereas, surgical jaundice demands invasive investigations and in many cases even early surgery.

DIAGNOSIS

Majority of cases can be diagnosed by history, physical examination and simple biochemical tests. Preliminary tests include urinalysis, examination of feces and biochemical and immunological tests of the serum. More definitive diagnostic tests to delineate the anatomy of the biliary tree are ultrasonography, radiological studies, liver

Textbook of Medicine

Table 83.2: Clinical differentiation of the types of jaundice

Clinical features	Hemolytic	Hepatocellular	Obstructive (cholestatis)
*Depth of jaundice	Usually mild	Variable	Usually deep
Pruritus	Absent	Variable	Present
Bradycardia	Absent	Absent	Present
Anemia	Present	Absent	Absent
Splenomegaly	Present	Variable	Absent
Palpable gallbladder	Absent	Absent	May be present
Bleeding tendency	Absent	Present	Present in the late stages
Features of hepatocellular failure	Absent	Present early in the disease	Present often late
Bile pigment in the urine	Absent	Present	Excessive
Urobilinogen	Excess	Present, may be in excess	Absent

*Not a reliable sign

Note: The depth of jaundice is not a reliable parameter to differentiate the types.

biopsy, isotopic investigations, endoscopic investigations, computed tomography (CT) scan, magnetic resonance imaging (MRI) and laparotomy.

Table 83.2 gives the clinical differentiation of the types of jaundice.

Biochemical Tests

Preliminary investigations: Laboratory investigations are necessary to determine the type of jaundice and its etiology.

Examination of feces: The stools are dark colored in hemolytic jaundice due to excessive bile pigment, whereas it is pale and chalky white (clay colored) in obstructive jaundice due to absence of bile. Ulcerating malignant lesions give rise to occult blood in stools. Silvery color of feces occurring in obstructive jaundice indicates the presence of altered blood.

Serum bilirubin: The total, conjugated and unconjugated fractions can be estimated. This helps in assessing the severity of jaundice and also in identifying the type. Van den Bergh reaction is a qualitative test used in detecting the type of bile pigment in the serum. Direct positive test is given by conjugated bilirubin, unconjugated bilirubin gives rise to the indirect reaction. When both pigments are present, the reaction is biphasic. A part of conjugated bilirubin in patients with cholestasis and hepatobiliary disorders may be covalently linked to albumin and this fraction is called delta bilirubin or biliprotein. This explains the reason for slow decrease of bilirubin values in these patients inspite of clinical improvement.

Enzyme Determination

- ***Increased levels of serum glutamic oxaloacetic transaminase (SGOT) aspartate transaminase (AST) and serum glutamic pyruvic transaminase (SGPT) alanine transaminase (ALT):*** Liver cells are rich in transminases, SGPT and SGOT. In the normal state, these enzymes are present in serum (10–40 U/L), but when hepatic cells may undergo necrosis, large amounts are released into circulation. The serum levels of these enzymes are raised in all forms of hepatocellular necrosis, irrespective of the etiology. Though these enzymes are not specific to the liver, when taken in conjunction with other tests of hepatic function, raised levels give a semiquantitative idea of the extent of liver cell necrosis in most cases. In fulminant hepatic failure where most of the liver cells have been lost the amount of enzyme released falls and so transaminase levels may fall despite very severe hepatic necrosis. In such a situation, the enzyme levels may be misleadingly low. Recently, it has been suggested that the upper normal limit (ULN) for ALT should be decreased to 30 IU/L for men and 19 IU/L for women by the American Association for the Study of Liver Diseases (AASLD) and National Institute of Health (NIH) in order to differentiate HBeAg negative chronic hepatitis B (CHB) patients from inactive chronic carriers better.

- ***Serum alkaline phosphatase (ALP)*** levels above 30 KA units/dL (210 IU/L) indicate cholestasis, if bone disease can be excluded. In extrahepatic biliary obstruction, it is disproportionately increased compared to plasma bilirubin. The raised levels are brought about by overproduction of hepatic alkaline phosphatase. Rise in serum alkaline phosphatase is even a more reliable parameter of biliary obstruction than serum bilirubin levels.

- ***Gamma glutamyl transpeptidase*** is a membrane bound enzyme that catalyzes the transfer of gamma glutamyl groups of peptides such as glutathione to other amino acids. It primarily arises from the liver and hepatobiliary system. Its levels are increased in cholestasis and hepatocellular disease and occur in the same spectrum of hepatobiliary diseases with elevated ALP.

- ***Lactate dehydrogenase*** is a cytoplasmic enzyme which has 5 isoenzyme types. The ALT: LDH ratio helps to differentiate between acute viral hepatitis (greater than 1.5) and ischemic hepatitis (less than 1.5).

Interpretation of Liver Function Test (LFT)

Cholestasis is diagnosed when there is an increase in ALP more than 2 times normal (N) and/or and ALT/ALP ratio <2. Hepatocellular injury is characterized by ALT/ALP ratio >5. Mixed liver injury is the intermediate between cholestasis and hepatocellular injury with and ALT/ALP ratio greater than 2 and less than 5.

LFT in Hepatitis and Cholestasis

Pattern	AST and ALT	GGT	ALP
Biliary obstruction	Mild increase	Moderate	Marked
Hepatitis	Marked	Mild	Mild
Alcohol and enzyme inducing drugs	Normal or mild	Moderate	Normal

Note: Mild = less than twice normal, moderate = 2–5 times normal and marked = more than 5 times normal.

Serum cholesterol: It is markedly elevated in obstructive jaundice, especially primary biliary cirrhosis. Several

Textbook of Medicine

other disorders lead to elevation of serum cholesterol and therefore, this test is not specific.

Serum albumin: It is lowered in hepatocellular failure. In hepatocellular disease, gamma globulin is elevated whereas in chronic biliary obstruction, alpha-2 and beta globulins are elevated.

Prothrombin time: In obstructive and hepatocellular jaundice, prothrombin time is prolonged. Shortening of the prothrombin time with parenteral administration of vitamin K_1 suggests that the jaundice is mainly obstructive. Total lack of response indicates gross liver cell damage.

Immunological Tests

Many hepatocellular disorders are immunologically mediated and so several antibodies can be demonstrated. Among them the most useful is the ***antimitochondrial antibody*** which is present in primary biliary cirrhosis. High titers of ***antinuclear and smooth-muscle antibodies*** suggest chronic active hepatitis. The different ***serological markers of hepatitis B infection*** such as HBsAg, HBeAg and their respective antibodies are most helpful in making specific diagnosis. Other viruses producing hepatitis give rise to specific diagnostic immunological markers (*See* Ch 55).

Ultrasonography

It is perhaps the most useful noninvasive method to delineate dilated bile ducts, dilated portal vein, pancreatic cysts and tumors, the gallbladder and the liver. This should be done as an initial imaging procedure to visualize the liver, gallbladder, biliary passage and the venous systems since, this can confirm the diagnosis in many cases and further expensive and invasive tests can be avoided.

Liver Biopsy

This may be necessary in long-standing jaundice when non-invasive investigations are unrewarding. In the presence of bleeding tendency, as revealed by prolonged prothrombin time, liver biopsy has to be undertaken with care. Percutaneous liver biopsies are now done with Trucut needles or biopsy guns. In liver failure with severe coagulation disturbances, only transjugular liver biopsy can be done. In focal lesions of the liver, guided biopsies are required, either ultrasound or CT scan guided biopsies.

Radiological Studies

Plain X-ray of the abdomen may reveal radiopaque biliary calculi in a minority of cases. Plain radiograph of the abdomen may show gallstones as a chance finding. Contrast radiography such as oral cholecystography, intravenous cholangiography and percutaneous tran-shepatic cholangiography (PTC) are seldom done now. But selective hepatic arteriography is useful for the diagnosis of focal lesions in the liver, planning hepatic resections and interventions such as embolization and local chemotherapy. For these, more elegant and non-invasive procedures employing ultrasound, CT scan and MRI principles are adopted at present.

Computed Tomography

CT scan is a very reliable method to demonstrate hepatic lesions. This should be employed when ultrasonography is not fully diagnostic. Structural lesions in the liver such as tumors, abscesses, vascular malformations, parasites, cirrhosis and others can be demonstrated by CT scan. When ultrasonography and CT scan are used in conjunction, diagnostic yield is much higher. Both these modalities can be employed for guided biopsies and aspirations.

Magnetic Resonance Imaging (MRI)

This gives more information than CT scan in the following conditions:

- Infiltrative disorders, especially fatty liver
- Accumulation of heavy metals such as copper and iron
- When hemangioma and metastatic deposits are suspected
- To determine the patency of blood vessels in the abdomen.

Computed tomography cholangiopancreatogram (CTCP) and magnetic resonance cholangiopancreatogram (MRCP) are useful non-invasive imaging modalities to delineate biliary and pancreatic ductular systems. They are equally informative compared to endoscopic retrograde cholangiopancreatogram (ERCP).

Isotopic Liver Scan

Technetium-99m (^{99m}Tc) labelled biliary analogues such as diisopropylamino diacetate, hepatobiliary iminodiacetic acid (HIDA) and paraisopropyl iminodiacetic acid (PIPIDA) when given IV are taken up by liver cells and excreted into bile. In obstructive jaundice this is delayed. These tests help to detect the cause of obstructive jaundice due to mechanical cholestasis (Table 83.3).

Endoscopy

Esophago-gastroscopy: This gives indirect evidence of portal hypertension. Presence of varices in the esophagus and stomach is due to rise in portal pressure, persisting over long periods.

Presence of spider nevi in the esophagus and/or stomach is suggestive of hepatic failure.

Endoscopic retrograde cholangiopancreatography (ERCP): This procedure helps in visualizing the biliary and pancreatic duct systems. In addition to diagnosis, the same method may be employed to dislodge obstructing stones or relieve a stricture or to deploy a stent (Fig. 83.2).

Peritoneoscopy (Syn: Laparoscopy): Direct inspection of the liver and gallbladder through the laparoscope and biopsies under vision from suspicious areas to improve diagnostic accuracy considerably.

Surgery

If the diagnosis is not clear by all these tests, laparotomy may have to be performed for initiating the treatment without further delay. Moreover, even in incurable malignant obstruction, drainage of bile through a cholecystojejunostomy helps to relieve symptoms and allay misery for considerable periods. At present, less traumatic procedures such as laparoscopic surgery are adopted.

COMPLICATIONS DUE TO JAUNDICE

Jaundice may give rise to further complications, apart from those caused by the primary disease.

Table 83.3: Differential diagnosis of jaundice

	Hepatocellular jaundice	*Intrahepatic cholestasis*	*Extrahepatic obstruction*
Common causes	Viral hepatitis spirochetal jaundice	Viral hepatitis, drugs biliary cirrhosis	Biliary stones, carcinoma of pancreas, carcinoma bile duct
Age	More in the young	Any age	Above 40 years
Duration of jaundice	Less than 3 months	Usually less than 3 months	Often more than 3 months
Itching	May be present	Common	Common
Color of feces	Slightly pale	Pale	Very pale (clay-colored)
Jaundice	Mild to moderate	Mild to moderate or deep	Very deep in the later stages
Pain	Mild discomfort	Nil	Characteristic pain in gallstones; constant radiating pain in pancreatic carcinoma
Liver	Tender and slightly enlarged	Variable	Enlarged and firm in long-standing jaundice
Gallbladder	Not palpable	Not palpable	Palpable in many cases of carcinoma head of pancreas and in some cases of bile duct obstruction
Bilirubin	Total and direct high	Total and direct high	Total and direct very high
Serum cholesterol	Normal	Raised	Markedly raised
Cephalin cholesterol flocculation	2 to 4+	1 to 2+	1+ in the early stages
Alkaline phosphatase (KA units)	10–15 KA units/dL	Over 15 KA units/dL	Over 3 KA units/dL
Transaminases	Markedly increases	Moderately increased	Only slightly increased in early stages
Obstruction to major bile ducts	Nil	Nil	Present

Note: Alkaline phosphatase—normal value 3 to 13 KA unit/dL or 21 to 91 IU/L.

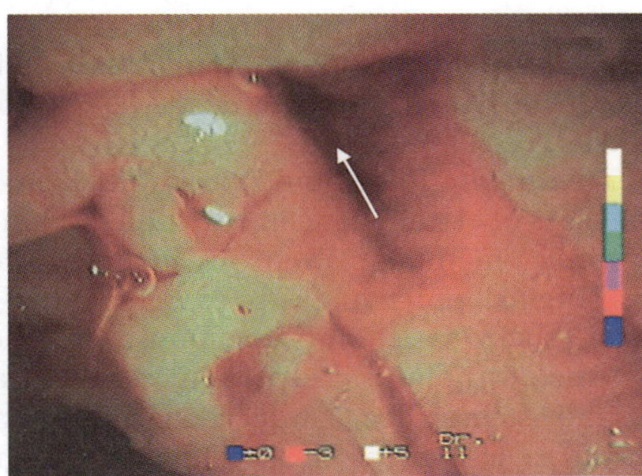

Fig. 83.2: Hemobilia. **Note:** The presence of blood in the opening of the bile duct during ERCP (arrow)

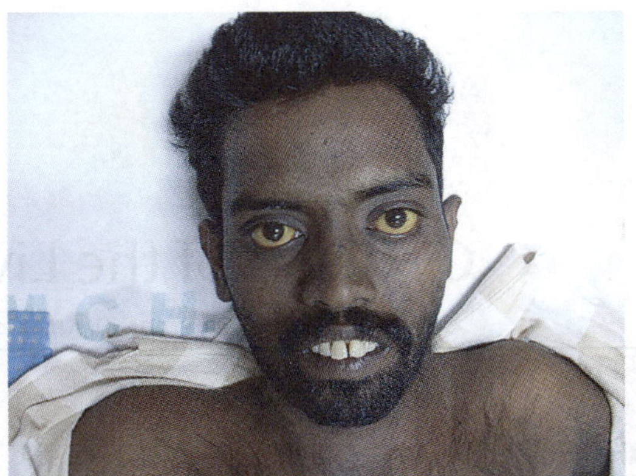

Fig. 83.3: Obstructive jaundice in viral hepatitis. **Note:** Deep yellow sclera

Obstructive Jaundice (Figs 83.3 and 83.4)

Skin: Skin changes include melanotic pigmentation, chronic pruritus, thickening and excoriation. Xanthomas develop due to hypercholesterolemia. Bleeding tendency manifests as purpura or bruising.

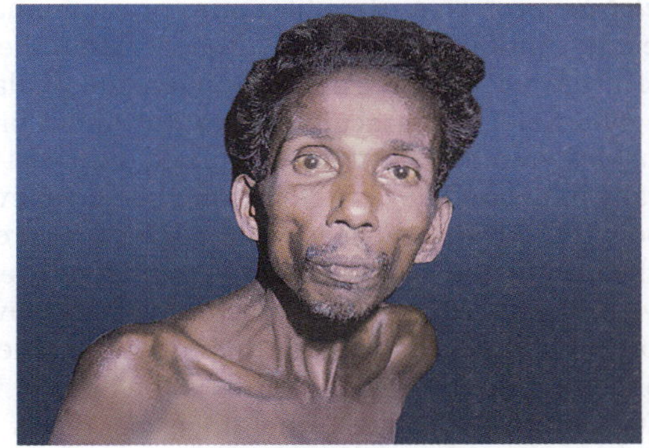

Fig. 83.4: Obstructive jaundice male aged 55—carcinoma head of pancreas. **Note:** Dark yellow pigmentation of sclera and skin

Malabsorption: Since bile does not reach to the intestine, absorption of fat and fat soluble vitamins is defective. This leads to steatorrhea and deficiencies of vitamins A, D, E and K and calcium.

Accumulation of copper: Copper is normally excreted in bile. In chronic obstructive jaundice, copper accumulates in the liver and may reach high values. Unlike, as in Wilson's disease in which copper is deposited in the lysosomes, in biliary cirrhosis the copper is present in the cytosol.

Hepatocellular failure: Back pressure of bile and prolonged obstruction leads to hepatocellular necrosis, secondary biliary cirrhosis and hepatic failure. Elderly, subjects are more prone to develop these complications.

Renal failure: This may develop during the icteric stage or after surgical relief of the obstruction.

Hemolytic Jaundice

Damage to nervous system: In the newborn, the blood-brain barrier for unconjugated bile pigment is not developed. The bilirubin is bound to albumin, but when the level exceeds 20 mg/dL binding capacity of albumin is exceeded. Bilirubin passes into the nervous tissues and gets fixed to the mitochondria whose function is impaired resulting in neuronal death. The basal ganglia are affected most but, no part of the central nervous system (CNS) is totally free. This used to be dreaded complication of hemolytic diseases of the newborn (kernicterus). The CNS of the newborn is most susceptible to this damage.

Pigment gallstones: Presence of excess of bilirubin in bile results in its precipitation and formation of pigment gallstones. Though, asymptomatic in many cases, rarely they may become symptomatic and lead to obstructive jaundice.

MANAGEMENT OF JAUNDICE

Definitive management depends upon the cause, but symptomatic treatment is necessary when the cause cannot be corrected.

Hemolytic jaundice: Treatment of the underlying disorder relieves the jaundice in most cases. In severe hemolytic disease of the newborn, measures such as exchange transfusion are necessary to lower serum bilirubin urgently and prevent neurological damage. Phototherapy [exposure to ultravoilet (UV) rays] benefits mild cases. Early detection of blood group incompatibility of the pregnant women with her husband and appropriate therapy helps to avoid severe hemolytic disease in the newborn.

Obstructive jaundice: Troublesome pruritus may be relieved by antihistamines like diphenhydramine in a dose of 50 mg twice daily. External application of calamine lotion gives relief. In intractable cases, the anion binding resin cholestyramine has to be given in a dose of 4–16 g/day orally in divided doses to lower the bile acid levels in the body. It binds the bile acids in the intestine, prevents their absorption and facilitate their elimination. The main dose (4–8 g) is mixed in water or fruit juice and given in the morning with breakfast, since this is the time when bile salt concentration in the duodenum is the highest. Since cholestyramine also binds other ingested drugs, such drugs should be given at least one hour before administering cholestyramine. Cholestyramine is of no use if bile does not reach the intestine as in complete obstruction.

In such cases, analogues of sex hormones may be effective. Methyltestosterone 25 mg is given sublingually for men and norethandrolone 10 mg is given orally for women. The antipruritic effect of these drugs will be manifested within a week of starting the drug.

Ursodexycholic acid (UDCA) promotes biliary flow and is useful in intrahepatic cholestasis.

Steatorrhea occurs in obstructive jaundice and this can be troublesome. This can be minimized by reducing the fat intake below 40 g/day. Since medium chain trigly cerides are absorbed even without the help of bile acids, administration of such fats helps to avoid steatorrhea. Parenteral injection of vitamin K (10 mg) and vitamin D (2.5 mg) should be given monthly. Calcium gluconate given in a dose of 2–4 g orally helps to prevent negative calcium balance.

Endoscopic Management

Interventional endoscopic procedures such as endoscopic cholangiopancreatography are the methods of choice for relieving biliary obstruction and these have eliminated the need for surgery to a great extent. Endoscopic interventions can be done by special instruments during the procedure. These include extraction of stones, division of strictures and stenting of the pancreatic and bile ducts. Stones can be extracted from the common bile duct, hepatic duct or even from intrahepatic portions of the smaller biliary ducts using baskets or balloons. Benign and malignant strictures can be dilated and stents deployed to restore the lumen (Refer Fig. 83.2).

Surgical treatment: This should be undertaken immediately in cases of extrahepatic obstruction not amenable to endoscopic methods. Even in incurable lesions, palliative surgical procedures to overcome the biliary obstruction such as cholecystojejunostomy, help in relieving the symptoms, especially the intractable pruritus and steatorrhea. Surgical decompression of the biliary tree also helps in arresting the progress of hepatocellular damage. Many years of symptom-free life can be achieved and hence, such procedures should be considered in suitable cases without delay.

CHAPTER

84

Cirrhosis of the Liver

KR Vinaya Kumar, KV Krishna Das

Chapter Summary

- Cirrhosis: General Considerations
  - Pathogenesis
- Special forms of Cirrhosis
  - Alcoholic Cirrhosis
  - Non-alcoholic Fatty Liver Disease
    - Biliary Cirrhosis
- Primary Sclerosing Cholangitis
- Liver in Wilson's Disease
- Hemochromatosis

CIRRHOSIS: GENERAL CONSIDERATIONS

Among the chronic parenchymal liver diseases, cirrhosis is most common. It is characterized by diffuse fibrosis and conversion of normal architecture into structurally abnormal nodules. At all times during the pathological process, there is evidence of liver cell necrosis, fibrosis and development of regenerative nodules which do not conform to normal anatomical pattern. The diffuse lesion involves the major portion of the liver. In many cases hepatocellular

Textbook of Medicine

Table 84.1: Etiological factors in cirrhosis

Chronic infections	Hepatitis B, C, D
Alcoholism	Alcoholic steatohepatitis
Drugs and toxins	Methotrexate, INH, methyldopa, arsenic
Metabolic	Hemochromatosis, Wilson's disease, galactosemia, glycogen storage disease type IV, alpha-1 antitrypsin deficiency
Immunological	Autoimmune hepatitis, primary biliary cirrhosis
Vascular	Hepatic venous obstruction, chronic congestive cardiac failure, constrictive pericarditis
Biliary obstruction	Gallstone, biliary atresia, biliary strictures, mucoviscidosis
Miscellaneous	Aflatoxins, hepatic steatosis
Cryptogenic	No definite cause detectable after full investigations

Note: There are suggestions that viral HEV may lead to cirrhosis in immunocompromised individuals.

Abbreviation: INH = Isoniazid (also known as isonicotinylhydrazide)

necrosis resulting from different pathological lesions initiate the process. In India, the common identifiable causes are hepatitis B and C virus infections and alcoholism. Malnutrition may act as an aggravating factor in the presence of other causes (Table 84.1).

Pathogenesis

When liver cells undergo necrosis, the hepatic lobules collapse and this leads to formation of diffuse fibrous septa. As a compensatory mechanism, nodular regeneration of hepatocytes occurs. When the necrosis is associated with collapse of the reticulin framework, cirrhosis results. If the reticulin framework is preserved, hepatocytes regrow and reproduce the normal histological pattern. Damage to the reticulin framework results in the formation of abnormal nodules which derive nourishment from the hepatic artery, but without portal and biliary connections. The nodules vary in size from a few millimeters to several centimeters. The liver surface becomes nodular. Hepatic vascular bed is distorted, truncated and obstructed, the obstruction being maximal at the level of sinusoids.

Several vascular abnormalities develop. These include:

- Generalized arterialization of the liver
- Formation of shunts between the branches of the hepatic artery, portal vein and hepatic vein
- Formation of arteriovenous (AV) shunts also in the pulmonary circulation
- Development of a hyperdynamic circulatory state with increased cardiac output and reduced peripheral vascular resistance.

Resistance to portal venous flow results in the development of portal hypertension. As the nodules grow, their centers are rendered ischemic. Once the disease process is initiated, other factors such as autoimmunity, continuing necrosis and chronic effect of toxins lead to progression of the pathological lesions.

Basement membrane forms in the **Disse space** and this interferes with the metabolic functions of the liver. The necrotic foci stimulate the proliferation of fibroblasts and collagen and fibrous septae develop in the portal zones and hepatic lobules. Hepatic fibrosis is a common sequel to chronic liver injury from various causes such as alcoholism.

Cirrhosis may be the end result of several unrelated conditions such as persistent viral and helminthic infections and hereditary copper or iron overload. In all these conditions the mechanism of fibrosis is similar, but the location varies. In chronic alcohol injury, the fibrosis is pericentral whereas in viral hepatitis it is periportal. The perisinusoidal **Ito cells** may also transform into fibroblasts and produce intralobular collagen. Though these cells produce at least five types of collagen, only types I and III are found in the final scar tissue. Fibronectin (FN), which is a soluble glycoprotein present in plasma, is rendered insoluble and deposited on the surface of the liver cells. FN binds collagen to form the extracellular matrix which replaces areas of liver cell necrosis. The matrix consists of proteoglycans, fibronectin-hyaluronic acid (FN-HA).

Cytokines initiate and perpetuate fibrogenesis. Among them platelet derived growth factor (PDGF) is most important. In the early stages fibrosis is reversible, but once established, it is not so.

Morphological Classification

The morphological types are:

- Micronodular (Laennec's cirrhosis)
- Macronodular
- Mixed.

In **micronodular cirrhosis**, the nodules are less than 3 mm in diameter, uniform and these are seen involving the whole liver. The fibrous bands are indistinct and fine. In **macronodular cirrhosis,** the nodules are coarse, irregular and may grow up to several centimeters. The liver surface is grossly distorted. The **mixed type** is a combination of the two. In some cases, at least the morphology may suggest the cause, though to a large extent this is decided by the extent of necrosis and other aggravating factors as well. In all types of cirrhosis in the later stages when fibrosis predominates, the organ shrinks.

Clinical Features

Early stages of the disease are asymptomatic. Vague ill health, anorexia, loss of weight, loss of libido, impotence, abdominal distention and dependent edema may bring the patient to the doctor. Night blindness is a common symptom in many and this results from the impairment of metabolism of vitamin A. Ascites is probably the most prominent feature which draws attention to the hepatic problem (Figs 84.1 and 84.2).

The major clinical features depend on the two main pathological processes, **hepatocellular failure** and **portal hypertension**. These processes often develop simultaneously in majority of cases but independent of each other. The liver is enlarged in the early stage due to infiltration but in the later stage it shrinks and becomes harder in consistency. The spleen enlarges in size due to portal hypertension and reticuloendothelial hyperplasia. Development of portal hypertension will lead to development of esophageal and gastric varices

Textbook of Medicine

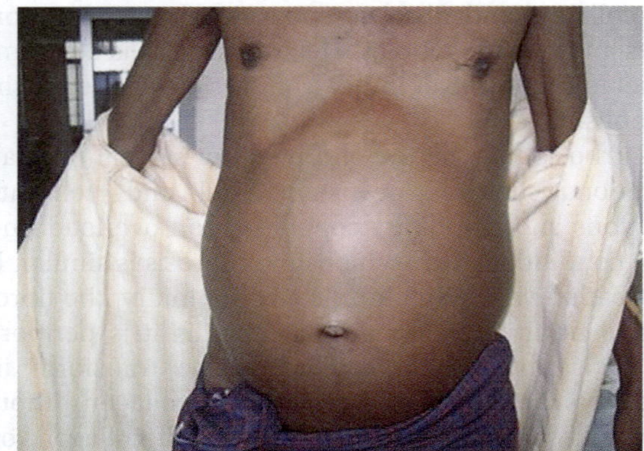

Fig. 84.1: Ascites with portal hypertension. **Note:** Prominent veins on the abdomen and eversion of the umbilicus

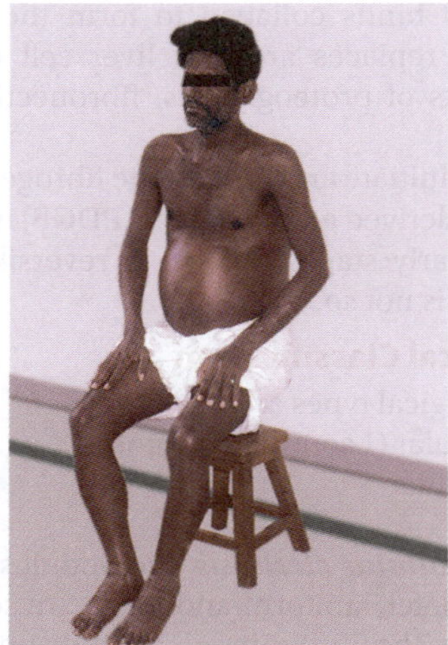

Fig. 84.2: Male 60-year-old—cirrhosis liver with gross ascites and edema. **Note:** The pale nails and shiny abdomen

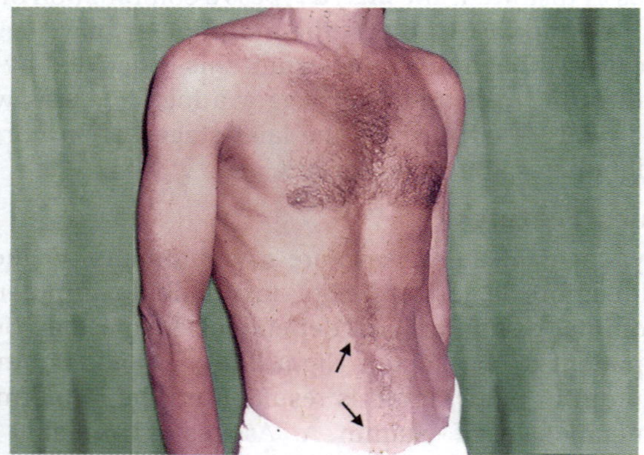

Fig. 84.3: Cirrhosis liver abdomen showing caput medusa. **Note:** The prominent veins on the abdominal wall, arrows point to the directions of blood flow

(Fig. 84.3) and later manifesting as hematemesis or malena. Some may present with altered sleep rhythm or altered sensorium, i.e. in the form of encephalopathy. **Clubbing of fingers** may develop in a few. **Dupuytren's contracture** has been found to be associated with cirrhosis, but this association is not strong in Indian subjects. Other causes of Dupuytren's contracture include trauma, diabetes, phenytoin intake and alcoholism. A

significant number of persons are at the risk of progression to hepatoma.

Compensated cirrhosis: Patient with chronic liver disease, but without any overt evidence of ascites or encephalopathy and normal liver function test (LFT).

Decompensated cirrhosis: Patient with chronic liver disease, but with evidence of ascites, bleed or encephalopathy with altered LFT.

Diagnosis

Cirrhosis has to be suspected clinically by the firm nodular feel of the liver, splenomegaly, signs of portal hypertension and hepatocellular insufficiency. The biochemical tests reflect parenchymal cell damage. Serum albumin is lowered with rise in gamma globulin, i.e. albumin/globulin reversal. Bromsulphthalein (BSP) retention is high. Transaminase levels are elevated if active necrosis is present. In all cases of doubt, liver biopsy should be performed for establishing the diagnosis and identifying the morphological pattern, since the diagnosis is based on hepatic morphology.

Since removal of the underlying cause is necessary to arrest progression of the disease, etiological diagnosis should be attempted. In conditions like Wilson's disease, hemochromatosis and autoimmune chronic hepatitis, specific measures can be employed for reversing the lesions.

European Association for the Study of the Liver Disease (EASL) Staging

Stage I: Absence of ascites and esophageal varices.
Stage II: Esophageal varices without ascites and without bleeding.
Stage III: Ascites with or without esophageal varices in a patient that has never bled.
Stage IV: Gastointestinal (GI) bleeding with or without ascites.

Model for End Stage Liver Disease (MELD)

This classification system was first devised by Mayo clinic to predict the outcome of cirrhosis patient undergoing shunt surgeries. It is based on a composite of three variables serum bilirubin, serum creatinine and prothrombin time (PT) and International Normalized Ratio (INR). It is calculated with the help of online calculator because of complex formulae. MELD score of more than 15 is an indication for listing the patient for liver transplantation.

Management of Hepatic Cirrhosis

All cases of cirrhosis should be carefully managed. Considerable symptomatic and functional improvement can be achieved and useful life-prolonged.

Uncomplicated Cases

Removal of the primary cause: If treatment is started early, the lesions can be reversed, as in alcoholism, hepatitis B virus (HBV) and hepatitis C virus (HCV) infection, drug toxicity, biliary obstruction and schistosomiasis.

Diet: The diet should contain 2500–2800 cal/day. Protein intake of 1.25–1.5 g/kg/bw should be attempted, if possible. The limiting factor is the development of hepatic encephalopathy. Vitamin and mineral supplements are indicated if there are overt or latent deficiencies.

Avoidance of precipitating factors: Factors that precipitate upper GI bleeding and hepatic failure should be strictly avoided. Drugs should be administered to cirrhotics only after taking into consideration these potential complications.

Management of Ascites

General Measures

- Bed rest helps the functional recovery of the liver and prevents deterioration of ascites. Low sodium diet 60–90 mmol/day of sodium (1500–2000 mg of sodium chloride) is ideal. If the serum sodium is < 130 mmol/L in the presence of ascites or edema, it suggests dilutional hyponatremia, due to impairment of water elimination by kidney, caused by syndrome of inappropriate antidiuretic hormone secretion (SIADH).
- In many advanced cases of cirrhosis, the urinary loss of sodium is generally less than 2 g/day. Therefore, dietary sodium has to be restricted. Apart from added salt at table, food containing excess salt such as pickles, bread, salted biscuits, salted canned food and salted butter should be avoided. The diet should contain moderate protein (50–70 g) and adequate calories. Since vegetable proteins are better tolerated than animal protein by patients with hepatic failure, these should be preferred. Failure to conform to a low salt diet is the most important cause of therapeutic failure. Fluid intake should be restricted to one liter a day.
- ***Diuretics*** are indicated if salt-restricted diet alone is not effective in clearing the edema and ascites. Loss of weight of at least 1 kg in 4 days is ideal. The diuretic has to be chosen depending on the severity and response to therapy. Powerful diuretics like furosemide, thiazides, ethacrynic acid and bumetanide cause loss of sodium and potassium. Potassium should be supplemented in a dose of 2 g/8 h. Combination of potassium sparing diuretics like spironolactone, triamterene or amiloride and the powerful diuretics enhances effectiveness and reduces the need for potassium replacement. An effective combination is furosemide with spironolactone or amiloride. Excessive diuresis may lead to hepatic failure, hypotension and uremia in 30–40% of cases and this should be avoided.

When potassium sparing diuretics are given, potassium intake should not exceed 50 mmol/day (3.75 g of KCl). Diuretic therapy may have to be continued over prolonged periods to get sustained benefits.

Diuretics should be started maintaining the ratio of spironolactone to furosemide as 50:20 and increasing the dose maintaining the ratio as this will maintain normokalemia.

Frequent determination of serum levels of creatinine, sodium, potassium and bicarbonate is necessary to detect acute kidney injury and avoid electrolyte disturbances.

Some of the resistant cases in whom the serum albumin level is below 2 g/dL, respond to intravenous (IV) infusion of salt-free human albumin, dextran or ascitic fluid itself. This temporarily raises the colloid osmotic pressure.

As the hepatic function improves and ascites clears up, dietary intake of salt can be increased and diuretics can be withdrawn in stages. Five to ten percent of patients with ascites become resistant to treatment. They do not respond even to high doses of diuretics (100–200 mg of spiranolactone and 40–160 mg of furosemide/day). In some others, complications such as hepatic encephalopathy, hyponatremia, hyperkalemia or azotemia preclude further increase in diuretic dosage. Risk of hepatorenal syndrome (HRS) occurs in 10% of cases of hepatic failure with ascites (Table 84.1). Prognostic factors in cirrhosis are listed in Table 84.2.

Refractory Ascites

Refractory ascites is defined as either:

- ***Diuretic-resistant ascites:*** Ascites that cannot be mobilized or the early recurrence of which cannot be prevented because of lack of response to dietary sodium restriction and intensive diuretic treatment.
- ***Diuretic-intractable ascites:*** Ascites that cannot be mobilized or the early recurrence of which cannot be prevented because of the development of diuretic-induced complications that preclude the use of an effective diuretic dosage.

Diagnostic Criteria of Refractory Ascites

- ***Treatment duration:*** Patients must be on intensive diuretic therapy (spironolactone 400 mg by mouth daily and furosemide 160 mg by mouth daily) for at

Table 84.1: Complications of cirrhosis

• Portal hypertension and its sequelae	• Hepatic encephalopathy	• Hepatocellular carcinoma
• Ascites	• Portal gastropathy	• Bleeding manifestations
• Spontaneous bacterial peritonitis	• Hepatorenal syndrome	• Cirrhotic cardiomyopathy
	• Hepatopulmonary syndrome	• Hepatic hydrothorax

Table 84.2: Poor prognostic factors in cirrhosis

Laboratory findings	*Clinical findings*
• Low serum albumin of less than 2.5 g/dL • Low serum sodium of less than 120 mmol/L • Rising serum creatinine • Prolongation of prothrombin time more than 1.5 times of control (> 6 seconds above normal)	• Persistent jaundice (serum bilirubin more than 20 mg/dL) • Ascites responding poorly to therapy • Encephalopathy not associated with an extensive collateral circulation • Hemorrhage from varices with poor liver function • Neuropsychiatric complications • Persistent hypotension • Small liver • Etiology (e.g. alcoholic cirrhosis, if the patient continues alcoholism)

least 1 week and on a sodium restricted diet of less than 90 mmol/L per day or 5.2 g of salt (NaCl) per day.

- *Lack of response:* Means weight loss of <0.8 kg over 4 days and urinary sodium output less than the sodium intake.
- *Early ascites recurrence:* Reappearance of grade 2 or 3 ascites within 4 weeks of initial mobilization.
- *Diuretic-induced complications:* Hepatic encephalopathy, acute kidney injury and electrolyte disturbances necessitating withdrawal of diuretics.

If the ascites tends to persist despite intensive general measures and diuretics, fluid should be removed by paracentesis.

Paracentesis: This is a short-term measure and the fluid reaccumulates rapidly. The loss of protein and electrolytes from the body may worsen hepatic function further. Paracentesis is indicated when ascites increases rapidly despite adequate general measures and causes severe embarrassment and pain. Only the minimum amount of fluid should be removed to relieve these symptoms. If the abdominal distention is severe and accompanied by dyspnea, removal of 4–5 L of fluid in 12–16 hours brings about temporary relief. Complications of paracentesis include shock, bleeding into the peritoneum, infection and precipitation of hepatic coma. Recently interest in this procedure has increased and controlled paracentesis is being employed more frequently. Regular removal of fluid by paracentesis helps to reduce the dose of diuretic. It is advisable to give albumin infusion to prevent hemodynamic alterations when the paracentesis exceeds 5 L of fluid [large volume paracentesis (LVP)].

It is possible to maintain patients for long periods in reasonable comfort with judicious abdominal tapping repeated at regular intervals.

Spontaneous Bacterial Peritonitis (SBP)

In advanced liver cirrhosis, bacterial translocation of gut microbes into the ascitic fluid occurs. This condition is called spontaneous bacterial peritonitis which is seen in about 50% of patients with cirrhosis and ascites. The ascitic fluid protein is typically low but more than 250 polymorphs/mm³ occur. Culture is positive for gram-negative enterobacteriaceae, usually a single type. The presentation is with mild fever or abdominal pain. Sometimes rapid worsening of cirrhosis may be the presenting feature. Untreated, the mortality is high with worsening of ascites, hepatorenal syndrome and encephalopathy. Treatment is with cefotaxime 2 g tid for 5 days. These patients also require secondary prophylaxis with norfloxacin.

Other forms of peritonitis in cirrhosis are:

- *Culture negative-neutrocytic ascites:* Where the polymorph count is > 250/mm³; but culture is negative.
- *Monomicrobial non-neutrocytic ascites:* In this the culture is positive for single type of microbial species; but polymorphonuclear count is less than 250/mm³.
- *Polymicrobial bacterial ascites:* In this condition culture is positive for multiple species of microbes. This usually results from needle puncture of the bowel while attempting paracentesis.

- *Secondary peritonitis:* In this condition polymorph count is very high, usually > 10000/mm³. This is a serious condition resulting from lesions such as bowel perforation, cholecystitis, appendicitis, diverticulitis, duodenal ulcer and others. Often surgical management is required.

Ascitic fluid ultrafiltration and reinfusion: Using an automated ultrafiltration apparatus (Rhodiascit) proteins of the ascitic fluid can be concentrated and infused IV. The equipment is expensive and the procedure demands special skills.

LeVeen peritoneovenous shunt: This surgical procedure establishes intermittent drainage of the peritoneal fluid into the superior vena cava through a valve. The respiratory movements of the diaphragm and the reciprocal pressure changes within the abdomen and thorax serve to operate the valve. Limited success has been reported in some cases.

The treatment of complications like hematemesis and hepatic failure is described in Chapters 85 and 87 respectively.

Intercurrent Infections

These are common and early treatment is essential to prevent hepatic failure. Ampicillin and amoxycillin are safe. Tuberculosis occurs more frequently in cirrhotics (4–6%). The lesions include pulmonary, lymph nodular or peritoneal tuberculosis. Such patients require standard chemotherapy. Cellulitis of legs is one of the important infections in cirrhotics and is caused by gram-negative bacteria in contrast to cellulitis in non-cirrhotics (Fig. 84.4).

Development of Primary Carcinoma

Cirrhosis predisposes to the development of primary carcinoma (hepatoma or hepatocellular carcinoma). Rapid enlargement of the liver, fever, pain, rapid loss of weight, development of massive hemorrhagic ascites or sudden hepatic or portal vein obstruction should suggest this possibility. Cirrhosis also predispose the patient to development of cholangiocarcinoma and other extrahepatic malignancies. In cirrhosis liver, obesity, diabetes, nonalcoholic hepatitis steatosis and nonalcoholic fatty liver diseases are independently associated with the risk of hepatocellular carcinoma.

In decompensated cirrhosis, into low systolic blood pressure should not receive anti-hypertensive drugs. In

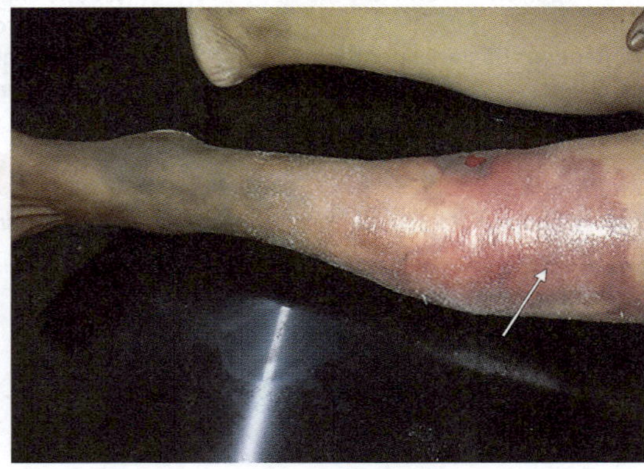

Fig. 84.4: Cellulitis in cirrhosis (arrow)

patients with cirrhosis and ascites mean arterial blood pressure of 82 mm Hg, or less is a single predictive factor related to a reduced probability of survival.

Source: Ge PS, Runyon BA. Treatment of Patients with Cirrhosis. N Engl J Med. 2016;375(8):767-77.

Prevention

Prevention of viral hepatitis, abstinence from alcohol, enforcement of laws on food adulteration and proper food hygiene to avoid contamination by toxins, serve to reduce the incidence of cirrhosis on a long-term basis. Widespread vaccination against hepatitis B has brought down the incidence of cirrhosis and carcinoma in many South East Asian countries.

SPECIAL FORMS OF CIRRHOSIS

ALCOHOLIC CIRRHOSIS

The final phase of alcoholic liver disease is alcoholic or Laennec's cirrhosis. This may result from repeated bouts of acute alcoholic hepatitis which is the more likely mechanism in most cases (50%). Presence of hepatic encephalopathy, deep jaundice with bilirubin above 20 mg/dL, prolongation of prothrombin time more than 5 seconds above normal, azotemia and severe hypoalbuminemia are associated with a higher risk of developing cirrhosis. The cirrhosis is micronodular and the liver is moderately enlarged, except in a few cases in whom it is shrunken.

Ascites, esophageal varices, muscle wasting and renal failure are common complications in alcoholic cirrhosis. Continued intake of alcohol leads to persistence of alcoholic hepatitis, progressive deterioration of liver function and death. Withdrawal of alcohol may arrest progress of the disease and in many cases even lead to regression. The inactive stage is compatible with prolonged survival.

NONALCOHOLIC FATTY LIVER DISEASE (NAFLD)

(*See* Ch 88 for details)

BILIARY CIRRHOSIS

This results from prolonged obstruction to the biliary passages anywhere between the canaliculi and the ampulla of Vater. This may be primary or more commonly secondary.

Secondary Biliary Cirrhosis

Obstruction to the larger bile passages by stones, strictures, growths or extrinsic pressure is the primary mechanism. Cirrhosis develops after a prolonged latent period. Biliary cirrhosis should be looked for if recurrent fever, chills, tender hepatomegaly, leukocytosis and features of obstructive jaundice develop.

Treatment

Early removal of the primary cause leads to regression. Secondary biliary cirrhosis is prevented by prompt relief of biliary obstruction. Elderly subjects are more prone to develop cirrhosis as a result of biliary obstruction and therefore in them, procedures to relieve obstruction should be undertaken without undue delay.

Primary Biliary Cirrhosis (PBC)

Recent reports from the west suggest that this disease is quite frequent in middle-aged and elderly women. The disease is still considered to be rare in India, accounting for 0.6–2% of all cirrhosis. PBC is characterized by chronic cholestasis, pigmentation, xanthomatous eruptions and histological features of chronic nonsuppurative, destructive cholangiohepatitis. The disease is immunologically mediated. There is a familial tendency, the incidence among close relatives is 1000 times more than in the general population.

Pathology

The liver is enlarged in the early stages, later it shrinks, portal hypertension develops late and the spleen enlarges. Forty percent show stones in the gallbladder. The pathology is one of lymphocytic cholangitis involving small intralobular bile ducts within the liver. The first step in pathogenesis is immunological attack on biliary radicles, the next step is hepatotoxicity caused by retention of toxic bile acids secondary to cholestasis and loss of bile ducts.

Histologically, the smaller bile ducts show epithelial damage and necrosis surrounded by granulomas consisting of histiocytes, CD8+ lymphocytes, plasma cells, eosinophils and giant cells. Fibrosis of the portal tracts progress (stage III) and give rise to frank cirrhosis (stage IV). The larger bile passages are normal. Antimitochondrial antibodies directed against a family of enzymes, especially pyruvate dehydrogenase complex which are inhibited *in vitro* are characteristic and are present in over 95% of cases.

Clinical Features

Classically, the disease affects middle-aged women and starts with fatigue, pruritus and jaundice. Male to female ratio is 1:9. Complications include malabsorption of fat-soluble vitamins, especially vitamin D, osteoporosis, progressive hepatic failure and portal hypertension. Copper accumulates in the liver. Unlike Wilson's disease in which copper accumulates in the lysosomes, in primary biliary cirrhosis it is in the cytosol. The disease progresses to end fatally within 5–7 years because of complications like hepatic failure or portal hypertension.

Diagnosis

Clinical suspicion is important in making a diagnosis. Conditions like chronic biliary tract disease, viral hepatitis, other causes of intra and extrahepatic biliary obstruction, toxic damage to the liver, systemic lupus erythematosus (SLE) and other forms of cirrhosis have to be excluded. Some cases are associated with other autoimmune disorders such as CREST syndrome (calcinosis, Raynaud's phenomenon, sclerodactyly and telangiectasia), Sjögren's syndrome, thyroid diseases and esophageal dysmotility.

In some cases, antimitochondrial antibodies may not be present but all other clinical features resemble PBC. In prognosis and response to ursodeoxycholic acid (UDCA), it is similar to that in classic PBC. Such cases are known as autoimmune cholangitis. It may lead to metabolic bone disease and hepatocellular carcinoma.

Textbook of Medicine

Laboratory diagnosis

Features of obstructive jaundice such as raised alkaline phosphatase and increased serum bilirubin may be obvious. Alanine transaminase serum glutamic-pyruvic transaminase (SGPT) may be elevated to different levels, sometimes it may be normal. Serum cholesterol is elevated. Since the high density lipoprotein (HDL) fraction is also considerably elevated, the risk of atherosclerosis is relatively less.

Specific test is the demonstration of ***antimitochondrial antibodies*** in the serum in titers above 1080 in over 95% of the cases. Titers above 1/40 are suggestive.

Other immunological phenomena such as presence of immune complexes [raised levels of immunoglobulin G (IgG) and immunoglobulin M (IgM)] and abnormalities of complement may be present, but are nonspecific. Around 70% of cases of primary biliary cirrhosis have raised levels of IgM.

Liver biopsy is confirmatory. Serum cholesterol may be high and xanthomas may develop. Median survival after diagnosis varies from 10 to 16 years.

Treatment

General measures include relief of pruritus by antihistaminics such as diphenhydramine 50 mg or hydroxyzine 25 mg given twice daily, or cholestyramine 4–8 g/day with breakfast. The diet is adjusted to contain less than 40 g fat per day, supplied as medium chain fatty acids, e.g. coconut. Monthly injection of vitamin D 2.5 mg and vitamin K 10 mg and oral supplementation of calcium gluconate 2–4 g/day serve to compensate for the malabsorption state.

Specific measures are directed:
- Towards the primary disease
- Towards the complications.

Attempts to treat the liver lesion with corticosteroids have given equivocal results and in many centers this drug is no longer given due to its tendency to worsen osteoporosis. D-penicillamine has shown promise in recent years. In addition to its copper chelating effect, it relieves inflammation in the liver. Dose ranges from 250 to 900 mg/day. An alternate drug is colchicine given in a dose of 0.6 mg twice daily. Cyclosporine has been employed with partial success. UDCA, given in a daily dose of 12–15 mg/kg/bw has been reported to arrest progress and bring about relief. Methotrexate given in a dose of 0.25 mg/kg twice a week orally produces resolution of lesions over a period of 6–12 months. The drug is toxic. Interstitial pneumonitis is one of the serious ill-effects of methotrexate. Portal hypertension, if already established, does not respond to medical therapy. This has to be treated on its own merits—if necessary by shunt surgery. If the condition is advanced, hepatic transplantation is indicated.

PRIMARY SCLEROSING CHOLANGITIS (PSC)

It is an idiopathic inflammatory disorder affecting the intra and extrahepatic biliary system resulting in fibrosis and stricture formation. Eighty percent of cases are associated with inflammatory bowel disease (IBD), especially ulcerative colitis. Despite the association between IBD and PSC, the latter appears to progress independent of each other.

Etiopathogenesis

The etiology and pathogenesis of PSC are unknown. A variety of causative mechanisms have been proposed, including toxins, infectious processes, ischemia and genetic and autoimmune factors.

Clinical Features

The median age of diagnosis of PSC is 39, males are affected more. The most common symptoms at the time of diagnosis are jaundice, pruritus and abdominal pain. The onset and progression of symptoms are usually insidious; rarely the disease can present as acute hepatitis like-illness. Loss of weight can occur at an alarming rate. Patients often experience chronic fatigue. Febrile episodes can occur, usually a manifestation of acute cholangitis. Symptoms and signs such as jaundice, pruritus, abdominal pain and fever may remit spontaneously and for prolonged periods. Rarely the initial presentation may be with complications such as cirrhosis and portal hypertension. About 20–40% of patients are asymptomatic. Jaundice and hepatomegaly are the most common abnormal physical findings and the spleen is enlarged in about one-third of patients.

Investigations

Typically, the serum alkaline phosphatase (SAP) level is increased three- to five-folds in PSC. Elevation in the SAP level is usually matched by increase in ***serum gamma glutamyl transpeptidase*** and ***5'-nucleotidase levels.*** Serum aminotransferases levels are usually elevated. Levels of conjugated bilirubin are increased in jaundiced patients. In others it may be normal. Serum albumin may be low and prothrombin time may be prolonged. Levels of immunoglobulin in the serum are often elevated. About 97% of patients with PSC have at least one autoantibody. The most common antibody is antineutrophil cytoplasmic antibody (ANCA). Other antibodies include anticardiolipin antibodies (ACA) and antinuclear antibodie. Non-specific markers of cholestasis such as increased serum cholesterol and lipoprotein X may also develop.

The most common characteristic histopathologic changes is 'onion skin' fibrosis, which describes the appearance of periductal concentric fibrosis around the interlobular and septal bile ducts. Ludwig has developed a histologc classification for PSC.
- ***Stage I:*** Portal hepatitis with or without bile duct abnormalities and cholangitis.
- ***Stage II:*** Periportal fibrosis or hepatitis may develop.
- ***Stage III:*** Characterized by septal fibrosis or bridging necrosis and stage.
- ***Stage IV:*** Biliary cirrhosis.

Non-invasive abdominal imaging can be suggestive but not diagnostic of PSC. Ultrasonography (USG) and computed tomography (CT) may detect extrahepatic and intrahepatic ductal dilation, lymphadenopathy and evidence of cirrhosis or mass lesion. Magnetic resonance

Table 84.3: Complications of primary sclerosing cholangitis
• Malabsorption of fat and fat-soluble vitamins • Secondary biliary cirrhosis • Biliary tract calculi • Pancreatic disease • Cholangiocarcinoma

imaging (MRI), and endoscopic retrograde cholangio-pancreatography (ERCP) is a useful investigation for PSC. ERCP is considered the gold standard for diagnosis. ERCP not only confirms the diagnosis of sclerosing cholangitis, but also provides information about the distribution of the disease and the presence of dominant strictures that may be amenable to interventional therapy.

Complications (Table 84.3)

The chronic cholestasis of PSC leads to malabsorption of fat and fat-soluble vitamins and secondary biliary cirrhosis, biliary tract calculi, pancreatic disease and possibly, cholangiocarcinoma.

Management

There is no definite medical, endoscopic or surgical therapy, except for liver transplantation, which improves the general health and well-being. Though several drugs including antibiotics, glucocorticoids and immuno-suppressants have been used from time to time, none showed any survival benefit. Results with UDCA are encouraging. Intervention such as balloon dilatation and stent placement for strictures are palliative and safe. This can allay acute exacerbations of jaundice, pruritus and cholangitis and improve the quality of life.

Liver transplantation is indicated for patients with complications such as portal hypertension, hepatic failure, worsening cholestasis with cirrhosis and recurrent cholangitis, refractory to medical or interventional therapy.

The median survival from diagnosis to death or liver transplantation has been estimated to be 12 years. A number of mathematical models have been developed to predict survival and optimal timing of liver transplantation. These are *CTP score, Modified Mayo Natural History Model, Cox regression model* and *Swedish prognostic index* which may be referred to for further reading.

Liver Transplantation

In severe cases not amenable to medical therapy liver transplantation is the ideal treatment of choice (for details *See* Ch 85 Hepatic failure).

Source: Lazaridis KN, LaRusso NF. Primary Sclerosing Cholangitis. N Engl J Med. 2016;375(12):1161-70.

LIVER IN WILSON'S DISEASE

Syn: Hepatolenticular degeneration

(*See* also Section 10, Ch 94, Wilson's Disease)

Wilson's disease is named after the British neurologist Samuel Kinnier Wilson who described the familial syndrome of cirrhosis liver with lenticular degeneration in the brain. Wilson's disease is an autosomal recessive disorder and a gene for Wilson's disease has been mapped to chromosome 13 (13q14). About 200 mutations in the Wilson's disease gene have been identified.

The fundamental abnormality is impairment of biliary excretion of copper which is the main mechanism to regulate body content of copper. Accumulation of copper in cells leads to cellular damage by free radicals, oxidative stress and depletion of glutathione. Though the metabolic defect is congenital, symptoms occur only after 5 years of age.

Pathology

Hepatic cirrhosis predominates in young subjects, while in older subjects neurological lesions predominate. The liver shows a variety of pathological changes such as periportal fibrosis, submassive necrosis and macronodular cirrhosis. Liver cells show fatty change, glycogen vacuolation and multinuclearity. Copper is deposited in the periportal regions in a patchy manner and this is demonstrable by staining with rubeanic acid or rhodamine. Wilson's disease is not rare among many communities in India and therefore all young subjects presenting with chronic parenchymal liver disease should be screened for this disorder.

Clinical features resemble those of cirrhosis, chronic active hepatitis, fulminant hepatitis or chronic hepatic failure. Presence of *Kayser-Fleischer ring* is diagnostic.

Serum ceruloplasmin is low (< 20 mg/dL), urinary excretion of copper exceeds 100 µg/day. Liver biopsy and estimation of hepatic copper are diagnostic. Hepatic copper > 250 µg/g of dry weight of liver tissue (normal < 35 µg/g liver tissue) is diagnostic.

Course of the disease is steadily downhill ending with cirrhosis, portal hypertension and hepatic failure. Early treatment arrests the progress and prolongs survival. Dietary articles rich in copper such as nuts, liver, shell fish and chocolates should be avoided. Severe cases may require liver transplantation.

Note: Management is described in Section 10, Ch 94.

HEMOCHROMATOSIS

(*See* also Section 10, Ch 94, Hemochromatosis)

This results from iron overload and the deposition of iron in several organs. The liver is enlarged, firm and tender. Histologically, deposits of iron can be demonstrated in the periportal liver cells. Fibrosis of the portal zone develops. Kupffer's cells are filled with iron. Macronodular cirrhosis develops if the condition proceeds. There is a high-risk of developing primary carcinoma. Removal of iron can be achieved by repeated venesection and use of iron chelating agents such as desferrioxamine.

CHAPTER
85

Hepatic Failure

KR Vinaya Kumar, KV Krishna Das

Textbook of Medicine

Chapter Summary
- Chronic Hepatic Failure
- Acute Hepatic Failure

Hepatic failure is a syndrome characterized by functional failure of hepatic parenchymal cells. It can result from various liver diseases with different pathological processes. Hepatic failure may be acute and fulminant or subacute and chronic.

CHRONIC HEPATIC FAILURE (CHF)

This may result from liver cirrhosis, carcinoma, drug toxicity, cholestatic jaundice and surgical obstruction of the biliary tree. Factors like high protein diet, hypotension, gastrointestinal (GI) bleeding, infections and overdose of sedatives like morphine precipitate the onset of symptoms (Table 85.1). Portal-systemic collateral circulation contributes to the development of encephalopathy. The clinical features differ in the acute and chronic forms.

Biochemical Disturbances in Hepatic Failure

In general, the biochemical abnormalities are more marked in acute fulminant hepatic failure than in the chronic form.

The failing liver is unable to convert ammonia into urea and hence ammonia accumulates. Glutamine is synthesized from ammonia and this is the major detoxification pathway to dispose ammonia. This occurs in the small intestine. Ammonia is converted into urea by the healthy liver. In hepatic failure this function suffers and so blood level of ammonia increases. Glutamine is synthesized in astrocytes and this causes brain swelling. The degree of brain swelling correlates with the neuropsychiatric abnormalities. Since amino acids are not further metabolized, aminoaciduria occurs. Synthesis of albumin is impaired. Hypoalbuminemia leads to ascites and dependent edema in chronic liver disease. Vitamin K-dependent coagulation factors (especially prothrombin) are reduced or not made functional and this leads to generalized bleeding tendency.

Table 85.1: Causes of chronic hepatocellular failure

Predisposing factors	*Precipitating factors*
• Cirrhosis—all types	• High protein diet
• Cholestatic jaundice	• Gastrointestinal bleeding, hypotension
• Drug toxicity	
• Surgical obstruction of biliary tract	• Hepatotoxic drugs or alcohol
	• Intense diuretic regimen leading to hypokalemia and hyponatremia
• Carcinoma—primary and metastatic	• Infections
	• Surgical intervention and trauma

Hepatic Encephalopathy (HE)

This is a neuropsychiatric syndrome that occurs in the presence of significant hepatocellular dysfunction and which has a full potential for reversal. The condition may be full-fledged or mild or even subclinical, occurring in 30–40% of cirrhotic patients.

This is associated with portal systemic shunting of blood. The blood is diverted through preformed collateral channels in portal hypertension. In acute hepatic failure, the liver cells do not metabolize the contents of the portal blood and hence these pass unaltered into the hepatic veins and further to the systemic circulation, thereby in effect producing a functional shunt. The nitrogenous products absorbed from the colon which reach the brain unaltered by hepatic metabolism lead to neurological dysfunction. The toxic products include ammonia and several pharmacologically active amines produced in the intestines by bacterial action and other products of protein digestion. Several of them have been implicated. The blood brain barrier is deranged. As a consequence these products reach the brain.

GABA and Endogenous Benzodiazepines

Gamma-aminobutyric acid (GABA) and endogenous benzodiazepines probably play their roles in the pathogenesis of this disorder. GABA and benzodiazepines are synthesized by the gut bacteria. The former has no major role in HE. It is possible that endogenous benzodiazepines which accumulated in HE play a major role in neuroinhibition.

The ill-effects of ammonia and other amines are further aggravated by alkalosis, hypoxia, hypokalemia, hypoglycemia and increase in the concentration of fatty acids in serum. Even though several biochemical abnormalities have been identified, the exact pathogenesis is still not clearly known. The blood levels of ammonia or other possible toxic metabolites do not correlate with the mental state, but serial estimations of blood ammonia can be used to monitor the effect of treatment. These metabolites do not cause neurological dysfunction in normal subjects. This fact suggests that an abnormal susceptibility of the brain to toxic metabolites is an important factor in leading to the clinical picture. The cerebrospinal fluid (CSF) is initially normal, but late in the disease, protein, glutamic acid and glutamine may be increased.

Clinical Features

The onset is insidious with general loss of health, fatigue and weight loss. Jaundice may occur, but this is not constant. The early stage may be missed if clinical suspicion is not high.

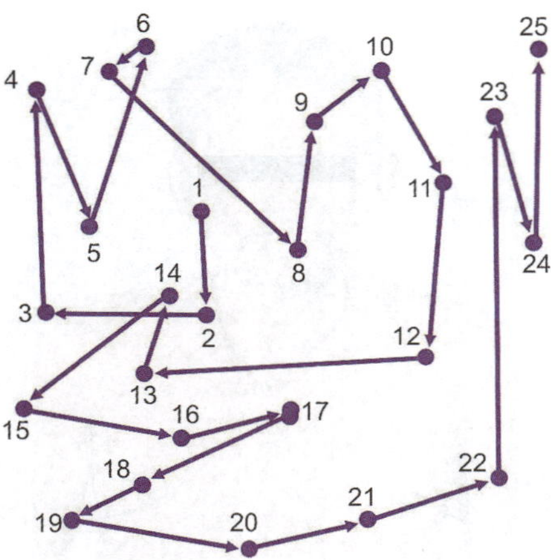

Fig. 85.1: Reitan number connection chart for trail making test

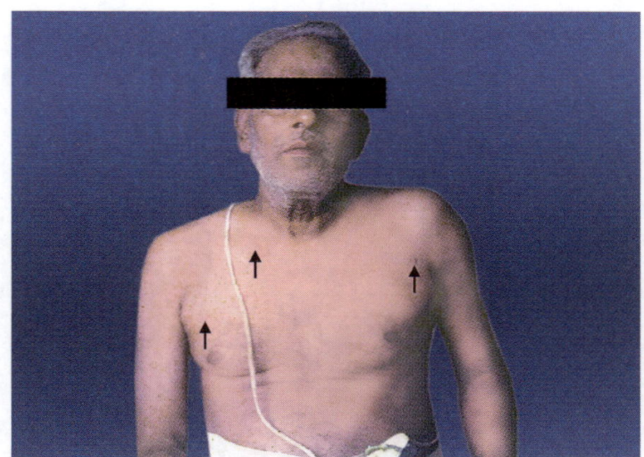

Fig. 85.2: Male 50-year-old alcoholic cirrhosis, hepatic failure. **Note:** Spider nevi on the chest (arrows)

Hyperkinetic circulation occurs which manifests as high volume pulse, warm extremities, tachycardia and ejection systolic murmur over the pulmonary area. It is likely that the circulatory disturbances are due to opening up of arteriovenous (AV) shunts and the effect of circulating vasodilator substances.

Neurological Manifestations Predominate

- *Alteration of consciousness* ranging from confusion to coma may develop. Sleep rhythm is altered early, with sleep during day and insomnia at night. Personality changes may be marked and these could be mistaken for primary psychiatric disorders.
- *Parkinsonian features*, especially akinesia may develop. Constructional apraxia develops which can be demonstrated by making the patient to draw along the Reitan number connection chart (Fig. 85.1).
- *A diagnostic physical sign is flapping tremor (asterixis)* elicited by holding the hands outstretched with extension of the wrist. The fingers and wrist show coarse tremors comparable to the flap of a bird's wing. In early cases, the tremor (flap) is confined to the extremities but later on it extends to the proximal joints of the limbs, trunk, jaw, neck and tongue. Flapping tremors are bilateral, asynchronous on both sides and absent at rest. The tremors fluctuate in severity with changes in hepatic function.
- *Electroencephalogram (EEG):* The EEG mainly shows slowing of rhythm from alpha (8–13 cps) to the delta (4 cps) range. Other abnormalities may also occur. Diffuse bilateral high voltage slow waves occur. The EEG changes closely reflect hepatic functional impairment. The EEG abnormalities can be precipitated by giving a high protein diet. As hepatic function deteriorates, coma sets in.

Magnetic resonance imaging (MRI) shows hyperintensity of globus pallidus on T_1 weighted imaging.

Vascular phenomena: Cyanosis occurs in one-third of patients due to hypoxia. Intrapulmonary AV shunts develop. The diffusing capacity of the lung is also impaired.

Finger clubbing, palmar erythema and *spider nevi* are common. Erythematous patches may occur over several parts of the body, especially the chest wall and supraclavicular regions. Arterial spiders are quite suggestive of chronic hepatic failure (CHF), though they can occur less commonly in other conditions such as pregnancy and estrogen therapy. A few may occur even in normal subjects. The upper limbs and the mucous membranes of the nose, mouth and gastrointestinal tract (GIT) are the sites of predilection. An arteriole comes to the surface and breaks up into capillaries which radiate like the legs of a spider. The central arteriole may pulsate in large nevi. Pressure over this vessel blanches the whole spider and on releasing the pressure blood fills from the center to the periphery (Fig. 85.2). Liver disease should be suspected when they are numerous and fresh spiders are appearing. The vascular phenomena of liver failure have been attributed to hyperestrogenism.

Other Features

Fetor hepaticus: It develops in some patients with severe hepatic failure. It is a slightly fecal odor attributed to the presence of methyl mercaptan and dimethyl sulfide in breath. This is present more often in acute hepatic failure. However, this sign is not prominent in Indian subjects when compared to those from the west.

Low grade fever: Attributable primarily to the liver disease, may be present. Gram-negative bacteremia and low grade septicemia are common due to shunting of the blood through collateral channels. Spontaneous bacterial peritonitis and endocarditis may occur with atypical presentations.

Skin changes: It occur in longstanding cases. They include appearance of white spots, white nails (leukonychia), loss of hair and pigmentation.

Endocrine disturbances: Males develop hypogonadism which presents as loss of libido and impotence and feminization manifested by gynecomastia (Figs 85.3 and 85.4) and loss of facial hair. In females, endocrine symptoms are less pronounced. The cause of feminization is still not fully understood.

Ascites: In CHF due to cirrhosis, when hypoalbuminemia and portal hypertension develop, ascites invariably occurs. The kidney plays a part in the development of ascites. Cirrhosis leads to a spectrum of renal abnormalities ranging from retention of sodium to fullfledged hepatorenal syndrome.

Textbook of Medicine

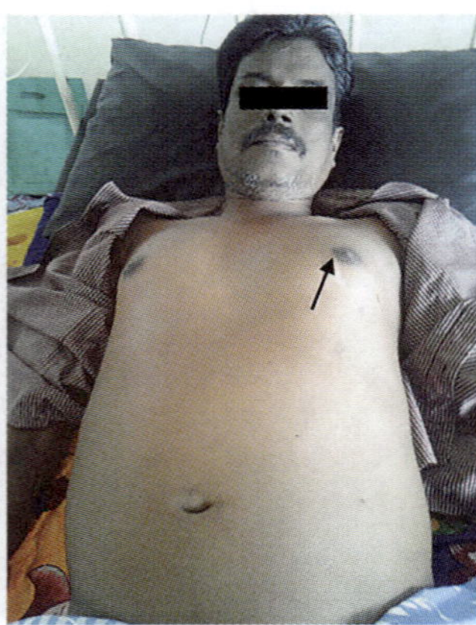

Fig. 85.3: Cirrhosis liver—hepatic failure ascites and gynecomastia (arrow)

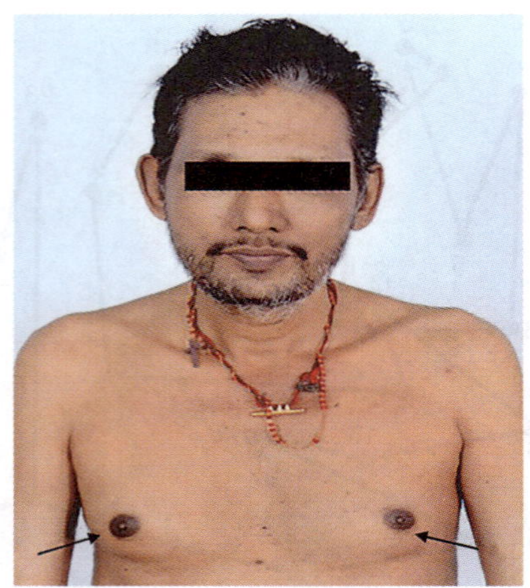

Fig. 85.4: Gynecomastia in chronic hepatic failure (arrows)

Drug metabolism: The detoxification function of the liver is impaired and elimination of drugs becomes defective. Even small doses of morphine produce profound sedation and tip the patient into hepatic coma. Several other drugs such as tetracycline may reach toxic levels in these patients. As the coma deepens, signs of upper motor neuron lesion, such as exaggeration of deep reflexes, patellar and ankle clonus and Babinski's sign develop.

Hepatic encephalopathy has been graded into four grades.

Clinical grading of hepatic encephalopathy	
Grade	**Characteristics**
1	Altered sleep patterns, altered mood, irritability, inability to maintain attention
2	Lethargy, altered speech, increased memory loss, dysarthria
3	Progressive stupor, decreased level of consciousness but responsive to stimuli
4	Coma, unresponsive to painful stimuli

Modified West-Haven criteria for hepatic encephalopathy		
Grade	**Intellectual function**	**Neuromuscular function**
0	Normal	Normal
1	Personality changes, attention deficits, irritability, depressed	Tremor and incoordination
2	Changes in sleep wake cycle, lethargy, behavioral changes, cognitive dysfunction	Asterixis, ataxic gait, speech abnormalities
3	Altered level of consciousness, confusion, disorientation and amnesia	Muscular rigidity, nystagmus, clonus, Babinski sign, hyporeflexia
4	Stupor and coma	Oculocephalic reflex, unresponsive to noxious stimuli

Prognosis

The prognosis depends upon the underlying condition, the presence of precipitating factors and the management of the case.

Precipitating Factors

- A diet with approximately 1–1.5 g of dietary protein/kg of bw/day can be administrated safely to a patient with HE. Branched-chain amino acids (BCAA) appear to be more acceptable with a positive nitrogen balance. However, supplementation with BCAA have failed to show any improvement in morbidity or mortality among patients with HE. Patterns of hepatic encephalopathy (HE) seen in clinical practice (Flowchart 85.1).
- GI or other hemorrhage, extravasated blood in the GIT acts as a source of nitrogenous products and is more harmful in this regard than other proteins on a weight for weight basis.
- Hepatotoxic drugs like morphine, ammonium salts and alcohol.
- Intense diuretic regimen which produces hypokalemia and hyponatremia.
- Infections—these may be systemic or infections of the peritoneum which are common in ascites.
- Minor or major surgery including liver biopsy and abdominal paracentesis.
- Progressive deterioration of hepatic function.

If the precipitating factors are avoided and the patient is properly managed, satisfactory physical and mental state can be maintained for prolonged periods. Cases with a removable precipitating factor do better than those in whom the hepatic failure is the result of advanced liver disease.

Management

The aim of treatment is to improve hepatic function, relieve symptoms and prolong useful life.

Symptomatic treatment: The patient should be put to bed rest in the acute and subacute stages.

Diet: The total dietary intake should be 2000–2500 Cal and the amount of protein has to be adjusted so as to give the maximum possible nourishment without precipitating portal systemic encephalopathy. This has to be determined by trial and error. Vegetable proteins are tolerated well than that of animal proteins and they may be preferred. On an average, many patients tolerate about 40 g proteins daily, 1–1.5 g of dietary protein/kg of bw/day can be administrated safely to a patient with HE if the patient tolerates. Proteins with BCAA are accepted better. Considerable persuasion may be necessary to make the patient eat despite the anorexia. Adequate intake of

Flowchart 85.1: Patterns of hepatic encephalopathy (HE) that may be encountered in clinical practice

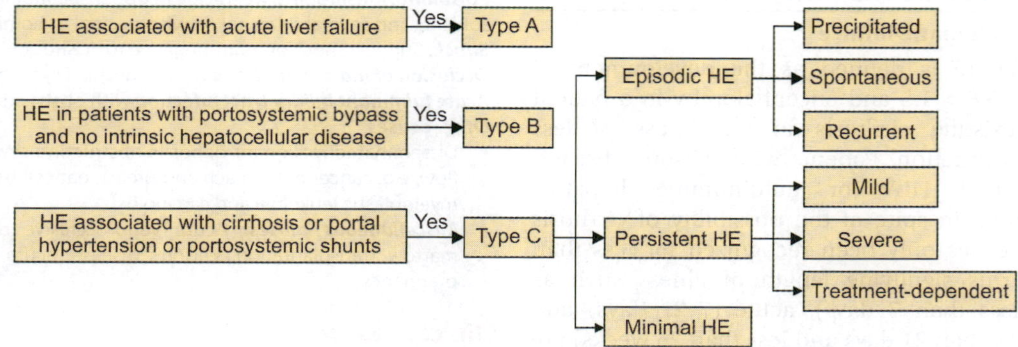

Abbreviation: HE = Hepatic encephalopathy

food definitely brings about improvement. Hematinics such as iron, folate and other vitamins should be given. The hemoglobin level has to be maintained around 10 g/dL, if necessary by packed cell transfusion.

Sedatives like morphine and paraldehyde precipitate coma and these should be avoided. While long-acting barbiturates like phenobarbitone which are mainly excreted by the kidney are tolerated, the short-acting ones like pentobarbitone and thiobarbital which are mainly metabolized by the liver should be avoided. Oxazepam and diazepam may be used.

Treatment of Hepatic Precoma and Coma

Diet: Proteins should be totally withdrawn. Carbohydrates are given orally or parenterally to supply 1500–1600 Cal in 24 hour. As the condition improves proteins are added to the diet.

Antibiotics: Broadspectrum antibiotics which sterilize the intestinal flora prevent bacterial breakdown of the products of protein digestion and the formation of toxic products. The ideal drug is neomycin 4–6 g/day given in divided doses. Being nonabsorbable, it reaches the colon in adequate concentrations to exert its effect. Ampicillin in a dose of 2 g/day in four divided doses is a suitable alternative.

Lactulose: This unabsorbable disaccharide is broken down by bacterial flora into lactic acid and small amounts of acetic acid when it reaches the ileum and cecum. The pH value of the colonic contents is lowered. At this low pH the lactose splitting organisms overgrow, suppressing the protein splitting organisms like ***bacteroides*** which produce ammonia. At a dose of 10–30 mL given thrice daily, lactulose is very effective in relieving chronic portal systemic encephalopathy. ***Lactitol***, which is a derivative of lactulose, has a better taste and is more acceptable. Oral antibiotics also have been used to treat hepatic encephalopathy, with the aim of modifying the intestinal flora and lowering stool pH to enhance the excretion of ammonia.

Rifaximin is a minimally absorbed oral broadspectrum antibiotic used for treatment of chronic HE. It has activity against gram positive, gram negative, aerobic and anaerobic enterobacteriae with low-risk of inducing resistance. It reduces recurrent episodes of HE. The dose is 400 mg orally three times daily. It is more effective than nonabsorbable disaccharides. If given continuously it reduces the chance for acute exacerbation of HE.

Purgatives: Proper evacuation of bowels helps in improving the mental state whereas constipation tends to worsen it. Purgation is achieved by the administration of magnesium sulfate 15–30 g orally. Lactulose itself acts as purgative. Enemas are employed to clear the bowels when purgation is contraindicated. The enemas should be at mildly acidic or neutral pH to prevent the absorption of ammonia. Bowel wash with saline or 1% dextran solution twice a day helps to clear the colon and this measure is effective in improving the mental state.

Attention to Precipitating Factors

- ***Intestinal blood loss*** should be treated by replacement of packed erythrocytes with fresh frozen plasma (FFP) or whole blood to maintain the hemoglobin around 10 g/dL. Blood should be removed from the intestines by aspiration and purgation. Oral broadspectrum antibiotics should be given to prevent the formation of ammoniacal products.
- If the coma has been precipitated by the use of sedatives, the appropriate antidote should be used, e.g. nalorphine in the case of morphine.
- ***Electrolyte imbalance*** should be corrected. Potassium deficiency can be prevented and mild cases treated by the use of copious administration of fruit juices and oral potassium chloride 2 g/6 hour. Intravenous (IV) administration of potassium is done if serum potassium is below 3.5 mmol/L.

Dopamine agonists: In some patients levodopa given in a dose of 0.5 g/6 hour brings about benefit. Similar effect has been seen with bromocriptine in a dose of 15 mg/day.

Flumazenil

Flumazenil is a GABA benzodiazepine receptor antagonist. In controlled trials it is found to improve HE significantly.

Follow-up: Improvement should be monitored clinically and by objective evaluation with EEG, trail making test (TMT) and blood ammonia levels. Irreversible hepatic failure is an indication for hepatic transplantation.

Subclinical HE

Clinically there is no change in the level of consciousness; but abnormality is detected during psychomotor testing such as TMT. The reaction time is prolonged and visual evoked potentials may be delayed. Such patients are unfit for handling fast mechanisms and for jobs such as driving vehicles and piloting aircraft.

ACUTE HEPATIC FAILURE (AHF)

Syn: Fulminant hepatic failure

Acute liver failure is defined as the development of coagulopathy INR > 1.5 and encephalopthy in a patient without pre-existing cirrhosis in an illness of less than 26 weeks duration. Patients with Wilson's disease, vertically-acquired HBV or autoimmune hepatitis may be included in spite of the possibility of cirrhosis if their disease has only been recognized for less than 26 weeks. Terms signifying length of illness such as hyperacute (less than 7 days), acute (7–21 days) and subacute (more than 21 days and less than 26 weeks) are not particularly helpful since they do not have prognostic significance distinct from the cause of the illness.

Acute on Chronic Liver Failure (ACLF)

This term refers to acute hepatic insult manifesting as jaundice and coagulopathy, complicated within 4 weeks by ascites and/or encephalopathy in a patient with previously diagnosed or undiagnosed chronic liver disease. The acute event may be infection with hepatotropic or non-hepatotropic viruses, flare up of chronic hepatitis B, autoimmune hepatitis, Wilson's disease, alcohol abuse, toxins or variceal bleed.

Acute insult in ACLF

- Infection—hepatotropic or nonhepatotropic viruses, reactivation of chronic hepatitis B
- Noninfectious
- Flares of autoimmune hepatitis or Wilson's disease
- Active alcohol use in the past 4 weeks
- Surgery
- Variceal bleed
- Hepatoxic drug or herbal medicines.

Pathology

Massive necrosis of liver cells leads to sudden impairment of liver function. Cerebral symptoms are caused by HE as well as development of cerebral edema which occurs in up to 80% of cases. Coning of brainstem may occur. Blood ammonia level increases.

Causes of Acute Hepatic Failure

Viral hepatitis: B, D, E and A and other viruses can cause AHF. Over 70% of cases of AHF are caused by viral infections. Overall incidence of AHF in viral hepatitis is around 1%. Frequency of AHF in different types of viral hepatitis is given below:

- ***Hepatitis A virus (HAV):*** 0.35%. AHF is more common in the elderly and drug users. Prognosis is relatively better with survival over 60%.
- ***Hepatitis B virus (HBV):*** 1%.
- ***Hepatitis C virus (HCV):*** By itself, it is rare to produce AHF. In combination with HBV, it predisposes to AHF.
- ***Hepatitis D virus (HDV):*** In combination with HBV it increases the frequency and severity of AHF.
- ***Hepatitis E virus (HEV):*** This is likely to cause AHF, especially in pregnant women.

  Other viruses such as cytomegalovirus (CMV), Epstein-Barr virus (EBV) and herpes viruses 1, 2 and 6 cause AHF especially in immunocompromised subjects.

Drugs: Paracetamol, halothane, monoamine oxidase-inhibitors such as iproniazid and phenelzine, isoniazid. Paracetamol, if given in doses of more than 4 g/day will lead to heptic ill effects. Drug induced liver failure is more common in older age groups.

Poisoning: Mushrooms, weedicides, copper sulfate, alcohol, organic solvents and several drugs taken with suicidal or homicidal intent.
Shock: Surgical shock or gram-negative toxic shock.
Occlusion of major hepatic veins (Budd-Chiari syndrome).
Acute fulminant biliary tract infection with obstruction.
Other causes

- Disseminated malignant deposits obstructing sinusoidal blood flow, e.g. cancer of stomach and breast, oat cell tumors of lung, myeloblastic leukemia and carcinoids.
- ***Miscellaneous causes:*** Acute veno-occlusive disease, bone marrow transplantation, Wilson's disease, acute fatty liver of pregnancy.

Clinical Features

Neurological manifestations predominate in this disorder. They are much more varied than in CHF. Flapping tremors, headache, change of personality and behavior, delirium, decerebrate rigidity, convulsions, abnormalities of ocular movements and coma occur in varying combinations. Finally the majority of cases go into coma. For clinical purposes, coma is graded from I to V (Table 85.2).

The light reflex and the plantar response are unaffected till late in the disease.

The patient is often jaundiced. Brainstem function is impaired and this manifests as irregularity of respiration, circulatory disturbances and hypotension. Generalized bleeding tendency occurs in most cases. This manifests as bleeding from the mucous membranes, GI, skin and injection sites. Prothrombin time is prolonged. Factors II, V, VIII, IX and X are reduced. Thrombocytopenia may develop in some. Other complications include pancreatitis, shock and circulatory failure.

Renal symptoms: Oliguric renal failure occurs as a result of hepatorenal syndrome in up to 50% cases.

Other general symptoms: Due to increasing intracranial pressure there is reflex hypertension and bradycardia (Cushing's reflex). Hypoglycemia is a common accompaniment. Superadded infections develop if the coma persists for a few days or more.

Depending on the duration, AHF can be subdivided into hyperacute, acute and subacute (Table 85.3).

Biochemical changes: Urine may show bile pigments, increased urobilinogen and amino acid crystals such as leucine and tyrosine.

The blood sugar is lowered. Serum bilirubin is increased. Serum albumin may be lowered as the disease progresses. Elevation of aspartate and alanine transaminases occurs in the early phase. As hepatic necrosis advances, the levels of these enzymes may even fall. Prothrombin time is prolonged. Blood ammonia level may be raised.

Table 85.2: Grading of coma (Sherlock S)	
Grades	
I	Confused, altered mood or behavior, psychometric defects
II	Drowsy, inappropriate behavior
III	Stuporous, but able to speak and obey simple commands, inarticulate speech, marked confusion
IV	Coma
V	Deep coma and no response to painful stimuli

Textbook of Medicine

Table 85.3: Clinical classification of acute hepatic failure

Clinical features	Hyperacute AHF	Acute AHF	Subacute AHF
Encephalopathy	+	+	+
Duration of acute disease	0–7 days	8–28 days	29–72 days
Cerebral edema	Common	Common	Infrequent
Prolongation of prothrombin time	+++	++	+
Rise in serum bilirubin	++	+ ±	+
Prognosis for recovery with treatment	Moderate	Poor	Poor

Table 85.4: Indicators of poor prognosis in acute liver failure (ALF)

- Etiology
- Idiosyncratic drug injury
- Acute hepatitis B (and other nonhepatitis A viral infections)
- Autoimmune hepatitis
- Mushroom poisoning
- Wilson's disease
- Budd-Chiari syndrome
- Indeterminate cause
- Coma grade on admission—III or IV

Table 85.5: King's College Criteria (KCC)

Acetaminophen
- Arterial pH < 7.3
- PT INR > 6.5 + serum creatinine > 3.4 mg/dL

Non-acetaminophen
- PT > 6.5
- Any 3 of the below mentioned
  1. Age < 10 or > 40 years
  2. Serum bilirubin > 17.6 mg/dL
  3. Etiology—non-A, non-B hepatitis, halothane hepatitis, idiosyncratic drug reaction, indeterminate
  4. Time taken from development of jaundice to encephalopathy > 7 days
  5. PT > 50 seconds INR 3.5

Complications

These include cerebral edema, renal failure, bacterial infections, circulatory failure, hemorrhage and hypoglycemia.

Course and Prognosis

If the coma is of grade IV or V, mortality is 75–80%. The prognosis is worse in females, older subjects and those with longer duration of coma. In those who recover, cirrhosis liver does not usually develop. It is essential to assess the prognosis early in the disease, in order to decide the need for liver transplantation (Tables 85.4 and 85.5).

Management

Recommendation in management of ALF are:
- Give activated charcoal within 4 hours just before starting N-acetylcysteine (NAC) (in suspected or known acetaminophen poisoning)
- Give NAC in suspected case of drug induced liver injury (DILI)
- H_2 blockers and proton pump should be administered
- Steroids should not be given to reduce cerebral edema
- Maintain serum sodium in between 145 and 155 mEq prophylactically in patients at high-risk for cerebral edema [serum ammonia >150 lM, grade 3/4 HE, acute renal failure (ARF), requiring vasopressors to maintain mean arterial pressure (MAP) using hypertonic saline.
- If dialysis support is needed for ARF, it is recommended that a continuous mode rather than an intermittent mode be used.
- The precipitating causes should be looked for and eliminated. Proteins are totally withdrawn from the diet. Neomycin, lactulose, magnesium sulfate and bowel washes should be started.
- The patient should be nursed as a case in deep coma. Nutrition is supplied parenterally. Continuous infusion of 10% glucose or intermittent administration of 50% glucose is necessary to prevent hypoglycemia. Sedation must be avoided, if possible. If the patient becomes restless, a sedative antihistaminic like diphenhydramine or buclizine may be used. Barbitone sodium has to be given parenterally if a patient becomes violent and unmanageable. Frequent neurological evaluation should be done to check for

development of intracranial hypertension and if it develops, mannitol should be administered. Measures to avoid rise in intracranial tension include artificial hyperventilation, infusion of IV mannitol 0.5 g/kg bw as a 20% solution within 10–15 minutes, hemodialysis and hemoperfusion.
- Infection has to be diagnosed early and treated with broadspectrum antibiotics like third generation cephalosporins such as cefotaxime, ceftriaxone, ceftazidime and others. Bacterial and fungal etiologies should be suspected.
- *Electrolytes:* Generally serum sodium and potassium are low. Hyponatremia may become severe as a preterminal phenomenon. Excess sodium should not be supplemented unless there is evidence of sodium loss, but potassium should be supplemented orally or parenterally. Serum calcium tends to be low and this is attributable to coexistent hypoalbuminemia and pancreatitis. IV calcium gluconate (10%) is administered to make up the serum calcium levels to normal. Glucose, potassium, phosphate and magnesium should be closely monitored.
- Renal failure may require dialysis.
- Bleeding due to vitamin K deficiency may be allayed by the IM administration of vitamin K 10 mg daily, but if the bleeding is due to hepatic functional impairment vitamin K is not beneficial. Such cases have a poor outcome. Fresh blood, coagulation factor concentrates or fresh plasma may be required at times. FFP, platelets and coagulation factors are given in case of active bleeding and while undertaking invasive procedures.
- The principles employed in the management of CHF have to be followed as the condition improves and the patient's chances of survival become brighter.

Textbook of Medicine

Artificial Liver Support

The principle is similar to hemodialysis in renal failure. The aim is to maintain or support liver function artificially till the patient's liver recovers or a donor liver is available for transplantation. The most effective bioartificial liver (BAL) model is based on the principle that viable hepatocytes are maintained in a chamber through which blood is passed through permeable artificial capillaries (to favor exchange of plasma components). Several of such extracorporeal devices are undertrial with encouraging results (Table 85.6).

Charcoal hemoperfusion (charcoal removes water soluble toxic metabolites) and Rhone-Poulenc hemodialysis system using special polyacrylonitrile membrane which removes middle molecules up to a molecular weight of 5000 kD.

Hepatocyte Transplantation

This is another procedure employed at times with favorable results. Unlike liver transplantation, donor hepatocytes can be obtained more readily and the procedure is technically easier. Hepatocyte transplantation helps to increase survival rate to > 35%.

In experienced hands and advanced centers all these have shown temporary benefit but none has been accepted universally. At present these are of value in tiding over a crisis in a patient with reversible hepatic disease and also for the preoperative preparation before hepatic transplantation. *Hepatic transplantation* should be considered as an emergency procedure if a donor organ and facilities for surgery are available.

Prognostication in cirrhosis liver which helps to determine the priority for liver transplantation is accepted by common consensus and in the national registries strict criteria are available for determining priority for surgery.

Liver Transplantation

First performed in 1963, this has become a standard therapeutic modality in several countries including India where it is available in several hospitals including government and private sectors.

Indications

As a curative therapy it is employed in cirrhosis, hepatobiliary neoplasms, biliary atresia, metabolic disorders such as glycogen storage disease (type II), Wilson's disease, α-1 antitrypsin deficiency, homozygous familial hypercholesterolemia, sclerosing cholangitis, hepatic vein occlusion and fulminant hepatic failure. In advanced centers, the one-year survival is about 70% and around 45% at 2 years. The perioperative mortality is 30%. Best results are obtained in subjects with primary biliary cirrhosis (PBC), sclerosing cholangitis and cryptogenic cirrhosis.

Contraindications include presence of extrahepatic malignant disease, active replication of HBV despite treatment, presence of irreversible disease in other organs and age above 55 years. The cost of hepatic transplantation is above $70,000.

Auxiliary liver transplant is the implantation of a partial liver draft either heterotopically or orthotopically leaving the diseased liver *in sito*. With recovery of the patient's liver, the draft either atrophies or can be removed.

Conventionally Child-Turcotte-Pugh (CTP): Classification is used where 1–3 scores are given to five parameters- serum bilirubin, serum albumin, ascites, encephalopathy and prothrombin time (Table 85.7). A score of 5 and 6 is classified as child's A—7, 8 and 9 as child's B—10 or more as child C. The prognosis for survival worsens as the class moves from A to C. It has disadvantage of lack of proper discrimination in later stages of liver disease for which another scoring system has been recently introduced. The modified end stage liver disease (MELD), score is based on serum bilirubin, prothrombin time and serum creatinine for which different weightages are given.

In case of hepatic cancer, additional points are given to facilitate early transplantation. At present this surgery is being done with greater success. Liver transplantation can be done with liver obtained from cadavers or living donors. In the latter case, part of the donor's liver from the right lobe is removed for transplantation. Postoperatively the donor's liver regrows and makes up the volume of the organ.

Major Indications for Liver Transplantation

- End stage liver disease
- Acute fulminant liver failure
- Hepatocellular carcinoma
- Large benign tumors such as hemangioma

Table 85.6: Extracorporeal liver support

Hemodiadsorption system	• Hemodialysis in combination with perfusion of the patients plasma or blood through charcoal, resins and albumin • Albumin dialysis-hemodialysis of whole blood with albumin dialyser and charcoal filter, like molecular adsorbent recirculating system (MARS)
Bioartificial liver	Patients plasma is perfused through the liver cells which are grown specialized hollow fibers

Table 85.7: Child-Turcotte-Pugh (CTP) scoring system to assess severity of liver disease

Points	1	2	3
Encephalopathy	None	Grades 1–2	Grades 3–4
Ascites	Absent	Slight (or controlled by diuretics)	At least moderate despite diuretics
Bilirubin	< 2	2–3	> 3
Albumin	> 3.5	2.8–3.5	< 2.8
PT INR	< 1.7	1.7–2.3	> 2.3
* For PBC, PSC or other cholestatic liver disease substitute following values of bilirubin (mg/dL)	< 4	4–10	> 10

- Score is calculated by adding points for each
- Score ranges from 5 to 15
- Patients are categorized into 3 child classes
  - Child A score: 5 to 6
  - Child B score: 7 to 9
  - Child C score: 10 to 15

Abbreviations: PT INR = Prothrombin time and International Normalized Ratio; PBC = Primary biliary cirrhosis; PSC = Primary sclerosing cholangitis

- Biliary cirrhosis with intractable pruritus
- Metabolic disorders.

Human leukocyte antigen (HLA) haplotyping and detailed immunological testing are not required. Blood group compatability and physical factors such as size of the transplant are of importance in cross-matching. Post transplantation immunosuppressant regimen consists of tacrolimus, cyclosporine, azathioprine or mycophenolate mofetil with or without corticosteroids. Operative mortality is around 5% and one year survival exceeds 80% in most centers. In the presence of renal failure, concomitant renal transplantation is also needed. The long-term survival depends also upon the primary condition for which transplantation was done.

Liver Transplantation

KR Vinaya Kumar

Chapter Summary

- Types of Liver Transplantation
- Indications for Liver Transplantation
- Patient Selection
- Transplantation Procedure
- Complications and Follow-up
- Future Perspectives

INTRODUCTION

The first human liver transplantation (LT) was performed in 1963 by a surgical team led by Dr Thomas_Starzl of Denver, Colorado, United States. Access to LT has profoundly altered the management of advanced liver disease. Management of decompensated cirrhosis and acute liver failure (ALF) before the advent of LT was limited to attempts to ameliorate complications. In contrast, successful LT extends life-expectancy and enhances quality of life. The first successful living donor liver transplantation (LDLT) in India was performed from an adult donor to a pediatric recipient in 1998. An 'Indian Transplant Registry' has been established over the past 2 years due to the efforts of the Indian Society of Organ Transplantation. This society is about 20 years old with over 450 members who are doctors and basic scientists. In India, 200–250 transplants are done every year at various centers. The Transplantation of Human Organs Act (THOA) was enacted in 1994. In Kerala, the first LT was done in 2004. In 2011, the Act was revised to promote cadaveric organ transplantation. Accordingly, the state government had revised the guidelines for implementation of deceased donor organ transplantation. According to the statistics provided by KNOS (Kerala Network for Organ Sharing), the number of deceased donor LT in Kerala in the past 2 years stands at 50.

TYPES OF LIVER TRANSPLANTATION

The term orthotopic liver transplantation (OLT) refers to placement of the new organ in the same location as the explanted liver. Although most LT recipients receive a whole organ from a deceased donor, an organ can be *split* with a pediatric recipient receiving a left lateral segment and an adult recipient the larger right lobe. Live donor transplant using the left hepatic lobe initially introduced for pediatric recipients has been extended into adult recipients using the donor's right lobe. The principle of auxillary LT is the implantation of a right or left hemiliver into the abdominal cavity to restore normal liver function temporarily, while the native liver recuperates. Once the native liver recovers, the graft can be removed or left in place without immunosuppression leading to atrophy. It is generally undertaken in ALF.

Recipients of live donor transplant have reduced waiting list mortality compared to potential recipients of deceased donor organs. Live donor transplant should only be contemplated when LT with a deceased donor is unlikely to occur within a reasonable time frame given the severity of the potential candidate's liver disease. In India, the rate of cadaveric LT was abysmally low initially, mainly because of lack of consensus in defining brain death and also by dearth of laws governing cadaveric organ donation. However, in the last few years, after the intervention by state government to promote cadaveric organ donation, the number of deceased donor LT have been on the rise.

INDICATIONS FOR LIVER TRANSPLANTATION

- Acute liver failure
- Complications of cirrhosis
- Ascites
- Chronic gastrointestinal (GI) blood loss due to portal hypertensive gastropathy
- Encephalopathy
- Liver cancer
- Refractory variceal hemorrhage
- Synthetic dysfunction.

Liver-based Metabolic Conditions with Systemic Manifestations

- Alpha-1-antitrypsin deficiency
- Familial amyloidosis
- Glycogen storage disease
- Hemochromatosis
- Primary oxaluria
- Wilson's disease.

Systemic Complications of Chronic Liver Disease

- Hepatopulmonary syndrome
- Portopulmonary hypertension.

CONTRAINDICATIONS TO LIVER TRANSPLANTATION

- Model for end-stage liver disease (MELD) score < 15
- Severe cardiac or pulmonary disease
- Acquired immune deficiency syndrome (AIDS)
- Ongoing alcohol or illicit substance abuse
- Hepatocellular carcinoma with metastatic spread
- Uncontrolled sepsis
- Anatomic abnormality that precludes LT
- Intrahepatic cholangiocarcinoma
- Extrahepatic malignancy
- Fulminant hepatic failure with sustained intracranial pressure (ICP) >50 mm Hg or cerebral perfusion pressure (CPP) <40 mm Hg
- Hemangiosarcoma
- Persistent noncompliance
- Lack of adequate social support system.

PATIENT SELECTION

For cirrhosis, the Child-Pugh score had been used to assess prognosis but has been increasingly superseded by the MELD. The MELD score is a mathematical score based on objective measures [serum creatinine and bilirubin levels and International Normalized Ratio (INR)] that quantify liver disease severity and is an accurate predictor of short-term mortality. It is calculated as MELD = 3.8 × log e [total bilirubin (mg/dL)] + 11.2 × log e (INR) + 9.6 × log e [creatinine (mg/dL)]. The MELD score is on a continuous scale from 6 to 40 that corresponded to a 3-month survival of 90–7%, respectively. The MELD score is now used to assess prognosis in cirrhosis in a variety of settings, including organ allocation for LT. Application of the MELD score has determined that the risk of deceased donor LT in patients with a MELD < 15 outweighs its benefits in most circumstances. Development of hyponatremia in cirrhosis is a marker of increased waiting list mortality, as well as neurological dysfunction post-LT. Incorporation of serum sodium into the MELD score has been proposed to increase priority for organ allocation to candidates with hyponatremia to reduce waiting list deaths. Since February 2002, all patients have been listed in descending order according to MELD score [or Pediatric End-Stage Liver Disease (PELD) score for candidates younger than 12 years)], with the highest scores receiving the highest priority for organ allocation. The PELD score utilizes serum albumin and bilirubin levels and INR but also includes components for growth retardation and age younger than 1 year to account for short-term survival disparities in such patients. Listing status and MELD scores are regularly reassessed by the listing transplant center at intervals determined by disease severity. Patients with MELD scores of 19–24 must recertify monthly and patients with MELD scores of 11–18 must be retested every 3 months.

Since the introduction of MELD for organ allocation the number of simultaneous liver kidney (SLK) transplants, has increased from less than 3% to nearly 5% in and continues to rise. SLK transplantation is indicated for LT candidates in whom renal failure reflects chronic kidney disease (CKD) with glomerular filtration rate (GFR) <30 mL/min or acute kidney injury (AKI) with dialysis >8 weeks or if extensive glomerulosclerosis is present.

Regarding LDLT, the person must donate on his/her own free will, should be between 18 and 55 years and weight between 50 and 85 kg, must be a close relative, the donor and recipient blood group must match, donor liver structure/function, as well as the other systems must be normal, half of the donor liver must be enough in volume for the recipient. LDLT from an unrelated donor is still a topic of debate.

The United Network for Organ Sharing (UNOS) facilitates organ allocation in the United States and also records graft and recipient outcomes. The UNOS database allows critical evaluation of center and disease-specific recipient outcomes with LT as well as guiding organ allocation policies.

TRANSPLANTATION PROCEDURE

At least two surgeons with significant experience in advanced hepatobiliary surgery and assistant surgeons are required for surgical team. The surgical team has to be actively supported by a group of highly skilled and experienced anesthetists, critical care physicians and transplant hepatologists with a round-the-clock access to diagnostic and interventional radiology, dialysis, endoscopy, immunology, pathology, transfusion, microbiology and biochemistry services of the highest quality.

The traditionally described OLT involves resecting the recipient native liver (hepatectomy) together with the retrohepatic inferior vena cava (IVC), a short anhepatic phase and implanting a whole deceased donor liver graft with the interposed donor IVC. Restoration of venous continuity during the implantation is achieved by an upper subdiaphragmatic and lower end-to-end donor-to-recipient IVC anastomosis; the donor-to-recipient portal vein and hepatic artery anastomoses are also performed in an end-to-end fashion. The biliary connections involve a primary duct-to-duct technique or the performance of a hepaticojejunostomy. The procedure duration ranges between 6 and 9 hours.

Liver ischemia/reperfusion (IR) injury during transplantation occurs at different periods. The first, after liver explantation from the donor and storage on ice at 0 to 4°C, is a variable but generally long-period of cold ischemia. The time of vascular anastomosis, when the liver is removed from ice until its implantation in the recipient, represents the second, relatively shorter period of warm IR injury. In this period of ischemia, the liver warms slowly up to a temperature of 12.5°C during the realization of suprahepatic cava and portal vein anastomoses and to a temperature of 34°C, once hepatic artery anastomosis is performed. Normothermic reperfusion of the implanted liver with the recipient's blood at 37°C delineates the third period. During the periods of IR of the liver, there is a microcirculatory failure, activation of Kupffer cells and production of reactive oxygen species, inflammatory responses and apoptosis of the hepatocytes. Static cold storage (SCS) is the standard method of liver preservation. It is based on the principle that hypothermia reduces the metabolism and enzymatic activity and slows down cell death, but during the process it causes cellular edema. Cellular edema is prevented by addition of various substances to the preservative fluid. EuroCollins (EC), University of Wisconsin (UW), Histidine-Tryptophan-Ketoglutarate (HTK), Marshall's hypertonic citrate (HOC) and Celsior are few of the perfusates being used in liver preservation.

COMPLICATIONS AND FOLLOW-UP

Within the first few days following LT, profound graft dysfunction suggests primary nonfunction or hepatic artery thrombosis and early diagnosis is critical as this entails consideration for retransplantation. Throughout the first few weeks, allograft function should be monitored closely in order to recognize acute cellular rejection (mostly occurs during first three months). It is widely known that LDLT recipients can potentially develop a specific syndrome known as 'small-for-size syndrome', when a small-for-size graft causes size mismatch in the presence of portal hypertension. The pathologic mechanism of small-for-size syndrome includes graft failure caused by excessive and destructive portal inflow into the small-for-size graft.

Immunosuppressive agents, based on specific protocols and on the patient's renal function, are started early after OLT. Doses are adjusted according to blood levels and functional status of the transplanted liver and renal function. Calcineurin inhibitors (CNI)—tacrolimus (TAC) and cyclosporine (CSA)—remain the cornerstone of immunosuppressive therapy; TAC is used in 90% of primary OLT recipients at the time of discharge. Administration of one of these agents at therapeutic doses is the key to preventing rejection of the liver allograft. The usual acceptable trough levels early after OLT are 8–12 ng/mL for TAC and 200 to 300 ng/mL for CSA. The most commonly used non-CNI immunosuppressive agents in OLT are corticosteroids. Adjunctive medications are usually prescribed in addition to a CNI and include the antiproliferative agents mycophenolate mofetil (MMF), azathioprine (AZA) and sirolimus (SRL). Common side effects related to immunosuppression agents include hypertension, renal insufficiency, diabetes and hyperlipidemia and these have a high impact on post-transplant morbidity and mortality if left untreated. Biliary tract abnormalities have been described in as high as 30% of LT recipients and these include biliary leak and stenosis. Overall 1 to 5 years survival rate post LT is 87% and 73% respectively.

FUTURE PERSPECTIVES

The cost of LT is significant, varying between ₹ 20 and 30 lakh in this country. This is one reason why it has mostly been confined to the private sector. All over world, the overall success rate of the procedure and the post LT patient care has improved dramatically. The advent of newer immunosuppressants have further added to the improvement of the overall survival rates. The participation of several nongovernmental organizations, support by medical insurance and welfare schemes have made LT more affordable to the patient population. With the increase in the number of cadaveric LT and availability of transplantation in the government sector, the future looks bright for patients with advanced liver disease.

Live donor's liver regrows and reaches normal volume and function within 6–12 months in most cases.

CHAPTER

87

Portal Hypertension

KR Vinaya Kumar, KV Krishna Das

Chapter Summary

- General Considerations
- Portal Hypertension in Cirrhosis
- Bleeding Esophageal Varices
- portopulmonary Syndrome
- Extrahepatic Portal Hypertension (EHPH)
- Noncirrhotic Portal Fibrosis

GENERAL CONSIDERATIONS

The superior mesenteric vein and the splenic vein join to form the portal vein which divides initially into the left and right branches and thereafter, in a dichotomous fashion. The portal blood is drained into the hepatic sinusoids. Major branches of the portal vein do not have valves. The abdominal parts of the alimentary tract, spleen, pancreas and gallbladder drain into the portal system. The portal venous flow is 1000–1200 mL of blood/minute. In the normal liver, the whole of the portal blood passes through the sinusoids and is drained by the hepatic veins into the inferior vena cava. When onward flow of blood is obstructed, portal vein radicles develop extensive collaterals with systemic veins so that even more than 80% of its blood can be drained into the systemic circulation without passing through the liver. Normal pressure in the portal vein is 7 mm Hg. Portal hypertension results from

Textbook of Medicine

obstruction to onward flow of portal blood. The term *portal hypertension* is applied when the portal venous pressure exceeds 12 mm Hg.

Classification

Portal hypertension can be classified in different ways. Depending on the site of obstruction in relation to the hepatic sinusoids, it may be divided into two types—*presinusoidal* and *postsinusoidal*.

Presinusoidal	Extrahepatic	Any cause of portal hypertension splenic vein occlusion
	Intrahepatic	All types of cirrhosis, noncirrhotic portal fibrosis schistosomiasis, myelofibrosis
Postsinusoidal		• Major hepatic vein obstruction (Budd-Chiari syndrome); obstruction to small radicles of hepatic vein-veno-occlusive disease • Generalized rise in inferior vena cava pressure, e.g. right sided heart failure, constrictive pericarditis and pericardial effusion.

The two most common causes of portal hypertension are mechanical obstruction to venous outflow in the liver by nodules developing in hepatic cirrhosis and extrahepatic occlusion of the portal vein. In many cases, portal hypertension remains silent till complications become visible. The portal blood normally carries oxygen and hepatotropic factors into the liver. When portal blood is shunted away, the liver depends more and more on hepatic arterial blood for oxygen supply and it undergoes functional impairment and atrophy. Bacteremias develop since the portal blood passes into the systemic circulation without being filtered by the hepatic macrophage barrier. Entry of the products of digestion directly into the systemic circulation without being metabolized by the liver hastens the onset of portal-systemic encephalopathy.

Rise in portal pressure tends to favor ascites when other factors like hypoproteinemia and sodium retention also develop.

PORTAL HYPERTENSION IN CIRRHOSIS

Fifty percent of patients with cirrhosis have gastroesophageal varices at the time of diagnosis. Development and growth of varices occur at a rate of 8% yearly. In cirrhosis, the development of portal hypertension is the result of complex mechanisms. The regenerating nodules of cirrhosis distort, obstruct and reduce the vascular bed. Obstruction occurs at all levels from the portal zones through the sinusoids to the hepatic venous outflow. The regenerating nodules derive their nourishment from the hepatic artery since they have no portal blood supply. Direct communication between the hepatic artery and portal radicles develop in cirrhosis and these serve to transmit arterial pressure to the portal venous system. Angiogenic factors modulate the development of varices.

Clinical Features

Signs of portal hypertension include asymptomatic splenomegaly, gradual development of portal-systemic collateral veins and bouts of hematemesis or melena. In some cases, chronic blood loss due to oozing of blood leads to iron deficiency anemia (IDA).

Common Sites for Portal-systemic Collaterals

- In the lower end of esophagus and gastric fundus, left and short gastric veins communicate with esophageal veins. These form esophageal and gastric varices (Fig. 87.1) that are responsible for fatal hematemesis.
- The veins of the abdominal wall become prominent and they radiate from the umbilicus. Rarely they may form ***caput medusae*** around the umbilicus. The direction of blood flow is the same as in the normal veins of the abdominal wall, but the flow is considerably increased. Blood from the portal vein is brought to the abdominal wall through the paraumbilical veins and other veins in the falciform ligament and these are drained by the abdominal veins (*See* Fig. 84.3).
- Communication between the inferior mesenteric veins and the hemorrhoidal veins results in the formation of varices in the rectum (Fig. 87.2). These varices are distinct from hemorrhoids. The former may regress when the portal hypertension is relieved.
- Hepatic veins communicate with diaphragmatic veins, veins in the lienorenal ligament, omentum and venous collaterals developing in the scars of previous laparotomies.
- Portal blood may be drained to the left renal vein from the splenic vein directly or through collaterals in the diaphragm, pancreas, stomach or left adrenal.

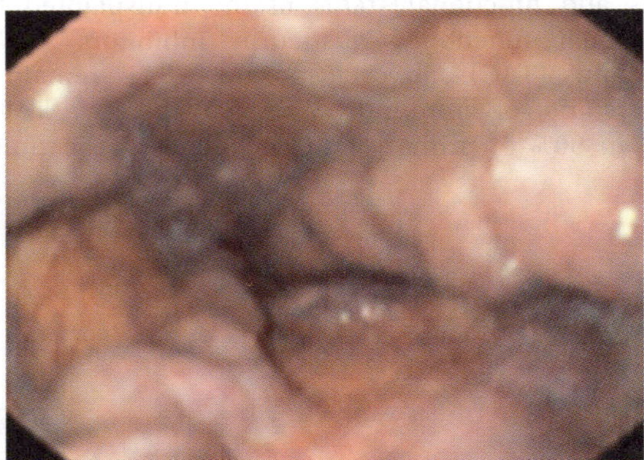

Fig. 87.1: Esophageal varices

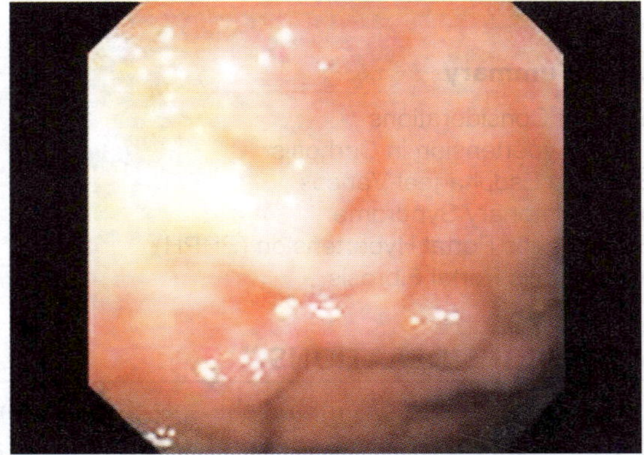

Fig. 87.2: Rectal varices

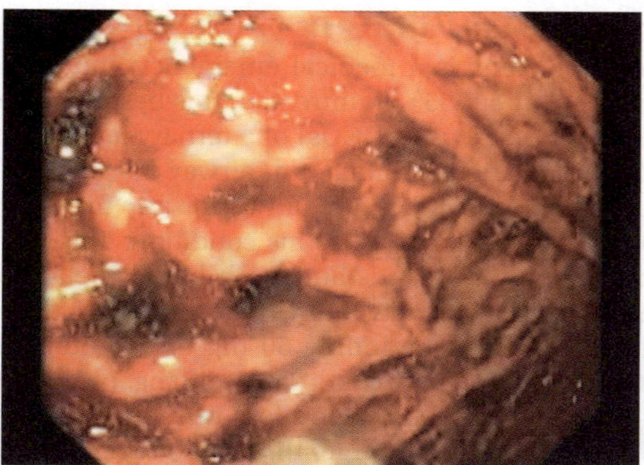

Fig. 87.3: Bleeding portal hypertensive gastropathy

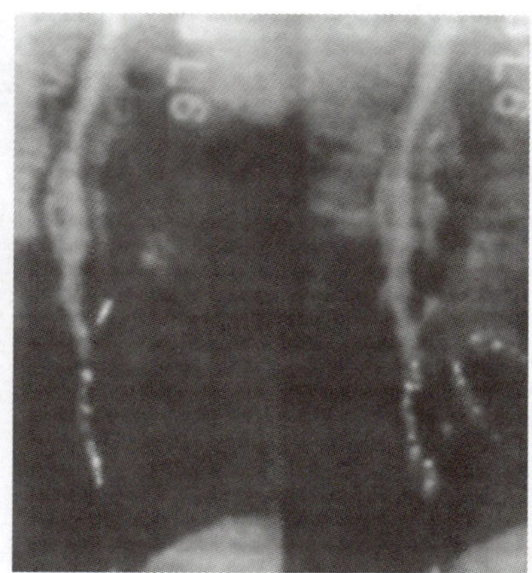

Fig. 87.4: Portal hypertension—barium swallow X-ray showing esophageal varices. **Note:** The longitudinal filling defects caused by the dilated veins

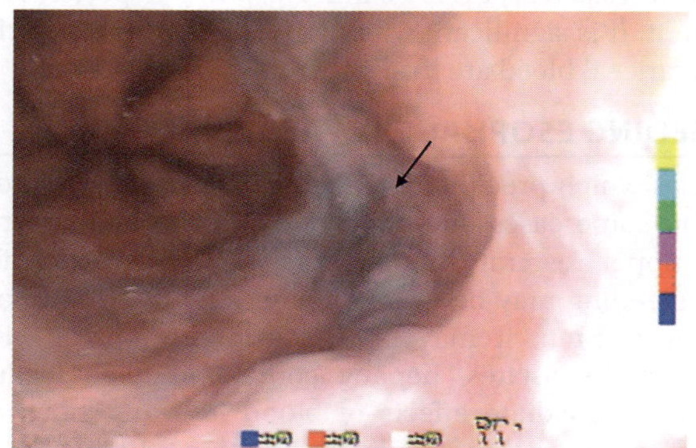

Fig. 87.5: Esophageal varices endoscopic view. **Note:** Dilated veins in the esophagus (arrow)

This blood passes mainly into the superior vena cava through the azygos and hemiazygos systems. A small quantity of blood enters the inferior vena cava and even into the pulmonary veins.

In addition to the classic sites, other venous collaterals may also develop in extrahepatic portal obstruction (ectopic portal-systemic collaterals). These may account for 5% of gastrointestinal (GI) bleeding in portal hypertension (Fig. 87.3). In a review of 169 cases, 17% occurred in the duodenum, 17% in the jejunum or ileum, 14% in the colon, 8% in the rectum and 9% in the peritoneum.

Source: Kinkhabwala M, Mousavi A, Iyer S, et al. Bleeding ileal varicosity demonstrated by transhepatic portography. AJR Am J Roentgenol. 1977;129(3):514-6.

The severity of portal hypertension and its cause have to be determined by investigations. The portal pressure can be measured by the following methods:

- ***Intrasplenic pressure*** can be directly measured by a needle introduced percutaneously or during surgery into the spleen.
- ***By umbilical vein catheterization (UVC).***
- ***By transhepatic portal vein puncture.***
- ***Wedged hepatic venous pressure (WHVP)*** can be measured by a catheter introduced through a hepatic venous radicle until it gets arrested. This pressure represents the sinusoidal venous pressure. Normal wedged hepatic pressure is 5–6 mm Hg which may go up to 20 mm Hg in portal hypertension.

The portal-systemic blood flow can be estimated by radioisotopic methods.

Demonstration of the Collaterals

- ***Esophageal varices:*** These stand out prominently in a properly made barium swallow picture (Fig. 87.4). These can be seen directly by endoscopy. Rectal varices can be visualized by proctoscopy (Fig. 87.5).
- ***Percutaneous trans-splenic portal venography:*** Radio-opaque dye is injected into the splenic pulp. This visualizes splenic and portal veins and their collaterals. The dye can be traced up by proper timing of the pictures. Deep jaundice and prolongation of the prothrombin time (PT) are contraindications for this procedure since the risk of bleeding is high.
- ***Scintiphoto-splenoportography (SSP):*** This is an isotopic method by which serial scans are made using a gamma camera after injection of ^{133}Xe (Xenon) or ^{99m}TcO$_4$ (technetium) into the spleen. The venous flow pattern can be traced.
- ***Selective visceral angiography (SVA):*** The celiac axis is catheterized and dye injected. The contrast material flowing into the splenic artery returns through the portal vein which is visualized. Similarly, superior mesenteric artery (SMA) can be catheterized.
- ***Selective venous catheterization:*** UVC and injection of contrast material visualizes the portal venous system.
- ***Transhepatic portography:*** The portal vein is visualized by injecting dye through a cannula introduced through the liver.
- ***Ultrasound study, Doppler and computed tomography (CT) scan:*** These are elegant methods which delineate the portal vein and its major branches. Dilatation, occlusion and deformity can be made out but the results are poorer in comparison to direct visualization by phlebography. In an ordinary case, all these advanced procedures are not necessary for diagnosis, but proper evaluation is essential when surgery is contemplated.
- ***Other modern investigations:*** The ratio of platelet count (PC)/mm^3 to spleen bipolar length in mm [as obtained by ultrasound scan (USS)], if above 909 has a high negative predictive value for varices.

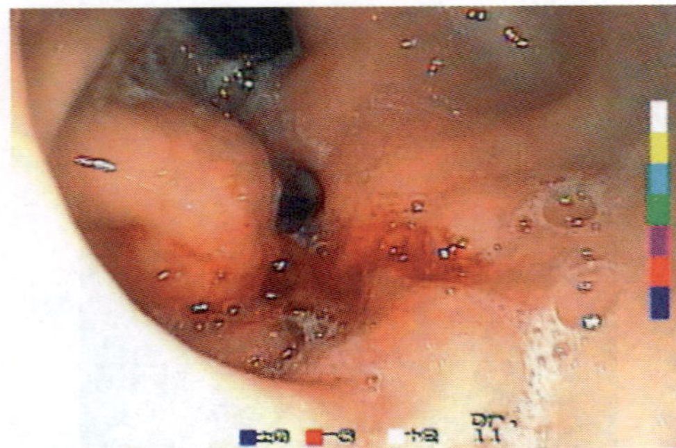

Fig. 87.6: Stomach bleeding in portal gastropathy

Liver Stiffness and its Role

Patients in child class C and hepatic venous pressure gradient (HVPG) are at high-risk. HVPG obtained by hepatic venous catheterization is a good parameter to quantify risk. If HVPG is > 5 mm Hg, portal hypertension is present. It is significant when HPVG > 10 mm Hg; varices and variceal bleed are likely.

BLEEDING ESOPHAGEAL VARICES

Causes which precipitate bleeding are not clearly known but in some cases, ingestion of aspirin or similar drugs and upper respiratory infections (URI) are responsible. The bleeding may be dramatic and fatal if left untreated or more often, it may be a continuous ooze. This is followed by ascites, hepatic coma and hepatocellular failure. Immediate effects of blood loss are shock and rapid deterioration of liver function. Reduction in hepatic arterial flow results in necrosis of liver cells which depend upon the hepatic arterial supply. Blood in the gastrointestinal tract (GIT) acts as a source of toxic nitrogenous products and this precipitates hepatic coma. The common site for rupture of the varices is within 7 cm of the lower end of the esophagus. Rupture is mostly caused by rise in the intravariceal pressure and disruption of the venous walls. Even in patients with esophageal varices, in about a third, bleeding may be from other sites such as peptic ulcers, gastric erosions and esophageal tears *(Mallory-Weiss syndrome)*. These have to be identified in order to institute effective therapy.

Portal hypertensive gastropathy (PHG): This is a change brought about in the gastric mucosa as a result of ectasia of submucous capillaries and veins, without any inflammatory change (Fig. 87.6). Relief of portal hypertension leads to regression of this condition as well.

Parameters which predict the development of esophageal varices and occurrence of variceal bleed have been identified. The ratio of PC/mm³ to bipolar length of the spleen in millimeters (as obtained by USS) if above 909, has a negative predictive value for varices. HVPG obtained by hepatic vein catheterization is a good parameter to quantify risk. If HVPG is > 5 mm Hg, portal hypertension is present. It is significant when HVPG is > 10 mm Hg since varices and variceal bleed are all more likely to be present. Liver stiffness which can be estimated non-invasively is a parameter which correlates well with HVPG, especially if HVPG is < 10 mm Hg.

Management of Variceal Bleeding

Variceal bleeding is a medical emergency and carries a mortality of about 35% if untreated. It is best managed in the intensive care units (ICUs) of a tertiary level hospital. Oxygen inhalation through an airway is started. The patient should be given first aid as for any major upper GI bleed in order to stabilize his condition. This consists of intravenous (IV) fluids and fresh blood replacement, sedatives to allay anxiety and IV injection of H_2 receptor antagonist such as ranitidine 50 mg or a proton pump inhibitor (PPI) such as pantoprazole 40 mg, over a period of 2–5 minutes. Sudden blood loss of more than 25% of the blood volume is an urgent indication for packed cell or fresh whole blood transfusion. Ideal is to make up the hemoglobin level to 100 g/L at which level adequate oxygen carrying capacity can be achieved with optimum benefit. Large doses of oral antacids such as aluminum hydroxide $[Al(OH)_3]$ and magnesium trisilicate $(Mg_2O_8Si_3)$ 1–2 g should be administered initially and repeated hourly to reduce bleeding from co-existing ulcers in the esophagus and stomach. The patient should be transported to a medical center with facilities for specialized care, as soon as possible, preferably with the blood transfusion in place. Portal hypertensive colonopathy which may give rise to bleeding may develops.

Principles of Management

- To stabilize the patient's vital functions
- To diagnose the site of bleeding
- To arrest the bleeding
- To prevent rebleeding
- Secondary prevention.

Stabilizing the patient

The patient requires rapid IV fluids, blood transfusion and oxygen inhalation to stabilize the vital functions. Central venous pressure (CVP) monitoring is essential. A moderate or severe bleed usually requires three units of fresh blood transfusion. Overtransfusion increases the risk of bleeding further. Systemic diseases such as diabetes, infections, electrolyte abnormalities and abnormalities of coagulation also require attention. Patient with Child-Pugh class C and those with HVPG > 20 are at higher risk.

Antibiotics like ceftriaxone, norfloxacin and ciprofloxacin should be started to prevent bacterial translocation during bleed. PPIs may also be started as infusion even though variceal bleed is high on the list, since other causes of bleed can also coexist in many cases.

Identifying the site of bleeding

After stabilizing, the patient should be taken up for emergency esophagogastroscopy. This is technically difficult during the emergency and should be done by a skilled endoscopist in a well-equipped center with therapeutic facilities. The bleeding sites may be single, multiple or diffused.

Arrest of bleeding

Methods include

- Pharmacotherapy
- Balloon tamponade
- Endoscopic interventions
- Surgery.

Textbook of Medicine

Pharmacotherapy—splanchnic vasoconstrictors

Somatostatin: It is given as an initial IV infusion for 3–5 days at the rate of 250 µg/hr. It controls bleeding in 80–85% of patients and prevents rebleeding also. ***Octreotide,*** which is the analogue of somatostatin is equally effective. The initial bolus dose is 50 µg followed by continuous infusion at the rate of 50 µg/hr. ***Vapreotide*** and ***lanreotide*** are newer analogues of somatostatin which have also been introduced. The dose is 250 µg as bolus followed by 250 µg hourly as continuous infusion for up to five days.

Vasopressin given in an IV bolus dose of 20 units over a period of 10–15 minutes at 4 hour intervals used to be the drug of choice prior to the use of somatostatin, which is more effective. ***Vasopressin*** also reduces portal pressure but troublesome side effects such as angina, bowel ischemia and gangrene of the toes may develop at times.

Terlipressin (triglycyl-lysine-vasopressin) is a vasopressin analogue which is more effective and has less of side effects. Terlipressin is started in a dose of 2 mg IV bolus followed by 1 mg every 4–6 hours for 3–5 days. It is the only drug which is shown to have mortality benefit in studies on variceal bleeding.

Contraindications for terlipressin: Age more than 70 years, chronic obstructive pulmonary disease (COPD), heart block, coronary artery disease (CAD), cardiomyopathy, cardiac arrhythmias and peripheral occlusive vascular disease.

Balloon tamponade

Sengstaken-Blakemore, Linton-Nachlas and Minnesota tube may be useful for temporary tamponade while the patient is being transported to a higher center. It is not as effective as somatostatin or endoscopic interventions. It is not used unless there are exceptional circumstances. It should only be used in massive bleeding as a temporary bridge (for maximum of 24 hours) until definite treatment can be instituted.

Endoscopic interventions

Endoscopic sclerotherapy (EST) can arrest 85–90% of active bleeding. The common sclerosants used for esophageal varies are sodium tetradecyl sulfate (STD), polidocanol and alcohol. The gastric varices require cyanoacrylate for injection. Endoscopic variceal ligation (EVL) is a better procedure than EST to prevent variceal bleeding (Figs 87.7A to C and 87.8A to C).

In this procedure, the varices are sucked into a hood attached to the distal end of the endoscope and a rubber band applied at its base. Transjugular intrahepatic portosystemic shunt (TIPS) is a catheter intervention procedure that may be undertaken to reduce portal venous pressure as an emergency measure. Preemptive TIPS is indicated in child class C patient with high-risk of re-bleeding. This is shown to reduce the mortality following variceal bleeding.

Surgery

The emergency surgical procedures to stop variceal bleeding carry high mortality. The same result can be achieved with endoscopic procedures. Hence, the role of surgery is limited.

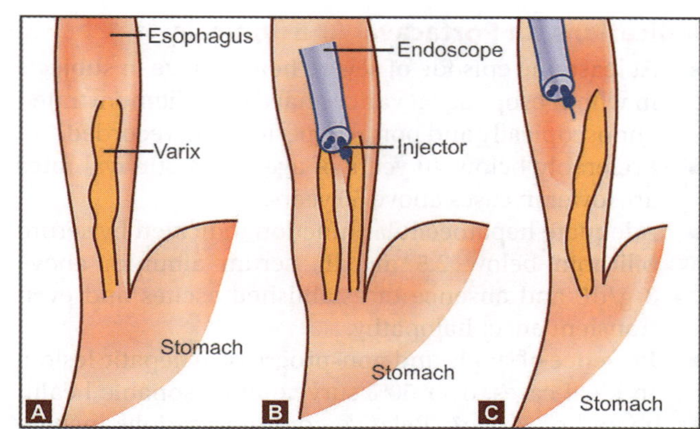

Figs 87.7A to C: Technique of sclerotherapy for esophageal varices. **A.** Esophageal varix; **B.** Intra-variceal injection; **C.** Para-variceal injection

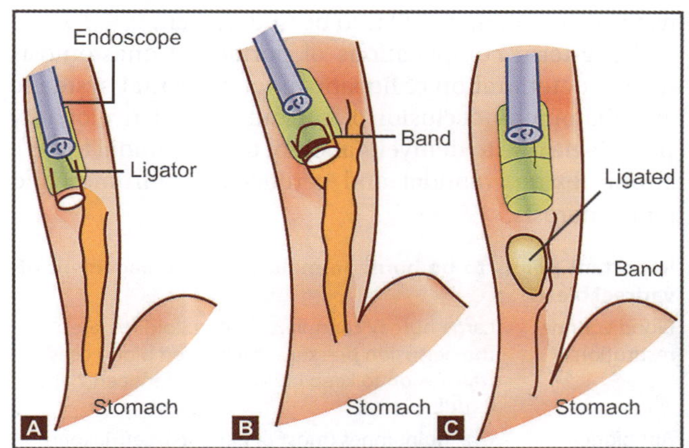

Figs 87.8A to C: Technique of variceal ligation of esophageal varices: B—Varix sucked into the housing cylinder

Newer Approaches

Self-expandable covered esophageal stents which can be used to treat refractory variceal bleed.

Management of Treatment Failure

Persistent bleeding despite continued pharmacological and endoscopic treatment is best managed by TIPS with ***polytetrafluoroethylene (PTFE)*** covered stents. Re-bleeding during first 5 days may be managed by a second attempt at endoscopy. If severe re-bleed occurs, PTFE covered TIPS may be the best option since thrombus formation and distal embolization are less common with these stents.

Long-term Prophylaxis

Large varices and varices which have bled previously require obliteration with EVL or EST. Drug therapy can lower portal pressure on a long-term basis. The drugs useful for prophylaxis are nonselective beta-blockers such as propranolol 80–160 mg/oral daily or nadolol 80 mg oral daily. Nonselective beta-blockers should be started on the 6th day following index bleed. Portacaval shunt surgery may be useful in selected cases of extrahepatic portal hypertension and noncirrhotic portal fibrosis (NCPF). This surgery is not done as a first-line procedure at present.

Textbook of Medicine

Indications for Portacaval Anastomosis

- At least one episode of severe hemorrhage in subjects in whom esophageal varices have been demonstrated endoscopically and portal hypertension, recorded.
- Preferably below 40 years of age, since survival rates are lower in cases above 50 years.
- Adequate hepatocellular function indicated by serum bilirubin below 2.5 mg/dL, serum albumin above 3 g/dL and absence of established ascites and even transient encephalopathy.
- Presence of stable and non-progressive hepatic lesion.

In ideal cases, over 50% survive in reasonable health at the end of 5 years. Relative contraindications include moderate or advanced hepatic failure and congenital or other acquired abnormalities of the portal vein. Portacaval shunting should not be undertaken if future liver transplantation (LT) is to be undertaken.

Long-term complications of portacaval anastomosis include deterioration of hepatic function, portal-systemic encephalopathy, occlusion of the shunt, shunt myelopathy (paraplegia due to demyelination of the pyramidal tracts), chronic extrapyramidal and cerebellar syndromes and hemosiderosis.

Important points to be borne in mind in the management of variceal bleed	
Blood volume restitution	Large bore IV cannula, saline, colloids to keep the perfusion pressure; packed red blood cells transfusion to keep hemoglobin between 7 and 8 g/dL
Antibiotic treatment	Oral quinolones (most of patients); ceftriaxone (who cannot take oral quinolones and with advanced cirrhosis)
Upper GI endoscopy	As soon as possible after admission (within 12 hours)
Pharmacological	Vasoactive drugs started as soon as possible before endoscopy and continued for 5 days
Therapeutic endoscopy	EVL for esophageal varices; sclerotherapy if ligation is technically difficult; therapy with tissue adhesive (n-butyl cyanoacrylate) for gastric varices
TIPS	Within 24 hours in patients with high-risk of treatment failure (child C <14 points or child B with active bleed) after initial pharmacological and endoscopic treatment

Abbreviations: TIPS = Transjugular intrahepatic portosystemic shunt; EVL = Endoscopic variceal ligation; GI = Gastrointestinal

PORTOPULMONARY SYNDROME

Significant pulmonary hypertension is seen in about 4–6% of cirrhosis patients with portal hypertension. Pulmonary vasculature shows medial hypertrophy, endothelial hyperplasia and luminal thrombosis. The changes may be due to the vasoconstrictors escaping hepatic metabolism in cirrhosis with portal-systemic anastomosis. Thromboembolism from the dilated and tortuous paraesophageal and mediastinal varices to the pulmonic vascular bed may be another mechanism.

Development of portopulmonary syndrome seriously shortens the lifespan in cirrhosis patients. There is no effective treatment. Epoprostenol (prostacyclin) and nitric oxide inhalations show some clinical benefit.

Portosystemic shunts (PSS) are also tried. Severe porto-pulmonary syndrome is a contraindication for LT.

Portal hypertensive enteropathy (PHE) is a manifestation of portal hypertensive intestinal vasculopathy (PHIV). Endoscopic findings include bleeding vascular ectasias, ulceration and small bowel varices. The stomach, small intestine and colon can be affected (Figs 87.9 and 87.10). Cirrhosis liver is the most frequent cause and the lesion is mainly related to the level of portal hypertension. The patients present with continuous GI blood loss, requiring repeated blood transfusions. Wireless capsule endoscopy is the investigative modality of choice to detect the bleeding lesions all along the GIT. ***Treatment*** consists of TIPS which promptly reduces the portal hypertension and arrests the bleeding.

EXTRAHEPATIC PORTAL HYPERTENSION (EHPH)

It is caused by portal or splenic vein thrombosis. This is a common cause of portal hypertension in India. The liver is normal. The disease starts in childhood and present for the first time between 11 and 25 years but sometimes symptoms may manifest even as early as 3–4 years.

Etiology

- Portal vein thrombosis (PVT) secondary to neonatal umbilical sepsis
- Intra-abdominal infections like acute appendicitis and peritonitis

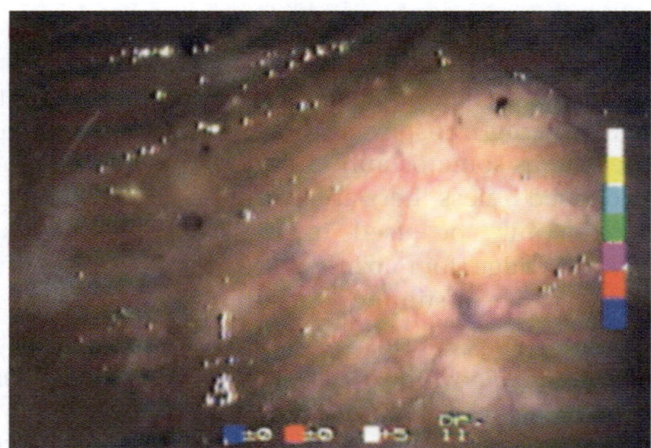

Fig. 87.9: Portal colonopathy. ***Note:*** The dilated submucous blood vessels. These may bleed during colonoscopy

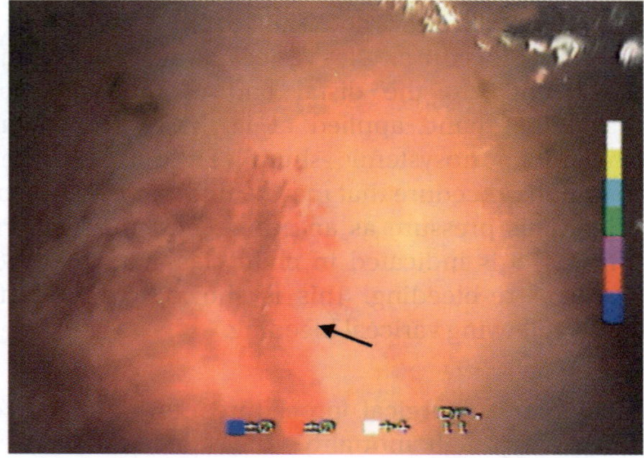

Fig. 87.10: Portal colonopathy colonoscopy. ***Note:*** Variceal bleeding (arrow)

- Abdominal trauma
- Malignant tumors of the pancreas, stomach, colon or periportal lymph nodes
- Acute pancreatitis and pancreatic cysts
- Hematological disorders like polycythemia, thrombocythemia and thrombophilic conditions such as deficiency of protein C and S and antithrombin may be present in a third of these cases
- Congenital anomalies of the portal veins
- Vascular lesions such as arteriovenous fistulae (AVF) in the spleen or hepatic artery-portal vein fistula in the liver. Hematemesis is the presenting symptom in the majority.

Management

It consists of emergency medical treatment of variceal bleeding followed by appropriate shunt surgery depending on the availability of suitable veins. Since the liver function is good, long-term prognosis is bright.

NONCIRRHOTIC PORTAL FIBROSIS (NCPF)

Syn: Idiopathic portal hypertension (IPH)

This disorder is frequently seen in India and the neighboring countries. It is characterized by gross splenomegaly and portal hypertension with patent extrahepatic portal veins. Hepatic function is normal. Histological and clinical features do not suggest cirrhosis. Liver biopsy may be normal or varying degrees of portal fibrosis and cellular infiltration may occur. Studies have suggested chronic arsenic intoxication as a probable cause.

The condition is most common in the third and fourth decades. Many patients complain of several attacks of hematemesis which are better tolerated by these patients than those with hepatic cirrhosis. Ascites and jaundice are uncommon.

Management

Since this condition may present with severe hematemesis, the treatment is that of bleeding esophageal varices.

CHAPTER

88

Other Hepatic Disorders

KR Vinaya Kumar, KV Krishna Das

Chapter Summary

- Hepatorenal Syndrome (HRS)
- Alcoholic Liver Disease
  - Alcoholic Hepatitis
  - Nonalcoholic Fatty Liver Disease (NAFLD)
- Chronic Hepatitis
  - Chronic HBV
  - Chronic HCV
- Autoimmune Hepatitis (AIH)
- Drug Toxicity on the Liver
- Hepatic Veno-occlusive Disease (VOD)
- Budd-Chiari Syndrome
- Liver Dysfunction in Circulatory Impairment
- Pyogenic Abscess of the Liver
- Carcinoma of the Liver
  - Primary Carcinoma
  - Secondary Carcinoma
- Reye's syndrome

HEPATORENAL SYNDROME (HRS)

Syn: Syndrome of functional failure

It is defined as functional renal failure (FRF) occurring in the setting of advanced liver disease but in the absence of intrinsic renal disease. The HRS is characterized by intense constriction of renal cortical vasculature with resultant diversion of blood flow from the renal cortex. As a result, glomerular filtration rate (GFR) comes down, plasma renin level increases, urine output decreases and sodium is avidly reabsorbed in the distal nephron.

Histologically, the kidneys are normal. Such kidneys can perform normally when transplanted into subjects without portal hypertension. In the same individual, correction of portal hypertension and liver failure by liver transplantation restores renal function too.

FRF occurs in 18% of decompensated cirrhosis and portal hypertension within one year. The three most important risk factors of HRS are low sodium concentration, high plasma renin activity (PRA) and absence of hepatomegaly. Other risk factors include ascites, poor nutritional status and esophageal varices.

Pathogenesis

It is characterized by sodium retention, water retention and renal vasoconstriction. It is associated with decrease in renal blood flow (RBF), GFR and urine output. These lead to azotemia. However, the pathophysiologic mechanisms are not fully defined, though several propositions are made.

Diagnostic Criteria

It should be suspected in any patient with acute or chronic liver disease and portal hypertension, when there is rise in serum creatinine above 1.5 mg/dL. The criteria are divided into different criteria, which must be present in all patients for diagnosis and minor criteria, which provide support for diagnosis (Box 88.1).

Clinical Types

It is divided into two types. ***Type 1 HRS*** is rapid in onset and progressive in course. Impairment of renal

Box 88.1: Criteria to diagnose HRS in patients with cirrhosis

- Cirrhosis with ascites
- Serum creatinine level ≥1.5 mg/dL
- No or insufficient improvement in serum creatinine level (remains ≥1.5 mg/dL) 48 hr after diuretic withdrawal and adequate volume expansion with IV albumin
- Absence of shock
- No evidence of recent use of nephrotoxic drugs
- Absence of intrinsic renal disease (proteinuria of > 500 mg/day, microhematuria, i.e. > 50 RBCs/hpf or abnormal renal ultrasound findings)

Abbreviation: RBCs/hpf = Red blood cells per high power field

function, defined as a doubling of the initial serum creatinine to a level higher than 2.5 mg/dL or a 50% reduction of the initial 24 hour creatinine clearance to a level lower than 20 mL/min occurs in less than 2 weeks. Patients with Type 1 HRS are usually very sick, with signs of advanced liver failure. **Type 2 HRS** is defined as the impairment in renal function evidenced by serum creatinine level more than 1.5 mg/dL, which does not meet the criteria for type 1 HRS. Commonly it manifests as refractory ascites.

Untreated, the median survival time for patients with type 1 HRS is less than 2 weeks.

Management of HRS

- Stop nephrotoxic drugs
- Antibiotics for infection
- Intravenous albumin (1 g/kg on day 1 and continue 20–60 g/day as needed
- In addition to albumin vasopressors like
  - Inj. terlipressin (1 mg q4h can increase up to 2 mg q4h)
  - Octreotide (100 µg q8h sc can increase up to 200 µg q8h)
  - Midodrine (2.5–5 mg q8h can increase up to 15 mg q8h)
- Evaluate for liver transplantation.

Note: Duration of vasopressors maximum for 2 weeks.

ALCOHOLIC LIVER DISEASE

(*See* also Section 4, Ch 23, Alcohol Intoxication)

Alcohol-related liver injury is common in places where alcohol consumption is high. It occurs if the intake is more than 40–80 g daily and 20–40 g daily for 10–12 years in males and females respectively. The three recognizable syndromes are *fatty liver, alcoholic hepatitis* and *Laennec's cirrhosis.* Alcoholic fatty liver is the most benign one. Infiltration of the liver with triglyceride is extremely common in men consuming alcohol regularly. The most frequent physical finding in such patients is hepatomegaly without any evidence of cirrhosis. Abstinence from alcohol at this stage leads to rapid regression within weeks.

Alcoholic Hepatitis

Approximately 25% of chronic alcoholics develop histological evidence of alcoholic hepatitis. This is characterized by hepatocellular necrosis affecting mainly the centrilobular zone. Remaining hepatocytes are often distorted and enlarged. In addition, inflammatory exudate consisting of polymorphs and perisinusoidal and perivenular fibrosis is usually present. Cytoplasmic inclusions known as *alcoholic hyaline* or *Mallory bodies* are seen. These changes may occur alone, but are usually accompanied by significant fatty infiltration and often by cirrhosis.

Clinically, alcoholic hepatitis tends to be more serious than fatty liver, although a few are asymptomatic. Anorexia, nausea, upper abdominal pain, weakness, vomiting, fever, jaundice and diarrhea may occur in various combinations. The pain may be in the right upper quadrant and closely resembles cholecystitis.

Biochemical abnormalities include elevation of transaminases, hyperbilirubinemia, hypoalbuminemia and prolongation of prothrombin time (PT). The ratio of serum glutamic oxaloacetic transaminase (SGOT)/serum glutamic pyruvic transaminase (SGPT) is usually >2/1 in alcoholic liver disease. Ratios >3/1 is more suggestive and significant. Alkaline phosphatase (ALP) is elevated in approximately 30% of such patients. Neutrophil leukocytosis is common (12000–20000 mm^3).

These are nonspecific changes, but in an alcoholic, these strongly suggest hepatitis. The diagnosis can be confirmed only by liver biopsy. It is to be remembered that the entire histological picture of alcoholic hepatitis may appear in conditions other than alcoholism, such as obesity, diabetes, short bowel syndrome, Indian childhood cirrhosis (ICC) and drug toxicity. The outcome in patients with alcoholic hepatitis is not nearly as benign as in those with alcoholic fatty liver alone. The reported overall acute mortality is 15–20% and approximately 50% cases develop alcoholic (Laennec's) cirrhosis.

Scores: There are different scoring systems to assess the severity and prognosis in alcoholic hepatitis. The most widely used among these is Maddrey's discriminant function (DF). It is calculated by the *formula* = [4.6 × (PT test – control time) + Serum bilirubin in mg/dL]. It is useful to predict the 30 day mortality in patients with alcoholic hepatitis. The other scoring systems used are Lille score, Glasgow alcoholic hepatitis score, model for end-stage liver disease (MELD) and age, serum bilirubin, INR and serum creatinine (ABIC).

Management: There is no specific therapy. Abstinence from alcohol is essential. Nutritional support, corticosteroids, propylthiouracil (PTU), glucagon, insulin, intravenous (IV) amino acids, pentoxifylline and colchicine have been tried with inconclusive results. Some of these agents seem promising but none has yet been established as an effective therapy.

Course: The healing of alcoholic hepatitis in survivors is slow, despite good nutrition, rest and abstinence from alcohol. Most patients show activity of the disease even after 3–4 months. Corticosteroids reduced mortality significantly in patients with a DF of at least 32 or hepatic encephalopathy. In patients with sepsis, gastrointestinal (GI) bleed, pancreatitis and renal failure pentoxifylline can be considered as first-line therapy. The final phase of alcoholic liver disease is alcoholic cirrhosis. Alcoholic cirrhosis is described in Chapter 84, pp 607. Pentoxyphylline, 400 mg tds for 4 weeks may help recoverery in 60% of cases.

Nonalcoholic Fatty Liver Disease (NAFLD)

It is a clinicopathologic syndrome encompassing a wide range of fatty liver disease in the absence of significant alcohol intake and other common causes of steatosis. Ongoing or recent alcohol consumption > 21 drinks on average per week in men and more 14 drinks on average per week in women is considered as significant alcohol intake (one alcohol drink is equal to 10 g of alcohol).

Epidemiology

At present, this has become a very common problem. The onset is insidious and course is progressive. Often it is detected when the patient is examined for vague abdominal symptoms or palpable hepatomegaly. Ultrasonography (USG) examination picks up excess fat deposit in the liver. This condition was initially recognized in women with diabetes with insulin resistance (IR).

The prevalence of NAFLD in population varies. Population based studies show NAFLD prevalence of 20–30% in western population and 12.2–22.6% in Indian population. Most cases of NAFLD are discovered in the fourth or sixth decade. However, it is being increasingly recognized in obese children and adolescents especially in the western population. Males may be affected as often as women and may be at higher risk of advanced forms of NAFLD. Hispanics demonstrated the highest prevalence of NAFLD compared with whites and African Americans.

Spectrum of Disease

NAFLD encompass the spectrum of disease, i.e. steatosis—steatosis with nonspecific inflammation or steatohepatitis (NASH)—NASH with fibrosis and cirrhosis.

Risk Factors Associated with NAFLD

Obesity, type 2 diabetes mellitus, dyslipidemia and metabolic syndrome (MS) are the conditions to be associated with NAFLD. Polycystic ovarian disease, hypothyroidism, obstructive sleep apnea (OSA), hypopituitarism, pancreato duodenal bypass and hypogonadism are the conditions with emerging association with NAFLD.

NAFLD is seen as hepatic manifestation of MS. When 3 of 5 of the listed characteristics are present, a diagnosis of MS can be made (Table 88.1).

Lean Nonalcoholic Steatohepatitis (NASH)

Nonalcoholic fatty liver in the absence of overweight and/or obesity, high body mass index (BMI), has been

Table 88.1: ATP III: Clinical identification of the metabolic syndrome	
Risk factor	**Defining level**
Central obesity	Waist circumference > 102 cm for men and > 88 cm for women
Triglyceride	> 150 mg/dL
HDL cholesterol	
• Men	< 40 mg/dL
• Women	< 50 mg/dL
Fasting blood sugar	< 100 mg/dL
Blood pressure	> 135/ > 85 mm Hg

Abbreviations: ATP = Adenosine triphosphate; HDL = High density lipoprotein

designated as *lean NASH*. While maintaining a close pathophysiological link with MS and IR, the presence of subtle alterations in measures of total body and regional adiposity not exceeding the designed cut-offs, are hallmarks of lean NASH.

Pathogenesis

The pathogenesis of NAFLD is poorly understood. The prevailing theory is the two hit hypothesis. According to this hypothesis, dysregulation of fatty acid metabolism leads to steatosis, which is the first hepatic insult (*first hit*) in NAFLD. Steatosis is associated with several cellular adaptations and altered signaling pathways which render hepatocytes vulnerable to a second insult (*second hit*). The second insult may be one or more genetic alteration which causes hepatocytes inflammation and necrosis and ultimately activate fibrosis cascade leading to cirrhosis. This condition may be mistaken for alcoholic liver disease (Fig. 88.1).

Histopathologic finding

- Steatosis—macrovesicular > microvesicular (predominates in zone 3)
- Hepatocellular injury—ballooning hepatocytes, apoptosis/necrosis, Mallory's hyaline, giant mitochondria
- Inflammation—mixed neutrophil and lymphocytes infiltrate (predominates in zone 3)
- Fibrosis—perisinusoidal and perivenular.

Clinical Features

Most patients are asymptomatic (48–100%). When symptoms occur, they are nonspecific including vague right upper quadrant pain, fatigue, malaise and others. On examination, obesity is the most common finding. Hepatomegaly may be seen in 75%. In advanced disease, stigmata of chronic liver disease including spider angioma, palmar erythema, splenomegaly and ascites may be noted.

Laboratory Finding

Lipid profile may be abnormal [elevated triglyceride and low high density lipoprotein (HDL)]. Elevation of hepatic transaminases levels to 2–4 times the normal are the most common abnormalities, with aspartate transaminase (AST)/alanine transaminase (ALT) ratio less than 1 in most of the patients. Serum alkaline phosphatase (ALP) and gamma glutamyl transferase (GGT) may be mildly elevated. Bilirubin, albumin and PT are normal unless advanced cirrhosis has set in. Elevated levels of ferritin, higher levels of transferrin saturation and presence of low titer antinuclear antibodies (ANA) are less common findings.

Imaging

USG shows bright hepatic echotexture, hepatomegaly and vascular blurring. USG is more sensitive than computed tomography (CT) for detection of fatty liver. In contrast-enhanced computed tomography (CECT), hepatic attenuation numbers are > 20 Hounsfield units (HU) less than the spleen.

Noninvasive Markers (for Measurement of Fibrosis)

- The NAFLD fibrosis score is based on six readily available variables (age, BMI, hyperglycemia, platelet

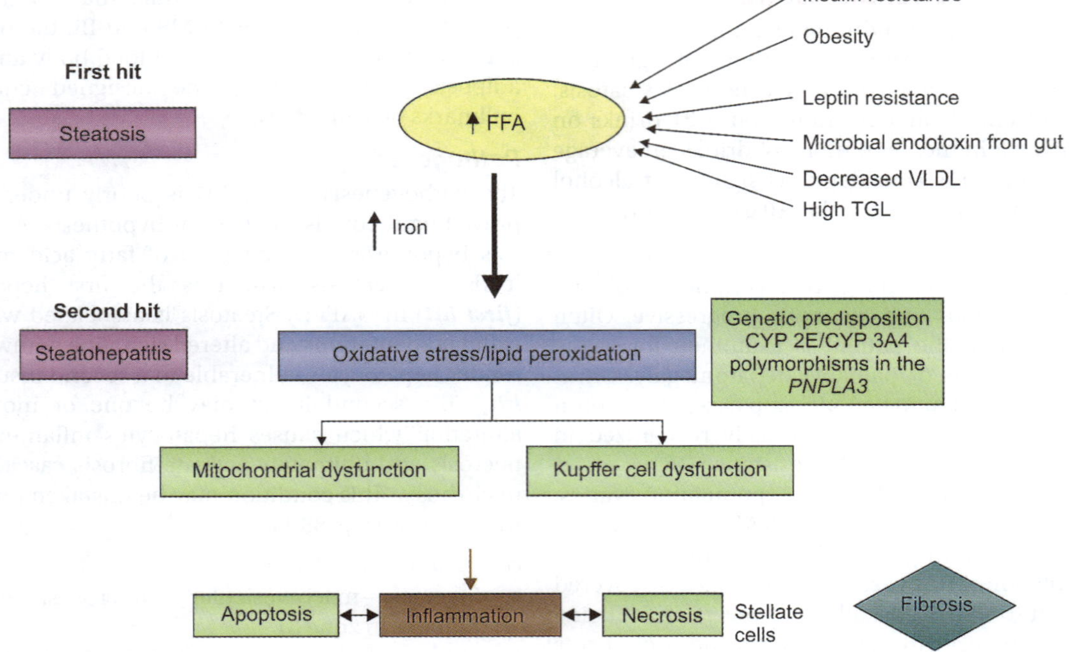

Fig. 88.1: Pathogenesis of nonalcoholic steatohepatitis (NASH)
Abbreviations: VLDL = Very low density lipoprotein; TGL = Triglyceride lipase; FFA = Free fatty acid; PNPLA3 = Patatin-like phospholipase domain-containing protein 3 gene

Textbook of Medicine

count, albumin, AST/ALT ratio) and it is calculated using the published formula (http://nafldscore.com).

- The enhanced liver fibrosis (ELF) panel consists of plasma levels of three matrix turnover proteins [hyaluronic acid, tissue inhibitor of metalloproteinases 1 (TIMP-1) and N-terminal procollagen III-peptide (PIIINP)].
- Transient elastography, which measures liver stiffness noninvasively, has been successful in identifying advanced fibrosis. Obesity interferes with interpretation.
- Circulating levels of cytokeratin-18 (CK18).

Liver Biopsy

It is the gold standard for diagnosis of NAFLD. Histology shows cytolytic changes in hepatocytes such as ballooning degeneration, Mallory hyaline and lobular inflammation. Increase in liver enzymes may occur. Variable degrees of fibrosis may be present (Table 88.2). This condition is not caused by alcoholism.

Treatment

Lifestyle modification

All patients with NAFLD should be encouraged for weight loss program by reducing calorie intake and/or increasing physical activity. Weight loss of 3–5% is necessary for improvement in the steatosis. However, greater weight loss (up to 10%) may be needed to improve necro-inflammation.

Drugs

- Vitamin E (alpha-tocopherol)—act by reducing oxidative stress. Vitamin E in dose of 800 mg/day is recommended in non-diabetic biopsy proven NASH, however, its role is not clear in NASH with diabetes,

Table 88.2: Grading and staging of histopathologic lesions of NAFLD (Brunt classification)

Grade 1: Mild

Steatosis: Predominantly macrovesicular, involves < 33 up to 66% of the lobules
Ballooning: Occasionally observed; zone 3 hepatocytes
Lobular inflammation: Scattered and mild acute (polymorphonuclear cells) and occasional chronic inflammation (mononuclear cells)
Portal inflammation: None or mild

Grade 2: Moderate

Steatosis: Any degree; usually mixed macrovesicular and microvesicular
Ballooning: Obvious and present in zone 3
Lobular inflammation: Polymorphonuclear cells may be noted in association with ballooned hepatocytes
Portal inflammation: Mild to moderate

Grade 3: Severe

Steatosis: Typically > 66% (paracinar) of lobules; commonly mixed steatosis
Ballooning: Predominantly zone 3; marked
Lobular inflammation: Scattered acute and chronic inflammation.
Portal inflammation: Mild or moderate

Staging: Fibrosis in NASH

Stage 1: Zone 3 perivenular, perisinusoidal/pericellular fibrosis, focal or extensive
Stage 2: As above with focal or extensive periportal fibrosis
Stage 3: Bridging fibrosis, focal or extensive
Stage 4: Cirrhosis

Grading for steatosis

Grade 1: 0–33% of hepatocytes affected
Grade 2: 33–66% of hepatocytes affected
Grade 3: > 66% of hepatocytes affected

NASH without liver biopsy, NASH cirrhosis or cryptogenic cirrhosis.

- Betaine—raises S-adenosylmethionine and decreases cellular oxidative damage.
- Metformin—reduces hyperinsulinemia and improves hepatic insulin sensitivity. However, results in human studies have been less impressive.
- Thiazolidinediones (pioglitazone)—it is a peroxisome proliferator-activated receptors (PPAR)-alpha agonist. It promotes insulin sensitivity and hyperinsulinemia by increasing glucose disposal in muscle and decreasing hepatic glucose output. Also decreases lipolysis and free fatty acid (FFA) release.
- Lipid lowering agents—atorvastatin showed improvement in lipid profile and hepatic steatosis.
- Ursodeoxycholic acid—cytoprotective agent.
- Other drugs—N-acetylcysteine (NAC), ragaglitazar, omega 3-fatty acids.

Newer drugs are undertrial for [N-acyl-homoserine lactone (NAHL)]

Obeticholic acid 25 mg orally daily was given to 141 patients between March 2011 and December 2012 and 142 patients given placebo were compared. Forty five percent of the treatment group showed improvement in liver biopsy at 72 weeks compared to 21% and 109 patients in the control group. Pruritis was the side effect in 23% of the treated group compared to 6% in the control further studies are continued.

Source: Neuschwander-Tetri BA, Loomba R, Sanyal AJ, et al. Farnesoid X nuclear receptor ligand obeticholic acid for non-cirrhotic, non-alcoholic steatohepatitis (FLINT): A multicentre, randomized placebo-controlled trial. Lancet. 2015;385(9972):956–65.

Many cases of NAHL have also features of the MS and thereby they have high-risk of cardiovascular disease (CVD)—peripheral, coronary and cerebrovascular diseases. Mortality in NAHL is higher than in general controls. Cardiovascular death is most common.

CHRONIC HEPATITIS

Definition

It is defined as chronic inflammatory activity in the liver continuing without improvement for more than six months. In asymptomatic patients, estimation of the duration may be difficult. Features such as spider angioma, firm irregular hepatomegaly and splenomegaly suggest a chronic process. Fibrosis seen in liver biopsy also suggest chronicity. The previously used terms, chronic persistent hepatitis and chronic active hepatitis are replaced by the term *chronic hepatitis*.

Etiology

- Hepatitis B and C are the most common causes
- Hepatitis delta virus (HDV) positive in 5–10% of hepatitis B virus (HBV) positive cases
- Autoimmune hepatitis
- Wilson's disease
- Drug toxicity—several drugs
- Chronic alcoholic hepatitis

- One-third of case are idiopathic, since no causative factor can be identified. They form a heterogeneous group.

Natural History

It depends on various factors such as the degree of necro-inflammatory activity, stage of the disease, etiology and the host response to treatment. Most of patients are asymptomatic and progress towards cirrhosis liver. The risk of hepatocellular carcinoma (HCC) is increased in HBV and hepatitis C virus (HCV) related chronic hepatitis. Some patients with high inflammatory activity present with jaundice and even liver failure.

Chronic HBV Hepatitis

(*See* also Section 6, Ch 55, Hepatitis B Virus, pp 388)

Clinical Features

Most of the patients are asymptomatic and present with elevation of AST and ALT or viral markers detected during routine check-up, especially during blood donation. Sometimes asymptomatic hepatomegaly is detected clinically or on USG for some other purposes. Rarely they may present with acute hepatitis and the jaundice fails to clear within six months. In some cases, the presentation is with acute onset of jaundice, but symptoms persist and the ALT and AST may remain high. Liver biopsy may reveal chronic hepatitis.

Pathogenesis

After an acute attack of hepatitis B, more than 95% of adults clear the virus completely. If the host immune response is inadequate, the virus tends to persist. Causes of poor immune defense response include: (i) Poor expression of human leukocyte antigen (HLA) class I antigens on the hepatocyte membrane, (ii) increased suppressor T-cell function (iii) defective cytotoxic (K) lymphocyte function and (iv) presence of blocking antibodies on the liver cell membrane.

Pathology

The entire disease activity spectrum caused by HBV has to be labeled as *chronic hepatitis B infection* and further classification should be based on histology. Necroinflammatory activity and fibrosis form the basis of histological classification.

Modified *Knodell classification* scores the necro-inflammatory activity which is the histologic activity index scored on a scale 0–18 and this forms the basis of Knodell's classification (Box 88.2). Presence of fibrosis is scored on a scale of 0 to 4 and this forms the basis of staging (Box 88.3).

Diagnosis

The viral etiology is established by viral markers—HBsAg, HBeAg, HBcAg and their antibodies. HBV virus can exist in the liver in a replicating stage or integrated stage.

Box 88.2: Knodell's histologic activity index (HAI)

Component	Score
Periportal necrosis with or without bridging necrosis	0–10
Intralobular necrosis	0–4
Portal Inflammation	0–4

Box 88.3: Staging (fibrosis)

		Score
Fibrosis	None	0
Portal expansion	+	1
Portal to portal tract fibrosis	+	2
Bridging fibrosis	+	3
Cirrhosis	+	4

Box 88.4: Factors with a prediction of favorable therapeutic outcome in chronic HCV hepatitis

Young age	Non-alcoholics
Females	Low viral load
Non-obese	Less fibrosis
Short duration of infection	Elevated transaminases
Hepatic iron content not raised	Virus genotype II or III

In the replicating stage, the virus multiplies actively. It is present in blood and the disease can spread. The histologic activity index is high and the patients require antiviral treatment.

Clinical feature	Replicating stage	Integrated stage
Infectivity	High	Low
HBsAg	Positive	Positive
HBeAg	Positive	Negative
Anti-HBe	Negative	Positive
HBV DNA	Positive	Negative

Abbreviations: HBsAg = Hepatitis B surface antigen; HBeAg = Hepatitis B envelope antigen; HBV DNA = Hepatitis B virus deoxyribonucleic acid.

The viral genome integrates with host hepatocyte deoxyribonucleic acid (DNA) and there is no independent viral replication or viremia in the integrated phase. Hepatic necrosis is minimal at this stage and the benefit of antiviral treatment is probably only slight.

Treatment and Prophylaxis

The goal of therapy is to improve quality of life and survival by preventing progression of the disease to cirrhosis, decompensated cirrhosis, end-stage liver disease, HCC and death.

The assessment of the severity of the liver disease should include: Biochemical markers, including AST and ALT, GGT, ALP, bilirubin, serum albumin and globulins, blood counts, PT and hepatic ultrasound.

Chronic HCV Hepatitis

(*See* also Section 6, Ch 55, HCV infection, pp 390)

Sixty to ninety percent hepatitis caused by HCV tend to become chronic. It is the most common cause of post-transfusion chronic hepatitis and cirrhosis. There is increased incidence of HCC.

Clinical Features

Most of the patients are asymptomatic or have only mild symptoms like anorexia and fatigue. The ALT and AST levels are often elevated. Periods of normal transaminase levels are characteristic of HCV infection. They may also present with extrahepatic manifestations such as lichen planus, thyroiditis or membranous glomerulonephritis (MGN). Mixed cryoglobulinemia may develop and lead to symptoms.

The course of the illness is slower compared to chronic HBV infection. Cirrhosis liver and liver failure develop only after 10 years or more.

Diagnosis

Third generation anti-HCV test [enzyme linked immuno-sorbent assay (ELISA)] is useful for screening. Radioi-mmunoblot assay (RIBA) is confirmatory. Hepatitis C virus-ribonucleic acid (HCV-RNA) can be detected by polymerase chain reaction (PCR) and can be quantified. Tests are available for genotyping also. Genotyping is helpful in predicting treatment response. PCR test done in reliable laboratories only should be accepted since several factors vitiate the test results.

Liver biopsy helps to assess the activity and the results are expressed according to Metavir scoring system. Lymphoid aggregation, fatty changes and bile duct injury are features of HCV infection.

In chronic liver disease, there is a general tendency to accumulate iron in the liver. Increased hepatic iron content is associated with poorer outcome. In such cases, phlebotomy and regular removal of blood improves the outcome if done along with anti-HCV treatment (Box 88.4).

HCV hepatitis leading to cirrhosis and carcinoma are common reasons for hepatic transplantation at present.

AUTOIMMUNE HEPATITIS (AIH)

It is encountered less commonly than the previously described types. Continuing hepatocellular necrosis and inflammation with fibrosis are characteristic. It can produce cirrhosis and hepatocellular failure. Many cases are associated with autoimmune diseases such as rheumatoid arthritis (RA), thyroiditis, hemolytic anemia, ulcerative colitis (UC), membranoproliferative glomerulonephritis and others.

Pathogenesis

Hepatitis results from cell-mediated cytotoxicity in the susceptible host. There is an aberrant display of class II HLA antigens on the hepatocyte surface which initiates cytotoxic response. The aberrant display may be due to viral infection or exposure to drugs or other environmental factors.

Pathogenic mechanisms include destruction of liver cells by sensitized lymphocytes. Antibodies to nuclei such as antinuclear antibodies (ANAs) and smooth muscle antibodies directed against actin and antibodies to antigens in the liver and pancreas and others are demonstrable. These may be causative of the extrahepatic manifestations such as arthritis, cutaneous vasculitis, glomerulonephritis (GN) and others. Histologically, liver shows rosette formation of cells, bridging necrosis, multilobar collapse and cirrhosis (Fig. 88.2).

Laboratory Features

In addition to the antibodies demonstrable in the serum, hypergammaglobulinemia (>2.5 g/dL) and

Textbook of Medicine

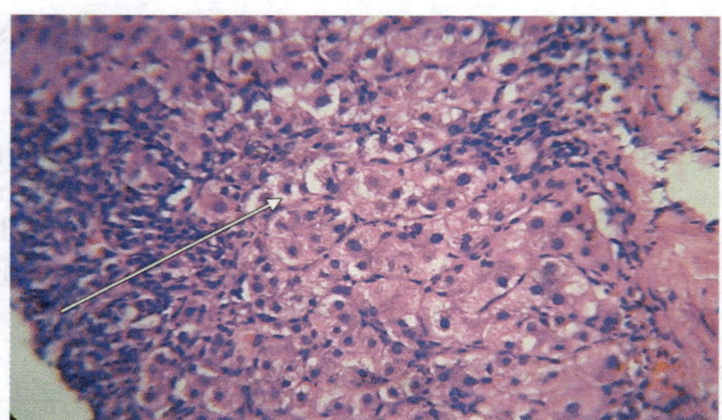

Fig. 88.2: Liver biopsy in autoimmune hepatitis. Rosette formation (arrow)

hypoalbuminemia (< 3 g /dL) occur. Hepatic enzymes AST, ALT and hepatic ALP may show moderate elevation. Serum bilirubin may be moderately elevated (2–10 mg/dL). PT is prolonged when hepatic failure sets in. Two types of AIH have been identified:

1. *Type 1 AIH* occurs in young women associated with lupoid features and marked hyperglobulinemia, they may show circulating ANAs, perinuclear-antineutrophilic cytoplasmic antibodies (p-ANCA) and HLA-DR3 or HLA-DR4 subgroups.
2. *Type 2 AIH* is more often seen in children. They show antibodies to liver cytosol type I and soluble liver antigens. They are less responsive to steroid therapy (Table 88.3).

Diagnosis

This is based on clinical features, laboratory tests and liver biopsy. The definite diagnosis of AIH requires not only periportal hepatitis, hypergammaglobulinemia and auto-antibodies, but also the absence of viral markers, chronic alcoholism, exposure to blood products, hepato-toxic drugs and biliary lesions. The serum gammaglobulin levels are usually more than twice the normal. The scoring system for AIH is given in Table 88.4.

Treatment

There is good response to steroids. Prednisolone is given initially in the dose of 30–60 mg/day orally in divided doses which is tapered to 5–15 mg after about 4 weeks depending upon the response. The exact duration of treatment is not well-defined and prolonged treatment may be necessary. Azathioprine should be added in the usual doses 50 mg/day in cases where steroids cannot be tapered or steroid monotherapy is not fully effective. Liver transplantation may be required if end-stage liver disease occurs.

DRUG TOXICITY ON THE LIVER

Liver is one of the main organs concerned with drug metabolism. Most of the drugs are converted into more water soluble, inactive and nontoxic compounds for elimination by the kidneys or through bile. The enzymes required for drug metabolism are present in the microsomes of the endoplasmic reticulum (ER). The enzymatic reactions occur in two steps. The *first step* includes oxidation, reduction or hydrolysis. The *second step* reactions are conjugation and excretion. Some drugs are directly conjugated. Though majority of the metabolites

Table 88.3: Clinical-pathological distinction between type 1 and 2 AIH

Features	Type I	Type II
Diagnostic antibodies	Smooth muscle nuclear	Liver kidney microsome I
Other antibodies	Atypical p-ANCA Actin	Liver cytosol type I Soluble liver antigen
Age	Infants to elderly	Children
Concurrent immune diseases	Autoimmune-thyroiditis UC	Autoimmune thyroiditis Vitiligo
Serum gammaglobulin level	+++	+
Steroid response	+++	++

Abbreviations: AIH = Autoimmune hepatitis; UC = Ulcerative colitis; p-ANCA = Perinuclear autineutrophilic cytoplasmic antibodies.

Table 88.4: Scoring system for diagnosis of AIH

Category	Variable	Score
ANA or ASMA	> = 1:40	+1
	> = 1:80	+2
Anti-LKM-1 Anti-SLA	> = 1:40	+2
	Positive	+2
Immunoglobulin G (IgG)	More than upper limit of normal	+1
	>110 times upper limit of normal	+2
Liver histology	Compatible with AIH	+1
	Typical of AIH	+2
Absence of viral hepatitis	No viral markers	0
	Yes	+2
Definite		> = 7
Probable		6

Abbreviations: ASMA = Anti-smooth muscle antibody; LKM-1 = Liver kidney microsomal antibody type 1; SLA = Soluble liver antigen; AIH = Auto-immune hepatitis.

are harmless, some are toxic, e.g. acetaminophen and isonicotinylhydrazide (INH). Some drugs induce enzymes which accelerate the metabolism of the same drug as well as others, e.g. barbiturates, alcohol, anesthetics, oral hypoglycemic drugs, anticonvulsants, griseofulvin, rifampicin, phenylbutazone, meprobamate and warfarin. Protein deficiency and pregnancy make the liver more vulnerable to toxic damage.

Drug injury to the liver is of two types—the injury is predictable and dose-dependent; the other type, which is due to idiosyncrasy to the drug, is unpredictable and independent of the dose. Hypersensitivity reaction is triggered off by the drug or its metabolites which act as complete antigens or haptens. The patterns of adverse reactions of the liver to drugs are limited. The general pattern of injury to the liver caused by some of the common drugs is listed (Table 88.5).

Several types of hepatic tumors have been associated with drug administration.

Textbook of Medicine

Hepatocellular adenoma	Oral contraceptives (OCPs), anabolic steroids
Focal nodular hyperplasia	OCPs
Hepatocellular carcinoma	OCPs, anabolic steroids, methotrexate androgens
Angiosarcoma	Diethylstilbestrol, vinyl chloride
Peliosis hepatis	Azathioprine, corticosteroids, diethylstilbestrol, fluoxymesterone, methyltestosterone, oxymetholone

Once a particular drug is identified as the potential cause of liver injury then it is graded for the likelihood of its implication and for the severity of liver injury. Roussel Uclaf Causality Assessment Method (RUCAM) is an objective numerical scoring system in which points are given for clinical, biochemical, serological and radiological characteristics of liver injury. The seven domains which are included are:

Seven domains of Roussel Uclaf Causality Assessment Method (RUCAM)

1. Time of onset of liver disease after initiation of the drug
2. Course of liver diease
3. Risk factors for developing liver disease
4. Potential for hepatotoxicity of concomitant drugs
5. Exclusion of non-drug causes of liver injury
6. Previous information regarding hepatotoxicity of the implicated drug
7. Response to readministration.

Each domain is given positive or negative numerical score, the total ranging from –9 to +14. Higher the score, more severe is the lesion.

Management

The primary approach for hepatotoxicity is to discontinue the offending agent immediately. In most, but not all situations, the liver injury will subside. When the

Table 88.5: Liver injury caused by drugs

Types of reactions	Causative drugs
Chronic hepatitis	Acetaminophen, tetracycline, acetylsalicylic acid, INH, alpha methyldopa, sulfonamides, nitrofurans, phenylbutazone aspirin
Cholestasis	INH, methyltestosterone, chlorpromazine, thiouracil, para-aminosalicylic acid
Granuloma formation	Phenylbutazone, long-acting sulfonamides, allopurinol, dilantin, diazepam, (granulomatous hepatitis) chlorpropamide, hydralazine, halothane, methyldopa, procainamide
Fulminant hepatitis	Acetaminophen, combination of INH and rifampicin
HVT (Budd-Chiari syndrome)	OCPs
Peliosis hepatis	Anabolic steroids, OCPs
AIP	Barbiturates
Cholelithiasis	Clofibrate
Cirrhosis	Oral antidiabetic drugs, alcohol
Tumor formation	OCPs, anabolic steroids

Abbreviations: INH = Isonicotinylhydrazide; HVT = Hepatic vein thrombosis; AIP = Acute intermittent prophyria; OCPs = Oral contraceptives

injury presents as AIH, corticosteroids may be used. Cholestyramine is used for those with pruritus.

Peliosis hepatis is a rare ill-defined lesion, the cause of which is unknown. The liver appears mottled blue and the section shows numerous small blood-filled lacunar spaces which may arise from sinusoids or portal or hepatic veins. Sometimes this may be a chance finding at autopsy in patients dying of tuberculosis.

HEPATIC VENO-OCCLUSIVE DISEASE (VOD)

(*See* also Section 4, Ch 24)

Though originally described from West Indies, it is reported from several parts of the world. In India, small outbreaks have occurred in Punjab, Rajasthan and Madhya Pradesh. Though the exact etiology is unknown, it is most likely caused by toxic phlebitis produced by **pyrrolizidine alkaloids** found in plants like **senecio, heliotropium** and **crotalaria**, consumed as local herbal remedies or accidentally in contaminated cereals. Pathological changes lead to occlusion and fibrosis of the central and sublobular veins. Cirrhosis may develop in the subacute and chronic forms.

The presentation may be acute, subacute or chronic. In children, it tends to be acute with sudden development of hepatomegaly and ascites. Hepatic failure develops in them and mortality is higher. Those who recover may pass into the subacute or chronic phase. In the subacute variety, ascites and hepatosplenomegaly tend to persist. The chronic form leads to cirrhosis of liver with portal hypertension.

Treatment

In the acute phase, general nutritional support, maintenance of fluid and electrolyte balance and symptomatic measures help in tiding over the crisis. There used to be no specific treatment. Defibrotide is a novel drug with antithrombotic and thrombolytic activity which has shown efficacy in treating this disease. Transjugular intrahepatic portosystemic shunt (TIPS) can be done for patients with refractory ascites or those who are candidates for liver transplantation.

BUDD-CHIARI SYNDROME (BCS)

It is caused by thrombotic obstruction of the hepatic venous outflow, usually at the level of inferior vena cava (IVC) or the major hepatic veins. Most of the cases are idiopathic. A membrane is seen in the IVC in some cases. This may be congenital or acquired.

In 75% of cases, there is a prothrombotic state. Myeloproliferative diseases, especially polycythemia vera and essential thrombocythemia account for over 50% of cases. Thrombophiliac states predispose to this syndrome (Box 88.5) (*See* also Ch 171).

Clinical Features

It may present in three forms:

1. ***Acute form:*** This constitutes 20%. The onset is acute with sudden onset presenting with occlusion of all the hepatic veins, characterized by abdominal pain, ascites and even fulminant hepatic failure.

Box 88.5: Prothrombotic conditions predisposing to BCS

- Factor V Leiden mutation
- Prothrombin mutation G20210A
- Antiphospholipid antibody syndrome
- Paroxysmal nocturnal hemoglobinuria
- Deficiency of protein C, S and AT-III
- Cancers such as HCC, adrenal and renal cancer, retroperitoneal sarcoma and thrombophlebitis migrans complicating distant neoplasms
- Oral contraceptives, Behcet's syndrome
- Local conditions such as liver abscess and ecchynococcal cysts
- 20% seem to be idiopathic, but many of them prove to be occult myeloproliferative diseases, on follow-up.

Latent myeloproliferative diseases can be identified by demonstrating mutations in the JAK2 gene.

Abbreviations: BCS = Budd-Chiari syndrome; HCC = Hepatocellular carcinoma; JAK2 = Janus kinase 2

Table 88.6: Pyogenic and amebic liver abscess: Clinical comparisons

Parameter	*Pyogenic liver abscess*	*Amebic liver abscess*
Number	Often multiple	Usually single
Location	Either lobe of liver	Usually right hepatic lobe, near the diaphragm
Presentation	Subacute	Acute
Jaundice	Mild	Moderate
Diagnosis	USG or CT aspiration	USG or CT and serology

Note: Also refer to Section 6, Ch 65, Hepatic Amebiasis

Abbreviations: USG = Ultrasonography; CT = Computed tomography

2. **Subacute form:** Occurs in 40%. The onset is slow and the signs and symptoms persist for over 6 months. Ascites is mild. Hepatic necrosis is minimal due to the development of collateral circulation.

3. **Chronic form:** This constitutes 40%. Duration exceeds 6 months. Cirrhosis may be associated. Compression to IVC by enlarged caudate lobe leads to BCS.

The hepatojugular reflux is abolished and this should raise the possibility of obstruction to hepatic veins.

Diagnosis

It has to be distinguished from occlusion of the portal vein and IVC. In portal vein thrombosis (PVT), ascites is rare and there is no tender hepatomegaly. Massive enlargement of caudate lobe is a characteristic feature of this syndrome. Inferior vena caval occlusion leads to edema of lower limbs and distention of abdominal veins without ascites. Often hepatic veins and the IVC may both be occluded by the same process. Doppler studies, CT and magnetic resonance imaging (MRI) demonstrate the lesion. Direct venography using transjugular techniques can confirm the diagnosis. The transaminases may show moderate elevation up to 4–5 times the normal levels. Ascitic fluid in BCS shows high serum/ascitic fluid albumin gradient with high ascitic fluid protein, often < 2.5 g/dL.

Prognosis is generally poor and to a great extent it depends on the primary condition. Acute cases terminate in hepatic coma. Only a few patients survive more than a year. Survivors may develop portal hypertension later.

Treatment

This consists of removing local causes if any, fibrinolytics and long-term anticoagulation. Stenting the hepatic veins and insertion of transjugular intrahepatic portosystemic shunt (TIPS) help to prevent further occlusion. Portacaval and mesocaval shunts can be done. In severe cases, liver transplantation may be required.

LIVER DYSFUNCTION IN CIRCULATORY IMPAIRMENT

Acute circulatory failure: Hepatic cells are very susceptible to anoxia caused by cardiac failure or fall in hepatic artery perfusing pressure as in shock. These reflect as functional derangement. The left lobe is more affected than the right. Microscopically, central veins and central zones show congestion. These zones show hemorrhage, focal necrosis, hydropic changes and polymorphonuclear (PMN) infiltration. The reticulin network is usually preserved.

Chronic congestive heart failure: The liver is enlarged, congested and dark purplish in color with rounded edges. The central vein is dilated and congested and the sinusoids are distended. Liver cell necrosis occurs, but there is no marked cellular infiltration. The degenerating cells may show pigmentary disturbance. Fibrous bridges form between central veins, leaving the portal zones relatively unaffected. The ill effects of hypoxia and back pressure are felt maximally in the central zones. A complex micronodular cirrhotic picture develops (**cardiac cirrhosis**).

Jaundice may occur in chronic congestive heart failure, due to hepatic necrosis and release of bilirubin from multiple foci of infarction such as the lungs. Right upper quadrant pain with hepatomegaly is commonly observed. Ascites may develop. The ascitic fluid is highly proteinaceous. Mild grades of hepatic dysfunction develop. Mild portal hypertension occurs in many. Though mild splenomegaly may occur, other features like esophageal varices are uncommon. Treatment of cardiac failure in long-standing cases partially reverses the functional derangement but the structural abnormalities persist.

PYOGENIC ABSCESS OF THE LIVER

Liver is a common site for pyemic abscess. In gram-negative septicemia, microscopic abscess are common and tender hepatomegaly is a common event. However, liver may be the seat of focal collection of pus which may be more often multiple. Bacteria can reach the liver through the portal vein, hepatic artery and bile ducts or by direct extension from contiguous organs and through penetrating injuries. Secondary infection of an amebic abscess or hydatid cyst converts it into pyogenic abscesses (Table 88.6).

The organismal flora is mixed, containing *Escherichia coli, Staphylococcus aureus, Enterococcus faecalis, Proteus vulgaris, Pseudomonas, Bacteroides* and anerobic streptococci. Continuous pain, high fever, chills, jaundice, toxemia, neutrophil leukocytosis and tender hepatomegaly should draw attention to the possibility of pyemic abscess. US, CT and MRI aid in making the diagnosis. Aspiration of the pus and microbiological examination confirm the diagnosis. **Treatment** consists of appropriate antibiotic therapy and supportive care. Needle aspiration and rarely surgical drainage is required. Surgical drainage of the pus is required if medical measures alone are inadequate. The source of infection should be removed to prevent recurrence.

CARCINOMA OF THE LIVER

Primary Carcinoma

Syn: Hepatoma

HCC is the third leading cause of cancer-related mortality globally. Primary carcinoma of the liver is a common neoplasm seen in India, South Africa, Malaysia and China. It is less common in Caucasians. HCCs form 75% of the primary tumors while cholangiocarcinomas form 20%.

Etiology

The etiological factors vary in different geographical regions. Carcinoma supervening on cirrhosis accounts for 20% of the total. The regenerating nodules in macronodular cirrhosis may become malignant. Hepatitis B and C and aflatoxins from *Aspergillus flavus,* alcoholism, hemochromatosis and clonorchiasis predispose to carcinoma. In many cases, the tumor arises *de novo* (Box 88.6).

Though the majority are unicentric, some are multiple. The right lobe is more affected. The hepatocytes show hyperchromatic nuclei and mitotic figures with only scanty stroma. The tumor spreads throughout the liver, involves the peritoneal surface and spreads to the peritoneum. It spreads locally through the portal vein, IVC and bile ducts causing obstruction to these channels. Distant metastasis is rare. Nodes in the porta hepatis, mediastinum and cervical chains may also be affected.

Clinical Features

In India, younger subjects (second and third decades) suffer more, though any age group can be affected. Vertical transmission of hepatitis B from mother to offspring and development of B hepatitis early in life accounts for this phenomenon. Males are four to five times more affected than females. The presenting complaints are pain, fullness in the right hypochondrium, feeling of a mass, fever or

---

Box 88.6: Risk factors for HCC
• Cirrhosis of any etiology • Chronic hepatitis B infection • Chronic hepatitis C infection • Aflatoxin exposure • Alpha-1 antitrypsin deficiency • Hemochromatosis • Membranous obstruction of IVC • Tyrosinemia • Type I and II glycogen storage disease

Abbreviations: IVC = Inferior vena cava; HCC = Hepatocellular carcinoma

jaundice. Auscultation may reveal arterial bruit and venous hum along the porta hepatis. This venous hum is referred to as *Cruveilhier-Baumgarten syndrome*. This may occur in cirrhosis liver with portal hypertension also. Portal hypertension and intraperitoneal hemorrhage are late features. Left supraclavicular nodes may be enlarged due to metastases. Liver function is maintained till late in the disease. Pleural effusion and atelectasis of the right lower lobe can occur. Occlusion of the portal vein or hepatic vein may present with acute symptoms of portal hypertension.

Diagnosis

Carcinoma should be suspected if massive enlargement of the liver occurs with fever, cachexia and hemorrhagic ascites. Jaundice is usually a late manifestation in hepatoma whereas it occurs early in cholangioma. Rarely, secondary polycythemia may develop.

Diagnosis of HCC

Imaging techniques such as, USG, CT and MRI are very useful. Lesions more than 2 cm in diameter to be HCCs. Triple phasic helical CT is diagnostic. The unenhanced phase, enhanced phase and arterial and portal venous phases can be studied (Fig. 88.3).

Alfa-fetoprotein (AFP) values above 200 ng mL (normal 0–8.5 ng/mL) are also diagnostic.

If the diagnosis is not possible by imaging and AFP levels, ultrasound-guided fine-needle aspiration biopsy (FNAC) is useful. Complications include hemoperitoneum, dissemination of the lesion and needle track seeding.

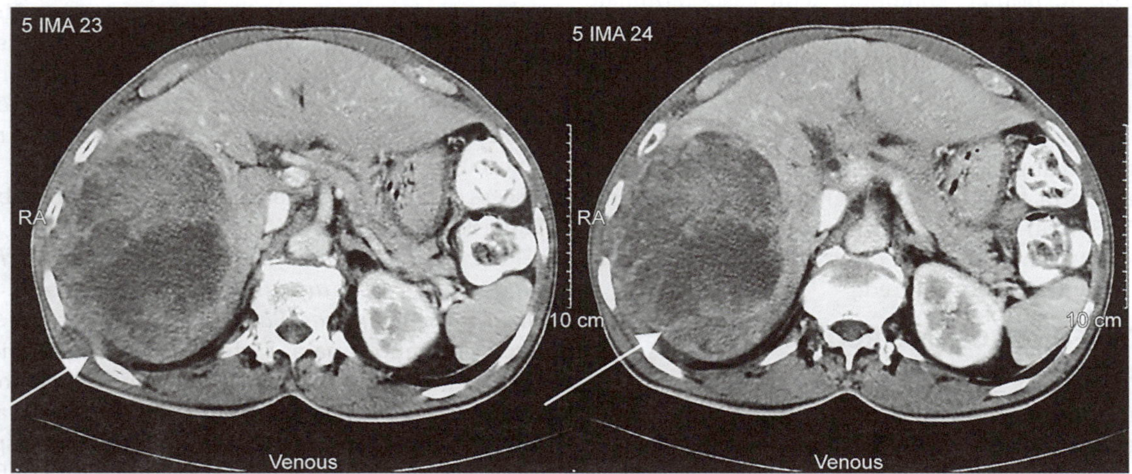

Fig. 88.3: CT image of HCC in the venous phase. ***Note:*** The tumor with heterogenous consistency (arrow)

Textbook of Medicine

Table 88.7: Barcelona Clinic Liver Cancer (BCLC) Staging

Stage	Characteristics	Treatment
0	Very early single HCC < 2 cm	No cirrhosis—resection Cirrhosis—liver transplantation Cirrhosis with other comorbidities RFA/PEI
A	Single HCC or 3 nodules < 3 cm each PS 0 CHILD A–B	Transplantation or PEI/RFA
B	Intermediate stage Multinodular PS 0 Child A–B	TACE
C	Advanced portal invasion N1 M1 PS 1–2 Child A–B	Sorafenib
D	End stage PS >2 Child C	Best suppportive care

Abbreviations: PS = Performance status scale; RFA = Radiofrequency ablation; PEI = Percutaneous ethanol injection; TACE = Transarterial chemoembolization

Liver biopsy confirms the diagnosis, if the selection of the site is proper. Celiac axis angiography reveals the abnormal branches of the hepatic artery feeding the tumor. Angiography is necessary if surgical excision is planned.

Management

It may be curative or palliative. Curative modalities may be surgical or interventional. Surgical resection and liver transplantation are the surgical procedures. Unfortunately, only around 15% of HCC are resectable at the time of diagnosis. Local resection has the advantage that transplantation is not needed. Liver transplantation is the surgical procedure of choice in the western world. It is especially useful for HCC with cirrhosis and hepatic failure. Several criteria have been employed to select cases for transplantation. The ***Barcelona Clinic Liver Cancer (BCLC)*** staging system is used for staging of HCC. It includes measures of liver function and performance status both of which are significant predictors of outcome (Table 88.7).

Radiofrequency ablation (RFA) is the most common type of ablation for local disease.

Performance status WHO

- 0-Asymptomatic fully active
- 1-Symptomatic but completely ambulatory
- 2-Symptomatic <50% bedbound during day
- 3-Symptomatic >50% bedbound during day
- 4-Bedbound (completely disabled).

Interventions

Transarterial chemoembolization (TACE): The hepatic artery is selectively catheterized and the chemotherapeutic agent is directly delivered into the tumor followed by gel occlusion. Occlusion of the artery will lead to necrosis of the tumor which is mainly dependent on arterial blood supply, whereas the normal liver parenchyma is supplied by the portal vein. ***Radiofrequency ablation (RFA)*** and ***alcohol injection into the tumor*** are the other interventions which are effective.

Chemotherapy

Sorafenib: It is a multikinase inhibitor including vascular endothelial growth factor (VEGF) and platelet-derived growth factor (PDGF) receptor kinases. It is given in a dose of 200–400 mg twice a day. In Sorafenib Hepatocellular Carcinoma Assessment Randomized Protocol (SHARP) trial, a 44% 1 year survival was seen in BCLC-C patients when compared to placebo. Sorafenib induces a clinically relevant improvement in time to progression and in survival. Possible complications include hematological abnormalities and desquamation of the skin (hand foot syndrome).

TARE (Transarterial radioembolization): It is the technique of selective catheterization of the feeding vessel to the tumor and injecting radioisotopes (e.g. Yittrium) directly to the tumor in order to destroying the tumor cells. Microwave ablation, laser ablation and cryoablation have been proposed for local ablation in HCC. All these treatments are still investigational.

Operability

To be operable, single lesions should be less than 5 cm in diameter and multiple lesions should be less than 3 in number and less than 3 cms in diameter. The rest of the liver parenchyma should be normal.

Surveillance for HCC in cirrhosis: Cirrhotic patients are at higher risk for developing HCC and hence, they have to be followed up. The current practice is to screen them with ultrasound scan and AFP at 6 month intervals. Follow-up at shorter intervals (every 3–4 months) is recommended for the following cases:

- Where a nodule of less than 1 cm has been detected.
- In the follow-up strategy after resection or loco-regional therapies.
- Operability is high in HCC detected by surveillance.

In persons with HCC, second carcinoma in the transplant may develop since the underlying chronic liver disease puts the patients at risk of second cancer.

SECONDARY CARCINOMA

Liver is a very common site for metastasis. These are thirty times more common than primary carcinoma. The usual primary sites are stomach, esophagus, other parts of the GI tract, bronchus, breast, thyroid, kidney, adrenal or melanoma of the skin. Biopsy from the secondaries may give clue regarding the primary.

Clinical examination reveals the irregular enlargement of the liver ***(hob-nail liver)*** in advanced cases. The nodules show umbilication due to necrosis in the center. Jaundice occurs early if any of the major biliary passage is obstructed. The secondaries are generally less vascular than primary tumors and therefore, arterial bruit is not heard. Splenomegaly may be present. Secondaries may lead to hypoglycemia. Ascites develops in due course. Ascitic fluid shows increase in proteins. Carcinoembryonic antigen (CEA) may be detectable in the fluid. Lactic dehydrogenase (LD) is elevated to thrice the normal value. Cytology of the fluid shows malignant cells. Liver biopsy confirms the diagnosis. The progress is rapidly downhill and death occurs within weeks or months. The extent of replacement of normal liver tissue by the metastases is the main determinant of prognosis. Causes of death include malignant cachexia, hepatic failure and bleeding esophageal varices.

Therapy is at best only palliative. 5-fluorouracil given singly or as a combination regimen given either systemically or by local infusion into the hepatic artery is beneficial in some cases. Surgical resection, liver transplantation and RFA are the other treatment options.

Benign tumors, which are rare, include adenoma and hemangioma.

HEPATIC ADENOMA

This may be associated with the administration of sex hormones and OCPs. This may present as local tumors or with peritoneal hemorrhage. Treatment is surgical resection.

HEMANGIOMA LIVER

It is the most common benign tumor. Two types are seen—cavernomas and the true hemangiomas. Some of them are associated with regular use of OCPs. These tumors may sequester platelets and lead to consumption coagulopathy, especially disseminated intravascular coagulation (DIC) (***Kasabach-Merritt syndrome***). X-ray may show calcification. The USS appearance is characteristic and in doubtful cases contrast CT may be diagnostic.

Treatment is largely aimed to reassure the patient and prevent injuries and bleeding. Definitive management includes surgery or angiographic embolization. Very large lesions which lead to consumption coagulopathy may have to resected with liver transplantation, if needed.

REYE'S SYNDROME

During the course of viral infections like influenza A and B, varicella and probably others, toxic damage to the liver occurs. The condition is more common in children, especially if given aspirin. The liver shows fatty infiltration. Clinically, it presents with hepatic failure, encephalopathy and rise in intracranial tension. Jaundice is usually absent. The mortality is high, if untreated (*See* Ch 52).

CHAPTER
89

Diseases of the Gallbladder and the Major Bile Ducts

KR Vinaya Kumar, KV Krishna Das

Chapter Summary

- General Considerations
- Investigations of the Gallbladder and Bile Ducts
- Cholecystitis
  - Acute Cholecystitis
  - Chronic Cholecystitis
- Carcinoma of the Gallbladder

GENERAL CONSIDERATIONS

The right and left hepatic ducts join to form the common hepatic duct. It joins the cystic duct to form the common bile duct (CBD) which ranges in length from 2 to 9 cm. It passes behind the duodenum through the head of the pancreas to join the pancreatic duct and opens into the second part of the duodenum at the ampulla of Vater.

The gallbladder, situated below and in close contact with the liver, is pear-shaped and has a capacity of 50 mL. Its fundus lies beneath the tip of the right ninth costal cartilage. In 10% of people, the gallbladder has a mesentery (floating gallbladder) and it is freely movable. The liver secretes 600–700 mL of bile in 24 hours at a pressure of 15–25 cm of water. The gallbladder concentrates the bile ten-fold by absorption of water and electrolytes. Bile secretion is inhibited when the pressure in the CBD exceeds 30 cm water. Vagus, which is the motor nerve, probably maintains the tone of the gallbladder. Gallbladder contracts in response to cholecystokinin (CCK) secreted by the duodenal mucosa. CCK also causes relaxation of the sphincter. Drugs like morphine and pethidine cause spasm of the sphincter of Oddi and glyceryl trinitrate relaxes it.

Symptomatology of Biliary Tract Disease

The most obvious sign is jaundice which may be constant and progressive or fluctuating. This may or may not be associated with pain. Acute inflammatory lesions cause severe pain in the right hypochondrium, referred to the right shoulder. Obstruction to the cystic duct or CBD causes colicky pain with periodic waxing and waning. Unlike as in renal colic, mild constant pain persists between spasms. Persistence of continuous pain for more than five hours should suggest complications such as infection or perforation of the gallbladder.

The fundus of an enlarged gallbladder can be palpated at the lateral border of the right rectus abdominis as a globular firm mass. Sometimes an elongated or floating gallbladder may reach as low as the right iliac fossa. Obstruction of the CBD due to external pressure as in carcinoma of the head of the pancreas causes enlargement of the gallbladder (***Courvoisier's law).*** Since the gallbladder may enlarge only intermittently, repeated examinations may be necessary to detect it. Gallstones lead to chronic infection and thickening of the gallbladder and this restricts enlargement. Tenderness over the gallbladder is elicited over the right hypochondrium. ***Murphy's sign*** is sudden catching pain felt on inspiration when the palpating finger exerts gentle pressure below the

Textbook of Medicine

liver edge at the right border of the right rectus abdominis. The ***Boas' sign*** is tenderness, sometimes elicited over the region of the right scapula. Gallbladder pain may occasionally radiate to the chest and this may be mistaken for anginal pain. Gallbladder disease and ischemic heart disease (IHD) coexist in many instances.

INVESTIGATIONS OF THE GALLBLADDER AND BILE DUCTS

Radiographs: Plain radiograph taken in the anteroposterior and right lateral positions may reveal radiopaque calculi. Only 10% of biliary calculi are radiopaque. Opacities due to renal calculi, calcified lymph nodes and fecolith have to be differentiated from gallstones. An enlarged gallbladder may throw a soft tissue shadow. Gas in the biliary tree and pancreatic calculi are also seen at times.

Ultrasonography (USG): It is the most useful noninvasive method to detect dilated biliary passages and gallbladder calculi. This is the investigations of first choice.

Computed tomography (CT) scan: It demonstrates dilated biliary passages, intra and extrahepatic lesions and the gallbladder. The neighboring organs can also be well-visualized.

Contrast radiography: With the advent of noninvasive procedures such as ultrasound, CT scan and magnetic resonance imaging (MRI) which are much more effective in bringing out the abnormalities, the cumbersome and less precise investigations such as oral cholecystogram, intravenous cholangiography (IVC) and blind percutaneous transhepatic cholangiography (PTC) are seldom performed at present. Still in particular situations, USG-guided or CT-guided needling procedures and biopsies are done.

Endoscopic retrograde cholangiopancreatography (ERCP): This is an elegant method for visualizing the biliary and pancreatic duct systems. It utilizes endoscopy and radiography simultaneously. The ampulla of Vater is cannulated through a side-viewing duodenoscope and the contrast is injected. The pancreatic duct, bile duct and their tributaries are visualized in over 80% of cases. The ERCP also facilitates the collection of specimens for biopsy, cytology and analysis of the juices. Therapeutically, ERCP has been employed to remove stones from the ducts and relieve strictures and even malignant obstructions. Endoscopic ultrasound scan (EUS) is a very sensitive imaging modality for terminal CBD lesions.

Operative cholangiography: The bile duct can be opacified during surgery by injecting contrast medium and its progress is followed.

Choledochoscopy: Visualization of the intra and extra-hepatic biliary system intraoperatively is possible by the choledochoscope which is introduced into the CBD. Stones and lesions missed by other investigations can be detected.

Barium meal: A properly conducted barium meal examination may give valuable clues in hepatobiliary disease. Distortion of stomach and duodenum, abnormalities of the duodenum produced by ampullary carcinoma or pancreatic tumors, presence of fistulae and regurgitation of the barium through the incompetent biliary sphincter are all useful diagnostic findings. This is seldom done at present since direct visualization is possible by endoscopy.

Radionuclide imaging: Scintiscans using ^{131}I-rose bengal or ^{99m}Tc-pyridoxylidene hepapobiliary iminodiacetic acid (HIDA) derivative when given IV is taken up by the liver and excreted in bile. The biliary tree can be visualized.

Duodenal biliary drainage: Bile can be collected for examination through a duodenal tube after injecting CKK.

CHOLECYSTITIS

This may be acute or chronic.

Acute Cholecystitis

Obstruction to the gallbladder neck or cystic duct by gallstones, mucus plugs, neoplasms or other foreign bodies leads to stasis and infection. Initially, the lesion is sterile but soon infected by *Escherichia coli* and *Streptococcus faecalis* supervenes. Anaerobes such as ***fusobacteria*** and ***bacteroides*** are also common. Inflammation may be mild or fulminant. The gallbladder may become filled with pus ***(empyema of the gallbladder)*** and the organ may burst after perforation, leading to severe biliary peritonitis and shock. Invasion by gas-forming organisms leads to the presence of gas in the wall of the gallbladder (emphysematous gallbladder) or in its cavity.

Clinical Features

The disease is more common in middle-aged women. Sudden severe pain in the epigastrium and right hypochondrium referred to right shoulder, fever, vomiting and restlessness should suggest acute cholecystitis. Deep jaundice is rare unless the biliary tree is diffusely involved or the CBD is blocked. Heavy fatty meals at night, violent exercise, travel or even abdominal palpation in some cases may precipitate the attack. Pain may be colicky or continuous. The abdomen may be rigid. In some cases, the gallbladder may be enlarged and palpable but local tenderness and rigidity preclude proper palpation. ***Murphy's sign*** and ***Boas' sign*** may be positive. General features of infection like fever, rigor and neutrophil leukocytosis accompany these attacks. The condition subsides with treatment but recurs after varying intervals. Perforation of the gallbladder, ascending cholangitis and shock occur in severe cases.

Differential diagnosis of acute cholecystitis includes hepatitis, cholangitis, gastric perforation, pancreatitis, appendicitis, acute intermittent porphyria (AIP) and peritonitis. Pain may radiate to the chest, which could be mistaken for angina pectoris.

Diagnosis

The condition should be suspected clinically. Polymorphonuclear (PMN) leukocytosis with a shift to the left is usually seen. The ultrasound scan may demonstrate stones in more than 90% of cases. Radionuclide scan (HIDA) is typical. It may demonstrate the bile ducts without visualizing the gallbladder.

Treatment

Conservative treatment consists of bed rest, analgesics and intravenous (IV) fluids to give symptomatic relief. Antibiotics like penicillin, cephalosporins and

Textbook of Medicine

cotrimoxazole reach the bile in adequate amounts and these have to be employed judiciously. Metronidazole is to be given if anaerobic infection is suspected. In more than 90% of cases, the condition subsides with conservative treatment within 3–4 days.

Surgical Management

Elective cholecystectomy can be done within three months after the acute phase subsides. The surgical mortality in conventional open laparotomy used with is about 0.5–1%. With the advent of laparoscopic cholecystectomy which is the preferred method at present, the operation has become simpler, less traumatizing and with reduced risk. Gallbladder surgery was one among the earliest laparoscopic surgeries in vogue for the past three decades. Advantages of laparoscopic surgery which is practiced for diseases of several (almost all) abdominal organs are:

- Less of surgical trauma
- Reduction in postoperative pain
- Shorter hospitalization
- Early mobilization.

Acute gangrenous cholecystitis is seen in the elderly and immunosuppressed individuals. The gallbladder may rupture at the fundus giving rise to local peritonitis, adhesions with other viscera or formation of internal biliary fistula. Acute gangrenous cholecystitis should be suspected in any individual if the pain and toxemia increase despite treatment and shock supervenes. The mortality is 15–20%. Initial treatment consists of massive antibiotic therapy and supportive measures. Emergency cholecystectomy and drainage of abscesses are indicated if the condition deteriorates inspite of adequate conservative measures.

Chronic Cholecystitis

This is the most common medical lesion affecting the gallbladder and it is invariably due to cholelithiasis. The gallbladder is thickened and fibrotic and the mucosa may be destroyed by scarring.

Clinical Features

Vague upper abdominal pain, colic, gaseous distension after fatty meal or recurrent episodes of acute cholecystitis should suggest the possibility of chronic cholecystitis. Peptic ulcer, hiatus hernia and chronic pancreatitis have to be excluded by investigations. Murphy's sign may be positive and in the absence of hepatic disease it is very suggestive of cholecystitis. Calculi may be seen in plain radiographs of the abdomen. Oral cholecystogram, cholangiogram, USG and ERCP help to localize the lesion.

Course and Prognosis

The condition persists for several years with exacerbations and remissions. There is increased risk of malignancy.

Treatment

Medical treatment consists of dietary adjustment, reduction of weight, antispasmodics, antacids and antibiotics. Early cases may subside completely. Drugs which dissolve cholesterol gallstones are worth a trial.

- *Chenodeoxycholic acid* in a dose of 13–15 mg/kg body weight given orally at bedtime is effective in dissolving these stones in a period of 6–24 months. Recurrence may occur on stopping therapy. Side effects include mild diarrhea and elevation of serum cholesterol.
- *Ursodeoxycholic acid* is a better drug in this class and in a dose of 10 mg/kg given twice daily, it acts faster. Troublesome diarrhea does not occur. Rowachol is a mixture of essential fatty acids capable of dissolving gallstones. Medical treatment is generally not preferred on along term basis.
- *Shock wave lithotripsy (SWL)* disintegrates the stones. This helps in quicker resolution. Surgical removal of the gallbladder is indicated if medical treatment fails. With the availability of laparoscopic cholecystectomy in many centers in India at reasonable cost, this has become more popular as the definitive long-term treatment.
- *Typhoid cholecystitis:* The biliary tract may become colonized by *Salmonella typhi*. Typhoid bacilli form a nidus around which calculi may form. The gallbladder becomes chronically infected with *Salmonella* and this perpetuates the fecal carrier state. More commonly, chronic cholecystitis may occur in typhoid carriers who are responsible for disseminating the disease for long periods (e.g. Typhoid Mary). Antibiotic treatment followed by cholecystectomy helps in clearing the focus of infection and the carrier state (*See* Section 6, Ch 39).

CARCINOMA OF THE GALLBLADDER

It is a rare condition in South India, but is more common in the Gangetic belt of India. It is seen more in people above the age of 50 years.

Risk factors are cholelithiasis, family history, primary sclerosing cholangitis (PSC) and inflammatory bowel disease (IBD).

Around 90% of cases are adenocarcinomas. It presents with progressive biliary obstruction. Chronic calculous cholecystitis predisposes to malignancy.

Diagnosis is by USG, CT scan and MRI scan. Surgery is the treatment of choice. Currently, chemotherapy and radiotherapy are not preferred due to unsatisfactory results.

CHOLANGIOCARCINOMA

This is a rare slow-growing adenocarcinoma arising from any part of the biliary tree from the bile canaliculi to the sphincter of Oddi.

Risk factors are cirrhosis, hepatitis C, PSC and infection by the flukes *Clonorchis sinensis* and *Opisthorchis felineus*.

Progressive jaundice occurs depending on the site of obstruction. CA 19-9 is a tumor marker of cholangiocarcinoma. It can be detected by fluorescent *in situ* hybridization (FISH) technique. The lesion can be further assessed by imaging CT or MRI scan.

Treatment is considered with the help of surgery only.

Chemotherapy in inoperable cases and for post-surgical management consists of *Gemcitabine* which is the only Food and Drugs Administration (FDA) approved drug at present. Inoperable cases can be palliated by endoscopic biliary stenting or percutaneous biliary stent placement.

CHAPTER
90

Diseases of the Pancreas

KR Vinaya Kumar, KV Krishna Das

Chapter Summary

- General Considerations
  - Pancreatic Function Tests
  - Tests for Exocrine Function
- Pancreatitis
  - Acute Pancreatitis
  - Chronic Pancreatitis
  - Cystic Fibrosis of the Pancreas
- Pancreatic Ascites
- Carcinoma of the Pancreas
- Cystic Neoplasms of Pancreas
- Endocrine Tumors of the Pancreas

GENERAL CONSIDERATIONS

Applied Anatomy

Pancreas is situated posteriorly in the upper abdomen. It contains both exocrine and endocrine cells. Since the head of the pancreas lies within the duodenal loop in close approximation, enlarging lesions of the head of the pancreas produce radiologically demonstrable changes in the inner margin of the duodenum. The common bile duct (CBD) passes through the head of the pancreas and tumors of this region compress the CBD to produce obstructive jaundice. Being deeply placed, lesions of the pancreas may remain without producing clinically demonstrable local physical signs for long periods.

The pancreas is made up of large lobules, each made up of smaller lobules containing *acini*. Each acinus contains two types of cells. The zymogen-containing cells secrete the digestive enzymes and these predominate. Cells situated near the center of the acini secrete water and bicarbonate. The main pancreatic duct is formed by the confluence of smaller ducts. It opens into the second part of the duodenum along with the CBD at the ampulla of Vater. The islets of Langerhans which are made up of four types of cells known as alpha, beta, gamma and delta, are scattered throughout the organ. These cells secrete glucagon, insulin and other peptide hormones. Endocrine tumors may arise from them.

Applied Physiology

The pancreas secretes 1.5–3 L of juice daily. It is alkaline with the pH 8–8.3. Trypsin, chymotrypsin, amylase and lipase form the main enzymes. Sodium bicarbonate ($NaHCO_3$), which is the major electrolyte, renders alkalinity to the secretion. Potassium, calcium, zinc, chloride, phosphate and sulfate are also present in smaller amounts. The secretion is under hormonal and neural control, the former being more important. When acidic gastric contents enter the duodenum and the pH goes down to 4.5, the duodenal and jejunal mucosa release secretin. Cholecystokinin

(CCK) (pancreozymin) is also secreted from the duodenal and jejunal mucosa when long-chain fatty acids, amino acids (especially tryptophan, phenylalanine, valine and methionine) and acidic gastric contents enter. Copious amounts of alkaline juice are produced in response to secretin. CCK stimulates the production of thick juice which is rich in enzymes. Gastrin is also a weak stimulus for pancreatic secretion. Vasoactive intestinal peptide (VIP) antagonizes the effect of secretin. Bile acids in the intestinal lumen also stimulate pancreatic secretion.

Neural control is through the vagus which exerts direct effect on the acinar cells. Indirectly, it influences pancreatic secretion through the mechanism of gastrin. ***Actions of pancreatic juice:*** Amylase secreted in the active form digests starches into oligosaccharides and to the disaccharide maltose. The lipolytic enzymes (***lipase*** and ***co-lipase***) breakdown fat into glycerol and fatty acids.

The proteolytic enzymes are ***trypsin, chymotrypsin, carboxypeptidases, aminopeptidases, elastase, ribonuclease*** and ***deoxyribonuclease.*** They are secreted as inactive precursors (zymogens) which are activated later. ***Trypsinogen*** is activated by ***enterokinase*** found in the intestinal mucosa to ***trypsin.*** Trypsin further activates the other proteolytic enzymes sequentially.

Pancreatic Function Tests

Enzyme Levels in Blood and Urine

Amylase, trypsin and ***lipase*** are present in normal serum in small amounts. In acute pancreatitis, within a short interval, the amylase reaches very high levels and this rise is suggestive of the diagnosis. Normal value of amylase is about 60–180 Somogyi units/dL (or 150–340 IU/L). The serum levels come down within a few days.

Since serum amylase levels are not specific for pancreatic disease, measurement of renal clearance of amylase from blood has been suggested as a more reliable test for diagnosis of acute pancreatitis. The clearance ratio is calculated by simultaneous estimation of amylase and creatinine in serum and urine. Normal amylase/creatinine clearance ratio is around 3:1. Value of more than five suggests the diagnosis of acute pancreatitis. The value of this test is also doubtful.

Analysis of feces: Steatorrhea and creatorrhea are seen commonly in pancreatic disease. Fecal fat estimation done on feces collected for 3 days on a high fat diet (about 75 g/day) helps in confirming the presence of steatorrhea. Normal subjects do not lose more than 6 g of fat in feces daily. Higher values suggest pancreatitis or malabsorption. In pancreatitis, feces contain neutral fat whereas in malabsorption states, it contains mainly fatty acids.

Estimation of fecal trypsin and chymotrypsin is useful in the diagnosis of chronic pancreatic insufficiency, particularly cystic fibrosis (CF).

Tests for Exocrine Function

Pancreatic juice can be collected by duodenal aspiration or by endoscopy. Exocrine function may be tested directly (secretin-pancreozymin test) or indirectly (Lundh test).

Direct tests involve collection of pancreatic secretions after IV administration of a secretagogue or a combination of secretagogues. Indirect tests of pancreatic secretory function include the measurement of pancreatic enzymes in duodenal samples after nutrient ingestion—the measurement of products of digestive enzyme action on ingested substrates, the measurement of pancreatic enzymes in the stool and the measurement of the plasma concentration of hormones or other markers that are altered in pancreatic insufficiency states (Box 90.1).

The ability to produce enzymes and bicarbonate is tested after giving secretin 1 unit/kg IV and pancreozymin 4 units/kg. This test is the gold standard for exocrine pancreatic function.

Normal Values

- Volume output should be more than 2 mL/min and amylase more than 6 units/kg.
- Bicarbonate concentration should be more than 80 mmol/L.
- Bicarbonate output should be more than 10 mmol in 30 min.

Enzymes are also estimated and compared with the norms for the population studied.

- **Lundh test:** This test is based on the effect of fatty acids and amino acids on the endogenous release of CCK which in turn stimulates secretion of pancreatic enzymes. This is an indirect test of pancreatic function since it depends on the endogenous release of pancreozymin from duodenal mucosa. The test may be misleading in the presence of duodenal mucosal disease. Normal value of tryptic activity by this test is 19.6 ± 3.5 mEq/mL per min.
- **Tubeless pancreatic function tests:** The principle is to estimate the urinary elimination of digestion products of substances given orally. This indirectly estimates the digestive function. The two tests in this group are the **bentiromide test** and **pancreolauryl test**.
  - **Bentiromide test:** N-benzoyl-l-tyrosyl-p-amino-benzoic acid test is administered orally and its urinary elimination product—para-amino benzoic

acid is estimated. Chymotrypsin is the enzyme concerned.

- In the **pancreolauryl test**, fluorescein laurate is given and then fluorescein eliminated in urine is estimated. Pancreatic esterases are the enzymes responsible.

- **Cytology of duodenal aspirate:** Cytological examination may reveal the presence of neoplastic cells.
- **Isotopic scanning of pancreas:** The isotopic scanning of pancreas can be done by using radioactive selenomethionine using ^{22}Se which is taken up by the pancreas.
- **Assessment of endocrine function:** Studies of glucose homeostasis and determination of serum levels of insulin, glucagon, CCK and other peptide hormones help to assess the hormonal activity of the pancreas.
- **Radiography:** Pancreatic calculi and calcification can be demonstrated in plain radiographs. In acute pancreatitis, indirect evidences like dilatation of small bowel loops due to ileus may be present.
- **Ultrasonography (USG) and computed tomography (CT) scan:** These are very helpful noninvasive methods for demonstrating deep-seated lesions. Ordinary method of USG is less reliable since the pancreas does not lend itself to proper imaging and, therefore, small lesions may be missed.
- **Endoscopic USG** is a more reliable method to detect lesions even as small as 1 cm or less. It is helpful in staging pancreatic cancers, differentiating benign from malignant cystic lesions, obtaining fine-needle aspiration cytology (FNAC) from pancreatic mass lesions and guiding endoscopic drainage of pseudocysts.
- **Hypotonic duodenography** and barium meal reveal the changes produced in duodenum and intestines by pancreatic lesions.

Endoscopic retrograde cholangiopancreatography (ERCP) is a very valuable tool in investigating the pancreas directly. ERCP shows ductal abnormalities such as dilation, obstruction and stones. It is the gold standard for the diagnosis and staging of chronic pancreatitis, with sensitivity of 75–95% and specificity of over 90%. Morbidity caused by ERCP is 3–4% and mortality 0.1–1%.

MRI cholangiopancreatography is a recently developed imaging modality with about 96–100% sensitivity to detect ductal stages in the pancreatic duct.

PANCREATITIS

Pancreatitis may be acute or chronic. The incidence varies in different ethnic groups. **Acute pancreatitis** is seen infrequently as a medical or surgical emergency in India. **Chronic pancreatitis** accounts for a significant proportion of malabsorption syndrome. Chronic calcific pancreatitis with secondary diabetes is seen in some endemic areas, especially in Kerala. Pancreatitis is closely associated with alcoholism and biliary tract disease.

ACUTE PANCREATITIS

Pathogenesis

It results from autodigestion of the pancreas by its own enzymes. The inactive precursors of proteolytic enzymes

Box 90.1: Causes of hyperamylasemia and hyperamylasuria	
Pancreatic disease	**Non-pancreatic disorders**
Pancreatitis	• Parotitis
• Acute	• Salpingitis
• Chronic: Ductal obstruction	• Papillary cystadenocarcinoma of the ovary
• Complications of pancreatitis	• Carcinoma lung
▪ Pancreatic pseudocyst	• Intestinal infarction
▪ Pancreatogenic ascites	• Perforated viscus
▪ Pancreatic necrosis	• Renal failure
▪ Pancreatic trauma	• Macroamylasemia
Pancreatic carcinoma	

are activated by regurgitated bile, viral infections, ischemia, anoxia, trauma or toxins, within the pancreas. Digestion of the tissues results in edema, hemorrhage, vascular damage, coagulation necrosis and fat necrosis. Secondary factors like liberation of activated enzymes, bradykinin and histamine-like substances into the pancreas result in vasodilation, exudation and disseminated intravascular coagulation (DIC). These factors lead to further damage.

Acute pancreatitis has been defined as an acute inflammatory process of the pancreas with variable involvement of other regional tissues or remote organ systems. In mild disease when organ dysfunction is minimal, prognosis for recovery is good. In severe disease, there are local lesions such as necrosis, abscess or pseudocyst formation and systemic complications such as respiratory distress, shock, gastrointestinal (GI) bleeding, renal failure and others. The extent of severity has been semiquantified by using clinicopathological criteria such as Ranson's criteria or APACHE II scores (*See* Ch 54).

Causes

- *Alcoholic bouts*
- *Biliary tract disease,* especially cholelithiasis in the CBD
- *Trauma*—blunt abdominal injuries, surgical trauma, post-ERCP reaction
- *Metabolic causes*—hyperlipidemia, diabetes, renal failure, hypothermia
- *Endocrine causes*—hyperparathyroidism, corticosteroid therapy, oral contraceptives pills (OCPs)
- *Infections*—mumps, viral hepatitis, coxsackie and echovirus, mycoplasma
- *Pancreatic ductal obstruction* due to migration of *Ascaris lumbricoides* and other causes
- *Inflammation spreading from neighboring tissues*, e.g. penetrating peptic ulcer
- *Connective tissue diseases*, e.g. systemic lupus erythematosus (SLE)
- *Drug-induced pancreatitis* caused by diuretics, anti-inflammatory drugs, azathioprine, 6-mercaptopurine, asparaginase, isoniazid, rifampicin, tetracycline, phenformin
- *Toxins*—methyl alcohol, scorpion venom, organophosphorus insecticide.
  In many cases, there may not be any identifiable cause.

Clinical Features

Onset is sudden with acute upper abdominal pain which may radiate to the chest, precordium, back or lower abdomen. An alcoholic bout or heavy eating may precipitate the attack. The patient adopts a stooping posture with pressure on the abdomen to get relief. Nausea, vomiting, dehydration and signs of shock occur in severe cases. Mild jaundice may be present in a few cases. Erythematous skin nodules may form due to fat necrosis. Secondary pleural effusion may develop on the left side.

Acute pancreatitis is subdivided into two types:

1. *Interstitial edematous pancreatitis (IEP):* Majority of patients have diffused enlargement of pancreas due to inflammatory edema. Contrast-enhanced computed tomography (CECT) shows relatively homogenous enhancement of pancreatic parenchyma and symptoms resolve within one week.

2. *Necrotizing pancreatitis (NP):* About 5% of patients develop necrosis of the pancreatic parenchyma and the peripancreatic tissue or both. This most commonly manifests as necrosis involving both the pancreas and peripancreatic tissues and less commonly as necrosis of only the peripancreatic tissue and rarely of the pancreatic parenchyma alone.

Diagnosis

Diagnosis of acute pancreatitis requires two of the following—typical abdominal pain, threefold or greater elevation in serum amylase and/or lipase level and/or confirmatory findings on cross-sectional abdominal imaging.

Examination of the abdomen shows rigidity, marked tenderness, mild distension due to ileus of the intestines and absence of peristaltic sounds. A bluish discoloration may be seen in the flanks *(Turner's sign)* or around the umbilicus *(Cullen's sign)* due to extravasation of blood into the abdominal wall. When present, these signs strongly suggest acute NP. Ascites may develop as a complication *(pancreatic ascites)*.

Course and Prognosis: The acute phase subsides within a week but recurrence may occur. In general, the mortality is 10–20%. In hemorrhagic pancreatitis with profound shock the mortality is high. Adverse factors include elderly age, severe shock, respiratory failure, fall of serum calcium below 8 mg/dL, azotemia and high fluid requirements.

Laboratory features: Serum amylase is increased early during the stage of acinar necrosis and it comes down in 3–4 days. Amylase levels may reach even 2000 Somogyi units/dL. Urinary amylase is raised initially during the illness and it remains so for 4–7 days. In acute pancreatitis, the renal clearance of amylase is higher than that of creatinine. The amylase/creatinine clearance ratio (Cam/Ccr) is increased in acute pancreatitis and this is a diagnostic feature. Serum amylase levels are elevated in other conditions such as cholecystitis, intestinal infarction, perforation and obstruction and mumps. Amylase level is increased in the ascitic fluid of pancreatic ascites.

Moderate neutrophil leukocytosis is common. Blood glucose is increased and calcium is lowered. Serum bilirubin may be transiently elevated, up to 4 mg/dL in a few cases. Electrocardiogram (ECG) abnormalities such as ST-T wave changes may develop in some cases and this may resemble myocardial ischemia.

Radiology: Calculi in the biliary and pancreatic duct systems may be seen in the plain radiograph of the abdomen. Loops of duodenum and jejunum are distended (sentinel loop) due to ileus. The inner wall of the duodenal loop may show pressure effects and widening on barium meal and hypotonic duodenography.

USG and CT scan help to assess the morphological abnormality in the pancreaticobiliary system. ERCP performed after subsidence of the acute phase helps to demonstrate the underlying abnormality.

CECT is a very good imaging modality to reveal morphological changes in the pancreas. MRI scan gives additional information.

Classification of Severity of Pancreatitis

Organ failure that develops during the early phase is set in motion by the activation of cytokine cascades resulting in systemic inflammatory response syndrome (SIRS). When SIRS is present and persistent, there is an increased risk that the pancreatitis will be complicated by persistent organ failure and the patient should be treated as if they have severe acute pancreatitis.

Grades of severity

Mild acute pancreatitis
- No local or systemic complications

Moderately severe acute pancreatitis
- Organ failure that resolves within 48 hour (transient organ failure)
- Local or systemic complications without persistent organ failure

Severe acute pancreatitis
- Persistent organ failure (>48 hour)

Single organ failure/multiple organ failure (MOF)

SIRS (*See* Section 6, Ch 36, Sepsis and Septic shock)

Defined by presence of two or more criteria	
Heart rate	> 90 beats/min
Core temperature	< 36°C or > 38°C
White blood count (WBC)	< 4000 or >12000/mm³
Respirations	20/min or PCO_2 < 32 mm Hg

Differential diagnosis: Acute emergencies like gastric or duodenal ulcer perforation, acute cholecystitis, renal colic, hepatitis, peritonitis, acute myocardial infarction and pleurisy have to be considered in the differential diagnosis.

General complications: These include shock, hyperglycemia, hypertriglyceridemia, hypocalcemia and DIC. Infection generally supervenes on the necrotic tissue in 40–60% of cases. 10–15% of patients develop SIRS leading to a fulminant course and multiorgan failure. SIRS is the result of activation of the inflammatory cascade mediated by cytokines, immunocytes and the complement system.

Local Complications

- Acute peripancreatic fluid collection (APFC) is peripancreatic fluid associated with IEP with no associated peripancreatic necrosis. This term applies only to areas of peripancreatic fluid seen within the first 4 weeks after onset of IEP and without the features of a pseudocyst.
- CECT criteria:
  - Occurs in the setting of IEP
  - Homogeneous collection with fluid density
  - Confined by normal peripancreatic fascial planes
  - No definable wall encapsulating the collection
  - Adjacent to pancreas (no intrapancreatic extension)
- ***Pancreatic pseudocyst:*** An encapsulated collection of fluid with a well-defined inflammatory wall usually outside the pancreas with minimal or no necrosis. This entity usually occurs more than 4 weeks after onset of IEP.

CECT Criteria

- Well-circumscribed, usually round or oval
- Homogeneous fluid density

- No non-liquid component
- Well-defined wall; that is, completely encapsulated
- Maturation usually requires > 4 weeks after onset of acute pancreatitis; occurs after IEP.

Treatment consists of endoscopic or surgical drainage into the stomach or the small intestine.

Surgical drainage of a pseudocyst is possible with a cystogastrostomy or cystoduodenostomy if the pseudocyst wall is broadly adherent to the stomach or duodenum. Other procedures are Roux–en–Y cyst-jejunostomy and pancreatic resection if the pseudocyst is in the tail.

Acute Necrotic Collection

This refers to a collection containing variable amounts of both fluid and necrotic material associated with NP. The necrosis can involve the pancreatic parenchyma and/or the peripancreatic tissues.

CECT Criteria

- Occurs only in the setting of acute NP.
- Heterogeneous and non-liquid density of varying degrees in different locations (some appear homogeneous early in their course).
- No definable wall encapsulating the collection.
- Location—intrapancreatic and/or extrapancreatic.

Walled-off Necrosis (WON)

A mature, encapsulated collection of pancreatic and/or peripancreatic necrosis that has developed a well-defined inflammatory wall. WON usually occurs > 4 weeks after onset of NP.

CECT Criteria

- Heterogeneous with liquid and non-liquid density with varying degrees of loculations (some may appear homogeneous).
- Well-defined wall that is completely encapsulated.
- Location—intrapancreatic and/or extrapancreatic.
- Maturation usually requires 4 weeks after onset of acute NP.

Other local complications of acute pancreatitis include gastric outlet dysfunction, splenic and portal vein thrombosis (PVT) and colonic necrosis. Other complications are:

- ***Pancreatic ascites*** develops due to the rupture of pancreatic duct into the peritoneum. Massive intraperitoneal hemorrhage may develop.
- ***Intestinal infarction***
- ***Obstructive jaundice***
- ***GI bleeding:*** This may occur due to different causes. In some cases, bleeding may not be related to the pancreatic lesion, but related to factors such as stress-induced mucosal gastropathy, Mallory-Weiss tear and alcoholic gastropathy. Pancreatitis related causes include splenic artery rupture or splenic artery pseudoaneurysm rupture, splenic vein rupture, portal vein rupture, thrombosis of the adjacent splenic vein which can lead to gastric varices with or without esophageal varices which can rupture.

Systemic Complications

It includes organ failure and exacerbation of pre-existing comorbidity, such as coronary artery disease (CAD) or chronic lung disease (CLD), precipitated by the acute pancreatitis. Organ failure can be transient or persistent.

It is termed ***transient organ failure*** if the organ failure resolves within 48 hour. ***Persistent organ failure*** persists for > 48 hour. If organ failure affects more than one organ system, it is termed ***multiple organ failure (MOF)***.

- ***Respiratory system:*** Atelectasis, left-sided pleural effusion, mediastinal abscess, adult respiratory distress syndrome (ARDS)
- ***Cardiovascular system (CVS):*** Myocarditis, pericardial effusion, sudden death
- ***Renal failure***
- ***Central nervous system (CNS):*** Fat embolism, psychosis
- ***Fat necrosis in several organs:*** This may involve skin, CNS, bones and other organs.

Predictors of Severity

Predicting severity of pancreatitis early in the course of disease is critical to maximize therapy and to prevent and minimize organ dysfunction and complications. Although severity is now defined by the presence of organ failure or anatomic complications of acute pancreatitis, such as pancreatic necrosis, several scoring systems have been developed to predict severity. These include:

- Ranson's score
- The Imrie or Glasgow score
- Acute Physiology and Chronic Health Evaluation II (APACHE II) score
- Bedside Index of Sererity in Acute Pancreatitis (BISAP)
- Organ failure
- Peritoneal lavage
- Laboratory markers like blood urea nitrogen, hematocrit, C-reactive protein (CRP), interleukin-6 (IL-6), polymorphonuclear leukocyte elastase (PMNE), phospholipase A2, urinary trypsinogen activation peptide, procalcitonin
- CT severity index
- Chest radiography.

Atlanta Criteria for Severe Acute Pancreatitis

Modified Marshall scoring system for organ dysfunction

Organ system	Scores				
	0	1	2	3	4
Respiratory; (PaO$_2$/FiO$_2$)	> 400	301–400	201–300	101–200	< 101
Renal; serum. creatinine mg/dL	< 1.4	1.4–1.8	1.9–3.6	3.6–4.9	> 4.9
Cardiovascular; systolic BP mm Hg	> 90	< 90, fluid responsive	< 90, not fluid responsive	< 90, ph < 7.3	< 90, ph < 7.2

A score of 2 or more in any system defines the presence of organ failure.

Bedside Index of Severity in Acute Pancreatitis (BISAP)

It incorporates five clinical and labarotory parameters obtained within the first 24 hours of hospitalization:

- (B) BUN > 22 mg%
- (I) Impaired mental status
- (S) SIRS: 2/4 present
- (A) Age > 60 years
- (P) Pleural effusion.

Presence of three or more of these factors is associated with substantially increased risk for in hospital mortality among patients with acute pancreatitis.

CT Findings and Grading of Acute Pancreatitis (CT Severity Index)

Grade	Findings	Score
A	*Normal pancreas:* Normal size, sharply defined, smooth contour, homogenous enhancement, retroperitoneal peripancreatic fat without enhancement	0
B	Focal or diffuse enlargement of the pancreas, contour may show irregularity, enhancement may be non-homogenous but there is no peripancreatic inflammation	1
C	Peripancreatic inflammation with intrinsic pancreatic abnormalities	2
D	Intrapancreatic or extrapancreatic fluid collection	3
E	Two or more large collections or gas in the pancreas or retroperitoneum	4

Necrosis Score Based on CECT

Necrosis %	Score
0	0
< 33	2
33–50	4
≥ 50	6

CT severity index is the total sum of unenhanced CT score plus necrosis score: Maximum = 10; ≥ 6 = Severe disease.

Treatment

Mild cases require only symptomatic measures.

Medical management: Analgesics like methadone 10 mg or pethidine 100 mg are used to relieve pain. In severe cases, morphine 10–20 mg may be required. Since morphine causes spasm of the sphincter of Oddi, it may be combined with atropine 0.5 mg or propantheline bromide 15–30 mg. Oral feeding is avoided in the acute stages. Food is gradually introduced when the condition subsides.

Shock: It is managed on general lines by replacing fluids and electrolytes and the use of pressor agents when required. IV administration of glucose and electrolytes has to be continued till the ileus disappears. Hypocalcemia is corrected by the administration of calcium gluconate IV. If diabetic state develops, insulin has to be administered. Broad-spectrum antibiotics are indicated to treat secondary infection.

If there is troublesome abdominal distension, continuous nasogastric aspiration may help. Necrotic lesions and local fluid collections should be evacuated by guided needle aspiration.

Surgery: It may be indicated at times in acute pancreatitis.

Indications

- Excision of necrotic tissue (necrosectomy) is needed if there is extensive necrosis as demonstrated by helical CT with pancreatic protocol.

Textbook of Medicine

- Drainage of pus is required if there is evidence of infection and abscess formation. Gram staining of FNAC specimen may reveal organisms.
- Pancreatic ascites may have to be drained at times.
- Relief of biliary obstruction if medical treatment by itself is not successful.

In the presence of biliary stones or other obstructive lesions, surgery is undertaken electively to prevent relapse of pancreatitis. Necrotic lesions and local fluid collections should be evaluated by guided needle aspiration. The material should be submitted for microbiological tests. Surgical debridement is indicated if there is infection and also in sterile abscesses which fail to improve with medical therapy.

Sometimes biliary obstruction may have to be relieved in the acute phase of pancreatitis itself if conservative measures fail to resolve the condition.

Endoscopic Therapy

- Severe acute gallstone pancreatitis with ascending cholangitis is an indication for urgent ERCP.
- Pancreatic ductal rupture leading to peripancreatic fluid collections in NP.
- Pancreatic ascites and pancreatic pleural effusions as a result of main pancreatic duct disruption which requires ERCP and bridging stent placement.

Recurrent Acute Pancreatits (RAP)

Whether RAP is a chronic disease is still debated. RAP can develop into chronic pancreatitis over time if the cause of the disease persists. Recurrent pancreatitis is defined as the presence of at least two documented episodes of pancreatitis during one year with complete or near complete resolution of symptoms and signs of pancreatitis between episodes in a patient without chronic pancreatitis at imaging.

Initial evaluation fails to detect the cause of RAP in 10–30% of patients and as a result, the term *idiopathic recurrent acute pancreatitis (IRAP)* is used. The principal causes of RAP are gallstones and alcohol, constituting around 70%. The causes of IRAP can be mechanical, toxic–metabolic, anatomical or miscellaneous. Microlithiasis commonly reported from the West is not a common cause of IRAP among Indian patients. Pancreas divisum (PD) is now believed as a cofactor, the main factor being associated is genetic mutations. The role of sphincter of Oddi dysfunction (SOD) as a cause of IRAP remains controversial. Malignancy should be ruled out in any patient with IRAP > 50 years of age. Early chronic pancreatitis can present initially as RAP. The work-up of patients with IRAP includes a detailed history and investigations.

Primary investigations include liver function tests (LFT), serum calcium and triglyceride, abdominal USG and CECT of abdomen. Endoscopic ultrasound (EUS), magnetic resonance cholangiopancreatography (MRCP) and possibly ERCP are indicated in the secondary phase if the work-up is negative after the primary investigations. EUS is advised usually 6–8 weeks after an acute episode. Treatment of patients with IRAP is aimed at the specific etiology. In general, empirical cholecystectomy should be discouraged with the availability and widespread use of EUS. Endoscopic sphincterotomy is advised if there is strong suspicion of SOD. Minor papilla sphincterotomy should be carried out in those with pancreas divisum but with limited expectations. Regular follow-up of patients with IRAP is necessary because most patients are likely to develop chronic pancreatitis in due course.

CHRONIC PANCREATITIS

In this condition, the pancreatic tissue is progressively destroyed and replaced by fibrosis.

Epidemiology

In a nationwide study of 1086 subjects from India, the frequency with idiopathic pancreatitis was 60.2%, alcoholic chronic pancreatic 38.71% and the rest 1.1% had rare causes. 3.58% were tropical pancreatitis, smoking was present in 28.3% of cases and cassava intake was significant in 18.3%. 40.5% had diabetes mellitus (DM) alcoholism and female gender are independent risk factors for DM.

Risk of malignancy in chronic pancreatic was 4.1% on follow-up. Smoking is a risk factor for chronic pancreatitis and it is a leading risk factor for pancreatic cancer as well.

Source: Balakrishnan V, Unnikrishnan AG, Thomas V, et al. Chronic Pancreatitis. A Prospective Nationwide Study of 1,086 Subjects from India. JOP. J Pancreas (Online). 2008;9(5):593-600.

Pathology

The pancreas is firm to hard, fibrotic and distorted. Calculi may develop inside the distorted ductal system. Acinar tissue may also become calcified. Exocrine pancreatic function suffers when 80–90% of the acini are destroyed. Though the islets are relatively spared, they are also affected finally, resulting in diabetes. In chronic relapsing pancreatitis seen in India, DM is a prominent feature.

Etiology

- Alcoholic
- Tropical
  - Tropical calcific pancreatitis (TCP)
  - Fibrocalculus pancreatic diabetes (FCPD)
- Genetic
  - Autosomal dominant
  - Hereditary pancreatitis (HP) (PRSS1 mutations)
  - Autosomal recessive or modifier genes
  - Cystic fibrosis transmembrane conductance regulator (CFTR) mutations
  - SPINK1 mutations
  - Others
- Metabolic
  - Hypercalcemia
  - Hyperlipidemia
  - Hypertriglyceridemia
  - Lipoprotein lipase deficiency (LPLD)
  - Apolipoprotein C-II deficiency
- Obstructive
  - Benign pancreatic duct obstruction
    - Traumatic stricture
    - Stricture after severe acute pancreatitis
    - SOD or stenosis
    - Duodenal wall cyst
    - Pancreatic divisum

- Malignant pancreatic duct stricture
  - Ampullary or duodenal carcinoma
  - Pancreatic adenocarcinoma
  - Intraductal papillary mucinous neoplasm (IPMN)
- Autoimmune pancreatitis (AIP)
  - Associated with autoimmune diseases [Sjogren's syndrome, primary biliary cirrhosis (PBC), primary sclerosing cholangitis (PSC), others]
- Postnecrotic chronic pancreatitis
- Idiopathic
  - Early onset
  - Late onset
- Asymptomatic pancreatic fibrosis
  - Chronic alcoholism
  - Old age
  - Chronic renal failure
  - Diabetes
  - Radiotherapy.

Causes of chronic pancreatitis: TIGAR-O classification system

Toxic-metabolic
- Alcohol abuse (~70%)
- Tobacco smoking
- Hypercalcemia (e.g. hyperparathyroidism)
- Chronic renal failure

Idiopathic (~20%)
- Early/late onset
- Tropical

Genetic
- Hereditary pancreatitis (cationic trypsinogen mutation)
- Cystic fibrosis due to cystic fibrosis transmembrane conductance regulator (CFTR) gene mutations
- SPINK1 mutations

Autoimmune
- Isolated autoimmune chronic pancreatitis
- Part of multiorgan problem (Sjogren's syndrome, PBC)

Recurrent and severe acute pancreatitis
- Postnecrotic (severe acute pancreatitis)
- Recurrent acute pancreatitis

Obstructive
- Duct obstruction (e.g. tumor)
- Pancreas divisum
- Stenosis of sphincter of Oddi

Clinical Features

Chronic pancreatitis is more common in the fourth and fifth decades. It presents with recurrent upper abdominal pain following alcoholic bouts or dietary excesses. The pain may be referred to the back between T_{10} and T_{12} segments. These patients adopt a characteristic squatting posture with pressure applied to the abdomen. When present, this feature may suggest the diagnosis. Overt diabetes develops in one-fifth of the cases. Except for vague tenderness over the epigastrium, physical examination may not reveal much. Less commonly, enlarged pancreas, pseudocyst or pancreatic abscess may be palpable.

Course and prognosis: Chronic pancreatitis tends to be persistent or recurrent, especially if accompanied by biliary tract disease. Complications include malabsorption state, malnutrition, obstructive jaundice, DM and higher risk of malignancy. Chronic pancreatitis carries a mortality of 50% in 20–25 years. Malabsorption develops when the exocrine function falls by 80%.

Diagnosis: Chronic pancreatitis should be suspected clinically in any alcoholic patient complaining of epigastric pain referred to the back.

Investigations: Plain X-ray of the abdomen may reveal pancreatic calculi and calcification of the substance of the gland in 30–40% of cases. USG reveals enlargement, cysts, abscesses and ductal abnormalities. Functional impairment can be assessed by undertaking exocrine function tests. The ERCP helps to delineate the biliary and pancreatic duct system and also in obtaining biopsies and to carry out procedures to relieve obstruction. Glucose tolerance test (GTT) brings out the diabetic state. Serum amylase is not constantly elevated in chronic pancreatitis but its level may increase during acute exacerbations. Stool fat is increased (above 7 g in 24 h), this is made up of neutral fat. This helps to distinguish the condition from intestinal malabsorption in which the lipids are in the form of fatty acids. Vitamin B_{12} malabsorption occurs since the vitamin is bound in the gut by proteins other than intrinsic factor and thus, rendered unabsorbable.

Endoscopic Ultrasound (EUS) Criteria for Chronic Pancreatitis

Ductal	Parenchymal
Stones	Echogenic strands
Echogenic ductal walls	Echogenic foci
Irregular ductal walls	Calcifications
Stricture	Lobular contour
Visible side branches	Cyst
Ductular dilatation	

Treatment: Abstinence from alcohol and smoking and reduction of weight help to reduce exacerbations. Analgesics and antispasmodics may be necessary to relieve pain. Reduction of dietary fat to 20–30 g/day helps to reduce the abdominal discomfort and relieve steatorrhea in mild cases. Fat soluble vitamins have to be supplemented orally or parenterally as required.

Digestion can be aided by the administration of pancreatic enzymes or enzymes derived from fungal or other plant sources given orally after food. Pancreatic extract—pankreon (pancreatin) is available commercially. Four to six tablets (2–3 g) have to be given with meals or more frequently. This measure helps in digestion, corrects the steatorrhea and also ameliorates pain. Vitamin B_{12} malabsorption is also corrected. Though this is generally safe, excessive use of pancreatic extracts leads to hyperuricemia. In moderate and severe cases, H_2 receptor blocker drugs such as ranitidine 150 mg bd or a proton pump inhibitor (PPI) such as omeprazole 20 mg bd are given orally to reduce gastric acidity and thereby limit the inactivation of pancreatic enzymes in the intestine.

Medium chain triglycerides are useful to reduce diarrhea. They require only small amounts of pancreatic enzymes for digestion. Moreover, bile salts are not required for their absorption. They are contained in oils such as coconut oil. Diabetes has to be treated on its own merits.

Surgery: Intractable pain, pancreatic cysts, pseudocysts and neoplasms are indications for surgery. In many cases, relief of obstruction and withdrawal of alcohol results in improvement of pancreatic function. In some cases, removal of the affected portion of the pancreas may be required.

Autoimmune Pancreatitis (AIP)

Syn: Autoimmune related pancreatitis

This was first described in 1955 by Yoshida, et al. to describe the form of pancreatitis that is associated with autoimmune manifestations revealed by clinical and laboratory parameters. AIP refers to a distinct chronic inflammatory and sclerosing disease of the pancreas. It is a form of chronic pancreatitis caused by autoimmune inflammation. It forms 5–11% of the total cases of chronic pancreatitis. The distinct characteristic of the disease is dense infiltration of the pancreas and often other organs, with lymphocytes and plasma cells, many of which express immunoglobulin G4 (IgG4) on their surface. This leads to lymphocytic infiltration with associated fibrosis of the pancreas leading to organ dysfunction. The autoimmune target of this IgG4 and the trigger for disease are unknown.

Many cases are caused by IgG4: The *International Society* proposed the following criteria for AIP–1:

- Parenchymal and ductal abnormalities revealed by imagin
- Elevated serum IgG4 concentration
- Pancreatic histologic abnormalities
- Extrapancreatic involvement
- Response to glucocorticosteroids.

Fibrosis, sclerosis and obliterative phlebitis are characteristically seen in association with the chronic inflammatory infiltrate. Although this inflammatory infiltrate is present in the pancreas, similar infiltrates may be seen in other organs such as the bile duct, salivary glands, retroperitoneum, lymphnodes, kidney, prostate, ampulla and others. Much of the information on this disease comes from a series of studies from Japan and other Asian countries. Male to female ratio is 2:1. The disease is present in India and formed 1% of a series from Vellore.

Source: Etiology and clinical profile of chronic pancreatitis the CMC Vellore experience. Ashok Chacko and Shajan Peter in chronic pancreatitis and pancreatic diabetes in India. Edited by V Balakrishnan and others, published by The Indian Pancreatitis Study Group, 2006.

AIP is characterized by the presence of autoantibodies, elevated levels of serum immunoglobulins IgG4, enlargement of the pancreas (diffuse or focal), pancreatic duct strictures and pathologic features of a dense lymphocytic infiltrate and rapid response to steroid therapy. One of the hallmarks of AIP is diffuse or segmental irregularity and narrowing of the pancreatic duct. The pathologic hallmark in the pancreas is infiltration of inflammatory cells and fibrosis around medium-sized interlobular ducts. Two histologic variants have been described. The first *lymphoplasmacytic sclerosing pancreatitis (LPSP)* is more common. The second variant, termed *idiopathic duct centric chronic pancreatitis (IDCP)*, is less common.

Some cases show association with other autoimmune diseases such as rheumatoid arthritis (RA), Sjögren's syndrome and inflammatory bowel disease (IBD).

Clinical Features

A wide variety of symptoms may occur. The disease commonly affects middle-aged men usually after the age of 50 year. They usually present with painless obstructive jaundice mimicking pancreatic adenocarcinoma. Additional symptoms may include weight loss, vomiting and glucose intolerance. Jaundice and mild to moderate abdominal pain are frequent. Additional clinical manifestations include sclerosing sialadenitis (usually presenting as bilateral symmetrical swelling of the salivary glands), retroperitoneal fibrosis (RPF) (most commonly presenting as hydronephrosis due to entrapment of the ureters), tubulointerstitial nephritis, lymphadenopathy (particularly mediastinal, cervical and abdominal), prostatitis and sclerosing cholecystitis, interstitial pneumonia, pseudotumors of the liver, lung and pituitary. Imaging studies shows biliary duct strictures which may resemble those of primary sclerosing cholangitis (PSC). Histology helps to confirm the diagnosis.

Diagnosis

The CT scan image is characteristic. Endoscopic USG is an important tool to diagnose AIP. Abdominal USG usually shows a diffusely enlarged and hypoechoic pancreas. The appearance on EUS is similar. CT most commonly reveals a diffusely enlarged sausage-shaped pancreas in which enhancement with the IV contrast agent is delayed and prolonged. MRI of the pancreas also may reveal this diffuse pancreatic enlargement, typically with decreased T1-weighted intensity and increased T2-weighted intensity. MRCP can be very helpful in identifying the biliary strictures and in visualizing the pancreatic duct. The disease may be suspected from the clinical and imaging features previously noted. AIP has to be differentiated from alcohol-induced pancreatitis and pancreatic cancer. Laboratory evaluation may reveal elevation of serum immunoglobulins (especially IgG4), seen in one half to two thirds of cases. In studies from Japan, an IgG4 level greater than 135 mg/dL has a sensitivity of 90% and a specificity of greater than 95% for AIP.

There are several proposals for diagnostic criteria for autoimmune chronic pancreatitis. The first widely used system proposed by the Mayo Clinic uses the mnemonic HISORT (*h*istology, *i*maging, *s*erology, *o*ther organ involvement and *r*esponse to steroid *t*herapy). Other one is Asian *C*onsensus *C*riteria.

Mayo Clinic HISORT Criteria for Diagnosis of AIP

Features	
Histology	At least one of the following: • Periductal lymphoplasmacytic infiltrate with obliterative phlebitis and storiform fibrosis • Lymphoplasmacytic infiltrate with storiform fibrosis with abundant IgG4 positive plasma cells (≥10/HPF)
Imaging	• Typical; diffusely enlarged gland with delayed rim enhancement, diffusely irregular and attenuated pancreatic duct • Other; focal pancreatic mass or enlargement, focal pancreatic duct stricture, pancreatic atrophy, calcification, or pancreatitis

Textbook of Medicine

Serology	Elevated IgG4 level
Other organ involvement	Hilar or intrahepatic biliary strictures, distal (intrapancreatic) bile duct stricture, parotid or lacrimal gland involvement, mediastinal lymphadenopathy, retroperitoneal fibrosis (RPF)
Response to glucocorticoid therapy	Resolution or marked improvement of pancreatic or extrapancreatic manifestations

Patients meeting criteria for one or more of the groups have AIP.

Group A:

- Diagnostic pancreatic histology
- Specimen demonstrating the full spectrum of LPSP or ≥10 IgG4 positive cells/high power field (HPF).

Group B:

- Typical imaging and serology
- CT or MRI showing diffusely enlarged pancreas with delayed and rim enhancement
- Pancreatogram showing diffusely irregular pancreatic duct
- Elevated IgG4 level.

Group C:

- Response to glucocorticoids
- Unexplained pancreatic disease after negative work-up for other causes
- Elevated serum IgG4 or other organ involvement confirmed by the presence of abundant
- IgG4 positive cells
- Resolution or marked improvement in pancreatic or extrapancreatic manifestations with glucocorticoid therapy.

Treatment

Corticosteroids form the mainstay of treatment. Prednisolone in a dose of 40 mg/day should be started orally and continued for a week, before tapering the dose. Autoimmune chronic pancreatitis may progress rapidly unless treated with steroids, which produces rapid resolution of symptoms and radiographic improvement. Usual starting dose is 30–40 mg prednisolone daily orally for 4–8 weeks. Once clinical response and pancreatic imaging (after 4 weeks) shows resolution prednisolone is tapered at the rate of 5 mg/week to the minimum effective level for maintenance.

Tropical Pancreatitis

It is used to be the most common form of chronic pancreatitis in some parts of India including Kerala. It is generally a disease of youth and early adulthood with a mean age of onset of 24 years. The disease classically manifests as abdominal pain, severe malnutrition and exocrine and/or endocrine insufficiency. Pancreatic calculi develop in more than 90% of patients. The pathology is characterized by large intraductal calculi, marked dilatation of main pancreatic duct and gland atrophy. With improvement in socioeconomic status and alteration in dietary habits, in many endemic areas the disease has become less common. For further details (*See* Section 10, Ch 93).

CYSTIC FIBROSIS (CF) OF THE PANCREAS

Syn: Fibrocystic disease of pancreas, Mucoviscidosis

It is the most common lethal genetic disease in whites. This disease is encountered in India occasionally. The incidence in Orientals is 1/90000 of population, compared to 1/20000 in Caucasians and 1/17000 in Negroid races. It is an autosomal recessive disease. The defective gene is located in the long arm of chromosome 7. Normally, this gene encodes for a 1480-amino acid protein called cystic fibrosis transmembrane regulator (CFTR). The CFTR is a protein that regulates and participates in the transport of electrolytes across epithelial cell membranes and probably across intracellular membranes as well. At least more than 1000 mutations in the CFTR has been identified. Several molecular abnormalities in the gene give rise to a wide spectrum of clinical features. CFTR mutations can be classified into six groups:

1. CFTR is not synthesized
2. The processing is defective
3. Defective regulation
4. Defective conductance
5. Partially defective production and processing
6. Defective regulation of other channels.

The primary defect in CF is one of disordered ion-transport in epithelial cells. This abnormality is manifested in almost all secretory glands particularly the sweat glands and mucus-secreting organs such as pancreas, liver, lungs, intestines, salivary glands, prostate, testes and others.

Normally, sweat is formed in the secretory coil of the sweat glands as an ultrafiltrate of plasma containing 135 and 100 mmol/L of sodium and chloride respectively. These ions are reabsorbed by the ductal epithelium and normal sweat contains only less than 50 mmol/L of sodium ion (Na^+) and chloride ion (Cl^+), when the flow rate is 10 nanoliter/gland/minute. One of the main abnormality which is highly diagnostic, is the increase in chloride in the sweat to levels above 60 mmol/L.

Bicarbonate content of pancreatic juice is less than normal. The mucus secreted by mucous glands in all organs is abnormally viscid. This is responsible for blocking the smaller duct system and impairing ciliary activity of several tubular organs.

Pathology

Pancreatic ducts are occluded and dilated to form cysts. Acini undergo atrophy. There is interstitial fibrosis. Islets of Langerhans are relatively unaffected. Intrahepatic bile ducts may show obstruction in 10% of cases. Cirrhosis with portal hypertension may develop. Lungs which are normal at birth, soon develop purulent bronchitis, bronchiectasis and cystic changes. Other glands which develop ductal obstructions are the sublingual salivary glands, prostate and testes.

Nonclassic forms of CF occur in which milder mutation of the CFTR gene occurs, with partial preservation of pancreatic function. In this form, malabsorption is rare.

Clinical Features

Earliest manifestation in the newborn is meconium ileus in which the meconium (initial feces of the newborn) is abnormally thick leads to intestinal obstruction. As the child grows, the intestinal symptoms take the form of recurrent subacute or acute intestinal obstruction, ileocolic intussusception and rectal prolapse.

Pancreatic lesion leads to varying degrees of pancreatitis and malabsorption. Glucose tolerance may be impaired, frank diabetes is less common. If diabetes occurs, it shows features of both types 1 and 2.

In comparison to the respiratory morbidity, pancreatic dysfunction is milder.

Respiratory Infection

Defective CFTR gene leads to poor clearance of bacteria deposited on the mucosal surface, reduce the volume of airway surface liquid and alters the pH of lower airway surface fluid. Microbes colonizing the respiratory tract in CF differ between individuals and with increasing age of the patients.

Occurrence of respiratory infection and sinusitis is also genetically related. The action of cilia is impaired by the thick secretion and so infection is precipitated. The age of onset and severity of the lesions vary, depending on the genetic abnormality. Respiratory tract lesions include chronic sinusitis, nasal polyps, chronic otitis media and conductive deafness. Respiratory findings include bronchiectasis, recurrent purulent infection, hemoptysis and pneumothorax. Main infective agents are *Hemophilus influenzae, Staphylococcus aureus* and *Pseudomonas aeruginosa*. The *Staphylococcus* is generally methicillin-resistant *Staphylococcus aureus* (MRSA). Other organisms include *Burkholderia cepacia* and atypical mycobacteria. Infection by *P. aeruginosa* is a **landmark which heralds a progressive downhill course**. The organisms produce protective biofilms for protection against antibiotics. More than 80% of deaths are due to respiratory failure. Deafness occurs due to blockage of Eustachian tubes. Proper deployment of antibiotics contribute to the increase in life expectancy of CF patients. Azithromycin is a common antibiotic given on a long-term basis for chronic respiratory infections in CF on account of its anti-inflammatory and antibacterial effort. Long-term administration suppresses the susceptible bacteria. Antibiotics can also be delivered by inhalations. Some strains of *P. aeruginosa, B. cepacia* complex, *Achromobater xylosoxidans, S. maltophilia* are intrinsically resistant.

Congenital absence of vas deferens is almost universal. Azoospermia occurs in 80–90% of males and almost all males are infertile. Women can bear children. The degree of subfertility is also related to the genetic mutation.

Diagnosis

This is established by determining sweat electrolytes. Sweat is collected by stimulating diaphoresis with pilocarpine iontophoresis. Major and minor diagnostic criteria are given below. Normal sweat chloride level is < 40 mmol/L. In the nonclassic form, it may be 40–59 mmol/L. Other causes of increase in sweat chloride levels include heavy tobacco smoking, chronic bronchitis, malnutrition, hereditary nephrogenic diabetes insipidus, adrenal insufficiency and ectodermal dysplasia.

When sweat tests are inconclusive estimation of electrical potential difference between the nasal mucosa and forearm skin is helpful. Genotyping the CFTR gene helps to make more precise diagnosis. Methods for detection of CFTR mutations are commercially available.

Diagnosis in Newborns

Elevation of levels of immunoreactive trypsinogen in blood spots suggests pancreatic injury.

Criteria for diagnosis of CF

Major criteria
- Sweat chloride exceeding 60 mmol/L in children and 80 mmol/L in adults.
- Evidence of pulmonary involvement.
- Obstructive azoospermia.

Minor criteria
- Sweat chloride 40 mmol/L in children and 60 mmol/L in adults.
- Family history of CF or azoospermia.

Definite diagnosis is made if two major criteria, or a combination of one major and one minor criterion from two different organ systems are present.

Course and prognosis: If untreated, 80% of cases die in the first year of life. With treatment, median survival has gone up to about 30 years. Death is mainly due to respiratory complications. CF is one of the causes of chronic obstructive pulmonary disease (COPD) and pancreatic insufficiency occurring before the age of 30 years.

Management

General treatment includes healthy lifestyle and maintenance of positive nutrition from early life with supplementation of pancreatic enzymes and fat soluble vitamins reduce the ill-effects of chronic pancreatitis and malabsorption.

Treatment of Respiratory Complications

Aggressive treatment of respiratory infection is needed. Daily inhalation of the mucolytic enzyme dornase alpha [recombinant deoxyribonucleic acid (DNA)] and inhalation of tobramycin 300 mg twice daily given in 28 days on-off cycles in patients with *P. aeruginosa* in the airways are beneficial.

In resistant cases, colistin 100 mg IV 8 hourly combined with another antipseudomonas agent may be required.

Macrolide antibiotics—thrice weekly azithromycin help to reduce the incidence of *P. aeruginosa*, reduces biofilm and also acts as an anti-inflammatory agent.

Nonsteroidal anti-inflammatory drugs (NSAIDs) like ibuprofen 400 mg oral started early in disease reduces deterioration and hospitalization.

Respiratory physiotherapy—clearance of sputum by percussion and postural drainage help to improve quality of life and prevent deterioration. Hypertonic saline nebulization for 48 weeks (4 mL 7% bd) improve lung function, improves mucociliary clearance and infection.

Intractable cases have to undergo lung-transplantation. Five years survival is 50–60%. Attempts to institute gene therapy are in progress. Relatives of CF patients should undergo genetic tests and sweat tests to enable diagnosis early.

Future Directions

Drug ***Ivacaftor*** developed by vertex pharmaceuticals of Cambridge MA—approved in USA—an oral drug taken

Textbook of Medicine

twice daily treats not only the symptoms but the underlying cause. The drug improves lung function markedly, lowers salt content of sweat and improves weight either by improved intestinal function or by reducing the effort of breathing. The drug uses a lipid to deliver the replacement gene—the lipid vector is used instead of viral vectors used in other gene replacement trials. CF gene has > 1500 mutations. This drug probably works in all the CF mutations. Commercial name of drug—Kalydeco, the present cost of one year's treatment is $294,000.

Source:

1. O'Sullivan PB, Freedman DS. Cystic fibrosis. The Lancet. 2009;373(9678):1819-1918.

2. Corbyn Z. Promising new era dawns for cystic fibrosis treatment. Lancet. 2012;379(9825):1475-6.

PANCREATIC ASCITES

It is due to leakage of pancreatic juice into the peritoneum from a ruptured duct or pseudocyst. The fluid is rich in proteins and enzymes. The fluid may leak into the pleura causing a pancreaticopleural fistula. Fifty percent of these cases can be managed nonsurgically by paracentesis, diuretics, carbonic anhydrase inhibitors or octreotide and parenteral nutrition. If these fail, surgical measures aimed at diversion of the pancreatic juice to jejunum or using stents in the pancreatic duct may be needed.

CARCINOMA OF THE PANCREAS

This neoplasm is seen in all parts of India not uncommonly. It is more common in women of the age group 55–70 years, but both sexes may be affected. Histologically, they are adenocarcinomas arising from the ductal epithelium and occasionally from the acini. In some cases, ductal carcinomas arise multicentrically.

Genetic analysis has revealed that several germline mutations of P16, BRCA1, BRCA2, Rb and APC genes are associated with increased incidence of pancreatic cancer. 5–10% of pancreatic cancer patients have a positive family history. Cigarette smoking, hereditary pancreatitis and hereditary nonpolyposis colorectal cancers (HNPCC) are associated with higher risk of pancreatic cancer.

Clinical features: Cancer arises from ductal epithelium and evolves from premalignant to fully developed cancer. Pancreatic carcinomas may remain asymptomatic for long periods. The lesion is generally advanced by the time, it becomes symptomatic. Early symptoms are vague such as nonspecific dyspepsia, epigastric pain and vomiting. ***Thrombophlebitis migrans*** (recurrent venous thrombosis occurring in different parts) may develop in carcinomas of the body and tail of the pancreas.

Many cases may be misdiagnosed as hysteria or other neurotic disorders, before the actual diagnosis reveals itself.

Growths arising from the head of the pancreas cause painless progressive obstructive jaundice because of pressure on the CBD. The gallbladder enlarges and becomes palpable. The tumor may become palpable in the epigastrium on rare occasions. Lesions affecting the body and tail which do not produce jaundice but diabetes may develop when the lesion is extensive. Cachexia sets in late. Severe boring pain referred to the back develops when the nerves are affected. Death follows within 6 months of the onset of obstructive jaundice in untreated cases. Only 10% survive one year.

In carcinoma of the ampulla of Vater, obstructive jaundice is an early symptom. Ulceration and bleeding from the growth give rise to melena or a silvery color to feces.

Investigations: Carcinoma of the pancreas should be suspected when elderly persons complain of vague upper abdominal symptoms, painless progressive obstructive jaundice with a palpable gallbladder, migrating thrombophlebitis or progressive cachexia. USG, CT scan and ERCP give diagnostic information. Pancreatic juice collected endoscopically may reveal malignant cells. Serum biomarker such as CA 19–9 is useful in diagnosis. Multiphase multidetector helical CT with IV contrast is the imaging procedure of choice for initial evaluation.

Spiral CT, MRI, cholangiopancreatography and endoscopic USG help to bring out even small tumors better. Angiography helps to visualize the mass and its blood supply.

Treatment: Operable tumors of the ampulla of Vater are treated by excision of the duodenum and head of the pancreas. In inoperable cases, biliary obstruction is relieved by cholecystojejunostomy or choledochojejunostomy. This drainage procedure gives immense symptomatic relief. Chemotherapy using gemcitabine and 5-fluorouracil (5-FU)shows promise. Effective palliation of jaundice can be achieved with endoscopic stenting of bile duct.

CYSTIC NEOPLASMS OF PANCREAS

These are uncommon lesions, constituting around 10% of all pancreatic neoplasms and 30% of pancreatic resections. Usually benign, but can be premalignant and malignant and most are detected incidentally. They are difficult to diagnose and treat.

WHO histological classification of neoplastic pancreatic cysts
Serous cystic tumors
• Serous cystadenoma
• Serous cystadenocarcinoma
Mucinous cystic tumors
• Mucinous cystadenoma
• Mucinous cystadenoma with moderate dysplasia
• Mucinous cystadenocarcinoma
Noninfiltrating or infiltrating
• Intraductal papillary mucinous adenoma
• IPMN with moderate dysplasia
• Intraductal papillary mucinous carcinoma
• Solid pseudopapillary tumors.

Source: Khalid A, Brugge W. ACG Practice guidelines for the diagnosis and management of neoplastic pancreatic cysts.

The uncommon pancreatic cystic neoplasms are listed below:

- Metastases sarcoma, melanoma, ovarian carcinoma
- Neuroendocrine tumor (NET)—functional or nonfunctional
- Cystic pancreatic teratomas—multilocular cyst mass

Textbook of Medicine

Table 90.1: Salient clinical characteristics of the various neoplasms

Type	Sex	Decade	% of cystic neoplasm	Malignant potential
Serous cystic neoplasm	F	7th	32–39	Extremely rare, resection curative
Mucinous cystic neoplasm	F	5th	10–45	• Resection curative • Poor prognosis when invasive adenocarcinoma positive
Intraductal papillary mucinous neoplasm	M = F	6–7th	21–33	• Excellent prognosis when adenoma or borderline atypia • Poor prognosis when invasive adenocarcinoma positive
Solid pseudopapillary tumor	F	4th	<10	• Indolent neoplasm with rare nodal and extranodal metastases • Excellent prognosis with complete resection
Cystic endocrine neoplasm	M = F	5–6th	<10	Similar to solid endocrine neoplasm
Ductal adenocarcinoma with cystic degeneration	M > F	6–7th	<1	Dismal prognosis
Acinar cell cystadenoma	M	6–7th	<1	Aggressive neoplasm, better than adenocarcinoma

Abbreviations: SCN = Serous cystic neoplasm; MCN = Mucinous cystic neoplasm; IPMN = Intraductal papillary mucinous neoplasm; SPT = Solid pseudopapillary tumor

■ Lymphangioma, multiloculated, benign (Table 90.1). Other tumors include adenocarcinoma, acinar cell carcinoma, sarcoma and lymphoma.

Diagnosis and Treatment

They are diagnosed by CT and MRI with MRCP which is the procedure of choice. ERCP, FNAC and cyst fluid analysis done with EUS, pancreatoscopy, intraductal USG and position emission tomography (PET) scan are all required in some cases for full diagnosis.

Cyst fluid caricino embryonic antigen (CEA) is elevated in mucinous neoplasms. It is low in pseudocysts and nonmucinous neoplasms. Cyst fluid amylase is elevated in pseudocyst and ***intraductal papillary mucinous neoplasm (IPMN)***, whereas it is low in mucinous cystic neoplasms and serous cystadenoma.

Treatment by resection, distal pancreatectomy and lymph node dissection with or without splenectomy depending on location of tumor.

ENDOCRINE TUMORS OF THE PANCREAS

These are rare, but characteristic clinical features develop when they occur.

Islet cell tumors: Benign adenomas are rare. They secrete insulin and give rise to spontaneous hypoglycemia, which develops in the morning on a fasting stomach or after heavy exercise. This condition is relieved by food.

Zollinger-Ellison syndrome: This is due to gastrin-secreting tumors arising from the islets of Langerhans.

They are more common in the body and tail of the pancreas. Sometimes they may be multicentric. They may form part of multiple endocrine adenomatosis (MEN type I-Werner's syndrome), the other lesion being parathyroid adenoma. Excessive gastrin leads to the secretion of large amounts of gastric acid and aggressive gastric ulceration (Refer Section 8, Ch 78, p. 563).

Other Non-beta Cell Pancreatic Tumors

■ ***Glucagonoma:*** This arises from the alpha cells which grow to form adenomas or carcinomas and secrete excessive glucagon. These patients present with DM, severe weight loss and a skin rash termed as ***necrolytic migratory erythema*** seen particularly over the face, buttocks, abdomen, perineum and distal parts of the limbs. Treatment involves surgical removal of the tumor.

■ ***Watery diarrhea, hypokalemia achlorhydria (WDHA) syndrome, Verner-Morrison syndrome, pancreatic cholera:*** This condition is caused by a non-beta cell pancreatic islet neoplasm which produces excessive quantities of VIP. In comparison to the other endocrine tumors, these are larger. The severe watery diarrhea gives rise to shock, renal shut down, fatal hypokalemia and metabolic acidosis. The VIP also causes hyperglycemia and hypercalcemia. When located, treatment is surgical removal.

■ ***Somatostatinoma:*** Tumors producing somatostatin have been described in a few cases. Somatostatinomas are associated with hyperglycemia, loss of weight, hypochlorhydria, steatorrhea and gallbladder disease.

■ ***Tumors secreting adrenocorticotropic hormone (ACTH):*** These may arise from pancreatic islets. Cushing's syndrome produced by these tumors is milder than the classical types. In many of the cases, several hormones may be produced, e.g. insulin, gastrin, serotonin, etc.

Diabetes Mellitus

AG Unnikrishnan, Anjali Bhatt

Chapter Summary

- General Considerations
- Classification
- Epidemiology
- Diagnosis
- Screening
- Physiology, Pathology and Etiopathogenesis
  - Pancreas
  - Insulin Synthesis, Secretion and Action
  - Pathogenesis of Type 1 Diabetes Mellitus
  - Pathogenesis of Type 2 Diabetes Mellitus
- Clinical Features
- Evaluation
- Treatment
  - Oral Antidiabetic Drugs
  - Insulin Therapy and Other Parenteral Therapeutic Agents
- Brittle Diabetes
- Prognosis
- Prevention
- Diabetes during Pregnancy
- Diabetics and HIV Infection
  - Neonatal Diabetes Mellitus

GENERAL CONSIDERATIONS

Diabetes mellitus (DM) is a chronic metabolic disorder characterized by hyperglycemia with or without glycosuria, resulting from an absolute or relative deficiency of insulin, its action or both. This is brought about by an impairment of insulin production or its release by the β-cells of the islets of Langerhans. More often, it is due to resistance to the action of insulin either due to a receptor/postreceptor defect or an imbalance between insulin and its counter-regulatory hormones. Clinically, diabetes is characterized by a wide-spectrum of disorders ranging from asymptomatic hyperglycemia to abnormalities in the various organs. Worldwide, diabetes is the major risk factor for cardiovascular and cerebrovascular disease and is the leading cause of end-stage renal disease (ESRD), nontraumatic lower-extremity amputation and adult blindness.

CLASSIFICATION

The classification suggested by American Diabetes Association (ADA) is the etiological classification of diabetes. It narrates two main types of diabetes labeled as *type 1 DM*

and *type 2 DM*, along with *gestational DM (GDM)* and the other specific types where a precise etiological factor is identified (Table 91.1). Patients with any form of diabetes may require insulin treatment at some stage of their disease; hence, use of insulin therapy in itself to classify the patients may create confusion and should not be practiced.

Table 91.1: Etiologic classification of diabetes mellitus (DM)

- *Type 1 DM* (β-cell destruction, usually leading to absolute insulin deficiency)
  - Immune-mediated
  - Idiopathic
- *Type 2 DM* (may range from predominantly insulin resistance with relative insulin deficiency to a predominantly secretory defect with insulin resistance)
- *Other specific types*
  - Genetic defects of β-cell function characterized by mutations in:
    - Chromosome 12, HNF-1α (MODY-3)
    - Chromosome 7, glucokinase (MODY-2)
    - Chromosome 20, HNF-4α (MODY-1)
    - Chromosome 13, IPF-1 (MODY-4)
    - Chromosome 17, HNF-1β (MODY-5)
    - Chromosome 2, NeuroD1 (MODY-6)
    - Mitochondrial DNA
    - Others
  - Genetic defects in insulin action:
    - Type A insulin resistance
    - Leprechaunism
    - Rabson-Mendenhall syndrome (RMS)
    - Lipoatrophic diabetes
    - Others
  - Diseases of the exocrine pancreas:
    - Pancreatitis
    - Trauma/pancreatectomy
    - Neoplasia
    - Cystic fibrosis
    - Hemochromatosis
    - Fibrocalculous pancreatopathy
    - Others
  - Endocrinopathies:
    - Acromegaly
    - Cushing's syndrome
    - Glucagonoma
    - Pheochromocytoma
    - Hyperthyroidism
    - Somatostatinoma
    - Aldosteronoma
    - Others
  - Drug- or chemical-induced DM:
    - Vacor
    - Pentamidine

Contd...

Contd...

- – Nicotinic acid
- – Glucocorticoids
- – Thyroid hormone
- – Diazoxide
- – β-adrenergic agonists
- – Thiazides
- – Dilantin
- – α-interferon
- – Others
- • Infections:
  - – Congenital rubella
  - – CMV
  - – Others
- • Uncommon forms of immune-mediated DM:
  - – Stiff-man syndrome
  - – Anti-insulin receptor antibodies
  - – Others
- • Other genetic syndromes sometimes associated with diabetes:
  - – Down's syndrome
  - – Klinefelter's syndrome
  - – Turner's syndrome
  - – Wolfram's syndrome
  - – Friedreich's ataxia
  - – Huntington's chorea
  - – Laurence-Moon-Biedl syndrome
  - – Myotonic dystrophy
  - – Porphyria
  - – Prader-Willi syndrome
  - – Others
- • GDM

Source: Adapted from American Diabetes Association, 2014.

Abbreviations: HNF = Hepatocyte nuclear factor; MODY = Maturity-onset diabetes of the young; IPF-1 = Insulin promoter factor-1; CMV = Cytomegalovirus; GDM = Gestational diabetes mellitus; DNA = Deoxyribo-nucleic acid

EPIDEMIOLOGY

The prevalence of diabetes has risen worldwide dramatically over the past few decades, from an estimated 30 million cases in 1985 to 285 million cases in 2010. Based on current trends, the International Diabetes Federation (IDF) projects that 438 million individuals will have diabetes by 2030, of which about 100 million will be in India (Table 91.2).

Diabetes Studies from India

There is a trend towards more young persons, especially women from rural areas to develop DM (10-year analysis 1994–2004).

Source: Sreedhar GR, et al. J Assoc Phys Ind. 2010;58(210): 290-4.

Type 2 DM is by far the most common type of diabetes encountered in India, accounting for more than 95% of the total diabetics (Table 91.3). It generally starts between the ages of 30 years and 40 years (Table 91.4). The incidence increases with age; males are more commonly affected and 58% of the Indian diabetics have a positive family history of diabetes. The incidence of type 1 DM in India is very low. In Asia, the onset of type 2 DM appears at lower body mass index (BMI) and at younger age compared to western counterparts, possibly because of greater abdominal adiposity, i.e. higher waist circumference despite of lower BMI, increased insulin resistance and reduced insulin secretory capacity. The prevalence of type 2 DM

Table 91.2: Estimated number of diabetes patients (in million)

Country	In 2011	Country	In 2030
China	90.0	China	129.7
India	61.3	India	101.2
United States	23.7	United States	29.6
Russian Federation	12.6	Brazil	19.6
Brazil	12.4	Bangladesh	16.8
Japan	10.7	Mexico	16.4
Mexico	10.3	Russian Federation	14.1
Bangladesh	8.4	Egypt	12.4
Egypt	7.3	Indonesia	11.8
Indonesia	7.3	Pakistan	11.4

Table 91.3: Break up of types of diabetes mellitus (DM) seen in a tertiary care hospital in Trivandrum (2005–7)

Types of DM	%
Type 2 DM	96
Type 1 DM	0.8
GDM	1.2
DM secondary to drugs, pancreatic disease and viral infections	±2

Source: Poulose KP. Total number of cases 8,206. Personal communication.

Abbreviations: DM = Diabetes mellitus; GDM = Gestational diabetes mellitus

Table 91.4: Age of onset of type 2 diabetes mellitus (DM)

Age group (years)	%
< 30	4
31–40	25
41–50	37
51–60	20
61–70	9
> 70	5

is increasing much more rapidly, presumably because of increasing obesity, reduced physical activity level and aging of the population. The multicenter National Urban Diabetes Survey (NUDS), done in year 2000 showed that the prevalence of type 2 DM was 12.1% in population of age more than 20 years in urban India. This survey revealed that the prevalence in the southern part of India is higher. The study also suggested that the prevalence of impaired glucose tolerance (IGT) was 14.0% with no gender difference in population of age more than 20 years. More recent studies have shown that the prevalence is increasing with rates of 10–13% in urban areas and 2.4% in rural areas.

Source: Nagpal J, Kumar A, Kakar S, et al. The development of Quality of Life Instrument for Indian Diabetes patients (QOLID): a validation and reliability study in middle and higher income groups. J Assoc Physicians India. 2010;58:295-304.

The present trend shows that type 1 DM in children also will rise by 100% in incidence by 2020 in European countries and the prevalence of DM will rise by 70%. Hyperglycemia and DM are rising globally, driven by population growth and ageing of the population.

Type 1 DM is more common among the Caucasian populations of Finland, Sweden, USA and UK accounting

Textbook of Medicine

for 25–150 per 100,000 populations. Its prevalence in India is less than 1% of all diabetics.

A survey conducted in Neyyattinkara taluk of Thiruvananthapuram district under the auspices of Health Action by People (HAP) on 8,300 persons revealed that the overall prevalence of type 2 DM in persons aged 20 years and above was 6.7% with higher prevalence in males. When adjusted to an internationally comparable population, the prevalence in those aged 30–64 years worked out to be 8.2%. The demographic pattern of type 2 DM is also changing with a shift to start in younger persons. In the USA where the overall prevalence increased by 33% between 1990 and 1998 and the prevalence in the age group 30–39 years rose by 70%.

DIAGNOSIS

The revised diagnostic criteria (Box 91.1) gives equal importance to fasting plasma glucose (FPG) and 2-hour post glucose-load plasma glucose (2hPG) for diagnosis of diabetes, thereby eliminating the need for a routine oral glucose tolerance test (OGTT) for diagnosis of diabetes. The cutoff level of FPG for diagnosis of diabetes has been fixed as 126 mg/dL, since this reflects the same degree of hyperglycemia as a 2hPG of 200 mg/dL in terms of susceptibility for development of microvascular complications. These criteria are expected to rationalize and simplify the diagnosis of diabetes and a larger number of people could be screened due to the simplification of the procedure of doing only FPG rather than an OGTT.

Recently, glycosylated hemoglobin (HbA1C) has been added as a third option to diagnose diabetes by an International Expert Committee. HbA1C is formed by glycation (nonenzymatic addition of a sugar residue to protein) of N-terminal valine residue of each β chain. The HbA1C test should be performed using a standardized

---

Box 91.1: Revised criteria for diagnosis of diabetes mellitus (DM)

- Symptoms of diabetes + Random blood PG ≥ 200 mg/dL
  OR
- FPG ± 126 mg/dL
  OR
- 2-hour post glucose-load plasma glucose (2h-PGBS) ± 200 mg/dL during OGTT
  OR
- HbA1C > 6.5%

Source: Adapted from American Diabetes Association, 2014.

Note:

- Random is defined as without regard to time since the last meal. The classic symptoms of diabetes include polyuria, polydipsia and unexplained weight loss.
- Fasting is defined as no caloric intake for at least 8 hours.
- The test should be performed as described by the World Health Organization (WHO) using a glucose load containing the equivalent of 75 g of anhydrous glucose dissolved in water, not recommended for routine clinical use.
- HbA1C should be performed in certified laboratory according to HbA1C standards of the Diabetes Control and Complications Trial (DCCT).
- In the absence of unequivocal hyperglycemia with acute metabolic decompensation, these criteria should be confirmed by repeat testing on a different day.

Abbreviations: PG = Plasma glucose; FPG = Fasting plasma glucose; OGTT = Oral glucose tolerance test; HbA1C = Glycosylated hemoglobin

---

Table 91.5: Criteria for diagnosis of prediabetes

Category	Normal	Prediabetes IFG/IGT
FPG (mg/dL)	< 100	100–125
2h-PG (mg/dL)	< 140	140–199
HbA1C (%)	< 5.6	5.7–6.4

Source: Adapted from American Diabetes Association, 2014.
Abbreviations: FPG = Fasting plasma glucose; 2hPG = 2-hour post glucose-load plasma glucose; HbA1C = Glycosylated hemoglobin; IFG = Impaired fasting glucose; IGT = Impaired glucose tolerance

method. Epidemiological data show a similar relationship of A1C with the risk of retinopathy as seen with FPG and 2hPG. The HbA1C has several advantages to the FPG and OGTT, including greater convenience (fasting not required) and less day-to-day variations during stress and illness. These advantages must be balanced by greater cost, the limited availability of HbA1C testing in certain regions of the developing world, and the incomplete correlation between A1C and average glucose in certain individuals.

An intermediate group of subjects are recognized whose glucose levels, although not meeting the criteria for diabetes are nevertheless too high to be considered altogether normal. This group is defined as having ***impaired fasting glucose (IFG)*** when FPG levels above 100 mg/dL but below 126 mg/dL and IGT when 2-hour values in the OGTT of 140 mg/dL or above, but below 200 mg/dL (Table 91.5). On the same grounds, subjects with HbA1C between 5.7% and 6.4% are classified as ***prediabetes***. These individuals are at relatively high risk for the future development of diabetes. IFG and IGT are not considered as clinical entities on their own right but rather risk factors for diabetes and cardiovascular disease (CVD) and are often associated with obesity (especially abdominal or visceral obesity), dyslipidemia with high triglycerides and/or low high-density lipoprotein cholesterol (HDL-C), and hypertension. Aggressive interventions and vigilant follow-up should be pursued for those considered at very high risk (e.g. those with HbA1C > 6.0%).

Screening

The same tests should be used for both screening as well as diagnosis of diabetes. Screening in asymptomatic people should be considered in adults of any age with BMI above 25 kg/m² (>23 kg/m² for people with Asian origin) with one or more additional risk factors for diabetes (Box 91.2). The testing should begin at age of 45 years even without any risk factors. The tests should be repeated every 3 years, if baseline results are normal. In the absence of the above criteria, testing for diabetes should begin at age of 45 years. If results are normal, testing should be repeated at least at 3 year intervals. More frequent testing should be considered depending on initial results (e.g. those with prediabetes should be tested yearly) and risk status.

PHYSIOLOGY, PATHOLOGY AND ETIOPATHOGENESIS

Pancreas

The endocrine component of the pancreas consists of different types of cells: α-cells, β-cells, δ-cells and

Box 91.2: Criteria for testing for diabetes in asymptomatic adult individuals

Additional risk factors warranting screening for diabetes in overweight/obese adults:

- Physical inactivity
- First-degree relative with diabetes
- High-risk race/ethnicity (e.g. African-American, Latino, Native-American, Asian-American, Pacific islander)
- Women who delivered a baby weighing > 4 kg or were diagnosed with GDM
- Hypertension (>140/90 mm Hg or on therapy for hypertension)
- HDL cholesterol level < 35 mg/dL (0.90 mmol/L) and/or a triglyceride level > 250 mg/dL (2.82 mmol/L)
- Women with polycystic ovarian syndrome
- HbA1C > 5.7%, IGT, or IFG on previous testing
- Other clinical conditions associated with insulin resistance (e.g. severe obesity, acanthosis nigricans)
- History of CVD

Source: Adapted from American Diabetes Association, 2014.
Abbreviations: GDM = Gestational diabetes mellitus; HDL = High-density lipoprotein; IFG = Impaired fasting glucose; IGT = Impaired glucose tolerance; CVD = Cardiovascular disease

pancreatic polypeptide (PP) cells contained in the islets of Langerhans which constitute 1% of its weight. There are 100,000 islets in the pancreas, and each islet contains 1,000–3,000 cells. Thus, altogether there are 100–300 million β-cells in the pancreas which are the only source of the polypeptide hormone insulin. Pancreatic β-cells can store 200 units of insulin and can release 30–50 units of insulin per day. Ninty-five percent of cells of the pancreas have exocrine function and 5% have endocrine function. The β-cells produce insulin, α-cells produce glucagon, δ-cells produce somatostatin and the PP cells produce pancreatic polypeptide.

Insulin Synthesis, Secretion and Action

Biosynthesis and Structure of Insulin

This is the hormone produced by the β-cells of the islets of Langerhans and is composed of two polypeptide chains. A and B linked together by two disulfide bonds. The genetic locus for insulin is on chromosome 11 and that for the receptors is on chromosome 19. Initially, preproinsulin (a single chain of 86 amino acid precursor polypeptide) is secreted into the endoplasmic reticulum. Subsequent proteolytic processing removes the amino terminal signal peptide, giving rise to proinsulin. Proinsulin is structurally related to insulin-like growth factors I and II (IGF), which can bind to the insulin receptor although weakly. It can cross-reacts with insulin antibodies but, has none of the metabolic effects of insulin. Lastly, the polypeptide is clipped at two positions to release the intervening C-peptide and the A (21 amino acids) and B (30 amino acids) chains of active insulin. Finally, the active insulin and C-peptide are packaged into secretory granules for storage and co-secreted under appropriate stimulus. C-peptide is a useful marker of insulin secretion and it allows discrimination of endogenous and exogenous sources of insulin. Testing of serum C-peptide levels has a diagnostic utility in the classification of diabetes, especially in young patients as well as in decision-making for initiation of insulin therapy.

Insulin Secretion

Insulin is released from secretory granules by the process of exocytosis. Glucose is the key nutrient which regulates insulin secretion by the pancreatic β-cell; although a variety of nutrient and non-nutrient products regulate endogenous insulin release. Amino acids, ketones and various other nutrients also influence insulin secretion. Non-nutrient regulators of insulin are islet products (mainly glucagon), neurotransmitters, gastrointestinal (GI) hormones and adipokines, like adiponectin. The rate of secretion increases progressively at extracellular glucose levels between 90 mg/dL and 270 mg/dL, with half of maximal stimulation at around 140 mg/dL. After glucose is transported into β-cells, it gets phosphorylated by ***glucokinase***, which is the rate-limiting step of glucose-regulated insulin secretion. Further, glycolysis of glucose-6-phosphate generates ATP (adenosine triphosphate), which causes rapid and reversible inhibition of the activity of an ATP-sensitive potassium ion (K^+) channel. Inhibition of permeability to potassium ions through K^+ channel depolarizes β-cell membrane opening voltage-dependent calcium channels. An influx of calcium inside the β-cells thus stimulates insulin secretion. The secreted insulin enters the portal circulation of which 50–60% is trapped by the liver. The remaining portion enters the peripheral circulation. This can be estimated as immunoreactive insulin (IRI). Basal value of IRI in health is 2–20 μU/mL. Since C-peptide is secreted in equimolar quantities with insulin, its level can be estimated to assess the functioning of β-cell reserve.

Insulin Action

The fuel homeostasis of the whole body is regulated by insulin via its specific effects in multiple target tissues which vary dramatically from tissue to tissue. These uniquely expressed effector systems are described in skeletal muscle, adipose tissue and liver, three organs primarily responsible for fuel storage and oxidation as well as counter-regulatory metabolism. These are often called 'insulin-sensitive tissues'. The insulin receptors are large molecular-weight proteins (500,000 Daltons), which mediate insulin action. The metabolic actions are together known as post receptor effect. Binding of insulin to its receptor promotes the uptake of glucose into skeletal muscle (where it is utilized for energy production) and adipose tissue (where it is converted into triglycerides for storage) by type 4 glucose transporters (GLUT4). This binding in turn stimulates a signal transduction cascade which induces glycogen synthesis, protein synthesis, lipogenesis and regulation of various genes in insulin-responsive cells. Sensitivity of insulin depends upon the number of unbound receptors. The number of receptors varies inversely with the levels of circulatory insulin. The sensitivity of the receptors to insulin has a major role to play in the causation of DM.

Plasma glucose levels are maintained within a physiological range by a balance between hepatic glucose production and peripheral glucose uptake and utilization depending on the external energy (in the form of food) intake. This is achieved by low-insulin levels in fasting state which increases hepatic gluconeogenesis and glycogenolysis, reduces glucose uptake by peripheral tissue and mobilizes stored precursors, such as amino acids (proteolysis) and free-fatty acids (FFA) (lipolysis). IRI level ranges from 5 IU/mL to 50 IU/mL in fasting normal subjects. Food intake elicits a rise in insulin and fall in glucagon resulting in a reversal of these processes. Insulin retards gluconeogenesis in the liver. Excess glucose entering the skeletal muscle is converted into glycogen. Insulin helps to build up adipose tissue by aiding the conversion of glucose into fat and blocks the escape of fatty acids from fat cells. In conjunction with growth hormone, insulin enhances the incorporation of amino acids into peptides in the liver and skeletal muscles. Insulin activates a series of lipid and protein kinase enzymes linked to the translocation of glucose transporters to the cell surface, for the synthesis of glycogen, proteins, messenger ribonucleic acid (mRNAs) and nuclear deoxyribonucleic acid (DNA) which affect cell survival and proliferation. Glucagon-like peptide (GLP-1) is a potent insulin-releasing hormone, which triggers insulin release in response to postprandial hyperglycemia. Substances having this property are listed as *incretins*.

Pathogenesis of Type 1 DM

Type 1 DM has been classified into type 1A in which cell-mediated autoimmune attack on the β-cells is more prominent and type 1B in which the mechanism is less clear. Type 1B is less frequent of the two. In Asians and Africans, type 1B is seen more frequently than in the whites. Human leukocyte antigen (HLA) DR/DQ confers 50% susceptibility whereas other genes confer 15%. Type 1 DM is a heterogeneous disorder in which several factors may play a role. These are the HLA system, viral infections and autoimmune processes.

Human Leukocyte Antigen Associations

Type 1 DM tends to be a familial disorder and there is a 25-fold increase in the risk amongst the siblings than the general population. Its inheritance is related to HLA locus on chromosome 6. It is seen that HLA B8, B15, B6, B21, BW3, DR3 and DR4 are associated with a higher risk of DM. On the other hand, a negative association has also been noted with HLA B7 (Table 91.6). In Asian Indians and Japanese, type 2 DM appears to be associated more with HLA BW21 and BW54 than with B8. HLA DR4 is associated with two alleles of the DQB1 locus—DQw8 and DQw7 and five alleles of DRB1 locus. 96% of type 2 diabetics are homozygous for the amino acid aspartic at position 57 of the DQ beta chain, compared with only 19% of the general

Table 91.6: Human leukocyte antigen (HLA) and the effects on type 1 diabetes mellitus (DM) susceptibility

HLA antigen	Effect on DM susceptibility
DQ2	Predisposes
DQ8	Predisposes
DQ7	Neutral/protects
DQ6	Protects
DQ18	Protects

Table 91.7: Other autoimmune diseases commonly associated with type 1 DM

Associated autoimmune diseases			
Autoantibody			
Disease	Type	Percentage	Disease prevalence (%)
Addison's disease	21-hydroxylase	1.5	0.5
Celiac disease	Transglutaminase	12	6
Pernicious anemia	Parietal cell	21	2.6
Thyroiditis or Graves' disease	Peroxidase or thyroglobulin	25	4

population. Both DQw8 (DR3 associated) and DQw2 (DR4 associated) have a neutral amino acid at position 57 rather than aspartic. DR3 and DR4 (DQw8 and DQw2) heterozygous individuals in the general population can now be identified who have an 8% risk of developing type 1 DM. DR2 and DQR1 afford strong protection. Among identical twins, only 50% show concordance for type 1 DM as against 100% for type 2 DM.

Despite current emphasis on genes within the major histocompatibility complex (MHC), it is likely that genetic susceptibility to type 1 DM in humans will be influenced by multiple genes. Genetic heterogeneity will not only influence the probability of autoimmune-β cell destruction but also the rate of damage and age of onset of type 1 DM. The DQB1 allele is associated with high levels of anti-GAD (glutamic acid decarboxylase) antibodies and the DR4 alleles are associated with elevated levels of anti-insulin antibodies (Table 91.7). For the development of type 1 DM, 50% susceptibility is conferred by HLA. Other genetic factors confer 15%. In the west, only 50–60% of type 1 diabetics are below the age of 18 years. The situation in India is not very clearly known.

The immunological and metabolic changes occur long before the development of symptoms of hyperglycemia. This period preceding the development of diabetes, is known as prediabetes during which there is an increase in the levels of pancreatic islet cell antibodies (PICA) and impaired first-phase insulin release (FPIR) and this is the stage where preventive strategies are being aimed at in interventional trials.

Autoimmunity

These are the antibodies produced against certain antigens of the β-cells. They have not been found to have any etiological role in type 1 DM, but mainly serve as markers of type 1 DM. These antigens are GAD, insulin antibodies, islet-associated antigen 2 (IA-2) antibody, islet cell antibody (ICA), zinc transporter 8 (ZnT8), etc. Based on the pathogenesis, type 1 DM has been divided into type 1A and type 1B. In the former, there is cell-mediated autoimmune attack on β-cells. Type 1B is less frequent. The cause is not clearly known. Type 1B is more seen in Asians and Africans.

Infections

Coxsackie B4 has been incriminated to play a causal role in the pathogenesis of type 1 DM. The other viruses known to play a role are mumps, cytomegalovirus (CMV), Epstein-Barr virus (EBV), varicella and the viruses causing infective hepatitis. An autoimmune etiology is suggested by its association with other autoimmune disorders, such as Hashimoto's thyroiditis, pernicious anemia and Addison's disease. PICA and cell surface antibodies are demonstrable in several patients with recent onset type 1 DM. It is possible that all the three factors, namely HLA status, viral infections and autoimmunity, interact to produce the disease. In type 1 DM, there is progressive loss of β-cell and in severe forms they may be totally absent. Insulin secretion progressively decreases to almost nil when the disease is fully established.

Latent Autoimmune Diabetes in the Adult

A slow onset form of type 1 DM has been described. In this subtype, subjects are initially well-controlled with oral drugs (mimicking type 2 DM) but have a rapid acceleration of β-cell failure, leading to a frank autoimmune β-cell failure and long-term dependence on insulin in later years.

Pathogenesis of Type 2 DM

Type 2 DM is considered as a 'multifactorial' or 'complex' disease due to the complex interaction between various genetic and environmental factors in its pathogenesis. Multiple evidences suggest that genetic factors play a major role in this condition. A genetic predisposition running through families is evident. Identical twins invariably develop type 2 DM when exposed to the same environmental factors. In genetically predisposed individuals, several environmental factors precipitate the onset of diabetes. Important among these are obesity, physical inactivity, repeated pregnancies, infections, physical or psychological stress and diabetogenic drugs. The interplay of genetic and environmental factors is well brought out by the studies on migrant Indians who have settled in affluent countries. These studies show that although the prevalence of diabetes in India is about 6–7%, it increases sharply to 10–12% in Indians who have migrated to the developed countries. Birth of large babies weighing above 4 kg is a strong pointer to the subsequent development of diabetes in the mother.

Pathogenesis of type 2 DM is characterized by impaired insulin secretion, insulin resistance, excessive hepatic glucose production and abnormal fat metabolism.

Obesity

The current obesity epidemic due to the modern sedentary life and caloric abundance is a major factor that predisposes to type 2 DM. Hence, it is invariably seen that type 2 DM is closely related to obesity. Obese subjects show a relative resistance to the action of insulin due to a reduction in the number of insulin receptors on the target cells. The full complement of receptors is restored on shedding the excess weight. There is an association between low-birth weight and occurrence of IGT or DM in young adulthood. Increase in the BMI after the age of 2 years is also associated with the chance of developing diabetes.

Physical Inactivity

Many of the diabetics are physically inactive. Physical exercise improves their insulin sensitivity and improves glycemic control.

Role of Insulin Antagonists

Glucose metabolism is delicately balanced by the coordinated effects of insulin antagonist hormones like glucagon, cortisol, catecholamines and growth hormone. Several other hormones also take part in the metabolism of carbohydrates. Imbalance of this hormonal profile results in carbohydrate intolerance. Fatty acids which compete with carbohydrate for metabolism in muscle lead to insulin resistance. In hyperlipidemia, insulin-dependent carbohydrate metabolism suffers and a relative insulin resistance develops. The problem of antibodies to insulin, especially to the animal insulin, is rarely encountered in the case of human insulin and analogue insulins.

Amylin

Another polypeptide cosecreted by pancreatic β-cells is islet amyloid polypeptide (IAPP) or amylin. The physiological role of IAPP is not completely defined, but due to several reasons it gets deposited as insoluble fibers in the islets of patients with type 2 DM. This islet amyloidosis, which is the main pathological hallmark, seen in 90% of patients with type 2 DM at autopsy studies, is considered to be one of the factors responsible for β-cell failure in addition to glucotoxicity and lipotoxicity. Its analogue is sometimes used in treating type 1 DM and type 2 DM.

Role of Genomics

Some information on genetic susceptibility is available for gene effects and is summarized in Table 91.8.

Source: McCarthy MI. Genomics, type 2 diabetes, and obesity. N Engl J Med. 2010;363(24):2339-50.

Pathological Changes

Pancreas

In type 1 DM, the β-cells of the islets of Langerhans show reduction in number, degranulation and hyalinization. In recent onset type 1 DM, lymphocytic infiltration of the islets occurs and this may be caused by viral infection. Inflammation is seen particularly around the β-cells only and not around the other types of cells. This inflammation causes progressive destruction of β-cells leading to absolute insulin deficiency.

In type 2 DM, during the early phase, β-cells are normal in number or only slightly reduced. The β-cells lose their sensitivity to the hyperglycemic stimulus for releasing insulin. As a result, insulin secretion loses its

Table 91.8: Effect of genes in glucose metabolism leads to types 2 DM

Gene	Effects
CDKN2A, CDKN2B, CDKAL1	Reduced β-cells mass, reduced insulin secretion
MTNR1B, TCF7L2, KCNJ11	β-cells dysfunction, reduced insulin secretion
FTO	Obesity and insulin resistance
IRS1, PPARG	Insulin resistance unrelated to obesity

Abbreviations: CDKN2A = Cyclin-dependent kinase inhibitor 2A; CDKN2B = Cyclin-dependent kinase inhibitor 2B; CDKAL1 = Cyclin-dependent kinase 5 regulatory subunit-associated protein 1-like; MTNR1B = Melatonin receptor 1B; TCF7L2 = Transcription factor 7 like 2; KCNJ11 = Potassium voltage-gated channel subfamily J member 11; FTO = Fat mass and obesity-associated

smooth and fine relationship with glucose level. It tends to be erratic. In the early stages of evolution of type 2 DM, the reduction in the sensitivity of the receptors is compensated by overproduction of insulin and accompanying hyperinsulinemia. Frank diabetes results when β-cells start failing, and insulin production comes down on the background of insulin resistance. Insulin resistance in muscle develops early in persons who would develop type 2 DM later. β-cell function starts deteriorating about 10 years before the onset of DM, by which time the β-cell function has fallen to 30% or less.

Vascular Changes

Diabetics show a predisposition to develop vascular lesions affecting both small and large blood vessels. In microangiopathy, there is specific involvement of the small blood vessels. Venules, capillaries and arterioles are affected in this process. There is deposition of PAS (periodic acid Schiff) positive material in the capillary basement membrane. Glycosylation of several proteins in the vessel wall results in increased permeability. The basement membrane is thickened. Ultimately, there is vascular occlusion.

Microangiopathy is most marked in type 1 DM, developing early in life but also occurs in type 2 DM. Various factors, like endothelial damage, increased plasma viscosity, erythrocyte aggregation, reduced red cell deformability and increased platelet adhesion, lead to microangiopathy. The problem is more complex and the entire process is still not fully understood. Microangiopathy affects several organ systems. The main lesions are seen in the retina, kidneys, peripheral nerves and heart giving rise to diabetic retinopathy, nephropathy, many forms of diabetic neuropathy and cardiomyopathy.

Macroangiopathy

A diabetic is prone to develop occlusive vascular disease in medium-sized arteries, such as the coronary, cerebral and peripheral limb vessels. The process is one of atheroma which sets in at younger ages and is more extensive than that occurring in nondiabetics. These lesions lead to increased risk of ischemic heart disease (IHD), cerebrovascular accidents (CVA) and ischemia to the limbs with intermittent claudication and peripheral gangrene. Macroangiopathy largely accounts for the steep rise in mortality in middle-aged diabetics.

Retinopathy

DM produces a classical retinopathy. A specific change occurs in the vessels leading to loss of mural cells (pericytes) and formation of microaneurysms. The occurrence of retinopathy is related more to the duration of the disease than to the severity. Once initiated, the fundus changes are usually progressive. The early changes are venous dilation and the appearance of small dot-like microaneurysms in the perimacular area. Arterial blood is shunted and this leads to ischemia of the retina. Increased vascular permeability accounts for the formation of exudates. In the next stage, dot and blot hemorrhages predominate. Large subhyaloid hemorrhages and vitreous hemorrhages may develop and vision is seriously impaired. Such hemorrhages are due to rupture of newly formed blood vessels. As these hemorrhages are absorbed, organization by fibrous tissue results and multiple bands of retinitis proliferans develop. These lead to permanent visual impairment. The fibrous bands may contract giving rise to retinal detachment; leaking vessels in the retina can be demonstrated by fluorescein angiography. Retinopathy is usually associated with advanced nephropathy. Sometimes in diabetic ketoacidosis (DKA) with severe hyperlipidemia, the fat gives a milky-white appearance to the retinal arteries called *lipemia retinalis*.

Renal Lesions
(*See* also Section 16, Ch 187)

These are commonly seen in subjects who have had diabetes for over 15–20 years. Vascular changes include—arteriosclerosis of the renal artery, sclerosis of the arterioles and glomerulosclerosis. Glomerulosclerosis may be nodular (***Kimmelstiel-Wilson lesion***) or diffuse. There is accumulation of PAS-positive eosinophilic material within the mesangium. There is thickening of the glomerular capillary basement membrane. The establishment of glomerulosclerosis is indicated by the presence of proteinuria. Further damage to the glomeruli results in the development of chronic renal failure.

Distinct stages can be defined in the evolution of diabetic nephropathy. In the initial stages, asymptomatic microalbuminuria in which up to 200 µg/min of albumin may be lost in the urine. Normal subjects do not lose more than 20 µg/min or 300 mg of protein in 24 hours. Microalbuminuria is not detectable by the ordinary laboratory tests. In type 1 DM, there is elevation of systolic blood pressure (BP) during sleep preceding microalbuminuria. This rise in BP is an important contributory factor in the development of structural changes in the kidneys. It is absolutely necessary to control BP also along with blood sugar to prevent deterioration.

In the early stage, the kidneys are enlarged, more vascular and the GFR is increased. In the second stage, there is microalbuminuria and in third stage, proteinuria is more pronounced and easily detectable by routine tests. Loss of 3.5 g or more of protein in 24 hours may lead to the development of nephrotic syndrome. Hypertension develops during this stage. In the fourth stage, further structural changes develop and the GFR comes down with gradual increase in the blood levels of metabolic waste products, such as creatinine and urea. The fifth stage is one of gross reduction of GFR and overt renal failure with azotemia, severe hypertension and complications, such as cardiac failure and end-stage renal failure. Autonomic neuropathy may lead to functional obstruction of the bladder, retention with overflow, urinary infection, and, further deterioration of renal functions. Another system of classification is based on creatinine clearance.

The diabetic patient is predisposed to develop urinary infection, and therefore, acute pyelonephritis and chronic pyelonephritis are very common. Fulminant urinary infection leads to ischemic necrosis of the renal papillary. This condition presents as acute anuric renal failure. Fleshy masses may be passed in the urine. These are the necrosed papillae and the condition is called papillitis necrotic and ulcerans. ***Emphysematous pyelonephritis (EPN)*** is another serious complication in which there is production of gas in renal and perinephric tissues. This occurs only in DM.

Peripheral Nerves

In the myelinated nerve fibers, axonal atrophy was considered to be the primary lesion, secondary to ineffective axonal transport. Axoglial dysfunction and abnormalities of paranodal connections between the terminal myelin loops and the axonal membrane have also been described. This could explain the reduction in nerve conduction velocity. This improves with therapeutic inhibition of ***aldose reductase***. More recent studies, however, provide evidence for the presence of demyelination and hence, Schwann's cell involvement is the primary lesion. As the myelinated fibers degenerate, there is an attempt to regenerate, which manifests in the form of regeneration clusters. With progress of the neuropathy, the density of the regeneration clusters also comes down.

Structural abnormalities have also been found in the vessels supplying the nerve fibers. The epineural vessels show arteriolar attenuation, venous distension, arteriovenous shunting and new vessel formation along with intimal hyperplasia and hypertrophy, denervation and reduction in neuropeptide expression. The perineural vessels also demonstrate basement membrane thickening and endothelial cell hypertrophy and hyperplasia. There is also a reduction in capillary density and occurrence of pericyte loss with reduction of endoneural oxygen tension and blood flow to the nerves. In a large series from South India, overall prevalence of diabetic neuropathy was 19.1% among a group of 1,000 consecutive diabetic patients. Age and the duration of diabetes were important risk factors.

CLINICAL FEATURES

The classically described clinical manifestations of diabetes are polyuria (excessive urination), polydipsia (increased thirst) and polyphagia (increased hunger). Though the symptoms are similar in both types of diabetes, in type 1 DM, they develop acutely whereas in the majority of the type 2 DM the onset is insidious. Type 1 DM patients are usually below the age of 30 years, thin and emaciated and unless promptly treated with insulin, they would develop ketoacidosis (Table 91.9).

Due to the high prevalence of obesity, type 2 DM is occurring at earlier ages as a global phenomenon, especially in developed countries. Type 2 diabetic patients are generally above the age of 30 years; obese, usually asymptomatic and may present directly with the vascular complications of diabetes. Around 50% of the cases present with classical symptoms of polyuria, polyphagia and weight loss. These symptoms can be directly correlated with hyperglycemia and glycosuria. Other clinical presentations, which warrant full investigation to exclude diabetes, are following:
- Nonhealing ulcers
- Recurrent respiratory or urinary tract infections (UTIs)
- Rapid changes in refraction of the eyes

Table 91.9: Clinical differences between type 1 DM and type 2 DM

Clinical features	Type 1 DM	Type 2 DM
Usual age at onset (years)	5–30	35–65
Sex	Male: Female = 1:1	Female > Male (in India)
Prevalence	15–18%	95–98%
Among diabetes	Caucasians 1% in Indians	Indians
Genetic	Heredity + Strong HLA association	Heredity +++ Weak HLA association
Insulin deficiency	Invariable	Relative
Insulin resistance	Rare	Common
Nutrition	Lean	Often obese
Usual onset	Rapid with classic symptoms	Slow, insidious, often detected on routine examination
Ketosis	Prone	Not prone
Islet cell antibodies	May be present within 1 year of onset	Absent
Treatment modality	Require insulin for survival	Majority can be controlled by lifestyle modifications ± oral antidiabetic medications
Common cause of death	Nephropathy, CHD, DKA	CHD, nephropathy, stroke and gangrene

Abbreviations: HLA = Human leukocyte antigen; CHD = Coronary heart disease; DKA = Diabetic ketoacidosis

- Steady and unexplained rapid weight loss
- Increased tendency for fungal infections, like moniliasis, balanoposthitis and vulvitis
- Unexplained peripheral neuropathy
- Premature onset of IHD, stroke or vascular occlusions
- History of overweight babies and recurrent fetal loss in women
- Premature cataract often below the age of 50 years and retinopathy
- Impotence in males
- Any vague ill-health.

In some cases, diabetics may present to the doctor for the first time with any of the major emergencies, without any apparent illness previously.

Acanthosis nigricans is a cutaneous marker of hyperinsulinemia; this manifests as darkish pigmentation and thickening of the skin, usually around the nape of the neck. Several factors account for the frequency and time of onset of complications in diabetes. These include the abnormalities of glucose levels, duration of diabetes, genetic factors, smoking, obesity, hypertension, hyperlipidemia and others.

Maturity-onset Diabetes of the Young (MODY)

It accounts for about 2–3% of all type 2 DM and about 27% of all diabetes in the young below 30 years of age in India. The clinical picture of type 2 DM and MODY is almost similar. Both are insidious in onset and nonketotic, but the latter develops at a much younger age. Family history is very prominent in MODY. BMI may be high in more

Table 91.10: Genetic and clinical features of MODY

Type	Gene defects	Prevalence	Signs
MODY-1	HNF-4α Chromosome 20q12, 13 involved	5%	Severe hyperglycemia Microvascular complications. They may need insulin
MODY-2	Glucokinase Chromosome 7p15	10%	Mild microvascular complications are mild. Diet control alone may be sufficient
MODY-3	HNF-1α Most common type chromosome 12q24	70%	Symptoms as in MODY-1
MODY-4	IPF-1 mutation chromosome 13q12	Rare	Like MODY-3
MODY-5	HNF-1β mutation chromosome 17q 12-21	Rare	Microvascular complications and renal failure are common
MODY-6	Chromosome 2q32	Very rare	

Abbreviations: MODY = Maturity-onset diabetes of the young; HNF = Hepatocyte nuclear factor; IPF-1 = Insulin promoter factor-1

than 40% of MODY cases and it may be low in 13%. The features suggestive of the insulin resistance are *Acanthosis nigricans*, hypertension and abdominal obesity, which are not found in MODY. Strong family history running into three generations with autosomal-dominant inheritance is the most characteristic feature of MODY.

Although six different forms of MODY (Table 91.10) have been identified (MODY-1 to MODY-6), each involving mutation of a different gene located in a different chromosome, only three are considered more important. The first MODY gene to be recognized was a glucokinase gene (GCK) followed by hepatocyte nuclear factors (HNF: 1α, 4α, 1β). HNFs are transcription factors that regulate the expression of several genes in the liver and β-cells of pancreas. In all types of MODY, there is defect in insulin secretion by the β-cells, but the clinical presentation may be different. Some may respond to oral hypoglycemic agents (OHAs), but others require insulin.

EVALUATION

Initial medical and laboratory evaluations to classify diabetes, detect the presence of diabetic complications, review previous treatment and risk factor control in patients with established diabetes should be performed to assist in formulating a management plan (Table 91.11). Frequent follow-up visits to monitor the glycemic status should be based on individual patient's need.

TREATMENT

The aim of treatment is to achieve normal blood glucose levels throughout day and night, to alleviate symptoms and to prevent complications. The four pillars of diabetic management are

- Diet
- Exercise
- Drugs
- Patient education, backed up by regular monitoring of glycemic control and early detection and treatment of complications.

Table 91.11: Scheme for the total evaluation of a diabetic before starting therapy

Parameters	Evaluation
Clinical history	<ul><li>Age and way of onset of diabetes (e.g. symptomatic or during routine checkup)</li><li>Diet patterns, physical activity and recent change in weight</li><li>Developmental history in children and adolescents</li><li>Diabetes education and awareness history</li><li>Review of previous medical and laboratory records (HbA1C records)</li><li>Current treatment of diabetes</li><li>Results of SMBG (by glucometer)</li><li>History of DKA</li><li>***Hypoglycemic episodes:***<ul><li>Hypoglycemia symptoms</li><li>Any severe hypoglycemia (hypoglycemia requiring assistance from another person)</li></ul></li><li>***History of diabetes-related complications:***<ul><li>***Microvascular:*** Retinopathy, nephropathy, neuropathy (sensory, including history of foot lesions; autonomic, including sexual dysfunction and gastroparesis)</li><li>***Macrovascular:*** CHD, cerebrovascular disease and peripheral vascular disease</li><li>***Other:*** Psychosocial problems, dental disease</li></ul></li></ul>
Physical examination	<ul><li>Height, weight, waist circumference</li><li>BP (sitting and orthostatic)</li><li>Fundus examination</li><li>Thyroid palpation</li><li>*Acanthosis nigricans*</li><li>Insulin injection sites</li><li>***Comprehensive foot examination:***<ul><li>Inspection for ulcer, callous, fungal infections, deformity, ingrown toe-nails</li><li>Palpation of dorsalis pedis and posterior tibial pulses</li><li>Presence/absence of patellar and Achilles tendon reflexes</li><li>Determination of proprioception, vibration and monofilament sensation</li></ul></li></ul>
Laboratory evaluation	<ul><li>HbA1C every 3–6 months</li><li>***Annually:***<ul><li>Fasting lipid profile, including total, LDL and HDL cholesterol and triglycerides</li><li>Liver enzymes</li><li>Test for urine albumin excretion with spot urine albumin to creatinine ratio or microalbumin</li><li>Serum creatinine and calculated GFR</li><li>TSH in type 1 DM, dyslipidemia, or women over age of 50 years</li></ul></li></ul>

Note: Several National Diabetic Associations including the Diabetic Associations of India have from time to time given indications for the overall management and follow-up of DM. A common direction for evaluation of the diabetic evolved by the American Diabetes Association (ADA, 2014) is widely in vogue.

Abbreviations: SMBG = Self-monitoring of blood glucose; DKA = Diabetic ketoacidosis; CHD = Coronary heart disease; BP = Blood pressure; HbA1C = Glycosylated hemoglobin; LDL = Low-density lipoprotein; HDL = High-density lipoprotein; GFR = Glomerular filtration rate; TSH = Thyroid-stimulating hormone; DM = Diabetes mellitus

Education of a Diabetic Patient

The management plan should recognize diabetes self-management education (DSME) and ongoing diabetes support as integral components of care. In developing the plan, consideration should be given to the patient's age, school or work schedule and conditions, physical activity, eating patterns, social situation and cultural factors, presence of diabetes complications, health priorities and other medical conditions. Education regarding various aspects of diabetes helps to achieve better compliance from the patients.

Dietary Management (Medical Nutrition Therapy)

American Diabetes Association (ADA) introduced the term medical nutrition therapy (MNT). It involves use of a specific nutrition advice to treat an illness, injury or condition. Nutrition is the cornerstone in the management of diabetes. The objective of dietary therapy is the optimization of glycemic control and to provide a nutritious and balanced diet (Table 91.12). In type 1 DM patients, the total energy input has to be relatively higher in order to regain ideal weight and growth. In type 2 DM patients, the calories need to be restricted in order to avoid obesity. Dietary products, such as saturated fats, excess salt and cholesterol which promote vascular complications, have to be avoided.

Goals of Medical Nutrition Therapy

Goals of MNT include:

- To achieve and maintain near normal glycemia (A1C < 7%)
- To achieve and maintain optimal lipid profile (LDL cholesterol < 100 mg/dL; triglycerides < 150 mg/dL; HDL cholesterol > 40 mg/dL for men; HDL cholesterol > 50 mg/dL for women)
- To achieve and maintain normal BP levels (<140/80 mm Hg)
- To adjust the energy intake to restore and maintain ideal body weight according age, sex and phases of life, e.g. during childhood and pregnancy adjustment for growth also should be provided
- To adjust the nutrient intake to avoid dyslipidemia, CVD, hypertension and nephropathy

Table 91.12: Proportion of proximate principles in a diabetic diet

Nutrient	Recommended intake
Carbohydrate	~50–60% of total calories
Protein	15–20% of total calories
Total fat	25–35% of total calories
Saturated fat	< 10% of total calories (< 7% in dyslipidemia)
Polyunsaturated fat	~10% of total calories
Monounsaturated fat	Up to 20% of total calories
Cholesterol	< 300 mg/day (<200 mg/day in dyslipidemia)
Total calories	Adjust based on age, weight and height: • Sedentary individuals: 30 kcal/kg/day • Moderately active individuals: 35 kcal/kg/day • Heavily active individuals: 40 kcal/kg/day

Table 91.13: Optimum daily needs in calorie intake per kg of desirable body weight

Body weight	Activity		
	Sedentary	Moderate	Heavy
Obese	20	25	30
Normal weight	30	35	40
Under weight	35	40	45

Note: Additional allowances are required in case of pregnancy, lactation and growing children.

- For elderly patients, provision for proper nutrition and psychosocial needs
- To address individual needs, such as personal or cultural preferences and lifestyle practices.

Calculating Total Caloric Intake

This is the first and the most important step while prescribing a diet. Total caloric intake depends on the patient's body weight, degree of physical activity and the presence of any other comorbid illnesses. Obesity is an important factor in terms of target cell resistance to insulin action. The recommended daily allowance is calculated by multiplying the constant as given in (Table 91.13), e.g. total calories per day required for an obese patients with sedentary activity will be equal to his desirable weight × 20. Desirable body weight can be readily calculated by using the formula:

Ideal body weight (in kg) = Height (in cm) – 100

Having calculated the number of calories required, they are distributed into at least three principal meals and two or three small snacks. These calories are derived from three principal sources: (1) carbohydrates, (2) protein and (3) fats. Each fraction has its own importance and should provide 60% of the calories from carbohydrates and 20% each from proteins and fats.

- ***Carbohydrates:*** The amount of carbohydrates to be permitted in diet of diabetic patients has been an area of controversy. Till recently, most people recommended restriction of carbohydrates in the diet to provide only 30–40% of the calories. Our diets in India are cereal based and have a high carbohydrate component (~70%). Several studies in India have shown that good metabolic control can be achieved with high carbohydrate diets, provided the caloric intake is optimized and simple carbohydrate with high glycemic index are avoided. Such diets provided better patient compliance and had no adverse effect on the long-term complications.

  The American Diabetes Association (ADA) and the European Diabetes Association Study Groups have also altered their dietary recommendations. In an attempt, to reduce cardiovascular morbidity and mortality, they now recommend a liberalized use of carbohydrates in the diet up to 50–60% of the calories. This also helps to reduce the intake of saturated fats. Modification in the type of carbohydrate can be achieved by increasing the intake of legumes and pulses, green-leafy vegetables and other vegetables, which will increase the content of complex carbohydrates and fiber.

- **Fats:** The fat content of diet should be 20–25% of the total calories. The distribution of the type of fat should be equal, i.e. saturated fats, monounsaturated and polyunsaturated fats should be equally distributed to make up the total fat intake. The dietary cholesterol should be less than 300 mg/day. Invisible fat is derived in a fair amount from cereals, legumes and seeds and contributes to 5–10% of the total energy intake. Milk and its products contribute approximately to 40–45% of the total fat content in vegetarian diets. Milk fat is a saturated fat.
- **Proteins:** Protein intake has been recommended as 0.8 g/kg body weight and should contribute to 12–20% of the total caloric intake. Vegetable proteins, derived from cereals and lentils, do not contain cholesterol. They have high-fiber content. Animal protein is rich in saturated fats and tends to increase cholesterol and triglycerides. Lean meat and fish are to be preferred to fatty meat in order to minimize the risk.

Other considerations: Dietary salt should be less than 6 g/day. In the presence of hypertension or renal failure, it should be reduced to around 3 g/day. Alcohol should be avoided as far as possible. Alcohol intake increases the risk of hypoglycemia by inhibiting gluconeogenesis. It may induce ketoacidosis, lactic acidosis and may contribute to peripheral neuropathy. Alcohol also induces hypertriglyceridemia and hyperuricemia. Alcohol is an additional source of calories, without any further nutritional values each milliliter providing 7 calories. If consumed, it should be taken only in moderate quantities (one drink a day for women of all ages and men > age of 65 years, and up to 2 drinks a day for men age < 65 years). When instructing on the diet regime, the following points should be stressed:

- It is not a reduction in the diet but it is a modulation to suit the particular need of an individual. This concept will help to reduce the psychological resistance in accepting the diet.
- The patient and his spouse should be counseled together, so that the latter will understand the principles and help to provide the diet appropriately.
- Whenever possible, the dietary products should be prescribed in terms of weight, so that at least on a few occasions the actual quantities would be determined and adopted.
- It is better to prescribe the diet in terms of the primary food articles, such as rice, meat, fish and others, so that the patient can determine various items of the menu in relation to the allowed foodstuff.
- Many patients are under the wrong impression that reducing the food, further than what is prescribed, may be beneficial and this should be avoided.
- Both the quantity of diet and its timing are important since other aspects of management, such as medication and exercise, are timed in relation to the diet. As far as possible, the diet should conform to the cultural habits and socioeconomic condition of the patient.
- Vast majority of treatment failure can be avoided by proper dietary instructions.
- At all follow-up visits, enquiry on the diet should be made and the need for strict adherence stressed.

Table 91.14: Benefits and possible ill-effects of exercise	
Parameters	**Effects**
Benefits of exercise	• It lowers blood glucose concentration • It improves insulin sensitivity • Decreases triglyceride, increases HDL-C and decreases LDL-C • It lowers BP in mild to moderate hypertension • It causes weight reduction by metabolizing adipose tissue • It helps in cardiovascular conditioning • It improves sense of well-being and quality of life
Risks of unsupervised exercise in uncontrolled diabetic	• Hypoglycemia • Hyperglycemia after very strenuous exercise, particularly in poorly controlled diabetes • Precipitation or exacerbation of CVD and acute cardiac events, like arrhythmias, sudden death and cardiac failure • Worsening of long-term diabetic complications, particularly proliferative retinopathy, nephropathy (increases proteinuria), peripheral neuropathy risk of soft tissue and joint injuries. Autonomic neuropathy (causes reduced exercise tolerance, impaired response to dehydration and postural hypotension)

Note: The exercise program for each patient should be prescribed by the physician taking into account the overall health status of the individual. At each follow-up visit details of exercise should be evaluated.

Abbreviations: HDL-C = High-density lipoprotein cholesterol; LDL-C = Low-density lipoprotein cholesterol; BP = Blood pressure; CVD = Cardiovascular disease

Exercise

In type 2 DM, regular exercise forms an important component of therapy along with dietary regulation and oral antidiabetic agents. However, a careful assessment of the expected benefits and associated risks of exercise in individual patients should be made while incorporating an exercise program in the treatment (Table 91.14). Appropriate monitoring should be done to avoid complications. Exercise should not be recommended indiscriminately in all type 1 diabetic patient but efforts should be made to make it possible for those who want to exercise to do so as safely as possible.

Endocrine/Physiological Responses during Exercise

- ***Suppression of insulin release:*** Directly as well as through epinephrine
- Sympathetic system activation, which inhibits insulin release (by α-receptor stimulation) and stimulates lipolysis
- Non-insulin-dependent glucose uptake in the periphery.

In both type 1 and type 2 diabetic patients who are under good control, response to exercise will be normal. In untreated type 1 diabetic patients there is an increased production of FFA from adipocyte lipolysis, which leads to decrease glucose uptake in the periphery. This can even precipitate DKA in some patients. In the well-controlled patients this does not occur.

While prescribing exercise, it should suit the social and economic condition of the patient and his work schedule (Box 91.3). Regular exercise as part of the therapeutic intervention should be taken by all diabetics, irrespective

Box 91.3: Pre-exercise checklist for diabetic patients

- Correct planning of exercise program (which includes duration and intensity of exercise)
- Review diabetic medications (need to alter dosage, timing/site of insulin injection)
- Perform necessary tests to rule out any long-standing, silent diabetic complications that may need a change in exercise pattern:
  - **Treadmill test/stress ECHO:** To rule out coronary artery disease and also to know the individual's exercise tolerance capacity
  - **Ophthalmic fundoscopy:** To rule out proliferative retinopathy; if present, anaerobic exercise has to be avoided
  - **Biothesiometry:**
    - This is the method to determine any impairment of vibratory sensation in the extremities accurately in order to assess the extent and severity of sensory loss
    - The patients should be advised on appropriate footwear which will ensure protection to the feet and avoid localized pressure and trauma
- The blood glucose should be checked before the exercise:
  - **Plasma glucose levels:**
    - If < 100 mg/dL— if advise pre-exercise snacks
    - If 100–250 mg/dL—can proceed with exercise
    - If > 250 mg/dL—check urinary ketones, if positive, insulin should be started. Resume exercise only after correction of ketosis.

of the physical activity entailed in their regular occupation. Maximum benefit is achieved by exercises, such as brisk walking (4–5 km/hour), swimming, cycling and such other aerobic exercises. At least five sessions a week should be performed in order to achieve optimal benefit. While, starting the exercise program in persons above the age of 35 years, clinical assessment of their cardiovascular status should be done and introduction of the exercise regimen should be gradual, so that not to precipitate any acute cardiovascular events.

For the average middle-aged Indian diabetic, the following exercise regimen is adequate:

- Walk 3 km on level ground over a period of 45 minutes
- Swim for 30 minutes at average speed without cardiovascular distress
- Cycle on level ground at 8 km/hour for 30 minutes.

Regular sports and games activities can be undertaken and should be encouraged by those who desire to do them, with special provision made for the diet and medications. Since such sport activities are likely to be intermittent rather than regular, in practice walking or cycling is more regularly available. Before an exercise program is initiated, a fair control of blood glucose is to be ensured, and a thorough clinical evaluation of the patient should be made, particularly in regard to complications of diabetes, such as hypertension, coronary artery disease (CAD), peripheral vascular disease, retinopathy and nephropathy. In all cases, carefully planned exercise regimen taking into consideration the age and morbid status of the patient, and done under periodic supervision is always beneficial, despite small risks which have to be eliminated by medical advice. On an average, a minimum of five sessions of brisk walk covering 3 km in 20–30 minutes weekly is needed to give optimal benefit. In addition, in patients who have near normal health status, other exercises and sports activities can be undertaken, if done systematically. Wide fluctuation in the quantity and rate of exercise should be avoided.

Yoga Exercises

Recently, several well-planned studies have demonstrated the beneficial effects of yogic practices in diabetics. Patients with diabetes demonstrated a significant fall in fasting and postprandial blood glucose values and HbA1C, with reduction in the requirements of OHA and insulin. Type 1 diabetic patients with brittle diabetes showed marked improvement with the practice of yoga. There was a salutary effect on the lipid profile, with a fall in serum cholesterol, triglycerides and an increase in HDL-C fraction. Certain **Asanas** (specific postural manipulations which have to be learnt under supervision) have been identified as useful in the control of diabetes. Thus, yogic practices have a useful role in the control of diabetes and prevention of its long-term complications.

Monitoring Control of Diabetes (Table 91.15)

Self-monitoring of blood glucose (SMBG) by glucometer is preferred over the laboratory sampling whenever possible for monitoring of fasting and postprandial sugar levels. Frequency of blood sugar examination varies with the type of diabetes, treatment of diabetes (patients on insulin require more frequent monitoring) and its severity. In type 1 DM patients, it should be done as frequently as possible. In well-controlled type 2 DM patients, the blood glucose levels should be done once in 4–6 weeks. During periods of stress, the patients need closer follow-up as in type 1 DM. It is preferable to control both fasting and postprandial blood glucose.

Glycosylated Hemoglobin

HbA1C should be checked every 3–6 months depending upon the level of control of the individual patient. HbA1C of 6.5% denotes excellent control but less than 7% is alright for most nonpregnant adults. Glycosylated fructosamine is a marker of medium-term control of glycemia over the preceding 2–3 weeks. This test is rarely done and most laboratories do not have standardization to perform this test (Table 91.16).

Monitoring the Progress of Complications

Factors other than glycemic control also determine the complication rate. These include the genetic make-up,

Table 91.15: Treatment goals for adults with diabetes

Parameters		Values
Glycemic control	Fasting blood glucose	70–130 mg/dL
	2-hour postprandial blood glucose	< 180 mg/dL
	HbA1C	< 7.0%
BP		< 140/90 mm Hg
Lipids	LDL	< 100 mg/dL
	Triglycerides	< 150 mg/dL
	HDL	> 40 mg/dL (men)
		> 50 mg/dL (women)

Source: Adapted from American Diabetes Association, 2014.

Note: Total cholesterol levels below 150 mg/dL are preferable, especially if there is concomitant elevation of BP and renal involvement evidenced by urinary microalbumin above 30 mg in 24 hours.

Abbreviations: BP = Blood pressure; HbA1C = Glycosylated hemoglobin; LDL = Low-density lipoprotein; HDL = High-density lipoprotein

Table 91.16: Relationships between the average glucose values and HbA1C

HbA1C	Average glucose value (mg/dL) = eAG (mg/dL) = (28.7*HbA1C) - 46.7
5.6	114.02
5.8	119.76
6	125.5
6.2	131.24
6.4	136.98
6.6	142.72
6.8	148.46
7	154.2
7.2	159.94
7.4	165.68
7.6	171.42
7.8	177.16
8	182.9
8.2	188.64
8.4	194.38
8.6	200.12
8.8	205.86
9	211.6
9.2	217.34
9.4	223.08
9.6	228.82
9.8	234.56
10	240.3
10.2	246.04
10.4	251.78
10.6	257.52
10.8	263.26
11	269
11.2	274.74
11.4	280.48
11.6	286.22
11.8	291.96
12	297.7

Abbreviations: HbA1C = Glycosylated hemoglobin; eAG = Estimated average glucose

tobacco smoking, obesity, hypertension, hyperlipidemia and presence of other precipitating factors. All these should be taken into account while monitoring complications.

Renal function tests (creatinine, urinary microalbumin) should be performed every 6–12 months and more frequently if baseline values are abnormal. Lipid profile, electrocardiogram (ECG), chest X-ray, biothesiometry and ophthalmic examination should be carried out annually. Biothesiometry is based on the pattern of electrical response of different regions of the feet to electric current. Typical abnormalities develop along with the development of neuropathy. Biothesiometry helps to objectively measure the vibration sense and quantify the severity, extent and progress of neuropathy.

Table 91.17: Classification of oral antidiabetic drugs (OADs)

Mode of action	Drugs
Insulin secretagogues	• SUs • Meglitinides • DPP-4 inhibitors
Insulin sensitizers	• Biguanides • Thiazolidinediones
Inhibitors of GI glucose absorption	• α-glucosidase inhibitors
SGLT2 inhibitors	• Canagliflozin, dapagliflozin

Abbreviations: SUs = Sulfonylureas; DPP-4 = Dipeptidyl peptidase-4; GI = Gastrointestinal; SGLT2 = Sodium-glucose co-transporter 2

Oral Antidiabetic Drugs

The oral antidiabetic drugs (OADs) or agents are indicated in type 2 DM when diet and exercise fail to achieve euglycemia. The major groups of drugs in use are listed in (Table 91.17.)

Sulfonylurea Compounds

Actions and indications

The sulfonylurea (SU) compounds stimulate the β-cells of the pancreas to release insulin, as evidenced by an increase in the plasma levels of both basal and postprandial insulin in type 2 DM patients. A minimum of 30% of β-cells is required for their optimal action. These drugs, therefore, are most effective in individuals with type 2 DM of relatively recent-onset (< 5 years), who have residual endogenous insulin production. They improve the sensitivity of β-cells to glucose and other secretagogues. There is no evidence, so that SU may cause β-cell exhaustion. However, continuous exposure to maximum doses may result in desensitization of β-cells. Therapy should be initiated with the smallest dose, taken 15–30 minutes before food, and small increments should be made at weekly intervals till the optimum dose is reached. The SUs are similar in effectiveness in equipotent doses and in the absence of any specific reason, such as adverse side effects, cost or nonavailability, there is no need to change the medication in patients who are adequately controlled. Also, there is no advantage in combining two or more SU drugs.

Choice of compound

Tolbutamide and chlorpropamide, which were among the initial SU drugs, have been almost replaced by the newer derivatives which are easier to administer, safer and predictable in action (Table 91.18). Glibenclamide has a better effect on FPG than glipizide as it causes greater suppression of hepatic glucose production. Glipizide and gliclazide induce greater insulin levels in the postprandial state. Glimepiride, sometimes referred to as the third-generation SU, differs from all other preceding members of its class in several important attributes. It has the highest weight for weight potency and long duration of action requiring once or twice daily dosage. Its onset of action is rapid. It has no pharmacokinetic or pharmacodynamic interaction with β-blockers, calcium-channel blockers (CCBs), H_2-receptor blockers, angiotensin-converting enzyme (ACE) inhibitors or anticoagulants. The effective dose is 1–8 mg/day. On the pancreatic β-cells, glimepiride binds to a different receptor site as compared to the other

Table 91.18: Dosage of sulfonylureas (SUs)

Drug	Relative potency	Maximum dosage	Duration	Peak action hours	Half-life (hours)	Significant effect (hours)
Glibenclamide	150	10 mg bd	Long	3–4	10–16	Up to 24
Glipizide	100	10 mg bd	Short	1	3–7	Up to 2
Gliclazide	80	160 mg bd	Medium	4	10–12	10–24
Glimepiride	450	8 mg od	Long	1	12–16	Up to 24

SU compounds. It also acts as an insulin sensitizer by promoting glucose utilization of peripheral tissues, by increasing the availability of the glucose transporters—GLUT 1 and GLUT 4, in the cell membranes. It brings about a comparable reduction of blood glucose levels as other SUs, with lower insulin and C-peptide levels. On long-term treatment, about 40–50% of patients develop resistance to the action of the particular SU (secondary SU failure). In this situation, other SUs may be tried but is rarely effective.

Adverse effects of SU

These insulin secretagogues are generally well-tolerated. These agents, especially the longer-acting ones, have the potential to cause profound and persistent hypoglycemia, especially in elderly individuals. Hypoglycemia is usually related to the peak action of the drugs, delayed meals, increased physical activity, alcohol intake and renal/hepatic dysfunction. Duration and severity of hypoglycemia varies depending upon the type of SU and the dose. If not diagnosed in time, SU-induced hypoglycemia can be fatal.

Weight gain, another common side effect of SUs therapy, results from the increased insulin levels and improvement in glycemic control. Most SU are metabolized in the liver to compounds that are cleared by the kidney. Thus, there be use in individuals with significant hepatic or renal dysfunction is not advisable.

Nonspecific GI symptoms ranging from dyspepsia to diarrhea can occur with SUs in 3–5% of patients. Minor skin reactions occur which readily resolve on stopping the drugs. However, occasionally severe reactions, like exfoliative dermatitis or Stevens-Johnson syndrome may occur. Cholestatics type of jaundice and bone marrow depression are rare complications. Occasionally, water retention with dilutional hyponatremia may occur with SUs.

Nonsulfonylurea Secretagogues: Meglitinides

This group includes repaglinide and nateglinide. These act through separate receptors on β-cell membrane, compared to SUs.

- **Repaglinide:** It is a benzoic acid derivative. It was the first meglitinide analogue to become available. It initiates insulin secretion by closing the K⁺ATP channels. It induces rapid postprandial insulin response. The drug's short half-life ensures that insulin concentrations peak at 1–2 hours, by 6 hours they are back at fasting concentrations. It does not have the risk of severe or prolonged hypoglycemia. It is given in doses of 0.5–4.0 mg/day in divided does, taken 15 minutes before meal.
- **Nateglinide:** It is a D-phenylalanine derivative. This drug has a unique property of fast association and

dissociation kinetics at the pancreatic β-cell. The other unique property of this drug is that it does not inhibit the K⁺ATP in the presence of low sugars. This glucose-sensitizing property explains the low incidence of hypoglycemia associated with nateglinide. It is given in doses of 60–240 mg/day in 3 divided doses, 10–15 minutes before the meal.

Biguanides

The biguanides lower the blood glucose levels in diabetics through their extrapancreatic effects, but do not reduce the blood glucose levels in normal individuals, unless they are starved. They do not stimulate endogenous insulin secretion and do not cause hypoglycemia. The glucose-lowering effect of these compounds has been shown to occur through three main mechanisms:

1. Inhibition of intestinal glucose absorption
2. Increase in utilization of glucose by peripheral tissues
3. Stimulation of anaerobic glycolysis in the liver, which inhibits hepatic gluconeogenesis and increases production of lactate.

The biguanides are rapidly and almost completely absorbed from the gastrointestinal tract (GIT). Occurrence of drug-induced gastric side effects can be reduced by giving the drug after food.

Metformin

This biguanide is most widely used since the longest duration. It is the first OAD started in all type 2 DM patients unless contraindicated. It reduces hepatic glucose production and improves peripheral glucose utilization by increasing insulin sensitivity. Metformin is neither metabolized by the liver, nor bound to serum proteins. It is excreted unchanged by the kidneys. Its plasma half-life of 1.5–2.8 hours is much shorter than that of phenformin. Daily dosage of metformin is 500–2,500 mg. Studies have shown that metformin can delay the onset diabetes in high-risk groups. Effects of metformin are potentiated by other hypoglycemic agents, such as SUs and salicylates.

Effects of metformin

- **Insulin-receptor effects:** Metformin may help us to improve insulin sensitivity in diabetic subjects by increasing insulin-receptor binding in individuals with a reduced number of insulin receptors. The effect of metformin on the post-receptor sites is much of greater importance for the potentiation of insulin action.
- **Lipid metabolism:** Circulating triglyceride concentrations are decreased by metformin in both normal and type 2 DM patients. This is largely due to reduction in LDL (VLDL). A small increase in HDL has been observed in patients treated with metformin (Box 91.4).

Box 91.4: Other indications for metformin

- This drug has been used for conditions other than diabetes mellitus (DM), e.g. polycystic ovarian syndrome (PCOS) in women, which is an insulin resistance state and metformin is the first-line of drug to be used in such patients. Since, metformin passes the placental barrier, it is not approved for use in pregnancy.
- Recent studies have shown that metformin reduces the risk of spontaneous abortion during the first trimester and reduce the incidence of fetal anomalies.
- It effectively reduces the development of gestational DM.

Phenformin: This was popular before the introduction of metformin. It is very effective. Adverse effects include severe lactic acidosis. Due to this adverse side effect, phenformin is not generally used at present.

Biguanide and SU combination: The addition of biguanide in cases where SU alone cannot normalize blood sugar levels has allowed the continuation of oral therapy in many patients. SU increases insulin release and causes greater suppression of hepatic glycolysis, whereas metformin increases peripheral insulin-mediated glucose disposal. Many diabetologists in India prefer to initiate treatment with combination of a SU and metformin.

Metformin and insulin combination: Addition of metformin decreased the daily insulin requirement by 16% in a group of insulin requiring type 1 DM patients. Due to their insulin-potentiating effects, the biguanides have also been used as adjuvants of insulin therapy in both type 2 DM and type 1 DM patients. Metformin monotherapy is not effective in type 1 DM patients.

Adverse effects of biguanides

These are usually mild and limited to the GIT. The side effect includes a bitter or metallic taste in the mouth, anorexia, nausea, occasional vomiting and intermittent diarrhea. These are usually dose-related and can be minimized by the use of timed disintegrating tablets or by very slowly increasing the dosage. Less frequent toxic effects include stress reactions and malabsorption of B_{12} and folic acid with resultant-macrocytic anemia. Pancreatitis has been reported with the use of phenformin. Undoubtedly, the most serious side effect associated with the use of biguanides is ***lactic acidosis***. This is more commonly encountered with phenformin therapy and led to its ban in the USA. Metformin is a less lipophilic drug than phenformin, and it is not metabolized in the body but excreted unchanged in the urine. On the other hand, phenformin is metabolized in the liver, so the chances of lactic acidosis increase with phenformin. The risk of developing lactic acidosis increases if the metformin level builds up in the blood. Since metformin is cleared primarily by the kidneys, patients with impaired kidney function (serum creatinine > 1.4 mg/dL in women and > 1.5 mg/dL in men) should not be treated with metformin. It should also be avoided in any form of acidosis, congestive heart failure (CHF), liver disease or severe hypoxemia. Metformin should be discontinued in patients who are seriously ill, and in patients who cannot take oral food or medication. Insulin should be used until metformin can be restarted in such patients. Metformin is also employed as a primary mode of therapy in obese type 2 diabetic patients without complications.

Dipeptidyl Peptidase-4 Inhibitors

Dipeptidyl peptidase-4 (DPP-4) inhibitors inhibit degradation of native GLP-1 and thus enhance the incretin effect by prolonging GLP-1 action. This enzyme is widely expressed on the surface of endothelial cells and some lymphocytes. This enzyme degrades a wide range of peptides and it is not specific for GLP-1 alone. DPP-4 inhibitors promote insulin secretion in a glucose-dependent manner and do not cause hypoglycemia. They are used either alone or in combination with other oral agents, mainly with metformin in patients with type 2 DM. Different DPP-4 inhibitors available in market are vildagliptin, sitagliptin, saxagliptin and linagliptin (Table 91.19).

Thiazolidinediones

The thiazolidinedione currently in use is ***pioglitazone***. These drugs act by improving insulin sensitivity by binding to the ***peroxisome proliferator-activated receptor gamma (PPAR-γ)***, a molecule implicated in the transcription of numerous genes controlling carbohydrate and lipid metabolism. PPAR-γ is the target for thiazolidinediones. They reduce insulin resistance, thereby acting as hypoglycemic agents on their own, as well as insulin-sparing agents. In addition, they improve the lipid profile, lower BP in hypertension, and reduce cardiovascular risk factors. They promote fatty-acid uptake and storage in adipose tissue, thereby increasing body fat and weight gain. They lead to fluid retention and cardiac failure in susceptible subjects, especially, if combined with insulin.

These can also be used to treat polycystic ovarian syndrome (PCOS), like metformin, however, they should be stopped if the women with PCOS becomes pregnant. These drugs are not approved for use in pregnancy because they pass the placental barrier and affect fetal growth and development. Unlike metformin, these drugs cause modest weight gain of approximately 1–3 kg. This is due to increased subcutaneous adipose tissue in the periphery and fluid-salt retention. Pioglitazone also increases the fracture risk in elderly. Long-term use of pioglitazone has been found to increase the risk of bladder cancer and that is why new guidelines have suggested use of low-dose pioglitazone. Pioglitazone is administered in the doses of 7.5–30 mg/day as a single daily dose.

Contraindications for use of thiazolidinediones

- CHF
- Hepatic dysfunction with alanine transaminase (ALT) more than 2 times the normal
- Obesity.

Table 91.19: Characteristics of dipeptidyl peptidase-4 (DPP-4) inhibitors

Drug	Maximum dose per day (mg)	Frequency of dosing	Dose adjustment in	
			Renal impairment	Hepatic impairment
Sitagliptin	100	od	Yes	No
Vildagliptin	100	bd or od	Likely	Unlikely
Saxagliptin	10	od	Likely	Unlikely
Linagliptin	5	od	Unlikely	Unlikely

Textbook of Medicine

Alpha-glucosidase Inhibitors

They competitively inhibit the enzyme α-glucosidase, which is present in the brush border of small intestine. This enzyme breaks down complex carbohydrates into glucose and favors its absorption. Use of α-glucosidase inhibitors as a supplement to SU therapy reduces postprandial hyperglycemia. Drugs belonging to this class are **acarbose**, **voglibose** and **miglitol**. The tablet has to be administered orally with the first bite of each meal. Use of acarbose permits slightly liberal use of complex carbohydrates in the diets without causing hyperglycemia. The currently recommended initial dose is 25 mg 3 times daily with the dose increased slowly, every 4 weeks to a maximum of 100 mg 3 times/day. Only 2% of the administered acarbose gets absorbed into systemic circulation. Acarbose is metabolized exclusively by the kidneys. Its use is contraindicated in the presence of hypersensitivity to the drug, severe renal failure, DKA, inflammatory bowel disease, colonic ulcers, partial bowel obstruction, chronic intestinal disease associated with impaired digestion or absorption and other disorders that may deteriorate with intestinal gas formation. These drugs should be avoided in pregnancy. Miglitol has lesser side effects than acarbose in doses of 25–50 mg 3 times a day. Another recently introduced drug is voglibose 0.2–0.3 mg just before the meal. It is more potent in action with less of side effects.

Sodium-Glucose Co-transporter-2 (SGLT2) Inhibitor

In this, inhibitors belong to a new class of antidiabetic drugs and have a novel mechanism of action. SGLT2 is a transport system that is specifically expressed in the kidney and plays an important role in renal glucose reabsorption in the proximal tubule. Glucose is freely filtered by the glomeruli and essentially completely reabsorbed from the proximal tubules via sodium-coupled transporters in the border membrane. Competitive inhibition of SGLT2 enhances glucose and energy loss through the urine. These agents are unique in that they increase glucose excretion, independent of insulin secretion, by inhibiting the renal reabsorption of glucose, inducing glycosuria.

Since this drug leads to heavy glycosuria (sometimes up to ~70 g/day), it can lead to rapid weight loss and tiredness. The glucose acts as an osmotic diuretic (this effect is the cause of polyuria in diabetes) which can lead to dehydration. The increased amount of glucose in the urine can also worsen the infections already associated with diabetes, particularly UTIs and genital mycotic infections (candidiasis).

The examples of this class of drugs are **dapagliflozin**, **canagliflozin** and **empagliflozin**. These drugs have completed phase 3 clinical trials and are waiting for approval from regulatory authority. Long-term data on these medications are not available.

Table 91.20, Flowchart 91.1, Table 91.21 and Fig. 91.1 for approach to drug management of diabetes.

Insulin Therapy and Other Parenteral Therapeutic Agents

The discovery of insulin at the University of Toronto in 1921 by Sir Frederick Banting and Charles Herbert Best

Table 91.20: Approximate glucose-lowering potential of oral type 2 DM therapies

Drug class	FPG reduction (mg/dL)	HbA1C reduction (%)
SU	50–60	1–2
Metformin	50–60	1–2
DPP-4 inhibitors	40–60	0.5–0.8
Meglitinide	~70	1–2
Thiazolidinediones	50–60	1–2
α-glucosidase	15–30	0.5–0.8
Combination of SU and metformin	100–120	3–4

Abbreviations: SU = Sulfonylurea; DPP-4 = Dipeptidyl peptidase-4; FPG = Fasting plasma glucose; HbA1C = Glycosylated hemoglobin.

Flowchart 91.1: Algorithm for antihyperglycemic therapy in type 2 DM

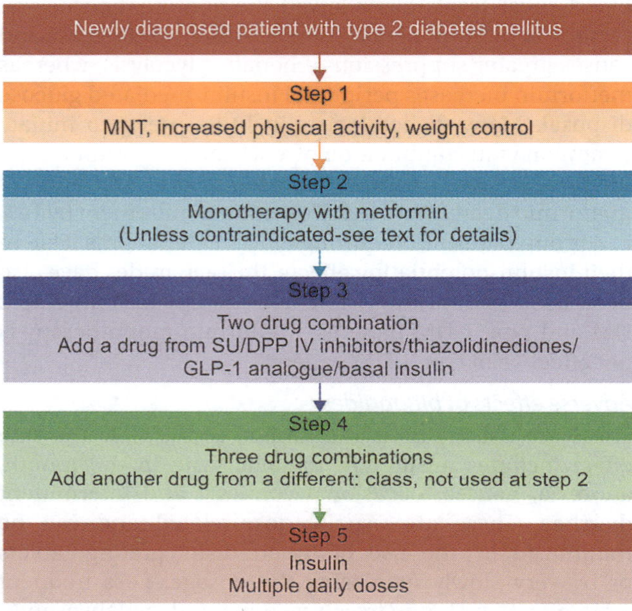

Note:
1. Drugs of same class should not be combined.
2. Caution should be taken while combining drugs with potential of causing hypoglycemia.

Abbreviations: MNT = Medical nutrition therapy; SU = Sulfonylurea; DPP-4 = Dipeptidyl peptidase-4; GLP-1 = Glucagon-like peptide-1; FPG = Fasting plasma glucose; HbA1C = Glycosylated hemoglobin

revolutionized the treatment of diabetes, extending the life expectancy of insulin-dependent diabetics. The early commercial preparations of insulin were from bovine and porcine pancreas. They were impure and of variable quality, still they dramatically improved the prospects of life in several thousand diabetics. Banting was awarded the Nobel Prize in 1923 along with McLeod, Professor of Physiology in whose laboratory, Banting and Best conducted their study.

During the past 5 decades, several developments have taken place in insulin production, purification and formulation, aimed at improving metabolic control, safety and convenience of its use. Improvement in insulin purity was the first challenge and has been the goal ever since. This resulted in the production of chromatographically-purified insulin and later insulin with the chemical and

Table 91.21: Agents used for treatment of type 1 and type 2 DM

Drugs	Mechanism of action	Generic names	A1C reduction (%)	Agent-specific advantages	Agent-specific disadvantages	Contra-indications
Oral						
Biguanides	Hepatic glucose production	Metformin	1–2	Weight neutral, do not cause hypoglycemia inexpensive	Diarrhea, nausea, lactic acidosis	Acute illness, CHF, liver failure, advanced renal failure
α glucosidase inhibitor	GI glucose absorption	Acarbose, miglitol	0.5–0.8	Reduce postprandial glycemia	GI flatulence, LFTs	
DPP-4 inhibitors	Prolong endogenous GLP-1 action	Saxagliptin, sitagliptin, vildagliptin	0.5–0.8	Do not cause hypoglycemia	Rare cases of pancreatitis, rare cases of medullary thyroid cancer	Family history of thyroid cancer, past history of pancreatitis
Insulin secretagogues—SUs	Insulin secretion	Glimepiride, gliclazide, glipizide, glibenclamide	1–2	Inexpensive	Hypoglycemia weight gain	
Insulin secretagogues—non-SUs	Insulin secretion	Repaglinide, nateglinide	1–2	Short onset of action, lower postprandial glucose	Hypoglycemia	
Thiazolidinediones	Insulin resistance glucose utilization	Rosiglitazone, pioglitazone	0.5–1.4	Lower insulin requirements	Peripheral edema, CHF, weight gain, fractures, macular edema; rosiglitazone may increase cardiovascular risk	CHF, liver disease, see text about rosiglitazone
Bile acid sequestrants	Bind bile acids mechanism of glucose lowering not known	Colesevelam	0.5		Constipation, dyspepsia, abdominal pain, nausea, triglyceri-des, interfere with absorption of other drugs, intestinal obstruction	Elevated plasma triglycerides
Parenteral						
Insulin	Glucose utilization, hepatic glucose production and other anabolic actions	See Table 91.23	Not limited	Known safety profile	Injection, weight gain, hypoglycemia	
GLP-1 receptor agonists	Insulin, glucagon, slow gastric-emptying satiety	Exenatide, liraglutide	0.5–10	Weight loss, do not cause hypoglycemia	Injection, nausea, risk of hypoglycemia with insulin secretagogues, pancreatitis, renal failure	Renal disease, agents that also slow GI motility
Amylin agonists	Slow gastric emptying, glucagon	Pramlintide	0.25–0.50	Reduce postprandial glycemia; weight loss	Injection, nausea, risk of hypoglycemia with insulin	Agents that slow GI motility
MNT and physical activity	Insulin resistance, insulin secretion	Low-calorie, low-fat diet, exercise	1–3	Other health benefits	Compliance difficult, long-term success, low	

Note: Added by editor

Abbreviations: SUs = Sulfonylureas; DPP-4 = Dipeptidyl peptidase-4; GLP-1 = Glucagon-like peptide-1; CHF = Congestive heart failure; MNT = Medical nutrition therapy; LFTs = Liver function tests; GI = Glucosidase inhibitors

Diabetes Mellitus

molecular composition of human insulin referred to as human insulin (Table 91.22). Similarly, attempts to retard the subcutaneous absorption of insulin to spare diabetics the discomfort of multiple-daily injections resulted in the development of intermediate and long-acting insulins (Table 91.23). Like other proteins, insulin is unstable and is susceptible to chemical degradation and inter- and intra-molecular transformations. The presence of contaminants and immunogenicity of bovine and porcine insulins used to give rise to problems, such as:

- Immunogenic insulin resistance
- Insulin allergy
- Insulin-induced lipoatrophy and lipohypertrophy
- Insulin-antibody complex-mediated complications.

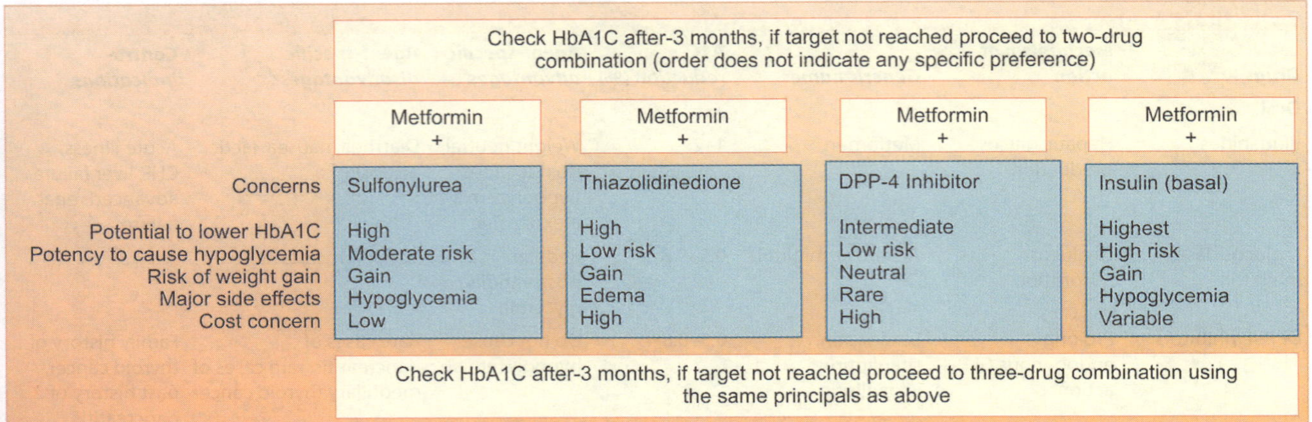

Fig. 91.1: Choice of antihyperglycemic drug to be added if control is not achieved with monotherapy. **Note:** It is generally preferable to start insulin in some form (at least basal) if the initial A1C is more than 9%.
Abbreviations: HbA1C = Glycosylated hemoglobin; SU = Sulfonylurea; DPP-4 = Dipeptidyl peptidase-4

Table 91.22: Differences between insulins from three species

| Species | A chain | | B chain |
	A_8	A_{10}	B_{30}
Bovine	Alanine	Valine	Alanine
Porcine	Threonine	Isoleucine	Alanine
Human	Threonine	Isoleucine	Threonine

Note: Bovine insulin is more different from human insulin, compared to the porcine variety. At present both bovine and porcine insulin are not manufactured and all available insulin is of the human variety.

Table 91.23: Human insulin preparations

Insulin preparation	Onset of action (hr)	Peak action (hr)	Total duration (hr)
Short-acting insulin			
Regular or soluble	0.5–1	2–4	4–6
Intermediate-acting insulin			
NPH	2–4	10–16	20–24
Lente	2–4	10–16	20–24
Long-acting insulin			
Ultralente	6–8	14–20	24–32
Premixed insulin			
Regular and NPH (30: 70 or 50: 50)	0.5	2–10	12–18

Note: Insulin manufacturers supply different formulations of insulin separately or in the premixed form containing regular and longer-acting preparations.
Abbreviations: NPH = Neutral protamine Hagedorn; hr = hours

Human Insulin

Human insulin is produced by recombinant DNA technology, the composition of the final product being identical to that of natural human insulin chemically and in molecular configuration. Being synthetic, the supply can be modified to meet the need, without shortage. It is more rapidly absorbed and has a somewhat shorter duration of action when compared with insulin of animal origin. Human insulin has a molecular weight of 5,807 Daltons and contains 51 amino acids arranged in two polypeptide chains. The A chain contains 21 amino acids and is linked to the B chain by two disulfide bridges.

Insulin Analogues

Insulin analogues are molecules which differ from insulin in their molecular structure, but produce the same biological response as insulin. Two types of insulin analogues are available—short-acting and long-acting analogues. Using genetic engineering technique, it is now possible to change amino acids at strategic locations in insulin polypeptide chain to produce insulin analogues that have different absorption and pharmacokinetic profile. Thus, it is possible to have fast- and short-acting or long-acting insulin analogues. The fast-acting insulin analogues are absorbed faster; achieve quicker peak and their level declines more rapidly as compared to short-acting human insulin. Similarly, by changing the amino acid sequence or structure, it has been possible to delay the breakdown of hexameric forms, and further enhance binding to albumin. It has been possible to produce long-acting insulin analogues that have slower and more predictable absorption and can provide basal insulin level throughout 24 hours. Several analogues are available worldwide.

Short-acting insulin analogues: They include insulin lispro, aspart and glulisine. These insulin analogues enter the bloodstream within minutes, so it is important to inject them within 5–10 minutes of eating. They have a peak action period of 60–120 minutes and fade completely after about 4 hours. Higher doses may last slightly longer, but will last no more than 5 or 6 hours. ***Rapid-acting insulin analogues*** are ideal for bolus insulin replacement. They are given at mealtimes and for high blood sugar correction. Rapid-acting insulins are also used in insulin pumps, also known as continuous subcutaneous insulin infusion (CSII) devices. When delivered through a CSII pump, rapid-acting insulins provide basal insulin replacement, as well as the mealtime and high blood sugar correction insulin replacement.

- ***Lispro:*** It was engineered through recombinant DNA technology in which the 28th and 29th amino acids (lysine and proline) residues on the C-terminal end of the B-chain have been reversed. This modification did not alter the insulin receptor binding, but have fewer tendencies for self-aggregation, resulting in more rapid absorption and onset of action and shorter duration of action to be available for postprandial use.

- ***Aspart:*** It was created through recombinant DNA technology so that the amino acid, B28, which is normally proline, is substituted with an aspartic acid residue. This analogue also prevents formation of hexamers, to create faster-acting insulin. It is approved for use in insulin pens and insulin pumps.
- ***Glulisine:*** It is newer rapid-acting insulin analogues, approved for use with a regular syringe, in an insulin pump or pen.

Long-acting insulin analogues: These include insulin glargine, detemir and insulin degludec. These long-acting insulin analogues have slower onset of action, less pronounced peak and longer duration of action. They are widely used for basal supplementation as add on therapy to oral drugs or along with short-acting insulin.

- ***Glargine:*** It was created by modifying three amino acids. The amino acid asparagine at position 21 in the A chain is replaced by glycine and two arginine residues were added to the C-terminus of the B chain, making glargine more soluble at a slightly acidic pH and less soluble at a physiological pH. These three structural changes and formulation with zinc result in a prolonged action when compared with biosynthetic human insulin. When pH 4.0 solution is injected, most of the material precipitates and is not bioavailable. A small amount is immediately available for use and the remainder is sequestered in subcutaneous tissue. Small amounts of the precipitated material will move into solution in the bloodstream and the basal level of insulin will be maintained up to 24 hours. The onset of action of subcutaneous insulin glargine is somewhat slower than neutral protamine Hagedorn (NPH) human insulin. Since this insulin has acidic pH, it should not be mixed with any other insulin.
- ***Detemir:*** The basal level of insulin may be maintained for up to 20 hours, but the time is clearly affected by the size of the injected dose. This insulin has a high affinity for serum albumin, increasing its duration of action.
- ***Degludec:*** This is an ultra-long-acting insulin analogue. Theoretically it can be given twice or thrice weekly instead of the daily administration, but presently it is approved for once-daily dosing. Data on twice or thrice weekly is not sufficient currently.

Therapeutics of Insulin

Insulin therapy aims at providing ideal physiological insulin profiles with peaks at mealtimes and maintenance of basal levels between meals and at night (Box 91.5).

Dosage of Insulin

There are no hard and fast rules to assess the optimal initial dose of insulin. It is ideal to start with a small dose and gradually increase at intervals of 2–3 days till the optimum dose is achieved as judged by the plasma

- All type 1 DM patients
- In type 2 DM patients:
  - During episodes of metabolic complications, like DKA, hyperosmolar nonketotic coma and lactic acidosis
  - During infections, myocardial infarction, stress, surgery, renal insufficiency or infective hepatitis
  - During pregnancy
  - When diet, exercise and OHAs fail to achieve euglycemia (primary and secondary SU failure)
  - Lean type 2 DM patients with very high blood glucose levels at onset
  - Pancreatic calculi patients most of whom require insulin
  - Even in nondiabetics, when the blood glucose level rises under stress, such as myocardial infection or septic shock, insulin is used to lower blood glucose.

Abbreviations: DM = Diabetes mellitus; DKA = Diabetic ketoacidosis; OHAs = Oral hypoglycemic agents; SU = Sulfonylurea

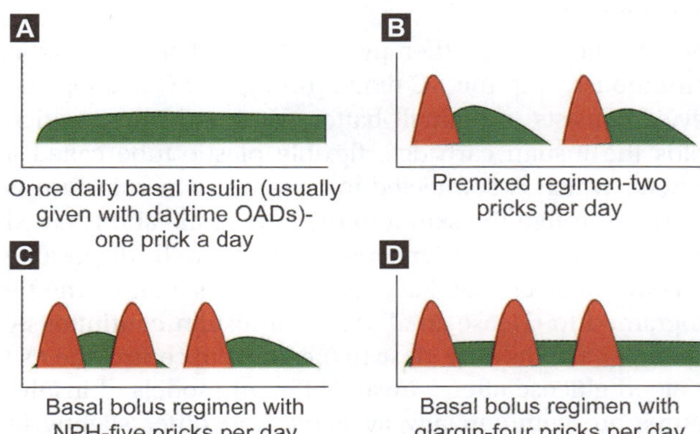

Figs 91.2A to D: Various insulin regimens (insulin replacement regimens)
Abbreviations: OAD = Oral antidiabetic drug; NPH = Neutral protamine Hagedorn

glucose levels. The initial dose required can be calculated at the rate of 0.5 U/kg/day for type 1 DM and 0.2 U/kg/day for type 2 DM. If the patient is not symptomatic, 50% of the calculated dose can be given initially and the dose can be gradually increased by 4 units every 4th day. If the patient is symptomatic, the calculated dose can be given in full at the start and adjusted subsequently (Figs 91.2A to D).

Site of Insulin Injection

Subcutaneous insulin can be given at one of the following sites—anterior abdominal wall, lateral aspects of the thighs and arms. Intramuscularly (IM), it can be administered over the deltoid or other regions. The rate of absorption of insulin from the injected site varies. More rapid absorption occurs from the abdominal wall compared to the deltoid region and the thighs when given subcutaneous (SC). IM injections are more rapidly absorbed and duration of action is only for several minutes. IV injections produce immediate effect, but only for a few minutes.

Storage

It should preferably be stored at 4–8°C. However, it is stable at room temperature for 3–4 weeks.

Intensive Insulin Therapy

Awareness of the significance of tight metabolic control in the prevention of long-term complications of diabetes has led to the development of newer insulin delivery systems and different types of insulin therapy. Intensive insulin therapy of type 1 DM uses either 3–4 injections daily or a CSII from an insulin infusion pump. Blood glucose determinations done prior to each meal and at bedtime helps to determine the dose of soluble insulin to be administered based on an adjustment schedule algorithm.

Insulin Injection Devices

This can be done using conventional disposable syringes, specially calibrated for insulin. Insulin pens using specially made insulin cartridges are available which are disposable or suitable for refilling. Availability of insulin pen facilitates the injection of insulin and also ensures the availability of the injection at the exact time, irrespective of the activity of the patient. The insulin pen with its insulin cartridge can be stored at room temperature (< 28°C) for 4 weeks.

Insulin pumps

The insulin pump therapy or CSII, delivers insulin continuously into the SC tissue through a SC needle. The device consists of a small battery powered pump which holds the insulin cartridge, flexible plastic tube called a catheter which is connected to a needle, which in turn is inserted through the skin into the fatty tissue and is taped in place. Catheter and needles are generally disposable and have to be changed at regular intervals. Pumps can be programed to release small doses of insulin continuously (basal), or a bolus dose close to mealtime to control the rise in blood glucose after a meal. Different models of insulin pumps are commercially available and differ slightly in terms of programing of insulin delivery, synchronization with continuous glucose monitoring device and automatic shutting down of insulin delivery, if hypoglycemia is detected. Insulin pumps closely resemble the physiological release of insulin but are not widely popular in India due to high cost of the device and disposables.

Artificial pancreas

In contrast to conventional insulin pumps, closed-loop insulin delivery system or 'artificial pancreas' delivers insulin at a rate that varies depending on the patient's interstitial glucose level. This requires an insulin pump with integrated continuous glucose monitoring device and a computer-generated control algorithm modulating the insulin delivery rate. Bihormonal closed loop devices that infuse both insulin and glucagon are also under investigation. Early results of short-term trials towards real-life clinical use of artificial pancreas in type 1 DM are promising in achieving improved glycemic control with reduced risk of hypoglycemia. But they are still facing technological and metabolic challenges.

Pancreatic Transplants

Pancreatic transplantation has been carried out in diabetics since 1966 with the aim to provide euglycemia and an insulin independent state. Such a state is achieved and maintained along with the use of immunosuppressant drugs. The clinical results have improved greatly after the Edmonton Protocol of using immunosuppressants published in 1999. Patients with type 1 DM suffering from recurrent severe hypoglycemia with hypoglycemia unawareness or glycemic lability leading to poor quality of life are currently considered for pancreatic transplant. These patients generally have uncontrolled hyperglycemia for more than 5 years and have no endogenous insulin production suggested by negative stimulated C-peptide levels.

Islet Cell Transplantation

It is done along with a renal transplant in most cases either simultaneously or after renal transplant depending upon the patients' kidney status. Simultaneous kidney pancreas transplant is the most commonly performed procedure.

In islet cell transplantation, cadaver pancreas is removed en bloc and their islets are separated out using collagenases. These isolated islets are then injected into the portal vein by percutaneous transhepatic procedure under fluoroscopic guidance. These injected islets get trapped in the hepatic sinusoids where they establish vascularity. This is associated with risks of liver failure, portal vein thrombosis and portal hypertension. Major indications for islet cell transplantation are cases of type 1 DM with any one of the following indications: (1) Unawareness of hypoglycemia, (2) brittle diabetes with frequent episodes of hypoglycemia and/or ketoacidosis and (3) progressive diabetic complications, such as retinopathy, nephropathy and neuropathy. Today, most islet transplants are done in conjunction with renal transplants, although people are focusing on solitary islet cell transplants. $2\text{–}7 \times 10^8$ islets cells are required to make effective transplantation. About 50% continue to have functioning pancreas without insulin dependence 5 years after transplantation.

Data from clinical trials suggests that even a partially functioning islet graft helps in reducing severe hypoglycemia in patients with type 1 DM. Numerous studies have also shown that islet transplantation may slow progression of microvascular complications including retinopathy and neuropathy in patients with type 1 DM but the limited data on renal function is contradictory. Therapeutic impact of human islet cell transplant is limited by few unsolved issues, namely: (1) Unavailability of donors compared to the large amount of potential recipients, (2) occurrence of instant inflammatory reaction after exposure of islet cells to recipient's blood requiring multiple transplants to achieve significant reduction of exogenous insulin dependence. Secondly, long-term use of immunosuppressants with their side-effects is weighted against the use of long-term use of insulin. With the advances in the field of regenerative medicine, mesenchymal stem cells are highlighted due to their additional anti-inflammatory potential. Experimental islet transplantation including mesenchymal stem cell transplantation is explored widely as one of the future options and also provides important knowledge regarding pathophysiology of diabetes but its clinical application is still a long way to go.

Noninvasive Insulin Delivery Methods

Due to the inconvenience of injections, there is an unmet need for a minimally invasive or noninvasive method of insulin delivery. Technological advances are being explored to investigate the possibility of insulin delivery though oral, buccal, nasal, peritoneal and transdermal approaches.

Inhaled insulin (Exubera) was the first approved noninvasive method but was withdrawn from the market within a year after its introduction due to high cost, bulky delivery device, concerns related to declining in pulmonary function and less preference by patients and physicians. Recently, another inhaled insulin (Afrezza) has completed phase 3 clinical trials and is in the Food and Drug Administration (FDA) approval process.

Noninsulin Parenteral Therapeutic Agents

GLP-1 Analogues

The incretin effect is the process by which stimulatory response of oral glucose on insulin secretion is more than IV glucose dose. Pathological alterations in endogenous incretins have major contribution towards development of type 2 DM. Native GLP-1 incretin has very short half-life (< 5 minutes) and degraded rapidly by DPP-4 enzyme. Incretin-based agents include GLP-1 receptor agonists, which mimic endogenous GLP-1 and DPP-4 inhibitors (as discussed above) which inhibit the breakdown of endogenous incretin hormones. Incretins, GLP-1 and glucose-dependent insulinotropic peptide (GIP) hormones are the peptide hormones secreted by L-type of cells at the terminal ileum in response to food intake. GLP-1 hormone reduces blood glucose level by increasing glucose-dependent insulin secretion by β-cells. In addition, it slows gastric emptying, suppresses glucagon release, and also acts at central level by increasing satiety level. Agents that either act as GLP-1 agonists or enhance endogenous GLP-1 activity are being used for treatment of type 2 DM. Agents in this class do not cause hypoglycemia because of the glucose-dependent nature of incretin-stimulated insulin secretion. Additionally they benefit by helping in weight reduction (Flowchart 91.2).

Pharmacology of different GLP-1 analogues (Table 91.24)

- **Exenatide:** If administered within 60 minutes of morning and evening meals, exenatide predominately lowers postprandial glycemic excursion while effect remaining for 5–7 hours. Effects on lunch hyperglycemia and on fasting blood glucose are modest. In view of GI side effects, it is recommended to start therapy with 5 µg twice daily for 1 month and subsequently to increase to 10 µg twice daily. Severe kidney failure (creatinine clearance < 30 mL/min) is a contraindication to use of exenatide as it is predominantly eliminated by kidneys.
- **Liraglutide:** Half-life of liraglutide is about 13 hours following a once daily SC injection. Steady-state concentrations are obtained after 3–4 days after initiation of treatment. Treatment is titrated on weekly increments form 0.6 mg/day to a maximum of 1.8 mg/day.
- **Exenatide LAR:** It represents as the first-once-a-week injectable antihyperglycemia. Pharmacological characteristics are similar to that of exenatide, except the convenient once a week dosing and a safer side-effect profile (reduced upper GI symptoms). It is slightly more effective in reduction of HbA1C and FPG than regular exenatide.
- **Dulaglutide:** It is recently approved as once a week GLP-1 analogue for management of diabetes, especially in obese subjects.
- **Lixisenatide:** It is a novel human GLP-1 receptor agonist and is under phase 3 trials. It is proposed to be 4 times more potent and more selective than human GLP-1 in stimulating GLP-1 receptor.
- **Albiglutide:** It is also currently in phase 3 trials. Common side effects include nausea, vomiting, headache,

Flowchart 91.2: Effects of glucagon-like polypeptide-1 (GLP-1) receptor agonists on glucose metabolism

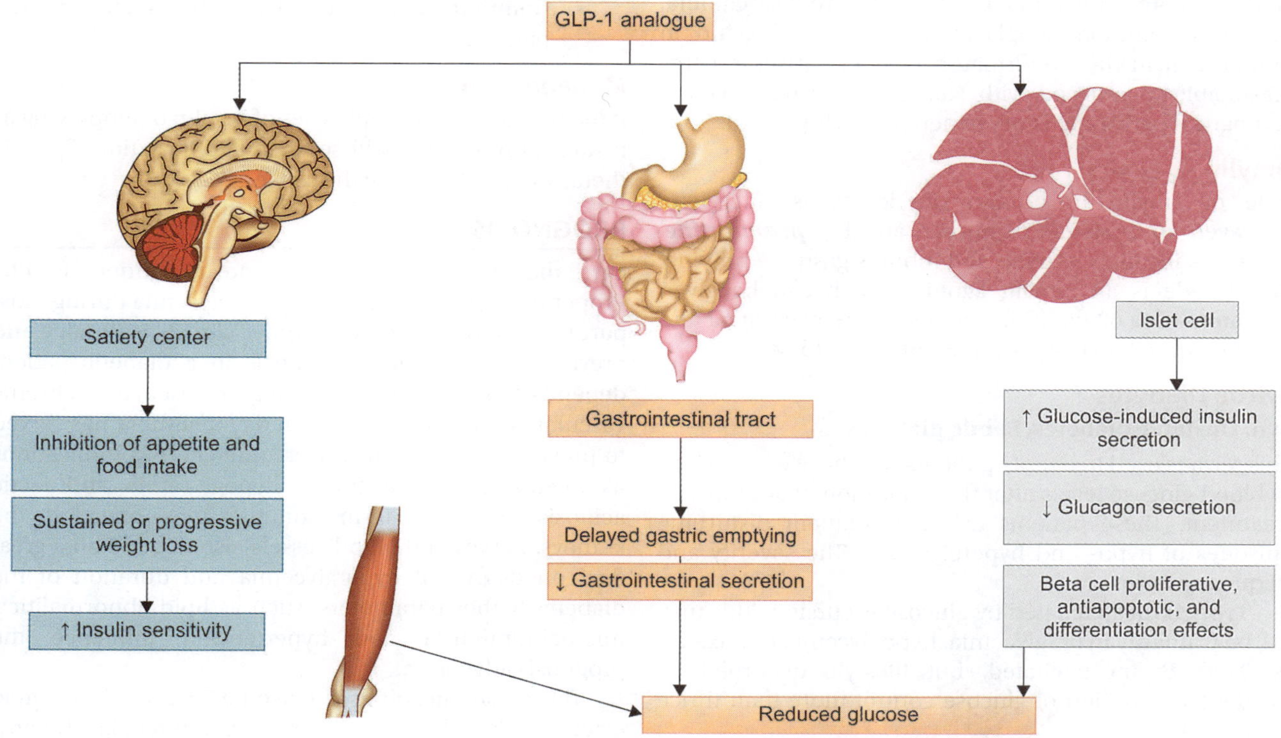

Table 91.24: Characteristics of different glucagon-like polypeptide-1 (GLP-1) analogues

Drugs	Approval status	Year of approval	Recommended dose	Frequency	Proposed A1C reduction	Effect on weight loss
Exenatide	USFDA	2005	5–10 μg	Twice a day	1.0–1.9%	Yes
Liraglutide	USFDA	2010	0.6–1.8 mg	Once a day	0.9–1.6%	Yes
Exenatide-LAR	USFDA	2011	2 mg	Once a week	1.5%	Yes
Dulaglutide	Awaited	2015	1.5 mg	Once a week	1–1.5%	Yes
Lixisenatide	Awaited	–	20 mg[†]	Once a day[†]	0.74%	Yes
Albiglutide	Awaited	–	30 mg[†]	Once a week[†]	0.57%	Yes[†]
Taspoglutide	Halted*	–	–	–	1.1%	Yes[†]

*Trial halted due to higher incidence of gastrointestinal side effects and hypersensitivity reactions.
[†]Uncertain.
Abbreviation: USFDA = United States of Food and Drug Administration

dizziness, nasopharyngitis, back pain, upper respiratory tract infections and local skin reactions.

- ***Taspoglutide:*** Further studies of this drug were halted due to higher incidence of GI side effects and hypersensitivity reactions.

Concerns regarding side effects of GLP-1 analogues

Most common side effects of GLP-1 analogues are GI—mainly nausea, which in most cases subsides with time. The fact that GLP-1 receptors are present throughout the human body tampering with the biology of these molecules could have a negative influence on certain conditions that could coexist with type 2 DM. Data obtained indicate that GLP-1 agonists could increase the risk of pancreatitis and pancreatic cancer, possibly due to their capacity to increase ductal cell turnover but there exists a contradictory data. There is a warning issued towards the rare complication of pancreatitis, and it can be strongly argued by most authors that the risk is more theoretical than practical. Exenatide and liraglutide are associated with medullary thyroid carcinoma in rat models. Concerns arise as GLP-1 receptors are found in papillary thyroid carcinoma, the most common neoplasm of the thyroid gland in humans. Till further confirmatory evidence arises it seems reasonable to proceed with caution while using GLP-1 analogue if personal history of neoplasms is present.

Amylin Agonists

Role of amylin in human physiology is uncertain. However, an analogue of human amylin, '*pramlintide*' enhances insulin secretion and inhibits gastric emptying. Pramlintide is an amylin agonist which can be given parenterally as 60 μg SC injections before each meal and may be titrated up to a maximum of 120 μg/day.

Brittle Diabetes

Syn: Unstable diabetes, Labile diabetes

This term is used to denote patients who have wide swings in blood glucose levels after the institution of appropriate treatment. These patients undergo frequent disturbing episodes of hypo- and hyperglycemia. The severity and frequency varies.

- ***Type A:*** Incapacitated by glucose excursion. This may be primarily hyperglycemia, hypoglycemia or mixed.
- ***Type B:*** Incapacitated, but lifestyle disturbed by decompensation of glucose control more than thrice a week.

Causes

Causes of brittle diabetes include the following:

- Disorders of glucose regulations
- Disturbances in other hormones, which influence glucose levels
- Disorders of insulin pharmacokinetics:
  - Insulin antibodies
  - Insulin-receptor antibodies
  - Renal insufficiency
  - Hepatic cirrhosis
  - Erratic absorption from SC injection of insulin
- Gastrointestinal disorders:
  - Gastroparesis diabeticorum
  - Malabsorption state
- Coexistent systemic illnesses
- Psychological problems:
  - Self-induced therapeutic problem
  - Bulimia (eating disorder)
  - Depression
  - Alcohol abuse
  - Communication gap between the doctor and the patients.

Management

It includes frequent small doses of insulin or employing as insulin pump which will self-regulate its action. Specific therapy aims at tracking the cause.

PROGNOSIS

Once diabetes is established, it tends to continue for life. Proper management can achieve euglycemia during most part of the day and thereby confer clinical normalcy and prevent complications. Prognosis in a diabetic patient depends largely on the presence or absence of chronic vascular complications. Present day treatment has served to prevent or successfully overcome acute complications like ketoacidosis, infections, hypoglycemia and lactic acidosis. The long-term complications affecting the kidneys, nerves and blood vessels also depend on a great deal on degree of hyperglycemia and duration of the diabetes. Other parameters, such as lipid abnormalities, microalbuminuria and hypertension influence the prognosis adversely.

These complications can also be prevented to a great extent by rigid diet control, exercise and regular therapy.

Once established, the degenerative complications progress relentlessly and lead to damage of vital organs, like the kidneys, heart and brain, unless properly managed. Death is mainly due to complications like myocardial infarction, CVA, end-stage of renal failure or acute diabetic complications, such as diabetic coma, hypoglycemia and infections. Cumulative morbidity occurs due to blindness, peripheral vascular disease and peripheral neuropathy which cripple the long-term survivors. Proper therapy also arrests the progression of established complications. Cardiovascular complications can be reduced further by elimination of other risk factors, like hypertension, cigarette smoking, obesity and hyperlipidemia.

The Diabetes Control and Complications Trial (DCCT) (1991-95), which was carried out at 14 different centers in the USA and Canada, had enrolled 1,441 patients with type 1 DM with the objective of assessing the role of intensive insulin therapy in the primary prevention of microangiopathic complications as well as in arresting the progression of these complications. The data has convincingly brought out the importance of tight metabolic control in preventing the development of microangiopathy and arresting its progression. The risk reduction of various measured outcomes ranged from 35 to 75%. A beneficial effect on the macroangiopathy was also demonstrated.

The United Kingdom Prospective Diabetes Study (UKPDS), a large study carried out in 23 centers all over the United Kingdom, followed 5,102 patients with newly diagnosed type 2 DM over 5 years (1987–91) and reported a significant decline in the incidence of macrovascular disease with strict glycemic control. Additional benefits were also obtained with control of BP. Strict control of BP also brought down the incidence of stroke and heart failure. Both of these trials and several other reports emphasize the role of strict biochemical control of all forms of DM in reducing the incidence of complications. Follow-up of patients included in the DCCT 1993 trial has shown that the benefits of strict control of the diabetic state continued even 4 years after the termination of the study. With proper motivation and education of the patient, considerable improvement in glycemic control can be achieved in almost all patients at relatively low cost.

PREVENTION

The prevalence of diabetes, especially type 2 DM, has increased considerably and reached epidemic proportions. It is likely to quadruple itself by the turn of the century. Such a situation the demands that we should contain this problem by concentrating on preventive strategies. Since, the two types of diabetes are different entities, the approach to their prevention would also be different.

Type 1 Diabetes Mellitus

Several advances have taken place in the understanding of the pathogenesis and natural history of type 1 DM, particularly in its preclinical phase. Coupled with this, the advances in the field of immunology and the development of the concept of immunomodulation and immunosuppression in autoimmune disorders have opened up newer vistas in its prevention. Recent experimental work on mice shows that autoimmune type 1 DM can be corrected by transplantation of islet cells along with splenic cells and immunomodulator adjuvants. Stem cells of the spleen can be home to the pancreas and develop into mature functioning islet cells. These landmark studies show promise for cure of type 1 DM in future.

Source: Melton DA. Reversal of type 1 diabetes in mice. N Engl J Med. 2006;355(1):89-90.

Type 2 Diabetes Mellitus

The potential for primary prevention of type 2 DM exists in the high-risk groups, such as: (1) Persons with a family history of diabetes, (2) obese individuals, (3) women with bad obstetric history and (4) hypertensive patients. In these populations, screening for IGT should be repeated at regular intervals. Enormous benefits could be achieved from preventive programs aimed at a balanced nutrition, avoidance of obesity, promotion of physical activity and reduction of smoking. Though studies have shown that administration of metformin, acarbose and thiazolidinediones during the stage of IGT and IFG all prevent the onset of florid diabetes, drugs are not generally recommended for this purpose as lifestyle modifications have been shown to be as effective and cheaper. Cases of prediabetes have to be managed on individual levels as the condition warrants.

DIABETES DURING PREGNANCY

DM encountered during pregnancy may be gestational diabetes mellitus (GDM) or pre-GDM. One should try to determine whether the woman had type 1 DM or type 2 DM before the onset of pregnancy. DM leads to serious complications during pregnancy. Not only the complications of the disease may get worse in the mother, but the fetus and neonate are also placed at a risk, leading to increased intrauterine death, perinatal morbidity and postnatal mortality.

GDM is defined as carbohydrate intolerance of variable severity with the onset or first recognition during the present pregnancy and which clears up spontaneously after delivery. Tissue sensitivity to insulin is slightly increased between 12 and 14 weeks of pregnancy and thereafter, it declines throughout the rest of the pregnancy. It returns to normal immediately after delivery. In normal pregnancy, development of insulin resistance is a mechanism to provide high energy substrate to the baby. Blood glucose and FFA levels increase. This in turn leads to higher insulin secretion. In 2–4% of women, the pancreatic insulin response is inadequate and GDM ensues.

If perinatal morbidity and mortality are to be reduced, GDM must be detected as early as possible and treatment instituted promptly. Screening of all pregnant women for GDM between 24 and 28 weeks of gestation with a 75 g oral glucose challenge is the most widely used method. The criteria for diagnosis of GDM by this method are summarized in Box 91.6.

All women with GDM should be screened for persistent diabetes at 6–12 weeks postpartum, using the OGTT and non-pregnancy diagnostic criteria. Women with a history of GDM should have lifelong screening

Box 91.6: Revised criteria for diagnosis of gestational diabetes mellitus (GDM)

- Fasting plasma glucose (FPG) ≥ 92 mg/dL

  OR
- 1-hour post-75-g glucose-load plasma glucose (1-hr PP) ≥ 180 mg/dL

  OR
- 2-hour post-75-g glucose-load plasma glucose (2-hr PP) ≥ 153 mg/dL

Source: Adapted from American Diabetes Association, 2014.

for the development of diabetes or prediabetes at least every 3 years. Women with a history of GDM found to have prediabetes should receive lifestyle interventions or metformin to prevent diabetes.

Maternal Complications

The most common obstetric complications include hydramnios, pre-eclamptic toxemia, UTIs, vaginal moniliasis and premature labor. Hyperemesis gravidarum and infections are associated with higher risk of ketosis in diabetic women. Diabetic retinopathy may worsen during pregnancy.

Fetal Complications

These include intrauterine death, prematurity and congenital anomalies. During the immediate postnatal period, maternal hyperglycemia makes the newborn prone for hypoglycemia, hypercalcemia hyperbilirubinemia or respiratory distress syndrome. Perinatal mortality is increased due to placental insufficiency, prematurity, or trauma during birth. The risk to fetus increases as the pregnancy advances and intrauterine death of fetus is more frequent towards the later stages. Incidence of intrauterine fetal death can be reduced by proper control of the diabetic state.

Management

Management of diabetes during pregnancy is a demanding task and can be best achieved through a team work approach involving the obstetrician, diabetologist, dietician and pediatrician. The management of pregnancy complicated by diabetes should begin before pregnancy is contemplated. Information about the potential complications of pregnancy for the mother and offspring should be explained to the couple. The importance of good stable metabolic control before conception should be highlighted. The aim of therapy should be to maintain the fasting blood glucose below 95 mg% and 1-hour postprandial blood glucose levels below 140 mg/dL. The insulin requirements may fall during the first trimester, and then there is a progressive increase in the requirements until about 34–36 weeks of pregnancy. The requirements come down soon after delivery. It is better to put on three doses of short-acting human insulin or two-split doses of soluble and intermediate-acting insulin. Recently, metformin has been shown to be safe and effective during pregnancy and may be added, especially if signs of insulin resistance are present.

Dietary Management

A meal plan is made to maintain euglycemia and to provide sufficient calories to sustain adequate nutrition for the mother and the fetus without excessive weight gain. Addition of 150 calories during the first trimester and 300 calories in the second and third trimesters above the basal requirements is adequate. Protein intake should be increased to 1.5–2 g/kg bw. Exercise should be advised as is compatible with the obstetric condition.

Monitoring Control

Preferably plasma glucose levels should be done by the patient before the main meals and also postprandially at least twice a day. Present day glucometers (available at ₹ 1,500) enable self-monitoring. The advent of glucometer and home blood glucose monitoring helps to achieve good glycemic control. Measurements of HbA1C at 4–6 weeks intervals help to confirm the status of long-term glycemic control. Urine examination for glucose does not give proper assessment of control, since renal threshold for glucose is lowered during pregnancy. It should be remembered that meticulous control of blood glucose levels and all others aspects of diabetes are extremely important to manage the women during pregnancy and any deficiency will result in complications for the mother and the baby. A trained pediatrician should be available to manage the baby during the first few hours of its birth, since wild fluctuations in blood glucose levels may develop giving rise to serious problems. This may be immediate or long time.

Fetal Monitoring Techniques

Ultrasound examination for evaluating fetal growth, estimating fetal weight, detecting hydramnios and malformations should be repeated at 4–6 week intervals. Determination of maternal serum α-fetoprotein at 16 weeks along with ultrasound at 18 weeks helps to detect neural tube defects and other anomalies. Fetal echocardiography (ECHO) at 20–22 weeks reveals cardiac defects. Amniocentesis is performed before elective delivery to document fetal pulmonary maturity.

Timing of Delivery

Delivery should be timed when fetal maturation is achieved. Maternal diabetes should be controlled meticulously. The route of delivery for the diabetic patient has to be decided individually. Diabetes as such is not an indication for cesarean section. The decision for cesarean section should be based on the obstetric indications. Termination of pregnancy at the optimum time is a combined decision of the team of doctors based on the:

- Degree of control of diabetes
- Fetal growth, maturity and viability
- General condition of the mother
- Outcome of previous pregnancies
- The neonatal services available.

In many instances, induction of labor and delivery are done by about 36–38 weeks by which time the risk of hyaline membrane disease of the lung is low.

Long-term Complications of GDM

Most women without pre-GDM become normoglycemic shortly after the delivery but on long-term follow-up more than 30% of GDM patients develop type 2 DM. Additionally, intrauterine exposure to maternal hyperglycemia conveys high risks for future obesity and type 2 DM in the offspring which is additional to the risk incurred by genetic predisposition due to history of diabetes to the mother and is independent of the type of diabetes during pregnancy.

DIABETES AND HUMAN IMMUNODEFICIENCY VIRUS INFECTION

Care of diabetes in human immunodeficiency virus (HIV) patients may involve patients with known diabetes acquiring HIV infection, concurrent diagnosis of diabetes and HIV infection or incident hyperglycemia after start of antiretroviral therapy. With increasing life-expectancy of HIV-infected adults, prevalence of diabetes and CVD is on rise. Prevalence of diabetes in patients infected with HIV is reported as high as 15%. HIV infection and antiretroviral treatment may both have adverse effects on glucose and lipid metabolism notably insulin resistance. General principles of the evaluation management of diabetes in HIV-infected patients are same with few specific considerations. HbA1C testing in HIV-infected individuals is considered less reliable for screening as well as follow-up due to increased red blood cell turnover and certain medications. It is also prudent to understand the interactions between antidiabetic medications, statins and antiretroviral therapy as well as the pathophysiological alterations of these medications on the disease processes, e.g. protease inhibitors increase insulin resistance and are strongly associated with developing diabetes. The choice and preferences of choosing antidiabetic medications are similar to that of patients without HIV infections. Some authorities recommend against using DPP-4 inhibitors, such as the gliptins due to possible adverse effects of these drugs on the molecular targets of immune cells. Insulin is generally the drug of choice in poorly controlled diabetes with multiple comorbidities. Concurrent treatment of the cardiovascular risk factors, such as antiplatelet therapy, BP control, cholesterol management and smoking cessation, should be emphasized. Routine screening of microvascular complications should be advised as per standard protocol same as non HIV-infected diabetes patients.

NEONATAL DIABETES MELLITUS (NDM)

It is defined as insulin-requiring hyperglycemia that is diagnosed within the first 3 months of life. It may be transient; subsiding by 3 months or may continue for longer periods. NDM is different from other forms of diabetes. It is caused by activating mutations of genes KCNJ11 which encodes kir 6, 2 subunit of the ATP-sensitive potassium channel (KATP) of the β-cell. The disease is rare with an incidence of 1/50,000 to 1/100,000 livebirths. Such children show intrauterine growth retardation (IUGR). The disease manifests in the first 3–6 months of life with glycosuria, polyuria, dehydration, failure to thrive and frank DKA. Serum levels of insulin and insulin-like growth factor are low. Treatment with insulin results in dramatic catch up growth and improvement. In 50% of cases, insulin can be discontinued, but DM may recur in the 2nd to 3rd decades of life. Fifty percent of cases of NDM develop permanent DM. Interestingly these cases respond to OHAs, such as glyburide. These are the cases which have mutations in the SUR regulatory subunit of KATP or Kir6 2 genes. Identification of these genetic mutations can predict cases which will respond to oral SU. This response may result from the closing of mutant KATP channels, thereby increasing insulin secretion in response to incretins and glucose metabolism.

Source: Sperling MA. ATP-sensitive potassium channels—neonatal diabetes mellitus and beyond. N Engl J Med. 2006;355(5):507-10.

CHAPTER
92

Complications of Diabetes Mellitus

AG Unnikrishnan, Anjali Bhatt

Chapter Summary

- Metabolic Emergencies in Diabetes
- Hypoglycemia
- Diabetic Ketoacidosis
- Hyperosmolar Nonketotic Coma
- Lactic Acidosis
- Diabetic Lactic Acidosis
- Other Acute Problems in the Diabetic
- Long-term Complications of Diabetes Mellitus
- Cardiovascular System
- Peripheral Vascular Disease
- Cerebrovascular Disease
- Diabetic Retinopathy
- Other Complications Affecting the Eye
- Diabetic Nephropathy
- Urinary Tract Infections
- Neuropathy
- Diabetic Foot
- Other Complications
- Future Prospects in Diabetology

INTRODUCTION

Diabetes mellitus (DM) is associated with several complications throughout the course of the disease. At present, short-term control of diabetes can be achieved in almost all cases by the use of dietary regimen, exercise and drugs. On long-term basis, majority of the patients fail to comply with the strenuous therapeutic regimen and the ideal control of blood sugar during day and night is compromised. Postprandial hyperglycemia is recognized to be an important factor contributing to vascular complications and increased mortality. Diabetes is more dreaded for complications, which invariably set in as the diabetic state continues. Though the Diabetes Control and Complications Trial (DCCT) and United Kingdom Prospective Diabetes Study (UKPDS) trials have demonstrated that the incidence and severity of all complications can be brought down, complete prevention cannot still be guaranteed in any particular case. On account of this, long-standing diabetic patients constitute a sizeable proportion of chronic morbidity requiring regular and expensive therapeutic interventions. In many diabetics, the disease may be first detected when the patient presents with a complication.

Acute Complications

- Metabolic derangements
  - Diabetic ketoacidosis (DKA) and coma
  - Hypoglycemia
  - Hyperosmolar nonketotic coma
  - Lactic acidosis.
- Infections
  - *Medical:* Acute infections such as skin infections, respiratory tract infections (RTI), urinary tract infections (UTI) (including emphysematous pyelonephritis), genital infections (such as balanophosthitis, vulvovaginitis), rhinocerebral mucormycosis and otitis externa.
  - *Surgical:* Boils, carbuncles, cellulitis, superficial and deep abscesses, gangrene, foot infections, necrotizing fasciitis.
- Acute events occurring as a result of long-term complications
  - Ischemic heart disease-acute
  - Renal failure
  - Peripheral vascular occlusion
  - Loss of vision.
- Obstetric complications
  - Intrauterine fetal death
  - Hydramnios, more frequent
  - Higher frequency of pre-eclamptic toxemia
  - Large baby (> 4 kg) giving rise to complications during delivery and perinatally
  - Infections of the genital tract
  - Worsening of the diabetic state during pregnancy and postpartum.

Long-term Complications

Cardiovascular: Earlier onset of atheroma, ischemic heart disease, cerebrovascular accidents (CVA), high incidence of hypertension (about 30% of diabetes have hypertension).

Neurological: Peripheral neuropathy, autonomic neuropathy and mononeuritis multiplex including cranial nerve palsies, urinary retention and incontinence, diabetic autonomic diarrhea.

Peripheral occlusive vascular diseases.

Renal: Recurrent urinary infections, chronic pyelonephritis, papillitis necrotians, diabetic glomerulosclerosis, end-stage renal failure.

Ocular: Cataract, retinopathy, iridocyclitis, glaucoma, refractive changes induced by treatment.

Respiratory: Pulmonary tuberculosis, other infections.

Alimentary: Xerostomia, stomatitis, gingivitis, dental sepsis, loosening of teeth, halitosis, hepatomegaly, gastric dilatation, nocturnal diarrhea and paralytic ileus.

Bone and joints: Osteoporosis, osteoarthritis and neuropathic joints (Charcot's joint).

Skin: Chronic fungal infections of skin, moniliasis of the mucous membranes of the genitalia and mouth, pruritus vulvae, necrobiosis lipoidica diabeticorum, trophic ulcers of the feet, scleredema.

Drug-induced complications: Hypoglycemia, drug allergy, toxicity to liver and bone marrow.

Even though the major long-term complications produce clinical deterioration in the patient, sometimes they may be ignored and the patient may not seek medical attention (Table 92.1).

METABOLIC EMERGENCIES IN DIABETES

All these situations are life-threatening. Hence, awareness, early diagnosis and appropriate management are necessary to cut down the morbidity and mortality. Metabolic emergencies in a diabetic can be classified as:

- Hypoglycemia
- DKA and coma
- Hyperosmolar nonketotic coma
- Lactic acidosis.

HYPOGLYCEMIA

Classically, hypoglycemia is the fall of blood glucose levels below 50–60 mg/dL associated with symptoms, which are relieved by glucose supplementation. However, development of symptoms also depends on the prevailing blood glucose levels and individual susceptibility. Factors such as age, medication and comorbid conditions influence the clinical manifestations. In those who have chronically elevated blood glucose levels, even reduction of glucose to normal values may precipitate symptoms. Clinically, it is characterized by a varying degree of neurological

Table 92.1: Major associated complications seen in longstanding diabetic subjects at the time of first examination in a tertiary care hospital at Trivandrum

Complications	%
Nephropathy	70
Hypertension (> 140/90)	50
Carotid artery disease	18
Peripheral vascular disease	21
Retinopathy	20
Coronary artery disease (ECG criteria)	12
Elevated LDL (> 150 mg%)	12
Hypertriglyceridemia (> 200 mg%)	18

Source: Poulose KP, personal communication (2004).

Abbreviations: ECG = Electrocardiogram; LDL = Low-density lipoprotein

dysfunction and is responsive to administration of glucose. The clinical manifestations are extremely varied and depend upon the rate of fall of blood glucose levels and the release of counter regulatory hormones.

Early recognition of the condition is essential since severe forms of hypoglycemia are life-threatening and delay in instituting therapy can result in permanent brain damage or loss of life. In many instances, slow onset hypoglycemia is recognized by the patient from his past experiences. Recent onset of episodes of hypoglycemia in a patient on therapy may be a pointer to renal insufficiency. The insulin requirements go down and necessary changes in doses have to be made. The excretion of oral hypoglycemic drugs is impaired and such drugs are better avoided in a diabetic with renal insufficiency.

Clinical Features

This varies from patient-to-patient and the circumstances in which an attack is provoked, generally depending on the rate of fall of blood glucose and the individual endocrine status. The hypoglycemic episodes with insulin usually occur at predictable time intervals in relation to their peak action. Hypoglycemia due to oral drugs can occur any time 30–60 minutes after ingestion. Unlike insulin induced hypoglycemia, it may present with bizarre symptoms and elude recognition. The presentation may mimic CVA at times. Persistence of hypoglycemia over prolonged periods is another feature which should be borne in mind. Recurrence after initial correction is also common.

With a rapid fall in the blood glucose, as happens during insulin therapy, manifestations due to epinephrine release are prominent, while with a gradual fall in blood glucose, the picture is predominantly due to decreased cerebral function presenting with varying neurological deficits (Box 92.1).

Symptoms of Hypoglycemia

- *Adrenergic symptoms:* Palpitation, sweating, tremors, anxiety.
- *Neuroglycopenic symptoms:* Tiredness, dizziness, drowsiness, seizures, coma.

Hypoglycemia usually manifests abruptly, unlike hyperglycemia which is more gradual in onset. Physical examination may reveal cold extremities, excessive sweating, tachycardia, elevated blood pressure (BP) and

Box 92.1: Precipitating factors for hypoglycemia

• Meal-medicine mismatch:
  ▪ Decreased food intake, missing a meal or its delay, diarrhea, vomiting.
  ▪ Increased physical activity (unplanned, excessive strenuous physical activity) without reduction of the dose of drugs or adjustments in food intake.
  ▪ Increased dose of either insulin or oral hypoglycemic agents.
• Decrease in insulin requirements, which can occur when a juvenile diabetic goes into remission *(honeymoon phase in type 1 diabetes)*, or soon after delivery in a pregnant woman (due to the drop in the placental hormones) or with the elimination of stress and control of infection.
• Renal and hepatic insufficiency which decrease the insulin requirements.
• Drug interactions, e.g. quinine, newer quinolones.
• Excessive alcohol consumption.

Table 92.2: Body's response to hypoglycemia	
Plasma glucose mg/dL	**Symptoms of hypoglycemia vs blood glucose levels**
66	Counter regulation starts
60	Autonomic symptoms
50	Neuroglycopenic symptoms such as difficulty to concentrate, confusion, weakness, drowsiness, blurring of vision, dizziness and dysphasia
40	Lethargy
31	Coma
20	Convulsions
11	Permanent brain damage
0	Death

mental agitation. As the condition proceeds, the patient becomes drowsy and comatose. Generalized convulsions may occur. The pupils are dilated and plantar response is extensor. Atypical features may occur at times.

At the suspicion of hypoglycemia, glucose should be administered after taking blood for glucose estimation. Venous blood glucose below 60 mg/dL suggests hypoglycemia. In severe cases, the value may be below 40 mg/dL and at times glucose may be undetectable. In any doubtful situation, the response to glucose can be taken as a reliable test for the diagnosis of hypoglycemia (Table 92.2).

The persistence of hypoglycemia for over six hours may lead to permanent central nervous system (CNS) damage. Recurrent attacks may also contribute to impairment of mental faculties in children and the elderly. Hypoglycemia impairs the quality of life. Sudden death due to cardiac arrhythmias ('dead in bed' syndrome) may occur due to the abrupt catecholamine surge associated with falling serum potassium levels, which can precipitate fatal arrhythmias. Electrocardiogram (ECG) may show QTc prolongation.

Management of Hypoglycemia

Management consists of emergency measures to correct the blood glucose levels and maintenance to avoid recurrence. If the patient can swallow, 50 g of glucose dissolved in 200 mL water should be given orally. Symptoms start improving within 5–7 minutes and patient becomes normal within 20–40 minutes. If glucose is not ready at hand, sucrose, sweet articles of food or even cereal foods can be given. Mild cases respond successfully. This method should be advised to all diabetic patients so as to avoid more serious consequences. If the patient is unconscious, parenteral glucose should be administered. About 15–20 g of glucose is usually needed. This is best administered by IV infusion of 200–250 mL of 10% dextrose, which is safe and effective.

An alternative is to give glucagon given IM in a dose of 1.0 mg and repeated 15 minutes later. It is effective in raising blood sugar. This is a useful method if the drug is available and in conditions, where IV injections are not possible due to technical reasons. Glucagon may be repeated after 15 minutes if response is poor. *Glucagon injections are ineffective in cases of alcohol-induced hypoglycemia.*

After initial correction of hypoglycemia, the patient is kept under observation for 3–4 hours, till he recovers completely and is fit for discharge. This is particularly important for those who are on long-acting sulfonylurea. Follow-up action consists of detecting the precipitating cause for hypoglycemia and avoiding these factors.

Prevention

All patients should be informed about the clinical picture of hypoglycemia and taught how to recognize an impending attack and take corrective steps. They should be given identity cards indicating the disease, medication received and the address of the personal physician. Hypoglycemic episodes are frightening to the patients and therefore, unless the warning symptoms are explained to them and corrective measures advised, many of them fail to comply with the prescribed regimen thereafter.

Recurrent Severe Hypoglycemia

Severe recurrent hypoglycemia is common among type 1 diabetes patients as well as among those with late stage of type 2 diabetes. ***The most frequent cause is exogenous insulin, which, unlike endogenous insulin does not get suppressed when the blood glucose starts falling.*** The other reason is the failure of the counter regulatory hormone response. The hypoglycemia is not recognized by the patient at its onset. This state is called as 'hypoglycemic unawareness'. A vicious circle develops and episodes of hypoglycemia recur.

Hypoglycemia Unrelated to Diabetes Mellitus

In resting adults, over 60% of glucose is used by the CNS and the remainder by other tissues such as muscles, bone marrow and kidneys. Fasting hypoglycemia may result from reduction in hepatic gluconeogenesis and/or excessive glucose utilization. The former is due to hepatic diseases. The latter is due to tumors, which use up large amounts of glucose or non-β-cell tumors, which produce one or other insulin like growth factors.

Tests

Plasma insulin is measured when blood sugar level is less than 45 mg/dL. In those in whom insulin levels are high, the probabilities are insulinoma, factitious hypoglycemia, ingestion of sulfonylurea drugs and the presence of anti-insulin antibodies. These can be differentiated by determining C-peptide, proinsulin and insulin antibody concentration. Insulinomas produce insulin and also proinsulin. The hallmark of insulinoma is failure to suppress insulin production in the presence of hypoglycemia.

Anti-insulin antibody: It is more commonly seen in systemic lupus erythematosus (SLE), rheumatoid arthritis, Graves' disease and benign monoclonal gammopathy. Rarely it may be an isolated disorder.

Antibody induced hypoglycemia: Autoimmune insulin syndrome is a rare cause of hypoglycemia. This is characterized by late postprandial hypoglycemia and polyclonal insulin-binding antibodies. The antibodies trap insulin and release it after varying intervals, giving rise to hypoglycemia.

DIABETIC KETOACIDOSIS (DKA)

It is caused by gross derangement of carbohydrate and fat metabolism brought on by severe deficiency of insulin.

This is characterized by hyperglycemia, presence of excess ketone bodies in blood and urine, and metabolic acidosis. In the early stages, the ketosis may be mild and easily correctable, but later it becomes clinically pronounced and resistant to therapy. DKA is a common medical emergency encountered in the medical casualties of all major general hospitals in India. The term diabetic coma was used to denote extreme ketoacidosis. This term is not commonly in vogue at present.

Pathogenesis

Insulin deficiency may be absolute or it may be a conditioned deficiency brought on by the precipitating factors. Severe insulin deficiency results in hyperglycemia. Hyperglycemia leads to hyperosmolarity of the plasma, which causes a shift of intracellular fluid to the extracellular compartment with consequent cellular dehydration. Osmotic diuresis leads to loss of water and sodium from the extracellular compartment. Severe loss of water and electrolytes result in the shrinkage of extracellular fluid volume and hypotension. Reduction of renal blood flow impairs renal function.

In the presence of insulin deficiency, fat cells undergo lipolysis. This releases excess of fatty acids which reach the liver but they are only incompletely metabolized. Due to this, large amounts of ketone bodies are formed.

Apart from insulin deficiency, other concomitant metabolic derangements also contribute to the severity of ketosis. Growth hormone and glucocorticoids which antagonize the action of insulin are produced in excess. These enhance gluconeogenesis, lipolysis and ketogenesis in the liver. Lipolysis leads to production of free fatty acids (FFA). Glucagon directs the FFA to enter the mitochondria for β-oxidation leading to excess production of ketone bodies such as acetone, acetoacetic acid and β-hydroxy butyrate. All the ketone bodies are excreted in urine. Acetone being volatile is present in the expired air and this imparts a fruity smell to the breath. Acidosis gives rise to peripheral vasodilatation which aggravates hypotension and leads to shock. The plasma bicarbonate level is reduced progressively as ketosis worsens. Another serious metabolic consequence is the abnormal shift of potassium. Potassium moves out of the cells into the extracellular compartments leading to hyperkalemia. Potassium is lost in urine, resulting in the net loss of potassium from the body even in the presence of hyperkalemia. When the metabolic abnormality gets corrected with insulin, fluids and electrolytes, the glucose and potassium re-enter the cells. This leads to severe hypokalemia, which may be fatal, if undetected and treated promptly. The anion gap is increased. Serum magnesium concentration falls. Total body phosphorous is also lowered. The erythrocyte 2,3-diphosphoglycerate levels are also lowered and as a consequence the oxygen dissociation curve is shifted to the left. This leads to tissue anoxia. Once ketosis develops, if left untreated, it proceeds to diabetic coma. Precipitating factors for DKA are given in Box 92.2.

Clinical Features

Since the metabolic derangement takes time to develop, the onset of ketosis is gradual over a few days, but in

Box 92.2: Precipitating factors for diabetic ketoacidosis (DKA)

- Withdrawal or reduction in insulin dosage
- Infections
- Trauma or surgery
- Medical emergencies like acute myocardial infarction (Acute MI) and cerebrovascular accidents (CVA)
- Large carbohydrate intake
- Drugs which aggravate the diabetic state, e.g. corticosteroids
- Psychological stress.

In majority of cases, the condition is precipitated by sudden withdrawal of insulin in the presence of an offending factor.

some young diabetics, it may occur more rapidly. The early symptoms are those of uncontrolled diabetes such as extreme fatigue, polyuria, vomiting and insomnia. Drowsiness and altered behavior should draw attention to the possibility of ketoacidosis. The clinical state steadily deteriorates. Some cases present with abdominal symptoms like severe pain and distension, which may be mistaken for surgical emergencies.

The fully established case presents a characteristic picture. The patient is dehydrated, drowsy or deeply comatose. The respiration is deep and sighing and this is known as *Kussmaul's respiration.*

Note: Adolf Kussmaul (1822–1902) was a German physician. He has described three important clinical phenomena-pulsus paradoxus, Kussmaul's sign in pericardial tamponade and Kussmaul's respiration in metabolic acidosis.

A fruity smell of acetone may be detectable in the breath. Eyeball tension is low and BP is low. The limbs are flaccid and deep reflexes are sluggish. Plantar response is upgoing. The abdomen may be distended due to gastric dilation or paralytic ileus, which results from autonomic neuropathy. Initially the pupils are normal, but they may dilate, when the coma becomes deep. In some cases

fundal examination may reveal *lipemia retinalis* (milky plasma in the retinal vessels).

Unchecked gluconeogenesis	→	Hyperglycemia
Osmotic diuresis	→	Dehydration
Unchecked ketogenesis	→	Ketosis
Dissociation of ketone bodies into hydrogen ion and anions	→	Anion gap metabolic acidosis

Diagnosis

Any deterioration of the general condition, loss of control of the diabetic state, bizarre symptoms, fatigue, vomiting and altered behavior occurring in a diabetic should be investigated for ketoacidosis. The diagnosis should be established by urine examination and blood biochemistry. Urine shows sugar and acetone. Acetoacetic acid and acetone can be detected by Rothera's test or Acetest tablets or Ketostix. The tests can be semi-quantitated by noting the speed of development and depth of color and also testing the urine in progressive dilutions. Acetone disappears on boiling. Plasma ketones can also be detected by Ketostix or chemical methods. Acetoacetic acid can be tested also by the Gerhardt's test (ferric chloride test). Drugs like captopril which are eliminated in urine, give rise to false positive tests for acetone. Blood sugar is considerably elevated in most cases, but in some the elevation may be only moderate. Serum triglycerides are elevated (Table 92.3).

Differential Diagnosis

The diagnosis is easily suspected if coma occurs in a known case of diabetes, but the previous history may not be forthcoming always. So also the diabetic may develop other disorders leading to coma, e.g. CVA. Diabetic coma has to be differentiated from hypoglycemic coma,

Table 92.3: Clinical and biochemical data to assess the severity of diabetic ketoacidosis

	Mild	Moderate	Severe
Symptoms	Increasing polyuria, thirst, weakness, tiredness	Severe polyuria, polydipsia, rapid breathing, smell of acetone in breath, weakness; somnolence, vomiting	Symptoms of moderate ketosis with drowsiness progressing to stupor and coma
Signs	Flushed face and skin tachycardia, slight smell of acetone in breath	Kussmaul's breathing, loss of skin turgor, soft eyeballs small pulse volume, heavy odor of acetone in breath, drowsiness, and weakness	Severe dehydration, hypotension, extreme tachycardia, air hunger, coma
Urine			
Glucose	2%	Above 2%	Above 2%
Acetone	+++	+++ in 1:4 dilution	+++ in 1:8 dilution
Serum			
Acetoacetate	Positive in undiluted serum (3–6 mmol/L)	Positive in 2–3-fold dilution (6–12 mmol/L)	Positive in 1:4 dilution (above 12 mmol/L)
Plasma bicarbonate	Above 18 mEq/L	10–18 mEq/L	Below 10 mEq/L
Potassium	Normal	Often elevated	Usually elevated
Sodium	Normal	Normal	Normal
Hematocrit	Normal	Elevated	Elevated
pH	Normal	7.2	7.1 or less
Approximate water	1–2 L	3–4 L	5–8 L
Approximate sodium deficit	Less than 100 mmol	100–250 mmol	250–480 mmol

CVA, other causes of metabolic coma, head injuries, poisoning and intracranial infections like meningitis and encephalitis. In CVA, diabetic ketosis may also develop as a complication. Another point to be remembered is that in cerebral hemorrhage and subarachnoid hemorrhage, temporary glycosuria may develop even in non-diabetics, but this passes off when the acute stage is over. Moreover, this is not usually associated with ketonuria and acidosis. Other common causes of ketoacidosis are starvation and severe vomiting. In this glycosuria does not occur and blood glucose levels are low. Other causes of metabolic acidosis such as renal failure, lactic acidosis, poisoning by acids and salicylates and circulatory shock has to be excluded.

Management of Diabetic Coma and Ketoacidosis

The principles of management include:

- Correction of dehydration
- Control of hyperglycemia
- Correction of electrolyte disturbances and acidosis
- Attention to precipitating factors like infection, injury or stress
- Supportive measures
- Long-term management.

DKA is a medical emergency requiring hospitalization for treatment. In comatose patients, nasogastric tube is introduced to aspirate the stomach contents. In many cases, stomach may contain large amounts of fluid due to gastroparesis and therefore it is advisable to empty the stomach to prevent aspiration into the respiratory tract. Oral feeds are not permitted due to the possibility of aspiration pneumonia. Milder forms of ketoacidosis can be treated by conservative measures and if the patients can tolerate oral food and fluids, this route can be employed for correction.

Correction of Dehydration

Fluid and electrolytes should be replenished by IV normal saline as early as possible and this is the most effective single step to arrest further deterioration and bring about recovery. The approximate fluid deficit ranges from 2 to 8 L depending on the severity of the condition. The speed of administration of isotonic saline for a moderately severe case is given below:

1st L	30 minutes
2nd L	1 hour
3rd L	1 hour
4th L	2 hours
5th L	3 hours
6th L	4 hours (total infusion of 6 L in 11–12 hours)

Blood glucose and plasma bicarbonate are estimated at 2-hourly intervals. When the blood glucose falls below 250 mg/dL, 5% glucose solution may be given instead of saline. This helps to prevent hypoglycemia and also provide water for correcting cellular dehydration. By this time, oral intake is increased and IV administration tapered off.

A serious complication that may develop during fluid and electrolyte replacement is cerebral edema which may even go on to coning of the brainstem. This is more frequent in children and newly diagnosed diabetics. Symptoms of increased intracranial tension usher in after the initial period of recovery. Unless this complication is kept in mind and promptly managed by the use of IV mannitol and other measures, mortality will be high.

Insulin

Diabetic coma is the most urgent indication for soluble insulin. Insulin has to be given IV in moderate and severe cases. In mild cases insulin may be given IM.

Dose: Since large intermittent doses may lead to complications such as late hypoglycemia, hypokalemia, hyperlactatemia and osmotic disequilibrium, the present trend is to use smaller doses, 2–10 units per hour continuously as slow IV infusion. In some cases higher bolus doses may be required. Action of insulin lasts only for few minutes if given IV. In mild cases the same dose can be given IM hourly.

Soluble insulin is diluted with saline to give 0.1 unit/mL and administered in the drip or by intermittent injections in a dose of 6 units/hour (0.1 unit/kg/h) till the blood glucose comes down to 180 mg/dL. Thereafter the dose of insulin is reduced to 3 units/hour. It is ideal to reduce the blood glucose to 90 mg/dL (5 mmol/L). In insulin-resistant cases as detected by blood sugar estimation at 1-hour and 2-hour intervals, larger doses should be started without delay. It should be the aim to correct the metabolic abnormality within the shortest period, since prolongation of the coma may give rise to irreversible cellular damage. Insulin infusion is continued till the patient is able to take oral feeds and is fit for subcutaneous insulin.

If IM injections of insulin are used, the dose is 20 units as loading dose and 6 units every hour to be reduced to 6 units every 2 hours when the blood glucose falls below 180 mg/dL. Once the emergency is tided over, the patient should be put back on his regular insulin regimen.

Electrolyte Disturbances

In addition to severe loss of sodium, there is also gross potassium deficit. The serum potassium level does not reflect the total body content since there is shift of intracellular potassium to the extracellular compartment. In the early phases, serum potassium level is high. With the normalization of metabolism with insulin and fluid replacement, potassium re-enters the cells. At this stage, serious hypokalemia may supervene. Administration of potassium early in the regimen prevents this complication. If serum potassium is above 4–5 mmol/L, potassium chloride administration is not started till the potassium falls with therapy. The dose and frequency are adjusted by 2-hourly serum potassium estimations. It is desirable to maintain the serum potassium levels between 4 and 5 mmol/L. Potassium replacement is crucial to prevent death due to hypokalemia during recovery. In a severe case, approximately 100–200 mmol of potassium may be necessary in the first 24 hours. ECG monitoring is a helpful bedside method to indicate the effects of hypo- and hyperkalemia on the heart.

Administration of bicarbonate: There is considerable controversy regarding the use of bicarbonates in diabetic ketoacidosis. It need not be given as a routine. Its use results in a fall of serum potassium, shift of oxygen dissociation curve to the left resulting in tissue hypoxia and cerebrospinal fluid (CSF) disequilibrium. The indications for use of bicarbonates are:

- Severe acidosis with plasma bicarbonate level less than 10 mmol/L
- Patients with DKA complicating acute MI
- Patients with associated lactic acidosis.

Sodium bicarbonate is given slowly in doses of 55–100 mmol (200–300 mL of 2.74% $NaHCO_3$ solution). As the condition improves, the dose is reduced. Foci of infection, which may act as the precipitating factor should receive attention from the beginning.

Other supportive measures include proper care of the mouth, attention to the bladder and bowels, maintenance of fluid balance charts and prevention of decubitus ulcers. When the patient improves, he is rehabilitated and his usual antidiabetic regimen is restored. With modern lines of therapy, almost all cases of diabetic coma can be saved if the condition has not advanced too far. Many of the deaths may be due to the underlying conditions, which have precipitated diabetic coma, such as myocardial infarction (MI), stroke or infections.

Mild forms of DKA if detected early, can be managed at home using soluble insulin and if needed, the insulin analogues such as insulin lispro, which are more prompt and predictable in action.

Prevention of recurrence: The patient should be advised on the regular use of insulin and other antidiabetes drugs. The fact that insulin should be continued during intercurrent illness has to be stressed. Frequent monitoring of blood glucose levels and urine examination for acetone should be done when the diabetic gets stressful situations, particularly infections.

HYPEROSMOLAR NONKETOTIC COMA

Syn: Hyperosmolar hyperglycemic nonketotic state (HHNS)

This is a serious emergency seen occasionally in the elderly diabetics. It is commonly precipitated by infections, myocardial infarction, burns, trauma, surgical stress, renal failure, pancreatitis and use of drugs like thiazide diuretics, steroids, phenytoin and propranolol. In this condition, probably small amounts of endogenous insulin are present so that lipolysis does not occur, but glucose metabolism is greatly deranged. Blood glucose levels often exceed 300 mg/dL and go up above 600 mg/dL. Ketosis is absent and this distinguishes HHNS from diabetic coma. Normal osmolarity of the plasma is ± 290 mOsm/L. In HHNS, the plasma osmolarity rises above 300 and in severe cases, may exceed 370 mOsm/L. There is profound cellular dehydration. The hematocrit value is high. When the fluid loss becomes severe, hypernatremia develops. Sodium ions are critically important in determining plasma osmolarity. Body potassium is lost and a total deficit of 200–300 mmols may occur.

Clinical Features

The condition starts with extreme weakness and drowsiness and the patient gradually sinks into coma. Other neurological manifestations such as seizures, ataxia, hemiparesis, aphasia and mental disturbances may be present. Though thirst is present in the early stages, it disappears later. Respiration is normal or depressed. Apart from these features, the picture may resemble diabetic coma.

Diagnosis

Hyperosmolar nonketotic coma should be suspected in all cases of coma occurring in diabetics, without demonstrable ketosis. Plasma osmolarity can be calculated from the plasma levels of sodium, potassium, glucose and urea using the following formula:

$$\text{Plasma osmolarity in mOsm/L} = 2\,(Na^+ + K^+) + \frac{\text{Glucose in mg/dL}}{18} + \frac{\text{Urea in mg/dL}}{5.6}$$

Note: Some authors do not include K^+ in the calculation.

Treatment

Principles of management include correction of extreme fluid depletion and the hyperosmolar state. Insulin is administered in small doses as soon as the condition is recognized. Small doses are preferable since these patients are very sensitive to even small doses of insulin. Soluble insulin is given in doses of 5–10 units/hour IV as an infusion till the blood sugar comes to normal. Alternatively, 20 units of soluble insulin may be given IM, followed by small doses of 5–10 units/hour IM.

Hypotonic fluids are administered to lower the osmolarity. Half normal saline is the fluid of choice. About 6–8 L may have to be given over 24 hours. Monitoring of central venous pressure (CVP) is essential in the elderly to avoid fluid overload and cardiac failure. In patients with shock, isotonic saline should be infused till the CVP begins to rise. Potassium should be replaced early during the treatment and it should be monitored with serum potassium estimations. The prognosis is grave and mortality may be 20–40%. Prompt and early treatment results in recovery. Differentiation between DKA and hyperglycemic hyperosmolar state are given in Table 92.4.

LACTIC ACIDOSIS

Normal level of serum lactate is between 0.4 and 1 mmol/L in the fasting state and it may go up to 2 mmol/L after meals (5–18 mg/dL). This is maintained by a balance between the production and utilization of lactate. Though lactate is produced in all the tissues; brain, red blood cells (RBCs) and skeletal muscles account for the major part of this metabolite. Lactate is used for energy metabolism by several tissues under different circumstances. Seventy percent of lactate is cleared by the liver and 30% by the kidneys. Lactic acidosis has been divided into types A and B. In type A there is hypotension and tissue anoxia. Lactic acidosis may be primary when tissue perfusion is poor as in shock states. It may occur secondary to metabolic derangements as in uncontrolled diabetes, especially when treated with phenformin. In diabetic lactic acidosis, the blood lactate level is increased above 5 mmol/L and the arterial pH is below 7.25 (Table 92.5).

Table 92.4: Differentiation between diabetic ketoacidosis and hyperglycemic hyperosmolar state

Features	Diabetic ketoacidosis	Hyperglycemic hyperosmolar state
Clinical features		
Type of diabetes	Both types 1 or 2 diabetes mellitus	Type 2 diabetes mellitus
Evolution/onset	Over hours	Over days
Fruity (acetone odor) of breath	Observed	Not present
Kussmaul's respiration	Seen	Not seen
Abdominal pain/tenderness	Present	Absent
Laboratory findings		
Blood glucose level	>250 mg/dL	>600 mg/dL
Serum sodium	Normal or low (<140 mmol/L)	Usually high (>155 mmol/L)
Blood/urine ketones	++++	Negative or trace
Blood pH	<7.3	>7.3
Serum bicarbonate	<18 mmol/L	>18 mmol/L
Serum osmolality	Variable	>320 mOsm/kg
Mortality rate	5–10%	Variable if not properly managed

DIABETIC LACTIC ACIDOSIS

The hypoxic state produced by aberration in tissue metabolism probably contributes to the lactic acidosis associated with severe diabetes. Biguanides, especially phenformin aggravate this condition by inhibiting gluconeogenesis and mitochondrial electron transport chain. Due to this complication, phenformin is not routinely used at present. Metformin can also rarely produce lactic acidosis in patients with renal failure but the risk is quite low in normal subjects.

Clinical Features

In 80% of the patients, the condition starts with gastrointestinal (GI) problems, followed by sudden alteration in the sensorium leading to loss of consciousness, hypotension, Kussmaul's breathing, hypothermia, severe dehydration and circulatory collapse. Diagnosis should be confirmed by estimating plasma lactate which is above 5 mmol/L. The lactate pyruvate ratio would be above 15. Arterial pH falls below 7.25 and plasma bicarbonate falls below 18 mmol/L. The anion gap which measures the unmeasured anions in blood would be above the normal range of 8–12 mmol/L. In the absence of ketonuria, an increased anion gap in a diabetic is almost diagnostic of lactic acidosis. Mortality exceeds 50% in most series, if untreated.

Treatment

The principles of treatment comprise correction of shock, tissue hypoxia and acidosis. Toxic metabolites may be removed by hemodialysis. Insulin therapy speeds up recovery from lactic acidosis. Thiamine has been used with benefits especially in alcohol induced lactic acidosis. However, its value remains doubtful. Sodium bicarbonate is given to counteract acidosis (buffer action). It should be used with great caution since volume overload, worsening of acidosis and rebound alkalosis may develop. The total dose of bicarbonate can be calculated from the formula:

$$\text{Total requirement of bicarbonate (mmol)} = (25 - \text{plasma bicarbonate}) \times \text{body weight in kg} \times 0.3$$

Note: Carbicarb (a mixture of sodium carbonate and sodium bicarbonate) can also be used as a buffering solution IV. It is seldom used in practice.

OTHER ACUTE PROBLEMS IN THE DIABETIC

Somogyi effect (posthypoglycemic hyperglycemia): Insulin treated patients may show wide fluctuation in blood glucose levels, especially hyperglycemic episodes following periods of hypoglycemic episodes. The counter regulatory hormones that are secreted abruptly give rise to this phenomenon.

Dawn phenomenon: This is hyperglycemia occurring around 3–4 am, which is due to partial insulin resistance caused by release of growth hormone. An additional bed time dose of insulin controls the hyperglycemia.

Rhinocerebral mucormycosis: This presents as a fulminant infection of the nasal cavity and paranasal sinuses with extension into the cranial cavity. This is seen more commonly in association with DKA. It gives rise to facial edema, cranial nerve palsies and coma. The organism belongs to the order mucorales in the class zygomycetes. Unless detected early and treated promptly, the condition is fatal. Strong clinical suspicion and demonstration of the fungus helps to make early diagnosis. Amphoterecin B is the drug of choice. The newer antifungals such as voriconazole are also effective.

Necrotizing fasciitis: It is fulminant infection in the fascial compartments of the limbs, caused by mixed bacterial flora. It presents as acute painful infection of the limb or other sites, rapidly leading to suppuration. The rise in pressure in the fascial compartments may lead to vascular occlusion and extensive gangrene, if not attended to early with antibiotic therapy and surgical decompression of the fascial compartment.

Table 92.5: Classification of lactic acidosis (Cohen and Woods, 1976)

Type A	Type B (without tissue hypoxia)		
(Tissue hypoxia)	B1 (common disorders)	B2 (drugs and toxins)	B3 (hereditary form)
• Cardiogenic shock • Endotoxic shock • Severe anemia • Left ventricular failure	• Diabetes mellitus • Renal failure • Liver disease • Infections • Leukemia	• Biguanides • Sorbitol • Xylitol • Salicylates • Methanol	• Type 1 glycogen storage disease • Fructose 1–6 diphosphatase deficiency • Methylmalonicacidemia (Leigh's syndrome)

LONG-TERM COMPLICATIONS OF DIABETES MELLITUS

GENERAL CONSIDERATIONS

The chronic complications of diabetes have been classified into microvascular and macrovascular complications. The microvascular complications are specific for diabetes and they constitute diabetic nephropathy, retinopathy, neuropathy and also dilated cardiomyopathy. The macrovascular complications on the other hand, are not exclusive to diabetes. They tend to start even before the onset of florid diabetes. These include coronary artery disease (CAD), cerebrovascular disease (CVD) and the peripheral vascular disease (PVD). Diabetes accelerates their progression and extent considerably.

PATHOGENESIS OF DIABETIC COMPLICATIONS

Several factors contribute to the total picture. These include:

Hyperglycemia: It raises the intracellular glucose concentration in insulin independent tissues such as nerves, glomeruli, lens and retina. Aldose reductase, the rate-limiting enzyme in the polyol pathway catalyzes the reduction of glucose to sorbitol, which is subsequently converted to fructose. Sorbitol does not easily cross the cell membranes. It accumulates intracellularly and leads to cellular damage through its osmotic effects (e.g. in the lens); by altering the redox state (the state of oxidation/ reduction equilibrium) of pyridine nucleotides (by increasing the NADH/NAD ratio) and by depleting the intracellular myoinositol levels.

Glycosylation of proteins: The attachment of glucose to amino groups of protein leads to the formation of Schiff base products or early glycation products. The glycation of proteins leads to alteration in the functions of proteins. It is also responsible for the free-radical mediated damage to the tissues. The early glycosylation products undergo *Amadori rearrangement* to form stable products termed *advanced glycosylation end products (AGE)*. Specific AGE receptors are found in several cells such as the macrophages and endothelial cells where they mediate the release of cytokines and reactive oxygen species leading to cellular damage.

The other important factors which are involved in the pathogenesis of both the microvascular and macrovascular complications of diabetes are hypertension, hyperlipidemia, smoking and hypercoagulability.

CARDIOVASCULAR SYSTEM

Atherosclerosis sets in early and it tends to be diffuse and extensive. Ischemic heart disease (IHD) is common. The single most frequent cause of death in diabetes is due to IHD, which in the diabetic differs from that in the non-diabetic by involvement of both the sexes in the same proportion and frequent occurrence of painless infarction. Some diabetics develop congestive cardiac failure in the absence of hypertension and demonstrable CAD. Such cases may be termed *diabetic cardiomyopathy*. Mortality from CVD is 2–3 times more common in the diabetics as compared with normal. The target levels for control of BP and lipids in the diabetics are lower than those in non-diabetics. The ideal levels to be achieved are: BP 130/80, LDL < 100 mg/dL, HDL > 40 mg/dL and HbA1C < 7%.

Management of acute MI in the diabetic is the same as in the non-diabetic. Since ketoacidosis may be precipitated by MI, strict control of diabetes using insulin is needed in the acute phase. Hypoglycemia should be avoided since it may lead to extension of infarct. Diabetes is not a contraindication for angiography, angioplasty or bypass grafting.

PERIPHERAL VASCULAR DISEASE (PVD)

It occurs in 20% of chronic diabetics. Affection of the upper limb is rare and the reasons for this not clear. Occlusion of femoral artery and its branches may occur. The foot becomes ischemic. Intermittent claudication may develop. Associated sensory neuropathy predisposes to minor trauma leading to fulminant infection and gangrene. Calcification of the arteries in the legs and feet may be demonstrable in X-ray. Monckeberg's arteriosclerosis affects several arteries.

Strict measures to control blood glucose and lipid levels and regulated exercise programs help to give symptom relief in the early stages. Cessation of smoking is absolutely necessary for recovery. Lipid lowering drugs such as atorvastatin 10–20 mg or more at bed time lowers the cholesterol levels and gemfibrosil normalize the triglyceride levels. Regression of the arterial narrowing does occur. Surgical measures include balloon angioplasty and bypass grafting. Once gangrene supervenes, the management of the local condition is essentially surgical.

CEREBROVASCULAR DISEASE (CVD)

In India, 8–32% of stroke patients have diabetes and CVD is encountered in about 10% of all diabetic patients. The most common age group for strokes in diabetics is the sixth decade. Study by Poulose KP from Trivandrum showed that carotid artery atherosclerosis was present in 18% of patients with type 2 DM above the age of 55 years. It was six times more common in diabetes compared to non-diabetic (IntJ: Diab. in developing countries 2002, vol 22). The presence of hypertension increases the risk of development of stroke. Thrombotic strokes are more common. The severity of neurological deficit is greater and the rate of recovery is poorer in a diabetic. The risk of a second episode within six months is very high and prophylactic use of antiplatelet agents is indicated.

DIABETIC RETINOPATHY

Diabetic retinopathy is now becoming the leading cause of blindness in most of the developing countries. The risk (8%) of developing diabetic retinopathy is directly related to the duration of the disease. In type 1 diabetes of 15 years or more duration, the chance of having any form of retinopathy is 98% and about one-third of such patients have proliferative disease. In type 2 DM of 15 years duration, the prevalence is 78%. One-third have macular

Complications of Diabetes Mellitus

Box 92.3: Classification of diabetic retinopathy

- Nonproliferative diabetic retinopathy (NPDR)
  - Mild
  - Moderate
  - Severe
  - Very severe
- Proliferative diabetic retinopathy (PDR)
- Clinically significant macular edema (CSME)—may exist by itself or along with NPDR and PDR.

edema and one in six have proliferative retinopathy. Insulin dependent diabetic patients have higher incidence of retinopathy compared to those controlled on diet and exercise without drugs.

Recent introduction of corneal confocal microscopy has helped to study the morphology of structures in the cornea including the nerves. The corneal structures are highly magnified up to a resolution of 1–2 μ. The lesions can be quantitated and followed up. The lesions of diabetic retinopathy can be divided into two broad categories namely nonproliferative diabetic retinopathy (NPDR) and proliferative diabetic retinopathy (PDR) (Box 92.3).

Fluorescein angiography is a reliable method to delineate retinal lesions. The earliest sign of retinal change is increased capillary permeability that is evidenced by the leakage of dye into the vitreous humor after fluorescein injection. Occlusion of the retinal capillaries follows with subsequent formation of saccular and fusiform aneurysms. Arteriovenous shunts also occur. There is proliferation of the lining endothelial cells with loss of pericytes that supports the vessels. Hemorrhages in the inner retinal areas are dot shaped, while bleeding in the more superficial nerve fiber layers appear flame shaped, blot shaped or linear. Preretinal hemorrhages are boat shaped. The exudates are of two types. The cotton-wool spots are microinfarcts. Non-perfused areas surrounded by a ring of dilated capillaries and hard exudates represent leakage of proteins and lipids from damaged capillaries, which can best be assessed by fluorescein angiography (Figs 92.1 to 92.4).

The increased capillary permeability leads to development of retinal edema and is often associated with hard exudates. If the edema involves the macular region, visual acuity may be affected severely and sometimes even permanently. The fundamental characteristic of proliferative retinopathy is new vessel formation and scarring. The stimulus for new vessel formation is retinal hypoxia secondary to capillary occlusion. Vascular endothelial growth factor (VEGF) plays a major role. Two serious complications of proliferative retinopathy are vitreal hemorrhage and retinal detachment, which can cause sudden loss of vision (Figs 92.1 and 92.2).

Treatment of diabetic retinopathy: This consists of retarding its progression by strict glycemic control, control of BP, cessation of smoking and correction of hyperlipidemia. Laser photocoagulation is used for decreasing the incidence of hemorrhage and scarring when new vessel formation occurs. Pan retinal photocoagulation is often used to diminish the retinal demands for oxygen in the hope that the stimulus for neovascularization may be decreased. Definite guidelines are available for the prevention and management of diabetic retinopathy. Persons who have no retinopathy as detected by fluorescein angiography should be screened by an ophthalmologist at intervals of three years. Those with retinopathy should be screened at intervals of 6–12 months for prophylactic and therapeutic photocoagulation of lesions.

Source: Younis N, Broadbent DM, Vora JP, et al. Incidence of sight-threatening retinopathy in patients with type 2 diabetes in the Liverpool Diabetic Eye Study: a cohort study. Lancet. 2003;361:195-200.

Surgical techniques used for treatment of non-resolving vitreal hemorrhage and retinal detachment include pars planavitrectomy. Newer, but experimental approaches include PKC (protein kinase C)-beta inhibitors like ruboxistaurin, which blocks the hyperglycemia-induced toxic PKC pathways.

OTHER COMPLICATIONS AFFECTING THE EYE

Refractive errors are common due to changes in osmolarity of the aqueous humor altering the convexity of the lens when the blood glucose levels change widely. This is a common phenomenon when an uncontrolled diabetic undergoes proper therapy, especially with insulin. This is called ***insulin presbyopia***. When the lens adjusts to the normal glucose levels, the vision corrects itself.

Cataract: Senile cataract is preponed by 10 years or more in the uncontrolled diabetic. Posterior capsular

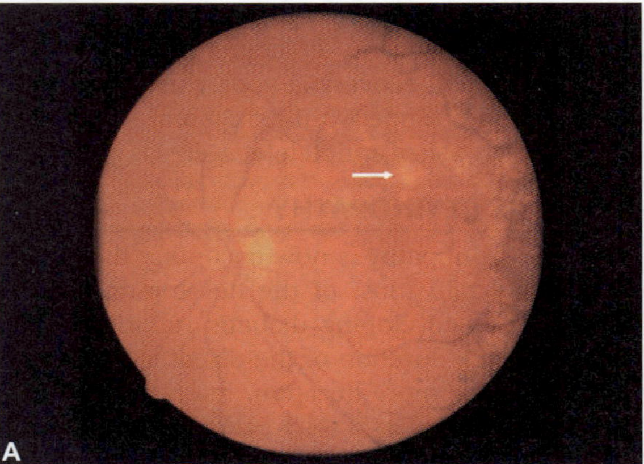
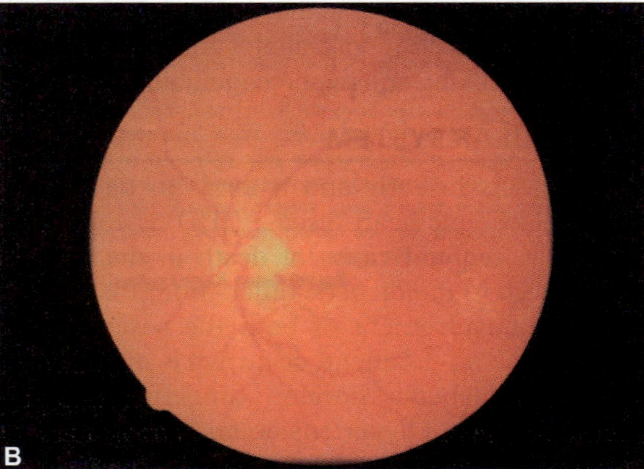

Figs 92.1A and B: Preproliferative retinopathy. Fundus—hard exudates (arrow)

Textbook of Medicine

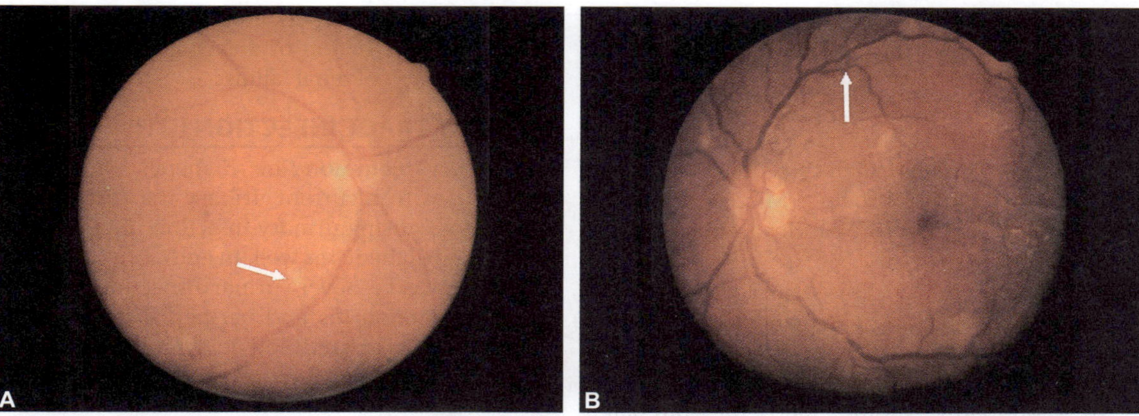

Figs 92.2A and B: Preproliferative retinopathy. **A.** Cotton wool patches (arrow); **B.** More advanced stage—neovascularization from veins (arrow)

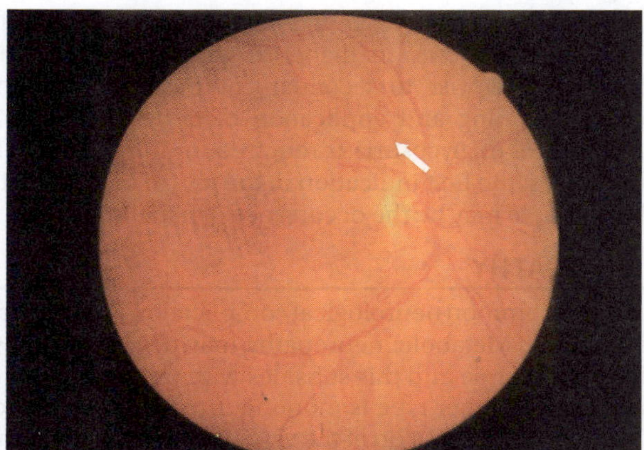

Fig. 92.3: Proliferative retinopathy. **Note:** Regular looped vessels arising from the disk and normal vessels (arrow)

cataract is more common. Management is similar to that of cataract in the non-diabetic. In type 1 diabetic patients, snowflake opacities may develop in the lens due to severe hyperglycemia.

DIABETIC NEPHROPATHY

Renal complications of DM have been studied extensively in both types of diabetes by close follow-up over prolonged periods. Five distinct phases in the course of the disease have been identified (*See* also Ch 187).

Stage I (hyperfiltration-hypertrophy stage): This stage is characterized by 20–40% increase in glomerular filtration rate (GFR) compared to normal age-matched controls, elevated renal plasma flow and an increase in kidney size by 30%. There is increase in the glomerular size and volume with elevated intraglomerular pressure. These changes are reversible with good glycemic control.

Stage II (with structural glomerular lesions): The hemodynamic changes of the earlier stage and structural glomerular changes begin to appear during this stage in the form of basement membrane thickening and mesangial expansion. During the later part of this stage, urinary albumin excretion may also increase transiently (normal < 7 µg/min) during periods of poor glycemic control and exercise.

Stage III (stage of microalbuminuria): This stage is characterized by the appearance of microalbuminuria, i.e. albumin excretion is in the range of 30–299 mg/day or 20–200 µg/minute. Estimation of urinary albumin/creatinine ratio is emerging as the best way to assess microalbuminuria since this will eliminate fallacies due to urinary dilution or concentration. Microalbuminuria appears primarily due to decreased concentration of anionic heparan sulfate proteoglycans in the glomerular basement membrane. The urinary albumin excretion varies greatly depending upon the time of the day, exercise, posture and glycemic control. Hence, it should

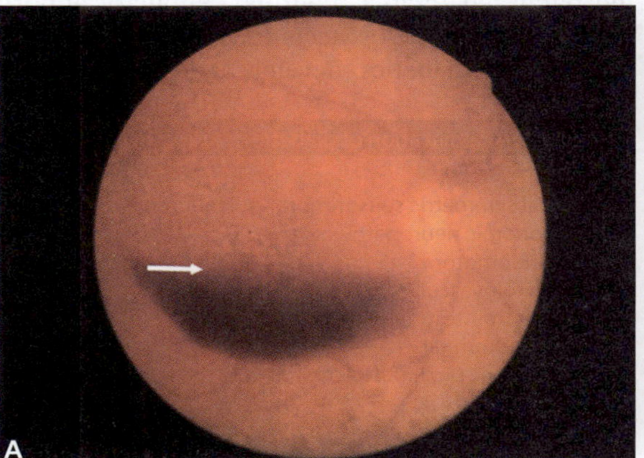

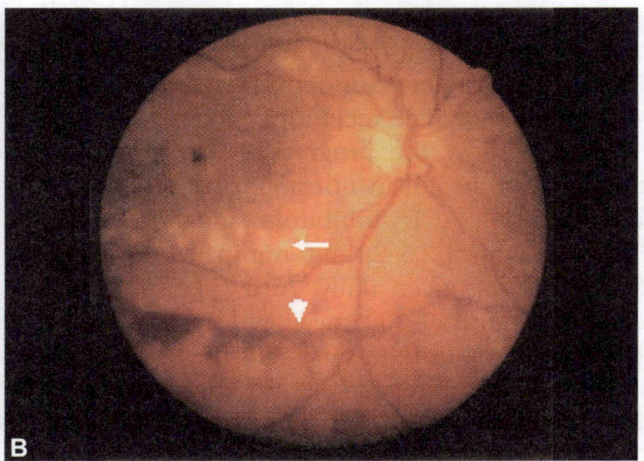

Figs 92.4A and B: **A.** Preretinal hemorrhage—horizontal upper border; **B.** Advanced diabetic retinopathy with laser scars (arrow). Also not absorbed preretinal hemorrhage (arrowhead)

be measured at least 2–3 times before microalbuminuria is confirmed. At this stage, the BP starts to rise. The risk of overt nephropathy increases 25–30 times once this threshold of albumin excretion is crossed. However, interventions such as strict glycemic control, aggressive antihypertensive therapy and dietary protein restriction have been shown to retard the progress. Microalbuminuria is an independent marker of cardiovascular risk of ischemic heart disease.

Stage IV (overt nephropathy): This stage is characterized by the appearance of dipstick positive proteinuria (>550 mg/day). Hypertension is invariably present and retinopathy is also present in over 90% of the patients. Absence of retinopathy should alert the physician towards a non-diabetic cause for the renal disease. Once overt proteinuric phase begins, there is a steady decline in renal functions with the GFR falling on an average by about 1 mL/min/month. A plot of the reciprocal of serum creatinine against time usually yields a straight line and allows the prediction of the rate of deterioration. Development of nephrotic range proteinuria portends a poor outcome.

Stage V (end stage renal disease): This stage is characterized by the presence of uremic symptoms, fluid retention and edema. At this stage, abnormalities of several other organ systems may be obvious. Cardiac insufficiency, peripheral neuropathy, gastroparesis, cystopathy and other extrarenal vascular disease may occur. Median survival in untreated patients is less than a year. Such patients require renal replacement therapy in the form of repeated hemodialysis, continuous ambulatory peritoneal dialysis or renal transplantation.

In type 2 diabetes, since the onset of the disease is not acute and since diabetes can remain unrecognized for a long period of time, many patients may present with nephropathy even at the time of first diagnosis. The presence of other disorder such as essential hypertension, UTI and other forms of kidney diseases hasten the progression of nephropathy.

Management

Even though there is no specific treatment for diabetic nephropathy, early detection and meticulous control of diabetes can reverse microalbuminuria and the progression of nephropathy can be slowed. Hypertension should be treated aggressively with the target BP being <130/85 mm Hg. Angiotensin converting enzyme (ACE) inhibitors and angiotensin receptor blockers (ARBs) have been shown to slow the progression of nephropathy. They may also be useful in normotensive subjects with microalbuminuria. ACE inhibitors include captopril 12.5–75 mg, lisinopril 2.5–20 mg, ramipril 1.25–5 mg, or perindopril 2–4 mg given daily. ARBs like losartan 25–100 mg, irbisartan 150–300 mg, candesartan 8–12 mg, valsartan 80–160 mg or telmisartan 40–80 mg are equally effective in retarding renal lesions. These drugs have been found to be useful to retard diabetic nephropathy also in normotensives. While administering them, renal function should be monitored in the initial phases to avoid hypotension and deterioration of renal function.

There is risk of hyperkalemia which should also be monitored. Restriction of dietary protein helps to retard the progression of renal failure.

URINARY TRACT INFECTION (UTI)

It is very common in diabetics since glucosuria predisposes to recurrent urinary infection. All common organisms causing urinary infection in non-diabetics are seen in the diabetics as well. In addition, candida may also become invasive. Severe urinary infection may give rise to pyelitis, pyonephritis and perinephric abscess. Papillitis necroticans is a condition in which the renal papillae undergo necrosis in the presence of fulminant infection. Fleshy bits are passed in the urine. At times these may give rise to urinary obstruction and reflex anuria.

Balanoposthitis: This is acute or chronic infection of the glans penis (balanitis) and prepuce (posthitis) occurring commonly in diabetics with glycosuria. This condition gives rise to secondary phimosis. In addition to local cleaning and application of nystatin ointment, strict control of glycosuria is required for full recovery. In many cases, the first indication of the loss of control of the diabetic state may be the occurrence of balanoposthitis.

NEUROPATHY

The most common neurological complication is peripheral neuropathy. Metabolic neuropathy may develop because of hyperglycemia and this subsides with proper control of diabetes. The other type is mononeuritis multiplex which is produced by occlusion of the vasa nervorum of the nerve trunks. This does not clear up promptly with treatment. Clinical presentation may be varied. Symmetrical distal sensory neuropathy with pain, numbness, paresthesia, glove and stockings sensory loss and areflexia is the common pattern seen in diabetics (Box 92.4).

Motor paralysis leads to foot drop, weakness and wasting of the quadriceps, wasting of small muscles of hands and feet and clawing of the feet. Entrapment neuropathies are also not uncommon. Patients may develop carpal tunnel syndrome. As a result of sensory motor neuropathy, pressure sores may develop over the metatarsal heads. In chronic cases with loss of sensation, the mid-tarsal and ankle joints may undergo degeneration (Charcot's joints). The third or sixth cranial nerves may be paralyzed (cranial neuritis). Pupillary abnormalities and disturbances of accommodation may also occur. Sometimes diabetics develop lancinating pain, motor

---

Box 92.4: Classification of diabetic neuropathy

Diffuse
- Distal symmetric sensorimotor polyneuropathy
- Autonomic neuropathy
  - Sudomotor
  - Cardiovascular
  - Gastrointestinal
  - Genitourinary
- Symmetric proximal lower limb motor neuropathy (amyotrophy)

Focal
- Cranial neuropathy
- Radiculopathy/plexopathy
- Entrapment neuropathy
- Asymmetric lower limb motor neuropathy

Textbook of Medicine

weakness and sensory ataxia and bladder derangements as in the case of tabes dorsalis (*diabetic pseudotabes*).

Diabetic amyotrophy consists of gross weakness and wasting of the proximal groups of muscles of the pelvic girdle, quadriceps and the iliopsoas. *Clinical features* are pain, paresthesia and loss of tendon jerks without any objective sensory loss. This is seen more commonly in elderly subjects. Diabetic amyotrophy has to be differentiated from a primary myopathy and neuropathy. With proper control of the diabetic state; amyotrophy clears off completely unlike myopathy and neuropathy. Diabetic amyotrophy is probably due to microvasculitis in the lumbosacral plexus.

The gold standard to detect and quantify the severity of diabetic neuropathy includes electrophysiological tests and quantitative sensory tests of thermal and pain perception by small fibers. Sural nerve biopsy and electron microscopy helps to demonstrate the morphological changes.

Autonomic neuropathy is common in diabetes. Presence of autonomic neuropathy should be looked for since the warning signs of hypoglycemia may not develop in such patients. Common manifestations of autonomic neuropathy are impotence in males, orthostatic hypotension, nocturnal diarrhea, disorder of sweating and atonia of the bladder. There is impairment of autonomic control of the heart. Absence of sinus arrhythmia and loss of normal response to Valsalva's maneuver clinically indicate autonomic dysfunction of the heart. Subjects with cardiac autonomic neuropathy are under high risk of sudden cardiac death.

Once established, diabetic neuropathy tends to persist. Meticulous control of diabetes is of definite benefit. Analgesics, antidepressants and antiepileptic drugs such as carbamazepine help to relieve the pain and insomnia. Empirically high dose of vitamins B_1, B_{12} and B_6 have been widely used based on clinical impression without much objective evidence. Electrical stimulation of the site of pain using a cutaneous nerve stimulator helps to relieve pain in some cases. More recently local application of capsaicin has been used with some benefit. Several drugs such as antioxidants, neurotropic peptides, nerve growth factor, prosaposin, memantine, gabapentin, frisium, duloxetine, pregabalin and erythropoietin have been employed from time to time with marginal benefit.

DIABETIC FOOT

Foot problems give rise to severe morbidity in diabetic patients. Diabetes accounts for up to 50–80% of non-traumatic amputations. The lifetime risk of developing foot lesions in a diabetic is 12–25%. The factors contributing to the foot problems are:

- Neuropathy—sensory, motor and autonomic
- Ischemia
- Trauma—physical, mechanical, thermal, continuous mechanical stress, uneven weight bearing
- Infection.

Ulceration of the foot in a diabetic usually results from the combination of neuropathic damage, tissue ischemia and excessive pressure loading, often with superimposed infections (Fig. 92.5).

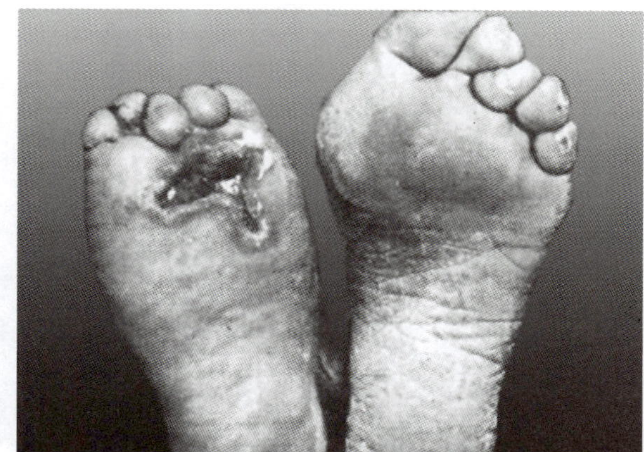

Fig. 92.5: Diabetic ulcer right foot—the indolent deep ulcer

Neuropathy predisposes to ulceration by reducing perception of pain and trauma inflicted by foreign bodies and walking with tight or ill-fitting shoes. Motor neuropathy leads to involvement of the small muscles of the feet altering the posture of the feet and leading to abnormal pressure distribution on to vulnerable areas, particularly over the metatarsal heads and heels. This leads to formation of callus which can breakdown and lead to ulceration. The other factors which contribute to abnormal distribution of foot pressure, in addition to motor neuropathy are limited joint mobility and local deformities, including Charcot's arthropathy. Removal of callus redistributes the pressure and reduces the risk of subsequent ulceration.

Ischemia: Tissue ischemia is a very important factor in the development of foot ulcers in the presence of neuropathy. Apart from major vascular occlusions, defects in microcirculation which occur in diabetes, contribute to the development of ulceration and failure of established ulcers to heal.

Infections: Infection in diabetic foot ulcers is commonly due to mixed pyogenic anaerobic organisms, some of which may be gas forming. Infection of the deeper tissue may lead to thrombosis in the vessels. Abscess formation may also occur which may compress the plantar arch and reduce blood supply to the forefoot and toes. This may lead to gangrene of the toes and osteomyelitis of the bones, necessitating amputation. Systemic signs such as fever may be absent even with deep-seated infections. X-ray may show resorption of bones (Fig. 92.6).

Management

Prevention of foot ulcers is very important and meticulous care has to be taken. The foot has to be inspected everyday for any evidence of injury, washed clean, wiped dry and powdered. Walking on barefoot should be avoided. Footwear has to be well-fitting and specially designed in case of deformity. Callosities or fissures in the skin have to be taken care of. Use of hot water, heating pads or corn plasters is to be avoided. Smoking should be stopped and meticulous control of hyperglycemia and hyperlipidemia is to be achieved.

If ulcers are present, specimens from the depth of the ulcer should be sent for bacterial culture and sensitivity.

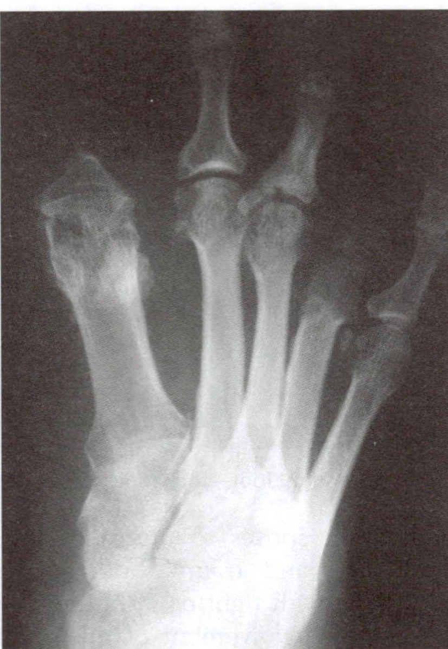

Fig. 92.6: X-ray of diabetic foot. **Note:** The resorption of the phalanges and distal parts of the metatarsals

Parenteral antibiotics are to be administered based on the organisms isolated. Local antibiotics are not very helpful. Delay in treatment will also cause rapid spread of infection leading to necrotizing myofasciitis resulting in large ulcers. X-ray of the foot is necessary to assess the involvement of bones and joints. Deep abscesses may need drainage. Full debridement of ulcers is required till granulation tissue is seen and they should be packed with gauze soaked in antiseptic cream. Deep infections with osteomyelitis and gangrene may require amputation.

OTHER COMPLICATIONS

Pruritus vulvae and ***recurrent vaginitis*** are distressing conditions associated with glycosuria. The common organism is *Candida albicans*. Strict control of diabetes and use of antifungal creams or tablets help to relieve the condition.

Tuberculosis: Diabetics are more susceptible to develop tuberculosis, especially pulmonary and pleural forms. Successful treatment should aim at simultaneous attention to both the diabetes and tuberculosis. The therapy for tuberculosis is the same as for non-diabetics.

Autonomic disturbances take the form of gastroparesis and paralytic ileus which give rise to bloating of the abdomen and this may mimic a surgical emergency. Correction of the diabetic state, especially ketoacidosis may relieve the condition. Prokinetic drugs such as domperidone may be of help at times.

Nocturnal diarrhea may occur in the uncontrolled diabetic and may be mistaken for infective diarrhea. Control of the diabetic state and antidiarrheal drugs such as codeine phosphate given in a dose of 30–40 mg oral bedtime may give relief. Loperamide which is an opiod derivative also reduces intestinal motility and this may be used as a short-term measure. Toxic megacolon is a serious side effect. Non-pharmacological measures such as dietary regulation and timing of the diet may help in some cases.

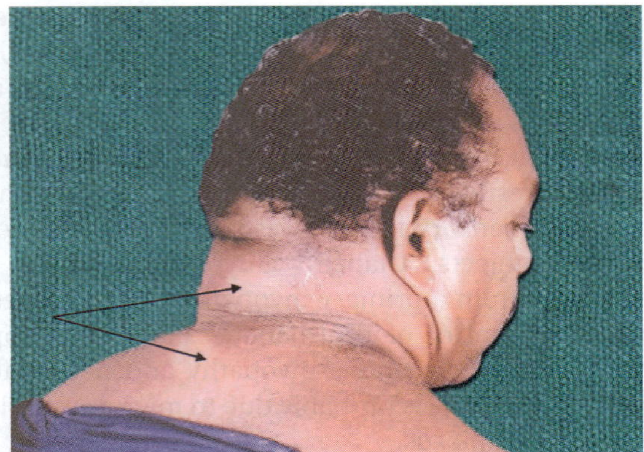

Fig. 92.7: ***Acanthosis nigricans. Note:*** The thickening of the skin along with velvety texture and mild pigmentation—nape of the neck (arrows)

Necrobiosis lipoidica diabeticorum: This is a skin condition associated with DM. It may occur only in less than 1% of diabetics, but above 80% of patients with necrobiosis may have diabetes. These lesions appear as shiny yellow plaques over the shin. There may be underlying telangiectasia. These lesions are susceptible to chronic ulceration as a result of repeated trauma.

Acanthosis nigricans, a velvety thickening and pigmentation of the nape of the neck, axilla and flexural zones, may be associated with insulin resistance and diabetes, especially in the obese. Indirectly it indicates excess insulin secretion (Fig. 92.7).

Scleredema diabeticorum diffuse non-pitting induration of skin over the nape of the neck.

Dupuytren's contracture may develop in some.

People with diabetes are prone to get repeated and troublesome infections both bacterial and fungal. These are not specific to diabetes but they are more common due to impaired local and general resistance.

Necrotizing fasciitis is the fulminant infection in the fascial compartments of the limbs caused by mixed bacterial flora. It presents as an acute painful infection of the limbs or other sites, rapidly leading to suppuration. The rise in pressure in the fascial compartments may lead to vascular occlusion and extensive gangrene, if not attended to early. Some other diabetic complications are given in Box 92.5.

Musculoskeletal complications that are more common in diabetes are given in Box 92.6.

FUTURE PROSPECTS IN DIABETOLOGY

In spite of advances in technology and analytical approaches, many facets in the pathogenesis and management of diabetes are still not well understood. Even though genetic susceptibility for β-cell dysfunction is a key factor for development of diabetes in an individual, the rapid increase in the epidemic of diabetes is not explainable by changes in the gene pool only. Apart from the traditionally known environmental factors like sedentary lifestyle, obesity and family history, certain chemical agents (air pollutants) are likely to emerge in the pathogenesis of β-cell dysfunction. Advance in laboratory methods are likely to provide better delineation of roles of emerging

Box 92.5: Other diabetic complications

- ***Skin infections:*** Due to immune dysfunction, e.g. carbuncles and furuncles
- ***Vaginal candidiasis:*** Due to immune dysfunction
- ***Diabetic ulcers:*** Due to peripheral neuropathy and ischemia
- ***Xanthomatosis:*** Due to hyperlipoproteinemia
- Necrobiosis lipoidica diabeticorum
    - One of the best known cutaneous markers for diabetes
    - Initially presents with well-circumscribed erythematous papules, which develop into large, irregularly delineated plaques with a waxy, yellow center
    - About 85% of necrobiosis lipoidica diabeticorum (NLD) cases occur on the legs bilaterally
    - Lesions can also appear on the face, scalp, hands, forearms, or abdomen
- ***Diabetic dermopathy:*** This may occur due to reduced vascularity of the underlying tissues. Shin spots are light brown or reddish oval or circular scaly patches on the surface of the shin
- Tight waxy skin the dorsum of the hands with joint contractures in type 1 DM—digital sclerosis
- Acanthosis nigricans
    - Hyperpigmented plaques
    - Most commonly found in armpits, neck and groin
    - Marker of insulin resistance
- ***Acrochordons/skin tags:*** Marker of insulin resistance
- ***Granuloma annulare***
- ***Diabetic blisters:*** Bullosis diabeticorum

Box 92.6: Musculoskeletal complications in diabetes

- Painful muscle swelling, usually in the thigh thought to be due to muscle infarction
- Neuropathic arthropathy (Charcot's joints)
- Carpal tunnel syndrome (CTS)
- Dupuytren's contracture
- Flexor tenosynovitis
- Adhesive capsulitis (frozen shoulder)
- Diabetic cherioarthropathy is a condition of thickened skin resembling scleroderma affecting small joints of the hands and leading to limitation of mobility and flexion deformities of the hand
- Diabetic sclerodactyly

factors like systemic inflammation, intestinal microbiome and hypothalamic contribution to glucose metabolism.

β-cell preservation therapies are thought to have important implications in treatment of type 2 DM. The ongoing follow-up of large clinical trials on the other hand have provided improved understanding of natural history of diabetes related complications. These results are also likely to provide information regarding varied response of different antidiabetic medications and metabolic surgeries (also called as bariatric surgeries) on different population. In many cases, bariatric surgeries have led to marked improvement in the diabetic state in addition to their benefit in obesity and related conditions. Substantial sustained weight loss and major improvements in glycemia control occur in obese type 2 DM. Several mechanisms other than malabsorption of food also play a part in the beneficial outcome. Weight loss improves insulin resistance and bariatric surgery is the best method to sustain the weight loss. β-cell function improves. Nutrition monitoring is necessary after bariatric surgery.

The knowledge from molecular as well as clinical trials has already resulted in subdivision of patients with diabetes into wide range of phenotypes in addition to traditionally described type 1 and type 2 DM. These phenotypes not only add up to the exhaustive classification of disorders related to chronic hyperglycemia but will also provide the directions for a more targeted therapy of diabetes and related complications in future. The day is not far when newer and apparently novel and surprising methodologies emerge to prevent and control the heterogeneous cluster termed diabetes in a more rational and effective manner.

Source:

1. Kahn SE, Cooper ME, Del Prato S. Pathophysiology and Treatment of Type 2 diabetes. Perspectives on the past, present and future. Lancet. 2014;383:1068-83.
2. Tuomi T, Santoro N, Caprio S, et al. The many faces of diabetes: a disease with increasing heterogenecity. Lancet. 2014;383:1084-94.

CHAPTER

93

Fibrocalcific Pancreatic Diabetes and Other Causes of Meliturias

KV Krishna Das, KP Poulose, RV Jaykumar

Chapter Summary

- Geographical Distribution
- Etiology and Pathogenesis
    - Complications
    - Prognosis
- Treatment
- Other Causes of Meliturias
    - Lactosuria
    - Fructosuria
    - Galactosemia
    - Pentosuria

Syn: Calcific pancreatitis, Tropical pancreatitis, Fibroc-alculous pancreatic disease

GEOGRAPHICAL DISTRIBUTION

Chronic relapsing pancreatitis is confined almost exclusively to the tropics, mainly Africa, India, Indonesia and Malaysia. In India, most of the cases have been reported from the midland and the hilly tracts of the southern districts of Kerala and Tamil Nadu. Smaller numbers have been reported from many other parts, especially Karnataka and Odisha. The incidence of fibrocalculous pancreatic diabetes (FCPD) seems to have come down in Kerala in recent years.

ETIOLOGY AND PATHOGENESIS

Almost all cases belong to the poor socioeconomic groups, which consume cassava as the staple food. The cyanide present in cassava is thought to be responsible for its toxic effects. However, some groups who did not consume cassava also had increased incidence of FCPD. This finding made the cassava theory unpopular. Currently, several genes are thought to be responsible for FCPD. The main gene incriminated is the serine protease inhibitor Kazal 1 (SPINK1) gene.

Pathology

The pancreas shows intra- and interacinar fibrosis with moderate round cell infiltration. The acini and islets undergo total atrophy and replacement by fat. The ducts are dilated and numerous intraductal calculi made up of calcium carbonate and traces of phosphate are seen to occupy the head and body of the organ. The calculi show a protein core with deposition of calcium in the interstices. The β-cells of the islets are reduced and this accounts for the diabetic state. The liver shows mainly glycogen infiltration and rarely fatty changes and cirrhosis. In long-standing cases, the kidneys, retina and peripheral nerves show lesions similar to those seen in maturity onset diabetes. The parotid glands are prominent and they show ductal dilation and round cell infiltration.

Clinical Features

The disease affects children and young adults in the age groups of 15–35 years. Both sexes are equally affected. In one-third cases, previous history of painful episodes of recurrent pancreatitis may be available. The pain is of a colicky or gnawing nature felt over the epigastrium. This differs from that of peptic ulcers in having no relation to food and not being relieved by antacids. Pressure over the epigastrium gives prompt relief. The physical appearance of these subjects is diagnostic. They show extreme emaciation (Fig. 93.1), distension of the upper abdomen, cyanotic hue of the lips, and bilateral painless parotid enlargement. Growth and development are reared. Women develop secondary amenorrhea. Urinary bladder is grossly distended and atonic. The patients generally seek treatment for diabetes or its complications (Fig. 93.2).

The diabetic state is often severe, requiring high doses of soluble insulin for control. In the majority of cases, the fasting and postprandial blood glucose levels are high. With the passage of time, the diabetes becomes brittle in many cases.

Laboratory Features

Fasting and postprandial blood glucose levels are in the ranges of type 1 diabetes. Pancreatic enzymes are lowered. Plasma immunoreactive insulin is reduced.

Diagnosis

The disease should be suspected when a young individual presents with abdominal pain and juvenile diabetes. Plain X-ray of the abdomen reveals radio-opaque calculi in the pancreas (Fig. 93.3). Computed

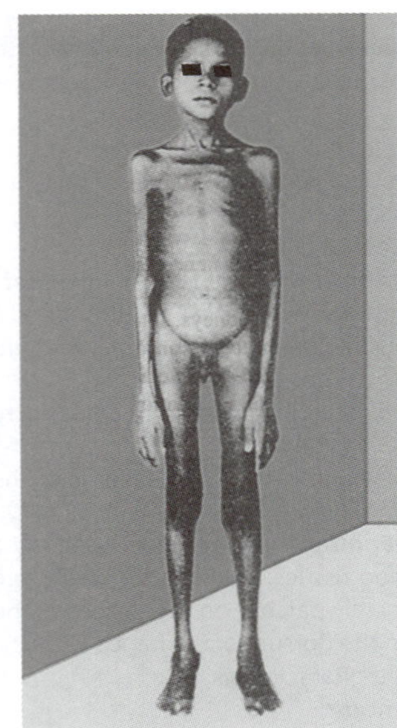

Fig. 93.1: Pancreatic diabetes—male aged 24 years

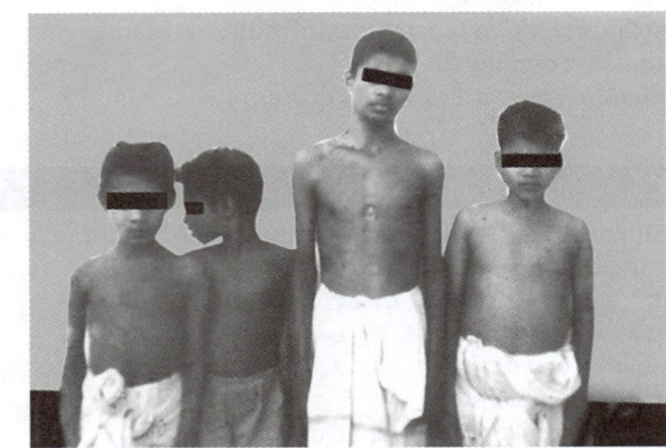

Fig. 93.2: Pancreatic diabetes—a group from a village

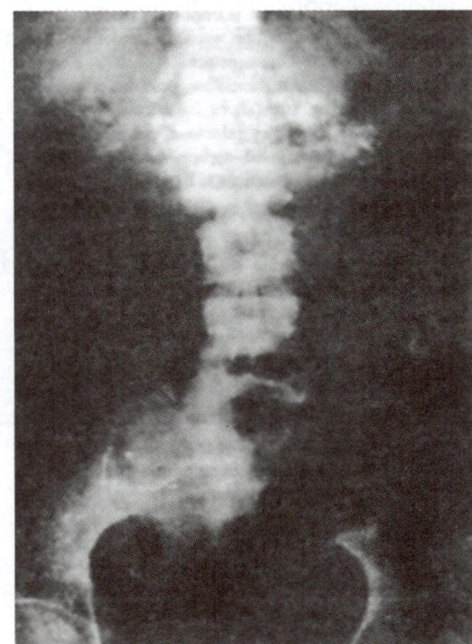

Fig. 93.3: Pancreatic diabetes—plain X-ray of abdomen. **Note:** Calculi across L1-L2 vertebrae

tomography (CT) scan of the abdomen confirms the diagnosis. The calculi are found mainly in the head and body of the organ. They are of varying size and shape and may show translucent centers.

Textbook of Medicine

Complications

Complications are due to diabetes, pancreatic calculi and pancreatic exocrine dysfunction.

- Diabetic complications are similar to the complications seen in maturity onset diabetes.
- Complications due to calculi and exocrine dysfunction include obstructive jaundice, recurrent attacks of pancreatitis and malabsorption state. Steatorrhea manifests if the diet contains normal amounts of fat or excess fat.
- Carcinoma pancreas.

Prognosis

With adequate control of diabetes by diet and insulin, many cases survive up to the fifth or sixth decade. With proper control of the disease, women resume menstruation. Pregnancy and normal childbirths can be achieved with proper management. The children born to such parents which do not have predisposition to develop the same disease. Early onset of microangiopathy shortens life considerably. Some develop pancreatic cancer on follow-up.

TREATMENT

The treatment is only symptomatic. Control of the diabetic state is similar to the other forms of juvenile diabetes. Since they are mostly insulin-dependent, oral hypoglycemic drugs are ineffective. Generally, insulin requirement is high and proper control can be achieved only by giving repeated doses of soluble insulin.

Abdominal pain of recurrent pancreatitis is very disabling and response to common antispasmodics like atropine and propantheline bromide is unsatisfactory. During acute attacks, the cases have to be managed on the same lines as acute pancreatitis. In intractable cases with demonstrable calculi, surgical removal of the stones and dilation of the sphincter of Oddi have been beneficial in many cases. When signs of malabsorption are present, dietary management and administration of pancreatic enzymes are indicated.

OTHER CAUSES OF MELITURIAS

Though glucose is the most common sugar present in urine, other sugars may be encountered at times. Some are present due to inborn metabolic errors whereas others are of the *overflow* type. In the latter type, sugars appear in urine whenever the blood levels rise above the renal threshold even in the absence of metabolic abnormalities.

Identification of the sugar is important since many cases of innocent meliturias may be wrongly treated as diabetes mellitus with disastrous consequences. A positive Benedict's test with negative diastix should suggest the possibility of non-glucose reducing substances in urine. These include sugars like lactose, fructose, galactose, pentose, and other substances like ascorbic acid, aspirin and para-aminosalicylic acid (PAS). The final identification of these substances is by chemical methods or chromatography.

Lactosuria

Newborn babies ingesting milk may develop lactosuria. The urinary level of lactose increases with the quantity ingested. Lactosuria is common in women during pregnancy and lactation. All these are nonpathological.

Fructosuria

After intake of large amounts of fructose-containing foods like berries, grapes, and honey, even normal persons develop fructosuria—alimentary fructosuria.

Rarely, fructosuria is due to deficiency of the specific enzyme, fructokinase in the liver. This is called ***essential fructosuria***. This condition is benign since most of the ingested fructose can be utilized by other metabolic pathways.

Hereditary fructose intolerance is a more serious metabolic error caused by the deficiency of ***hepatic fructose-1-phosphate aldolase.*** This is transmitted as an autosomal recessive. These subjects develop postprandial hypoglycemia. The clinical picture varies with age. The severe form presents in infancy. The baby is normal when breastfed, but vomiting and diarrhea occur when fructose-containing foods, or sucrose and sorbitol (which yield fructose on digestion) are introduced into the diet. The baby fails to thrive. Other accompaniments of the condition are hepatomegaly, jaundice, evidence of hepatic dysfunction, postprandial hypoglycemia, renal tubular acidosis (RTA), amino acidurias and lactic acidosis. If left untreated, the condition proceeds to portal or biliary cirrhosis. If the abnormality is recognized early and fructose is avoided, all the lesions clear up. In older children and adults, the disease presents with nausea, abdominal pain, distension and diarrhea. Since sugar and sweets precipitate these attacks; such persons learn to avoid these items. Hepatic involvement is less marked, but uricosuria and renal stones are more common.

Diagnosis

This should be suspected clinically from the history. Precipitation of hypoglycemia by small doses of fructose (0.25 g/kg bw in adults or 3 g/m^2 body surface in children) establishes the diagnosis. In normal subjects, hypoglycemia is induced only by large doses of fructose.

Hereditary fructosuria has to be distinguished from other metabolic disorders like galactosemia and tyrosinosis.

Galactosemia

Normally, lactose present in milk is converted into glucose and galactose by intestinal lactase. Galactose is absorbed and converted to glucose in the liver. Conversion into glucose is defective in galactosemia and hence, the concentration of galactose-1-phosphate and galactose increase in blood and tissues such as liver, brain, kidneys, intestines and lens.

Galactosemia is transmitted as an autosomal recessive trait. In the fully developed form, classical galactosemia presents with cataract, mental retardation, hepatic cirrhosis and death in early life. The enzyme galactose-1-phosphate uridyltransferase (GALT) is deficient. The severe form manifests within a few days of birth with intolerance to milk, vomiting, refusal to feed and failure to thrive. Jaundice, hepatomegaly and hepatic dysfunction develop early. Cataracts develop within weeks or months. As the child grows up, mental deficiency becomes evident. Recurrent bacterial infections (*Escherichia coli*) are common and may be fatal.

In the atypical form of galactosemia, the enzyme galactokinase is deficient. Galactokinase is required to convert galactose into galactose-1-phosphate and in its absence galactose accumulates in blood and tissues. The only complication in this disorder is cataract formation.

Diagnosis

Urine shows galactose. Diagnosis is established by demonstrating the deficiency of GALT in erythrocytes.

Treatment

This consists of dietary measures to avoid milk and milk products, and this results in dramatic improvement. Even in advanced cases, dietary management leads to regression of symptoms except the cataract.

Pentosuria

Pentosuria can be due to ingestion of excessive pentoses found in grapes, cherries, plums, etc. and this is known as *alimentary pentosuria*. The pentoses are arabinose, apiose, rhamnose, ribose and xylose. Essential pentosuria is an inherited disorder transmitted as an autosomal recessive trait and the urinary pentose is L-xylulose. It is caused by the deficiency of xylitol dehydrogenase. This condition is clinically silent and no treatment is required. The pentosuria is controlled by avoiding fruits.

CHAPTER

94

Other Metabolic Disorders

KV Krishna Das, TK Suma

Chapter Summary

- Inborn Errors of Metabolism
- General Considerations
- Metabolic Syndrome
- Hyperlipidemias
- Hemochromatosis
- Wilson's Disease
- Porphyrias
- Acute Intermittent Porphyria (AIP)
- Disorders of Amino Acid Metabolism
  - Phenylketonuria (PKU)
  - Alkaptonuria

INBORN ERRORS OF METABOLISM

GENERAL CONSIDERATIONS

Inborn errors of metabolism (IEM) are a group of disorders in which a single gene defect causes a clinically significant block in one or several related metabolic pathways. Clinical symptoms result from several abnormal metabolic processes. These include:

- Toxic accumulations of substrates before the block or intermediates from alternative metabolic pathways
- Defects in energy production and use caused by a deficiency of products beyond the block
- Organomegaly
- Profound central hypotonia
- Malformations
- A combination of these metabolic deviations. Nearly every metabolic disease has several forms that vary in age of onset, clinical severity and often, mode of inheritance.

All IEMs are genetically transmitted typically in an autosomal recessive or X-linked recessive fashion. The genetic defects involve mutations in genes encoding proteins with single enzymatic function. Though individually the inborn metabolic disorders are rare, when considered collectively, their incidence is higher.

The mode of presentation may give a clue to the metabolic disorder. Positive family history helps in diagnosis. Parental consanguinity and neonatal death of siblings or maternally related male members are factors which support diagnosis of IEM.

Acute presentations of IEM in neonates could be any one of the following:

- During the prenatal period baby is apparently normal, but soon after birth, starts deteriorating to a life-threatening situation, especially when external feeding is established
- *Energy deficient conditions:* These result from recurrent hypoglycemia and/or lactic acidosis
- Prominent visceral involvement, i.e. isolated hepatic, or cardiac failure
- Floppy baby from birth often associated with seizures
- Multiple malformations.

Metabolic defect should be suspected when an infant which is normal at birth fails to thrive, or develops metabolic acidosis. Other features are persistent vomiting, organomegaly, developmental abnormalities, convulsions and urinary abnormalities such as peculiar odor, color change and others. In some instances, the defect occurs in several children in the same family. It is important to make an early diagnosis since in many cases dietary modification and supplementation with the missing cofactor help to overcome the defect and prevent permanent damage.

Box 94.1 gives a list of the important metabolic disorders. For full description, the student may consult larger textbooks on the subject.

It is now possible to identify the abnormal gene and its product which leads to the clinical abnormality.

Many of the inherited metabolic disorders are correctable by bone marrow or stem cell transplantation. In some cases, replacement of the missing enzyme therapy using recombinant enzyme is possible but such treatment is expensive. In Hurler's syndrome, stem cell

Textbook of Medicine

Box 94.1: Some important inherited metabolic disorders

Abnormalities of glycogen metabolism
- Glycogenoses
- Glycogen storage disease (GSD)
- Type I (Von Gierke's)
- Type II (Pompe's)
- Type III (Cori's, Forbes)
- Type IV (Andersens)
- Type V (McArdle's)
- Type VI (Hers)
- Type VIa

Abnormalities of purine metabolism
- Gout
- Lesch-Nyhan syndrome
- Myopathy
- Combined immunodeficiency

Abnormalities of pyrimidine metabolism
- Orotic aciduria

Lysosomal storage diseases
- **Mucopolysaccharidoses (MPS)**
  - MPS IH-Hurler' syndrome (Gargoylism)
  - MPS IS (Scheie's syndrome)
  - MPS II (Hunter's syndrome)
  - MPS III (Sanfilippo-A, B and C)
  - MPS IV (Morquio)
  - MPS VI (Maroteaux-Lamy)
  - MPS VII (Sly)
- **Mucolipidoses (ML):** Types I, II, III and IV, mannosidosis, fucosidosis and aspartylglucosaminuria.

Lipid storage disorders
- Gaucher's disease
- Niemann-Pick disease
- Farber's lipogranulomatosis
- Krabbe's disease
- Metachromatic leukodystrophy
- Multiple sulfatase deficiency
- Fabry's disease
- GM1 gangliosidosis
- GM2 gangliosidosis infantile
- Tay-Sachs disease
- Juvenile Tay-Sachs diseases (Sandhoff's)

Disorders of amino acid metabolism
- Hyperphenylalaninemia [phenylketonuria (PKU)]
- Tyrosinemia
- Histidinemia
- Disorders of enzymes concerned with the urea cycle leading to increase in citrulline, argininosuccinic acid and ornithine in blood
- **Disorders of lysine metabolism:** Periodic hyperlysinemia, persistent hyperlysinemia and hyperpipecolatemia
- **Disorders of branched-chain amino acid metabolism:** Maple-syrup-urine disease, isovaleric acidemia, propionic acidemia, methyl malonic aciduria and biotin responsive multiple carboxylase deficiency
- **Disorders of sulfur-containing amino acids:** Homocystinuria, cystinosis, and alkaptonuria

Disorders of fat metabolism
- Hyperlipidemias-Fredrickson's types 1, 2a, 2b, 3, 4 and 5
- Hemochromatosis
- Wilson's disease

Disorders of heme metabolism
- Porphyrias

transplantation using cord blood alters the natural history of the disease, if undertaken early in life.

METABOLIC SYNDROME

Syn: Syndrome X, Reaven's syndrome

Metabolic syndrome is a risk factor for coronary heart disease (CHD), diabetes mellitus (DM), fatty liver, and several

Box 94.2: Five criteria for diagnosis of the metabolic syndrome

1. Fasting plasma glucose (FPG) ≥ 100 mg/dL (or receiving drug therapy for hyperglycemia)
2. Obesity with the waist circumference ≥ 102 cm in males and ≥ 88 cm in females
3. Plasma triglycerides ≥ 150 mg/dL (or receiving drug therapy for hypertriglyceridemia)
4. HDL cholesterol < 40 mg/dL in men and < 50 mg/dL in women (or receiving drug therapy for reduced HDL-C)
5. Blood pressure ≥ 130/85 mm Hg (or receiving drug therapy for hypertension)

Abbreviation: HDL-C = High-density lipoprotein cholesterol

cancers. It arises from insulin resistance accompanying abnormal adipose deposition and function.

Signs and Symptoms

This condition has gained prominence in modern times since it is a common forerunner of caronary artery disease (CAD), DM and atherosclerosis. This condition is amenable to lifestyle modifications and has been extensively studied and criteria for early diagnosis have been laid out by WHO, International Diabetes Federation (IDF) and American Association of Endocrinologists. As per the current guidelines revised in 2005, the metabolic syndrome is diagnosed when the patient has three out of the following five criteria (Box 94.2). The clinical presentations of metabolic syndrome include:

- Hypertension
- Hyperglycemia
- Hypertriglyceridemia
- Reduced high-density lipoprotein cholesterol (HDL-C)
- Abdominal obesity
- ***Chest pain or shortness of breath:*** Suggesting the rise of cardiovascular and other complications
- ***Acanthosis nigricans, hirsutism, peripheral neuropathy and retinopathy:*** In patients with insulin resistance and hyperglycemia or with DM
- ***Xanthomas or xanthelasmas:*** In patients with severe dyslipidemia.

Indians express this syndrome in an exaggerated manner, and this is probably one of the reasons for the increasing prevalence of type 2 diabetes and CAD in the Indian subcontinent and especially those who have settled in more affluent countries. The exact genesis of the syndrome is not well-understood. Inheritance of polygenic predisposition, abnormal intrauterine programming and sedentary lifestyle are but some of the hypotheses put forward to explain the syndrome. The central underlying feature of this syndrome is insulin resistance. Individuals with metabolic syndrome are at increased risk of developing diabetes, cardiovascular events (accelerated atherosclerosis), hypercoagulability and endothelial dysfunction.

The association between metabolic syndrome and abdominal obesity is well-proven. It is possible that in metabolic syndrome, various endocrine secretions of adipocytes could play a role in the pathogenesis. Recent reports also reveal a link between both high-birth weight as well as low-birth weight amongst infants as predisposing factors for the development of metabolic syndrome and type 2 DM in adulthood.

Several other manifestations are linked to insulin resistance. These include:

- Polycystic ovarian syndrome (PCOS)
- Fatty liver
- Hyperuricemia
- Microalbuminuria
- Markers of reduced fibrinolysis such as plasminogen activator inhibitor-1 (PAI-1)
- Endothelial damage.

In subjects who have any one component of this syndrome, it is important to look for other components also since they cluster together. Management consists of full investigations for all the component abnormalities, dietary regulation, physical exercise, control of lipid abnormalities and regular monitoring. Lifestyle change and weight loss are considered the most important initial steps in treating metabolic syndrome. With the achievement of ideal weight and regular exercise, the syndrome regresses. The exercise regime should include at least five sessions of brisk walk for 3 km weekly. With the reduction of weight and exercise, the metabolic abnormalities revert to normal. If full correction is not achieved, drug therapy may be required.

HYPERLIPIDEMIAS

General Considerations

Exogenous lipids: A liberal diet supplies about 100 g of triglycerides and 1 g of cholesterol daily. After absorption they circulate in blood as chylomicrons from which the fatty acids pass to muscle cells and fat cells where they are utilized for energy or re-esterified into triglycerides. The remaining portion of the chylomicron which is rich in cholesterol esters is taken up by the liver for formation of bile acids and the rest passes unaltered in bile. Free fatty acids liberated from fat depots are also metabolized in the liver to form triglycerides, phospholipids and cholesterol which circulate in blood as lipoproteins.

Endogenous lipids: The liver synthesizes triglycerides from surplus carbohydrates obtained from diet. The triglycerides are esterified and released into circulation as very low-density lipoproteins (VLDLs). The triglyceride is split off and it enters the adipocytes. The VLDL remnant which contains mainly cholesterol esters gets physically transformed into low-density lipoprotein (LDL). Around 75% of circulating cholesterol is present in the form of LDL, and this is the form in which cholesterol is supplied to extrahepatic tissues like the adrenal cortex, muscle cells, renal cells, and lymphocytes for the formation of cell membranes and hormones. Unesterified cholesterol which is liberated into plasma from disintegrating hepatic parenchymal and phagocytic cells constitutes high-density lipoproteins (HDLs). The levels of cholesterol and triglycerides in plasma show considerable variation in health. Cholesterol levels above 200 mg/dL and triglyceride levels above 150 mg/dL indicate hyperlipidemia in adults. The cholesterol of atheromatous lesion is derived principally from plasma.

HDL is protective whereas LDL favors atherogenesis. Lipoprotein abnormalities are particularly marked in the metabolic syndrome (syndrome X) in which the HDL level is reduced. In the presence of hypertriglyceridemia,

Table 94.1: Properties of the major lipoprotein fractions

Lipoprotein	Major lipid	Major apoproteins	Specific gravity	Electrophoretic mobility
Chylomicron	Dietary triglyceride	AI, AII, BI, CI, CII, CIII	Below 1.006	No movement
VLDL	Endogenous triglyceride	B, CI, CII, CIII, E	Below 1.006	Pre-beta
LDL	Cholesterol esters	B	1.019 to 1.063	Beta
HDL	Cholesterol esters	AI, AII	1.063 to 1.210	Alpha
Remnants and triglyceride	Cholesterol esters	B, CIII, E	Less than 1.019	Slow pre-beta

Abbreviations: VLDL = Very low-density lipoprotein; LDL = Low-density lipoprotein; HDL = High-density lipoprotein

a decrease in cholesterol content of HDL results from decrease in the cholesteryl-ester content of HDL lipoprotein core making the particle small and dense. This leads to increase in the clearance of HDL from the circulation and the serum level of HDL falls.

Small dense LDL: This form of LDL increases when the triglyceride levels rise. This leads to depletion of unesterified cholesterol and phospholipids with either no change or/an increase in LDL triglyceride.

Small dense LDL is more atherogenic than buoyant LDL due to the following reasons:

- It is more toxic to the endothelium
- It is able to pass more easily through the endothelial basement membrane
- It adheres to glycosaminoglycans (GAGs)
- It has increased susceptibility to oxidation
- It is more selectively bound to scavenger receptors on monocyte derived macrophages. Presence of small dense LDL is common in syndrome X (Table 94.1).

Clinical Considerations

The blood levels of cholesterol and triglycerides give valuable information for the assessment of errors of lipid metabolism. LDL and HDL together account for 90% of the cholesterol in the plasma. Lipids are present in circulation as lipoproteins and free fatty acids (nonesterified fatty acids) bound to albumin. The lipoproteins are formed by combination of lipids, triglycerides, phospholipid and cholesterol with specific apoproteins. These have been classified as VLDLs (pre-beta), LDLs (beta lipoproteins) or HDLs (alpha lipoproteins) based on ultracentrifugal studies and electrophoretic patterns. The LDL and HDL particles are heterogeneous. The terms ***pre-beta***, ***beta*** and ***alpha*** refer to the bands seen on electrophoresis.

The role of HDL is probably to transport cholesterol and remove lipids from the arterial walls. The HDL reduces uptake of LDL by cells. Increase in levels of LDL and VLDL and decrease of HDL are associated with higher incidence of atheroma and its complications. Specific subclasses are selectively related to CHD. HDL has a protective role against atherogenesis. In CHD, the concentration of HDL fraction is particularly low. Raised concentration of LDL is readily decreased by controlled diet and appropriate drugs. Reduction of saturated fats in the diet and increase in the proportion of mono- and polyunsaturated fats help to lower LDL levels. Regular physical exercise helps to lower LDL cholesterol (LDL-C) and raise HDL cholesterol (HDL-C) to a limited extent. High levels of LDL (above 500–700 mg/dL) lead to acute pancreatitis.

Lipoprotein (LP) (a): It is a genetically determined fraction, with less of environmental influences. In Asian Indians, it is a very powerful predictor of CAD. Concurrent high levels of triglycerides and LDL increase the risk. LP (a) is highly thrombogenic, atherogenic and antifibrinolytic. Its atherogenic risk is 10 times that of LDL. Due to this high risk, LP (a) is called the ***deadly cholesterol***. Measurement of LP (a) is advisable for all persons with family history of premature atherosclerosis.

Classification

Hyperlipidemias may be primary or secondary. In the primary hyperlipidemias, genetic factors may be prominent. Environmental factors such as obesity, high saturated fat diet and smoking aggravate the disorder. Primary hyperlipidemias may be further classified into three groups.

Primary Hyperlipidemias

Group I: This consists of hypercholesterolemia (280–400 mg/dL, 7–10 mmol/L) with a clear serum, normal triglyceride levels, and increase in LDL (beta lipoproteins). In the majority of cases, environmental factors like high saturated fat diet and smoking are seen to aggravate the condition. For a long time, the condition is asymptomatic, but 50% develop ischemic heart disease (IHD) by the age of 50 years.

The condition occurs as an autosomally dominant inherited disorder in 5% of subjects. They show very high serum cholesterol levels (320–640 mg/dL in heterozygotes and 640–1,280 mg/dL in homozygotes). Xanthomas and arthritis are common. Xanthomas are deposits of cholesterol seen as yellowish nodular masses which vary in size from a few millimeters to several centimeters. They develop insidiously and are painless. The common types are *Xanthoma tendinosum* (over the tendo-achilles, extensor tendons of the hand, etc.), *Xanthoma tuberosum* over the bony prominences (around the elbow, knees, iliac crest, etc.), *Xanthoma planum* (plaque-like), striate xanthoma along the palmar creases, or as papular eruptions ***(Eruptive xanthoma)***. Sometimes they ulcerate and discharge greasy material. Some may be calcified. Histology shows collections of lipid-laden cells.

Many subjects may show ***xanthelasma***. These are yellowish plaque-like lesions seen on the medial aspects of the upper and lower eyelids. Though, these show a strong association with hypercholesterolemia, they may also be seen in persons with normal cholesterol levels.

Corneal arcus occurs as a grayish ring along the periphery of the cornea. A clear zone of cornea can be seen outside the arcus and this feature distinguishes the corneal arcus from other lesions like ***Kayser-Fleischer ring***. Corneal arcus is seen to develop in the majority of persons with age, but premature occurrence of arcus has been associated with the presence of hypercholesterolemia,

Table 94.2: Frederickson's classification

Types	Lipoproteins	Groups
Type 1	Chylomicron	Group III
Type 2a	LDL	Group I
Type 2b	LDL and VLDL	
Type 3	Remnants	Group II
Type 4	VLDL	
Type 5	VLDL and chylomicrons	

Abbreviations: LDL = Low-density lipoprotein; VLDL = Very low-density lipoprotein

especially LDL cholesterol, but in several reports from India this association has not been seen.

Group II: In this type of disorder, there is predominantly hypertriglyceridemia. The serum is cloudy, triglycerides and pre-beta-lipoproteins are increased but cholesterol is normal or only moderately increased. Common associations are obesity, DM and gout. There is a strong tendency to develop CAD.

Group III: It consists of chylomicronemia and this results from the deficiency of extrahepatic lipoprotein lipase and this is rare.

Fredrickson's classification: He has suggested a classification of hyperlipidemia which includes six groups based on the serum levels of lipids and lipoproteins, estimated in the fasting state (Table 94.2).

Management of Primary Hyperlipidemias

Many cases can be controlled by dietary management. Excess weight should be reduced. Groups I and II benefit by the avoidance of dietary cholesterol and restriction of fat to supply less than 15% of the total calories. Lipids should be supplied as polyunsaturated fats. Foods such as egg yolk, butter, margarine, hydrogenated oils, lard, suet, cakes and biscuits made with these fats, whole milk, cream, fatty meat, chocolates, coconut oil and foods fried in saturated fats should be avoided. Some cases show an abnormal elevation of serum lipids with the intake of alcohol and refined carbohydrates. Such cases benefit by restriction of alcohol and refined carbohydrates. Group III hyperlipidemias respond to reduction of fat below 15% of their dietary intake.

As important as the diet are exercise programs. Weight reduction and aerobic exercises help to normalize several of the hyperlipidemias. Proper exercise regimen and avoidance of smoking reduce the coronary risk further.

The desirable level of total cholesterol for Indians is ideally 150–200 mg/dL. In persons with risk factors for cardiovascular disease (CVD) such as strong family history, evidence of vascular disease, hypertension, diabetes and others, the desirable levels of total cholesterol and LDL cholesterol have to be lower. Decreased level of HDL below 35 mg/dL is an independent risk factor for atherosclerosis. Presence of low HDL levels is an indication for active lowering of total cholesterol and LDL. Levels of triglycerides above 200 mg/dL especially when accompanied by a low HDL/LDL ratio increases the risk of coronary atheroma sixfold. The LDL particle size also influence the risk factor, smaller size being more harmful.

Drug therapy

The different groups of drug used to treat high cholesterol levels are the following:

- 3-hydroxy-3-methylglutaryl coenzyme A (HMG-CoA) reductase inhibitors (statins—atorvastatin, fluvastatin, lovastatin, pravastatin, rosuvastatin and simvastatin)
- Bile acid sequestrants (cholestyramine, colesevelam and colestipol)
- Cholesterol absorption inhibitor (ezetimibe), nicotinic acid (niacin) and fibrates
- Cholestyramine, which is an anion exchange resin, in a daily dose of 16–32 g in 3–4 divided doses helps to control the hyperlipidemia in group I. It acts by inhibiting the absorption of bile acids and cholesterol. It is very effective in type 2 hyperlipidemia, but is contraindicated in types 3, 4 and 5.
- Clofibrate, which is a branched chain fatty acid, reduces VLDL and it is effective in lowering plasma triglycerides in types 3 and 4, when given in doses of 0.5 g 3–4 times a day. Clofibrate is indicated in severe hyperlipidemia where the risk of atheromatous occlusions, xanthomatosis and pancreatitis is high (Fredrickson's types 3, 4 and 5). Adverse side-effects of clofibrate include gastrointestinal (GI) upsets, increased incidence of cholelithiasis, and increased frequency of malignant neoplasms. Fenofibrate given in a dose of 145 mg qid is an effective lowering agent for triglycerides. Nicotinic acid in a dose of 0.5–1 g or more thrice daily augments the lipid lowering effects of other drugs in groups I and II hyperlipidemias. Gemfibrozil in a dose of 0.8 g bd is an effective lipid lowering agent.
- ***Exercise and cessation of smoking*** help to increase HDL cholesterol, and reduce triglycerides and VLDL. High-fiber diet, guar gum powder, fenugreek seeds and bittergourd (*Karela*) are known to lower serum LDL levels.
- ***The statins:*** These are inhibitors of hydroxymethyl glutaryl (HMG) coenzyme reductase. They inhibit cholesterol biosynthesis in the liver thereby reduce LDL cholesterol. Other actions of statins include modulation of macrophage activity, changing immune functions of lymphocytes, reduction of inflammatory activity and improvement in hemorrheological factors. There are several members in this group— lovastatin, simvastatin, pravastatin, rosuvastatin, atorvastatin and others. The newer members have got greater clinical activity. The dose range from 10 mg to 80 mg once a day or more depending on the target level of cholesterol suppression. Effective lowering of cholesterol and LDL reduce the risk of thromboembolic occlusions of coronary and cerebral arteries. Maintenance of serum lipids at lower normal levels has also been shown to lead to regression of atheroma.

    Statins are indicated to normalize lipid levels in both genetic and secondary hyperlipidemias. They are very effective in reducing atherosclerotic cardiovascular events. Every 1 mmol/L reduction in LDL-C with statin therapy is associated with a proportional reduction of about 20% in major vascular events defined as coronary death, nonfatal myocardial infarction, coronary revascularization, or stroke.

    In addition to their remarkable beneficial effects in CVD, statin treatment safely improves liver function tests (LFTs) and reduces cardiovascular morbidity in patients with mild to moderate abnormal LFTs that are potentially attributable to nonalcoholic fatty liver disease (NAFLD).

- ***As per the current management guidelines***, statins are used as the first-line therapy in achieving the goal of reduction in LDL cholesterol. Large doses of up to 80 mg daily are used for this purpose. The ***side effects*** include muscle toxicity including myopathy and rhabdomyolysis, neuropathy, reversible elevation of liver enzymes alanine transaminase (ALT) and aspartate transaminase (AST), new onset DM and a small increase in occurrence of hemorrhagic stroke.

Diabetes and statins relationships

Statins increase risk of new onset DM type 2. This increased risk is at least partly attributable to the inhibition of HMG-CoA reductase (HMCGR) which is the intended drug target. Despite this minor disadvantage of statins, their potential to protect against hyperlipidemia and CHD far exceeds the minor ill-effect and statins should be used in all indications wherever necessary.

Probucol

This drug lowers LDL-C predominantly. It is an alternate drug in those whose response to statins is inadequate or those who cannot tolerate statins. The dose is 500 mg bd oral.

Probucol has no effect on triglycerides. It may lower HDL slightly. ***Side effects*** are mild, mainly GI. Rarely, prolongation of the QT interval and cardiac arrhythmias may develop. Therefore regular electrocardiography (ECG) monitoring is required.

Cholesterol absorption inhibitor

Ezetimibe selectively inhibits the absorption of cholesterol by the brush border of the small intestinal epithelium. Triglycerides, fatty acids and fat soluble vitamins are not affected. Its main use is in combination with statins when their effect is suboptimal. Ezitimibe in doses 10 mg/day oral inhibits absorption of cholesterol from the intestine leading 23–24% reduction of serum cholesterol. The levels are further lowered with coadministration of statins.

- ***Omega-3 fatty acids:*** Eicosapentaenoic acid (EPA) and docosahexaenoic acid (DHA), 2–7 g/day given orally reduces blood levels of triglycerides and cholesterol and thereby lower the coronary risk. Fish oils and fish products have similar beneficial effects.
- ***Newer drugs in hypercholesterolemia:*** Monoclonal antibody to proprotein convertase subtilisin/kexin type 9 (PCSK9) in combination with a statin produces better results than statins given alone. PCSK9 builds LDL receptors targeting them from degradation. AMG-145, a human monoclonal antibody against PCSK9 is beneficial and phase 3 clinical trails are in progress. ***Doses***—70 mg, 105 mg, or 140 mg were given subcutaneously once in 4 weeks and the results are encouraging; phase 3 clinical trials are in progress. A few drugs in this class include alirocumab,

bococizumab, evolocumab and others. These have to be given subcutaneously about 150 mg once in 2 weeks continuously. When added to statin therapy, further reduction of LDL-C levels occurs adverse events but these are mild.

Secondary Hyperlipidemias

Secondary hyperlipoproteinemias outnumber the primary type. In the majority of cases, LDL-C is increased in the serum. The risks of coronary, cerebral, renal and peripheral arterial disease are high irrespective of the primary cause and this risk can be brought down by appropriate therapy.

Causes

The secondary types are seen in DM, hypothyroidism, nephrotic syndrome, biliary obstruction, pancreatitis or as a side effect of drugs such as estrogens and corticosteroids.

In all subjects with hyperlipidemias, primary causes should be looked for and attended to.

HEMOCHROMATOSIS

Syn: Bronzed diabetes

This is a metabolic disorder associated with marked accumulation of iron in parenchymal organs. Two forms are—*genetic* and *acquired*. The genetic homochromatosis is an autosomal recessive disorder showing varied phenotype manifestations and varying expressivity in different families. Homozygous disease occurs in 3–5/1,000. Carrier frequency is 1/10–1/5 among the Caucasian population and this is one of the more common genetic abnormality in them. The human leukocyte antigen (HLA)-A3 and B14 are more frequently associated with genetic hemochromatosis.

Underlying defect is the pronounced increase in intestinal absorption of iron through an up regulation of the duodenal metal transporter gene caused by these mutations of *HFE* gene, which is located on chromosome 6 near the HLA locus. Its product is widely expressed in several tissues. More than 80% of affected subjects show a homozygous point mutation (G-A at nucleotide 845) in *HFE* gene. This results in a cytosine to tyrosine replacement at amino acid 282 (C282 Y). Another mutation is H63D, aspartic acid is substituted for histidine in position 63. These abnormalities can be demonstrated in the laboratory and is used for genetic screening. The *HFE* product binds to transferrin receptor. Several mutations are known to produce hemochromatosis. Mainly four types of hereditary hemochromatosis are identified. These include:

1. HFE-related
2. Juvenile type
3. Transferrin receptor 2 (TfR2)-related
4. Ferroportin-related iron overload.

Normal iron absorption is 1–2 mg/day. In hemochromatosis, it goes up to 6 mg/day and the body stores may reach up to 60 g against the upper limit of normal of 4 g.

The acquired or secondary type is due to iron overload caused in disorders of erythropoiesis including thalassemia, sickle-cell anemia (SCA), X-linked sideroblastic anemia (XLSA), pyruvate kinase deficiency, hereditary spherocytosis and congenital dyserythropoietic anemia (CDA).

Pathogenesis

The main defect is loss of regulation of intestinal absorption of iron resulting in increased absorption of dietary iron. This iron is taken up by several parenchymal tissues and macrophages which results in toxic damage. The pathological changes include cellular dysfunction, necrosis and fibrosis. Liver and pancreas are most severely affected. The skin, myocardium, and endocrine glands like the adrenal cortex, testes, pituitary and thyroid are affected with varying severity. The condition remains asymptomatic till the total body stores of iron reach 15–20 g.

The liver is enlarged, firm to hard in consistency, and the cut section is brown. The hepatocytes and Kupffer's cells show stainable iron. Eventually, portal cirrhosis develops. Cirrhosis develops when the hepatic iron content exceeds 400 µmol/g, i.e. 22.4 mg/g of dry liver tissue. Acinar cells of the pancreas and less frequently the islet cells show hemosiderin. Diabetes may develop. There is an increase in iron in several organs. Skin shows increased pigmentation due to deposition of melanin.

Clinical Features

Males are affected five times more frequently than females. Symptoms generally start in the 4th and 5th decades. These include lethargy, loss of libido and impotence, pigmentation, hepatomegaly and diabetes. The combination of pigmentation and diabetes is referred to as *bronzed diabetes.* Cirrhosis of liver and testicular atrophy occur in advanced cases. Severity of the diabetes is variable. Cardiac enlargement, cardiac failure, heart block and arrhythmias occur in 10–15% of cases. Arthropathy develops due to deposition of calcium pyrophosphate and hemosiderin in the synovium. In long-standing cases, hepatocellular carcinoma may develop.

Course and Prognosis

Mean survival in untreated cases is 5 years after diagnosis. Death is caused by infection, cardiac failure, hepatic failure, hepatic carcinoma or diabetic complications. Modern treatment has improved the outcome considerably.

Diagnosis

Hemochromatosis should be considered in all patients presenting with hepatic cirrhosis, diabetes, skin pigmentation and cardiac abnormalities. In hepatic cirrhosis due to any cause, there is an accumulation of iron in the liver and this should be distinguished from primary hemochromatosis.

Serum iron is usually above 175 µg/dL, total iron binding capacity (TIBC) is 200 µg/dL and transferrin saturation is about 60% and often even 100%. Serum ferritin may be increased to 1,000 ng/mL in severe cases and in the absence of significant hepatocellular damage, this reflects the enormous iron load.

The 24-hour urinary excretion of more than 2 mg iron following intramuscular (IM) injection of 0.5 g of desferrioxamine is suggestive of excessive iron stores. Values greater than 10 mg indicate idiopathic hemochromatosis.

Treatment

Simple venesection to remove 500 mL blood once in 2 weeks or at shorter intervals help to prolong life by a mean of 8.2 years and improves hepatic function. Venesection is indicated when the serum ferritin level exceeds 1,000 ng/mL. The hematocrit is adjusted to around 35% by venesection. Each venesection removes 250 mg of iron. When the iron stores become normal (ferritin drops to 50 ng/mL), progression of cirrhosis may halt. Rarely it may regress and the pigmentation may also come down. There is a general reluctance to do venesection at frequent intervals in them. An established case may require removal of several liters of blood at regular intervals of 5–7 days before the clinical benefits become evident.

The iron-chelating agent—desferrioxamine has been used when venesection is contraindicated by the presence of anemia, but the drug is less effective. Diabetes is controlled on its own merits. In secondary hemochromatosis, desferrioxamine is effective. (For details refer to thalassemias *See* Section 15, Ch 161).

WILSON'S DISEASE

Syn: Hepatolenticular degeneration; Westphal-Strumpell pseudosclerosis

It is an IEM of copper inherited as autosomal recessive. The abnormal gene is present in chromosome 13 and it is identified as ATP7B. This disease is present not uncommonly in many communities in India. Normally, copper which is absorbed from the gut is initially bound loosely to albumin, but very soon it binds firmly with ceruloplasmin, which is a globulin and produced in the liver.

In Wilson's disease, absorption of copper is normal or increased. There is defect in excretion of copper into the bile. Ceruloplasmin in the plasma is absent or considerably reduced. Production of ceruloplasmin is normal but its degradation is accelerated. Therefore, the serum copper remains loosely bound to albumin and gets deposited in various organs such as the liver, brain, cornea, kidneys, heart and muscles. This leads to damage of parenchymal tissues. The most prominent lesions are cirrhosis of the liver and damage to basal ganglia and renal tubules. Cirrhosis of liver is more common in children.

Clinical Features

The presentation may be predominantly hepatic, neurological or mixed. ***Hepatic manifestations*** include chronic active hepatitis, acute fulminant hepatic failure and cirrhosis liver which are the most common hepatic presentation. Hematemesis, portal-systemic encephalopathy and coma may follow.

In the brain, copper is deposited mainly in the basal ganglia, cerebellum and cerebral cortex. This manifests as involuntary movements, extrapyramidal features, dystonias, dementia, cerebellar disturbances and convulsions. Emotional lability, impulsiveness and disinhibition are the common psychiatric manifestations. Most patients presenting with neuropsychiatric manifestations also have cirrhosis liver. Renal tubular damage results in generalized aminoaciduria. Phosphaturia occurs resulting in osteomalacia and renal rickets. Other renal functions remain unaffected (*See* also Chapters 84 and 203).

Deposition of copper in the Descemet's membrane layer of the cornea appears as a brownish yellow ring (Kayser-Fleischer ring) which merges to the limbus without a clear intervening zone. This has to be distinguished from corneal arcus in which a clear zone of cornea intervenes between the ring and the limbus. Kayser-Fleischer ring is best studied by slit-lamp examination. Presence of Kayser-Fleischer ring is associated with definite neurological damage. At times, Wilson's disease may present with acute viral hepatitis like picture.

Diagnosis

Wilson's disease should be suspected in all young patients below the age of 40 years who present with hepatic dysfunction and/or neurological disorder, especially affecting the extrapyramidal system and cerebellum. Presence of Kayser-Fleischer ring is not considered pathognomonic unless accompanied by neurological manifestations. Diagnosis should be confirmed by estimating serum copper and ceruloplasmin and demonstrating high copper content in liver tissue obtained by biopsy.

Serum ceruloplasmin is low (<20 mg/dL). Normal value is 18–65 mg/dL. Total serum copper is below 80 µg/dL. Normal value is 100–200 µg/dL. Amount of copper bound to ceruloplasmin is low whereas the unbound copper is higher than normal. Urinary copper excretion is high—more than 100 µg/24 hours (Normal: 0.32 µg/24 hours). Hepatic copper is elevated—often above 250 µg/g dry weight (Normal: 20–45 µg/g).

Computed tomography (CT) scan in Wilson's disease shows general cerebral atrophy with basal ganglia having low attenuation signals. Magnetic resonance imaging (MRI) is more sensitive. Subtle changes in signal activity occur in the basal ganglia in symptomatic and even presymptomatic stages. Positron emission tomography (PET) scan shows diffuse reduction of glucose metabolism.

Course and Prognosis

The disease steadily progresses to end fatally in 5–14 years. Hepatic failure, hematemesis, or neurological deterioration accounts for majority of deaths. The natural history of Wilson's disease may be considered in four stages, as follows:

1. ***Stage I:*** The initial period of accumulation of copper within hepatic binding sites.
2. ***Stage II:*** The acute redistribution of copper within the liver and its release into the circulation.
3. ***Stage III:*** The chronic accumulation of copper in the brain and other extrahepatic tissue, with progressive and eventually fatal disease.
4. ***Stage IV:*** Restoration of copper balance by the use of long-term chelation therapy.

Treatment

Treatment aims at increasing the elimination of excess copper that is stored in tissues. Elimination is increased by chelating agents like penicillamine (dimethyl cysteine-distamine, cuprimine). The dose is 1–4 g daily given orally before food and at bedtime. It leads to urinary loss of copper. Adverse side effects include nephrotoxicity, agranulocytosis, arthralgia, lupus-like syndrome, lymphadenopathy, rashes and thrombocytopenia. These are seen on starting the therapy. ***Side effects*** may necessitate temporary withdrawal of the drug. Many toxic effects are dose-related. Interruption of therapy leads to relapse of symptoms and therefore treatment has to be life-long. Even during pregnancy, penicillamine can be continued.

Textbook of Medicine

Triethylenetetramine (Trientine) dihydrochloride is another chelating agent given in a dose of 400–800 mg orally thrice daily before food. It is not freely available.

Trientine enhances copper excretion and decreases intestinal absorption. Zinc given as zinc acetate blocks intestinal absorption by inducing metallothionein synthesis in intestinal cells. The dose is 150 mg oral daily in divided doses. Zinc is safe and can be given on a long-term basis for treatment as well as prevention in susceptible subjects. Potassium sulfide given orally is effective in inhibiting absorption of copper from foods. Therapy can be monitored clinically and by biochemical tests for free copper in the serum, urinary copper and hepatic transaminases. Another drug is tetrathiomolybdate which prevents absorption of copper and also makes the circulating copper unavailable to be deposited in tissues. Side effects include anemia which is due to overzealous elimination of copper from the body. Liver transplantation may be needed in some cases.

Screening of Relatives

Since asymptomatic siblings show abnormality of copper transport, they have to be investigated with estimation of serum ceruloplasmin and hepatic copper. Early treatment helps to prevent the development of organ damage.

PORPHYRIAS

These are rare metabolic errors involving enzymes concerned with the heme synthetic pathway. Heme is synthesized in every cell, 85% being in erythroid cells. Out of this, 85% is used for the creation of different cytochromes. The synthesis of heme involves eight steps and each step is enzymatically-mediated. These are:

1. Glycine
2. Delta-aminolevulinic acid (δ-ALA)
3. Porphobilinogen (PBG)
4. Polypyrrole (PPy)
5. Uroporphyrinogen III
6. Coproporphyrinogen III
7. Protoporphyrinogen III
8. Protoporphyrin III.

Heme

This pathway begins in the mitochondria and after three cytoplasmic stages ends at the mitochondrial level. The porphyrias include eight different inherited metabolic disorders each resulting from a specific enzymatic alteration in this heme synthetic pathway. Heme is produced in liver for synthesis of cytochrome and hemoproteins and in erythropoietic cells for hemoglobin synthesis. The rate limiting step for heme synthesis in liver is the first enzyme aminolevulinic acid (ALA) synthase, whereas in erythropoietic cells it depends on availability of iron.

The term 'porphyria' is derived from the Greek word 'porphura' which means 'purple'. Dominant clinical features of porphyria are two. *Photosensitivity* due to presence of porphyrin compounds in the skin—leading to pain, erythema, burn-like lesions, vesicles and bullae, skin erosions, hyperpigmentation, hirsutism skin infections and loss of tissues due to infection and minor trauma exposure to sunlight triggers off *acute symptoms*. These are prominent in the erythropoietic and erythrohepatic porphyrias. In them, *neuropsychiatric* manifestations are less pronounced or absent. In most of the cases of the different forms of porphyrias, precipitating factors include alcoholic bouts, stress and use of estrogens. *Porphyrias can be classified in different ways based on:*

- The organ in which the excess heme precursors accumulate, e.g. hepatic porphyria and erythropoietic porphyria (Table 94.3)
- Clinical manifestations
- Specific enzyme defects.

Table 94.3: Summary of the enzyme defects and salient clinical features of the various forms of porphyria

Porphyria	Deficient enzyme	Principal symptoms	Elevated porphyrins and precursors		
			RBCs	Urine	Stool
Hepatic porphyrias					
5-ALA dehydratase-deficiency porphyria (ADP)	ALA-dehydratase	Neurovisceral	Zn-Protoporphyrin	ALA, Coproporphyrin III	
Acute intermittent porphyria (AIP)	HMB-synthase	Neurovisceral		ALAa, PBG, Uroporphyrin	
Porphyria cutanea tarda (PCT)	URO-decarboxylase	Cutaneous photosensitivity		Uroporphyrin, 7-carboxylate porphyrin	Isocoproporphyrin
Hereditary coproporphyria (HCP)	COPRO-oxidase	Neurovisceral and cutaneous photosensitivity		ALA, PBG, Coproporphyrin III	Coproporphyrin III
Variegate porphyria (VP)	PROTO-oxidase	Neurovisceral and cutaneous photosensitivity			Coproporphyrin III Protoporphyrin
Erythropoietic porphyrias					
Congenital erythropoietic porphyria (CEP)	URO-synthase	Cutaneous photosensitivity	Uroporphyrin I Coproporphyrin I	Uroporphyrin Ib Coproporphyrin Ib	Coproporphyrin I
Erythropoietic protoporphyria (EPP)	Ferrochelatase	Cutaneous photosensitivity	Protoporphyrin	—	Protoporphyrin
X-linked protoporphyria (XLP)	ALA-synthase 2	Cutaneous photosensitivity			

Note: Classification based on the enzymatic abnormality.

Abbreviations: ALA = Aminolevulinic acid; PBG = Porphobilinogen; RBCs = Red blood cells; HMB = Hydroxymethylbilane; URO = Uroporphyrinogen; COPRO = Coproporphyrinogen; PROTO = Protoporphyrinogen

Textbook of Medicine

Clinical Classification

- ***Cutaneous manifestation without neurological features:*** Congenital erythropoietic porphyria (CEP), erythrohepatic porphyria [erythropoietic protoporphyria (EPP)], porphyria cutanea tarda (PCT).
- ***Neurological features without skin lesions:*** Acute intermittent porphyria (AIP).
- ***Those that produce either cutaneous or neurological or combined manifestations:*** Variegate porphyria (VP) (porphyria variegata), hereditary coproporphyria (HCP).

Among the porphyrias the most commonly encountered one in medical practice is AIP. In dermatological and pediatric practice, the cutaneous forms may be more frequently encountered.

'Porphyria with ALA (δ-ALA) dehydratase deficiency'—it is rare and it is transmitted as autosomal recessive. Symptoms resemble AIP, but starts in childhood. ALA dehydratase (ALAD) is reduced to 1–2% of normal. ALA is excreted in urine, and coproporphyrin III is excreted through bile and it appears in feces.

AIP-autosomal dominant. The enzyme PBG deaminase (previously known as uroporphyrinogen I synthase) is reduced by 50% or more. This is the most common porphyria seen in clinical practice.

CEP-autosomal recessive caused by deficiency of uroporphyrinogen III cosynthase (Fig 94.1). The condition is rare. Type 1 porphyrin isomers are produced in excess reflecting a hemolytic state. Excess porphyrins in circulating erythrocytes predispose to hemolysis. Splenomegaly may occur.

Severe cutaneous photosensitivity and reddish urine occur from early life. Later, bullae and vesicles occur on the skin and they tend to get infected. Skin may show hyper- or hypopigmentation and hypertrichosis. Porphyrins may get deposited in the teeth making them reddish brown. Life is shortened by hemolysis, infections or hematological complications.

Treatment is supportive. Regulated blood transfusion may be necessary in addition to infection management. This disease can be detected *in utero* and pregnancy can be terminated if necessary.

Porphyria Cutanea Tarda (PCT)

This is a common form of porphyria caused by deficiency of uroporphyrinogen decarboxylase (UPD) in the liver. Several forms of this disease have been identified. The term tarda denotes slow onset of clinical features:

- ***Sporadic form***—most adult cases of PCT belong to this group, the enzyme UPD is deficient in the liver but not in the erythrocytes
- ***Familial form termed type II***—the UPD deficiency affects the liver, erythrocytes and other tissues. It is transmitted as an autosomal dominant
- ***Type II PCT***—enzyme deficiency affects the liver not the other tissues
- ***Type IV hepatoerythropoietic porphyria***—the clinical picture resembles that of CEP.

Clinical manifestation

Men are more affected and women may get affected if there is alcoholism and use of estrogens, cutaneous photosensitivity occurs in variable degree and severity; often less severe than in CEP. The skin may become thickened, pigmented or scarred and calcified (pseudoscleroderma). Older patients develop hepatic cirrhosis and hepatic carcinoma.

Diagnosis

Skin lesions of PCT and VP are not distinguishable from other cutaneous forms of porphyria. Other forms of porphyria are HCP, VP and EPP, all have photosensitivity in different degrees.

Treatment

Management of cutaneous forms: This consists of avoidance of skin exposure and use of sun barrier creams containing zinc or titanium oxide. Beta-carotene given in high dose may be of benefit in erythropoietic porphyria.

A synthetic analog of alpha-melanocyte stimulating hormone (alpha-MSH)—(Afamelanotide) given in repeated doses as subcutaneous implants may be of benefit in EPP.

In PCT, repeated venesections to remove blood helps to reduce the iron stores in the body and bring about symptomatic benefit, especially if combined with avoidance of precipitating factors.

Acute attacks warrant hospitalization and supportive care with IV glucose solution and heme. Nutrition is maintained by high carbohydrate intake and vitamins. Heme therapy is given in the form of lyophilized hematin preparation (hydroxy–heme) which is available for use. This is reconstituted with sterile water and should be given without delay since the solution is unstable. Dose is 1–1.5 mg/kg given once or twice a day. Other preparations which are more stable include heme arginate and heme albumin. Heme therapy should be given only to patients with confirmed diagnosis. Heme therapy relieves the neurologic symptoms, if they are not far advanced.

Prevention: Family members of index cases can be screened *in utero* tests undertaken and preventive measures adapted. Patients and their relatives should avoid precipitating events and drugs.

ACUTE INTERMITTENT PORPHYRIA (AIP)

It occurs worldwide and in India; the condition has been reported from all parts of the country. It is inherited as autosomal dominant. Other porphyrias with autosomal dominant inheritance are VP and HCP. In AIP, women suffer more than men. Basic defect is a gross reduction of uroporphyrinogen I synthase (below 50%) which is required for the conversion of PBG to PPy (step 3). Urine contains the porphyrin precursors PBG and δ-ALA even when the patient is asymptomatic. During an acute attack, levels of porphyrin precursors such as δ-ALA and PBG increase and these are excreted in large amounts in urine. These precursors are neurotoxic, especially to the autonomic and peripheral nervous systems. In addition, urinary uro- and coproporphyrins also may increase.

Clinical Features

This condition may remain latent for long periods without recognition. Acute episodes are precipitated by several factors. Important among them are:

- Drugs—barbiturates, sulfa drugs, griseofulvin, phenytoin, female sex hormones and several others
- Dietary factors—starvation or excess eating
- Infections.

The acute attack is characterized by acute abdominal pain sometimes associated with pain over the back and thighs. Nausea, vomiting and constipation are common. Excitement, behavioral disturbances, depression, suicidal tendency, delirium, convulsions and coma are frequent. Peripheral neuropathy and mononeuropathies may be prominent in some cases. Autonomic neuropathy results in GI dysfunction, urinary retention, hypertensive crises, disordered sweating and tachycardia. Acute attacks are very rare before puberty and after menopause, the peak incidence being in the third decade.

Abdominal pain may be so severe as to be mistaken for a surgical emergency. Severe diarrhea may contribute to weight loss. GI fluid losses lead to hyponatremia and dehydration. Acute attacks could be life-threatening due to neurological complications. Muscle weakness can progress to tetraplegia and respiratory and bulbar paralysis. Motor neuropathy and proximal weakness can also occur.

Mental symptoms such as psychosis, mania, delirium, depression and suicidal tendencies may develop.

Diagnosis

AIP should be considered in the differential diagnosis of all bizarre—neurological and neuropsychiatric disorders, severe abdominal pain and autonomic disturbances.

Diagnosis is established by urine examination. Freshly passed urine is colorless but on standing for a few hours at room temperature it becomes portwine in color and this should be looked for in all cases. PBG in urine can be demonstrated by Watson-Schwartz test, i.e. the urine gives a pink color with Ehrlich's aldehyde reagent just as in the case of urobilinogen. On extracting the pigment with chloroform, PBG is not extractable whereas urobilinogen is. The amount of PBG can be estimated quantitatively.

Apart from AIP, PBG may occur in urine in hepatic diseases, drug toxicity, porphyria variegata and HCP. Specific diagnostic test is the demonstration of diminution of uroporphyrin I synthase in erythrocytes.

Treatment

Symptomatic management during an attack: The offending drugs should be stopped. Phenothiazine (chlorpromazine) administered in a dose of 50 mg IM relieves abdominal pain and hypertension. Maintenance of fluid and electrolyte balance helps to tide over the crisis. High carbohydrate intake and propranolol give symptomatic relief. This may be repeated, if necessary. Aspirin, morphine, guanethidine, reserpine and penicillin can be safely used for suitable indications.

IV hemin is the specific treatment of choice. Hemin inhibits upregulated ALA synthase-1 and curtails urinary excretion of 5-ALA and PBG. Single dose of human, hemin contains 22.7 mg of iron. So if regular doses are given, there will be a risk of iron overload. Liver transplantation is considered in selected patients with severe AIP.

Prophylaxis should be in the form of avoidance of precipitating factors. Relatives should be screened for the enzyme deficiency and susceptible persons should be warned to avoid the offending drugs.

DISORDERS OF AMINO ACID METABOLISM

These are a heterogeneous group of rare disorders clinically characterized by mental retardation and a shortened lifespan, generally inherited as autosomal recessive and ranging in severity from mild to very severe forms.

PHENYLKETONURIA

Syn: Hyperphenylalaninemia

This is one of the most widespread metabolic errors occurring in infancy. Frequency is one in 100,000 livebirths. Untreated children develop convulsions and restriction of mental faculties. It is an autosomal recessive disorder caused by deficiency of hepatic phenylalanine hydroxylase which is required for conversion of phenylalanine into tyrosine. In a well-developed case, there is severe mental retardation, seizures, microcephaly, hypopigmentation of skin and hair and eczema. Phenylacetic, phenylpyruvic, and phenyllactic acids, which are metabolites of phenylalanine, occur in excessive quantities in the urine which impart a musty odor to the urine and give a green color with 5% ferric chloride solution within 2–3 minutes. Ingestion of phenylalanine in milk and milk products aggravates the symptoms. Death occurs due to intercurrent infections.

Avoidance of milk and other phenylalanine containing diet from the first month of life prevents the development of symptoms. Even in established cases withdrawal of dietary phenylalanine improves the symptoms. Phenylketonuria (PKU) is one of the disorders included in neonatal screening program.

Diagnosis

The urine is screened by ferric chloride test for metabolites of phenylalanine. The Guthrie test which is a filter paper spot test using one drop of blood is done as a screening test for the presence of excess amounts of phenylalanine in blood. In infants with a positive Guthrie test quantitative, estimation of amino acids in blood is done. Serum phenylalanine is above 20 mg/dL in severe PKU, whereas normally the levels of phenylalanine and tyrosine do not exceed 1 mg/dL.

Treatment

Dietary measures using diets which are low in phenylalanine (200–800 mg/day) help to keep the serum level below 12 mg/dL. This is continued for the first 8–10 years of life. Restriction of phenylalanine in the diet forms the mainstay of treatment. Foods rich in protein are to be avoided. A protein derived from cheese which is rich in amino acids but deficient in tyrosine, tryptophan, and phenylalanine is available as a food supplement to children with the disease. Tetrahydrobiopterin has been tried as an alternate treatment for mild forms of PKU. Tetrahydrobiopterin is a natural cofactor of aromatic

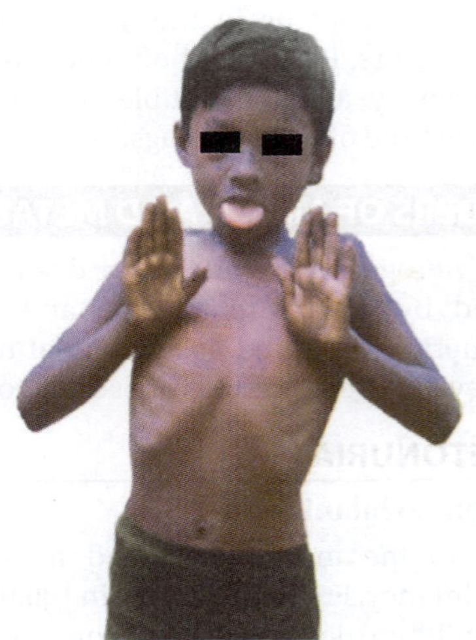

Fig. 94.1: Ochronosis. **Note:** The dark pigmentation of the hands, face and pinna of the ears in alkaptonuria

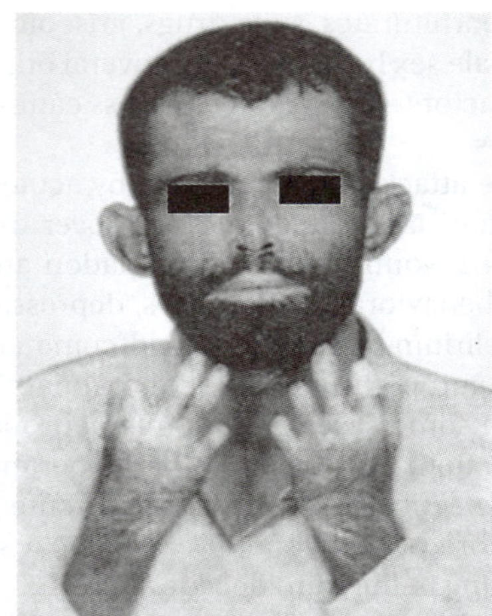

Fig. 94.2: Congenital erythropoietic porphyria. **Note:** (1) Ulceration and scarring face, (2) Ulceration and mutilation of ears and (3) Mutilation of hands and fingers

amino acid hydroxylases and nitric oxide synthase. Mild cases may respond but many of the severe cases do not. This depends on the specific genotypes. Gene therapy has been tried to restore function of the missing enzyme.

ALKAPTONURIA

This is caused by deficiency of homogentisic acid (HGA) reductase (homogenetisate 1, 2 dioxygenase). HGA is a metabolic product of tyrosine. The urine turns black on standing due to oxidation of HGA. 'Ochronosis' is dark pigmentation of cartilage tissues (Fig. 94.1).

Clinical features of alkaptonuria include arthralgia, arthropathies, pigmentation of the sclera and cartilages, especially of the pinna of the ear, renal stones, cardiac dysfunction and others. In spondylitis occurring in alkaptonuria, the sacroiliac joints are not affected. This feature distinguishes the condition from ankylosing spondylitis (Fig. 94.2).

A new drug has been introduced 'nitisinone'. The dose is 0.7 mg/day for 7 days followed by 2.8 mg/day for 3 days. It reduces the level of HGA in urine. Long-term results are awaited.

Inherited Disorders of Connective Tissue

KV Krishna Das

Chapter Summary

- General Considerations
- Major Disorders of Collagen
  - Osteogenesis Imperfecta
  - Ehlers-Danlos Syndrome (EDS)
  - Marfan's Syndrome
  - Homocystinuria and Hyperhomocysteinemia

GENERAL CONSIDERATIONS

The term connective tissue includes cartilage, bone, tendons, fascia, ligaments and vascular walls. The connective tissue consists mainly of the fibrous proteins—collagen and elastin and the amorphous complex carbohydrates, hyaluronic acid, proteoglycans and glycoproteins, together called the *ground substance*. Functions of connective tissue include:

- Formation of an elastic covering, e.g. dermis
- Protection of vital structures, e.g. skull
- Acting as levers for aiding muscular action, e.g. long bones
- Provision of deformable elastic cushions to bear stress and aid in joint movement, e.g. cartilage.

Collagens are a class of proteins, each being determined by a single gene. Two major types of collagens—*pericellular* and *interstitial collagens.* Pericellular collagen (types IV and V) occurs in basement membranes and intercellular tissues. The major collagen of skin, bones, articular cartilage, tendons, and fascia is interstitial collagen (types I, II, III). The collagens are formed from procollagens by complex enzymatic processes.

Developmental disorders involving the collagens may be hereditarily transmitted. The manifestation and severity differ on account of differences in penetrance and expression of single genes or genetic heterogenicity.

MAJOR DISORDERS OF COLLAGEN

Osteogenesis Imperfecta

This disorder is described in Section 12, Ch 116.

Ehlers-Danlos Syndrome (EDS)

This is a disorder of types I and III interstitial collagen. EDS comprises of at least eleven heritable disorders of connective tissue leading to defects in synthesis or structure of collagen. The abnormality is in the metabolism of fibrillar collagen. Mutations in the *type V collagen gene* account for up to 50% of classic EDS. Other abnormalities such as defects in tenascins which are extracellular matrix (ECM) proteins can lead to clinically distinct recessive forms of the syndrome. *Clinical features* include hyperextensibility of the skin, laxity of joints with tendency to subluxate, purpura, bruises, subcutaneous nodular calcification, and violaceous subcutaneous nodules called *molluscoid pseudotumors*, delayed wound healing and kyphoscoliosis. The genetics of this disorder is heterogenous and on this basis EDS may be subclassified into *autosomal dominant, autosomal recessive* and *X-linked types*.

Marfan's Syndrome

This name is derived from the first description of the disease by the French pediatrician Antoine Jean-Bernard Marfan (1858–1942). The main *pathology* is caused by quantitative deficiency of fibrillin-1 which is an ECM protein. This deficiency sets in motion structural changes in later life and results in multisystem connective tissue abnormalities. The skin texture and elasticity are normal. The basic mechanism is altered regulation of transforming growth factor-beta (TGF-β)—a family of cytokines that affect cellular performance. The gene is located on chromosome 15q21. More than 500 mutations have been reported. In this disorder, a wide spectrum of clinical abnormalities exists. The condition is inherited as autosomal dominant. Twenty-five percent give a family history and 25% is sporadic.

Clinical Features

- **Bony abnormalities:** These include disproportionately long limbs compared to the trunk (dolichostenomelia), arachnodactyly (spider fingers), pectus excavatum, pectus carinatum, kyphoscoliosis, increased joint laxity, recurrent dislocations, genu recurvatum and flat feet. The arm span is greater than height by 7.5 cm. Arm span/height ratio is more than 1.05 cm.
- **Ocular lesions:** The classic feature is ectopia lentis occurring in 60% of cases, the displacement of the lens is upwards, unlike as in traumatic dislocation in which the dislocation is downward. Other features include high myopia and retinal detachment.
- **Cardiovascular lesions:** Dilation of the aortic root, aortic regurgitation, aneurysms of the ascending aorta and sinus of Valsalva, dissecting aneurysms of descending aorta, mitral valve prolapse, mitral regurgitation and cardiac failure may occur. Respiratory manifestations include lung cysts and recurrent pneumothorax.

Differential Diagnosis

Marfan's syndrome closely resembles homocystinuria which may present with skeletal and ocular abnormalities similar to those of Marfan's syndrome. The urine shows homocysteine in the latter.

Eunuchoid features: These may be mistaken for marfanoid features. In the former, there is no arachnodactyly and other features of hypogonadism are present.

Diagnosis

Strong clinical suspicion is essential for diagnosis. If the terminal phalanx of the thumb projects beyond the medial border of the closed fist, it suggests Marfan's syndrome. The wrist sign is overlap of the thumb and little finger when wrapped around the wrist. Clinically, there should be involvement of two out of three systems (bony, ocular and cardiovascular) to diagnose Marfan's syndrome.

Diagnostic criteria have been postulated. Metacarpal index measured on X-ray of the hand is diagnostic.

Prognosis

Progressive dilation of the aortic root, aortic and mitral incompetence, aneurysm of descending aorta and heart failure account for death.

Treatment

There is no curative treatment. The orthopedic, ocular and cardiovascular lesions demand special attention. *Medical treatment* consists of β-adrenergic blockers such as atenolol given in doses of 25–50 mg od or bd. This reduces the tension on the aorta and delays dilation.

Enalapril and other antihypertensive drugs may be employed. Patients with Marfan's syndrome should avoid isometric exercises and competitive sports since sudden death may occur.

Surgery on the aortic aneurysm and valves are indicated during the course of the disease. Ectopia lentis has to be treated surgically.

Homocystinuria and Hyperhomocysteinemia

Homocystinuria is a disorder of methionine metabolism. Genetically determined homocystinuria occurs in 1/100,000 livebirths and leads to a 40-fold increase in total serum homocysteine (tHcy). The total pool is the sum of all forms of homocysteine.

In the plasma, homocysteine occurs in four forms:

1. Free thiol—1%
2. Disulfide bound to plasma proteins, especially albumin—70–80%
3. Dimer homocysteine
4. Combination with other thiols including cysteine to produce homocysteine-cysteine mixed disulfide (20–30%).

During the metabolism of methionine, homocysteine is formed. It is metabolized further in two ways:

1. In the liver, it is remethylated by betaine-homocysteine methyltransferase (BHMT). Betaine (trimethylglycine) acts as the donor of the methyl group.
2. In most of the other tissues, the *remethylation* is catalyzed by methionine synthase and N-methyltetrahydrofolate acts as the donor. The latter depends on dietary folate for its formation. Vitamin B_{12} is an essential cofactor for methionine synthase activity.

Textbook of Medicine

Normal fasting plasma level of tHcy is 5–15 µmol/L. The arbitrary value for hyperhomocysteinemia elevation is above 15 µmol/L of homocysteine after the methionine loading. The levels in the different grades of hyperhomocysteinemia are:

- Mild—16–30 µmol/L
- Moderate—31–100 µmol/L
- Severe—above 100 µmol/L.

The term ***homocystinuria*** refers to a group of rare inborn metabolic disorders resulting in high level of circulating homocysteine more than 100 mmol/L and urinary homocysteine.

Homocysteine in urine can be detected in many metabolic abnormalities. Most common among them is ***cystathionine beta-synthase deficiency,*** which is an autosomal recessive disorder. This deficiency leads to failure of homocysteine to react with serine to form cystathionine and further conversion to cysteine. Two molecules of homocysteine get converted to homocysteine by disulfide oxidation. Normally, homocysteine is not detectable in plasma or urine by ordinary chemical methods. In cystathionine β-synthase deficiency, plasma and urinary levels of homocysteine increase and become detectable. In some genetic variants of homocystinurias, the metabolic abnormality can be corrected by administration of large doses of pyridoxine whereas the others are not correctable. Increased levels of homocysteine interferes with normal cross linking of collagen and this may be a likely mechanism for the production of the ocular and skeletal abnormalities. Excess homocysteine reacts with cysteine residues thereby disrupting the structure and function of fibrillin-1, the main component of the lens zonules (suspensory ligaments). Four vitamins: (1) Folic acid, (2) Vitamin B_{12}, (3) Vitamin B_6 and (4) Vitamin B_2, are involved in the intermediate metabolism of homocysteine.

Pathological homocystinuria is characterized by disruption of the zonular fibers of the lens, osteoporosis and thromboembolism affecting arteries and veins.

Causes of Hyperhomocysteinemia

- Genetic enzyme defects in homocysteine metabolism.
- Nutritional deficiencies of vitamin cofactors, e.g. folate, vitamins B_{12} and B_6.
- Diseases—pernicious anemia, hypothyroidism, renal failure, malignancies such as acute lymphatic leukemia, breast cancer and severe psoriasis.
- Drugs—folate antagonists such as methotrexate, phenytoin and carbamazepine vitamin B_6 antagonists such as theophylline, tobacco smoke.
- Elderly age.

Measurement of plasma homocysteine is done by high performance liquid chromatography (HPLC).

The patient should fast for at least 12 hours to avoid variations caused by the meal. In chronic renal disease, hyperhomocysteinemia occurs. This acts as an independent risk factor for cardio vascular complications.

Hyperhomocysteinemia leads to a prothrombotic state by the following mechanisms:

- Increases platelet aggregation
- Activates factors V, X and XII
- Inhibits protein C.

In addition, hyperhomocysteinemia is a strong independent risk factor for osteoporotic fractures in elderly men and women. The exact mechanism is not clear, possibly, homocysteine-related collagen cross-linking in bone may be responsible.

Clinical Features

In some of the western societies, hyperhomocysteinemia is reported to be around 5%. Vitamin B_{12} deficiency leading to hyperhomocysteinemia, venous thrombosis and pulmonary embolism has been reported from India. Higher prevalence (13–47%) has been reported among groups of patients having symptomatic atherothrombotic disease. Genetically determined type is characterized by marfanoid body features, subluxation of the lens and mental retardation. Vascular thrombotic episodes are more frequent.

Acquired hyperhomocysteinemia has assumed great epidemiological importance on account of its association with coronary, cerebral and other vascular thrombotic episodes.

Pyridoxine responsive patients have milder forms of the disease compared to pyridoxine nonresponders. Bony abnormalities include osteoporosis of the spine and long bones, scoliosis, marfanoid features, pectus excavatum and pectus carinatum. Some children may develop mental retardation and seizures.

The characteristic feature is premature vascular disease. If the condition remains untreated, 20% die before 30 years of age. The homocysteine levels show relationship with coronary artery disease (CAD), peripheral artery disease, stroke or venous thrombosis. The vascular damage is mediated by oxidative injury to the endothelium. The embolic complications predominate over atherosclerotic complications.

Diagnosis is suggested by presence of homocysteine in urine detected by cyanide-nitroprusside reaction which is a simple way of detecting increased amounts of sulfhydryl compounds. This test is not specific.

Management

Several attempts are being made to reduce the risk of vaso-occlusive diseases by lowering plasma homocysteine levels by dietary supplementation with folic acid, 400 µg/day, vitamin B_{12}, 100 µg/day and vitamin B_6, 25 mg/day. Several studies are at present looking into the effect of this vitamin supplementation on the risk of atherogenesis and stroke in the young.

In genetic homocystinuria, dietary restriction of methionine and oral supplementation of folate and pyridoxine are beneficial. Cysteine and betaine are found to lower plasma homocysteine levels.

Food articles such as egg, milk and meat are rich in methionine and these should be avoided.

Low methionine dietary formulas are available for treating affected children.

Source: Dani SI, Thanvi S, Shah JM, et al. Hyperhomocysteinemia masquerading as pulmonary embolism. J Assoc Physicians India. 2003;51:914-5.

CHAPTER

96

Endocrinology: General Considerations

KP Poulose, B Jayakumar

Chapter Summary

- General Considerations
- Hormone Metabolism
- Hormone Actions
- Genetics and Endocrinology
- Clinical Aspects of Endocrine Disorders
- Types of Hormones and their Patterns of Secretion

GENERAL CONSIDERATIONS

Endocrinology continues to be a lead science. Many Nobel prizes have recognized the contributions of endocrinologists. The cloned gene products to reach the clinical pharmaceutical market were endocrine substances. Many advances in our understanding of cellular transduction systems, receptor binding and physiologic regulation are the results of studies conducted in endocrine laboratories. Why is this so? A likely answer is found by understanding that endocrinologists study the actions of specific chemicals that cause cells to undergo specific and (usually) easily quantifiable and regulated responses. These are very simple, basic and well-defined processes.

An estimated 108 million people in India suffer from endocrine and metabolic disorders, with the poor mainly bearing the brunt of the disease. Clinical endocrinology is a specialized branch of internal medicine. The discovery of immunoassay technology which permitted reliable measurement of picomolar or femtomolar concentrations of hormones in body fluids led to phenomenal growth of this specialty during the past four decades.

Introduction of investigative procedures like, ultrasound abdomen, computed tomography (CT), magnetic resonance imaging (MRI), positron emission tomography (PET), radioimmunoassay (RIA), immunoradiometric assay (IRMA), immunofluorescent assay (IFA) and enzyme linked immunosorbent assay (ELISA) techniques have revolutionized the diagnosis and treatment of endocrine diseases.

Personal Experience of the First Author

Barring diabetes mellitus (DM), thyroid diseases is the most common endocrine disease in my experience for the last 50 years. Ninety percent of endocrine diseases are either related to DM or thyroid. Adrenal diseases, pituitary diseases, gonadal problems like precocious puberty, hermaphroditism and hormone resistance syndromes belong to the remaining group.

Hyperfunction of the pituitary gland is more common than hypopituitarism.

Among the thyroid problems, hypothyroidism is about 10 times more common than hyperthyroidism; autoimmune thyroiditis is the most common cause for hypothyroidism in adolescents and adults. Iodine deficiency disorders are very rare in the community now. The prevalence of thyroid antibodies like thyroid peroxidase (TPO) and antithyroglobulin (anti-Tg) are very high in Kerala (around 80%). Twenty-nine percent of pregnant patients have thyroid auotantibodies and placental transfer of these antibodies from the mother to the child is also well-established (75%). Subclinical hypothyroidism is about five times more common than overt hypothyroidism. Screening for thyroid antibodies is must in pregnant women besides assessment of thyroid function. Neonatal screening of the babies born to mothers with autoimmune hypothyroidism is absolutely necessary. Screening includes TPO and anti-Tg antibodies besides thyroid-stimulating hormone (TSH). Some thyroid-related complications like ophthalmopathy and dermopathy have no curative medical treatment.

Papillary thyroid carcinoma is also associated with autoimmune thyroiditis. The high thyroid antibody prevalence could be due to excess dietary iodine (iodized salt consumption) as reported from other countries like China. This hypothesis needs further substantiation by prospective studies.

Other than thyroid carcinoma, malignancy of other endocrine organs is rare. Congenital adrenal hyperplasia (CAH), multiple endocrine neoplasia (MEN) syndrome, autoimmune polyendocrinopathy (hypofunction of multiple endocrine organs) are rarely encountered in our practice. Rare manifestations like scleredema (not sclerodema) involving the back of the neck and chest may be an indicator or forerunner of type 2 DM, occurring only in less than 1% of type 2 DM patients.

Source: Personal Communication and Consensus Statement Book of the API Kerala Chapter; published and edited by KP Poulose and Sajith Kumar.

Approximately 10% of the population in India suffers from endocrine/metabolic diseases other than DM and the proportion of various endocrine/metabolic diseases is given as follows:

Goiter	54%
Diabetes mellitus	20%
Hormone-related reproductive disorders	10%
Adrenal/pituitary disorders	4%
Nutritional/metabolic disorders	10%

Endocrine diseases account for 7–10% of patients admitted in hospitals. The prevalence varies from states to states as well as cities and villages.

PHYSIOLOGY

Endocrine system consists of specialized tissue organized in different anatomical sites in the form of glands such as thyroid and adrenals or distributed diffusely as identifiable cells in various organ systems, such as the gut, brain, kidneys, lungs and others. The latter are called *paracrine cells*. Hormones secreted by the former group reach the circulation directly since these glands are devoid of ducts. Their main action is at distant sites, and many have generalized systemic effects in addition to specific effects on the target tissues, e.g.

- Thyroid hormone stimulates general metabolism, growth and maturation.
- Glucocorticoids act as stress hormones, take part in several immunological functions and also influence the blood sugar level.

Effects of hormones on target tissue are mediated through the action on specific receptors which modulate cellular processes, often through the medium of several chemical messengers.

Hormones from the paracrine cells diffuse out and their action is mainly on the neighboring cells, but they can also have distant effects. The paracrine tissue consists of amine precursor uptake and decarboxylase (APUD) cells. Some of the hormones produced by this system are listed below:

- *Gut:* Gastrin, cholecystokinin (CCK), vasoactive intestinal peptide (VIP), motilin, bombesin, substance P and others.
- *Kidneys:* 1,25-dihydroxycholecalciferol, erythropoietin, renin, prostaglandins (PGA and PGE), kallikrein, insulin-like growth factors (IGF) and others.
- *Lungs:* Dopamine, substance P, prostaglandins, thromboxanes, adrenocorticotropic hormone (ACTH), parathyroid-hormone (PTH), antidiuretic hormone (ADH), melanocyte-stimulating hormone (MSH) and others.

Other hormones such as inhibin, ghrelin and leptin are newly discovered, they also becomes integrated into the science and practice of medicine on the basis of their functional roles rather than their tissues of origin; leptin acts centrally to control appetite.

Hormones can be divided into five major classes:

1. Amino acid derivatives such as dopamine, catecholamine and thyroid hormone.
2. Small neuropeptides such as gonadotropin-releasing hormone (GnRH), thyrotropin-releasing hormone (TRH), somatostatin and vasopressin.
3. Large proteins such as insulin, luteinizing hormone (LH) and PTH produced by classic endocrine glands.
4. Steroid hormones such as cortisol and estrogen that are synthesized from cholesterol-based precursors.
5. Vitamin derivatives such as retinoids (vitamin A) and vitamin D.

A variety of peptide growth factors, most of which act locally, share actions with hormones. As a rule, amino acid derivatives and peptide hormones interact with cell surface membrane receptors. Steroids, thyroid hormones, vitamin D, and retinoids are lipid-soluble and interact with intracellular nuclear receptors.

Functions of the endocrine system may be considered under the following headings:

- Maintenance of cellular constancy of the body
- Maintenance of the constancy of body fluids (micro-homeostasis)
- Control of metabolic processes
- Growth and differentiation of tissues
- Reproduction
- Adaptation to changes in the external environment (fluid, food and electrolyte availability).

Hormones or chemical messengers which are secreted by endocrine cells are released into circulation in response to specific signals. Endocrine dysfunction may manifest as overt clinical disorders such as Cushing's syndrome and acromegaly or silent biochemical abnormalities like hyperglycemia or failure of control mechanisms as in gonadal disturbances.

Biological responses are also under control of other substances such as the neurotransmitters like cate-cholamines and acetylcholine, prostaglandins, histamine, kinins, cytokines and several others. Intracellular chemicals like cyclic 3',5'-adenosine monophosphate (cyclic AMP), cyclic 3',5'-guanosine monophosphate (cyclic GMP) and calcium act as second messengers for exerting the biological activity of hormones on cells.

Developmentally, origin of the endocrine system can be traced back to all the three germ layers. The endocrine glands can be broadly grouped into:

- *The pituitary-thyroid-gonadal-adrenal axis (classical endocrine system).* These glands act in unison through feedback control and modulate biological activity of distant target cells and organs.
- *The neuroendocrine system derived from neuro-ectoderm:* This is composed of neurosecretory cells. The central component of this system is formed by the brain-pituitary system and the peripheral component is made up of diffusely scattered paracrine cells in many organs. The paracrine system is seen mainly in the gastrointestinal tract (GIT), adrenal medulla and the C cells of thyroid. These paracrine cells are APUD cells which are necessary for the formation of amine or peptide hormones.
- *Several tissues produce humoral substances which circulate along with the known hormones, e.g. prostaglandins and kinins:* These exert strong physiological responses and tend to modulate hormone effects.

HORMONE METABOLISM

Synthesis, storage, release and transport to the site of action are the processes undergone before a hormone activates its target. After exerting their effects, the hormones are metabolized to inactive products or they are continually excreted. The concentration of a hormone in blood is governed by its rate of synthesis, release, metabolism and elimination. Many hormones function in closed loop systems, i.e. rise in level of the hormone in the blood exerts feedback inhibition on its controlling hormone. Many endocrine glands exhibit diurnal rhythmicity (sleep-wake cycle), pulsatility with regular periodicity and regulation of secretion in response to substrate augmentation. Hormones like steroid hormones and thyroid hormones are bound to carrier proteins of high affinity for transport. The hormone is biologically inactive in the bound form and it has to be split to restore its activity.

HORMONE ACTIONS

Hormones modulate both the intracellular and extracellular activities of cells so that the different cells in an organ or tissue behave as a synchronous macrocellular complex. As a general rule, hormones do not initiate biochemical processes primarily, but they only regulate the rate of the reactions in responsive cells. Hormones produce measurable specific effect in organs, cells, cellular organelles, enzymes, genes or membranes. The specificity of hormone response is achieved by three mechanisms such as (1) specific target tissue, (2) appropriate receptor stimulation, and (3) the capacity of the cells to respond specifically to receptor activation. Hormone effects are generally brought about by conformational changes in protein molecules of the receptors or enzymes in the target cell. The receptors show increase and decrease in number (up regulation and down regulation) and alteration in their sensitivity to the hormone. Alteration in number and the sensitivity of the receptor also grossly influences the final result produced by the hormone. In type 2 diabetes, the basic abnormality is the resistance of the receptors to secreted insulin. Modification of receptor function to increase the sensitivity to insulin by drugs brings about relief. The hormonal effects often lead to acceleration of some biochemical reactions or metabolic pathways with inhibition of others.

One of the main functions of the endocrine system is communication of information between cells. Polypeptide hormones and catecholamines act on the cell surface through specific receptors and activate intracellular second messengers like cyclic AMP, calcium or enzymes. These in turn regulate the activities of the cell. Peptide hormones bring about rapid responses in tissues within seconds or minutes.

Steroid hormones exert their action within the cell by influencing specific receptors which bind to nuclear chromatin. The hormone receptor complex regulates protein synthesis. Thyroid hormones enter the target cells and bind directly to receptor proteins in the chromatin. Such interactions which affect nuclear processes are relatively slow, taking a few hours at times.

Hormone Receptors

The responsive cells contain specific sites of binding of active hormones. The hormones bring about their effect or response in target cells through the receptors. The binding to receptors takes place very quickly. Changes in receptor affinity or number also modify the magnitude of hormone responses. The biological effects of a hormone depend on:

- Its affinity for receptors
- Intrinsic agonist property
- Its concentration at the site of action
- Its rate of degradation.

The number of hormone receptors on a cell far exceeds that required for bringing about a response. When 5–10% of available binding sites on the cells are occupied, the hormones exert their maximal effect. The remaining number act as spare receptors. Receptors have strict structural specificity, saturability, high affinity and often tissue specificity for target cell responsiveness. The surface receptors are regulated by metabolites such as cyclic GMP within the cell. At times, the receptors may become antigenic and stimulate the production of antibodies. These antibodies react with the receptors and interfere with their functions.

Hormone agonists (optimal inducers) are substances which directly stimulate hormone action by stabilization of hormone-receptor complex in an active conformational state. Hormone antagonists (anti-inducers) specifically block the effect of an agonist by binding with hormone receptors.

Endocrine disorders result from excessive or diminished secretion of hormones, or abnormalities in responsiveness of tissues. Progressive rise in hormone levels may reduce tissue sensitivity (negative cooperativity).

GENETICS AND ENDOCRINOLOGY

Genetic components contribute to virtually all disorders. Many chromosomal and monogenic disorders can now be explained at the molecular level, permitting us to establish the diagnosis by mutational analysis (Tables 96.1 and 96.2). It is important to recognize that genetic and environmental modifiers may also strongly influence the phenotype in monogenic disorders, which simply present the least complex form in a continuum of complex disorders. For example, siblings with identical mutations in the transcription factor PROP1, which lead to combined pituitary hormone deficiency (CPHD), may have variable constellations of anterior pituitary hormone deficiencies, and the onset of hormonal defects may differ. In phenylketonuria, development of neurologic defects is dependent on the amount of phenylalanine in the diet. In complex disorders, also referred to as polygenic or multifactorial disorders, several or multiple genes contribute to the pathogenesis, typically in conjunction with environmental and lifestyle factors such as in DM type 2.

The information about the human genome sequence through the Human Genome Project (HGP) is facilitating genetic analyses substantially, and the ongoing advances in the functional characterization of the human genome, transcriptome, and proteome are fundamentally changing our understanding of the molecular mechanisms underlying pathophysiologic processes. Ongoing efforts such as the haplotype map (HapMap) project will facilitate

Table 96.1: Chromosomal disorders with endocrine manifestations

Disorder	Phenotype	Chromosomal defects
Turner's syndrome	Ovarian failure, short stature, autoimmune thyroid disease	45, XO
Klinefelter's syndrome	Hypogonadism, tall stature	47, XXY
Prader-Willi syndrome	Short stature, obesity, hypogonadism	Del 15q11-13 (paternal copy) maternal uniparental disomy

Table 96.2: Molecular basis of selected endocrine disorders

Disorder/Phenotype	Gene	Inheritance
Hypothalamic and pituitary disorders		
CPHD (GH, PRL, TSH, LH, FSH)	PROP1	AR
Short stature	GH	AR, AD
Neurohypophyseal DI	AVP-NPH	AD, AR
Obesity	Leptin receptor	AR
Thyroid		
Congenital hypothyroidism with thyroid hypoplasia	PAX8	AD
Bamforth–Lazarus syndrome: Congenital hypothyroidism, cleft palate, spiky hair	TTF2 (FOXE1)	AR
Pendred syndrome: Sensorineural deafness, impaired iodide organification	PDS (SLC26A4)	AR
Congenital hypothyroidism, thyroglobulin defects	TG	AR
Resistance to thyroid hormone	THRB	AD, AR
Parathyroid and bone disorders		
Familial benign hypocalciuric hypercalcemia	CaSR	AD
Familial hypoparathyroidism	CaSR	AD
Albright hereditary osteodystrophy	GNAS1	AD
Adrenal gland		
CAH, 21-hydroxlyase	CYP21	AR
Glucocorticoid-remediable aldosteronism	CYP11B2-CYP11B1 fusion gene	AD
Adrenal hypoplasia, congenital hypogonadism	DAX1 (NROB1)	X
Pancreas		
MODY 1	HNF4α	AD
MODY 2	GCK	AD (inactivating mutations)
MODY 3	HNF1α	AD
MODY 4, renal cysts	IPF1	AD
MODY 5	HNF1β	AD
MODY 6	NEUROD1	AD
Pancreas agenesis	IPF1	AR
Gonads		
Androgen insensitivity, androgen-receptor inactivation	AR	AR
Androgen insensitivity, five-reductase deficiency	SRD5A2	AR
Aromatase deficiency, female genitalia with masculinization during puberty	CYP19A1	AR
Water and salt metabolism		
Nephrogenic DI (X-linked form)	AVPR2	X
Nephrogenic DI	AQP2	AR, AD
Liddle syndrome: Hypokalemic metabolic acidosis, hypertension	SCNN1B or SCNN1G	AD
Lipid metabolism		
Obesity	LEP	Leptin
Familial hypercholesterolemia	LDLR	AD
Tumor syndrome		
MEN1	MEN1	AD
Parathyroid adenoma, pituitary adenoma, pancreas tumors	RET	AD
MEN2		AD
• Medullary thyroid cancer, pheochromocytoma, parathyroid hyperplasia		
• + Ganglioneuromas, Von Hippel-Lindau disease (VHL)	VHL	
Renal carcinomas, pheochromocytomas, other tumors		
Somatic mosaicism		
McCuneâ Albright syndrome (precocious puberty, fibrous dysplasia, cafe-au-lait spots, hyperthyroidism)	GNAS1	Mosaic somatic mutation acquired in early development

Contd...

Complex syndromes		
Autoimmune polyglandular syndrome type 1: Adrenal insufficiency, hypoparathyroidism, candidiasis	AIRE	AR
DM type 1 and type 2 also have several genetic abnormalities		

Note: This list contains only selected examples. In addition, the reader should be aware that the same or similar phenotype can be caused by mutations in other genes.

Source: Modified from Kopp P. Genetics, genomics, proteomics, and bioinformatics. In: Brook GD, Brown R (eds). Clinical Pediatric Endocrinology, 5th edition. Blackwell Science: Oxford; 2005. pp. 18-44.

Abbreviations: AD = Autosomal dominant; AR = Autosomal recessive; X = X-chromosomal; CPHD = Combined pituitary hormone deficiency; PRL = Prolactin; DI = Diabetes insipidus; MODY = Maturity onset diabetes; MEN1 = Multiple endocrine neoplasia1; DM = Diabetes mellitus; CAH = Congenital adrenal hyperplasia; PROP1 = PROPHET OF PIT1; GH = Growth hormone; AVP-NPH = Arginine-vasopressin-neurophysin; TTF2 (FOXE1) = Thyroid transcription factor 2 (Forkheadbox E1); PAX8 = Paired box gene 8; PDS = Pendred syndrome; TG = Thyroglobulin; THRB = Thyroid hormone receptor beta; CaSR = Calcium-sensing receptor; IPF1 = Insulin promoter factor 1; HNF1β = Hepatic nuclear factor 1 beta; SRD5A2 = Steroid-5-alpha-reductase type 2; AQP2 = Aquaporin 2 gene; AVPR2 = Arginine vasopressin V2 receptor gene; RET = Rearranged during transfection

the understanding of complex disorders. The HapMap project has determined single-nucleotide polymorphisms (SNPs), variants that occur on average every 300 base pairs throughout the genome in deoxyribonucleic acid (DNA) samples from multiple individuals from four different ethnic backgrounds.

Because somatic mutations in genes controlling cell growth, survival and differentiation are key elements in the pathogenesis of neoplasia, benign and malignant tumors can also be viewed as genetic disorders. The MEN1 and MEN2 are excellent examples to illustrate this (Table 96.2). MEN2 also highlights the impact of genetic analysis for carrier detection in the clinical management of families with this tumor syndrome. A thorough understanding of the molecular pathogenesis of cancer also is of paramount importance for the development of novel therapeutic modalities. The mutations in the tyrosine kinase rearranged during transfection (RET) causing MEN or the serine/threonine kinase B-Raf found frequently in papillary thyroid cancers, make them attractive targets for therapy with kinase inhibitors.

ETIOLOGY

Mutations in DNA cause alterations and abnormal function in the encoded ribonucleic acid (RNA) and protein products, thereby leading to disease. Mutations can occur randomly or through factors such as radiation and chemicals. Somatic mutations conferring a growth advantage to cells, or a decrease in apoptosis, can be associated with neoplasia.

Structurally, mutations are extremely diverse. They can involve the entire genome, as in triploidy, or gross numeric or structural alterations in chromosomes or individual genes. Large deletions may affect a part of a gene, an entire gene or several genes (contiguous gene syndrome).

PATHOPHYSIOLOGY

Very broadly, endocrine disorders can be categorized into four major types of conditions:
1. Hormone excess
2. Hormone deficiency
3. Hormone resistance
4. Tumors of endocrine glands without alterations of hormone secretion.

Numerous conditions in these categories have recently been explained by mutations in genes involved in growth or function of endocrine tissues, thereby leading to a better understanding of the pathophysiology at the molecular level, and often providing a means for accurate diagnosis.

DIAGNOSIS

Approach to the Patient

It cannot be emphasized enough that a careful clinical examination with thorough phenotyping, using appropriate biochemical and ancillary tests, is absolutely essential. One should always be aware of the possibility of phenocopies, i.e. a phenotype that is identical or similar to the suspected disorder, but that has a distinct genetic or nongenetic pathogenesis. The family history is of great importance for the recognition of a hereditary component. The history, in combination with the pedigree, may become of practical relevance for genetic counseling, carrier detection, quantitative risk estimation for individuals within the kindred, or early intervention and prevention of a disease in relatives of the index patient(s). The ethnic background is relevant because certain alleles are more common in certain populations.

When evaluating relatives of an index patient with a genetic disorder, the phenomena of variable expressivity and incomplete penetrance should always be considered. Incomplete penetrance is characterized by a disease phenotype skipping generations, with unaffected carriers transmitting the mutant gene. Expressivity describes the degree to which a phenotype is expressed, the phenotypic spectrum. The mechanisms resulting in variable expressivity and incomplete penetrance include the need for modifiers such as genetic background, gender, and environmental factors, emphasizing again that these factors play a prominent role not only in complex disorders, but also in Mendelian traits. This is well-illustrated by mutations in the androgen receptor; mild mutations may cause epispadias, whereas severe inactivation of the receptor results in complete resistance to testosterone with testicular feminization.

CLINICAL ASPECTS OF ENDOCRINE DISORDERS

Symptomatology

Endocrine disorders may manifest with dysfunction of the gland at fault or secondary disturbances in other endocrine glands. Sometimes the presenting symptom may be a remote effect due to defective regulation of a metabolic process, e.g. secondary amenorrhea in hypopituitarism or Cushing's syndrome. The structural changes in the endocrine glands do not always correlate with the severity of dysfunction. For example, gross functional defects may result from microadenomas of the pituitary whereas large tumors may remain silent.

- **Abnormalities of growth:** The rate of growth may be altered in physiological (e.g. puberty) or pathological conditions. Heredity and environmental factors playing a major role in determining growth are common in endocrine disorders. Growth is brought about by increase in number and size of body cells. When considering disorders of growth, rate of growth is a more reliable parameter, than the actual size of an individual. The maturation of organs and systems in the body constitutes development.
  - **Endocrine dwarfism:** It may be accompanied by abnormalities of sexual characteristics, e.g. hypothyroidism, hypopituitarism, gonadal dysgenesis (XO), pseudohypoparathyroidism and adrenogenital syndrome. Hypothalamic syndromes and Cushing's syndrome are causes of impaired growth. Disparity between age and height, disparity in bone age, alteration of skeletal proportions and disorder in sexual development are features which suggest endocrine etiology. Endocrine causes of dwarfism have to be differentiated from constitutional dwarfism, primary bone diseases, malnutrition, metabolic disorders and severe systemic diseases like renal and hepatic failure.
  - **Excessive height:** It may result from accelerated GH activity or abnormalities of adrenal, ovarian or testicular hormones. Pituitary disorders cause gigantism or acromegaly. Hypogonadism causes abnormal increase in height and is associated with eunuchoidism (arm span considerably greater than height and lower segment longer than upper segment). Disorders like Marfan's syndrome and homocystinuria cause abnormally tall stature with other associated congenital abnormalities. Though gigantism is commonly the result of excessive GH activity occurring in young age, rarely it may be secondary to other cerebral disorders as well.
- **Obesity:** Increase in weight by 10% or more above the ideal weight caused by excessive accumulation of fat is called obesity. Endocrine causes include Cushing's syndrome, hypothalamic syndromes, insulinomas, hypothyroidism, polycystic ovarian syndrome (PCOS) and familial hyperlipidemia (type VI). Obesity is associated with delayed puberty in children. It is now known that many cases of apparently dietary obesity in young persons may have abnormalities of adrenocortical function.

- **Polyphagia:** Polyphagia or increased appetite is a common feature of DM and hyperthyroidism and it is accompanied by loss of weight. Polyphagia leading to gain in weight is seen in acromegaly and insulinomas. Hypothalamic disorders like craniopharyngioma and Laurence-Moon-Biedl syndrome may give rise to polyphagia, galactorrhea, hypogonadism and somnolence.
- **Loss of weight:** Significant weight loss (> 5 to 6%) in spite of increased intake of food is suggestive of DM, thyrotoxicosis and pheochromocytoma. Loss of weight is accompanied by loss of appetite in disorders like Addison's disease, panhypopituitarism, anorexia nervosa and psychiatric illnesses.
- **Nonspecific symptoms:** Like anorexia, nausea, vomiting and diarrhea with considerable weight loss may be the features of metabolic disturbances occurring in diabetic ketoacidosis, adrenal crisis, thyroid storm or hypercalcemia.
  - **Fatigue and weakness:** These are the presenting symptoms in DM, Addison's disease, hypothyroidism, hypopituitarism, hyperthyroidism, Cushing's syndrome, hyperparathyroidism and hypogonadism.
- **Polyuria:** Polyuria of more than 3 L/day of recent onset should suggest DM, diabetes insipidus (DI) or hypercalcemia. Other rare endocrine causes include primary hyperaldosteronism and hypokalemic nephropathy. Polyuria is generally accompanied by polydipsia. Psychogenic polydipsia has to be distinguished from a primary endocrine abnormality.
- **Skin changes:** Several endocrine disorders lead to characteristic abnormalities of the skin and mucous membranes. In many cases, these precede other features of endocrinopathies. Hyperpigmentation affecting skin folds, pressure points, and oral mucous membranes and gums is seen in Addison's disease. Cushing's syndrome is accompanied by increased pigmentation. Pregnancy, thyrotoxicosis, and use of oral contraceptives lead to spotty brown pigmentation over the face (chloasma). *Acanthosis nigricans* which appears as velvety hyperpigmented thickened plaques in the flexural areas and nape of the neck occurs in Cushing's syndrome and juvenile myxedema.
  - **Vitiligo (hypopigmentation of the skin)** may occur in many endocrine disorders like Addison's disease, hypothyroidism and hypopituitarism which have an autoimmune basis. Vitiligo may be localized or generalized.
  - **Pallor** of the skin may occur in hypothyroidism or myxedema. Panhypopituitarism also leads to hypodepigmentation and loss of hair and the skin does not tan on exposure to sunlight.
- **Abnormalities of hair:** Hirsutism is excessive hair growth in women and children occurring over the androgen sensitive areas such as face, axilla and pubis. Hirsutism may be primary (idiopathic) or secondary to endocrine disorders. Growth of hair is determined by genetic, endocrine and other factors. Hirsutism commonly occurs in women at puberty,

Textbook of Medicine

pregnancy or menopause. In hyperandrogenism, it is an early symptom. In such cases, it may be accompanied by other features like virilism in which there is change of voice, clitoromegaly, baldness and malodorous perspiration. Secondary hirsutism occurs in hyperfunction of the adrenal cortex, polycystic ovaries (Stein-Leventhal syndrome), testicular and ovarian tumors, and bronchogenic carcinoma with endocrine manifestation. Therapy with glucocorticoids and other drugs such as phenytoin and diazoxide also give rise to hirsutism.

- ● ***Loss of hair (alopecia):*** Androgenic tumors and hyperfunction of the adrenal cortex give rise to frontal baldness. Generalized loss of hair over the head and eyebrows is suggestive of myxedema. Hypopituitarism and hypogonadism are accompanied by absence or loss of facial, axillary, and pubic hair. Many nonendocrine disorders like cirrhosis of liver and malnutrition are also characterized by loss of hair.

For descriptions of alopecia *See* Section 18, Ch 230.

- ■ ***Gynecomastia:*** Benign glandular enlargement of male breast is called gynecomastia. The glandular tissue is hypertrophied in true gynecomastia. Accumulation of fat in the region of the breasts is called pseudogynecomastia. Bilateral breast enlargement (usually painless, at times tender) occurs physiologically during adolescence. Pathologically gynecomastia occurs in testicular disorders like dysgenesis, atrophy and tumors, systemic diseases associated with disturbances of gonadal hormones (e.g. hepatic failure) and as adverse side effects of drugs like estrogens, spironolactone, digitalis, reserpine phenothiazines, cimetidine, ketoconazole, busulfan and several others. In most instances, gynecomastia recedes when the cause is removed, but sometimes it tends to persist.

- ■ ***Galactorrhea:*** This refers to a condition where there is abnormal (unphysiological) secretion of milk. Normal secretion of milk occurs only during lactation and pregnancy. Galactorrhea is a common finding which may not be disclosed by the patient and, therefore, this has to be specifically looked for. Newborn infants may show galactorrhea at times (witch's milk). Hyperprolactinemia, acromegaly, thyroid disorders (hypothyroidism and rarely thyrotoxicosis), feminizing adrenal tumors, corpus luteum cysts, and rarely choriocarcinoma may present with galactorrhea. Drugs like phenothiazines, metoclopramide, digoxin and many others may give rise to galactorrhea.

- ■ ***Disorders of sexual maturation:*** Normally boys attain sexual maturity before the age of 18 years and girls do so before the age of 16.

- ■ ***Precocious puberty:*** Sexual maturation before the age of 8 years constitutes precocious puberty. Though rarely this may be a familial trait, more often it is due to some serious organic disease. Hypothalamic disturbances, congenital virilizing adrenal hyperplasia, adrenal tumors and gonadal neoplasms are commonly associated with sexual precocity. Androgen therapy gives rise to sexual precocity in boys. Juvenile hypothyroidism in boys may be associated with pituitary enlargement and sexual precocity. Precocious puberty leads to premature fusion of the epiphyses and this results in dwarfism.

- ■ ***Delayed puberty (infantilism):*** When there is failure to attain sexual development by the age of 18 years in boys and 16 years in girls, it is delayed puberty. Though it may be a familial trait in some, often it is a manifestation of genetic or gonadal disturbances. In India, nonendocrine causes like malnutrition or undernutrition are also responsible for delayed puberty. Hypothalamic lesions, pituitary lesions and gonadal dysgenesis (Klinefelter's syndrome) are common causes of infantilism in boys. Failure to attain puberty by the age of 18 years is seen in girls with gonadal dysgenesis (Turner's syndrome), pituitary and hypothalamic disease and PCOS. Rare causes include congenital absence of uterus and vagina and pseudohermaphroditism.

- ■ ***Disturbances of sexual function:*** Impotence is the inability to get penile erection sufficient to perform the sexual act. Proper penile erection is a complex process requiring vascular, neural and endocrine mechanisms. The sex drive is termed libido. Impotence and loss of libido are commonly caused by psychogenic factors, but endocrine disturbances like testicular atrophy, Addison's disease, thyrotoxicosis and feminizing tumors of the adrenal cortex may be associated with this symptom. Autonomic neuropathy occurring in DM, chronic alcoholism, central nervous system lesions and therapy with several drugs are other common causes of impotence.

- ■ ***Skeletal manifestations:*** Several endocrine disorders give rise to changes in bones which may be the presenting manifestations. The predominant manifestations of metabolic bone disorders are bone pains and muscular weakness. When patients present with bone pains, bone cysts, pathological fractures, bony deformities or X-ray evidence of bony abnormalities, hyperparathyroidism, osteomalacia, rickets and osteoporosis should be looked for. Cushing's syndrome and hyperthyroidism may occasionally manifest with severe osteoporosis. The appearance of ossification centers and their fusion follow a strict chronological order if the nutrition is normal and the baby is healthy otherwise. Endocrine disorders can alter the appearance and fusion of the various ossification centers (Table 96.3).

- ■ ***Urinary calculi:*** Several metabolic disorders lead to recurrent stone formation in the kidneys or other parts of the urinary tract. Calcium stones are seen in hyperparathyroidism, hypervitaminosis-D and sarcoidosis. Idiopathic hypercalciuria is a common cause of recurrent calcium stones in male children. Metabolic abnormalities such as cystinuria, renal tubular acidosis, gout and oxaluria may all be associated with urolithiasis.

Textbook of Medicine

Table 96.3: The time of appearance of the ossification center and its fusion in normal subjects

Bone	Epiphyseal appearance	Fusion with diaphysis
Head of humerus	1st year	18–20th year
Medial epicondyle of humerus	4–6th year	18–20th year
Lower end of radius	End of 1st year	17–19th year
Lower end of ulna	5–6th year	17–19th year
Head of femur	1st year	14–17th year
Lower end of femur	Before delivery	20th year
Patella	Before 2–6 year	Puberty
Lower end of tibia and fibula	1st year	17th year

Box 96.1: Endocrine symptoms

- Abnormalities of growth
- Obesity
- Polyphagia
- Polyuria
- Polydipsia
- Weight loss
- Skeletal manifestations
- Urinary calculi
- Tetany
- Psychiatric symptoms
- Fatigue and weakness
- Skin changes:
  - Hirsutism
  - Pallor
  - Vitiligo
  - Alopecia
- Gynecomastia
- Galactorrhea
- Disorders of sexual maturation

■ **Tetany:** It may occur classically in hypocalcemia and less commonly in hypomagnesemia. It is clinically characterized by carpopedal spasm, Chvostek's sign and Trousseau's sign. Tetany is commonly seen in hypoparathyroidism, pseudohypoparathyroidism, osteomalacia, rickets, alkalosis and acute pancreatitis. Tetany is rapidly correctable by intravenous administration of 10 mL of 10% calcium gluconate. Tetany unresponsive to the administration of calcium should suggest the possibility of hypomagnesemia.

■ **Psychiatric symptoms:** Psychiatric symptoms may be prominent in several endocrine disorders. Confusion, behavioral disturbances, somnolence or coma may develop in hypopituitarism, hypothyroidism, Addison's disease, water intoxication and hypercalcemia. Mental changes are also common in hyperthyroidism, Cushing's syndrome and hypoparathyroidism. In many cases, the higher functions return to normal when the endocrine disorder is controlled, but this need not be so in all cases.

The common endocrine symptoms are given in Box 96.1.

PHYSICAL EXAMINATION

The total clinical effect produced by an endocrine disturbance is determined by the age of onset, severity of hormone dysfunction, duration of the disorder, compensatory mechanisms, and behavior of the target organs. Several other factors like generic behavior, nutritional status, intercurrent illnesses and therapy modify the expression of symptoms. Familial incidence is seen in disorders like DM, thyroid disorders, pure gonadal dysgenesis, Kallmann's syndrome, Laurence-Moon-Biedl syndrome and multiple endocrine adenomatosis.

■ **Growth and development:** Disorders of growth are common in many endocrine disorders.

■ **Secondary sexual characters:** Disorders of sexual development may take the form of sexual precocity, heterosexual signs (appearance of features of the opposite sex), delayed puberty or regression of secondary sexual characters.

■ **Anthropometry:** In addition to height and weight, measurement of skeletal proportions is of great value in diagnosis. At birth, the ratio of the upper segment to the lower segment is 1.7:1 with the pubic symphysis taken as the reference point. The two segments become equal by the age of 10 years and this proportion is maintained throughout. The arm span equals the height in adults. The infantile proportion is retained in conditions such as juvenile hypothyroidism and chondrodystrophies which interfere with growth in early age. In hypopituitarism and other causes of generalized short stature, growth retardation is proportional and the ratio is maintained. The lower segment and arm span are disproportionately increased in eunuchoidism, because of delay in closure of the epiphyses.

■ **Cardiovascular abnormalities:** Various grades of hypertension may be present in pheochromocytoma, hyperaldosteronism and CAH. The hypertension may be paroxysmal as in the case of pheochromocytoma or persistent as in the others. Malignant hypertension occurring in young subjects should raise the possibility of an endocrine cause.

Orthostatic hypotension may be a prominent symptom in Addison's disease, hypopituitarism and diabetic neuropathy. It may also occur less commonly in pheochromocytoma. Cardiovascular manifestations may be prominent in thyrotoxicosis and myxedema.

■ **The integument:** The texture and pigmentation of the skin should be looked for. Black freckles and 'café au lait' (Fr. coffee with milk) spots are seen in gonadal dysgenesis, neurofibromatosis, and some types of sexual precocity. Hirsutism is common in virilizing conditions. Presence of acne is a sensitive index of excessive androgen activity.

■ **Breasts:** Careful examination of breasts for recent change in size, tenderness, pigmentation and galactorrhea is absolutely essential in all cases. Enlargement and hyperpigmentation of breasts occur in pregnancy, trophoblastic tumors, luteinizing tumors, Cushing's syndrome and estrogen therapy. Though the breasts are large in size in testicular feminization, the nipples and areola are immature. In Sheehan's syndrome, the areola may undergo depigmentation.

■ **Musculoskeletal system:** Several endocrine disorders give rise to characteristic abnormalities. Excessive muscle weakness, hypotonia and localized hypertrophy or atrophy are suggestive of diseases of the thyroid or adrenal cortex. In juvenile myxedema, hypertrophy of the calf muscle may be present in a few, e.g. **Hoffmann's syndrome**. **Adrenogenital syndrome** is characterized by hypertrophy of the muscles in children—**(Infant Hercules)**. Myopathy is characteristic of thyrotoxicosis.

- **Periodic paralysis** (episodes of paralysis mainly involving peripheral muscles lasting for a few minutes to hours) may occur in thyrotoxicosis, hyperaldosteronism and others.

- **Ocular manifestations:** Exophthalmos (abnormal protrusion of eyeball) and ophthalmoplegia may be present in thyrotoxicosis and pituitary tumors. Cataract occurring prematurely may point to DM or hypoparathyroidism. Visual field defects are common in space occupying lesions in the region of the pituitary and hypothalamus.

- **External genitalia:** State of development of the external genitalia gives an indication of the hormonal status in the early developmental period. Fusion of the labia and enlargement of the clitoris in female babies with or without formation of a penile urethra at birth, are indicative of excessive androgenic activity during early fetal development. Development of clitoromegaly is the result of androgen overactivity later in life. Pelvic examination is necessary for assessment of the size of the uterus and ovaries and vaginal development. Examination of vaginal epithelium and cervical mucus gives evidence of activity of the ovarian hormones.

  Defective development of the penis (less than 2.5 cm in length and flaccid) may be due to abnormalities of testosterone biosynthesis, organ unresponsiveness, gonadal dysgenesis, hypothalamo-pituitary disorders or rarely defective development.

Box 96.2: Clinical examination

- Growth and development
- Secondary sexual characters
- Anthropometry
- Cardiovascular abnormalities
- Skin changes
- Musculoskeletal system
- Ocular manifestation
- External genitalia

Testicular size is objectively assessed by measurement. Normal adult testis measures 5 cm in length and its volume is 15–25 mL. The testes are small and firm in Klinefelter's syndrome whereas they are small and soft in acquired testicular atrophy.

- **Bone age:** This is a common parameter used for assessing the maturity of the skeleton. Appearance of the centers of ossification and fusion of epiphyses occur regularly at definite periods during the growth of the individual. These are under hormonal control. Abnormalities in the growth of the skeleton provide evidence of endocrine dysfunction. Radiography of selected bones is routinely done for this purpose. In hypothyroidism occurring in early life, centers of ossification fail to appear. Cushing's syndrome, hypopituitarism and hypogonadism lead to delay in epiphyseal fusion. The epiphyses appear and fuse prematurely in hyperthyroidism and sexual precocity. Table 96.4 lists some nonspecific symptoms which may accompany endocrine disorders. Box 96.2 showing the salient points in clinical examination.

Table 96.4: Nonspecific symptoms which may accompany endocrine disorders

Abdominal pain	Addisonian crisis, diabetic ketoacidosis, hyperparathyroidism
Amenorrhea or oligomenorrhea	Adrenal insufficiency, adrenogenital syndrome, anorexia nervosa, Cushing's syndrome, hyperprolactinemic states, hypopituitarism, hypothyroidism, menopause, ovarian failure
Anemia	Adrenal insufficiency, hypothyroidism, hyperparathyroidism, panhypopituitarism
Anorexia	Addison's disease, diabetic ketoacidosis, hypercalcemia (e.g. hyperparathyroidism), hypothyroidism
Constipation	Diabetic neuropathy, hypercalcemia, hypothyroidism, pheochromocytoma
Depression	Adrenal insufficiency, Cushing's syndrome, hypercalcemic states, hypothyroidism
Diarrhea	Hyperthyroidism, metastatic carcinoid tumors, metastatic medullary thyroid carcinoma
Fever	Adrenal insufficiency, hyperthyroidism
Hair changes	Decreased body hair (hypothyroidism, hypopituitarism, thyrotoxicosis); hirsutism (androgen excess states, Cushing's syndrome, acromegaly)
Headache	Hypertensive episodes with pheochromocytoma, hypoglycemia, pituitary tumors
Hypothermia	Hypothyroidism
Libido changes	Adrenal insufficiency, Cushing's syndrome, hypercalcemia, hyperprolactinemia, hyperthyroidism, hypokalemia, hypopituitarism, hypothyroidism, poorly controlled DM
Nervousness	Cushing's syndrome, hyperthyroidism
Polyuria	DI, DM, hypercalcemia, hypokalemia
Skin changes	Acanthosis nigricans (obesity, insulin resistance, Cushing's syndrome, acromegaly), acne (androgen excess), hyperpigmentation (adrenal insufficiency, Nelson's syndrome), dry (hypothyroidism), hypopigmentation (panhypopituitarism), striae, plethora, bruising, ecchymoses (Cushing's syndrome), vitiligo (autoimmune thyroid disease, Addison's disease)
Weakness and fatigue	Addison's disease, Cushing's syndrome, DM, primary aldosteronism, hypothyroidism, hyperthyroidism, hypercalcemia (e.g. hyperparathyroidism, panhypopituitarism, pheochromocytoma)
Weight gain	Cushing's syndrome, hypothyroidism, insulinoma, pituitary tumors, type 2 DM
Weight loss	Adrenal insufficiency, anorexia nervosa, cancer of endocrine glands, hyperthyroidism, type 1 DM, panhypopituitarism, pheochromocytoma

Abbreviations: DM = Diabetes mellitus; DI = Diabetes insipidus

LABORATORY INVESTIGATIONS

The function of any endocrine gland can be assessed by:

- Quantitative estimation of its hormones and their metabolites
- Biochemical tests which reflect the metabolic abnormality, e.g. blood glucose in DM, serum calcium in parathyroid disorders
- Imaging procedures which reveal the morphology and function of the endocrine glands and other tissues
- Assessment of the functional reserve of the glands by appropriate stimulation and suppression tests.

Estimation of Hormones and their Metabolites in Body Fluids

The levels of hormones in blood and body fluids are very low. Nonpeptide hormones are present in body fluids in microgram (10^{-6} g) concentration whereas peptide hormones are present only in the range of nanogram (10^{-9} g) or picograms (10^{-12} g) per unit volume. Several techniques are used for their estimation. These are:

- Bioassay
- Spectrophotometric and fluorometric assay
- RIA (radioimmunoassay)
- ELISA (enzyme-linked immunosorbent assay)
- Chemiluminescent assay.

Adrenal steroids like plasma cortisol and its metabolites—17-ketosteroids, 17-ketogenic steroids and 17-hydroxysteroids are estimated by spectrophotometric analysis.

RIA which has revolutionized the diagnosis and management of endocrine diseases is the most extensively used method for quantitation of hormones in clinical practice. By this method almost all hormones which exist even at picogram levels can be estimated. This method was devised by Berson and Yallow in 1959 and they were awarded the Nobel Prize in medicine in 1977.

ELISA is used instead of RIA in many cases. Though ELISA has some advantages over RIA, so far ELISA has not been able to achieve the type of exquisite sensitivity required for measuring picogram quantities of substances and, therefore, many hormones cannot be estimated by this technique.

Imaging of endocrine glands is done in several ways. Imaging techniques are employed when surgical or other methods of ablative therapy are contemplated.

Commonly used imaging procedures are given in Box 96.3.

The hormone secretion from these glands can also be estimated by selective catheterization of their efferent veins.

Textbook of Medicine

Box 96.3: Imaging procedures in endocrine diseases

- Radiography—plain and contrast studies
- Isotope scanning—dynamic[*] and static studies
- Ultrasonography of neck, abdomen and pelvis
- Computerized tomography
- Magnetic resonance imaging (MRI)
- Angiography to detect abnormal vascularity
- Positron emission tomography (PET)

[*] After the injection of the appropriate isotope, images of the organ are taken at 1 second or at shorter intervals (perfusion phase or vascular phase) and later, after minutes or hours (static phase). Isotope scans give structural and functional details.

Stimulation and suppression tests: These are useful to assess the functional reserve and autonomy of the different endocrine glands and integrity of their feedback control.

TYPES OF HORMONES AND THEIR PATTERNS OF SECRETION

- *Polypeptides:* GHRH, GHRIH, TRH, ADH, oxytocin, GH, IGF-1
- *Single chain peptide:* CRH, ACTH, PRL
- *Glycoproteins:* LH, FSH, TSH, hCG
- *Steroids:* Cortisol, estrogen and androgens
- *Amines:* Dopamine
- *Iodinated tyrosine:* T3, T4.

Pattern of Secretion of Hormones

- *Continuous secretion:* T3, T4
- *Intermittent pulsatile:* LH, FSH, GH, PRL
- *Circadian rhythm:*
  - *Highest at early morning:* Cortisol
  - *Highest at midnight:* Melatonin
  - *Low at midnight:* ACTH
- *Variable secretion rate:* Stress-related hormones.

Acronyms

Acronyms commonly used in endocrinology are:

- ACTH: Adrenocorticotropic hormone
- ADH: Antidiuretic hormone
- CRH: Corticotropin releasing hormone
- FSH: Follicle stimulating hormone
- GH: Growth hormone
- GHRH: Growth hormone releasing hormone
- GHRIH: Growth hormone release inhibiting hormone
- GnRH: Gonadotropin releasing hormone
- hCG: Human chorionic gonadotropin
- IGF-1: Insulin-like growth factor-1
- LH: Luteinizing hormone
- PIH: Prolactin inhibiting hormone
- PRH: Prolactin releasing hormone
- TRH: Thyrotropin releasing hormone
- TSH: Thyroid stimulating hormone
- T3: Tri-iodothyronine
- T4: Tetra-iodothyronine

CHAPTER 97

Hypothalamus, Pituitary and their Disorders

KP Poulose, B Jayakumar

Chapter Summary

- Physiological Considerations
- Pituitary Gland
- Hypothalamic Hormones
- Hypothalamic Disorders
- Diseases of the Posterior Pituitary
- Diabetes Insipidus
- Vasopressin Excess
- Anterior Pituitary and its Disorders
- Diseases Affecting the Pituitary
- Pituitary Hyperfunction
- Hyperprolactinemia
- Gigantism and Acromegaly
- Cushing's Disease
- Hypopituitarism
  - Adult Panhypopituitarism
  - Childhood Hypopituitarism
- Dwarfism
- Empty Sella Syndrome

PHYSIOLOGICAL CONSIDERATIONS

The main seat of neuroendocrine coordination is the hypothalamus. The higher neural centers influence it through the monoaminergic pathways. Physical and chemical stimuli also influence the hypothalamus through the blood perfusing it. The supraoptic and paraventricular nuclei respond to these stimuli by the production of hormones vasopressin and oxytocin. These are bound to carrier proteins—neurophysins, and in this form they travel down the pituitary stalk to be stored in the posterior pituitary. The releasing hormones which help to release the tropic hormones of the anterior pituitary are secreted by the hypothalamus. These pass down the hypothalamohypophyseal portal circulation to exert their action on the anterior pituitary.

The ***pituitary gland weighs*** 0.5–1 g (usually 0.6 g). It consists of two portions: (1) Adenohypophysis which is composed of columns of epithelial cells derived from the primordial foregut and (2) neurohypophysis which is formed from a diverticulum arising from the floor of the third ventricle. The neurohypophysis (posterior pituitary) stores the secretions of the supraoptic and paraventricular nuclei of the hypothalamus.

Blood supply to the hypothalamus and the pituitary is derived from the superior and inferior hypophyseal arteries which are branches of the internal carotid artery. The radicles of these vessels lie in close relation to the axons of the peptidergic neurons of the hypothalamus which transfer their secretions into the blood that perfuse them. From these radicles the hypothalamohypophyseal

portal system arises and it terminates around the epithelial cells of the anterior pituitary. The releasing and inhibiting hormones secreted by the hypothalamus reach the pituitary through this system and exert their control. Blood-returning from the pituitary reaches the hypothalamus and the pituitary secretions are able to influence the hypothalamus through this pathway.

PITUITARY GLAND

Histology

This consists of three types of cells: (1) Acidophils, (2) basophils and (3) chromophobes. The acidophil cells (eosinophilic cells) which form about 60–75% of the total number of epithelial cells are situated in the posterolateral aspect of the gland. They secrete growth hormone (GH) and prolactin (PRL). The basophils secrete follicle-stimulating hormone (FSH), luteinizing hormone (LH), thyroid-stimulating hormone (TSH), adrenocorticotropic hormone (ACTH) and melanocyte-stimulating hormone (MSH). The chromophobe cells are either precursors of secretory cells or are cells which are depleted of their secretions. Based on electron microscopic findings, the cells of the pituitary can be classified as somatotrophs, lactotrophs, thyrotrophs, gonadotrophs, corticotrophs, and melanotrophs.

Lactotrophs form 15–20% of the total number of cells and they are distributed throughout the gland. Their number increases during pregnancy. Somatotrophs make up about 50% of the cells of the anterior pituitary. Corticotrophs form less than 10% of cells and are situated anteromedially. Gonadotrophs which form 10% of cells are mainly distributed in the lateral wings and thyrotrophs are found mainly in the inferomedial and superior parts of the gland.

Hormones of the Pituitary

Type of cells	Percentage	Secretion
Acidophils (eosinophils)	60–75	
Lactotrophs	15–20	Prolactin
Somatotrophs	50	GH
Basophils	25	
Corticotrophs	10	ACTH
Gonadotrophs	10	FSH, LH
Thyrotrophs	5	TSH
Melanotrophs	—	MSH

Abbreviations: GH = Growth hormone; ACTH = Adrenocorticotropic hormone; FSH = Follicle-stimulating hormone; LH = Luteinizing hormone; TSH = Thyroid-stimulating hormone; MSH = Melanocyte-stimulating hormone

HYPOTHALAMIC HORMONES

Alcmaeon, a sixth century BC Italian physiologist philosopher, introduced the brain as the center of human thinking, organizer of the senses and coordinator for survival. However, the need for a visible connection between the brain and rest of the body to explain a rapid and effective way of communication that would maintain homeostasis led Aristotle to the erroneous conclusion that the heart was the central coordinating organ and blood, the means of information transmission. In contemporary medicine, the two ancient concepts are integrated in the exciting field of neuroendocrinology. The traditional distinctions between neural (brain) and hormonal (blood) control have become blurred. Endocrine secretions are influenced directly or indirectly by the central nervous system (CNS) and many hormones influence brain function. The hypothalamic-pituitary unit is the mainstay of this nonstop, interactive and highly efficient connection between the two systems. Its function is mediated by various stimulating and inhibitory hormones including gonadotropin-releasing hormone (GnRH), thyrotropin-releasing hormone (TRH), growth hormone-releasing hormone (GHRH), growth hormone-releasing inhibiting hormone (GHRIH) [somatostatin (SS), or somatotropin release-inhibiting factor (SRIF)], corticotropin-releasing hormone (CRH), PRL inhibiting hormones and the neurotransmitter dopamine.

Growth Hormone-releasing Hormone

In contrast to GnRH and TRH, a decapeptide and tripeptide, respectively, GHRH is larger and exists in more than one isoform in the human hypothalamus. The first evidence for a hypothalamic substance with GH-releasing action was available in 1960, when it was shown that rat hypothalamic extracts could release GH from pituitary cells *in vitro*. It was not until 1980 that part of the peptide was purified. Subsequently, three isoforms of peptide were identified and sequenced from pancreatic islet cell adenomas with ectopic GHRH production. It stimulates the release of GH from the anterior pituitary.

Corticotropin-releasing Hormone

The idea that the hypothalamus controlled pituitary corticotropin (ACTH) secretion was first suggested in the late 1940s, whereas experimental support for the existence of a hypothalamic-pituitary-adrenal axis was obtained in 1955. In 1981, the sequence of a 41-amino acid peptide from bovine hypothalami, designated as CRH, was reported. In the pituitary, CRH acts by binding to membrane receptors (CRH-Rs) on corticotrophs, which couples to guanine nucleotide-binding proteins and stimulate the release of ACTH in the presence of calcium ions by a cyclic adenosine monophosphate dependent mechanism.

Thyrotropin-releasing Hormone

TRH was the first hypothalamic-releasing factor to be is isolated in 1969. Its discovery was followed by the description of GnRH, somatostatin, CRH and GHRH, all in the early 1970s. TRH is a tripeptide (pGlu-His-Pro-NH2), synthesized as a part of a large prohormone termed prepro-TRH. The latter contains repeating sequences (Gln-His-Pro-Gly), found in the median eminence of the hypothalamus and in several other parts of the nervous system. This stimulates the pituitary to enhance the secretion of TSH and PRL in normal individuals. Only TRH modulates the release of PRL.

Gonadotropin-releasing Hormone

The existence of GnRH as a hypothalamic factor was demonstrated in 1960. The structure of GnRH was elucidated in 1971. The decapeptide pyroGlu-His-Trp-Ser-Tyr-Gly-Leu-Arg-Pro-Gly-amide was named luteinizing hormone-releasing hormone (LHRH)/(LH) from the adenohypophysis. The term has been supplanted by GnRH, since this peptide not only releases LH from gonadotropes, but also FSH. An FSH-specific hypothalamic-releasing hormone, however, may also exist and be similar to the LHRH/GnRH protein, explaining the difficulty researchers have met with its purification. GnRH plays a pivotal role in reproduction. Sex steroids exert a negative feedback on the hypothalamus and pituitary and influence the secretion of FSH and LH. However, estrogens from the developing Graafian follicles exert a positive feedback on the hypothalamus and pituitary and thereby enhance the secretion of GnRH and gonadotropins.

Growth Hormone-releasing Inhibiting Hormone or Somatotropin-releasing Inhibiting Hormone or Somatostatin

The first evidence for the existence of SS was provided in 1968, when hypothalamic extracts were shown to inhibit GH secretion from pituitary cells *in vitro*. The term SS was applied to the originally described cyclic peptide (S-14), but today it is used for other members of this family of proteins, which in mammals include the 28 amino acid form (S-28) and a fragment corresponding to first 12 amino acids S-28 (S-28[1-12]). The hormone exerts a general inhibiting effect on the surrounding endocrine and exocrine tissue. SS has a short biological life and hence it is unlikely to exert its effect on distant tissues. The GH response brought about by stimuli like exercise, hypoglycemia, arginine and sleep is inhibited by SS. It also reduces the TSH response to injected TRH. In the stomach and intestine, the production of gastrin, gastric inhibitory polypeptide, hydrochloric acid and vasoactive intestinal polypeptide is diminished. The secretion of insulin and glucagon from islet cells is reduced. The exocrine pancreatic secretions like bicarbonate and enzymes are inhibited (Table 97.1).

Antidiuretic Hormone or Arginine Vasopressin

AVP is the natural ADH in humans, whereas in the pig it is lysine vasopressin. This is stored in the posterior pituitary. The term **vasopressin** denotes its ability to raise the blood pressure (BP) of experimental animals and humans in pharmacological doses. The synthesis and release of vasopressin are regulated by osmotic and nonosmotic stimuli. During periods of fluid deprivation the release of ADH increases 3–5 times the basal levels and this helps to conserve fluid by the kidneys. Half-life of ADH in circulation is 7–20 minutes. Under basal conditions, osmotic mechanisms predominate over nonosmotic

Textbook of Medicine

Table 97.1: Hypothalamic hormones, their action on the pituitary and the peripheral hormones liberated

Hypothalamic hormones	Action on pituitary	Peripheral hormones released (or) peripheral effect
Thyrotropin-releasing hormone (TRH)[1]	Thyroid-stimulating hormone (TSH)[1]	T_3, T_4 and prolactin[1]
Gonadotropin-releasing hormone (GnRH), (LHRH)[1]	Releases luteinizing hormone (LH), and follicle-stimulating hormone (FSH)[1]	Estrogens and androgenic steroids[2]
Growth hormone-releasing hormone (GHRH)	Growth hormone[1] secreted	Somatomedin (IGH-1)[1]
Growth hormone-releasing inhibiting hormone (GHRIH-somatostatin)[1]	GH inhibited TSH response to TRH reduced	
Prolactin inhibiting factor (PIF)[3]	Prolactin (PRL)[1] inhibited	Prolactin level kept at normal levels
Corticotropin-releasing hormone (CRH)[1]	Adrenocorticotropic hormone (ACTH)[1]	Cortisol mainly[2]
Vasopressin [antidiuretic hormone (ADH)][1]	–	Action on the renal tubules
Oxytocin[1]	–	Uterine contraction

Note: (1) Peptide, (2) Steroids, (3) Amine

mechanisms. Changes in serum osmolality by 1–2% lead to alteration in the volume of the osmoreceptors in the anterior hypothalamus and this triggers the supraoptic nucleus. However, under conditions of stress, volume receptors in the atrium and pulmonary veins are also activated. When there is a fall in BP, receptors in the carotid and aortic sinuses are stimulated and they augment the secretion of vasopressin. Other factors which stimulate vasopressin secretion are psychological and physical stresses. Once triggered, the nonosmotic mechanisms are capable of stimulating the synthesis and secretion of vasopressin.

Vasopressin exerts its main effect on the distal convoluted tubules and collecting tubules of the kidney and increases the reabsorption of water. The hormone activates the adenylate-cyclase system in the cells lining the tubules and makes them more permeable to water by increasing the size and number of pores. In addition, vasopressin stimulates the smooth muscles of the arterioles in the mesentery, coronary circulation and skin. Intestinal smooth muscle is also stimulated to activity. The main source of vasopressin for therapeutic use is synthetic and the preparation is 1-deamino-8-D-arginine vasopressin (DDAVP). It is used mainly for the treatment of diabetes insipidus. In other conditions like hemophilia, DDAVP is finding increasing use. In conditions of intractable hypotension, vasopressin is used with benefit. Vasopressin is also employed to reduce portal hypertension and esophageal variceal bleeding.

In addition to its hormonal role, DDAVP is also used in the management of one form of von Willebrand's disease (a bleeding disorder).

Oxytocin

This hormone enhances uterine contraction during labor and also in the postpartum period. This helps in delivery and postpartum hemostasis. Oxytocin also enhances the release of milk from the breast during suckling.

The production of oxytocin is controlled mainly by stimuli arising from the breast during suckling. The impulses reach the hypothalamus through the spinal cord and stimulate the production of oxytocin. Distension of the female genital tract stimulates oxytocin production whereas stress and emotional disturbances inhibit it.

Oxytocin is used mainly to induce labor and stimulate uterine contraction after delivery. Estrogens also stimulate the release of oxytocin.

HYPOTHALAMIC DISORDERS

Hypothalamic disorders result from destruction of the neurons which secrete the hormones or from alterations in the afferent impulses from the higher neural centers into the hypothalamus (defects in KAL gene discovered in 1991.)

Reduction of hypothalamic neurons may either be due to lack of development as in *Kallmann's syndrome* or destruction by disease processes such as encephalitis, meningitis, tumors or ischemia. Hypothalamic disturbances may lead to deficiency of the releasing hormones and consequent hypothyroidism, hypogonadism, hypoadrenocorticism and dwarfism. In general, hypothalamic lesions induce only partial failure of the target glands unlike lesions of the pituitary. Hypothalamus exerts a tonic inhibitory control on PRL secretion, hypothalamic lesions result in uncontrolled production of PRL. This may lead to galactorrhea, amenorrhea and hypogonadism.

Hypothalamic function is regulated by feedback impulses from the target glands and also by impulses from higher neural centers. Other stimuli arising from the osmoreceptors and glucoreceptors situated in hypothalamus and alteration in the physical and chemical characteristics of blood influence hypothalamic activity. Functions such as temperature regulation, eating, satiety, and thirst are controlled by regulatory centers situated in the hypothalamus. Important disorders of the hypothalamus are psychogenic *amenorrhea, anorexia nervosa* and *deprivation dwarfism* in children. Impairment of inhibitory inputs from other areas of the brain may lead to precocious puberty and excessive secretion of ADH [the syndrome of inappropriate secretion of ADH secretion (SIADH)] (Fig. 97.1).

DISEASES OF THE POSTERIOR PITUITARY

DIABETES INSIPIDUS (CRANIAL DIABETES INSIPIDUS)

Normally, ADH is secreted in response to physiological stimuli such as osmolality, hypovolemia, hypotension and

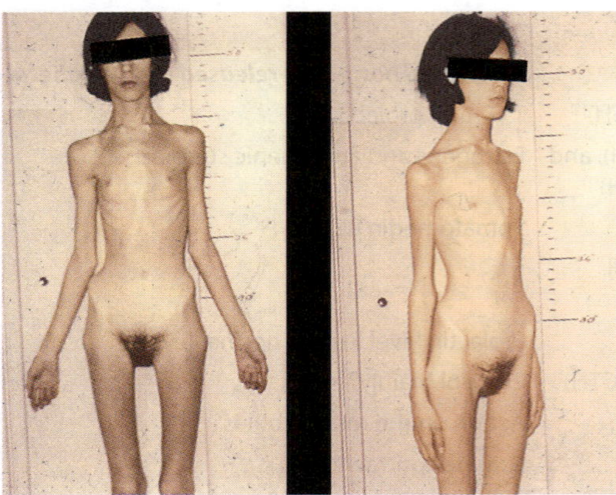

Fig. 97.1: Anorexia nervosa. ***Note:*** Emaciation, breast is developed pubic hair is present, refusal to eat

Table 97.2: Causes of pituitary diabetes insipidus	

• Head trauma (closed and penetrating)
• Neoplasms
  ▪ Primary
    – Craniopharyngioma
    – Pituitary-adenoma (suprasellar)
    – Dysgerminoma
    – Meningioma
  ▪ Metastatic deposits (lung, breast)
    – Hematological (lymphoma, leukemia)
• Granulomas
  ▪ Neurosarcoidosis
  ▪ Histiocytosis
  ▪ Xanthoma disseminatum
• Infections
  ▪ Chronic meningitis
  ▪ Viral encephalitis
  ▪ Toxoplasmosis
• Inflammatory
• Lymphocytic infundibuloneurohypophysitis
• Wegener's granulomatosis
• Lupus erythematosus
• Scleroderma
	• Chemical toxins
	  ▪ Tetrodotoxin
	  ▪ Snake venom (envenomation sequel)
	• Vascular
	  ▪ Sheehan's syndrome
	  ▪ Aneurysm (internal carotid)
	  ▪ Aortocoronary bypass
	  ▪ Hypoxic encephalopathy
	  ▪ Pregnancy
	  ▪ Idiopathic
	• Congenital malformations
	  ▪ Septo-optic dysplasia
	  ▪ Midline craniofacial defects
	  ▪ Holoprosencephaly
	  ▪ Hypogenesis, ectopia of pituitary
	  ▪ Genetic causes
	• Autosomal dominant (AVP-neurophysin gene)
	• Autosomal recessive (AVP-neurophysin gene)
	• Autosomal recessive-Wolfram-(4pWFS 1 gene) disease
	• X-linked recessive (Xq28)
	• Deletion chromosome 7q

psychological stress. This hormone (ADH) plays a major role in maintaining serum osmolality within a narrow range. Normal blood level of AVP is 1–3 IU/mL. Failure of secretion of ADH from the supraoptic nucleus leads to the development of central diabetes insipidus. The clinical abnormality becomes evident only when about 99% of the neurons in this region are lost. Several conditions may lead to diabetes insipidus.

Causes of pituitary diabetes insipidus are listed in Table 97.2.

Clinical Features

Diabetes insipidus presents with gross polyuria, thirst and polydipsia. The urine volume may vary from 2.5 to 10 L or more in 24 hours and the osmolality may fall below 200 mOsm/kg. Majority of those patients have normal

thirst mechanisms and they make up the fluid loss by taking adequate quantity of water and salt and thus prevent the development of dehydration and hyponatremia. In this condition, plasma osmolality is raised whereas the urinary osmolality is low. When the free intake of water and salt is diminished as in coma or due to other causes, severe dehydration and hypovolemia develop. In moderately severe cases, the osmolality of plasma ranges from 400 to 600 mOsm/kg. In well-compensated patients, apart from the history and gross polyuria with dilute urine (specific gravity around 1,004), no other abnormality may be evident. In those subjects in whom the disease is secondary to other disease processes, the primary abnormality may be evident. In idiopathic cases, magnetic resonance imaging (MRI) may reveal evidence of neurohypophysis.

Diagnosis

Diabetes insipidus should be diagnosed by history and presence of polyuria with fall of specific gravity of urine. The urine volume does not fall and the specific gravity does not rise with fluid deprivation. Since fluid restriction may be hazardous in these subjects, it has to be done only under close supervision. Other conditions producing polyuria with low specific gravity of the urine such as nephrogenic diabetes insipidus and psychogenic polydipsia have to be differentiated.

Differential Diagnosis

Nephrogenic diabetes insipidus: The renal tubules are refractory to the actions of normal levels of circulating ADH. This may be congenital as in primary nephrogenic diabetes insipidus or secondary to diseases such as chronic renal failure, diabetes mellitus (DM), hypercalcemia, hypokalemia and sickle cell anemia or due to drugs such as lithium and demeclocycline.

Primary polydipsia (psychogenic polydipsia): Compulsory water drinking is a part of complex psychiatric disturbances in which the patient drinks large amounts of water. The disorder may show remission and exacerbation.

Investigations

Cranial or central diabetes insipidus can be distinguished from nephrogenic diabetes insipidus and primary polydipsia by simple laboratory tests.

- ■ ***Measurement of 24 hours urine volume:*** If the urine volume is less than 2 liters, diabetes insipidus is unlikely. It is to be remembered that mild cases may present with lower urine volumes, but in times of stress such as diarrhea or excessive sweating, hypovolemia, shock and hyponatremia ensue early.
- ■ ***If the osmolality of early morning urine*** exceeds 800 mOsm/kg, it almost rules out diabetes insipidus.
- ■ ***Water deprivation test and vasopressin administration:*** Fluid deprivation for 8 hours is done under medical supervision, only dry food is given. Since this is hazardous, it should not be continued if the body weight falls by 5% or 2 kg. Urine osmolality is measured hourly till steady values are obtained in three consecutive samples. Then 5 units of aqueous vasopressin or desmopressin 1 mg is given parentally. Osmolality of plasma and urine is determined hourly

Textbook of Medicine

for further 3 hours. In central diabetes insipidus, the rise in urine osmolality after vasopressin exceeds 9% whereas in patients with nephrogenic diabetes insipidus the rise is less than 9%. With desmopressin 1 µg intramuscular (IM) or 20 mg intranasal, the increase in urine osmolality exceeds 50% whereas in nephrogenic diabetes insipidus it is below 45%. Patients with psychogenic polydipsia require longer periods of fluid deprivation for obtaining steady urine osmolality, since they tend to be fluid overloaded. Fluid deprivation results in rise of urine osmolality in this condition.

X-ray of the skull may reveal conditions such as histiocytosis, secondary deposits or hematological malignancies which cause destructive lesions of skull bones. Computed tomography (CT) or MRI scan will be more specific in delineating the lesion.

The prognosis of diabetes insipidus depends upon the primary cause. As such, diabetes insipidus does not shorten life-expectancy if it is identified and promptly managed.

Treatment

Cases with moderate or severe disease require specific therapy.

- ***Vasopressin analogues:*** At present, the synthetic analogue DDAVP (desmopressin) is used. It is given as nasal spray or instillation. It has duration of action for 12–24 hours and many cases require only one or two doses daily. Moreover, DDAVP is devoid of the pressor activity. It is absorbed even in the presence of nasal congestion. Parenteral preparations are available for use in more severe cases or in emergencies. Dose of DDAVP is 5–10 µg as nasal installation twice a day.

Several nonhormonal substances which act on the nephrons by different mechanisms effectively reduce the urine volume in pituitary dibetes insipidus. These are listed below. Many of them are quite effective in practice.

- ***Chlorpropamide*** (250–500 mg/day), clofibrate and carbamazepine bring about reduction in urine volume in mild and moderate cases.
- ***Thiazide diuretics*** are effective in bringing down urine volume.

These drugs, being cheaper and more easily available, are generally used except in rare occasions when hormonal replacement becomes inevitable.

VASOPRESSIN EXCESS (SIADH)

Normally secretion of ADH depends upon plasma osmolality and blood volume. When this mechanism fails or ectopic sources secrete ADH, ***SIADH*** results. This syndrome is not rare in clinical practice. Adults and children may be affected. This is an important cause of hyponatremia in many chronically ill-patients.

Causes of SIADH are shown in Box 97.1.

Clinical Features

The symptomatology is vague and it is likely to be missed unless the condition is strongly suspected. There is

Box 97.1: Causes of SIADH

- ***Tumors:*** Carcinoma lung, carcinoid, leukemia, lymphoma and thymoma
- ***Drugs:*** Vasopressin, chlorpropamide, carbamazepine, clofibrate, vincristine, cyclophosphamide, thiazides, nicotine and demeclocycline
- ***Pulmonary disorders:*** Pneumonia, pleural effusion and tuberculosis
- ***Neurological disorders:*** Meningitis, encephalitis, Guillain-Barré syndrome
- Metabolic acute intermittent porphyria
- ***Endocrine disorders:*** Addison's disease
- AIDS and AIDS related complex
- Idiopathic

Abbreviation: AIDS = Acquired immunodeficiency syndrome

dilutional hyponatremia. When the level of serum sodium falls (120–125 mmol/L), somnolence, anorexia, confusion and depression may be observed. These are manifestations of cerebral edema when the serum sodium suddenly falls to 125 mmol/L or less. When the sodium level falls below 120 mmol/L, coma, convulsions and focal neurological deficits may develop. Severe hyponatremia with serum sodium below 110 mmol/L is usually fatal if undetected, due to brainstem herniation.

Diagnosis is by estimating serum sodium level, which is below 125 mmol/L with high urine sodium level above 20 mmol/L. Plasma osmolality must be less than 270 mOsm/kg with normal renal, adrenal and thyroid functions. Urine osmolality is more than 100 mOsm/kg.

Treatment

SIADH is only a manifestation of other serious underlying diseases and, therefore, the problem should receive total attention. Mild hyponatremia responds to fluid restriction of 0.5–1 L/day in addition to the previous days' urine output. Administration of demethylchlortetracycline (demeclocycline) which produces nephrogenic diabetes insipidus is effective in some cases. The dose is 600–1,200 mg/day. In severe cases presenting with convulsions, coma or hemiparesis, urgent infusion of hypertonic saline (3–5%) is indicated. Too rapid a correction results in central pontine myelinolysis. IV saline containing 500 mmol/L is infused slowly till the plasma sodium rises above 125 mmol/L, thereafter oral supplements are continued. One hundred mL of 3% saline contains 50 mmol of sodium chloride.

Tolvaptan is a selective nonpeptide oral vasopressin V2-receptor antagonist which promotes aquaresis (excretion of electrolyte-free water). This drug is useful in the management of hyponatremia (Na^+ level below 135 mmol/L) which is a predictor of death in chronic heart failure and cirrhosis liver. The excretion of water is not associated with electrolyte excretion. The dose is 15 mg daily orally to start with and increased up to 60 mg/day. The effect wanes off if tolvaptan is stopped. Adverse side effects include increased thirst, dryness of mouth and polyuria.

Tolvaptan is indicated in SIADH and severe fluid overload states such as chronic heart failure, cirrhosis liver and others.

GENERAL CONSIDERATIONS

Hormones of the anterior pituitary are polypeptides with one or more chains. They can be grouped into three groups.

1. ***Corticotropin group***
   - ACTH
   - Melanocyte-stimulating hormone, lipotropins (LPH)

   Corticotropin and lipotropins form the major bulk, MSH is present only in small quantities. Endogenous opioid peptides (endorphins) are derived from the lipotropins. The adenohypophysis can maintain its functional capacity even if 50% of its tissue is lost, but beyond this its function suffers.

2. ***Glycoprotein hormones***
   - FSH
   - LH or interstitial cell-stimulating hormone
   - TSH

3. ***Somatotropin-mammotropin group:***
   - GH
   - PRL.

ADRENOCORTICOTROPIN HORMONE

It is a single chain polypeptide with 39 amino acids formed from pro-opiomelanocortin (POMC) a precursor polypeptide with 241 amino acid residues. POMC is synthesized from 285 amino acid long polypeptide precursor pre-POMC, by removal of a 44 amino acid long signal peptide sequence during translation synthesized mainly in corticotroph cells of the anterior pituitary. The hormone can be estimated by radioimmunoassay (RIA). Blood levels show considerable variation, values being highest early in the morning (40–80 pg/mL). ACTH release is facilitated by the corticotropin-releasing factors of the hypothalamus and inhibited by increasing levels of circulating plasma cortisol. ACTH production goes on independent of feedback inhibition and diurnal variation during periods of stress. It exerts action on the adrenal cortex and extra-adrenal tissues. ACTH promotes the synthesis of glucocorticoids and androgens by the adrenal cortex. Aldosterone secretion is only marginally affected.

Other effects of ACTH include lipolysis and increase in pigmentation brought about by stimulation of the melanocytes. Normally these extra-adrenal effects of ACTH are not pronounced, but when ACTH production is increased as in Addison's disease and Nelson's syndrome, pigmentation becomes prominent. The role played by lipotropins in man is not understood.

GLYCOPROTEIN HORMONES

The pituitary glycoprotein hormones are TSH, FSH, and LH. The placental glycoprotein hormone ***human chorionic gonadotropin*** (hCG) resembles LH in function. All these hormones act through the adenylate cyclase mechanism.

Thyroid-stimulating Hormone (Thyrotropin)

The TSH acts mainly on the thyroid to increase its vascularity and size. It enhances all aspects of thyroid function such as iodine uptake, synthesis of thyroglobulin, and release of thyroxine. TSH secretion is increased by TRH and inhibited by increasing levels of circulating thyroxine and tri-iodothyronine. The inhibitory effect of circulating thyroid hormones on TSH is stronger than the stimulatory effect of TRH on the pituitary. Plasma TSH level is about 0–5 µU/mL. Basal TSH levels are considerably increased and TSH response to TRH is amplified in primary hypothyroidism. The TSH levels are very low and often undetectable in primary thyrotoxicosis. Moreover, the TSH response to TRH is also negligible.

Gonadotropins

GnRH produced by the hypothalamus influences the synthesis and secretion of LH and FSH. LH is stimulated to a greater degree than FSH. Secretion of LH and FSH is inhibited by rising levels of estrogens, progesterone and testosterone in blood, except during the preovulatory phase. During the preovulatory phase, high-level of estrogens produces a positive feedback on the hypothalamus and pituitary, and this result in excessive production of LH.

Gonadotropins increase the synthesis and secretion of sex steroids and promote gametogenesis. The pituitary produces FSH and LH, and HCGs are produced by the placenta. FSH and LH secretion occurs in spurts in females. FSH facilitates the maturation of Graafian follicles by acting on the granulosa cells of the ovary. LH also acts on the granulosa cells to enhance estrogen production. Acting on the interstitial cells of the testes, it increases the secretion of testosterone. Spermatogenesis is stimulated. Increase in LH levels in the midcycle phase leads to rupture of the mature follicle and liberation of ovum. In addition, it leads to luteinization of the ruptured follicle. LH is responsible for continued development of the corpus luteum till the placenta takes over this function during pregnancy. LH also maintains the steroidogenic function of the placenta.

SOMATOMAMMOTROPIN GROUP OF HORMONES

Growth Hormone

GH is a single polypeptide with 191 amino acids. The quantity of GH exceeds that of the other pituitary hormones. Human pituitary contains 6–10 mg of extractable GH. Normal daytime circulating level of GH is less than 0.5 µg/L.

Postmortem pituitary was a major source of this hormone used for diagnostic and therapeutic purposes. This has led to the spread of disease such as slow virus infections of the CNS.

GH is secreted by the acidophilic somatotrophs of the anterior pituitary, the secretion is controlled by regulatory hormones released by the hypothalamic neurons into the hypothalamic pituitary portal system. The 44 amino acid GHRH stimulate GH release via its receptor (GHRH receptor) while its release is inhibited by SS from the hypothalamus; another stimulant of GH release is the gastric derived hormone ***ghrelin***.

Textbook of Medicine

Fasting level of GH in the plasma is below 4 ng/mL. Secretion occurs in bursts lasting 1–2 hours. Maximal secretion occurs during the stages III and IV of nonrapid eye movement (NREM) sleep. Factors such as exercise, hypoglycemia and rise in amino acid levels enhance secretion.

GH promotes linear growth in prepubertal children by its anabolic activity and effect in cartilage growth. Another metabolic effect includes lipolysis which leads to the increase of serum free fatty acids, which in turn inhibit glucose uptake by cells. This partly accounts for the anti-insulin activity of GH.

GH acts on the liver and other tissues to stimulate the production of *insulin-like growth factor-1 (IGF-1,* also known as *somatomedin-C)* which is responsible for growth promoting activity. Serum level of IGF-1 is an indicator of overall GH secretion. Whereas GH secretion occurs in spurts, IGF-1 level does not show marked diurnal variation.

Prolactin

PRL resembles GH closely. PRL level can be estimated by RIA. This hormone is also secreted in bursts lasting for a few minutes to hours, maximal secretion occurring during sleep. Hypothalamus exerts an inhibitory effect on PRL secretion through *prolactin inhibitory factor*. It is most likely that PRL-releasing factors also exist. TRH also stimulates release of PRL. Neuroendocrine reflexes caused by suckling and stimulation of breast in females also help to release PRL. PRL exerts its main action on the breast which is primed by the action of estrogens, progesterone, GH and cortisol. PRL stimulates the synthesis of milk proteins. The physiological role of PRL in male is not clearly known.

Basal PRL level is about 10–20 ng/mL in men and nonpregnant women. Towards the end of pregnancy, levels as high as 200 ng/mL are observed. During puerperium, values fall to nonpregnant levels even though lactation is continued. PRL is released during suckling and this prepares the breast for the next feeding.

INSULIN LIKE GROWTH FACTORS (SOMATOMEDIN-C)

Insulin like growth factors are substances which act as intermediaries to exert the action of other hormones like GH and insulin. IGF participates in the growth and functions of almost all organs in the body. The three peptide hormones or growth factors namely insulin, IGF-1 and IGF-2 have approximately 50% of the amino acids in common. Interaction of GH with its hepatic cell receptors stimulates the expression of IGF-1 gene and release of IGF-1. Levels of IGF-1 in the liver and serum inhibit further GH release. The mechanisms of regulation of IGF-2 are not known.

Whereas insulin which is secreted by the β-cells of the islets of Langerhans as a prohormone initially proinsulin, gets cleaved at the C-peptide level, the IGFs which are synthesized primarily in the liver retain the C-peptide moiety. Insulin present in picomolar concentrations in plasma has a half-life of minutes, whereas IGFs circula-

ting in nanomolar concentrations bound to IGF binding proteins is secreted by the liver. This binding limits the availability of IGFs to the target cells. They act in an autocrine or paracrine manner.

Physiological Role and Mechanism of Action

Insulin acts primarily on the liver, muscles and adipose tissue. IGF take part in the metabolism of all tissue cells. Both the IGFs are important for embryonic development. After birth, IGF-1 seems to have a predominant role in regulating growth. The exact function of IGF-2 is not known. IGFs bind specifically to IGF receptors which are distinct from insulin receptors. Once the insulin receptor or IGF receptor is activated, similar metabolic processes are evoked within the large cells. Insulin regulates metabolic functions whereas IGF-1 regulates growth and differentiation in postnatal life. Mechanisms of action of insulin and IGF-1 differ. Liver and fat express both insulin and IGF-1 receptors. Insulin controls hepatic glucose production and lipolysis by signaling exclusively through insulin receptors. So, also insulin stimulated uptake of glucose by cells is solely meditated by insulin receptors.

Insulin like growth factor-1 mediates many, if not most of the metabolic actions of GH. It stimulates bone formation, protein synthesis, glucose uptake in muscle, neuronal survival and myelin synthesis. It also reverses negative balance during starvation and inhibits protein degradation in muscles.

Locally produced IGFs have important actions in several organs. GH, parathyroid hormones and sex-steroids regulate the production of IGFs in bone, whereas sex-steroids are the main regulators of IGFs in the reproductive system. The exact role of the locally produced IGFs has not been fully elucidated.

Pathological conditions associated with abnormalities of IGF-1 include Laron's dwarfism, type 2 DM, type 1 DM, insulin resistance states and others. IGF-1 is secreted by some tumors whose growth rate is modified by this hormone.

Insulin-like Growth Factor-1 in Therapy

- *Dwarfism:* Laron's dwarfism is a GH deficiency syndrome in which insensitiveness to GH exists as a result of unresponsiveness of the receptors. In these subjects IGF-1 150 μg/kg bw/day given subcutaneously (SC), increases height velocity by three times that of normals, i.e. 10.8 cm versus 3 cm/year.
- *Insulin resistant states:*
  - *Type 2 DM:* IGF-1 has been proposed as therapy for severe insulin resistance states since its actions resemble those of insulin and may therefore bypass the defects that block the action of insulin. In doses of 100 μg/kg bw given SC, it decreases serum insulin levels by 60–80% and improves glucose utilization both in DM and impaired glucose tolerance. In type 2 DM, the resistance is overcome.
  - *In type 1 DM, IGFs exert their action by:*
    – Decreasing the secretion of GH
    – Increasing the sensitivity to insulin
    – Decreasing insulin requirements.

- **Osteoporosis:** IGF-1 which has anabolic activity has been used as an adjunct in the management of osteoporosis.
- **Regulation of growth of baby after birth by mediating the metabolic effects of GH:**
  - Stimulates bone formation
  - Protein synthesis
  - Glucose uptake in muscle
  - Myelin synthesis.

Side Effects of Insulin-like Growth Factor-1

IV injection may cause anaphylaxis and cardiovascular problems including asystole and hypertension which are secondary to hypophosphatemia. Multiple SC doses given for more than 10 days may give rise to temporomandibular pain, facial and hand edema, weight gain, dyspnea, tachycardia, raised intracranial tension, gynecomastia and Bell's palsy. All of these regress on withdrawal of therapy.

INVESTIGATIONS IN HYPOTHALAMO-PITUITARY DISORDERS

These are designed to detect the morphological and functional abnormalities. Tumors may present as space occupying lesions with pressure effects on neighboring neural structures. Endocrine disturbances resulting from increased or decreased secretion of hormones are also seen commonly, but these may not be constant. Some tumors secrete excess of hormones while others compress normal tissue and suppress its function. The investigations may be grouped under three heads: (1) Neurological, (2) imaging and (3) hormonal studies (Table 97.3).

1. **Neurological investigations**
   - **Perimetry:** Pressure of tumors in the region of the pituitary causes compression of the optic chiasma and leads to defects in the visual field. These can be documented by perimeter.

Table 97.3: Tests of pituitary function

Hormone to be estimated	Test	Blood samples	Interpretation
Growth hormone	**Insulin tolerance test:** Regular insulin (0.05–0.15 U/kg IV)	−30, 0, 30, 60 minutes for glucose and GH	Glucose < 40 mg/dL; GH should be >3 µg/L
	GHRH test: 1 µg/kg IV	0, 15, 30, 45, 60, 120 minutes for GH	Normal response is GH >3 µg/L
	L-arginine test: 30 g IV over 30 minutes	0, 30, 60, 120 minutes for GH	Normal response is GH >3 µg/L
	L-dopa test: 500 mg PO	0, 20, and 60 minutes for TSH and PRL	Normal prolactin is >2 µg/L and
Prolactin	**TRH test:** 200–500 µg IV		Increase >200% of baseline
ACTH	**Insulin tolerance test:** Regular insulin (0.05 U/kg IV)	−30, 0, 30, 60, 90 minutes for glucose and cortisol	Glucose <40 mg/dL; cortisol should increase by >7 µg/L or to >20 µg/dL
	CRH test: 1 µg/kg bovine CRH IV at 0800 hours	0, 15, 30, 60, 90, 120 minutes for ACTH and cortisol	Basal ACTH increase two to four-fold and peaks at 20–100 pg/mL; cortisol levels >20–25 µg/dL
	Metyrapone test: Metyrapone (30 mg/kg) at midnight	Plasma 11-deoxycortisol and cortisol at 8 AM ACTH can also be measured	Plasma cortisol should be <4 µg/dL to ensure an adequate response Normal response is 11-deoxycortisol >7.5 µg/dL or ACTH > 75 pg/mL
	Standard ACTH stimulation test: ACTH 1–24 (cosyntropin) 0.25 mg IM or IV	0, 30, 60 minutes for cortisol and aldosterone	Normal response is cortisol >21 µg/dL and aldosterone response of >4 ng/dL above baseline
	Low-dose ACTH test: ACTH 1–24 (cosyntropin) 1 µg IV or 3-day ACTH stimulation test consisting of 0.25 mg ACTH 1–24 given IV over 8 hours each day	0, 30, 60 minutes for cortisol 3rd day	Cortisol should be >21 µg/dL
Thyroid function test (TFT)	**Basal thyroid function tests:** T_4, T_3, TSH, free T_3, free T_4	Basal tests	
	TRH test: 200–500 µg IV	0, 20, 60 minutes for TSH and PRL	TSH should increase by >5 mU/L unless thyroid hormone levels are increased
LH, FSH	LH, FSH testosterone, estrogen	Basal tests	Basal LH and FSH should be increased in postmenopausal women Low testosterone levels in the setting of low LH and FSH
	GnRH test: GnRH 100 µg IV	0, 30, 60 minutes for LH and FSH	In most adults, LH should increase by 10 IU/L and FSH by 2 IU/L
Multiple hormones	**Combined anterior pituitary test:** GHRH (1 µg/kg), CRH (1 µg/kg), GnRH (100 µg) TRH (200 µg) are given IV	−30, 0, 15, 30, 60, 90, 120 minutes for GH, ACTH, cortisol, LH, FSH and TSH	Normal responses are variable Combined or individual releasing hormone responses must be elevated in the context of basal target gland hormone values and this may not be diagnostic (see text)

Abbreviations: IV = Intravenous; GH = Growth hormone; TSH = Thyroid-stimulating hormone; PRL = Prolactin; TRH = Thyrotropin-releasing hormone; PO = Postoperative; ACTH = Adrenocorticotropic hormone; CRH = Corticotropin-releasing hormone; FSH = Follicle-stimulating hormone; LH = Luteinizing hormone; GnRH = Gonadotropin-releasing hormone; GHRH = Growth hormone-releasing hormone; IM = Intramuscular

- ***Visual evoked potential*** studies will be of further help to record involvement of the optic nerve and its pathway.

2. ***Imaging studies***
   - Lateral view diagrams of the skull may show enlargement of sella, double flooring, destruction of clinoid processes or suprasellar calcification. More detailed information of this area may be obtained by cone views of the pituitary fossa.
   - ***Computed tomography scanning coupled with contrast studies:*** These studies give definite information in almost all cases.
   - Isotope scanning procedures help to reveal regional vascularity and focal lesions.
   - MRI with gadolinium contrast is superior to CT to detect smaller lesions especially in the posterior fossa.

3. ***Hormonal studies***
   - ***RIA:*** Anterior pituitary hormones and secretion of its target glands can be measured precisely by RIA.
   - ***Feedback control:*** Integrity of hypothalamo-hypophyseal system can be assessed by tests involving suppression or stimulation tests.
   - ***Indirect indices of hormonal disorders:*** When the measurement of hormones in blood is not practical, e.g. ADH, the functions of the target organs are studied. For example in diabetes insipidus, studies of concentrating function of the kidney give valuable information.

DISEASES AFFECTING THE PITUITARY

PITUITARY HYPERFUNCTION

Excessive activity of pituitary hormones may result from several causes. These are:

- ***Tumors of the pituitary:*** Tumors can arise from different cellular constituents of the pituitary. Pituitary tumors may be isolated or they may form part of multiple endocrine adenomatosis in which the parathyroid and pancreatic islets may also show tumors.
- ***Defective regulatory control by the hypothalamus:*** Diseases of the hypothalamus may result in increased secretion of the release hormones or decreased secretion of inhibitory hormones acting on the pituitary.
- ***Ectopic secretion of pituitary hormones:*** Hormones of the pituitary or their analogues may be secreted by malignant neoplasms as a paraneoplastic phenomenon, e.g. chorionic gonadotropin and LH may be secreted by hepatoblastoma and PRL, GH and ACTH may be produced by carcinoma of the bronchus. Well-defined clinical syndromes are common and can occur due to excess of PRL, GH and ACTH. TSH, FSH and LH are less commonly involved and they may not produce typical clinical syndromes at times.

HYPERPROLACTINEMIA

Prolactin excess is the most common disorder resulting from overactivity of the pituitary. About one-third of

Box 97.2: Causes of hyperprolactinemia

- Prolactinoma
- Chest wall injury and spinal cord lesions
- Lactotroph hyperplasia
- Chronic renal failure
- Cirrhosis
- Empty sella syndrome
- Drugs, e.g. chlorpromazine and oral contraceptives
- Increased prolactin

women with long-standing menstrual disorders show excessive PRL activity. Hyperprolactinemia is less common in males. PRL is released sparingly into circulation, because its secretion is under-inhibition by a hypothalamic PRL inhibitory factor.

Causes (Box 97.2)

- Lactotroph adenomas (prolactinomas) arising from the pituitary—the most common pituitary tumor.
- Chest wall injury and spinal cord lesions—several lesions of the thoracic wall and conditions which stimulate the breasts leading to oversecretion of PRL.
- Lactotroph hyperplasia—tumors and inflammatory lesions of the hypothalamus may result in excessive liberation of PRL by the pituitary. In empty sella syndrome, the pituitary stalk is compressed due to cisternal herniation into the pituitary fossa and the inhibitory factor for PRL secretion falls.
- Chronic renal failure—patients suffering from chronic renal failure has three-fold increase in secretion in PRL levels, owing to decreased clearance.
- Cirrhosis—basal PRL levels are increased in 5–20% of patients with cirrhosis, possibly because of alterations in hypothalamic dopamine generations.
- Adrenal insufficiency—glucocorticoids have a suppressive effect on PRL gene transcription and release.
- Several drugs such as chlorpromazine, oral contraceptives, reserpine, haloperidol and digoxin may lead to the release of excess amounts of PRL.
- Increased amounts of PRL are seen in other endocrine disorders such as hypothyroidism. Pregnancy may be associated with PRL overactivity.

Other rare cases are idiopathic hyperprolactinemia (cause unknown) and macroprolactinemia.

Clinical Features

About 50% of patients with hyperprolactinemia develop galactorrhea and menstrual irregularities. Hirsutism may develop. Women show anovulation and infertility.

Signs of local pressure on the neural structures such as optic chiasma, optic tract and third ventricle lead to focal neurological defects such as visual field defects, obstructive hydrocephalus and others. Generalized increase in intracranial tension gives rise to headache and papilledema. PRL suppresses the release of LH and therefore prolactinomas are associated with loss of libido, impotence and azoospermia in men. Ninety-five percent of prolactinomas are benign. The ratio of incidence of microadenoma in females and males is about 20:1, while no gender difference is seen with macroadenoma.

Hook effect (prozone effect): Measurement of serum PRL levels is important in the differentiation of prolactinomas

Textbook of Medicine

from nonfunctioning adenomas. Immunoradiometric assay is frequently used for measurement of serum PRL levels. The sensitivity and the precision of the assay are good, with a short incubation time. Falsely low values have been reported with this technique when a large amount of PRL is present that saturates the antibodies present in the test solution. This is known as the hook effect.

Diagnosis

Basal serum PRL levels above 20 ng/mL which fail to increase with the administration of TRH, suggests the possibility of prolactinomas. In moderate or large-sized tumors, the value may go up above several hundred ng/mL. There is generally a direct relationship with the level of PRL and tumor size. Serum PRL levels also help to assess the improvement with therapy. Hyperprolactinemia is often associated with thyroid dysfunction. Hence such cases should also be investigated for abnormalities of thyroid function. Other tests of pituitary function should also be done when macroadenomas bigger than 1 cm in diameter are present, in order to assess the degree of suppression of other hormones by the tumors.

CT and MRI may reveal almost all the macroadenomas. MRI can detect only over 70% of the microadenomas. In patients with clinical features and raised hormonal levels suggesting prolactinoma, about 30% of microadenomas may not be readily demonstrable by direct imaging. CT combined with positron emission tomography (PET) is very useful in the detection of functioning tumors.

Treatment

Dopamine agonists arrest the growth of the tumor, lower the secretion of PRL and bring about clinical and biochemical relief in more than 80% of cases. Among the dopamine agonists, ***bromocriptine*** which is a derivative of ergot is most popular in India.

The drugs have to be given on a long-term basis, often for several years. After 2 years of successful therapy, the dose can be reduced on a trial and error basis.

In case of microadenomas medical treatment may be sufficient, but in cases of macroadenomas, if tumor regression is not complete or if local complications develop, surgical or radiation therapy may have to be undertaken. Irradiation with a dose of 3.5–5 Gy over 4–6 weeks is effective, but it is only rarely required.

Other dopamine agonists include ***cabergoline, quinagolide*** and ***pergolide*** (Table 97.4).

If with treatment of prolactinomas the sexual function does not recover, accompanying hypogonadism or menopause has to be suspected.

Usually medical treatment is very satisfactory. Macroadenomas shrink to a considerable extent in more than 70% of cases. Those who desire pregnancy should be informed that there is a small chance of the tumor enlarging during the early weeks of pregnancy.

When the tumor produces pressure effects and threatens vision, surgical removal is the treatment of choice. The procedure commonly employed is trans-sphenoidal microsurgery.

Even in patients with focal neurological deficits, medical treatment can be given a fair trial since dramatic improvement is the rule.

Radiotherapy is limited to patient with macroprolactinomas that are refractory to medical treatment and surgery.

Prolactinomas and pregnancy: Patients with prolactinomas wishing to become pregnant should be referred to specialists in obstetrics and endocrinology because they may need to be pretreated with bromocriptine to achieve fertility. The therapy should be discontinued on conception.

GIGANTISM AND ACROMEGALY

Effects of excessive amount of GH depend on the age of onset of the disease. Onset before closure of the epiphyses leads to gigantism and later onset after closure of epiphyses results in acromegaly.

Causes: Hyperplasia or adenoma of the pituitary affecting the acidophils, chromophobes or both lead to hypersecretion of GH. In 80% of cases, the underlying tumor is a somatotroph adenoma, in 10% it is nonsomatotroph adenoma and in 10% it is of mixed type. Rarely, it is due to abnormality of the hypothalamus or ectopic hormone production. The total clinical picture results from the local effects of the tumor and endocrine effects of GH. The tumor compresses the neighboring cells in the pituitary and leads to suppression of gonadotrophs and thyrotrophs. Mixed acidophil adenoma produces both GH and PRL. Large-sized tumors may present as space occupying lesions.

Gigantism

Onset of GH excess before the age of 10 years leads to gigantism. This disorder is caused in the majority of cases by hyperplasia of the eosinophilic cells of the pituitary. There is disproportionate growth in height and

Table 97.4: Dopamine agonist drugs		
Dopamine agonist drugs	**Dose orally**	**Side effects**
Bromocriptine	2.5–15 mg/day given in divided doses daily	Gastrointestinal intolerance, fatigue, postural hypotension and nasal blockage
Cabergoline	250–1,000 µg/week given as two doses in a week, maximum dose up to 3.5 mg/week	This is also an analogue of bromocriptine. Better than bromocriptine with fewer side effects, but more expensive, can be given weekly
Quinagolide	50–150 mg once daily	This is a nonergot drug
Pergolide	25–50 mg daily	Long acting ergot derivative with potency 100 times that of bromocriptine, side effects are few

Table 97.5: Causes of tall stature	
Nonendocrine causes	**Endocrine disorders**
• Constitutional tall stature • Genetic tall stature • Syndromes of tall stature • Cerebral gigantism • Marfan's syndrome • Homocystinuria • Beckwith-Wiedemann syndrome • XYY and XYYY syndromes	• Pituitary gigantism • Sexual precocity • Thyrotoxicosis • Infants of diabetic mothers • Klinefelter's syndrome

size. Maximal linear growth occurs in the bones of the extremities so that the arm span exceeds the height and the lower segment exceeds the upper segment (Table 97.5). Early during the disease, muscular hypertrophy and sexual precocity may be evident. Later, features of acromegaly may also develop. GH exerts its effect on tissue cells through the medium of IGFs.

Acromegaly

Acromegaly develops when GH excess develops after the fusion of the epiphyses. This is seen in adults, between the ages of 20 and 50 years. Both sexes are affected. The hormone level may go above 30 mU/L (normal 2 mU/L) (Figs 97.2 to 97.5).

Clinical Features

The onset is insidious. There is enlargement of soft tissues and bones of the hands, feet and skull. The face is elongated and the features are coarse. Lips, tongue, nose, salivary glands and lacrimal glands are enlarged. The mandible is prominent and prognathic. Growth of the mandible leads to separation of the lower incisors. The larynx is enlarged and the voice becomes husky. Thyroid may enlarge under the influence of GH, but there is no hyperfunction. During the active stage, excessive sweating occurs. Spine may show kyphosis, enlargement of vertebrae and osteoarthrosis.

Arthritis with hypertrophy and edema of periarticular tissues may occur around the peripheral joints. Bony prominence and attachments of muscles to bone become hypertrophied. Though the bones increase in thickness, unlike in gigantism, the length does not increase. There is generalized enlargement of all viscera. The changes in the heart include enlargement, specific cardiomyopathy and congestive cardiac failure. The nerves are also thickened which may lead to entrapment neuropathies such as carpal tunnel syndrome. Increase in collagen fibers in the nerves may result in peripheral neuropathy. Though the muscles are hypertrophied, they may be weak due to proximal myopathy. Glucose intolerance develops in 25–30% of cases and many proceed to overt DM. Males complain of loss of libido and impotence. Females develop amenorrhea. Gynecomastia and galactorrhea may be seen in some cases.

Course and Prognosis

The endocrine disturbances and local pressure effects progress in cases with pituitary tumors. Death occurs due

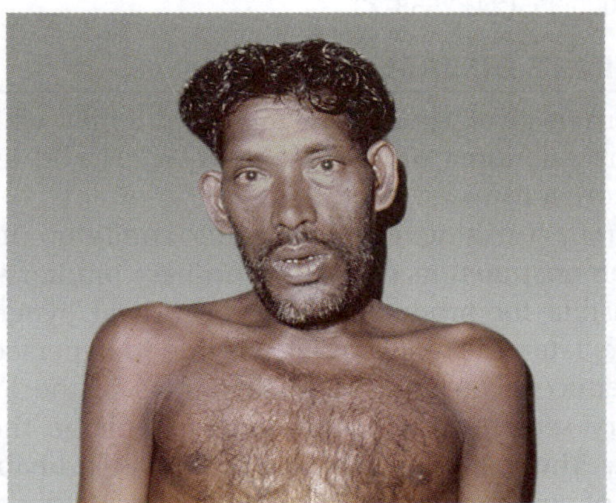

Fig. 97.2: Acromegaly male (45 years)

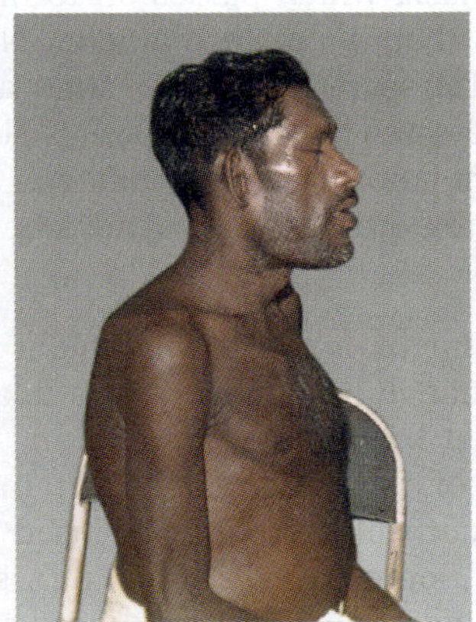

Fig. 97.3: Acromegaly male (side view). *Note:* Prognathic mandible

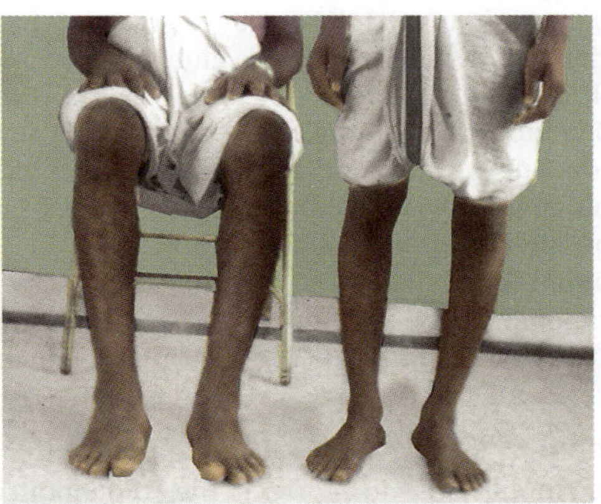

Fig. 97.4: Acromegaly large legs and feet. *Note:* Normal for comparison

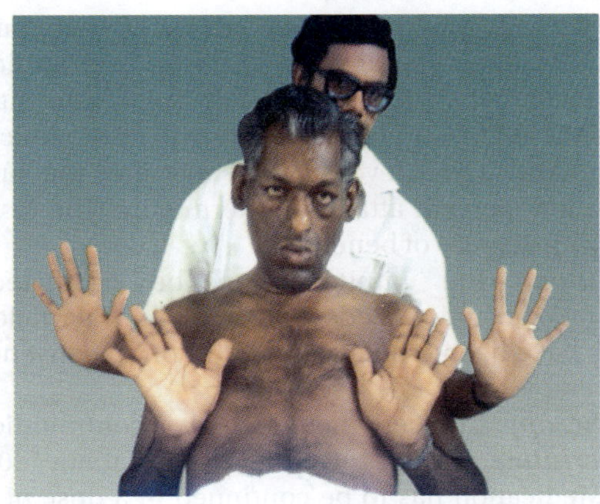

Fig. 97.5: Acromegaly large hands. *Note:* Normal for comparison

to raised intracranial tension, diabetic complications, cardiac failure or infections. The course depends on the nature of the pituitary tumor and its growth. In many cases, the conditions may burn out. Factors which contribute to increased mortality include higher prevalence of hypertension, diabetes, cardiomyopathy and sleep apnea.

Diagnosis

Acromegaly should be suspected clinically from the appearance of the patient. The diagnosis has to be established by investigations.

- *Imaging procedures:* X-ray of skull reveals enlargement of the sella turcica. Anterioposterior (AP) or transverse diameter of more than 16 mm is diagnostic of pituitary fossa widening. Prominence of the bony points of the skull and enlargement of the frontal air sinuses are suggestive points. X-ray of chest may reveal cardiomegaly. X-ray of mandible reveals separation of teeth especially incisors. Hands and feet show tufting of the phalanges and enlargement of soft tissues.

  CT or MRI gives definite localization of the lesions. MRI of pituitary with contrast administration is the most sensitive method for diagnosis. Adenomas greater than 2 mm in size can be visualized. More than 75% of patients with acromegaly have macroadenomas greater than 1 cm diameter at the time of diagnosis.

- *GH estimation:* Basal GH levels in blood are elevated. The diagnostic finding is the failure of suppression of GH levels by a glucose load. The patient undergoes an oral glucose tolerance test with 75–100 g glucose and blood is collected over 120 minutes. In normal subjects, the GH levels fall below 2 µg/L. The blood glucose and GH are estimated simultaneously. Other pituitary hormones may also show alterations like PRL, IGF and TSH.

- Estimation of IGF-1 is helpful. IGF-1 levels also correlate with the activity of the disease. Normal levels of IGF-1 range from 0.35 to 1.9 U/mL in men and 0.45 to 2.2 U/mL in women.

Treatment

Aim of therapy is to correct the biochemical and morphological abnormalities and remove the tumor if pressure effects are evident.

Surgery is the method of choice if there are no contraindications. Impairment of vision is an indication for urgent surgery. The GH levels fall rapidly after surgery. Trans-sphenoidal surgery is the treatment of choice, the GH level and IGH-1 level falling soon after the surgery. Forty to fifty percent attain long-term cure. The rest may get varying degrees of benefit.

Irradiation: The pituitary can be irradiated by implantation of radon seeds or yttrium. Alpha particles and protons have been employed in addition to conventional radiotherapy.

Drug therapy: In cases where surgery is contraindicated, *bromocriptine* reduces GH levels in about 50% of cases. Medication has to be continued in a dose of up to 10 mg/day for several months. Unlike in the case of prolactinomas, drug therapy is less effective than surgery. Hence its main role is in cases unsuitable for surgery or surgical failures.

Several newer modalities of drug therapy have been introduced recently. These include:

- *Somatostatin receptor ligands: Octreotide* which is a synthetic analogue of SS is 45 times more potent than the latter in inhibiting GH release. It is given in doses of 100–200 µg as SC injections 8 hourly. Continuous medication is required. Cholelithiasis is one of the major adverse side effects. The physical abnormalities regress with successful therapy. Though the diabetic state may improve, in many cases, it may persist in some. Total blindness may not recover. Complications like cardiomyopathy, DM and neuropathy can be avoided by early treatment. Other preparations include:
  - *Octreotide long-acting release (LAR)* 10–40 mg IM injection once in 4 weeks
  - *Lanreotide* 30 mg IM every 10–14 days or
  - *Lanreotide gel* 60–120 mg deep SC injection once in 4 weeks.
- *GH receptor antagonist: Pegvisomant* 10–40 mg SC injection daily. This is a pegylated GH analogue.
- *Dopamine agonists: Cabergoline* 1–4 mg oral weekly.

The choice of the preparation and monitoring of therapy are highly specialized procedures to be undertaken by trained endocrinologists.

Source: Melmed S. Medical progress: Acromegaly. N Engl J Med. 2006;355(24):2558-73.

CUSHING'S DISEASE

This term is given specifically to a condition in which the pituitary adenoma produces excess ACTH and leads to hypercortisolism.

Harvey Cushing described this condition in 1912 and demonstrated its cause as a primary pituitary tumor responsible for producing adrenal cortical hyperplasia, 20 years later. Cushing's disease is due to hypersecretion of adrenocorticotropin. Microadenomas of the anterior pituitary secrete ACTH. They do not enlarge the sella turcica. The pathological mechanism is probably the failure of negative feedback exerted by circulating cortisol on the hypothalamus. In most of the cases, the lesions start as hyperplasia which passes on to microadenomas which are less than 1 cm in diameter. Normal diurnal rhythm of ACTH secretion is abolished and the ACTH response to stress and hypovolemia is also lost.

Due to stimulation by ACTH, bilateral hyperplasia of the adrenal cortex and Cushing's syndrome result.

Treatment

The ideal treatment is trans-sphenoidal microadenectomy. An alternative line of therapy is bilateral adrenalectomy followed by pituitary irradiation. When surgery and irradiation of the pituitary are contraindicated, drugs which inhibit cortisol secretion are used (*metyrapone, ketoconazole*). Some cases of Cushing's syndrome due to ACTH secreting tumors of the pituitary may respond to *bromocriptine* or *cyproheptadine*.

In some cases of Cushing's disease, bilateral adrenalectomy may be followed by enlargement of the pituitary tumor and associated hyperpigmentation. This is called **Nelson's syndrome**.

Pituitary incidentalomas: The term incidentaloma refers to an incidentally detected lesion with no symptoms. Autopsy studies show an incidence of 10–20%.

HYPOPITUITARISM

When there is failure of one or more cell types of the pituitary to secrete normally, hypopituitarism results. It is unusual to get deficiencies of single hormones. More often several hormones are deficient. The condition commonly presents as dwarfism in children and as hypogonadism in adults.

Hypopituitarism may result from primary lesions of the pituitary or secondary to lesions of the hypothalamus (Box 97.3). Head injury, surgery, irradiation, chronic infections and tumors in the suprasellar region may lead to damage to the hypothalamus. Congenital lesions of the hypothalamus leading to diminution or absence of GnRH and GHRH may occur. **Kallmann's syndrome** is a congenital deficiency of LHRH associated with anosmia and demonstrable defects in midline neural structures. Sheehan's syndrome is hypopituitarism resulting from infarction of the adenohypophysis, usually precipitated by massive hemorrhage, particulary associated with hemorrhagic complications of pregnancy. Simmonds' disease described by Morris Simmonds a German Physician (1855–1925) is panhypopituitarism caused by complete atrophy of the adenohypophysis.

Adult Panhypopituitarism

Symptoms depend on the type and severity of cell failure, age of the patient and the age of onset of the disease. The condition becomes overt only when more than 75% of cells are destroyed. In panhypopituitarism, GH is affected first followed by gonadotropins, TSH and ACTH deficiency and consequent secondary adrenal deficiency occur only when the pituitary function is grossly affected. Hypoprolactinemia manifests only during the puerperium as failure of lactation.

Clinical Features

One of the common modes of presentation is **Sheehan's syndrome** in which the hyperplasic pituitary of pregnancy which is vulnerable for ischemic damage undergoes infarction due to postpartum hemorrhage and shock. The earliest manifestation is failure of lactation. The patient develops amenorrhea, genital atrophy, loss of axillary and pubic hair and loss of libido. Men with hypopituitarism present with testicular atrophy, loss of libido and absence of spermatogenesis. Failure of ACTH secretion leads to secondary adrenal cortical failure. As the hypopituitarism advances, thyroid hormone deficiency also manifests. It is rare to get classical myxedema. The symptoms of GH deficiency are usually evident clinically. The symptoms of GH deficiency include lack of strength due to reduction in muscle mass, increased insulin sensitivity and mild refractory anemia (Fig. 97.6).

Differential Diagnosis

Panhypopituitarism has to be differentiated from other causes of dwarfism, general debility and asthenia. In **anorexia nervosa,** which affects young women between the age of 15 and 30 years, may mimic hypopituitarism. In **anorexia nervosa,** all the pituitary hormones except GH are decreased. With weight loss of more than 20%, amenorrhea may also develop. Unlike hypopituitarism, the pubic and axillary hairs are retained. Moreover, emaciation is more suggestive of **anorexia nervosa** (*See* Fig. 97.1).

Box 97.3: Etiology of hypopituitarism

- **Developmental/structural causes**
  - Transcription factor defect, pituitary dysplasia/aplasia
  - Congenital CNS mass, encephalocele
  - Primary empty sella syndrome
- Congenital hypothalamic disorders (septo-optic dysplasia, Prader-Willi syndrome, Laurence-Moon-Biedl syndrome, Kallmann's syndrome)
- **Traumatic**
  - Surgical resection
  - Radiation damage
  - Head injuries
- **Neoplastic**
  - Pituitary adenoma
  - Parasellar masses (meningioma, germinoma, ependymoma and glioma)
  - Rathke's cyst
  - Craniopharyngioma
  - Hypothalamic hamartoma, gangliocytoma
  - Pituitary metastases (breast, lung, colon, carcinoma)
  - Lymphoma and leukemia
  - Meningioma
- **Infiltrative/inflammatory diseases:** Hemochromatosis, lymphocytic hypophysitis, sarcoidosis, histiocytosis X, granulomatous hypophysitis
- **Vascular causes**
  - Pituitary apoplexy
  - Sheehan's syndrome due to massive intrapartum hemorrhage resulting in pituitary infarction
  - Sickle cell disease
- Atrophy of the pituitary—Simmonds' disease
- **Infections**
  - Fungal (histoplasmosis)
  - Parasitic (toxoplasmosis)
  - Tuberculosis
  - Pneumocystis carinii

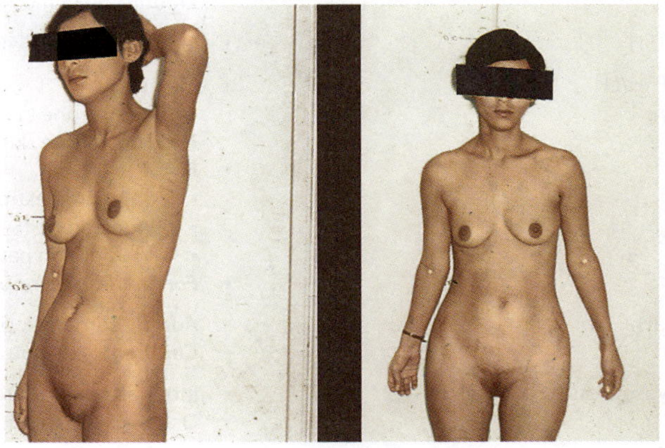

Fig. 97.6: Sheehan's syndrome. **Note:** The absence of hair in the axilla and pubic region

Textbook of Medicine

Investigations

The diagnosis of panhypopituitarism is established by estimating the pituitary hormones and the hormones of the target glands.

Stimulation tests reveal the functional integrity of the target glands.

- **ACTH:** When adrenal response to ACTH is established, insulin induced hypoglycemia may be used to test the pituitary reserve of ACTH. If plasma cortisol rises above 20 µg/dL following insulin, there is normal reserve of ACTH in pituitary.
- **Thyroid-stimulating hormone reserve:** This can be easily assessed by administration of TRH. This could also elucidate the PRL secretory status of pituitary.

Management

This consists of replacement of the hormones of the target organs.

Cortisol deficiency is corrected with 12.5–25 mg of cortisol or its equivalent of other synthetic steroids. Glucocorticoids should be replaced before supplementation of thyroxine and gonadotropins in order to avoid the development of adrenal crisis. Glucocorticoid replacement should be increased during periods of acute stress like operations and infections. Mineralocorticoid replacement is not usually needed since this hormone is not markedly deficient in hypopituitarism. Thyroid replacement is best achieved with synthetic thyroxine started in a dose of 50–100 mg/day and raised to a dose of 150–200 µg slowly.

Testosterone replacement improves vigor, vitality, and libido. The oral preparation is methyl testosterone. Alternatively, testosterone can be given IM as depot injections. Estrogens and progesterone therapy prevent atrophy of breasts and vaginal mucosa and also osteoporosis. **Gonadotropin therapy:** Gonadotropin replacement is essential for return of ovulation and spermatogenesis. Short courses of admixture of FSH and LH (menotropins) followed by hCGs are used to induce ovulation (Table 97.6 and Box 97.4).

Box 97.4: Replacement therapy for adult hypopituitarism

- **Adrenocorticotropic hormone:** Hydrocortisone 10–20 mg daily in divided doses
- **Follicle-stimulating hormone/luteinizing hormone**
- **Female patients**
  - Conjugated estrogen 0.65 mg/day
  - Micronized estradiol 1 mg/day
  - Ethinyl estradiol 0.02–0.05 mg/day
  - Estradiol skin patch 4–8 mg twice weekly
  - Estradiol plus testosterone
- **Male patients**
  - Testosterone enanthate 200 mg IM every 2–3 weeks
  - Testosterone skin patch 2.5–5.0 mg/day; can increase dose up to 7.5 mg/day
  - Testosterone gel 3–6 g daily
- **Growth hormone**
  - **Adults:** Somatotropin 0.2–1.0 mg SC daily
  - **Children:** Somatotropin 0.02–0.05 mg/kg/day
- **Thyroid-stimulating hormone:** l-Thyroxine 0.05–0.2 mg daily according to T_4 levels
- **Vasopressin**
  - Intranasal desmopressin-rhinal tube 5–20 µg twice daily
  - Oral DDAVP 300–600 µg daily, usually in divided doses

Protracted hypopituitarism can lead to premature atherosclerosis and increase in cardiovascular mortality.

Source: Kovacs K. Sheehan syndrome. Lancet. 2003;361 (9356):520-2.

Childhood Hypopituitarism

Hypopituitarism starting in childhood presents with a wide spectrum of disorders such as dwarfism (GH deficiency), hypogonadism (LH and FSH deficiency), hypothyroidism (TSH deficiency) or a combination of these.

Etiology

In general, the etiological factors operating in adults are seen in children as well. In addition, hypopituitarism may be part of a general abnormality in the CNS like absent septum pellucidum. GH deficiency may develop as a familial trait transmitted as an autosomal recessive disorder. Vaginal breech delivery may be complicated

---

Table 97.6: The details of pituitary hormone therapy

Hormone deficit	Hormone replacement
ACTH	• Hydrocortisone (10–20 mg AM; 10 mg PM) • Cortisone acetate (25 mg AM; 12.5 mg PM) • Prednisone (5 mg AM; 2.5 mg PM)
TSH	• L-thyroxine (0.075–0.15 mg daily)

FSH/LH	• Males
	  ▪ Testosterone enanthate (200 mg IM every 2 weeks)
	  ▪ Testosterone skin patch (5 mg/d)
	• Females
	  ▪ Conjugated estrogen (0.65–125 mg qd for 25 days)
	  ▪ Progesterone (5–10 mg qd on days 16–25)
	  ▪ Estradiol skin patch (0.5 mg, every other day)
	• **For fertility:** Menopausal gonadotropins, hCG

GH	• **Adults:** Somatotropin (0.3–1.0 mg SC qd) • **Children:** Somatotropin (0.02–0.05 mg/kg per day)
Vasopressin	• Intranasal desmopressin (5–20 mg twice daily) • Oral 300–600 mg qd

Abbreviations: GH = Growth hormone; TSH = Thyroid-stimulating hormone; TRH = Thyrotropin-releasing hormone; ACTH = Adrenocorticotropic hormone; FSH = Follicle-stimulating hormone; LH = Luteinizing hormone; IM = Intramuscular; SC = Subcutaneous; hCG = Human chorionic gonadotropin

by GH deficiency in the child as a result of mechanical distortion of the skull and consequent damage to the pituitary stalk.

Clinical Features

The child is normal at birth. Growth retardation is evident at the age of 2–3 years when the growth rate falls to 50% of the normal. Such children are obese with abnormal, deposition of body fat. When there is associated hypothyroidism, retardation of bone growth is more severe. In spite of growth retardation, these children have normal intelligence, but they may develop psychological disturbances due to their physical appearance. Hypogonadism leads to delay in the fusion of epiphyses. Such children continue to grow for longer periods, thus attaining taller stature than children whose gonadal function is normal.

Hypopituitarism has to be distinguished from other common causes of growth retardation. Pathological causes of dwarfism include malnutrition, severe systemic illnesses, malabsorption state, skeletal disorders, corticosteroid therapy and deprivation dwarfism. Deprivation dwarfism occurs in children brought up in family circumstances under great stress, especially without maternal care.

DWARFISM

This is defined as shortness of stature that is below the third percentile for children of similar age and ethnic group. Genetic and environmental factors influence growth. This is a common problem in pediatric practice. In many cases short stature is seen in families without any demonstrable pathology. Pathologically dwarfism may result from several groups of conditions (Fig. 97.7 and Table 97.7).

- **Major constitutional disorders:** Generalized malnutrition, rickets, malabsorption states, congenital cyanotic heart disease, severe respiratory, hepatic or renal disease and long-term corticosteroid therapy.
- **Inherited and genetic disorders:** Achondroplasia, fragilitas ossium, aminoacidurias, other metabolic defects, Turner's syndrome, pseudohypoparathyroidism and renal tubular acidosis.
- **Endocrine disorders:** Cretinism, juvenile hypothyroidism, adrenogenital syndrome, precocious puberty, hypopituitarism, hypothalamic disturbances, idiopathic hypoparathyroidism. The term **Fröhlich's syndrome (dystrophia adiposo genitalis)** refers to

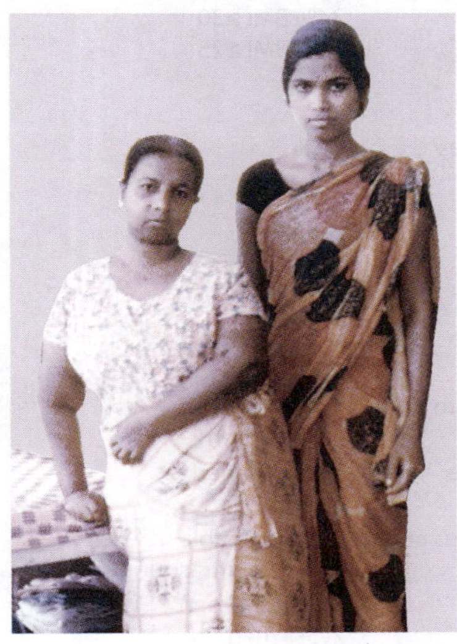

Fig. 97.7: Dwarf normal age-matched woman for comparison (30 years)

Table 97.7: Causes of short stature	
Nonendocrine causes	**Endocrine disorders**

• Constitutional short stature
• Familial short stature
• Genetic short stature
• Intrauterine growth retardation and SGA
• **Syndromes of short stature**
  ▪ Turner's syndrome and its variants
  ▪ Noonan's syndrome
  ▪ Prader-Willi syndrome
  ▪ Laurence-Moon and Bardet-Biedl syndromes
• **Chronic disease**
  ▪ Cardiac disorders (left-to-right shunt, congestive heart failure)
  ▪ Pulmonary disorders (cystic fibrosis, asthma)
  ▪ **Gastrointestinal disorders:** Malabsorption (e.g. celiac disease)
  ▪ **Hematologic disorders**
    – Sickle cell anemia
    – Thalassemia
  ▪ **Renal disorders**
    – Renal tubular acidosis
    – Chronic uremia
  ▪ **Immunologic disorders**
    – Connective tissue disease
    – Juvenile rheumatoid arthritis
  ▪ **Chronic infection (TB)**
• Malnutrition
• Voluntary dieting
• Anorexia nervosa
• Cancer chemotherapy
	• **GH deficiency and variants**
	  ▪ Congenital GH deficiency
	  ▪ With midline defects
	  ▪ With other pituitary hormone deficiencies
	  ▪ Isolated GH deficiency
	  ▪ Pituitary agenesis
	  ▪ Acquired GH deficiency
	  ▪ Hypothalamic-pituitary tumors
	  ▪ Histiocytosis X
	  ▪ Central nervous system infections
	  ▪ Head injuries
	  ▪ GH deficiency following cranial irradiation
	  ▪ Central nervous system vascular accidents
	  ▪ Hydrocephalus
	    – Empty sella syndrome
	    – Abnormalities of GH action
	• GH insensitivity (Laron's dwarfism)
	• Pygmies
	• Psychosocial dwarfism
	• Hypothyroidism
	• Glucocorticoid excess (Cushing's syndrome)
	• Pseudohypoparathyroidism
	• Disorders of vitamin D metabolism
	• Diabetes mellitus (DM), uncontrolled
	• Diabetes insipidus, untreated

Abbreviations: GH = Growth hormone; SGA = Small for gestational age; TB = Tuberculosis

Textbook of Medicine

the combination of dwarfism, obesity, hypogonadism and diabetes insipidus and is produced by craniopharyngioma or chromophobe adenoma.

- ***Psychogenic dwarfism or deprivation dwarfism:*** This is probably an emotionally-mediated disorder unassociated with malnutrition, in which maternal deprivation leads to a selective deficiency of GH. Provision of maternal care and emotional support improves GH levels and promotes growth.
- ***Laron's dwarfism:*** This is an autosomal recessive disorder characterized by small face and mandible, prominent forehead, saddle nose, discoloration of teeth, sparse hair, retarded growth of hair and teeth, and small hands and feet. Serum GH levels are increased, but IGF are lower than normal. Receptor insensitivity is the mechanism underlying this disorder.

Investigation and Treatment

Management of a case of dwarfism depends upon the clinical findings and endocrine investigations (Table 97.8).

When dwarfism is due to deficiency of GH, the treatment of choice is human recombinant growth hormone given

Table 97.8: Prevalence of endocrine and metabolic disorders in the adults with dwarfism

Disorder	Approximate prevalence in adults[a]	Screening/testing recommendations[b]
Obesity	34% BMI ≥30 68% BMI ≥25	• Calculate BMI • Measure waist circumference • Exclude secondary causes • Consider comorbid complications
Type 2 diabetes mellitus	>7%	Beginning at age of 45 years, screen every 3 years or earlier in high-risk groups: • Fasting plasma glucose (FPG) >126 mg/dL • Random plasma glucose >200 mg/dL • An elevated HbA1C • Consider comorbid complications
Hyperlipidemia	20–25%	• Cholesterol screening at least every 5 years; more often in high-risk groups • Lipoprotein analysis (LDL, HDL) for increased cholesterol, CAD, diabetes • Consider secondary causes
Hypothyroidism	5–10% women 0.5–2% men	• TSH; confirm with free T_4 • Screen women after age 35 and every 5 years thereafter
Graves' disease	1–3% women 0.1% men	TSH, free T_4
Thyroid nodules and neoplasia	2–5% palpable >25% by ultrasound	• Physical examination of thyroid • Fine-needle aspiration biopsy
Osteoporosis	5–10% women 2–5% men	• Bone mineral density measurements in women >65 years or in postmenopausal women or men at risk • Exclude secondary causes
Hyperparathyroidism	0.1–0.5% women > men	• Serum calcium PTH, if calcium is elevated • Assess comorbid conditions
Infertility	10% couples	• Investigate both members of couple • Semen analysis in male • Assess ovulatory cycles in female • Specific tests as indicated
Polycystic ovarian syndrome	5–10% women	• Free testosterone, DHEA-S • Consider comorbid conditions
Hirsutism	5–10%	• Free testosterone, DHEA-S • Exclude secondary causes • Additional tests as indicated
Menopause	Median age 51 years	FSH
Hyperprolactinemia	15% in women with amenorrhea or galactorrhea	PRL level MRI, if not medication-related
Erectile dysfunction	20–30%	• Careful history, PRL, testosterone • Consider secondary causes (e.g. diabetes)
Gynecomastia	15%	• Often, no tests are indicated • Consider Klinefelter's syndrome • Consider medications, hypogonadism, liver disease
Klinefelter's syndrome	0.2% men	• Karyotype • Testosterone
Vitamin D deficiency	10%	Measure serum 25-OH vitamin D; consider secondary causes
Turner's syndrome	0.03% women	Karyotype; consider comorbid conditions

[a] The prevalence of most disorders varies among ethnic groups and with aging. Data based primarily on the United States population.

[b] See individual chapters for additional information on evyaluation and treatment. Early testing is indicated in patients with signs and symptoms of disease and in those at increased risk.

Abbreviations: BMI = Body mass index; LDL = Low-density lipoprotein; HDL = High-density lipoprotein; CAD = Coronary artery disease; HbA1C = Hemoglobin A1C; TSH = Thyroid-stimulating hormone; PTH = Parathyroid hormone; DHEA-S = Dehydroepiandrosterone sulfate; FSH = Follicle-stimulating hormone; PRL = Prolactin; MRI = Magnetic resonance imaging

in a dose of 0.02–0.2 IU/kg twice a week or 150–300 ug IM injection daily. GH therapy has different goals in children and adults. In children it increases linear growth, restores body composition and improves the quality of life and self-image. In adults, the main effects are restoration of body composition, reduction of fat tissue, improvement of muscular and cardiac function, beneficial effects on serum lipids and improvement in the quality of life.

Side effects include arthralgia, myalgia and edema. Initial spurt of growth is remarkable and a linear growth of 12–15 cm may be obtained in 1 year, but the growth rate slows down later and at this stage higher doses of hormone are needed.

Concurrent use of anabolic steroids helps to improve growth and bring about a positive anabolic response. Commercially available GH is prepared by recombinant deoxyribonucleic acid (DNA) technique or synthetic processes.

EMPTY SELLA SYNDROME

Syn: Subdiaphragm cistern, Intrasellar-subarachnoid space, Intrasellar cyst

This is a rare disorder in which the pituitary fossa is enlarged with accumulation of cerebrospinal fluid (CSF) at the expense of pituitary tissue, which may be reduced to a small remnant. The condition may be primary in which anatomical defects occur in the diaphragm sellae or secondary to surgery or irradiation in the region of the pituitary. The suprasellar subarachnoid space herniates through defects in the diaphragm sellae. The sella turcica becomes filled with CSF enclosed in an arachnoid-lined sac. This causes pressure effects on the pituitary stalk resulting in hyperprolactinemia and galactorrhea.

Diagnosis

The condition may be associated with normal endocrine profile in 60% of cases. In 40% of cases GH response to stimuli and levels of gonadotropins may be reduced.

X-ray skull may show either a normal sella or an enlarged sella with thinned out dorsum sellae. Bony erosion is absent. The diagnosis is confirmed by air-encephalography which shows absence of diaphragm sellae and presence of CSF in the sella turcica. CT scan with metrizamide cisternography or MRI confirms the diagnosis.

Treatment

Hormonal replacement is undertaken if endocrine deficiency exists.

Pineal Gland and its Disorders

KP Poulose, B Jayakumar

Chapter Summary
- General Considerations
- Disorders

GENERAL CONSIDERATIONS

Syn: Pineal body

The pineal gland, or epiphysis cerebri, a neuroendocrine organ, is one of the major parts of the cardiac system, which also includes the eyes and the suprachiasmatic nuclei of the hypothalamus. The pineal gland exerts important regulatory influences by secreting its hormone, melatonin, in variable amounts, depending on the time of the day, the animal's age and in some species, the time of year. The daily rhythm in circulating melatonin is characterized by very low concentrations during the day and high levels at night. This rhythm persists in constant darkness but can be altered by night-time light exposure, because light can actually suppress melatonin production. Normally, daily variations in melatonin secretion synchronize numerous body rhythms and, in diurnal species, probably are important for night-time sleep initiation and maintenance. Since the onset and offset of melatonin production by pineal gland occur at dusk and dawn, respectively, the length of time per 24-hour period that plasma melatonin levels are elevated can synchronize physiologic processes to seasonal changes and, in seasonal animals, can affect season-dependent functions, such as body temperature, locomotor activity and reproductive behavior.

Anatomy

The pineal gland which weighs 120 mg lies beneath the posterior border of the corpus callosum and between the superior colliculi. Embryologically, it develops from the ependyma lining the roof of the third ventricle.

Two types of cells are found in the pineal gland: (1) Pinealocytes which form the majority and (2) neuroglial cells. The pinealocytes produce indoleamines mainly ***melatonin*** and peptides such as vasotocin. Melatonin diffuses into the bloodstream. Secretion increases soon after the onset of darkness, peaks between 2 AM and 4 AM and falls off thereafter.

In infancy, melatonin levels are high (325 pg/mL). They fall off with age to 10–60 pg/mL in young adults. Exposure to light inhibits secretion. The effects on tissues are receptor mediated. Possible physiological effects of melatonin include:
- Hypnotic—increased propensity to sleep
- Control of circadian rhythm, e.g. temperature regulation

Textbook of Medicine

- Possible role in cyclical mood changes
- Sexual activity and reproductive function
- Antiproliferative action in cancer
- Enhancement of the immune response
- Modulation of aging response and protection of cells and damage.

Diminished levels of melatonin may be associated with acceleration of the aging process.

In addition to melatonin, three hypothalamic hormones [thyrotropin-releasing hormone (TRH) luteinizing-hormone-releasing hormone (LHRH) and somatostatin] and an octapeptide, arginine vasotocin (AVT) (vasopressin), have also been detected in the pineal gland. During infancy, the pineal gland is relatively large. With age, it involutes.

Clinical Implications

The pineal gland, through the rhythmic secretion of its hormone, melatonin, is part of a complex neuroendocrine mechanism that controls the temporal organization of physiologic, biochemical and behavioral processes within the organism and synchronizes the patterns of their activities to that of environmental cycles. The characteristic time course of nocturnal melatonin secretion, together with the somnogenic effect of exogenous melatonin in physiologic doses, underlies its involvement in processes that generate normal sleep and its potential use as a treatment of insomnias, including difficulty in falling or remaining asleep.

DISORDERS

Calcification

This occurs in the matrix of ground substance secreted by pinealocytes. Calcification begins in early childhood and is completed by about puberty. Calcification is not associated with any functional disturbance.

Tumors

The pineal may be a seat of tumors. These may be pinealoma, teratoma, glial tumors or vascular tumors.

Tumors lead to mechanical effects due to pressure and endocrine disturbances. Pressure effects include rise in intracranial tension, internal hydrocephalus due to pressure on the aqueduct of Sylvius, and paralysis of upward gaze due to oculomotor involvement (Parinaud's syndrome). Ataxia, visual disturbances and signs of hypopituitarism may occur.

Endocrine disturbances manifest as abnormalities of sexual maturation such as sexual precocity, delayed puberty and hypogonad states, evidence of hypothalamic involvement like diabetes insipidus (DI), polyphagia, somnolence, obesity or behavioral disturbances are seen in 70% of patients with pinealomas and precocious puberty.

Treatment

Surgical treatment is beneficial in trained hands, though the procedure is difficult. Pineal tumors are partially radiosensitive and irradiation is effective. Chemotherapy with carboplatin, etoposide, vincristine and bleomycin has also been found to be successful. Prognosis is good with a 5-year survival of 70–85%.

CHAPTER
99

Thyroid and its Disorders

KP Poulose, B Jayakumar

Chapter Summary

- General Considerations
- Goiter
- Hyperthyroidism
  - Diffuse Toxic Goiter
- Hypothyroidism
  - Cretinism
- Myxedema
- Thyroid Hormone Resistance Syndrome (THRS)
- Thyroiditis
- Solitary Thyroid Nodule
- Tumors of the Thyroid

GENERAL CONSIDERATIONS

At present, thyroid diseases are the second most common endocrine disorders in India next only to diabetes mellitus (DM). If asymptomatic endemic goiter is also included, thyroid diseases may even rank as the most common endocrine disease. The prevalence of iodine deficiency disorders (IDD) is very high. With the introduction of iodized salt, the prevalence of IDD is coming down.

Anatomy

The thyroid gland weighs 15–25 g, and it is made up of an isthmus and two lateral lobes. The isthmus lies just below the cricoid cartilage. The gland lies deep to the strap muscles of the neck enclosed in the pretracheal fascia which anchors it to the trachea, so that the thyroid moves up on swallowing. The width and length of isthmus averages 20 mm, thickness 2–6 mm. The lateral lobes from superior to inferior pole measure 40 mm, breadth is 15–20 mm and thickness 20–39 mm. The parathyroid glands which are four in number are embedded in the substance or sheath of the thyroid, behind the lateral lobes. The thyroid develops as early as the third or fourth week of gestation. The thyroid is formed as an outgrowth on the ventral wall of the pharynx in association with the parathyroids which are derived from the third and fourth branchial arch. The 'C' cells which produce calcitonin are formed from the cells of the ultimobranchial body. Persistence of the remnants of the thyroid stalk may give rise to the pyramidal lobe, which lies just to the left of the midline extending upwards from the isthmus or to thyroglossal cyst. Failure of the thyroid stalks to descend results in the formation of lingual thyroid.

In the fetus, the thyroid hormones are synthesized under the influence of thyroid-stimulating hormone (TSH) only by about the 11th or 12th week of gestation. Hence, in the first trimester, the fetus is totally dependent on maternal thyroxine. For proper development of mental and motor skills, adequate thyroid hormone concentration is necessary, whose synthesis depends on the availability of maternal iodine status. Initially, there is synthesis of thyroxine (T4) only in the fetus (TSH dependent) and inactive tri-iodothyronine (reverse T3) is formed from T4. ***Iodine metabolism and hormone synthesis:*** The average Indian diet contains variable quantities of iodine ranging from very low values to more than 200 µg/day. Ingested iodine is reduced to iodide in the gastrointestinal tract (GIT) and absorbed throughout the gut, the maximum being in the small intestine. Thyroid traps this iodine.

Daily dietary requirement of iodine varies with age
- Children < 5 years of age   90 µg
- 6–12 years   120 µg
- > 12 years   150 µg
- Pregnancy and lactation   200 µg

In iodine deficiency, the level of iodine in urine is less than 100 µg/L.

Iodine uptake is mediated by sodium-iodide symporter (NIS) against a concentration gradient which is expressed at the basolateral margins of the cell. NIS also transports ClO_4^- (chlorate) and SCN^- (thiocyanate) and $^{99m}TcO_4^-$ (pertechnetate). Another protein involved in iodine transport in pendrin, which is a product of PDS gene. Iodine is oxidized by the enzyme thyroid peroxidase (TPO) followed by iodination of tyrosine molecules in thyroglobulin (Tg). Monoiodotyrosines (MIT) and diiodotyrosines (DIT) are then coupled to form T4 and T3 with the help of TPO. There are many molecules (3–4) of T4 in each Tg molecule, while only one-fifth of Tg molecule contain T3. T3 and T4 are released from Tg by proteolytic enzymes while the uncoupled MIT and DIT are recycled back to iodine by deiodination.

About 90% of the total body iodine is in the thyroid gland.

T4 and T3 are formed by sequential reactions occurring in the Tg molecule under the control of TSH. The follicular cells synthesize Tg and store it within the follicles as colloid. This colloid acts as a reservoir of thyroid hormones. ***Release of thyroid hormones from Tg:*** The follicular cells take up Tg colloid droplets and release T3 and T4 by their degradation. The Tg molecule is split by proteases and peptidases into T3 and T4 which are released into circulation and this is controlled by TSH. The total T4

Table 99.1: Binding of thyroid hormones to various protein fractions in blood%

	TBG	TBA	TTH
T4	68	20	11
T3	69	11	9

Note: 3–6% of plasma T3/T4 are bound to lipoproteins. TBG affinity for T4 is 20 times more than that for T3.

Abbreviations: TBG = Thyroid-binding globulin; TBA = Thyroid binding albumin; TTH = Transthyretin

secretion is about 60–120 µg and T3 is 20–30 µg per day. In the peripheral tissues, T4 is converted into T3. Eighty percent of circulating T3 is derived from deiodination of T4 in the peripheral tissues and the rest from the thyroid gland. The turnover of T4 from Tg is only 1% per day and thus the large store of hormone provides prolonged protection against disorders of thyroid hormone synthesis. Total T4 stored in the thyroid gland is about 500 µg while the total body pool is only l mg (1000 µg).

Plasma transport: Around 75% of T4 circulates in blood bound to ***thyroxine-binding globulin*** (TBG) which is an alpha-globulin, 15% is bound to pre-albumin, now called ***transthyretin (TTR)*** and the rest to albumin (Table 99.1). T3 also remains bound to TBG in the plasma. The plasma level of T4 is 5–10 µg/dL and that of T3 is 150–250 ng/dL. The sum total of T4 and T3 bound to the carrier protein is referred to as plasma protein-bound iodine (PBI). The normal range is 4–8 µg/dL. In serum, the free T4 is 0.03% of total T4 and free T3 is 0.3% total T3. The levels of T4 and T3 are regulated by the TSH from the anterior pituitary and thyrotropin-releasing hormone (TRH) from hypothalamus. Rising levels of thyroid hormones inhibit TSH secretion. Both T4 and T3 are deiodinated in the cells by the microsomal enzymes (deiodinases types 1, 2 and 3) and the iodides are excreted in urine (70 µg/day). T3 is bound to specific nuclear DNA thyroid hormone receptors and it is carried by cystosolic binding proteins into the cell nucleus.

Deiodinases are expressed in liver, kidney, pituitary and thyroid. The metabolic effects of thyroid hormone are initiated by the binding of T3 to the nuclear receptors. T3 has 15-fold higher binding affinity to intranuclear receptors compared to T4.

Actions of Thyroid Hormones

- Increases cellular oxidation in all tissues
- Increase of protein breakdown
- Increases the turnover of carbohydrates and lipids
- Calcium is mobilized from bone
- The cardiovascular effects consist mainly of increase in heart rate and cardiac output.

Calcitonin

It is a 32 amino acid peptide hormone formed in the parafollicular cells (C cells) of the thyroid. It inhibits bone resorption and release of calcium from bone, thereby helping to lower calcium levels in blood. Catabolism of bone is significantly reduced. Levels of calcitonin increase during hypercalcemia and the secretion stops when the calcium levels fall. High levels of calcitonin are seen in

Textbook of Medicine

patients with medullary carcinoma of the thyroid, however, in this condition there is no hypocalcemia. Human calcitonin gene is located in the short arm of chromosome 11. Glucocorticoids, glucagon and gastrin increase calcitonin secretion. It is also secreted by insulinomas, Vasoactive Intestinal Peptide Tumor (VIPoma) and some lung tumors. Calcitonin has therapeutic use in the management of acute hypercalcemia, osteoporosis, and Paget's disease of bone.

Calcitonin Gene-related Peptide (CGRP)

This is a 37 amino acid peptide formed from the pre-procalcitonin gene located on chromosome 11. Final targets of action of this peptide are the C-cells of the thyroid and neural tissue. In the C-cells, the product is calcitonin, whereas in neural tissue the product is pro-CGRP, which is a neurotransmitter influencing the sensory system. It is also a very powerful vasodilator which is concerned with the regulation of regional blood flow.

ASSESSMENT OF THYROID FUNCTION

Clinical examination is most valuable in all cases. Though several classic features such as lid lag and thyroid bruit specifically point to florid hyperthyroidism, in marginal cases, the clinical symptomatology shows considerable overlap with normals or other nonthyroid disorders. Many tests are available to assess thyroid function but no single test is totally satisfactory.

Thyroid Function Tests

Isotopic Tests

- Estimation of T3, T4 and TSH by radioimmunoassay (RIA) or enzyme-linked immunosorbent assay (ELISA)
- Estimation of free T3 and T4
- TRH stimulation test
- Thyroid scan ^{131}I, ^{125}I and TCO$_4$
- ^{131}I uptake studies, TSH stimulation and T3 suppression tests. These are seldom done at present.

Nonisotopic Tests

- T3, T4, TSH can also be assessed by ELISA tests
- Estimation of thyroid autoantibodies and serum Tg
- Perchlorate discharge test
- Imaging procedures of the neck, ultrasound scan (USS), computed tomography (CT), magnetic resonance imaging (MRI) and positron emission tomography (PET) scan
- Biopsy of thyroid—fine-needle aspiration cytology (FNAC) or open biopsy.

Radioactive iodine uptake test: The amount of radioactivity concentrated by the thyroid, following oral administration of ^{131}I, after 2 and 24 hours is measured. In Indians, the normal ranges are 10 ± 5% at 2 hours and 42 ± 7% at 24 hours. The uptake values are high in hyperthyroidism and are low in hypothyroidism. Since this test is likely to be altered in several nonthyroidal diseases, and by drugs containing iodides, this is not routinely done except under special circumstances. These include:

- Factitious hyperthyroidism
- Acute and subacute thyroiditis

Table 99.2: Alteration of T3, T4 and TSH values in common thyroid disorders

Total or free	T3	T4	TSH
Graves' disease	High	High	Low
T3-toxicosis	High	Normal	Low
Primary hypothyroidism	Low	Low	Very high
Secondary and tertiary hypothyroidism	Low	Low	Low

Abbreviations: T3 = Tri-iodothyronine; T4 = Thyroxine; TSH = Thyroid stimulating hormone

Table 99.3: Results of various isotopic tests in thyroid disorders

Diseases	RAIU	T4 (RIA)	T3 (RIA)	TSH
Graves' disease	H	H	H	L
Iodine deficiency—goiter	H	N	N/M	N
Primary hypothyroidism	L	L	L	H
Suprathyroidal hypothyroidism	L	L	L	L
Subacute thyroiditis	L	N/H	N/H	N/L
Factitious hyperthyroidism	L	H	H if T3 is taken	L
T3 toxicosis	H/N	N	H	L

Abbreviations: RAIU = Radioactive iodine uptake; RIA = Radioimmune assay; N = Normal; H = High; M = Marginal change; L = Low

- Hashitoxicosis
- For calculating the therapeutic dose of ^{131}I in thyrotoxicosis.

Normally, iodine uptake is suppressed by exogenous administration of T3 or T4. In Graves' disease (primary hyperthyroidism), T3 and T4 fail to suppress iodine uptake. In hypothyroidism, in order to identify the site of lesion as the thyroid, pituitary or hypothalamus, the effect of TSH or TRH respectively on iodine uptake by the thyroid is studied. In primary hypothyroidism, the values do not change, whereas in pituitary or hypothalamic disease, the iodine uptake is increased by TSH or TRH, respectively (Tables 99.2 and 99.3).

Estimation of T4, T3 and TSH: These hormones can be directly estimated by RIA or ELISA. The total plasma level of T4 is 4–8 µg/dL and T3 is 150–250 ng/dL. Normal range of TSH is up to 5 µIU/mL.

Free T3/T4 estimation: The values of total serum T3 and T4 may be altered by many drugs, which interfere with TBG binding (estrogen increases, androgen decreases) and in conditions like pregnancy and hypoproteinemic states. In these situations, free hormone concentrations correlate better with the metabolic state than the total hormone concentrations because they are unaffected by changes in binding protein concentration or affinity. Free T3/T4 is the preferred test now and can be measured by RIA/ELISA.

Table 99.4 shows the thyroid function tests and their normal values.

Table 99.4: Thyroid function tests and their normal values

Test	Abbreviation	Typical ranges
Serum thyroxine	T4	4.6–12 µg/dL
Free thyroxine fraction	FT4F	0.03–0.005%
Free thyroxine	FT4	0.7–1.9 ng/dL
Thyroid hormone binding ratio	THBR	0.9–1.1
Free thyroxine index	FT4I	4–11
Serum tri-iodothyronine	T3	80–180 µg/dL
Free tri-iodothyronine I	FT3	230–619 pg/dL
Free T3 index	FT3I	80–180
Radioactive iodine uptake	RAIU	10–30%
Serum thyrotropin	TSH	0.5–6 mIU/mL
Thyroxine-binding globulin	TBG	12–20 µg/dL T4 +1.8 µg
TRH stimulation test peak	TSH	9–30 µIU/mL at 20–30 min
Serum thyroglobulin I	Tg	0–30 ng/mL
Thyroid microsomal antibody titer	TMAb (TPO) AMA	Varies with method
Thyroglobulin antibody titer	TgAb (ATg)	Varies with method

Abbreviations: AMA = Antimicrosomal antibody; ATg = Antithyroglobulin antibody; (AMA and TPO are the same); TPO = Thyroid peroxidase; TRH = Thyrotropin-releasing hormone

Commonly Observed Thyroid Function Tests Abnormalities in Practice

FT4↑, FT3↑, TSH↓	Graves' toxic multinodular goiter (MNG), toxic adenoma, excess thyroid ingestion, thyroiditis (postpartum, postviral) drugs (camiodarone, iodides), gestational hyperthyroidism.
FT4↓, FT3↓, TSH↑	Hypothyroidism (post-surgical, post iodine therapy, drugs [lithium, antithyroid drugs (ATDs)], amiodarone, neck irradiation, congenital hypothyroidism, Riedel's thyroiditis
FT4 and FT3 ↔ TSH↑	Subclinical hypothyroidism, poor compliance with T4, TSH resistance, T4 malabsorption, drugs (amiodarone), nonthyroidal illness
FT4↓, FT3 ↔ TSH↓	Subclinical hyperthyroidism, nonthyroidal illness, drugs like steroids and dopamine, recent treatment for hyperthyroidism
FT4↓, FT3↓, TSH ↔ or ↓	Nonthyroidal illness, central hypothyroidism, Isolated TSH deficiency
FT4↑, FT3↑, TSH ↔ or ↑	Familial dysalbuminemic hyperthyroxinemia, drugs (heparin), non-thyroidal illness, TSH secreting pituitary adenoma and disorders of thyroid transport

Note: ↑ elevated, ↓ low, ↔ normal.

TRH stimulation test: 100–200 µg of TRH is injected intravenously (IV) after estimation of basal TSH level in the serum. At 20, 40 and 60 minutes post-injection, TSH levels are estimated. Normally, there is a two-fold rise. In Graves' disease, the TSH response to TRH is minimal. In hypothalamic hypothyroidism, the basal level of TSH is low, but TRH causes more release of TSH. In pituitary disease, the basal as well as post-injection level of TSH remains the same at a low level.

Thyroid scintiscanning: Scanning offers a visual display of the size and shape of the thyroid gland. It is employed in different situations.

- It provides an objective assessment of the morphology of the gland
- It locates ectopic foci of thyroid tissue
- The functional activity of thyroid nodules can be evaluated (hot or cold nodules)
- In the investigation of masses in the neck or mediastinum, scintiscanning is useful to detect their nature (e.g. retrosternal thyroid)
- Postsurgical residual thyroid tissue can be assessed
- Metastasis from thyroid carcinoma can be visualized.

Originally, ^{131}I was used for visualizing the thyroid, the scan being done after 24 hours of oral administration. At present, technetium pertechnetate (^{99m}TcO$_4^-$) which has a half-life of 6 hours is used for this purpose. With technetium, scanning can be done soon after the injection of the radioisotope.

Additional laboratory investigations include hematological tests and estimation of the levels of serum calcium, sodium, creatine phosphokinase (CPK) and proteins.

Fine-needle aspiration biopsy is a very valuable preoperative procedure done routinely. A correct diagnosis can be obtained in over 80% of cases. False-negative results occur more frequently than false-positive ones. The diagnostic accuracy of FNAC is about 95%, specificity 92% and sensitivity is around 83%. Aspiration from multiple sites are required to avoid false-negative results. In select cases, ultrasound-guided FNAC can be done.

Ultrasound/CT/MRI Scanning: Ultrasound scan provides an accurate indication of the size and is useful for differentiating cystic from solid lesions. CT and MRI are useful in the evaluation of retrosternal and retrotracheal extension of the gland, so also compression of trachea, extent of intrathoracic extension of thyroid malignancy and infiltration to adjacent structures. MRI gives better delineation of soft tissue involvement like infiltration of nerves.

Demonstration of thyroid autoantibodies: Different types of antibodies are demonstrable in patients with thyroid diseases. These include antibodies against Tg, intracellular microsomal antigen (TPO) and TSH-receptors. Their presence is diagnostic in many disorders, especially chronic lymphocytic thyroiditis (Hashimoto's disease) and ***postpartum thyroiditis (PPT)***.

All autoantibodies against thyroid cells are IgG. Some antibodies are stimulatory, whereas others are inhibitory with reference to thyroid function [TSH-receptor antibodies (TSHRAb)].

Blood Tests

- TSHRAb are of two types:
  1. Stimulating antibodies [thyroid stimulating immunoglobulin (TSI)]
  2. Blocking antibodies as seen in myxedema
- Other antibodies
  - ***TPO or antimicrosomal antibodies:*** The antigen is TPO

Table 99.5: Frequency (%) of the presence of antibodies in various thyroid disorders

	TSH receptor antibodies (%)	hTgAb (%)	hTPOAb (%)
Normal	0	5–20	8–27
Graves' disease	80–95	50–70	50–80
Autoimmune thyroiditis	10–20	80–90	90–100
Thyroid cancer	0	20–40	+
Pregnancy	0	14	14
Type 1 DM	0	40	40

Note: Serum thyroglobulin (Tg) estimation is done as a follow-up in patients with well-differentiated thyroid follicular carcinoma. However, serum Tg can also be elevated in goiter, hyperthyroidism and inflammatory conditions of the thyroid.

Abbreviations: hTgAb = Human thyroglobulin antibodies; hTPOAb = Human thyroid peroxidase antibodies; TSH = Thyroid stimulating hormone; DM = Diabetes mellitus

- ***anti-thyroglobulin antibodies (ATG) Antithyroid microsomal antibody (AMA):*** Antibodies are estimated by various methods immunofluorescence, hemagglutination, RIA (more precise) and ELISA techniques. Antibodies are produced due to secondary response to a thyroid injury. The thyroid antibodies most frequently estimated are those directed against Tg and TPO. The latter correlates better with thyroid dysfunction and its presence tends to correlate with damage to thyroid tissue and lymphocytic infiltration. The mechanisms of autoimmune destruction of the thyroid probably involve both cellular and humoral components (Table 99.5).

Other Tests

Serum Tg: In acute/subacute thyroiditis, Tg will be increased. Serial measurements are useful for the follow-up of patients with differentiated thyroid carcinoma (DTC). Antithyroglobulin antibodies (anti-TgAbs or ATg) may interfere with the measurement of serum Tg and may give false low serum Tg values.

Special Tests

- **Perchlorate discharge tests:** This test is used to demonstrate disordered organification of iodine in thyroid gland. When sodium iodide transporter inhibitors like perchlorate is given orally, after giving oral ^{131}I or ^{123}I, unorganified radioactive iodine in the thyroid leaks into circulation resulting in rapid fall of radioactivity over the thyroid gland.
- **PET scan:** For this test, in addition to sophisticated equipments, positron emitters like fluorine 18 is used, as a constituent of fluorodeoxyglucose which has higher avidity to a tissue with hyperactive metabolism (malignant tumors). This can be combined with a CT scan to give more structural information in addition to increased metabolic activity and thus commonly used in the differentiation of benign from malignant tumors.

TPO antibodies may be present in normal elderly women in up to 20% of cases. TSI are thyroid-stimulating hormone receptor antibodies (TSHR).

Since low levels of antibodies are present in normal individuals, the absolute concentration becomes more important.

GOITER

Enlargement of the thyroid gland is known as **goiter**. A benign diffuse enlargement not caused by inflammation or tumor is called **simple goiter** or **nontoxic diffuse goiter (NTDG)**.

Diagnosis and management of thyroid enlargement have been explained in Flowchart 99.1.

Causes of Goiter

- **Simple (nontoxic) goiters** may occur due to different causes:
  - **Physiological goiter:** This is simple enlargement of the thyroid in puberty and pregnancy. It generally subsides when the physiological stress is over or it may persist. The term physiological goiter is being questioned.
  - **Parenchymatous goiter or colloid goiter:** Iodine deficiency, iodine excess, dyshormonogenesis and intake of goitrogens cause thyroid enlargement, the acini being filled with colloid. In some, the cause may not be evident.
- **Goiter due to thyroiditis:** Acute, subacute or chronic.
- **Nodular goiter:** Single or multiple nodules.
- **Toxic goiter:** Primary (Graves' disease) or secondary (Plummer's disease).

Simple Goiter

This may be endemic or sporadic. Puberty goiter, colloid goiter and parenchymatous goiter are included in this group. The thyroid gland is diffusely enlarged, painless and nontender. It may be soft or firm in consistency. The term physiological goiter is being discarded since it is doubtful whether the thyroid enlarges due to physiological reasons. Many of these show occult or overt iodine deficiency. Similarly, many of the previously labelled puberty goiters were actually due to autoimmune thyroiditis.

Etiology

It is the result of relative iodine deficiency which occurs during periods of increased demand for thyroid hormones, such as menarche and pregnancy. Diffuse colloid goiters are common in younger subjects and are unusual above the age of 40 years. By the age of 35–40 years, the diffuse goiter becomes multinodular. Retrosternal extension may be present occluding the thoracic inlet.

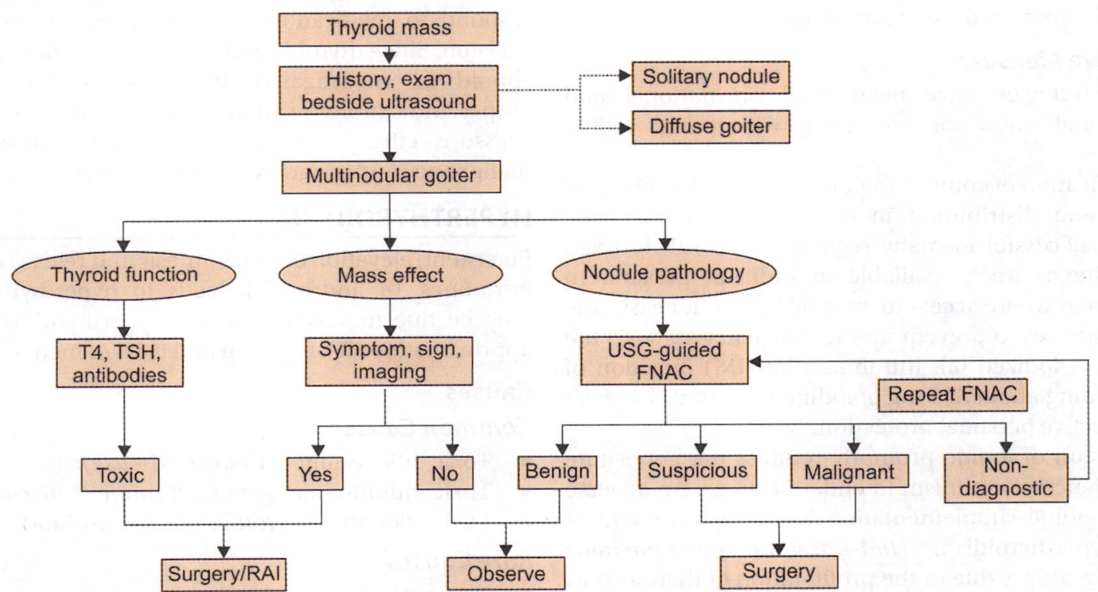

Abbreviations: TSH = Thyroid stimulating hormone; FNAC = Fine-needle aspiration cytology; RAI = Radioactive iodine; USG = Ultrasonography

The gland enlarges due to hyperplasia and hypertrophy. When the stress is over or it is corrected, the cells undergo hyperinvolution and this leads to the formation of colloid goiter. These subjects are clinically euthyroid. Thyroid function is preserved by the preferential production of excess T3 instead of T4. In many cases, the thyroid gland reaches large sizes.

Treatment

Administration of T4 (up to 0.3 mg/day) brings about a favorable response in 60% of subjects. The gland shrinks within 3 months of starting treatment. Treatment has to be continued for 1–2 years or more. Complete regression of the goiter is rare. Abrupt withdrawal of the drug causes rapid enlargement of the gland.

Endemic Goiter

This is a major public health problem all over the world, especially in India. Iodine deficiency manifests in various ways and goiter is the most easily recognized form. Endemic cretinism, which is also common, leads to severe morbidity in these zones. It is also estimated that there are 2.2 million cretins and 6.6 million children with mild neurological defects in India attributable to iodine deficiency. The spectrum of abnormalities due to iodine deficiency is now grouped under the title *IDD*. About 54 million people in India have goiter and the number at risk is estimated to be above 167 million.

Result of sample surveys in 325 districts covering all union territories and states in India showed a prevalence of iodine deficiency in more than 10% of people in 263 districts. Seventy-one million persons are suffering from goiter and IDD. The Indian Government introduced the National Iodine Deficiency Disease Control Programme (NIDDCP) with compulsory provision of iodized salt in 2006. IDD includes goiter, cretinism, deaf-mutism, paralytic squint, neurological deficits (spastic diplegia) and cognitive defects.

An area is termed endemic for goiter when 10% or more of the population is affected. Important among the well-recognized goiter belts of the world are the high mountain regions of Andes, Alps and Himalayas, region of the Great lakes of USA and several pockets in Africa (Zaire). The broad belt covering the mountain ranges of Afghanistan to the sub-Himalayan regions of India, Pakistan, Nepal, Bangladesh and Myanmar extends up to Malaysian archipelago and Indonesian islands. Apart from these well-recognized regions, many other states in India, such as Haryana, Rajasthan, Uttar Pradesh, Odisha, Madhya Pradesh, Tamil Nadu and Kerala also show areas of iodine deficiency. In these endemic belts, the daily iodine intake is generally less than 50 µg. The drinking water is very low in iodine content. Normal daily requirement of iodine is 150–200 µg for adults.

Dietary sources of iodine such as sea fish, milk and eggs may be absent in the diet of the people in these areas.

Pathology

The thyroid gland is enlarged with hypertrophy and hyperplasia of the cells. The euthyroid state is maintained in many subjects because of the increased production of T3. The plasma inorganic iodide levels are low. The absolute iodine uptake by the thyroid is maintained normal by increasing the plasma clearance rate of iodide. PBI is also normal. Urinary iodide excretion is low. Plasma T4 is normal but T3 may be high. Correction of iodine deficiency leads to resolution of the goiter. Alternatively, the cells may undergo hyperinvolution. In this case, the acini become filled with colloid and diffuse colloid goiter may develop. With repeated episodes of iodine depletion and repletion, multinodular goiter may develop.

Iodine deficiency during pregnancy leads to abnormalities in the mother and baby. Neonatal and infantile iodine deficiency leads to a spectrum of clinical abnormalities ranging from latent to overt thyroid disorders. Cretinism occurring as a result of iodine deficiency is widespread and this is one of the correctable causes of abnormality in growth and development in the endemic areas.

Preventive Measures

Several strategies have been tried on national and international basis for correcting widespread iodine deficiency.

Fortification of common salt with iodide (15–30 parts/million) and distribution in endemic areas has been partially successful in many regions. Table salt fortified with iodine is freely available in India at present. In remote areas where access to medical help is not easy, one of the strategies to prevent iodine deficiency states is the injection of iodized oil. Intramuscular (IM) injection of oil containing about 500 mg of iodine once in three years offers effective personal protection.

Provision of iodide promptly reduces the goiter rate and incidence of cretinism in endemic areas. An adverse effect of iodine supplementation is the development of acute hyperthyroidism **(Jod-Basedow phenomenon)** very rarely. This is due to the proliferation of thyroid cells during the iodine deprivation period and also the formation of hyperfunctioning nodules leading to hyperthyroidism on supplementing iodine.

Excessive supplementation of iodine in regions with only marginal iodine deficiency may lead to subclinical hypothyroidism and autoimmune thyroiditis rarely (*See also Ch 32*).

Sporadic Goiter

The etiology of sporadic goiter is not fully clear. The possible causes include increased iodine demand during pregnancy or puberty, presence of goitrogens in the diet and genetic factors.

Exogenous goitrogens include common drugs such as thiocarbamides [ATDs], chlorpropamide, amiodarone, glutethimide, iodine on a long-term basis, reserpine, phenylbutazone and lithium carbonate. Items of food like cabbage, turnips, soyabean flour, and cassava may act as goitrogens. Cabbage contains thiocyanates which inhibit iodine uptake by the thyroid. Cassava (tapioca) contains cyanogenic glycosides such as linamarin and lotaustralin, which liberate hydrocyanic acid on acid hydrolysis in the stomach.

Goiter may be the result of defective hormone synthesis. Such defects may involve pathways like oxidation, organification, coupling of iodine or proteolysis. The condition manifests as large goiters which show increased iodine uptake. Features of hypothyroidism or cretinism may be evident in some cases. Clinically, retrosternal extension of the goiter can be demonstrated by asking the patient to raise both arms above the head for 30 seconds, when the neck veins will engorge with plethoric appearance of face **(Pemberton's sign)**.

In cases of dyshormonogenesis, MIT or DIT may be elevated in blood depending upon the enzymopathy. In many cases, the goiter is familial.

Management

It is essential to detect the cause and tackle the same. Mild iodine deficiency and drug-induced goiters respond to medical therapy. Established goiters which do not respond to medication have to be treated by surgical excision. Since thyroid carcinomas are not rare, all goiters should be investigated, including needle aspiration biopsy. Indications for surgery include cosmetic disability, pressure effects, retrosternal extension, suspicion of malignancy and progressive enlargement.

HYPERTHYROIDISM

Persistent, elevation of the synthesis and release of thyroid hormones T4 and/or T3, leads to hyperthyroidism. It may be due to several causes. Hyperthyroidism affects approximately 2% of women and 0.2% of men.

Causes

Common Causes

- Toxic diffuse goiter **(Graves' disease):** 80%
- Toxic multinodular goiter **(Plummer's disease):** 5%
- Toxic adenoma **(autonomous hot nodule).**

Rare Causes

- Neonatal hyperthyroidism due to transplacental transfer of long-acting thyroid stimulator (LATS), now designated as TSI.
- Thyrotoxicosis factitia caused by self-administration of thyroid hormones.
- Iodide-induced hyperthyroidism (Jod-Basedow phenomenon), rarely seen in regions where iodized salt is distributed, or also with the use of drugs like amiodarone and radiopaque contrast dyes.
- Hashimoto's thyroiditis may be associated with thyrotoxicosis (Hashitoxicosis).
- Ectopic secretion of TSH like substances by trophoblastic tumors, e.g. hydatidiform mole or choriocarcinoma.
- TSH-secreting tumors of the pituitary.
- Transient gestational hyperthyroidism seen in hyperemesis gravidarum due to increased choriogondotropins which are functionally similar to TSH.
- Tumors such as ovarian teratomas containing thyroid tissue (struma ovarii) and metastases from follicular carcinoma of thyroid.
- Acute or subacute thyroiditis may give rise to transient hyperthyroidism. PPT occurring as enlargement of the thyroid within 6 months of delivery may also be accompanied by hyperthyroidism.
- Pituitary resistance to thyroid hormone.

TOXIC DIFFUSE GOITER

Syn: Graves' disease, Parry's disease, Basedow's disease

The disease is quite common in general practice, but the severity may vary. Females are affected more with a peak incidence between 20 and 40 years. Though neonates of thyrotoxic mothers may suffer from hyperthyroidism, usually the condition subsides within 3–6 weeks of birth.

Etiology

The exact etiology is not fully understood. The consensus is that Graves' disease is an autoimmune disorder. Several genetic susceptibility loci and environmental factors are likely to contribute to the development of the disease,

Textbook of Medicine

for example, human leukocyte antigens (*HLA-138, HLA-DR3, HLA-DR2), CTLA-4* (cytotoxic T-lymphocyte associated-4) gene regions. There is a 50% concordance in monozygotic twins and 5% in dizygotic twins. There is also strong association with other autoimmune diseases like pernicious anemia, type 1 DM, myasthenia gravis, Addison's disease, systemic lupus erythematosus (SLE), idiopathic thrombocytopenic purpura (ITP) and rheumatoid arthritis (RA). Various immunoglobulin (Ig) antibodies are found directed against antigens in the thyroid cells, orbital tissues and dermis. In some cases, TSI (autoantibodies) are demonstrable. These are immuno-globulins of IgG class and have TSH-like action. They cross the placenta and lead to hyperthyroidism in the fetus and neonates as well. TSI are of two types:

1. TSHRAb compete with TSH at TSH-receptor sites in the thyroid cell membrane and behaves like TSH. The serum levels of TSI correlate with the severity of hyperthyroidism, more the level of TSI, more severe is the disease.
2. Inhibiting or blocking antibodies such as TSHRAb which may block the ligand binding site and act as TSH antagonists. TSH-receptor is an autoantigen and its gene structure and chromosomal location is identified now as antagonists (14q31). TSHRAb is seen in 15% of patients with myxedema.

Pathology

Thyroid is diffusely enlarged due to hyperplasia of acinar cells and increased vascularity. Histologically, the acinar cells are hyperplastic, with accumulation of the colloid. Varying degree of lymphocytic infiltration is also seen. Microsomal and anti-TgAbs are also found in many patients with Graves' disease, but in lower levels than in Hashimoto's disease.

Thyroid-associated eye disease is a frequent manifes-tation of thyroid disorders, particularly hyperthyroidism. Extraocular muscles are the target of autoimmune response. There is evidence of retro-orbital inflammation characterized by focal edema, glycosaminoglycan (GAG) protein deposition, followed by fibrosis. Retro-orbital tissue may act as an autoantigen which has immune reactivity similar to the TSH-receptor. GAGs are secreted by the fibroblasts under the influence of cytokines from local lymphocytes.

The present consensus is that the immune system in the body recognizes an antigen common to the thyroid gland, retro-orbital tissues and skin and this is likely to be TSHRAb and the level of TSHRAb correlates with the severity of ophthalmopathy and dermopathy. The interstitium shows diffuse mononuclear infiltration, primarily by activated T-cells with some B-cells and occasional macrophages. The retrobulbar fibroblasts and skin fibroblasts are affected by the autoimmune processes. Graves' ophthalmopathy and dermopathy are strongly associated. Dermopathy is uncommon.

Clinical Features

Graves' disease is more frequent in young women. The effect of thyroid hormone is to increase metabolism and sensitize the tissues to catecholamines. The condition is

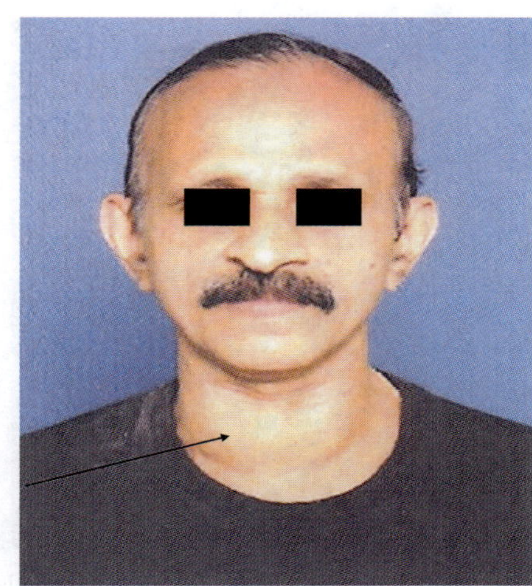

Fig. 99.1: Primary hyperthyroidism. ***Note:*** The smooth diffuse enlarge-ment of the thyroid (arrow).

florid and easily detectable in many cases. The symptoms may be less obvious in others. The general symptoms attributable to hypermetabolic state include loss of weight, intolerance to heat, increased sweating, excessive appetite, palpitation, tachycardia, exertional dyspnea, nervousness, tremor, diarrhea, easy fatigability, apprehension and insomnia. Rarely mental changes like severe agitation and frank psychosis may be the presenting features.

Examination of the neck shows the thyroid to be diffusely enlarged, but sometimes it may be asymmetrical. It is soft, warm, pulsatile and tender. Arterial thrills and bruit may be detectable. These phenomena indicate increased vascularity (Fig. 99.1).

- ***Thyroid-associated eye disease may present*** in several ways, 90% have overt hyperthyroidism. Ten percent have no obvious thyroid dysfunction. Those with no signs of thyrotoxicosis are known as ***ophthalmic*** or ***euthyroid Graves' disease***. Among them, 50% have autoimmune hypothyroidism and the remaining 50% have no detectable clinical or biochemical dysfunction of the thyroid. Main clinical features include diplopia with vertical separation of visual images, asymmetry of palpebral fissures, disorders of movement of the eyes and lids, and compression of the optic nerve.
- Sympathetic overactivity leads to lid lag, stare, increased watering and infrequent blinking. These subside with correction of thyroid function.
- There is abnormal protrusion of the eyeball (exoph-thalmos) and partial or complete ophthalmoplegia.
- Exophthalmos is generally bilateral, but can be unilateral or asymmetrical. It may precede overt hyperthyroidism. Exophthalmos is assessed by measuring the distance between the lateral angle of the bony orbit and the anterior part of cornea by Hertel exophthalmometer (Fig. 99.2).
- Papilledema may develop in advanced cases. Some cases may show optic atrophy.

Werner's classification of eye changes in Graves' disease is explained in Table 99.6.

- ***Skin changes:*** The skin is soft and moist. The hair is soft. Sweating is excessive. The nails show thinning

Textbook of Medicine

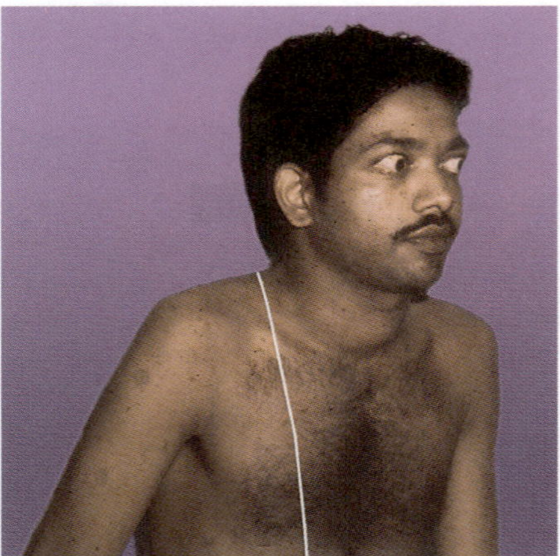

Fig. 99.2: Bilateral exophthalmos in a male thyrotoxic patient

Table 99.6: Werner's classification of eye changes in Graves' disease 'NO SPECS'

Class	Definition
0	**N**o signs or symptoms
1	**O**nly signs, no symptoms (signs limited to upper lid retraction, stare, lid lag)
2	**S**oft tissue involvement (symptoms and signs)
3	**P**roptosis
4	**E**xtraocular muscle involvement
5	**C**orneal involvement
6	**S**ight loss (optic nerve involvement)

(onycholysis) and may get separated from the nailbed *(Plummer's nails)*.

Sometimes localized myxedematous deposits may occur. The common site is the front of the leg *[hence, called pretibial myxedema (PTM)]*. Over this site, the skin is raised, nodular, indurated, and reddish brown in color. The lesions may be pruritic. Examination reveals *peau de orange* (orange peel-like) appearance. In addition to the pretibial regions, thighs, genitalia and lower abdomen may be affected. PTM is attributed to local nonresponsiveness of tissues to the thyroid hormones.

Some cases show clubbing of fingers and toes, and hypertrophic osteoarthropathy *(thyroid acropachy)*.

- ***Changes in skeletal muscles:*** There is excessive fatigue and weakness. The proximal muscles of pelvic and pectoral girdles show myopathy characterized by selective weakness, atrophy and this may incapacitate the patient. The condition recovers completely when thyrotoxicosis is controlled. This is an example of reversible endocrine myopathy. Myasthenia gravis may coexist with Graves' disease and the relationship is more of a see-saw phenomenon—myasthenia abating when thyrotoxicosis is active and vice versa. Both conditions demand management on their own merits. Hypokalemic periodic paralysis may occur more frequently in thyrotoxic subjects.
- ***Cardiovascular system (CVS):*** Cardiac output increases out of proportion to the rise in basal metabolic rate (BMR). T4 has a direct chronotropic effect on cardiac tissues. Increase in workload leads to cardiac hypertrophy. Combination of excessive demand in the presence of reduction of reserve capacity of the myocardium leads to high output cardiac failure. Atrial fibrillation occurs in up to 25% of cases and this is resistant to drug therapy and cardioversion, till the thyrotoxicosis is also controlled.

  Other arrhythmias such as paroxysmal tachycardia and atrial flutter are also common. Some patients develop effort angina.
- ***Alimentary system:*** Abdominal cramps, diarrhea and vomiting are common features. The diarrhea is due to intestinal hurry. In many cases, it takes the form of increased frequency of bowel movements, especially after food.
- ***Reproductive system:*** In women, the periods become scanty and fertility is reduced. In men, libido and potency may be altered variably. Gynecomastia may develop. Oligospermia may occur.
- ***Bones:*** Osteoporosis may develop as a result of increased resorption of bones. Hypercalcemia and hypercalciuria may be demonstrable.

The general clinical picture produced by toxic diffuse goiter and toxic nodular goiter is similar in many respects. However, eye changes and PTM are more common in toxic diffuse goiter. Association with other autoimmune diseases is more characteristic of Graves' disease, which is the more frequent form in younger age groups. Toxic adenomas occur usually at later age groups. In them, cardiovascular manifestations are more prominent and sometimes may be the only clinical presentation. In toxic adenoma, local examination of the thyroid may not reveal generalized hypervascularity and bruit, but the condition can be easily diagnosed by palpating the nodules.

Sometimes the thyroid gland may produce excessive quantities of only T3. Such a condition is called T3 toxicosis, mostly seen in autonomous hot, nodules or in iodine deficient areas.

Diagnosis

In florid cases, clinical diagnosis is easy. Subclinical cases may be missed if thyrotoxicosis is not kept in mind. In all cases, it is advisable to confirm the diagnosis and establish its severity by investigations.

Differential Diagnosis

When the symptoms are mild, hyperthyroidism may be mistaken for anxiety state, tuberculosis, diabetes or primary muscle disease. In anxiety state, the palms are cold and moist whereas in hyperthyroidism, they are warm and moist.

Euthyroid Graves' disease: This is a condition in which exophthalmos is present with or without thyroid enlargement. There may not be the signs of overt hyperthyroidism. [131]I uptake is increased or normal, but the uptake is not inhibited by administration of T3. Moreover, administration of TRH does not lead to elevation of TSH. T3 and T4 levels will be normal.

Laboratory Investigations

[131]I-uptake by the thyroid gland and levels of T4 and T3 are all increased (Fig. 99.3). TSH is low and there is no increase in TSH levels when TRH is administered.

Treatment

Thyrotoxicosis may be treated with antithyroid drugs, irradiation by radioactive iodine or surgery.

Drug Therapy

Drugs form the first line of management in the ordinary case. Antithyroid drugs block the synthesis of thyroid hormones by inhibiting thyroid peroxidase (TPO) enzyme, thus blocking iodination of tyrosine. The drugs are started in a small dose and worked up to optimum response, and maintained for a period of 18–24 months. With improvement in the condition the dose can be tapered and maintained at a lower level. In 50% of cases remission is obtained during drug therapy. Many cases may relapse on withdrawal of therapy. Thiocarbamides, potassium perchlorate, and Lugol's iodine are also employed as antithyroid drugs.

- ***Thiocarbamides: Carbimazole, methylthiouracil*** and ***propylthiouracil*** are the drugs in this class, of which methylthiouracil is seldom used at present. Carbimazole (Neomercazole) is most widely used on account of its effectiveness, relative safety and free availability. It is started in a dose of 10–15 mg 6 hourly as tablets. Carbimazole has mild immunosuppressive effects while PTU in addition blocks the conversion of T4–T3. As the desired effect is obtained, the dose is reduced and continued at a lower level to maintain euthyroid state.

  Propylthiouracil is used at times when carbimazole is not tolerated. The daily dose is 150 mg 6 hourly as tablets. Both these drugs promptly block the formation of thyroxine and tri-iodothyronine, but do not prevent the release of hormone stored in the colloid. Therefore, it takes 2–3 weeks for the effect to be fully established. If found effective, the therapy should be continued for 12–18 months before reducing the dose and withdrawing it. Early withdrawal may lead to relapse. Even after the full course some cases may still relapse.

  Adverse effects: Thiocarbamides are toxic drugs and therefore, close watch should be instituted when administering them. Adverse effects include fever, lymphadenopathy, splenomegaly, jaundice, leukopenia, thrombocytopenia and agranulocytosis. Generally, adverse effects manifest during the early part of treatment. Reversible enlargement of the thyroid may occur during therapy and this subsides on stopping the drug. Enlargement of the thyroid may be troublesome at times. Another untoward side effect is the worsening of exophthalmos. Concurrent use of T4 sodium in a dose of 0.05–0.1 mg daily helps to reduce these side effects and continue antithyroid medication more smoothly (block replace regimen).

- ***Potassium perchlorate ($KClO_4$):*** It is an ion inhibitor which inhibits the transport of iodine to the thyroid. In an initial dose of 800 mg daily, drug is very effective. As the condition improves, dose is reduced. The action is rapid. Potassium thiocyanate (KSCN) is another drug in this category.

- ***Iodine*** (inorganic or organic) given in pharmacological doses promptly blocks iodine uptake by the thyroid, formation of T4 and also release of preformed hormone from colloid. Iodine blocks the peripheral conversion of T4–T3. For immediate effect, iodine or iodides are preferable. Since the vascularity of the thyroid also comes down, it becomes less friable during surgery. Therefore, iodine is given as a preoperative drug for thyroidectomy and also for the management of thyroid storm.

Dose: Lugol's iodine (iodine dissolved in potassium iodide solution containing 10 mg iodine in each drop) or saturated solution of potassium iodide which contains 50 mg iodine per drop is given in a total dose of 500 mg/day. Effect of iodine on the thyroid is not permanent. With continued use exceeding 2–3 weeks, the antithyroid activity wanes (Wolff-Chaikoff effect). Therefore, iodine or iodides are used only for short-term treatment. Sodium iodide can be given IV 1g/day.

Inorganic iodine is not routinely used because of toxicity and high incidence of recurrence. Organic iodine such as oral cholecystography dye can be used on a short-term basis. Iodine blocks the peripheral conversion of T4–T3. Because of the rapid action, iodides are most useful in the management of thyroid crisis. Since the entero-hepatic circulation of T3 and T4 is higher in thyrotoxi-

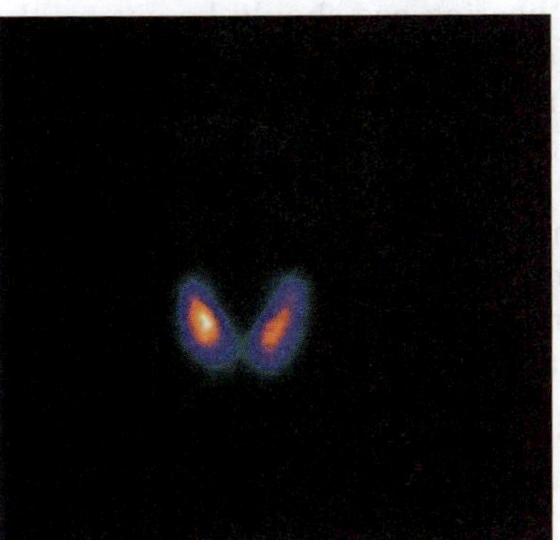
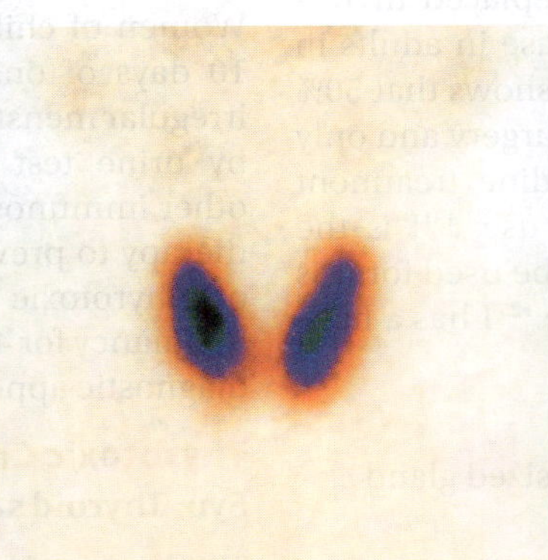
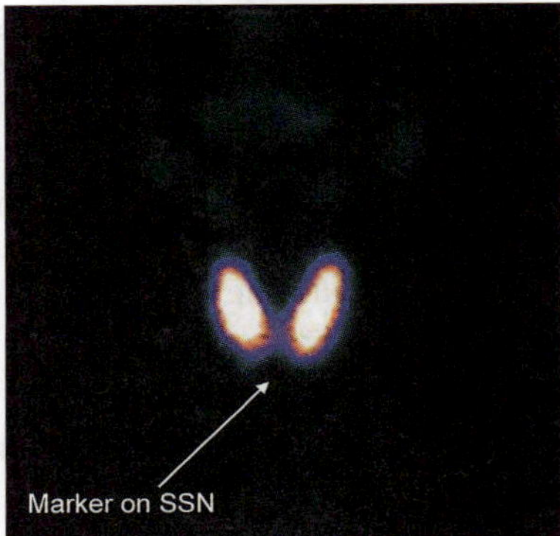

Fig. 99.3: TcO₄ scan of thyroid in hyperthyroidism. ***Note:*** The increased uptakes in both the lobes; suprasternal notch (SSN) the violet colored in first picture is due to very high uptake.

cosis, it may be beneficial to use bile salt sequestrants like colestipol hydrochloride along with carbimazole in the initial phase of treatment of resistant cases of thyrotoxicosis.

- Steroids like dexamethasone which suppresses the peripheral conversion of T4–T3 and secretion of T4/T3 are also found to be useful especially in thyrotoxic crisis.
- *PTM* responds to the local application of triamcinolone cream under occlusive dressing.
- *Beta blockers:* T4 has a half-life of about 5 days in the body. Therefore, the effect of ATDs is not immediately evident. There is a latent period of 7–10 days before the symptoms are controlled. In order to reduce the distressing symptoms immediately, beta-adrenergic blockers like propranolol (up to 120 mg/day) may also be used. This promptly controls the tachycardia, palpitation, diarrhea, tremor and exertional dyspnea. Excitement and insomnia are indications for drugs like phenothiazines (100 mg/day) or diazepam (20–30 mg/day). Other beta blockers like atenolol, esmolol and metaprolol can be used. Beta blockers may also block the conversion of T4–T3 like iodides.

Surgery

Subtotal thyroidectomy is the operation of choice. Indications for surgery are:

- Large goiter with pressure effects
- Nodular toxic goiter
- Failure of drug therapy or serious toxicity of drugs
- Poor drug compliance, socioeconomic factors, cosmetic reasons and desire for quick response.

The patient is given drug therapy before surgery to make him euthyroid. This is necessary to prevent *thyrotoxic crisis*. Two weeks prior to surgery carbimazole is replaced by potassium iodide 60–100 mg per day in order to reduce the size and vascularity of the gland. Surgery is effective in reducing toxic symptoms in almost all cases. Recurrence after surgery occurs in 10% cases. The immediate complications include recurrent laryngeal nerve palsy and damage to the parathyroid glands (2%). 40–45% of cases may develop hypothyroidism in 10 years, requiring thyroid supplementation.

Radioiodine Treatment

Currently, ^{131}I treatment has practically replaced thyroidectomy in the treatment of Graves' disease in adults in many countries. Data from major centers shows that 50% of patients are treated with ^{131}I, 35% with surgery and only 15% with ATDs alone. In India, radioiodine treatment is available in many centers for routine use. [131]I is the commonly used preparation. [125]I can also be used for this purpose. [131]I has a half-life of 8 days, while ^{125}I has a half-life of 60 days.

Indications for radioiodine treatment

- Thyrotoxicosis with small or moderate sized gland
- Recurrent thyrotoxicosis
- Masked hyperthyroidism
- Thyrotoxic heart failure
- Poor surgical risk

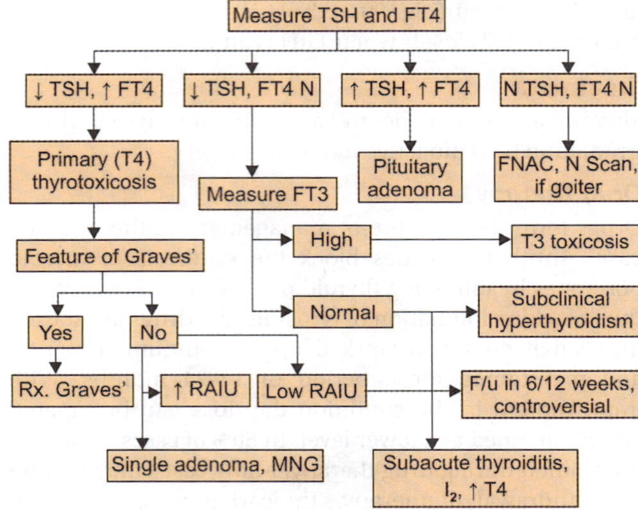

Flowchart 99.2: Hyperthyroidism—diagnostic approach to thyroid testing

Abbreviations: FT4, FT3 = Free T4, free T3; FNAC = Fine-needle aspiration cytology; F/u = Follow-up; TSH = Thyroid stimulating hormone; RAIU = Radioactive iodine uptake; MNG = Multinodular goiter; N = Normal

Contraindications

- Pregnancy is an absolute contraindication since the isotope may reach the fetus and destroy its thyroid as well.
- In severe thyrotoxic patients, ^{131}I treatment may precipitate thyroid storm. Hence, treatment has to be undertaken with caution.

[131]I dose: The thyroid will be effectively irradiated with 7000 rads. For this dose, each gram of thyroid tissue should receive 150 microCuries (µCi) of [131]I. The average total dose is 8–10 milliCuries (mCi) (300–400 MBq). However, this dose leads to hypothyroidism in 30–70% of cases within 2–10 years. Hence, lower doses are preferred in many centers. After an initial dose of 4–5 mCi (150–200 MBq), the dose is repeated after 3–6 months. Even among those who were given the lower dose hypothyroidism may develop in 50% within 25 years. [131]I can be administered orally as a solution on an outpatient basis, but the urine and feces which contain high amounts of radioactivity have to be disposed safely. Antithyroid medication should be withdrawn four days before administering ^{131}I and this can be continued thereafter till the patient becomes euthyroid. Women of child bearing age should be given ^{131}I within 10 days of onset of menstrual bleeding. In those with irregular menstrual periods pregnancy should be excluded by urine test before drug administration. Steroids or other immunosuppressant drugs are given along with ^{131}I therapy to prevent radiation thyroiditis and exacerbation of thyrotoxic ophthalmopathy. They should avoid pregnancy for 4 months thereafter. Flowchart 99.2 shows a diagnostic apporach to thyroid testing (hyperthyroidism).

Thyrotoxic Crisis

Syn: Thyroid storm

This is caused by sudden release of thyroid hormones from the gland, spontaneously or immediately after surgery. Thyroid crisis is more frequent if surgery is undertaken during active thyrotoxicosis. Thyroid storm can be precipitated by ^{131}I treatment also.

Thyroid crisis should be suspected if the patient develops high fever, severe tachycardia, restlessness, heart failure, peripheral vascular collapse or psychotic behavior.

Treatment

This is a medical emergency, demanding urgent specific treatment.

- Diazepam is given in doses of 5–10 mg IV to allay the agitation and quieten the patient. Tepid sponging helps to keep the temperature down from rising to hyperpyrexia levels.
- IV glucose saline drip is started and hydrocortisone 100 mg is given at 4–6 hour intervals to combat shock.
- Sodium iodide is given IV in a dose of 300–600 mg 8 hourly till the metabolic crisis is controlled.
- Beta-adrenergic blockers are very effective in reducing tachycardia and adrenergic symptoms. Propranolol is given IV in doses of 1–4 mg stat over a period of 5 minutes is very effective and effect lasts for 3–4 hours, after which it is to be repeated. In less severe cases, propranolol can be given orally, in doses ranging from 120–240 mg in 24 hours up to 600–1200 mg.
- If IV sodium iodide is not available, an effective anti-thyroid regimen is to give, PTU 100 mg 6 hourly along with potassium iodide 50–100 mg orally, rectally or through a Ryle's tube as the case may be. Iodine containing radio-contrast dyes such as sodium iopodate 500 mg orally daily will restore the serum T3 to normal in 2–3 days. Propranolol and sodium iopodate can be withdrawn after 14 days. Carbimazole can also be given 15–20 mg 6 hourly through a Ryle's tube.

Hyperthyroidism During Pregnancy

Both PTU and carbimazole are effective. These drugs cross the placenta and appear in breast milk. PTU is preferred in pregnancy since the fetus receives only 0.025% of the administered dose whereas with carbimazole it receives 0.2%. Aplasia cutis of scalp can develop in neonates with carbimazole. The minimum dose of these drugs required to keep the mother's T4 level at the upper limit of normal and should be continued. After delivery, baby should be fully investigated for thyroid function and appropriate management instituted. Up to 20 mg neoMercazole or 200 mg of PTU can be safely given during lactation. Acute hepatitis with liver failure has been reported with PTU. In general, hyperthyroidism naturally remits during pregnancy and relapses after delivery. In pregnancy, the T4 requirement goes up by 40% due to increase in TBG.

Toxic adenomas: These are usually autonomous and thyrotoxicosis, due to this cause tends to be permanent and prolonged, without any natural remission. Specific ATDs are less effective. Beta-adrenergic blocking drugs may control the adrenergic symptoms. [131]I is the more effective therapy, but larger doses up to 10–50 mCi may be required at times. Surgical removal is the better alternative.

Hyperthyroidism due to thyroiditis: Usually, this is a transient phenomenon occurring in subacute thyroiditis or Hashimoto's thyroiditis. The condition is self-limiting,

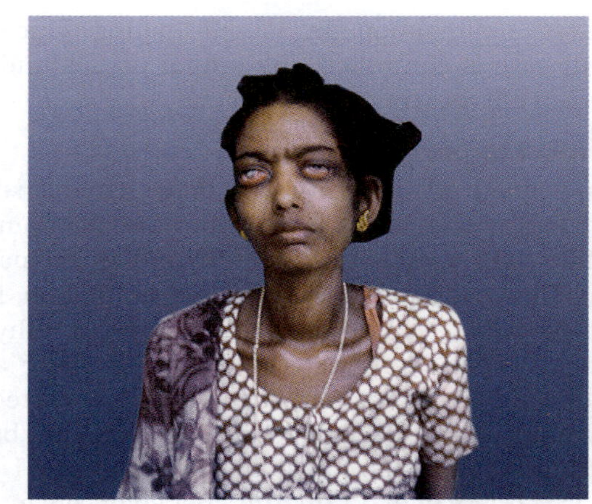

Fig. 99.4: Female thyrotoxicosis with exophthalmic ophthalmopathy

but some cases may go on to hypothyroidism, later becoming euthyroid. Specific ATDs may not be needed in many. Often beta-adrenergic blocking drugs are sufficient to control the symptoms.

Exophthalmos

There is no specific treatment for exophthalmos. During treatment of Graves' disease, the exophthalmos subsides in some, but in others it remains unchanged or worsens. The treatment of exophthalmos is only empirical since the pathogenesis is not fully understood. Radioiodine treatment aggravates ophthalmopathy.

Irritation and watering of the eyes are benefited by the use of eyedrops containing corticosteroids, methyl cellulose or 5% guanethidine. Use of sunglasses with side shields and adoption of semi-upright position help to give further relief. Use of prismatic glasses helps to overcome diplopia. Injection of botulinum toxin (BTX) to paralyse selected extraocular muscles has been tried as a measure to avoid diplopia. Diuretics are also beneficial in some cases.

Malignant Exophthalmos

When exophthalmos is associated with reddening, edema and bulging of conjunctiva from under the lids and around the corneal limbus it is called *malignant exophthalmos* (Fig. 99.4). If left untreated, this may lead on to corneal ulceration and blindness. This is also treated on the same line as for exophthalmos but prednisolone orally 90–120 mg daily or methyl prednisolone 1 g daily for 3 days IV followed by oral steroids is found to be beneficial. The eyes are protected from exposure keratitis by performing lateral tarsorrhaphy. Surgical decompression of the retro-orbital space (orbital decompression) is undertaken when the vision is threatened or papilledema develops. Irradiation of retro-orbital tissues may arrest the progression of exophthalmos and this is tried in severe cases where vision is in danger.

The dose required may be up to 2000 cGy given in 10–12 sittings. Plasmapheresis has been used as a temporary measure, with limited success.

Long-term use of octreotide in a dose of 100–200 µg daily by subcutaneous injection is beneficial in the management of troublesome exophthalmos.

Graves' ophthalmopathy is self-limiting. Once the active disease is controlled, the orbital tissues undergo fibrosis but full recovery may not occur.

Subclinical Hyperthyroidism

This is defined as the condition in which the serum level of TSH is undetectable but with normal serum T4/T3. Subtle signs and symptoms of thyrotoxicosis may be present. Some patients may have atrial fibrillation. Even if asymptomatic, some authors advocate antithyroid medication especially in elderly to prevent future atrial fibrillation and osteoporosis, in addition to correcting the thyroid status, especially if the TSH levels are below 0.1 μIU/mL. Progression to overt hyperthyroidism is also high if TSH is less than 0.1 μIU/mL. Beta blockers may be given to patients with subtle signs.

HYPOTHYROIDISM

Insufficient synthesis and release of thyroid hormones give rise to hypothyroidism. This may be congenital or acquired, later in life. Congenital hypothyroidism leads to developmental abnormalities resulting in cretinism. When hypothyroidism occurs in juveniles or adults, a characteristic clinical picture develops in which there is accumulation of hydrophilic mucopolysaccharides in the ground substance of the dermis and several other tissues resulting in induration and coarsening of the skin and enlargement of organs like the tongue. This is called *myxedema*. Women are affected more with 10% prevalence in adult women and 3% in adult men. Myxedema which is very rarely seen now is associated with other autoimmune disorders like DM, RA and pernicious anemia.

There is another entity called subclinical hypothyroidism which is defined as mild TSH elevation with normal T3 and T4. Symptomatic patients require treatment. (TSH below 10 mIU/mL). *Clinical features*—depend on the age of onset of the disorder and the types.

Cretinism

The incidence of neonatal hypothyroidism in India is nearly 1 in 2500, whereas it has a worldwide incidence of 1 in 4000 on neonatal screening.

This results from hypofunction of the thyroid from birth. This may result from iodine deficiency occurring in endemic goiter belts. Babies born to hypothyroid women or those taking ATDs during pregnancy may develop cretinism. Though the abnormality is present at birth in many babies, symptoms manifest only after several months and therefore, the condition may remain undetected in the newborn. There are two types of endemic cretinism.

1. Myxedematous (prominent features of hypothyroidism)
2. *Neurological cretins central nervous system (CNS) features.* The infant is dull and lethargic. Growth is retarded. Other features include large protruding tongue, broad flat nose, widely set eyes, sparse hair, dry skin, protuberant abdomen and umbilical hernia. Abnormal persistence of physiological jaundice, croaky voice, constipation, somnolence and problems in feeding should raise the possibility of cretinism in

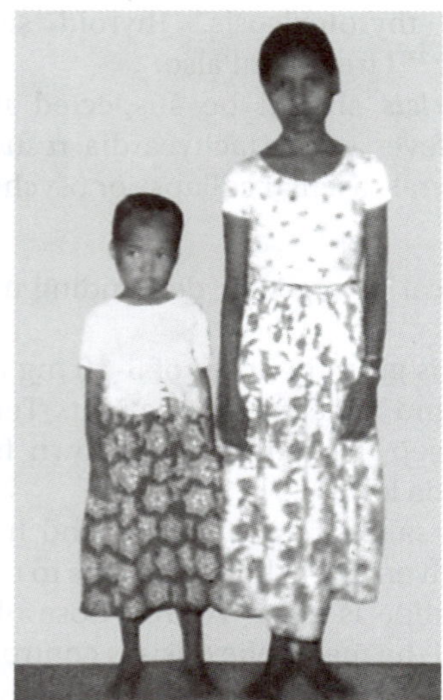

Fig. 99.5: Cretin. **Note:** The retardation of growth and dull facies—normal of the same age for comparison on the right.

the newborn. As the baby becomes older, retardation of growth and milestones become evident (Fig. 99.5).

Neurological abnormalities are prominent in some cases. These include deafness, spastic limbs, abnormal, coma. Mental development is severely retarded. If replacement T4 treatment is not given within the first 6–12 months, the newborn will lose 3–5 intelligence quotient (IQ) points every month from birth.

The appearance and ossification of several epiphyseal centers are delayed. Delay in the appearance of epiphyseal centers for carpal bones and delay in the eruption of teeth are useful diagnostic features to diagnose florid cretinism but for best results the diagnosis should be made much earlier with biochemical tests as early as possible in the child's life. Delay in diagnosis of even mild hypothyroidism in infancy leads to permanent impairment of the cognitive faculties in the child even though other functions may recover to varying degrees. TSH screening is a must in all neonates especially if the mother is hypothyroid. Antibodies (TPO, anti-Tg) also may be estimated in mothers with positive antibodies. Cretinism may be present with goiter or no goiter.

Treatment

The development of normal mental function in cretinism depends almost solely on the institution of treatment early in the neonatal period. Any delay in starting thyroid hormone replacement will lead to permanent disability. Therefore, need to make an early diagnosis cannot be overemphasized. The dose for infants is 10–15 μg/kg daily, the average infant may require 50 μg/day and this may go up to even 0.1–0.2 mg/day as the child grows. The child's growth and bone development should be monitored by regular clinical and radiological examination. Undetected congenital hypothyroidism is one of the most frequent causes of remediable mental retardation in later life.

Routine estimation of TSH, T4 and T3 in neonates is undertaken in many centers to exclude neonatal hypothyroidism. As a screening test, estimation of TSH alone is carried out at times. The prospect for normal

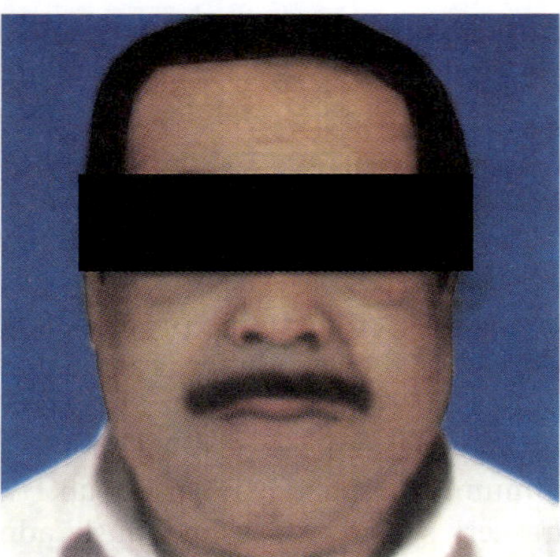

Fig. 99.6: Myxedema—50-year-old male

mental development is poor if treatment is not started before the first few months of life.

MYXEDEMA

Primary hypothyroidism occurring in juveniles and adults leads to myxedema.

Clinical Features

Clinical features depend upon the degree of impairment of thyroid function and its duration. The onset is insidious and often unnoticed by the patient or relatives. Early manifestations include slowing of activities, lethargy, somnolence, constipation and generalized disinterestedness. Due to lowering of metabolism and accumulation of fluid and adipose tissue, considerable weight gain occurs. The patient becomes intolerant to cold and patient prefers to sit in the sun or near the fire. The hair is coarse, dry and sparse. The scalp and eyebrows may become bald. The skin is lusterless, thick, and dry with scanty hair. Puffiness, coarseness and skin thickening are due to deposition of GAG. This is a diagnostic feature in a well-developed case. The voice is croaky due to thickening of the vocal cords. Generalized non-pitting edema is common. Many people show periorbital edema and macroglossia (Fig. 99.6). There is no thyromegaly.

- **Neurological features predominate in many cases:** Common presentations are slowness of mental and physical activity, slowed speech, muscle cramps, muscle hypertrophy, paresthesia and entrapment neuropathies. **Carpal tunnel syndrome** is common. The tendon reflexes are altered. The relaxation phase is delayed. This abnormality is best seen in the ankle jerk. Nerve conduction velocity is reduced. Psychiatric disturbances **(myxedema madness)** are common. Unless treated early, severe cases go into somnolence, stupor and coma. Myxedema coma is precipitated by exposure to cold, infections, trauma or sedatives. Hypothermia and respiratory depression may develop. Sleep apnea may occur at times. It carries a high mortality rate.
- **Cerebellar dysfunction** may develop, manifesting as truncal or limb ataxia and intention tremor. Unless hypothyroidism is kept in mind, these cases may be missed.

- **Cardiovascular manifestations** include cardiomegaly, pericardial effusion, angina pectoris, mild or moderate hypertension and predisposition to ischemic heart disease (IHD) due to dyslipidemia. Cardiac failure is not uncommon.
- **Abnormalities of sexual function:** Impotence occurs in men. Women may develop menorrhagia and girls may attain precocious puberty.
- **Hoffman's syndrome:** Muscle dysfunction is common in hypothyroidism. Hypertrophy of muscles associated with pseudomyotonia (slowness of contraction and relaxation) are diagnostic features of Hoffman's syndrome. Calf muscles are affected very frequently.
- **Pendred syndrome:** In this congenital condition, there is permanent deafness or deaf-mutism in addition to goitrous hypothyroidism. The defect is a block in the synthesis of thyroid hormone (dyshormonogenesis).

Laboratory Investigations

- Both total and free serum T3 and T4 levels are low.
- The TSH level is very high in primary hypothyroidism. Raised TSH level is the most readily available indicator for primary hypothyroidism. Levels of TSH above 20 mU/L and lowered levels of T4 are virtually diagnostic. T3 levels may be unreliable. TSH is low in pituitary or hypothalamic hypothyroidism. In hypothalamic hypothyroidism, administration of TRH leads to the production of TSH and increase in T4 and T3 levels. Normal serum TSH is 0.4–4.0 mIU/mL.
- TSH may be elevated in adrenal cortical (glucoroticoid) deficiency, renal failure and exposure to cold without hypothyroidism.
- ^{131}I uptake by the thyroid is low.
- **Immunological markers:** Titers of anti-Tg and antimicrosomal TPO antibodies are high, especially if the disease is of autoimmune origin. TSHR blocking antibodies may be present. Anti-TPOAbs are more consistently elevated.
- Serum cholesterol level is raised above 300 mg/dL in many cases of myxedema. In pituitary hypothyroidism, the cholesterol level is normal.
- CPK level is increased.
- Electrocardiography (ECG) shows slow rate, low voltage and ST and T wave changes.
- The BMR is low. Since low BMR occurs in many other conditions, this finding is not specific and hence, not used as a diagnostic test at present.

Diagnosis

Hypothyroidism should be suspected in all cases of rapid increase in weight without obvious edema, slowing of activity, tendency to fall asleep often, hoarseness of voice, recent onset of constipation and psychiatric disturbances, especially depression. Uncommon presentations include vague aches and pains, non-articular rheumatism, neurological phenomena such as carpal tunnel syndrome and cerebellar disturbances.

The clinical suspicion of hypothyroidism should be strong in all infants and children who fail to thrive and in whom milestones of development are delayed. Since hypothyroidism is a common cause of growth retardation in many communities in India, even a therapeutic trial with 0.05 mg T4 will not be out of place in areas where access to specialized endocrinology services are not available.

Differential Diagnosis

Myxedema has to be distinguished from other causes of edema such as nephrotic syndrome and chronic congestive cardiac failure (CCF).

Obesity due to any cause may mimic hypothyroidism. In many cases of obesity, subclinical thyroid dysfunction may coexsist.

Secondary Hypothyroidism

It is caused by hypopituitarism and to be distinguished from primary hypothyroidism. In the former, there is no myxedema, the skin is fine and hair is silky. There is no cardiomegaly. Evidence of hypoadrenocorticism and hypogonadism may be present in varying degrees. Diagnosis is established by estimating the level of TSH in serum, which is low in secondary hypothyroidism and typically high in primary hypothyroidism. T3 and T4 are low. Functions of the adrenal cortex and gonads may also be affected frequently.

Course and Prognosis

The course of hypothyroidism is slowly progressive with fluctuations in thyroid function. Myxedema coma, IHD or cardiac failure may prove fatal in some. Myxedema promptly responds to replacement therapy, but the condition recurs on cessation of medication. *Delay in instituting treatment in children results in permanent retardation of mental faculties, even though the physical and sexual characteristics may recover to variable extent with medication.*

Treatment

The principle of therapy is life-long replacement of thyroid hormone so as to produce full clinical remission and achieve normal biochemical parameters as far as possible. Replacement therapy is started with synthetic *levothyroxine sodium,* available as 0.05 and 0.1 mg tablets given orally once or twice a day as required. The drug is freely available, cheap and free from serious side effects and very satisfactory for prolonged use. T3 is available as tablets containing 25 µg. It is more rapid in action and therefore, employed in emergency situations like myxedema coma.

Dosage: T4 is given in a dose of 1.6 µg/kg in adults orally as single daily doses. Average daily dose for adults is 0.1–0.2 mg of L-thyroxine sodium. T4 should be preferred for treatment of an ordinary case. T4 and T3 are available both for oral and parenteral use. In complicated myxedema, monitoring of treatment can be done by clinical assessment and TSH levels which should be kept at the lower levels of normal. When treating children, biochemical monitoring is necessary to achieve full success, whereas in the case of adults clinical assessment is adequate in most cases. But in those with coexisting lipid abnormalities, more meticulous correction of the hypothyroid state is beneficial. Failure to achieve full improvement with T4 supplementation should raise suspicion about concomitant diseases such as hypoadrenal corticism.

Since myxedema tends to be permanent, thyroid supplementation has to be life-long. With effective treatment, the clinical abnormalities subside within 4–6 weeks, but they promptly return within weeks to months on stopping therapy. During periods of other intercurrent illness and other forms of stress, T4 supplementation should not be interrupted.

In elderly subjects, due to the presence of coexistent IHD, overdose of T4 may precipitate angina. It is essential to exclude IHD by ECG before starting therapy. In the presence of IHD, the initial dose of T4 should be smaller and the optimum dosage has to be worked up. Hypothyroid subjects are very sensitive to exogenously administered T4. Concurrent administration of beta blockers in doses which reduce the heart rate helps to avoid angina. The optimum dosage has to be worked out. Overdose may lead to hyperthyroid symptoms.

Treatment of myxedema coma is a medical emergency. Coma is the result of a combination of factors such as heart failure, cerebral ischemia, hypothermia and hypothyroidism.

The patient should be hospitalized. The drug of choice is T3 given IV in a dose of 20 µg stat and repeated 4 hours later. At present, parenteral preparation of L-thyroxine sodium is also available for use. The dose is 500 µg IV stat and thereafter 100 µg/day. Hydrocortisone should be given along with T4 replacement, in order to prevent hypoadrenal crisis and to help recovery from shock. The dose is 100 mg IV, 3–4 times a day. Dexamethasone 2 mg IV 6 hourly is a suitable alternative.

Supportive measures include gradual warm up of the patient, IV glucose drips, maintenance of proper ventilation and treatment of coexisting infections. Myxedema coma is a condition associated with high mortality and therefore best results are obtained if treatment is undertaken in well-equipped centers. If parenteral preparations of T4 are not available, administration of T4 through a nasogastric tube in doses of 0.1 mg 3 or 4 times a day is advised till the coma clears, and thereafter the dose is modified suitably.

Subclinical Hypothyroidism

This is more common than subclinical hyperthyroidism. In this situation, T3, T4 will be normal and TSH is above normal (>5 µIU/mL). Majority of the patients are asymptomatic and this state is usually found among pregnant patients with positive thyroid autoantibodies, whether to treat this condition in non-pregnant patients is controversial. However in pregnancy, there is no controversy regarding treatment especially because thyroid hormones influences neuronal and astrocytes proliferation and migration in the fetus. T4 is taken up by receptors in the fetal brain astrocytes and is deiodinated to produce T3. In early pregnancy, TSH is normally low and because the fetus is dependent on mother's T4/T3. T4 therapy is indicated to maintain TSH is level below 2.5 mIU/mL in the first trimester and below 3 mIU/mL in subsequent trimesters. Women with positive TPO antibodies have a 15% risk of developing subclinical hypothyroidism.

THYROID HORMONE RESISTANCE SYNDROME (THRS)

This was first described in 1967. It is defined as an impaired response of the target tissues to thyroid hormone despite increased levels of T3 and T4, with normal TSH levels usually. These patients often present with symptoms of hypothyroidism. About 90% of THRS result from mutations in the gene encoding TR-B (thyroid hormone-beta) and mutant receptors have reduced affinity for T3 and are functionally deficient. Pattern of inheritance is autosomal dominant. Three types have been described:

1. Generalized resistance to thyroid hormone by all tissues including the pituitary.
2. Pituitary resistance to inhibition by thyroid hormone. TSH may be normal or increased in this type. Such patients may show thyrotoxic symptoms.
3. Selective peripheral tissue resistance to circulating thyroid hormone. They are clinically hypothyroid but T3, T4 and TSH levels are normal.

Treatment is difficult because thyroid hormone analogs designed to suppress TSH and relieve the hypothyroid symptoms lead to worsening of the cardiovascular manifestations.

All these patients may respond better to analogues of T4. Patients with selective pituitary resistance may respond to dextrothyroxine or 3, 5, 3-tri-iodothyroacetic acid (TRIAC). It may be that a higher circulating concentration may initiate some degree of receptor binding to T4. Analogs of thyroid hormone with TR-B may eventually prove useful in treatment.

Octreotide and bromocriptine are also used to suppress TSH secretion in patients with high TSH.

THYROIDITIS

Different types of classifications are in vogue now:

- *Painful thyroiditis:* Acute, subacute, radiation thyroiditis, trauma
- *Painless thyroiditis:* PPT, sporadic painless thyroiditis, autoimmune thyroiditis (Hashimoto's), fibrous thyroiditis.
- *Drug-induced thyroiditis:* Lithium, amiodarone, alpha-interferon, interleukin IL-2, kinase inhibitors, tumor necrosis factor (TNF) inhibitors, alemtuzumab.

Depending on the onset of symptoms and signs, thyroiditis can also be classified as acute, subacute and chronic. Of late autoimmune thyroiditis has become the most common thyroid disease in Southern Kerala comprising about 66% of the total thyroid cases, and the diagnosis is by the presence of antimicrosomal and or anti-Tg antibodies in the blood. An epidermiological study done in Trivandrum showed a positivity of 89% in asymptomatic young females and 72% in males. 29% of pregnant patients had positive antibodies, more TPO than anti-Tg. A significant majority of pregnant patients with hypothyroidism had positive antibodies (90%) and in 75% neonates born to mothers with positive antibodies also showed antibodies in blood. Familial autoimmune thyroiditis is also prevalent here. In one study of first degree relatives of hypothyroid patients with thyroid autoantibodies, 86% had positive antibodies and 66% were hypothyroid (22% were newly detected in this study). If Hürthle cells are present in the thyroid gland, the name Hashimoto's disease is given, otherwise labeled as autoimmune thyroiditis. In fact, Graves' disease and myxedema are also autoimmune thyroid diseases however, they are not included in the above classifications. These diseases (Graves' disease and myxedema) will have presence of TSHR antibodies.

Acute Suppurative Thyroiditis

Syn: Acute bacterial or Pyogenic thyroiditis

In general, the thyroid gland is resistant to suppuration on account of (1) its capsule, (2) rich blood supply, (3) rich lymphatic supply and (4) high iodine content. Pre-existing thyroid disease may predispose to suppuration.

Acute suppurative thyroiditis is caused by direct invasion by *pneumococcus, Staphylococcus aureus* or *haemolyticus.* Local symptoms include painful enlargement of the thyroid with other signs of acute inflammation. Clinical examination and ultrasonography (USG) will confirm the diagnosis. Systemic manifestations include fever and leukocytosis. Treatment is with appropriate antibiotics, sometimes requiring incision and drainage.

Subacute Thyroiditis

Mainly two forms are known as:

1. Granulomatous thyroiditis
2. Lymphocytic thyroiditis.

Subacute Granulomatous Thyroiditis

Syn: Giant cell thyroiditis, De Quervain's thyroiditis

It may follow an episode of upper respiratory infection. *Subacute granulomatous thyroiditis* is most probably viral in origin caused by coxsackie, mumps or adeno-viruses.

This is painful and the pain radiates to the mandible, neck or the ears. Low grade fever, myalgia and dysphagia may be present. Fifty percent of patients show hyperthyroid features. The thyroid is tender, firm and asymmetrically enlarged. The erythrocyte sedimentation rate (ESR) is elevated.

T4 and T3 levels are elevated, but radioactive iodine uptake is low. Antiviral antibodies may be demonstrable. Mainstay of treatment is to use analgesics and corticosteroids.

Initial dose of prednisolone is 10–20 mg tid for a few days, soon tapered off as a maintenance dose.

In the present acquired immunodeficiency syndrome (AIDS) era, *Pneumocystis carinii* thyroiditis which may occur in association with pneumocystis pneumonia has to be borne in mind.

Subacute Lymphocytic Thyroiditis or Painless Thyroiditis

It is also known as silent or painless thyroiditis. This is characterized by an abrupt onset of hyperthyroidism, elevated T3 and T4 levels, low radioactive iodine uptake and a painless non-tender goiter. Autoimmunity is considered to be the cause and there is a high prevalence of

Textbook of Medicine

thyroid autoantibodies in these patients. Viral antibodies are absent.

Since the hyperthyroidism is transient in both of these types, only beta blockers are required to control hyperthyroid symptoms. Antithyroid drugs are not given.

Postpartum Thyroiditis (PPT)

Thyroid dysfunction occurring within the first 6 months postpartum is called PPT. The prevalence varies from 5 to 7%. PPT develops in 30–50% of women who have TPO antibodies. Most of the patients go into complete remission. PPT is twice as common in patients with type 1 DM and other autoimmune disorders compared to normals. Thyroid gland is enlarged and painless in the majority of cases, with elevated levels of T3/T4. Histology shows lymphocytic infiltration. Sometimes overt thyrotoxic symptoms develop. More than 80% of patients recover thyroid function within an year. Recurrence in subsequent pregnancies is common.

Unlike as in postpartum Graves' disease ^{131}I uptake is low in this condition.

Management

Thyrotoxic symptoms may have to be treated with beta adrenergic blockers. Later, if hypothyroid symptoms develop, T4 has to be supplemented.

Chronic Thyroiditis

- Hashimoto's diseases, Syn: ***Struma lymphomatosa***
- Riedel's thyroiditis also known as Riedel's struma.

Chronic Lymphocytic Thyroiditis

Syn: Hashimoto's disease-Autoimmune thyroiditis

Hashimoto's disease is an autoimmune disorder which has close relationship with Graves' disease. Autoimmune diseases like Sjögren's syndrome, pernicious anemia, myasthenia gravis and RA may co-exist. Other associations include multiple endocrine neoplasia (MEN) type II, polyneuropathy, organomegaly endocrinopathy, monoclonal, gammopathy and skin changes (POEMS) syndrome, Turner's syndrome, Down syndrome and Addison's disease. The peak incidence occurs in the fourth and fifth decades of life. Females are affected more than males.

The thyroid is diffusely enlarged, lobulated, firm or hard in consistency and painless. More commonly it is associated with hypothyroidism. Rarely thyrotoxicosis may occur in Hashimoto's disease ***(Hashitoxicosis)***. The thyroid is infiltrated with lymphocytes. Large hyperplastic lymphoid follicles with germinal centers may be present. The thyroid cells tend to be slightly larger and have an acidophilic staining character (Hurthle or Askanazy cells).

The follicles contain very little colloid. Varying degrees of fibrosis may occur.

Most characteristic laboratory feature is the presence of high titers of circulating antibodies which include ***anti-TgAbs*** and ***AMAs***. Asymptomatic relatives of the patients may show low titers of the antibodies. ESR is markedly elevated and serum gammaglobulin is high.

Radioactive studies show irregular uptake of the isotope in different parts of the gland (Fig. 99.7).

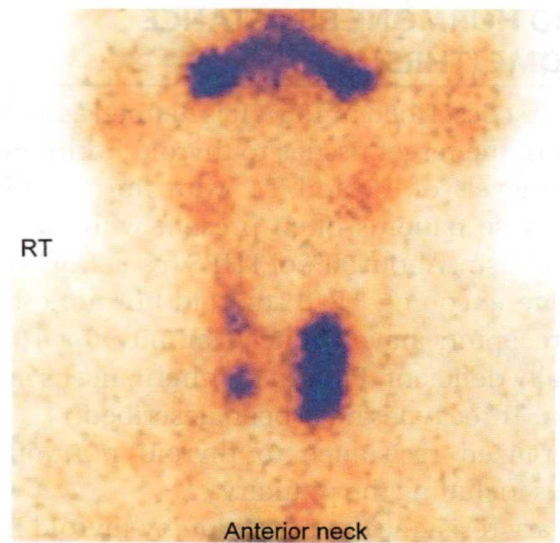

Fig. 99.7: Focal autoimmune thyroiditis right lobe. ***Note:*** The irregular uptake of the isotope in the right lobe as compared to the left lobe

Course: The condition may persist as such for many years. As a sequel, hypothyroidism may develop in many cases.

Treatment

Long-term suppressive medication with T4 in a dose of 0.1–0.2 mg daily may lead to resolution of the goiter.

Hashimoto's Encephalopathy

First described in 1966, Hashimoto's encephalopathy (HE) is an uncommon autoimmune syndrome, characterized by subacute onset of confusion/altered level of consciousness, seizures/and myoclonus. Cerebrospinal fluid (CSF) will show increased protein and up to 25% show lymphocytic pleocytosis. Pathogenesis is due to autoimmue vasculitis and/or other inflammatory processes associated with immune complex deposition. Thyroid autoantibodies (APO/ATG) will be present in serum as well as in CSF. Response to steroids is dramatic. Thyroid function tests (TFTs) tests are variable. Oral prednisolone 50–150 mg/daily can be started and tapered gradually. IV methyl prednisolone can be given in emergencies.

Riedel's Thyroiditis

Syn: Fibrous thyroiditis; Woody thyroiditis

This is extremely rare. The patients present with pressure symptoms due to the enlarged thyroid gland which is hard and immobile. Twenty five percent of patients may have hypothyroidism. Treatment is surgical removal.

Euthyroid Sick Syndrome (ESS)

It is not a thyroid disorder, but a group of changes in serum TSH and thyroid hormones and tissue thyroid hormone levels that result from proinflammatory mediators produced during nonthyroid illnesses. These mediators inhibit the thyroid axis at multiple levels including TSH secretion, response to TSH, transport and peripheral conversion of T4.

Deiodinase D1 activity may be reduced and D3 activity may be increased with low serum TSH and high T3 (reverse T3 activity); Therapy is not routinely recommended except in patients with chronic heart failure (CHF).

Trauma, stress and severe illness may induce alterations in the production, transport and metabolism of thyroid hormones especially the peripheral conversion of T4–T3. The regulation of TSH secretion also becomes altered. These manifest as abnormalities of the serum levels of both bound and free T4, T3 and TSH. This condition is known as sick-euthyroid syndrome. The most consistent features are the low levels of T3 in the serum, with decreased, normal or elevated T4.

Different functional abnormalities may be encountered. Correction of the primary disorder helps to correct the thyroid dysfunction as well. The importance of recognizing this condition is to differentiate it from primary thyroid disorders.

SOLITARY THYROID NODULE

Many patients may present with solitary thyroid nodule which demands investigation and appropriate management. Thyroid nodules may be solid or cystic. True solitary nodules may occur in 4–7% of the adult population.

Generally, functioning adenomas tend to be benign, whereas the chance of malignancy is more in the case of non-functioning nodules, often referred to as *cold nodules*, by isotope scanning. The problem is to distinguish benign lesions from malignant ones and to assess the functional status of the nodule. Clinical examination should include careful local examination of the thyroid, cervical lymph nodes, evidence for pressure effects on cervical structures, and mediastinal obstruction. Thyroid nodules occurring after irradiation of the neck may be papillary adenocarcinomas. Physical findings suggestive of malignancy include a firm or hard nontender nodule, a recent history of mild or moderate enlargement, fixation to adjacent tissues and the presence of regional lymphadenopathy. Rapid painful enlargement occurring within days or weeks is suggestive more of hemorrhage into a nodule rather than malignancy.

Investigations should include USG, ^{131}I or ^{99m}Tc scintiscanning and FNAC (Fig. 99.8). Solid nodules detected by USG are more likely to be malignant than cystic lesions. FNAC gives histological diagnosis in most of the cases. In case of doubt, open biopsy of the nodule is required.

In order to distinguish whether a hyperfunctioning nodule is autonomous or thyrotropin dependent, T3 in a dose of 25 μg tds is administered for 5 days and scintiscanning is repeated. Autonomous nodules are not suppressed.

TPO cytoimmunochemistry with a monoclonal antibody (MoAb47) significantly increases the accuracy of FNAC in follicular lesions.

Treatment

The management of a solitary nodule is still a matter of controversy. Early surgery is recommended for solitary cold nodules and hard rapidly growing nodules. For normally functioning and nonautonomous nodules, a course of thyroid hormone 0.3 mg/day is given and in many cases the nodule may reduce in size. Thyroid hormone is of no use in the treatment of autonomous hyperfunctioning nodules. Such nodules can be irradiated with ^{131}I given preferably after a course of T3/T4 for 5 days. T3 suppresses iodine uptake by the normal tissue and thus ^{131}I gets concentrated only in the autonomous nodule.

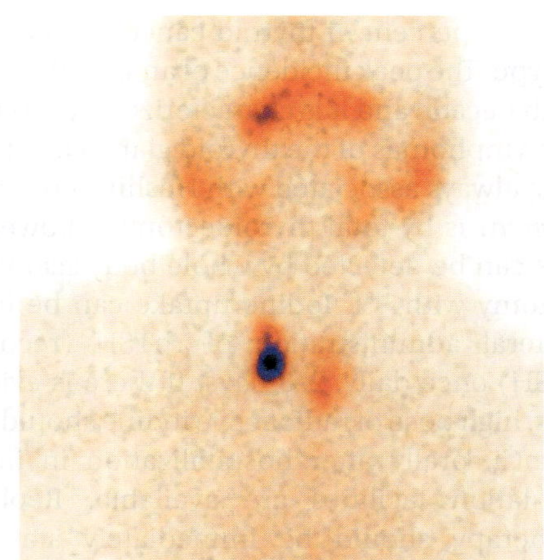

Fig. 99.8: The autonomous hot nodule. The remaining thyroid gland is suppressed by raised T4 from the nodule in the right lobe and hence not visualized.

Table 99.6:	Data from Regional Cancer Center, Trivandrum on carcinoma thyroid	
Papillary Ca		65%
Follicular Ca		24%
Anaplastic Ca		5%
Medullary Ca		6%

Source: Poulose KP. Personal observation, on 350 patients seen between 1990 and 1994.
Abbreviation: Ca = Carcinoma

Autonomous thyroid adenomas may respond to local repeated injection of ethanol (0.4–2 mL) under ultrasonic guidance. Repeated injections may be necessary. Cystic nodular lesions require repeated aspiration followed by injection of sclerosing agents like tetracycline diluted in normal saline (100 mg/mL). Subcutaneous leakage may produce pain. Surgical removal is necessary if other measures fail.

TUMORS OF THE THYROID

Thyroid may be the seat of benign or malignant neoplasms. Most of the malignant tumors are primary, rarely metastases from the kidneys, breasts and lungs may occur. Benign tumors are adenomas. Carcinomas are less common. They may be differentiated or undifferentiated. Irradiation to the tonsils, thymus, lungs or cervical lymph nodes during childhood may predispose to carcinoma of thyroid after a latent period of 10–20 years. Therapy with ^{131}I has not been associated with increase in thyroid carcinoma, but follow-up of children in Marshall's islands where atomic bombs were tested and in the vicinity of the Chernobyl accident, external irradiation has been found to increase the incidence of papillary adenocarcinoma of the thyroid. Rarely thyroid may be the seat of lymphoma or sarcoma. The frequency of thyroid cancer is higher in females. It varies from 0.92% to 1.99% of cases in males and 0.9–5.71% in females. The highest frequency in India is observed in Kerala State as compared to other states according to the National Cancer Registry Programme of the Indian Council of Medical Research (ICMR) (Table 99.6).

Textbook of Medicine

Eighty-five percent of thyroid cancers in children are papillary type. The peak incidence of anaplastic carcinoma is in the 7th decade and it is characterized by rapid growth of tumor. Lymphomas of the thyroid gland can also occur, and almost always associated with Hashimoto's disease.

Treatment is by total thyroidectomy followed by [131]I. Metastasis can be detected by whole body scanning after thyroidectomy with [113]I. Iodine uptake can be increased by parenteral administration of rhTSH (recombinant human TSH) once daily, 2–3 days. If there is evidence of metastasis, high dose of radioactive iodine should be given 150–200 mCi, orally after hospitalization in institution where isolation facilities are available. Replacement thyroid therapy should be immediately started after surgery or radiation. The average dose is 150–200 pg daily. TSH should be around 0.1 mIU/mL in high risk patients and 0.1–0.5 in low-risk patients. Periodic estimation of serum Tg which is a precursor protein for thyroid hormone is useful to detect subsequent recurrence or metastases. Metastases have been reported even 22 years after the primary thyroid surgery. If patient is already on thyroid medications T4 has to be stopped for at least 4 weeks before whole body scan. [123]I can be used instead of ^{131}I for whole body scanning.

In inoperable DTC, doxorubicin, multikinase inhibitors like sorafenib and levatinib are under trial.

[131]I has no role in the treatment of anaplastic carcinoma. Thyroidectomy is the treatment of choice. External beam radiation therapy and multitargeted kinase inhibitors are tried in anaplastic carcinoma. In cases of thyroid cancer, the 5-year survival rate is above 80%. Although the incidence of some forms of thyroid cancer is related to radiation, studies in Kerala did not show any relationship of thyroid cancer to the higher background irradiation from the monazite sands of Kerala sea shores.

Medullary carcinoma of thyroid (MCT): Around 10–15% of malignant lesions of the thyroid are medullary carcinomas. The disease may be familial. Relatives of patients may show elevation of serum calcitonin levels, if they are harboring latent tumors. Medullary carcinoma arises from the 'C' cells or parafollicular cells. Metastasis is common. Elevation of serum calcitonin level is diagnostic in the presence of a palpable thyroid nodule. Medullary carcinoma may secrete serotonin, prostaglandins and even adrenocorticotropic hormone (ACTH). Such cases are associated with flushing and diarrhea. [111]Indium octreotide scintigraphy is useful in detecting MCT.

Medullary carcinoma may coexist with other endocrine tumors MEN such as bilateral pheochromocytoma and hyperparathyroidism (MENIIa and IIb).

Treatment consists of surgical removal of the carcinoma. Medullary carcinoma does not respond to ^{131}I therapy. Kinase inhibitors like vandetanib and cabozantinib are under trial. The different types of MEN are given in below box.

I. Tumors of anterior pituitary, adrenal cortex, parathyroid and pancreas
IIa. Tumors of adrenal medulla, parathyroid, and medullary Ca thyroid
IIb. Tumors of adrenal medulla, medullary Ca thyroid and neurinomas

Abbreviation: Ca = Carcinoma

CHAPTER

100

Parathyroids and their Disorders

KP Poulose, B Jayakumar

Chapter Summary

- General Considerations
- Parathyroid Hormone (Parathormone)
- Primary Hyperparathyroidism
- Secondary and Tertiary Hyperparathyroidism
- Hypoparathyroidism
- Pseudohypoparathyroidism

GENERAL CONSIDERATIONS

Collip identified the active principle of the parathyroid glands in 1924. There are two superior and two inferior parathyroids together weighing 120 mg. The superior parathyroids develop along with the thyroid and the inferior parathyroids develop along with the thymus. Twigs from the superior and inferior thyroid arteries supply the parathyroids. Aberrant parathyroids may be seen at the tracheoesophageal groove, substance of the thyroid gland or thymus, retroesophageal space, anterior mediastinum, surface of the pericardium, carotid bifurcation, jugular foramen or pharyngeal mucosa. The parenchyma consists of chief cells arranged in trabecular, alveolar or acinar patterns with mature fat cells interspersed. Parathyroid hormone (PTH) is secreted by chief cells. In addition, the glands contain large polyhedral oxyphil cells with bright eosinophilic cytoplasm which appear after puberty. Pre-PTH and pro-PTH are precursors formed during the synthesis of PTH.

PARATHYROID HORMONE (PARATHORMONE)

This is a single chain polypeptide having 84 amino acids. PTH is secreted as a pre-pro-hormone with 115 amino acid residues in the endoplasmic reticulum. It is converted into a prohormone containing 90 amino acid residues. The active hormone contains 84 amino acid residues. In circulation, PTH is metabolized to biologically inactive fragments. The circulating PTH is a mixture of polypeptide chains of different biological activity. Therefore, the biological activity does not correlate strictly with the total levels of PTH. The secretion of PTH is controlled by several factors. Circulating ionized calcium exerts the major control on PTH secretion and release. Fall in ionized serum calcium stimulates and rise inhibits PTH secretion. This reciprocal relationship is maintained as long as the serum calcium level ranges between 7 and 15 mg/dL (1.74–3.75 mmol/L; 1 mmol/L Ca = 4 mg/dL). Rise in serum phosphate in renal failure stimulates PTH secretion indirectly by decreasing calcium levels. Extracellular magnesium concentration can also influence secretion of PTH. The half-life of PTH is less than 2 minutes.

Ninety-nine percent of total body calcium remains as hydroxyapatite in bones. In the plasma, 50% of the circulating calcium is in ionized form (i.e. free calcium), 40% is protein bound and 10% is complexed with citrate and phosphate ions. Calcium and phosphorus constitute 65% of the weight of bones. Hypoalbuminemia is the most common cause of hypocalcemia. Therefore, it is necessary to estimate the levels of serum albumin along with serum calcium levels before a diagnosis of hypocalcemia is made.

Calcium homeostasis: Normal calcium concentration is essential for bone formation, blood coagulation, cardiac contractility, neural function and secretory activities. Calcium stabilizes biological membranes and serves as a cofactor in cellular reactions. The plasma calcium level is maintained within a narrow range of 9–11 mg/dL.

Actions of Parathormone

The ultimate effect of this hormone is to conserve body calcium and increase its level in extracellular fluid. It exerts its influence in several ways. The action is receptor mediated.

- PTH increases calcium resorption from bone and raises serum calcium.
- It increases tubular reabsorption of calcium.
- It increases absorption of calcium from the intestine.
- It increases the renal excretion of phosphate and hydroxyproline, resulting in decreased plasma phosphate.
- It enhances the formation of $1,25(OH)_2D_3$ (calcitriol) in the kidneys.
- It increases the secretion of acid and pepsin in the stomach.
- It activates cyclic adenosine monophosphate (cAMP)-adenyl cyclase system in its target cells (PTH receptors in kidney, osteoblasts and intestines).

PTH acts on bones to modulate both osteoblastic and osteoclastic activity, thereby controlling both formation and resorption. PTH acts on bone to modulate osteoblastic activity directly and osteoclastic activity indirectly. Only the osteoblasts have receptors for PTH. Indirect activity on the osteoclasts is brought about by releasing cytokines which activate the osteoclasts to increase bone resorption. PTH does not have any direct effect on the intestine. With excess of PTH levels as in hyperparathyroidism, bone remodeling is increased and there is increased release of calcium resulting in hypercalcemia. Enhanced absorption of calcium and phosphate is due to increase in the levels of $1,25(OH)_2D_3$ caused by increased formation of $1,25(OH)_2D_3$ by the renal tubules under the action of PTH.

The net effect on bones depends on factors such as the bone involved, the dose of PTH and the duration of exposure. In small doses, osteoblastic activity is promoted. Higher levels of PTH result in increased osteoclastic activity in bone, inhibition of collagen formation by osteoblasts and accelerated osteolysis. The net result is the resorption of bone with release of calcium, products of collagen breakdown and alkaline phosphatase (ALP) into blood stream. Kidney tubules possess PTH receptors. PTH acts on the kidneys to conserve calcium and eliminate phosphate, bicarbonate and sodium. The net effect on bone depends on the complex interplay of PTH, vitamin D and renal function (Box 100.1 and Table 100.1).

Tests of Parathyroid Function

Biochemical Studies

Serum calcium: In normal adults, the total serum calcium level is maintained between 9 mg/dL and 11 mg/dL, regardless of the intake. As age advances, serum calcium level gradually falls in men but it increases in women. Several factors affect serum calcium level. These are serum protein concentration, pH of blood, postural variations, and the actions of PTH and vitamin D. While interpreting serum calcium values, all these factors have to be taken into account. Ionized calcium levels in plasma usually range from 4 to 5 mg/dL. When serum albumin

---

Box 100.1: Main actions of parathyroid hormone

- Increases bone resorption—serum calcium increased
- Increases calcium reabsorption from distal nephrons—urinary calcium decreased
- Inhibits phosphate reabsorption from proximal tubules—urinary phosphate increased
- Increases calcium absorption from gut indirectly by stimulating the production of 1,25-vitamin D_3 from kidneys
- Osteoblastic activity—increased in smaller dose and shorter duration
- Osteoclastic activity—increased in larger doses on prolonged exposure.

Table 100.1: Actions of parathyroid hormone (PTH), vitamin D and calcitonin

Hormone	Serum Ca	Serum PO_4
PTH	↑	↓
Vitamin D	↑	↑
Calcitonin	↓	↓
Sites of calcium absorption		
Proximal convoluted tubules	50–60%	Not under PTH influence
Henle's loop	20–30%	Not under PTH influence
Cortical distal nephrons	15–20%	Under PTH influence

Abbreviations: Ca = Calcium; PO_4 = Phosphate

levels rise above normal, serum calcium levels also rise at a rate of 0.8 mg/dL for every 1 g of albumin/dL. While collecting blood for calcium estimation, venous stasis should be avoided, i.e. blood should be collected from a free-flowing vein.

Serum phosphorus: In adults, the level of serum phosphate ranges from 2.5 to 4.8 mg/dL. The levels are higher in children (5.0 ± 1.6 mg/dL). Serum phosphate level shows marked diurnal variation. Several factors such as serum protein levels, calcium, renal function, age, sex and diets rich in carbohydrates influence serum phosphate level. Blood has to be collected in the fasting state for phosphorus estimation. In hyperparathyroidism, serum phosphorus is low. Approximately 85% of body phosphate is in bones and 15% either in the inorganic or organic form is distributed in the intra- and extracellular compartments. Phosphate is an integral part of nucleic acids, adenosine triphosphate (ATP), phospholipids and creatinine phosphokinase (CPK).

Serum ALP: Total serum ALP, especially bone ALP reflects bone turnover in metabolic bone diseases. The normal adult value is 30–110 IU/L [3–13 King-Armstrong (KA) units/dL]. The isoenzyme bone ALP is elevated in osteoclast overactivity.

PTH levels in serum can be estimated by radioimmunoassay (RIA). In hyperparathyroidism, PTH is elevated and in hypoparathyroidism, it is reduced. PTH levels estimated by RIA may not reflect true biological activity since a part of the estimated hormone may not be biologically active. It is more advantageous to estimate PTH and ionized calcium simultaneously. Elevated PTH levels in the presence of low calcium levels suggest pseudohypoparathyroidism (PHP), calcium and vitamin D deficiency (osteomalacia) and renal failure. In magnesium deficiency also, PTH levels are low.

Serum vitamin D: In healthy subjects, total vitamin D level is 35.0 ± 3.4 ng/mL, $25(OH)D_3$ is 28.5 ± 2.0 ng/mL and $1,25(OH)_2D_3$ is 35.0 ± 3 pg/mL. In hypoparathyroidism and chronic renal failure, circulating levels of $1,25(OH)_2D_3$ are low. Dietary intake of calcium and phosphate also influences serum vitamin D levels.

Serum electrolytes: Since PTH inhibits the tubular absorption of bicarbonate excess, PTH may lead to renal tubular acidosis (RTA). Hypercalcemia of primary hyperparathyroidism (PHPT) is often associated with hyperchloremic acidosis. This feature helps to distinguish PHPT from hypercalcemia occurring in bony metastases or hypervitaminosis D in which there is mild alkalosis.

Urinary calcium: In health, more than 95.0% of filtered calcium is reabsorbed by the tubules. If the intake of calcium is steady, urinary loss of calcium is less than 3–4 mg/kg of ideal body weight in 24 hours. In hyperparathyroidism, with sustained hypercalcemia, the daily urinary loss of calcium exceeds 300 mg. This gives a positive ***Sulkowitch test***.

Urinary phosphate: PTH facilitates the excretion of phosphates in urine. Approximately 88% of the filtered phosphate is reabsorbed in the proximal and distal tubules and only 12% is excreted. When the dietary intake of phosphates is 1–1.5 g/day, the daily urinary loss is less than 1 g. Dietary phosphate is mostly absorbed and it tends to raise serum phosphate level. The urinary excretion therefore varies directly with dietary intake. Normal phosphate clearance, determined by simultaneous measurement of urinary and serum phosphate is 10.8 ± 2.7 mL/minute. The tubular reabsorption of phosphates exceeds 75–85% of the filtered load. Tubular reabsorption is reduced in hyperparathyroidism and thereby phosphate clearance is increased at least by 50%.

Urinary hydroxyproline: Normal adults eliminate 15–42 mg of hydroxyproline in 24 hours. This is increased in hyperparathyroidism and osteomalacia. Other conditions in which urinary hydroxyproline is altered include growth spurt and bone resorption.

Urinary cyclic adenosine-3′, 5′-monophosphate (cAMP): Measurement of urinary cAMP levels gives useful clues regarding parathyroid function. Normal adults excrete 10 micromoles of cAMP in 24 hours (1.8–4.5 nmol/dL of glomerular filtrate). In PHPT, urinary cAMP levels are high. Administration of PTH raises urinary cAMP levels in normal. This response is absent in PHP. Urinary cAMP levels are elevated in hypercalcemia secondary to bony metastases.

Suppression tests: Tests to determine the suppressibility of PTH are employed to differentiate various hypercalcemic states from hyperparathyroidism. Rarely used now—calcium infusion test, cortisone test.

Ellsworth-Howard test: Normal subjects respond to the administration of 200–400 USP units PTH or by increasing the urinary levels of phosphate and cAMP by about 100%. Subjects with hypoparathyroidism show exaggerated increase in these parameters. In patients with PHP, this response is blunted.

Indirect tests of parathyroid function include estimation of bone mineral density and isotopic bone scans.

- Estimation of bone mineral density by radiography and dual-energy X-ray absorptiometry (DEXA).
- Isotopic bone scans using [99m]technetium (^{99m}Tc) phosphate compounds.

Imaging the parathyroids: This can be done by subtraction techniques using [207]thallium chloride and [99m]technetium ($^{99m}TcO_4^-$) pertechnetate radionuclides. Initial scan with technetium delineates the thyroid. Thallium is taken up both by thyroid and parathyroids. Computerized subtraction techniques allow localization of parathyroids. Scanning with ^{99m}Tc-sestamibi is used now for parathyroid imaging; however, this substance is also taken up by Hürthle cell adenomas and other thyroid tumors.

Computed tomography (CT)/magnetic resonance imaging (MRI) is also helpful. Selective venous blood sampling for PTH is also useful for localizing the source of abnormal function. Ultrasound of the neck is also helpful with a sensitivity of 80%.

PRIMARY HYPERPARATHYROIDISM

When pathological hypersecretion of PTH occurs persistently, it results in hyperparathyroidism. It is characterized by hypercalcemia, hypophosphatemia, metabolic bone disease, recurrent nephrolithiasis, renal damage, peptic ulceration and other complications. Adult women are more affected than men. Peak incidence is in the sixth decade and two to three times more in women. Rarely, PHPT may occur in neonates. A wide spectrum of severity ranging from an asymptomatic illness to fatal hypercalcemic crisis may be seen. Though hyperparathyroidism is one of the common endocrine disorders, many patients may remain asymptomatic.

Causes

The main causes are:

- Benign adenoma of one parathyroid gland seen in 85% of cases
- Hyperplasia of all the parathyroid glands (15%)
- Carcinoma of one of the glands (1%).

In 85% of cases, the lesion is an **adenoma** which may vary in weight from 0.5 to 5 g. Histologically, the adenoma is composed of chief cells in vast majority, but at times oxyphil cells or mixed cells may predominate. Adenomas remain well-encapsulated within a rim of normal tissue. Ectopic foci for parathyroid adenomas include thymus, thyroid, pericardium or retroesophageal space.

About 15% of cases are due to diffuse or nodular hyperplasia affecting all or most of the parathyroid glands. **Carcinoma** is rare forming only about 1%. When present, it affects only one gland. The degree of malignancy is low. Adenoma or carcinoma may be part of the multiple endocrine neoplasia (MEN) syndromes. MEN1 (pituitary and pancreas) and MEN2 (medullary carcinoma of thyroid and pheochromocytomas) are genetically-mediated autosomal dominant disorders.

Clinical Manifestations

Classic description of hyperparathyroidism is that it is *a disease of bones, stones, abdominal groans and psychic moans*. The presenting symptoms may vary depending on hypercalcemia, renal involvement, bone involvement or other complications. Sometimes, a tumor may be palpable in the neck or visualized radiologically in the mediastinum.

Hypercalcemia

Hypercalcemia manifests in several ways. Common symptoms include lethargy, polyuria, polydipsia, drowsiness, confusion, weight loss, generalized muscle weakness, hypertension and autonomic dysfunction such as anorexia, uncontrolled vomiting and constipation. Proximal muscle weakness may be prominent. Severe cases go into stupor and coma. Long-standing hypercalcemia leads to metastatic calcification in the lungs, cornea, kidneys, blood vessels and other organs. The corneal lesion is **band keratopathy** in which calcium deposition is best demonstrated by slit-lamp examination. Cardiac dysfunction occurs. Ventricular systole is shortened. Electrocardiogram (ECG) shows shortened QT interval and other nonspecific changes.

Skeletal Manifestations

Osteitis fibrosa cystica (OFC) or diffuse loss of bone tissue such as osteoporosis or osteomalacia may occur.

It is accompanied by severe localized bone pain, marked deformities and pathological fractures. In OFC, the bone trabeculae are reduced. There is increase in multinucleated osteoclasts and fibrovascular tissue. Radiological abnormalities of bone include subperiosteal erosion of cortical bone, demineralization, local destructive lesions such as cystic changes (bone cysts and brown tumors) and calcification of fibrocartilage. The phalanges show loss of bone tuft and subperiosteal erosions and these are diagnostic. Acromioclavicular joints, symphysis pubis and sacroiliac joints also show similar changes. Osteopenia is seen characteristically as punched out and mottled areas in the skull (pepper pot skull). The lamina dura of the teeth is lost. Joints may show chondrocalcinosis and degenerative changes. With successful treatment of hyperparathyroidism, all the radiological abnormalities clear-up.

Renal Manifestations

Nephrolithiasis, nephrocalcinosis and disorders of glomerulotubular function are common in long-standing cases. Renal calculi are made up of a mixture of calcium oxalate (CaC_2O_4) and calcium phosphate ($Ca_3O_8P_2$). Renal stones tend to be recurrent. Hypercalcemia predisposes to urinary infection. Nephrocalcinosis is usually associated with bony changes such as OFC. Glomerular filtration rate (GFR) is reduced. Blood urea and serum creatinine are elevated. Tubular dysfunction also occurs. Correction of hypercalcemia reverses the functional defects in the kidneys.

Alimentary Manifestations

Hypercalcemia increases gastric acid production and thus predisposes to peptic ulceration. Zollinger-Ellison syndrome (ZES) may coexist MEN1. Hypercalcemia leads to chronic pancreatitis, pancreatic calcification or acute hemorrhagic pancreatitis.

Diagnosis

PHPT should be suspected in all cases of hypercalcemia, recurrent urinary calculi, OFC, peptic ulcer, pancreatitis, myopathy, chondrocalcinosis and vague constitutional symptoms. All cases presenting with dehydration, polydipsia, nocturia, anorexia, confusion, joint stiffness and hypertension, in which other causes are not evident, should also be investigated for PHPT.

Biochemical Tests

The diagnosis is confirmed by the presence of hypercalcemia and hypophosphatemia. Serum ALP, urinary hydroxyproline, osteocalcin and collagen telopeptide excretion are elevated. Urinary cAMP excretion is elevated. PTH levels are elevated. Higher levels of 1,25-vitamin D are also present.

Demonstration of Tumor or Hyperplasia

Large parathyroid tumors may produce indentation on the barium-filled esophagus, demonstrable by barium swallow examination. Ultrasonography (USG), CT scan with contrast imaging and MRI demonstrate the lesion in most cases. Radioactive thallium-technetium subtraction or technetium (MIBI) scanning may be employed to locate the tumor. Selective venous blood sampling from the veins draining the parathyroids to detect a gradient in PTH levels helps to assess the functional status of the lesion as well.

Intraoperative parathyroid localization can be done using technetium sestamibi (MIBI). A handheld gamma probe after ^{99}Tc injection over the parathyroid can locate an abnormal gland. Similarly, intraoperative USG performed by experienced surgeon has also proved successful in localization of parathyroid tumors.

Virtual neck exploration is CT-based imaging technique which can delineate the minute anatomy of the neck including various glands. In areas where this is available, it facilitates surgical management. Its adverse effects include high cost, irradiation and thyroid storm caused by iodinated contrast.

Differential Diagnosis

PHPT has to be distinguished from secondary hyperparathyroidism and all other causes of hypercalcemia. In secondary hyperparathyroidism, though PTH levels are high, serum calcium values are not elevated, but phosphate is elevated, e.g. renal rickets.

Common causes of hypercalcemia are disseminated malignancy involving bone, hypervitaminosis D, thyrotoxicosis, Addison's disease and prolonged immobilization. Rarely hypervitaminosis A, sarcoidosis, multiple myeloma and thiazide drugs may be the cause of hypercalcemia. Sometimes hypercalcemia runs in families (familial hypocalciuric hypercalcemia). This is due to an autosomal dominant mutation of calcium sensor that results in inappropriate secretion of PTH and enhanced renal calcium reabsorption. Idiopathic hypercalcemia is a rare disorder of infancy, often associated with congenital cardiovascular defects. Hypercalcemia of malignancy seen in bony metastasis and multiple myeloma is either due to local osteolytic lesions releasing cytokines [interleukin-6 (IL-6) and tumor necrosis factor-beta (TNF-β)] which enhance bone reabsorption or due to release of PTH-related polypeptide (PTHrP) which is a PTH-like humoral factor (Table 100.2).

Changes in blood levels of PTH, serum calcium, phosphorus and creatinine in various parathyroid disorders have been shown in Table 100.3.

Prognosis

The course of hyperparathyroidism tends to be progressive. If detected and treated early, the condition subsides.

Skeletal changes revert to normal but advanced renal lesions fail to clear up and, therefore, it is essential to start treatment before renal damage is established.

Points to Remember
Primary hyperparathyroidism
- Increased PTH is associated with hypercalcemia, osteoporosis, nephrolithiasis.
- Surgery is indicated in PHPT (asymptomatic) if the serum calcium is greater than 1 mg% above the upper normal limit, GFR < 60 mL/min, nephrolithiasis and osteoporosis.
- Most surgeons prefer perioperative localization especially in suspected bilateral disease.

Treatment

Surgical removal of the adenoma is the treatment of choice. Indications for surgical intervention in PHPT have been depicted in Box 100.2.

In the case of hyperplasia, all the glands are removed except for a portion of one gland which is left behind. All cases should be investigated for MEN and appropriate treatment is indicated if this is detected. Serum calcium level above 11 mg/dL, evidence of bone disease, recurrent renal stones, reduction of GFR below 60 mL/min and uncontrollable peptic ulcer are indications for early surgery.

After successful parathyroidectomy, serum PTH falls by 50% within 10 minutes and serum calcium falls to normal within 24–36 hours. This does not happen if surgical removal is inadequate. Some cases develop postoperative tetany due to hypocalcemia. This is managed by giving intravenous (IV) infusions of calcium gluconate or calcium chloride (1 mg/mL of fluid), the total dose and duration of therapy being decided by clinical progress. One ampoule of calcium gluconate contains 10 mL, each mL containing 137.5 mg of the drug. If hypocalcemia tends to persist, it is managed on the lines indicated for hypoparathyroidism.

At times, magnesium deficiency may be the cause of postoperative tetany. Serum magnesium levels are low (Normal values: 0.7–1.2 mmol/L or 2–3 mg/dL). Mild cases respond to oral supplementation with magnesium chloride ($MgCl_2$). In severe cases, magnesium sulfate ($MgSO_4$) can be given intramuscularly (IM) repeatedly or as IV infusion lasting for 8–12 hours. The total dose is decided by the serum magnesium levels. A severe case may require 2 mmol/kg/bw. $MgSO_4$ is available as 20% solution or 50% solution. Parenteral magnesium therapy should be closely monitored, since serum levels above 4 mmol/L lead to neuromuscular paralysis.

Medical Treatment

Mild cases with moderate hypercalcemia, elderly patients, and those who are at poor surgical risks have to be managed medically. In such cases, the intake of calcium should be restricted to 200 mg or less by avoiding dairy products. Serum calcium can be lowered by the regular administration of potassium phosphate (K_2SO_4) 1–2 g daily. The patient should be carefully followed up for detecting metastatic calcification. Peptic ulceration should be managed on its own merits. Liberal intake of fluids (3.5–4.5 L/day) and calcitonin injections at intervals help to reduce the risk of urinary calculi.

Table 100.2: Different mechanisms lead to hypercalcemia	
Due to increased bone resorption	Hyperparathyroidism, humoral hypercalcemia of malignancy (HHCM), thyrotoxicosis, vitamin A toxicity (> 25,000 IU/day), immobilization, lithium carbonate
Increased renal absorption or decreased renal clearance	Milk-alkali syndrome, rhabdomyolysis, thiazide diuretics, familial hypocalciuric hypercalcemia, renal failure
Increased gut absorption	Excessive vitamin D (> 10,000 IU/day), fungal infections, sarcoidosis, eosinophilic granuloma, HIV, lymphomas

Abbreviation: HIV = Human immunodeficiency virus

Textbook of Medicine

Table 100.3: Changes in blood levels of parathormone (PTH), serum calcium, phosphorus and creatinine in various parathyroid disorders

Diagnosis	PTH	Calcium	Phosphorus	Creatinine	Congenital abnormalities
Primary hyperparathyroidism	H	H	L	N	Nil
Secondary hyperparathyroidism	H	L/N	H	H	Nil
Tertiary hyperparathyroidism	H	H	H	H	Nil
Hypoparathyroidism	L	L	H	N	Nil
Pseudohypoparathyroidism	N/H	L	H	N	Present
Pseudopseudohypoparathyroidism	N	N	N	N	Present

Abbreviations: H = High; N = Normal; L = Low

Box 100.2: Indications for surgical intervention in primary hyperparathyroidism

- Serum calcium > 2.85 mmol/L (1 mmol calcium = 4 mg/dL)
- Renal manifestations
  - Marked hypercalciuria
  - Creatinine clearance < 30% of normal
- Gastrointestinal manifestations
  - Peptic ulcer disease
  - Pancreatitis
- Bone manifestation
  - Reduction of bone mineral density (BMD) by 2 standard deviations from age- and sex-matched mean
  - Soft tissue calcification
- Age < 50 years; patient choice or when regular follow-up is difficult or impossible

Acute Hypercalcemia and its Management

Normal serum calcium levels range around 2.6 mmol/L (10.4 mg/dL) when the serum albumin levels are normal, i.e. 4 g/dL. Acute hypercalcemia usually results from hyperparathyroidism or disseminated secondaries in bones. Serum calcium levels above 3.5 mmol/L (14 mg/dL) lead to life-threatening situations demanding emergency management.

In hyperparathyroidism, PTH is elevated. In bony secondaries, PTHrP secreted by the tumor is elevated whereas PTH values are normal or reduced. Both PTH and PTHrP lead to resorption of bone by osteoclasts, increase in the renal tubular absorption of calcium and decrease in the reabsorption of sodium and water. As a result, polyuria and dehydration develop. Clinical abnormalities are referable to gastrointestinal (GI), cardiovascular, renal and central nervous systems (CNS).

GI system: Anorexia, nausea, vomiting, constipation and at times acute pancreatitis.

Cardiovascular system (CVS): ECG abnormalities such as QT prolongation and increased sensitivity to digoxin.

Excretory system: Polyuria, polydipsia, nephrocalcinosis and renal failure.

CNS: Apathy, drowsiness, confusion, coma.

Treatment (Table 100.4)

- The patient is rehydrated by IV infusion of normal saline. Often 2.5–4 L may be needed.
- Furosemide given in a dose of 20–40 mg IV helps to increase urinary excretion of calcium. Thiazide diuretics are contraindicated since they enhance distal tubular absorption of calcium.

Drugs which Inhibit Osteoclast Activity (Table 100.5)

- *Calcimimetics:* Calcimimetics bind to the calcium-sensing receptors (CaSRs) on parathyroid cells and increases chief cell sensitivity to extracellular calcium (suppressive effect). Oral cinacalcet is the only drug available now. Cinacalcet also decreases the calcium reabsorption from the renal tubules. Dose is 30 mg daily.

Table 100.4: Therapy for hypercalcemia

Therapy	Dose	Route	Monitor/Comment
Saline	250–1,000 mL/h	IV	Cardiopulmonary functions, central venous pressure/pulmonary capillary wedge pressure and chest radiograph
Furosemide	20–80 mg every 2–4 h or 40 mg/h CI	IV	Serum and urine electrolytes, replace K, Mg and PO_4 based on serum levels and urinary losses
Salmon calcitonin	4–8 IU/kg every 6–12 h	IM, SC	Allergic reaction. Give a skin test of 1 IU intradermally before treatment. Effective only during first 48–72 h
Prednisolone/ methylprednisolone	20 mg 2–3 times a day	PO/IV	Possible adjunct to calcitonin. Effective in $1,25(OH)_2D_3$ associated hypercalcemia
Zoledronic acid	4 mg IV over 15 min every 2–4 weeks PRN	IV	Drug of choice for malignancy associated hypercalcemia. Caution with chronic kidney disease and myeloma
Pamidronate	39–90 mg over 2–24 h every I–3 weeks PRN	IV	Infuse over at least 4 h in severe renal failure (glomerular filtrating rate < 30 mL/min)
Cinacalcet	30–90 mg bd-qid	PO	Take with meals. Monitor PTH, Ca and PO_4 at least 12 h after dose

Abbreviations: bd = Twice daily; CI = Continuous infusion; IM = Intramuscular; IV = Intravenous; K = Potassium; Mg = Magnesium; Na = Sodium; PO = Orally; PO_4 = Phosphate; PRN = As needed; qid = Four times daily; SC = Subcutaneously; PTH = Parathyroid hormone

Textbook of Medicine

Table 100.5: Mechanisms of action of drugs used in hypercalcemia

Drug	Mechanism(s) of action
Saline	Dilutes serum calcium by volume expansion and increases urinary flow and calcium excretion
Furosemide	Impairs renal sodium and calcium reabsorption in Henle's loop, increasing urinary flow and calcium excretion
Calcitonin	Binds to receptors on osteoclasts, inhibiting osteoclastic activity and decreasing bone resorption; also decreases renal reabsorption
Glucocorticoids	Antagonism of vitamin D causing decreased calcium absorption; in tumoral states, may decrease production of osteoclast activating factors and vitamin D
Bisphosphonates	Impair osteoclast differentiation, recruitment, motility and attachment; incorporate into bone matrix making the matrix resistant to hydrolysis; overall effect is decreased bone resorption
Cinacalcet	Calcimimetic that binds to the CaSR

Note: For long-term hypocalcemic effects, drug used for hypercalcemia almost antagonize one of the three main mechanisms for hypercalcemia, i.e. (1) bone resorption; (2) renal reabsorption or (3) gut absorption. Any one of these three mechanisms should be considered for the choice of drug therapy. Most drugs used for hypercalcemia impair bone resorption.

Abbreviation: CaSR = Calcium-sensing receptor

- **Calcitonin:** Both salmon calcitonin and human calcitonin are available for use. Calcitonin is given in a dose of 4 Medical Research Council (MRC) units/kg subcutaneously (SC) or IM every 12 hours. It is rapid in action but weaker compared to bisphosphonates. If the response is inadequate the dose may be increased to 8 MRC units/kg. Preparations for nasal spray IV and rectal use are also available.
- **Bisphosphonates:** Etidronate, pamidronate and alendronate are available for use as oral/IV preparations.

Dose	
Etidronate	7.5 mg/kg daily orally for 6 months
Pamidronate	15–45 mg IV daily for 6 days
Alendronate	40 mg/day orally before food—10 mg tablets are available

- Other analogs such as **ibandronate** (oral) and **zoledronate** (IV) are also available at present. They also lower serum calcium levels. On a long-term basis, they also suppress osteoclastic activity.
- Recombinant PTH analogs such as teriparatide SC injection 20 mcg daily up to 18 months.
- **Glucocorticoids:** Hypercalcemia caused by lesions other than hyperparathyroidism temporarily responds to corticosteroids.

In life-threatening emergencies, calcium can be removed from the system by dialysis procedures using calcium-free dialyzing fluids.

- **Denosumab:** This is a monoclonal antibody that decreases osteoclastic bone resorption which is already approved for treatment of osteoporosis.

SECONDARY AND TERTIARY HYPERPARATHYROIDISM

These are seen in conditions where there is resistance to the action of PTH. Increased levels of PTH are seen in the presence of persistent hypocalcemia. Increased secretion of PTH is the result of chronic stimulation by hypocalcemia.

Secondary hyperparathyroidism is seen in rickets, osteomalacia, malabsorption syndrome, chronic renal failure and skeletal fluorosis. Removal of the primary cause early in the disease may correct the parathyroid dysfunction also but this is not invariably so. Though, in the initial stages, the parathyroids are stimulated by hypocalcemia, later on, the glands become autonomous because of the development of adenomas. This condition is known as ***tertiary hyperparathyroidism***.

Biochemical profile includes normal or low serum calcium with elevated serum phosphate. In tertiary hyperparathyroidism, serum calcium may rise. Bone changes are the result of excessive parathyroid activity and calcium deficiency. Serum ALP is high.

Therapy is intended to correct hypocalcemia which is the chronic stimulus for stimulation of the parathyroids. Surgical removal of the adenoma may be indicated in tertiary hyperparathyroidism.

Humoral Hypercalcemia of Malignancy

This refers to the condition in which PTH like substances (peptides or prostaglandins) are secreted by other tumors like carcinomas of the breast, kidneys, lungs and uterine cervix, lymphomas, and also leukemias. Often this leads to severe and fulminant hypercalcemia. Malignancies may also cause hypercalcemia by local bone destruction (e.g. myeloma, breast cancer) or by release of PTHrP (e.g. lung, kidneys, squamous cell cancers) or by activating lymphocytes to release IL-1 and TNF. Serum PTH level is suppressed in this condition which clinches the diagnosis.

HYPOPARATHYROIDISM

Deficiency in the secretion of PTH leads to hypoparathyroidism. This is characterized by hypocalcemia, hyperphosphatemia and low levels of circulating PTH. The hyperphosphatemia leads to calcification of the basal ganglia in 50% of cases. Soft tissue calcification may also occur.

Etiology

- Accidental surgical removal of parathyroids or interference with their blood supply during surgery in the neck
- Idiopathic atrophy of the parathyroids
- Destruction of the parathyroid by carcinomatous secondaries, infarction, radioiodine therapy or irradiation of the neck
- Neonatal hypoparathyroidism may occur as a transient phenomenon in premature infants and infants of mothers with hyperparathyroidism or diabetes mellitus (DM)
- PHP
- Developmental defects as in DiGeorge syndrome

- Rare causes—hemochromatosis, Wilson's disease with copper deposition in the parathyroids
- Hypomagnesemia
- Vitamin D deficiency, renal failure
- Hungry bone syndrome
- Pancreatitis.

Postoperative hypoparathyroidism may be transient or permanent. Idiopathic hypoparathyroidism may run in families. It may be associated with other congenital abnormalities involving maldevelopment of the third and fourth pharyngeal pouches such as *DiGeorge syndrome* in which the thymus and parathyroids are absent. Other immune-mediated endocrinopathies such as Addison's disease, hypothyroidism, hypofunction of ovaries and pernicious anemia may coexist. Antibodies against parathyroids and other organ-specific antibodies may be present.

Clinical Manifestations

Clinical features depend upon the onset, duration and the severity of hypocalcemia. Prominent features include tetany, dental abnormalities, subcapsular cataracts, myocardial dysfunction and neurological abnormalities.

Tetany is due to hypocalcemia. It manifests as muscle cramps, paresthesia of the hands, feet and mouth, spasmophilia (carpopedal spasm, bronchospasm and laryngospasm) and severe neuromuscular irritability. Physical exertion, emotional stress, hyperventilation, vomiting and ischemia to the limb may precipitate tetany. In less severe and chronic forms of hypocalcemia, tetany may remain latent.

Latent tetany can be identified by eliciting the *Chvostek's sign, Trousseau's sign*, and also by *electromyography*. Hyperexcitability of the facial muscles manifesting as contraction of the facial muscles on gentle tapping over the facial nerve in front of the tragus of the ear is the *Chvostek's sign*. *Trousseau's sign* is elicited by making the forearm ischemic by applying a sphygmomanometer cuff to the arm and keeping the pressure above systolic blood pressure for 5 minutes. The hand goes into painful carpopedal spasm and assumes the *Accoucheur's hand position*. Laryngeal spasm gives rise to inspiratory dyspnea or stridor (*Laryngismus stridulus*).

Hypocalcemic tetany has to be differentiated from tetany occurring in alkalosis, hypokalemia and hypomagnesemia. When serum magnesium falls below 0.8 mmol/L, PTH secretion is depressed and this leads to secondary hypoparathyroidism. Parenteral replacement of magnesium restores parathyroid function.

Common neurological manifestations of hypocalcemia include convulsions which are unresponsive to conventional anticonvulsant therapy, paresthesia and psychiatric behavior. Other manifestations such as papilledema and extrapyramidal disturbances like chorea, Parkinsonism and athetosis may develop. Soft tissue and basal ganglia calcification can occur.

The skin is dry and scaly. The hair is brittle and coarse. Deformity and moniliasis of the nails are common. The enamel of the teeth is pitted, dental roots are short and blunt and early loss of teeth is common. Subcapsular posterior or anterior zonular cataracts develop.

Cardiac abnormalities may occur. Chronic hypocalcemia may lead to cardiac failure and tetany. Diuretics further aggravate the hypocalcemia. The ECG shows prolonged QT interval. The acute manifestations of hypoparathyroidism are corrected dramatically by the IV administration of calcium. IV administration of 10% calcium gluconate, calcitriol and oral maintenance doses of calcium gluconate restore cardiac function.

Causes of Hypocalcemia

The causes of hypocalcemia have been depicted in Box 100.3.

Diagnosis

Presence of hypocalcemia with hyperphosphatemia should arouse suspicion of hypoparathyroidism, if renal disease can be excluded. Other causes of hypocalcemia are rickets, malabsorption states, hypoproteinemia, acute pancreatitis and extreme dietary deficiency of calcium. The total serum calcium is low in hypoproteinemia since the fraction bound to albumin is reduced, even though the ionized calcium is kept normal. Tetany does not occur in this condition. In acute pancreatitis, transient hypocalcemia develops which is self-limiting. In rickets and osteomalacia, both calcium and phosphorus are low. Diagnosis of hypoparathyroidism can be confirmed by demonstrating low levels or absence of PTH. The response to therapeutic administration of PTH is dramatic. In vitamin D deficiency and renal failure, PTH is elevated.

PSEUDOHYPOPARATHYROIDISM

Syn: PTH resistance syndrome

The term *pseudohypoparathyroidism (PHP)* refers to a condition in which the target tissues become resistant to the action of PTH. As a result, there is overactivity and hyperplasia of the parathyroids with excessive secretion of PTH. In spite of the raised blood levels of PTH, the clinical and biochemical features are those of hypoparathyroidism. In most cases, it is an inherited disorder associated with short stature, brachydactyly, round face, obesity and webbing of the neck.

Box 100.3: Causes of hypocalcemia

Increased phosphate levels
- Chronic renal failure (common)
- Phosphate therapy—hypoparathyroidism
- Surgical—after neck exploration [thyroidectomy, parathyroidectomy (common)]
- Congenital deficiency (DiGeorge syndrome)
- Idiopathic hypoparathyroidism (rare)
- Severe hypomagnesemia

Vitamin D deficiency
- Osteomalacia/rickets
- Vitamin D resistance

Resistance to pseudohypoparathyroidism (PHP)

Drugs
- Calcitonin
- Bisphosphonates

Other
- Acute pancreatitis (quite common)
- Citrated blood in massive transfusion (not uncommon)
- Low plasma albumin, e.g. malnutrition, chronic liver disease
- Malabsorption, e.g. celiac disease

This is characterized by biochemical features of genuine hypoparathyroidism with elevated PTH levels. In the two major forms of this (type I and type II) disorder, correction of hypocalcemia results in alteration of symptoms and suppression of PTH levels; however, the resistance continues. The common disorder, PHP type Ia is characterized by short stature, brachydactyly, round facies, obesity, short fourth metacarpal bone, webbing of the neck, mental retardation and subcutaneous calcification. The term ***Albright's hereditary osteodystrophy (AHO)*** has been used to describe the somatic features of type Ia. This is due to defective functioning of guanine nucleotide-coupling protein (G protein). These patients may also have resistance to other hormones like thyroid-stimulating hormone (TSH), glucagons, luteinizing hormone (LH) and antidiuretic hormone (ADH). Diagnosis is made by estimation of G protein in red cells. In type Ib PHP, the somatic features of type Ia are absent. Physical appearance is normal, and there is normal cAMP response to PTH stimulation despite the high levels of PTH.

Pseudopseudohypoparathyroidism: Some of the relatives of subjects with PHP show skeletal changes, but none of the biochemical abnormalities of hypoparathyroidism. Osteoma cutis may be present. Both PHP and pseudo-PHP may involve the same GNAs gene. This condition is called pseudo-PHP.

Treatment of Hypoparathyroidism

Aim of treatment is to normalize serum calcium levels without increasing urinary loss. Though correction of hypocalcemia is easy, in the absence of PTH, considerably large amounts of calcium are lost in urine. Therefore, even with low-normal levels of serum calcium, nephrolithiasis may develop. Intestinal absorption of calcium can be enhanced by administration of vitamin D. This corrects hypocalcemia, but not other metabolic abnormalities. It is desirable to keep serum calcium levels between 8.5 and 9 mg/dL by adjusting the dose of vitamin D. Several preparations are available. Vitamin D_3 50,000–100,000 IU/day or the metabolically active product $1,25(OH)_2$ cholecalciferol (calcitriol) in doses of 0.25–0.5 µg given orally daily helps to improve serum calcium level. Vitamin D preparations take a few weeks to exert

Table 100.6: Elemental calcium in the commonly available preparations		
Oral	**Each tablet strength**	**Elemental calcium (mg)**
Calcium citrate	950 mg	200
Calcium acetate	667 mg	169
Calcium carbonate	500 mg	200
Injections		
Calcium chloride	2.5 mL of l0%	90
Calcium gluconate	10 mL of 10%	90
Calcium gluceptate	5 mL of 22%	90

their full effect. Loss of control may develop even after long periods of satisfactory control. Along with vitamin D_3, approximately 1.0 g of elemental calcium should be provided in the diet. Elemental calcium in the commonly available preparations has been shown in Table 100.6.

Hypomagnesemia confers resistance to vitamin D which clears up on supplementation of magnesium orally or parenterally.

Treatment of Tetany

Slow IV injection of 20 mL of 10% calcium gluconate solution promptly relieves tetany. The relief is maintained by giving an IV drip containing calcium gluconate 15 mg/kg body weight. IV calcium injection is quite safe even though it may cause a feeling of heat over the body, which could be disturbing to the patient, unless informed beforehand. In subjects receiving digitalis therapy, it may precipitate fatal arrhythmias like ventricular fibrillation. Supplementation of oral calcium carbonate or gluconate along with alfacalcidol serves to increase serum calcium on long-term basis.

Alkalotic Tetany

In hysterical subjects who hyperventilate, alkalotic tetany may develop. Alkalosis enhances neuromuscular excitability. This can be prevented by inhalation of 5% carbon dioxide or rebreathing into the same bag. For tetany due to metabolic alkalosis, infusion of isotonic saline is the most effective measure. In alkalosis produced by excessive administration of alkalies, relief is obtained by giving ammonium chloride (NH_4Cl) orally in a dose of 2 g 6 hourly.

CHAPTER 101

Disorders of the Adrenal Cortex and Adrenal Medulla

KP Poulose, Mathew John, AG Unnikrishnan

Chapter Summary

- General Considerations
- Adrenal Cortical Hormones
- Diseases of the Adrenal Cortex
  - Cushing's Syndrome
  - Nelson's Syndrome

- Abnormalities of Sex Hormones caused by Adrenocortical Lesions
  - Congenital Adrenal Hyperplasia
  - Adrenocortical Insufficiency
  - Addison's Disease
  - Adrenal Crisis
  - Primary Hyperaldosteronism

- Disorders of Adrenal Medulla
  - Pheochromocytoma
  - Adrenal Incidentaloma

INTRODUCTION

The adrenal glands are two paired glands, which produce hormones necessary for metabolism as well as hemodynamic stability. Several disorders of the adrenals exist and these range from autoimmune adrenal damage to neoplastic transformations of the glands.

GENERAL CONSIDERATIONS

Anatomy

The adrenals are paired glands each weighing about 4.7 g. Section of the gland shows an outer cortex and inner medulla. Histologically, three zones are visible in the cortex—(1) the zona glomerulosa, (2) zona fasciculata and (3) zona reticularis from without inward (Fig. 101.1). The arterial supply is derived from several branches of the phrenic, renal, ovarian or spermatic arteries and aorta. Venous drainage on the left is into the left renal vein and on the right to the inferior vena cava (IVC).

Embryology

The fetal adrenal cortex is formed during the fourth to sixth week of gestation from the celomic mesoderm of the posterior abdominal wall. The permanent adrenal cortex is formed from the small basophilic cells, which appear 5 weeks later. The adrenal medulla develops in the seventh week from sympathogonia that migrate from the neural crest into the fetal adrenal cortex. The adrenals are relatively bigger at birth, but with the passage of time, the size reduces since the inner zone of acidophilic cells undergoes involution.

Physiology

Several hormones are produced by the adrenal cortex. The cortex synthesizes cholesterol and also takes cholesterol from the circulation for the production of its hormones. Synthesis of hormones takes place in several steps. The tropic hormone produced by the anterior pituitary—***adrenocorticotropic hormone (ACTH)*** stimulates the adrenal cortex to secrete hormones. Adrenal medulla secretes adrenaline and noradrenaline.

ACTH secreted by the anterior pituitary stimulates secretion of adrenal cortical hormones (glucocorticoids and sex hormones) by acting on specific receptors present on the adrenal cortex through the mechanism of cyclic adenosine monophosphate (cAMP) (Fig. 101.2).

Steroid Synthesis Pathway

The intramitochondrial delivery of cholesterol is the rate-limiting step for steroid biosynthesis and is mediated by steroid acute regulatory protein (StAR). Cholesterol is released and enters steroid hormone synthesis by the action of the enzyme cholesterol esterase. The conversion of cholesterol to pregnenolone requires the action of cytochrome P450 side-chain cleavage enzyme (P450scc, CYP11A1), which is present in the inner

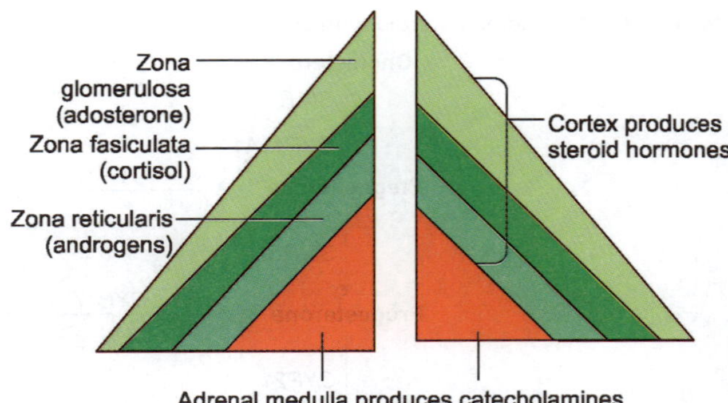

Fig. 101.1: Diagrammatic representation of the layer of the adrenal gland

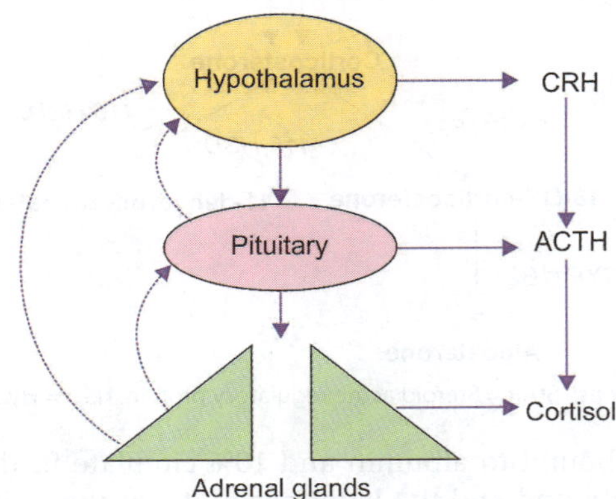

Fig. 101.2: Hypothalamopituitary axis controlling the adrenal gland. ***Note:*** Broken lines indicate negative feedback loops that exist.
Abbreviations: CRH = Corticotropin-releasing hormone; ACTH = Adrenocorticotropic hormone

mitochondrial membrane of all steroidogenic cells. The biosynthetic pathway of cortisol and aldosterone share a number of intermediates and enzymes, becoming exclusive only at 11-deoxycortisol (DOC, cortisol pathway) and 11-deoxycorticosteroid (aldosterone pathway) (Flowchart 101.1).

Steroid Hormone Secretion, Role of ACTH, Transport and Metabolism

The secretion of cortisol (the most physiologically important steroid hormone) occurs only in response to stimulation by ACTH. In health, the levels of cortisol are highest in the morning. Plasma cortisol reciprocally influences ACTH, i.e. higher cortisol levels inhibit and lower levels stimulate production of ACTH and also stimulate the melanocytes and activates tissue lipase. Within 2–3 hours of falling asleep, the ACTH levels progressively rise and reach the highest level about an hour or so before waking up. During waking hours, ACTH levels progressively fall to reach the minimum before falling asleep. The secretion of ACTH and cortisol is increased in response to different stress factors such as trauma, fever, surgery, hypoglycemia, severe anxiety and several others. The circadian rhythm disappears during periods of stress and in adrenal tumors.

About 75% of cortisol circulates in blood bound to transcortin, which is a glycoprotein. Nearly 15% is

Flowchart 101.1: Adrenal steroid synthesis pathway

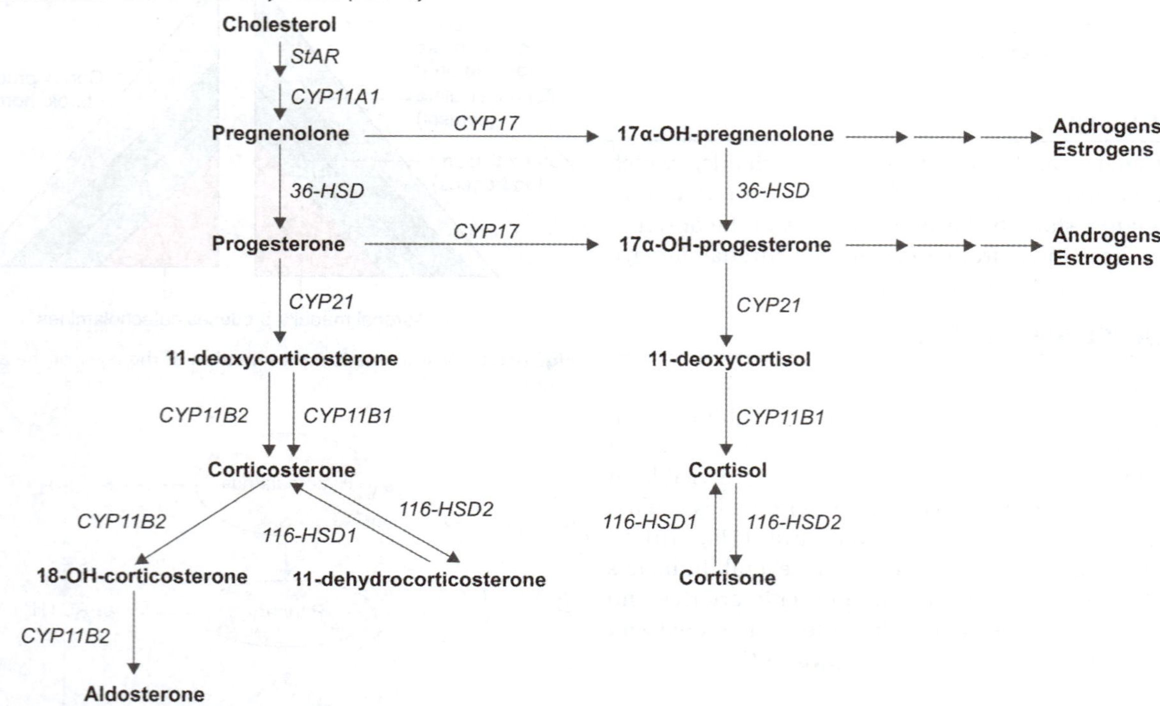

Abbreviations: StAR = Steroid acute regulatory protein; HSD = Hydroxysteroid dehydrogenase; CYP = Cytochrome P450

loosely bound to albumin and 10% circulate in the free state unbound and the latter accounts for the metabolic activities of the hormone. When plasma cortisol level is high (e.g. Cushing's syndrome), plasma transcortin is saturated and the level of unbound cortisol increases. This appears in excessive amounts in urine. Steroid hormones are inactivated mainly in the liver. Other tissues such as muscles, skin, fibroblasts, intestine and lymphocytes also metabolize them.

Glucocorticoids act via the glucocorticoid receptor (GR). The human GR is ubiquitously expressed in all human tissues and organs. In humans, the GR protein is encoded by NR3C1 (nuclear receptor subfamily 3, group C, member 1) gene which is located on chromosome 5 (5q31). It has a single polypeptide chain of 777 amino acids and belongs to the steroid/sterol/thyroid/retinoid/orphan receptor superfamily of nuclear-translocating factors. It resides primarily in the cytoplasm complexed to heat-shock proteins (HSP). The endogenous glucocorticoid hormone cortisol diffuses through the cell membrane into the cytoplasm and binds to the GR resulting in release of the HSP. The resulting activated form GR has two principle mechanisms of action: (1) transactivation and (2) transrepression.

ADRENAL CORTICAL HORMONES

Based on their main functional activity, cortical hormones can be grouped as glucocorticoids, mineralocorticoids and sex hormones (androgens and estrogens). *Glucocorticoids* are secreted by zona fasciculata, *mineralocorticoids* by zona glomerulosa and *sex hormones* by zona reticularis (Table 101.1). The adrenal medulla produces the catecholamines, adrenaline and noradrenaline.

Table 101.1: Secretory rates of adrenal cortical hormones

Adrenal cortical hormones	Secretory rate in mg/day
Cortisol (hydrocortisone)	12–30
Corticosterone	1–4
Aldosterone	0.05–0.15
Deoxycorticosterone	0.05–0.2
Dehydroepiandrosterone	15–50

Glucocorticoids

The important members of this group are cortisol (hydrocortisone), corticosterone and 11-dehydrocorticosterone. Normal cortisol level at 8 AM is 140–700 nmol/L (5–25 µg/dL) and it falls to 0.8 µg/dL at midnight, highest concentration is around 4 AM.

Glucocorticoids promote gluconeogenesis and lead to hyperglycemia. Other major effects include increase of protein catabolism, suppression of ACTH, anti-inflammatory and antiallergic action, immunosuppressant effects and reduction in the size of circulating lymphocyte pool and lymphatic organs (lympholysis). In addition, glucocorticoids exert minor effects such as induction of several enzymes, stimulation of hematopoiesis, fat deposition over the trunk, uricosuria, elimination of water load, production of a feeling of well-being, reduction in circulating eosinophils and maintenance of the capacity for muscular work. Glucocorticoids are used therapeutically for replacement therapy and in many other conditions. Several synthetic analogs are available for therapeutic use.

Mineralocorticoids

Aldosterone is the most important member in this group, the other being deoxycorticosterone (DOC). These exert

<table>
<tr><td colspan="3">Table 101.2: Relative potency of the different corticosteroid for selective activity</td></tr>
<tr><td>Steroid preparation</td><td>Glucocorticoid activity</td><td>Mineralocorticoid activity</td></tr>
<tr><td>Cortisol (hydrocortisone)</td><td>1</td><td>1</td></tr>
<tr><td>Cortisone</td><td>0.7</td><td>0.7</td></tr>
<tr><td>Aldosterone</td><td>0.3</td><td>300</td></tr>
<tr><td>Fludrocortisone</td><td>—</td><td>125</td></tr>
<tr><td>Prednisolone</td><td>4</td><td>0.25</td></tr>
<tr><td>Dexamethasone</td><td>25</td><td><0.1</td></tr>
<tr><td>Betamethasone</td><td>25</td><td><0.1</td></tr>
<tr><td>Triamcinolone/methyl prednisolone</td><td>5</td><td><0.1</td></tr>
<tr><td>Deflazacort</td><td>5</td><td>0.25</td></tr>
</table>

their main action on epithelial membranes of the skin, gastrointestinal tract (GIT) and kidney. The main action is conservation of sodium and chloride, and elimination of potassium. Excessive activity of these hormones causes retention of sodium and chloride, edema and potassium loss. Aldosterone secretion is stimulated by angiotensin II which is the final product of the renin-angiotensin system (RAS) initiated by the afferent arterioles of the renal glomeruli. ACTH does not exert any appreciable effect on the secretion of aldosterone. Details of the RAS are given in Chapter 188.

All available preparations of adrenocortical hormones are synthetic products. Comparison of the potency of natural and synthetic corticosteroids (for equivalent dose) is given in Table 101.2. Betamethasone and dexamethasone differ structurally by a single methyl group and hence, their pharmacological effects are also slightly different. Both have the same bioavailability. Betamethasone has a longer half-life and larger volume distribution.

Sex Hormones

Adrenal cortex secretes sex steroids (both androgens and estrogens), which are small in amount compared to the secretion of gonads. Under normal conditions, they play only a minor role in the development of secondary sex characters. When the secretion is increased under pathological conditions, they may produce virilization and less commonly feminization, which is more evident in the male. Adrenal estrogen-secreting tumors can lead to gynecomastia in males and precocious puberty in girls. In adult women, excessive secretion of adrenal androgens leads to amenorrhea, hirsutism and infertility.

Investigation of Adrenal Cortical Disorders

Serum Cortisol

This is the simplest examination and can be carried out by radioimmunoassay (RIA). The test results depend on the time of sampling. Normally, serum cortisol levels are highest early in the day and then decline over a period of time to reach a nadir in the late night. If measured at 8 AM, the normal cortisol levels in the serum range from 5 to 25 µg/dL. However, if measured at 4 PM, the

normal values would range from 2 to 8 µg/dL. Neither the 8 AM cortisol nor the ratios of 8 AM to 4 PM cortisol are sensitive enough to serve as a diagnostic test for Cushing's syndrome. A low 8 AM cortisol in a patient with clinical features of Cushing's syndrome suggests iatrogenic Cushing's syndrome.

Midnight Cortisol

Midnight cortisol either as serum cortisol or salivary cortisol can be used in screening for Cushing's syndrome. There is a circadian rhythm of circulating cortisol with values less than 1.8 µg/dL after 2 hours of sleep. Loss of circadian rhythm occurs early in Cushing's syndrome. Properly collected late night cortisol in an unstressed patient with an indwelling venous line with values more than 1.8 µg/dL is suggestive of Cushing's syndrome. Biologically, active cortisol in the serum is in equilibrium with cortisol levels in the saliva and would serve as a marker of Cushing's syndrome.

Urinary-free Cortisol

Urinary-free cortisol (UFC) is an integrated index of circulating free cortisol over a 24-hour period. Normal range is 55–193 nmol (20–70 µg) in 24 hours. This is a very sensitive test for the diagnosis of Cushing's syndrome in which the urinary cortisol is increased. If performed correctly with optimum urine collection, 24-hour UFC has a high sensitivity of 95% for diagnosing Cushing's syndrome. At least, 24-hour collections are required. Fourfold elevations of UFC are strongly suggestive of Cushing's syndrome.

Aldosterone and its Derivatives

Normal plasma concentration estimated by RIA is 10 ng/dL and urinary excretion is 5–19 µg/day.

Other Hormones

Dehydroepiandrosterone sulfate (DHEAS) can be estimated by RIA. The values of DHEAS are extremely high if there is a DHEAS-producing adrenal tumor. DHEAS estimation helps to differentiate androgen secretory tumor of adrenal from that of an ovarian tumor.

Basal ACTH

Estimations of ACTH levels are helpful in various situations. ACTH is collected at 9 AM with a sample of cortisol. In a subject with Cushing's syndrome suppressed ACTH confirms that lesion is ACTH independent, i.e. the cortisol is from primary adrenal source. Basal ACTH is elevated in primary adrenal insufficiency.

ACTH Testing

This is a useful test to detect the adrenal reserve. While a simple serum cortisol level might suffice to pick up adrenal insufficiency, if the value is less than 3 µg/dL at 8 AM, many time the serum cortisol level could be normal, but the adrenal may be damaged and might therefore lack the capacity to augment the adrenal secretion in response to stress or conditions of increased hormone requirement. In order to pick up these cases, where the adrenal reserve capacity is compromised, ACTH testing is useful. The estimation of plasma and/or urinary steroids before and after ACTH administration

Table 101.3: Interpretation of diagnostic tests in hyperadrenocortical states

Test	Normal subjects	Pituitary cause (Cushing's disease)	Adrenal tumor	Ectopic ACTH production
Basal cortisol	N	H/N	H/N	H/N
Plasma ACTH	N	H	L	H
Suppression by dexamethasone 1 mg screening test	Suppression of plasma cortisol	No suppression	No suppression	No suppression
• Low dose 0.5 mg 6 h for 2 days • High dose 2 mg 6 h for 2 days	• do • Suppression	• do • Suppression	• do • No suppression (tumor)	• do • No suppression
24 h urine-free cortisol	N	H	H	H

Abbreviations: ACTH = Adrenocorticotropic hormone; H = High; N = Normal; L = Low

reveals the responsiveness of the adrenal cortex to ACTH. A simple method is to administer 250 μg of synthetic ACTH (Synacthen) intramuscularly (IM) and to sample serum cortisol at 30 and 60 minutes. Levels greater than 20 μg/dL exclude impairment of adrenal reserve (double the baseline value).

Dexamethasone Suppression Test (DST)

Exogenous or endogenous glucocorticoids normally suppress ACTH secretion. This feedback inhibition is lost in Cushing's syndrome. Dexamethasone is given in a dose of 0.5 mg 6 hourly for 2 days. Urinary 17-hydroxycorticosteroid (17-OHCS) comes down below 2.5 mg/day in normals and plasma cortisol falls below 2 mg/dL on the second day of the test. In the overnight version of the DST, plasma cortisol is estimated at 8 AM after taking 1 mg of dexamethasone during the previous night at 11 PM. If plasma cortisol is less than 2 μg/dL, Cushing's syndrome can be excluded. Several other modifications of this test are available at present. Normal subjects show prompt suppression even when small doses of dexamethasone (single dose of 1 mg) are administered. In adrenal hyperplasia, suppression can be achieved only with higher doses (8 mg/day for 2 days) while in the case of adrenal adenoma, carcinoma and ectopic sources of ACTH, cortisol production is not suppressed even by higher dose of dexamethasone. After the estimation or basal cortisol values in the high-dose DST—2 mg dexamethasone is given every 6 hours for 2 days and cortisol estimations are repeated and in the overnight high-dose DST—8 mg of dexamethasone is given at 11 PM and serum cortisol measured at 8 AM on the next day—values more than 50% of the basal value indicate nonsuppression (Table 101.3).

Demonstration of the Lesion

Adrenals can be visualized radiologically especially if they are calcified. In many cases, the tumors are 4–6 cm in diameter by the time they show endocrine abnormalities. Adrenals can be well-visualized by computed tomography (CT) scanning and magnetic resonance imging (MRI) and these should be done to demonstrate the anatomy of the gland. Even much small tumors can be visualized. Isotope scanning after administration of ^{123}I or ^{131}I metaiodobenzylguanidine (MIBG) helps to show up the adrenals. Sampling of blood from the adrenal veins helps to identify the abnormal gland in cases where there is a difficulty in localizing which adrenal (right or left) is the source of excess hormone production.

DISEASES OF THE ADRENAL CORTEX

CUSHING'S SYNDROME

Syn: Hypercortisolism

Hypercortisolism may develop either due to primary disease of the adrenal cortex such as adenoma, carcinoma or hyperplasia or due to stimulation of the gland by ACTH secreted by the pituitary or ectopic ACTH-like substances which are produced in paraneoplastic processes. The term *Cushing's disease* refers specifically to pituitary-dependent hyperadrenal corticism. In addition, corticosteroids administered therapeutically can give rise to iatrogenic Cushing's syndrome. It is caused by persistent oversecretion of glucocorticoids. In addition to increased levels of cortisol in blood, loss of the normal diurnal rhythm is also a prominent feature.

Causes (Box 101.1)

- Pituitary Cushing—ACTH dependent.
- Adrenal Cushing—non-ACTH dependent.
- Ectopic Cushing—ACTH or ACTH-like substances dependent.
- Iatrogenic Cushing—externally administered gluco-corticoids.

Box 101.1: Etiology of Cushing's syndrome

- ***ACTH-dependent causes:***
  - ***Bilateral adrenal hyperplasia:*** Nearly 70% of these are secondary to a small adenoma involving the basophils (Cushing's disease) or chromophobes in the pituitary. Sometimes the abnormality is in the production and release of corticotropin-releasing factor (CRF) from the hypothalamus.
  - ***Ectopic ACTH secretion:*** This is seen as a paraneoplastic syndrome in bronchogenic carcinoma, medullary carcinoma of thyroid (MTC), carcinoids, pancreatic carcinoma, ovarian carcinoma, neuroblastoma and ganglioma.
- ***ACTH-independent causes:***
  - Adenomas or carcinomas of the adrenal cortex and micro-nodular hyperplasia.
  - ***Iatrogenic:*** Use of physiological or pharmacological doses of glucocorticoids over prolonged periods.
  - Cushing's syndrome is not uncommon in India. It has been reported from all parts of the country. Pituitary-dependent adrenal hyperplasia and adrenal tumors are more frequent in women in the fourth and fifth decades.

Textbook of Medicine

Clinical Features

The symptoms are mainly due to excessive production of glucocorticoids. Almost all features can be attributed to gluconeogenesis, excessive protein catabolism and androgenic effects of cortisol.

General Features

The affected subject is plethoric with rounded appearance of the face (moon face). There is a characteristic obesity with deposition of fat over the neck, shoulders, abdomen and hips. Often, this results in a typical crest of fat on the nape of the neck and this is referred to as *buffalo hump* (Fig. 101.3).

Integument

Hirsutism develops in many cases and it is particularly disturbing in women. Face, chest and other regions are affected most. Acne may develop. The hairline may recede over the temporal regions (temporal baldness) or even general baldness may result. Skin shows painless striae, which develop as reddish streaks over the thighs, gluteal regions, abdomen, axillae and outer aspect of the arms (Fig. 101.4). Striae are formed as a result of rupture of subcutaneous collagenous tissue. In severe cases, the overlying skin may be stretched and thinned out and it tends to rupture and ulcerate. Repair of wounds is considerably delayed. Wound dehiscence is common after surgery. Scar formation is poor. Bruising, purpura and melanotic pigmentation are seen in some cases. Some cases show secondary polycythemia.

Other Features

Hypertension and its complications are common. Muscles are easily fatigable, flabby and atrophic. Proximal muscles show myopathic changes. Psychiatric symptoms like depression and melancholia may be the presenting features in some. Amenorrhea and clitoromegaly develop in women. In women with overproduction of androgen hormones, infertility may occur. Males show loss of libido and impotence. Bones show osteoporosis, which is more prominent in the axial skeleton. Fractures are common (Fig. 101.5).

Biochemical abnormalities: Secondary diabetes develops in many of these patients. Hypokalemia and fluid retention may develop.

Pituitary Cushing's Syndrome (Cushing's Disease)

This is the common variety of Cushing's syndrome, next only to iatrogenic Cushing's syndrome. Usually, it is caused by pituitary microadenoma. Insidiously developing diabetes, hypertension and cushingoid habitus, with mild hyperpigmentation are characteristic. Rarely pituitary macroadenoma (>1 cm in size) may occur and in this situation, features of tumor enlargement like visual field defects and headache may be present.

Carcinoma of the adrenal cortex: These tumors are rapidly progressive with local invasion and distant metastases early in their course. Some tumors do not produce hormones whereas others produce both cortisol and sex hormones. Over 80% of estrogen-producing tumors are malignant.

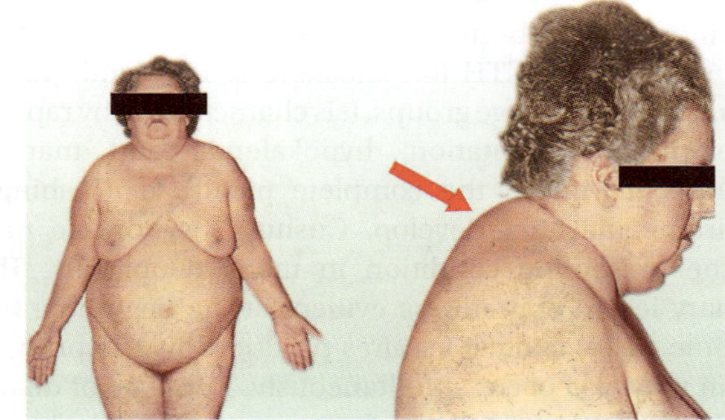

Fig. 101.3: Cushing's syndrome. ***Note:*** Truncal obesity and buffalo hump (arrow)

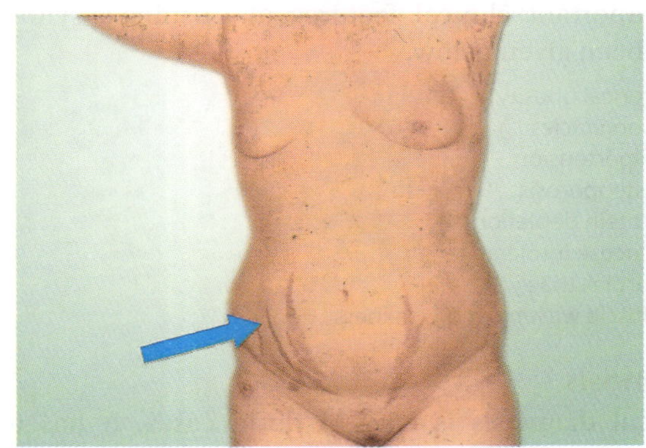

Fig. 101.4: Cushing's syndrome: Striae on abdominal wall (arrow)

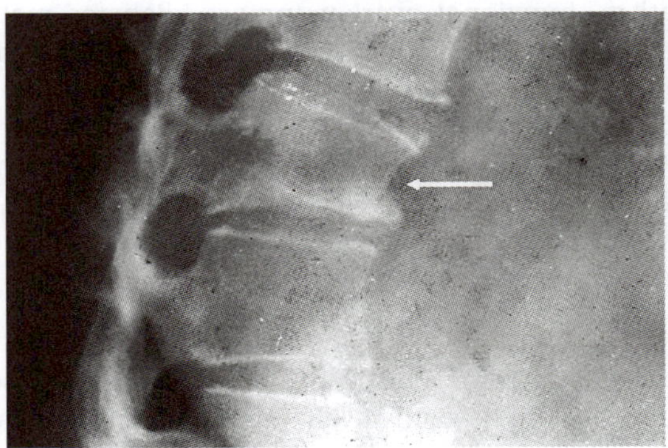

Fig. 101.5: Cushing's syndrome osteoporosis compression fracture (arrow)

Iatrogenic Cushing's Syndrome

This may occur at all ages in both sexes but it is more prominent in young adults. Daily administration of 5–10 mg or more of prednisolone or its equivalent for a period of more than 3–6 months can give rise to Cushing's syndrome. Though it was considered that only moderate or high doses of glucocorticoids led to hypercortisolism, now it is known that even small doses given as aerosols or surface applications can at times lead to the condition, on prolonged use. The full-fledged case resembles classic Cushing's syndrome. The clinical features are variable in many cases. Regression of symptoms occurs within months of withdrawal of the drug, but established diabetes may not clear up promptly, especially so if there is a family history of diabetes.

Textbook of Medicine

Ectopic ACTH Secretion

Carcinomas of the bronchus, neural tissue, ovaries and GIT may give rise to ACTH-like substances. This syndrome is seen more in older age groups. It is characterized by rapidly developing pigmentation, hypokalemia and marked alkalosis. In many, the complete picture of Cushing's syndrome may not develop. Cushing's syndrome may be the presenting condition in many neoplasms. The primary lesion may not be evident at the beginning but in some cases, clinical features produced by the primary lesion may also occur simultaneously. Presence of digital clubbing and osteoarthropathy in any case of Cushing's syndrome should suggest pulmonary malignancy as the underlying cause.

Important clinical features of Cushing's syndrome have been given below.

- Truncal obesity
- Moon facies
- Hypertension
- Osteoporosis
- Protein depletion
- Glucose intolerance
- Purple striae
- Muscle wasting and weakness

Diagnosis

Clinical diagnosis is easy in florid cases. It has to be supported by biochemical investigations. Cushing's syndrome has to be differentiated from simple obesity, hirsutism, functional ovarian tumors, diabetes mellitus (DM) and hypertension. In borderline cases, continued observation and repetition of tests might be required to establish the diagnosis.

Workup of Cushing's syndrome is shown in Flowchart 101.2. Radiological studies, ultrasonography (USG), CT scan, MRI and estimation of cortisol levels in the adrenal veins identify the site of tumor or hyperplasia.

Course and Prognosis

Cushing's syndrome due to primary adrenal disease or pituitary lesions is fatal if left untreated, though rarely spontaneous remissions may occur. Death is due to diabetic complications, hypertension, hypokalemia, infections or the physical effects of the underlying neoplasm.

Flowchart 101.2: Workup of Cushing's syndrome

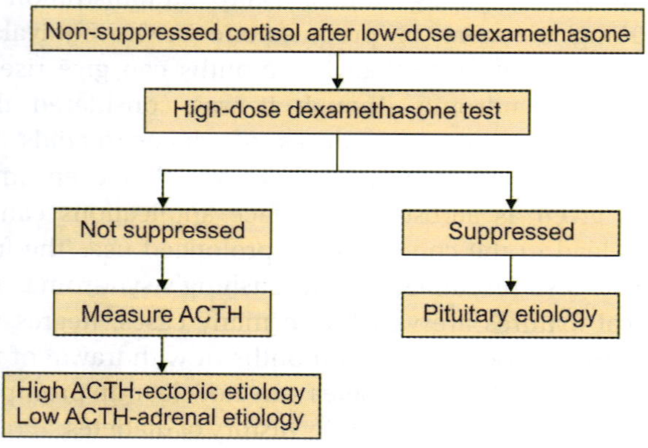

Treatment

Surgical removal of the adrenal tumor is the treatment of choice. Since the normal portions of the glands may be atrophic, substitution therapy is needed in the postoperative period to prevent adrenal crisis. Cushing's syndrome due to pituitary adenoma resolves after surgical removal of the microadenomas. Initial results are good. Trans-sphenoidal surgery is preferred in pituitary adenomas. Ten percent develop postsurgical complications. These include cerebrospinal fluid (CSF) rhinorrhea, diabetes insipidus (DI) and infection. Recurrence occurs is 15–25% of cases. They may require irradiation. An alternative is to do bilateral adrenalectomy and life-long hormone replacement.

Medical Management

Symptomatic management of diabetes, hypertension and electrolyte disturbances is indicated as the conditions warrant. Specific drugs are rarely used.

- **Metyrapone** in a dose of 250–750 mg thrice daily blocks the synthesis of cortisol and abolishes the effects of hypercortisolism. Medical therapy is indicated if the primary cause is not correctable surgically.
- **Aminoglutethimide** given orally in a total daily dose of 0.5–2 g daily, blocks the synthesis of aldosterone, cortisol and other adrenal hormones. It may cause side effects such at ataxia, rashes, fever and drowsiness.
- **Ketoconazole** in a dose of 800–1,000 mg/day inhibits cortisol secretion. Given on a long-term basis, it controls the symptoms.
- **Pasireotide** has been approved for use of Cushing's disease patients who are not cured following transphenoidal therapy or in those in whom surgery carries excessive risks.

Irradiation

Pituitary tumor may respond to local irradiation with 40–50 Gy using a cobalt-60 source or yttrium-90 implantation. However, the features of Cushing's syndrome take about one year to resolve even after successful therapy. Cushing's syndrome seen as a paraneoplastic manifestation of advanced malignancy does not generally respond to surgery. The improvements in pituitary surgery have resulted in far fewer patients being treated by irradiation and hence, irradiation is not recommended as the primary treatment.

NELSON'S SYNDROME

Some patients who undergo bilateral adrenalectomy develop enlargement of the pituitary, pressure effects on the optic chiasma and raised intracranial tension. They also show increased pigmentation due to hypersecretion of melanocyte-stimulating hormone (MSH). This syndrome follows after a few years of bilateral adrenalectomy.

ABNORMALITIES OF SEX HORMONES CAUSED BY ADRENOCORTICAL LESIONS

Adrenal cortex may be the source of excessive androgen production if the lesion is a tumor or congenital enzyme defect interfering with the synthesis of cortisol. Excessive

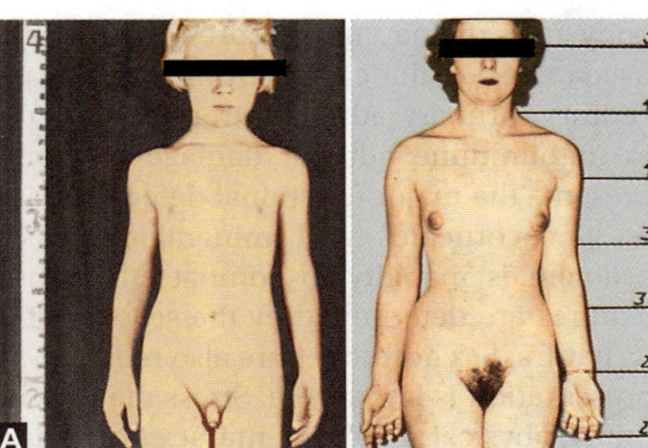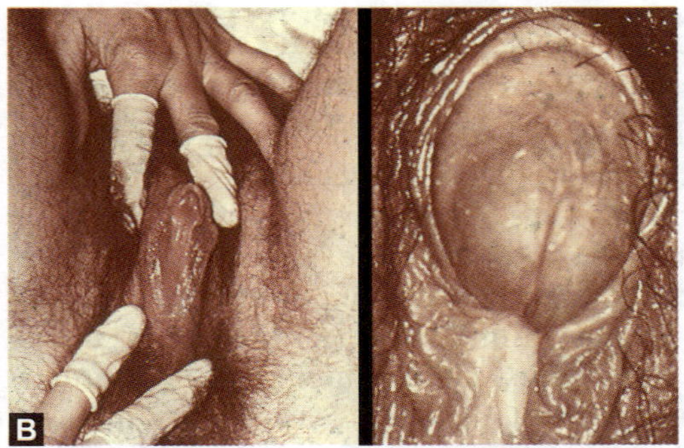

Figs 101.6A and B: A. Virilizing adrenal hyperplasia. *Note:* Enlarged clitoris in the girl on the left and normal girl of same age on the—right; **B.** Close-up view of enlarged clitoris

androgens influence the secondary sexual characters. The final clinical picture is determined by the sex of the patient, age of onset of the disorder and its severity. The condition may remain unnoticed in adult males. Women develop virilization. Boys show precocious puberty. Girls develop clitoromegaly and other signs of hyperandrogenism. The classic example of this situation is congenital adrenal hyperplasia (CAH) (Figs 101.6A and B).

Congenital Adrenal Hyperplasia

This rare disorder is characterized by virilization in female and precocious puberty in male children. The underlying defect is congenital deficiency of enzymes leading to metabolic block in hormone synthesis. This results in the accumulation of intermediary metabolites with andro-genic activity. Deficient synthesis of glucocorticoids and mineralocorticoids results in functional adrenocortical deficiency.

Etiology

The enzyme defect is transmitted as an autosomal recessive disorder, with clinical expression in the homozygous state. Females are affected more than males. The severity of enzyme defect determines the age of manifestation. Severe defects manifest earlier in life. At least, six different enzyme defects are known, but five of these are more frequent. These are—*C-21 hydroxylase defect, C-11, C-17 and C-18 hydroxylase defects* and *3-beta dehydrogenase defect*. Though the clinical effects are grossly similar, minor differences exist between them. C-21 hydroxylase defect accounts for 95% of the cases.

Clinical Features

In some cases, the newborn female infant shows pseudohermaphroditism due to androgen effect on the genitalia. Male infants show precocious sexual development after birth. Manifestations of adrenal insufficiency are failure to thrive, vomiting, hyponatremia and hypotension. Death may occur due to adrenal insufficiency unless the condition is recognized and treated. Milder cases manifest as virilization in girls and sexual precocity in boys. Due to the premature fusion of epiphyses, growth is retarded. Hyperandrogenism causes testicular atrophy and infertility in adult males.

Diagnosis

This disease should be considered in the differential diagnosis of all cases of hermaphroditism or ambiguous sexual development. In Western countries, CAH is diagnosed by neonatal screening program which measures 17-hydroxyprogesterone (17-OHP) in dried blood spots. Diagnosis of patients with suspected CAH-21-(OH) deficiency is done with basal and ACTH stimulated 17-OHP tests. The other forms of CAH are diagnosed by measurement of other intermediates in the adrenal steroidogenesis pathway. Genetic testing may be done in appropriate individuals.

Treatment

Deficiency of glucocorticoids and mineralocorticoids should be corrected by supplementation. Liberal intake of salt helps in mild cases. Fludrocortisone in a daily dose of 0.05–0.1 mg orally is given to correct mineralocorticoids deficiency. Prednisolone in a dose of 5 mg/day serves to overcome glucocorticoid deficiency. Surgery may be required for cosmetic correction of the genitalia. In those cases in which adrenal tumors or hyperplastic glands are demonstrable, surgical removal is indicated.

ADRENOCORTICAL INSUFFICIENCY

Hypofunction of the adrenal cortex may be due to a primary disorder of the gland or secondary to hyposecretion of the tropic hormone. The causes are listed below.

Primary adrenocortical insufficiency—lesions in the adrenal cortex:
- Atrophy of the adrenal cortex due to autoimmune adrenalitis.
- Tuberculosis, fungal infection, cytomegalovirus (CMV) infection, sarcoidosis and other granulomas
- Infiltration by metastatic carcinoma
- Hemochromatosis
- Amyloidosis
- Postsurgical (total or subtotal adrenalectomy)

Secondary adrenocortical insufficiency—
- *Hypothalamic causes:* Tumors of the third ventricle, meningitis, encephalitis, injury to the base of the brain, corticosteroid therapy, sarcoidosis and histiocytosis
- *Pituitary causes:* All causes of panhypopituitarism, especially tumors, basal meningitis, viperine snake bite, hypophysectomy or irradiation and empty sella syndrome.

Majority of the cases are due to autoimmune adrenal atrophy. The classic features include hypotension, increased skin pigmentation, low levels of serum sodium ion (Na$^+$) and chloride, high levels of bicarbonate (HCO$_3^-$) and potassium ion (K$^+$) and lower levels of plasma glucose.

ADDISON'S DISEASE

Syn: Primary adrenocortical insufficiency

Thomas Addison described this condition first in 1855. It was due to tuberculosis of adrenal glands.

Among the diseases of the adrenal cortex, this is the most treatable one. Autoimmune adrenal destruction (previously called idiopathic or primary atrophy) is more common in women. Antibodies against adrenal tissue may be demonstrable. Other autoimmune disorders like myxedema, type 1 diabetes, Hashimoto's disease, thyrotoxicosis, pernicious anemia, vitiligo, idiopathic ovarian failure and hypoparathyroidism may be associated. There is association between Addison's disease and human leukocyte antigen (HLA-B38 and HLA-DR3).

Causes

Causes of primary adrenocortical insufficiency and secondary adrenocortical insufficiency have been shown below.

Primary adrenocortical insufficiency

- Autoimmune
- Metastatic malignancy (lung, breast, stomach carcinomas) or lymphoma
- Adrenal hemorrhage
  - Waterhouse-Friderichsen syndrome
  - Anticoagulation therapy
- Infectious
  - Tuberculosis, CMV, fungi (histoplasmosis, coccidioidomycosis), human immunodeficiency virus (HIV)
- Adrenal infarction
  - Antiphospholipid antibody (APLA), systemic lupus erythematosus (SLE)
- Adrenoleukodystrophy
- Infiltrative disorders
  - Amyloidosis, hemochromatosis, sarcoid
- Bilateral adrenalectomy
- CAH
- Familial glucocorticoid deficiency and hypoplasia
- Drugs
  - Ketoconazole, metyrapone, aminoglutethimide, trilostane, mitotane, etomidate, rifampin, cyproterone acetate

- Autoimmune polyglandular syndrome 1 and 2
- Kearns-Sayre syndrome (oculocraniosomatic disorder or oculocraniosomatic neuromuscular disorder with ragged red fibers, which is a mitochondrial myopathy occurring before 20 years of age).

Secondary adrenocortical insufficiency

- Exogenous glucocorticoid therapy
- *Hypopituitarism:* Selective removal pituitary
- Pituitary apoplexy
- Granulomatous disease of pituitary (tuberculosis, sarcoid, eosinophilic granuloma)
- Secondary tumor deposits in pituitary (breast, bronchus)
- Postpartum pituitary infarction (Sheehan's syndrome)
- Pituitary irradiation.

Pathology

The adrenal glands show total cortical atrophy involving all three zones. The medulla is normal. In the primary form, histology shows lymphocytic infiltration and increase in fibrous tissue. In the other types, evidence of underlying disease may be demonstrable. In tuberculosis of the adrenals, evidence of tuberculosis elsewhere in the body may or may not be present. Though tuberculosis used to be a major cause during the early part of the 20th century, primary adrenal atrophy, most commonly due to autoimmune adrenal damage is more common at present. The major functional defect is marked reduction of glucocorticoids and mineralocorticoids. The main problem is inability to combat stress and the clinical features are determined by the severity of the stress and its nature. Sex hormones are also reduced, but the clinical presentation is less severe. Stress may include infections, injury, physical factors, mental stress and drugs which lead to hypoglycemia or hypotension and opioid narcotics.

Clinical Features

Generally, the onset is slow and may be unnoticed but many patients present for the first time in acute adrenal failure precipitated by stress. Initial symptoms may be vague such as weakness, tiredness, lethargy, weight loss and GI upset, especially vomiting. Sooner or later, dark pigmentation develops. When fully developed, the pigmentation is characteristic and in most cases, diagnostic of primary adrenal failure. Face, palms, soles extensor aspects of limbs, flexures, and mucous membranes of the mouth, tongue and genitalia show pigmentation. In severe cases, the complexion becomes dark (Figs 101.7A and B). Pigmentation is mediated by the melanocyte-stimulating effect of ACTH and also secretion of MSH. Unlike primary hypoadrenalism in the secondary type, there is no hyperpigmentation. On the other hand, these subjects are pale and light colored. Vitiligo is seen in some cases of Addison's disease. Premature graying of hair may occur which reverts to normal with treatment.

Women develop amenorrhea and men develop impotence. Addison's disease confers abnormal sensitivity to drugs like morphine or pethidine. Hypoglycemia leads to extreme fatigue, sweating and coma.

Cardiovascular abnormalities include low blood pressure especially postural hypotension and diminution of heart size.

Laboratory Investigations

- Hypoglycemia is common. Blood glucose falls further during periods of stress.
- Hyponatremia and hyperkalemia may occur.
- Plasma cortisol levels are low and the diurnal rhythm is lost.
- *ACTH stimulation test (Synacthen stimulation):* There is no response to ACTH stimulation in primary and long-standing secondary adrenal insufficiency. Loss of ACTH from the pituitary leads to gradual atrophy of the adrenals. During the initial 4 weeks after loss of endogenous ACTH stimulus, the adrenal undergoes atrophy. Hence, the adrenals may continue to respond to exogenous ACTH (Synacthen) during this initial 4 weeks and hence, give a false-positive response to Synacthen stimulation.
- In Addison's disease, plasma ACTH levels are high. In secondary hypoadrenocorticism, ACTH levels are low.
- Adrenal antibodies may be demonstrable in autoimmune adrenal damage.

Textbook of Medicine

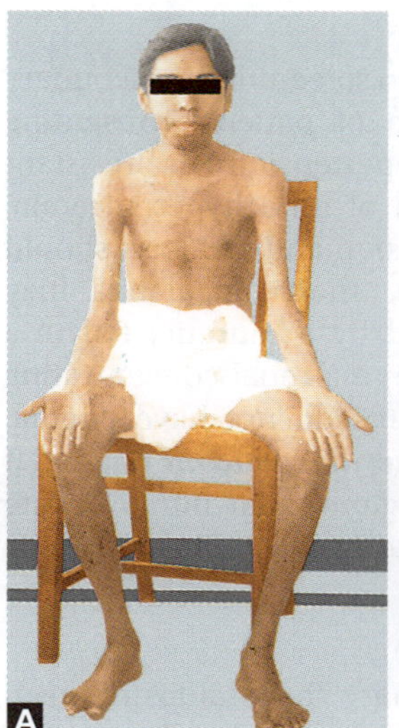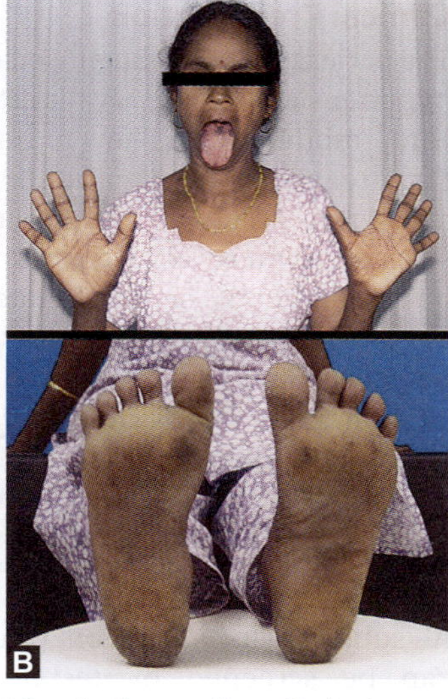

Figs 101.7A and B: A. Male Addison's disease. ***Note:*** Dark pigmentation of the whole body—particularly palms, soles and face; **B.** Female Addison's disease. ***Note:*** Pigmentation

- X-ray of abdomen may show adrenal calcification. More often calcification is the sequel of tuberculosis of the gland.
- CT/MRI of abdomen visualizes the anatomy quite clearly. Radionuclide imaging of adrenals gives information of morphology and function.

Diagnosis

Addison's disease should be suspected clinically and confirmed by investigations. Chronic malnutrition, malabsorption states, megaloblastic anemia, tuberculosis, disseminated malignancy and psychiatric disorders should be considered in the differential diagnosis.

Diagnosis is established by estimating plasma cortisol level before and after ACTH injection. The normal level of plasma cortisol at 8 AM is 5–25 mg/dL and ACTH is less than 80 mg/mL.

Secondary hypoadrenocorticism is a part of hypopituitarism.

In patients with primary adrenal insufficiency, the adrenal glands need to be imaged with CT or MRI if autoimmunity is not evident. In patients with secondary adrenal insufficiency, the pituitary needs to be imaged with MRI.

Course and Prognosis

Severe Addison's disease is fatal if untreated. Adrenal crisis occurring during periods of stress causes death. Severe hyponatremia, shock, hypoglycemia or toxic reactions to drugs like morphine are common in them and these may prove fatal.

The prognosis has been completely changed with modern therapy. Apparent clinical and biochemical normalcy can be restored with adequate hormonal supplementation and fairly with normal life span can be ensured. In many of them, DM may develop on prolonged therapy with glucocorticoids.

Management

The aim of therapy is to replace glucocorticoids and mineralocorticoids for life, with increase in dosage during periods of stress. Initially, hydrocortisone is given in a dose of 100–200 mg/day IV in a crisis-like situation, the exact requirement is determined based on clinical and biochemical parameters. The optimum dosage required to keep the patient symptom-free with normal blood glucose and electrolyte levels is determined by trial and error. The treatment is started with 2.5 mg of prednisolone once or twice a day and the dose is increased till the patient becomes clinically normal and biochemical results also become normal.

Once a state of equilibrium is reached, long-term maintenance is by giving any one of the more potent preparations such as prednisolone, betamethasone or dexamethasone. Timing of the dosage is adjusted to coincide with the normal diurnal variations, i.e. the equivalent of 20 mg cortisol at breakfast and 10 mg at about 6 PM. Peak serum levels are obtained 30–50 minutes after oral administration and the action lasts for 6–8 hours. In general, the dose required for replacement therapy is much lower than that required for immunosuppression. Though glucocorticoids bring about considerable benefit, full health will be restored only with the replacement of mineralocorticoid preparations as well. ***Mineralocorticoids:*** In all cases with moderate or severe adrenal deficiency, mineralocorticoids have to be supplemented. Fludrocortisone is the most potent preparation in this class and it is given in a dose of 0.05–0.15 mg orally as a morning dose. Adequacy of therapy is assessed by the restoration of blood pressure to normal and corrected serum aldosterone levels. ***Side effects*** of overdose include hypertension, edema and hypokalemic alkalosis.

Importance of stress dosing: During periods of stress and other medical or surgical emergencies, the dose of corticosteroids should be stepped up to avoid the development of adrenal crisis. All subjects with hypoadrenocorticism should carry identity cards giving details of the disease, the treatment schedule and the doctor who treats him.

ADRENAL CRISIS

Syn: Acute adrenal insufficiency (adrenal apoplexy)

Sudden development of adrenal cortical failure leads to adrenal crisis. It is a medical emergency, which is fatal if undiagnosed. Prompt recognition and replacement of glucocorticoids and mineralocorticoids with other supportive measures gives prompt relief and saves life. Adrenal crisis may complicate chronic adrenal insufficiency or it may occur acutely in subjects who develop fulminant infections.

Causes

- Sudden withdrawal of ACTH or glucocorticoid therapy.
- Infections, trauma, surgery, drugs like morphine, diarrhea, vomiting, physical or psychological stress, and obstetric accidents precipitate acute adrenal failure in patients with chronic adrenocortical insufficiency.
- During meningococcal septicemia occurring in otherwise normal subjects, hemorrhagic necrosis of

Textbook of Medicine

the adrenal may develop (Waterhouse-Friderichsen syndrome) leading to shock. Infarction of the adrenal, accidental destruction of the adrenal by trauma or surgery and neonatal adrenogenital syndrome are rare causes.

Clinical Features

Severe vomiting, diarrhea and profound shock are the prominent symptoms. Blotchy purpura develops in septicemia. If untreated, coma supervenes and death follows within hours.

Diagnosis

It is based mainly on clinical features. Estimation of serum Na$^+$, K$^+$, chloride (Cl$^-$) and bicarbonate HCO$_3^-$ give the electrolyte status. Estimation of plasma cortisol and aldosterone will help to assess the severity.

Management

Normal saline with 10% glucose should be started immediately. The rate is adjusted to maintain normal blood pressure, serum electrolytes and blood glucose level. IV infusion may have to be continued for days. Drug of choice in an emergency is hydrocortisone hemisuccinate sodium in a dose of 100 mg given IV initially and repeated every 4–6 hours. Parenteral medication is continued till the patient is fit for oral therapy. If the blood pressure does not come up promptly, or it tends to drop, fludrocortisone 0.1 mg oral is given in addition. After tiding over the crisis, long-term management for adrenal failure is instituted. When the condition is secondary to sepsis or other causes, these should receive prompt attention.

PRIMARY HYPERALDOSTERONISM

Syn: Conn's syndrome

The classical syndrome of primary aldosteronism is characterized by hypertension, unprovoked hypokalemia and low-plasma renin activity (PRA). Around 0.5% of cases of hypertension present with this typical syndrome. However, screening of hypertensive patients with biochemical tests yields a prevalence of 5–10% among all patients with hypertension.

Around 60–75% of cases are due to aldosterone-producing adenoma (APA) of the adrenal cortex. In women, aldosteronomas are more common. The second type called *idiopathic hyperaldosteronism* is probably due to bilateral adrenal hyperplasia. Idiopathic hyperaldosteronism is more common in men. Other rare groups are also described.

Classification of Primary Hyperaldosteronism

- Aldosterone-producing adenoma: 35% (Conn's syndrome)
- Bilateral idiopathic hyperplasia: 60%
- Primary (unilateral) adrenal hyperplasia: 2% of cases
- Aldosterone producing adrenocortical carcinomas (<1%)
- Familial hyperaldosteronism (FH):
  - Glucocorticoid remediable aldosteronism (FH type I) less than 1%
  - FH type II less than 2%
- Ectopic APA less than 0.1%.

Clinical Presentation

The patients may be diagnosed on screening for secondary hypertension in the evaluation of patients presenting with moderate to severe hypertension or resistant hypertension. The combination of mild hypernatremia, low serum potassium, hypertension and alkalosis should suggest primary aldosteronism. The hypokalemia may be spontaneous or precipitated by a diuretic. Polyuria or nocturia may be present due to a renal concentrating defect. Conn's syndrome patients do not have edema. This phenomenon is called *mineralocorticoid escape*. It is probably due to increase in glomerular filtration rate (GFR) and by the activity of both atrial and brain natriuretic peptides (BNP).

Diagnosis

A subject suspected of primary hyperaldosteronism can be screened by testing for plasma aldosterone concentration (PAC) and PRA in a morning sample. The patient be seated or ambulant. A PAC level of greater than 20 ng/dL per hour in the presence of PRA greater than 15 ng/dL is suggestive of primary hyperaldosteronism . The diagnosis can be confirmed by oral sodium loading followed by 24-hour urinary aldosterone levels, IV saline loading test or fludrocortisone suppression tests.

CT imaging of the adrenals would help to localize the adrenal adenoma. Since adrenal incidentalomas are not uncommon, adrenal venous sampling (AVS) from the adrenal veins would help to categorize the type of primary hyperaldosteronism and the side which has to be chosen for surgical treatment.

Differential diagnosis includes malignant hypertension uni- or bilateral renal ischemia and potassium losing nephropathies.

Treatment

Adenomas have to be treated by surgery. Those with idiopathic hyperaldosteronism have to be treated medically with spironolactone 50–100 mg thrice daily. In intractable cases, bilateral adrenalectomy can be done. The blood pressure returns to normal after several months in aldosteronomas, in the other types results are variable.

Secondary hyperaldosteronism can occur due to high-renin production occurring in renal artery stenosis, congestive heart failure (CHF), prolonged use of diuretics and others.

DISORDERS OF THE ADRENAL MEDULLA

PHEOCHROMOCYTOMA

Tumors arising from chromaffin tissue produce excess of catecholamines and give rise to hypertension and other effects. Tumors may occur at several sites. Common locations are the adrenal medulla (90%), Zuckerkandl's bodies adjacent to the abdominal aorta (8%), paraganglionic cells of the sympathetic nervous system, urinary bladder, aortic and carotid bodies and the mediastinum. It is seen that 0.1–0.3% hypertensive patients may have a pheochromocytoma. The disease may be familial in 10% of cases and show autosomal dominant inheritance. The familial form may occur in association with the syndromes of multiple endocrine neoplasms (MENs) particularly MEN2 in which primary hyperparathyroidism and medullary carcinoma of the thyroid may also occur. Pheochromocytomas secrete large amounts of adrenaline and noradrenaline. In pheochromocytomas at nonadrenal sites, noradrenaline is the major component constituting up to 80% of the total. Some tumors produce only one of these products of the pheochromocytomas, 90% are benign and 10% are malignant and these may metastasize. The secondary sites also produce catecholamines.

It can occur in association with von Hippel-Lindau (VHL) disease, neurofibromatosis type 1 and familial paraganglioma (associated with mutations in succinate dehydrogenase).

Clinical Features

The most prominent feature is hypertension, which is paroxysmal in the initial stages, but later becomes persistent. Headache, flushing, excessive sweating, tachycardia, fever, glycosuria and postural hypotension accompany hypertensive paroxysms. Abdominal palpation, minor surgery and parturition may precipitate hypertensive attacks. The common hypotensive drugs like guanethidine, hydralazine, beta-adrenergic blockers and methyldopa lead to paradoxical elevation of blood pressure. Many develop malignant hypertension which may prove fatal. Hypertensive attacks triggered by micturition should suggest pheochromocytoma of urinary bladder.

For practical purposes, *rule of tens* is relevant in pheochromocytoma.

- 10% extra-adrenal
- 10% bilateral
- 10% malignant
- 10% familial
- 10% children.

Diagnosis

Pheochromocytoma has to be clinically suspected in subjects developing paroxysmal hypertension associated with other manifestation of sympathetic overactivity.

Investigations

Metanephrine and normetanephrine are the 3-methoxy metabolites of epinephrine and norepinephrine, respectively. Metanephrine and normetanephrine are both further metabolized to vanillylmandelic acid (VMA). One of the most reliable methods is to measure a 24-hour urine sample for fractionated metanephrines and catecholamines (sensitivity 98% and specificity 98%). Plasma-free catecholamines as well as plasma metanephrines are the tests that offer the best diagnostic value and a high value of either strongly suggests the diagnosis. However, the specificity of these tests is in the order of 85–88% and reduces further in patients older than 60 years. 24-hour urinary metanephrines are better for the diagnosis of pheochromocytomas compared to the traditional VMA which has poor diagnostic sensitivity and specificity. Quantitative determinations are done in 24-hour collection of urine. Spot tests are also available for screening. Several drugs and food articles such as bananas, chocolate, coffee, nuts and vanilla produce false-positive tests when urinary VMA or catecholamine determination are done and therefore, these have to be avoided preferably for 5 days before doing the test. Provocative testing involving clonidine, phentolamine, glucagon, histamine and metoclopromide has limited roles.

Localization of the tumor is achieved by CT scanning, MRI, USG or radionuclide imaging using MIBG and adrenal angiography. MRI is especially useful—a bright signal on T2-weighted image is highly suggestive of a neuroendocrine tumor like pheochromocytoma. Selective sampling of adrenal venous blood for estimating catecholamines is a very useful confirmatory test. All these tests should be undertaken only in well-equipped centers since there is the risk of sudden hypertensive crisis.

Pheochromocytoma multisystem crisis (PMC) is a rare but life-threatening complication precipitated by a variety of drugs, foods, exercise, investigations and infection. Clinical features of PMC include the following:

- Presence of hypertension or hypotension
- Temperature above 40°C
- Encephalopathy
- Multiorgan failure.

Pheochromocytoma causes the production of interleukin (IL-6) which causes inflammatory response. Glucocorticoids worsen the condition. Timely surgery saves the patient. Mortality is more than 50%.

Treatment

Once the diagnosis is established, treatment is to remove the tumor surgically. Rapid fluctuations in blood pressure occur during premedication, anesthesia, surgical manipulation and postoperative period.

Preoperatively, the blood pressure should be controlled by giving phenoxybenzamine or other alpha-blockers like prazosin or doxazosin in doses of 1–4 mg/day. It is important to give adequate fluid intake during this preoperative phase. Beta-blockers may be added a few days prior to surgery, especially if there is tachycardia. IV diazoxide, sodium nitroprusside or phentolamine can control hypertensive episodes if judiciously administered.

Preoperative Preparation Regimens

- Combined α + β-blockade to be started at least 2 weeks preoperatively to control the hypertension. Antihypertensive agents used are:
  - Phenoxybenzamine
  - Selective α_1-blocker (e.g. prazosin)
  - Propanolol
  If uncontrolled add;
- Metyrosine
- Calcium channel blocker (CCB)—nicardipine
- Avoid diuretics if the extracellular fluid (ECF) volume is contracted
- Intraoperative blood pressure needs to carefully monitored and controlled. Postoperatively, patients may become normotensive free

Textbook of Medicine

- If excision is not possible, long-term treatment with α- and β-adrenoreceptors blocking drugs (phenoxybenzamine and propranolol or labetalol) is advocated. β-blockers should never be given alone. Patients can be subjected to radionuclide therapy with ^{131}I. MIBG, if the lesion is malignant.

ADRENAL INCIDENTALOMA

There is an increasing trend to do abdominal imaging for diverse purposes, ranging from evaluation of abdominal pain to searches for occult or evident masses. This has resulted in the 'incidental' detection of adrenal masses, aptly called **adrenal incidentalomas**. A patient with an incidentaloma needs careful evaluation to rule out a malignancy. A tumor size more than 4–6 cm and a heterogeneous consistency strongly suggests malignancy. However, benign adenomas of this size can also occur as incidentalomas without hormonal abnormalities. In addition, in every case, hormonal abnormalities must be ruled out by biochemical tests. This should include tests to look for medullary tumors such as pheochromocytomas as well as cortical tumors that produce excess cortisol or androgens. A contrast-enhanced CT (CECT) scan with delayed washout images helps to characterize the masses as benign or malignant and give important decisions in management.

CHAPTER
102

Gonads and their Disorders

Mathew John, KP Poulose, KV Krishna Das

Chapter Summary

- General Considerations
- Gonadogenesis
- Reproduction in Males
- Gonadal Disorders in Males
  - Hypogonadism
  - Impotence
- Gonadal Disorders Affecting Both Sexes
  - Delayed Puberty
    - Sexual Precocity
    - Infertility
    - Hermaphroditism
- Gonadal Disorders in Females
  - Hypogonadism in Women
  - Ovarian Hormonal Disorders
  - Medical Problems of Menopause
  - Hormone Replacement Therapy (HRT) in Women
- Disorders of Sexual Differentiation

GENERAL CONSIDERATIONS

Sexual reproduction requires three types of differentiation:

1. **Gonadal:** For production of gametes
2. **Genital:** For transfer of gametes to the site of fertilization
3. **Behavioral:** For the urge to behave sexually.

The most important gene for gonadal differentiation is **SRY gene** situated in the short arm of the Y chromosome. This gene induces the gonad to differentiate into a testis.

The gonads and genital ducts intended for reproduction develop under the influence of genetic and hormonal factors. The sex chromosomes X or Y determine the genetic sex or gonadal sex of the offspring. Phenotypic sex (also called somatic sex) comprises the external genitalia and the secondary sex characters. The translation of gonadal sex into phenotypic sex is the direct consequence of the type of gonad formed and the endocrine secretion of the fetal gonads resulting in the formation of male or female urogenital tract. The development of the genitalia, breasts, body build, voice, facial and pubic hair, and other pubertal changes constitute secondary sexual development. The term 'psychological sex' and the 'gender role' refers to the behavioral and psychosocial aspects of two sexes.

GONADOGENESIS

The genetic composition XX or XY determines the morphological development of the gonads and other structures. The germ cells present in the intermediate mesoderm of the developing embryo transforms into the bipotential gonad, which can differentiate into testes or ovary. The important event in gonadal differentiation is the commitment of the bipotential gonad to become either an ovary or a testis. Testis determination occurs at about the sixth week of gestation. SRY gene that is located on the Y chromosome (Yp11.3) initiates sex determination by downstream regulation of sex-determining factors. The essential genes affecting this process are as follows: WT1, SF1, CBX2, SOX9, fibroblast growth factor 9 (FGF9), prostaglandin D2 (PGD2), DAX1, WNT4, forkhead box L2 (FOXL2), R-Spondin 1 (RSPO1) and β-catenin. While SOX9, FGF9 and PGD2 have more testis-promoting activity, AX1, WNT4, FOXL2, RSPO1 and β-catenin are predominantly ovary-promoting genes.

In the testes, the production of anti-Mullerian hormone (AMH) by Sertoli cells and androgens by Leydig cells in a critical concentration-dependent and time-dependent manner induces the process of male sexual differentiation. Testosterone secreted by the testes directs the Wolffian ducts to differentiate into the male internal reproductive tract. The epididymis, vas deferens and seminal vesicles develop from the Wolffian ducts. The Mullerian ducts degenerate under the influence of AMH. The Leydig cells also produce insulin-like factor 3 (INSL3, relaxin-like factor), which causes the testes to descend to the scrotum.

In the absence of Y chromosome (SRY gene), the gonad differentiates into an ovary. However, the development of ovary is not a default process and requires the adequate expression of genes like DAX-1, FOXL2, RSPO1 and β-catenin. Mullerian ducts give rise to the fallopian tubes, uterus and the upper two-third of the vagina. In the female, the genital tubercle becomes the clitoris, the labioscrotal folds become the labia majora, and the urethral folds become the labia minora. The development of external genitalia is controlled to a great extent by the hormonal profile of the individual. Sexual differentiation should be considered anomalous in any patient with ambiguous genitalia, cryptorchidism, inguinal masses in apparent females, inguinal hernia, clitoromegaly or gynecomastia.

Pubertal changes: Puberty is a period of rapid physical and sexual development during which a sexually immature child is transformed into a mature adult. Pubertal development is preceded by adrenarche, which is characterized by the enhanced secretion of adrenal androgens—dehydroepiandrosterone (DHEA) and androstenedione. The factors that determine the onset of puberty are poorly understood, but the sequence of events is well-characterized. The earliest sign of puberty is the sleep-related pulses of luteinizing hormone (LH), secretion and episodic follicle-stimulating hormone (FSH) secretion. Later on, a persistent and sustained secretion of gonadotropins ensues throughout the day resulting in elevated plasma levels of sex hormones that result in sexual maturation.

Sexual maturation in males and females occurs in stages and this has been divided into five grades. Changes in male include increase in testicular volume, growth of penis and glans, appearance of scrotal rugosity and scrotal pigmentation. The pubic hair appears and spreads to the medial surface of the thighs and the linea alba as an inverted triangle (pubarche). In girls, the breasts and areola enlarge and papillae project on the areola. The pubic hair appears and spreads. Mean age for menarche in girls is 12 years, and this is 1–2 years earlier than the age of puberty for boys. The gonadal hormones are essential for the maintenance of fertility, sexual behavior and systemic effects in both sexes. In addition, in the female, ovulation, menstruation and nidation of ovum are maintained by gonadal steroids. Later axillary hair develops (adrenarche). Pubarche and adrenarche are under the influence of androgens (Table 102.1).

Tanner's classification of pubertal development (Figs 102.1 to 102.3).

Ovulation: The ovary increases in size after birth. In the years preceding menarche, the medullary stroma hypertrophies. When puberty develops, cyclic gonadotropin rhythm is established and under the influence of gonadotropins, a group of primary follicles are recruited and after the 6–8th day of menses,

Table 102.1: Sequential changes in pubertal development in both sexes

Girls		Boys	
Signs	**Age (in years)**	**Signs**	**Age (in years)**
Breast budding	8–13	Growth of scrotum and testis	10.5–17
Growth of pubic hair	8–14	Change in voice	10.5–18
Growth spurt	10–14 (peak 11–13.5)	Lengthening of penis	11–15
Menarche	10–16	Growth of pubic hair	11–14
Axillary hair growth	10.5–16.5	Growth spurt	12–16 (peak 13–15)
Change in body shape	11–14.5	Change in body shape	12–17
Adult breast size	12.5–16.5	Growth of facial/axillary hair	13–17

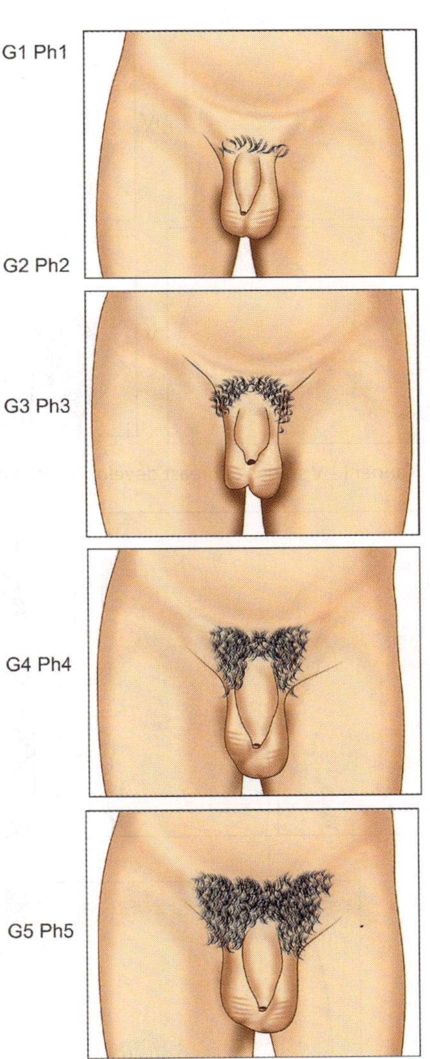

Fig. 102.1: Tanner 1–5 phase of external genitalia development in boys

one follicle becomes mature and dominant with accelerated growth of granulosa cells, and this results in ovulation. With the approach of menopause, the ovary becomes less sensitive to gonadotropin stimulation.

Textbook of Medicine

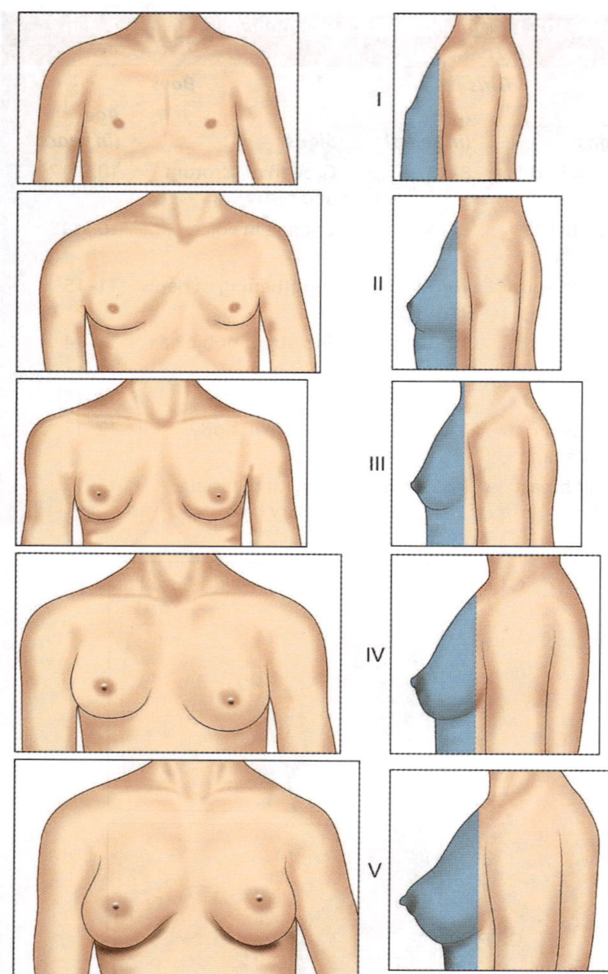

Fig. 102.2: Tanner I – V stages of breast development in girls

Maturation of follicles and ovulation stops. The levels of pituitary gonadotropin increase considerably and remain so for life.

REPRODUCTION IN MALES

The male reproductive system comprises of testes, vas deferens and accessory sex glands. The bulk of the testes is made up of seminiferous tubules embedded in a connective tissue matrix which also contains Leydig cells, blood vessels and lymphatics. Spermatogenesis takes place in the epithelium of the seminiferous tubules and it takes about 74 days. Spermatozoa are stored in the epididymis. Sertoli cells present in the seminiferous epithelium secrete an androgen-binding protein under FSH control. Interstitial tissue of the testes contains the Leydig cells, which secrete the principal testicular hormone—testosterone.

Androgens are steroid hormones, which are responsible for conferring male characteristics. They are responsible for the development of male reproductive organs, secondary sexual characters and masculine behavior. The testicular androgens include testosterone, androstenedione and DHEA. Androgens are secreted by the testes under the influence of the LH of the pituitary. Testosterone is converted into its active metabolite dihydrotestosterone (DHT) enzymatically by 5-alpha reductase. This conversion takes place both in blood and the target tissues.

The testicular hormones show variation with age. About 4–7 months after birth, male infants show a substantial increase of circulating testosterone and LH levels. The levels of testosterone fall to low range by one year, so also FSH and LH. Puberty occurs by the age of 10–15 years. The FSH reaches adult levels by the age of 15 years and LH reaches adult levels by the age 17

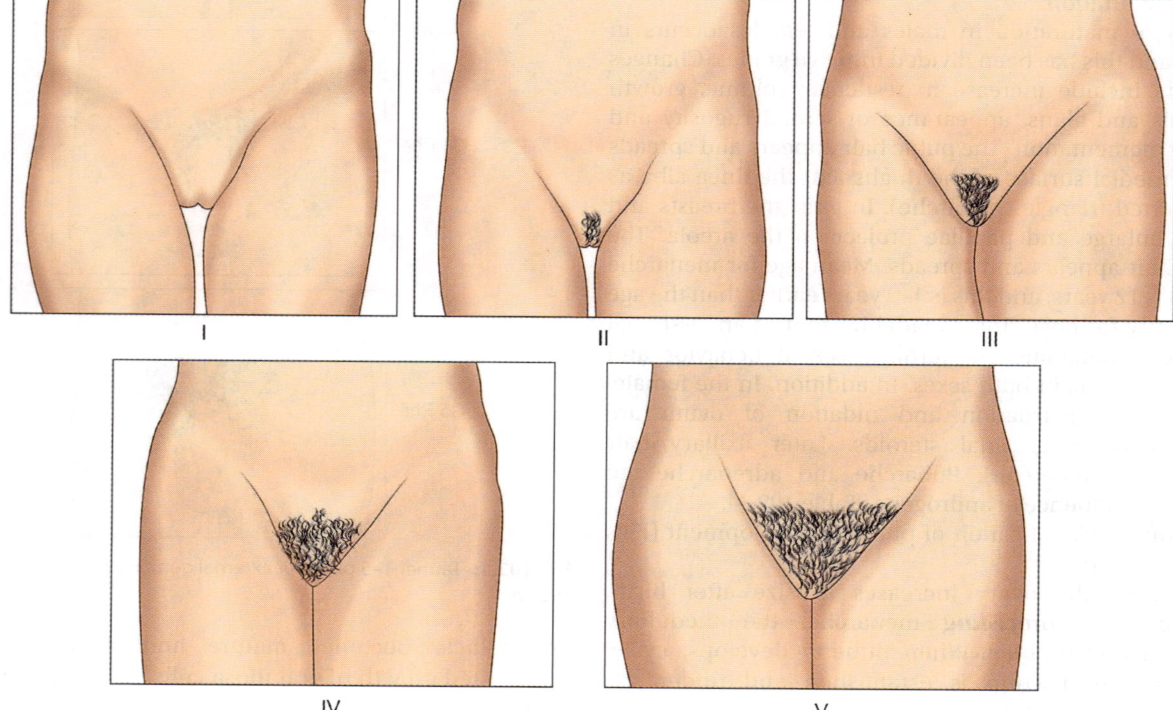

Fig. 102.3: Tanner I–V for pubic hair development in girls

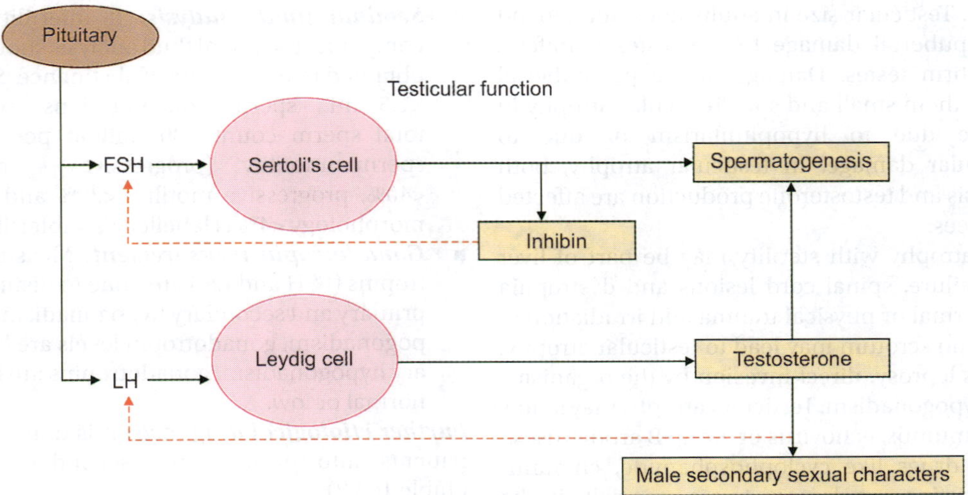

Fig. 102.4: An overview of testicular function. The gonadotropins, follicle-stimulating hormone (FSH) and luteinizing hormone (LH) are secreted from the pituitary, and they control the Sertoli and Leydig cells respectively, which carry out testicular functions. ***Note:*** Dotted arrows represent inhibitory pathways, while straight lines represent stimulatory pathways

years. During puberty, gonadotropin output occurs in spurts related to sleep. After completion of puberty, the gonadotropin levels become steady. After the age of 40 years, marked changes in gonadal function occur in women but only to a lesser extent in men. Plasma levels of testosterone gradually decline in men. There is a gradual decline in libido and reduction in size of the testes.

Testicular function is essentially under a dual gonadotropin control. The LH stimulates the Leydig cells and FSH stimulates seminiferous tubules (Fig. 102.4).

Functions of Androgens

Androgens regulate gonadotropins secretion by the hypothalamo-pituitary axis, initiate and maintain spermatogenesis and are also responsible for the development of secondary sexual characters during puberty, and control of libido. Testosterone is necessary for linear growth and muscular development. It enlarges the larynx, including vocal cords, and is responsible for change of voice in the male. Testosterone is converted to an active metabolite DHT in target tissues by the action of 5-alpha reductase and DHT is responsible for the terminal hair growth of the beard, trunk, limbs, nostrils and external ears (Fig. 102.4).

GONADAL DISORDERS IN MALES

HYPOGONADISM

Testicular hypofunction at any age leads to functional and morphological abnormalities depending upon the age of onset and duration of the disorder. This may be primary or secondary depending upon whether the defect is in the gonads or it is in the endocrine glands controlling gonadal function.

Primary Hypogonadism in Males
Disorders Involving Male Sexual Differentiation

- Chromosomal sex disorders:
  - Klinefelter's syndrome (XXY)
  - XX male
  - Mixed gonadal dysgenesis (X/XY)

- True hermaphroditism (XX/XY)
- Ullrich-Turner syndrome (XO/XY)
- Heredofamilial disorders (e.g. Noonan's syndrome).
- Developmental disorders occurring in normal genotypic males (46 XY):
  - Anorchism
  - Hypospadias
  - Cryptorchidism
  - Germinal cell aplasia
  - Abnormalities in the outflow tract for sperms.
- Male pseudohermaphroditism:
  - Dyshormonogenesis (androgen biosynthetic defects)
  - Androgen insensitivity disorders
  - Persistent Mullerian duct syndrome.

Adult Testicular Failure (Acquired)

- Idiopathic type
- Primary testicular disease
- Orchitis occurring in mumps, lepromatous leprosy and other infections
- Neurological diseases, e.g. paraplegia, dystrophia myotonica
- Acquired disorders like varicocele
- Drugs, e.g. cyclophosphamide, spironolactone, cyproterone, furosemide, cimetidine, heroin, medroxy-progesterone, phenothiazines, estrogens
- Hepatic and renal failure
- Autoimmune disorders
- Accidental or surgical trauma and irradiation.

Secondary Hypogonadism

- ***Hypothalamic causes:*** Tumor, trauma, radiation
- ***Pituitary causes:*** Tumor, trauma, isolated gonadotropin deficiency.
- Postsurgical and Postradiation

Testicular Atrophy

The seminiferous tubules account for the size and volume of the testes. Normally, the adult testes measures 15–25 mL in volume. In the prepubertal period, its volume

Textbook of Medicine

is only 2–3 mL. Testicular size in adults does not depend upon age. Prepubertal damage to the testes manifests as small and firm testes. Damage in the postpubertal period renders them small and soft. Testicular atrophy in adult may be due to hypopituitarism or due to primary testicular damage. In testicular atrophy, both spermatogenesis and testosterone production are affected to varying degrees.

Testicular atrophy with sterility may be part of liver failure, renal failure, spinal cord lesions and dystrophia myotonica. Thermal or physical trauma and irradiation of the abdomen and scrotum may lead to testicular atrophy. In lepromatous leprosy, direct invasion by the organisms results in panhypogonadism. Testicular atrophy may follow orchitis due to mumps, echovirus or group B arboviruses.

Anticancer drugs like cyclophosphamide, chlorambucil and vincristine can damage testes especially in the prepubertal period.

Clinical Manifestations

The clinical manifestations of hypogonadism depend on the stage of sexual development at which the dysfunction develops.

Fetal Androgen Deficiency

Ambiguous genitalia (various degrees, from females—looking external genitalia to cryptorchidism and micropenis).

Prepubertal

- Poorly-developed external genitalia
- Small testes
- Lack of androgen dependent hair
- Female type of pubic hair
- Poor muscle mass
- Arm span greater than height
- High-pitched voice
- Gynecomastia.

Adult

- Sexual dysfunction
- Gynecomastia
- Infertility
- Loss of androgen dependent hair
- Hot flushes
- Low bone mass.

Investigations

In a male suspected to have hypogonadism, investigations are done to establish the diagnosis of hypogonadism, classify it as primary or secondary, and finally to reach an etiology for the same.

- **Testosterone levels:** Consistently and unequivocally, low testosterone levels on at least two occasions are required to confirm a diagnosis of androgen deficiency. Testosterone is preferably estimated in the morning hours. Lower limit of normal values for total testosterone in healthy young men is 2.8–3 ng/mL.

Criteria for male hypogonadism in adults:
- Testosterone levels normal values—morning
- Total testosterone—normal >3.2 ng/mL (11 nmol/L)
- Free testosterone levels—normal >64 pg/mL (220 pmol/L)
- Levels below this and three symptoms indicate clinical hypogonadism.

- **Seminal fluid analysis:** If infertility is the main complaint, a seminal fluid analysis should be done. It is obtained after 48 hours of abstinence. Semen volumes <1.5 mL, sperm concentrations <15 million/mL, total sperm count <39 million per ejaculate, total sperm motility (progressive + nonprogressive) <40%, progressive motility <32% and normal sperm morphology <4% is labelled as subfertile.
- **Gonadotropin measurement:** Measures of gonadotropins (FSH and LH) are done to distinguish between primary and secondary hypogonadism. In primary hypogonadism, gonadotropin levels are high. In secondary hypogonadism, gonadotropins are inappropriately normal or low.

Further etiological diagnosis: It is done after classifying patients into primary and secondary hypogonadism (Table 102.2).

Androgen therapy: Orally administered testosterone is rapidly degraded in the liver, so that only a fraction of the administered dose reaches the systemic circulation. Similarly, injected testosterone is rapidly absorbed and metabolized. So, for effective androgen therapy, the testosterone must be administered in a slowly absorbable form, e.g. transdermal or slow-release oral preparations or by injection of chemically modified testosterone preparations.

Oral preparations of testosterone include mesterolone acetate in doses of 25 mg/day and testosterone undecanoate. Of these, the latter is absorbed through lymphatic systems into the circulation and physiological blood levels may be attained by a dose of 120 mg/day, given in divided doses. Transdermal preparations are also effective; a scrotal patch of testosterone is able to deliver 4–6 mg of testosterone over 24 hours. Of the injectable forms, testosterone propionate is short acting. It is given in doses of 20 mg intramuscular (IM) injection. Testosterone caproate (60 mg IM) and enanthate are long acting. They have to be given once every 2–3 weeks. Troublesome side effects of androgens are the development of precocious puberty (PP), premature fusion of the epiphyses in children, dyspepsia, polycythemia, suppression of endogenous androgens, and temporary cessation of spermatogenesis. Prostatic carcinomas may spread under the influence of androgens. Rarely androgens produce hepatic adenoma on prolonged therapy. Androgen withdrawal leads to tiredness, loss of libido, impotence, and hot flushes.

Testosterone (T) replacement is contraindicated in men with metastatic prostate and breast cancer. In men above 40 years of age, a digital rectal examination (DRE)

Table 102.2: Investigations that distinguish between primary and secondary hypogonadism

Primary	Secondary
• Karyotype (Klinefelter's, Turner's syndrome)	• Prolactin in females
	• Iron studies (exclude hemochromatosis)
• Medical history review (mumps, testicular trauma, gonadotoxic drugs)	• Cortisol/thyroid axis estimations (to look for anterior pituitary deficiency)
	• MRI (sellar and suprasellar regions)

Abbreviation: MRI = Magnetic resonance imaging

and prostate-specific antigen (PSA) level should be done before initiating T therapy. PSA levels more than 4 ng/mL or abnormal DRE should have a urologic assessment including transrectal ultrasound study and prostate biopsy, before initiating testosterone therapy. Relative contraindications to testosterone therapy include untreated obstructive sleep apnea, baseline hematocrit more than 50, benign prostatic hyperplasia and edematous states. There is no evidence that testosterone causes prostate cancer.

Gonadotropin therapy: This restores fertility in subjects with hypopituitarism. Since prolonged therapy can cause antibody production, this is reserved for inducing spermatogenesis. The commonly available preparations include human menopausal gonadotropin (HMG), which has 75 IU each of LH and FSH activity. hCG has got mainly LH activity and only slight FSH activity. hCG is supplied in vials containing 2,000–10,000 units. Usually, treatment is begun with hCG and later HMG is added on to stimulate the FSH-dependent phases of spermatogenesis. Human pituitary gonadotropin (HPG) has strong FSH and weak LH activity. One miligram is equivalent to 500–750 IU. It can also be used with hCG to promote spermatogenesis.

GnRH therapy: Usually, GnRH stimulates gonadotropin release, and when given in a pulsatile manner every 90–120 minutes, it is the ideal treatment for purely hypothalamic GnRH deficiency. Eventhough this condition is rare, some of the cases of isolated gonadotropin deficiency may be due to GnRH deficiency. Interestingly, if given continuously, GnRH can produce the opposite effect and suppress gonadotropin release.

Klinefelter Syndrome (KS)

(*See* also Section 1, Ch 2)

It is the most common sex chromosomal anomaly and most common cause of primary hypogonadism in males. The prevalence is 1 in 2,500 males. The main chromosomal abnormality is 47,XXY (90%) due to meiotic nondisjunction. In addition to hypogonadism, individuals with KS may demonstrate learning disability, behavioral problems, tall stature and gynecomastia. At puberty, testes may fail to increase in size and there is progressive loss of germ cell and seminiferous tubule hyalinization and fibrosis.

Azoospermia and infertility is the rule but testicular epididymal sperm extraction permits identification of seminiferous tubules that contain active spermatogenesis and may be harvested for intracytoplasmic sperm injection.

Idiopathic Hypogonadotropic Hypogonadism

Idiopathic hypogonadotropic hypogonadism (IHH) is a clinically heterogeneous group of disorders characterized by isolated gonadotropin deficiency of varying degree with otherwise normal pituitary hormones. Gonadotropin deficiency is caused by a defect in normal gonadotropin-releasing hormone (GnRH) production or action. In approximately 60% of cases, IHH is associated with anosmia or hyposmia and is known as Kallmann syndrome. Development failure of the olfactory bulb is responsible for anosmia.

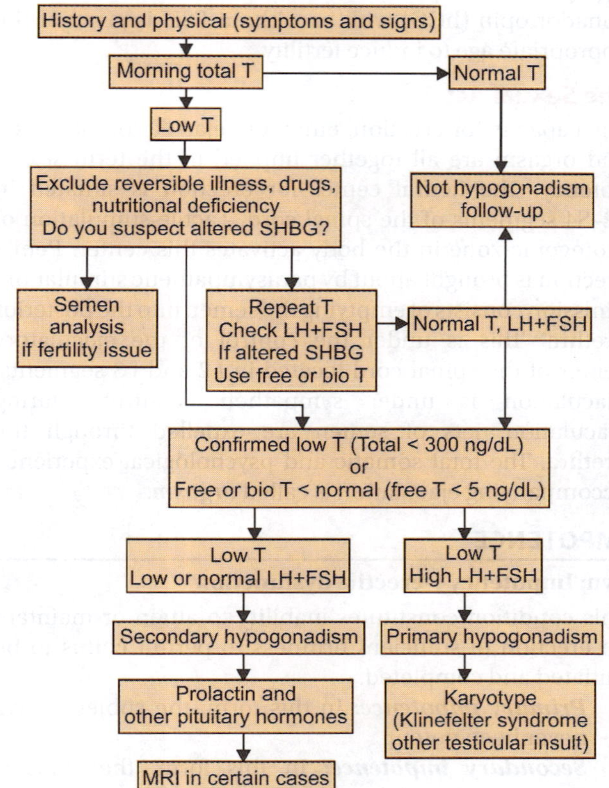

Flowchart 102.1: Algorithm for investigating a case of gonadal dysfunction in males

Abbreviations: T = Testosterone; LH = Luteinizing hormone; FSH = Follicle-stimulating hormone; SHBG = Sex hormone binding globulin; MRI = Magnetic resonance imaging

The prevalence of Kallmann syndrome is 1 in 8,000–10,000 men with a male predominance (male-to-female ratio, 4:1 to 5:1).

The inheritance pattern is X-linked recessive, autosomal dominant or autosomal recessive. Mutations of KAL1 (10–20%), FGFR1, KAL2, PROK2 and PROKR2 are associated with hypogonadotropic hypogonadism (HH). In 30% of cases, GnRHR, GnRH receptor, KISS1R, TAC3 or TAC3R mutations are associated. They present with normosmic IHH.

Hypogonadism in males can be understood with the help of Flowchart 102.1.

Treatment of Hypogonadism

The aim of treatment of hypogonadism is to replace androgens and to stimulate spermatogenesis. In primary hypogonadism, androgen replacement can be done successfully, but there is limited opportunity for stimulating spermatogenesis.

In pubertal boys with hypogonadism, androgen replacement therapy (ART) helps growth of penis and scrotum, increases strength and muscle mass, improves bone mass, and stimulates libido, mood and energy. In adults, ART helps to improve sexual function, muscle mass and strength, hematocrit, bone density, energy and mood.

While inducing puberty in males with hypogonadism, testosterone enanthate is started at 50 mg every 4 weeks and doses gradually increased over 3–4 years to an adult dose of 200 mg every 2–3 weeks. In secondary hypogonadism, pulsatile GnRH or human chorionic gonadotropin (hCG) with or without FSH is given at the appropriate age to induce fertility.

The Sexual Act

The capacity for erection, emission, ejaculation of semen and orgasm are all together implied in the term sexual potency. The neural center for erection is situated in S2–S4 segments of the spinal cord. Tactile stimulation of erotogenic zone in the body activates this center. Penile erection is brought about by parasympathetic stimulation. Emission consists of emptying the semen into the posterior urethra. This is under the control of the ejaculatory center of the spinal cord located in L2 and L3 segments. Ejaculation is under sympathetic control. During ejaculation, jets of semen are expelled through the urethra. The total somatic and psychological experience accompanying ejaculation is called *orgasm*.

IMPOTENCE

Syn: Impotency—erectile dysfunction

This condition constitutes inability to attain or maintain an erection of sufficient firmness to permit coitus to be initiated and completed.

- **Primary impotence:** In this form, the subjects have never been potent.
- **Secondary impotence:** In this form, the subjects experience impotence after a period of normal potency. The term *apareunia* indicates inability to perform the sexual act.

Even in normal individuals, transient episodes of impotence may occur as a result of fatigue, distraction, acute illnesses, or anxiety. These recover spontaneously.

Impotence is a common disorder after the age of 40 years. The prevalence is given below:

Men <40 years	1–10%
40–49 years	2–9%
60–69 years	20–40%
Above 70 years	50–100%

Erectile dysfunction below 40–50 years occurring spontaneously is a strong predictor of coronary artery disease (CAD) and therefore, it is a major health problem demanding appropriate investigations and management.

Etiology

Eighty-five to ninety percent of cases are due to organic causes. In 10–15% cases, the condition is psychogenic. In all types of impotence, it is common for psychological or behavioral abnormalities to supervene.

Organic Causes

- All cases of primary and secondary hypogonadism.
- **Other endocrine disorders:** Acromegaly, hyper- and hypothyroidism, Cushing's syndrome and Addison's disease.
- Neurological disorders involving the lumbosacral segments of the spinal cord, nervi erigentes and autonomic neuropathy occurring in diabetes mellitus (DM)
- **Chronic systemic illnesses:** DM, hepatic cirrhosis, chronic renal failure, obesity, starvation, disabling

Table 102.3: Difference between organic and psychogenic impotence

Organic	Psychogenic
Impotence is always present	Conditional and situational
Begins insidiously and slowly progressive	Usually sudden onset
The onset of impotence coincides with any significant illness like myocardial infarction	There may be a temporal association to a stressful event as the death of a parent or child
There is no reflex penile erection in the early hours of the morning	Morning erections are present (nocturnal tumescence)

arthritis, connective tissue diseases, chronic obstructive airway disease and systemic malignancy.

- **Iatrogenic:** Antihypertensive drugs, estrogens, H_2 receptor blockers, tranquilizers, sedatives, alcohol, psychedelic drugs and anticancer drugs.
- **Occlusive vascular disease:** Atherosclerotic and otherwise (normal diameter of the penile artery is 1–2 mm).

Psychogenic Causes

- Affective disorders like depression, mania, schizophrenia, hysteria and antisocial personality
- Alcoholism and other drug addictions
- Organic brain syndromes
- Personality disorders
- Trans-sexualism (a strong desire to change to the opposite sex)

Diagnosis

It should be determined whether the impotence is primarily psychogenic or organic. The essential differences between the two are given in Table 102.3.

Investigations include local palpation, pharmacoarteriography, pharmacocavernosometry, neurological tests and studies on nocturnal penile tumescence (NPT).

Treatment

Organic impotence must be managed according to its cause. In many cases, the patient or his sexual partner may benefit from counseling or by psychotherapy. Drugs like androgens and replacement hormones are indicated only if the condition is secondary to an endocrine disorder. Important lifestyle modification include avoidance of smoking, regular exercise, management of obesity, treatment of underlying chronic diseases, social interactions with the spouse and involvement in leisure activities.

Drugs

Several drugs are available which increase penile tumescence.

Sildenafil is a selective inhibitor of cyclic guanosine monophosphate (cGMP)—specific phosphodiesterase type 5, which is present in the cavernosa tissue. By selectively inhibiting this enzyme, the catabolism of cGMP is arrested and the normal erectile response of sexual stimulation is restored. Relaxation of smooth muscle allows inflow of blood into the corpora cavernosa and gives rise to penile erection, in response to sexual stimulation.

Textbook of Medicine

Table 102.4: Dose and onset of action and duration of effect of cyclic guanosine monophosphate inhibitor drugs given orally				
Drug	**Dose**	**Onset of action**	**Duration**	**Efficacy**
Sildenafil	25, 50 and 50 mg	30–60 minutes	4–8 hrs	65%
Vardenafil	2.5–20 mg	30 minutes	4–8 hrs	65%
Tadalafil	2.5–20 mg	45 minutes	36 hrs	> 65%
Udenafil	100–200 mg	30–60 minutes	12 hrs	> 65 %
Mirodenafil	50–100 mg	30–60 minutes	6–12 hrs	–

Sildenafil citrate is rapidly absorbed when given orally, blood levels peak at one hour and the mean half-life is 3–5 hours. Dose varies from 25 to 100 mg to be taken one hour before the desired sexual activity. The drug should not be used concurrently with nitrates or nitric-oxide donor drugs. Adverse effects include headache, flushing, dyspepsia, nasal congestion, diarrhea and impairment of platelet function.

Tadalafil is a drug with marginally better benefit and risk profile as compared with sildenafil.

Vardenafil is another analogue which can be used in a dose of 5–20 mg/day for impotence.

Other drugs include ***udenafil*** and ***mirodenafil***, which are less easily available in India (Table 102.4).

Contraindications include advanced cardiac, hepatic and renal disease. In the Indian context, since a good proportion of elderly women desire to avoid sexual intercourse, the drug should be given to elderly patients only after proper counseling of the sexual partners.

Testosterone is indicated in cases with hypogonadism. Repeated testosterone injection may give rise to erythrocytosis with consequent thrombotic tendencies, virilization and oligospermia.

In cases which are not amenable to these general measures and in whom impotence leads to severe impairment in the quality of life and disruption of family relationships, local measures to ensure penile tumescence are available. ***Sexual medicine*** has attained a high degree of specialization and several methods of treatments are in vogue to achieve penile erection and the sexual act. These are generally used by specialists in sexual medicine. Some common procedures include:

- Intracavernosal injection of papaverine as self-injection by the patient or spouse
- Vacuum suction devices and inflatable balloons implanted in the corpora cavernosa
- Penile prosthesis, and penile stimulators which can be operated by the couple.

Source: Shamloul R, Ghanem H. Erectile Dysfunction. Lancet. 2013;381(9861):153-65.

CRYPTORCHISM

Syn: Cryptorchidism

Cryptorchidism is the failure of one or more testes to descend naturally from within the abdomen through the inguinal canal to the scrotum. It is the most common congenital disorder in children affecting 2–4% of full-term male births. It is more common in premature and low birth weight (LBW) infants. Spontaneous descend of testes occurs during the first few years in most infants. Ectopic testes is located outside the normal path of testicular descend. Bilateral cryptorchidism may be associated with various disorders causing primary hypogonadism (Klinefelter syndrome and Noonan syndrome) and secondary hypogonadism like IHH, Kallmann syndrome and congenital syndromes like Prader-Willi syndrome.

There is reduced spermatogenesis in cryptorchidism. It is also associated with 2.5–8-fold risk of testicular cancer. If clinical examination does not detect the undescended testes, USG or magnetic resonance imagining (MRI) should be used to detect its location.

Recent recommendations suggest that treatment should be initiated between 6 and 12 months or up to 24 months of age. Hormonal treatment with hCG or GnRH in prepubertal boys is effective in 10–20%. Orchiopexy is performed if hormonal therapy fails or is not attempted.

AZOOSPERMIA

Absence of sperms in the semen is called ***azoospermia***. This is common in primary testicular disorders, which are developmental or endocrine in nature. In addition, several structural abnormalities also lead to this condition. These include congenital absence of vas deferens acquired occlusion of the epididymis and vas deferens, and absence of seminal vesicles. Varicosity of the pampiniform plexus may lead to oligospermia or azoospermia in about 15% of cases.

GONADAL DISORDERS AFFECTING BOTH SEXES

DELAYED PUBERTY

When sexual maturity is delayed beyond 14 years in boys and 13 years in girls, puberty is delayed. The first sign of puberty in male is the increase in testicular size and the first sign in female is the larche. Some of these subjects may have constitutional delay and some of them may need extensive investigations to arrive at a diagnosis.

Causes of Delay in Puberty

- Idiopathic delay of growth and development
- Neuroendocrine disorders:
  - Tumors of the central nervous system (CNS)—craniopharyngioma, pinealoma
  - Congenital malformations of the CNS
  - Hypopituitarism
  - Kallmann's syndrome
  - Laurence-Moon-Biedl syndrome
  - Prader-Willi syndrome
  - Functional gonadotropin deficiency
- Chronic systemic diseases:
  - Malnutrition
  - Anorexia nervosa
  - Hypothyroidism
  - Debilitating illnesses like uncontrolled diabetes, renal failure, hepatic cirrhosis, thalassemia, malignancies and others

Textbook of Medicine

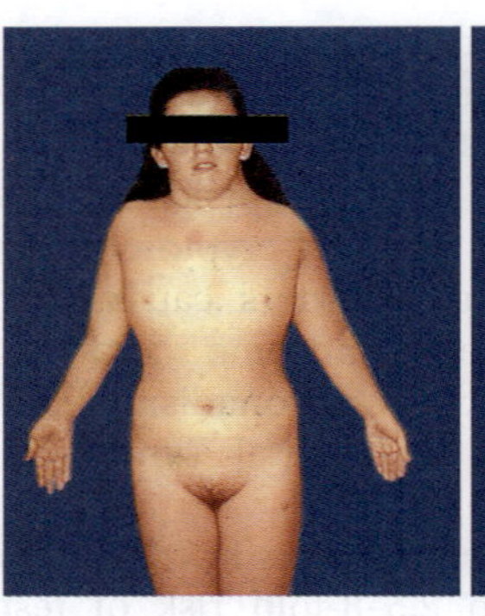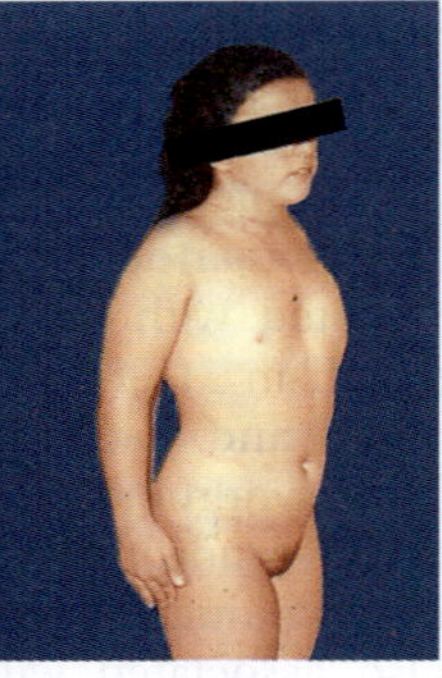

Fig. 102.5: Girl aged 18-year-old with Turner's syndrome

- Primary gonadal failure:
  - Chromosomal disorders—Klinefelter's and Turner's syndromes and their variants (Fig. 102.5)
  - Developmental agenesis—anorchia, cryptorchidism
  - Other causes of primary gonadal failure.

Laurence-Moon-Biedl syndrome: In this rare congenital disorder which is characterized by obesity, dwarfism, hypogonadism, mental retardation, retinitis pigmentosa and polydactyly, a strong familial tendency is noticeable. It is inherited as autosomal recessive.

Prader-Willi syndrome: In this rare anomaly, intrauterine and postnatal hypotonia, obesity, mental deficiency and hypogonadism are seen. The hands and feet are small. There may be mild retardation of growth. There will be feeding difficulty in the first few years of life followed by severe hyperphagia and uncontrolled obesity later in life.

Evaluation

There are many causes of delayed puberty. A detailed history and clinical examination will help narrow down the differential diagnosis. Detailed history should include birth history, milestones, nutritional state and neonatal history. Family history of endocrinopathies, infertility, anosmia or hypogonadism should be noted. Pubertal onset and growth pattern in siblings and parents should be noted.

Physical examination include height, weight, segments (upper/lower segment). These parameters should be plotted on a growth chart and height velocity should be calculated. Puberty should be assessed by the sexual maturity rating with Tanner's method. Pubic hair and axillary hair should be assessed. Signs of raised intracranial tension, fundus and anosmia should be noted. Physical findings suggestive of Turner syndrome, Noonan syndrome, Prader-Willi syndrome and Laurence-Moon-Biedl syndrome should be noted. Clinical examination should also look for systemic diseases which may delay pubertal development.

Investigation should include tests for excluding systemic disease. Testosterone, FSH and LH levels should be done in boys, and estradiol, FSH and LH should b done in girls. Thyroid function test and prolactin should be done based on clinical features. X-rays should be done for bone age. MRI of the sellar and suprasellar region is to be done if clinical or biochemical evaluation suggests an intracranial lesion. Karyotype should be done in all girls who are short with delayed puberty, especially if FSH is elevated.

Constitutional delay in growth and puberty (CDGP) is the most common cause in boys presenting with delayed puberty. Family history may show male members with similar history. Growth charts will show short stature with growth velocity appropriate for the skeletal age.

Treatment

The main aim of investigation is to establish a diagnosis. Treatment is targeted at diagnosis, e.g. an intracranial lesion. In male patients with suspected CDGP, and age more than 14 years, 3 to 6 month course of testosterone enanthate 50–100 mg is given once every 4 weeks. Follow-up of these patients shows that pubertal development starts and progresses following this. In girls, ethinylestradiol 5µ/day or conjugated equine estrogen (CEE) 0.3 mg/day will help start the pubertal development.

SEXUAL PRECOCITY

The appearance of secondary sexual characters before 7 years of age in boys and 8 years in girls constitutes sexual precocity. True precocious puberty is due to premature maturation of pituitary gonadal axis. Disorders of puberty may also result from increased secretion of testosterone or estrogen, independent of pituitary control. This leads to incomplete isosexual precocity (Figs 102.6A and B).

Causes

- ***True precocious puberty (both sexes):***
  - Idiopathic type
  - CNS tumors in the region of the hypothalamus
  - Other CNS disorders, e.g. encephalitis, trauma, tuberculoma, hydrocephalus, neurofibromatosis
  - Severe primary hypothyroidism.
- ***Incomplete isosexual precocity in boys:***
  - Ectopic hormone secretion, e.g. hepatomas, chorionepitheliomas, congenital adrenal hyperplasia (CAH) (21 or 11 hydroxylase defects)
  - Adrenal carcinoma, Leydig cell adenoma and drugs such as androgens, anabolic steroids
- ***Incomplete isosexual precocity in girls:***
  - Ovarian diseases, e.g. follicular cysts, granulosa or theca cell tumors, gonadoblastoma, Albright's syndrome
  - Gonadotropin-producing tumors, e.g. teratoma, hepatoma and drugs such as estrogens, gonadotropins.

Precocious Puberty

The appearance of any form of sexual maturation before the normal age of puberty (9 years for boys, 7 years for girls, 6 years for African American girls) is called precocious puberty. If sexual precocity is due to premature activation of the hypothalamic GnRH pulse generator or pituitary hypothalamic gonadal axis, it is called GnRH dependent or central precocious or true precocious puberty. If the gonadal secretion of steroids is independent of pituitary gonadotropins, it is called GnRH-independent precocious puberty or pseudoprecocious puberty. If there is excessive estrogen secretion in males or androgen secretion in females, it is called contrasexual precocity.

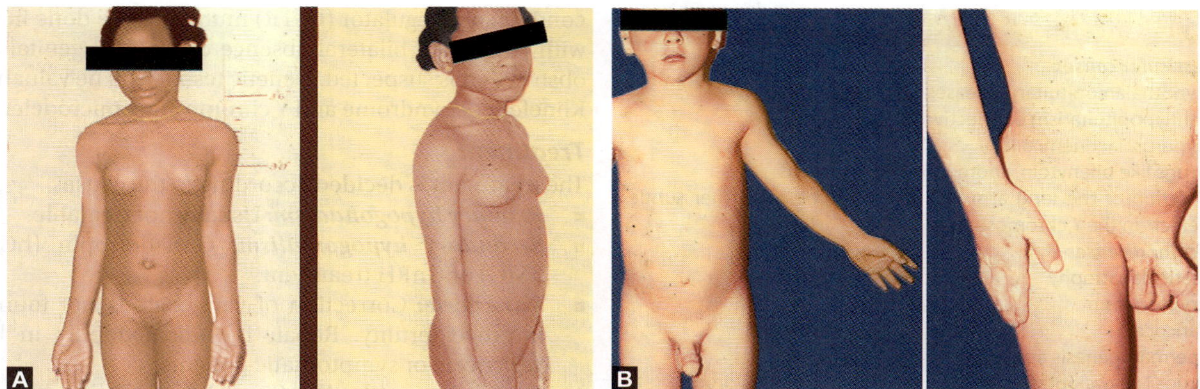

Figs 102.6A and B: A. Sexual precocity girl aged 7 years; **B.** Sexual precocity boy aged 8 years, normal (left), precocious (right)

In all forms of sexual precocity, gonadal steroids increase height and this accelerates somatic development and rate of sexual maturation. There is premature fusion of epiphysis and short adult height.

Central precocious puberty (GnRH dependent): There is a female predominance in central precocious puberty (CPP). It may be idiopathic or associated with intracranial lesions like hypothalamic hamartoma, optic glioma, encephalitis, head trauma or hydrocephalus.

GnRH-independent precocious puberty: In males, it can be due to hCG secreting tumors, CAH, virilizing adrenal tumors, Leydig cell adenoma and familial testotoxicosis. In girls, it can be due to estrogen-producing lesions of the ovary or McCune-Albright's syndrome (both sexes).

Diagnosis and Management

Patients with precocious puberty have elevated levels of gonadal steroids (estradiol in girls and testosterone in boys). Levels of gonadotropins help to decide if it is GnRH dependent (elevated basal levels of LH or stimulated LH levels) or GnRH independent (suppressed basal LH levels or failure of stimulated LH to increase). Subjects with GnRH dependent puberty (true/central) should have MRI of the sellar regions to exclude intracranial lesions. Subjects with GnRH dependent puberty can be managed by long-acting GnRH agonists. Following initial stimulation of GnRH receptor, these agents suppress the pulsatile LH and FSH release, gonadal steroid output and gametogenesis. For GnRH-independent puberty, the offending condition should be managed. Surgical removal of tumors producing hCG (in males) and estrogen (in females) will help resolve puberty.

Albright's syndrome (polyostotic fibrous dysplasia of bone): This is a rare disorder, which may be associated with precocious puberty due to inappropriate activation of the gonadotropins receptor. Other abnormalities include irregular pigmentation and dysplasia of several bones.

Treatment: Drugs inhibiting gonadotropins are partly successful in avoiding premature fusion of epiphyses and arresting sexual precocity. Drugs like medroxyprogesterone acetate 100 mg given IM once a week or 200–300 mg as depot injections, suppress gonadotropin secretion. For central or true precocity, GnRH agonists given continuously can delay puberty.

INFERTILITY

It is defined as the inability of a sexually-active couple to achieve conception despite 1 year of unprotected intercourse. ***Primary infertility*** refers to the inability to give birth either because of not being able to become pregnant or carry a child to live birth, which may include miscarriage or a stillborn child. ***Secondary infertility*** refers to the inability to conceive or give birth while there was a previous pregnancy or live birth. Thirty percent of infertility is due to female factor alone, 30% due to male factor alone and in the rest due to problems in both or unexplained causes. Approximately 15% of couples in the reproductive age are infertile.

Causes of Male Infertility

- ***Isolated impairment of sperm production or function hypogonadism—80–90%***
  - Androgen deficiency and impaired sperm production
  - Androgen resistance.
- ***Disorder of sperm transport (15–20%)***
  - ***Genital tract obstruction***
    - Congenital bilateral absence of vas deferens
    - Cystic fibrosis
    - Congenital defects
    - Vasectomy.
  - ***Accessory gland dysfunction associated with***
    - Androgen deficiency or resistance
    - Infection or inflammation
    - Antisperm antibody.
  - ***Sympathetic nerve dysfunction:*** Associated with autonomic neuropathy and spinal cord injury.
- ***Ejaculatory dysfunction:*** For example, premature ejaculation, retrograde ejaculation or reduced libido.
- ***Coital disorders:*** Erectile dysfunction, defects in coital technique (Table 102.5).

There is an 8–10-fold increase in prevalence of chromosomal abnormalities among infertile men with impaired spermatogenesis, specifically Klinefelter's syndrome or Robertsonian translocation involving chromosome 13 and 14 or 14 and 21. Small deletions in the azoospermia factor region (Y chromosome microdeletions) are the most common genetic cause of impaired sperm production and male infertility.

Gonads and their Disorders

Textbook of Medicine

Table 102.5: Causes of male infertility

Pretesticular causes
- Hypothalamopituitary diseases
- Panhypopituitarism or selective FSH deficiency
- Hyperprolactinemia
- Drugs like phenytoin, androgens and estrogens
- Deletion of the long arm of Y chromosome and other subtle defects in the Y chromosome

Testicular diseases
- Testicular atrophy
- Cryptorchism
- Varicocele
- Spermatogenesis arrest
- Drugs like cyclophosphamide and other antimitotic drugs
- Autoimmune disorders giving rise to antibodies against testicular basement membrane and sperms

Post-testicular causes
- Infection of the genitourinary tract with bacteriospermia, congenital or acquired ductal obstruction, varicocele
- Disorders of ejaculation, e.g. retrograde ejaculation
- Anatomical defects such as hypospadias

Abbreviation: FSH = Follicle-stimulating hormone

Table 102.6: WHO criteria for normal semen analysis

Criteria	Parameters
Volume	2.0–5.0 mL
pH	7.2–7.9
Sperm concentration	20 million/mL or more
Total sperm count	40 million spermatozoa or more
Motility	50% or more with forward progression or 25% or more with rapid linear progression within 60 min after collection
Morphology	30% or more with normal morphology (WHO)/>4% strict morphology (Tygerberg)
Viability	75% or more live (i.e. excluding dye)
White blood cells	Fewer than 1 million/mL
IBT (antisperm Ab)	<20% of sperm with adherent particles
MAR (antisperm Ab)	<10%
Fructose (total)	13 mol or more per ejaculate (for seminal vesicle presence/function and ejaculatory duct obstruction)

Note: Can be repeated in 3 weekly intervals according to the specific findings and history if abnormal.

Abbreviations: IBT = Immunobead binding test; MAR = Mixed erythrocyte-spermatozoa antiglobulin reaction; Ab = Antibody

Diagnosis

The diagnosis of male infertility is established with analysis of the seminal fluid (2–3 analysis over a period of few months). Normal values in a semen analysis are summarized in Table 102.6.

The following terminologies describe characteristic of sperms:

Oligospermia: Sperm concentration less than 20 million/mL
Asthenospermia: Forward motility <50%
Teratospermia: <30% with normal morphology by WHO
Azoospermia: Complete absence of sperm in the specimen
Aspermia: No ejaculate (zero volume) after masturbation

Serum testosterone and gonadotropin levels are done to exclude hypogonadism. Cystic fibrosis transmembrane conductance regulator (CFTR) mutations are done in men with congenital bilateral absence of vas or if genital tract obstruction is suspected. Genetic testing will be valuable in Klinefelter's syndrome and Y chromosome microdeletion.

Treatment

The treatment is decided according to the cause:
- **Primary hypogonadism:** Usually not treatable.
- **Secondary hypogonadism:** Gonadotropin (hCG + hMG) or GnRH treatment.
- **Varicocele:** Correction of varicocele is not found to improve fertility. Repair is indicated only in large varicocele or symptomatic patients.
- **Antisperm antibodies:** Steroids.

Intracytoplasmic sperm injection (ICSI) can be done with ejaculated sperm or sperm obtained by testicular biopsy [testicular sperm extraction (TESE) or from epididymis (microsurgical epididymal sperm aspiration—MESA)]. With ICSI, fertilization rates are about 60% and pregnancy rates are around 20%.

Female Infertility

The various causes of female infertility are:
- **Ovulatory dysfunction:** Polycystic ovarian syndrome (PCOS), hyperprolactinemia, hypopituitarism, HH.
- **Fallopian tubular dysfunction:** Pelvic inflammatory disease (PID) (like chlamydia, gonorrhea), endometriosis, sterilization, pelvic surgery (adhesion).
- **Cervical and/or uterine dysfunction:** Congenital abnormality, fibroids, Asherman's syndrome, cervical cancer treatment.

Investigations

In women with regular periods, ovulation can be documented by follicular studies and progesterone levels more than 10 ng/mL on day 21 (of 28-day cycle). Transvaginal ultrasound can be used to assess the uterine and ovarian anatomy. Tubal patency can be assessed by a hysterosalpingogram. Inhibin B levels on day 3 of the periods is a marker of ovarian reserve.

Treatment

In women with ovulatory dysfunction, ovulation is induced by:
- **Antiestrogen therapy:** Clomiphene citrate
- **Gonadotropins:** hCG and FSH (or HMG)
- Pulsatile GnRH therapy.

Monitoring is done by serial ultrasound and estradiol levels. Ovarian hyperstimulation syndrome (OHSS) is an emergency characterized by enlarged ovary with multiple follicles, capillary leak, ascitis and pleural effusion. Liver dysfunction, hemoconcentration, high WBC count and oliguria/anuria are features of severe OHSS.

HERMAPHRODITISM

Syn: Intersex

Intersex refers to a condition when the external genitalia are ambiguous; that is neither truly female nor truly male. It could be a male child whose genitalia are not adequately masculinized or a female child whose genitalia are virilized. Intersex is classified into the following categories.

True Hermaphroditism

It is characterized by the presence of both ovarian and testicular tissues in one or both gonads. Variable differentiation of the internal and external genitalia is seen. The external genitalia sometimes resembles that of a male or female, but mostly they are ambiguous. Chromosomal analysis reveals the common karyotypes as 46XX.

Pseudohermaphroditism

In pseudohermaphroditism, the gonadal sex is at variance with the gender sex. The terms male or female denote the corresponding gonadal sex. Thus, in *male pseudohermaphroditism,* the gonads are exclusively testes with XY karyotype, but phenotypic characteristics are to varying degrees female (failure of virilization). Causes include defective testicular stimulation due to gonadotropin resistance or deficiency, suboptimal testosterone and/or AMH secretion and failure of tissue response to androgens and/or AMH.

In *female pseudohermaphroditism,* the gonad is an ovary and the karyotype is XX. Varying degrees of virilization of external organs may be present. Ambiguity of external genitalia is usually caused by androgenic influences. Often there is no abnormality of internal genital development or functional capacity of the ovaries. The uterus, tubes and ovaries may be normally present and reproductive function may become possible after suitable correction of the external genitalia, which are masculine. Several causes may lead to female pseudohermaphroditism. The most common cause is CAH due to 21-hydroxylase deficiency. Patients have impaired cortisol synthesis, high adrenocorticotropic hormone (ACTH) levels and adrenal androgen hypersecretion. Steroid therapy can inhibit the ACTH drive and correct androgen excess.

It is preferable to investigate these cases in the first year of life so that the sex of the child can be assigned before the second year. Therapy is based on thorough clinical, psychological and genetic analysis. In female pseudohermaphroditism, the external genitalia should be surgically corrected during the first year of life. In male pseudohermaphroditism and intersexual genitalia, sex is assigned according to the state of external genitalia. Prolonged therapy may be necessary to achieve reasonably satisfactory results. Therapy includes hormone supplementation, surgical correction and psychological rehabilitation.

GYNECOMASTIA

It is a benign enlargement of the male breast (usually bilateral but sometimes unilateral) resulting from a proliferation of the glandular component of the breast.

It is defined clinically by the presence of a rubbery or firm mass extending concentrically from the nipples. Gynecomastia should be differentiated from pseudogyne-comastia (lipomastia), which is characterized by fat deposition without glandular proliferation. The causes of gynecomastia are given in Table 102.7.

The principal complaint is unilateral or bilateral concentric enlargement of breast glandular tissue. Breast

Table 102.7: Causes of gynecomastia	
Physiological factors	**Psychoactive agents**
Neonatal	Diazepam
Pubertal	Haloperidol
Involutional	Phenothiazines
Drug-induced	Tricyclic antidepressants
Hormones	**Drugs of abuse**
• Androgens and anabolic steroids	• Alcohol
• Chorionic gonadotropin	• Amphetamines
• Estrogens and estrogen agonists	• Heroin
• Growth hormone	• Marijuana
Antiandrogens or inhibitors of androgen synthesis	**Other**
• Cyproterone	• Highly active antiretroviral therapy (HAART)
• Flutamide	• Phenytoin
Antibiotics	• Penicillamine
• Isoniazid	**Endocrine**
• Ketoconazole	• Primary hypogonadism with Leydig cell damage
• Metronidazole	• Hyperprolactinemia
Antiulcer medications	• Hyperthyroidism
• Cimetidine	• Androgen receptor disorders
• Omeprazole	• Excessive aromatase activity
• Ranitidine	
Cancer chemotherapeutic agents (especially alkylating agents)	**Systemic diseases**
Cardiovascular drugs	• Hepatic cirrhosis
• Amiodarone	• Uremia
• Captopril	**Neoplasms**
• Digitoxin	• Testicular germ cell or Leydig cell tumors
• Enalapril	• Feminizing adrenocortical adenoma or carcinoma
• Methyldopa	• hCG-secreting nontrophoblastic neoplasms
• Nifedipine	
• Reserpine	
• Spironolactone	
• Verapamil	**Idiopathic**

pain is present in one-fourth of patients and objective tenderness in about 40%. A complaint of nipple discharge can be elicited in 4% of cases.

Patients with gynecomastia may have a slightly increased risk of development of breast carcinoma.

Treatment

Medical Treatment

The underlying disease should be corrected if possible and offending drugs should be discontinued. Antiestrogens or selective estrogen receptor modulators, such as tamoxifen or raloxifene, have been found useful in relieving pain and reversing gynecomastia in some patients. Aromatase inhibitors have also been tried but are not as beneficial as tamoxifen.

Surgical Treatment

Reduction mammoplasty should be considered for cosmetic reasons.

Radiotherapy

Patients with prostatic carcinoma may receive low-dose radiation therapy (900 cGy or less) to the breasts before initiation of estrogen therapy. This may prevent or diminish the gynecomastia that usually results from

Textbook of Medicine

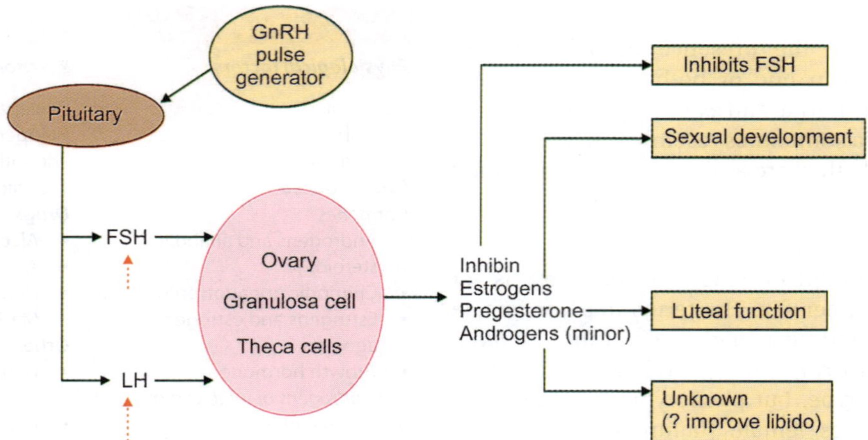

Fig. 102.7: Diagrammatic representation of ovarian function. This figure shows the gonadotropin-releasing hormone (GnRH) pulse generator in the hypothalamus that controls the pulsatile secretion of follicle-stimulating hormone (FSH) and luteinizing hormone (LH), which act on the ovarian cells to produce the sex hormones

such therapy. Radiotherapy should not be given to other patients with gynecomastia.

GONADAL DISORDERS IN FEMALES

Ovarian hormones: Estrogens stimulate sexual heat (estrus) in female animals. Major estrogens produced by the ovary are estradiol and estrone. The former is the main and more powerful hormone. Estrogens are inactivated by the liver and several metabolites are excreted in urine and bile as the conjugated products (Fig. 102.7).

Actions of estrogens: Estrogens bring about pubertal changes occurring in females. They are responsible for development of the breasts, formation of the feminine body contour, proliferation of uterine endometrium, vaginal keratini-zation and epiphyseal closure.

Progestogens and their action: These hormones prepare the uterus for reception and development of the fertilized ovum. The corpus luteum does this function normally and its main secretion is progesterone which is under the control of LH of the pituitary. Synthetic progesterone with high potency is available for therapeutic uses. Progesterone makes the endometrial glands coiled and secretory (secretory phase). They are prepared for nidation of the ovum. The rise of temperature at ovulation is mediated by progesterone. Withdrawal of progesterone results in menstrual bleeding.

Assessment of ovarian function: Clinically, ovarian function can be assessed by the development and maintenance of the breasts and the internal and external genitalia. Hypofunction of the ovaries manifests as delay in sexual development, menstrual irregularities and disorders of ovulation. Several conditions give rise to such a clinical picture. These include primary ovarian disease, hypothalamopituitary abnormalities, unresponsiveness of the target organs, systemic diseases and gonadal dysfunction occurring in other endocrine diseases.

HYPOGONADISM IN WOMEN

Hypogonadism in women is associated with anovulation with or without estrogen deficiency. They may be characterized under the following heads:

- ***Hypothalamic anovulation:*** Maybe functional or associated with lesions in the pituitary and suprasellar region.
- ***Hyperprolactinemia:*** Associated with prolactin secreting tumors and drug-induced hyperprolactinemia
- ***Androgen excess:*** PCOS, androgen secreting tumors, drugs
- Premature ovarian insufficiency
- ***Chronic illness:*** Chronic liver disease, chronic kidney disease and AIDS.

Investigations

These include: (1) Determination of levels of FSH/LH and ovarian hormones, (2) studies of the effect of ovarian hormones on vaginal epithelium such as cornification, cervical mucus and changes in the endometrium and (3) tests of ovulation such as measurement of basal body temperature which goes up at the time of ovulation and serial ultrasound measurements of follicle maturation.

OVARIAN HORMONAL DISORDERS

Ovarian dysfunction manifests clinically as amenorrhea, infantilism or sexual precocity. In primary ovarian failure, the levels of pituitary gonadotropins are high. Ovarian failure may be due to primary disease of the ovaries in 60% and extraovarian causes in 40% of cases. For proper development and functioning of the ovaries, the essential requirements are:

- Presence of two genetically active X-chromosomes
- Absence of Y-chromosome
- Proper endowment of germ cells (oogonia)
- Development of germ cells into primary oocytes
- Adequate gonadotropin stimulation in fetal life.

Abnormalities of any or all of these factors lead to ovarian failure.

Ovarian Failure

Causes of ovarian failure are shown in the box below. When it occurs due to a disease of the ovary, it is called *primary ovarian failure;* when it is secondary to gonadotropin deficiency, it is called ***secondary ovarian failure.***

Primary ovarian failure

- Dysgenesis or agenesis of the ovaries
- Resistant ovary syndrome—the ovaries are resistant to the action of pituitary gonadotropin even though they are morphologically and genetically normal
- Polycystic ovaries
- Prepubertal infections like tuberculosis and mumps, which give rise to oophoritis
- Systemic diseases like thalassemia, mucopolysaccharidoses, dystrophia myotonica and autoimmune disorders such as primary Addison's disease

- Female pseudohermaphroditism
- Isolated enzyme deficiencies such as 17-alpha hydroxylase deficiency and 21-hydroxylase deficiency
- Genetic disorders, e.g. Turner's syndrome.

Secondary ovarian failure

- Panhypopituitarism
- Prolactinomas–prolactin reduces ovarian response to FSH and LH and pituitary response to luteinizing hormone-releasing hormone (LHRH)
- Acromegaly
- Isolated gonadotropin deficiency.

Premature Ovarian Insufficiency

Early depletion of ovarian follicles before the age of 40 years is called premature ovarian insufficiency (or premature ovarian failure).

Clinical features

These women have a normal puberty followed by oligomenorrhea or amenorrhea after a variable period of time. They have hot flushes and urogenital atrophy.

Investigations

- FSH levels >40 IU/L on 2 occasions
- TSH may be elevated in autoimmune polyendocrine syndromes in association with hypothyroidism
- Karyotype.

Causes

- Autoimmune polyglandular endocrinopathy
- Chemotherapy
- Radiation
- Mumps orchitis
- ***Chromosomal anomalies:*** Fragile X syndrome, FMR1 mutations.

Management

The chance of recovery of ovarian function and pregnancy is low once premature ovarian failure (POF) sets in. Replacement of estrogen and progesterone with a low dose oral contraceptive pill is the treatment of choice.

Amenorrhea

Primary amenorrhea is delay of menarche beyond 18 years of age and secondary amenorrhea denotes cessation of menstruation for 6 months or more in normally menstruating women.

Gynecological Causes

- Diseases of the endometrium
- Obstruction to the outflow tract of the uterus
- Imperforate hymen.

Endocrine Causes

- Primary or secondary ovarian hypofunction
- Other endocrine disorders like Cushing's syndrome, adrenogenital syndrome, Addison's disease and thyrotoxicosis.

Systemic Disease

Disorders such as chronic liver disease, renal disease, DM and malnutrition.

Drugs

Several drugs which include hormonal and nonhormonal preparations are capable of producing amenorrhea, e.g. corticosteroids, androgens, estrogens, contraceptive pills, psychotropic drugs, antihypertension drugs and others.

Hypothalamic Causes

Anorexia nervosa, psychiatric disorders, hypothalamic tumors and developmental neurologic defects such as Kallmann's syndrome.

Diagnosis

The most common physiological cause of secondary amenorrhea in the young is pregnancy. This should be excluded in all cases. Other common causes include menopause, drug therapy, systemic illnesses and psychiatric disturbances. Signs and symptoms of estrogen deficiency such as vasomotor instability and drying up of vaginal secretions should suggest the possibility of primary ovarian failure or menopause. The investigations and management of amenorrhea are the realm of the gynecologist.

Polycystic Ovary Syndrome

Syn: Stein-Leventhal syndrome, Cystic disease of the ovary

Polycystic ovary syndrome (PCOS) is a heterogeneous disorder, clinically characterized by ovulatory failure, hirsutism, obesity, glucose intolerance, resistance to insulin, dyslipidemia and infertility. The ovaries are enlarged, multicystic and show hyperplastic theca cells around the cysts. Only very small amounts of estradiol are produced by immature follicles. Excessive amounts of androgens are produced by the hyperplastic theca cells and stromal cells. The enlarged cystic ovaries on both sides can be made out by bimanual examination, by ultrasonography or by diagnostic laparoscopy. Therapeutic measures are designed to restore fertility, normalize menstruation and reverse hirsutism. Signs of insulin resistance like acanthosis nigricans may be looked for in these patients.

The three key features of PCOS are:

1. Oligomenorrhea
2. Hyperandrogenesis (clinical and laboratory parameters)
3. Absence of other endocrinological disorders, such as CAH, hyperprolactinemia, thyroid dysfunction and androgen-secreting tumors. Two of the three criteria should be present (Rotterdam criteria, 2003, 2006).

The exact etiology is not known but the main biochemical abnormality in PCOS is hyperinsulinemia secondary to insulin resistance. This leads to varian overproduction of testosterone and adrenal over-production of DHEA and androstenedione. Increased testosterone affects the pituitary ovarian axis leading to decrease in production of estrogen, abnormal production of progesterone, and overproduction of testosterone, LH and FSH.

Those with PCOS are at higher risk of diabetes and cardiovascular disease later in life. The diagnosis of PCOS is by demonstration of the cystic ovaries, exclusion of other hyperandrogenic disorders in women with chronic anovulation and androgen excess. PCOS is considered as a part of the metabolic syndrome.

Investigation

In a patient with a phenotype of PCOS, investigations are done to document metabolic derangement and to exclude other conditions.

- Glucose tolerance test, lipid profile
- Testosterone, prolactin and thyroid functions—testosterone levels are usually high normal or mildly elevated
- 17-hydroxyprogesterone (17-OHP) (to exclude CAH), post dexamethasone suppression cortisol (to exclude hypercortisolemia) can be done if indicated.

Pathogenesis

The pathogenesis of PCOS is not well-understood. The various pathophysiological changes in PCOS are:

- Increased LH frequency due to increased sensitivity of pituitary to GnRH stimulation
- LH stimulated increased androgen production by the ovary
- Chronic anovulation leads to steady state increased estrogen production
- Reduced sex hormone binding globulin (SHBG) levels
- Follicular growth is continually stimulated but not to the point of full maturation or ovulation.

Treatment

Treatment of this condition depends on the patient's main concerns. Bilateral wedge section of ovaries were done previously to induce ovulation. Metformin is commonly used to reverse the endocrine abnormalities in PCOS by reducing the resistance to insulin, and correcting the other endocrine abnormalities. Dose of metformin is 500–750 mg bd. Metformin can be continued during pregnancy also, especially in the first two trimesters. Other treatment modalities include antiandrogens like cyproterone acetate, spironolactone and finasteride for controlling virilizing signs, and cyclical estrogen and progesterone for regularizing the menstrual cycles. For inducing ovulation and fertility, clomiphene citrate can be used in doses of 50 mg daily for 5 days, preferably from the fifth to the ninth day of the menstrual cycle. Clomiphene increases the output of gonadotropins from the pituitary. Cyproterone acetate which is an androgen antagonist relieves hirsutism. Application of hair removing preparations improves cosmetic results. Regularization of periods with oral contraceptive pill or progesterone is also advised.

Dysfunctional Uterine Bleeding

Excessive or more frequent menstrual bleeding resulting from functional disturbances, but without other obvious pathological causes is called *dysfunctional uterine bleeding (DUB)*. Hormonal imbalance and nutritional, psychological and hematologic factors play contributory roles. This is a common gynecological problem in women in the fourth and fifth decades of life, often requiring hysterectomy.

Medical Problems of Menopause

Women attain menopause usually between 40 and 47 years. Menopause is considered to be complete when a woman has not had periods for one year in the absence of any pathological condition or obvious features of ovarian deficiency.

Physiological changes: Menopause represents a form of primary ovarian failure. The number of ovarian follicles steadily declines with age and these follicles become less and less sensitive to the action of FSH as age advances. As women reach menopause, the FSH or LH reach high levels and the estrogen levels fall. Because of diminishing number of follicles in the ovary, production of estrogen is reduced. In many subjects, the development of menopause may be quite uneventful and asymptomatic.

The following four groups of symptoms may develop in those who become symptomatic:

1. *General symptoms:* These include insomnia, nervousness, anxiety, depression, irritability, headache, dizziness, and joint pains. These affect the quality of life considerably.
2. *Vasomotor symptoms:* These consist of hot flushes, inappropriate perspiration and palpitation, occurring frequently as sudden burning feeling all over the body followed by sweating, faintness, and palpitation. In 10–20% of women, these symptoms are very frequent and disabling. Low body weight, sedentary habits and smoking increase the risk of developing these symptoms.
3. *Atrophic changes in the genitals:* The main symptoms are urinary stress incontinence, vaginal atrophy, vaginal discharge and irritation, dryness, dyspareunia, pruritus and burning.
4. *Cosmetic effects:* Characteristic changes include development of fine folds and marks radiating from the mouth, sagging of the infraorbital fold of skin on the face, sagging and atrophy of the breasts, and generalized wasting of adipose tissue. Osteoporosis is common and this may lead to fractures of the vertebrae and limbs.

Hormone Replacement Therapy (HRT) in Women

The Women Health Initiative (WHI) study changed the approach of HRT in postmenopausal women. Results from the WHI study indicated that a combination of CEE and medroxyprogesterone acetate (2.5 mg/day) should not be initiated or continued in women for primary prevention of coronary heart disease in postmenopausal women. There was modest increase in thromboembolic disease and stroke. There was a

Textbook of Medicine

slight increase in coronary heart disease risk which was not significant. There was a borderline statistically increased risk of breast cancer. The women in WHI study started HRT at an average of 12 years after menopause. In postmenopausal women, short-term HRT may be considered for hot flushes or dyspareunia. It is absolutely contraindicated in those with cerebrovascular disease, recent myocardial infarctions, carcinoma breast, pancreatitis, cholecystitis, venous thromboembolism and endometrial carcinoma.

In women with POF, early surgical menopause and gonadal dysgenesis, HRT is indicated to reduce hot flushes and long-term prevention of osteoporosis and target organ atrophy. This is achieved with a low dose oral contraceptive pill till the age of 45 years. Further continuation of HRT is decided on a case-to-case basis with lowest dose of estrogen with or without cyclical progesterone. The risk of thromboembolic complications on long-term continuation of HRT should be weighed against the risk of osteoporosis and target organ atrophy in the absence of estrogen. Recent work has shown that starting HRT early after onset of menopause is more effective in reducing the incidence of CAD than late onset of therapy.

DISORDERS OF SEXUAL DIFFERENTIATION

Disorders of sexual differentiation (DSD) encloses the spectrum of disorders in which chromosomal, gonadal or anatomical sex is atypical. The terminology of DSD replaces the previous terms of intersex disorders or pseudohermaphroditism. Many DSD are associated with ambiguous genitalia. DSD is classified into:

- Sex chromosome DSDs [45,X Turner and variants, 47,XXY Klinefelter and variants, 45X/46XY mixed gonadal dysgenesis (MGD) and chromosomal ovotesticular DSD 46XX/46XY chimeric type or mosaic type]
- 46,XY DSDs (disorders of testicular development or disorders in androgen synthesis/action)
- 46,XX DSDs (disorders of ovarian development or fetal androgen excess).

Optimal care of patients with DSD requires a multidisciplinary team including endocrinologists, geneticists, pediatric surgeons and counsellors. A family history, prenatal history, a general physical examination with attention to any associated dysmorphic features, and an assessment of the genital anatomy are the first steps towards a correct diagnosis. The diagnostic evaluation of DSD includes hormone measurements, imaging, cytogenetic and molecular studies and in some cases endoscopic, laparoscopic and gonadal biopsy. Reaching a proper diagnosis would help in choosing the appropriate sex of rearing in a subject with DSD and ambiguous genitalia. Surgical procedures for 'feminization' and 'masculinization' should be undertaken by teams with extensive experience in this area. Functional outcome should be taken into consideration rather than a strictly cosmetic appearance.

CHAPTER

103

Miscellaneous Endocrine-related Conditions

B Jaykumar, KP Poulose

Chapter Summary

- Endocrine Disorders of the Breast
  - Atrophy of Breasts
  - Hypertrophy of Breasts
  - Gynecomastia
  - Galactorrhea
- Prostaglandins
- Endocrine Syndromes Produced by Cancer
  - Ectopic Cushing's Syndrome
  - Hypercalcemia
  - SIADH Production
  - Rare Endocrine Syndromes due to Tumors

ENDOCRINE DISORDERS OF THE BREAST

GENERAL CONSIDERATIONS

The breasts develop from the mammary crest of the ectoderm called the *milk line*. Though the mammary gland is rudimentary at birth, sometimes the high prolactin (PRL) levels derived from the mother may induce transient milk secretion in the newborn *(witch's milk)*. The breasts grow and areolae enlarge with puberty depending on the influence of estrogens and progesterone. The mammary glands develop fully with the formation of alveoli and they start functioning only during pregnancy. During early pregnancy, the breasts enlarge and become nodular. The areolae become pigmented with the development of Montgomery's tubercles. Later, colostrum is secreted.

Hormonal Interactions

Estradiol stimulates growth of mammary ducts and nipples and the formation of progesterone receptors. Cortisol and growth hormone (GH) potentiate the effects of estrogens. Further development of lobules and alveoli are mediated by four hormones—estradiol, progesterone, GH and PRL. Progesterone inhibits the formation of estrogen receptors. Lactation is initiated by increase in PRL and the sudden reduction in progesterone level on expulsion of the placenta. Oxytocin facilitates ejection of milk by contraction of myoepithelial cells of the alveoli. Regular suckling stimulates PRL secretion by a neuroendocrine reflex and this is responsible for maintenance of lactation. Other hormones like GH, adrenocorticotropic hormone (ACTH), thyroxine (T4), human placental lactogen (hPL) and insulin also play their role in the maintenance of optimal milk secretion. In health, the size of the breasts varies.

During menstrual cycles, premenstrual pain and tenderness of the breasts may develop even in normal women. These symptoms are promptly relieved by diuretics, progesterone or bromocriptine. Lactation can be suppressed by high doses of estrogens or bromocriptine.

ATROPHY OF BREASTS

This commonly occurs when the estrogen levels fall as in hypogonadism or menopause. Disorders occurring before puberty lead to abnormal breast development. Lesions occurring thereafter result in regression of the size of the breasts. Breast atrophy is also common in hyperandrogenism due to any cause—adrenal, ovarian or iatrogenic.

HYPERTROPHY OF BREASTS

Hyperprolactinemia may give rise to bilateral hypertrophy of breasts with galactorrhea. This may be idiopathic in some rare cases. Unilateral breast enlargement is usually due to juvenile fibroadenoma, malignant tumors, infections like tuberculosis or infiltrations as in acute leukemia. Bilateral fibroadenosis is associated with premenstrual pain and it commonly develops after puberty.

GYNECOMASTIA

The increase of glandular and stromal tissue of male breast is termed *gynecomastia*. True glandular enlargement has to be differentiated from adipose tissue deposition (pseudogynecomastia), carcinoma or neurofibromatosis by careful examination. Increased levels of estrogens with or without reduction of androgens lead to gynecomastia. If PRL is also increased, galactorrhea follows.

Causes of Gynecomastia

- About 50–70% of normal boys develop transient gynecomastia during puberty
- Primary testicular failure as in Klinefelter's syndrome, cryptorchidism, leprosy
- Testicular tumors—seminoma or teratoma
- Hepatic cirrhosis
- Endocrine disorders like hyperthyroidism, hypothyroidism, adrenal cortical overactivity
- Paraneoplastic syndromes, e.g. bronchogenic carcinoma, renal carcinoma, Hodgkin's disease
- Drugs, e.g. estrogens, digitalis, spironolactone, reserpine, marijuana, metoclopramide, methyldopa, H_2-receptor antagonists, phenothiazines and others
- Trauma to chest wall
- Idiopathic.

The serum levels of testosterone, 17-estriol and gonadotropins are normal in idiopathic gynecomastia. High serum luteinizing hormone (LH) levels indicate primary testicular failure or human chorionic gonadotropin (hCG) secreting choriocarcinoma of the testes. A very high level of serum 17-estradiol should suggest a feminizing adrenal carcinoma.

Treatment

Pubertal gynecomastia is often self-limiting and this may be left alone after assuring the individual of its benign nature. In others, the cause should be detected and treated. In some cases, surgical excision is done for cosmetic reasons and to prevent neoplasia later.

GALACTORRHEA

Nonphysiological secretion of milk from the breast is known as galactorrhea. It is seen in both sexes and the amount of milk may vary from a few drops to large volumes. Amenorrhea accompanying galactorrhea suggests a hypothalamo-pituitary disorder.

Causes

- Hypothalamo-pituitary diseases
  - Hypothalamic lesions, e.g. tumors, granulomas, histiocytosis X, postencephalitic sequelae, trauma, pituitary stalk section.
  - Pituitary disease, e.g. prolactinoma, acromegaly, empty sella syndrome (ESS), Cushing's syndrome.
- Functional hyperprolactinemia
  - Drugs, e.g. oral contraceptives, digoxin, chlorpromazine, reserpine, methyldopa and several others.
  - Chest wall lesions, surgery, herpes zoster, burns.
- Other endocrine disorders, e.g. myxedema, adrenal cortical disorders
- Ectopic PRL secretion and paraneoplastic syndromes, e.g. bronchogenic carcinoma, hypernephroma, Hodgkin's disease
- Chronic renal failure
- Idiopathic.

Diagnosis

Galactorrhea may be an isolated symptom or this may be part of other endocrine manifestations. Many patients do not volunteer this symptom and, therefore, it is likely to be missed if not carefully looked for.

Management

Therapy depends upon the cause. Endocrine disorders should be treated appropriately. Drug-induced galactorrhea responds promptly to drug withdrawal. When the cause is obscure, bromocriptine in a dose of 5 mg/day may be tried. It stops galactorrhea within a few weeks. Adverse side effects of bromocriptine include nausea, vomiting and hypotension.

PROSTAGLANDINS

PK Jabbar, KP Poulose

Ulf von Euler of Sweden first discovered and isolated prostaglandins from human semen in the 1930s. Attributing origin from the prostate gland, he termed them prostaglandins (in fact these are produced from seminal vesicle). Now it is known that prostaglandins are present and are synthesized in all tissues in the body. Prostaglandins are biologically synthesized from arachidonic acid. Essentially, they are unsaturated carboxylic acids, like classic hormones, they act as chemical messengers, but with the difference that they act within the cells which produce them without being transported to distant sites for their action. As per very rigid nomenclature systems, only the compounds produced by the cyclo-oxygenase pathway and prefixed as *PG* are termed *prostaglandins*, but all the other molecular derivatives of arachidonic acid which are called eicosanoids, belong to the prostaglandin family and will be discussed together.

PHYSIOLOGICAL ROLE

The most important role is in the modulation of the immune response. Leukocytes flock to areas of tissue destruction and release local prostaglandins that cause inflammatory reaction. In addition, prostaglandins have effects on vascular system. For instance thromboxane A2, a potent prostaglandin, causes vascular construction and aggregation of platelets. Another prostaglandins stimulate smooth muscles contraction. For instance, leukotrienes cause bronchoconstriction and prostaglandin E2 (PGE2) stimulates uterine contractions.

CLINICAL APPLICATIONS

PGE2 as mentioned earlier, can stimulate uterine contractions and it is used for inducing labor. Aspirin inhibits the action of cyclo-oxygenases (COX-1) and COX-2 which can convert arachidonic acid to prostaglandins. By this effect, aspirin suppresses prostaglandin-induced inflammation and pain. This is the main mechanism by which aspirin and nonsteroidal anti-inflammatory drugs (NSAIDs) agents act as anti-inflammatory and analgesic agents. Some prostaglandins that have beneficial effects on blood flow, like PGEl have been used to improve the microcirculation. Administration of PGEl helps to occlude a patent ductus arteriosus (PDA) if administered to a baby in the perinatal and neonatal periods. In addition, leukotriene antagonists like montelukast have been used in the therapy of bronchial asthma. Prostacyclin (PGl2) reduces pulmonary artery pressure and therefore it is used, in the treatment of pulmonary hypertension. Glucocorticoids exert their anti-inflammatory effects through the enzyme phospholipase A, which converts phospholipids into arachidonic acid, thereby reducing prostaglandin and leukotriene production (Flowchart 103.1).

Aspirin exerts its antiplatelet effect by irreversibly inhibiting action of thromboxane which favors platelet aggregation and promotes thrombosis.

Clinical uses of Prostaglandin

- Induce labor
- Promote closure of patent ductus in newborn
- Treatment of peptic ulcer
- Raynaud's phenomenon
- Treatment of glaucoma
- Erectile dysfunction
- Cosmetic purpose.

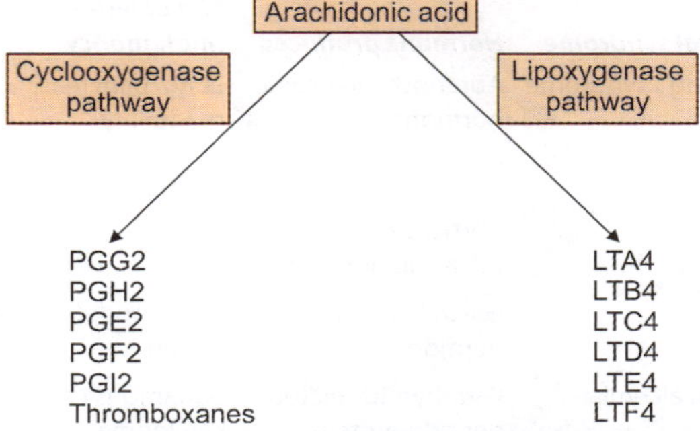

Flowchart 103.1: Eicosanoid family prostaglandins (PG) and leukotrienes (LT)

ENDOCRINE SYNDROMES PRODUCED BY CANCER

PK Jabbar, KP Poulose

Neoplastic tissues can infiltrate and metastases to various tissues. Neoplastic cells can also produce a variety of products which can induce hematological, dermatological, neurological and hormonal response. Wherever a hormone is abnormally produced from a source that is different from the tissue of its usual origin, the production is called ectopic. Since most of the conditions are malignant, these are called *paraneoplastic syndromes*. An example of this is small cell lung cancer which can produce ACTH in excess quantities. Usually, ectopic hormones produce significant clinical manifestations because the hormones are produced in excess and in an unregulated manner. Some of the ectopic hormones producing various clinical situations are listed in Table 103.1. The common syndromes amongst them are discussed below. The appropriate therapy is to treat the hormonal abnormality and attend to the tumors which produce these hormones.

ECTOPIC CUSHING'S SYNDROME

Ectopic ACTH production can stimulate the adrenal glands to produce excess cortisol and this result in Cushing's syndrome. The most common neoplasms that result in ectopic Cushing's syndrome are carcinomas of the lung, thymus and pancreas. Rarely, pheochromocytomas, medullary carcinoma thyroid, bronchial carcinoids and adenomas can cause this syndrome. The diagnosis should be suspected clinically if features which suggest malignancy such as weight loss, severe hyperpigmentation, muscle weakness, hypokalemia, alkalosis, lack of cortisol suppressibility to low and high dose (8 mg) of dexamethasone and ACTH levels more than 1,000 pg/mL are noted. Recent studies have yielded an insight into the molecular basis of this syndrome. Usually, ACTH is a part of a larger precursor molecule called pro-opiomelanocortin (POMC). POMC gene is stimulated by three promoter genes: P1, P2 and P3. In the pituitary, P2 is the promoter gene, while in all peripheral tissues, usually P3 (which results in a weak activity of the POMC gene) is the dominant one. In ectopic ACTH syndromes, it has been shown that P1 replaces P3, P2 and promotes the formation of a large transcript with

Table 103.1: Clinical syndromes, hormone produced and the site of lesion

Clinical syndrome	Hormone produced	Site of lesion (malignancy)
Cushing's syndrome	Adrenocorticotropic hormone	Lung, pancreas, medullary thyroid carcinoma thymus
	Corticotropin-releasing hormone	Pancreas, carcinoid, lung
	Gastric inhibitory peptide	Macronodular adrenal hyperplasia
Hypercalcemia	Parathyroid-related peptide protein Vitamin D_3	Squamous cell carcinoma Lymphoma
Syndrome of inappropriate antidiuretic hormone	Vasopressin	Lung, gastrointestinal tract and neurological tissues
Male feminization	Human chorionic gonadotropin	Testis, lung, choriocarcinoma
Hypoglycemia	Insulin-like growth factor	Mesenchymal tumors, small cell lung cancers
Diarrhea	Calcitonin	Medullary carcinoma thyroid
Oncogenic osteomalacia	Phosphatonin (phosphate regulatory protein)	Hemangio-pericytomas, osteoblastomas

identical product as P2 of the normal pituitary. Thus, while normal peripheral tissues have P3, a weak promoter, the ectopic peripheral tissue has P1, which is a strong promoter resulting in Cushing's syndrome.

The treatment of this syndrome is the excision of the tumor. Adrenalectomy may be needed symptomatically if Cushing's syndrome is very severe. Ketoconazole which is an antifungal drug has effect in suppressing the symptoms if given in sufficient doses. Ketoconazole is effective for long-term control of hypercortisolism both of pituitary or adrenal cause. Ketoconazole inhibits adrenal 11beta-hydroxylase and 17,20-lyase, and it prevents the expected rise in ACTH secretion in patients with Cushing's disease, the mechanism of which is not quite clear. Dose is 600–800 mg daily for long periods.

HYPERCALCEMIA

Hypercalcemia of malignancy may be either parathyroid hormone (PTH) dependent or independent. Usually, there is release of PTH or PTH-like protein. PTH or PTH-like protein-dependent syndromes result in hypercalcemia with hypophosphatemia, as in the classic form of hyperparathyroidism. PTH-independent syndromes in malignancies can cause severe hypercalcemia and hyperphosphatemia through different mechanisms like extensive bony metastases, tumor lysis syndrome or overexpression of 1-alpha hydroxylase enzyme, which activates vitamin D at the 1-alpha position in an unregulated manner, resulting in extreme hypercalcemia with hyperphosphatemia, hematological malignancies like lymphoma, and solid tumors like bronchogenic carcinoma may be associated with hypercalcemia.

SYNDROME OF INAPPROPRIATE ANTIDIURETIC HORMONE PRODUCTION

Antidiuretic hormone (ADH) or vasopressin decreases free water excretion and retains free water, resulting in dilutional hyponatremia. Unregulated and excess production of ADH is called syndrome of inappropriate antidiuretic hormone (SIADH). Lung carcinoma, predominantly small or oat cell carcinoma is the most important cause of SIADH. Usually, the patient appears euvolemic and hyponatremic. Plasma osmolality is low and urine osmolality is high.

Vaptans are new classes of drugs which are useful in the management of dilutional hyponatremia. Vaptans are particularly useful in hypervolemic hyponatremia and in the long-term management of SIADH. They are effective and safe. Drugs in this class include tolvaptan, conivaptan and others. Conivaptan is given in a loading dose of 20 mg in 100 mL of 5% dextrose intravenously (IV) over 30 minutes. This should be followed by 20 mg in 250 mL of 5% dextrose administered in a continuous IV infusion over 24 hours. Conivaptan treatment should be accompanied by fluid restriction. Severe hyponatremia needs IV fluid (hypertonic saline) administration under supervision. Tolvaptan is available for oral use. The dose is; initial dose—15 mg orally once a day. Maintenance dose—increase the dose to 30 mg once a day, after at least 24 hours, to a maximum of 60 mg once a day, as needed to achieve the desired level of serum sodium. Maximum dose—60 mg once a day. Duration of therapy—maximum of 30 days.

RARE ENDOCRINE SYNDROMES DUE TO TUMORS

- ***Growth hormone (GH):*** There have been a few reported cases of acromegaly due to excess GH or growth hormone releasing hormones (GHRH) from islet carcinoids. These patients will present as classical acromegaly.
- ***Erythropoietin:*** Production of excessive quantity of erythropoietin by tumors can result in secondary polycythemia, as erythropoietin stimulates erythropoiesis.

  Tumors of the kidney, liver, cerebellum and others organs may rarely produces erythropoietin-like substances. Thrombocytosis may be seen in renal cell carcinoma.
- ***Insulin-like growth factors (IGF):*** Some carcinoids can produce IGF or even insulin, causing hypoglycemia. Rarely, large retroperitoneal tumors, especially sarcomas cause excess utilization of glucose resulting in hypoglycemia. Certain tumors like hemangiopericytomas can lead to phosphate depletion due to the elaboration of phosphaturic factors called phosphatonins. In these situations, metabolic activation of vitamin D into its active form is also inhibited. This syndrome is rare. It results in a particular variety of osteomalacia known as ***oncogenic osteomalacia***.
- ***Human chorionic gonadotropin (hCG):*** Production of hCG in dysgerminomas can lead to stimulation of the testes by hCG which, in turn produces high estrogen level and cause breast enlargements in boys.

PK Jabbar, KP Poulose

CHAPTER 104

Multiple Endocrine Neoplasia

Chapter Summary

- MEN1 Syndrome (Werner's Syndrome)
  - Management of Parathyroid Surgery
- MEN2 Syndrome

INTRODUCTION

Multiple endocrine neoplasia (MEN) syndromes are defined as tumors arising from two or more endocrine glands in many members of the same family. In general, two types of MEN syndromes are described in literature.

MEN1 SYNDROME (WERNER'S SYNDROME)

MEN1 is an autosomal dominant familial tumor syndrome in which persons develop tumors of the multiple endocrine glands (parathyroid, pancreatic neuroendocrine system, pituitary gland and the skin). The most common endocrine tumors arise from parathyroid, that cause hyperparathyroidism. Other tumors include insulinomas, gastrinomas, prolactinomas and carcinoid tumors. The cutaneous tumors include multiple angiofibromas, collagenomas and lipomas.

Pathophysiology involves a mutation in a tumor suppressor gene called MEN1 which codes for the protein, menin.

Clinical Features (Table 104.1)

Primary hyperparathyroidism is the earliest and most common manifestation of MEN1. Hypercalcemia may develop during the early years and most individuals are affected by the age of 40. Clinical presentation of hyperparathyroidism in MEN1 is similar to those in sporadic hyperparathyroidism and includes calcium-containing kidney stones, nephrocalcinosis, bone abnormalities, gastrointestinal (GI) and musculoskeletal symptoms. *Parathyroid hyperplasia* is the most common pathological features of hyperparathyroidism in MEN1.

- *Gastrinomas* are the most common enteropancreatic tumors seen in MEN1 and produce *Zollinger Ellison syndrome (ZES)*. ZES is caused by excessive gastrin production and occurs in more than one-half of MEN1 patients. The increased acid production may cause esophagitis, ulcers in unusual sides (throughout the duodenum, ulcers involving the proximal jejunum) and diarrhea.
- *Insulinomas* are the second most common pancreatic tumors in patients who have MEN1. Hypoglycemia caused by insulinomas is observed in about one-third of MEN1 patients. The tumors may be benign or malignant.

Table 104.1: Endocrine abnormality and laboratory features in MEN1

Endocrine abnormality	Laboratory features
Hyperparathyroidism	Calcium, phosphorous, alkaline phosphatase, PTH, subtraction scan, USG, CT, MRI scan
Gastrinoma	Basal gastrin, stimulated gastrin
Insulinoma	Blood sugar, insulin, C-peptide, proinsulin, DSA (digital substraction angiography) imaging
Pituitary hormones	PRL, IGF-1, cortisol
Pheochromocytoma	Metanephrine/catecholamine, imaging, MIBG scan
Medullary carcinoma thyroid	Calcitonin (basal and stimulated)

Abbreviations: PTH = Parathyroid hormone; USG = Ultrasonography; CT = Computed tomography; MRI = Magnetic resonance imaging; MIBG = Metaiodobenzylguanidine; IGF-1 = Insulin-like growth factor-1; PRL = Prolactin; MEN = Multiple endocrine neoplasia

- *Glucagonoma,* which is seen occasionally in MEN1, causes a syndrome of hyperglycemia, classical skin rash (necrolytic migratory erythema), anorexia, glossitis, anemia, depression, diarrhea and venous thrombosis.
- *Angiofibromas* are telangiectatic, skin-colored, pink or light-brown papules that are 1–4 mm in diameter and mostly located on the central parts of the face.
- *Lipomas* are soft, compressible, subcutaneous nodules that are generally 0.5–5 cm in diameter. They are solitary or multiple and they occur on the trunk, the extremities and the scalp.

Additional skin findings include 'cafe au lait' macules, hypopigmented macules, gingival papule and solitary periungual fibroma.

Genetic testing (MEN1 gene) can be performed in individuals at risk for development of MEN1. Management of hyperparathyroidism is challenging because of early onset, significant recurrence rates and parathyroid gland involvement.

Management

Individuals with serum calcium levels 12 mg/dL or above, evidence of calcium nephrolithiasis or renal dysfunction, neuropathic or muscular symptoms or bone involvement (including osteopenia) in individuals less than 50 years of age should undergo parathyroid surgery.

When parathyroid surgery is indicated in MEN1, there are two approaches. In the first, all the parathyroid tissue is identified and removed at the time of primary operation and parathyroid tissue is implanted in the nondominant forearm. If reoperation for hyperparathyroidism is necessary at a later date, transplanted parathyroid tissue can be resected from the implanted sites.

Textbook of Medicine

Another approach is to remove three parathyroid glands from the neck, carefully marking the location of residual tissue so that the remaining tissue can be located easily during subsequent surgery.

The ***diagnosis of*** gastrinoma is made by documenting elevated basal serum gastrin levels more than 100 pg/mL and an exaggerated response of gastrin to either secretin or calcium.

Treatment of prolactinomas with dopamine agonists (bromocriptine, cabergoline and others) usually returns the serum prolactin (PRL) level to normal and relieves the symptoms. Insulinoma needs excision of the tumor and hypoglycemia may be controlled with medications.

MEN2 SYNDROME

MEN2 is a rare familial (autosomal dominant) cancer syndrome caused by mutations in the RET proto-oncogene. MEN2 has three distinct subtypes MEN2A, MEN2B and familial medullary thyroid carcinoma (FMTC) only. The subtypes are defined by the combination of tissues affected (Table 104.2).

- ***Medullary thyroid carcinoma:*** Almost all patients with MEN2A develop medullary thyroid carcinoma (MTC). This is often the first expressed abnormality and usually occurs in the second or third decade of life. The MTC in patients with MEN2A is typically bilateral and multicentric, in contrast to sporadic MTC, which is unilateral.
- ***Pheochromocytoma:*** They are present in approximately half of MEN2A patients. They are bilateral in two-thirds of patients compared with 10% of patients with sporadic pheochromocytomas. Pheochromocytomas tend to be diagnosed at the same time as MTC or several years later (with both occurring primarily in the second or third decade). The pheochromocytomas of MEN2A patients are usually benign.
- ***Parathyroid hyperplasia:*** They are present in nearly half of patients with MEN2A but are less common than pheochromocytomas. In many patients, such hyperplasias can be clinically silent. However, as in other cases of hyperparathyroidism, symptoms can be very mild.

Investigations

Perform genetic screening for RET mutations in all index patients. If a mutation is identified, screen family members who are at risk.

Biochemical screening consists of assessment of baseline calcitonin levels, serum calcium and parathyroid hormone (PTH) levels for hyperpara-thyroidism; urine and serum catecholamines and metanephrine levels for pheochromocytoma. If these are elevated, imaging studies of the adrenals are done. If a patient's calcitonin level is normal, a pentagastrin and/or Ca^{++} stimulation test may be used as a guide to assess the necessity of a central compartment or modified neck dissection. Patients who have been diagnosed with MTC require serial calcitonin and carcinoembryonic antigen (CEA) testing to assess for persistent or recurrent disease. The same investigations may be used for the screening purpose in suspected MEN syndromes.

Table 104.2: Main features of MEN1 and MEN2

MEN1	MEN2

• Hyperparathyroidism
• Islet cell tumors
• Pituitary growth
• Carcinoids
• Pheochromocytoma lipomas
	• MEN2A
	  ▪ MTC
	  ▪ Hyperparathyroidism
	  ▪ MEN2A with amyloidosis
	  ▪ MEN2A familial MTC
	• MEN2B
	  ▪ MTC
	  ▪ Pheochromocytoma
	  ▪ Neurinomos
	  ▪ Marfanoid features

Abbreviations: MEN = Multiple endocrine neoplasia; MTC = Medullary thyroid carcinoma

Avoid fine needle cytology in patients with type 2 (MEN2) who have had their diagnosis previously confirmed by either genetic analysis or elevated calcitonin levels.

Treatment

MEN type 2A (MEN2A) is treated by excision of the affected glands.

Medullary Thyroid Carcinoma

Total thyroidectomy with central lymph node dissection should be performed in children who carry the mutant gene. In adults with MTC more than 1 cm in size, metastases to regional lymph nodes are common (>75%). Total thyroidectomy with central lymph node dissection and selective dissection of other regional chains provide cure in most. In patients with extensive local metastatic disease in the neck, external radiation may prevent local recurrence or reduce the tumor mass. Chemotherapy with combinations of adriamycin, vincristine, cyclophosphamide and dacarbazine may provide palliation. Preoperative medical treatment may consist of prostaglandin inhibitors to alleviate diarrhea that may be associated with MTC. Evaluation for pheochromocytomas is important because, these should be removed before any surgical intervention. Thyroid hormone supplementation is necessary following total thyroidectomy.

Pheochromocytoma

Most clinicians recommend removing only the affected gland. Preoperative preparation is very important for uneventful surgery. This may be achieved by treating with an alpha-blocker or a tyrosine hydroxylase inhibitor, such as metyrosine for 1–2 weeks, after which administration of a beta-blocker can be considered.

Hyperparathyroidism

This is described in the context of hyperparathyroidism associated with MEN1. Medical management of severe hypercalcemia should be hydration, after which they should be treated with furosemide. If they remain severely hypercalcemic, consider treatment with calcitonin, glucocorticoids or bisphosphonates. Cinacalcet, a calcimimetic, can also be effective in reducing serum calcium levels.

Monitoring the patients for recurrence of MTC with calcitonin is essential. Annual screening for hyperparathyroidism with serum calcium and PTH; and catecholamine levels to assess for recurrence of pheochromocytoma in MEN2A patients is usually done.

CHAPTER
105

Polyglandular Autoimmune Syndromes

PK Jabbar, KP Poulose

Chapter Summary

- Polyglandular Autoimmune Syndrome Type 1
- Polyglandular Autoimmune Syndrome Type 2
- IPEX (Immune Dysfunction, Polyendocrinopathy, Enteropathy, X-Linked)

INTRODUCTION

Polyglandular autoimmune (PGA) syndromes are combinations of multiple endocrine gland insufficiencies. Thomas Addison first described the clinical and pathologic features of adrenocortical failure in patients who also had features of pernicious anemia. Thorpe and Handley recognized the association of mucocutaneous candidiasis with glandular failure; Neufeld and colleagues distinguished two major types of PGA syndromes in 1981.

In clinical setting, two types of PGA exist; type I and the more common type II, also known as Schmidt syndrome. A third type (type III), which occurs in adults has been described. Type III does not involve the adrenal cortex, but it includes two of the following—thyroid deficiency, pernicious anemia, type 1A diabetes mellitus (DM), vitiligo and alopecia (Table 105.1).

POLYGLANDULAR AUTOIMMUNE SYNDROME TYPE 1

PGA 1, also known as autoimmune polyendocrinopathy-candidiasis-ectodermal dystrophy (APECED) or as Whitaker syndrome, is associated with candidiasis, hypoparathyroidism and adrenal failure.

At least two components have to be present in an individual for fulfilling PGA 1. Additional manifestations include type lA diabetes, hypogonadism, pernicious anemia, malabsorption, alopecia and vitiligo.

Mucocutaneous candidiasis is the most common of the three main components of PGA 1. Candidiasis is the first clinical manifestation, mostly occurs before 5 years of age. Most of the lesions are limited to the skin, nails, oral and anal mucosa.

Hypoparathyroidism is the first endocrine manifestation to occur during the natural course of PGA 1, usually developing after candidiasis and before Addison's disease. Hypoparathyroidism usually occurs in people younger than 10 years. *Clinical features* may include carpopedal spasm and paresthesias of lips, fingers, and feet; seizures, laryngospasm, leg cramps, diffuse mild encephalopathy, cataracts and papilledema. Addison's disease typically occurs in people aged 10–30 years. Mineralocorticoid and glucocorticoid deficiencies usually develop simultaneously, but their onset can be

Table 105.1: Manifestations of polyglandular autoimmune (PGA) syndrome 1 and 2

PGA 1	PGA 2
• Autosomal recessive	• Polygenic
• Early onset	• Adult onset
• Mucocutaneous candidiasis	• Addison's disease
• Hypoparathyroidism	• Autoimmune thyroiditis
• Addison's disease	• Type lA diabetes
• Hypogonadism	• Hypogonadism
• Pernicious anemia	• Myasthenia gravis, celiac disease

Table 105.2: Antibodies and associated diseases

Antibody	Associated disease
TPO antibody	Thyroiditis
Islet cell antibody	Type 1 Diabetes
GAD antibody	Type 1 Diabetes
Insulin antibody	Type 1 Diabetes
IA2-antibody	Type 1 Diabetes
Parietal cell antibody	Pernicious anemia
Adrenal antibody	Addison disease

Abbreviations: GAD = Glutamic acid decarboxylase; TPO = Thyroid peroxidase

dissociated by up to 3 years. The symptoms of Addison's disease are essentially same as usual primary adrenal deficiency. Presence of hyperpigmentation may serve as a differentiating sign from secondary hypoadrenalism.

Less common clinical association in PGA 1 are hypergonadotropic hypergonadism (HH), type 1 DM, autoimmune thyroid disease, pernicious anemia, chronic atrophic gastritis, chronic active hepatitis, enamel hypoplasia, asplenia, keratoconjunctivitis, cholelithiasis, malabsorption, alopecia, vitiligo and interstitial nephritis.

Laboratory Studies

A detailed clinical evaluation may suggest evidence of more than one endocrine gland deficiency.

Serum endocrine autoantibody is useful for screening family members who may develop autoimmune endocrine disease in the future (Table 105.2).

The endocrine status should be done for confirming hormone deficiency. Reduced calcium and elevated phosphorus are suggestive of hypoparathyroidism and increased blood glucose is the hallmark of DM. Altered thyroid hormones will determine the thyroid status. The reduced levels of serum cortisol and elevated adrenocorticotropic hormone (ACTH) are diagnostic of Addison's disease.

Management

The treatment for PGA syndrome type I is targeted at the affected organ. It is always better to identify and treat the respective autoimmunity before any significant morbidity develops.

Mucocutaneous candidiasis may be treated with oral antifungal agents.

The onset of hypoparathyroidism is usually gradual and permanent. Oral calcium and vitamin D are the usual standard treatment for hypoparathyroidism. Doses of vitamin D range from 50,000 to 100,000 U/day. Calcitriol (1,25-dihydroxyvitamin D3) is a better choice—0.25 µg orally once daily is the usual dose.

Addison's disease: The treatment may be started with hydrocortisone (20 mg in the morning and 10 mg in the evening). Prednisolone is an alternative drug for them. Most of the time, a mineralocorticoid (e.g. fludrocortisone) is also added to the regimen. The glucocorticoid dose is adjusted according to the patient's symptoms.

Other associations may be managed by appropriate medications, e.g. hypothyroidism can be corrected by appropriate replacement therapy.

POLYGLANDULAR AUTOIMMUNE SYNDROME TYPE 2

This is the most common type of the immune endocrinopathy syndromes. It is characterized by the obligatory occurrence of autoimmune Addison disease in combination with thyroid autoimmune diseases and/or type I DM. Primary hypogonadism, myasthenia gravis and celiac disease also are commonly observed in these patients. The most frequent clinical combination is Addison's disease and Hashimoto's thyroiditis, while the least frequent clinical combination is Addison's disease, Graves' disease and type 1 DM. PGA 2 occurs primarily in adulthood, usually around the third and fourth decades of life. Middle-aged women have an increased prevalence of PGA 2. It is associated with human leukocyte antigen-DR3 (HLA-DR3) and/or HLA-DR4 haplotypes and the pattern of inheritance is autosomal dominant with variable expression.

Pathophysiology

A genetic susceptibility is often present in the individuals. After a subclinical phase of active production of organ-specific autoantibodies, there is progressive glandular destruction. The individual is still asymptomatic. Overt clinical disease subsequently develops when extensive organ damage occurs. Manifestations of hormonal deficiency do not differ substantially from those symptoms which occur in general population.

Laboratory Studies

Measuring annual thyroid stimulating hormone (TSH) levels in individuals with type 1 DM is recommended.

Screening for autoantibodies is helpful to verify the autoimmune etiology of the disease.

Evaluation of end-organ function is necessary to confirm the diagnosis in patients with positive autoantibodies. Even if these antibodies are negative, testing is needed if clinical suspicion is high. Gonadotropins [follicle-stimulating hormone (FSH), luteinizing hormone (LH)] and appropriate sex hormones (testosterone, estradiol) estimations are needed for assessment of hypogonadism. TSH, free thyroxine (T4) and free tri-iodothyronine (T3) are done to detect hypothyroidism. ACTH level and cosyntropin stimulation test for assessing the cortisol axis will give clue about the pituitary adrenal interactions as well. Plasma renin activity and serum electrolytes, calcium, phosphorus, fasting blood glucose, complete blood count (CBC) with mean cell volume (MCV) and vitamin B_{12} levels are performed in appropriate settings.

Management

With the exception of celiac disease and Graves' disease, the mainstay of treatment is primarily hormonal replacement.

Treatment of hypothyroidism remains the same and the aim is to achieve euthyroidism with thyroxin (1.7 µg/kg).

A diabetes patient requires lifelong treatment with exogenous insulin. Replacement with cyanocobalamin is the treatment for pernicious anemia.

Graves' disease needs antithyroid medications till euthyroidism is achieved and the final treatment (radioactive iodine/medical/surgical) may be decided after discussing the treatment options with the patient and relatives.

Addison's disease requires replacement therapy with hydrocortisone and fludrocortisone.

IPEX (IMMUNE DYSFUNCTION, POLYENDOCRINOPATHY, ENTEROPATHY, X-LINKED)

- It is also called XLAAD (X-linked autoimmunity-allergic dysregulation).
- Often it presents as a fatal autoimmune lymphopro-liferative disease.
- Rarely, it may be X-linked recessive.
- Genetic background is due to the absence of normal forkhead box P3 (FOXP3) expression.
- The onset is in the neonatal period with type 1 diabetes, dermatitis, enteropathy, thyroiditis, hemolytic anemia, and thrombocytopenia.
- Long-term immunosuppression or bone marrow transplantation appears to be the only effective therapy for IPEX.

CHAPTER

106

Disease of Locomotor System

Binoy J Paul, KV Krishna Das

Chapter Summary

- Rheumatoid Disorders
- General Considerations
- Symptomatology
- Disease Pattern Affecting the Locomotor System in India
- Laboratory Investigations
- Synovial Fluid Examination
- Arthroscopy
- Synovial Biopsy

RHEUMATOID DISORDERS

GENERAL CONSIDERATIONS

Rheumatic disorders are probably the most common ailments affecting mankind. They are the most common cause of severe long-term pain and morbidity, having a substantial influence on health and quality of life by imposing an enormous burden of cost on the healthcare system. World Health Organization (WHO) estimates that 40% of people over the age of 70 years suffer from osteoarthritis knee. At any time, about 80% of the people in their life have low back pain. Osteoporotic hip fracture, injuries and other diseases of the musculoskeletal system account for more than 20% of patient visits to primary care physicians. The global prevalence of musculoskeletal diseases (MSDs) ranges from 14% to as high as 42%.

The term rheumatology denotes the branch of medicine which deals with the medical disorders of the musculoskeletal or locomotor system. The term *rheuma* is first encountered in the portion of the Hippocratic Corpus titled *on the locations in the human body* written in about the 4th century BC. It belongs to the humoral theory of diseases and literally meant 'flowing'. It is the French physician Guillaume de Baillou (1538–1616) known as the father of rheumatology, who introduced the term *rheumatism* for joint ailments, through his posthumously published work, *The Book on Rheumatism and Back pain*.

Rheumatology developed as a well-recognized specialty in the early half of 20th century. The term rheumatologist was coined in 1940 by two American physicians—Comroe Bernard Isaac (1906–1945) and Joseph Lee Hollander (1910–2000). Three events made the year 1948 the *annus mirabilis* (year of miracles) for rheumatology. First, the agglutination of sensitized sheep erythrocytes by sera of patients with rheumatoid arthritis (RA) was reported by Harry M Rose and Erik Waaler. Second, was the discovery of lupus erythematosus (LE) cells reported by Hargraves and his colleagues. Third, Philip Hench (1896–1965) and his co-workers introduced corticosteroids in the treatment of RA.

The existing knowledge on musculoskeletal conditions comprise over 150 diseases and syndromes usually associated with pain.

The common disorders include:

- Inflammatory diseases of joints, periarticular tissue, muscles, tendons and fascia
- Degenerative joint diseases, like osteoarthritis
- Problems of the vertebral column produced by local pathological lesions, postural abnormalities and trauma
- Diffuse connective tissue diseases
- Systemic vasculitides
- Several other multisystem diseases.

Assessment of diseases of musculoskeletal system requires a basic knowledge of the structure and functions of bone, joint and related connective tissues.

Bones

The human body contains about 206 bones. Structurally, they can be divided into spongy and compact bones. In spongy bone, the lamellae are stacked one above the other as trabeculae. In compact bone, the lamellae are arranged closely in concentric circles around a central canal containing the osteocyte. Spongy bones house the bone marrow whereas compact bones do not. During bone formation and repair, different cells such as osteocytes, osteoblasts and osteoclasts act in a coordinated and orderly manner under the influence of several humoral factors. Periosteum covers bones. It has an outer fibrous layer and an inner cellular layer capable of producing bone—the osteogenic layer.

Trabecular bone has a greater turnover than cortical bone. Bone matrix consists of type 1 collagen which is laid down in lamellae. These give tensile strength to bones. Mineralization of the bone matrix with deposition of hydroxyapatite $Ca_{10}(PO_4)_6(OH)_2$ between the collagen fibrils bestows rigidity to the bones.

Bone remodeling occurs throughout life and it replaces worn-out bone by new bone. About 10% of the skeletons participate in this process at any one time. It starts with the arrival to the site of osteoclasts, which are derived from the monocyte macrophages system. These contain the enzyme tartrate resistant alkaline phosphatase. They reabsorb bone matrix and the minerals. At the end of this, the process of osteoclasts undergo apoptosis. Then osteoblasts, which are derived from marrow stromal cells, arrive to lay down bone matrix, which is subsequently mineralized. Osteoblasts are small cuboidal cells, which actively lay down bone matrix. They are stimulated by parathormone, platelet-derived growth factor (PDGF) and prostaglandins. They are inhibited by corticosteroids. Some osteoblasts remain embedded within bone matrix. They differentiate into osteocytes. They act as a sensors of mechanical strain. They also secrete prostaglandins and nitric oxide, which are signaling molecules concerned with the functions of neighboring bone cells. ***Osteoprotegerin*** is a key regulator of osteoclasts activity by inhibiting its action. The receptor activator of nuclear factor kappa-B (RANK), its ligand (RANKL) and osteoprotegerin constitute a critical mechanism for signaling between osteoblasts and osteoclasts.

Cytokines participate in the process of bone remodeling. Parathormone, activated vitamin D, 1,25-dihydroxy-vitamin D3 [1,25$(OH)_2D_3$] thyroid hormone and growth hormone increase bone remodeling whereas, it is suppressed by calcitonin, estrogens and androgens. In conditions like Paget's disease of bone, where bone remodeling is very rapid, lamellae formation may be distorted and the resultant bone, though larger, may be brittle.

Long bones transmit bodyweight and act as levers for movement. The middle part of the tubular shaft is the diaphysis, which is flanked on either end by the metaphyseal regions. The ends are expanded to form the particular areas, the epiphyses. Long bones derive their blood supply from diaphyseal, metaphyseal, epiphyseal and periosteal nutrient arteries. Short bones like the carpal bones function as a point of absorption of pressure and distribution of shearing forces. They are made of compact bone.

Joints

Joints may be classified as fibrous, cartilaginous or synovial.

Types of joints	Range of movement	Examples
Fibrous	Nil	Cranial sutures, tibiofibular joint
Cartilaginous	Limited	Intervertebral joint, symphysis pubis
Synovial	Wide	Hip, knee and elbow

In a synovial joint, the bone ends are capped by hyaline cartilage. At the osteochondral junction, synovium is attached to bone and reflected from it to line the joint cavity outside. The synovium is a tough fibrous capsule, which is thickened in some areas to form ligaments. The capsule and ligaments prevent excess movement at the joint. In joints, like the knee there are fibrocartilaginous pads or menisci, which serve to appose the articulating surfaces properly. The synovial fluid and synovium reduce friction during movement. Bursae prevent friction between tissues around a moving joint. These are similar to synovium in structure, function and disease susceptibility.

Synovium is highly vascular. Structurally, the synovium presents an ideal stage for humoral and cellular immune reactions. Synovium has only very few nerve endings, while cartilage has none. Articular cartilage is avascular. It derives its nutrition from materials passing into it from bone or synovial fluid. Articular branches of blood vessels enter at the joint margin.

The articular cartilage consists of chondrocytes, embedded in a matrix and it is provided with a framework of type 2 collagen which imparts its tensile strength. It does not contain nerves. It provides a low-friction surface to the articular ends of bones.

Synovial membrane that lines the inner surface of joint capsules consists of fibroblasts, which secrete synovial fluid and macrophage-like cells with phagocytic activity. The synovial fluid is an ultrafiltrate of plasma, to which materials, which increase its viscosity such as hyaluronan and lubricin are locally added. Hyaluronan is responsible for lubrication of the joint surface during movement, whereas lubricin acts as the lubricant during static stress. In addition to its lubricating function, synovial fluid provides nutrition to the avascular articular cartilage and helps to perform other metabolic functions. The synovium is supplied by unmyelinated nerve fibers, which transmit pain.

The capsules, ligaments and periosteum around the joints are supplied with myelinated nerves for proprioception and unmyelinated nerves for conducting pain.

The points of attachment of tendons and ligaments to bone are called ***entheses***. The joint capsule, entheses, ligaments and tendons are rich in nerve endings that perceive pain and proprioception. When a joint is inflamed, reflexogenic nerve endings cause reflex contractions of neighboring muscles leading to painful stiffness.

The main function of all synovial joints is to allow stable, controlled movements. Muscles of the locomotor system are all striated muscles. They are all under voluntary control.

SYMPTOMATOLOGY

Rheumatology is still a preeminently clinical discipline depending heavily on laboratory and other types of investigations. Since the joints and bones respond in a stereotyped clinical manner to different and multiple diseases process, clinical distinction between the various rheumatological syndromes may not be perfect. So also the laboratory parameters usually undertaken in these diseases are of a more general character rather than being absolutely specific, so that considerable overlap occurs between health and disease. Many of the laboratory investigations such as antistreptolysin O (ASO) titer, rheumatoid factor (RF), erythrocyte sedimentation rate (ESR) and almost all others show prevalence in low titers even in apparently normal population, so that the interpretation of an equivocal laboratory value has to be made in the context of clinical features, and the characteristics in general population.

Main symptoms pertaining to locomotor system include pain in and around joints or other parts of axial or appendicular skeleton, deformities of bones and joints,

Table 106.1: Symptomatology in articular and extra-articular lesions

Joint tissues	Lesions around the joint or unconnected with the joint
Pain occurs during active and passive movements	Pain occurs during active movement, but not on passive movement
Swelling and tenderness limited to the anatomy of the joint	Not confined to the joint
Crepitus, instability and locking of joint in particular positions present	Not present

Table 106.2: Prevalence of musculoskeletal diseases (MSDs) in India

MSDs (overall prevalence)	7.08–11.52%
Rheumatoid arthritis	0.17–0.62%
Osteoarthritis	3.28–6.52%
Spinal disorder	4.8–5.76%
Inflammatory arthritis-undifferentiated	0–0.05%
Soft tissue rheumatism	0.14–0.85%
Nonspecific body ache and pain	0.59–1.89%
Gout	0.02–0.13%

Source: Epidemiology of musculoskeletal conditions in India (ICMR Task-Force Project Report, 2012).

Box 106.1: World Health Organization (WHO) has categorized rheumatological disorders

The WHO has categorized rheumatological disorders into seven major categories:

1. Arthropathies—infectious arthropathies, inflammatory polyarthropathies, degenerative joint diseases (osteoarthrosis)
2. Systemic connective tissue disorders
3. Spinal disorders (dorsopathies)
4. Soft tissue disorders, disorders of muscles, synovium and tendon
5. Osteopathies (bone diseases)
6. Chondropathies
7. Other disorders of the musculoskeletal system and connective tissue

loss of functions of joints and systemic manifestations such as fever, loss of weight, anemia and involvement of several organ systems. There may be considerable overlap in the clinical manifestations between the different rheumatic diseases. Therefore, it is very necessary to do investigations to pinpoint the diagnosis and follow-up the case.

The main clinical presentation of musculoskeletal disorders is with joint pains, stiffness of muscles, swelling, bone pains and muscle weakness. The source of the symptom can be clinically assessed by examination (Table 106.1).

The distribution of joint lesions gives some clue. Predominent affection of the joints of the lower segment of the body occur in various spondyloarthropathies, such as ankylosing spondylitis, Reiter's syndrome, psoriatic arthropathy and early stages of polyarticular gout. In RA and systemic lupus, the upper segment is more often affected. Morning stiffness is a frequent finding in many joint diseases. This term refers to pain on waking up from sleep or prolonged recumbency, felt especially in the lower limbs and spine, which takes 30–60 minutes to get maximum relief. This is a usual feature of inflammatory joint disease.

DISEASE PATTERN AFFECTING THE LOCOMOTOR SYSTEM IN INDIA

In India, at any period of time, around 10% of adults suffer from one or other of the rheumatic disorders. Recent Indian Council of Medical Research (ICMR) study on MSDs from various states of the country shows a prevalence varies from 7.08 to 11.52% (Table 106.2). It is possible that about 50 million people suffer from these disorders at any one time. Degenerative joint diseases, like osteoarthritis, inflammatory diseases, like RA and spinal disorders forms the major burden of chronic MSDs in our country. Traumatic fractures, dislocations are also common. These fall in the realm of orthopedics.

The patterns of rheumatological disorders differ in different age groups (Box 106.1). In children, the common problems seen are growing pains, hypermobility, hip pain due to several causes, traumatic lesions of knees, rheumatic fever, postviral arthritides, osteomyelitis, pyarthrosis, juvenile rheumatoid arthritis (JRA), rickets and others. In the young adult male, seronegative spondyloarthritides are common. During the sexually active periods of life, arthritic complications of sexually transmitted diseases are more common. In pregnancy and the puerperium, low back pain is nearly universal and sciatica is common enough. The postmenopausal age is associated with bone and joint symptoms. Osteoporosis proceeds rapidly after menopause. Hypothyroidism, depressive illness and osteoarthritis are common causes of rheumatic symptoms in this group. Degenerative joint diseases such as osteoarthritis of several joints, cervical spondylosis, sciatica and lumbar canal stenosis are more common in the elderly. Those exposed to repeated occupational trauma during work develop osteoarthritic changes of particular joints early.

Occupation and environment can modify joint diseases, particularly osteoarthritis, e.g. *goal-keeper's fingers*, *bass player's thumb, Zulu dancer's hip*, teno-synovitis, like the Achilles tendinitis of long distance runners and prepatellar bursitis in housemaid's knee are other examples of occupation-related rheumatism. Enthesopathies, like lateral and medial epicondylitis of elbow (syndrome: tennis elbow and golfer's elbow) are common in Indian housewives who do clothes washing, grain grinding and pounding. Factory workers inhaling metal or polymer fumes can get fever associated with arthralgias.

Disease burden of rheumatic diseases in India Community Oriented Program for Control of Rheumatic Disease (COPCORD) perspective (2015) is shown in Table 106.3.

Immunological principles dominate the practice of present day rheumatologists. A sound understanding of immunology will go a long way in interpreting the evolution, course and management of rheumatological diseases.

Textbook of Medicine

Table 106.3: The distribution of cases in different studies (all figures in percentages)

Diseases	COPCORD study (Bhigwan no—4092)	Bone and joint decade (India study 2004–2010)
Rheumatoid arthritis	0.67 (0.57–0.79) In Trivandrum 0.4	0.34 (0.08–0.79)
Undifferentiated inflammatory arthritis	0.76	0.22
• Spondyloarthritis	0.3	0.23
• Ankylosing spondylitis	0.10	0.03
• Osteoarthritis	6.25	4.39
Osteoarthritis knee	4.42	3.34
Gout	0.13	0.04
Any form of soft tissue rheumatism	3.77	1.31
Nonspecific arthralgias	6.25	4.25
Lupus and connective tissue diseases	Nil identified	0.02 (0.01–0.03)

Source: Chopra A. Disease burden of rheumatic diseases in India: COPCORD perspective. Ind J Rheumatol. 2015;10(2):70-7.

Abbreviation: COPCORD = Community Oriented Program for Control of Rheumatic Disease

Box 106.2: Spectrum of cases seen in India

- Degenerative joint disease—osteoarthritis
- Spondyloarthropathies—ankylosing spondylitis, psoriatic arthritis reactive arthritis
- Diffuse connective tissue diseases—rheumatoid arthritis, systemic lupus erythematosus, systemic sclerosis, polymyositis, dermatomyositis, Sjögren's syndrome, mixed connective tissue disease and primary systemic vasculitis
- Infective arthropathies—by direct infection, e.g. tuberculosis or syphilis or indirectly by immunological mechanisms, e.g. rheumatic fever, chikungunya
- Crystal induced arthropathies gout, pseudogout, chondrocalcinosis
- Nonarticular rheumatism—tendonitis, enthesitis, fibromyalgia and others
- Bone and joint manifestations associated with systemic diseases, e.g. osteomalacia, osteoporosis, Marfan's syndrome, endocrine disorders, malignancies, fluorosis and others.

Note: Almost all the varieties of bone and joint diseases are seen in India, in varying proportions in all age groups and in different geographical regions.

The rapid strides in rheumatology during the last 60 years heavily depends on the progress in immunology, molecular biology and genetics, which leads to the development of newer immunological tests for accurate diagnosis of these complex, confusing and sometimes overlapping spectrum of connective tissue diseases (Box 106.2). The scientific advances in biomedical engineering and clinical pharmacology helped in the development of newer imaging modalities and targeted therapies with biological agents.

LABORATORY INVESTIGATIONS

There are many laboratory tests available for the diagnosis of rheumatological disorders, but no single laboratory marker has proved sufficiently reliable or specific to be used in *isolation*. The diagnosis always depends on the symptoms and clinical signs in combination with the laboratory tests.

Blood

Acute Phase Reactants

Acute phase response is a major pathophysiological phenomenon, which accompanies inflammation resulting from tissue damage. Acute phase reactants get altered both in acute and chronic inflammation. The major acute phase reactants are ESR, chronic renal failure (CRF) and plasma viscosity.

Erythrocyte Sedimentation Rate

Normal value is up to 10 mm/hour in men and 20 mm/hour in women. Rise in ESR suggests inflammatory processes. Levels above 100 mm/hour should suggest RA, systemic lupus erythematosus (SLE), tuberculous arthritis and polymyalgia rheumatica or giant cell arthritis. ESR is raised in a wide range of diseases and therefore, the test is nonspecific for diagnosis. In many cases, the level of ESR may reflect the severity of the inflammatory process and this can be used as an easily available laboratory parameters for follow-up of the diseases, provided there are no coexisting conditions, which modify the ESR. Joint manifestations caused by allergic processes and osteoarthritis are not accompanied by high rise in ESR.

The disadvantages of ESR is that it is affected by age and gender, by red cell morphology and numbers, and according to the levels of many kinds of plasma proteins all of which are not acute phase reactants.

C-reactive Protein (CRP)

It is a beta-globulin present in serum, capable of reacting with the outer coat of pneumococci. Normally, it is absent in human plasma. When inflammatory processes occur in any part of the body, the liver produces an identical protein, which can be detected by a slide test using readymade reagents. This test is also nonspecific. The test can be performed quickly within 5 minutes. CRP is unaffected by age or gender and reflects the value of a single acute phase protein. It is more expensive than determining ESR.

Advantages of study of CRP are:

- Shorter time to perform
- CRP is positive even before the ESR starts rising
- CRP can be quantified by determining dilution titers
- It helps to distinguish between RA and SLE. In RA, CRP is elevated, whereas in uncomplicated SLE, CRP will be normal.

Note: CRP in modified forms have been used in other subspecialties of medicine.

Epidemiologic studies have demonstrated that CRP when measured with high-sensitivity assays (HSAs) CRP is more strongly and independently predictive of the risk of myocardial infarction, stroke, peripheral arterial disease and sudden cardiac death in apparently healthy individuals even in the absence of conventional risk factors like elevated low-density lipoprotein (LDL) cholesterol.

Routine Blood Counts

Hemoglobin and Erythrocyte Count

Reduction of hemoglobin level is seen in chronic rheumatoid disease. This anemia may be due to impairment of utilization of iron, hemolysis or toxic effects of antirheumatic drugs. SLE may be associated with hemolytic anemia.

Leukocyte Count

Total leukocyte count (TLC) is elevated in the acute phase of inflammatory arthritides. Considerable elevations of TLC with marked preponderance of neutrophils suggest septic arthritis, acute rheumatoid disease or acute gout. In chronic forms of these diseases and in tuberculous arthritis, lymphocytes may show relative preponderance. TLC and differential count are absolutely essential to diagnose acute leukemia, which may masquerade as polyarthritis on initial presentation. In active SLE, leukopenia is common.

Platelet Count

Generally, platelet count is not diagnostic of the primary condition. Thrombocytopenia may occur in SLE as part of the disease. More often thrombocytopenia is an early sign of drug induced bone marrow aplasia. Several drugs such as the nonsteroidal anti-inflammatory drugs (NSAIDs), methotrexate and cyclophosphamide are known to produce bone marrow aplasia.

Serological Tests

Serological tests to detect several immune markers in the serum of patients with poly, pauci and monoarthritis are employed almost universally for the diagnostic work-up, assessment of prognosis and follow-up of response to therapy. Several markers are available for diagnostic work-up.

Antistreptolysin O Titer

This is an easily performed slide test. Positive tests with titer above 1/200 Todd units indicate recent streptococcal infection. Rising titers are more reliable. Presence of ASO alone does not confirm the diagnosis of rheumatic fever unless the clinical setting is appropriate. Streptolysin is one of the components of streptococcal antigens. Antibodies formed against streptolysin (ASO) are another marker of recent streptococcal infection.

Rheumatoid Factor

Presence of RF can be detected by several tests such as sheep cell agglutination test (Rose-Waaler), latex fixation test and nephelometry. Later on it is easier to perform, since commercial kits are available and, therefore, they are more popular. RF, which consists of different types of immunoglobulins, is present in 70–80% of cases of RA. Since, the usual tests detect only IgM antibodies, negative results are obtained in about 25% of cases. The presence of RF has assumed great importance because RA can be broadly divided into seropositive and seronegative varieties. Presence of RF has been associated with poorer prognosis in RA.

Presence of RF is not specific for RA. Other conditions in which RF is present in a smaller proportion of cases include SLE, progressive systemic sclerosis, mixed connective tissue disease (MCTD) and others. False positive RF may be seen in several other conditions such as infective endocarditis, leprosy or tuberculosis. If RF is present in high titers (above 1/40) and the clinical points favor a diagnosis of RA, the test can be taken as diagnostic.

Antibodies to Cyclic Citrullinate Peptides (Anti-CCPs)

This is a new antibody test for early diagnosis of RA. Citrulline is found in synovial joints of RA patients. Formations of anti-CCP are highly specific for RA patients (96% specific, 70% sensitive). Anti-CCP antibodies are present early in RA patients even before developing arthritis. High titer also correlates with erosive changes in bone.

Antinuclear Antibodies

These are present in many of the connective tissue diseases. For the sake of convenience, certain anticytoplasmic antibodies are also clubbed with the antinuclear antibodies (ANAs) as they have a similar role in pathogenesis in these diseases. Autoantibodies in serum can be detected by flocculation tests, immunohistochemistry, radioimmunoassay (RIA), immunodiffusion or immunoblotting. Immunohistochemistry can be done by indirect immunofluorescence (IIF), enzyme-linked immunosorbent assay (ELISA) or RIA. The IIF is most commonly used to detect ANAs, which are associated with different diseases and often react in different IIF patterns giving further clues to the diagnosis. A diffuse homogenous nuclear pattern detects antibodies to double-stranded deoxyribonucleic acid (dsDNA) and suggest SLE. A speckled pattern occurs in Sjögren's syndrome and MCTD. A nucleolar pattern occurs often in scleroderma. A peripheral pattern also occurs typically in SLE.

Different autoantibodies are seen in different connective tissue diseases. Specific antibodies to dsDNA and single-stranded DNA (ssDNA) are seen most commonly in SLE. Antibodies to dsDNA are seen particularly in SLE with nephritis and central nervous system (CNS) involvement and the titers falls as the disease activity comes down. These antibodies are usually absent in drug induced lupus and discoid lupus. Specific antihistone antibodies are almost always present in drug induced lupus. This can be used as a reliable screening test to detect drug induced lupus at an early stage in patients receiving drugs such as phenytoin, hydralazine or isoniazid (INH). Anticentromere antibodies occur in scleroderma, and CREST (calcinosis, Raynaud phenomenon, esophageal dysmotility, sclerodactyly, and telangiectasia) syndrome. Nonhistone nuclear proteins can be extracted as they are soluble and hence they are called extractable nuclear antigens. These are detected by immunodiffusion or immunoblotting. Anti-Smith (Anti-Sm) antibodies are specific for SLE. Antibody to ribonucleoprotein (RNP) was thought to be specific for MCTD, but now it is clear that many of these patients also progress to develop RA or scleroderma. Antibodies to SSA (anti-Ro) are seen in SLE and Sjögren's syndrome. Antibodies to an antigen named Scl-70 are seen in scleroderma and antibodies to JO–1 are seen in polymyositis. It must be remembered that overlap does occur and therefore, a firm diagnosis should take into account the clinical features, immunological markers and other investigations.

Antineutrophil Cytoplasmic Antibodies

Antibodies to cytoplasmic antigens, which develop in several forms of vasculitides are employed for diagnosis. The most important ones are antineutrophilic cytoplasmic antibodies (ANCAs). These are immunoglobulin G (IgG) antibodies. When they react with proteinase 3, present in the cytoplasm of neutrophils they are called cytoplasmic-ANCA (c-ANCA).

When the reaction is perinuclear, it is called p-ANCA. When the staining is atypical, it is called a-ANCA. c-ANCA is specific for Wegener's granulomatosis, p-ANCA is more characteristic of vasculitides such as Churg-Strauss syndrome, polyarteritis nodosa and idiopathic crescentic rapidly progressive glomerulonephritis (RPGN). p-ANCA and a-ANCA may be positive in a variety of conditions such as glomerulonephritis, SLE, RA, polyarteritis nodosa, ulcerative colitis, Crohn's disease, tuberculosis, human immunodeficiency virus (HIV) infection and others.

Antiphospholipid Antibodies

These are directed against negatively charged phospholipids. These include anticardiolipin antibodies and circulating lupus anticoagulant. Lupus anticoagulant is directed against the coagulation factors X and V and the platelet phospholipids. The presence of these antibodies has been linked to a syndrome known as the antiphospholipid antibody syndrome (APS) characterized by recurrent multiple arterial and venous thrombosis leading to transient ischemic attacks, cerebrovascular accidents (CVA), myocardial infarction, recurrent abortions, thrombocytopenia and livedo reticularis in the skin. APS may occur as a primary condition or it may be seen also in other connective tissue diseases.

The lupus anticoagulant is detectable in 30% of SLE. Among clinically normal individuals tests for these antibodies may be weakly positive in a small proportion. Therefore, the significance of the tests has to be correlated with the clinical presentation.

Serum Complement Levels

Components of the complement system such as C3 and C4 consumed during antigen antibody reactions occurring in collagen vascular diseases. Elevated titers of anti-dsDNA antibodies are typically accompanied by hypocomplementemia. Reduction in levels of C3 suggests active SLE.

Demonstration of Lupus Erythematosus Cell Phenomenon

Presence of LE cells is suggestive of SLE. The LE cells can be demonstrated in active SLE. The LE cells are also rarely seen in RA, allergic states, drug induced lupus and others. Due to low sensitivity and low specificity, it is replaced by ANA in modern laboratories (Table 106.4).

Serological Tests for Syphilis-VDRL

Though syphilitic arthropathy is not very common, syphilis is a curable cause of bone and joint disease. Arthritis may occur in the secondary stage of syphilis. In the tertiary

Table 106.4: Antinuclear antibodies (ANAs) in connective tissue disorders

dsDNA	SLE	High specificity, moderate sensitivity
SmB	SLE	High specificity, low sensitivity
Ro/SSA	Skin LE, Sjögren's syndrome	Complete heart block in newborn
La/SSB	Sjögren's, LE	Minor salivary gland biopsy
snRNP	MCTD	Also seen in SLE Scleroderma, RA
Scl-70	Diffuse scleroderma	Lung involvement in scleroderma
Centromere	CREST syndrome	Also seen in limited scleroderma
Histone	Drug induced SLE	Positive in 100% cases
Jo-1	Dermatomyositis	Low sensitivity

Abbreviations: dsDNA = Double stranded deoxyribonucleic acid; SmB = Small nuclear ribonucleoprotein polypeptides B And B1; SnRNP = Small nuclear ribonucleoprotein; SLE = Systemic lupus erythematosus; LE = Lupus erythematosus; MCTD = Mixed connective tissue disease; RA = Rheumatoid arthritis

stage, gumma may develop. In congenital syphilis, syphilitic epiphysitis may be seen.

Apart from syphilis, false positive venereal disease research laboratory (VDRL) reaction may occur in SLE. With treatment of the primary disorders, the VDRL test also becomes negative. False positive VDRL is more frequently associated with antiphospholipid antibodies.

Serum Uric Acid

It is raised (normal 5–6 mg/dL) in hyperuricemia and gout, should be examined after overnight fasting.

Each laboratory should standardize its results and give its normal values for comparison. Administration of NSAID reduces serum uric acid level. Therefore, false negative values may be seen even in gouty subjects receiving NSAIDs. In chronic tophaceous gout, serum uric acid is elevated, often above 8 mg/dL, but in active gout, the serum uric acid may be normal. Moreover, all cases of hyperuricemia may not present with gouty arthritis. Table 106.5 summarizes the diagnostic relevance of ANAs in connective tissue diseases.

Synovial Fluid Examination

Examination of the synovial fluid is a very reliable and cost effective test for diagnosis of joint disease. When the diagnosis is in doubt, this should be done early. It can be done as a bedside procedure. Normal synovial fluid is a thick viscous yellow liquid. Fluid from inflamed joints is thin, watery and opalescent (Table 106.6).

The fluid can be examined as a fresh wet preparation under the microscope after staining with methylene blue. Other tests include cell count, cytocentrifugation to detect microorganisms and culture, and polarized microscopy for crystals.

Determination of Human Leukocyte Antigen (HLA) Status

In humans, the short arm of chromosome 6 contains the genes that regulate immunological processes and these

Table 106.5: Clinical relevance of autoantibodies

Antibody	Antibody prevalence (%)	*Major clinical features*
SLE		
dsDNA	70–80	Renal or skin disease
Smith	10–30	Renal disease
Nucleo-some	60–90	Renal or skin disease
U1RNP	15–20	Raynaud's syndrome, puffy fingers, myositis hypergamma-globulinemia
α-actinin	20	Renal disease
C$_1$q	40–50	Active disease, renal disease
SLE or Sjögren syndrome		
Ro/SSA	30–40	Kidney disease, skin disease, photosensitivity, congenital heart block, neonatal lupus
La/SSB	15–20	Heart block, Sicca symptoms Subacute cutaneous lupus
α-fodrine	30–100	Sicca symptoms
Inflammatory myositis		
Jo-1	20–30	Antisynthetase syndrome
Mi-2	8–12	Dermatomyositis or polymyositis
TRIM 33	10–30 (dermatomyositis)	Malignancy
U1RNP	8–15	MCTD, SLE
PM/Scl	12–16	Systemic sclerosis or overlap syndrome
Progressive systemic sclerosis		
Centromere	15–40	Limited scleroderma, pulmonary hypertension
Scl-70	10–40	Diffuse cutaneous scleroderma, ILD
RNA polymerase III	5–25	Renal crisis, pulmonary hypertension

Abbreviations: SLE = Systemic lupus erythematosus; dsDNA = Double-stranded deoxyribonucleic acid; MCTD = Mixed connective tissue disease; RNA = Ribonucleic acid; ILD = Interstitial lung disease.

are called the major histocompatibility complex (MHC). It extends over about 4 million base pairs. These codes for the HLA proteins, which are of two types, i.e. HLA class I antigens and HLA class II antigens. HLA class I molecules are distributed widely among most somatic cells of the body with the exception of erythrocytes. HLA class II molecules are seen mainly in the cells of the immune system such as B-lymphocytes, macrophages, dendritic cells and a group of T-cells. One of their main functions is concerned with the presentation of antigens to CD4 positive T-cells, which activate further immunological processes. Certain HLA types have strong association with different rheumatological diseases. HLA-B27 is often positive in ankylosing spondylitis and other seronegative spondyloarthritis. HLA-DRA may be positive in RA and DR2 or DR3 in SLE.

In routine clinical rheumatological practice, only detection of HLA-B27 has become a standard investigation due to its very strong association with ankylosing spondylitis. It is not needed in a definite case of ankylosing spondylitis. But HLA-B27 is useful in suspected spondyloarthritis, acute uveitis with low back pain and normal X-ray, asymmetrical oligoarthritis or recurrent enthesitis, and in women with inflammatory backache and normal radiology.

X-Ray Examination

This is a very simple, reliable, easily available and cheap investigation giving diagnostic information in most of the diseases associated with structural changes in bones and joints. X-ray examination is routinely done in almost all rheumatic diseases for the following purposes:

- To exclude bone and joint lesions
- To establish the diagnosis by the presence of typical changes
- To confirm the clinical diagnosis and the stage of disease for follow-up.

Characteristic abnormalities, which are themselves diagnostic may occur in osteoarthritis, cervical spondylosis, ankylosing spondylitis, RA, gout, tuberculous arthritis, osteomalacia, fluorosis and others. Serial X-rays form the most reliable records for follow-up of the cases. In traumatic lesions, skiagrams are mandatory to detect fractures and dislocations.

Other Imaging Techniques

Apart from plain X-ray examination, several imaging techniques are available to study bone and joint problems. These may be required at times when other investigations fail to confirm the diagnosis. These include computerized tomography (CT) scan, musculoskeletal ultrasonography (USG), magnetic resonance imaging (MRI), bone densitometry-dual energy X-ray absorptiometry (DEXA) scan and radioisotope bone scintigraphy.

CT scan gives clear pictures of bony abnormalities and soft tissues. Discrimination between bone and joint disease is generally clear. CT scan and MRI are very useful to pick up sacroiliitis in early ankylosing spondylitis. It detects periarticular and ligamental thickening and calcifications and also detects early changes in bone and adjacent soft tissues.

The indications for CT scan are increasing. Multi-detectors CT scanning gives better details and hence this may be done when facilities are available.

MRI: This is the ideal imaging for diarthrodial joints when diagnostic information cannot be obtained by other modalities. MRI can detect pre-erosive inflammatory changes, synovial hyperplasia and joint effusion. It is also very useful to detect bony erosions early in RA. MRI clearly delineates soft tissue changes, like thickening or rupture of tendons, meniscal tear inside the knee joint and others. Changes in the spine and intervertebral disc are also better imaged with MRI. It is also considered as the gold standard imaging of brain in neuropsychiatric lupus and vasculitis. MRI can detect infarcts, hemorrhage, demyelination and vasculitic brain damage.

Table 106.6: Synovial fluid analysis

Feature	Normal	Noninflammatory arthritis	Inflammatory noninfectious arthritis	Infective arthritis
Volume	< 1 mL	>1 mL	>1 mL	< 1 mL
Viscosity	High	High	Low	Variable
Color	Colorless	Straw to yellow	Yellow	Yellow
Clarity	Transparent	Transparent	Translucent	Opaque
WBC count	<220/mm³	50–1,000/mm³	1,000–75,000 mm³	> 100,000/mm³
Neutrophils	<25%	<25%	Often > 50%	> 85%
Culture	Sterile	Sterile	Sterile	+
Mucin clot	Firm	Firm	Friable	Friable
Glucose	Nearly equal to blood glucose	Nearly equal to blood glucose	Low (< 50 mg%)	Very low (< 20 mg%)
Crystals	–	±	±	–

Abbreviation: WBC = White blood cell

Early inflammatory changes are picked up on MRI scans before they become evident in conventional X-rays or CT scans. Dynamic contrast enhanced MRI is even more efficient in this respect. Inflammatory changes reflecting active sacroiliitis include bone marrow edema, synovitis, enthesitis and capsulitis.

Diffusion weighted imaging (DWI) can quantify the diffusion coefficients of lesions, which can discriminate between normal and affected subchondral bone.

Ultrasonography with high frequency linear probe is being employed in rheumatological work more and more. With modern development in transducer technology, it is possible to image neuromuscular structures with good resolution. USG can be used for diagnosis and follow-up during management. It is useful in diagnosing synovitis, erosions, tenosynovitis, tendon rupture, minimal effusions and others. It is widely used in the management of RA, crystal induced arthropathy, spondyloarthropathies, osteoarthritis connective tissue disorders, like Sjögren's syndrome, vasculities and for detection of periarticular and soft tissue lesions. Crystal induced arthropathy can be detected early from its beginning, USG detects ankylosing spondylitis earlier than X-rays with a sensitive 87% and specificity of 96%. Arteritis-temporal arteritis, Takayasu arteritis and other forms of arterial diseases can be detected with precision. The present limitations of USG include the inability to imaging structures deep to bones, gas-filled areas and deeper tissues.

Joint aspiration or injection done under ultrasound guidance in sacroiliac joint, hips, shoulders and others markedly increase the accuracy and effectiveness of the procedure. Specialized ultrasonographic studies are being employed more and more in rheumatology practice.

Radionucleotide scanning of bone shows areas of increased or decreased activity related to vascularity, metabolism or inflammation of bone and joints. It is very sensitive to changes in tissue activity but highly nonspecific. Technetium-99m (^{99m}Tc) scintigraphy commonly employed in our country is very useful to detect bone metastasis, occult infections, like septic discitis and stress fractures.

Bone Densitometry

This is the measurement of bone mass or bone mineral density (BMD), which is the most reliable parameter to diagnose osteoporosis and to predict the chances for fragility fractures in future. Several types of bone densitometers are available worldwide. In India, the two types available are ultrasound densitometers and dual-energy X-ray absorptiometry (DEXA) densitometers. The latter is more reliable and results are more reproducible, though it is more expensive.

The results of DEXA are quantitative values expressed in two forms—T-scores and Z-scores. T-scores compare the BMD of the patient with the mean peak BMD of the normal young adult population using standard deviation (SD).

Z-score compares the BMD of the patient with the mean BMD of patients of the same age. The sites commonly measured are the lumbar spines (L1–L4) including the intervertebral discs, hips and forearm. BMD of any other part of the skeleton or that of the whole skeleton can also be determined.

ARTHROSCOPY

This is endoscopic visualization of joints by an arthroscope. Arthroscopy is done for biopsy, therapeutic debridement of diseased joint structures, synovectomy and arthroscopic fixation of intra-articular structures following injury, e.g. knees and shoulders are the most frequently arthroscoped joints. As a therapeutic measure, it has given the best results in osteoarthritis. Removals of loose bodies and debridement have given significant improvement in joint function and pain reduction. In skilled hands and well-chosen cases, arthroscopic treatment is very useful to give relief.

SYNOVIAL BIOPSY

It is a useful procedure to make a definite diagnosis of undiagnosed chronic monoarthritis. In conditions like synovial malignancies and tuberculosis, it gives a definite diagnosis.

MICROBIOLOGICAL INVESTIGATIONS

Depending upon the clinical probability, microbiological tests are done which includes:

- Studies on exudates and skin lesions
- Blood culture serology
- Synovial fluid biochemistry, staining and culture

Textbook of Medicine

- Studies on cerebrospinal fluid (CSF) in selective cases such as secondary syphilis, generalized septic arthritis, relapsing fever, borreliosis and others.

INFLAMMATORY VERSUS NONINFLAMMATORY ARTHRITIS

In general, rheumatic diseases can be broadly divided into inflammatory and noninflammatory lesions.

Examples of the former include rheumatoid disease, systematic lupus, tuberculous arthritis and others.

Noninflammatory lesions include—osteoarthritis, allergic arthritis, sarcoidosis, drug-induced lesions and systemic vasculitis. The clinical features of the two types differ and help to make clinical diagnosis.

Patients with an inflammatory arthritis usually complain of pain and stiffness in involved joints; typically these symptoms are worse in the morning or after periods of inactivity (the so-called 'gel phenomenon'), lasts for more than 1 hour and improve with mild to moderate activity. On examination, the larger joints can be warm, and when severely inflamed as in acute gout or septic arthritis, can have erythema of the overlying skin. Laboratory investigations often reveal an elevated ESR and a high CRP level.

In contrast, patients with noninflammatory arthropathy have pain that worsens with activity and improves with rest. Stiffness is generally mild and usually not a prominent symptom. The ESR and CRP are usually normal.

The most reliable means for making this distinction is analysis of the white blood cell (WBC) count in the synovial fluid. The synovial fluid WBC count is more than 2,000/mm^3 in inflammatory arthritis and is less than 2,000/mm^3 in non-inflammatory arthritis.

CHAPTER
107

Rheumatoid Arthritis and its Variants

Binoy J Paul, KV Krishna Das

Chapter Summary

- Rheumatoid Arthritis
- General Considerations
- Clinical Features
- Laboratory Investigations
- Diagnosis
- Prognosis
- Modern Concept of Therapy of Rheumatoid Disease
- Management
- Variants of Rheumatoid Arthritis
- Juvenile Idiopathic Arthritis
- Felty's Syndrome
- Sjögren's Syndrome
- Palindromic Rheumatism

RHEUMATOID ARTHRITIS

GENERAL CONSIDERATIONS

Rheumatoid arthritis (RA) is one of the most common chronic inflammatory arthritis affecting 0.5–1.0% of the general population worldwide. Epidemiological surveys by WHO-COPCORD (World Health Organization-Community Oriented Program for Control of Rheumatic Diseases) shows a prevalence of 0.45% in urban India and 0.7% in rural population. RA in India is predominantly with arthritic manifestations with lower frequency of extra-articular features and rheumatoid nodules. The frequency of positive rheumatoid factor (RF) varies from 45% in a rural community to 80% in the hospital setting. The frequency of antibody to anti-cyclic citrullinated peptide (anti-CCP) positivity in this survey varies from 59 to 100%. RA in the Indian rural setting is much more disabling and is related to work conditions and methods, and popular Indian customs of squatting and sitting cross legged in floor. The disease is 3 times more common in women than men with a peak incidence in 3rd and 4th decades.

ETIOLOGY

RA is multifactorial in its etiology consisting of genetic and environmental factors. Interaction of these factors cause altered post-transcriptional regulation and self-protein citrullination leading to loss of self-tolerance.

Genetic Factors

Overall, the contribution of genetic factors is to the order of 10–15%. The strongest genetic association is with the class II major histocompatibility complex (MHC) gene containing the susceptibility epitope (SE) which is a specific 5 amino acid sequence in the hypervariable region of human leukocyte antigen (HLA)-DR4. Presence of SE causes a 4–5-fold increase risk of developing RA. Recently other genes, like $PTPN_{22}$, $PADI_4$ are also found to increase the risk of RA by two-fold, suggesting that the genetic association of RA are complex and may involve many genes.

Environmental Factors

Many environmental triggers, like smoking, infection, chronic gingival disease, diet and hormonal factors, can precipitate RA in genetically susceptible persons.

- ***Smoking*** is a strong stimulus for protein citrullination and generation of anti-CCP antibodies. The SE has increased ability to bind to citrullinated protein. A smoker with two copies of HLA-SE has 40-fold chance of developing RA than a nonsmoker without HLA-SE.

- ***Infections*** by viruses, like Epstein-Barr virus, parvovirus and chikungunya virus can act as a triggering agent to develop RA. Chronic periodontitis is found to be risk factor for RA as the bacteria *Porphyromonas gingivalis* commonly associated with this disease stimulate protein citrullination and development of autoantibodies of RA.

Hormonal Factors

Breastfeeding increases the risk of RA due to the surge of proinflammatory hormone prolactin. Nulliparity also found to increase the risk of RA.

PATHOLOGY

RA is an autoimmune disease of unknown etiology. It evolves through a multistep pathogenic process starting with break in self-tolerance with production of antibodies, like RF and antibodies to anti-CCP. There is increased production of proinflammatory cytokines, like tumor necrosis factor-alpha (TNF-α), interleukin-1 (IL-1), interleukin-6 (IL-6), etc. which leads to influx of immune cells into the synovial compartment. This process results in synovial cell proliferation and angiogenesis which leads into the formation of pannus. The pannus consists of fibroblast like synoviocytes mixed with macrophages surrounding newly formed blood vessels. Enzymes, like proteases and elastases released by the cells in the pannus, cause cartilage erosion. The proinflammatory cytokines, like TNF-α, IL-1 and IL-6, activate the osteoclast causing bone erosions also.

The articular cartilage is eventually destroyed with loss of joint space. Fibrosis develops across the joint space to produce ankylosis. The joint is deformed and secondary degenerative changes develop. Infection may supervene in these joints to convert them into septic arthritis.

Extra-articular Lesions

Other tissues are affected to varying degrees. Basic pathology is the same as in the synovium. Lesions are seen in the skin, lungs, heart, liver, nervous system and eyes. The small blood vessels may be affected. They show intimal hyperplasia, perivascular round cell infiltration and occasionally necrotizing panarteritis. Subcutaneous nodules consist of a central area of fibrinoid necrosis surrounded by mononuclear cells arranged in a palisade manner.

Source: McInnes IB, Schett G. Pathogenesis of rheumatoid arthritis. N Engl J Med. 2011;365:2205-19.

CLINICAL FEATURES

Females are affected more than males in a ratio of 3:1. The disease is more common in the 4th and 5th decades. The disease passes through different stages:

- Onset to 6 months—early RA
- 6 months to 2 years—established RA
- Above 2 years—advanced RA.

Early symptoms are nonspecific and they include undue fatigability, weight loss, poor appetite, transient myalgias and paresthesia.

Articular Involvement

The onset is generally insidious and the disease presents as a chronic symmetrical polyarthritis. Less common presentations include:

- Acute polyarthritis
- Oligoarthritis
- Acute monoarticular arthritis
- Chronic monoarticular arthritis
- Systemic disease with fever, sweating, leukocytosis and pleural effusion in addition to arthritis.

Any diarthrodial joint may be inflamed. Arthralgia, arthritis, muscle wasting, tendonitis, tendon rupture and deformities constitute the main lesions. The affected joints are warm, painful and swollen. Movements are restricted, especially in the morning after sleep (morning stiffness) and after periods of resting. Classic findings are seen in the joints of the hands and feet. Metacarpophalangeal (MCP), metatarsophalangeal (MTP) and proximal interphalangeal (PIP) joints are inflamed most frequently (Figs 107.1 and 107.2). Wasting of the small muscles of hand may develop due to disuse and direct muscle involvement.

In the hands, there is typical ulnar deviation of the MCP joints and wrists. Sometimes, there is anterior subluxation of metacarpal heads and medial dislocation of the extensor tendons. Swan neck deformity (Fig. 107.3) of the fingers consists of hyperextension of the PIP joints and flexion of the distal interphalangeal joints. This deformity impairs effective handgrip. Sometimes, the extensor expansion overlying the PIP joint ruptures

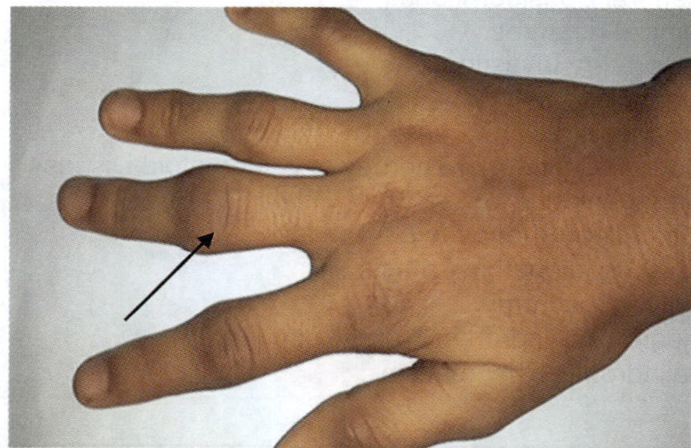

Fig. 107.1: Spindling of fingers at proximal interphalangeal (PIP) joint in early rheumatoid arthritis (RA) (arrow)

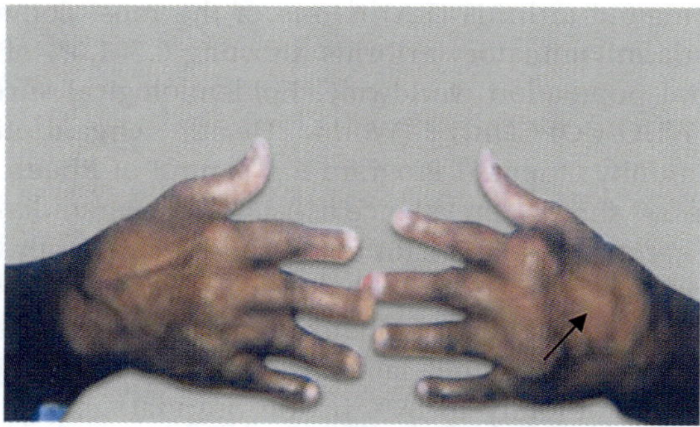

Fig. 107.2: Symmetrical arthritis of wrists, proximal interphalangeal (PIP) joints and metacarpophalangeal (MCP) joints in moderately advanced rheumatoid arthritis (RA). ***Note:*** The muscle wasting (arrow)

Textbook of Medicine

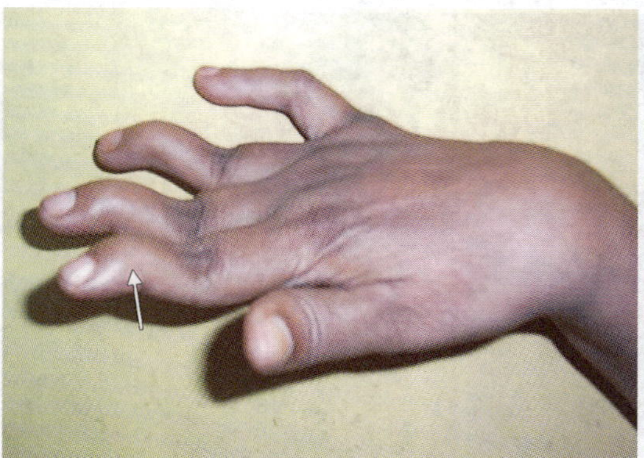

Fig. 107.3: Swan neck deformity of fingers (arrow)

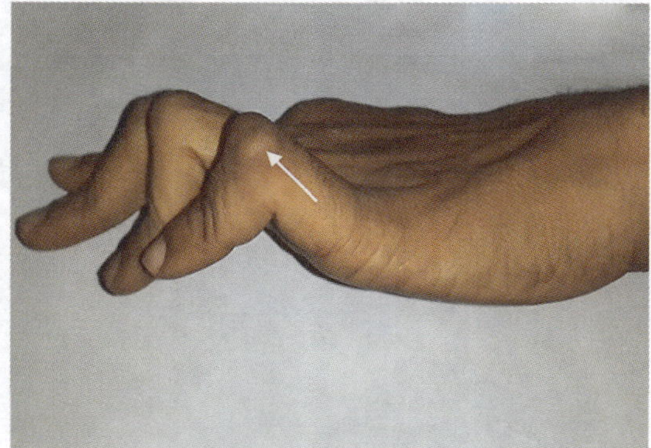

Fig. 107.4: Boutonnière (button hole) deformity (arrow)

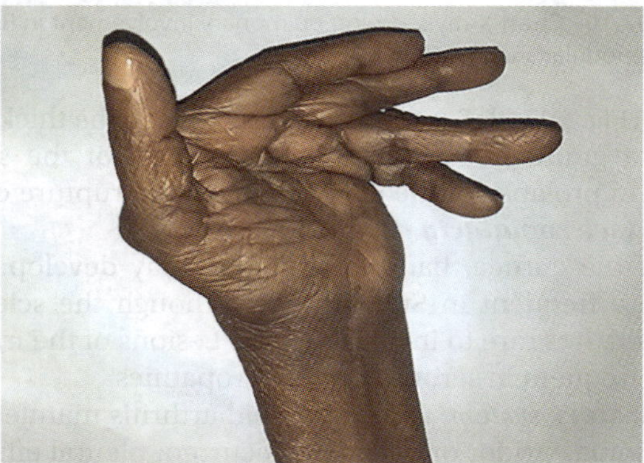

Fig. 107.5: Ulnar deviation of fingers

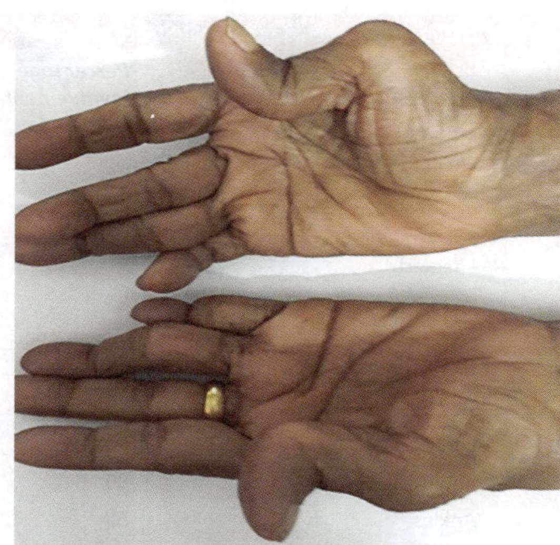

Fig. 107.6: Z-shaped deformity (Hitchhiker's thumb)

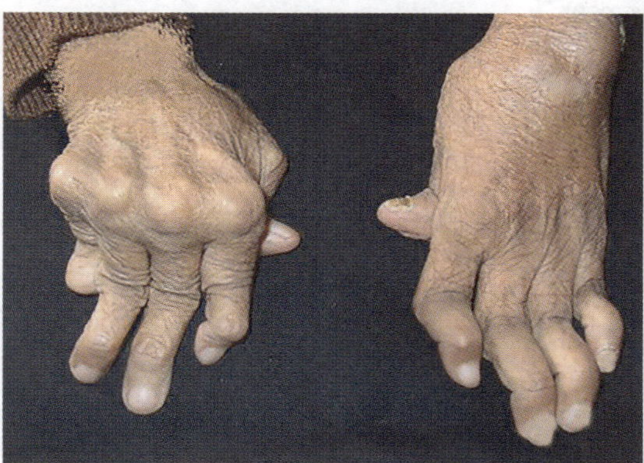

Fig. 107.7: Advanced rheumatoid arthritis (RA). ***Note:*** The deformities in all the fingers

resulting in the dorsal protrusion of the head of the proximal phalanx. This leads to flexion of the PIP joint and hyperextension of the distal interphalangeal joint (boutonnière or button hole) deformity (Fig. 107.4).

The extensor tendons may undergo attrition, these result in loss of extension of the ***fingers (dropped fingers)*** (Fig. 107.5). The thumb may show a Z-shaped deformity ***(Hitchhiker's thumb)*** (Fig. 107.6). Large joints, like the knees, wrists, ankles, elbows and shoulders, may also be involved. Tense synovial effusions may develop in the knees. ***Baker's cysts*** are tense cysts developing in the popliteal fossae as a result of collection of synovial fluid. These may occasionally rupture giving rise to a painful and tender swelling on the calf. Lateral subluxation of the knee joint is also very common. Chronic arthritis develops

which leads to permanent deformities (Fig. 107.7). Deformities are also common in the feet. ***Hammer toe*** is flexion at the PIP joint and hyperextension at the MTP joint. ***Hallux valgus*** (lateral deviation of the big toe) may also develop. The arches of the feet may be lost due to affection of the joints and ligaments. Callosities develop over prominent bony points.

Less commonly, the cervical spine and temporomandibular joints are affected, but when they occur, the lesions are characteristic. At the atlantoaxial joint, the transverse ligament of the atlas may be weakened leading to ***atlantoaxial subluxation***. This leads to pain in the neck and pain referred to the temporal and retro-orbital regions. There may also be a ***clunking sound*** in the neck on flexion. It is dangerous to manipulate the neck to elicit this sign. Atlantoaxial subluxation produces a host of neurological manifestations. The risk of sudden compression of the spinal cord is high in such subjects. Hence, tracheal intubation and similar procedures, which require manipulation of the neck, should be done only with caution. ***Temporomandibular arthritis*** leads to pain on mastication. Other portions of the spine, such as the dorsolumbar regions and sacroiliac joints are usually not affected in RA.

Textbook of Medicine

Table 107.1: Tissue involvement in rheumatoid arthritis (RA)

Parameters	Involvement of tissue	Percentage of involvement (%)
Number of joints affected	Monoarticular (only 1 joint affected)	3
	Oligoarticular (< 5 joints affected)	34
	Polyarticular (5 or more joints affected)	63
Joints affected	Proximal interphalangeal (PIP) joints	85
	Metacarpophalangeal (MCP) joints	70
	Wrists	70
	Elbows	50
	Knees	80
	Ankles	65
	Metatarsophalangeal (MTP) joints	30
Nonarticular involvement	Pulmonary interstitial fibrosis	3
	Episcleritis	1
	Sjögren's syndrome	2
	Pleural effusion	1

Note: As reported from Chennai, India.

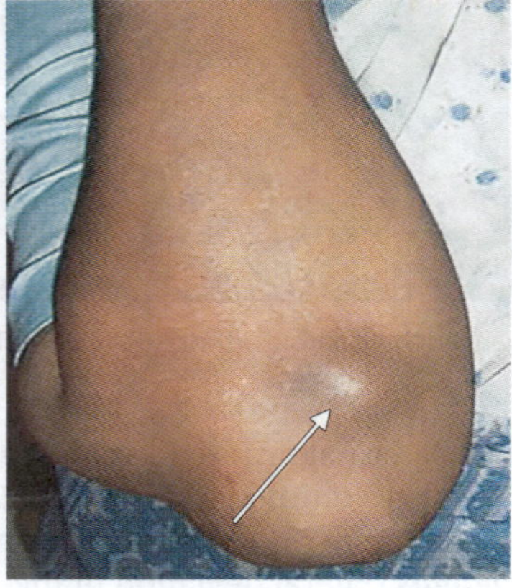

Fig. 107.8: Rheumatoid nodule at the elbow

Tissue Involvement in RA (Table 107.1)

Systemic Involvement

Extra-articular manifestations

Skin: Painless and nontender subcutaneous nodules ranging in size from a few millimeters to a few centimeters develop around the extensor aspects of the elbow (Fig. 107.8) and other subcutaneous bony surfaces and over tendons in 20–30% of cases.

They are almost always associated with a positive serology. They persist for considerable periods. Involvement of blood vessels gives rise to Raynaud's phenomenon, vasculitis of the nailbeds and finger pulps, nonhealing ulcers of the finger, palmar erythema and hyperhidrosis of the extremities.

Eyes: Ocular lesions develop in a few cases and these may become disabling. Scleritis is common. In some cases, it becomes nodular. In necrotizing scleritis, the nodules degenerate and the underlying dark uvea imparts a blue

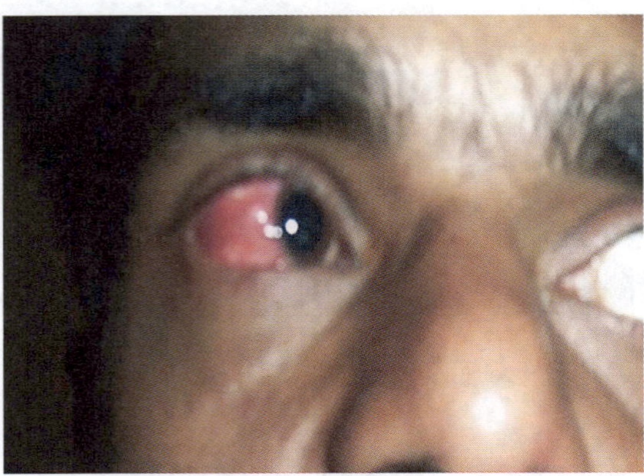

Fig. 107.9: Scleritis in rheumatoid arthritis (RA). ***Note:*** The congestion of the sclera

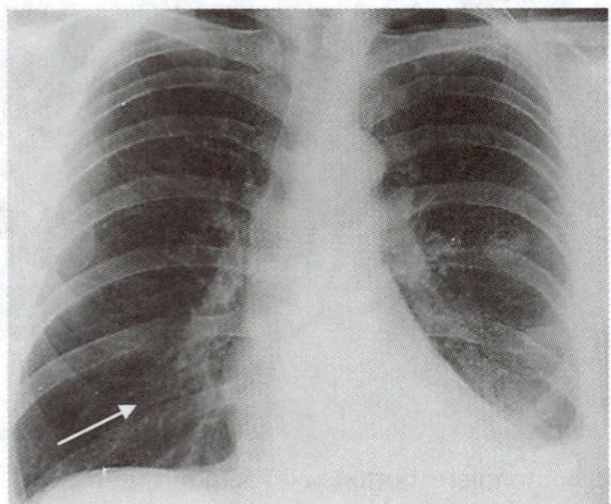

Fig. 107.10: Chest X-ray showing pulmonary involvement in RA. The reticulonodular shadows (arrow)

color (Fig. 107.9). Sometimes the sclera may be thickened due to granuloma formation. Perforation of the sclera leads to prolapse of the uvea and eventual rupture of the globe ***(scleromalacia perforans)***.

In the cornea, band keratopathy may develop. This is more frequent in Still's disease. Though the sclera is affected, it is rare to involve the iris. Lesions of the iris are more frequent in seronegative arthropathies.

Respiratory system: Cricoarytenoid arthritis manifests as dysphonia, stridor or dyspnea. Recurrent pleural effusion may occur which is usually unilateral. Rheumatoid nodules may develop in the lungs and these may cavitate (Figs 107.10 and 107.11). Interstitial fibrosis may develop and this may be indistinguishable from the idiopathic type. ***Caplan's syndrome*** is a special phenomenon occurring in subjects with rheumatoid disease who develop pneumoconiosis. Large coalescing nodules develop in the lungs. These are demonstrable by X-rays.

Cardiovascular system: It is only rarely involved. Lesions include pericarditis, mitral/aortic regurgitation and conduction defects. There is increased incidence of atherosclerosis and ischemic heart disease with higher mortality in RA.

Nervous system: Neurological involvement is not uncommon in chronic cases. ***Entrapment neuropathy***, such as carpal tunnel syndrome and tarsal tunnel syndrome, may be the presenting lesions or they may develop during the course. ***Symmetrical polyneuropathy*** develops which

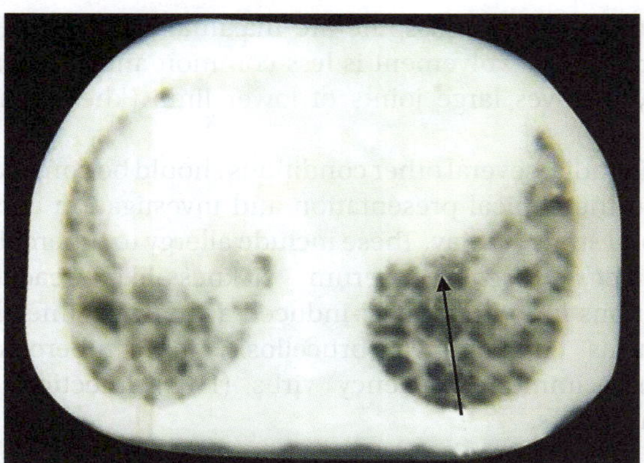

Fig. 107.11: Computed tomography (CT) scan thorax in advanced rheumatoid lung showing cavitation and honey comb appearance (arrow)

improves with treatment. ***Mononeuritis multiplex*** also occur in severe cases of rheumatoid disease (malignant RA) and leads to foot drop or wrist drop. These are generally resistant to treatment. ***Cervical cord compression*** due to atlantoaxial subluxation is a less common complication in long-standing RA. Mild cases present with transient neck pain radiating to the back of the head. It can rarely lead to subluxation of the odontoid process with compression of the cord which may end fatally. Progressive clinical ***myelopathy*** at a lower level may develop insidiously. This is characterized by gradual onset of limb weakness, inability to hold the head erect and quadriparesis. The lesion is due to subluxation at lower levels of the cervical cord.

Renal involvement: Type 1 renal tubular acidosis and analgesic nephropathy can rarely occur.

Secondary amyloidosis is a late complication in some cases of chronic rheumatoid disease (*See* also Section 16, Ch 187).

LABORATORY INVESTIGATIONS

Erythrocyte sedimentation rate (ESR) is markedly raised in the active disease and may exceed 100 mm/hour in the majority. Normochromic normocytic anemia, iron-deficiency anemia or rarely hemolytic anemia may be present in the acute phase. Serum protein electrophoresis may show elevation of α- and γ-globulins. C-reactive protein (CRP) will also be high.

Serology

Rheumatoid Factor

Antibodies in rheumatoid disease, especially the immuno-globulin M (IgM), can be demonstrated by the ***Rose-Waaler test, latex fixation test*** or ***nephelometry***. RF is positive in 70–80% of adults with RA. In 20–30% of cases, antinuclear antibodies may be demonstrable. To establish seropositivity, the test should be positive at least on two occasions separated by 3–6 months. If negative, it should be repeated at least once more after 6–12 months. Five to ten percent of normal individuals, especially elderly, may show RF positivity in low titers.

Antibody to Anti-Cyclic Citrullinated Peptide

It is a new antibody test for the early diagnosis of RA. Formations of anti-CCP antibodies are highly specific for RA patients (96% specific, 70% sensitive). Anti-CCP antibodies are present early in RA patients even before developing arthritis. High titer also correlates with disease activity and erosive changes in bone.

Antinuclear Antibody

Antinuclear antibody (ANA) of unknown specificity may be positive in 30% of RA.

Synovial Fluid Aspiration

This reveals a turbid fluid with low viscosity and poor mucin clot. The white cell count in the fluid exceeds 1,500/mm³. The cells are mostly neutrophils even though the synovial membrane is not infiltrated by them. Complement levels are low. The protein content will also be high.

Radiology

Characteristic lesions, which have been graded from I to IV, are seen on radiological study.

- ***Grade I:*** Soft-tissue swelling which indicates synovitis with or without juxta-articular osteoporosis which indicates active inflammation.
- ***Grade II:*** Narrowing of joint space due to cartilage destruction.
- ***Grade III:*** Erosions which may be of two types:
  1. Surface erosion at joint margins
  2. Cystic erosion of the bone shaft.
- ***Grade IV:*** Marked irregularity of articular surfaces with subluxation and secondary degenerative changes. Bony ankylosis occurs only very rarely (Fig. 107.12).

DIAGNOSIS

The diagnosis is to be made on clinical examination and laboratory criteria. Since, clinically several conditions resemble RA, new diagnostic criteria have been laid down by the Joint Committee for American College of Rheumatology (ACR) and European League Against Rheumatism (EULAR) in 2010. This score is based on:

- Joint involvement
- Autoantibody status
- Acute phase reactants
- Duration of joint symptoms (Table 107.2).

A score with six or more points supports the diagnosis of RA. Patients with typical bony erosion or long-standing disease previously satisfying the criteria can also be labeled as RA.

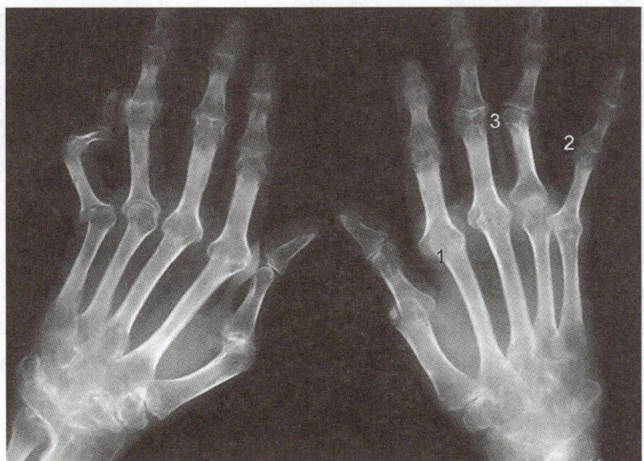

Fig. 107.12: X-ray of hands and wrist in RA: (1) Narrowing of joint space, (2) Cartilage erosions, (3) Subluxation and ulnar deviation of PIP joints, MCP joints and wrists

Table 107.2: ACR/EULAR classification criteria for RA-2010

Parameters	Score
Joint involvement	**(0–5)**
1 medium to large joint	0
2–10 medium to large joint	1
1–3 small joints (large joint not counted)	2
4–10 small joints (large joint not counted)	3
> 10 joints (at least 1 small joint)	5
Autoantibody status	**(0–3)**
Negative: RF and ACPA	0
Low-positive: RF and ACPA	2
High-positive: RF and ACPA	3
Acute phase reactants	**(0–1)**
Normal: CRP and ESR	0
Abnormal: CRP and ESR	1
Duration of joint symptoms	**(0–1)**
<6 weeks	0
≥6 weeks	1
A score with 6 or more points can be classified as RA.	

Abbreviations: ACR = American College of Rheumatology; EULAR = European League Against Rheumatism; RF = Rheumatoid factor; ACPA = Anti-citrullinated protein antibody; CRP = C-reactive protein; ESR = Erythrocyte sedimentation rate; RA = Rheumatoid arthritis

DIFFERENTIAL DIAGNOSIS

RA has to be distinguished from ***rheumatic arthritis*** in which children are more affected, the joint lesions are migratory, large joints are affected, effusion is prominent and ASO (antistreptolysin O titer) titer is high (> 1/200 Todd units).

Psoriatic Arthritis

In psoriatic arthritis, there is invariably evidence of psoriasis of the skin or nails and the arthritis involves the small joints of the hands (especially distal interphalangeal joints) and feet more. The hand may be severely mutilated ***(arthritis mutilans)***. Involvement of the sacroiliac joints and spine is not uncommon.

Gout

Several joints may be affected in gout. The MTP joint of the big toe is characteristically affected more frequently, though any joint may be involved. In chronic tophaceous gout, tophi may be seen as nodules around the joints, especially the elbow.

Osteoarthritis

It affects elderly subjects. Most common joints affected are the spine, hips, knees and distal interphalangeal joints. ***Heberden's nodes*** may be seen at the base of the distal phalanges. The condition is progressive. The ESR is generally normal or only mildly elevated. In many cases, rheumatoid and osteoarthritis may coexist in different joints.

Other Conditions

Other conditions, which may mimic RA, are ***syphilitic arthritis, gonococcal arthritis, reactive arthritis*** and ***ankylosing spondylitis***. In ankylosing spondylitis, the sacroiliac joints and spine are maximally affected. Peripheral joint involvement is less common and predominantly involves large joints of lower limb (knees, ankles and hips).

In India, several other conditions should be considered when the clinical presentation and investigation are not helpful straight away. These include allergy to tuberculosis (***Poncet's disease***), serum sickness-like reactions, reactions in leprosy, drug-induced arthralgias, infections such as chikungunya, brucellosis, joint tuberculosis, human immunodeficiency virus (HIV) infection and many others.

PROGNOSIS

In general, the disease tends to become recurrent and chronic and in many cases it leads to considerable disability and deformity. Severe RA shortens life. It leads to severe impairment of the quality of life. A third of the patients with RA deteriorate clinically by consumption of food articles, such as trout, fishes, peas, carrots, bottled mineral water, sea salt, milk, dairy products, wheat, coffee, chocolate, citrus fruits, corn and others. Free amino acids and oligopeptides contained in some of them are weakly antigenic and they may be responsible for this adverse effect.

TREATMENT

Early Intervention

Early use of disease-modifying antirheumatic drugs (DMARDs) preferably, methotrexate with low-dose steroids for 2–3 months started within 3–6 months of onset of RA has achieved marked clinical benefits. Combination of synthetic DMARDs with low-dose steroids are widely useful in patients with poor prognostic factors, like early erosion, strongly positive RF or anti-CCP or high-disease activity [disease activity score (DAS) > 5.1].

Treat-to-target or Tight Control Strategy

Targeting no- or low-disease activity by regular monitoring using primary composite measures of disease activity and adhering to a predefined treatment strategy when compared with unstructured treatments conveys better outcome. In the past this was not possible primarily because of the complexity of measures assessing disease activity in RA and insufficient knowledge of optimal treatment strategies. DAS28, simplified disease activity index (SDAI), clinical disease activity index (CDAI), routine assessment of patient index data 3 (RAPID3) are all validated and these functioning measures now used in every day case allowing physicians to treat-to-target (Table 107.3).

Disease activity score is a frequently used scoring system for classifying activity in RA for clinical research purposes and therapeutic decision-making and prognostication as well, since the development of DAS in 1990. It has gained immense importance. At present DAS based on 28 joints (DAS28) is in vogue. The DAS28 score combines number of swollen and tender joints in addition to a measure of general health and the acute phase reactants with scores ranging from 0 to 9.4. The

Table 107.3: Measures included in composite score commonly used in RA

Parameters	DAS28	SDAI	CDAI	RAPID3
Swollen joint	+	+	+	
Tender joint	+	+	+	
Physicians global assessment		+	+	
Patients global assessment	+	+	+	+
Functional score pain				+
ESR/CRP	+	+		

Abbreviations: RA = Rheumatoid arthritis; DAS28 = Disease activity score 28; SDAI = Simplified disease activity index; CDAI = Clinical disease activity index; RAPID3 = Routine assessment of patient index data 3; ESR = Erythrocyte sedimentation rate; CRP = C-reactive protein

acute phase reactants used for calculating the DAS28 are ESR and less commonly CRP. DAS28 ESR values are categorized as follows:

- More than 5.1: High-disease activity
- Less than 3.2: Low-disease activity
- Less than 2.6: Remission.

Recent studies encourage the application of DAS28 using CRP (DAS28 CRP) compared to DAS ESR. Since ESR usually reflects disease activity of the past few weeks whereas CRP tends to reflect more short-term changes in disease activity. The reader may access website: das-score.nl/das28/en/for the formula to calculate DAS28 score (Table 107.4).

Favorable Criteria

Favorable criteria are:

- Acute onset
- Male sex
- Onset at late age
- Asymmetrical or monoarticular involvement
- Negative RF
- Negative anti-CCP
- Absence of subcutaneous nodules
- Absence of vasculitis
- Prompt response to therapy early in the disease.

Prognostic Factors

Unfavorable prognostic factors:

- Female gender
- More than 1 year of synovitis without remission
- High titers of RF and/or anti-CCP
- Early development of nodules and bony erosions
- Extra-articular features
- High DAS28.

Table 107.4: Activity level cut-off for composite indices

Activity level	DAS28 (0–10)	SDAI (0–86)	CDAI (0–76)	RAPID3 (0–30)
High	>5.1	>26	>22	>12
Moderate	3.2–5.1	11–26	10.1–22	6.1–12
Low	2.6–3.2	3.3–11	2.9–10	3.1–6
Remission/near remission	≤2.6	≤3.3	≤2.8	≤3

Abbreviations: DAS28 = Disease activity score 28; SDAI = Simplified disease activity index; CDAI = Clinical disease activity index; RAPID3 = Routine assessment of patient index data 3

Aim of Therapy

The aims of therapy are:

- Relief of pain
- Control of disease activity
- Prevention of joint damage and disability
- Maintenance and recovery of function
- Improvement in the quality of life.

The modalities employed include:

- Patient education
- Supportive measures
- Pharmacotherapy
- Physiotherapy and occupational therapy
- Surgical measures.

General Measures

The approach to treatment of RA has seen three major advances in the last 10–15 years that has changed the outcome of the disease. They are:

1. Early intervention with DMARDs and low-dose steroid bridging
2. Treat-to-target or tight control strategy
3. Use of biological response modifiers (BRMs).

Bed rest is essential during the acute phase of the disease. Local rest is ensured by splints which reduce muscle spasm and deformities. In the stage of deformity, splints are used as corrective measures. Physiotherapy to relieve muscle spasm and maintain joint mobility is an essential component of management during all stages of the disease.

Articles of diet such as fish or fish oils, which are rich in eicosapentaenoic and docosahexaenoic acids, are reported to give relief of inflammation and clinical symptoms, when combined with other modalities of treatment. These polyunsaturated fatty acids suppress the inflammatory response and platelet activation. They may be tried in suitable cases. The dose of fish oils required for the beneficial effects varies from 10 to 20 g daily.

Drugs

There is no curative drug. Hence several groups of drugs are used symptomatically. Some also suppress inflammation and bring about resolution of the disease process.

- Analgesics, e.g. paracetamol, tramadol
- Nonsteroidal anti-inflammatory drugs (NSAIDs), like aspirin, indomethacin, naproxen, ibuprofen, ketoprofen, etodolac, mefenamic acid, aceclofenac, diclofenac and the selective cyclooxygenase 2 inhibitors (COX-2 inhibitors), such as celecoxib and etoricoxib
- DMARDs, such as chloroquine, hydroxychloroquine, salazopyrin and low-dose methotrexate.

Antimalarial drugs, like chloroquine and hydroxychloroquine, act as antirheumatic drugs by the following mechanisms. They are immunosuppressants. This action is brought about by the following processes:

- They act in autoimmune conditions by inhibiting lymphatic proliferation, action of phospholipase A, antigen presentation to dendritic cells, release of enzymes by lysozymes, release of oxygen species from macrophages and reduction in the production of cytokines such IL-1 and IL-6.

Textbook of Medicine

- They influence the metalloproteinase network, thereby contributing to their immunoregulatory and anti-inflammatory properties.
- They suppress toll-like receptor, thereby suppressing the inflammatory activity.
- In systemic lupus erythematosus (SLE) and antiphospholipid antibody syndrome (APAS), antimalarials protect against thrombotic complications.

- ***Corticosteroids:*** Prednisolone, methylprednisolone, deflazacort, dexamethasone, triamcinolone.
- ***Biological agents***, such as infliximab, etanercept, rituximab, tocilizumab and abatacept.
- Immunosuppressants, like azathioprine, cyclosporine, cyclophosphamide and others.
- Janus kinase (JAK) inhibitors—tofacitinib.

Aspirin

Aspirin being very effective and cheap used to be the drug of first choice in earlier days. This is given as calcium aspirin or the other preparations in doses of 3–6 g/day and an antacid is prescribed concurrently to reduce gastric upset. Troublesome side effects include abdominal pain, upper gastrointestinal (GI) bleeding, allergic rashes, tinnitus and vertigo. Due to weaker action and availability of more potent drugs, aspirin is rarely used as the drug of first choice at present.

Nonsteroidal Anti-inflammatory Drugs

These are the most widely used drugs in view of their analgesic and anti-inflammatory actions and free availability. The analgesic effect of NSAIDs is prompt within hours, whereas the anti-inflammatory effects manifest only after 1–2 weeks of therapy. They can be given orally after food (Table 107.5).

All of them share the same GI side effects of aspirin but to a lesser degree and these are indicated when adequate relief is not obtained with rest, splinting and use of disease-modifying drugs. They are several times more expensive than aspirin. NSAIDs are effective in relieving pain and acute manifestations. As a maintenance therapy they help to suppress symptoms and make the patient ambulant. They have only little effect in modifying the course of disease, so that the disease flares up on withdrawing the NSAID. Therefore, they have to be combined with DMARDs. **GI complications** induced by the ingestion of NSAIDs have assumed importance in recent times since hematemesis and melena occurring in day-to-day

Table 107.5: Nonsteroidal anti-inflammatory drugs (NSAIDs)

Drugs	Dosage
Indomethacin	25–50 g 3 times daily
Naproxen	250–500 mg 3 times daily
Ibuprofen	200–800 mg 3 times daily
Mefenamic acid	250–500 mg 4 times daily
Diclofenac	50–75 mg 3 times daily
Aceclofenac	100 mg 2 times daily
Piroxicam	10–20 mg daily
Meloxicam	7.5–15 mg daily

Note: Many others newer drugs are entering the market frequently

practice are commonly induced by these drugs. One to three percent of patients consuming NSAIDs develop a major GI problem annually. The manifestations include overt or occult GI bleeding, acute and chronic gastritis and progressive anemia. *Helicobacter pylori* infection is an independent risk factor which also aggravates hematemesis. ***NSAID-related hematemesis has a mortality of 5–10%, if not treated promptly***. NSAIDs inhibit the synthesis of prostaglandins. Prostaglandins are protective to the mucosa. Even as small a dose as 30 mg of aspirin can inhibit gastric prostaglandin synthesis. The spectrum of lesions includes subepithelial hemorrhage, erosions and ulcers in the stomach and duodenum. NSAIDs should not be taken on an empty stomach, since this favors GI complications, especially pain and bleeding. These can be prevented to some extent by the concurrent use of a H_2-receptor blocker, such as ranitidine 150 mg bd or a proton-pump inhibitor, such as omeprazole 20 mg od or bd. Antacids and mucosal protective agents, like sucralfate and prostaglandins, augment the benefit partially.

The different NSAIDs vary in their propensity to cause GI bleeding. Aspirin is highly ulcerogenic to the gastroduodenal mucosa. None of the NSAIDs is totally safe. All NSAIDs cause serious impairment of renal function in those with underlying kidney disease.

COX-2 inhibitors: They have been introduced with the claim that they do not produce GI bleeding, e.g. celecoxib 100 mg bd, etoricoxib 60–120 mg daily. They are more expensive. They are effective pain relievers but, long-term use has revealed serious adverse effects including the precipitation of myocardial infarction and sudden death. Some of the COX-2 inhibitors, such as rofecoxib, have been withdrawn from the market due to their adverse effects on the cardiovascular system. They are also not totally devoid of adverse GI side effects, and some patients do not tolerate these drugs.

Disease-modifying Antirheumatic Drugs

Even though DMARDs used to be administrated as the second-line drugs when the analgesics and NSAIDs proved inadequate, the present trend is to employ them early in the course of the disease in order to modify the disease activity and prevent progression and permanent disability. The drugs included in this class are chloroquine, hydroxychloroquine, sulfasalazine, methotrexate and immunosuppressants and biological disease modifiers. DMARDs should be introduced early during therapy. They are effective in more than 80% of cases.

- ***Chloroquine diphosphate:*** 250 mg twice daily or once at bedtime orally is effective in controlling pain, swelling and stiffness in chronic cases. This drug is to be used over long periods. It helps to suppress the inflammatory process and prevents further deterioration. Serious side effects include retinopathy and deposition of the drug in the cornea. These are indications for stopping the drug.
- ***Hydroxychloroquine***: It is more effective and has much less retinal toxicity than chloroquine and it is to be preferred. The dose is 200–400 mg/day orally. This is more expensive than chloroquine.

- **Salazopyrin (sulfasalazine)**, which is used for ulcerative colitis, is an excellent drug to bring about relief in RA and a few other autoimmune diseases as well, and modify their progression also. The dose is 0.5–1.0 g thrice a day orally. The effect is manifested 4–8 weeks after starting the drug. It may have to be continued for several months or years. The common adverse side effects include GI upsets, elevation of liver enzymes, allergic manifestations and blood dyscrasias.
- **Methotrexate**: This drug at low doses is considered as a DMARD in rheumatic disorders. It is an immunosuppressive anti-malignancy drug at higher doses. It is found to be the most useful drug in active RA, with predictable benefit and relatively good safety and tolerability. The drug is given at a dose of 7.5–25 mg once weekly. Folic acid 5–10 mg/week is supplemented to avoid mucositis and bone marrow toxicity including suppression. The drug is well tolerated and can be used for prolonged periods. A cumulative dose of 2.5–3.0 g can be given safely in most cases. In unusual situations when the disease is aggressive and unresponsive to other measures the higher doses can be employed with close monitoring for adverse effects. The drug is teratogenic and should be stopped 3 months prior to conception.
- **Leflunomide:** It is a drug which is an isoxazole derivative. It is a prodrug which is converted into its active metabolite in the system. It blocks the enzyme dihydroorotate dehydrogenase which is needed for the synthesis of pyrimidines. Its DMARD activity is comparable to that of methotrexate. It is given as a loading dose of 100 mg/day orally for 3 days followed by 10–20 mg daily as a maintenance dose. It is contraindicated in pregnancy due to teratogenicity. Serious side effects include hepatotoxicity and Stevens-Johnson syndrome.

Systemic Corticosteroids

These are very helpful in bringing about dramatic relief in acute cases and during exacerbations. Due to their undesirable side effects, they should be employed only when other drugs fail and that too for only short periods, if higher doses are employed. In situations in which the disease is subacute or acute with severe pain and disability, glucocorticoids have to be given in appropriate doses orally or parenterally in order to get quick relief. With the attainment of relief, the dosage has to be adjusted.

Indications for systemic corticosteroids are:

- Bridge therapy
- Extra-articular disease
- Severe disease flares
- Pregnancy and lactation
- Intra-articular and intralesional administration.

In bridge therapy with steroids, low-dose prednisolone (7.5–10 mg/day) is given for 8–12 weeks in the beginning of pharmacotherapy, along with DMARDs to get rapid relief of symptoms. Once the DMARDs started their action, steroid will be withdrawn. Recently, it also found that low-dose steroids have disease-modifying action and can be given for a period of 1–2 years at the onset of RA, monitoring the adverse effects.

In life-threatening or sight-threatening visceral or eye disease, high-dose systemic steroids (40–60 mg/day of prednisolone) are given and slowly tapered-off, e.g. rheumatoid vasculitis, interstitial lung disease (ILD) or scleritis of the eye. In established RA with severe disease flares, short course of high-dose steroids are indicated.

In uniarticular or oligoarticular flares, it is advantageous to use intra-articular steroids. Intra-articular dose is 50–100 mg of cortisone acetate for large joints and 5–10 mg for small joints. In tendonitis or tenosynovitis also (e.g. tennis elbow or plantar fasciitis), local steroid injections are useful. In pregnancy and lactation, low-dose prednisolone (< 10 mg/day) is safe. A few patients who are not responding to other drugs require small doses of corticosteroids for symptom relief (steroid-dependent cases).

Immunosuppressant Drugs

Cyclophosphamide and azathioprine are potent drugs which suppress the immunological injury and help to arrest the disease process. Due to toxicity, these drugs are used when methotrexate is contraindicated (e.g. RA with ILD). They are also useful in rheumatoid vasculitis. Dose of cyclophosphamide is 1 g/m^2 surface area once in a week and that of azathioprine is 50–100 mg oral daily. Rarely, other immunosuppressants, like cyclosporine, chlorambucil and others, may have to be given.

Biological Therapies

Biological agents are structurally engineered versions of naturally occurring molecules which have the ability to inhibit cytokines or prevent cellular activation. These include monoclonal antibodies, soluble cytokine receptors and natural antagonists.

Despite aggressive treatment strategies and early use of synthetic DMARD, treatment failures are not uncommon in RA and other rheumatic diseases. Eighteen to twenty-eight percent of patients fail to achieve satisfactory disease control. Hence, better therapeutic agents are needed for these patients. Laboratory research in the understanding of immunopathogenesis, especially the cytokine milieu and their network in RA, contributed heavily towards the development of biological agents (BRMs). In RA, the proinflammatory cytokines, like TNF-α, IL-1 and IL-6 levels, are high and drugs are available against these cytokines.

Antitumor necrosis factor agents: Inhibiting the cytokine, TNF-α can cause remission in RA, blocking the action of TNF-α is highly effective in the treatment of early and advanced RA. The available anti-TNF biologicals are following:

- **Infliximab:** It is a chimeric monoclonal antibody that binds TNF-α with high affinity. The dose is 3–5 mg/kg intravenous (IV) at 0 week, 2 weeks and 6 weeks followed by maintenance infusion once in 8 weeks. It predisposes to reactivation of tuberculosis.
- **Adalimumab:** It is a fully humanized antibody that binds TNF-α, made by rDNA technology. It is given in doses of 20–80 mg SC weekly. Adverse side effects

include severe infections, neurological defects and lymphoid malignancies.

- **Etanercept:** This is a recombinant fusion protein which binds to TNF-α molecule. It is given in a dose of 25 mg SC twice a week or 50 mg once a week. Adverse effects include local irritation at injection sites and predisposition to infection. Indian biosimilars are now available at much lower cost.
- **Golimumab:** It is a human monoclonal antibody to immunoglobulin G1 (IgG1), that is specific for human TNF-α. It is available in abroad.
- **Certolizumab:** Pegylated certolizumab is also highly effective when other anti-TNF agents have failed. It is not available in India.

Anti-interleukin drugs

- **Anakinra:** It is a recombinant form of non-glycosylated human IL-1 receptor antagonist. The dose is 1–2 mg/kg SC daily. It is found to be less effective than anti-TNF agents.
- **Tocilizumab:** It is an anti-IL-6 receptor monoclonal antibody given at a dose of 8 mg/kg every 4 weeks. It is found to be very effective in active RA.

Anti-β-cell agents: The β-cells are responsible for the production of autoantibodies, like RF and anti-CCP in RA. Suppression of β-cells is also effective to bring about clinical remission in RA. The drug rituximab which is an anti-CD 20 monoclonal antibody when used in RA brings about marked relief. Two doses of 1,000 mg given at 15 days interval give prolonged remission in many patients.

Co-stimulation blockers: Agents that block the co-stimulatory pathways of T-cells cause partial suppression of T-cell function without profound immunosuppression. The biological agent **abatacept** which is a CTLA4 (lymphocyte-associated antigen 4 T cytotoxic C5a fraction complement 5a)-IgG1 fusion protein acting as a T-helper cell, co-stimulatory blocker, is given in a dose of 10 mg/kg IV monthly for 6–12 months to produce sustained benefit.

Indications for biological agents: Biological agents are indicated in patients with active RA who had no response to at least two conventional DMARDs. Patients should be screened for infections, like tuberculosis prior to the onset of therapy. *Vaccination using live vaccines should be avoided during the therapy.* They should be used in combination with DMARDs preferably methotrexate. Pregnancy should be avoided during therapy. If TNF inhibitors are found to be ineffective within 3–6 months of therapy or if they produce severe toxic effects, they should be withdrawn.

Indian experience on these biologicals is limited, though a few studies are available. Effect in RA is good, but there are several reports of exacerbation of hidden tuberculosis. These drugs are very expensive, but biosimilars of etanercept and rituximab manufactured indigenously in India are now available and are cheaper.

At present, this group of drugs is reserved for patients who do not respond to the more easily available conventional drugs which are cheaper, safer and are capable of inducing remission in the vast majority of patients over long periods. In a small proportion of patients who suffer from severely disabling disease with crippling deformities and rapid progression, judicious use of these drugs under close supervision can bring about dramatic relief. Therefore, despite the high cost and adverse side effects, biological should be employed for their appropriate indications.

Janus Kinase Inhibitors

Tofacitinib: It is a new drug approved by the Food and Drug Administration (FDA) of the USA for RA. At present it is not freely available in India. It is a cytoplasmic tyrosine kinase (JAK) inhibitor which acts by altering the intracellular signaling pathways that can be given orally at a dose of 5–10 mg twice daily. It is generally well-tolerated. Increased incidence of infections, dyslipidemia and dose-dependent cytopenias are reported adverse effects. If the response to tofacitinib is poor, addition of methotrexate improves the response. This combination is safe.

Pregnancy and Antirheumatic Drugs

NSAIDs are better to avoid in pregnancy. If absolutely necessary, short-acting NSAIDs like ibuprofen and naproxen are preferred. NSAIDs should not be given during the last 4 weeks of pregnancy, since they may give rise to bleeding complications and delay in labor. Low-dose prednisolone, sulfasalazine, hydroxychloroquine and azathioprine are safe during pregnancy. Leflunomide and methotrexate are absolutely contraindicated due to teratogenic effects.

During lactation, a short-acting NSAID, such as ibuprofen is preferable, taken just before feeding the baby and feeding interval should be 4 hours or more.

Modern Concept of Therapy of Rheumatoid Disease

It is now established that use of disease-modifying agents which will arrest progress of the disease and prevent joint damage should be introduced from the start of therapy. DMARDs can be used singly or in combination determined by trial and error and the experience of the physician. However, methotrexate is considered as the drug of choice in moderate-to-severe RA. Hydroxychloroquine or sulfasalazine are tried in mild disease with low-disease activity. The effects produced by these drugs are slow. Therefore, NSAIDs and low-dose steroids have to be given for immediate symptomatic relief of acute cases. The present approach is as follows in Table 107.6.

MANAGEMENT

Physical Modalities of Treatment

These play a major role in the total management of all cases of moderately advanced and advanced rheumatoid disease. The aims of physiotherapy are:

Table 107.6: Modern concept of therapy of rheumatoid disease		
Steps	**Conditions**	**Approaches**
Step 1	Early cases	NSAIDs, DMARD monotherapy, short course of low-dose steroids, physical modalities
Step 2	Moderately advanced cases	Combination therapy with two or more DMARDs plus steroids and/or biological agents
Step 3	Disabling deformities	Drug combinations, surgical correction of deformities and rehabilitation

Abbreviations: NSAIDs = Nonsteroidal anti-inflammatory drugs; DMARDs = Disease-modifying antirheumatic drugs

- To provide comfort, relieve pain and aid in recovery.
- To prevent deformities and loss of function of joints.
- To help in functional and corrective rehabilitation.

Physical modalities of treatment include various forms of superficial and deep heating devices, ultrasound, short-wave, exercises, manipulation of joints, splinting and others. During the acute and subacute stages of the disease, rest, splinting and various forms of heat give relief. As the pain subsides, exercises are started with a view to maintain normal range of movement in all joints and prevent wasting of muscles. These have to be accepted as a lifestyle by the patient. Surgical measures and rehabilitatory procedures are to be instituted in crippled patients.

Surgical Correction

When permanent joint deformities develop, surgical measures have to be employed. These help to relieve morbidity and hasten recovery. Occupational therapy, social rehabilitation and re-education constitute the remedial measures necessary to bring the cripple back to the stream of almost normal day-to-day activities. Surgical measures include surgical decompression of the joint and synovectomy, especially at the wrists and carpal tunnel, reconstructive tendon surgery, osteotomies, excision arthroplasty, arthrodesis and joint replacement.

Medical Synovectomy

Synovial obliteration can be achieved by the instillation of osmic acid or a variety of radioactive colloids into the synovial cavity. Due to the wide availability of other modes of effective treatment and expertize with arthroscopic synovectomy this procedure is seldom done at present.

Ayurveda and Several Types of Herbal Medicine Prevalent in India

In *Ayurveda* and several types of herbal medicine prevalent in India, there are modalities of treatment which are preferred by many patients. Their role in the management of RA has to be evaluated by modern methods.

Source: Mukherjee S, Ghosh A (Eds). Monograph on RA. Mumbai, India: Indian College of Physicians, 2012.

VARIANTS OF RHEUMATOID ARTHRITIS

Several arthritic syndromes occur which show some resemblance to RA, but also show distinguishing features with overlap into other conditions. These include:

- Juvenile idiopathic arthritis (JIA)
- Felty's syndrome
- Sjögren's syndrome (SS)
- Palindromic rheumatism.

JUVENILE IDIOPATHIC ARTHRITIS

Juvenile idiopathic arthritis is an acute inflammatory and not autoimmune disease. It is the most common cause of chronic arthritis in childhood. This term encompasses all idiopathic arthritis affecting children below 16 years of age and lasting for more than 6 weeks. This may be oligoarticular, polyarticular or systemic varieties. In the oligoarticular types, lower limb joints-knees, hips, ankles and tarsal joints are affected asymmetrically. In the polyarticular type both small and large joints are affected, usually in a symmetrical manner. The clinical features may be confined 0–9 skeletal system but in 10%, the onset and course are characterized by systemic manifestations such as high fever (> 38.5°C), transient erythematous rash, generalized lymphadenopathy, hepatosplenomegaly, anemia and weight loss. This is known as **Still's disease**. Fever is intermittent with periods of normal temperature in between, during which period the child appears to be normal. The serious complications include macrophage activation syndrome (MAC) characterized by onset of thrombocytopenia, anemia, liver dysfunction and rapid downhill course which may end fatally. Gene expression profiling has identified different forms of the disease.

No antibodies are demonstrable. The pathological features distinguish two different types:

1. Oligoarticular less than 4 joints affected after 6 months of onset
2. Enthesitis-related arthritis.

In JIA, proinflammatory cytokine is excessively produced.

Treatment

In addition to all general measures required for polyarthritis, specific medications include methotrexate in relatively high doses and biological therapies, such as tocilizumab or etanercept. NSAIDs and corticosteroids relieve symptoms and may even modify the course of the disease.

About 50–60% of children recover by the time they reach adulthood, whereas 40% continue to have active disease even after 10 years. The monoclonal antibody tocilizumab is effective.

Source: Rajendran CP. Juvenile idiopathic arthritis. In: Rao URK (Ed). Manual of rheumatology: Rheumatic disease of childhood, 4th edition. Gurgaon, Haryana: Indian Rheumatology Association; 2014. pp. 390-406.

Macrophage Activation Syndrome

This is a complication which can develop in chronic rheumatic disorders, particularly in systemic onset JIA occurring in 5–10% cases. It is a hemophagocytic syndrome characterized by excessive activation of well differentiated macrophages, clinically manifesting as fever, hepatosplenomegaly, lymphadenopathy, peripheral blood cytopenias, liver involvement, intravascular coagulation and neurological lesions. This entity has been described from India, mostly associated with other connective tissue diseases or malignancy. Untreated, the mortality is high reaching up to 40%.

Classification

- ***Familial macrophage activation syndrome (MAS):*** It is caused by gene mutations.
- ***Secondary or acquired:*** It is seen in viral infections and malignancy.
- ***Reactive:*** It is also secondary to rheumatic diseases.

Pathogenesis

Macrophage activation occurs as a result of Th-1 type of T- cell activity. The T-cells augment the phagocytic capacity of the macrophages and also recruit the macrophages to the site of inflammation or infection. Bone marrow is stimulated to produce macrophages. Th-2 cells inhibit the processes.

Strong immunological activation may result from infection, malignancy or autoimmune disease. The viruses particularly incriminated include herpes viruses, especially Epstein-Barr virus, cytomegalovirus and adenoviruses.

The pathological findings in infection-associated histiocytosis include:

- Infiltration of all organs by benign-looking lymphocytes and histiocytes
- Atrophy of the germinal centers of lymph nodes and spleen.

The immunological abnormalities include hyperstimulation by infective agents, immunosuppression by drugs or HIV or immune dysregulation as in autoimmunity and malignancy.

Clinical Features

It includes fever, cutaneous rash, lymphadenopathy, hepatosplenomegaly and a downhill course. Failure of the liver and central nervous system (CNS), disseminated intravascular coagulation (DIC) and overwhelming infections may supervene. If untreated, the disease is fatal in about 2 weeks.

Investigations reveal cytopenias, rise in liver enzymes such as transaminases, at times alkaline phosphatase, lactate dehydrogenase (LDH) and high serum ferritin levels often exceeding 10,000 ng/dL. Blood picture is one of normocytic normochromic anemia, low reticulocyte counts and sometimes, atypical lymphocytes. ***The ESR is characteristically low due to hypofibrinogenemia***.

Bone marrow shows varying cellularity, with normal or at times, megaloblastic erythropoiesis. There is infiltration by histiocytes accounting for more than 2% of the cells. Many show hemophagocytosis, i.e. phagocytosis of erythrocytes. Phagocytes specific S100 proteins act as biomarkers helpful in diagnoses and follow-up.

Treatment

This includes supportive care and attention to the underlying disease. Two lines of treatment are available.

1. Interruption of function of the activated macrophages and histiocytes by drugs, such as etoposide, glucocorticoids and IV immunoglobulin (IVIG).
2. Interruption of function of the activated lymphocytes by glucocorticoids, cyclosporine, antithymocyte globulin (ATG) and biological drugs against TNF-α.

Source: Joshi VR, Kaushik B. Macrophage activation syndrome. In: Mukherjee S (Ed). Recent trends in connective tissue disorders. Mumbai, India: Indian College of Physicians; 2005. pp. 161-9.

FELTY'S SYNDROME

This is seen in older age groups. In addition to the classic features of seropositive RA, splenomegaly and neutropenia also occur. Splenomegaly may lead to hypersplenism. Splenectomy may have to be considered to correct hypersplenism, in addition to treatment for the rheumatoid state.

SJÖGREN'S SYNDROME (SS)

This is a chronic inflammatory autoimmune disease characterized by mixed cellular infiltration of the exocrine glands, particularly the lachrymal and salivary glands—a form of autoimmune exocrinopathy. This results in dryness of the eyes (***xerophthalmia***), dryness of the mouth (***xerostomia***) and frequently, dryness of the nose, throat and vagina due to the absence of secretions from the exocrine glands. This condition predisposes to increased risk of ***mucosa-associated lymphoid tissue lymphoma*** (MALT lymphoma).

Sjögren's syndrome may be primary in which it is the only demonstrable abnormality. Secondary SS, known also as sicca complex may be associated with any of the other autoimmune diseases. Radiation therapy of the head and neck for Hodgkin's disease, sarcoidosis, amyloidosis and tuberculosis may lead onto secondary SS.

Epidemiology

The disease is rare. Two precent of cases of RA and 0.73% of SLE may have associated SS. Almost all patients are females.

Immunology

At least one of the following autoantibodies will be present in the serum. These are antibodies to Ro/SSA LA/SSB, ANAs or RF. Levels of these antibodies correlate with the degree of cellular infiltration of the salivary and other glands. β-cell activation is the consistent immunoregulatory aberration. Viral infections may trigger-off the condition.

Clinical Features (Table 107.7)

A wide spectrum of clinical features may be present. These are:

- Ocular dryness and consequent symptoms
- Oral dryness with consequent symptoms
- Arthralgias in 75%, arthritis in 50%
- Skin manifestations—annular erythema on the face and trunk
- Vascular involvement—leading to Raynaud's phenomenon in 35–50%
- Gastrointestinal symptoms—dysphagia, atrophic gastritis
- Renal tubular acidosis
- Hypothyroidism in 10–15%
- MALT lymphoma.

Diagnosis

Schrimer's test is positive. This test is based on the wetting of a piece of filter paper by tears when applied to the palpebral conjunctiva. It is positive if the length of the

Table 107.7: Clinical features of Sjögren's syndrome (SS)

Glandular features	Extraglandular features
• Xerostomia	• Arthralgia/arthritis
• Dry eyes	• Skin manifestations
• Parotid enlargement	• Raynaud's phenomenon
• Organ involvement	• Lungs, kidneys, liver, peripheral nerves, muscles, central nervous system (CNS) and vasculitis

wetting is more than 5 mm in 5 minutes. Biopsy of the parotid gland, salivary gland scintigraphy and parotid sialography are helpful in diagnosis.

Treatment

The disease follows a benign prolonged course over 10–12 years or more. The conjunctival sac and mouth are kept moist. Hypromellose [hydroxypropyl methylcellulose (HPMC)] helps to moisten the conjunctival sac.

Strict oral hygiene is advised. Bromhexine 40 mg/day oral in divided doses and pilocarpine hydrochloride 5 mg TDS helps the dryness of the mucous membranes. Drugs, such as hydroxychloroquine 200 mg oral daily, corticosteroids, cyclosporine and interferon, have been tried with modest benefit. High-dose IVIG and plasma exchange may produce limited benefit.

Secondary Sjögren's Syndrome

This can occur as a complication of RA, primary Sjögren's syndrome (pSS), SLE, mixed connective tissue disease (MCTD) and primary biliary cirrhosis, polymyositis (PM)/dermatomyositis (DM), chronic active hepatitis (CAH) and mixed cryoglobulinemia. The underlying disease generally manifests earlier.

Prognosis: The condition is generally benign. Purpura, glomerulonephritis, decrease in complement levels and mixed monoclonal cryoglobulinemia are adverse prognostic factors.

Treatment: Eye care, sugar-free lozenges for xerostomia and lubricating jellies for vaginal dryness give symptomatic relief. Hydroxychloroquine 200 mg is effective to relieve arthralgia and myalgia. Systemic corticosteroids and immunosuppressants may be required for the treatment of systemic manifestations.

Source: Clair EW. Sjögren's syndrome. In: Firestein GS, Budd RC, Gabriel SE, McInnes IB, O'Dell JR (Eds). Kelley's Textbook of Rheumatology, 9th edition. 2013. pp. 1169-92.

PALINDROMIC RHEUMATISM

In this condition, repeated attacks of joint pains, redness and swelling occur. The attacks occur suddenly within hours and may affect one joint usually. The affected joint shows signs of inflammation. These last for a few days and subside without any residual lesions. The ESR is raised during the attacks and remains high even during the intervals. After varying periods of time, typical RA supervenes in many cases, whereas spontaneous remission occurs in some. Patients who are positive for RF or anti-CCP are likely to progress to RA. When the attacks are frequent, DMARDs, like sulfasalazine or hydroxychloroquine, are indicated.

CHAPTER 108

Systemic Lupus Erythematosus and Antiphospholipid Antibody Syndrome

Binoy J Paul, KV Krishna Das

Chapter Summary

- General Considerations
- Pathology
- Clinical Features
- Laboratory Investigations
- Systemic Lupus Erythematosus and Pregnancy
- Management
  - Drug-induced SLE
- Antiphospholipid Antibody Syndrome

SYSTEMIC LUPUS ERYTHEMATOSUS (SLE)

GENERAL CONSIDERATIONS

It is an inflammatory disease of autoimmune nature involving the connective tissue of several organ systems and associated with a variable course.

Systemic lupus erythematosus (SLE) is worldwide in distribution. In India, it constitutes 1–2% of the major rheumatological problems. Females predominate and the male to female proportion is 1:18. The disease is rare below the age of 5 years, but children account for 20%. More than 60% of cases are between the ages of 30 and 60. SLE results from a gross disturbance of immune mechanisms. Normal body constituents are rendered immunogenic by various damaging factors such as exposure to ultraviolet rays, infection, tissue injury, emotional stress, drugs or female sex hormones. Several autoantibodies are produced against the host's own tissues. There is suppression of T-lymphocytes function and overactivity of B-lymphocytes, leading to formation of autoantibodies, mainly belonging to immunoglobulin G (IgG) and immunoglobulin M (IgM) classes. Antigen-antibody complexes are formed with the utilization of complement factors. Deposition of immune complexes on tissues stimulates further inflammatory processes and this accounts for most of the lesions. C3 and C4 components of complement are mainly used up and, therefore, their levels fall.

Genetic Factors

These probably play an important role in many. This is evidenced by simultaneous occurrence of the disease in monozygotic twins, higher incidence of SLE and other connective tissue disorders in the relatives of SLE patients and the presence of several autoantibodies and low serum complement levels in many of them. Human leukocyte antigen (HLA) types B8, DR3 and DR2 and inherited deficiency of C1q, C4 and C2 complements are known to be associated with a higher incidence of SLE.

Pathogenesis

SLE develops in genetically susceptible individuals after trigger by environmental factors. The precise molecular mechanisms leading to autoimmune process is still not clear. The environmental factors seem to act via cellular pathways containing disease associated to polymorphisms. The environmental factors cause apoptosis of cells and the apoptotic material is not cleared by the phagocytes. The accumulated apoptosis-related endogenous nucleic acids stimulate the production of type 1 interferon (IFN) and promote autoimmunity by breaking the self-tolerance through activation of the dendritic cells. The stimulated dendritic cells act as antigen presenting cells, activating the B cells. The dendritic cells also promote differentiation, e.g. CD8+ T lymphocytes into cytotoxic T lymphocytes which are capable of cell lysis and generation of autoantigens. Hyperactive B cells also produce autoantibodies against several self-components. Activated T and B cells infiltrate several tissues and produce autoantibodies and immune complexes. Immune complex deposition leads to further inflammation and tissue damage. The progression of the disease occurs in distinct stages.

- **Stage 1:** Accumulated apoptosis-related endogenous nucleic acids stimulate the production of type 1 IFN.
- **Stage 2:** Activation of B cells and autoreactive T cells by type 1 IFN.
- **Stage 3:** Invasion of tissues by the hyperactive T and B cells, producing autoantibodies and immune complexes.
- **Stage 4:** Immune complexes and autoantibodies causing inflammation of tissues.
- **Stage 5:** Tissue damage, organ destruction and fibrosis.

Source: Wahren-Herlenius M, Dorner T. Immunopathogenic mechanisms of systemic autoimmune disease. Lancet. 2013;382(9894):819-31.

PATHOLOGY

The lesions of SLE are widespread and all tissues may be affected. Basically, four types of histological pictures are seen. These are:

1. Fibrinoid change
2. Collagen sclerosis
3. Formation of hematoxylin bodies
4. Inflammatory changes in arterioles and capillaries.

Tissue damage occurs in two different ways. These are: (1) Direct cytotoxicity (type II reaction) caused by antibody and complement, e.g. brain damage and abortion and (2) type III immune reaction caused by immune complexes and complement, e.g. renal and vascular lesions. Though the full spectrum of autoimmunity in SLE is not clear, several abnormalities have been observed. Among the tissues which become antigenic, nuclear components, especially nucleosomal histone complex, are important. Antinuclear antibodies (ANAs) are important demonstrable diagnostic markers occurring in over 95% of cases.

Table 108.1: Clinical manifestation of systemic lupus erythematosus (SLE)

Clinical manifestation	Frequency
Arthralgia/arthritis	89.3%
Skin rashes	64%
Malar rash	40%
Discoid lupus	5.3%
Photosensitivity	32%
Oral ulcers	64%
Alopecia	60%
Renal disease	33.3%
Neuropsychiatric symptoms	13.3%
Pleuropulmonary lesions	8%
Cardiac lesions	5.3%
Raynaud's phenomenon	2.7%

CLINICAL FEATURES

SLE presents a wide spectrum of clinical presentation depending upon the system affected maximally. Data collected from authors series is given in Table 108.1.

Source: Paul BJ, Farsaludeen M, Kumar N, et al. Clinical profile of SLE in Northern Kerala. J Indian Rheumatol Assoc. 2003;11:94-7.

In many cases, the presenting symptom is fever which may take several forms, from mild or subacute illness to severe hectic fever.

Arthritis and Arthralgia

Joint manifestations occur in 90% of subjects with SLE in the early stages. Large joints are affected more than others. Severity of joint involvement varies widely. Permanent deformities do not occur. Jaccoud's arthropathy may affect the hand in up to 50% of cases. It is characterized by reducible, nonerosive joint deformities with preservation of hand function. The pathogenesis of this condition is probably extra-articular, secondary to inflammation of and fibrosis of the periarticular tissue or tendons.

Hip pain may suggest the development of avascular necrosis and is usually a complication of corticosteroid therapy. It may be a manifestation of active SLE, most of which are associated with the presence of antiphospholipid antibodies (APLAs).

Skin Lesions

These occur in 64% of patients at some stage or other. The classic lesion is the erythematous, photosensitive, butterfly rash affecting the cheeks and nose and this is diagnostic. Discoid lupus, maculopapular rashes and purpura may occur in some. Frontal baldness may develop. Alopecia occurs due to breaking up of the hair. Painful ulcers may develop in the mouth and pharynx (Figs 108.1 to 108.4).

Discoid lupus is the form in which the only manifestation of the disease is confined to the skin for a few years. The lesions show scaling, atrophy, telangiectasia and keratotic plugging. They heal with considerable scarring. Some patients develop systemic lupus (Fig. 108.3).

Textbook of Medicine

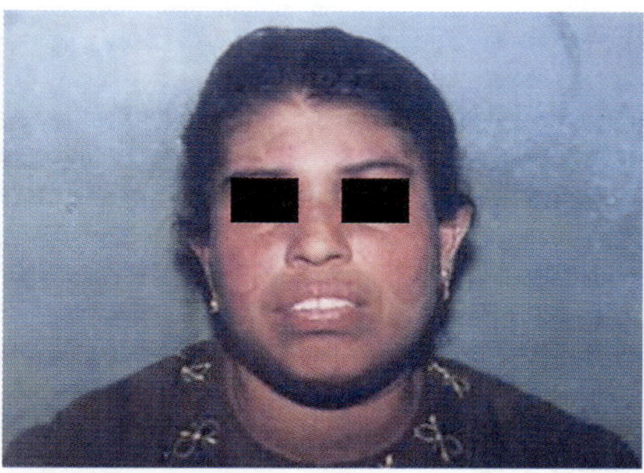

Fig. 108.1: Malar rash in SLE

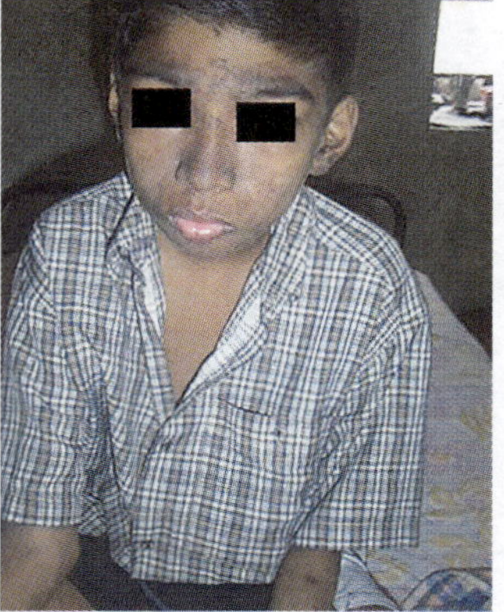

Fig. 108.2: Child with SLE—facial rash

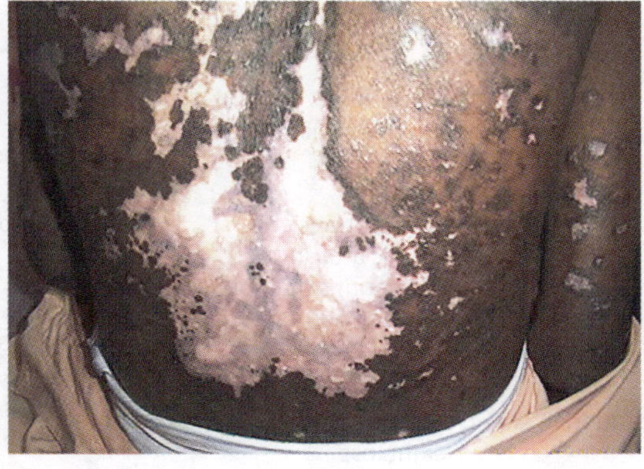

Fig. 108.3: Discoid lupus erythematosus (back)

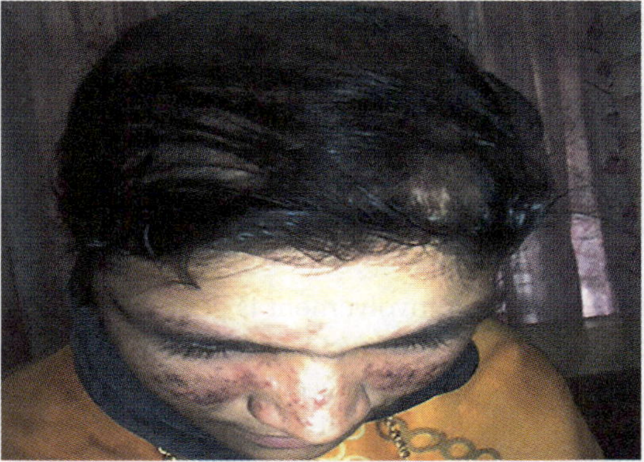

Fig. 108.4: Alopecia in SLE. ***Note:*** The rashes over the face, forehead and scalp

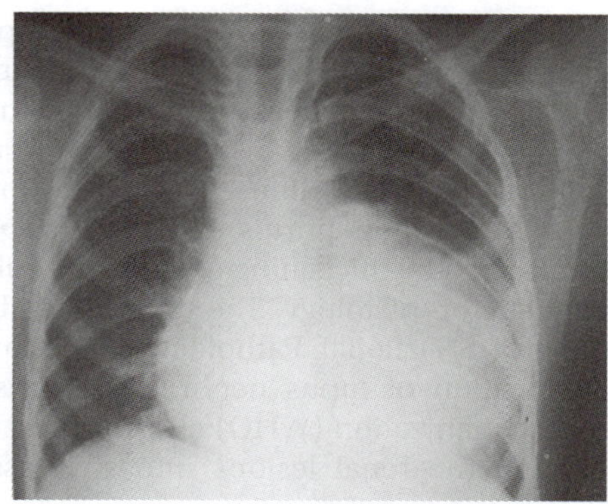

Fig. 108.5: Pericardial effusion (in the chest X-ray)

Cardiovascular System (CVS)

Cardiovascular lesions develop in 25–40% of cases. Cardiac lesions include pericarditis, pericardial effusion (Fig. 108.5), myocarditis with cardiac failure and valvulitis involving the mitral valve. ***Libman-Sacks endocarditis*** is a nonbacterial verrucous endocarditis affecting the mitral valve which is occasionally seen. It results in mitral incompetence. Cardiac abnormalities in the form of valvular thickening, vegetations and stenosis develop in decreasing order of frequency. Cardiac involvement does correlate with either the duration or the presence of other clinical manifestations, and its presence increases the morbidity. Early treatment clears the lesions if treatment is delayed, the structural abnormalities tend to persist.

Vasculitis leads to ***Raynaud's phenomenon***, necrotic ulcers of the finger pulp and chronic ulcers (Fig. 108.6). Patients with SLE have increased risk of ischemic heart disease (IHD) and major cardiac events apart from the risk factors posed by the disease and its treatment. Proper control of SLE brings down the cardiovascular risk as well.

Respiratory System

Common lesions are dry pleurisy, pleural effusion, fibrosing alveolitis and lupus pneumonitis. A ***syndrome of shrinking lung*** is uncommon but virtually pathognomonic of SLE. It is characterized by progressive reduction in lung volume with evidence of diaphragmatic weakness.

Kidney

This organ is affected in one-third of cases. Renal involvement used to be the most important lesion deciding the

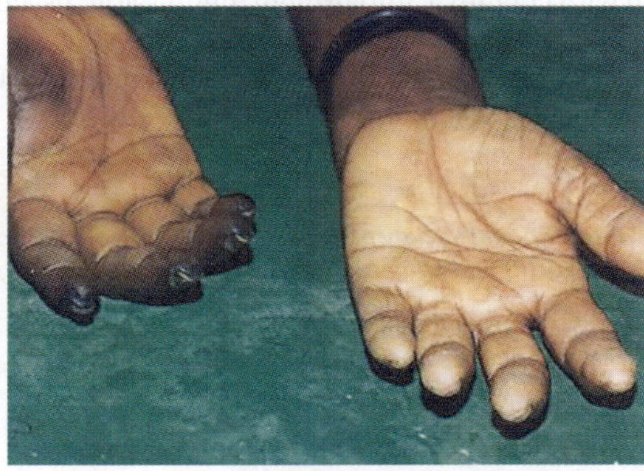

Fig. 108.6: SLE with antiphospholipid antibody syndrome. ***Note:*** The gangrene of the left fingers

prognosis. Renal involvement may remain asymptomatic with only proteinuria for long intervals or may manifest as nephrotic syndrome, hematuria, acute nephritic syndrome or renal failure. The histological pattern is that of focal glomerulonephritis, diffuse glomerulonephritis or membranous glomerulonephritis. The **wire loop lesions** which are produced by thickening of the glomerular walls are characteristic on histology. The International Society of Nephrology (ISN)/Renal Pathology Group proposed a new classification of lupus nephritis by revising the World Health Organization (WHO) classification in 2003. It has classified the renal lesions into six classes I–VI (Table 108.2).

Smith (Sm) antibodies are associated with membranous nephritis. Renal tubular acidosis (RTA) is occasionally seen in patients with anti-Ro or anti-La antibodies particularly and is due to tubulointerstitial disease. APLAs may be associated with renal vein thrombosis (RVT). Treatment instituted early in the disease helps to avert renal involvement. Indian experience is that 33% of adults and 80% of children develop renal lesions. Among them 14.3% had class II lesions, 22.8% had class III, 17.2% had class IV. Compared to the West, the progress of renal lesions appears to be more severe in Indian subjects. Fifty percent of class IV develop renal failure and 25% develop end-stage renal disease (ESRD) (*See* also Section 16, Ch 187).

The varied symptomatology in SLE has been shown in Table 108.3.

Nervous System

Neuro Lupus

This is clinically characterized by neuropsychiatric symptoms. The frequency probably varies between individuals and involves antibodies, immune complexes and cytokines. About 20 antibodies have been detected in the serum or cerebrospinal fluid (CSF) of these patients. Eleven of them are brain-specific and the rest are system-specific. The brain-specific autoantibodies are those binding neuronal tissue, N-methyl-D-aspartate (NMDA) receptor-specific, gangliosides microtubule-associated protein-2 (MAP-2), neurofilament and glial fibrillary acidic proteins (GFAP) specific. The most common auto-antibodies in patients with active neuropsychiatric lupus are anticardiolipin (aCL) antibodies. These antibodies correlated with cognitive, impairment, depression, psychosis, chorea, seizures and migraine.

Source: Lisnevskaia L, Murphy G, Isenberg D. Systemic lupus erythematosus. Lancet. 2014;384(9957):1878-88.

Table 108.2: Classification of renal lesions in SLE

Class	International Society of Nephrology (ISN)/Renal Pathology Society (RPS)—nomenclature
I	Minimal mesangial lupus nephritis
II	Mesangial proliferative lupus nephritis
III	Focal lupus nephritis
IV	Diffuse lupus nephritis
V	Membranous lupus nephritis
VI	Advanced sclerosing lupus nephritis

Table 108.3: The varied symptomatology in systemic lupus erythematosus

System	Common	Rare
Head and neck	• Alopecia • Oral ulcers • Nasal ulcers • KCS • Dry mouth • Episcleritis, scleritis	• Angioedema • Polychondritis • Retinitis • Optic neuritis • Uveitis
Skin	• Malar rash • Discoid rash • Maculopapular rash • Panniculitis (lupus profundus) • Nailfold capillary changes • Livedo reticularis	• Bullous lupus • Cutaneous vasculitis
Cardio-pulmonary	• Pleurisy/pleural effusion • Pericarditis/pericardial effusion • Interstitial pneumonitis (acute or chronic) • PH	• Myocarditis • Libman-Sacks endocarditis • Pulmonary hemorrhage • Coronary arteritis/aneurysm
Gastrointestinal (GI)	• Esophageal dysmotility • Hepatomegaly • Splenomegaly • Elevated liver enzymes	• Mesenteric vasculitis (with or without ischemia) • Colitis • Protein-losing enteropathy • Primary biliary cirrhosis • Budd-Chiari syndrome • Ascites
Nervous system	• Cognitive impairment • Seizures • Psychosis • Stroke (or transient ischemic attack) • Mononeuritis multiplex • Peripheral neuropathy	• Cranial neuropathy • Chorea • Pseudotumor cerebri • Transverse myelitis • Encephalopathy/coma
Constitutional	• Fever • Weight loss • Fatigue • Lymphadenopathy	
Musculoskeletal	• Polyarthralgias/arthritis • Myalgias	Myositis
Hematology	Anemia, hemolysis, thrombocytopenic purpura, LE cell phenomena	

Abbreviations: KCS = Keratoconjunctivitis sicca; PH = Pulmonary hypertension; LE = Lupus erythematosus

Nervous system involvement is generally a late manifestation, even though psychiatric symptoms may occur early. Lesions are caused by vasculitis and occlusive vascular phenomena. Patients with APLAs are more prone to develop stroke. Other manifestations include psychosis, convulsions, cranial nerve palsies, peripheral neuropathy, mononeuritis multiplex, chorea and cerebellar disturbances.

The total neurological picture may be the result of central nervous system (CNS) lupus or the secondary effects of complications or drugs. Infection, uremia and malignant hypertension are not uncommon. Patients with neurological involvement have a poor prognosis. ***Muscle involvement*** manifests as myalgia, rarely polymyositis and muscle wasting.

Hematology

Most of the cases show normocytic normochromic anemia. Other abnormalities include Coombs' positive autoimmune hemolytic anemia, leukopenia and thrombocytopenia. ***Lupus erythematosus (LE) cells*** are demonstrable by suitable techniques. These are polymorphonuclear leukocytes (PMNL) which have phagocytosed nuclear material under the influence of antibodies. Their number increases with the activity of the disease. Their presence and numbers generally correlate with the activity of the disease. In a marginally positive case, their diagnostic value is not absolute since a few other conditions such as rheumatoid arthritis (RA), drug allergy, and drug-induced lupus may also show this phenomenon. These cells are called LE cells.

SLE may be the primary lesion in at least 10% of cases of immune thrombocytopenic purpura (ITP). For considerable periods of time, the diagnosis may masquerade as ITP till other features of SLE manifest (Fig. 108.7).

Antiphospholipid Antibody Syndrome (APS) in SLE

It gives rise to additional features such as strokes, portal vein thrombosis (PVT), thrombophlebitis, pulmonary embolism and recurrent abortions in the later part of the second trimester or in the third trimester. Recurrent abortions with or without phlebothrombotic episodes should raise the possibility of this syndrome. The three types of APLAs seen in SLE are lupus anticoagulant (LAC) and/or aCL antibodies and beta 2-glycoprotein 1 which are demonstrable in over 30% of cases of SLE. Those that show aCL also give false-positive venereal disease research laboratory (VDRL) test.

About 40 APLAs have been described out of which at least triple positivity for LAC, aCL antibodies and beta-2 glycoprotein 1 antibodies must be positive on two or more occasions, 12 weeks apart for making a firm diagnosis. APLAs also predispose to atherosclerosis. In addition to anticoagulants to prevent thrombosis, statins, hydroxychloroquine (HCQ) and rituximab have been found useful in treatment. Statins are beneficial in APS. HCQ acts by inhibiting platelets aggregation thereby preventing thrombosis, suppresses disease activity and modifies lipid profile. HCQ and low-dose glucocorticoids are safe in pregnancy.

Presence of APLA imposes 30% lifetime risk of venous thromboembolism (VTE). ***Other features*** of this syndrome include thrombocytopenia and immune hemolytic anemia. Nearly 1–2% of young and 2–12% of elderly among the general population show low levels of APLAs without any other demonstrable disease.

Hepatosplenomegaly and lymphadenopathies also seen in active SLE. Abdominal emergencies may be produced by the development of acute peritonitis, perisplenitis or pancreatitis.

Eyes: These may be affected in a few cases, lesions include dryness of the conjunctiva and retinal abnormalities such as hemorrhage and exudates known as ***cytoid bodies***.

LABORATORY INVESTIGATIONS

SLE gives rise to an array of abnormalities, some being specific and the other nonspecific. The nonspecific features include, markedly elevated erythrocyte sedimentation rate (ESR) (above 100 mm), moderate anemia, leukopenia, thrombocytopenia and moderate to severe proteinuria. The specific tests depend upon the immunological abnormalities and they are described as follows.

Serological Abnormalities in SLE

Antinuclear Antibodies (ANAs)

They occur in around 95% of cases. Though the ANAs are not specific for SLE, their absence makes the diagnosis of SLE very unlikely. ANA done by indirect immunofluorescence (IIF) which is more specific than done by enzyme-linked immunosorbent assay (ELISA) method. Low levels of ANAs occur in RA (20%), Sjögren's syndrome (60%), scleroderma (40%), dermatomyositis (30%) and drug reactions in a variable number. Anti-dsDNA (double stranded-deoxyribonucleic acid) and anti-Sm antibodies are highly specific for SLE. Their titers are high during exacerbation and low during remission (Table 108.4).

LE Cell Phenomenon

The phenomenon is due to ANAs. Since the titer required for LE cell formation is high, the positivity for LE cells is less

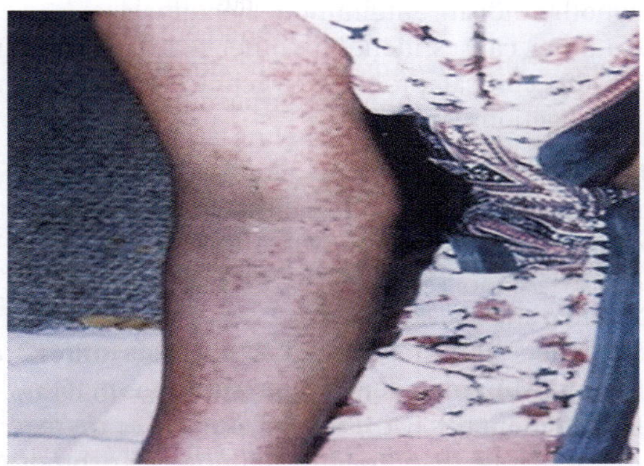

Fig. 108.7: SLE with thrombocytopenic purpura

Table 108.4: Frequency of antibodies in SLE	
ANAs	95%
Anti-dsDNA	60%
Anti-Sm	35%
False-positive VDRL	15%
Low level of C3	60%
Low level of C4	70%
APLAs	30%
Rheumatoid factor	25%

Abbreviations: ANAs = Antinuclear antibodies; Anti-dsDNA = Anti-double stranded deoxyribonucleic acid; VDRL = Venereal disease research laboratory; APLAs = Antiphospholipid antibodies

than that for ANA (Fig. 108.8). Due to the low sensitivity and low specificity, this test is almost replaced by ANA.

Other immunological markers which are nonspecific are antibodies against red blood cell (RBC), white blood cell (WBC) and platelets, circulating anticoagulants, antithyroid and other organ-specific antibodies, rheumatoid factor, false-positive Wassermann reaction and VDRL, cryoglobulins and circulating immune complexes. Levels of complements C3 and C4 are reduced. Cryoglobulins are IgG and IgM proteins which precipitate when cooled to 37°C and redissolved when warmed. They get deposited on the walls of blood vessels. They may be monoclonal, polyclonal or both.

Presence of ANAs and anti-dsDNA or anti-Sm should make the diagnosis reasonably certain if the clinical setting is appropriate.

Immunofluroscent antibody patterns have been shown in Figures 108.9 and 108.10.

DIAGNOSIS

The diagnosis of SLE should be suspected if there are febrile episodes with multisystem involvement and high ESR which is not responding to general lines of treatment. The American College of Rheumatology (ACR) has laid down criteria for diagnosis of SLE. These help to distinguish SLE from the other rheumatic disorders (Box 108.1). Presence of four or more of these features is highly suggestive for the diagnosis.

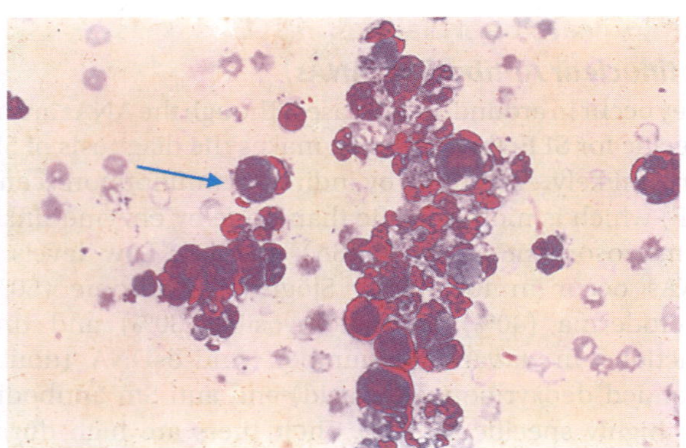

Fig. 108.8: Lupus erythematosus cell—a neutrophic leukocyte engulfing amorphous eosinophilic material—its own nucleus pushed to the periphery (arrow)

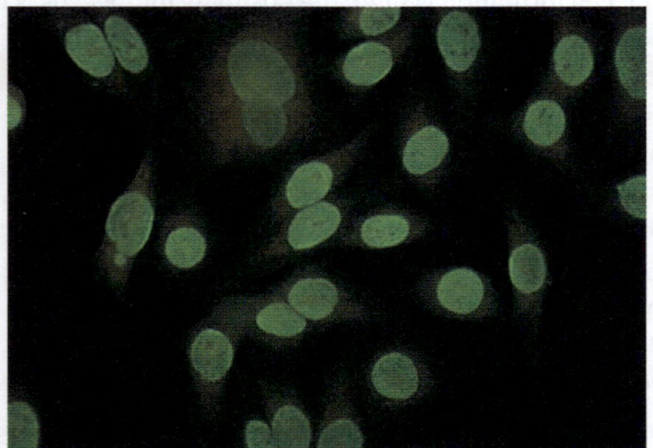

Fig. 108.9: Homogenous pattern (dsDNA)

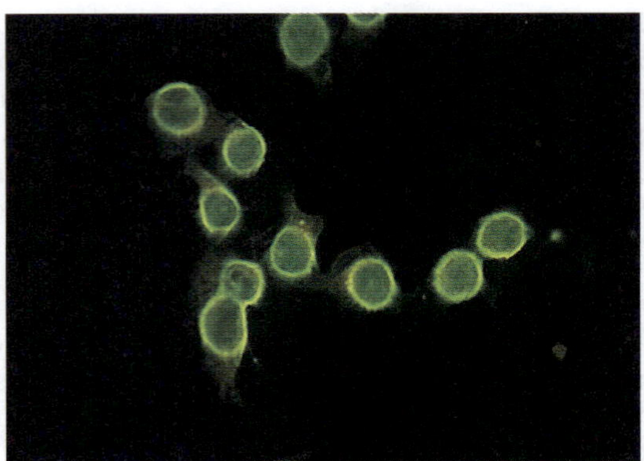

Fig. 108.10: Rim pattern (dsDNA)

Box 108.1: 1997 Revised ACR criteria for SLE

1. Serositis—pleuritis or pericarditis
2. Oral ulcers
3. Arthritis (nonerosive)
4. Photosensitivity
5. Blood disorders—hemolytic anemia, leukopenia, thrombocytopenia
6. Renal disorders—proteinuria (>0.5 g/day) or cellular casts
7. ANA
8. Immunological disorders—positive anti-ds DNA, anti-Sm, APLA or VDRL
9. Neurological disorders—seizure, psychosis
10. Malar rash
11. Discoid rash

Note: Presence of four out of the above eleven criteria is suggestive of SLE.

Abbreviations: ANA = Antinuclear antibody; Anti-dsDNA = Anti-double stranded deoxyribonucleic acid; anti-Sm = anti-Smith; APLA = Antiphospholipid antibody; VDRL = Venereal disease research laboratory

Several other workers have brought out criteria for diagnosis of SLE, a recent one brought out from Kozhikode Medical College is given here.

Source: Arathi N, Sasidharan PK, Geetha P. Kozhikode criteria for diagnosing systemic lupus erythematosus as a hematological disorder. J Blood Med. 2016;7:13-8.

Kozhikode Criteria for Diagnosis of SLE

Major/Essential Criteria

- Presence of an unresolved autoimmune disorder, which is known to occur with SLE [chronic ITP, autoimmune hemolytic anemia (AIHA) autoimmune hypothyroidism, autoimmune hepatitis].
- No other causes identified other than autoimmunity for the clinical problem by clinical reasoning and investigations if required.

Minor Criteria

- Another coexisting autoimmune disorder/any other evidence of autoimmunity
- Positive ANA
- Positive anti-dsDNA
- Sustained and definitive response to steroid and immunosuppressant even after 6 months of follow-up.

If the patient has two essential and two or more minor criteria, it can be diagnosed as SLE. Comparison of ACR criteria and Kozhikode criteria (Table 108.5).

Table 108.5: Comparison of ACR criteria and Kozhikode criteria

ACR criteria	*Kozhikode criteria*
Classification criteria only. It cannot be used for diagnosing SLE	Diagnostic criteria
Requires at least 4 out of the 11 criteria most of which are not present at the time of initial presentation, it could be at any time in a patient's history—delays diagnosis	Requires 4 out of 6, easily available features occurring early on, as the diagnosis of SLE is based on clinical suspicion. Useful helps early diagnosis
Under-representation of hematological manifestations, which is more common in at least our subset of patients	Adequate representation of hematological manifestations
Presence of ANAs is given equal weightage as other criterion	ANA is only a minor criteria, and helps in identification of ANA-negative SLE

Abbreviations: ACR = Americen College of Rheumatalogy; ANAs = Antinuclear antibodies; SLE = Systemic lupus erythematosus

COURSE AND PROGNOSIS

The course is variable, but in general, the prognosis is grave, if untreated. Treatment improves the outlook for morbidity and mortality considerably. At present, the majority of cases are detected early and they respond to treatment. More than 60–80% survive over 10 years. The main causes of death are renal failure, hypertension secondary to proliferative or membranous glomerulonephritis (MGN), cardiovascular events and CNS complications leading to strokes, coma or seizures. With modern therapy, the renal lesions can be arrested to a great extent, but neurological complications pose a major threat to life.

SYSTEMIC LUPUS ERYTHEMATOSUS AND PREGNANCY

(*See* also Section 16, Ch 189)

SLE does not affect fertility. SLE may flare up during pregnancy and this may cause deterioration of renal function. During pregnancy, there is increased risk of pre-eclampsia (5–38%). Presence of pre-existing hypertension, nephritis and APS increases the risk further. It may be difficult to distinguish between the renal-flare of SLE from pre-eclampsia; since both conditions are associated with hypertension, proteinuria, edema and deterioration of renal function. Complement C3 and C4 levels fall in SLE flare up whereas they remain unchanged in pre-eclampsia. In SLE, anti-dsDNA levels increase whereas they are unaffected in pre-eclampsia.

Abortion rates are high, 6–35% and stillbirths, 0–22%. Active SLE, presence of APLAs and history of previous fetal deaths are worse prognostic factors. Both LAC and aCL are associated with higher rates of fetal loss.

Neonatal lupus erythematosus (NLE) may develop in the baby; caused by maternal antibodies to the 52KD SSA/RO, 60KD SSA/RO or 48 KD SSB/La ribonucleoproteins. The baby may present with skin rash and **congenital complete heart block**. Except the heart block, the other features disappear in a few days.

Aspirin and nonsteroidal anti-inflammatory drugs (NSAIDs) should be avoided during the last weeks of pregnancy due to risk of hemorrhage.

HCQ, NSAIDs, prednisolone and azathioprine can be continued during pregnancy if the mother's condition warrants. Breastfeeding is safe for the baby if the mother is taking prednisolone and HCQ. Breastfeeding is contraindicated if the mother is on azathioprine, cyclophosphamide, methotrexate or cyclosporine A.

The chance of SLE being transmitted to the offspring is low (± 10%). Contraceptive pills do not flare up SLE.

MANAGEMENT

Since there are no curative measures, the main aim is to induce remission and prevent relapses. General management consists of avoidance of direct sunlight and offending drugs and prompt attention to complications (Box 108.2).

Drug treatment depends upon the stage and severity of the disease. Mild SLE with only cutaneous and joint involvement without constitutional symptoms respond to HCQ 200 mg od or bd given orally. Symptomatic relief for arthritis and constitutional features like fever can be provided by the use of NSAIDs and analgesics. Arthritis not responding to HCQ and low-dose steroids may need methotrexate or leflunomide. In moderately severe SLE in which major systems are affected, steroids are used as the mainstay of treatment with immunosuppressants as add-on drugs. In severe SLE, there is gross affection of vital organs, particularly the heart, kidneys, lungs and brain. In them, immunosuppressants are almost always required.

Corticosteroids are indicated as the first-line drugs in major organ lupus (renal, CNS, lung or cardiac involvement). On an average, the dose is 1 mg prednisolone/kg/bw given orally daily. Once the symptoms are controlled, the dose can be slowly tapered off over a period of months or years. The activity of the disease is assessed clinically and by the fall in ESR, dsDNA titer and complement levels. Many cases will require maintenance dose of steroids for several years.

Immunosuppressant Drugs

The commonly used drugs are **cyclophosphamide** and **azathioprine**. They are indicated in severe life-threatening disease, failure to respond to steroids or intolerance to steroids. However, infections, severe anemia and leukopenia are relative contraindications. The usual daily dose of cyclophosphamide is 2–3 mg/kg orally or monthly pulse 15 mg/kg IV monthly for 6 months and followed by azathioprine is 1–3 mg/kg given in divided dosage. Several dosage schedules of cyclophosphamide have been advocated. High doses such as 0.5–1 g/m² given once a month for 6 months, followed by smaller doses at longer intervals for 2 years have been found to be beneficial in severe cases. Some individuals have genetic defects which lead to severe marrow suppression following exposure to azathioprine. Therefore, persons receiving this drug should be monitored by regular blood tests.

Mycophenolate mofetil: It is a potent suppressor of lymphocyte proliferation by its inhibitory effect. The drug is found to be effective in lupus nephritis and lung involvement. Dose is 500–1,000 mg twice daily. Most common adverse side effects are nausea, vomiting and leukopenia.

Box 108.2: Summaries of the action of drugs used in SLE

- Glucocorticoids
  - Induce anti-inflammatory cytokines IL-10, IL-1 receptor antagonist and annexin-1
  - Decrease production of the adhesion molecules and inflammatory cytokines (IL-2, IL-6 and TNF)
  - Inhibit processing of antigens by monocytes for presentation to lymphocytes
  - Inhibit cyclo-oxygenase (COX) 2 and inducible NOS. Steroids are used for all features of SLE.
- NSAIDs have analgesic, antipyretic, anti-inflammatory properties. They inhibit COX 1 and 2. They are used for fever, arthritis and serositis.
- Hydroxychloroquine (HCQ)
  - It has immunomodulating properties without immuno-suppression. It increases lysosomal pH and interferes with antigen processing and possible modulation of the immune response mediated by the TLR9. It is used for arthritis, skin rashes and fatigue.
  - Other possible effects include: (1) Reduction of nephritis, (2) antithrombotic properties and (3) reduction of cholesterol concentration.
- Cyclophosphamide
  - Action:
    - It forms active alkylating metabolites (4-hydroxycyclo-phosphamide, phosphoramide mustard and acrolein).
    - It prevents cell division by suppressing DNA synthesis. It is used for lupus nephritis and severe SLE.
- Azathioprine (a purine analog that suppresses DNA synthesis)
  - Used for systemic features of lupus and maintenance therapy lupus nephritis class III and IV
  - Used for induction of remission of lupus nephritis in cases where cyclophosphamide which causes sterility is to be avoided
  - Steroid sparing effect.
- Biological treatments available or potentially available for the treatment of SLE.
  - ***Targeting B cells:***
    - B cell depleting therapy through rituximab
    - B cell modulating therapy—epratuzumab
    - Inhibition of B cell survival—belimumab, atacicept
    - Other potential B cell (plasma cell) targeting strategies—bortezomib.
  - ***Targeting T cells:*** Inhibition of T cell function—abatacept, ruplizumab, toralizumab and lupuzor (this is a new non-immune suppressant peptide drug undergoing clinical trials)
  - ***IL 6:*** Tocilizumab
  - ***TNF-alpha inhibitors:***
    - Infliximab
    - Etanercept
  - ***Type 1 IFN inhibitors:***
    - Sifalimumab
    - Rontalizumab
  - ***Complement inhibitors:*** Eculizumab.

Abbreviations: IL = Interleukin; TNF = Tumor necrosis factor; NOS = Nitric oxide synthase; DNA = Deoxyribonucleic acid; SLE = Systemic lupus erythematosus; TLR9 = Toll-like receptor 9; IFN = Interferon

Rituximab: It is an anti-CD20 monoclonal antibody (mAb). CD20 is a cell surface antigen seen on the B cells not on plasma cells. Rituximab is found to be useful in resistant lupus nephritis by selectively eliminating peripheral B cells. Two doses of 1,000 mg of the drug are given at 2 weeks interval IV. If needed, it can be repeated after 6–12 months.

Belimumab: It is a mAb to soluble B cell stimulator B lymphocyte stimulator (BLyS) also known as B cell activating factor (BAFF) which is a key survival factor for B lymphocytes. It is approved for clinical use by US Food and Drug Administration (FDA) (not yet available in India) for active SLE with musculoskeletal or cutaneous manifestations not responding to conventional drugs. Dose is 10 mg/kg IV at 2 weeks interval for first 3 doses and 4 weeks interval thereafter. The drug is not approved for lupus nephritis or other major organ involvement.

Autologous stem cell transplantation has been used as a therapeutic strategy in SLE and other autoimmune rheumatic diseases in patients who are refractory to conventional treatment. The reported overall survival is 81% with 18% mortality recorded at 2 years. Despite high morbidity and mortality, the ability to achieve a sustained disease-free state in patients with poor prognosis supports autologous stem cell transplantation in patients with refractory lupus.

General supportive measures include maintenance of nutrition, management of infection, prevention of direct exposure to sunlight using sunscreens, analgesics and hematinics. Specific clinical symptoms like convulsions, psychosis, pericardial effusion and cardiac failure require appropriate management.

For maintenance therapy in mild cases, especially with localized skin lesions, HCQ in a dose of 200–400 mg given oral daily is effective. Long-term therapy may lead to ocular complications which very rare.

In severe cases with rapid deterioration of renal function or neuropsychiatric manifestations, high doses of methylprednisolone 1 g given IV daily for 3 days with pulse doses of cyclophosphamide 0.5–1 g daily IV may be required to tide over the crisis. Intravenous immunoglobulin (IVIG) at a dose of 400 mg/kg for 5 days is tried with success in resistant thrombocytopenia and massive proteinuria.

Source:

1. Bertsias GK, Salmon JE, Boumpas DT. Therapeutic opportunities in systemic lupus erythematosus: state of the art and prospects for the new decade. Ann Rheum Dis. 2010;69(9):1603-11.

2. Gulati A, Bagga A. Management of lupus nephritis. Ind J Rheumat. 2012;7:69-79.

Drug-induced SLE

Several drugs like hydralazine, procainamide, dilantin, mesantoin, oral contraceptives (OCPs), phenothia-zines isoniazid (INH), para-aminosalicylic acid (PAS), methyldopa, levodopa, penicillin and sulfonamides lead to a syndrome of fever, arthritis, skin rashes and lymphadenopathy which closely resembles SLE. The clinical and biochemical profile are identical with natural SLE but the course is mild and renal and CNS manifestations are rare. In these patients, ANA will be positive but anti-dsDNA will be negative, antihistone antibody will be positive in majority of drug-induced lupus. Withdrawal of the offending drug leads to resolution. If resolution is delayed, short course of corticosteroids (20–30 mg prednisolone oral daily) will accelerate remission. The patient should be informed about drug toxicity in future.

ANTIPHOSPHOLIPID ANTIBODY SYNDROME (APS)

Syn: Hughes syndrome (Refer to Ch 178)

This condition is seen not uncommonly in all parts of India and several case reports and studies are available.

It is characterized by the presence of a family of autoantibodies termed APLAs. These are a family of 20 antibodies that are directed against phospholipid-binding plasma proteins. These include ***aCL antibodies, LAC, beta 2-glycoprotein 1*** and others. These antibodies are directed against anionic phospholipids participating in the coagulation cascade. These antibodies are detected by radioimmunoassay (RIA) and ELISA tests. APS shows overlap between systemic autoimmune connective tissue diseases and coagulapathies, particularly thrombophilic states. Moderate to high positivity of two readings (>20 units) at 12 weeks apart confirms the lab diagnosis.

It may be primary or secondary. In ***primary APS***, there is no evidence of underlying connective tissue disease. ***Secondary APS*** occurs in association with other connective tissue diseases, particularly SLE in which 15–34% have LAC and 12–30% have aCL.

Several surveys done worldwide show the presence of APLAs in small quantities in 2–5% of the general population. LAC and aCL may occur together in the same individual or only either of them may be present. Persons with aCL also show the presence of LAC in 20%. On the other hand, the presence of aCL in those with LAC is 80%.

CAUSES OF SECONDARY APS

- ***Connective tissue diseases:*** SLE, Sjogren's syndrome, mixed conective tissue disease (MCTD), PSS, progressive systemic sclerosis, primary SS, discoid lupus, RA and AS.
- ***Other immunological disorders:*** Crohn's disease, systemic vasculitis, ITP, Behcet's syndrome and others.
- ***Malignancy:*** Lymphomas, cancers of kidney, lung and ovary.
- ***Drug-induced:*** OCPs, quinine, quinidine, phenytoin, hydralazine, procainamide, beta-adrenergic blockers, biologics like alpha IFN.

These antibodies predispose to venous and arterial thrombosis and consequent complications. They also lead to fetal loss in pregnancy. The hallmark of APS is the presence of the antibodies aCL and LAC, false-positive VDRL and Wassermann reaction and other antibodies against cofactors associated with anionic phospholipids.

Common Presenting Features

- Deep vein thrombosis (DVT) 32%
- Thrombocytopenia which is mild and subclinical 22%
- Livedo reticularis 20%
- Stroke 13%
- Superficial thrombophlebitis 9%
- Fetal loss 8%
- Transient ischemic attacks (TIA) 7%
- AIHA 7%
- Arterial thrombosis in limbs and several organs. This may lead to gangrene of the limbs and superficial structures or infarcts in deep organs. Others include osteonecrosis, pulmonary hypertension, renal lesions and catastrophic antiphospholipid antibody syndrome (CAPS) (*See* Section 15, Ch 178).

APS and Pregnancy

Fetal loss occurs around the 10th week of pregnancy. Placental venous thrombosis is a contributory factor. Presence of LAC antibodies or IgG class of aCL antibodies confers a risk of 50% for fetal loss. The central role for thrombosis and fetal death is played by endothelial cells. Proper management leads to successful outcome in over 75% of such cases (Table 108.6).

Causes of Miscarriage in APS

- Thrombosis and infarction of the uteroplacental vasculature.
- Interference with signal induction mechanisms which control endometrial cell decidualization, promotion of trophoblast apoptosis, decrease in trophoblast fusion and impairment of trophoblast invasion.

Management

Unfractionated or low-molecular weight heparin (LMWH) and low-dose aspirin improve the fetal survival in 80–85% of cases. Heparin should be given when pregnancy is confirmed or when the cardiac activity of the fetus is demonstrable. Heparin dose should be individualized. Heparin, in addition to its anticoagulant effect, can bind to APLAs and antagonize the action of Th1 cytokine IFN-gamma, thereby protecting the fetus from injury. Aspirin is also given to prevent thrombotic events.

CATASTROPHIC ANTIPHOSPHOLIPID ANTIBODY SYNDROME (CAPS)

In CAPS, widespread vascular occlusions in multiple vital organs may develop. Vascular occlusion occurs in three or more organs simultaneously within a period of 1 week. APLAs are present. Histology of the organs reveals noninflammatory thrombotic lesions.

Table 108.6: Revised criteria for APS

Clinical	*Laboratory*
Vascular thrombosis • One or more episode of arterial venous or small vessel thrombosis • Exclusion of other causes • Exclusion of male >55 years; female >65 years **Pregnancy morbidity** • Three or more abortion <10 weeks • One or more abortion >10 weeks • One or more premature birth before 34 weeks due to PET/eclampsia/placental insufficiency	• Positive lupus anticoagulant • aCLA IgG/IgM in titer >40 units • Anti-b Gp1 (IgG/IgM) (>99th percentile titer) • Antibodies should be positive for two or more occasions at least 12 weeks apart

Note: Patient is classified as APS if one clinical plus one lab criterion is present.

Source: Miyakis S, Lockshin MD, Atsumi T, et al. International consensus statement on an update of the classification criteria for definite antiphospholipid syndrome (APS). J Thromb Haemost. 2006;4(2):295-306.

Abbreviations: aCLA = Anticardiolipin antibody; IgG = Immunoglobulin G; IgM = Immunoglobulin M; PET = Pre-eclampsia toxemia

Infections, pregnancy or surgery may trigger off this syndrome. If untreated, mortality exceeds 50%, usually due to cardiopulmonary failure. CAPS has to be distinguished from disseminated intravascular coagulation (DIC), thrombotic thrombocytopenic purpura (TTP), other forms of systemic vasculitis and severe infections. ***Laboratory investigations*** help to distinguish between them.

Condition	Diagnostic features
Systemic vasculitis	Thrombocytosis
DIC	Thrombocytopenia and low fibrinogen levels
TTP	Low platelets and presence of schistocytes

Coexistence of APS with SLE worsens the clinical features of the latter.

Management of APS

Elective long-term anticoagulant therapy with heparin and later on, coumarin drugs to keep INR at 2.5–3 depending on the severity and frequency of thrombotic episodes is effective in preventing thrombotic complications. HCQ is also found to reduce the level of APLA in primary and secondary APS and is usually given along with oral anticoagulants.

Normalization of LAC or aCL is not on indication for stopping therapy. Treatment has to be continued indefinitely. There is no firm indication for using glucocorticoids or immunosuppressant drugs unless the APS is associated with active SLE or immunological diseases.

Statins upregulate endothelial nitric oxide and also block the thrombogenic tendencies of APS.

Thrombocytopenia: Corticosteroids and/or IVIG should be considered.

Management of CAPS: It is a life-threatening emergency. A combination of high-intensity anticoagulation, corticosteroids, plasma exchange and IVIG form the cornerstone of therapy.

Treatment of Asymptomatic Antiphospholipid Positivity

There is no consensus of opinion on this matter. Prophylactic low-dose aspirin is recommended by some workers.

At times, clinical features of APS occur, without demonstrable antibodies. Anticoagulation therapy, given on presumptive grounds, has helped such patients. Each case has to be managed on individual merits.

Source: Lim W, Crowther MA, Eikelboom JW. Management of antiphospholipid antibody syndrome: a systematic review. JAMA. 2006;295(9):1050-7.

CHAPTER 109

Progressive Systemic Sclerosis
(Syn: Scleroderma)

KV Krishna Das, Binoy Paul

Chapter Summary

- General Considerations
- Pathology
- Clinical Features
- Diagnosis
- Overlap Syndrome
- Undifferentiated Connective Tissue Disease
- Mixed Connective Tissue Disease

GENERAL CONSIDERATIONS

In this generalized disorder of connective tissue, fibrosis and degenerative changes predominate. The skin, synovium, digital arteries, gastrointestinal tract (GIT), lungs, heart, kidneys and other organs may be affected. The most conspicuous feature is thickening and hardening of the skin, which becomes 'hide-bound'. The term scleroderma is derived from the Greek word 'scleros', which means 'hard' and 'derma', which means skin. The two major categories are: (1) Limited cutaneous scleroderma where sclerosis is confined to the extremities distal to the elbows and knees with or without facial involvement and (2) diffuse cutaneous systemic sclerosis (SSc).

The extent of skin involvement and presence of lesions in internal organs form the basis of classification into diffuse and limited diseases.

- ***Localized scleroderma (morphea):*** The lesion is restricted to a localized area on the skin
- ***Linear scleroderma:*** The skin involvement is linear. It leads to atrophy of underlying tissues. In the face, it gives a characteristic appearance
- ***Disseminated morphea:*** There are multiple skin lesions, but systemic involvement is minimal or absent
- ***CREST syndrome:*** This consists of calcification of subcutaneous tissues, Raynaud's phenomenon, esophageal hypomotility, sclerodactyly and telangiectasia
- ***Progressive systemic sclerosis (PSS):*** There is progressive involvement of skin and other internal organs leading to systemic manifestations. This carries the worst prognosis.

Even in the limited cutaneous disease occlusive vascular lesions, gastrointestinal (GI) lesions, interstitial pulmonary fibrosis and pulmonary hypertension may occur. Scleroderma occurs all over the world and is occasionally seen in Indian subjects.

PATHOLOGY

The three cardinal features are excessive collagen production and deposition, vascular damage and inflammation or autoimmunity. Small vessel inflammation and injury leads to obliteration vasculopathy. The prominent pathological abnormality is overproduction and cross-linking of collagen and vasculitis. The vascular lesion consists of structural damage to small vessels occurring extensively, resulting in proliferative changes and luminal narrowing. The humoral arm also shows abnormalities. The presence of antinuclear antibodies (ANAs), inflammatory lesions in the skin and lung and increased amounts of profibrotic chemokines in circulation and in tissues are the consequences of immune activation. ANA is positive in 50% of cases; antibodies to single stranded ribonucleic acid (ssRNA) develop. Scl-70, also known as anti-topoisomerase is an antibody against an extracellular nuclear antigen. It may be detectable in 50% of cases of diffuse scleroderma. Its presence is a predictive marker for pulmonary involvement. In 75% cases of limited scleroderma, anti-centromere antibody (ACA) are found to be positive. There is activation of T lymphocytes and complement. Advanced lesions show atrophy of the dermis, loss of hair follicles and sweat glands, depigmentation and calcinosis.

Skin

The dermal collagen is increased leading to fibrosis. Endarteritis and calcinosis supervene in some cases. Collagen types 1 and 3 are increased, the former being more abundant.

Joints

Synovium shows infiltration with lymphocytes and plasma cells and deposition of fibrin. The changes may resemble those of rheumatoid disease, but pannus formation is unusual.

Kidneys

Changes occur in the interlobular arteries. These comprise intimal hyperplasia, fibrinoid necrosis of afferent arterioles and glomerular tufts, and thickening of glomerular basement membrane (GBM). These changes lead to cortical infarctions and glomerulosclerosis. The lesions may resemble those seen in malignant hypertension (*See* Section 16, Ch 187).

Muscles

The histological lesions resemble those seen in myopathy such as fragmentation and loss of striation of muscle fibers and nuclear changes. Affected muscles are replaced by fibrosis.

Vasculitis

Affection of small arteries leads to intimal thickening and narrowing of lumen. The lesions are particularly demonstrable in the digital arteries of patients showing Raynaud's phenomenon.

CLINICAL FEATURES

The disease is seen more in the 4th and 5th decades and male to female ratio is 1:4. Onset is insidious. The initial symptoms are variable. These include Raynaud's phenomenon, tightness of the extremities, arthralgia and vague manifestations.

Cutaneous Manifestations

Three stages can be distinguished during the evolution of the disease. These are edematous, indurative and atrophic stages. Initial manifestations are edema of the hands and feet, which may extend more proximally. The edema is followed by thickening and tightening of the skin. Skin loses its normal pliability and ultimately becomes 'hide-bound' and nonpinchable. Appendages are lost over the affected areas. Affection of the face gives rise to the 'mouse head' appearance with microstomia, beaked nose, mask-like expression and difficulty in opening the mouth (Fig. 109.1A).

Pigmentary changes develop over the extremities and anterior chest wall. These consist of hyperpigmentation or a combination of spotty hyper- and hypopigmentation (salt and pepper skin), and telangiectasia over the fingers, palms, face, lips and tongue (Fig. 109.1B). The tight atrophic skin is particularly vulnerable to trauma. Painful, nonhealing, chronic, indolent ulcers are common over the fingers and toe tips. When the extremities are predominantly affected, the condition is called ***acrosclerosis***. Over the palmar aspect of the terminal phalanges, subcutaneous calcification occurs. These ulcerate and extrude calcareous material. Ischemia aggravates this tendency. Paroxysmal vasospasm of digital blood vessels leads to Raynaud's phenomenon, which is present in 25% of cases, when exposed to cold environment. Raynaud's phenomenon may also occur during emotional disturbances or even spontaneously.

Raynaud's Phenomenon

It is the term used to describe the episodic events of vasoconstriction of the digital arteries, precapillary arterioles and cutaneous arteriovenous shunts. Raynaud's phenomenon may be primary or secondary.

Features of primary Raynaud's phenomenon:
- Vasospasm is precipitated by cold or emotional stress
- Symmetrical in distribution
- Absence of necrosis and gangrene
- Normal nail fold capillaries
- Normal erythrocyte sedimentation rate (ESR) and negative tests for dyscollagenoses.

Secondary Raynaud's phenomenon is characterized by:
- Age over 30 years
- Presence of tissue necrosis
- Evidence of connective tissue diseases (CTDs)
- Abnormal nail fold capillaries and presence of autoantibodies.

Limited cutaneous forms, often confined to the skin may be seen at times. These include morphea, linear scleroderma and limited cutaneous SSc syndrome, also known as ***CREST (consists of calcinosis, Raynaud's phenomenon, esophageal dysmotility, sclerodactyly*** and ***telangiectasia) syndrome***. Morphea and linear scleroderma give rise to well-demarcated pale, indurated lesions of the skin and subcutaneous connective tissue. Pitted scar of pulp of the fingers secondary to digital vasculopathy is also common in long-standing cases

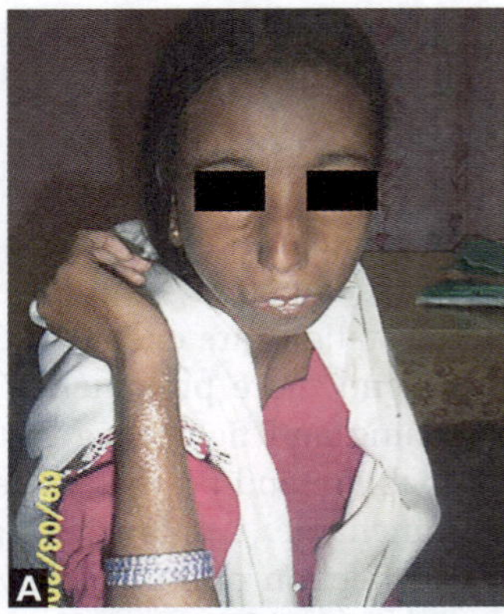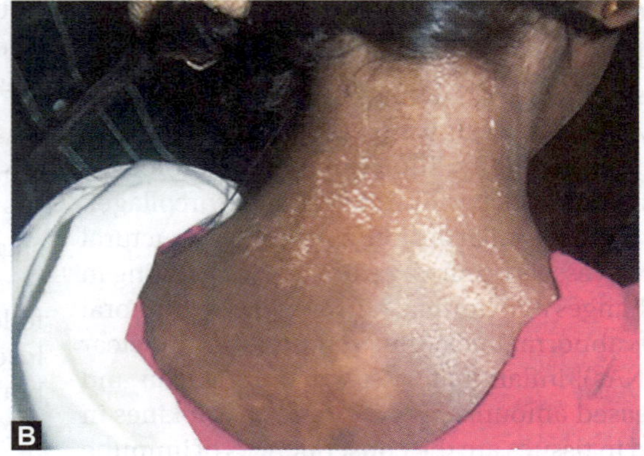

Figs 109.1A and B: Progressive systemic sclerosis (PSS). **A.** Pinched nose, purse-like mouth and hypopigmentation over the forearm; **B.** Hypo- and hyperpigmentation and thickening of skin

(Fig. 109.2). Even in the absence of systemic involvement, the serological markers may be present.

In patients with Raynaud's phenomenon, two markers viz abnormal cutaneous capillaries in the nailfold (detectable by an ophthalmoscope) and presence of ANAs predict the subsequent development of scleroderma.

Raynaud's phenomenon may be part of SSc, without evidence of cutaneous scleroderma (***scleroderma sine scleroderma***) but with only systemic lesions. In this form, the humoral markers such as antinuclear factor (ANF) and Scl-70 are detectable, and these help in diagnosis.

Systemic Manifestations

The pattern of involvement reported in Indian series is acrosclerosis (53%), arthralgia (83%), arthritis (20%), upper GI lesion (66%), lower GI lesion (33%), lungs (20%) and kidneys (25%).

PSS overlaps with other connective tissue disorders such as systemic lupus erythematosus (SLE) (14%), rheumatoid arthritis (RA) (8.4%) and mixed connective tissue disease (MCTD) (2.8%).

Bones and Joints

Mobility is restricted due to fibrosis of soft tissue. Primary articular involvement can occur in many. Crepitus can be palpated over major joints and tendons and 50% develop deformities. Long-standing cases show erosion and absorption of the terminal phalanges.

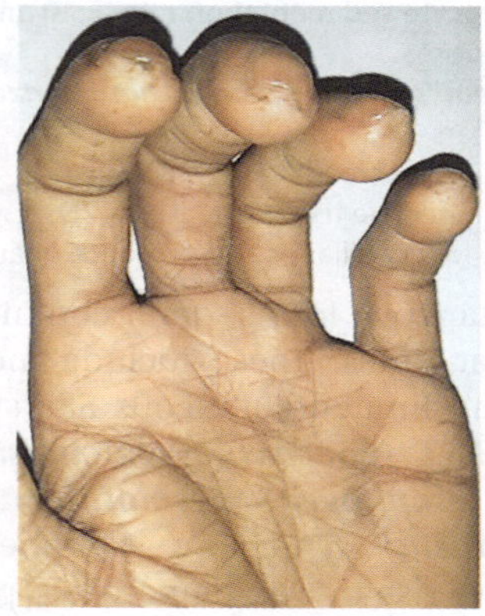

Fig. 109.2: Digital pitting scar on the pulp of index, middle and ring finger in a patient with progressive systemic sclerosis (PSS) due to vascular necrosis

Other Systems

Gastrointestinal tract: Affection of the GIT can be demonstrated by investigations even in the asymptomatic cases. Esophagus and intestines are affected most frequently. Common symptom is dysphagia, which is initially due to esophageal spasm and later fibrosis. Barium swallow reveals dilated esophagus resembling achalasia cardia. The small and large intestines show dilatation, impaired peristalsis and malabsorption.

Involvement of the lungs results in progressive interstitial fibrosis and alveolocapillary block syndromes. Cystic changes are seen occasionally. Secondary pulmonary hypertension and cor pulmonale develop in long-standing cases.

Cardiovascular system (CVS): Heart is enlarged with myocardial dysfunction and rarely conduction defects. Malignant hypertension is more common.

Renal involvement: Secondary hypertension and renal failure may follow. Scleroderma renal crisis is the rapid development of malignant hypertension and oliguric renal failure during the course of SSc.

Nervous system involvement: This manifests as cranial or peripheral neuropathy at times.

DIAGNOSIS

This is mainly clinical—the most important finding is the hard skin, which is not pinchable and is also devoid of hair. Laboratory investigations help to rule out other conditions. Skin biopsy helps to confirm the diagnosis and rule out other conditions, like eosinophilic fasciitis and scleroderma.

Laboratory Investigations

ESR is moderately raised but it may be normal in early cases and in cases where only the skin is affected. During the active phase, immunoglobulin G (IgG) may be elevated. Muscle enzymes are elevated when myopathy occurs. Rheumatoid factor (RF) is positive in 20–25% and atrial natriuretic factor (ANF) in about 95% cases in low titers Scl-70 are detectable in 50% patients with diffuse disease. ACA is positive in 75% cases of limited scleroderma (Table 109.1).

Nailfold capillaroscopy is a noninvasive method to detect vascular changes of scleroderma. The typical

Table 109.1: Relationship between the prevalence of specific antibodies in relation of the clinical features

Autoantibody	Prevalence (%)	Associated clinical features
Antinuclear antibody	>95	—
Anti-Scl-70 (anti-topoisomerase I)	20–40	Lung disease, diffuse skin involvement, African-Americans, worse prognosis
Anticentromere	20–40	CREST syndrome, digital ulcerations or digital loss
Anti-RNA polymerases	4–20	Diffuse skin involvement, scleroderma renal crisis, cardiac disease, worse prognosis
Anti-B23	10	Pulmonary hypertension
Anti-Pm-Scl	2–10	Limited cutaneous involvement, myositis
Anti-U3-RNP (antifibrillarin)	8	Lung disease, diffuse skin involvement, African-American males
Anti-U1-RNP	5	MCTD
Anti-Th/To	1–5	Limited cutaneous involvement, pulmonary disease

Abbreviations: RNA = Ribonucleic acid; RNP = Ribonucleoprotein; CREST = Calcinosis, Raynaud phenomenon, esophageal dysmotility, sclerodactyly, and telangiectasia; MCTD = Mixed connective tissue disease

changes include decrease in number of capillary loops and giant loops.

Differential Diagnosis

PSS must be distinguished from other collagen disorders such as dermatomyositis and MCTD. Thickening and tightness of the skin may occur in other disorders, like eosinophilic fasciitis, scleredema adultorum Buschke, myxedema and acromegaly.

- ***Scleredema adultorum Buschke:*** This condition is characterized by painless edematous induration with an abrupt onset over a short period of time occurring in young subjects. Face, scalp, trunk and proximal parts of the extremities are extensively affected. Though the exact cause is not clear, some cases are seen to follow streptococcal infection. There is accumulation of mucopolysaccharides in the dermis and in the underlying muscles. The condition resolves spontaneously over a period of 6–12 months even without specific treatment. Systemic manifestations of PSS are not present.

- ***In eosinophilic fasciitis***, which starts in the form of painful and tender swellings over the extremities, there is fasciitis, myositis, eosinophilia and hypergammaglobulinemia. The skin is indurated and tight. Etiology is unknown. Onset is acute or subacute starting as symmetrical swelling and pain of the extremities followed by induration and joint contractures. Forearms, legs, hands and feet are affected. These parts become shiny and erythematous, which later become taut and woody. The skin is restricted by the subcutaneous tissue. Systemic involvement may develop at times. There is no evidence of autoimmunity.

  Biopsy reveals perivascular infiltration by eosinophils, histiocytes, lymphocytes, and plasma cells in the skin, fat and even underlying muscles. These lesions are self-limiting. Raynaud's syndrome does not occur. Carpal tunnel syndrome may develop. Histology shows inflammatory exudate consisting mainly of eosinophils. Fibrosis is prominent. The condition is self-limiting. Excessive consumption of L-tryptophan in health foods has been associated with the development of eosinophilic fasciitis. Corticosteroids bring about remission promptly.

- ***Myxedema and acromegaly*** are conditions, which may show skin changes mistaken for scleroderma. They are associated with other endocrine abnormalities as well.

Course and Prognosis

PSS is a slowly progressive disease. Widespread skin involvement, lesions of the kidneys, lungs and heart, and onset earlier in life are unfavorable factors. More than 70% survive 5 years or more.

TREATMENT

At present, there is no drug, which will arrest the progression of the disease. The use of corticosteroids is controversial. The renal lesions may even be aggravated by corticosteroids. Nonsteroidal anti-inflammatory drugs (NSAIDS), like indomethacin or ibuprofen may help to relieve arthralgia and arthritis. D-penicillamine may help in the early stages on account of its ability to inhibit cross-linking of collagen. Blood flow in the digital arteries can be improved by infusion of low-molecular weight dextran. This may prevent ischemic ulcers and help in their recovery. Early use of angiotensin-converting enzyme (ACE) inhibitors helps to delay the progress of renal lesions and hypertensive complications. Calcium channel blockers have found use in complications such as pulmonary hypertension, Raynaud's phenomenon and calcinosis. Nifedipine in usual dosage relieves Raynaud's phenomenon. Severe and disabling Raynaud's phenomenon may respond to infusion of prostacyclin. Epoprostenol 0.5–0.6 ng/kg/bw is infused intravenous (IV) for 6–24 hours for 2–5 days. The drug is expensive. Intractable Raynaud's syndrome is relieved by cervical sympathectomy.

Since the potential role of cells, cytokines, paracrine signaling and role of immunity have been known; treatment targeted against these processes is possible. Best results are obtained in case of vascular complications.

ACE inhibitors prevent renal crisis and these drugs are the preferred choice in the treatment of renal crisis.

The following drugs have been approved by the Food and Drug Administration (FDA) for the treatment of pulmonary artery hypertension (PAH). These include:

- ***Epoprostenol, treprostinil, iloprost:*** They supply prostacyclin to the vascular endothelium

- **Sildenafil and tadalafil:** These are phosphodiesterase inhibitors. They can generate nitric oxide (NO), which leads to vasodilation
- **Bosentan:** It is an endothelin receptor antagonist (ERA).

These drugs reduce vasospasm and increase the walking distance and quality of life. Epoprostenol and bosentan may prolong survival. Nifedipine is given orally, iloprost and epoprostenol are given IV and nitroglycerine is given as an ointment. Bosentan and tadalafil reduces the frequency of new digital ulcers and necrosis.

Drugs targeted against immune activation include, methotrexate and cyclophosphamide. They improve skin lesion and a few other manifestations, but not the visceral lesions. Cyclophosphamide given in doses of 3–5 mg/kg or higher doses IV monthly for 6 months with prednisolone 20 mg on alternate days showed improvement in interstitial lung disease (ILD). Azathioprine and mycophenolate are also effective in ILD.

OVERLAP SYNDROME

Multisystem diseases of varied pathogenesis and clinical features are difficult to be compartmentalized precisely. This is particularly true of the CTDs. Some distinct entities include SLE, PSS, polymyositis dermatomyositis (PM-DM), RA and others. Some patients show overlapping features of more than one CTD and these are included under the terms *overlap syndrome*.

UNDIFFERENTIATED CONNECTIVE TISSUE DISEASE

Patients with incomplete features of a defined CTD are encountered from time to time, (e.g. a patient with Raynaud's phenomenon, arthritis and weakly positive ANA). About 35% of such patients differentiate into a definite CTD usually within the first 2 years after onset of symptoms. Complete remissions of symptoms occur in 12% of cases. Management of such patients has to be individualized and this consists of periodic follow-up and essential laboratory tests to assess progress of the disease. Once specific differentiation is evident, the appropriate treatment has to be started. Till that time, management has to be symptomatic and supportive.

It should be borne in mind that paraneoplastic manifestations of malignancy may present as vague rheumatic disorders and they have to be excluded by clinical examination and laboratory tests.

MIXED CONNECTIVE TISSUE DISEASE

Overlap syndrome combining features of SLE, PSS and PM associated with a specific antibody directed against a specific extractable nuclear antigen (ENA) called U1 ribonucleoprotein particle (U1RNP) is known as MCTD.

A set of patients show features combining the manifestations of SLE, PSS, PM-DM and RA. This combination is termed MCTD. Presenting symptoms are given below:

- Hand edema or puffy fingers
- Raynaud's phenomenon
- Sclerodactyly
- Skin changes of dermatomyositis or scleroderma or SLE
- Arthralgia or arthritis
- Prolonged fever
- Myositis
- **Lung involvement**: ILD or pulmonary hypertension
- **Renal involvement** (*See* Section 16, Ch 187).

Symptomatic measures to relieve Raynaud's phenomenon and arthralgia give relief. Hydroxychloroquine given in a dose of 200–400 mg oral daily is beneficial in mild and moderate cases. Corticosteroids and immunosuppressants are indicated in severe cases.

CHAPTER
110

Systemic Vasculitis

Binoy J Paul, KV Krishna Das

Chapter Summary

- Vasculitis
  - General Considerations
  - Takayasu's Arteritis
  - Giant Cell Arteritis
  - Polymyalgia Rheumatica
- Medium Vessel Vasculitis
  - Polyarteritis Nodosa
  - Kawasaki Disease
- Small Vessel Vasculitides
  - Cryoglobulinemic Vasculitis
- Variable Vessel Vasculitis
  - Behçet's Disease (Behçet's Syndrome)
- Single-Organ Vasculitis
  - Hypersensitivity Vasculitis

VASCULITIS

General Considerations

The term *vasculitis* refers to inflammation occurring primarily in the blood vessel wall. It can affect arteries, arterioles, capillaries, venules and veins which often lead to

Table 110.1: Frequency distribution of vasculitic disorders in India (N = 1,064)

Disease	%
Henoch-Schönlein purpura	22
Aortoarteritis	20.2
Wegener's granulomatosis	13.8
Behçet's disease	13.6
Polyarteritis nodosa	8.8
Small vessel vasculitis	5.7
Microscopic polyangiitis	3.9
Giant cell arteritis	3.4
Churg-Strauss syndrome	1.8
Kawasaki disease and miscellaneous conditions	0.5
Undiagnosed	5.9
Others [Cogan, Bazin's, central nervous system (CNS) vasculitis]	0.56

Source: Joshi VR, Mittal G. Vasculitis–Indian perspective. J Assoc Physicians India. 2006;54(Suppl):12-4.

destruction of the vessel wall and/or aneurysm formation. Epidemiological studies from India are sparse. The data available shows that Henoch-Schönlein purpura (HSP) is most commonly followed by aortoarteritis. Recently, there are several case series about Kawasaki disease in children from South Indian states like Kerala and Karnataka (Table 110.1).

Etiology

Vasculitis could be primary (primary systemic vasculitis) where the etiology is unknown or secondary to different causes are given in Box 110.1.

Classification

In 2012, International Chapel Hill Consensus Conference modified the classification of vasculitis (Box 110.2). The classification depends mainly on the size of the blood vessel that is predominantly affected. Large vessels are the aorta and its major branches and the analogous veins. Medium vessels are the main visceral arteries and veins and their initial branches. Small vessels are intraparenchymal arteries, arterioles, capillaries, venules, and veins (Fig. 110.1).

Box 110.1: Causes of secondary vasculitis

Infections	**Connective tissue diseases**
• Tuberculosis	• Systemic lupus erythematosus
• Infective endocarditis	• Rheumatoid arthritis
• Hepatitis B, C	• Progressive systemic sclerosis
• Syphilis	**Coagulopathies/microangiopathies**
• Disseminated gonococcal infection (DGI)	• Thrombotic thrombocytopenic purpura (TTP)
• Pulmonary histoplasmosis	• Antiphospholipid antibody syndrome
• Coccidioidomycosis	**Drugs**
• Lyme disease	• Penicillins
Neoplasms	• Sulfonamides
• Lymphoma	• Thiazides
• Leukemia	• Allopurinol
• Carcinomas	**Miscellaneous**
	• Cryoglobulinemia
	• Sarcoidosis

Box 110.2: 2012 International Chapel Hill Consensus Conference nomenclature

Large vessel vasculitis (LVV)
- Takayasu arteritis
- Giant cell arteritis

Medium vessel vasculitis
- Polyarteritis nodosa (PAN)
- Kawasaki disease

Small vessel vasculitis (SVV)
- Antineutrophil cytoplasmic antibody (ANCA) associated vasculitis
  - Granulomatosis with polyangiitis (Wegener's granulomatosis)
  - EGPA (Churg-Strauss syndrome)
  - Microscopic polyangiitis

Immune complex SVV
- Anti-glomerular basement membrane disease
- Cryoglobulinemic vasculitis
- Immunoglobulin A vasculitis (Henoch-Schönlein)
- Hypocomplementemic urticarial vasculitis (anti-C1q vasculitis)

Variable vessel vasculitis
- Behçet's disease
- Cogan's syndrome

Single-organ vasculitis
- Cutaneous leukocytoclastic angiitis, cutaneous arteritis, primary central nervous system vasculitis, isolated aortitis, others

Vasculitis associated with systemic disease
- Lupus vasculitis, rheumatoid vasculitis, sarcoid vasculitis, others

Vasculitis associated with probable etiology
- Hepatitis C virus-associated cryoglobulinemic vasculitis
- Hepatitis B virus-associated vasculitis
- Syphilis-associated aortitis
- Drug-associated immune complex vasculitis
- Drug-induced ANCA-associated vasculitis
- Cancer-associated vasculitis, others

Abbreviation: EGPA = Eosinophilic granulomatosis with polyangiitis

Fig. 110.1: Caliber of vessels affected by the different types of vasculitides

Abbreviations: IgA = Immunoglobulin A; GBM = Glomerular basement membrane; ANCA = Antineutrophil cytoplasmic antibody

Source: Special article: Jennette JC. 2012 Revised International Chapel Hill Consensus Conference Nomenclature of Vasculitides Arthritis & Rheumatology. 2013;65(1);1-11.

Pathology

There is an inflammation of blood vessels causing endothelial damage. This leads to inflammatory cell infiltration of the blood vessels. This vascular necrosis,

Textbook of Medicine

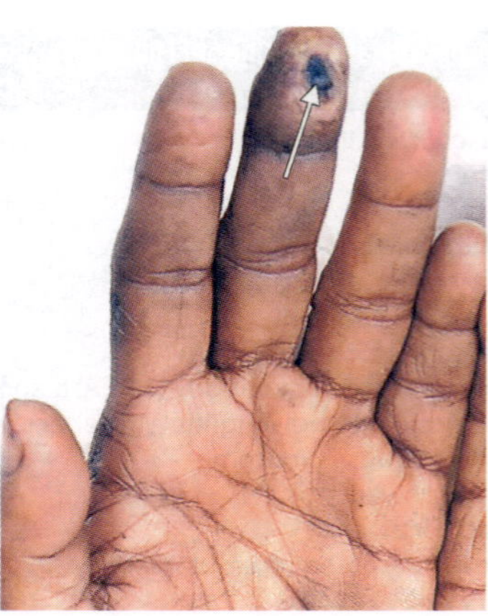

Fig. 110.2: Necrotic ulcer pulp of middle finger in small vessel vasculitis (arrow)

granuloma formation or fibrosis of vessel wall causes partial or total occlusion of the vessels (Fig. 110.2).

There are different pathological subsets like systemic necrotizing vasculitis (SNV), e.g. eosinophilic granulomatosis with polyangiitis (EGPA), granulomatous vasculitis like Takayasu and giant cell arteritis (GCA), and necrosis and granuloma formation as in granulomatosis with polyangiitis (GPA) or leukocytoclastic vasculitis (LCV), hypersensitivity vasculitis and cryoglobulinemic vasculitis.

Clinical Features

Features common to all vasculitis syndromes include fever, anorexia, weight loss, arthralgia and/or arthritis. Other clinical manifestations vary with the vessels affected (Table 110.2).

LARGE VESSEL VASCULITIS

Takayasu Arteritis

Syn: Aortoarteritis, Pulseless disease, Harbitz-Rendu syndrome

(*See* Section 16, Ch 187 and Section 13, Ch 131)

It is a large vessel vasculitis (LVV) where there is granulomatous inflammation of the aorta and its major branches. Usually it occurs in females below the age of 40 years. It is the most common LVV in India and is often associated with vascular occlusion. Pathologically, there is aortic wall thickening with intimal wrinkling. There

is prominent granulomatous infiltrates with giant cells restricted to media and adventitia. The inflammation in the vascular wall heals with collagenous fibrosis.

Clinical Features

Patients present with limb claudication or features of uncontrolled hypertension. One-third of patients are present with systemic features like fever, fatigue, arthralgia, myalgia or weight loss. In some of them, the disease is diagnosed when present with stroke, renal failure or hypertensive encephalopathy. Clinical examination reveals asymmetric or absent pulse. Hypertension or blood pressure difference between limbs is not uncommon. Arterial bruit is often heard over major vessels like brachial and femoral artery or carotid vessels. When the aortic arch is affected, cerebrovascular manifestations and upper limb ischemia may manifest. The pulses in the upper limbs may be absent, with hypertension in the lower limbs caused by affection of the renal arteries (***reversed coarctation***) (Fig. 110.3).

Investigation

The erythrocyte sedimentation rate (ESR) is high. Aortography shows stenosis or occlusion of aorta or its major branches. Magnetic resonance (MR) angiography or computed tomography (CT) angiography is often preferred. Arterial biopsy is not required routinely for diagnosis.

Treatment

Glucocorticoids—prednisolone (1–2 mg/kg/day) is helpful in reducing the systemic symptoms and vascular inflammation. Methotrexate 10–15 mg/week or azathioprine 1–2 mg/kg/day are useful adjuncts to steroids for long-term control of vascular inflammation. Surgery or angioplasty may be required in addition to aspirin and other anti-platelet drugs to prevent and relieve vascular occlusion.

Giant Cell Arteritis

Syn: Temporal arteritis, Cranial arteritis

It used to occur more frequently in the 6th and 7th decades in elderly. It is a less common LVV present in India. It is characterized by panarteritis with giant cell infiltration, predominantly affecting the cranial vessels.

Table 110.2: Common clinical manifestations of vasculitis		
Large vessel vasculitis	*Medium vessel vasculitis*	*Small vessel vasculitis*
• Limb claudication • Asymmetric blood pressures • Absence of pulses • Bruits • Aortic dilation/ aneurysms	• Cutaneous nodules • Skin ulcers • Livedo reticularis • Digital gangrene • Mono-neuritis multiplex • Micro-aneurysms	• Purpura • Glomerulo-nephritis • Alveolar hemorrhage • Vesiculobullous lesions • Urticaria • Cutaneous extravascular necrotizing granulomas • Splinter hemorrhages • Uveitis/episcleritis/ scleritis

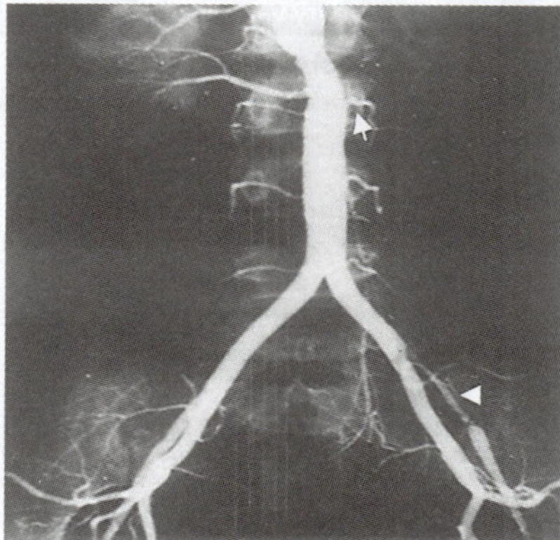

Fig. 110.3: Aortogram showing narrowing of proximal descending aorta with left renal artery and external iliac artery stenosis (arrow heads) reversed coarctation

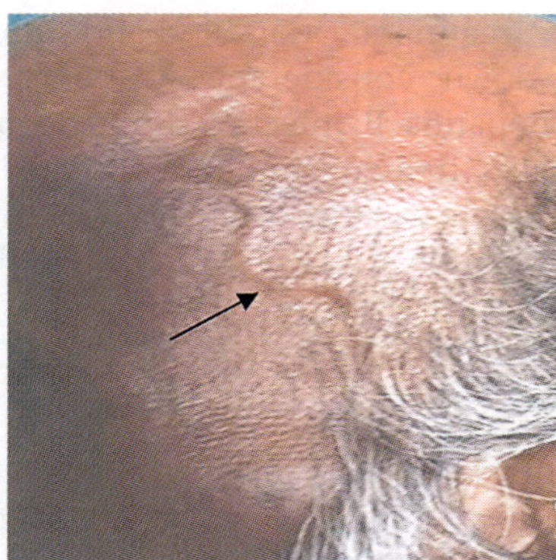

Fig. 110.4: Temporal arteritis. **Note:** Thickened, prominent and nonpulsatile temporal artery (arrow)

Pathology

The arterial wall normally contains dendritic cells in the adventitia. The inflammation is T-cell mediated. The activation of the dendritic cells sets in motion a complex cascade consisting of cytokine activation, intimal proliferation supported by neoangiogenesis, oxidative injury to smooth muscles and effects of systemic inflammation. The larger arteries such as internal and external carotids, temporal, occipital and ophthalmic arteries are usually involved, though any other artery may show lesions. The lesions are segmental with intervening normal areas. The media of the artery is infiltrated by round cells and giant cells. The vessels may be occluded by thrombus which recanalized later.

Clinical Features

Both sexes are equally affected. Onset is with severe—unilateral or bilateral headache in the temporal or less commonly in the occipital regions, associated with vomiting. **Diagnostic feature** is the palpably thickened, tender and nonpulsatile temporal arteries (Fig. 110.4).

Loss of vision due to occlusion of the ophthalmic artery is a dreaded complication. Rarely patients present as facial neuralgia with **jaw claudication** on chewing (caused by ischemia to pterygoid muscles), deafness, necrosis of the tongue, or an associated widespread necrotizing arteritis of small vessels which presents as peripheral neuropathy.

Laboratory Diagnosis

ESR often exceeds 100 mm and all immunoglobulin (Ig) fractions are elevated. Temporal artery biopsy which reveals the characteristic histology is diagnostic. However, a negative biopsy does not rule out the diagnosis, since the lesions may occur segmentally.

Treatment

Corticosteroids are indicated in high doses. Prednisolone (50–60 mg/day) may be started initially and tapered off slowly to the minimum maintenance dose required to keep the ESR below 20 mm/hr. This treatment must be continued for at least one year. Once blindness occurs, it is irreversible and it has to be prevented by early diagnosis and institution of steroid treatment. Relapse occurs in 20–30% on stopping treatment. This is an indication for restarting treatment with addition of immunosuppressants such as azathioprine or methotrexate in their usual dosage.

Table 110.3: Differential features between giant cell and Takayasu's arteritis

Features	Giant cell	Takayasu's arteritis
Female-male ratio	2:1	8:1
Age range (year)	50	< 40
Average age of onset (year)	72	25
Visual loss	10–30%	Rare
Involvement of aorta or its major branches	25%	100%
Pathology	Granulomatous arteritis	Granulomatous arteritis
Pulmonary artery involvement	No	Possible
Renal hypertension	Rare	Common
Claudication	Uncommon	Common
Ethnic groups with highest incidence	Scandinavians	Asians
Corticosteroid responsive	Yes	Yes
Bruits present	Minority	Majority
Surgical intervention	Rarely needed	Commonly needed

Low-dose aspirin is useful in long-term management for preventing vascular occlusion.

Table 110.3 shows differential features between giant cell and Takayasu's arteritis.

Polymyalgia Rheumatica (PMR)

This is a syndrome rarely seen in India, characterized by severe pain and stiffness in the neck, back, shoulder, upper arms and thighs, particularly worse in the morning. Periarticular and articular inflammatory changes may occur. This condition may be associated with GCA which may coexist, or in some cases, develop later. The ESR is elevated, muscle enzymes are normal and this finding helps to differentiate this condition from polymyositis.

Diagnosis is clinical since laboratory tests may be nonspecific. Diagnostic criteria have been proposed. Magnetic resonance imaging (MRI) may show subacromial and subdeltoid bursitis.

Treatment with corticosteroids gives prompt relief. The dose is 15–20 mg of prednisone to start with, later to be tapered off. In resistant cases, methotrexate and biologicals such as infliximab may be tried with benefit.

MEDIUM VESSEL VASCULITIS

Polyarteritis Nodosa (PAN)

General Considerations

It is characterized by formation of multiple nodules along blood vessels, mainly affecting the smaller arteries, arterioles and adjacent veins. Capillaries are spared. Pathologically, the lesion consists of polymorphonuclear infiltration, necrosis and aneurysmal dilatation of the arterial wall. Thrombotic occlusions may occur. The lesions are widespread and all tissues may be involved. Main impact is on the arteries of the muscles, kidneys, heart, mesentery, and vasa nervorum. The disease is more common in people who are infected with hepatitis

B virus (HBV). Circulating immune complexes containing hepatitis B surface antigen may be present in them. In view of this finding, PAN may be classified as HBV-related and HBV-unrelated.

Clinical Features

Polyarteritis is rare compared to the other connective tissue disorders. Though all ages may be affected, adults suffer more frequently. Males predominate. The onset is variable. The condition may be precipitated by drugs or upper respiratory infections.

The onset is with general symptoms like fever, muscle pains, arthralgia, rash and anorexia. Inflammatory nodules ranging in size from 5–10 mm may be palpable over the superficial arteries. These nodules are tender. Symptoms referable to organ systems develop depending on the lesions. In about 50% cases, the kidneys are affected leading to the clinical picture of acute nephritic syndrome or glomerulosclerosis with secondary hypertension and renal failure. Vascular occlusion leads to distal gangrene of extremities (Fig. 110.5A). Occlusion of vasa nervorum leads to mononeuritis multiplex (Figs 110.5B and C). Retina may show hemorrhages and exudates. Pericarditis, pleurisy, myocardial infarction (MI), ulceration, and bleeding from intestines and necrosis of the liver and gallbladder may be encountered at times.

Diagnosis

The condition has to be suspected clinically. There are no specific laboratory tests. The ESR is markedly elevated. Neutrophil leukocytosis is common. Diagnosis is confirmed by demonstrating the lesions on biopsy specimens. Muscle, kidney or liver or sural nerve is selected for biopsy depending on the presentation. Angiography of abdominal vessels may show aneurysms, especially, in renal vessels. Tests for infection by hepatitis B and C are indicated in all cases.

Differential diagnosis includes allergic vasculitis, Goodpasture's syndrome and microscopic polyangiitis (MPA).

Prognosis

PAN is a serious illness with a mortality ranging from 50 to 60% in one year. Common causes of death are renal failure, MI, infections, congestive heart failure (CHF) and gastrointestinal (GI) bleeding.

Treatment

Corticosteroids may cause symptomatic improvement. Immunosuppressants are of benefit if used judiciously.

With proper treatment, mortality and morbidity can be brought down considerably. Patients who show evidence of hepatitis B infection improve better if the infection is also treated simultaneously with antiviral agents. Appropriate use of these drugs is highly rewarding and the 5-year survival is well above 80%. Relapses are generally rare.

Kawasaki Disease (Mucocutaneous Lymph Node Syndrome)

It is a medium vessel vasculitis first reported from Japan, affecting children below 5-years of age. Most of the initial cases from India are reported from coastal districts of Karnataka and Kerala. The prevalence is progressively rising.

This is an acute or subacute exanthema-like disease, often affecting children, characterized by onset of abrupt fever, conjunctival congestion, erythematous rash over the face, mouth, palms and soles, nonsuppurating cervical lymphadenopathy and vasculitis affecting particularly the coronary arteries. The arterial lesion leads to aneurysms in the coronary arteries. The coronary arterial lesion can be demonstrated by color Doppler echocardiography after the first week of illness. The diagnostic criteria for kawasaki disease are listed in Box 110.3.

Treatment

During the acute febrile phase it consists of aspirin given in a dose of 80–100 mg/kg body weight (bw)/day to be tapered off later. Ig is given as IV infusion in a dose of 2 g/kg bw and it is considered as the drug of choice in severe disease. Five percent of children who develop Kawasaki disease develop coronary aneurysms.

Source: Singh S, Kawasaki T. Kawasaki disease-an Indian perspective. Indian Pediatr. 2009:46(7):563-71.

SMALL VESSEL VASCULITIDES

This group of vasculitis is broadly divided into those with production on antineutrophil cytoplasmic antibodies (ANCA) or immune complex deposition.

ANCA-associated Vasculitis

These are clinical entities corresponding to necrotizing inflammation of small vessels. There are three known entities in this group, two are recently renamed—(1) GPA (Wegener's granulomatosis), (2) EGPA (Churg-Strauss syndrome), (3) MPA.

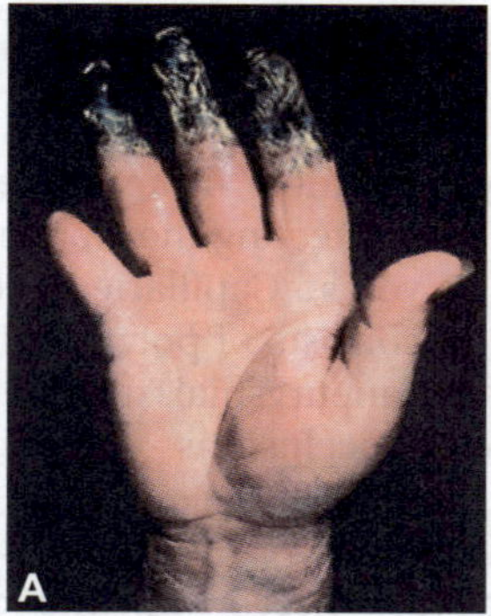
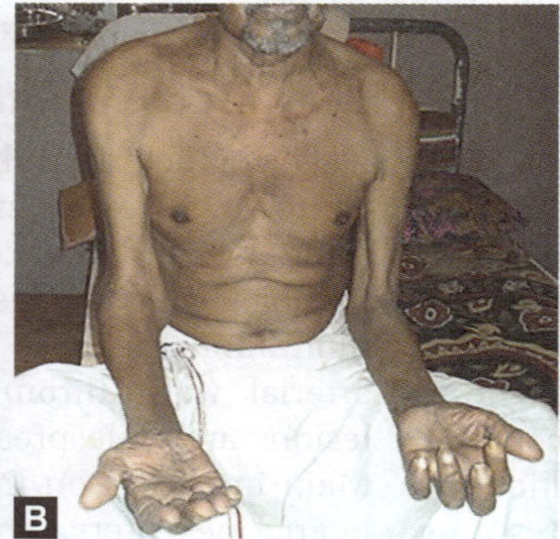
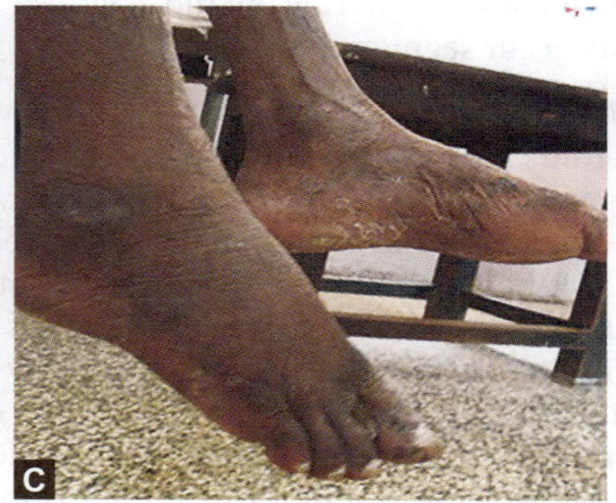

Figs 110.5A to C: Polyarteritis nodosa: **A.** Gangrene of fingers, discoloration of hands; **B.** Mononeuritis multiplex (left clawhand); **C.** Right foot drop

Textbook of Medicine

Box 110.3: Diagnostic criteria for Kawasaki disease

- Fever of five or more days duration plus
- Presence of at least four of the following five clinical signs:
  1. **Changes in extremities**
     - **Acute:** Erythema and edema of hands and feet
     - **Convalescent:** Membranous desquamation of fingertips
  2. Polymorphous exanthema
  3. Bilateral, painless bulbar conjunctival injection without exudate
  4. **Changes in lips and oral cavity:** Erythema and cracking of lips, strawberry tongue, diffuse injection of oral and pharyngeal mucosae
  5. Cervical lymphadenopathy (≥1.5 cm in diameter), usually unilateral
- Exclusion of other diseases with similar findings

Pathogenesis of ANCA-associated vasculitis is not clear. Support for autoimmunity is evident by the production of ANCA antibodies and occasional association with other autoimmune diseases. Death in this group of diseases is generally due to renal failure or pulmonary hemorrhage. Different genotypes are described which differ in therapy and its outcome.

Granulomatosis with Polyangiitis (GPA) (Wegener's Granulomatosis)

(*See* also Section 14, Ch 152 and Section 16, Ch 187)

It is a rare vasculitis characterized by granulomatous infiltration or necrotizing vasculitis of upper and lower respiratory tract, eyes, kidneys or peripheral nerves. Patient present with upper airways involvement in the form of recurrent sinusitis, nasal obstruction, nasal septal perforation or saddle nose deformity. Lower airway involvement leads to cough and hemoptysis and cavitary lung nodules. Vasculitic skin rashes are also common. Uveitis, keratitis and scleromalacia can occur in the eye. Renal involvement is common in the form of glomerulonephritis or renal failure. Rarely mononeuritis multiplex can also occur. Limited disease affecting lung and the eyes alone sparing the kidneys are also reported.

Investigations show high ESR or C-reactive protein (CRP). **Cytoplasmic ANCA (c-ANCA)** will be positive in 90% of patients with diffuse active disease. X-ray of the paranasal sinuses show evidence of sinus involvement. X-ray chest shows pulmonary infiltration or multiple cavitating nodules. Biopsy of the affected tissue from nasal cavity, lung or kidney shows granuloma formation and necrotizing vasculitis. Figures 110.6A to D shows GPA (Wegener's granulomatosis).

Eosinophilic Granulomatosis with Polyangiitis (EGPA) (Churg-Strauss Syndrome)

It is a small vessel vasculitis characterized by infiltration of the vessels with eosinophilic granulomas. There is previous history of asthma and eosinophilia antedating the vasculitic manifestations by 3–4 years. Pulmonary infiltrates with eosinophilia may be present. Necrotizing vasculitis occurs in several organs leading to skin nodules or rashes, mononeuritis multiplex, myocarditis, pericarditis and renal involvement (Refer to Section 16, Ch 187).

Peripheral blood eosinophilia is common. Perinuclear anti-neutrophil cytoplasmic antibodies (p-ANCA) are present in high titers in this disease. Biopsy of the affected tissues shows infiltration with eosinophil rich granulomas and necrotizing vasculitis (Figs 110.7A and B).

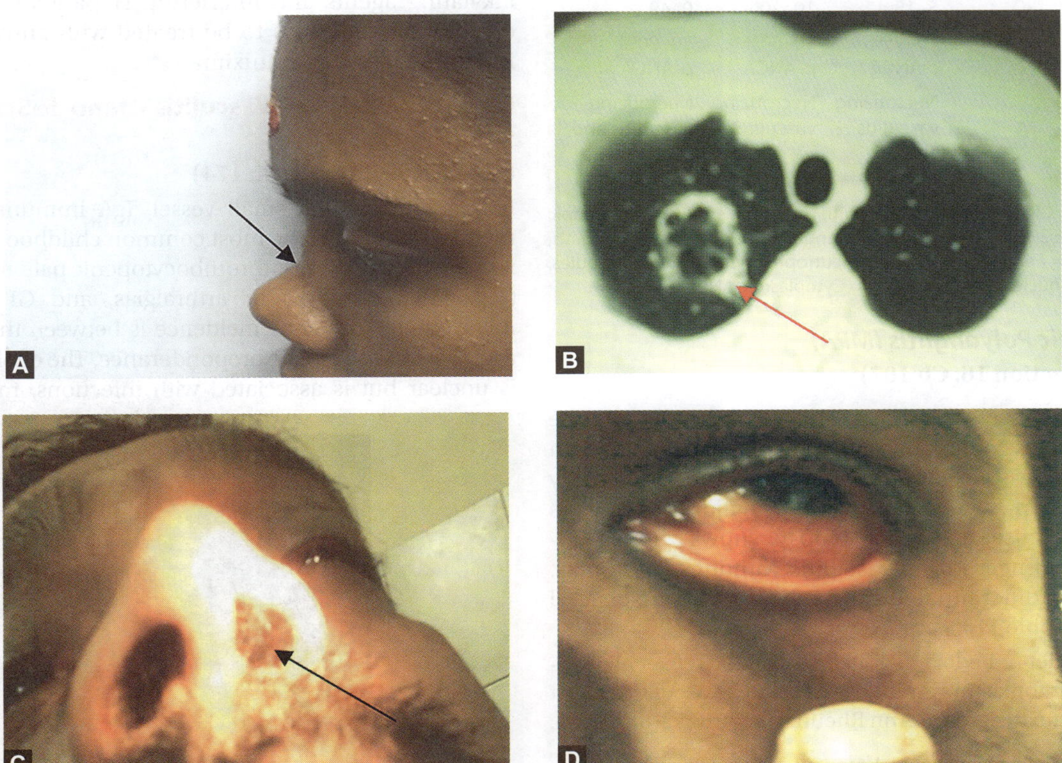

Figs 110.6A to D: **A.** Saddle nose deformity; **B.** CT scan of thorax showing cavitating pulmonary nodule; **C.** Sinus infection with nasal crusting (*see* arrows); **D.** Scleritis. **Note:** The hyperemic sclera

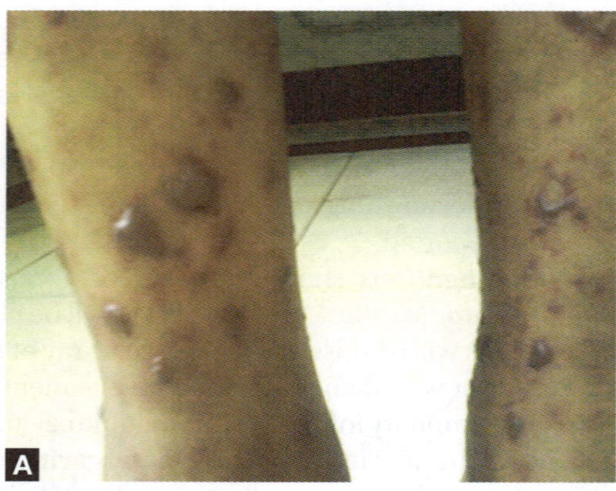
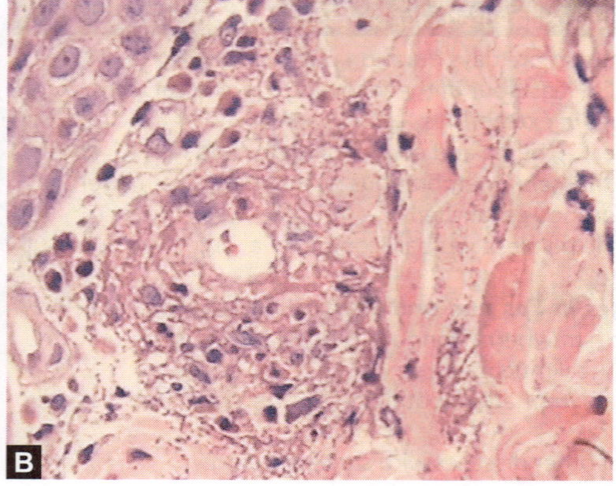

Figs 110.7A and B: **A.** Vasculitic skin rashes; **B.** Skin biopsy showing eosinophil rich granuloma (Churg-Strauss syndrome)

Table 110.4: Comparative details of ANCA-associated vasculitis

Patient characteristics	GPA	MPA	EGPA
Gender	M > F	M > F	M = F
Peak age of onset (years)	64–74	64–74	40–60
Pattern of appearance	Cyclical	Random	Not applicable
Organ involvement (%)			
Skin	30–60	40–70	51–67
Kidneys	50–80	90–100	4–51
Lungs	60–80	20–60	34–76
Ear, nose, throat	80–90	20–30	53–78
Joints	50–80	30–70	30–40
Peripheral nerves	10–50	20–30	42–84
Eyes	30–60	10–30	<10
Bowel	<10	10–30	0–42
Heart	5–15	10–20	0–49
ANCA	70–95% c-ANCA	30–80% p-ANCA	30–90% p-ANCA
Histopathology	Necrotizing vasculitis and granuloma	Necrotizing vasculitis	Necrotizing vasculitis and eosinophilic granuloma

Abbreviations: GPA = Granulomatosis with polyangiitis; MPA = Microscopic polyangiitis, EGPA = Eosinophilic granulomatosis with polyangiitis; M = Male; F = Female; ANCA = Antineutrophil cytoplasmic antibodies; p-ANCA = Perinuclear ANCA; c-ANCA = Cytoplasmic ANCA

Microscopic Polyangiitis (MPA)
(*See* also Section 16, Ch 187)

It is a small vessel vasculitis predominantly affecting the kidneys and less often, lungs. Patient usually present with rapidly progressive glomerulonephritis and pulmonary hemorrhages. p-ANCA is positive in the majority of patients with active disease. Renal biopsy shows glomerulo-nephritis and necrotizing vasculitis without granulomas. It should be differentiated from other ANCA- associated vasculitis (Table 110.4).

Source: Millet A, Pederzoli-Ribeil M, Guillevin L, et al. Anti-neutrophil cytoplasmic antibody-associated vasculitides: is it time to split up the group? Ann Rheum Dis. 2013;72(8):1273-9.

Cryoglobulinemic Vasculitis
Cryoglobulinemic vasculitis is characterized by the deposition of cryoglobulins in small and medium sized blood vessels which precipitate at low temperatures (4–10°C). Serological classification defines type I as isolated monoclonal Ig without rheumatoid factor, predominantly associated with malignant conditions of the immune system such as multiple myeloma. Types II and III are polyclonal containing polyclonal IgG and monoclonal IgM and are also known as *mixed cryoglobulinemias*. Ninety percent of type II is associated with chronic hepatitis C infection. In the remaining cases, etiology is unknown (essential mixed cryoglobulinemia). Type III is associated with polyclonal IgG and IgM. The disease is due to autoimmune diseases or infections.

Clinical manifestations include palpable cutaneous purpura, arthralgia, myalgia or Raynaud's syndrome. More severe vasculitis involving renal and neurological systems may be seen. ***Treatment*** consists of corticosteroids, alkylating agents and interferon. Hepatitis C-associated cryoglobulinemia has to be treated with antiviral drugs, interferon alpha and rituximab.

Immunoglobulin A Vasculitis (Henoch-Schönlein Syndrome)
(*See* also Section 15, Ch 174)

It is a multisystem, small vessel, IgA immune complex-mediated LCV. It is the most common childhood vasculitis, is characterized by nonthrombocytopenic palpable purpura (Fig. 110.8), arthritis or arthralgias, and GI and renal involvement. The peak incidence is between the ages of 4 and 8 years with a male preponderance. The etiology of HSP is unclear but is associated with infections, medications,

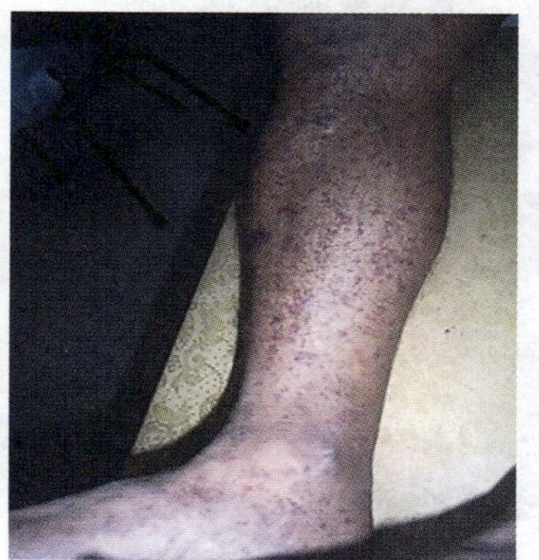

Fig. 110.8: Immunoglobulin A vasculitis, Henoch-Schönlein purpura

Textbook of Medicine

<table>
<tr><td colspan="2">Table 110.5: Classification criteria for Henoch-Schönlein purpura (EULAR/PRES)–2010</td></tr>
<tr><td>Criterion</td><td>Definition</td></tr>
<tr><td>Purpura (mandatory)</td><td>Purpura (palpable, in crops) or petechiae, with lower limb predominance, not related to thrombocytopenia</td></tr>
<tr><td colspan="2">And at least one of four of the following</td></tr>
<tr><td>Abdominal pain</td><td>Diffuse, acute, colicky pain. May include intussusception and GI bleeding</td></tr>
<tr><td>Arthritis or arthralgias arthritis</td><td>Acute joint swelling or pain with limitation of movement</td></tr>
<tr><td>Arthralgia</td><td>Acute joint pain without joint swelling or limitation on movement</td></tr>
<tr><td>Renal involvement</td><td>Proteinuria, >0.3 g/24 hour; spot urine albumin to creatinine ratio, >30 mmol/mg; or ≥2 + on dipstick</td></tr>
<tr><td>Hematuria, red cell casts</td><td>Urine sediment showing >5 red cells per high power field or red cell casts</td></tr>
<tr><td>Histopathology</td><td>LCV with predominant IgA deposit; or proliferative glomerulonephritis with predominant IgA deposit</td></tr>
</table>

Abbreviations: GI = Gastrointestinal; LCV = Leukocytoclastic vasculitis; IgA = Immunoglobulin A

vaccination, tumors (non-small-cell lung cancer, prostate cancer and hematological malignancies), alpha-1-antitrypsin deficiency (A1AD) and familial Mediterranean fever. The classification criteria has been updated in 2010 by the European League Against Rheumatism (EULAR) and Pediatric Rheumatology European Society (PRES) which is given in Table 110.5.

The ***diagnosis*** is often clinical, but can be confirmed by demonstration of IgA deposits in the skin or kidney by immunofluorescence. Majority of cases has a benign course, but in some the mesangial IgA nephropathy may progress to chronic renal failure.

Treatment

In mild disease, nonspecific symptomatic treatment is all that is needed. Patients with significant renal involvement require corticosteroids, immunosuppressives like cyclophosphamide, azathioprine or mycophenolate mofetil.

VARIABLE VESSEL VASCULITIS

Behçet's Disease (Behçet's Syndrome)

This disease was originally described by Hulusi Behçet, a Turkish dermatologist. It is a vasculitic disorder of unknown cause which can affect blood vessels of any size, characterized by recurrent aphthous ulceration in the mouth, genital ulcers, uveitis and skin lesion or nervous system involvement. The uveitis tends to recur and leads to blindness, whereas most of the other manifestations are self-limiting.

Pathologically, it is a recurrent acute inflammatory disease rather than a chronic inflammatory process. Persons with human leukocyte antigen (HLA) B51 have a strong predilection to develop Behçet's disease. This disease is present in India rarely and it may masquerade as other multisystem diseases.

The basic pathophysiological process is small vessel vasculitis, autoimmune responses and hyperfunction of neutrophils. The neutrophils are overactive with increased lysosome production and chemotaxis. Clinically, this can be demonstrated by the ***pathergy test*** in which a needle prick area is infiltrated by neutrophils to produce a visible papule or pustule seen at 48 hours. Lymphocyte function is also abnormal.

Clinical Features

Recurrent genital ulcers (Fig. 110.9A), eye lesions, skin lesion especially erythema nodosum, folliculitis, pustules or acneiform lesions.

- ***Mucous membrane lesions:*** Recurrent painful oral aphthous ulceration (Fig. 110.9B) is the most common lesion in Behçet's syndrome. Recurrent ulcers over the scrotum, penis or vulva are also common.
- ***Skin lesions:*** Erythema nodosum, pseudofolliculitis, papulopustular or acneiform lesions (Fig. 110.9C) may occur.
- ***Ocular lesions:*** Anterior or posterior uveitis and retinal vascular occlusions may develop. Hypopyon uveitis (Fig. 110.10) is characteristic.
- ***Joint lesions:*** Mono- or polyarthritis; major joints are affected.

Systemic Vasculitis

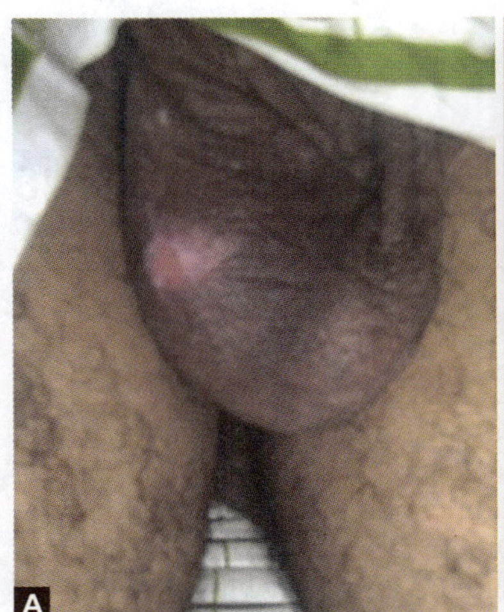
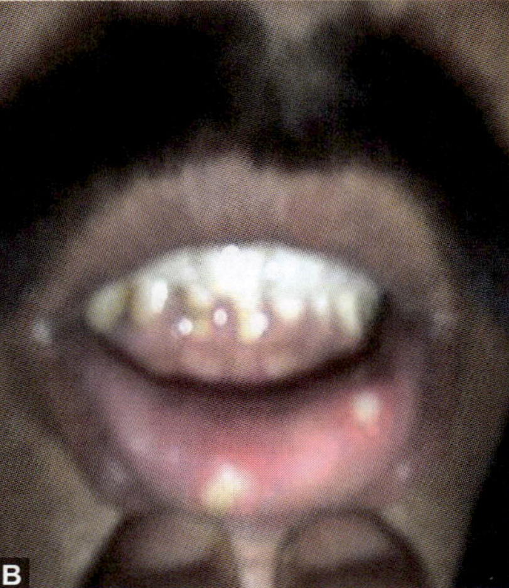
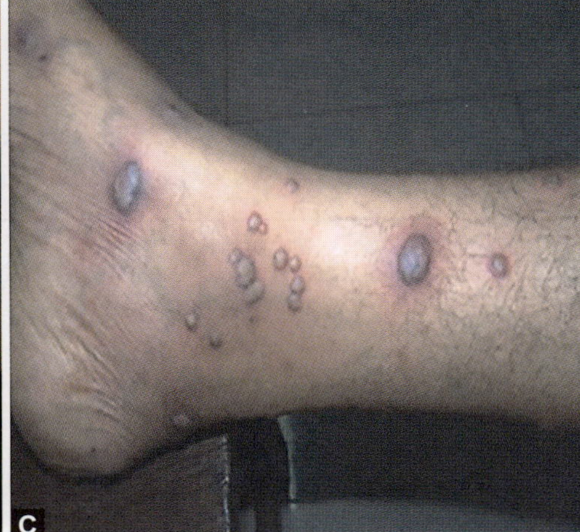

Figs 110.9A to C: Clinical manifestations of Behçet's disease. **A.** Scrotal ulcer; **B.** Oral aphthae; **C.** Vesiclular skin lesions

Textbook of Medicine

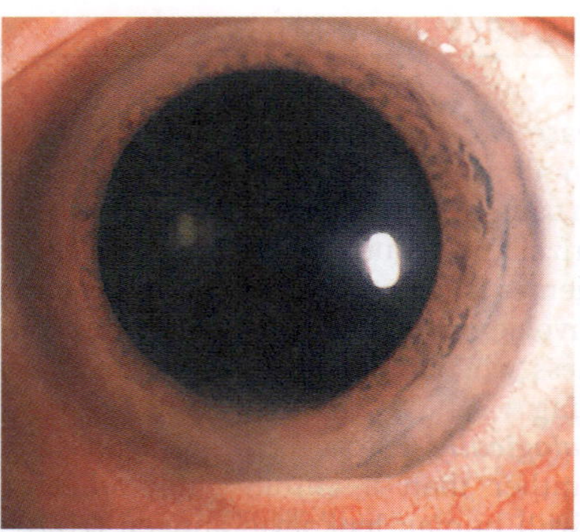

Fig. 110.10: Hypopyon uveitis

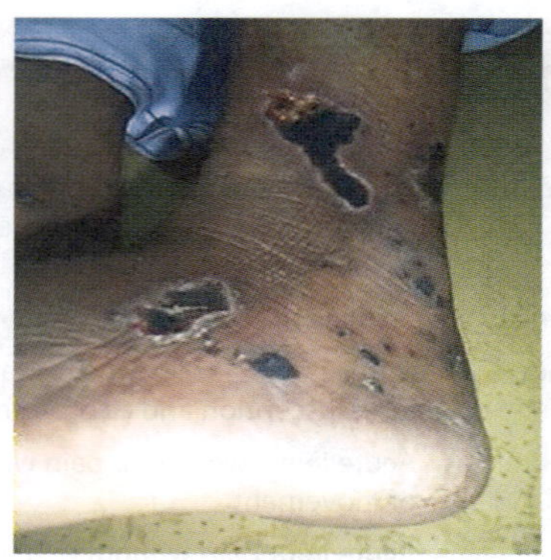

Fig. 110.11: Cutaneous leukocytoclastic angiitis (hypersensitivity vasculitis)

Box 110.4: International study group criteria for Behçet's syndrome

Recurrent oral ulcerations
Minor aphthous, major aphthous or herpetiform ulceration observed by physician or patient that recurred at least three times in 12 months.
Ulcerations plus two of the following criteria:
1. ***Recurrent genital:*** Aphthous ulcer or scarring, observed by physician or patient
2. ***Eye lesions:*** Anterior/posterior uveitis or cells in the vitreous on slit lamp examination or retinal vasculitis observed by ophthalmologist
3. ***Skin lesions:*** Erythema nodosum, pseudofolliculitis or papulo-pustular lesions or acneiform nodule observed by physician in post adolescent patient not on steroids
4. ***Positive pathergy test:*** Read by physician at 24–48 hours.

Gastrointestinal features include abdominal pain, hematemesis, melena and perforation of viscera.

Neurological manifestations include meningitis, meningoencephalitis, motor disturbances, brainstem symptoms and psychiatric disturbances.

Box 110.4 shows International study group criteria for Behçet's syndrome.

Treatment

Arthritis and oral ulcers can be treated with colchicine (1–2 mg) day and nonsteroidal anti-inflammatory drugs (NSAIDs). Mainstay of treatment of severe disease is corticosteroids. Immunosuppressants such as azathioprine and cyclosporine and cytotoxic drugs such as cyclophosphamide and chlorambucil are required in cases resistant to corticosteroids. Ocular lesions are treated with local corticosteroid drops and colchicine 0.51–0.5 mg/day orally. In intractable cases, interferon alpha and anti-TNF (tumor necrosis factor) agents are used with success. Deep vein thrombosis (DVT) or arterial occlusions may warrant anticoagulation.

SINGLE-ORGAN VASCULITIS

Hypersensitivity Vasculitis (Cutaneous Leukocytoclastic Angiitis)

It is a small vessel LCV involving the skin without affecting internal organs. It can occur secondary to infections, drugs or malignancies. Patients present with vasculitic lesions on the trunk or lower extremities. ***Treatment*** is symptomatic with control of the underlying cause. Steroids may be required in severe cases. Immunosuppressives are not indicated (Fig. 110.11).

Source: Konttinen YT, Pettersson T, Matucci-Cerinic M, et al. Roadmap to vasculitis: a rheumatological treasure hunt. Indian J Rheum. 2007;2(2):55-64.

CHAPTER
111

Polymyositis and Dermatomyositis

Binoy J Paul, KV Krishna Das

Chapter Summary

- General Considerations
- Inflammatory Muscle Disease
  - Polymyositis
  - Dermatomyositis
  - Inclusion Body Myositis
    - Pathology

GENERAL CONSIDERATIONS

Myopathies are diseases which are characterized by acute, subacute or chronic weakness, wasting, myalgia, muscle cramps, stiffness, fatigability and such features. Many of them are hereditary. Others are acquired. Most of them have a neurological basis. They are dealt with in Section 17 on Neurology.

Rheumatological affection of muscles, tendons, entheses and soft tissues are inflammatory lesions and hence, they are termed *myositis*. Myositis may be primary (idiopathic) or secondary to other factors.

- **Idiopathic inflammatory myositis (IIM):**
  - Polymyositis
  - Dermatomyositis
  - Inclusion body myositis (IBM)
- **Secondary myopathies:**
  - Connective tissue diseases
  - Malignancy
  - **Drugs:** Statins, penicillamine, zidovudine
  - **Infections:** Human immunodeficiency virus (HIV), dengue fever.

INFLAMMATORY MUSCLE DISEASE (IDIOPATHIC INFLAMMATORY MYOSITIS)

POLYMYOSITIS

It is a diffuse immune-mediated IIM in which predominantly muscles show nonsuppurative inflammatory lesions associated with weakness and atrophy. Some are associated with changes in the skin, manifesting as rash, pigmentation or others. These are included under the term dermatomyositis. In India, this disease may be seen in skin clinics, rheumatology services, neurology clinics or internal medicine departments. Majority of them are primary without any underlying disease. Secondary form occurs in the course of other connective tissue diseases or as a paraneoplastic manifestation of malignancy.

DERMATOMYOSITIS

It is the least common among the connective tissue disorders. It consists of inflammatory and degenerative lesions involving the skin, striated muscles and other connective tissues in varying combinations. Dermatomyositis is more common in the 2nd, 5th, and 6th decades. Women are more affected than men. It can occur in association with connective tissue diseases and as paraneoplastic manifestation of malignancies arising from ovaries, gastrointestinal tract (GIT), breast, lungs, nasopharynx and also in lymphomas.

INCLUSION BODY MYOSITIS (IBM)

It is an IIM occurring in adults above the age of 50 years. It can be seen in association with Sjögren's syndrome. Systemic features like fever and fatigue are not usual. Skin changes are not seen. There is early involvement of finger flexors, wrist flexors and wrist extensors. Quadriceps weakness is also common to develop early.

Analysis of 87 patients with inflammatory myositis seen over a 10-year period at the Madras Medical College gave the following break up:

- Adult polymyositis—24
- Adult dermatomyositis—26
- Juvenile myositis—5
- Carcinomatous myositis—1
- Amyopathic dermatomyositis—1
- Overlap connective lesions—30

Male to female distribution was 1.2:3.5.

Source: Porkodi R, Shanmuganandan K, Parthiban M, et al. Clinical spectrum of inflammatory myositis in South India—a ten year study. J Assoc Physicians India. 2002;50:1255-8.

Pathology

The muscles show fragmentation, loss of cross-striation, cellular infiltration of interstitial connective tissue, increase in sarcolemmal nuclei and rarely calcification. Perivascular inflammatory changes are present. Skin shows swelling and edema of dermal collagen, atrophy of epidermis and flattening of rete pegs.

In IBM, muscle biopsy shows vacuolated fibers and tubulofilamentous inclusions in the muscle.

Clinical Features

Polymyositis and *dermatomyositis* patients present with muscle pain and symmetrical muscle weakness. A wide spectrum of clinical severity ranging from an acute, extensive rapidly fatal paralytic syndrome to a very slowly progressive muscle disease closely resembling a muscular dystrophy may be seen. Proximal muscles are affected more than others in the early stages. Muscle tenderness is prominent in the acute stages. Eventually fibrosis and contractures occur. The muscles are hyper-reflexic. Though in one-third of patients, the esophageal and pharyngeal muscles are affected, the ocular muscles are spared. Muscle enzymes creatine phosphokinase (CPK) and lactic dehydrogenase (LDH) are increased. The electromyogram (EMG) shows myopathic pattern.

In dermatomyositis, in addition to muscle involvement, characteristic skin lesions are seen. The diagnostic skin lesion of dermatomyositis is a **heliotrope rash** on the face, associated with periorbital edema (Fig. 111.1). Another pathognomonic skin lesion is **Gottron's papules** which are erythematous plaques over the metacarpophalangeal joints and, proximal or distal interphalangeal joints (Fig. 111.2). Skin lesions may precede, coexist or follow the muscular involvement. Cutaneous lesions may ulcerate and leave behind depressed scars. Subcutaneous and periarticular calcification may be seen. Around 35% of cases show a nonerosive arthritis, particularly small joints of the hands.

In IBM, skin lesions are absent. Muscle weakness is often asymmetrical. There is early involvement of finger flexors and wrists. Weakness of quadriceps femoris also

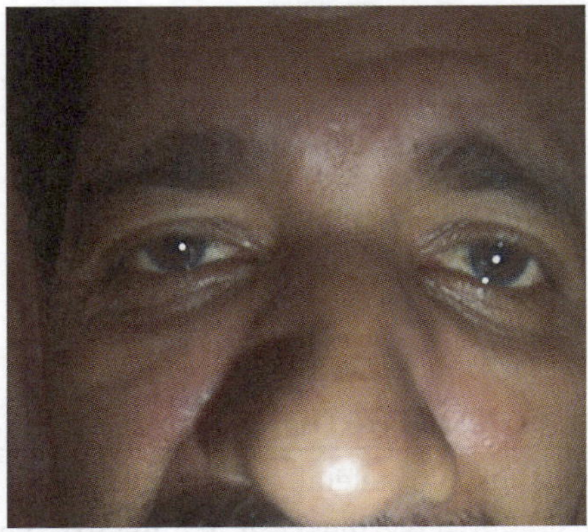

Fig. 111.1: Heliotrope rash on the face associated with periorbital edema and erythema in dermatomyositis

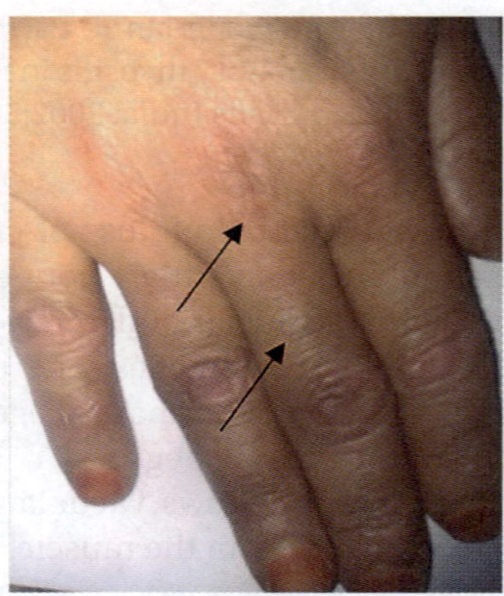

Fig. 111.2: Gottron's papules. **Note:** The erythematous plaques over the metacarpophalangeal and proximal interphalangeal joints (arrow)

may occur. Muscle enzymes may show normal or high values, but EMG will be usually abnormal. Muscle biopsy shows vacuolated fibers and tubulofilamentous inclusions in the muscle fibers.

Diagnosis

The diagnosis is made on clinical grounds, electromyography, raised levels of CPK, aldolase, serum glutamic oxaloacetic transaminase (SGOT) and LDH. **Rheumatoid factor** is present in many cases and antinuclear factor in 30% cases. EMG shows myopathic potentials. Muscle biopsy confirms the diagnosis.

The course is variable. In some, it is rapidly progressive and fatal due to cardiac, renal or pulmonary complications (myocarditis, interstitial lung disease and others). Many follow a slowly progressive course extending over 10–15 years leading to muscle weakness, contractures and deformities. Spontaneous remission is seen in some cases.

The clinical picture of dermatomyositis may develop in the course of other connective tissue disorders like rheumatoid disease, Sjögren's syndrome, scleroderma or lupus erythematosus. In such cases, the occurrence of muscle weakness out of proportion to the primary condition should suggest the possibility of superadded dermatomyositis. Death in dermatomyositis is mainly due to respiratory complications.

Management

Corticosteroids are the mainstay of treatment in polymyositis/dermatomyositis. Prednisolone in a dosage of 1–2 mg/kg/day to start with and subsequently tapered off, is effective in the majority of cases. Immunosuppressive agents like methotrexate and azathioprine are indicated when the response to corticosteroids is unsatisfactory. The dose of azathioprine is 2–3 mg/kg/day, to start with and tapered off to 1 mg/kg daily for varying periods depending on the response. Mycophenolate mofetil is a good drug which may be tried in resistant cases. The dose is 2 g/day. Cyclosporine given in a dose of 3–5 mg/kg/day is effective in many cases. Physiotherapy is indicated to prevent disuse atrophy and contractures.

The response to steroids is poor for IBM. Intravenous (IV) immunoglobulin is found to be useful in these cases. In refractory cases, rituximab and tacrolimus can be tried. Dose of rituximab is 1,000 mg IV on days 0 and 14.

Since dermatomyositis may occur as a paraneoplastic phenomenon, an underlying malignancy should be excluded in all cases. Factors like age of onset more than 50 years, mild or no elevation of muscle enzymes, lack of muscle weakness in spite of characteristic skin lesions and progressive weight loss are pointers towards underlying malignancy. Removal of the tumor brings about remission.

CHAPTER
112

Miscellaneous Rheumatic Syndromes

KV Krishna Das, Binoy J Paul

> **Chapter Summary**
>
> - General Considerations
> - Lumbago-Sciatica Syndrome
> - Frozen Shoulder
> - Shoulder-hand Syndrome
> - Tennis Elbow
> - Golfer's Elbow
> - Fibromyalgia

GENERAL CONSIDERATIONS

In many musculoskeletal syndromes, no definite disorders of bone, cartilage or connective tissue may be demonstrable. These present with pain and varying grades of disability due to local inflammatory changes but follow a self-limiting course. **Precipitating factors** include exposure to inclement weather, unaccustomed exercise, infections, faulty postures and mild trauma. These disorders are more common in the older age groups. In many cases, underlying diseases such as diabetes may be present, which have to be specially looked for.

LUMBAGO-SCIATICA SYNDROME

Pain is vaguely located in the low back, it may radiate to the lower limbs. Signs of nerve root compression do not occur.

Even though the condition is not life-threatening and apparently trivial without positive physical findings except anxiety and depression, low back pain of obscure etiology is one among the most common pain syndromes, accounting for absenteeism, loss of work force and disability benefits. *Management* consists of elimination of organic disease, analgesics, physiotherapy, psychotropic drugs and counseling. In many patients, the disability tends to persist.

FROZEN SHOULDER

This is a condition of painful limitation of movement of the shoulder. In the initial stages, the shoulder is tender and painful, but later on it becomes painless. It is most probably caused by lesions of the rotator cuff. Myocardial infarction (MI), hemiplegia, herpes zoster or surgery on the chest wall may be followed by the syndrome of 'frozen shoulder'.

SHOULDER-HAND SYNDROME

This is a condition in which shoulder movements are restricted and it is associated with pain and swelling of the hand. Conditions which lead to frozen shoulder also may give rise to this syndrome. The incidence is more in epileptics and those on barbiturates and anti-tuberculosis drugs. *Treatment* consists of judicious administration of analgesics, anti-inflammatory drugs, corticosteroids, local shortwave diathermy and manipulation and in some cases sympathetic nerve block may be required. In many cases, shoulder-hand syndrome may be the first manifestation of diabetes mellitus (DM) or impaired glucose tolerance.

Other Painful Conditions Around the Shoulder

These include supraspinatus tendinitis, subacromial bursitis, bicipital tendinitis and periarthritis of the shoulder joint. These result from overuse of the joints or faulty positions. They are more common in diabetics and elderly persons.

Management

Though these various rheumatic syndromes are not serious, they can lead to painful limitation of movement, prolonged morbidity and atrophy of shoulder muscles. *Treatment* consists of nonsteroidal anti-inflammatory drugs (NSAIDs), local physiotherapy and manipulation of the joint to restore mobility. Local injection of cortisone acetate into the affected tissue gives immediate relief.

TENNIS ELBOW

This condition is caused by tendinitis of the common origin of the extensor tendons at the lateral epicondyle.

GOLFER'S ELBOW

This condition is caused by the inflammation of the common flexor tendon from the medial epicondyle.

FIBROMYALGIA

Pain and stiffness arising in muscles or other soft tissues may occur in the absence of any definable musculoskeletal pathology. It is a syndrome of widespread chronic muscular pain and tender points. Widespread pain is defined as pain on the axial spine together with pain in at least two contralateral quadrants of the body; *chronic* is defined as more than three months of pain; high-tender count was defined as 11 or more tender points out of a specified set of 18 points to be examined. These tender points may have physical lumps of all sizes ranging from the size of wheat grain to that of an apple. Associated symptoms such as fatigue, poor sleep and stiffness are also recognized as common. They are also more likely to report depressive symptoms, anxiety and difficulty with sleep. There are other associations with diseases such as irritable bowel syndrome and chronic fatigue.

The *etiology* of this condition is unclear. The relationship with psychological factors suggests an abnormal sensitivity to pain. Analgesic therapy is of questionable benefit. Cognitive therapies are being assessed.

Whether we label patients as having fibromyalgia or not, there is no doubt that many patients have diffuse pain, sleep disturbances, fatigue and tender points. There is no specific treatment, but individual patients may be helped by tricyclic antidepressants such as fluoxetine or analgesics like tramadol. Adequate explanation of the condition to learn to live with it and avoid further unnecessary investigations are very important. Regular exercises, physiotherapy, group exercises and alternate forms of therapy such as yoga, acupuncture may also help.

CHAPTER

113

Seronegative Spondyloarthropathies

Binoy J Paul, KV Krishna Das

Chapter Summary

- General Considerations
- Ankylosing Spondylitis
- Enteropathic Arthritis
- Psoriatic Arthropathy
- Reactive Arthritis and Reiter's Syndrome
- Undifferentiated Spondyloarthritis

GENERAL CONSIDERATIONS

Seronegative spondyloarthropathies (SSpA) are a group of heterogeneous joint disorders sharing certain common characteristics (Table 113.1). These are predilection to affect the axial skeleton (sacroiliac joint and lumbar spine), oligoarthritis of large joints of lower limbs, enthesitis, extra-articular manifestations (skin, eyes, gut,

Table 113.1: Salient clinical features of the common seronegative spondyloarthropathies

	Ankylosing spondylitis	*Psoriatic arthritis*	*Reactive arthritis*	*Enteropathic arthritis*
Prevalence[a]	0.1%	0.1%	>0.05%	>0.05%
Male:female ratio	3:1	1:1	9:1	1:1
Axial arthritis				
Frequency	100%	20%	20%	15%
Radiographic features				
Sacroiliitis	Bilateral	Unilateral	Unilateral	Bilateral
Syndesmophytes	Symmetric Marginal	Asymmetric Bulky	Asymmetric Bulky	Symmetric Marginal
Peripheral arthritis				
Frequency	25%	60–95%	90%	20%
Typical distribution	Monoarticular, oligoarticular	Oligoarticular, polyarticular	Monoarticular, oligoarticular	Monoarticular, oligoarticular
Typical affected joints	Hip, knee, ankle	Knee, ankle, DIPs	Knee, ankle	Knee, ankle
Uveitis frequency	30%	15%	15–20%	5%
Dactylitis frequency	Uncommon	25%	30–50%	Uncommon
Cutaneous findings	Nonspecific	Psoriasis Onycholysis, Nail pitting	Oral ulcerations Keratoderma blennorrhagica	Erythema nodosum Pyoderma gangrenosum
HLA-B27 positivity[a]				
All cases	90%	40%	50–80%	30%
With axial disease	90%	50%	90%	50%
Pulmonary involvement	Upper lobe fibrosis, chest expansion decreased	Nil	Rare	Nil
GI involvement	Nil	Nil	Nil	Yes
Genitourinary involvement	Nil	Nil	Genital lesions, urethritis	Nil
Cardiac involvement	Aortic regurgitation, conduction abnormalities	Rare	Rare	Nil

Abbreviations: DIPs = Distal interphalangeal joints; HLA-B27 = Human leukocyte antigen-B27; GI = Gastrointestinal

urogenitals), negative rheumatoid factor (RF) and high association with human leukocyte antigen B27 (HLA-B27). The major members are ankylosing spondylitis (AS), reactive arthritis, psoriatic arthritis, enteropathic arthritis and undifferentiated spondyloarthritis (USpA).

The positivity rates for HLA-B27 in the different forms of arthritis are:

- Ankylosing spondylitis—90–95% (white population) and 50% in blacks
- Reactive arthritis—75%
- Psoriatic arthropathy—less than 50%
- Enteropathic arthritis—50%.

Association with HLA-B27 is one of predispositions to the disease, but only 1–6% of adults who are HLA-B27 positive develop AS. There is 6–16 times increased chance of developing the disease in first degree relatives of patients who are HLA-B27 positive.

ANKYLOSING SPONDYLITIS (MARIE-STRÜMPELL DISEASE, BAMBOO SPINE, POKER BACK)

This is an inflammatory arthropathy predominantly involving the axial skeleton and in the advanced stages the entire vertebral column undergoes bony ankylosis. This disease entity is considered as the prototype of SSpA (Fig. 113.1).

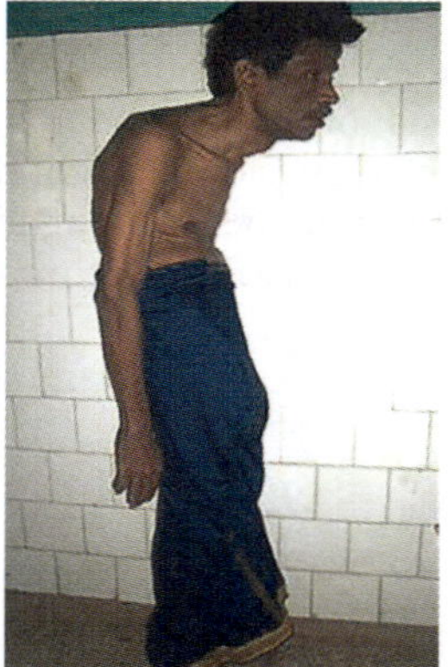

Fig. 113.1: Ankylosing spondylitis. **Note:** The kyphosis and fixed flexion deformity of the neck and upper thoracic spine

Prevalence and Epidemiology

This disease is rare compared to rheumatoid arthritis (RA). It is not an uncommon disease in India. Male to female ratio is 7:3.

Genetic Factors

The histocompatibility antigen type HLA-B27 is positive in over 90% of white and 50% of black population. The presence of the HLA-B27 antigen predisposes such individuals to develop arthritis in response to several environmental factors. The triggering event is probably an infection. In many cases, the organism is *Klebsiella pneumoniae*. Maximal lesions are in the **enthesis** (area of ligament or tendon that attaches to a bone) which show edema and infiltration by lymphocytes, plasma cells and polymorphonuclear leukocytes (PMNs). The adjacent bone marrow also shows edema and inflammation.

Pathology

The sacroiliac joints and vertebral joints are maximally affected, but the manubriosternal joints, symphysis pubis, costovertebral and sternocostal joints, shoulders, hips, and very rarely the joints of the hands and feet may also be affected. The joints show mild synovitis. Periarticular fibrous tissue, ligaments and articular cartilage also show inflammation. Extra-articular lesions develop in various ligaments, tenoperiosteal junctions (enthesis), the ascending aorta, uveal tract and the upper lobes of the lungs. Ankylosis develops in the joints on account of the tendency for calcification and ossification. The new bones formed are known as **syndesmophytes** which form the characteristic feature of the disease. Calcification and ossification of the annulus fibrosus and proliferative bony outgrowths from the vertebral borders result in ankylosis of the spine. The spinal column becomes a rigid pillar giving the radiological appearance of **bamboo spine**.

Clinical Features

The clinical severity ranges from partial forms (formes frustes) to the classic picture of severe ankylosis of the spine and other joints. The disease is more common in the 2nd, 3rd and 4th decades. Bouts of **inflammatory low backache**, felt mostly in the morning and aggravated by periods of rest are the early manifestations. Activity reduces the back pain in contrast to mechanical backache. Later, the pain becomes constant. At this stage, obliteration of lumbar lordosis and generalized limitation of movements of the lumbar spine due to muscular spasm are detectable. Later, ankylosis of spinal joints *(poker back)* occurs. The whole spine becomes a single rigid column.

Tenderness over the sacroiliac joints is elicitable by deep palpation. Pain from the sacroiliac joints is elicited by the **pump handle test**, the pelvic compression test and hyperextension test.

Other joints may be involved in 50% of cases, the most common being the root joints, viz. hips and shoulders, and hence, the term **rhizomelic spondylitis**. It is rare to get affection of the peripheral small joints. When it occurs, it is **asymmetrical** and milder compared to RA. Later on, they also may be ankylosed.

The patient with advanced AS develops forward craning of the neck, high dorsal kyphosis, rounding of the shoulders, obliteration of the normal lumbar lordosis, wasting of the glutei, flattening of the chest and ballooning of the abdomen. Forward vision is impaired due to the stooping posture.

A simple but reliable test to diagnose AS is the **modified Schober test**. A 10 cm long line is drawn perpendicularly up from the midpoint of a line joining the posterior superior iliac spines. In normal persons, this line stretches to 16–22 cm when the patient fully bends forwards. In established AS, this line does not stretch more than 1 or 2 cm.

Extra-articular Features

These include unilateral anterior uveitis (20%), aortic incompetence, heart block, pericarditis and fibrosis of the upper lobes of the lung.

Recurrent enthesopathy occurs in many cases. This manifests as plantar fasciitis, tennis elbow, costochondritis or Achilles tendonitis.

Complications

Fracture dislocations of the spine and other bones, and secondary amyloidosis constitute the main complications.

Though in the majority of cases the picture of AS is typical, less commonly the presentation may be atypical. These are—(1) isolated sacroiliitis, (2) asymmetrical peripheral polyarthritis and (3) uveitis.

Laboratory Data

The erythrocyte sedimentation rate (ESR) and C-reactive protein (CRP) are elevated in the early phases of inflammation, but it returns to normal levels in the later stage when ankylosis is complete.

Imaging

X-ray

Early abnormality is in the sacroiliac joints which shows an appearance of widening *(pseudowidening)* and erosions (Fig. 113.2). As the disease progresses, the adjacent zones become sclerosed and the joint space is obliterated by bony fusion. The vertebrae appear square due to a combination of osteitis of the borders and filling up of the anterior concavity. The fully developed stage gives the typical picture of **bamboo spine** (Fig. 113.3).

Magnetic Resonance Imaging

Sacroiliitis can be identified in magnetic resonance imaging (MRI) in early stage much before changes occur in plain X-ray. Soft tissue edema, tendinitis and joint effusions can also be identified in MRI.

Diagnosis

Clinical diagnosis has to be confirmed by radiology and the diagnosis is strengthened by demonstration of

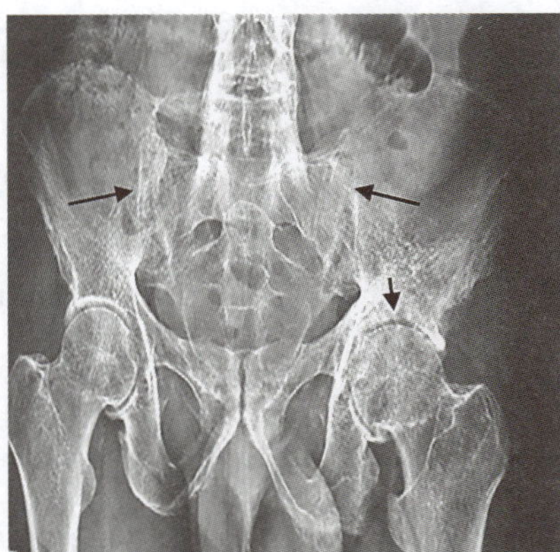

Fig. 113.2: X-ray pelvis and hip in ankylosing spondylitis. **Note:** The bilateral sclerosis of sacroiliac joints (arrows) and erosive changes in the left hip joint (arrowhead)

Textbook of Medicine

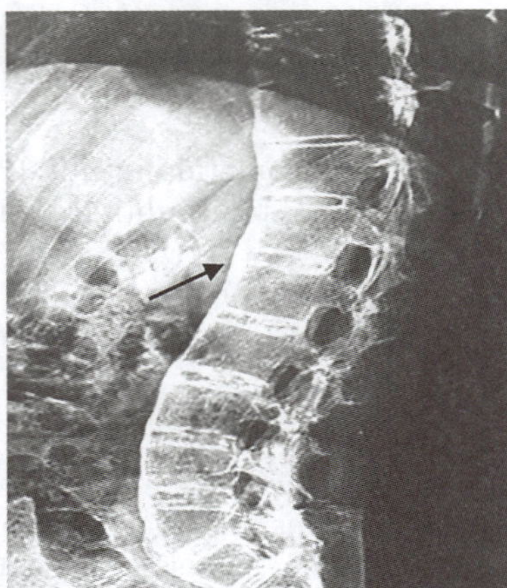

Fig. 113.3: X-ray lumbar spine in ankylosing spondylitis (AS). **Note:** Calcification of anterior longitudinal ligament leads to the appearance of bamboo spine (arrow)

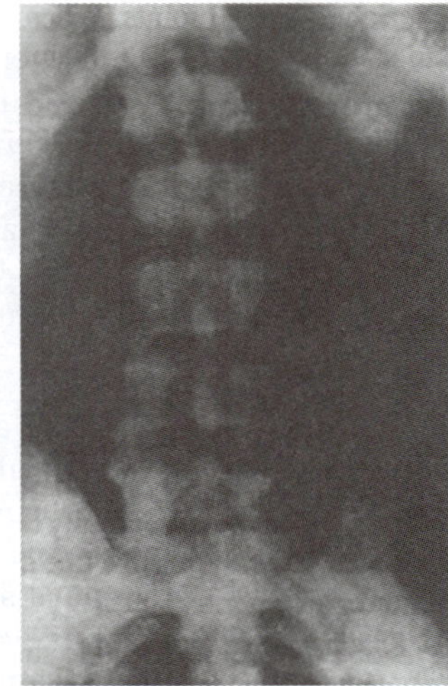

Fig. 113.4: X-ray spine—fluorosis. **Note:** SI joints are free

HLA-B27. When the age of onset is below 20 years, other forms of arthritis which involve this age group have to be distinguished. The diagnosis is likely to be delayed in such cases. Assessment of Spondylo-Arthritis International Society (ASAS) developed a classification criteria which is widely used now (Flowchart 113.1).

Differential Diagnosis

This includes osteoarthritis, lumbar spondylosis, other causes of sacroiliac arthritis like tuberculosis, brucellosis, and also endemic fluorosis. In endemic fluorosis, radiology may show lesions of the spine resembling AS but the sacroiliac joints are normal (Fig. 113.4).

Management

Treatment is aimed at improving spinal mobility, preventing ankylosis and giving symptomatic relief. The modalities of treatment include physical measures and appliances, medications, irradiation or surgery.

Flowchart 113.1: Assessment of Spondylo-Arthritis International Society (ASAS) classification criteria for axial spondyloarthritis in patients with back pain of more than 3 months duration and age of onset less than 45 years

Sacroiliitis on imaging plus* One or more SSpA features**	or	HLA-B27 plus two or more other SSpA features**

*Sacroiliitis on imaging
- Active (acute) inflammation on MRI, suggestive of sacroiliitis associated with SpA
  or
- Definite radiographic sacroiliitis according to modified criteria

**SSpA features
- Inflammatory back pain
- Arthritis
- Enthesitis (heel)
- Uveitis
- Dactylitis
- Psoriasis
- Crohn's disease/ulcerative colitis
- Good response to NSAIDs
- Family history of SpA
- HLA-B27
- Elevated CRP

Note: Elevated CRP is considered a SpA feature in the context of chronic back pain

Abbreviations: SSpA = Seronegative spondyloarthropathies; HLA-B27 = Human leukocyte antigen B27; MRI = Magnetic resonance imaging; NSAIDs = Nonsteroidal anti-inflammatory drug; SpA = Spondyloarthropathies; CRP = C-reactive protein

Physical Measures and Appliances

Regular spinal exercises help to correct postural abnormalities and strengthen the spinal ligaments and paraspinal muscles. Prolonged immobility tends to accelerate ankylosis and this should be avoided. Spinal braces help to correct postural defects partly. Prismatic spectacles enable the patient with severe kyphosis to see objects in front.

Drugs

Commonly used drugs are indomethacin and other nonsteroidal anti-inflammatory drugs (NSAIDs). Systemic corticosteroids are not useful. Intra-articular or intra-lesional steroid injections are tried in recalcitrant enthesitis, persistent peripheral synovitis and severe sacroiliitis. Topical steroids are useful in anterior uveitis.

Sulfasalazine in doses of 500–1,000 mg 8 hours orally, given over prolonged periods help to relieve pain of peripheral arthritis and possibly of the axial lesion too. In peripheral arthritis, methotrexate is also useful in doses of 7.5–25 mg/week. In axial disease, these disease modifying agents are not very effective. Pamidronate and thalido-mide were also tried with limited success.

Anti-tumor necrosis factor (anti-TNF)-alpha biological agents like ***infliximab***, ***etanercept*** and ***adalimumab*** are very useful to control the disease activity and maintaining the mobility of spine.

Infliximab given in a dose of 5 mg/kg intravenous (IV) at weeks 0, 2 and 6 produced remarkable improvement when followed up to 1 year. Etanercept 50 mg weekly was also equally useful (*See* Ch 118 for anti-TNF agents).

Surgery

Permanent deformities of the spine, hip and other joints can be corrected by orthopedic procedures. The disability has been considerably reduced by total hip replacement which has improved the outlook for patients with AS.

ENTEROPATHIC ARTHRITIS

A heterogeneous group of arthritic syndromes develop secondary to primary lesions in the gastrointestinal tract (GIT). The primary GI disorders leading to arthritis are: (1) Chronic inflammatory bowel diseases (IBD) such as ulcerative colitis (UC), Crohn's disease (regional ileitis) and Whipple's disease (intestinal lipodystrophy); (2) acute infective disorders such as salmonellosis, bacterial dysenteries and *Yersinia enterocolitica* infection; (3) intestinal bypass surgery and (4) gut-associated neoplasms which produce arthritis as paraneoplastic manifestations.

Arthritis-associated with Chronic Inflammatory Disease of Bowel

Even though UC, Crohn's disease and Whipple's disease are separate entities, arthritis produced by all the three and are similar clinically. Two types are seen—(1) a ***peripheral polyarthritis*** and (2) secondary ***AS*** with sacroiliitis.

The peripheral arthropathy manifests as asymmetric affection of the major joints of the lower limbs. Distal interphalangeal (DIP) joints may be affected. The arthritis is self-limiting and residual damage is unusual. With subsidence of the intestinal lesion, the arthritis also subsides.

A clinical picture identical with idiopathic AS may develop in some cases but there is no male preponderance. Unlike the peripheral arthritic syndrome, the spondylitic variety does not bear any relation to the severity or extent of the bowel disease.

Investigations

Neither the synovial fluid nor the synovial biopsy shows diagnostic features. Radiology of the joints remains essentially normal except for the soft tissue swelling and minimal osteoporosis. The diagnosis is based on the clinical picture, temporal relation with bowel disease and exclusion of other forms of arthritis.

Management

Since the peripheral type of arthritis is self-limiting, only symptomatic and supportive measures are required for the joint disease. ***Treatment*** is directed toward the bowel disorder. Sulfasalazine is highly useful for bowel and joint diseases. In the spondylitic type, line of management is similar to that of idiopathic AS.

Arthritis-associated with Other Forms of Intestinal Disease

Whipple's Disease

This is a rare disorder affecting several systems characterized predominantly by diarrhea, steatorrhea, malabsorption, fever, anemia, pigmentary disturbances and joint lesions.

The causative agent is most probably a gram-positive bacillus belonging to the ***Actinobacter*** group and designated *Tropheryma whipplei*. Histologically, the small intestine shows characteristic lesions. Large macrophages containing glycoprotein-rich lysosomes are seen to infiltrate the lamina propria and submucosa. The bacilli are seen within the macrophages. The mucosal and submucosal lymphatics are dilated and obstructed. Other tissues may be involved. These include mesenteric and peripheral lymph nodes, liver, spleen, heart, lung and central nervous system (CNS).

Clinical features

Clinical features are protean, depending upon the predominant pathological process. Joint symptoms occur in about 60% of cases. These may predate the intestinal symptoms, or coexist with them. Joint symptoms include episodic inflammatory arthritis of abrupt onset involving large joints mainly, but also the joints of the hands at times. Diagnosis is established by demonstrating the intestinal lesion by mucosal biopsy. The joint fluid shows only signs of nonspecific inflammation.

Treatment

Whipple's disease responds to antibiotics such as cotrimoxazole, chloramphenicol or tetracyclines. Symptomatic measures are instituted for joint symptoms.

Infective Disorders of the Intestines

A migratory polyarthritis may develop up to 3 weeks after the occurrence of bacillary dysentery, *Salmonella* infections and *Yersinia enterocolitica* infection. This is an immunologically-mediated reactive arthropathy.

Gastrointestinal Bypass Surgery

Jejunocolic or jejunoileal anastomosis done as a therapeutic measure for severe obesity may be followed by a polyarthritic syndrome 2–3 months later. Restoration of normal bowel anatomy clears the arthropathy.

Arthritis associated with malignancies of the GIT may precede or accompany the neoplasm. Removal of the tumor clears the joint lesions too.

PSORIATIC ARTHROPATHY

Joints may be affected in psoriasis in one of the following five ways:

1. Predominantly distal arthritis involving the interphalangeal joints
2. Asymmetrical oligoarthritis
3. Classic arthritis mutilans with digital telescoping and sacroiliac involvement
4. Symmetrical arthritis closely resembling RA
5. Spondylitis with or without peripheral arthritis.

Clinical Features

Pain and disability are less severe than in RA. Psoriatic lesions may be demonstrable in the skin or nails along with the arthritis. Rarely the joint lesion may precede or follow the skin lesion and in such cases diagnosis may be presumptive for long periods. Involvement of the DIP joint has to be distinguished from RA, osteoarthritis, hypertrophic osteoarthropathy and enteropathic arthropathy (Figs 113.5A to D). Extensive psoriasis is a risk factor for metabolic syndrome, cardiovascular risk factors and subclinical atherosclerosis.

Source: Karoli R, Fatima J, Shukla V, et al. A study of cardiometabolic risk profile in patients with psoriasis. J Assoc Physicians India. 2013;61(11):798-803.

Management

Disease modifying antirheumatic drugs are highly useful for control of disease activity in psoriatic arthritis. The commonly used agent is methotrexate (10–25 mg/

Textbook of Medicine

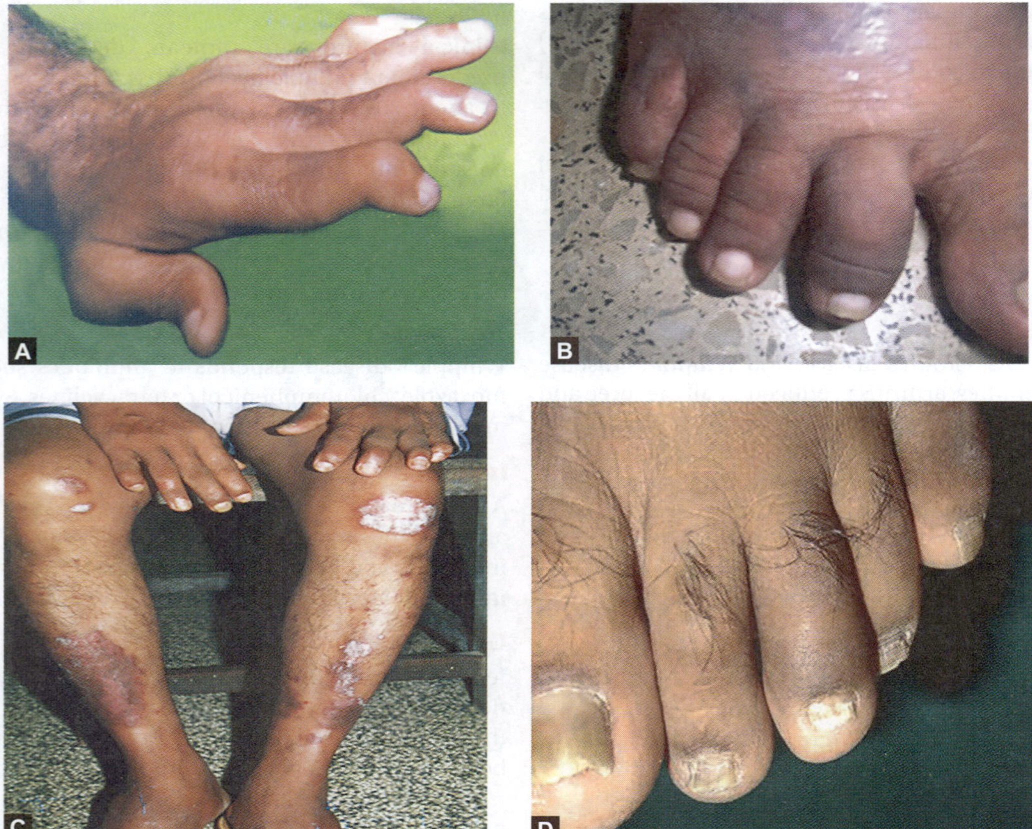

Figs 113.5A to D: **A.** Psoriatic arthritis. Involvement of distal interphalangeal joints; **B.** Sausage-shaped second toe due to dactylitis in psoriasis; **C.** Psoriatic skin lesions, arthritis of knees and distal interphalangeal (DIP) joints; **D.** Nail dystrophy in psoriasis

week). Leflunomide and sulfasalazine are also useful. Chloroquine and hydroxychloroquine are better avoided due to risk of exacerbating the skin lesion. Corticosteroids bring about dramatic relief in an acute case of arthritis but can cause flare up of skin lesions on withdrawal and are not preferred agents. In resistant cases, anti-TNF agents like etanercept and infliximab are very useful.

The retinoid—***etretinate*** 20 mg daily is an effective adjuvant to treat the joint as well as the skin condition. A newer analog is ***acitretin*** which is cleared faster from the system the dose is 25–50 mg/day, to be given for several months. It should be avoided in young women due to risk of teratogenicity. The primary treatment for psoriasis, i.e. photochemotherapy with methoxypsoralen and long wave ultraviolet light, while relieving the skin condition may benefit the arthritis as well. (For further details *See* Section 18, Ch 223, Psoriasis).

REACTIVE ARTHRITIS AND REITER'S SYNDROME

Reactive arthritis is a sterile joint inflammation occurring following a distant infection. Common sites of infection are genitourinary tract and the gut.

The triad of symptoms—nonspecific urethritis, conjunctivitis and arthritis—which follow an attack of urethritis is termed ***Reiter's syndrome***. It is a type of reactive arthritis. The etiology is unknown. Reiter's syndrome develops as a complication of nongonococcal urethritis. Over 80% of subjects have HLA-B27.

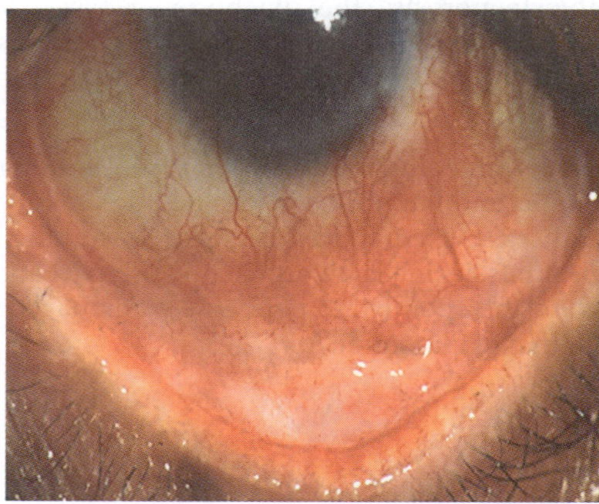

Fig. 113.6: Conjunctivitis in Reiter's syndrome

Age and Sex

Reiter's syndrome develops more frequently in males following nongonococcal urethritis. This gender difference is less striking in the postdysenteric group. The organisms implicated in reactive arthritis are chlamydia, *Shigella*, *Campylobacter*, *Yersinia*, *Salmonella enteritidis* and *Salmonella typhimurium*.

Clinical Features

Patients with reactive arthritis present with acute oligoarthritis of lower limb joints. The clinical spectrum of Reiter's syndrome may vary from the fully developed picture of urethritis, arthritis and conjunctivitis (Fig. 113.6)

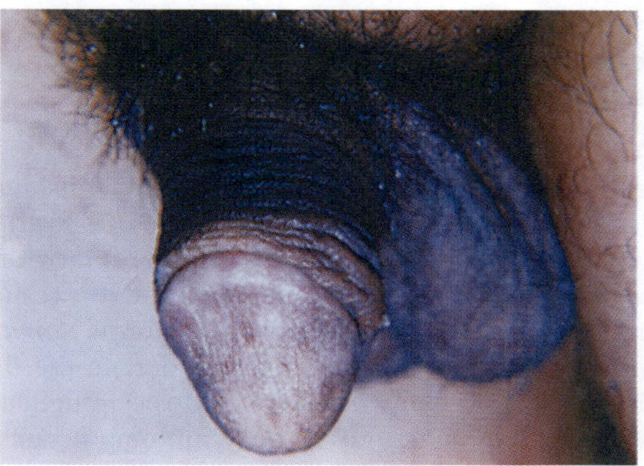

Fig. 113.7: Circinate balanitis in Reiter's syndrome

to less complete forms with only urethritis and arthritis. The clinical spectrum includes recurrent episodes of tenosynovitis, plantar fasciitis, enthesopathies and frank arthritis. Twenty percent may develop lesions of the sacroiliac joints and secondary spondylitis. In Reiter's syndrome, other common features include stomatitis, circinate balanitis (Fig. 113.7), and ***keratoderma blennorrhagica*** (hyperkeratotic lesions of the palms, soles, and other regions) which may proceed to pustulation and scaling. The oral and cutaneous lesions are painless. The ESR is elevated up to 100 mm and this is a common finding. Anterior uveitis may develop in some of the patients. In many cases, the disease tends to become chronic and progressive, leading to spondyloarthritis.

Diagnosis

Clinical features and the presence of the precipitating cause should suggest the diagnosis. RF is negative. X-ray changes are unusual except in chronic or recurrent cases.

Presence of the primary causative lesion supports the diagnosis.

Management

Management is symptomatic, since there is no specific curative treatment. Doxycycline is employed to treat the urethritis. NSAIDs give symptomatic relief. Intra-articular corticosteroids have been tried with temporary benefit. Patients with persistent peripheral arthritis (>3 months) often respond to sulfasalazine. Methotrexate is also useful which can be given safely under supervision in chronic cases.

UNDIFFERENTIATED SPONDYLOARTHRITIS

It is a type of spondyloarthritis where the patient does not fulfill the criteria for any specific form of SSpA. It may be an early phase or atypical form of AS or any other type of SSpA in some cases. But the majority of these patients remain in the undifferentiated form even on long-term follow up. This entity is very common in India.

Diagnosis

A patient with either inflammatory back pain or peripheral arthritis who also has evidence of current or previous enthesopathy or alternating buttock pain would be classified as USpA. There are no pathognomonic clinical features for USpA. Diagnosis has to be made on a combination of history, clinical examination and supportive laboratory tests. Inflammatory back pain, unilateral or alternating buttock pain, enthesitis, peripheral arthritis, dactylitis (sausage digit), acute anterior uveitis, elevated ESR or CRP, HLA-B27 positivity, family history of spondyloarthritis, imaging showing sacroiliitis and good response to NSAIDs are points in favor of USpA.

CHAPTER

114

Metabolic Arthropathies
Osteoporosis, Gout and Other Forms of Crystal-induced Arthropathies

Binoy J Paul, KV Krishna Das

Chapter Summary

- Osteoporosis
- Gout
- Other forms of Crystal-induced Arthropathy
  - Calcium Pyrophosphate Crystal Deposition Disease
  - Basic Calcium Phosphate Crystal Arthropathy
  - Calcium Oxalate Arthropathy

OSTEOPOROSIS

It is defined as a systemic skeletal disease characterized by lowered bone mass and microarchitectural deterioration of bone tissue with consequent increase in fragility and susceptibility to fractures. World Health Organization (WHO) has defined osteoporosis based on bone mineral content and bone mineral density (BMD). In simple terms, osteoporosis can be described as a reduction in bone mass without gross alteration in its chemical composition. Osteopenia is reduction in bone mass or disruption of bone architecture leading to increased risk of fractures. Osteoporosis can also be defined in terms of BMD studies as a dual energy X-ray absorptiometry (DEXA) score of 2.5 or less at the spine, hip and forearms. BMD studies of the hips are the most reliable parameters to predict fracture risk.

The bone matrix itself is deficient but osteoid is normally mineralized. Bone formation and resorption are in equilibrium in adults up to the age of 50 years and, therefore, up to this age the bone mass is fairly constant. The bone mass declines steadily but slightly after the age

Textbook of Medicine

of 50 years. Osteoporosis results from excessive resorption compared to formation. The precise mechanism leading to osteoporosis is not clear. In the majority, an etiological factor is demonstrable while in a few, this is not so. Genetic factors play a role. Several potential candidate genes have been described especially the one for vitamin D receptor.

Common Causes

Generalized Osteoporosis

Primary osteoporosis
- Type I (postmenopausal)
- Type II (senile)

Secondary osteoporosis
Endocrine abnormalities
- Diabetes mellitus (DM)
- Cushing's syndrome and corticosteroid therapy
- Hypogonadism
- Hypopituitarism
- Thyrotoxicosis
- Hyperparathyroidism

Renal causes
- Chronic kidney disease (CKD)
- Renal tubular acidosis (RTA)
- Idiopathic hypercalciuria

Gastrointestinal (GI)
- Malabsorption syndrome
- Inflammatory bowel diseases (IBD)

Chronic inflammatory diseases
- Rheumatoid arthritis (RA)
- Systemic lupus erythematosus (SLE)

Drugs
- Glucocorticoids
- Phenytoin

Hereditary connective tissue diseases
- Ehlers-Danlos syndrome
- Marfan's syndrome
- Homocystinuria and osteogenesis imperfecta

Miscellaneous
- Prolonged immobilization
- Disuse, paralysis, malnutrition

Localized Osteoporosis

- Localized immobilization following fractures
- Periarticular, e.g. RA
- Reflex bone dystrophy, e.g. shoulder-hand syndrome
- Secondary to irradiation therapy.

Pathogenesis

The resorption rate is high in osteoporosis, even though bone formation proceeds normally. Particular areas of the skeleton such as the metacarpals, femoral neck and vertebral bodies show higher rates of resorption. Maximum impact is on the axial skeleton. The peripheral bones are affected to a varying extent. Two types of bone loss are seen—type I and type II which are due to different mechanisms:

- ***Type I*** is seen mainly in women in the age group 50–70 years. It is due to accelerated bone loss with fracture sites mainly in the vertebrae, distal part of the radius and intracapsular part of hip.
- In ***type II***, trabecular bone is not affected. Cortical loss of bone occurs. It is seen above the age of 70 years in women and above 80 years in men. It presents with multiple wedge fractures of the vertebrae and extracapsular fracture of hip, proximal humerus and tibia.

Clinical Features

Osteoporosis remains asymptomatic for considerable periods till bone loss has become advanced. The vertebral bodies become soft and compressed. The intervertebral discs herniate into the vertebral bodies and this results in shortening of the vertebral column. The terms ***dowager's hump*** or ***widow's hump*** are used to denote the dorsal kyphosis with exaggerated cervical lordosis brought about by vertebral compression. When symptoms occur, they include vague muscular aches and pains, loss of height of the spine, and kyphoscoliosis. Vertebral collapse, fracture neck of the femur and Colles' fracture (fracture distal end of the radius) develop as a result of trivial trauma or even spontaneously. In general, the fractures heal within 4–6 weeks with simple treatment.

These sites may become painful and even tender for varying periods before demonstrable fractures develop. Early institution of treatment of this stage may relieve this symptom.

Skiagram reveals reduction in density of the vertebral bodies in the early stages and the vertical trabeculations appear more prominent. The vertebra becomes biconcave and this is referred to as ***cod fish vertebra*** (Fig. 114.1). The intervertebral disks herniate into the vertebral bodies. Vertebral collapse in the late stages results in anterior wedging of the vertebral bodies. The medullary cavities of long bones are expanded with thinning of the cortex. Sometimes differentiation from osteomalacia can be extremely difficult but pseudofractures which are present in osteomalacia are not seen in osteoporosis.

The most reliable investigation is to measure BMD by DEXA scan. Quantitative values of BMD are given, expressed in two forms—T score and Z score. T score compares the BMD of the patient with the mean peak BMD of the normal young adult population and expressed in terms of standard deviation (SD) (Box 114.1). Z score compares the BMD of the patients of the same age.

Quantitative computed tomography (CT) scan is also a sensitive test to pick up early osteoporosis but high

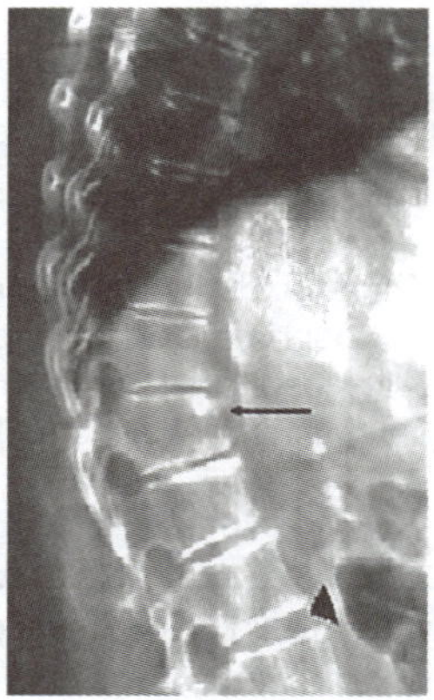

Fig. 114.1: X-ray osteoporosis spine. **Note:** Kyphosis, loss of density of vertebrae compression fracture (arrow) cod fish vertebrae (arrow head)

Metabolic Arthropathies

Box 114.1: WHO criteria for osteoporosis in adult women using T score by dual energy X-ray absorptiometry (DEXA)

- **Normal:** BMD is within 1.0 SD of the young adult reference mean
- **Osteopenia:** BMD 1–2.5 SD below the young adult mean
- **Osteoporosis:** BMD more than 2.5 SD below the young adult mean
- **Severe osteoporosis:** Osteoporosis with the presence of one or two fragility fractures.

Abbreviations: BMD = Bone mineral density; SD = Standard deviation

cost and exposure to ionizing radiations are drawbacks of this investigation.

BMD values of 0.72 suggests fracture threshold in South Indian elderly persons.

The sites commonly measured are the lumbar spine (L1–L4) including the intervertebral disks, hips and forearms. BMD of any other part of the skeleton or that of the whole skeleton can also be determined.

Before accepting the diagnosis as osteoporosis, a careful search for primary bone malignancies such as multiple myeloma and bone secondaries from the female genital organs, breasts and other sites should be excluded by appropriate investigations.

Laboratory Findings

The serum calcium, phosphorus and alkaline phosphatase (ALP) are normal and this distinguishes osteoporosis from osteomalacia in which calcium and phosphorus are low and ALP is elevated. As a result of excessive resorption of bone, urinary hydroxyproline is elevated above normal range (6.42 mg/g of creatinine up to 55 years of age), during the active phase of the disease.

Treatment

Acute episodes of fracture should be managed in the usual orthopedic lines.

General Measures

Adequate nutrition should be ensured, especially with supplements of calcium, vitamin D and proteins. Calcium supplementation (Table 114.1) given as calcium gluconate, lactate or carbonate 500–1,000 mg/oral/day helps to improve bone mineralization (Table 114.2). Active vitamin D_3 analogs such as calcitriol and alfacalcidol stimulate the formation and action of osteoblasts. A small but definite risk of urolithiasis occurs. Supplementation of vitamin D 800 units/day reduces the risk of fracture. Vertebral collapse usually heals satisfactorily with bed rest and analgesics. Early ambulation and exercise help to improve muscle tone. Provision of weight-bearing appliances or corsets helps to relieve pain and prevent further damage in the acute phase.

There is a slight risk of nephrolithiasis (1.17) in those taking calcium supplement and the risk is dose-dependent.

Table 114.1: Calcium supplementation—recommended intake for fracture prevention (Institute of Washington DC)

	Age (years)	Calcium recommended (mg/day)
Women Men	19–50 19–70	1,000
Women Men	> 50 > 70	1,200

Table 114.2: Elemental calcium content of calcium salts

Formulation	Dose	Elemental Calcium Content (%)	Comments
Calcium carbonate	1–2, 500 mg tablet taken oral two to three times/day with meals	40	Acidity improves absorption
Calcium citrate	1–2, 500 mg tablet taken two to three times a day	21	Need not be taken with meals, can be used in patients taking long-term acid suppression
Calcium gluconate	500, 642 or 972 mg	9	
Calcium lactate	300–325 mg tablet	13	
Bone meal, oyster shell, dolomite	Varies	30	May contain lead as a contaminant

Bisphosphonates

They are synthetic analog of inorganic pyrophosphate. They are deposited on bone surfaces. When ingested by osteoclasts during bone turnover their main action is anti-resorptive. These are excellent drugs which help to restore BMD in both sexes, relieve bone pains and possibly reduce the progression of osteoporosis (Table 114.3). They are indicated for treatment of established cases with demonstrable X-ray or DEXA criteria, on a short-term (a few months) or a long-term basis depending on the individual case. Though several preparations are available, one acceptable drug is **alendronate sodium** which is an aminophosphate. It inhibits osteoclastic activity. Given over periods up to 3 years in daily doses of 10 mg, it relieves the symptoms of postmenopausal osteoporosis and restores bone density. An alternative is to give 75 mg orally on an empty stomach once a week. Since the drug causes esophageal ulceration by local contact, the patient should maintain the erect posture for 15–30 minutes after taking the tablet. **Side effects** include heartburn, nausea, abdominal pain and vomiting. The drug is freely available in India. Other drugs in this class include etidronate, pamidronate, ibandronate, risedronate and zoledronic acid. Follow-up studies exceeding 10 years in osteoporosis have shown continued benefit with these drugs. On stopping bisphosphonates, the bone density falls gradually. In a trial of glucocorticoid-induced osteoporosis, alendronate in a dose of 10 mg/oral daily was more effective than alfacalcidol.

Apart from osteoporosis, bisphosphonates have been used for the treatment of hypercalcemia, malignant secondaries in bones and multiple myeloma.

Calcitonin: It is an excellent drug for osteoporosis. It acts by inhibiting the osteoclasts. Calcitonin nasal sprays are available which also relieve the bone pain of osteoporotic fractures due to release of beta endorphins, but long-term use is to be avoided due to the risk of developing malignancies like basal cell carcinoma of skin.

Table 114.3: Pharmacological interventions for osteoporosis

Intervention	Dosing regimen	Route of administration	Licensed indication
Alendronate	70 mg once weekly, or 5 mg or 10 mg once daily	Oral	Postmenopausal osteoporosis; glucocorticoid-induced osteoporosis and in men
Zoledronate	5 mg yearly for 3 years	Intravenous	Postmenopausal osteoporosis; glucocorticoid-induced osteoporosis
Ibandronate	150 mg once monthly; 3 mg once every 3 months	Oral Intravenous injection	Postmenopausal osteoporosis
Risedronate	35 mg once weekly, or 5 mg once daily	Oral	Postmenopausal osteoporosis; glucocorticoid-induced osteoporosis
Raloxifene	60 mg once daily	Oral	Postmenopausal osteoporosis
Strontium ranelate	2 g once daily	Oral	Postmenopausal osteoporosis
Teriparatide	20 µg once daily	Subcutaneous injection	Postmenopausal osteoporosis
Denosumab	60 mg once in 6 months	Subcutaneous injection	Postmenopausal osteoporosis

Parathyroid hormone: Parathyroid hormone (PTH) given in doses of 100 µg/day by subcutaneous (SC) injection increases bone strength, primarily by stimulating bone formation, especially of trabecular bones like the vertebrae and other sites. Both intact PTH as well as the 1-34-amino acid peptide, known as ***teriparatide*** are effective in reducing fracture risk, as long as the drugs are continued. The risk for fracture in postmenopausal women is also reduced. In smaller doses, PTH promotes osteoblastic activity, whereas in higher doses osteoclastic activity predominates. Continued elevation of PTHs, as is seen in hyperparathyroidism gives rise to bone demineralization and bone loss.

Hormone Replacement Therapy (HRT)

It was an accepted regimen for prevention of osteoporosis and fragility fractures in postmenopausal women. Menopause before the age of 45 years, surgical menopause, lean body mass, presence of nutritional inadequacy, lack of aerobic exercise and concurrent use of drugs such as corticosteroids aggravate the tendency and prepone the onset of osteoporosis. Benefits of HRT are several, including the feeling of well-being, reduction in progression of ischemic heart disease (IHD) and cosmetic effects. In postmenopausal osteoporosis, administration of 0.625–1.25 mg of conjugated estrogen daily for 3 weeks every month helps to arrest the progression of bone loss. Since estrogens may increase the tendency to develop endometrial cancer, it is advisable to give intermittent therapy with estrogens and progesterone. A popular regimen is 0.625 mg conjugated estrogen and 2.5–5 mg medroxyprogesterone daily. Withdrawal bleeding may be a troublesome side effect in some. It has been reported that early institution of HRT after the onset of menopause is more effective in preventing the risk of IHD and starting the drug later.

The possible adverse effects include slight, but statistically significant increase in cancer of the breast and endometrium, increase in venous thrombosis, especially in these with thrombophilia. Women on HRT should have regular gynecological check-up once a year and also self-palpation of the breasts.

With the availability of evidence that female hormones will increase the risk of cancers of the endometrium and breasts and venous thrombosis, their use has come down markedly.

Selective Estrogen Receptor Modulators (SERM)

Raloxifene is a SERM which reproduces the beneficial effect of estrogen without the negative effect on breast and endometrium. Raloxifene is an alternative for women not tolerating bisphosphonates. It is given as 60 mg/day orally along with calcium and vitamin D_3.

Strontium Ranelate

This drug has anabolic and antiresorptive properties. This drug is used when the patient is not tolerating or has contraindications for bisphosphonates.

Denosumab

It is a human monoclonal antibody against receptor activator of nuclear factor kappa-B ligand (RANKL). Precursors to osteoclasts (preosteoclasts) express surface receptors called receptor activator of nuclear factor (RANK). RANK is activated by RANKL (the RANK-ligand), which exists as cell surface molecules on osteoblasts. Activation of RANK by RANKL promotes the maturation of preosteoclasts to osteoclasts. Denosumab inhibits the maturation of osteoclasts by binding and inhibiting RANKL. This protects bone from degradation, and helps to counter the progression of the disease. It is given as a dose of 60 mg SC every 6 months.

Prevention

Incidence of generalized osteoporosis can be reduced by ensuring regular exercises and proper intake of proteins, vitamins, calcium and avoidance of alcohol and tobacco. Regular exposure to sunlight for 20–30 minutes on at least 5 days a week, preferably on bare skin ensures adequate supplementation of vitamin D, which helps to preserve bone mineralization.

GOUT

It is a clinical syndrome which occurs as a result of deposition of monosodium urate (MSU) monohydrate crystals from hyperuricemic body fluids. The crystals may be deposited in joints or in soft tissues like cartilage or connective tissue at various sites. In the joints this leads to inflammatory changes whereas in the other sites inflammation does not occur.

The term ***gout*** includes a heterogeneous group of diseases characterized by hyperuricemia. This can be the result of several metabolic errors operating singly or in combination. Plasma levels of uric acid vary from 2–7 mg/dL (0.12–0.42 mmol/L) in health. The term hyperuricemia denotes values above 7 mg/dL (0.42 mmol/L) in men and 6 mg/dL (0.36 mmol/L) in women.

Uric acid metabolism follows different pathways. It is the end product of purine metabolism. Purines are derived partly from the diet and partly from endogenous metabolism. In the liver, nucleic acids and purine nucleotides are degraded to form the purine bases—**xanthine** and **hypoxanthine**. These are oxidized to form uric acid by the enzyme ***xanthine oxidase***. The urates circulate in the plasma to be excreted mainly by the kidneys. A smaller amount is secreted into the gut.

Precursors of uric acid can be utilized by endogenous metabolism to synthesize purine nucleotides, through pathways involving several enzymes, including ***5-phosphoribosyl 1-pyrophosphate synthetase*** and ***hypoxanthine-guanine phosphoribosyltransferase (HGPRT).***

In normal men taking purine-free diets, the daily urinary excretion of uric acid is 350–500 mg. Increased production of uric acid reduced urinary elimination or a combination of both these processes lead to hyperuricemia.

Causes

Primary Gout

The exact defect in the pathogenesis of primary gout is still not known, but is likely to be due to a genetic defect in the renal urate-handling. Around 90% of these patients are found to have a decreased renal clearance of uric acid and in 10% overproduction of uric acid is the causative factor.

Secondary Gout

Hyperuricemia results from a demonstrable disorder, leading either to overproduction or defective excretion of uric acid.

Causes of secondary gout

Increased urate production

- Inherited enzyme defects
  - HGPRT deficiency (Lesch-Nyhan syndrome)
  - Glucose-6-phosphatase (G6P)deficiency
  - Phosphoribosyl pyrophosphate synthetase overactivity
- Myeloproliferative disorders
- Psoriasis
- Hemolytic diseases
- Malignancies, tumor lysis syndrome
- High-purine diet
- Alcohol

Decreased renal clearance

- ***Renal:*** Chronic renal failure, polycystic kidney disease, lead nephropathy
- ***Endocrine:*** Hyperparathyroidism, hypothyroidism, diabetes insipidus (DI)
- Metabolic lactic acidosis, ketoacidosis, starvation
- Severe dehydration
- ***Metabolic syndrome:*** Obesity, dyslipidemia
- Hypertension
- Drugs diuretics low-dose aspirin, pyrazinamide
- Cyclosporin, ethambutol
- ***Miscellaneous:*** Sarcoidosis, toxemia of pregnancy Down syndrome

Pathogenesis

Hyperuricemia is the central abnormality in gout but this may not lead to gout in all cases.

Arthritis is caused by the deposition of MSU crystals in the synovium. Polymorphonuclear leukocytes (PMNL) ingest the crystals. They release lysosomal enzymes which cause inflammation. Kinins and related cytokines lead to increased vascular permeability. Crystals are demonstrable in the synovium and articular cartilage in the stage of acute arthritis. In the chronic stage, erosion of articular cartilage, proliferation of synovial membrane, pannus formation, cystic erosions of bones and secondary osteoarthritic changes develop.

Tophi are nodular urate deposits found in and around the joints and in articular cartilage. Histologically, these consist of MSU crystals surrounded by mononuclear cell infiltration and foreign-body giant cells. These lead to osteoarthritic changes, ankylosis of joints and tissue destruction.

Urate deposition and inflammatory reaction in the parenchyma of the kidneys lead to hyalinization or fibrosis of glomeruli. Multiple urate calculi, chronic pyelonephritis, and arteriolosclerosis are other changes seen in long-standing gout.

Clinical Features

Gout passes through three clinical stages, namely—(1) Asymptomatic hyperuricemia, (2) acute gouty arthritis and (3) chronic tophaceous gout. Gout is seen predominantly in men during middle life. The M:F ratio is 7:1 to 9:1. Onset of gout in the 2nd or 3rd decade of life should raise the possibility of other metabolic disorders of purine metabolism such as ***HGPRT*** deficiency.

Acute Gout

Classically, intensely painful monoarticular arthritis of the metatarsophalangeal joint of the big toe develops within minutes to hours (Fig. 114.2). The joint is red and swollen and this may be mistaken for septic arthritis. The term ***podagra*** denotes painful affection of the foot occurring as a result of metatarsophalangeal arthritis. Later other joints are involved. This may be associated with fever and other constitutional disturbances. The initial attack subsides with treatment or spontaneously to recur periodically, due to precipitating factors like dietary excess, alcoholic bouts, infections, trauma, undue physical exercise, surgery or withdrawal of drugs.

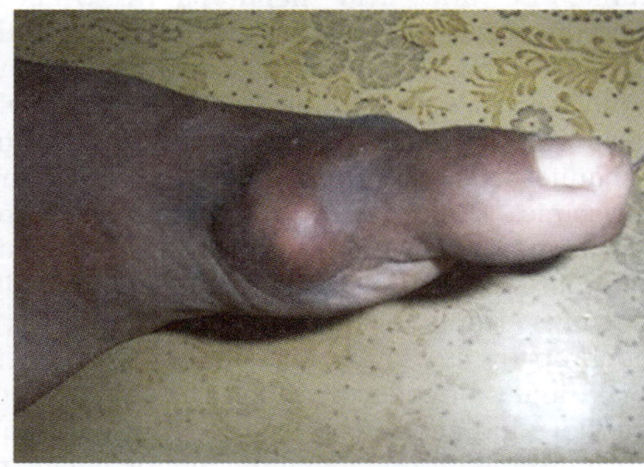

Fig. 114.2: Acute gouty arthritis of first metatarsophalangeal joint

Metabolic Arthropathies

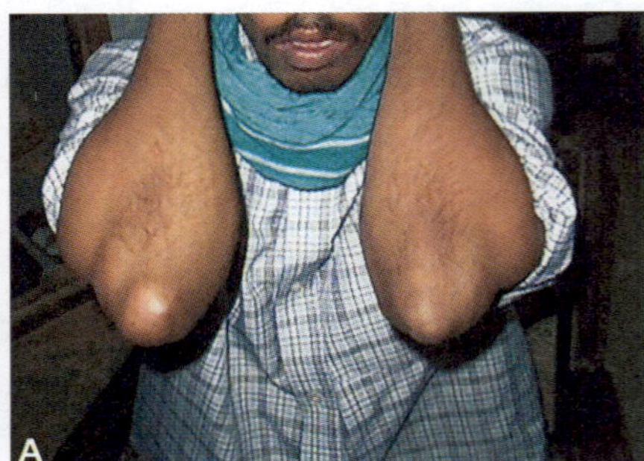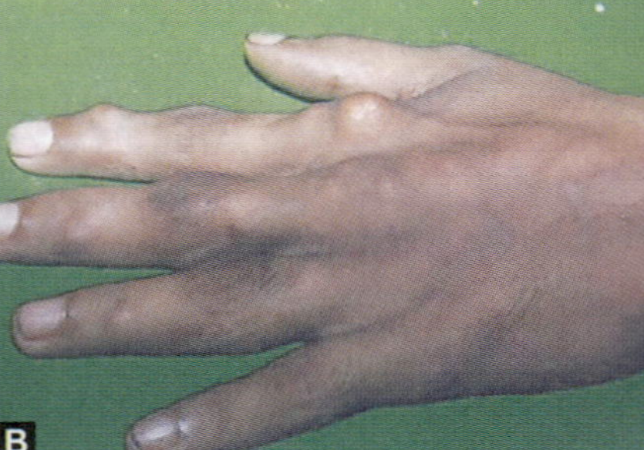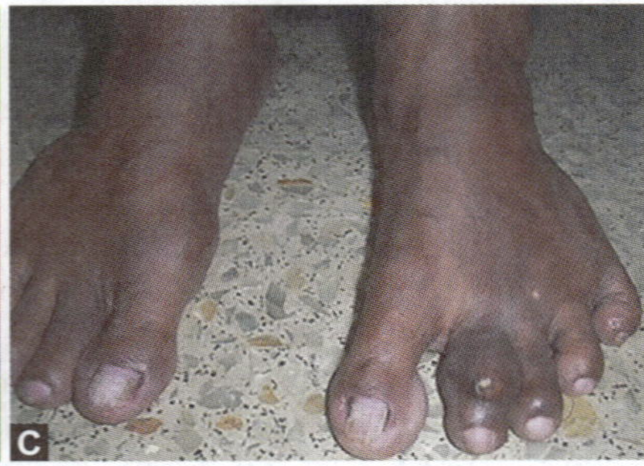

Fig. 114.3A to C: **A.** Right olecranon bursitis in a patient with gout; **B.** Multiple gouty tophi over the dorsum of the hand; **C.** Gouty tophus on the left second toe

Intercritical (Interval) Gout

The interval between two gouty attacks is called intercritical gout. The patient will be totally asymptomatic, but uric acid crystals can be demonstrated by aspiration of synovial fluid from previously inflamed joint. Progressive bony erosions can also develop during this period which can be demonstrated by serial radiographs of the affected joint. The duration of intercritical gout varies. Without diet control, lifestyle modification or drugs, most patients experience a second episode of arthritis within 2 years and thereafter, more frequently.

Chronic Tophaceous Gout

The acute attacks do not remit completely and the joints become constantly painful and swollen. Tophi develop as subcutaneous nodular masses around the joints and on tendons (Figs 114.3A to C). They are soft and small initially but later on become hard and may reach up to 7 cm in diameter. They may ulcerate discharging the chalky material. Most common sites for tophi are around the olecranon, ankles, tendo-Achilles, helix of the ear and over other joints. Osteoarthritis and ankylosis supervene.

Atypical forms may develop in addition to the typical gouty arthritis. Subacute polyarthritis similar to rheumatoid disease or isolated joint lesions may occur. Sometimes the initial presentation may be with soft tissue involvement such as Achilles tendonitis or olecranon bursitis (Fig. 114.3A). Tophi may be seen in organs such as the cornea, heart, tongue, bronchi and pleura.

Complications

Renal Damage

Persistently high uric acid level can lead to urolithiasis and urate or uric acid nephropathy. Urolithiasis precedes the onset of gouty arthritis in many patients with hyperuricemia. The uric acid may act as a nidus on which other crystals like calcium oxalate can precipitate. Uric acid stones can develop in individuals without other manifestations of gout, only 20% of whom are hyperuricemic. Urate nephropathy (urate nephrosis) is a late manifestation of severe hyperuricemia due to deposition of MSU crystals in the medullary interstitium and pyramids leading to chronic renal insufficiency. Uric acid nephropathy is due to precipitation of uric acid in the renal tubules or collecting ducts causing obstruction of urine flow and acute renal failure. This is a frequent complication of aggressive chemotherapy for malignancies with antitumor drugs given without proper attention

to maintain positive fluid balance and adequate urine output. Untreated hyperuricemia patients may develop uric acid nephropathy if severe dehydration or acidosis develops (*See* also Section 16, Ch 192).

Cardiovascular System

There is higher incidence of hypertension and IHD in gouty subjects. Gout is associated with insulin resistance.

Diagnosis

Strong clinical suspicion is required to make prompt diagnosis. Gout should be considered in all cases of obscure monoarticular or polyarticular disease. Presence of positive family history, hyperuricemia and radiological findings strengthen the diagnosis. Whereas hyperuricemia is invariably present in chronic gout, the serum uric acid may be normal at times in acute gout. Urate crystals can be demonstrated in synovial fluid or from tophi by their birefringence under polarized light. This is diagnostic of gout.

Radiological Changes

Radiological changes occur in chronic recurrent gout. In well-developed chronic gout, plain X-ray shows periarticular small punched out erosions with overhanging margins (Figs 114.4 and 114.5). In the late phases, there will be osteoarthritic changes, and destruction and subluxation of joints (Fig. 114.6). Dual energy computed tomography (DECT) is a new technique, which can demonstrate MSU crystal deposition. Magnetic resonance

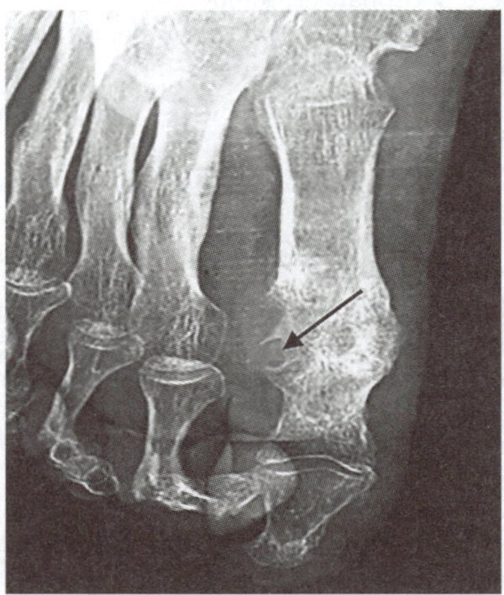

Fig. 114.4: X-ray foot in gout. *Note:* The punched out lytic lesions with overhanging margin (arrow) on the proximal phalanx of big toe

Textbook of Medicine

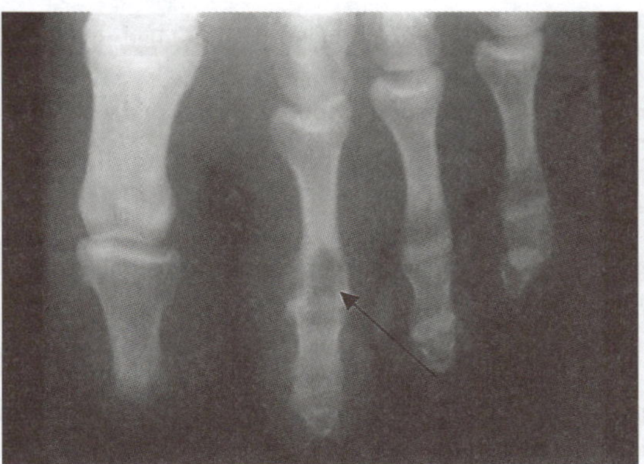

Fig. 114.5: X-ray of the same left foot showing soft tissue swelling and lytic lesion on the proximal phalanx of second toe (arrow)

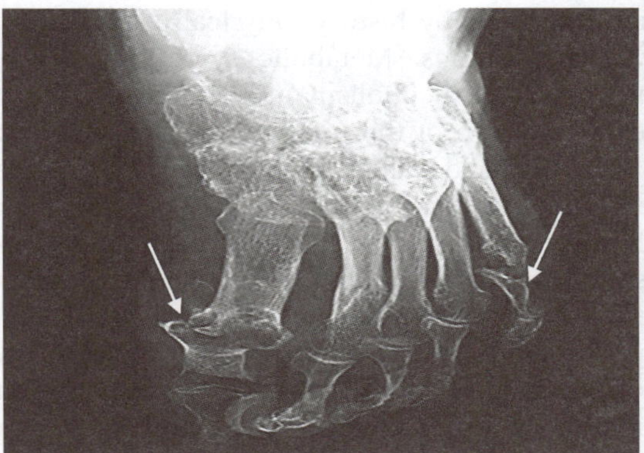

Fig. 114.6: X-ray foot in chronic tophaceous gout. **Note:** The destruction and subluxation of first and fifth metatarsophalangeal joints (arrows)

imaging (MRI) can demonstrate joint effusion, synovitis, tendon abnormalities, tophi, cartilage disorder and bone edema in gout.

Treatment

Treatment of gout has to be considered under two heads—(1) Treatment of the acute attack and (2) management of chronic tophaceous gout.

Management of the Acute Attack

The affected part is immobilized with a splint and bandage. Indomethacin 25 mg thrice daily initially and then reduced to a maintenance dose is very effective in relieving pain and arthritis. Other nonsteroidal anti-inflammatory drugs (NSAIDs) are also effective in appropriate dosage, given after food along with antacid medication, in order to prevent gastric irritation.

Colchicine in an initial dose of 1 mg orally followed by 0.5 mg after 1 hour is specific in relieving the acute attack but sometimes the response may be delayed. This drug is freely available in India at present.

In patients with contraindication for NSAIDs or colchicine, oral or parenteral steroids are useful alternatives to relieve the pain. In resistant monoarticular involvement, intra-articular hydrocortisone is highly useful. Dose of the drug and volume of the injection depend on the joint affected. The injection can be given as an outpatient procedure. All precipitating factors should be meticulously avoided.

Blocking interleukin-1 (IL-1) is a novel concept in the treatment of acute gout because MSU crystals stimulate the inflammation in gout leading to IL-1b secretion. IL-1 inhibitors prevent IL-1b secretion via this mechanism and also block IL-1 secretion by macrophages via a toll-like receptor dependent mechanism. The anti-IL-1 drugs like **anakinra, canakinumab** and **rilonacept** have been found to be useful in patients with acute gout. However, they are extremely expensive when compared with traditional agents and therefore, their place in the management of gout is only in an occasional and exceptional case.

Treatment of Chronic Gout

Diet: Acute attacks can be avoided by omitting purine-rich diets like red meat, liver, testes, sea foods and alcohol. Though vegetable articles of diet such as lentils, peas, beans, spinach, mushrooms, cauliflower and oatmeal are rich in purines they generally do not provoke acute attacks. Obese individuals should reduce their weight gradually.

Drugs: The drugs used for chronic gout can be divided in three categories:

1. *Uricostatic drugs:* Allopurinol, febuxostat
2. *Uricosuric agents:* Probenecid, sulfinpyrazone Losartan, amlodipine, fenofibrate
3. *Uricolytic drugs:* Uricase, rasburicase, polyethylene glycol (PEG)-uricase.

Uricostatic drugs

- *Allopurinol* inhibits *xanthine oxidase* which is required for the conversion of xanthine and hypoxanthine to uric acid and is a very effective drug to lower the serum uric acid. In addition, allopurinol also helps in urinary elimination of urates. The advantages of this drug are its low toxicity and sustained therapeutic effect even in the presence of renal disease or diuretic therapy. The starting dose is 100 mg thrice daily, to be increased up to 500 mg/day if required, to achieve the effect. Later the dose is reduced to a maintenance level. Diarrhea, dyspepsia, and skin rashes are untoward side effects. Dose-dependent toxic effects consisting of hypersensitivity reactions such as fever, eosinophilia, dermatitis, hepatic dysfunction, renal failure and vasculitis may develop in persons taking more than 400 mg/day. If allowed to proceed, the condition can be fatal. Treatment is to desensitize the patient and use lower doses of the drug. Dose of allopurinol has to be adjusted depending on the renal function, as indicated by serum creatinine levels.

- *Febuxostat:* This new drug is a nonpurine xanthine oxidase inhibitor with high oral absorption (85%) and high affinity to serum proteins (Box 114.2). It has a half-life of 4–9 hours. It is metabolized by liver and renal excretion is insignificant. It selectively inhibits both oxidized and reduced forms of xanthine oxidase without inhibiting other enzymes in purine

Box 114.2: Indication of febuxostat in gout

- Patients with renal impairment
- Patients allergic to allopurinol
- Allopurinol failure (as a second-line drug)
- Concomitant use of oral anticoagulants like warfarin

metabolism. The major adverse effects of febuxostat are hepatic (transaminase elevation), nausea and dizziness. It is contraindicated in patients treated with azathioprine, mercaptopurine or theophylline which are metabolized by xanthine oxidase. The initial dose of febuxostat is 40 mg/daily taken with or without food. If the target serum uric acid level is not achieved, dosage may be increased 80–120 mg/day. Like allopurinol, the drug should be started after subsidence of acute attack of gout and prophylactic therapy with low-dose colchicines or NSAIDs is required to reduce the incidence of paradoxical gout flares. It can be safely given without dosage reduction in patients with renal impairment and moderate hepatic impairment.

Uricosuric agents

Uricosuric agents are useful to correct hyperuricemia and gout caused by inadequate renal excretion of urates. The drugs are contraindicated if there is a history of urolithiasis or if there is oliguria. They are less effective in presence of renal disease with low glomerular filtration rate (GFR).

Probenecid and *sulfinpyrazone* are well-tolerated uricosuric agents but are not freely available in India. Hence, there is increasing interest in the uricosuric effects of commonly used antihypertensives like losartan and amlodipine and lipid-lowering drugs like fenofibrate. *Losartan*, an angiotensin-2 receptor blocker has moderate uricosuric properties by decreasing the renal tubular reabsorption of uric acid. It is particularly useful as an adjunct therapy in patients with gout and hypertension. It is also useful to control the hyperuricemia caused by thiazides. The usual dose needed is 50 mg/day. *Amlodipine* and other calcium channel blockers given in a dose of 5–10 mg/day are also found to be useful in reducing the urate levels in patients with cyclosporine-induced hyperuricemia. *Fenofibrate*, the lipid-lowering agent increases the renal urate clearance. 25–30% reduction of uric acid level is possible with a dose of 200 mg/day and this drug is a good choice in patients with gout and dyslipidemia.

Uricolytic agents

Humans are prone to hyperuricemia due to lack of functional *uricase (urate oxidase)*, unlike lower animals. Natural *uricase* from *Aspergillus flavus* effectively reduces uric acid levels in humans, but is highly antigenic. A biosynthesized recombinant *A. flavus* *uricase (rasburicase)* is available in the United States of America for tumor lysis syndrome in patients allergic to allopurinol. The drug is highly antigenic. PEG-uricase is another potentially powerful agent for treating refractory gout in those who are unable to tolerate other drugs. It has the advantages of prolonging the drug half-life and decreasing antigenicity. It has been tried to debulk tophi in advanced gout before switching on to other agents for maintenance treatment.

Asymptomatic Hyperuricemia

There are many individuals with uric acid level higher than that of normal controls (more than 7 mg in males and 6 mg in females) who are totally asymptomatic and hyperuricemia is detected incidentally. Few of them can

Box 114.3: Indication for treatment of asymptomatic hyperuricemia

This warrants drug treatment if there is:
- Previous history of recurrent gouty arthritis
- Presence of tophi
- Presence of uric acid stones
- Urate nephropathy
- Serum uric acid greater than 12 mg/dL
- During chemotherapy of cancer to prevent tumor lysis syndrome
- Inherited enzyme defects.

have musculoskeletal pain but not directly related to hyperuricemia. But mere presence of hyperuricemia is not an indication for specific uric acid lowering treatment (Box 114.3). Instead meticulous search for the cause of hyperuricemia should be made. In more than 70% of hyperuricemia patients, an underlying cause can be readily found out by history, physical examination and a few investigations. Metabolic syndrome, renal and thyroid diseases, alcoholism and drugs are the usual causes. Correction of the underlying cause often brings back the uric acid values to normal levels. Currently, there is no evidence of benefit to be obtained from treating sustained asymptomatic hyperuricemia unless it is severe (more than 12 mg/dL) or in situations where there is acute or massive urate overproduction. Hence, it seems prudent to not treat asymptomatic hyperuricemia with specific antihyperuricemic agents unless symptoms attributable to hyperuricemia like arthritis, urolithiasis or nephropathy develops. The rare exceptions to this rule include individuals with a known hereditary cause of uric acid overproduction or at potentially high-risk for acute uric acid nephropathy as in tumor lysis.

OTHER FORMS OF CRYSTAL-INDUCED ARTHROPATHY

Calcium pyrophosphate (CPP) dihydrate crystals may be deposited in joint tissues and this leads to acute gout like attacks. This is known as *pseudogout*. Basic calcium phosphates (BCPs) (hydroxy apatite and octacalcium phosphate) may be deposited in joint tissues mainly affecting shoulders and knees. Calcium oxalate crystals may be deposited in cartilage, synovium, bone and other tissues in renal failure patients treated with dialysis regimen and those with primary oxalosis.

CPP Crystal Deposition Disease (Pseudogout)

CPP crystals are seen in synovial fluid and these are derived from articular cartilage. Processes that lower solubility of the CPP crystals lead to their precipitation. The condition may be familial, sporadic or caused by metabolic disorders such as hyperparathyroidism, hemochromatosis, hypothyroidism, hypomagnesemia, hypophosphatasia and others. CPP crystals are deposited in hyaline cartilage and fibrocartilage, the latter is affected more. The menisci of the knees, articular disks of distal radioulnar joints, acetabulum, symphysis pubis and annulus fibrosus of lumbar and dorsal intervertebral disks are sites of predilection. Men above 50 years are more affected though both sexes are susceptible. The patients may fall into one of three categories.

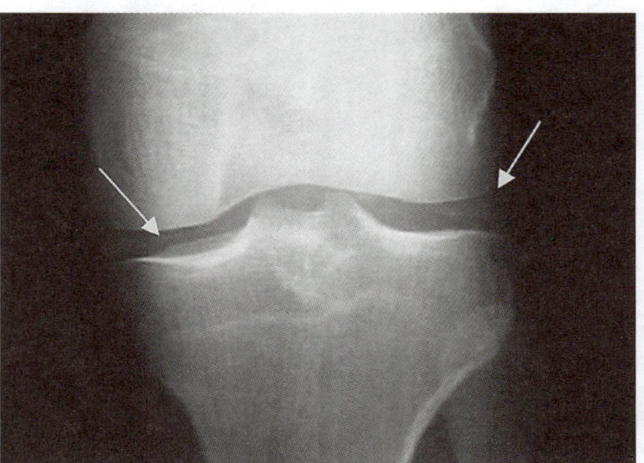

Fig. 114.7: X-ray of knee showing chondrocalcinosis (arrows) in calcium pyrophosphate crystal deposition (CPPD) disease

1. Familial
2. Those associated with metabolic disease, trauma or joint surgery
3. Sporadic.

Though many cases may be silent, some present with recurrent attacks of subacute inflammation and progressive degeneration of joints. Once the degenerative process starts, it proceeds relentlessly, despite treatment.

The presentation may resemble gout, RA, osteoarthritis or neuropathic joints.

Differential diagnosis includes all other types of mono-arthritis or polyarthritis, depending upon the presentation. X-ray of the joints reveals calcification in distinctive locations and this is diagnostic (Fig. 114.7). Microscopy of the synovial fluid is confirmatory.

Management

During acute attacks, NSAIDs may be tried. Colchicine is also very effective. Aspiration of synovial fluid and injection of microcrystalline cortisone (cortisone acetate) gives rapid relief.

BCP Crystal Arthropathy (Calcium Apatite Deposition Disease) (Milwaukee Shoulder/Knee Syndrome)

This condition affects elderly persons, mostly women. BCP crystals get deposited at sites of trauma or tissue damage. The crystals are present in the joint fluid. They are also deposited primarily on the matrix vessels. The shoulder or knee may be affected. Many cases may be asymptomatic, despite the deposition of crystals. Symptoms include pain in the shoulders or knees after exertion and at night. Progressive destruction of joints occurs. The term ***Milwaukee shoulder*** refers to the common affection seen in elderly patients caused by BCP arthropathy. ***Treatment*** is symptomatic.

Calcium Oxalate Arthropathy

This is a complication occurring in renal failure when the serum creatinine levels exceed 8 mg/dL, especially so in patients undergoing dialysis regimen. Crystals of calcium oxalate may be deposited in joints, skin, blood vessels and other tissues. Joint manifestations include subacute, chronic or acute painful episodes. Several other substances may get deposited in joints and lead to crystal-induced arthropathy. These include xanthine, cholesterol, cystine, aluminum phosphate, Charcot-Leyden crystals and possibly others.

CHAPTER
115

Osteoarthritis

Binoy J Paul, KV Krishna Das

Chapter Summary

- General Considerations
- Clinical Features
- Management
- Course and Prognosis

GENERAL CONSIDERATIONS

Syn: Osteoarthrosis, Degenerative joint disease

Osteoarthritis (OA) is the most common form of arthritis. It is predominantly a disease of the elderly but no age is exempt. It is caused mainly by wear and tear of the joints. It may be primary or secondary. Presence or absence of ***Heberden's nodes*** on the distal interphalangeal (DIP) joints helps to distinguish two forms of primary osteoarthrosis, the nodal and non-nodal types. The former indicates the presence of generalized disease.

Epidemiology

Reported prevalence of OA from India (studies from Lucknow and Pune) shows 4.2–5.7% in rural population and 11.5% in urban areas. OA forms about 25–35% of the joint diseases seen in clinical practice. Major risk factors are age, obesity, previous joint trauma, abnormal joint mechanics and occupations causing excessive bending or overstrain to joints. Heredity plays a role in primary nodal OA affecting interphalangeal joints.

Etiology

The most regular association of OA is with aging. Beyond the age of 50 years, OA is demonstrable in one or more joints invariably, but it may be asymptomatic. Several factors predispose to the disease and accelerate its progression. These include pre-existing joint disease, obesity, hypermobility, orthopedic deformities, endocrine disorders like diabetes mellitus (DM), acromegaly, hyperparathyroidism and sensory neuropathies which impair joint sensations. Overuse of any joint and adoption of unusual postures for long periods predispose to the condition, e.g. OA of the knees of obese subjects and long distance walkers and OA of the neck in computer professionals.

Pathogenesis and Pathology

Normal hyaline cartilage consists of chondrocytes embedded in the extracellular matrix. The cartilage remains stable with active degeneration and regeneration in equilibrium. In OA, there is excessive degeneration in comparison to regeneration. The chondrocytes secrete numerous matrix metalloproteinases which can destroy the cartilage. In OA, there is increased production of interleukin-1 (IL-1) also which suppresses proteoglycan synthesis. Proteoglycans are essential for cartilage repair. IL-1 also stimulates the production of osteoblast like cells leading to osteophyte formation.

Primary lesion starts in the articular cartilage. The basic pathology can be defined as a loss of focal areas of hyaline cartilage with increased activity in marginal and subchondral bones in synovial joints. Due to mechanical stress, the collagen fiber network of the articular cartilage is disrupted. This leads to alteration in the composition of the ground substance with resultant loss of resilience. The chondrocyte function and number change. Bone turnover is less in OA, but cartilage turnover is more. Crystals may be present in synovial fluid, especially in the knee. These include hydroxyapatite, octacalcium phosphate and tricalcium phosphate, and calcium pyrophosphate dihydrate (CPPD). Presence of crystals in synovial fluid is strongly associated with cartilage degeneration.

Wear and tear leads to further disruption of collagen fibers. The lubricating mechanism of the joint is impaired. The normal surface matrix is lost, resulting in exposure and fibrillation of the cartilage fibers and later cleft formation. Synovial fluid gains access to the deeper layers of the cartilage. This leads to further destruction of load-bearing cartilage. The cartilage undergoes calcification. The exposed weight-bearing bones undergo eburnation. Osteophytes grow at the margins of articular bones. Still later, subchondral bone may fracture to form cysts. Crystals are liberated into the synovial cavity. These add to the inflammatory process. Though synovial inflammation and effusion occur, these process are generally mild compared to the primary inflammatory arthropathies.

CLINICAL FEATURES

Many cases are asymptomatic though abnormalities are detectable radiologically. Knees, cervical spine, lumbar spine, hips, shoulder and DIP joints are affected most frequently. Weight bearing joints such as the knees develop deformities (Fig. 115.1). Osteophyte formation at the DIP joints leads to the formation of **Heberden's nodes** (Fig. 115.2) which may sometimes be painful. In the knees, movement of the patella sideward causes pain (Fig. 115.3). Vague pain and stiffness in the knee, especially, after getting up from the sitting posture are the

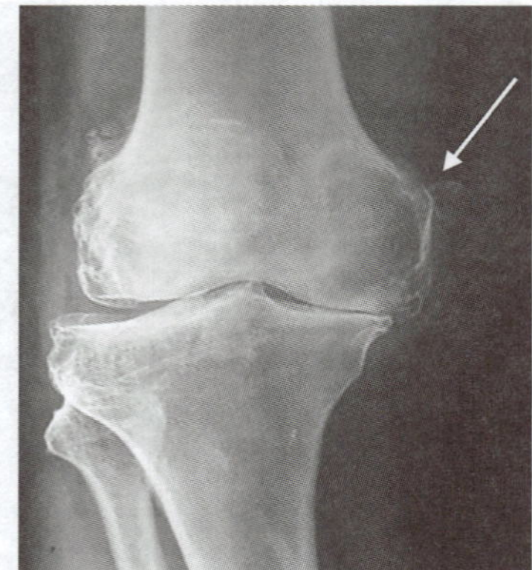

Fig. 115.1: X-ray knees—osteoarthritis. **Note:** Narrowing of joint space and calcified loose bodies (arrow)

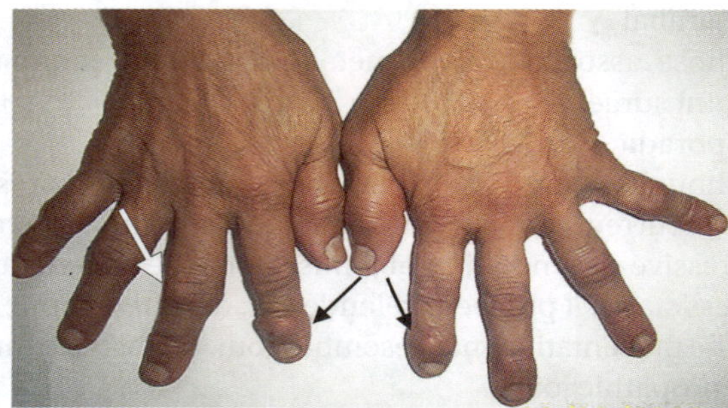

Fig. 115.2: Primary nodal osteoarthritis of hand. **Note:** Herberden's nodes (black arrows) and Bouchard's nodes (white arrow)

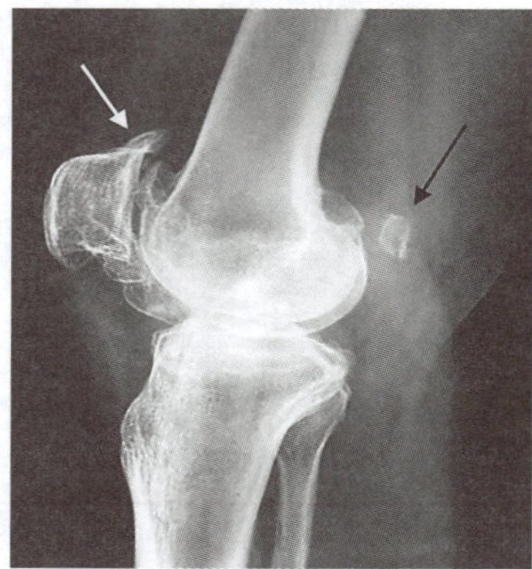

Fig. 115.3: Osteoarthritis knees lateral view. **Note:** Patellar osteophytes (white arrow) and calcified loose body (black arrow)

early symptoms. Cartilage is aneural and therefore, it does not contribute to pain. The tissues from which pain arises are osteophyte growths, localized areas of increased intraosseous pressure, synovitis and periarticular structures. Subchondral bone and synovium may be responsible for nociceptive stimuli. Sensitization of peripheral neuronal elements aggravates the pain response. The processes of attempted joint repair lead to osteophyte growth as well as subchondral bone changes which are nociceptive. Production of secondary particles and chemical mediators from the cartilage give rise to secondary synovitis. In addition, altered mechanics of the joints give rise to periarticular phenomena such as strain on muscles and ligaments and inflammation of bursae which are all painful. These lesions which cause pain lower

Textbook of Medicine

the pain threshold centrally either at the spinal cord level or cortical level, or both.

The patients experiencing disability while walking downstairs or slopes. The quadricep undergoes atrophy. Transient effusions may occur even in asymptomatic cases. Osteophytes may be palpated around the joints. Crepitus may be elicited on movement. Deformities may develop OA of the cervical spine (cervical spondylosis) leads to a group of clinical manifestations. These are described in Section 17, Ch 211. Affection of the lumbar spine leads to low backache and sciatica (Figs 115.4 and 115.5).

DIAGNOSIS

Laboratory Investigations

Blood tests are not diagnostic. They help to exclude other forms of inflammatory arthropathies. The acute phase reactants are not elevated. The leukocyte pattern is not altered. **Synovial fluid** study shows normal viscosity, normal mucus content and cell count below 2000/cm^2. Fragments of cartilage or bone and crystals of hydroxyapatite and CPPD may be seen.

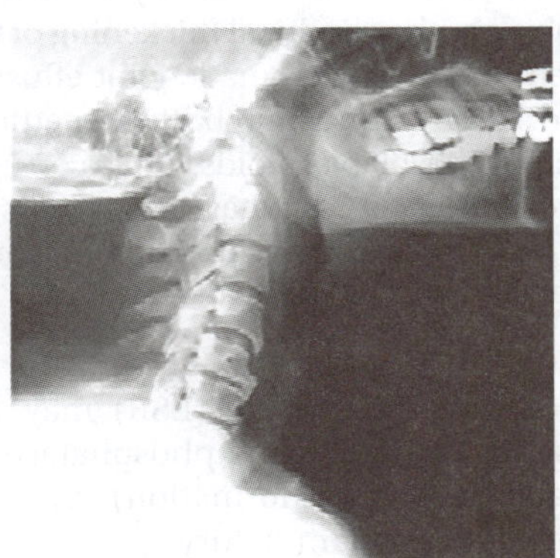

Fig. 115.4: Osteoarthritis cervical spine. **Note:** Osteophytes in front and back of the vertebral bodies, narrowing of disc spaces and loss of cervical lordosis

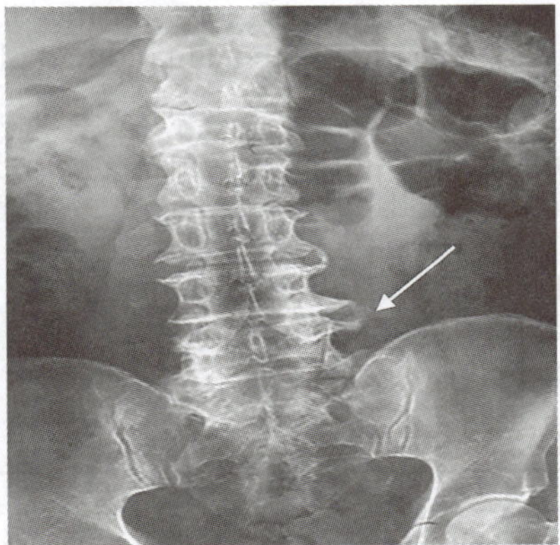

Fig. 115.5: X-ray of lumbosacral spine showing osteophytes in lumbar spondylosis (arrow)

Imaging

- **X-rays:** The bones show subchondral sclerosis, narrowing of joint spaces, osteophyte formation, joint destruction, cyst formation in the cortical bone and loose bodies (joint mice) within the joints.
- **Magnetic resonance imaging (MRI):** Cartilage surface defects, meniscus and ligamentous damage occurring in the joints are picked up early by the MRI of the affected joint.
- **Computed tomography (CT) scan** is useful in assessing the axial joints and spine.

Arthroscopy

Using appropriate arthroscopes, the interior of many of the peripheral joints can be directly inspected and this helps to confirm the diagnosis. Arthroscopic surgery is also practiced widely. Arthroscopy is available in many centers in India.

MANAGEMENT

The principles of management include prevention of overuse of the affected joint, limitation of activity to reduce pain and physiotherapy to strengthen the muscles around the joint. Application of heat and graded movement help to reduce pain.

- **Symptomatic treatment:** Paracetamol and nonsteroidal anti-inflammatory drugs (NSAIDS) relieve pain and inflammation. Reduction of weight and management of metabolic and endocrine disorders may serve to arrest the progress of the joint lesions.
  - **Intra-articular steroids:** Intra-articular methylprednisolone or triamcinolone may be given as temporary measures to relieve acute pain and disability. Intra-articular corticosteroids may accelerate degenerative changes in the joint, if given repeatedly.
  - **Viscosupplementation:** Intra-articular hyaluronic acid which increases the joint lubrication is useful in early stages of OA.
  - **Nutraceuticals:** Glucosamine and chondroitin sulfate are nutraceutical agents used extensively for OA, though their effectiveness is debated. Glucosamine 1,500 mg/day and chondroitin 1,200 mg/day may provide symptom relief in knee OA on prolonged use when combined with other symptomatic measures.
  - **IL-1 inhibitors:** Diacerein, an IL-1 inhibitor at a dose of 50 mg twice daily is also found to be useful in early OA.
- **Surgical treatments:** Joint replacement should be considered for OA of the hip and knee if medical measures fail to relieve pain and disability and to restore mobility. The mechanical impairement caused by OA lesions in the knees can be properly assessed by simple tools. The results of knee and hip replacement are excellent in most of the cases. Therefore, replacement surgery should be advised without undue delay. In good centers, the success rate is high. The average life for a prosthetic knee is more than 10 years and that for a hip is 10–15 years. Second operations can be undertaken.
  - **Chondrocyte transplantation:** Chondrocytes obtained from the patient can be cultured and transplanted to the site of cartilage defects. This procedure is useful

Osteoarthritis

Textbook of Medicine

in large defects of cartilage after injury to the joint. It is not currently recommended in the treatment of primary OA.

COURSE AND PROGNOSIS

OA is a slowly progressive disease which leads to considerable morbidity with passage of time, if allowed to proceed unchecked. The rate of progress and morbidity can be considerably retarded by lifestyle changes such as weight reduction, use of appropriate footwear on walking and regular exercises for strengthening the weight bearing muscles in and around the joints and for preserving the range of movements. Any postural or orthopedic deformity should be corrected to prevent progress of the arthritis.

CHAPTER
116

Other Bone Diseases

KV Krishna Das, Binoy J Paul

Chapter Summary

- Hypertrophic Osteoarthropathy (HOA)
- Paget's Disease of Bone
- Achondroplasia
- Osteogenesis Imperfecta (OI)
- Bone and Joint Tuberculosis
- Sports Injuries

HYPERTROPHIC OSTEOARTHROPATHY (HOA)

Syn: Hypertrophic pulmonary osteoarthropathy, Marie-Bamberger syndrome

It is a syndrome which is characterized by abnormal proliferation of the skin and osseous tissues at the distal part of extremities, clinically manifesting as clubbing, periostosis of tubular bones and synovial effusions. HOA is classified as primary or secondary and the latter having very diverse etiologies as shown in Box 116.1. There is now evidence to sustain the belief that clubbing and HOA represent different stages of same disease process. In majority of cases, the finger deformity is the first manifestation and as the syndrome progresses periostosis becomes evident (Figs 116.1A and B).

Box 116.1: Classification of hypertrophic osteoarthropathy (HOA)

- ***Primary (pachydermoperiostosis)***
- ***Secondary***
  - Pulmonary
    - Bronchogenic carcinoma, lung abscess, emphysema, bronchiectasis
    - Pulmonary fibrosis, mesothelioma of pleura, arteriovenous (AV) fistula
  - Cardiovascular
    - Congenital cyanotic heart disease, bacterial endocarditis
    - Aortic aneurysm, Eisenmenger's syndrome
  - Hepatic
    - Cirrhosis, hepatoma, amoebic liver abscess
  - Intestinal
    - Inflammatory bowel disease, esophageal and colonic carcinoma
  - Miscellaneous
    - Graves' disease, thymoma, thalassemia, connective tissue diseases (CTDs)

Clinical Features

Primary HOA (pachydermoperiostosis) is an autosomal dominant condition characterized by insidious development of clubbing with cylindrical thickening of forearm and legs. Recurrent mildly symptomatic joint effusions may be accompanied. Facial features may be thickened and furrowed with prominent nasolabial folds and corrugated scalp known as ***Leonine*** facies. Skin may show excessive sweating and a greasy feel. Other features include gynecomastia, acne vulgaris, striae and cranial suture defects.

Investigations

Erythrocyte sedimentation rate (ESR) may be elevated with increase in serum alkaline phosphatase (ALP) (due to considerable new bone formation). Synovial fluid is characteristically noninflammatory.

Radiological examination shows periosteal new bone formation often seen in the tibia, radius, ulna, fibula and femur. The coarse layered appearance is most evident along the diaphysis. Radionucleotide bone scan and magnetic resonance imaging (MRI) are more sensitive in detecting periosteal reaction earlier than plain radiography

Treatment

For patients with painful osteoarthropathy, nonsteroidal anti-inflammatory drugs (NSAIDs) are effective in alleviating pain. Treatment of the underlying disease results in dramatic regression of all features of secondary HOA. Vagal block and vagotomy are also helpful in symptomatic relief.

PAGET'S DISEASE OF BONE

Syn: Osteitis deformans

This is a rare disease of unknown etiology, characterized by enlargement, softening and deformity of several bones, seen after the age of 40 years, more commonly in men. Though this disease is common in the West, it is seen only rarely in Indians. The involvement is localized in majority of cases but may be widespread, involving several bones. The disease tends to repeat in family members and genetic patterns have been described. Virus infections like respiratory syncytial virus are implicated in the causation of the disease.

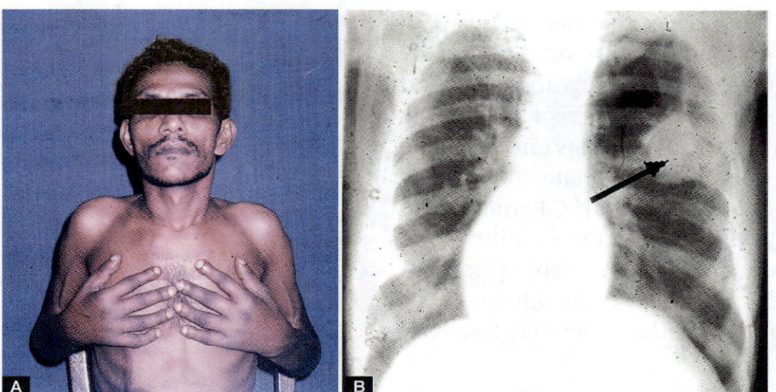

Figs 116.1A and B: **A.** Hypertrophic pulmonary osteoarthropathy male (52 years). ***Note:*** Clubbing of fingers; **B.** Chest X-ray of the same patient showing cancer left lung (arrow)

Pathology

There is increased and disorderly formation and destruction of bone. This results in a high rate of bone turnover. There is increase in the number and activities of osteoclasts. The osteoblasts try to compensate by adding more bone, but osteoclastic activity preponderates. The bone is highly vascular and functional arteriovenous (AV) shunts develop, resulting in a high-output cardiac state. The marrow is replaced by highly vascular fibrous tissue. Pelvis, femur, skull, tibia and vertebrae are affected in the order of frequency.

Clinical Features

Many cases are asymptomatic and detected on routine radiological examination. Symptoms include pain in weight-bearing joints, progressive enlargement of the skull, deformities of the affected bones, pressure on the nerves which pass through bony canals (cranial nerves, spinal nerves and spinal cord) and rarely the development of high-output cardiac failure state. Though the bones are thickened, they are weaker than normal. The femur and tibia undergo bowing and other deformities due to weight-bearing. The overlying skin is warm due to increased vascularity. Deafness, optic atrophy and paraplegia are rare neurological complications. Serum ALP is grossly elevated. Bone specific ALP is the iso-enzyme that is diagnostic. Serum calcium and phosphorus are normal. Urinary hydroxyproline is increased during the active phase of the disease.

Complications

These include fractures, progressive deformities, cranial nerve palsies (especially deafness), spinal cord compression, degenerative joint disease, high-output cardiac failure if the disease is extensive and in long-standing cases, osteogenic sarcoma.

Diagnosis

The diagnosis is based on clinical features and is confirmed by radiography (Figs 116.2A and B). The bone appears larger, chalky white and nonhomogenous in the skiagram. Localized enlargement and hyperdensity of bones is suggestive. This feature helps to differentiate from multiple osteosclerotic secondaries and other osteosclerotic conditions such as myelosclerosis and endemic fluorosis.

Treatment

Asymptomatic localized lesions have to be left alone. Symptomatic relief of pain is achieved by aspirin, indomethacin or corticosteroids. Human calcitonin in a daily dose of 0.5 mg subcutaneously (SC) for 6 months [or salmon calcitonin 100 Medical Research Council (MRC) units/day] promptly relieves bone pains and helps to reduce the turnover of bone with improvement in the condition, the serum level of ALP also comes down. Mithramycin (now called plicamycin) in a dose of 25–50 μg/kg given intravenously (IV) for 10–14 days is effective. This drug inhibits bone resorption. It produces

Other Bone Diseases

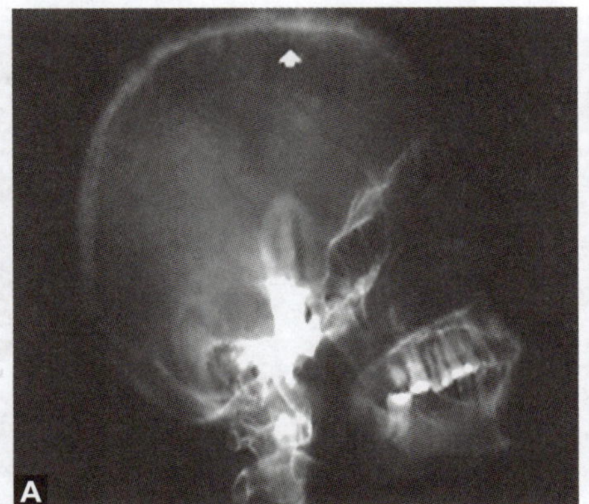
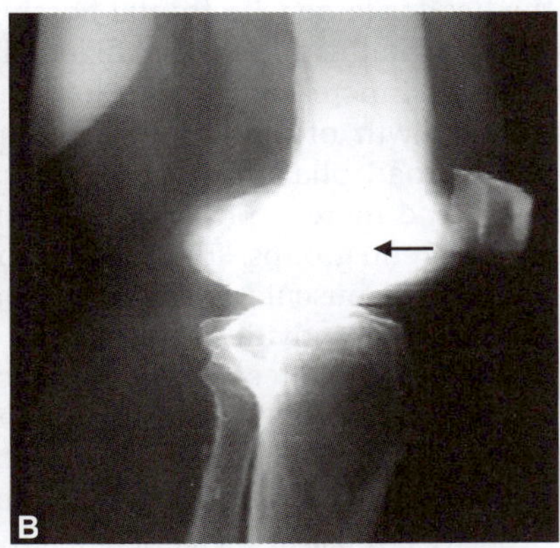

Figs 116.2A and B: **A.** X-ray of Paget's disease of bone skull. ***Note:*** Non-homogenous mouth eaten appearance (arrowhead); **B.** X-ray of Paget's disease of bone. ***Note:*** Dense enlarged deformed lower end of femur; normal tibia (arrow)

Textbook of Medicine

myelosuppression and a hemorrhagic tendency. Bisphosphonates (disodium etidronate) in a dose of 5–10 mg/kg/day also reduce bone turnover and bring about clinical relief in some cases. Bisphosphonates correct the chaotic bone formation by inhibiting the osteoclasts and inducing the formation of lamellar bone. Alendronate, 10 mg may be given orally daily on a long-term basis. Pamidronate may be given by slow IV infusion. 30 mg IV infusion is given for 3 consecutive days. Newer bisphophonates include zolendronic acid 5 mg given IV as infusion over 15 minutes or at longer intervals. The effect may last even as long as 6 months.

Since vitamin D deficiency is rampant in the Indian population, it is worthwhile to exclude deficiency of vitamin D and calcium and institute supplement therapy if there is deficiency, even though there is no direct role for vitamin D or calcium nutrition in the pathogenesis of Paget's disease of bone.

Juvenile Paget's Disease of Bone

Syn: Hyperostosis corticalis deformans, Familial idiopathic hypophosphatasia

This is a rare autosomal recessive disorder causing bony deformities. A homozygous deletion of **tumor necrosis factor receptor superfamily member 11B (TNFRSF11B)** gene which controls osteoprotegrin is seen to be causative. There is uncontrolled osteoclastic activity and bone resorption. Nerve deafness may occur due to compression of the 8th nerve in the petrous temporal bone. It usually starts in infancy or early childhood. It is characterized by painful debilitating fractures and deformities. Accelerated bone remodeling occurs throughout the skeleton. Juvenile Paget's disease is different from the adult form of the disease.

Treatment

Recombinant osteoprotegrin is effective in treating Juvenile Paget's disease.

ACHONDROPLASIA

It is the most common skeletal dysplasia, which is due to mutation in the gene expressing the fibroblast growth factor receptor 3 (FGFR3). It is transmitted as an autosomal dominant disorder. The distinguishing features are present at birth, although the diagnosis is seldom made at that time. The head is large with frontal bossing, midface hypoplasia and prognathism. There is rhizomelic shortening of arms and legs, increased lumbar lordosis, bowing of the legs, overgrowth of fibula and a trident shaped hand with short broad phalanges. The physical appearance is diagnostic and there is physical similarity among patients from different groups. The trunks and heads are normal. They have muscular strength, sexual ability and are capable of normal activities of life.

Radiograph shows a very small sacrosciatic notch of pelvis, changes in the epiphysis of distal femur and constriction at the base of the skull. Adult life may be shortened if there is spinal canal stenosis causing spinal cord compression. Otherwise most of these persons live healthy productive and independent lives. Limb lengthening involving bilateral femoral and tibial distraction

Table 116.1: Classification of OI phenotype according to Sillence et al. (1979)

OI type	Inheritance	Clinical characteristics
I	AD	Normal stature, little or no deformity, blue sclerae, hearing loss
II	AD (new mutations)	Lethal in perinatal period, beaded ribs, long bone fractures
III	AD, AR (rare)	Progressively deforming, short stature, multiple fractures, triangular facies, hearing loss
IV	AD	Moderately severe, variable short stature, dentinogenesis imperfecta, osteoporosis, bowing of long bones

Abbreviations: AD = Autosomal dominant; AR = Autosomal recessive

osteotomies may add up to 12 inches to the adult height. The procedures are best done in the second decade.

OSTEOGENESIS IMPERFECTA (OI)

Syn: Fragilitas ossium, Brittle bone disease

It is a genetic syndrome of abnormal bone matrix with secondary osteoporosis. This is a generalized connective tissue abnormality inherited as an autosomal dominant disorder, manifesting as peculiar brittleness of the bones, making them vulnerable to recurrent pathological and traumatic fractures. This disease is present in India, but seen infrequently. OI is one of the most common heritable disorders of connective tissue. It is inherited as autosomal recessive or autosomal dominant manner depending on the disease subtype. It is associated with abnormalities of structure or synthesis of type I collagen (Table 116.1).

The severity of the disease ranges from a slight increase in susceptibility to bone fractures to forms that are lethal *in utero*. In addition to fracture susceptibility, there is marked osteoporosis secondary to osseous matrix abnormality. The skeletal abnormalities vary with the type.

OI is associated with variable non-osseous features like blue sclera, dentinogenesis imperfecta, deafness, pectoral deformities, kyphoscolyosis, mitral valve prolapse and growth retardation (Fig. 116.3). The ***diagnosis*** of OI can be usually made clearly on clinical and radiological basis. It has been classified into nine groups based on inheritance pattern, color of the sclera, neurological abnormalities like deafness and the clinical pattern (Sillence classification).

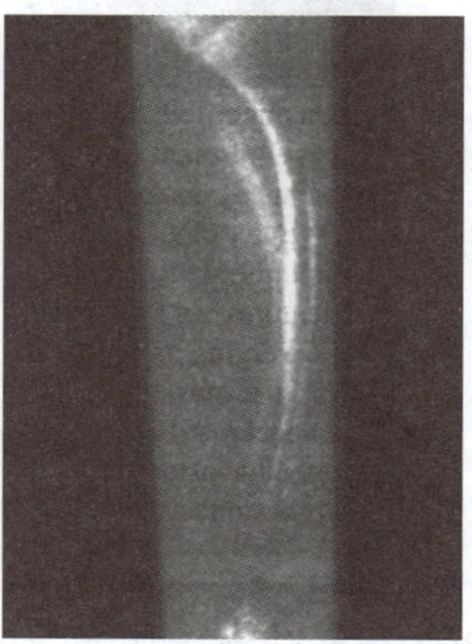

Fig. 116.3: Osteogenesis imperfecta—bowing of leg bones

Treatment with bisphosphonates may be beneficial to prevent vertebral compression and long bone fractures and to delay the development of scoliosis. Bisphosphonates, especially pamidronate given IV in short courses with intervals in between, may produce clinical improvement and also reduce the frequency of fractures. These drugs also reduce bone pains. Long-term management requires expert physical therapy or orthopedic surgery. Counseling and emotional support are important for patients and their parents. With treatment considerable improvement occurs and many of these patients can lead a normal (but protected) life.

BONE AND JOINT TUBERCULOSIS

(Refer also Section 6, Ch 49 Tuberculosis)

This is common in India. Bone tuberculosis is generally secondary to established tuberculosis in other parts such as lungs, lymph nodes or kidneys. The organisms reach the synovium or subchondral bone by hematogenous or lymphatic spread. In vast majority of cases, a single large joint like the hip or knee is affected. Involvement of the vertebrae is common. In addition to the general symptoms of tuberculosis, severe local pain and restriction of movement of the affected region occur. If left untreated, the joint may be destroyed. Tuberculosis of the vertebrae leads to cold abscess formation and compression of the spinal cord. This used to be a frequent cause of paraplegia in India. However with the control of tuberculosis, the incidence has fallen considerably.

Diagnosis

Strong clinical suspicion is necessary for making early diagnosis. X-rays show periarticular osteoporosis and soft tissue swelling in the early stages. Later, there is narrowing and irregularity of joint space and erosion of the cartilage and subchondral bone. Cold abscess may be seen (Figs 116.4 and 116.5). The Mantoux test is often strongly positive. X-ray of the affected joint and synovial biopsy help in confirming the diagnosis.

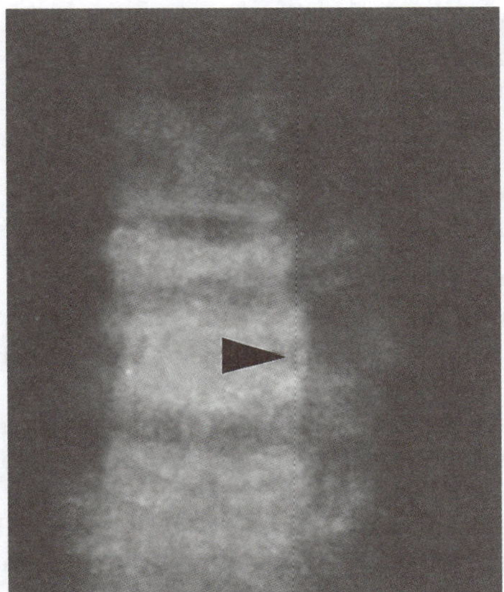

Fig. 116.4: X-ray PA view—tuberculosis spine. ***Note:*** Cold abscess (arrow)

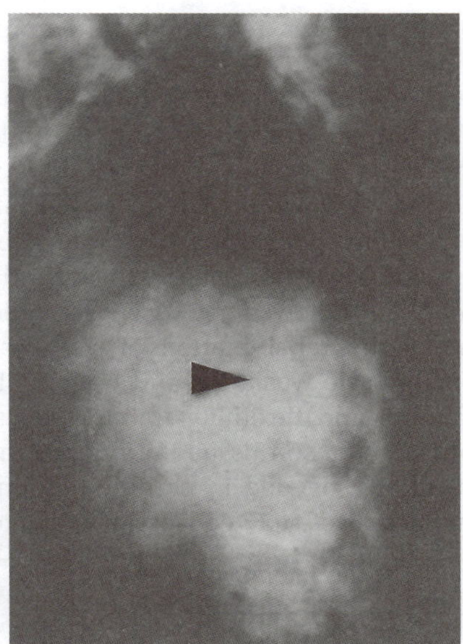

Fig. 116.5: X-ray lateral view—tuberculosis spine. ***Note:*** Compression of vertebra (arrow)

Treatment

Standard systemic anti-tuberculous therapy is indicated for durations ranging from 9 to 12 months. Local measures include immobilization of the spine to reduce pain and spinal compression. Supplementation with vitamin D, calcium and proteins hastens the recovery. Surgery may be indicated to relive spinal cord compression and gross vertebral destruction.

SPORTS INJURIES

In modern times, several persons (young and old) take to sporting activities which expose them to repeated injuries. These include growth plate fractures, epiphyseal fractures, osteochondritis dissecans and traction apophysitis. Sports injuries are becoming increasingly common. Most of them are soft tissue lesions and are often managed inadequately. Many of them are preventable. There are two major mechanisms of injury—trauma and overuse. Overuse may be due to intrinsic factors like malalignment of joints or limbs. Extrinsic factors are related to equipment and environment.

Excessively strenuous training, especially for competitive sports leads to injuries associated with overuse and growth problems. Negligence on the part of the children and parents, such as failure to wear protective equipment like helmet, knee guards, face shields predispose to injury. They may also not care to follow proper techniques which will minimize injuries to themselves and others. Competitive sports at all levels should be supervized by trained experts in order to avoid injuries and also to improve performance. Evidence-based preventive measures are available which have to be followed by those in training.

Principles of General Management

Prevention is by addressing the contributory factors like malalignment of joints which should be corrected and the equipment used should be reviewed. Management of acute phase involves treatment of inflammation, the NICER approach.

- **N**SAIDs is used to reduce pain and inflammation
- **I**ce is an analgesic and it limits excessive inflammation
- **C**ompression
- **E**levation of the injured area reduces swelling
- **R**est for 24 hours and supportive protective strapping may be helpful to relieve muscle spasm and pain.

This may be followed by exercise which is the cornerstone of the rehabilitation of soft tissue injury. This prevents muscle weakness and wasting. It includes strength training and flexibility training. Local steroids have no role in acute soft tissue injury even though they may be useful and needed in chronic tendon insertion injury unresponsive to conservative management.

Arthroscopic surgery procedures may have to be performed with minimal invasiveness for faster rehabilitation.

Specific structural injuries to tendon, ligament, muscle and bone may require special management. Commonly affected tendons are the Achilles tendon and supraspinatus. The most common ligament injury in sport is the sprained lateral ligament of the ankle. Muscle injury results from trauma or overstretching. Rupture is uncommon and hematoma may be complicated by myositis ossificans in which the muscle may undergo change to calcification and even formation of bones. Stress fracture of bone may be missed unless a high degree of suspicion is maintained.

In many countries, athletes in training for major sports events are subjected to appropriate investigations to rule out the known causative factors.

CHAPTER
117

Rheumatological Manifestations of Systemic Diseases

Binoy J Paul, KV Krishna Das

Chapter Summary

- General Considerations
- Endocrine Diseases
- Hematological Disorders
- Renal Disorders
- Other Disorders
- Infective Conditions
- Drug-induced Joint Manifestations

GENERAL CONSIDERATIONS

Many systemic illnesses can present with musculoskeletal symptoms as the initial presentation. In some of the systemic diseases, rheumatological problems can occur in the course of the illness. The major systemic illnesses with rheumatological manifestations are given in Table 117.1.

Table 117.1: Major systemic illnesses with rheumatological manifestations

Endocrine diseases	*Renal disorders*
• Diabetes mellitus (DM)	• Chronic renal failure (CRF)
• Hypo/hyperthyroidism	• Renal tubular acidosis (RTA)
• Hypo/hyperparathyroidism	*Malignancies*
• Cushing syndrome	• Primary malignancies
• Acromegaly	• Secondary deposits
Hematological problems	• Paraneoplastic syndrome
• Hemophilia	*Others*
• Sickle cell disease (SCD)	• Sarcoidosis
• Leukemia	• Hemochromatosis
• Lymphoma	• Amyloidosis
• Multiple myeloma	• Infections
	• Human immunodeficiency virus (HIV), tuberculosis, Lyme disease, brucellosis
	• Drugs

ENDOCRINE DISEASES

Diabetes Mellitus (DM)

Diabetes can affect the locomotor system in many ways. Long-standing diabetes produce changes in the connective tissues and bones. Rheumatological manifestations of DM:

- Diabetic cheiroarthropathy
- Neuropathic joint
- Diabetic osteolysis
- Diabetic muscle infarction (DMI)
- Diffuse idiopathic skeletal hyperostosis (DISH)
- Adhesive capsulitis
- Shoulder-hand syndrome
- Dupuytren's contracture
- Trigger finger
- Plantar fasciitis
- Diseases with possible association:
  - Gout
  - Osteoarthritis
  - Pseudogout

Diabetic Cheiroarthropathy or Limited Joint Mobility

Patients with long-standing diabetes present with restriction of movement of hand and fingers. It is seen in approximately 25–50% diabetics, equally common in both sexes; and commoner in patients on insulin, juvenile onset and longer duration of the diabetes. It usually involves small joints of hand, range of movements reduced at metacarpophalangeal joint and proximal interphalangeal joints. Fingers are swollen with tight, thick and waxy skin mimicking scleroderma. Blood tests for autoimmunity like rheumatoid factor (RF) and antinuclear antibody

Textbook of Medicine

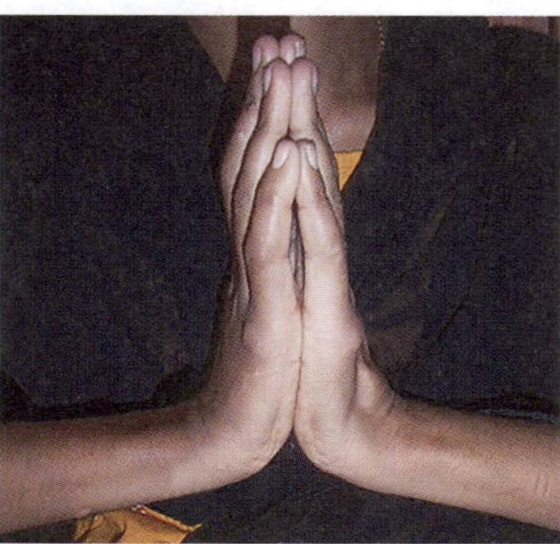

Fig. 117.1: *Prayer sign* in diabetic cheiroarthropathy

(ANA) will be negative. Radiographs will be normal. Diabetic cheiroarthropathy has direct correlation with microvascular complications.

Pathophysiology

Sorbitol and other polyols can cause movement of water into the cells leading to skin thickening. Microangiopathy of dermal or subcutaneous vessels also causes fibrosis of connective tissue. Non-enzymatic glycosylation of collagen and collagen cross linkage also occur.

Diagnosis

The diagnosis is clinical. Demonstrating ***prayer sign*** where the patient is asked to put his or her hands together in a praying position with the fingers fanned and to press together the palmar surfaces of the interphalangeal joints and the palms. Normally, an individual is able to oppose both hands together (Fig. 117.1), but a patient with limited joint mobility (LJM) fails to do. Inflammatory markers like erythrocyte sedimentation rate (ESR) and tests for autoimmunity like RF, anti-cyclic citrullinated peptide (CCP) and ANA will be negative. Biopsy of the skin and periarticular tissues may show abnormal thickening of the dermis and fibrosis of subcutaneous tissue.

Treatment includes strict control of blood glucose, passive stretching and digital extension and occupational therapy. No drugs are approved for treatment; however, injection of corticosteroids in the palmar flexor tendon sheath, ***aldose reductase inhibitors*** like ***epalrestat*** which prevent eye and nerve damage in people with diabetes, and penicillamine, have been tried.

Neuropathic Arthritis (Charcot's Joint)

Neuropathic joint disease (Charcot's joint) is a progressive destructive joint disease associated with sensory loss. The common cause today is DM. Other causes are leprosy, tabes dorsalis, syringomyelia, hereditary sensory neuropathies, amyloidosis and spinal cord trauma.

Clinical features

The distribution of the joint involvement depends on the underlying neuropathy as shown in Table 117.2. The onset of neuropathic arthropathy is usually gradual. The joint will be swollen and warm. As there is relatively little pain, patient often do not seek medical consultation until progressive deterioration has occurred. Arthralgia is well-documented in 50% of patients though the symptoms are usually less than expected from the degree of joint destruction.

Table 117.2: Joint involvement in neuropathic arthropathy (Charcot's joints)

Disease	Site of involvement
Diabetes mellitus	Metatarsophalangeal, tarsometatarsal, intertarsal joints
Leprosy	Tarsal, tarsometatarsal joints
Syringomyelia	Shoulder, elbow, wrist
Hereditary sensory neuropathy	Knee, ankle, intertarsal, metatarsophalangeal joint
Tabes dorsalis	Knee, hip, ankle
Amyloidosis	Knee, ankle

Investigations

Plain radiography in early stages shows joint effusion, periosteal calcification or minimal subluxation. Subsequently fragmentation of articular surface occurs leading to complete joint disorganization. This is associated with prominent periosteal new bone formation. Osteocartilaginous bodies of synovial origin and fragments from articular surface lead to a great deal of osseous debris inside the joint. Osteosclerosis and osteophytosis are very prominent radiological features. Synovial fluid may be serous, serosanguineous and lipid crystals secondary to subchondral bone lesions may be seen.

Treatment

The management of Charcot's joint consists of joint immobilization and rest for stabilization of the joint. Weight-bearing may be avoided and orthotic devices like plaster cast, crutches, stabilizing splints or braces are used as required to permit limited mobilization. The treatment of basic neurological disease usually does not improve the condition. Recently, bisphosphonates like pamidronate have been used successfully to halt the underlying bone resorption in neuropathic arthropathy.

Thyroid Disorders

Hypothyroidism is classically associated with muscle stiffness, cramps or calf muscle hypertrophy (Hoffman's syndrome). Carpal tunnel syndrome is also common in hypothyroidism and could be a presenting manifestation. Hyperuricemia is also not uncommon in hypothyroidism due to reduced uric acid clearance and can cause joint pain. Autoimmune thyroiditis, a common cause of hypothyroidism, can be associated with connective tissue disease (CTD) like systemic lupus erythematosus (SLE) or rheumatoid arthritis (RA).

Hyperthyroidism can cause proximal muscle wasting and respiratory muscle weakness. Occasionally, myositis or myasthenia with periodic paralysis can occur. ***Thyroid acropachy*** is a rare condition characterized by soft tissue swelling of hand and feet with clubbing. Generalized osteoporosis is also common in long-standing thyrotoxicosis.

Parathyroid Diseases

Hyperparathyroidism can cause articular and periarticular disorders or additional bone resorption. Patients may present with generalized aches and pains, stiffness or tenderness at enthesis or tendon rupture. Subperiosteal bone resorption can lead to erosive arthropathy of the small joints of fingers and wrists. Proximal muscle weakness and chondrocalcinosis are also not uncommon.

Hypoparathyroidism can cause spondylitis due to extensive calcification of paraspinal ligament. Hypocalcemia can lead to myopathy or myotonia.

Other Endocrine Disorders

Cushing's syndrome can cause proximal muscle weakness, osteoporosis and avascular necrosis of femoral head. Tendinitis or tendon rupture can also occur with increased frequency. ***Acromegaly*** can lead to synovial thickening, bursae hyperplasia and bony proliferation. Acromegalic limb arthropathy affects large joints like knee, shoulders and hip. Joint effusions can develop. Ultimately, cartilage degeneration occurs leading to severe destructive osteoarthritis. Spine involvement in acromegaly causes chronic dorsilumbar pain, kyphosis or spinal canal stenosis. Entrapment neuropathies like carpal tunnel syndrome and proximal myopathy are also common.

HEMATOLOGICAL DISORDERS

Several hematological disorders may present with bone and joint symptoms. Unless these are borne in mind, the primary condition may be missed.

Leukemias: In acute lymphatic leukemia, arthralgia, arthritis and bone pains are common. These may be mistaken for rheumatic fever or RA. Secondary gout is common in all forms of leukemias either in the florid stage or this may be precipitated by treatment.

Sickle cell anemia: Involvement of finger joints and other periarticular tissues and severe bone pains are common especially during crisis. Bone infarction and avascular necrosis of the head of femur or humerus and tibial condyles can also occur.

Hemophilia and other coagulation defects: Bleeding into weight-bearing joints is common. The knees, ankles and elbows are frequently affected. In the early stages, particularly in toddlers, a primary joint disease may be suspected. Later, due to recurrent bleeding, the joint is damaged and secondary osteoarthritis results. Radiography of the affected knee may show widening of femoral intercondylar notch and degenerative changes (Figs 117.2 and 117.3).

Multiple myeloma: This disorder commonly presents with bone pain and fractures, especially in the axial skeleton. It may also lead to secondary gout.

Malignant lymphoma: This disorder may involve bones directly or indirectly by giving rise to secondary gout.

Renal Disorders

Chronic kidney disease causes various musculoskeletal manifestations. The various skeletal disorders are collectively known as renal osteodystrophy. They are characterized by bone pain, extraskeletal calcification, osteomalacia and osteitis fibrosa cystica.

Distal ***renal tubular acidosis***, secondary Sjögren's syndrome or SLE can also rarely cause renal osteodystrophy in addition to hypokalemia.

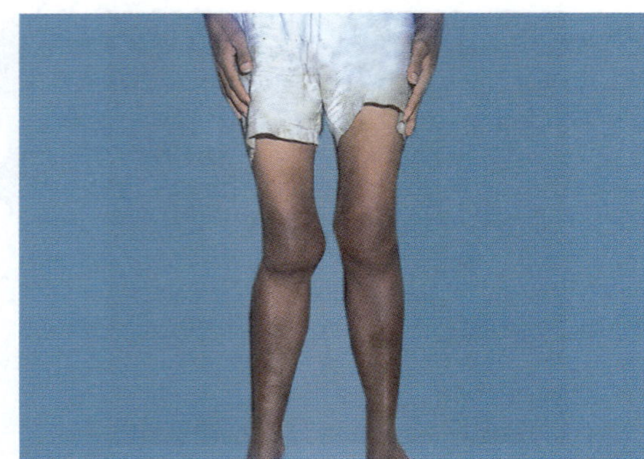

Fig. 117.2: Hemophilial arthritis knees (male)

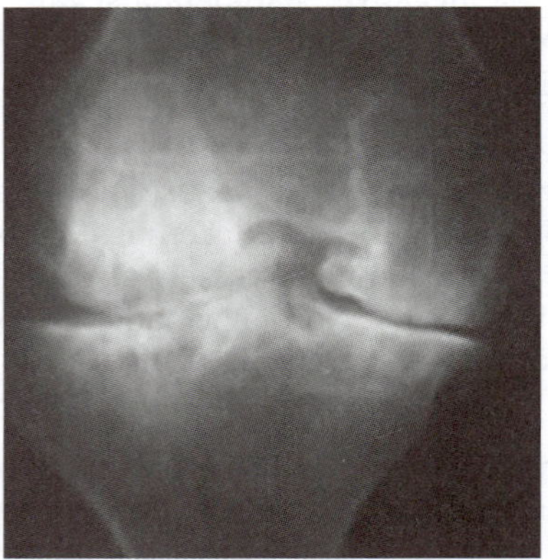

Fig. 117. 3: X-ray of knee showing widening of femoral intercondylar notch in hemophilic arthritis

OTHER DISORDERS

Malignancies

Primary or ***metastatic neoplasms*** in the juxta-articular site or synovial membrane can simulate. Monoarthritis, metastasis in the small joints of hand can mimic RA. Synovial cell sarcomas are usually located in the knee, foot or ankle. In hematological and lymphoreticular malignancies, periarticular infiltration causes joint symptom. Multiple myeloma can present with small joint arthritis like RA. ***Carcinomatous polyarthritis*** is a paraneoplastic manifestation seen in association with malignancies of breast, lung, colon, ovarian cancers and lymphomas. It usually occurs in older patients with explosive onset. It has a predilection for lower limb joints and is often asymmetrical. These patients may present with polyarthritis and vague arthralgias which may be mistaken for any of the common rheumatological disorder. Arthritis symptoms improve with successful treatment of the malignancy.

Sarcoidosis

Joint manifestations develops in 25–30% of systemic sarcoidosis. The musculoskeletal manifestations include inflammatory arthritis, dactylitis, tenosynovitis, periarticular soft tissue swelling or myopathy. Patients may present with ***Löfgren's syndrome***, an acute variant of sarcoidosis characterized by hilar adenopathy, erythema nodosum and arthritis. The arthritis in Löfgren's syndrome predominantly affects the lower limb joints, especially ankles. This oligoarthritis is often self-limiting. The other variety of sarcoid arthropathy is a chronic polyarthritis which is rare but has a prolonged course with bony erosions and cystic lesions affecting in the small bones of hand and feet. Arthritis in Löfgren's syndrome often responds to nonsteroidal anti-inflammatory drugs (NSAIDs) or colchicine. Chronic polyarthritis may need disease-modifying antirheumatic drugs (DMARDs) like methotrexate, hydroxychloroquine or corticosteroids.

Hemochromatosis

Twenty five to forty percent patients with hemochromatosis can develop arthropathy after the age of 50 years. It is a degenerative joint disorder usually starting in the second and third metacarpophalangeal joints of both hands. Later, larger joints like knee, hip, ankle and shoulder may be involved. The picture is similar to that of osteoarthritis. Chondrocalcinosis of hands and wrists are also common. Radiographs show joint space narrowing, subchondral, sclerosis and hook-like osteophytes. *Treatment* consists of NSAIDs and other measures. Phlebotomy done to reduce erythrocyte volume has little effect on the arthropathy. Joint replacement is successful in advanced osteoarthritis of knee and hip.

Amyloidosis

It can cause carpal tunnel syndrome, alopecia, nasal changes. Amyloid arthropathy can present like polyarticular RA or asymmetrical arthritis affecting hip and shoulder. Infiltration of amyloid deposits into the glenohumeral (GH) joint and surrounding soft tissue produce characteristic ***shoulder pad sign***.

INFECTIVE CONDITIONS

Several infections give rise to joint symptoms either as allergic manifestations or due to direct involvement. Polyarthritis occurring in systemic tuberculosis ***(Poncet's syndrome)*** and reactions in leprosy fall in the former group. Joints may be directly involved by pyogenic organisms, *Mycobacterium tuberculosis, Treponema pallidum, gonococci, meningococci, Salmonella typhi, Brucella, Lyme borreliosis,* rubella, hepatitis B virus (HBV), mumps, chickenpox, smallpox, HIV infection and several others. Unless clinical suspicion is strong these conditions may be mistaken for primary rheumatic diseases for long periods.

DRUG-INDUCED JOINT MANIFESTATIONS

Several drugs give rise to arthralgia and possibly arthritis as adverse side effects. These include immune serum and vaccines, penicillin and other antibiotics, antihypertensive drugs, parenteral iron, iron chelators, interferons and others. Detailed drug history is important to diagnose these conditions. Serum sickness and immunological reactions are similar problems which present with major joint involvement.

CHAPTER
118

Newer Diagnostic and Therapeutic Modalities in Rheumatology

Binoy J Paul

> **Chapter Summary**
>
> - Newer Autoantibodies in Rheumatic Diseases
> - Recent Advances in the Therapy of Rheumatic Diseases
> - Rheumatoid Arthritis
> - Systemic Lupus Erythematosus
> - Seronegative Spondyloarthritis
> - Osteoporosis
> - Biological Agents
> - Biosimilars

NEWER AUTOANTIBODIES IN RHEUMATIC DISEASES

There is refinement of classification criteria for various rheumatic diseases like rheumatoid arthritis (RA), vasculitis, Sjögren's syndrome in the past few years which help the clinician to establish early diagnosis and therapy. When specific diagnosis is in doubt, clinicians resort to immunological tests for arriving at firm diagnosis. A growing number of autoantibodies, which have specificity for particular clinical phenotypes, are being identified. They can also offer prognostic information in addition to specific diagnosis.

In many patients with autoimmune rheumatic diseases like RA, systemic lupus erythematosus (SLE) or progressive systemic sclerosis, the autoantibodies precede the clinical symptoms by many years. Patients with RA might have detectable anti-cyclic citrullinated peptide (CCP) many years before the onset of arthritis. In SLE, antinuclear antibody (ANA) or double stranded deoxyribonucleic acid (dsDNA) may be detectable in the patient's serum, months or years before the clinical onset of the disease. Patients with Raynaud's phenomenon and positive anti-topoisomerase-1 antibody are more likely to progress to systemic sclerosis than those without this autoantibody. In myositis patients, antisynthetase myositis specific antibodies like anti-Jo-1 can develop. These antibodies are associated with lung fibrosis, mechanics hands, nonerosive polyarthritis and Raynaud's phenomenon collectively called antisynthetase syndrome in addition to myositis.

RECENT ADVANCES IN THE THERAPY OF RHEUMATIC DISEASES

Significant advances have been made in our understanding of autoimmune rheumatic diseases and its management in the past decade. The limit of what conventional drugs like nonsteroidal anti-inflammatory drugs (NSAIDs), steroids and disease-modifying antirheumatic drugs (DMARDs) can achieve has probably been reached. Improved understanding of the pathogenesis of these diseases with the introduction of more targeted biological treatment is beginning to show encouraging signs of improvement in the outlook of these patients.

RHEUMATOID ARTHRITIS

The approach to treatment of RA has seen three major advances in the last 10–15 years that has changed the outcome of the disease. They are:

1. Early intervention with DMARDs and low dose steroid bridging
2. Treat-to-target or tight control strategy
3. Use of biological response modifiers (BRMs).

Early Intervention

Early use of DMARDs preferably methotrexate with low dose steroids for 2–3 months started within 3–6 months of onset of RA has achieved marked clinical benefits. Combination of synthetic DMARDs with low-dose steroids are widely useful in patients with poor prognostic factors like early erosion, strongly positive rheumatoid factor or anti-CCP or high disease activity [disease activity score (DAS) > 5.1].

Treat-to-target or Tight Control Strategy

Targeting no or low-disease activity by regular monitoring using primary composite measures of disease activity and adhering to a predefined treatment strategy when compared with unstructured treatment conveys better outcome. In the past this was not possible primarily because of the complexity of measures assessing disease activity in RA and insufficient knowledge of optimal treatment strategies. DAS28, simplified disease activity index (SDAI), clinical disease activity index (CDAI), routine assessment of patient index data (RAPID3) (Tables 118.1 and 118.2) are all validated and these functioning measures now used in every day case allowing physicians to treat-to-target.

Biological Response Modifiers (Biological Agents)

Despite aggressive treatment strategies and early use of synthetic DMARDs, treatment failures are not uncommon

Table 118.1: Measures included in composite score commonly used in RA

	DAS28	SDAI	CDAI	RAPID3
Swollen joint	+	+	+	
Tender joint	+	+	+	
Physicians global assessment		+	+	
Patients global assessment	+	+	+	+
Functional score pain				+
ESR/CRP		+	+	

Abbreviations: DAS28 = Disease activity score 28; SDAI = Simplified disease activity index; CDAI = Clinical disease activity index; RAPID3 = Routine assessment of patient index data3; ESR = Erythrocyte sedimentation rate; CRP = C-reactive protein; RA = Rheumatoid arthritis

Table 118.2: Activity level cut off for composite indices

Activity level	DAS28 (0–10)	SDAI (0–86)	CDAI (0–76)	Rapid3 (0–30)
High	>5.1	>26	>22	>12
Moderate	3.2–5.1	11–26	10.1–22	6.1–12
Low	2.6–3.2	3.3–11	2.9–10	3.1–6
Remission/near remission	<2.6	<3.3	<2.8	< 3

Abbreviations: DAS28 = Disease activity score 28; SDAI = Simplified disease activity index; CDAI = Clinical disease activity index; RAPID3 = Routine assessment of patient index data3

in RA and other rheumatic diseases. A significant minority of patients (18–28%) fails to achieve satisfactory disease control. Hence better therapeutic agents are needed for these patients. Laboratory research in the understanding of immunopathogenesis especially the cytokine milieu and their network in RA contributed heavily towards the development of biological agents (BRMs).

SYSTEMIC LUPUS ERYTHEMATOSUS

The improved understanding about the pathogenesis, more judicious use of pharmacological agents which are potentially toxic, invention of newer therapeutic agents like mycofenolate and belimumab, early detection and prompt treatment of infection and renal replacement therapies resulted in considerable improvement in the prognosis of SLE. In 1956, the 4-year survival with SLE was 50%, but in 2013 the 15-year survival is 85%. It is shown that mycofenolate in comparison with cyclophosphamide is an equally useful induction agent in lupus nephritis and is much less toxic. It is also more beneficial than azathioprine for maintenance treatment. ***Eurolupus project*** showed equivalent efficacy of low dose IV cyclophosphamide [(six fortnightly pulses of 500 mg) to National Institute of Health (NIH) protocol 750 mg/m²/monthly IV cyclophosphamide for 6 months followed by quarterly infusion for 2 years].

Increased recognition of multifaceted role of B cells in SLE led to the development of novel drugs notably rituximab and belimumab. In SLE, B cells produce autoantibodies that causes T cell activation, cytokine secretion and modulation of dendritic cells. They also act independently as antigen presenting cells. CD20 is a β lymphocyte specific antigen that is expressed by pre β cells and mature β cells. ***Rituximab*** is a chimeric monoclonal immunoglobulin G1 (IgG1) antibody to CD20. Administration of rituximab causes β cell depletion lasting for 6–12 months. Rituximab has been used mainly in refractory lupus nephritis, when conventional drugs have failed. In addition to RA and SLE, rituximab is used in refractory antineutrophil cytoplasmic antibodies (ANCA) associated vasculitis like Wegener's granulomatosis type II mixed cryoglobulinemia and dermatomyositis. Two doses of 1000 mg is usually given at 15 day interval as slow IV infusion.

B cells rely on several different cytokines for its proliferation, activation and maturation. B lymphocyte stimulator (BlyS) also known as B cells activating factor (BAFF) is a cytokine of tumor necrosis factor (TNF) family is a notable example. Belimumab is a monoclonal human antibody that inactivates BlyS causing inhibition of B cell maturation. The drug is appropriate for use in patients with antibody positive active SLE who are receiving standard treatment. The drug is found to have a steroid sparing effect, also reduce constitutional symptoms like fatigue, skin lesions and joint disease. It is not approved for the use in major organ lupus like nephritis or central nervous system (CNS) involvement.

B cell modulating treatment inhibiting costimulatory molecules like epratuzumab (anti-CD22 monoclonal antibody) is under clinical trial. Atacicept, a drug inhibits interaction between BlyS and a proliferation inducing ligand-APRIL with their receptors. It suppresses the differentiation and survival of B cells and could be an emerging therapeutic agent in the treatment of lupus.

Although pathogenic autoantibodies in SLE are derived from B cells, evidence suggests that T cell dysfunction also exists in SLE. The main target of T cell direct treatment has been the inhibition of costimulation of T cells. ***Abatacept*** is a fusion protein consisting of T lymphocyte associated antigen (CTLA4) and modified Fc portion of human Ig. CTLA4 competes with CD28 for binding to CD80/86; thus abatacept down regulates T cell activation. Initial clinical trials with abatacept and low-dose cyclophosphamide followed by maintenance treatment with azathioprine are promising.

Interleukin 6 (IL6) inhibition with ***tocilizumab***, a monoclonal antibody that inhibit IL6 receptors showed improvement in mild to moderate lupus. Anti-TNF agents are well-known to cause lupus and may cause flare up of disease and hence are not generally recommended in SLE.

Autologous stem cell transplantation has been used as a therapeutic strategy in SLE and other autoimmune rheumatic diseases in patients who are refractory to conventional treatment. The reported overall survival is 81% with 18% mortality recorded at 2 years. Despite high morbidity and mortality, the ability to achieve a sustained disease free state in patients with poor prognosis supports autologous stem cell transplantation in patients with refractory lupus.

SERONEGATIVE SPONDYLOARTHRITIS

Response to therapy with synthetic DMARDs like sulfasalazine and methotrexate in seronegative spondyloarthritis (SSpA) like ankylosing spondylitis was quite unsatisfactory as these drugs are not very effective in axial disease. Thalidomide and biphosphonates like pamidronate has been used with limited benefits. Dramatic improvement has been noticed with the use of anti-TNF agents in early ankylosing spondylitis, psoriatic arthritis and other types of SSpA. Infliximab, etanercept and adalimumab demonstrated effectiveness in these conditions. There is rapid resolution of sacroilitis and spondylitis. As anti-TNF therapy is highly effective for axial, peripheral and entheseal diseases, these agents should be used in all patients refractory to NSAIDs and conventional synthetic DMARDs like sulfasalazine or methotrexate.

OSTEOPOROSIS

Biological agents like teriperatide and denosumab open new avenues in the management of refractory osteoporosis. An array of pharmacological agents like biphosphonates, raloxifene, salmon calcitonin and strontium in addition to calcium and vitamin D supplementation is already available for therapy of osteoporosis.

Teriparatide (1–34) produced using recombinant DNA technology retains all biological activity of intact parathyroid hormone (PTH) peptide and is recommended for treatment of severe osteoporosis in men and women at a dose of 20 µg/day/SC.

Denosumab is a human monoclonal antibody against RANK (receptor activator of nuclear factor kappa B). Osteoblasts express ligand of RANK, a member of TNF superfamily of ligands and receptors. Osteoclast precursors express RANK denosumab reduces bone resorption by inhibiting formation, function and survival of osteoclasts. It is given at a dose of 60 mg in 1 mL subcutaneously every 6 months.

BIOLOGICAL AGENTS

They are molecules produced biotechnologically and are used to neutralize or nullify action of any physiological molecule or cellular receptors.

Classification

Anticytokine BRMs

- ***Anti-TNFα agents:*** Infliximab, etanercept, adalimumab, golimumab, PEGylated certolizumab
- ***Anti-interleukin agents***
  - ***IL1 antagonists:*** Anakinra, rilonacept, canakinumab
  - ***IL6 antagonists:*** Tocilizumab

Nonanticytokine BRMs

- ***Anti B cell agents:*** Rituximab
- ***Costimulation blockers***
  - ***CTLA4Ig***: Abatacept
  - ***BlyS inhibitor:*** Belimumab
- ***Anti RANK ligand drugs:*** Denosumab.

Anti-TNF agents tried in RA are given below but these agents are also useful in ankylozing spondylitis, psoriatic arthritis and other spondyloarthropathies. In rheumatoid arthritis and other autoimmune rheumatic diseases like SLE and vasculitis, newer BRMs acting against IL, anti-B cell agents and BlyS inhibitors are found to be useful. Comparative merits of the different drugs have been explained in Tables 118.3 to 118.5.

BIOSIMILARS

Biosimilars are biotherapeutic products which is similar in terms of quality, safety and efficacy to an already available biological disease modifying drug, several pharmaceutical companies in the developing nations like India developed biosimilar versions of originator (reference) product. The biosimilars or ***follow on biologics*** are new biopharmaceutical products and not the generic versions of innovator biopharmaceuticals. The active ingredient in the biosimilar is not identical to the innovator (reference) product. The properties of biopharmaceutical products, dependent on the manufacturing process, protein source of extraction, purification process and others, result in heterogeneity of the resulting follow-on biologics.

In India, biosimilars of ***rituximab (Reditux RA)*** and ***etanercept (Etacept)*** are available. These agents are markedly cheap in comparison to the originators and are broadening the access of these drugs to more needy patients in our country. Because there is limited clinical database at approval of these biosimilars, switching or substitution between innovator product and biosimilar is often viewed actually as a change in clinical management. The efficacy and safety of these drugs are very similar

Table 118.3: Anti-TNF agents: Comparative merits of the different drugs

Name	Infliximab	Etanercept	Adalimumab	Golimumab	Certolizumab
Structure	Mouse-human chimeric monoclonal antibody again TNFα	TNFα receptor IgGE Fe region dimeric fusion protein	Fully humanized monoclonal antibody against TNFα	Fully humanized mAb agent TNFα	PEGylated Fe free Fab monoclonal antibody
Dose and route of administration	3–5 mg/kg slow IV every 2 weeks for 3 doses then once monthly	25 mg twice weekly SC	40 mg every two weeks SC	50 mg monthly SC	400 mg monthly SC
Indications	RA, ankylosing spondylitis, psoriatic arthritis, inflammatory bowel diseases	RA, ankylosing spondylitis, psoriatic arthritis, juvenile, idiopathic arthritis	RA	RA	RA

Abbreviations: RA = Rheumatoid arthritis; TNFα = Tumor necrosis factor alpha; SC = Subcutaneously; mAb = Monoclonal antibody

Table 118.4: Anti-interleukin agents: Comparative merits of the different drugs

Name	Anakinra	Rilonacept	Canakinumab	Tocilizumab
Structure	IL1 receptor antagonist	Dimeric fusion protein directed against IL1	Fully humanized monoclonal antibody directed at IL1β	Humanized recombinant monoclonal antibody against IL6
Dose and route of administration	100 mg daily SC	80–120 mg weekly SC	150 mg SC	8 mg/kg monthly
Indications	RA (less effective than TNF agents), JIA, adult onset stills disease, refractory gout	CAPS, Muckle Wells syndrome, refractory gout	Refractory gout	RA, systemic onset JIA, SLE, large vessel vasculitis

Abbreviations: JIA = Juvenile idiopathic arthritis; CAPS = Cryopyrin associated periodic syndromes; SLE = Systemic lupus erythematosus; RA = Rheumatoid arthritis; SC = Subcutaneously; IL1 = Interleukin1

Table 118.5: Non anti-cytokine biological response modifiers: Comparative merits of the different drugs

Name	Rituximab	Abatacept	Belimumab
Structure	Chimeric (human-mouse) monoclonal antibody against CD20 + molecule on the surface of B cells	A fusion protein consisting of IgG1 and CTLA4	A monoclonal human antibody that inactivate B lymphocyte stimulator
Dose and route of administration	Two infusions of 1000 mg at 15 days apart (can be repeated after 6 months) IV infusion	3 doses of 10–12 mg/kg at 15 days apart then once in a month IV infusion	10 mg/kg at 15 days apart then once in a month as IV infusion
Indication	RA, refractory lupus nephritis primary systemic vasculitis	RA, refractory SLE	Active SLE without major organ involvement

Abbreviations: CTLA4 = Cytotoxic T lymphocyte associated antigen 4; SLE = Systemic lupus erythematosus, RA = Rheumatoid arthritis; IV = intravenous

though the experience is limited. The immunogenicity of biosimilars is another concern.

Definition of Therapeutic Product

Terms used in the studies of biological products

Product	Alternative name	Definition
Generic	Intended copy	Exact copy of the drug synthesized by a similar or differentiated process with structural and therapeutic identity to the reference product
Biosimilar	Follow-on biologic (USA) Subsequent entry biologic (Canada) Similar biotherapeutic product (WHO)	A biological product that is highly similar to reference product in terms of quality and efficacy
Second generation biological	Bio better	A structurally, or functionally alternated product resulting in improved or different biological activity from the reference product
Me-too biological	Non innovator biological	A biological product developed with the same target antigen but without demonstrated comparability to the reference product

COMMENT

These innovations are exciting and they have been made possible by constant report of their producers. At present, all the biological are extremely expensive (beyond the capacity of the vast majority of the patients suffering from rheumatological diseases). In addition, due to interference with normal biological immune processes they lead to susceptibility to infections like tuberculosis and also malignancies especially the immunological system. Hence, even in countries of their origin, these drugs are kept in reserve for those who do not respond to all the conventional drugs used in combination and/or in sequence. The immediate response caused by these drugs is so dramatic that the benefit should not be denied to the deserving patients when needed.

Editor's Note: These drugs are expensive, but very effective when used in specific indications. Being drugs acting on the immunological system, they depress the body's immune mechanisms, predisposing to infections and also promoting neoplasia. Hence, they are best used by specialists who have special skills to use them with confidence. Despite all the disadvantages, they are very potent drugs which will improve the quality of life and deterioration in many of the chronic disabling rheumatic conditions and also immune mediated diseases affecting other systems.

A

Abadie's sign 1354
Abatacept 736, 789
Abciximab 913, 1185
Abdominal compartment syndrome 520
Abdominal form 383
Abdominal pain 475
Abducent nerve 1321
  palsy 1323
Abetalipoproteinemia 1437
ABO
  hemolytic disease 1078
  system 1097
Abortus fever 243
Abram's pleural biopsy punch 968
Abreaction 1584
Absence seizures 1382
Absolute reticulocyte count 1056
Abstinence 951
Acamprosate 1570
Acanthamoeba 410
Acanthocytes 1056
Acanthosis nigricans 71, 614, 1540
  malignant 1541
Acarbose 592
Accident, management of 123
Accidental hypothermia 108
Accommodation reflex 1319
ACE inhibitors 809
Acetaminophen 140
Acetazolamide 1389
Acetic acid 139
Acetohydroxamic acid 1260
Acetylcholine receptor antibodies 1469
Acetylcholine test 915
Achalasia cardia 486
Achondroplasia 782
Achylia gastrica 1069
Acid maltase deficiency 1479
Acid phosphatase 71
Acid-base
  balance 453
    abnormalities of 452
  disorder 454
    mixed 452, 462
  profile 1484
Acne 1509
  conglobata 1510
  excoriée 1510
  keloidalis nuchae 1536
  occupational 1510
  variants of 1510
  vulgaris 1509
Acneiform eruptions 1530
Acoustic neuromas 1420
Acquired aplastic anemia 1089
Acquired cystic kidney disease 1246
Acquired cysts 1026
Acquired epileptic aphasia 1381
Acquired hemolytic anemias 1075
Acquired hemophilia 1189
Acquired hypertrichosis lanuginosa 1536, 1542
Acquired immune deficiency syndrome 287, 290, 1075
  dementia 293
    complex 293
  encephalopathy 293
Acquired PRCA in adults 1092
Acquired renal cystic disorders 1246
Acquired syphilis 274
Acquired thrombophilia 1204
Acquired von Willebrand disease 1191

Acrochordon 1543
Acrodermatitis
  chronica atrophicans 259
  continua of Hallopeau 1513
Acrokeratosis 71
Acromegaly 650, 651, 786, 936
ACTH 646, 654
  stimulation 692
  testing 687
Actinic keratoses 1543
Actinomyces 382
Actinomycosis 382
Acute attack, management of 775
Acute leukemias, treatment of 1114
Acute malnutrition, moderate 164
Acute myeloid leukemia treatment, high-risk 1121
Acute pharyngitis, microbial causes of 974
Acute poisoning, symptoms of 144
Acute respiratory failure, management of 970
Acute tachycardias, management of 872
Acyanotic congenital heart defects 818, 819
Acyclovir 57, 333, 336
  ointment 336
Acylcarnitine 1487
Acylglycines 1487
Adalimumab 735, 766, 1515
Addison's disease 448, 692, 936
Addisonian pernicious anemia 1069
Adductor reflex, crossed 1291
Adefovir 57
  dipivoxil 348
Adenocarcinomas 1020
Adenoma, bronchial 1019
Adenomatous polyps 509
Adenovirus infections 357
Adie's pupil 1464
Adjustment disorders 1566
Adrenal cortex
  diseases of 688
  disorders of 684
Adrenal cortical
  disorders 687
  hormones 686
    secretory rates of 686
Adrenal crisis 693
Adrenal gland 1145
Adrenal hyperplasia, congenital 691
Adrenal incidentaloma 696
Adrenal medulla, disorders of 684, 694
Adrenergic system, inhibitors of 890
Adrenocortical insufficiency 691
  primary 691
Adrenocortical lesions 690
Adrenocorticotropin hormone 646
Adrenomyeloneuropathy 1430
Adriamycin 1142
Adult personality, disorders of 1567
Adverse drug event 45
Adverse prognostic indicators in stroke 1413
Adverse reactions, management of 100
Aedes aegypti 371
Aerosol
  drug delivery 988
  inhalation 967
  vaccines 330
Aflatoxicosis 145
African river blindness 439
African trypanosomiasis 402
African tumbu fly 90
Agnivesa 1
  tantra 1

Agnogenic myeloid metaplasia 1161
Agonist drugs 40
Agoraphobia 1561
Agranulocytosis 1135
  drug-induced 1135
Air inadvertently during aspiration 1031
Air travel, medical problems of 121
Airway
  clearance 1041
  disease, small 997
  diseases of 1003
    lower 996
  maintenance of 970, 1337
  mechanisms of 955
  resistance 958
    syndrome, upper 1016
  secretion of 954
Akinetic mutism 1337
Alastrim 331
Albendazole 416, 418, 420, 438, 441
Albiglutide 597
Albright's hereditary osteodystrophy 684
Albright's syndrome 705
Albuminocytologic dissociation 1310, 1455
Albuminuria 1214
Alcohol 188, 1349
  acts 1349
  exposure 939
  injection into tumor 561
  intoxication 137
  related disorders 1569
  septal ablation 946
  withdrawal syndrome 137
Alcoholic beverages 951
Alcoholic cirrhosis 533
Alcoholic dementia 1350
Alcoholic hallucinosis 1569
Alcoholic hepatitis 347, 552
Alcoholic hyaline 552
Alcoholic liver disease 552
Alcoholic myopathy 1350
Alcoholic paranoia 1569
Alcoholism 446, 448, 1350, 1438
  chronic 1569
Aldermoniac posture 1474
Aldose reductase inhibitors 785
Aldosterone 687
  antagonists 810
Aldrin 132
Alefacept 1515
Alemtuzumab 1129
Alendronate sodium 771
Aleppo boil 400
Alfa-fetoprotein 560
Alien hand 1291, 1367
Alimentary disorders 476, 1592
  symptoms in 475
Alimentary endoscopy, upper 478
Alimentary manifestations 679
Alimentary pentosuria 618
Alimentary symptoms 176
Alimentary system 666, 1064, 1588
Aliskiren 892
Alkalies 140
Alkalotic tetany 684
Alkaptonuria 628
Alleles 6
Allergen
  identification of 986
  immunotherapy 991
Allergic bronchopulmonary aspergillosis 996

Allergic contact dermatitis 1521
Allergic rhinitis 993
    treatment of 973
Allergic to penicillin, treatment of patients 277
Allodynia 1302
Allogenic stem cell transplantation 1157
    in myeloma 1143
Allogenic transplantation 1116
Alopecia 637, 1535
    areata 1535
    totalis 1535
    universalis 1535
Alpha-1 antitrypsin deficiency 1004
Alpha-adrenergic receptor blocking drugs 890
Alpha-fetoprotein 70
Alpha-glucosidase inhibitors 592
Alpha-interferon 57
Alpha-synucleinopathies 1395
ALS-parkinsonism dementia complex 1434
Alternate cover test 1323
Alternative regimen 281, 284
Alveolar hypoventilation, causes of 957
Alveolar membrane 958
Alveolar ventilation 958
Alzheimer's disease 1370, 1371
Amanita muscaria 143
Amanita phalloides 144
Amantadine 57, 324, 1394, 1428
    hydrochloride 56
Amblyomma 94, 267
    americanum 267
Ambrisentan 835
Ambulatory electroencephalogram 1303
Ambulatory peritoneal dialysis, continuous 1280
Ameba rare 1357
Amebiasis 405
    treatment of 408
Amebic dysentery, acute 406, 409
Amebomas 407
Amenorrhea 709
American cutaneous and mucocutaneous
        leishmaniasis 401
American trypanosomiasis 403
Amifostine 77
Amikacin 50
Amino acids 1487
Aminoglutethimide 690
Aminoglycosides 50, 1285
Aminophylline 992
Amiodarone 867, 868
Amlodipine 776, 892
Ammonia 456
Ammonium 456, 1486
    chloride 456
Amnesia 1548, 1564
Amnesic syndrome 1569
Amnestic disorders 1553
Amnestic syndrome 1569
Amebic meningoencephalitis 1357
    primary 409
Amotivational syndrome 1570
Amoxicillin 48
Amphoric breathing 966
Amphotericin B 58, 59, 399, 410
Ampicillin 48
Amplified Mycobacterium tuberculosis detection 303
Amylin 474, 582
    agonists 598
Amylnitrate 144
Amyloid
    A, secondary 1146
    light-chain 1264
    type of 1146
Amyloidosis 448, 938, 1144, 1146, 1264
    localized 1145
    secondary 731
Amyotrophic brachial diplegia 1433
Amyotrophic lateral sclerosis 457, 1431
Anacrotic pulse 848
Anaerobes 268
Anaerobic
    bacteria, role of 61
    food poisoning 143
    infections 268
    organisms 981

Anagen 1535
    phase 1544
Anagrelide 1167
Anakinra 736, 775
Anal canal 476
Anamnestic reaction 231
Anankastic personality disorder 1567
Anaphylactic
    reaction, type I 29
    shock 817
Anaphylactoid purpura 1264
Anaplasma 267
    phagocytophilum 267
Anaplasmataceae 267
Anaplasmosis 263, 267
Anastrozole 78
Anca-associated vasculitis 756
Ancylostoma duodenale 417
Ancylostomiasis 413, 417
Andreas Vesalius 2
Androgen
    excess 708
    functions of 699
Androgenic alopecia 1536
Anemia 1057, 1089
    aplastic 346, 1089, 1091
    based etiopathogenesis, classification of 1058
    correction of 1066
    etiology of 1059
    in rheumatoid arthritis 1070
    in systemic diseases 1070
    management of 1060
    of chronic diseases 1071
    of infections 1071
    severe 389
    treatment of 1241
Anesthesia dolorosa 1302
Anesthetic risk 1018
Anetoderma 1538
Aneuploidy 16
Aneurine 174
Aneurysmectomy 812
Angioedema 1526
Angiofibromas 715
Angiogenesis 72
Angioimmunoblastic
    lymphadenopathy 1159
    lymphoma 1157
Angioplasty, primary 946
Angiosarcomas 944
Angiostrongyliasis 441
Angiostrongylus
    cantonensis 441
    costaricensis 441
Angiotensin converting enzyme 448
    inhibitors 891
Angiotensin receptor blockers 447, 809, 891
Angiotensin-converting enzyme inhibitors 1285, 1286
Angiotensinogen 1211
Angiotensin-receptor blockers 908
Angular chelitis (perleche) 1506
Anhedonia 1555, 1559
Anhidrotic heat exhaustion 104
Anidulafungin 59
Animal rabies 362
Anisakiasis 441
Anisocoria 1319
Anistreplase 906
Ankylosing spondylitis 513, 764, 1027, 1035
Ankyrin 1046
Annual influenza vaccination 1000
Anomalous origin 829
Anomalous pulmonary venous connection 834
Anorectal lesions 282
Anorexia 475
    nervosa 653, 1571
Anosmia 1367
Anosognosia 1297
Anoxic damage to liver, acute 347
Antagonist drugs 40
Anterograde amnesia 1553
Anthracosis 1007
Anthrax 239, 240
Anthropometry 154, 638

Antianginal
    agents 911
    therapy 910, 914
Antianxiety drugs 1582
Antiarrhythmic 811
    drugs 880
Antibacterial
    agents 47, 1500
    drugs 327
    spectrum 50
Antibiotic 61, 76, 271, 539, 970, 983, 1286
    misuse of 61
    regimens, start initial 980
    resistance, future strategies in 61
Antibody 1374
    against viruses 322
    demonstration of 1074
    dependent immunity 29
    response 25
    to clotting factors 1192
Antibody-based therapies 1117
Antibody-detection tests 398
Anticholinergic agents 990, 999
Anticoagulant 811, 908, 913, 1194
    detection of circulating 1174
    indications of 1194
    rodenticides 134
    therapy 174
Anticoagulation, initial 927
Antidepressant 152
    drugs 1581
Anti-diphtheritic serum 224
Antidiuretic hormone 442, 642
Antidotes 127
    to cyanides 134
Antiepileptic drugs 1386
Antifolates 75
Antifungal drugs 58
Anti-GBM disease 1225
Antigen 25
    detection 363
Antiglomerular basement membrane disease 1028
Anti-GPIIB/IIIA antibodies 1185
Antihypertensive
    drug choices 894
    therapy 892
Anti-idiotype therapy 74
Anti-IGE treatment 994
Anti-immunoglobulin E 991
Anti-inflammatory agents 213, 1000, 1499
Anti-ischemia therapy 910
Antimicrobial
    agents 47
    drugs 249
    regimen 232
    resistance 194
    spectrum 51
    therapy 235, 244
Antimicrosomal antibody 661
Antimitochondrial antibody 526, 534
Antimutagens 70
Antimycobacterial drugs 55
Antineutrophil cytoplasmic antibodies 724
Anti-n-methyl-d aspartate syndrome 1377
Antinuclear 526
    antibodies 723, 724, 731, 743, 1262
Antiparkinsonism drugs 1583
Anti-pellagra vitamin 175
Antiphospholipid antibody 724
    syndrome 739, 743, 747
Antiplatelet
    agents 910, 913
    drug 913
        in stroke 1412
        therapy 1185
    therapy 1185
Antipruritic agents 1499
Antipsychotic
    atypical 1580
    conventional 1580
    drugs 1556, 1580
    side effects of 1580
Antipurines 75
Antipyrimidines 75
Antirabic serum 364

Antiretroviral therapy 295
Antirheumatic drugs 736
Anti-snake venom 99
Anti-sterility vitamin 173
Antistreptolysin O titer 723
Antitetanus serum 271
Antithrombin 1172
Antithrombotic mechanisms 1172
Anti-thyroglobulin antibodies 662
Anti-TNF agents, biological 1010
Antitrypsin deficiency 1003
Antituberculous drugs 1286
Antitumor necrosis factor agents 735
Antiviral drugs 56
Antiviral therapy in special population 349
Anti-voltage gated potassium channel syndrome 1376
Anti-β-cell agents 736
Anton's syndrome 1297
Anuria 1212
Anxiety
    acute 1578
    disorders 1560
    neurosis 1560
Anxiolytics 1582
Anxious personality disorder 1567
Aorta
    aneurysms of 930
    diseases of 928
Aortic diseases 928
Aortic incompetence 850
Aortic regurgitation 850
    acute 853
    causes of 850
    signs of 852
Aortic stenosis 847, 848
    congenital 819, 847
    severity of 849
Aortic syndrome, middle 929
Aortic valve, degenerative calcification of 848
Aortoarteritis, type III 929
Aortography 1219
Aphasia
    conduction 1300
    management of 1481
Aphthous ulcers
    major 481
    minor 481
Aplastic anemia
    congenital 1089
    moderate 1090
    severe 1090
    treatment of 1091
    very severe 1090
Aplastic crisis 1084
Apnea test 1338
Apnea-hypopnea index 1016
Apocrine glands 1497
Apoptosis 69
Appendages, infection of 1500
Appetite 475
Apraxic gait 1303
Aprotinin 1194
Aquagenic pruritus 1164
Aquagenic urticaria 1526
Aquaporin channels 465
Arabic medicine 1586
Arbovirus 365, 1360
    group B 370
Arenaviridae 359
Arenavirus 358
    infections 358
Argas persicus 258
Argatroban 1198
    dabigatran 914
Argemone mexicana 145
Argentine 359
Arginine vasopressin 443, 642
    role of 804
Argyll Robertson pupil 1319, 1354, 1367
Armadillo gait 1303
Arnold-Chiari malformation 1450
Arrhythmias 811, 902, 942, 1413
Arrhythmogenic right ventricular
    cardiomyopathy 917
    dysplasia 872

Arsenical keratoses 1544
Artemether 392
Arterial blood
    gases 452, 454, 926
    pressure 792
Arterial embolism 902
Arterial pulse 793
Arterial strokes 1406
Arterial wall, examination of 794
Arteriographic studies 915
Artery
    peripheral 857
    syndrome, basilar 1410
Artery-to-artery embolism 1407
Artesunate 393
Arthralgia 377, 740
Arthritis 210, 377, 513, 767, 740
    inflammatory 727
Arthropod bites 91
Arthroscopy 726, 779
Articular involvement 728
Asbestosis 1007
Ascariasis 413
Ascites 518, 537
    management of 531
    prognosis of 519
Ascitic fluid ultrafiltration 532
Asclepid hippocrates 1
Ascorbic acid 178, 1347
Aseptic meningitis 355
Ashworth scale 1291
Asian opticospinal multiple sclerosis 1428
Asiatic schistosomiasis 431
Aspartate transaminase 901
Aspergillosis 378
Aspergillus 1361, 1362
    flavus 145
Aspermia 706
Aspiration 409, 1031
    elective 1031
    emergency 1030
    pneumonia 979, 981
Aspirin 734, 903, 1185
    in dose 915
Astanga hridaya 1
Astanga sangraha 1
Asterixis 1405
Asthenopia 1297
Asthenospermia 706
Asthma 985, 993, 1042
    acute severe 992
    atopic 985
    bronchial 984
    complications of 994
    controller drugs in 988
    exacerbation, acute 993
    management of 991
    reliever drugs in 988
    severity of 988
    signs to assess severity of 992
Astringents 1499
Astrocytoma 1420
    high-grade 1420
Astrovirus 250
Asymptomatic bacteriuria 1250, 1254, 1273
    in pregnant women 1254
Asymptomatic coronary artery disease 915
Asymptomatic cyst passers 409
Asymptomatic hyperuricemia 776
    treatment of 776
Asymptomatic microscopic hematuria 1220
Asymptomatic non-nephrotic proteinuria 1220
Ataxia 1366, 1437, 1484
    telangiectasia 1438
Ataxic dysarthria 1300
Ataxic gait 1302
Atherosclerosis 896
Atherosclerotic
    complication 885
    renovascular disease 1268
Athetosis 1400
Athletics heart 919
Atlantoaxial dislocation 1449
    types of 1450
Atlantoaxial subluxation 729

Atonic seizures 1382
Atrial fibrillation 843
Atrial flutter 868
Atrial natriuretic peptide, detect 1464
Atrial premature beats 863
Atrial septal defect 823, 947
Atrophic candidiasis, chronic 1506
Atrophic gastritis, chronic 490
Atropine 131
    toxicity 131
Attacks, acute 626
Attention deficit hyperactivity disorder 1577
Atypical pneumonia, primary 319, 320, 979
Auchmeromyia luteola 90
Auditory hallucinations 1548
Auditory nerve 1328
Auscultation 796
Austin flint murmur 851
Autistic disorder 1576
Autoimmune 1425
    diseases 32, 581, 1075
        treatment of 32
    encephalitis 1374, 1376
    encephalopathies 1370, 1375
    hemolytic anemia 1075
    hepatitis 556
    neonatal thrombocytopenia 1180
    polyglandular syndrome 32
    thyroiditis 674
Autoimmunity 581
Autoinfection 419
Autologous
    peripheral stem cell transplantation 1157
    stem cell transplantation 789, 1143
Autonomic function, tests of 1464
Autonomic nervous system
    alterations in 804
    disorders of 1460
Autonomous bladder 1465
Autosomal chromosomes 7
Autosomal disorders 16
Autosomal dominant
    inheritance 12
    polycystic kidney disease 1244
Autosomal recessive
    inheritance 12
    polycystic kidney disease 1245
Autosomes 6
Autosplenectomy 1083
Autotransfusion 1102
Aversion therapy 1585
Avian embryo vaccines 364
Avian flu 325
Avicenna 1
Axon reflex 1463
Ayurveda 1, 1586
Azathioprine 1471
Azidothymidine 57
Azithromycin 51, 235, 266, 281
Azoles 59
Azoospermia 703, 706
Azotemia 810
Aztreonam 49

B

B cell lymphoma, diffuse large 1156
B. novyi 258
B$_{12}$ deficiency, effects of 177
B$_2$-agonists 989
Babinski's reflex 1300
Bacillary angiomatosis 253
Bacillary dysentery, acute 512
Bacillus
    anthracis 240
    cereus 142
Bacitracin 55
Back leak theory 1232
Baclofen 1428
Bacteremia 236, 237, 238, 255
Bacterial endocarditis, subacute 855
Bacterial index 317
Bacterial infection 1075, 1500
    of childhood 223
    secondary 324

Textbook of Medicine

Bacterial meningitis 1364
Bacterial nephritis, acute 1243
Bacterial prostatitis
    acute 1254
    chronic 1255
Bacterial vaginosis 284
Bacteriological tests 966
Bacteriuria 1250
    significant 1250
Bacteroides 539
Baghdad boil 400
B-agonists 999
Bainbridge reflex 863
Baker's cysts 729
Balamuthia mandrillaris 410
Balanced diet 161
Balanoposthitis 1506
Balantidiasis 405, 411
Balantidium coli 411
Bald tongue 484
Ballism 1402
Ballistic movements 1400
Balloon
    atrial septostomy 947
    kyphoplasty 1143
    mitral valvotomy 843
    procedures 946
    tamponade 548, 549
Bamboo spine 764
Band forms 1048
Banded krait 96
Banding techniques 19
Bangarus caeruleus 96
Bangarus fasciatus 96
Barbara Wartenberg's sign 1328
Barbiturates 135
Barcelona clinic liver cancer 561
Bariatric surgical techniques 191
Barium
    enema 478, 512
    meal 477, 563
    swallow 477
Barlow's syndrome 846
Barometric pressure 109, 121
    alterations in 109
    increased 109
Barotrauma 109
Barr bodies 18
Barthel's index 1594
Bartonella bacilliformis 253
Bartonella henselae 253
Bartonella quintana 253
Bartonellosis 253
Bartter's syndrome 446, 459, 1249
Basal cell layer 1496
Basal ganglia
    circuits 1398
    physiology of 1391
Basedow's disease 664
Basedow's paraplegia 1493
Basement membrane 1261
Basilar invagination 1448
Basket cells 1128
Basophilic leukemia, chronic 1127
Basophils 1050
Bass player's thumb 721
Batista procedure 812
B-cell origin 1149
BCG vaccination 309
BCP crystal arthropathy 777
Beau's nails 1537
Becker muscular dystrophy 1476
Bedside peak flow meter 987
Bedside testing methods 1299
Bed-wetting 1577
Beef tapeworm 423
Bees 92
Beevor's sign 1441
Behavior theory 1568
Behavior therapy 1584
Behavioral symptoms, adjunctive therapies for 1371
Behavioral syndromes 1571
Behavioral therapy technique 1570
Behçet's disease 759
Behçet's syndrome 759, 760

Bell's palsy 1326
    prognosis of 1327
Belly tendon method 1304
Belt system 1328
Bender visual motor gestalt test 1551
Bentiromide test 566
Benzene 1090
Benzodiazepines poisioning 136
Bereitschafts potential 1289
Bernard-Soulier syndrome 1182
Berry aneurysms 1414
Beta 2-agonists, long-acting 990
    inhaled 994
Beta adrenergic blockers 914
Beta blockers, treatment with 810
Beta interferon 57
Beta thalassemia major 1086
Beta-adrenergic
    blockers 904
    blocking drugs 891
    receptor pathway, alterations in 804
Beta-blockers 668, 809, 910, 915, 1286
    benefits of 809
Betaine 555
Bethlem myopathy 1473, 1474
Bhatia's battery of intelligence scale 1551
Bicarbonate, administration of 606
Biermer's anemia 1069
Biguanides 590
    adverse effects of 591
Bile acid diarrhea 499
Bile culture 230
Bile ducts 563
    major 562
Bilharziasis 430
Biliary cirrhosis 533
    primary 533
    secondary 533
Biliary disorders 499
Biliary obstruction, acute 347
Biliary tract disease 562
Binet-Simon intelligence scale 1551
Binswanger's disease 1373
Bioactive phytochemicals in food 158
Biochemical
    abnormalities 523, 689
    changes 171, 540
    disorders 1383
    feedback 152
    investigation 1234, 1484
    tests 476, 519, 525, 679, 1217, 1464
Biofilm formation 61
Biological agents 734, 736, 788, 789
Biomarkers 926
Biomphalaria 430
Biopsy 201, 479, 1132, 1313
    role of 201
    studies 502, 968
Biosimilars 789
Biosynthesis 580
Biot's breathing 957
Bioterrorism 194
Biotin 176, 1346
    metabolism, defects of 1485
Bipyridyl herbicides 133
Birbeck granules 1497
Birth defects 1347
Bisferiens pulse 794, 851
Bites, local treatment of 364
Bithional 429
Bivalirudin 1198
BK virus 1243
Black fever 397
B-lactam antibiotics 49
B-lactamase resistant penicillin 48
Bladder
    automatic 1440, 1465
    care of 1337
Blalock-Taussig-Thomas shunt 832
Blastic transformation 1124
Blastomyces 1362
Blatchford scores 497
Bleeding 1197
    arrest of 548
    during delivery, serious 1180
    episodes 1188
        acute 1188

esophageal varices 548
    from gums 475
    into pleural cavity 1031
    tendency 1055
    time 1173
Blindness 1084
    denial of 1297
Blink reflex 1305
Blistering disorders, classification of 1523
Block vertebrae syndrome 1450
Blood
    bank procedures 1098, 1103
    chemistry 1060
    component 368
        therapy 1112
    counts 1059
    culture 230, 858
    examination 501
    film
        examination, peripheral 1106
        peripheral 1074, 1120
    findings 359
    formation 1044
    gases 958, 1484
    group
        antibodies 1097
        antigens 1046, 1096
        system 1097, 1098
    losses 1063
    pressure 1413, 1463
        control of 1461
        rapid control of 893
        recording 796
        regulation of 1266
    smear 1059
    substitutes 1102
    supply 522, 1289, 1440
    transfusion 368, 497, 1084, 1087, 1096
    urea 1217
        nitrogen 1217
    vessels 1591
        disorders of 1531
B-lymphocytes 25, 1051, 1052
Boas' sign 563
Body buffers 453
Body fluids, metabolites in 640
Body myositis, inclusion 761, 1473, 1479
Body's response to hypoglycemia 603
Bogorad's sign 1327
Bolivian hemorrhagic fevers 359
Bombay blood group 1098
Bombesin 474
Bone 236, 243, 666, 719, 750, 1592
    age 639
    changes 1139
    densitometry 726
    diseases 780
    lesions 275
    marrow 1093, 1120, 1428
        aspiration 201, 1132
        culture 230
        examination of 1056, 1059, 1140
        transplantation 1084, 1110, 1115, 1143
    resorption 77
        inhibiting agents 1143
    tuberculosis 783
Boogards angle 1446
Bornholm's disease 356
Borrelia duttoni 258
Borrelia recurrentis 94, 257
Borrelial infections 257
Bortezomib 78, 1142
Bosentan 752, 835, 1015
Boston memory scale 1551
Bosutinib 1125
Boswellia carteri 258
Botulism 142
Boutonnière or button hole 729
Bovine cough 962, 976
Bowel
    care of 1337
    disease, inflammatory 511, 1490
    enema, small 477
    infarction of 509
Bowen's disease 1544
Bowenoid papulosis 1544

Brachial
neuralgia 1457
plexitis 1457
plexus 1447
Brachytherapy 73
Bradycardiac agents 911
Bradyphrenia 1368
Brain
biopsy 1315
death 1333, 1338
imaging, role of 1475
parts of 1288
stimulation in epilepsy, deep 1390
Brainstem
auditory evoked response 1305
encephalitis 71
lesions 1328, 1332, 1410
Break bone fever 365
Breasts 638
atrophy of 712
Breath
sounds 965
tests 502
Breathing 956
capacity, maximal 961
chemical control of 956
control of 956
techniques, deep 1463
Brittle asthma 993
Brittle bone disease 782
Broad spectrum 1387
penicillins 48
Broca's aphasia 1299
Brock's syndrome 1002
Broken heart syndrome 920
Bromhexine hydrochloride 1000
Bromocriptine 650, 652
Bronchial asthma, management of 988
Bronchial obstruction 977
Bronchial thermoplasty 991
Bronchial tree, divisions of 953
Bronchiectasis 1001, 1043
sicca 1002
Bronchioloalveolitis, types of 994
Bronchitis
acute 996
chronic 997, 1004
emphysema syndrome, chronic 997
Bronchoalveolar lavage 968
Bronchoconstriction 457
Bronchodilator 999
response 1001
Bronchogenic carcinoma 1019, 1025
Bronchography 967, 1005
Bronchophony 966
Bronchopleural fistula 1031
Bronchopneumonia 980
Bronchopulmonary segments 953, 954
Bronchoscopy 968
Brown induration 1013
Brownell-Oppenheimer variant 1374
Brown-Sequard syndrome 1441
Brucella
abortus 243
canis 243
melitensis 243
suis 243
Brucellosis 239, 243, 1354
chronic 244
treatment of complicated 244
Brudzinski's leg sign 220
Brugia malayi 432
Brugia timori 432
Bruxism 475
Bubonic plague 242
Budd-Chiari syndrome 540, 558
Buffer systems 453
Bulbar palsy 1332, 1433
Bulimia nervosa 1571
Bulinus 430
Bull's angle 1449
Bulla spread sign 1524
Bullous disease of childhood, chronic 1525
Bullous emphysema 1004
Bullous impetigo 1501

Bullous pemphigoid 1524
Bumetanide 459
Bundle branch block 877
partial 877
Buprenorphine 1570
Burkholderia pseudomallei 244
Burkitt's lymphoma 1158
Burtonian line 146
Busse-Buschke's disease 380
Busulfan (myleran) 1126
Buthidae 92
Byssinosis 1008
Bythinia species 429

C

C_3 glomerulopathy 1230
Ca-199 71
Cabergoline 650, 652
Cabot's rings 1045, 1068
Cachexia 1026
Cacosmia 1316
Cadaveric position 976
Cafe coronary 976
Calciferol 169
Calcific pancreatitis 615
Calciphylaxis 1239
Calcitonin 450, 659, 677, 682, 771
gene-related peptide 660
Calcitriol 1,25-dihydroxyvitamin 450
Calcium 179
absorption 677
antagonists 911, 915
channel 861
blockers 868, 1014, 1341
blocking drugs 892
free phosphate binding resin 451
homeostasis 442
disorders of 449
oxalate arthropathy 777
receptor agonists 450
stones 1257
Calcium-channel blockers 914
Callitroga 90, 91
Caloric test 1322, 1329, 1335
Calpainopathy 1473
Calymmatobacterium granulomatis 282
Campylobacter jejuni 251
Canakinumab 775
Canals of Lambert 954
Cancer 938, 1591
prognosis in 72
screening programs 78
therapy, adjuvants in 77
Candida 1361, 1362
Candidiasis 378, 1505
Cangrelor 1185
Canities 1536
Cannabis-related disorders 1570
Cannon waves 795
Capillaria philippinensis 441
Caplan's syndrome 730
Capsule endoscope 478
Captopril 891
Caput medusae 546
Carbamazepine 1325, 1582
Carbenicillin 49, 459
Carbimazole 667
Carbohydrate 156, 586
absorption of 473
digestion of 473
intolerance 504
Carboxylase deficiency, multiple 1346, 1437
Carbuncle 214, 1501
Carcino-embryonic antigen 71
Carcinoid syndrome 510
Carcinoid tumors syndrome 510
Carcinomatous polyarthritis 786
Cardiac aneurysm 903
Cardiac arrest 878
management 878
Cardiac arrhythmias 861
Cardiac assist devices 950
Cardiac cachexia 808
Cardiac catheterization 801, 849

Cardiac cirrhosis 559
Cardiac complications 324
Cardiac cycle 791
Cardiac disease 1494
Cardiac electrophysiology, development in 862
Cardiac failure 803
complications of 807
treatment of 843
Cardiac lesions 856
Cardiac lymphomas 944
Cardiac manifestations 259, 942
Cardiac muscle 453
Cardiac output 792
Cardiac pain, control of 904
Cardiac physiology 791
Cardiac resynchronization therapy 947
Cardiac rupture 903
Cardiac surgery 948
Cardiac transplantation 812, 950
Cardiac tumors 942
malignant 944
secondary 944
Cardiac-specific troponins 901
Cardioembolic stroke, causes of 1407
Cardiogenic shock 814-816, 902
compressive 815
intrinsic 815
Cardiology 791
preventive 951
Cardiomyopathy 917, 946, 952
unclassified 917
Cardiopulmonary exercise test 961
Cardiorenal syndrome 937
Cardiospasm 486
Cardiovascular
abnormalities 638
affection 244
changes 1588, 1591
disease 122, 792, 871
drugs in pregnancy 941
lesions 629
manifestations 671, 1238, 1560
system 293, 609, 666, 681, 730, 741, 774
changes in 885
Carditis 211
Carey-Coomb's murmur 211
Carfilzomib 1142
Carney syndrome 936
Carotene, overdosage of 169
Carotenoids 168
Carotid artery stroke syndrome 1409
Carpal tunnel syndrome 671, 1458
Carphology 229
Carrion's disease 253
Carvallo's sign 853
Caspofungin 59
Cassava toxicity, acute 144
Catagen 1535
Catalepsy 1549
Cataract 610
Catastrophic antiphospholipid antibody syndrome 747
Catatonia 1291
Catatonic stupor 1334
Cathepsin 1000
Catheter-based techniques 822, 825, 827, 828, 927
Catheterization 820, 826
Cat-scratch disease 253
Cauda equina 1441
Causalgia 1454
Causative organism 288
Cave disease 379
Cavernous 965
Cefaclor 50
Cefadroxil 49
Cefamandole 50
Cefazolin 49
Cefepime 50
Cefixime 50
Cefoperazone 50
Cefotaxime 50
Cefotetan 50
Cefoxitin 50
Cefpirome 50
Cefradine 49
Cefsulodin 50

Ceftazidime 50
Ceftizoxime 50
Ceftriaxone 50, 1376
Cefuroxime 50
  axetil 50
Celiac disease 502, 1489
Cell
  based treatments 813
  carcinoma, large 1021
  counts 1055
  culture vaccines 364
  large 1156
  lung cancer
    non-small 1021
    small 1021, 1025
    subtypes, non-small 1021
  lung carcinoma, small 1021
  types of 1045
  wall polysaccharide 379
Cell-mediated immunity 26
Cellular casts 1216
Cellular immunity, deficiency of 33
Cellulitis 208, 1501
Centipedes 94
Central anticholinergic agents 1394
Central cord syndrome 1442
Central core disease 1474
Central hypoventilation syndrome, congenital 1335
Central monoamines 1557
Central nervous system 226, 244, 275, 681, 857,
  1026, 1561
  changes in 886
  gumma of 1354
  infection of 238, 1351
  lymphomas, primary 293
  manifestations 1489
    in respiratory disease 1491
    in systemic disorders 1489
  viral infections 1357
Central neurofibromatosis 1459
Central osmotic demyelination 469
Central pontine myelinolysis 445, 464, 469
Central precocious puberty 705
Central scotoma 1320
Central sleep apnea 1016
Centrifugal devices 812
Cephalexin 49
Cephalic tetanus 270
Cephaloridine 49
Cephalosporins 49
Cephalothin 49
Cerbera odollam 138
Cerberin 138
Cercariae daily 430
Cercarial dermatitis 431
Cerebellar ataxias responsive to specific therapy 1437
Cerebellar cortical degeneration, subacute 1438
Cerebellar dysfunction 671
  causes of 1438
Cerebellar hemorrhage 1416
Cerebellar homunculus 1436
Cerebellar nystagmus, classical 1324
Cerebellar tumors 1438
Cerebellopontine angle tumors 1420
Cerebellum
  diseases of 1435
  inflammatory lesions of 1438
Cerebral artery
  stroke, middle 1409
  syndrome
    anterior 1410
    posterior 1410
Cerebral form 111
Cerebral hemorrhage 1176
Cerebral malaria 388, 1356
Cerebral paraplegia 1447
Cerebral thrombosis 1407
Cerebral toxoplasmosis 293
Cerebral vasculitis 1370
Cerebral venous thrombosis 1413
  treatment of 1414
Cerebrospinal fever 220
Cerebrospinal fluid 1307, 1309
  examination 1308
Cerebrotendinous xanthamatosis 1438

Cerebrovascular accidents 122, 1481
Cerebrovascular disease 609, 1406, 1493
Certolizumab 736
Cervical
  cord compression 731
  dysfunction 706
  radiculopathy 1451
  spondylosis 779, 1343, 1451
Cervicofacial form 383
Cestodiasis 423
Chaddock's sign 1301
Chagas disease 403, 936
Chagoma 404
Chamberlain's line 1446
Chancroid 283
Chandipura virus 1361
  encephalitis 361
Charaka samhita 1
Charcoal, activated 126
Charcot's joint 785, 1354, 1446
Charles Bonnet phenomena 1298
Chelated iron 1066
Chemical carcinogens 69
Chemical pleurodesis 1034
Chemokines 26
Chemoprophylaxis 43, 62, 309, 393
Chemotherapy 74, 317, 561, 1025
  adverse effects of 938
Chenodeoxycholic acid 564
Chest
  examination of 796
  syndrome, acute 1083
  wall, diseases of 1034
Cheyne-Stokes
  breathing 957
  respiration 1335
Chiasm 1317
Chickenpox 332
Chiclero's ulcers 401
Chiggers 266
Chigoe flea 95
Chikungunya 370
  virus 1361
Childhood absence epilepsy 1380
Childhood autism 1576
Childhood epilepsy 1380
  benign 1380
Childhood hypopituitarism 654
Chilopoda 94
Chimerism 16
Chinese liver fluke 429
Chipmunk facies 1086
Chlamydia, lifecycle of 280
Chlamydial respiratory infections 319
Chloasma 1533
Chloramphenicol 52, 1089
Chloride
  resistant metabolic alkalosis 459
  responsive metabolic alkalosis 459
Chlorinated diphenyls 132
Chloroquine 408, 1010
  diphosphate 734
Chlorpropamide 645
Cholangiocarcinoma 564
Cholecystitis 563
  acute 563
  chronic 564
Cholecystokinin 471, 474
Choledochoscopy 479 563
Cholera 246
Cholestasis 346, 525
Cholesterol crystal embolism 932
Cholinergic syndrome, acute 130
Cholinergic urticaria 1526
Cholinesterase inhibitors 1470
Chondrocyte transplantation 779
Chordoma 1419
Chorea 1400
  minor 211
Choroidal artery syndrome, anterior 1410
Christmas disease 1189
Chromatin 7
Chromones 994
Chromosomal disorders 15
Chromosomal translocation 68
  syndromes 18

Chromosome 7
  components of 7
Chronic carriers, treatment of 232
Chronic liver disease, systemic complications of 544
Chronic obstructive pulmonary disease
  acute exacerbation of 1001
  infection in 997
Chronic tobacco addiction, therapy of 149
Chronic undernutrition, severe 164
Chronic valvular diseases, surgery for 949
Chrysomya 90, 91
Churg-Strauss syndrome 757, 935
Cicatricial alopecia 1535
Cidofovir 376
Cigarette smoking 952
Ciliospinal reflex 1319
Cilnidipine 892
Ciprofloxacin 54, 235
Circadian rhythm, exaggerated 199
Circle of Willis 1289
Circulating anticoagulants 1193
Circulatory failure, acute 559
Cirrhosis 346, 533, 561
  of liver 528
  patients 349
Cladribine 1129, 1131
Clarithromycin 51, 52
Claviceps purpurea 146
Cleistanthus collinus leaf 138
Climatic bubo 281
Clindamycin 53, 413
Clinico-pathological correlates, causes of 1236
Cloaca 1207
Clobazam 1388
Clofazimine 318
Clonal origin of neoplasms 69
Clonic phase 1382
Clonidine 890, 1464, 1570
Clonorchiasis 429
Clonorchis sinensis 429
Clonus 1291
Clopidogrel 1185
Clostridia, diseases caused by 269
Clostridial myonecrosis 272
Clostridium
  botulinum 142
  difficile 252
  perfringens 142, 143
  tetani 269
Clot retraction 1173
Clotrimazole 58
Clotting cascade 1171
Clotting time 1173
Cloxacillin 48
Clozapine 1395
Clunking sound 729
Clutton's joints 276
Cnidae 95
Coagulase negative staphylococci 214
Coagulation after warfarin 1197
Coagulation defects 1175
Coagulation disorders 1191
  rare 1193
Coagulation vitamin 173
Coal worker's pneumoconiosis 1007
Coarctation of aorta 820, 947
Coarse hair 1539
Coat hanger phenomena 1462
Cobra 96, 97
  bite 98
Coccidioides 1362
Cochlear system 1328
Cochliomyia 91
Cockroft-Gault formula 1588
Cod fish vertebra 770
Codox-M 1159
Coenurus cerebralis 441
Cogan's twitch sign 1467
Cognition, disturbance of 1546, 1547
Cognitive behavior therapy 1585
Cognitive disturbances 1555
Cognitive enhancers 1553, 1583
Cognitive functions 1296, 1583
Cognitive impairment, mild 1372
Cognitive rehabilitation 1481

Textbook of Medicine

Cognitive theory 1558
Cognitive therapy 1585
Coin shadow 1023
Coital headache 1342
Colchicine 775
Cold
    agglutinin-positive pneumonia 979
    agglutinins diseases 1075
    areas 801
    injuries to 107
    sore 336, 1503
    urticaria 1526
Colistin 55
Collagen
    diseases 1027
    disorders 1075
    fiber 1538
        disorders of 1537
    major disorders of 629
Collapsing pulse 794
Collaterals, demonstration of 547
Collet-Sicard syndrome 1331
Colon 472
    cancer, genetics of 516
    carcinoma of 512
    diseases of 511
Colonic mucosa 472
Colonic stricture 512
Colonoscopy 478, 512
Color anomia 1298
Color vision 1318
Column disease, lateral 1442
Coma 388, 1333, 1334, 1336
    causes of 1334
    diagnosis of 1336
    grading of 540
Comatose patient 1334
    management of 1337
Combination therapy 399, 1130
Communication system 89
Community acquired pneumonia 320
Community water, fluoridation of 483
Community-acquired pneumonia, causes of 978
Compensatory emphysema 1003
Complement system, deficiency of 34
Complete heart block 876, 877
Complete left bundle branch block 877
Complete right bundle branch block 877
Complete transverse section 1441
Complex partial seizure 1380, 1381
Complex tremor 1405
COMT inhibitors 1394
Conation, disturbance of 1547, 1549
Conchotome biopsy 1312
Condyloma acuminata 286
Condylomata acuminata 1502
Cone shells 95
Congenital aregenerative anemia, chronic 1092
Congenital heart disease, burden of 817
Congenital myasthenia syndromes, treatment of 1471
Congenital syphilis, diagnosis of 277
Congestive heart failure, chronic 559
Congo maggot fly 90
Conidae 95
Conjunctival reflex 1325
Conn's syndrome 459, 936
Connective tissue disease 747, 752
    mixed 752, 1263
Connective tissue disorders 724
Consciousness 1295
    alteration of 537
    disturbance of 1546, 1549
    levels of 1333
Consecutive optic atrophy 1320
Constipation 476, 1595
    predominant 506
Constitutional symptoms 508
Constructional apraxia 537
Consumer Protection Act 3
Contact dermatitis 1521
Contact urticaria 1527
Continend by rhazes 1
Contractile apparatus, changes in 805
Convalescence 225, 372
Conversion disorders 1563

Convulsions, control of 272
Convulsive status 1389
Cooley's anemia 1086
Coomb's test 1074, 1098
Cope's needle 968
Copper 185, 1348
    accumulation of 527
Coprinus species 144
Coral snake 96
Cord blood 1112
    banking 1102
    transfusion 1102
    transplantation 1088
    uses of 1102
Cordylobia anthropophaga 90
Core system 1328
Corkscrew esophagus 488
Corneal reflex 1325
Corneomandibular reflex 1301, 1325
Coronary
    angiography 802, 913, 915
    heart disease 951
    revascularization 906
    stents 945
Coronary artery
    bypass
        graft 900, 907, 914
        surgery 949
    disease, prevention of 915
Coronavirus 250
Corpus callosum 1298
Corrigan's pulse 794
Corrosive acids 138
Cortical arousal 1463
Cortical blindness 1367
Cortical dementia, mixed 1372
Corticobasal degeneration 1373, 1396
Corticosteroid 327, 687, 734, 745, 1110
    therapy, adverse side effects of 65
    withdrawal 66
Corticotropin group 646
Corticotropin-releasing hormone 642
Corynebacterium diphtheriae 223
Coryza 323
Cosmetic effects 710
Co-stimulation blockers 736
Co-trimoxazole 52
Cough
    fracture 962
    reflex 955
    syncope 962
    variant asthma 993
    with expectoration 962
    without expectoration 962
Councilman bodies 342
Cover test 1323
Cowpox 1503
    virus 1503
COX-2 inhibitors 734
Coxa vara 171
Coxiella burnetii 94, 267
Coxsackieviruses infections 355
CPP crystal deposition disease 776
Crab louse 1509
Crab yaws 256
Crackles 965
Cramps 1453
Cranial arteritis 754
Cranial diabetes insipidus 643
Cranial form 355
Cranial nerve 1316, 1330
    eighth 1328
    palsy 1495
    signs 1367
Craniopharyngioma 1419, 1421
Craniotabes 171
Craniovertebral anomalies 1448
    management of 1450
C-reactive protein 722, 897
    high level of 952
Creatine kinase 901
Creatinine clearance 1217
Creatorrhea 500
Crepitations 965
Crest syndrome 748

Cretinism 670
Creutzfeldt-Jakob disease 1373, 1374
Crigler-Najjar syndrome 524
Crimean-congo hemorrhagic fever 360
Crohn's disease 506
    acute exacerbation of 507
Cross reacting antibodies 31
Crotalaria 145, 558
Crotalidae 96
Croup 975
Crunching sounds 966
Crusted scabies 1508
Cryoglobulinemia
    essential mixed 344
    mixed 758, 1264
Cryoglobulinemic vasculitis 758
Cryoprecipitate 1100, 1188
    infusions 1191
Cryptococcal meningitis 293
Cryptococcosis 380
Cryptococcus 1362
    neoformans 1362
Cryptogenic 1380, 1381
    polycythemia 1163
    stroke 1410
Cryptorchidism 703
Cryptorchism 703
Cryptosporidiosis 294, 405, 413
Cryptosporidium parvum 413
Ctenopharyngodon idellus 144
Cubam receptor 1068
Culex tritaeniorhynchus 372
Culicoides 439, 440
Cultural bond syndromes 1563, 1565
Culture negative-neutrocytic ascites 532
Cupids bow sign 1473
Cupping 171
Curb-65 rule 981
Cushing's disease 652, 688, 689
Cushing's syndrome 459, 688, 786, 936
Cushing's vasomotor phenomena 1419
Cutaneous
    amebiasis 407
    anthrax 240
    candidiasis 1506
    diphtheria 224
    drug reactions 1528
    embolism 857
    forms, management of 626
    horn 1544
    larva migrans 422
    leishmaniasis 400
        diffuse 401
    leukoclastic vasculitis 344
    manifestations 291, 749
        of systemic disorders 1539
Cutis laxa 1538
Cyanide
    poisoning 134
    routes of entry of 134
Cyanocobalamin 177, 1347
Cyanosis 793, 964
Cyanotic CHD, management for 836
Cyanotic congenital heart disease 818, 830
Cyanotic heart disease, congenital 836
Cyclical neutropenia 1049
Cylindroma 1543
Cymevene 57
Cyproheptadine 652
Cystathionine beta-synthase deficiency 630
Cystatin 1234
    C 1217
Cystic disease
    congenital 1244
    of kidneys 1244
    of ovary 709
Cystic disorder 1246
Cysticercosis 424, 425, 1355
    eradication of 426
Cysticercus cellulosae 424
Cystine stones 1257, 1258
Cystitis 1250
    in women, acute uncomplicated 1251

Cystourethrography 1219
Cysts 1040
    congenital 1026
    of kidney 1246
Cytisine 152
Cytokines 1052
    role of 804
Cytomegalovirus 374, 1075, 1359, 1377
    infection 376
        reactivation of 293
Cytotoxic hypersensitivity, type II 30
Cytotoxic test 37

D

Da Costa's syndrome 934
Dabigatran 1198
Daclizumab high-yield process 1428
Danazol 1527
Dancing gait 1401
Dandy fever 365
Dandy-Walker malformation 1450
Dapsone 317
    syndrome 318
Daptomycin 53
Darbepoetin-α 1047
Darling's disease 379
Dasatinib 77, 1125
Dawn phenomenon 608
De Motu Cordis 2
De Quervain's thyroiditis 673
Dead hand 120
Death adder 96
Decadron 1142
Decerebrate posture 1336
Decorticate posture 1336
Decubitus ulcers 1413
Deferiprone 1088
Deficiency
    pathology of 174
    states 174
Degenerative joint disease 777
Dehydration, correction of 606
Deliberate self-harm 1577
Delirium 1552, 1596
    tremens 137, 1350
Delivery, timing of 600
Delta sign, empty 1414
Delusion 1547
    primary 1548
Delusional disorders 1554
Demeclocycline 468
Dementia 1377, 1553
    cortical 1368
    drug in 1553
    praecox 1554
    reversible 1369
    subcortical 1368
    with lewy bodies 1373
Demodarans gait 1303
Demyelinating lesions 1425
Dengue 1361
    attacks of 366
    classification 366
    fever 936
    first attack of 366
    shock syndrome 367
Denosumab 682, 772, 789
Dense deposit disease 1230
Dental
    caries 482
    fluorosis 147
    procedures 860
Denture stomatitis 1506
Deoxyribonucleic acid, antidouble standard 1262
Dependence syndrome 1569
Depression 934, 1413, 1557, 1558
    major 1558
Depressive mutism 1559
Depressive stupor 1559
Deprivation dwarfism 656
Depth electrodes recording 1303
Derealization 1548
Dermacentor 94
    marginatus 361
    reticulatus 361

Dermal vasculature, expansion of 1512
Dermatitis
    atopic 1518
    herpetiformis 502, 1524
    management of contact 1522
Dermatobia hominis 90
Dermatome 1439
Dermatomyositis 760, 761, 1479
Dermatophytosis 1504
Dermis 1497
Dermoepidermal junction 1497
Dermographism 1526
Desferrioxamine 1087
Desmopressin 645, 1188
Detemir 595
Detoxification 1570
Detrusor-external sphincter dyssynergia 1465
Developmental anomalies 1438
Devic's disease 1428
Dexamethasone
    high dose 1178
    suppression test 688
Dexrazone 77
Dextrocardia 836, 837
Dextro-transposition of great arteries 833
Dextroversion 836
Dhat syndrome 1565
Di Guglielmo's syndrome 1118
Diabetes 601, 602, 1260
    during pregnancy 599
    in asymptomatic adult, testing for 580
    insipidus 643
    mellitus 577, 604, 784, 935, 1018, 1539
        and pregnancy 1270
        complications of 601, 609
        type 1 577, 599
        type 2 577, 578, 599
        types of 578
    monitoring control of 588
    patients, estimated number of 578
Diabetic cheiroarthropathy 784
Diabetic coma, management of 606
Diabetic complications, pathogenesis of 609
Diabetic dermopathy 1540
Diabetic dyslipidemia 935
Diabetic foot 613
Diabetic ketoacidosis 604, 605
Diabetic lactic acidosis 608
Diabetic nephropathy 611, 1260
Diabetic neuropathy 1456
    classification of 612
Diabetic patient, education of 586
Diabetic retinopathy 609
    classification of 610
    treatment of 610
Diabetic ulcers 1540
Diabetic, acute problems in 608
Diabetology, future prospects in 614
Dialysis 126, 1276
    adequacy 1279
    dementia 1493
    disequilibrium syndrome 1238, 1492
    in acute kidney injury 1278
    monitor 1277
Diamond on quadriceps sign 1474
Diamond-Blackfan anemia 1092
Diaper dermatitis 1506
Diaphragmatic dysfunction, causes of 1037
Diaphragmatic flutter 1039
Diaphragmatic hernia 1037
Diaphragmatic paralysis 1036
    causes of 1037
Diaphragmatic tic 1039
Diarrhea 476
    antibiotic associated 252
    predominant 506
Diarrheal disease 357
    of children, acute 250
    of infective origin 245
Diastolic heart
    dysfunction 805
    failure 805
Diazepam 1428
Diazoxide 891
Dicobalt-acetate 144

Diet 69
    and environmental factors 44
Dietary advice 1259
Dietary iron, metabolism of 181
Dietary management 502, 586
Dietary modification 951
Dietary sources 178
Dietetic management 249
Diethylcarbamazine 437
Diffusion 465, 1277
Difluoromethylornithine 403
Digastric line 1446
DiGeorge syndrome 33, 939
Digestive organs 470
Digestive symptoms 1462
Digestive system, radiological examination of 477
Digital subtraction angiography 86, 802
Digitalis purpurea 810
Digitorum brevis, extensor 1473
Digitoxicity, treatment of 811
Digoxin 810, 811
Dihydroartemisinin 392
Dilated cardiomyopathy 917
Diloxanidefuroate 408
Diltiazem 892
Diminished hematopoiesis 1095
Dipeptidyl peptidase-4 inhibitors 591
Dipetalonema
    perstans 432
    streptocerca 432
Diphtheria 223, 936
    antitoxin 224
Diphyllobothriasis latum 427
Diphyllobothrium latum 427
Diplococcus pneumoniae 216
Diploid cells 6
Diplopia 1323
    crossed 1322
Dipylidium caninum 428
Direct immunofluorescent antibody 363
Direct thrombin inhibitors 1198
Direct toxicity 1284
Directly acting antivirals 350
Directly observed treatment 306
Disaccharidase deficiency 504
Discoid eczema 1520
Discoid lupus 740
Disease modifying therapy 1427
Disease modifying treatments 1435
Disease states 1592
Disease-modifying antirheumatic drugs 734
Disequilibrium syndrome 1279
Disinfection 1101
Disorders, autonomic 1461
Dispermic chimeras 16
Dissecting aneurysms of aorta 931
Disseminated encephalomyelitis, acute 1425, 1443
Disseminated gonococcal infection 279, 280
Disseminated intravascular coagulation 1200
Disseminated morphea 748
Dissocial personality disorders 1567
Dissociated anesthesia 1446
Dissociative disorders 1563, 1564
Dissociative identity disorder 1564
Disturbances, autonomic 614, 1462
Diuretic 531, 810, 813, 889, 1286
    intractable ascites 531
    resistant ascites 531
    therapy 446, 810
    urogram 1219
Diverticulitis 514
Dizziness 1595
DNA polymorphism 19
Dobutamine 816
Dog tapeworm 426
Doll's eye movements 1335
Domiciliary treatment 305
Donepezil 1371, 1395
Donor feces infusion 252
Donor marrow, infusion of 1111
Donor selection 1282
Donovania granulomatis 282
Donovanosis 282
Dopa-agonist responsive dystonia 1399
Dopamine 816
    agonists 539, 652, 1394

Textbook of Medicine

Dopa-responsive dystonia 1399
Dornase alpha 1000
Dowager's hump 770
Down's syndrome 16, 939, 1575
Doxazosin 890
Doxycycline 51, 266, 410
Dracontiasis 440
Dragon worm 440
Dressler's syndrome 903
Dropped fingers 729
Drowning 113
Drowsiness 1333
Drug 188, 485, 554, 702, 709, 733, 766, 770,
    775, 910, 1142, 1438, 1512, 1559
    acting against filarial parasite 437
    administration 40, 43
        during pregnancy 44
        in elderly 43
        in special groups 43
        routes of 40
    alternative 66
    and dialysis 1286
    and kidney 1284
    and toxins 461
    availability 1568
    combinations 868, 889
    distribution 42
    dosage of 1402
    elimination of 42
    emergency 893
    eruption, fixed 1530
    first-generation 905
    in renal failure, dosage of 1286
    interaction 46
        prevention of 46
    L-interactions ataxia behavioral 1387
    metabolism 538
    prophylaxis 1341
    related adverse effects 44
    related problem 45
    reserve 306
    resistance 238, 306
        of microbes 59
        primary 306
    therapy 440, 492, 498, 652, 667, 903, 1088,
        1272, 1327, 1403, 1561, 1580
        in elderly 1595
    to improve memory 1583
    toxicity on liver 557
Drug-drug interactions 44
Drug-resistant
    epilepsy, surgery for 1390
    tuberculosis, extensively 307
Dry beriberi 174
Dry drowning 113
Dual personality 1564
Duchenne muscular dystrophy 933, 1476
Duct occluder device 828
Duction movements 1323
Duke's criteria for diagnosis 857
Dulaglutide 597
Duodenal aspirate, cytology of 566
Duodenal biliary drainage 563
Duodenal ulcer 491
Dupilumab 994
Duplex ultrasound 82
Dupuytren's contracture 614
Dura producing, side of 1334
Duration of fever 196
Dwarf tapeworm 427
Dwarfism 647, 655
Dyken criteria for diagnosis 1360
Dynamic cardiomyoplasty 812
Dysbarism 109
Dysesthesias 1302, 1453
Dysfunction, autonomic 1592
Dyskinesias 1405
Dyslipidemia, treatment of 1241
Dysmyelination 1425
Dyspepsia 1595
Dysphagia 475, 485
    causes of 485
    lusoria 485
Dyspnea 792, 963
Dysprosody 1299

Dysreflexia, autonomic 1291
Dysthymia 1557
Dysthymic disorders 1559
Dystonia 1399
    management of 1400
    primary 1399
    with myoclonus 1399
Dystonia-plus syndromes 1399
Dystonic tremors 1404
Dystrophia
    adiposo genitalis 655
    myotonica 1478
Dystrophinopathies 1478
Dystrophy 1472
Dysuria 1212

E

Ear
    infections 238
    middle 120
Eardrum 120
Eating disorders 1571
Eaton agent pneumonia 979
Ebola vaccine 360
Ebola virus
    disease 360
    infections 359
Ebstein anomaly 836
EBV infection, chronic active 375
Ecallantide 1527
Eccrine glands 1498
Echinocandins 59
Echinococcosis 426
Echinococcus granulosus 426
Echinococcus multilocularis 426
Echo Doppler 947
Echocardiography, uses of 800
Echoing 1299
Echolalia 1549
Echopraxia 1549
Echoviruses 355
E-cigarette 152
Eclampsia 1271, 1495
Econazole 58
Ecthyma 214, 1501
Ectopic ACTH secretion 690
Ectopic adrenocorticotropic hormone 71
Ectopic beats 863
Ectopic Cushing's syndrome 713
Ectopic parathyroid hormone 71
Eculizumab 1096
Eczema 1517
    herpeticum 336, 1503
    management of 1518
Edema 792, 793, 1212, 1237
Edmonston B strains of measles virus 330
Edmonston-Zagreb strains 330
Edward's syndrome 17
Efalizumab 1515
Effusion
    complicated 1029
    uncomplicated 1029
Eflornithine 403
Ehlers-Danlos syndrome 629, 1538
Ehrlichia 267
    chaffeensis 267
    ewingii 267
Ehrlichiosis 267
Eight-and-a-half syndrome 1328
Eisenmenger syndrome 828, 835
Elapidae 96
Elastin fiber, disorders of 1537
Elastin fibers 1538
Elastography 82
Electric shock-like sensation 1451
Electrical injuries 116
Electroconvulsive therapy 1557, 1579
Electrocorticography 1303
Electrodiagnostic tests 1469
Electroencephalogram 537, 1303
Electroencephalography 1338
Electrolyte abnormality 938
Electrolyte balance, abnormalities of 442
Electrolyte depletion 810
Electrolyte disturbances 606

Electrolyte imbalance 539
Electromyography 1304
Electron microscopy 1229, 1475
Electrophoretic study 1141
Electrophysiology study 947
Elephantiasis
    treatment of 438
    verrucosa nostra 1532
Eleventh cranial nerve 1331
Elicit memory 1551
Elicit plantar response 1300
ELISA test, capture 371
Ellsworth-Howard test 678
Elsberg pattern 1441
Eltrombopag 1055, 1179
Embolic episodes 856
Embolic phenomenon 857, 942
Embolic stroke 1407
Embolism 1592
Embryo
    damage to 116
    during renal development 1207
Embryology 685
Emergency management 125, 497, 991
Emery-Dreifuss
    muscular dystrophy 934, 1478
    myopathy 1473, 1474
Emollients 1499
Emotional disorders 1576
Emotions 1461
Emphysema 457, 996, 1003, 1004
    atrophic 1004
Emphysematous cystitis 1255
Empirical therapy 859
Empyema 209, 1029, 1031
    necessitans 1031
    of gallbladder 563
Enalapril 891
Enanthems 328
Encephalitic stage, acute 372
Encephalitis 333, 1373
    acute 1360
Encephalomyelitis 329
    ventriculitis 333
Encephalomyelopathy 337
Encephalopathy
    acute 1483
    chronic 1483
Endemic fluorosis 147
    prevention of 149
Endemic gastroenteritis 250
Endemic goiter 663
Endemic typhus 265
Endocardial involvement 294
Endocarditis 221, 238, 267, 1494
    infective 855, 856
    prophylaxis 860
Endocrine 1267, 1558
    abnormalities 770
    causes 709, 1370
    cells 471
    diseases 784
    disorders 636, 786, 935, 1493
        of breast 711
    disturbances 537
    dwarfism 636
    function 566
        of gut 473
    myopathy 1479
    neoplasia, multiple 715
    organ 1211
    syndromes 713, 714
    system 1592
Endocrine-related conditions 711
Endocrinology 631
Endogenous
    benzodiazepines 536
    eczema 1518
    lipids 620
Endorphins 474
Endoscopic interventions 548, 549
Endoscopic management 528
    elective 498
Endoscopic retrograde
cholangiopancreatography 479, 526, 563, 566

Index

Textbook of Medicine

Endoscopic sclerotherapy 549
Endoscopy 408
Endothelin
  receptor antagonists 1015
  role of 804
Endotheliomas 1420
Endovascular intervention 1412
Endrin 132
End-stage of Alzheimer's disease 1375
Energy deficient conditions 618
Enkephalins 474
Entacapone, dose of 1394
Entamoeba histolytica 405, 406, 409
Entecavir 57, 348
Enteral feeding 163
Enteric cytopathogenic human orphan viruses 355
Enteroaggregative *Escherichia coli* 236
Enterobacteriaceae group 237
Enterobiasis 420, 477
Enterococci 209
Enterocolitis 233
Enteroglucagon 474
Enteroinsular axis 473
Enterokinase 473
Enteropathic arthritis 766
Enteropathy 718
Enterovirus 352, 355, 1359
  caused diseases 356
  treatment of 357
  type 70 355
Entrapment neuropathy 730, 1456, 1458
Entry inhibitors 295
Enuresis 1577
Enzyme 76, 97
  determination 525
  levels in
    blood 565
    urine 565
  studies 1487
Enzyme-linked
  immunosorbent assay test 32, 231
  immunospot 303
Eosinophilia 1050
  causes of 1050
Eosinophilic
  esophagitis 486
  fasciitis 751
  gastritis 490
  gastroenteritis 1050
  granulomatosis with polyangiitis 757, 1263
  leukemia 1126
  myocarditis 1050
Eosinophils 1049
Epalrestat 785
Ependymomas 1420
Epidemic dropsy 145
Epidemic gastroenteritis 250
Epidemic keratoconjunctivitis 357
Epidemic myalgia 356
Epidemic spastic paraplegia 146
Epidemic typhus 263
Epidermal proliferation 1512
Epidermis 1496
Epidermoid carcinoma 1020
Epigenetics 11
Epilepsy 122, 1379, 1381
  and pregnancy 1383
  management of 1386
    women with 1384
  primary 1380
  sudden death in 1386
  syndrome 1381
    classification of 1380
  with myoclonic 1381
    absences 1381
Epileptic myoclonus 1403
Epileptic seizures, classification of 1380
Epileptic syndrome 1382
  classification of 1380
Episodic apnea 1468
Epistasis 13, 973
  causes of 973
Epitopes 31
Eplerenone 810, 909

Epoprostenol 751
Epratuzumab 1117
Epstein-Barr virus 339, 374, 1359
Eptifibatide 913
Epworth sleepiness scale 1017, 1018
Eratyrus 404
Erectile disorder 1573
Ergonovine test 915
Ergotamine 146, 1340
Ergotism 146
Eruptive xanthomas 1540
Erysipelas 208, 1501
Erythema annulare centrifugum 1541
Erythema gyratum repens 1541
Erythema multiforme 1528
Erythema nodosum 1009, 1542
  causes of 1542
  leprosum 317
Erythematous 1506
Erythremia 1163
Erythrocyte 1044
  count 723
  preparations 1099
  production, defective 1089
  sedimentation rate 722
Erythroderma 1517
Erythrodermic psoriasis 1514
Erythrogenesis imperfecta 1092
Erythrohepatic porphyria 626
Erythroleukemia 1118
Erythromycin 51, 281
Erythroplakia 483
Erythroplasia of Queyrat 1544
Erythropoietic porphyria, congenital 626
Erythropoietin 714, 1046
Escherichia coli 234, 236, 1075
  enterohemorrhagic 236
  enteropathogenic 236
  infections 236
Esmolol 905
Esophageal
  candidiasis 294
  disease, symptoms in 484
  dysphagia 485
  hiatus hernia 488
  pain 484
  spasm, diffuse 488
Esophagitis 486
Esophago-gastroscopy 526
Esophagus 470
  carcinoma of 489
  diseases of 484
Established neuroleukemia, treatment of 1117
Esthiomene 282
Etanercept 736, 766, 1515
Ethacrynic acid 459
Ethanol 135, 460
Ethical committees 3
Ethylene
  dibromide poisoning 132
  glycol 460
Euglobulin lysis time 1174, 1193
Eunuchoid 629
European blastomycosis 380
European Burkitt's lymphoma 1159
Euthyroid Graves' disease 665, 666
Euthyroid sick syndrome 674
Euvolemic hyponatremia 444, 468
Evan's syndrome 1078
Everolimus 510
Evoked responses 1305
Exacerbating factors 1518
Exacerbations
  severity of 999
  treatment of 1427
Exanthems 328
Excessive fibrinolysis, causes of 1193
Exemestane 78
Exenatide 597
  lar 597
Exercise, benefits of 587
Exfoliative dermatitis 1517
Exfoliative drug eruption 1529
Exhibitionism 1573
Exocrine function, tests for 566

Exogenous eczema 1521
Exophthalmos 669
  malignant 669
Expiratory reserve volume 960
Extra-articular
  features 765
  lesions 728
  manifestations 730
Extra-axial tumors 1420
Extracampine hallucination 1548
Extracellular fluid 442
Extracorporeal liver support 542
Extracorporeal membrane oxygenator 812
Extradural hematomas 1422
Extrahepatic manifestations 344, 346
Extrahepatic portal hypertension 550
Extraintestinal amebiasis 406
Extraintestinal infection 236
Extra-intestinal lesions 406
Extraintestinal manifestations 513
Extrapulmonary complications 983
Extrapyramidal disorders 1398
Extrapyramidal dysfunction 1377
Extrapyramidal movement disorders 1484
Extrapyramidal signs 1366
Extrathoracic manifestations 1023
Extreme pica 1064
Extrinsic allergic alveolitis 994
Exudate pleural effusions 1030
Exudative effusion 1030
Eye 730
  movement 1335
    abnormal 1367
    control 1321
  signs 1462, 1556
Eyelids, movement of 1335
Ezogabine 1388

F

Fabry's disease 938
Facial colliculus 1326
Facial nerve 1326
Facial pains 1339
Facial palsy
  bilateral 1328
  chronic 1328
Facioscapulohumeral dystrophy 1473
  muscular 934, 1478
Factitious disorder 1565
Factitious fever 198
Faint 793
Falciparum malaria 347
  treatment of 392
Fallacies of tests 295
Fallopian tubular dysfunction 706
False localizing sign 1419, 1440
Famciclovir 336
Familial colonic polyposis 509
Familial macrophage activation syndrome 737
Familial spastic paraparesis 1430
Fanconi's anemia 1091
Fanconi's syndrome 451
Fannia 90, 91
Fasciculation 1368, 1432, 1453
Fascioliasis 428
Fat 156
  absorption of 472
  digestion of 472
  functions of 156
Fatal insomnia 1376
Fatigue 636, 1435
Fatigue syndrome, chronic 1463
Fat-soluble vitamins 167
Fatty acid
  diarrhea 499
  oxidation, defects of 1479, 1485
Fatty casts 1216
Fatty liver 552
  of pregnancy, acute 1274
Febrile convulsions 1381, 1383
Febrile encephalopathy, nonspecific 1359
Febrile respiratory illness, acute 357
Fecal fat estimation 501
Fecal immunochemical testing 476

Fecal protein loss 501
Feces 565
    culture 230
    examination of 407, 476, 500, 525
Feigned insanity 1565
Felbamate 1388
Felodipine 892
Felty's syndrome 738
Female infertility 706
Female orgasmic disorder 1573
Female pseudohermaphroditism 707
Female purpura over legs 1177
Fenofibrate 776
Ferri reductase enzyme 181
Ferric carboxymaltose 1067
Ferric gluconate 1066
Ferroportin 181, 182
Festinating gait 1303
Fetal alcohol syndrome 1350
Fetal hemoglobin 1088
Fetal life, irradiation in 116
Fetal monitoring techniques 600
Fetishism 1573
Fetor hepaticus 537
Fever 194, 939, 1055, 1413
    blister 336
    in immunocompromised host 35
    of unknown origin 197
    patterns of 196
    undifferentiated 367
    with joint pain 230
Fiber electromyography, single 1305, 1469
Fibrin degradation products, estimation of 1174
Fibrinogen levels, increase in 952
Fibrinolytic system 1172
Fibrocalcific pancreatic diabetes 615
Fibrocalculous pancreatic disease 615
Fibromas 943
Fibromyalgia 763
Fibrothorax 1029
Fibrous pial 1288
Fibrous thyroiditis 674
Fifth cranial nerve 1324
Fighter aircrafts 122
Filarial infections 439
Filariasis 413, 432
    control of 438
    prevention of 438
Filovirus infections 358
Fine-needle aspiration biopsy 661
Finger clubbing 537
Fingolimod 1428
Fire ants 92
First aid 114
    prevention and 131
Fish poisoning 144
Fish tapeworm 427
Fishgold's line 1446
Fissured tongue 484
Flaccid dysarthria 1300
Flail chest 1036
Flapping tremor 537
Flash pulmonary edema 1268
Flea typhus 265
Flexibilitas cerea 1549
Flexural psoriasis 1513
Floppy valve syndrome 846
Flow cytometry 1133
Flucytosine 58, 59
Fludarabine 1129
Fluent aphasia, progressive 1372
Fluid
    transudation, evidence of 841
    treatment of 1240
Fluke infections 428
Flumazenil 539
Fluorescein angiography 610
Fluorescence
    antibody, indirect 398
    in situ hybridization 19, 1107
Fluorine 184
Focal fibrosis 1010, 1011
Focal segmental glomerulosclerosis 1227
Focal signs 1415
Foix-Alajouanine syndrome 1444

Folate deficiency, causes of 178
Folic acid 177, 1346
    deficiency anemia 1071
Follicular impetigo of Bockhart 215
Folliculitis 1501
    decalvans 1536
Fomepizole 135
Fondaparinux 1195, 1196
Food poisoning 142
    chronic 143
    infection type of 143
    type of 142
Food, function of 156, 158
Foot disease 356
Forced acid diuresis 126
Forced alkaline diuresis 126
Forced diuresis 126
Forced expiratory
    flow 961
    time 960
Formal cognitive assessment 1366
Formic acid 139
Forrest classification 497
Forward heart failure 805
Foscarnet 57, 376
Fossa ovalis 823
Foster Kennedy syndrome 1316
Fothergill's disease 1325
Foville's syndrome 1328
Fractional excretion of sodium 1233
Fragile X-associated tremor ataxia 1405
Fragilitas ossium 782
Fragmentation hemolysis 1199
Frailty syndrome 1589
Fraying 171
Freckles 1533
Fredrickson's classification 621
Free living cycle 419
Free radicals and apoptosis, role of 805
Freezing cold injury 107
Frequent respiratory infections 171
Fresh blood in stools 498
Fresh frozen plasma 1100, 1188
Frey's sign 1327
Friedlander's pneumonia 979
Friedreich's ataxia 934, 1436
Fröhlich's syndrome 655
Frontal lobe
    epilepsies 1380
    hemorrhage 1416
Frontotemporal lobar degeneration 1372
    complex 1434
Frozen shoulder 763
Fructosuria 617
Fulminant hepatic failure 540
Fulminant hepatitis 346
Fulminant meningococcemia 221
Fulvestrant 78
Functional residual capacity 960
Fundamental symptoms 1556
Fundus examination 1320
Fungal infections 292, 382, 1361
    superficial 1504
Furosemide 459
Furuncle 214, 1501
Fusidic acid 53
Fusiform bacilli 483
Fusion toxins 74

G

G6PD deficiency, hemolysis in 1080
Gabapentin 1325, 1388, 1428
Gadolinium diethylenetriaminepentaacetic acid 89
Gag reflex 956
Gait cycle 1302
Galactomannan 379
Galactorrhea 637, 712
Galactosemia 617
Galantamine 1371
Gallbladder 563
    carcinoma of 564
    diseases of 562
Gallium nitrate 450
Gallop 797
    rhythm 797

Gallstone disease 347
Gamma glutamyl transpeptidase 525
Gamma interferon 57
Gamma irradiation of blood 1102
Ganciclovir 56, 57, 376
Gander cough 962
Gangrenous cholecystitis, acute 564
Gaol fever 263
Garcin syndrome 1332
Gardnerella vaginalis 284
Gas exchange 958
    in alveoli 958
Gas gangrene 268, 272
Gas mixing within alveoli 961
Gas transfer across alveolar membrane 961
Gas transport down the airways 959
Gasserian ganglion 1324
Gastric
    acid analysis 477
    drainage, continuous 446
    inhibitory polypeptide 471, 474
    juice 471
    lavage 125
    lesions 1060
    outlet obstruction 496
    surgery 1490
Gastrin 471, 474, 1589
Gastrinomas 715
Gastritis 489
    acute 137, 490
    chronic 490
        superficial 490
Gastroenteritis 229, 255
Gastroesophageal reflux disease 488, 993
Gastrointestinal
    anthrax 240
    bleed, upper 1413
    complications 734
    disease 1489
    endoscopy 478
    hormones 473
    infections 238
    manifestations 1238
    motor function 1588
    symptoms 1560
    system 681, 1461
    tract procedures 860
Gatifloxacin 54
Gaze paralysis 1324
Geftinib 77
Gemcitabine 564
Gene 7, 8
    expression profiling 1107
    mapping 19
    therapy 21, 813, 1084, 1088, 1189
        limitations of 22
General paralysis of insane 1353
Genetic
    aspects of cancer 68
    causes, classification of 1430
    changes 1476
    constitution 1475
    counseling 21, 952
    disorders 18, 1267
    effect 31
    epidemiology 22
    factors 188, 495, 727, 739, 764, 1431, 1557
    newer developments in 19
    role of 1475
    syndromes 939
    testing 919
Geniculate bodies 1317
    lateral 1318
Geniospasm 1404
Genital
    atrophic changes in 710
    warts 286, 1502
Genitalia, external 639
Genitourinary
    infection 221
    schistosomiasis 431
    symptoms 1462, 1560
    system 244
    tract procedures 860
    tuberculosis 1255

Textbook of Medicine

Genomics, role of 582
Gentamicin 50
Geographical tongue 484
Geriatric 1586
  assessment
    comprehensive 1594
    multidimensional 1593
  diseases 1590
  giants 1593
  health services, development of 1596
  medicine 1586
  symptoms 1595
    management 1595
German measles 336
Gerstmann-Straussler-Scheinker
    syndrome 1373, 1376
Gestational diabetes mellitus 1270
Gestational hypertension 1271
GH estimation 652
GH receptor antagonist 652
Ghrelin 188, 1589
Giant cell 755
  arteritis 754, 935
  thyroiditis 673
Giant platelet syndromes 1182
Giardia intestinalis 410
Giardia lamblia 410
Giardiasis 405, 410
Gigantism 650
Girdle sensation 1302, 1440
Gitelman syndrome 1249
Glabellar tap 1325
Glanders 245
Glargine 595
Glasgow Coma Scale 1336
Glatiramer acetate 1428
Gleevec 1125
Glioblastoma 1420
  multiforme 1420
Gliomas 1420
Global aphasia 1300
Global initiative for asthma 984
Glomerular proteinuria 1221
Glomerulonephritis 1212, 1222, 1225
  acute 230, 1508
  chronic 1223
Glossodynia 484
Glossopharyngeal
  nerve 1330
  neuralgia 1343
Glucagon 471, 474
  like polypeptide-1 474
Glucagonoma 715
Glucocorticoid 65, 213, 682, 686, 1010
  advantages of 64
  in typhoid, role of 232
  resistance 66
    in inflammatory diseases 66
  therapeutics of 63
  therapy 65
Gluconeogenesis, disorders of 1485
Glucose 1310, 1484
  metabolism 522
Glucose-6-phosphate dehydrogenase deficiency 1080
Glulisine 595
Glutamate decarboxylase antibody 1374
Glutaminase 456
Glutamine 456
Gluten-induced enteropathy 502
Glyceryl trinitrate, side effects of 904
Glycogen storage
  disease 938, 1479
  disorders 1485
Glycogenolysis defects 1479
Glycolysis defects 1479
Glycoprotein hormones 646
Glycosylated hemoglobin 588
Glycosylation of proteins 609
Gnathostoma spinigerum 441
GnRH-independent precocious puberty 705
Goalkeeper's fingers 721
Goblet cells 471
Goiter 662
  causes of 662
Goitrous cretinism 184

Golden 's' sign 1023
Goldmann perimetry 1317
Golfer's elbow 763
Golimumab 736
Gonadal disorders
  affecting both sexes 703
  in females 708
  in males 699
Gonadogenesis 696
Gonadotropin 646
  releasing hormone 642
  therapy 654
Gonads disorders 696
Gonda's sign 1301
Gonococcal infection in newborn 279
Gonorrhea 278
  in female 279
  in male 279
Goodpasture's syndrome 1028, 1225
Gopalan's syndrome 1346
Gordon's sign 1301
Gottron's papules 761
Gout 732, 772
  acute 773
  causes of secondary 773
  primary 773
  treatment of chronic 775
Gowers sign 1474
Graded physical activity 951
Graft disease 37
Graft rejection 1283
Graham little syndrome 1515
Graham steell murmur 840
Gram staining 1364
Granular casts 1215
Granular layer 1497
Granulocyte 1048
Granulocyte-macrophage colony-stimulating
    factor 1047
Granulocytic sarcomas 1124
Granuloma
  annulare 1540
  inguinale 282
  pyogenicum 1543
  venereum 282
Granulomatosis
  infantiseptica 255
  with polyangiitis 757, 1263
Granulomatous
  colitis 506
  gastritis 490
  thyroiditis, subacute 673
Graves' disease 664
Green pit viper 96
Green symptoms 153
Gregor Mendel 2, 6
Griseofulvin 58
Groove sign of Greenblatt 282
Group psychotherapy 1584
Growth hormone 646, 714
  releasing
    hormone 642
    inhibiting hormone 642
Growth of baby, regulation of 648
Growth, abnormalities of 636
Guarnieri bodies 330
Guillain-Barre syndrome 374, 457, 933, 1310, 1454
Guinea worm 440
Gustatory experience 1589
Gustatory sweating 1327
Gut flora in health and disease 473
Gut hormones 1589
Guttate psoriasis 1512
Gynecological causes 709
Gynecomastia 637, 707, 712
  causes of 707, 712

H

H_2 receptor blocker 492
Habitual hyperthermia 199
Hachinski ischemic score 1417
Hemophilia, complications of 1189
Haemophilus influenzae 1363
  frequently causes pharyngitis 227
  infections 223, 227
  meningitis 227
  type B 227

Haff disease 143
Hair 1498, 1544, 1587
  abnormalities of 636
  disorders of 1534
  loss of 637
  pigmentation, variation in 1535
  shaft abnormalities 1535
Hairy cell leukemia 1130
Hairy tongue 484
Halitosis 475
Hallucination 1548
Hallux valgus 729
Ham acid 1095
Hammer toe 729
Hampton's hump 925
Hand and foot warts 1502
Hand disease 356
Hansen's disease 312
Hantavirus infections 359
Haploid cells 6
Hapten 25, 31
Harmful cannabis 1570
Harmful use 1569
Harrison's sulcus 171
Hartmann's pouch 522
Hartmannella 410
Hartnup disease 1437
Hashimoto's disease 674
Hashimoto's encephalopathy 674, 1377
Hashitoxicosis 674
HBV
  hepatitis, chronic 555
  infection 294, 341, 349
HCV
  hepatitis, chronic 556
  infection 294
    acute 343
    chronic 343
Head louse infestation 1509
Headache 1339, 1342
  chronic daily 1341
  drug-induced 1343
  secondary 1339
  syndromes, primary 1339
Health problems 1551
  in elderly 1591
  occupational 153
Healthcare personnel through counseling 152
Healthcare-associated pneumonia 978
Healthy carrier 192
Hearing 1588
  impairment 1588
  loss, age-related 1347
Heart 114, 210, 1591
  block 874
    etiology of 876
    first degree 876
    second degree 876
    third degree 876
  disease 939, 941
    congenital 817, 837, 947, 948, 952
    critical congenital 838
  failure 803, 808
    acute 805
    backward 805
    chronic 805
    diagnosis of 807
    pathophysiology of 803
    types of 805
  malpositions of 836
  muscle disease, specific 920
  rate related tests 1463
  rate, controlling 842
  sounds 791
Heat cramps 106
Heat hyperpyrexia 102
Heat stroke 102
  first aid for 104
Heat syncope 105
Heat-shock proteins 103
Heavy chain estimation 1140
Hebephrenia 1556
Heberden's nodes 777, 778
Heidenhain variant 1374
Heimlich maneuver 976

Heine-Medin disease 352
Heinz bodies 1074, 1081
Helicobacter heilmannii 491
Helicobacter pylori 491
    diagnosis of 491
    eradication of 493
    infection, treatment of 491
Heliotrope rash 761
Heliotropium 558
Heller's operation 487
HELLP syndrome 1271
Helmet cell 1200
Helminthiasis 413
Helminthic infestations 441
Helper function 26
Helper T-cells 1051
Hemangioma liver 562
Hemaphasalis leachi 267
Hemaphysalis 94
Hematemesis 496
Hematochezia 476, 498
Hematogenous tuberculosis, acute 310
Hematological abnormalities 389
Hematological diseases 122
Hematological disorders 786, 1055, 1154, 1494, 1592
Hematological manifestations 1238
Hematological values, normal 1057
Hematology 743, 1044, 1132, 1139
Hematomyelia 1445
Hematopoietic growth factors 1046
Hematuria 1212
Heme iron 181
Hemidesmosomes 1496
Hemiplegic syndromes, crossed 1410
Hemisphere functions 1296
Hemochromatosis 535, 623, 937
Hemodialysis 1276
    complications of maintenance 1279
Hemodynamic 819, 820, 822, 823, 825, 827, 829,
        831, 833
    alterations 803
    changes 845, 857
    of pregnancy 940
    theory 1233
Hemodynamically-mediated renal failure 1284
Hemoglobin 181, 453, 723
    E disease 1085
    estimation 1055
Hemoglobinometry 1059
Hemoglobinopathy 1081, 1088
Hemogram 1234
Hemolytic anemia 1071, 1072, 1095
    secondary 1076
    type of 1075
Hemolytic disease of newborn 1076
Hemolytic jaundice 527
Hemolytic uremic syndrome 1202, 1273
Hemoperfusion 126
Hemophilia
    A 786, 1185
    B 1189
    defects 786
Hemoptysis 962
    in mitral stenosis, causes of 840
    management of 963
Hemopumps 812
Hemorrhage 226
Hemorrhagic conjunctivitis, acute 355
Hemorrhagic disease of newborn 174
Hemorrhagic disorders 1173
Hemorrhagic fever 358, 361
Hemorrhagic thrombocythemia 1166
Hemosiderin 182
Hemosiderosis 1102
Hemostasis 1169, 1192
    normal 1169
Henderson Patterson bodies 1502
Henderson-Hasselbalch's equation 453
Henoch-Schonlein
    purpura 759, 1264
    syndrome 758, 1183
Hepar lobatum 275
Heparin 1194, 1195
    in ischemic stroke 1412
Heparin-induced thrombocytopenia 1195

Hepatic adenoma 562
Hepatic amebiasis 407, 409
Hepatic cirrhosis, management of 530
Hepatic coma, treatment of 539
Hepatic disease 937
Hepatic disorders 551
Hepatic encephalopathy 536, 538, 1490
Hepatic failure 536
    acute 540, 541
    biochemical disturbances in 536
    causes of acute 540
    chronic 536
Hepatic function 1018
Hepatic precoma, treatment of 539
Hepatic transplantation 542
Hepatic veno-occlusive disease 145, 558
Hepatitis 525
    A virus 339
    B 351
        chronic 349
        infection 526
        virus 340
    C 350
        chronic 349
        virus 342
    chronic 346, 555
    delta virus 344
    drug induced 347
    E virus 344
    viruses 345
Hepatobiliary system 521
Hepatocellular
    carcinoma 346
    failure 527
Hepatocyte 453
    transplantation 542
Hepatojugular reflux 795
Hepatolenticular degeneration 535, 624
Hepatorenal syndrome 540, 551
Hepatosplenomegaly 171, 1055
Hepcidin 181, 182
Hephaestin 182
Hereditary angioedema 1527
    treatment of 1527
Hereditary ataxias 1436
Hereditary connective tissue diseases 770
Hereditary coproporphyria 626
Hereditary disorders 1425
Hereditary elliptocytosis 1079
Hereditary hemochromatosis gene product 182
Hereditary hemorrhagic telangiectasia 1184
Hereditary motor sensory neuropathy 1458
Hereditary myelopathies 1444
Hereditary nonspherocytic hemolytic anemias 1080
Hereditary spastic paraplegia 1438, 1444
Hereditary spherocytosis 1078
Hereditary thrombasthenia 1182
Heredity 1554
Heredodegenerative dystonias 1399
Heredofamilial ataxias 1436
Hermaphroditism 706
Herniation 1334, 1419
Herpangina 356
Herpes febrilis 336
Herpes genitalis 285
    in newborn 285
Herpes gestationis 1545
Herpes gladiatorum 336, 1503
Herpes simplex 1503
    virus 336
        encephalitis 336
        type 1 1357
        type 2 1359
Herpes viruse 1357
Herpes zoster 334
Herpesvirus hominis 336
Herpetic whitlow 1503
Hess tourniquet test 1173
Heterophyes heterophyes 429
Heterophyiasis 429
Heteroplasmy 20
Hexachlorobenzene compounds 132
Hexadecylphosphocholine 399
Hiatus hernia 488
HIB infection 227

Hiccough, causes of 1038
Hiccup 1038
High altitude
    disease 113
    pulmonary edema 112
Hippocratic fingers 963
Hippocratic oath 2
Hip-up sign 1474
Hirsutism 1535, 1536
Hirudo medicinalis 95
His bundle electrography 799
Histamine headache 1342
Histopathologic lesions, staging of 554
Histoplasma 1362
Histoplasmosis 379, 1362
Histrionic personality disorder 1567
Hitchhiker's thumb 729
Hockey stick sign 1375
Hodgkin's disease 1148
Hoffman's syndrome 638, 671, 1473, 1474
Holiday heart syndrome 939
Holmgren's wool 1318
Holter monitoring 799
Homeopathic system 2
Homeostenosis 1590
Homme rouge 1128
Homocysteine, total 1070
Homocystinuria 629, 630
Homoplasmy 20
Homunculus 1289
Hormonal abnormalities 1025
Hormonal disorders, indirect indices of 649
Hormonal factors 728
Hormonal interactions 711
Hormonal metabolism 523
Hormonal studies 649
Hormone 76, 687
    actions 633
    estimation of 640
    metabolism 632
    of pituitary 641
    receptors 633
    replacement therapy 772
        in women 710
    secretion of 640
    types of 640
Horn, anterior 1442
Horner's syndrome 1319, 1446, 1464
Horny envelope 1497
Horny layer 1497
Horton's syndrome 1342
Hospital staff, infection control precautions for 325
Hospital treatment 114
Hospital-acquired pneumonia 977
Host disease 37
Host parasite interaction 414
Hot cross bun skull 276
Howell-Jolly bodies 1045, 1068
Hughes syndrome 747
Hughlings Jackson syndrome 1331
Human anaplasmosis 267
Human brain, adult 1288
Human chorionic gonadotropin 714
Human ehrlichiosis 263, 267
Human genome
    mapping project 2
    project 9, 69
Human herpes
    virus-types 6 and 7 1359
    virus-types 7 and 8 1359
Human immunodeficiency virus 278, 287, 936, 1075
    associated cognitive motor complex 293
    co-infection 397
    infection 287, 316, 601
        management of 295
    test 294
Human insulin 594
Human leukocyte antigen
    associations 581
    status, determination of 724
    system in humans 36
Human metapneumovirus 327
Human monocytotropic ehrlichiosis 267
Human placental lactogen 71
Human polymicrobial infections 193

Textbook of Medicine

Human rabies 362
    immunoglobulin 364
Human T-cell lymphocytotropic virus 1361
Human-to-human transmission 362
Humming bird sign 1396
Humoral hypercalcemia of malignancy 682
Humoral immunity 27
    deficiency of 33
Huntington's disease 1401
Huntington's like diseases 1401
Hutchinson's pupillary reaction 1422
Hutchinson's teeth 276
Hyaline casts 1215
Hyalomma 267
Hybrid techniques 87
Hydantoin-linked lymphoma 1159
Hydatid worm 426
Hydralazine 811, 891
Hydrazine derivatives 76
Hydrocele 434
    surgery for 438
    treatment of 438
Hydrocephalus 1423
    developing in infancy, causes of 1423
    in adults, causes of 1424
Hydrophidae 96
Hydrophobia 361, 363
Hydropneumothorax 1033
Hydrops fetalis 1077
Hydrostatic pressure gradient 1277
Hydroxy
    indole acetic acid 71
    proline 71
Hydroxycarbamide 1126
Hydroxychloroquine 734
Hydroxyurea 1084, 1126, 1165, 1167
Hymenolepis diminuta 428
Hymenolepis nana 427
Hyperadrenocorticism 1493
Hyperaldosteronism 446, 936
    classification of primary 694
    primary 694
Hyperalgesia 1302
Hyperalimentation 504
Hyperamylasemia, causes of 566
Hyperamylasuria, causes of 566
Hyperbaric oxygen 110
Hypercalcemia 180, 442, 450, 679, 680, 714, 938
    acute 681
        management 681
Hypercapnia 969
    manifestations of 970
Hyperchloremic metabolic acidosis 460
Hypercholesterolemia, newer drugs in 622
Hypercortisolism 688
Hypereosinophilia 1050
Hypereosinophilic syndrome, management of 1050
Hyperesthesias 1453
Hyperglycemia 587, 609
Hyperhomocysteinemia 629, 952
    causes of 630
Hyperkalemia 442, 448, 938, 1285
    management of 448
    treatment of 1240
Hyperkalemic distal RTA 460
Hyperkinetic circulation 537
Hyperkinetic movement disorders 1399
Hyperkinetic syndrome 1577
Hyperlipidemias 620
    management of primary 621
    primary 621
    secondary 623
Hypermagnesemia 442, 451, 939
Hypernatremia 442, 445
    management of 445
Hyperosmolar
    hyperglycemic nonketotic state 607
    nonketotic
        coma 607
        diabetic coma 445
    states 464, 466
Hyperparathyroidism 716, 1238, 1493
    primary 678
    secondary 682
    tertiary 682

Hyperpathia 1302, 1453
Hyperphenylalaninemia 627
Hyperphosphatemia 442, 451
Hyperpigmentation 1530, 1544
Hyperpigmented palms 71
Hyperplasia, demonstration of 679
Hyperplastic type 1506
Hyperprolactinemia 649, 708
Hyperpyrexia 195
Hypersensitivity, delayed 27
Hypersomnia 1572
Hypersplenism 1168
    causes of 1169
Hypertension 882, 938, 952, 1213, 1238, 1266,
    1268, 1269
    accelerated 887, 1269
    causes of secondary 883, 1267
    chronic 1271
    classification of 1266
    complications of 885
    drug in 889
    essential 883, 885, 1267, 1269
    in children 894
    in pregnancy 894, 1272
    malignant 887
    secondary 883, 885, 1267
        causes of 1268
Hypertensive
    emergencies 893
    encephalopathy 886
    nephrosclerosis 1269
    urgencies 893
Hyperthermia, malignant 199
Hyperthyroidism 664, 936, 1493
    during pregnancy 669
    to thyroiditis 669
Hypertransfusion 1087
Hypertrichosis 1535, 1536
Hypertrophic
    cardiomyopathy 917, 918
    gastritis 490
    osteoarthropathy 71, 780
        classification of 780
    pulmonary osteoarthropathy 780
Hypertrophy of breasts 712
Hyperuricemia 1143
Hyperventilation 957
Hyperviscosity
    state, management of 1126
    syndrome 1143
Hypervitaminosis D 173, 450
Hypervolemic hyponatremia 444, 468
Hypesthesia 1453
Hypnagogic hallucinations 1548
Hypnic headache 1342
Hypnopompic hallucinations 1548
Hypoadrenocorticism 1493
Hypoaldosteronism 448
Hypocalcemia 180, 442, 450, 938
Hypocomplementemia 1262
Hypofrontality 1558
Hypoglossal nerve 1331
Hypoglycemia 388, 587, 602-604, 1484
    management of 603
    symptoms of 603
Hypogonadism 699
    in women 708
    secondary 699
    treatment of 701
Hypokalemia 442, 446, 939
    antibiotic induced 446
    management of 447
Hypomagnesemia 442, 448, 452, 939
Hyponatremia 442, 1413
    causes of 467
    hypovolemic 444, 468
    management of 444
Hypo-osmolar disorders 464, 467
Hypoparathyroidism 682, 1493
    treatment of 684
Hypophosphatemia 180, 442, 448, 451
Hypopituitarism 653, 1493
Hypoplastic anemia 1071
    congenital 1092
Hypopnea 1016
    syndrome 1018

Hyposmia 1316
Hyposplenism 1169
    causes of 1169
Hypostatic
    congestion 1013
    pneumonia 980
Hypotension 810
Hypothalamic
    anovulation 708
    causes 709
    disorders 643
    hormones 642
Hypothalamo-pituitary
    adrenal axis, suppression of 65
    disorders 648
Hypothalamus
    defective regulatory control by 649
    disorders 641
Hypothermia 108, 939
Hypothyroidism 670, 936, 1493
    secondary 672
Hypotonia 1291
Hypotonic duodenography 478, 566
Hypoventilation syndromes 1492
Hypoxanthine-guanine phosphoribosyltransferase 773
Hypoxia 969
    correction of 970
    manifestations of 969
Hypoxic form 111
Hypsarrhythmia 1382
Hysterical attacks 1384
Hysterical coma 1334
Hysterical fever 199
Hysterical neurosis 1563

I

Iatrogenic Cushing's syndrome 689
Ibandronate 682
Icatibant 1527
Ice-cream headache 1343
Icepack test 1467, 1469
Ice-pick scars 1510
Icroangiopathy hemolytic anemia 1200
Icterus gravis neonatorum 1077
Ideal body
    mass index 951
    weight 586
Idiopathic hypereosinophilic syndrome 1050
Idiopathic hypogonadotropic hypogonadism 701
Idiopathic inflammatory myositis 761
Idiopathic intracranial hypertension 1424, 1495
Idiopathic polyneuropathy, acute 1454
Idiopathic portal hypertension 551
Idiopathic thrombocytopenic purpura 1175
Idiopathic thrombocytosis, primary 1166
Idiopathic ulcerative colitis 511
Idoxuridine 56, 57
IGF-1, estimation of 652
Ill patients, chronically 122
Illnesses with treatable dementia 1369
Iloprost 751
Imatinib 77, 1125
Imidazole derivatives 54, 76
Imiquimod 286, 1544
Immersion syndrome 113
Immune
    complex mediated tissue damage, type III 30
    dysfunction 718
    reconstitution inflammatory syndrome 308
    response 25, 362
        secondary 26
    system 1589
    therapy
        long-term 1470
        short-term 1470
    thrombocytopenic purpura 1175
Immune-mediated damage 1284
Immunity 230, 246
    active induced 37
    against
        infections 26
        malaria 387
        tuberculosis 300
Immunity-based therapeutic innovations in cancer 74
Immunization, active 350, 351

Immunoblastic lymphadenopathy 1150
Immunochromatographic test 436
Immunocompetent individuals 335, 1359
Immunocompromised individuals 335
Immunoconjugate 1122
Immunocytes 1051
Immunodeficiency states 33
    combined 33
    primary 34
    secondary 34
Immunoglobulin A
    nephropathy 1224
    vasculitis 758
Immunological (immune) tolerance 32
Immunological changes 69
Immunological disorders 747
Immunological disturbances 857
Immunological tests 526
Immunologically-mediated paraneoplastic
        neurological syndromes 1025
Immunology 434, 738
Immunomodulation 1110
Immunomodulatory drugs 1142
Immunopathogenesis 1426, 1511
Immunosuppressant drugs 735, 745
Immunosuppressed hosts 1359
Immunosuppression 1204
Immunotherapy 93
Immunotoxins, therapy with 74
Impetigo contagiosa 1501
Impetigo herpetiformis 1513, 1545
Implantable cardioverter defibrillator 812, 947
Implantable devices 812
Implosion 1585
Impotence 702, 1573
Impulse noise, effects of 120
Inappropriate antidiuretic hormone 71
    secretion 51
Inborn errors of metabolism 618
Incontinentia pigmenti 1533
Incretins 581
Incubation period 362
Indeterminate leprosy 314
Indian Council of Medical Research 1293
Infant botulism 143
Infant hercules 639
Infantile acne 1510
Infantile autism 1576
Infantile B$_{12}$ deficiency 1068
Infantile paralysis 352
Infantile spasms 1381, 1382
Infantilism 637
Infarct, core of 1408
Infection 192, 312, 581, 728, 936, 1075, 1092,
        1370, 1413, 1425, 1443, 1512, 1591
    abdominal 236, 237
    mixed 389, 393
    primary 1503
    secondary 335
    severe 43
    subacute 857
    types of 192
Infection-associated stones 1257
Infectious mononucleosis 374
Infective agent, isolation of 200
Infective endocarditis, acute 855
Infective episodes, treatment of 1000
Infertility 705
Inflammation 1051
Inflammatory
    demyelinating polyneuropathy
        acute 1454
        chronic 1455
    disease
        chronic 770
        nonspecific 481
        of bowel, chronic 767
    myelopathy 1443
    response, inhibitors of 1000
Infliximab 735, 766, 1515
Influenza 323
    A viruses, emergent 325
    virus 1075
        pneumonia, primary 324
Influenzal pneumonia 324

Infusion urogram 1219
Ingested poisons 125
Ingrowing toenail 1537
Inhalation anthrax 240
Inhaled corticosteroids 994
Inhaled glucocorticoids 1000
Inhaled steroids 989
Inheritance pattern 1082
Inheritance, types of 12
Inherited disorders 1185
    of connective tissue 628
    of erythrocytes 1078
Inherited forms of rickets 172
Inhibit neutrophil elastases 1000
Inhibit osteoclast activity 681
Inosine pranobex 58
Insomnia 1572
Inspiratory
    capacity 960
    reserve volume 960
Insulin 474, 606
    action 580
    analogues 594
        long-acting 595
        short-acting 594
    antagonists, role of 582
    combination 591
    degludec 595
    injection 595
        devices 596
    like growth factors 647
    presbyopia 610
    pumps 596
    rapid-acting 594
    release 587
    resistant states 647
    secretion 580
    structure of 580
    synthesis 580
    therapeutics of 595
Insulin-like growth factor 647, 714
    side effects of 648
Insulinomas 715
Insulin-receptor effects 590
Integrase inhibitors 295
Intelligence quotient 1549
Intelligence scale for children 1551
Intelligence, disturbance of 1549
Intensity
        conditioning allografts, reduced 1116
        modulated radiation therapy 1152
Intensive insulin therapy 595
Intention tremors 1404
Intercalated cells 446
Intercritical gout 774
Intercurrent infections 532
Interferon 27, 57, 322, 1110
    alfa 348, 1126
    beta 1b 1427
    gamma release assays 303
Interferon-alpha 76
Interleukin 27, 76, 1000
Intermediate syndrome 130
Intermittent porphyria, acute 353, 626
International Physician for Prevention of
        Nuclear War 118
International prognostic index 1155
Interstitial
    edema 1363
    fibrosis 1010, 1011
    fluid 442
    keratitis 278
    nephritis, acute 1242
Interstitium, diseases of 1242
Interval gout 774
Intervention, type of 825
Interventional cardiology 802, 948
Interventional radiology 87
Intestinal absorption 501
Intestinal amebiasis 406
    chronic 409
Intestinal angina 510
Intestinal blood loss 539
Intestinal capillariasis 441
Intestinal contents 477, 502

Intestinal diseases 499
Intestinal hemorrhage 230, 232
Intestinal myiasis 91
Intestinal nematodes 415
Intestinal pathogenic strains 236
Intestinal perforation 230, 232
Intestinal polyposis 508
Intestinal schistosomiasis 431
Intestinal tuberculosis 508
Intestine
    infective disorders of 767
    large 472, 1060
    small 471, 509
    ulceration of 508
Intolerant to methotrexate 1010
Intoxication 1349
    acute 1568, 1570
Intra-aortic balloon
    counter-pulsation 947
    pump 914
Intra-articular steroids 779
Intracardiac repair 832
Intracellular
    compartment 448
    fluid 442
    to extracellular compartment 448
Intracerebral hemorrhage 1415
Intracranial hematomas 1422
Intracranial hemorrhagic stroke, causes of 1407
Intracranial hypertension, benign 1320, 1424
Intracranial neoplasms 1420
    primary 1420
Intracranial space-occupying lesions 1417
Intracranial structures, traction on 1342
Intractable cardiac failure 813
Intraluminal bacterial proliferation in intestines 504
Intraoral bite wing X-rays 482
Intrasellar cyst 657
Intrasellar-subarachnoid space 657
Intrasplenic pressure 547
Intrathecal drugs 1115
Intravascular
    fluid 442
    hemolysis 1074
    ultrasound 82, 946
Intravenous
    drug users 288
    immunoglobulin 1178, 1455, 1470
    urography 1218
Intrinsic factor deficiency, congenital 1070
Inulin clearance 1234
Invasive tests 491
Involuntary movements 1366
Iodine 183, 667, 1349
    induced hyperthyroidism 184
    nutrition in community 184
Ionizing radiations 118
    injuries to 115
Iothalamate 1234
Ipratropium bromide 992
Ipsilateral hemiparesis 1419
Irbesartan 892
Iron 181, 1348
    chelating agents 1087
    deficiency
        anemia 1063, 1494
        development of 183
        effects of 183
    preparations 1066
    sorbitol citrate 1066
    sucrose 1066
Irritable bowel syndrome 505
Irritable heart syndrome 934
Irritant contact dermatitis 1521
Ischemic cardiomyopathy 915
Ischemic heart disease 895, 1493
Ischemic imbalance 900
Ischemic neurological deficit, reversible 1406
Ischemic penumbra 1408
Ischemic stroke
    in young 1407
    management of 1411
    syndromes 1409
Ischemic syndromes 938
Ishihara pseudoisochromatic plate 1318

Islet cell transplantation 596
Isolated demyelinating syndromes 1425
Isolated joint 513
Isomerism 837
Isometric handgrip test 1463
Isonicotinylhydrazide 1287
Isoprenaline 816
Isoprenaline-B 1464
Isopropyl alcohol 460
Isosexual precocity in boys, incomplete 704
Isosorbide dinitrate 811, 904
Isotope renography 1219
Isotope studies 1060
Isotopic liver scan 526
Isotopic tests 660
Itraconazole 58
Ivabradine 812, 912
Ivermectin 416, 419, 420, 437, 441
Ixodes 94
    scapularis 267

J

Jaccoud's arthritis 210
Jacksonian motor seizures 1381
Jacobson's triad 1316, 1326
Janeway lesions 857
Janus kinase 1161
    inhibitors 736
Japanese encephalitis 372, 1360
Japanese river fever 266
Jarisch-Herxheimer reaction 258, 277
Jaundice 389, 523, 1055
    classification 523
    complications to 526
    management of 528
    types of 524
Jaw jerk 1325
Jellife's syndrome 1345
Jellyfish 95
Jeryl-lynn strain 339
Jigger 95
Jod-Basedow phenomenon 184, 664
Joint 243, 720, 749, 750, 1592
    manifestations, drug-induced 787
    tuberculosis 783
Jones criteria, exceptions to 212
Jugular vein, engorgement of 806
Jugular venous pulse 794
Junctional premature beats 863
Juvenile absence epilepsy 1380
Juvenile delinquency 1577
Juvenile idiopathic arthritis 737
Juvenile myoclonic epilepsy 1382
Juvenile neutrophils 1048
Juvenile Paget's disease 782
Juvenile polyposis 509

K

Kala-azar 397
Kallikrein-kinin system 1211
Kallmann's syndrome 643, 653
Kampavata 1391
Kanamycin 50
Kaposi's sarcoma 292, 1075
Kaposi's varicelliform eruption 336, 1503
Karokampam 1391
Kartagener's syndrome 1002
Karyotyping 8, 19
Kasabach-Merritt syndrome 562, 1201
Katayama disease 431
Katayama syndrome 431
Kawasaki disease 757, 935, 756
Kayser-Fleischer ring 535
Kearns-Sayre syndrome 20
Keloid and hypertrophic scar 1538
Keratinization 1496, 1497
Keratoacanthoma 1543
Keratoderma blennorrhagica 1516
Keratolytic agents 1499
Kerley B lines 841
Kernicterus 1077
Kernig's sign 220
Keshan disease 186, 1349
Kestenbaum's number 1319

Ketoacidosis 452, 461, 606
Ketoconazole 58, 59, 652, 1505
Ketogenic diet 1390
Ketolides 52
Ketones 1485
Ketotifen 994
Kidney 114, 741, 749, 1260, 1266, 1268
    artificial (dialyzers) 1277
    changes in 886
    development of 1207
    disease 1231
        chronic 786, 937, 1236
    disorders 1540
    function of 1207, 1210, 1211
    injury
        acute 1212, 1230
        in pregnancy, acute 1272
        intrinsic acute 1233
    structure of 1207
    transplantation 1282
        immunosuppression in 1283
    vulnerability of 1284
Kiel classification 1153
Killed vaccine 373
Killer cells 1051
Killing function 1049
King cobra 96
Klebsiella granulomatis 282
Klebsiella pneumoniae 234, 979
    infections 237
Klinefelter's syndrome 17, 701, 1445, 1450
Knee syndrome 777
Knidosis 1526
Knock knees 171
Knodell classification 555
Kocher-Debre-Semelaigne syndrome 1473
Koebner's phenomenon 1502, 1512
Koilonychia 1064
Köllner's rule 1318
Koplik's spots 328
Korotkoff's sounds 796
Korsakoff's psychosis 1569
Korsakoff's syndrome 1345, 1554
Krait 96, 97
    bite 98
    venom 99
Kreb's tricarboxylic acid cycle 174
Kupffer's cells 522, 1051
Kuru 1374, 1376
Kussmaul's breathing 460, 957
Kussmaul's respiration 605
Kwashiorkor 163, 166, 1349
Kyasanur forest disease 370, 1360
Kyphoscoliosis 1034

L

LA appendage exclusion 947
Labile diabetes 598
Lacosamide 1390
Lactate dehydrogenase 525, 901
    deficiency 1479
Lactate infusion test 1561
Lactic acidosis 452, 460, 607, 1485
    type A 461
    type B 461
Lactitol 539
Lactose absorption 501
Lactosuria 617
Lactulose 539
Lacunar stroke syndromes 1409
Lacunar syndromes 1410
Laennec's cirrhosis 552
Lafora body disease 1383
Lambert-Eaton myasthenic syndrome 1468
Lamellar granules 1497
Lamina propria 471
Lamivudine 57, 348
Lamotrigine 1387, 1388
Langerhan's cells 1051
Language disorders 1300
Lanreotide 652
Lanthanum carbonate 1241
Laparoscopy 479, 519, 526
Laparoscopy-assisted panendoscopy 478
Larva migrans 422

Larval migration 420
Laryngeal
    diphtheria 224
    obstruction, acute 976
    paralysis 976
Laryngitis
    acute 975
    chronic 975
Laryngysmus stridulus 171
Lasegue's sign 1452
Lassa fever 359
Latent syphilis 274, 277
Latent tuberculosis 299
Late-onset rubella encephalitis 1361
Latex agglutination tests 1311
Lathyrism 146
Latrodectus mactans 91
Lazy leukocyte syndrome 1049
Lead poisoning 146
    acute 146
    chronic 146
Lean nonalcoholic steatohepatitis 553
Leech infestations 95
Leeuwenhoek 2
Leflunomide 735, 1010
Leg raising test 1452
Legionella pneumophila 267
Legionellosis 253, 254
Legionnaires disease 254
Leiomyosarcomas 944
Leishmaniasis 384, 394
    prevention of 401
Lenalidomide 1142
Lenegre's disease 876
Lennox-Gastaut syndrome 1381, 1382
Lentigines 1533
Lepore hemoglobins 1088
Lepra reaction 316
Lepromatous
    borderline 314
    leprosy 313
Lepromin test 314
Leprosy 298, 316
    borderline 314
    reactions in 316
Leptins, role of 188
Leptospirosis 260, 347, 936, 1243
Leptotrombidium deliense 266
Leser-Trélat sign 1541
Lesion 254, 268
    at chiasm 1318
    demonstration of 688
    in optic pathway 1318
    of conus medullaris 1441
    of peritoneum, malignant 520
    of vestibular division 1329
    outside
        brainstem 1332
        cranial cavity 1332
    primary 1498
    produced by staphylococci 214
    secondary 1498
    structural 504
    superficial 214
Letermovir 376
Letrozole 78
Leukapheresis 1100, 1126
Leukemias 786, 1103
    acute 1104, 1113, 116
    chronic 1104, 1122
    classification of 1104
    congenital 1109
    diagnosis of 1106
    drug in 1109
    treatment trials 1122
Leukemic reticuloendotheliosis 1130
Leukemoid reaction 1108
Leukocyte
    alkaline phosphatase score 1123
    count 723
    groups 1098
    patterns 196
Leukoerythroblastic blood picture 1134
Leukomyelitis 1443
Leukonychia 537, 1537

Textbook of Medicine

Leukopenia 231
Leukoplakia 483
Leukotriene 27
    modifiers 990, 994
Lev's disease 876
Levamisole 77
Leveen peritoneovenous shunt 532
Levodopa 1393
Levofloxacin 54
Levosalbutamol 992
Levothyroxine sodium 672
Lewis system 1098
Lewy body dementia 1375
    diffuse 1395
Lhermitte's sign 1302, 1354, 1440
Lice 94
Lichen planus 1515
Lichenoid eruptions 1530
Liddle's syndrome 459
Life support measures 874
Life-threatening
    bleeding 1179
    Clostridium difficile infection, chronic 252
    complications 1235
Lightning pains 1354
Limb girdle
    muscular dystrophy 1478
    weakness 1473
Limbic encephalitis 1369, 1377
    common infections 1377
Limbs, temperature of 793
Linagliptin 591
Linamarin 144
Lincomycin 53
Linear immunoglobulin A disease 1525
Linear scleroderma 748
Linezolid 53
    optic neuropathy 53
Lingual dystonia 1300
Lipid
    lowering agents 555
    metabolism 523, 590
    storage-related disorders 1479
Lipid-lowering agents 908, 910
Lipomas 715, 944
Lipoprotein, increase in 952
Liposomal amphotericin B 399
Lipoxygenases 1000
Liquorice ingestion 459
Lispro 594
Listeria monocytogenes 254
Listeriosis 253, 254
    during pregnancy 255
Lithium 935, 1582
    toxicity 1375
Live attenuated
    measles vaccine 330
    varicella zoster virus vaccines 334
Live vaccine 65
Liver 42, 535, 1145, 1540
    abscess, complications of 407
    biopsy 201, 526, 534, 554, 561
    carcinoma of 560
    disease 44
        chronic 1070
        end stage 530, 612
    dysfunction in circulatory impairment 559
    failure
        acute 540, 541, 1491
        chronic 540
    function
        test 525
        zones in 523
    involvement 244
    pyogenic abscess of 559
    structure of 521
    support, artificial 542
    transplantation 535, 542–544
        types of 543
Liver-based metabolic conditions 543
Lixisenatide 597
Loa loa 432
Lobar hemorrhage 1416
Lobar pneumoniae 217
Lobe syndrome, middle 1002

Local radiation injury 116
Local reactions 93, 98
Localized myeloma, treatment of 1143
Locked-in syndrome 1337
Locomotor system 344
    disease of 719
Löfgren's syndrome 1009
Loiasis 438
Lomefloxacin 54
Long-chain fatty acids 1487
Losartan 892
Louse borne
    relapsing fever 257
    typhus 263
Low backache, inflammatory 765
Low birth weight 884
Low grade fever 537
Low tension headache 1343
Lower cranial nerves 1332
Lower GIT bleeding, management of 498
Lower motor neuron 1291
Low-molecular-weight heparin 1195
Lucio leprosy 316
Lucio phenomenon 317
Lues venerea 274
Lugol's iodine 667
Lumbago-Sciatica syndrome 762
Lumbar canal stenosis 1452
Lumbar disc lesions 1452
Lumbar puncture 311, 1415
Lumbosacral plexus 1448
Lumefantrine 392
Lundh test 566
Lung 114
    abscess 981
    allergic disorders of 984
    biopsy 968
    cancer 1541
        classification of 1020
        manifestations of 1022
        signs of 1022
        symptoms of 1022
    capacity 960
        total 960
    circulatory disturbances in 1012
    diseases, occupational 1005
    microbiome 956
    neoplasms of 1019
    perfusion 961
    purpura 1028
    transplantation 1001
    ventilation of 957
    volume 959
        reduction surgery 1000
Lupus erythematosus cell phenomenon 724
Lupus nephritis 1225
Lyme arthritis 32
Lyme borreliosis 253
Lyme disease 936
Lymnaea truncatula 429
Lymph node 508
    biopsy 968
    moderate enlargement of 1055
Lymphangitis 208
    carcinomatosa 1023
Lymphatic drainage 955
Lymphatic filariasis 432, 438
    in children 435
Lymphatic leukemia
    acute 1113
    chronic 1127
Lymphatic organs 1591
Lymphatic structures 1151
Lymphatics, disorders of 1531, 1532
Lymphedema 1532
    treatment of 438
Lymphoblastic leukemia, acute 1113
Lymphocyte 1051
    tumors 1159
Lymphocytic choriomeningitis 359
Lymphocytic lymphoma 1156
Lymphocytic thyroiditis
    chronic 674
    subacute 673
Lymphocytotoxic crossmatch 1282

Lymphogranuloma
    inguinale 281
    venereum 281
Lymphoid cells, malignant disorders of 1147
Lymphoid stem cell 1149
Lymphoid tissue lymphoma, mucosa-associated 738
Lymphokines 26
Lymphoma 450, 1147, 1150, 1157
    in cancer statistics 1148
    malignant 786
    staging of 1151
    types of 1159
Lymphoproliferative malignancies 1494
Lymphorrhage 434
Lymphoscintigraphy 436
Lynch syndrome 495
Lyssa 361

M

Maccallum's patch 210
Macro electromyography 1305
Macroangiopathy 583
Macrocytic anemias 1067
Macrolides 51
Macrophage activation syndrome 737
Macropolycytes 1068
Macroscopic hematuria 1221
Macular atrophy 1538
Macular degeneration, age-related 1347
Macular splitting 1318
Maculopapular 1528
Mad cow disease 1374
Madame-Louis-Bar syndrome 1438
Madura foot 383
Maduramycosis 383
Magnesium 185, 1349
    homeostasis 442
        disorders of 451
    salts 908
    sulfate 992
Magnetic resonance spectroscopy 85, 1306
Magnetic susceptimetry 1087
Maintenance therapy 1115
Major tranquilizers 1580
Malabsorption 527
    causes of 499
    states 499
    syndromes 1489
Malaria 384, 1075
    in pregnancy 390, 393
    treatment of severe 393
    vaccines 394
Malarial hepatopathy 389
Malassezia furfur 1519
Male infertility, causes of 705
Male pseudohermaphroditism 707
Malignant pustule 240
Mallory bodies 552
Mallory-Weiss syndrome 496, 548
Malnutrition 155
    mild acute 164
    severe acute 163, 164
    treatment of 1241
Malt lymphoma 1157
Malta fever 243
Mania 1557
Manioc 144
Mansonella ozzardi 432, 440
Mansonella perstans 439
Mantle cell lymphoma 1157
Mantoux test 200
Mao-B inhibitors 1394
Maple syrup urine disease 1437
Marasmic kwashiorkor 166
Marasmus 166
Marburg virus 359
Marchiafava-Bignami disease 1350
Marcus Gunn pupil 1319
Marfan's syndrome 629, 939
Marginal zone lymphoma 1157
Marie's quadrilateral space 1299
Marie-Bamberger syndrome 780
Marie-Strümpell disease 764
Marine animals, injuries to 95
Marrow cells, ablation of recipient's 1111

Masked hypertension 882
Maternal problems during pregnancy 941
Mature erythrocyte 1046
Maturity-onset diabetes of young 584
Maxillary sinusitis, causative organism in acute 975
Maximal voluntary ventilation 961
May-Hegglin anomaly 1182
McConnell's sign 926
McGregor's line 1446, 1449
MDR-TB, treatment of 307
MDT regimens, alternative 318
Measles 328, 329, 1360
    atypical 329
    inclusion body encephalitis 329, 1360
Measly pork 424
Mebendazole 418, 419
Mechanical ventilation 971
Medial medullary syndrome 1332, 1410
Mediastinal lymphadenopathy 1009
Mediastinal tumors 1039
Mediastinoscopes 968
Mediastinum, diseases of 1039
Medical disorders 1575
Medical errors 45
Medical genetics 5
Medical nutrition therapy 586
Medical Research Council Breathlessness Scale 963
Medical Research Council Modified
        Dyspnea Scale 1001
Medical synovectomy 737
Medical termination of pregnancy 337
Medically active stones 1257
Medication overuse headache 1341
Medicinal iron 1066
Medicine
    computers in 5
    evidence-based 5
    history of 1
Medium vessel vasculitis 755
Medullary cystic kidney disease 1245
Medullary sponge kidney 1246
Medullary syndrome, lateral 1410
Medullary thyroid carcinoma 716
Medulloblastoma 1420
Medulloepithelioma 1419
Mee's nails 1537
Megakaryoblast 1053
Megakaryoblastic leukemia, acute 1118, 1120
Megakaryocyte 1053
Megakaryocytic myelosis 1166
Megaloblastic anemias, congenital 1070
Megaloblasts 1067
Melanonychia, longitudinal 1537
Melarsoprol 403
Melasma 1533, 1544
Melatonin 657
Melioidosis 239, 244
Melituias, causes of 615, 617
Melkersson-Rosanthal syndrome 1328
Melphalan 1142
Membranoproliferative glomerulonephritis 1229
Membranous nephropathy 1228
Memory
    disturbance of 1546, 1548
    disturbances 1595
    impaired patient, examination of 1365
    testing 1299, 1551
    types of 1365
MEN1 syndrome 715
MEN2 syndrome 715, 716
Mendel-Bekhterev sign 1301
Mendelson's syndrome 1013
Ménétrier's disease 490
Menghini's needle 968
Ménière's disease 1330
Ménière's syndrome 1330
Meningeal
    anthrax 241
    irritation 1343
Meningiomas 1420
Meningitis 255, 333, 338, 1360
    etiology of 1363
Meningococcal infections 219
Meningococcal meningitis 220
Meningococcemia 221
    chronic 221

Meningoencephalitis 255, 374, 1360
Menopause 1384
    medical problems of 710
Mental disorders
    classification of 1551
    signs of 1546
    symptoms of 1546
Mental retardation 1575
    causes of 1575
Mental status examination 1550
Mental stress 934
    ischemia 934
Mental symptoms 1560
Mepolizumab 994
Meralgia paresthetica 1458
Meropenem 49
Mesobuthus tamulus 92
Mesonephros 1207
Metabolic acidosis 388, 452, 460
    treatment of 1240
Metabolic agents 911
Metabolic alkalosis 452, 459
Metabolic arthropathies 769
Metabolic causes 1370
Metabolic disorders 618, 938, 1182
Metabolic disturbance 1438
Metabolic emergencies 602
Metabolic functions, zones in 523
Metabolic muscle diseases 1479
Metabolic syndrome 619, 952
    diagnosis of 619
Metabolism 185
Metanephros 1207
Metastasis 71, 943
Metastatic
    neoplasms 786
    tumors 1421
Metformin 555, 590, 591
    effects of 590
Methacholine test 915
Methanol 460
    poisoning 135
Methisazone 331
Methotrexate 735, 766, 1010, 1514
Methyldopa 890
Methylprednisolone 1178
Methylthiouracil 667
Methylxanthines 990
Metolazone 459
Metrifonate 431
Metronidazole 54, 408
Metyrapone 652, 690
Meyer's loop 1317
Micafungin 59
Miconazole 58
Microalbuminuria 611, 1221, 1261
Microarray analysis 19
Microbial flora 855
    normal 1250, 1500
Microbial virulence factors 1251
Microbiology 1251, 1252, 1253, 1254
Microdermabrasion 1510
Microfilaria detection tests 435
Micropsia 1548
Microscopic polyangiitis 758
Microscopic polyarteritis nodosa 1263
Micturating cystogram 1219
Midnight cortisol 687
Mid-systolic click syndrome 846
Miglitol 592
Migraine 1339-1341
    classic 1340
    drug in 1340
    management of transformed 1341
    with aura 1340
    without aura 1340
Migrating motor complex 471
Migrating thrombophlebitis 1542
Miliary tuberculosis 310
Milk-alkali syndrome 459
Milker's nodule 1503
Millard-Gubler syndrome 1328, 1410
Millennium development goals 3
Miller-Fisher syndrome 1455
Miltefosine 399

Milwaukee shoulder 777
Mimicking coma 1337
    clinical conditions 1337
Mimicking dementia 1368
Minamata disease 143
Mineral bone disease, treatment of 1240
Mineralocorticoid 686, 693
    excess 1267
    hypertension 894
    receptor antagonist 810, 909
Minerals 179
Minimally conscious state 1337
Mini-mental state examination 1296, 1366
Minnesota multiphasic personality inventory 1551
Minocycline 51
Minoxidil 891
Minute sequence pictures 1219
Miracidia 430
Mirodenafil 703
Mirror movements 1450
Miscellaneous infections 294
Mite
    fever 266
    typhus 266
Mitgehen 1291
Mithramycin 450
Mitochondria 20
Mitochondrial diseases 1397, 1473, 1479
Mitochondrial encephalomyopathy 1383
Mitochondrial genetics 20
Mitochondrial inheritance 20
Mitochondrial myopathy 934
Mitotic pool 1048
Mitoxantrone 1428
Mitral annuloplasty 812
Mitral incompetence 844
Mitral regurgitation 844
    acute 845
    cause of 844
    surgery in chronic 846
Mitral restenosis 843
Mitral stenosis 839-941
Mitral valve
    apparatus 839
    prolapse syndrome 846
    repair 812
    replacement 843
Mitral valvotomy, closed 843
Miyoshi myopathy 1474
MMR vaccines 339
Mobile phone radiation 1495
    complications 1495
Mobiliferrin 182
Mobiluncus 284
Mobitz type
    I block 875
    II block 875
Moderately severe patients, treatment of 513
Modern ultrathin fiber-optic bronchoscopes 1024
Modified jones criteria 212
Modified Schober test 765
Molecular characteristics of lymphomas 1158
Molecular genetic
    of epilepsy 1380
    studies 1488
Molecular mimicry 32
Molecular pathogenesis 1123
Molluscum body 287, 1502
Molluscum contagiosum 1502
Mönckeberg's sclerosis 794
Monge's disease 113
Mongolism 1575
Monoamine oxidase inhibitors 935, 1582
Monoclonal antibodies 77, 1130
Monoclonal gammapathy 1143, 1144
Monocytes 1050
Monocytic leukemia, chronic 1127
Monomelic atrophy 1434
Mononeuritis 1456
    multiplex 731, 1454, 1456
Mononeuropathy 1454
Mononuclear phagocytes 1050
Monosomy 16
Montelukast 994
Montenegro skin test 399

Mood
disorders 1557
disturbance of 1546, 1547
elation of 1558
stabilizers 1582
Morbid anatomy 138
Morphea 748
Morphine 140, 904
Morphology 417, 418, 424, 426, 432, 440
life cycle 421, 429, 430
pathogenesis 429
Mosaic wart 1502
Motilin 474, 1589
Motion sickness 121
Motor activity 1558, 1559
Motor denervated bladder 1465
Motor disturbances 1555
Motor functions 1289
Motor impersistence 1400
Motor neuron disease 1430, 1473
Motor polyneuropathy, acute 353
Motor predominant 1454
Motor symptoms 1563
Motor system
disease 1430
examination of 1300
Mountain sickness
acute 111
chronic 113
Mouth
disease 356, 480
dryness of 475
Movement disorders 1350, 1482, 1495
drug-induced 1405
Moxifloxacin 54
Mucocutaneous lymph node syndrome 756
Mucopolysaccharides 1487
Mucor 1361
Mucormycosis 1362
Mucous membrane lesions 275
Muehrcke's nails 1540
Multiceps multiceps 441
Multicystic dysplastic kidneys 1246
Multifocal atrial tachycardia 865
Multifocal leukoencephalopathy 293, 1361
Multiple personality 1564
Multiple systems atrophy 1395
Mumps 338, 937, 1075, 1361
Munro microabscess 1512
Murine typhus 265
Murmurs 797
Murphy's sign 563
Muscle 749, 1592
action potential, compound 1304
biopsy 1311, 1312
disease 1472
inflammatory 761, 1479
tests for 1311
problems 1482
stretch reflexes 1301
training 1041
Muscular atrophy, progressive 1432
Muscular dystrophy 933
classification of 1476
congenital 1475, 1477
diagnosis of 1475
distal 1478
Musculoskeletal
system 638
tissue 860
Mushroom poisoning 143
Myasthenia 1473
congenital 1468
gravis 1466, 1468
diagnosis of 1469
in pregnancy 1471
Myasthenic crisis 457
treatment of 1471
Myasthenic reactions 1472
Myasthenic syndrome, congenital 1468
Mycetoma 383
Mycobacterial infections, atypical 294
Mycoplasma 1075
hominis 284
pneumonia 979, 1075

Mycosis fungoides 1159
Myelin, role of 1425
Myelitis 333
Myelodysplastic syndrome 1131
Myelofibrosis 1161
causes of secondary 1163
primary 1161
Myeloid leukemia
acute 1117
chronic 1122
Myeloid metaplasia 1161
Myeloma 450, 1141
evolution of 1138
genetics of 1138
multiple 786, 1075, 1138, 1264, 1494
staging of 1141
variant forms of 1143
Myelomatosis 1138
Myelomonocytic leukemia
acute 1118
chronic 1127
Myelopathy 731, 1444
compressive 1441, 1451
Myelophthisic anemia 1071
Myeloproliferative disorders 1160
Myiasis 90
Myoadenylate deficiency 1479
Myocardial disease 938
Myocardial infarction 900, 901
acute 898
classification of 900
Myocardial involvement 294
Myocardial ischemia 1413
Myocardial scanning 801
Myocardial stunning 902
Myocarditis 916
acute 916
chronic 917
Myocardium, diseases of 916
Myoclonic epilepsy
progressive 1383
severe 1381
Myoclonic jerks 1382
Myoclonus 1366, 1377, 1403
Myopathy 933, 1484, 1493
secondary 761
Myositis 1473
Myotome 1439
Myotonia 1473
congenta 1478
Myotonic disorders 1478
Myotonic dystrophy 934, 1478
Myxedema 671, 751, 1473
coma, treatment of 672
madness 671
Myxomas 943

N

N-acetylcysteine 1000
NADH oxidation, defects of 1485
Naegleria gruberi 1357
Nail 857, 1498, 1587
changes 1064
diseases of 1536
disorders of 1534
half 1540
infection 1506
psoriasis of 1513, 1537
Nailfold capillaroscopy 750
Naja bangarus 96
Naja hanna 96
Naja naja 96
Nakayama yoken strain 373
Nalorphine 539
Naloxone 1570
Naltrexone 1570
Narcoanalysis 1584
Narcolepsy 1572
Narcotics 140
Nasal diphtheria 224
Natalizumab 1428
Nateglinide 590
National Institute of Virology 361
National Leprosy Control Program 319
National Leprosy Eradication Program 319

Natriuretic peptides, role of 804
Natural immunity, active 37
Natural killer cells 25
Nausea 475
Near reflex 1319
Nebulizers 989
Necator americanus 417
Necrobiosis lipoidica diabeticorum 614
Necrolytic migratory erythema 1541
Necrotizing fasciitis 208, 608, 614
Necrotizing myelopathy 1444
Necrotizing ulcerative gingivitis, acute 483
Needle biopsy 1312
Negative phenomena 1453
Neglect syndromes 1296
Negligent adverse event 45
Neisseria gonorrhoeae 278
Neisseria meningitides 219, 1363
Nelson's syndrome 653, 690
Neologism 1547
Neonatal
alloimmune thrombocytopenia 1180
diabetes mellitus 601
gonococcal conjunctivitis 280
infection 236, 286
myasthenia gravis 1468
seizures 1381
thrombocytopenia 1179, 1180
Neoplasia 1265
Neoplasms 1071
malignant 1071
Neoplastic cells, characteristics of 70
Neoplastic syndromes 1375
Neorickettsia 267
Neostigmine injection test 1469
Nephritic syndrome 1221
acute 1212, 1220
Nephrogenic diabetes insipidus 443, 1249
Nephrolithiasis 1213, 1256
Nephron 1208
Nephronophthisis 1245
Nephropathy, contrast-induced 948
Nephrotic syndrome 1212, 1220, 1221, 1285
Nerve
biopsy 1313
conduction 1304
disease, peripheral 1454
of arnold 1331
of hering 1330
peripheral 584
problems 1482
roots, diseases of 1439
stimulation studies 1468
Nervous involvement 1145
Nervous system 344, 730, 742, 1288, 1344,
1349, 1589
damage to 527
in pregnancy 1495
peripheral 1026
Netilmicin 50, 51
Neural mechanisms 884
Neuralgia 1453
Neuralgic
amyotrophy 1457
headache 1343
Neuraminidase inhibitors 57
Neurilemmoma 1420
Neurinoma 1420
Neuritic leprosy, pure 316
Neuro lupus 742
Neuroacanthocytosis 1405
Neurocirculatory asthenia 934
Neurocysticercosis 425
treatment of 425
Neurodegenerative disorders 1310
Neuroendocrine 1267
Neurofibroma 1420
Neurofibromatosis 1458
peripheral 1458
Neurogenic
dysphagia 1482
pulmonary edema 356
Neurohumoral activation 810
Neurohumoral alterations 804
Neuroleptic malignant syndrome 199

Textbook of Medicine

Neuroleptics 1580
Neuroleukemia 1114
Neurologic disorders 933
Neurologic manifestations of liver disease 1490
Neurological causes 1334
Neurological complications 100, 324, 329, 333,
    1451, 1492, 1494
Neurological cretins 670
Neurological disorders 1037, 1307, 1381, 1592
Neurological examination 1294
Neurological investigations 1294
Neurological lesions 356
Neurological manifestations 293, 1139
Neurological system 1366
Neuroma 1420
Neurometabolic disorder 1483
Neuromuscular junction, function of 1466
Neuromyelitis optica 1428
    spectrum disorders 1425
Neuromyopathy, critical illness 1493
Neuromyotonia 1453
Neuron specific enolase 71
Neuronal cell 453
Neuronal ceroid lipofuscinosis 1383
Neuronal plasticity 1292
Neuroparalytic syndromes 144
Neuropathic arthritis 785
Neuropathic ulcers 1532
Neuropathology 1347, 1555
Neuropathy
    critical illness 1457
    drug-induced 1456
    peripheral 293, 1368, 1454, 1459, 1493
Neuroprophylaxis 1115, 1117
Neuropsychiatric manifestations 1238
Neurosyphilis 1353
    diagnosis of 1354
    treatment of 1354
Neurotensin 474
Neutralizing antibodies 1188
Neutropenia 1049
    diagnosis of 1136
    idiopathic benign 1049
    severe 1135
Neutropenic patients 62
Neutrophil 1048
    counts, alteration in 1049
    leukocytosis 1049
Neutrophilic leukemia, chronic 1123
Neutrophils
    functional defects of 1049
    functions of 1048
New immune strategies 1117
New therapeutic regimens 1121
Newer antiamyloid treatment studies 1147
Newer antiplatelet drugs 913
Newer drugs 392, 507
Nezelof's syndrome 33
Niacin 175, 1345
Niclosamide 425
Nicorandil 911
Nicotinamide 175
Nicotine replacement therapy 152
Nicotine-related disorders 1571
Nicotinic acid 175, 1345, 1346
Nicotinic receptor partial agonists 152
Nifedipine 892
Night terror 1572
Nightmare 1572
Nikolsky sign 1524
Nilotinib 1125
Nipah virus 327
    encephalitis 1361
Nitazoxanide 250
Nitrates 904, 911, 914
Nitrofurantoin 54
Nitrosoureas 76
Nocardia 382
    brasiliensis 383
Nocardiosis 383
Nocturia 1212
Nocturnal diarrhea 614
Nodular encephalitis 1359
Noise 119
    pollution 120

Nonalcoholic fatty liver disease 553
Nonanticoagulants rodenticides 134
Nonanticytokine BRMs 789
Nonatopic asthma 985
Noncardiogenic pulmonary edema 389
Non-cholera vibrios 250
Noncirrhotic portal fibrosis 551
Non-communicable disease burden, chronic 4
Non-compressive myelopathies 1444
Noncoronary vascular interventions 947
Nondysenteric amebiasis 407
Non-enzyme peptides 97
Nonepileptic seizure 1384
Nonfluent aphasia, progressive 1372
Non-freezing cold injury 107
Nongonococcal genital infections in women 281
Nongonococcal infections in
    children 281
    infants 281
Nongonococcal urethritis 280
Non-heme iron 181
Non-Hodgkin's lymphoma 1153, 1154, 1159
Noninfantile neuronopathic Gaucher's
    disease 1383
Noninflammatory arthritis 727
Noninsulin parenteral therapeutic agents 597
Noninsulin-dependent glucose 587
Noninvasive insulin delivery methods 596
Noninvasive tests 491
Nonisotopic tests 660
Nonlymphocytic leukemia, acute 1117
Nonmetastatic syndrome 1495
Nonmotor manifestations 1392
Nonmyeloablative transplants 1116
Non-nephrotic proteinuria, fixed 1221
Nonobstructive pyelonephritis, acute 1252
Nonparalytic polio 353
Non-polio enteroviruses 1360
Non-Rh hemolytic anemias 1078
Nonsecretory myeloma 1138, 1144
Nonseptic cerebral venous thrombosis 1414
Nonskeletal manifestations 148
Nonsteroidal anti-inflammatory drugs 448, 734,
    1284, 1286
    related hematemesis 734
Nonsulfonylurea secretagogues 590
Nontuberculous mycobacteria 298, 312
Non-typhoid Salmonella infections 233
Non-uremic renal osteodystrophy 1239
Non-Wilsonian cerebral degeneration 1491
Noonan's syndrome 939
Normoblasts 1200
Norovirus infections 251
Norwalk viruses 250
Norwalk-like agents 251
Norwegian scabies 1508
Novartis 1125
Novel target visualization 1322
Novel therapeutic approaches 991
Novel therapies 1262
Nuclear angiocardiography 801
Nuclear explosion, dangers of 118
Nuclear imaging 902
Nuclear medicine techniques 86
Nuclear winter 118
Nucleoproteins 7
Nucleus ambiguous, rostral part of 1330
Nummular eczema 1520
Nutraceuticals 779
Nutrient solutions 504
Nutrition 154, 156, 1042, 1591
Nutritional amblyopias 1349
Nutritional anemia, causes of 1070
Nutritional deficiencies 1438
Nutritional disorders 916, 1344
Nutritional inadequacy 1063
Nutritional megaloblastic anemia 1067
Nutritional recovery syndrome 1349
Nutritional science 154
Nutritional status 154
    maintenance of 1235
Nystagmoid movements 1324
Nystagmus 1324
    congenital 1324
Nystatin 58

O

Obesity 186, 457, 582, 636, 884
    hyperventilation syndrome 1016
Obeticholic acid 555
Objective vertigo 1329
Obliterative cardiomyopathy 920
Obsessive compulsive disorders 1562
Obsessive phobia 1562
Obsessive-compulsive personality disorder 1567
Obstruction 1017
    jaundice 527, 528, 937
Obstructive lesions 818, 819
Obstructive lung disease, chronic 997
Obstructive nephropathy 1259
Obstructive pulmonary disease, chronic 937,
    996, 1001, 1042
Obstructive shock 814
Obstructive sleep apnea 937, 1017, 1018, 1492
    syndrome 1015
Obstructive uropathy 1273, 1284
Occipital lobe epilepsies 1380
Occipital paroxysms 1380
Ochronosis 628
Octreotide 549, 652
    long-acting release 652
Ocular lesions 629
Ocular manifestations 639
Oculocephalic reflex 1335
Oculomotor nerve palsy 1322
Oculo-orogenital syndrome 175
Odland bodies 1497
Odynophagia 475
    causes of 485
Oestrus 90, 91
Ofatumumab 1130
Offspring, complication in 1383
Ofloxacin 54
Ogilvie's disease 513
Ogilvie's syndrome 367
Oil drop sign 1513
Olfactory nerve 1316
Oligodendrogliomas 1420
Oligosaccharides 1487
Oligosecretory myeloma 1144
Oligospermia 706
Oliguria 1212
Olmesartan candesartan 892
Omalizumab 991, 994
Omega-3 fatty acids 622
Onchocerca volvulus 432
Onchocerciasis 439
Oncogenes 68
Oncogenic osteomalacia 714
Oncogenous osteomalacia 71
Oncology 67
Oncomelania 430
Oncoproteins 68
Onco-suppressor genes 69
Ondine's curse 1335
Onyalai 145
Onychomycosis 1536
Oophoritis 338
Opaque nerve fibers 1320
Open biopsy 1311
Open mitral valvotomy 843
Operative cholangiography 563
Ophthalmic herpes 335
Ophthalmic myiasis 91
Opioids 140
Opioids-related disorders 1570
Oppenheim's sign 1301
Opsoclonus 1324
Optic atrophy 1320, 1354
    secondary 1320
Optic disk pallor 1367
Optic fundus, examination of 1335
Optic nerve 1316, 1317
Optic neuritis 1320
Optical coherence tomography 946
Oral
    antidiabetic drugs 589
        classification of 589
    cancer 484
    cinacalcet 681

corticosteroid therapy, short-course 989
hairy leukoplakia 483
mucosa 484
submucous fibrosis 481
Orally administered drugs 40
Orbital lymphoma, female with 1155
Orchitis 338
Organic acid 1487
metabolism, defects of 1485
Organic causes 702
Organic disorders 1558
Organic laryngeal paralysis, causes of 976
Organic mental disorders 1552
Organic reflexes 1301
Organism, isolation of 322
Organochlorine insecticides 132
Organophosphorus compounds 130
Ornithodoros lahorensis 258
Ornithodoros tholozoni 258
Orofacial granulomatosis 481
Oropharyngeal
anthrax 240
candidiasis 1505
dysphagia 485
causes of 485
infections 279
Oroya fever 253
Orthopnea 792, 964
Orthostatic
hypotension 894, 1462
intolerance 895, 1462
proteinuria 1214, 1221
tremors, primary 1404
Oseltamivir 57, 324
Osler's disease 1163
Osler's nodes 857
Osmolality, disorders of 466
Osmolar gap 461
Osmole 465
Osmometer 465
Osmoreceptors 442
Osmosis 465
Osmotic demyelination 464
Osmotic equilibrium, disturbances of 464
Osmotic fragility of erythrocytes 1056
Osteitis
deformans 780
fibrosa 1239
Osteoarthritis 732, 777
Osteoarthrosis 777
Osteogenesis imperfecta 629, 782
Osteomalacia 172, 1239
Osteomyelitis 215, 221
variolosa 331
Osteoporosis 648, 769, 770, 789
localized 770
primary 770
secondary 770
Osteosclerotic myeloma 1144
Ostium
primum defect 823
secundum 823
Otitic barotrauma 109
Otogenic reflex cough 962
O-toluidine blue 476
Ovarian cancer antigen 71
Ovarian failure 708
primary 709
secondary 708, 709
Ovarian function 708
Ovarian hormonal disorders 708
Overlap syndrome 752
Overt nephropathy 612
Ovulatory dysfunction 706
Oxamniquine 431
Oxantel pamoate 419
Oxcarbazepine 1387, 1582
Oxybutinin 1428
Oxygen 904
therapy 1000
Oxytocin 643
Oxyuriasis 420

P

Pacemaker implantation, temporary 947
Packed cell volume 1059
Paget's disease of bone 780

Pain 78, 1595
management 78
chronic 1482
Painful cranial neuropathies 1339
Painful thyroiditis 673
Painless thyroiditis 673
Palatal tremor 1404
Palindromic rheumatism 739
Palinopsia 1298
Palla's sign 925
Palliative care 78, 1596
Pallidotomy 1394
Palmar erythema 537, 1545
Palmomental reflex 1301
Palmoplantar psoriasis 1513
Palmoplantar pustular psoriasis, chronic 1513
Pamidronate 77, 766
Pancoast's syndrome 1022
Pancoast's tumor 1022
Pancreas 579, 582
artificial 596
diseases of 565
isotopic scanning of 566
Pancreatic
disorders 499
function tests 565
polypeptide 474
transplants 596
Pancreatitis 338, 566
acute 566
Pancreolauryl test 566
Pancytopenia, congenital 1091
Paneth cells 471
Panhypopituitarism, adult 653
Panic disorder 1561
Panic episode 1578
Pantothenic acid 176, 1346
Papanicolaou's staining 966
Papanicolaou's method 1023
Papillary dermis 1497
Papillary fibroelastomas 944
Papillary muscle dysfunction 903
Papillary necrosis 1285
Papilledema 1320, 1367, 1418
Papular dermatitis of spangler 1545
Papulosquamous disorders 1511
Paracentesis 532
Paracetamol 140
Paracoccidioides 1362
Paradoxical aciduria 447
Paradoxical embolism 828
Paradoxical split 797
Parainfluenza 326
Parakinesia 1400
Paralytic form 363
Paralytic polio 353
Paramyotonia 1478
Paraneoplastic 1375
limbic encephalitis 1374
pemphigus 1524
syndromes 71, 1025
Paranoid 1556
personality disorder 1567
Paraphilias 1573
Paraplegia in
extension 1447
flexion 1447
Paraproteinemias 1182
Paraproteinemic neuropathies 1456
Parasite
detection 398
life cycle of 385, 395
malignancy of 428
Parasitic infections 1354
Parasitology 405
Parasomnias 1572
Parasylvian 1300
Parasympathetic system 1461
Parathormone 450, 676
actions of 677
Parathyroid 676, 678
diseases 785
disorders 676
function, tests of 677
hormone 676, 677, 772
actions of 677
hyperplasia 715, 716

Paratonia 1291
Paratyphoid fever 233
Parenteral iron 1066
side effects of 1066
Parenteral nutrition 162, 392, 504
Parenteral routes 40
Paresthesias 1301, 1453
Parietal lobe 1296, 1318
epilepsies 1380
Parietal pain 476
Parkinson's disease 1391
disorders 1391
Parkinsonian syndromes 1395
Parkinsonian tremors 1404
Parkinsonism syndromes 1398
Paromomycin 399
Paronychia 1536
acute 1536
Parosmia 1316
Parotid enlargement, causes of 480
bilateral 480
Paroxysmal atrial tachycardia 865
Paroxysmal dyskinesia, part of 1399
Paroxysmal hemicranias, chronic 1342
Paroxysmal nocturnal
dyspnea 792, 964
hemoglobinuria 1095
Paroxysmal tachycardias 864
Parrot's fever 320
Parrot's nodes 276
Parry's disease 664
Partial pressure of oxygen 121
Partial seizures 1380, 1381
Parvovirus 374
infection 376, 377
Paschen bodies 330
Passive immunization 350, 351, 364
Passive induced immunity 37
Passive natural immunity 38
Passive smoking 151
Patau's syndrome 17
Patch test 1521
Patent ductus arteriosus 827, 947
Patent foramen ovale 947
Pathological fibrinolysis 1193
Pathological nystagmus 1324
Pathological tremors 1403
Paton's lines 1320
Paul-Bunnell test 375
Peak expiratory flow rate 960
Pectus carinatum 1035
Pectus deformities 1035
Pectus excavatum 1035
Pediatric autoimmune neuropsychiatric disorders 32
Pediculidae 94
Pediculosis 1509
capitis 1509
corporis 1509
pubis 1509
Pediculus humanus
capitis 94
corporis 94, 257
Pedophilia 1573
PEEP sign 1467
Pegvisomant 652
Pegylated interferon 58
Peliosis hepatis 558
Pellagra 176, 1345
sine pellagra 176
Pelvic infection 236
Pemberton's sign 664
Pemphigoid gestationis 1545
Pemphigus
drug-induced 1524
erythematosus 1524
foliaceus 1524
neonatorum 215
vegetans 1524
vulgaris 1523
Pendred syndrome 671
Pendulum breathing 1036
Penicillin 47
adverse effects of 277
Penicilliosis 294
Pentamidine isothionate 382

Index

Textbook of Medicine

Pentavalent antimonials 399
Pentostatin 1129, 1131
Pentosuria 618
Pepper pattern in skull 1239
Peptic esophagitis 488
Peptic ulcer 490, 491
Peptic ulceration
    acute 490
    chronic 490
Perception, disturbances of 1555
Perchlorate discharge tests 662
Percutaneous biopsy 1312
Percutaneous coronary intervention 900, 914
Percutaneous left ventricular assist device 947
Percutaneous transluminal coronary angioplasty 906
Pergolide 650
Pericardial aspiration 923
Pericardial disease 294, 938
Pericardial effusion 922
Pericardiectomy 924
Pericardiocentesis 947
Pericarditis 902
    acute 921
    constrictive 923
Pericardium, diseases of 921
Perineal warts, large 1502
Perinephric abscesses 1255
Periodic alternating nystagmus 1324
Periodic fevers 199
Periodic paralysis 457, 639, 934
Peripheral nervous system, diseases of 1453
Peripheral neuropathy, causes of 1454
Peripheral vesicles 1525
Peritoneal dialysis 1280
    adequacy of 1281
    automated 1281
Peritoneoscopy 479, 526
Peritoneum, diseases of 518
Peritonitis 519
    acute 519
    chronic 519
    in cirrhosis 532
    secondary 532
Permanent pacemaker implantation 946
Pernicious anemia 1069
Persistent delusional disorders 1557
Persistent vegetative state 1337
Personal prophylaxis 249
Personality
    changes 1567
    disorders 1567
    factors 1568
    tests 1551
    type A 934
    type D 934
Pertussis infections 223, 225
Pervasive developmental disorders 1576
Petit mal 1382
Petroleum products 141
Peutz-Jeghers syndrome 495, 509, 1534
Phagocytes, deficiency of 33
Phagocytic function 1168
Phagocytosis, defective 1049
Pharmacotherapy 548
Pharyngeal diphtheria 224
Pharyngitis 974
Pharyngoconjunctival fever, acute 357
Phenformin 460, 591
Phenoxybenzamine 890
Phentolamine 890
Phenylketonuria 627
Pheochromocytoma 694, 716, 936
    multisystem crisis 695
Philadelphia chromosome 1107, 1122
Phlebothrombosis 902, 1592
Phlebotomus papatasi 369
Phobia, simple 1561
Phobic anxiety disorders 1561
Phoma sorghina 145
Phosphate homeostasis 442
    disorders of 451
Phosphide poisoning 132
Phosphodiesterase inhibitors 1000
Phosphonoformate 56
Phosphorus 180

Phosphorylase B deficiency 1479
Photochemotherapy 1514
Photosensitive
    dermatitis 1522
    drug reaction 1530
Photostress test 1317
Phototoxicity 1522
Phrynoderma 1348
Phthirus 94
Physical activity, resumption of 909
Physical examination 495, 507, 638, 793, 806, 910,
        913, 932, 965, 1003, 1022, 1029, 1176, 1551
Physical inactivity 582
Physiological changes 710, 1587
Physiological functions of liver 523
Physiological nystagmus 1324
Physiological proteinuria 1214
Physiological reward theory 1568
Physiological skin changes in pregnancy 1544
Physiological tremor, enhanced 1403
Pickwickian syndrome 1016
Piece meal vision 1298
Pierre marie's three paper test 1299
Pigeon chest 1035
    deformity 171
Pigment casts 1216
Pigment gallstones 528
Pigmentation
    disorders of 1533
    of tongue 484
Pineal body 657
Pineal gland 657
    disorders 657
Pineal tumors 1421
Pinworm 420
Pioglitazone 591
Pipecolic acid 1487
Piperaquine 392
Pironella conica 429
Pit vipers 96
Pitless vipers 96
Pituitary
    anterior 646
    apoplexy 1493
    Cushing's syndrome 689
    disorders 641
    fossa tumors 1421
    gland 641
    hormones, ectopic secretion of 649
    hyperfunction 649
    tumor of 649, 1493
Pityriasis rosea 1516
Pityriasis versicolor 1507
Plague 239, 241
Plantar warts 1502
Plasma
    cell
        dyscrasias 1137
        leukemia 1138, 1143
        proliferative disorders, classification of 1137
    exchange 1203, 1470
    lipids 951
    protein binding 42
Plasmacytoma 1140
Plasmapheresis 1100, 1455
Platelet 1053, 1170
    adhesion, tests for 1173
    aggregometry 1173
    antigenicity of 1170
    count 723, 1202
        even women with 1180
    disorders 1174
    dysfunction 1238
    function 1181
        acquired disorders of 1182
    functional disorders, treatment of 1182
    groups 1098
    plug, formation of 1170
    transfusion 1099, 1100
    ultrastructure of 1170
    vascular diagnosis 1175
Plateletpheresis 1100
Platinum complexes 76
Platybasia 1449
Pleiotropy 13

Pleura 955
    diseases of 1028
    tumor of 1032
Pleural biopsy 968
Pleural effusion 1028
    bilateral 457
    malignant 1022
Pleural friction rub 966
Pleural shock 1031
Pleurisy 1028
    etiology of 1028
Pleuropericardial sounds 966
Pleuropulmonary amebiasis 981, 983
Plexopathy 1454
Plexuses, diseases of 1439
Plumbism 146
Plummer-Vinson syndrome 484
Plus minus sign 1467
Pneumococcal infection 216, 1085
    treatment of 219
Pneumococcal meningitis 218
Pneumococcal peritonitis 219
Pneumococcal pneumonia 217
Pneumoconiosis 1005
    types of 1006
Pneumocystis jirovecii
    infection 381
    pneumonia 290
Pneumomediastinum 1040
Pneumonia 209, 221, 236, 357, 977, 978
    nonspecific 979
Pneumonic plague 242
Pneumothorax 1032
Podoconiosis 437
Podophyllin resin 286
Podophyllotoxin 75, 286
Poems syndrome 1144
Poikilocytosis 1056
Poisoning
    acute 124
    prognosis of 127
Poisonous snakes, identification of 96
Poisons 130
    classification of 124
Polioencephalitis 353
Poliomyelitis 352, 457, 1443
Poliovirus 1359
Poly hill sign 1473
Polyarteritis nodosa 755, 935, 1263
Polycystic kidney disease 1244
Polycystic ovary syndrome 709
Polycythemia 71
    causes of secondary 1164
    rubra vera 1163
    secondary 1165
    vera 1165, 1494
Polydipsia, primary 644
Polyendocrinopathy 718
Polyene antibiotics 55
Polyglandular autoimmune syndrome 717
    type 1 717
    type 2 718
Polymerase chain reaction 19, 231, 322, 1311
Polymicrobial bacterial ascites 532
Polymorphism, restriction site 19
Polymyalgia rheumatica 755
Polymyositis 760, 761, 1479
Polymyxin B 55
Polyneuropathy 337, 1454
Polyopia 1298
Polyostotic fibrous dysplasia of bone 705
Polyphagia 636
Polysomnography 1303
Polyuria 636, 1212
Pomalidomide 1142
Pompholyx 1520
Poncet's disease 732
Poncet's syndrome 302, 787
Pontiac fever 254
Pontine hemorrhage 1416
Porch index of communicative ability 1299
Pores of kohn 954
Porphyria 625
    cutanea tarda 626
Portacaval anastomosis 550

Portal hypertension 545
  in cirrhosis 546
  signs of 546
Portal hypertensive
  colonopathy 548
  enteropathy 550
  gastropathy 548
Portopulmonary syndrome 550
Posaconazole 58, 59
Positive inotropes 812
Post kala-azar dermal leishmaniasis 400
  of brahmachari 400
Postencephalitic parkinsonism 1397
Postexposure prophylaxis 297, 364
Post-gonococcal urethritis 281
Posthepatitis syndrome 346
Postherpetic neuralgia 335, 1343
Posthyperventilation apnea 1335
Postinfectious measles encephalitis, acute 329
Postinfective polyneuropathy 1454
Post-lumbar puncture headache 1343
Postmitotic maturation pool 1048
Postobstructive diuresis 445, 1275
Postpartum blues 1573
Postpartum psychiatric disorders 1573
Postpartum psychosis 1573
Postpartum thyroiditis 661, 674
Postpolio syndrome 354
Postprimary tuberculosis 300
Postrenal failure 1233
Poststreptococcal glomerulonephritis 214, 1223
Post-traumatic stress disorder 1565
Postural drainage 983
Postvaccinal encephalitis 332
Postviral encephalomyelitis 1360
Potassium
  channel antibodies 1369
  homeostasis 442
    disorders of 446
  perchlorate 667
Potential favorable effects 894
Poverty of thinking 1547
Pradhan's sign 1474
Pralidoxime hydrochloride 131
Pramlintide 598
Prasugrel 913, 1185
Praziquantel 425, 429, 431
Prazosin 890, 915
Prebiotics 475
Precancerous lesions 72
Precocious puberty 637, 704
Precordial pain 793
Precordium, examination of 806
Prediabetes, diagnosis of 579
Predisposing to infection 238
Pre-eclampsia 1271, 1495
  management of 1271
Pre-excitation syndrome 867
Pre-exposure immunization 364
Pregnancy 278, 335, 650, 736, 745, 747, 840,
    939-942, 1274, 1544
  associated diseases 1495
  complicating aids 296
  first trimester of 1383
  high-risk 940
  indicators of high-risk 940
  mask of 1544
  plaques of 1545
  specific dermatoses of 1545
Pregnant asthmatic 993
Pregnant patients 277
Pregnant women, active rubella in 337
Prehemorrhagic phase 361
Preherpetic neuralgia 335
Premature ejaculation 1573
Premature ovarian insufficiency 709
Prenatal diagnosis 19
Prenatal management 1077
Prescription of drugs 46
Presinusoidal 546
Pressure hydrocephalus, normal 1370, 1424
Pressure natriuresis 1269
Presystolic gallop 797
Prevention-vaccination 219
Prevotella 284

Priapism 1084
Primary tumor, location of 1022
Primordial T-cells 1051
Principal cells 446
Prinzmetal's angina 914
Prion disease 1373
Prion protein disease 1374
Prion transmitted diseases 1376
Probable tuberculous meningitis 1352
Probenecid 776
Producing stomatocytosis 1080
Prognostic factors, unfavorable 1112
Progressive ataxia, chronic 1437
Prolactin 647
  inhibitory factor 647
Prolactinomas 650
Prolonged fever, causes of 198
Prolymphocytic leukemia 1131
Promyelocytic leukemia, acute 1110, 1118, 1206
Pronephros 1207
Propagation of clot 1171
Propantheline 1428
Prophylactic
  antibiotics 62
  management 1386
  measures 1084
  treatment 280
Prophylaxis 239, 326, 334, 350, 364, 418, 517,
    860, 1026, 1067
  active 228
  antibiotic regimen for 860
  long-term 549
  primary 1188
  secondary 213, 927
  treatment and 285, 556
Propranolol 868, 1341
Propylthiouracil 667
Prosopagnosia 1298
Prostacyclin 1014
Prostaglandin 712, 1211
  clinical uses of 713
Prostate specific antigen 71
Prostatitis, chronic 281
Prosthetic valves 942
Protease inhibitors 295, 1000
Proteasome 77
  inhibitors 1142
Protein 587, 1310
  absorption of 473
  binding 42
  C 1172
  digestion of 473
  energy malnutrition 163, 1349
  metabolism 522
  S 1172
  utilization 157
Proteinuria 1214, 1221
  fixed 1214
  functional 1221
  significant 1221
Proteolytic enzymes 473
Proteomic 11
  account on 11
  finger printing methods 304
Proteus infections 234, 239
Protodiastolic gallop 797
Protozoal diseases 384, 1075
Proximal neuropathy 1456
Prozone effect 649
Prurigo gestationis 1545
Prurigo of pregnancy 1545
Pruritic urticarial papules 1545
Pruritus 1539
  vulvae 614
Prussian blue stain 1093
Pseudobulbar palsy 1332
Pseudocholinesterase in serum 131
Pseudodementia 1368, 1553, 1559
Pseudodystonias 1400
Pseudogout 776
Pseudohemophilia 1190
Pseudohermaphroditism 707
Pseudohyperphosphatemia 181
Pseudohyponatremia 443
Pseudohypoparathyroidism 683, 1493

Pseudolym 1150
Pseudolymphoma 1159
Pseudomembranous colitis 252
Pseudomonas 234
  aeruginosa 238
Pseudomyxoma peritonei 520
Pseudopseudohypoparathyroidism 684
Pseudothrombocytopenia 1175
Pseudotumor cerebri 1424
Pseudoxanthoma elasticum 1538
Psittacosis 319, 320
Psoriasis 1511
  treatment of 1515
  vulgaris 1512
Psoriatic arthritis 732
Psoriatic arthropathy 767
Psychiatric conditions 1569
Psychiatric disorders 934, 1334, 1575, 1576
  in adolescence 1576
  in childhood 1576
  management of 1579
Psychiatric emergencies 1577
Psychiatric patient, clinical examination of 1550
Psychiatric pharmacotherapy 935
Psychiatric problems 1484
Psychiatric symptoms 638
Psychiatry 1546
  evolution of 1546
Psychoanalysis, principles of 1583
Psychoanalytic psychotherapy 1583
Psychogenesis 1563
Psychogenic
  blindness 1321
  causes 702
  dwarfism 656
  fevers 199
  headache 1343
  tremors 1404
Psychological changes 1592
Psychological development, disorders of 1576
Psychological methods of treatment 1583
Psychological testing 1551
Psychometry 1551
Psychosocial treatment 1557
Psychosomatic disorders 1574
Psychosurgery 1580
Psychotherapy 1559, 1561, 1583
Psychotropic drugs, abnormal reactions to 1578
Pteroylglutamic acid 177
PTH resistance syndrome 683
Ptyalism 475
Puberty
  causes of delay in 703
  delayed 637, 703
Puerperal psychosis 1573
Pulfrich phenomena 1317
Pulmonary angiography 967
Pulmonary arterial hypertension 1014
  causes of 1014
Pulmonary arteriovenous fistula 836
Pulmonary artery 829
Pulmonary blood flow
  increased 819
  reduced 818
Pulmonary circulation 955
Pulmonary collapse 1005
Pulmonary compliance 958
Pulmonary complications 982
Pulmonary cysts 1026
Pulmonary diseases 122
Pulmonary edema 1012, 1031
  acute 1012
  chronic 1013
  emergency treatment of acute 813
Pulmonary embolism 857, 902, 924, 1413
Pulmonary eosinophiliosis 995
Pulmonary fibrosis 1010
Pulmonary function 959
  tests 959
Pulmonary hypertension 937, 1084
Pulmonary infections 237
Pulmonary manifestations 1021
Pulmonary mechanics 958
Pulmonary physiology 956
Pulmonary rehabilitation 1000, 1041, 1042

Textbook of Medicine

Pulmonary response 815
Pulmonary stenosis 822
Pulmonary thromboembolism 1013
Pulmonary tuberculosis, complications of 302
Pulmonary tumors, isotopic localization of 967
Pulmonary valve, acquired lesions of 854
Pulmonary vasculature abnormalities 841
Pulmonary wedge pressure 801
Pulsatile devices 812
Pulsating empyema 1031
Pulse oximetry 838
Pulseless disease 929
Pulsus
    alternans 794
    paradoxus 794
    parvus 794, 848
Pulvinar sign 1375
Pump handle test 765
Pupil 1319, 1335
    abnormal 1320
Pupillary dilatation, relative afferent 1319
Purgatives 126, 539
Purpura over palate 1177
Purpuric disorders 1173
Pursuit system 1322
    abnormalities of 1322
Purulent conjunctivitis 221
Pustular psoriasis 1513
    of pregnancy 1513
Putaminal hemorrhage 1416
Pyelonephritis 1255
    acute 1250, 1273
Pyloric obstruction 496
Pyloric stenosis 446
    congenital 496
Pyoderma 1500
    gangrenosum 1531
    primary 1500, 1501
    secondary 1500
Pyogenic thyroiditis 673
Pyramidal dysfunction 1377
Pyramidal signs 1367
Pyramidal tract syndrome 1442
Pyrantel pamoate 416, 418
Pyrethroid
    exposure, effects of 133
    poisoning 133
Pyrexia 197
Pyridoxine 176, 1346
    dependency, congenital 1346
Pyrimethamine 412
Pyrrolizidine alkaloids 558
Pyruvate kinase deficiency 1081
Pyruvate metabolism, defects of 1485
Pyuria 1250

Q

Q fever 263, 267
    acute 267
    chronic 267
Quantitative sudomotor axon reflex test 1464
Quetiapine 1395
Quinagolide 650
Quincke needle 1308
Quinidine 868
Quinine 393
Quinolones 54
Quinupristin-dalfopristin 53

R

Rabies 361, 1360
    diagnosis, rapid 363
Rachitic rosary 171
Radiation hazards 948
Radiation sickness 74
Radiation syndrome, acute 115
Radiation therapy, adverse effects of 938
Radioactive iodine uptake test 660
Radioactive rain 118
Radiocontrast agents 1285
Radiofrequency ablation 561, 947
    catheter 868
Radioimmunotherapy 74
Radioiodine treatment 668

Radioisotopic investigations 967
Radiosensitivity 73
Raloxifene 772
Ramp movements 1399
Rampant caries 482
Ramsay-Hunt syndrome 1328
Ranolazine 912
Rational therapeutics 45
Raven's progressive matrices test 1551
Raynaud's phenomenon 120, 741, 749
    secondary 749
Rayport clamp 1311
Reactions, treatment of 318
Reactive arthritis 768
Readiness potential 1289
Reaven's syndrome 619
Rebound nystagmus 1324
Recombinant tissue plasminogen activator,
    dose of 1412
Rectum 476
Recurrent acute cystitis 1252
Recurrent aphthous ulcer 480
Recurrent ataxia, acute 1437
Recurrent infection 1254
Recurrent lesions 1503
Recurrent severe hypoglycemia 604
Recurrent vaginitis 614
Red blood cell 1059, 1487
Red cell
    aplasia in children 1092
    aplasia, pure 377, 1092
    enzymopathies 1080
    indices 1056
    membrane 1046
        disorders 1079
    plasmalogens 1487
    production 1044
Red flag signs 506
Red pulp 1168
Reduvid bugs 403
Referred headache 1343
Referred pain 476
Reflex epilepsy 1383
Reflex eye movements 1335
Refractive errors 610
Refractory ascites 531
Refractory cardiac failure 813
Refractory cases, relapse of 1143
Refsum's disease 1438
Regional enteritis 506
Regulatory peptides 473
Regurgitant lesions 818
Rehabilitation 167, 1569
    in neurology 1481
Rehydration therapy 248
Reinfection 1250
Reiter's syndrome 768, 1516
Relapse, treatment of 233, 1117
Relapsing fevers 253, 257
Relapsing-remitting type 1426
Relaxation techniques 1041
Renal abscesses 1255
Renal artery stenosis 937
Renal biopsy 1219, 1234
Renal causes 770
Renal cell carcinoma 1246
Renal changes 98
Renal complications 1143, 1269
Renal cystic neoplasms 1246
Renal damage 774, 1284
    drug-induced 1284
Renal denervation 893
Renal disease 344, 937, 1212, 1213, 1269,
    1272, 1492
    intrinsic 1267
Renal disorders 786
Renal dysfunction
    causes of 1240
    treatment of complications of 1240
Renal failure 101, 389, 527, 1139, 1286
    acute 144, 1070
    chronic 1070, 1212
Renal glycosuria 1247
Renal hormones 884
Renal hypertension 894

Renal indices 1233
Renal infarction 857
Renal involvement 731, 1084, 1270
Renal lesions 583, 1265
    classification of 742
Renal manifestations 679
Renal parenchymal hypertension 1268
Renal replacement therapies, continuous 1279
Renal replacement therapy 1235, 1276
Renal response 815
Renal stones, types of 1257
Renal sympathetic denervation 947
Renal symptoms 540
Renal system 1588
Renal transplantation 1272
    complications of 1283
Renal tubular acidosis 446, 1248
    distal 460
Renal tubules
    diseases of 1242
    functional disorders of 1247
Rendu-Osler-Weber syndrome 1184
Renin angiotensin system, alteration in 804
Renin-angiotensin 1211
    system 1266
Renovascular disease 1267
Repaglinide 590
Reperfusion 909
Repetitive nerve stimulation 1469
Replacement fibrosis 1010
Reproductive system 666
Reserpine 890
Resistant hypertension 893, 1269
    causes of 893
Resistant malaria, new drug for 393
Respiratory
    acidosis 452, 457
    alkalosis 452, 458
    centers 1335
    chain diseases 20
    diseases 937, 962, 966
    distress syndrome 972
        acute 971
    effort related arousal 1016
    failure 968
        acute 1491
        causes of 969
        chronic 971, 1492
        type I 969
        type II 969
        type III 969
        type IV 969
    lesions 356
    manifestations 1239
    physiotherapy 1041
    re-education 1041
    symptoms 1560
    syncytial virus 326
    syndrome
        middle east 327
        severe acute 326
    system 244, 290, 730, 741, 953, 1588, 1592
    tract 323, 1145
        procedures 860
Restarting warfarin after bleeding 1198
Restless leg syndrome 1405
Restrictive cardiomyopathy 917
    classification of 920
Reticular dermis 1497
Reticulocyte count 1055
    corrected 1055
Reticulocyte proliferation index 1056
Retigabine 1388
Retina
    changes in 887
    macula 1320
Retinal lesions 1318
    inner 1318
Retinoids 168
Retinol 168
Retinopathy 583
Retrograde pyelography 1219
Retroperitoneal fibrosis 520
Retroviral syndrome, acute 290
Retroviruses 1361

Rett syndrome 1405
Revascularization procedures 912
Revised National Tuberculosis Control Programme 306
Rexed laminae 1439
Reye's syndrome 332, 562
Rh incompatibility 1076
Rhabdomyomas 944
Rhabdomyosarcomas 944
Rhagades 276
Rhesus system 1098
Rheumatic aortic stenosis 847
Rheumatic chorea 211
Rheumatic fever
    acute 209
    prophylaxis 843
Rheumatic heart diseases 952
Rheumatic manifestations 212
Rheumatic syndromes 762
Rheumatoid arthritis 727, 788, 935, 1262
    variants of 737
Rheumatoid disease, therapy of 736
Rheumatoid disorders 719
Rheumatoid factor 723, 731, 762
Rheumatoid nodules 730
Rheumatological disorders 721, 1075
Rhinitis 973
Rhinocerebral mucormycosis 608
Rhinophyma 1511
Rhinosporidiosis 381
Rhipicephalus 94
    sanguineus 267
Rhodnius 404
Rhonchi 965
Ribavarin 57, 175, 327, 361
Richter's syndrome 1129
Richter's transformation 1129
Rickets 170
Rickettsia akari 267
Rickettsia mooseri 265
Rickettsia prowazekii 263
Rickettsia typhi 265
Rickettsial diseases 263
Rickettsial pox 267
Riedel's thyroiditis 674
Rifabutin 55
Rifampicin 55, 318, 410
Rifapentine 55
Rifaximin 504, 539
Right isomerism 837
Right ventricular
    infarction 909
    physiology 792
Rigid spine syndrome 1474
Rilonacept 775
Rimantadine 57, 324
Rinne's test 1329
Ristocetin cofactor activity 1190
Ritter's disease 215
Rituximab 788, 1130, 1179
Rivaroxaban 914
Rivastigmine 1371, 1395
Road accidents 121, 122
    injuries caused by 123
Rockall scoring system 497
Rocky mountain spotted fever 267
Rodenticides 134
Roflumilast 1000
Rogers sign 1326
Rolandic epilepsy, benign 1382
Romaña sign 404
Romiplostim 1055, 1179
Rorschach Test by Hermann Rorschach 1551
Rosacea 1509, 1511
Rosenbach's sign 1334
Rossolimo's sign 1301
Rotablator 946
Rotavirus 250
Roth's spots 857
Routine blood counts 723
Roxithromycin 51
Rubella 937, 1075, 1361
    congenital 1361
    embryopathy 337
    in adults 337
    in baby, congenital 337
    syndrome, congenital 337

Rufinamide 1388
Rugger jersey spine 1239
Russel's viper 96
    venom 1174
Rusven-clotting time 1174
Ruxolitinib 1163, 1166
Rytand's murmur 851

S

Sabre tibia 276
Saccadic system 1321
Saddle nose 276
Salaam spasm 1382
Salaam seizures 1381
Salazopyrin 52, 735
Salbutamol 992
Salicylate 460
Saline 469
Salivary glands, inflammation of 480
Salmonella 142
    enteritidis 143, 233
    infections 228
        prevention of 233
    typhimurium 143, 233
Salt and water
    intake 884
    retention 1285
Salt balance 1240
Salt depletion heat exhaustion 105
Sarcoglycanopathy 1473
Sarcoidosis 450, 786, 935, 1008
Sarcomas 944
Sarcopenia, age-related 1587
Sarcophaga 90, 91
Saw-scaled viper 96
Saxagliptin 591
Scabies 1507
Scalded skin syndrome 215
Scalene fat pad biopsy 1024
Scalp psoriasis 1513
Scarlet fever 208
Schaefer's sign 1301
Schirmer's test 1464
Schistocytes 1200
Schistosoma haematobium 430, 431
Schistosoma japonicum 430
    infection 431
Schistosoma mansoni 430
    infection 431
Schistosomiasis 413, 430
Schizoaffective disorder 1557
Schizoid personality disorder 1567
Schizophrenia
    classification of 1556
    disorders 1554
Schizophrenic thought disorders 1555
Schmidt's syndrome 1331
Schwabach's test 1329
Schwartzman phenomenon 221
Scleredema Adultorum Buschke 751
Scleredema diabeticorum 614
Scleroderma 748, 935
    localized 748
Scleromalacia perforans 730
Sclerosing cholangitis, primary 534
Sclerosing panencephalitis, subacute 329, 1360
Sclerosis
    multiple 1425, 1427, 1438
    primary lateral 1433
Scopophilia 1573
Scorpion 92
Scrombotoxicity 144
Scrotal tongue 484
Scrub typhus 266
Scurvy 178
Sea snake 97
    bites 99
Seat worm 420
Sebaceous glands 1497
Seborrheic dermatitis 1519
Seborrheic keratoses 1542
Secondary delusion 1548
Secondary drowning 113
Secondary drug resistance 306

Secondary gout 773
Secondary granules 1048
Second-generation drugs 905
Secretin 471, 474
Sedative drug poisoning 136
Segmental bronchi 954
Seizures
    in stroke 1412
    unclassified 1380
Selenium 186, 1349
Sella syndrome, empty 657
Semantic dementia 1372
Semen analysis, normal 706
Senear-Usher syndrome 1524
Senile plaques 1370
Senile purpura 1184
Sensations, abnormal appreciation of 1301
Sensorimotor peripheral neuropathy 1026
Sensory 1454
    assessment 1325
    denervated bladder 1465
    system 1291, 1301
Sentinel headache 1415
Sepsis 62, 236, 1413
    shock 202
Septal defects, atrioventricular 828
Septic cerebral venous thrombosis 1413
Septic shock 202
Septicemic plague 242
Seriously ill patients, treatment of 514
Serologic diagnosis 503
Serological tests 231, 276, 408, 723, 724, 1220, 1234
    frequency of 276
Seronegative spondyloarthritis 789
Seronegative spondyloarthropathy 763, 764
Serotonin reuptake inhibitors 935, 1582
Serpent worm 440
Serum 452, 455
    albumin 526
    alkaline phosphatase 525
    bilirubin 525
    calcium 1218
    cholesterol 525, 1218
    complement levels 724
    cortisol 687
    creatinine 1217
    electrolytes 1217
    gamma glutamyl transpeptidase 534
    late 101
    sickness 33
    uric acid 724
Serum-free light chain estimation 1140
Sevelamer carbonate 1241
Sevelamer hydrochloride 1241
Sex chromosomal disorders 17
Sex chromosome 7
    related disorders 13
    trisomy of 18
Sex hormones 687
    abnormalities of 690
Sexual act 702
Sexual characters, secondary 638
Sexual differentiation, disorders of 711
Sexual dysfunction 1239, 1462, 1573
Sexual function
    abnormalities of 671
    disturbances of 637
Sexual masochism 1573
Sexual maturation, disorders of 637
Sexual medicine 703
Sexual precocity 704
Sexual preference, abnormalities of 1573
Sexual sadism 1573
Sexually transmitted
    diseases 273
    viral diseases 284
Sézary's syndrome 1159, 1160
Shanchol 249
Shank sign 1474
Sheehan's syndrome 653
Sheep liver fluke 428
Sheep-cell agglutination 375
Shigella 143, 234
    boydii 234
    dysenteriae 234

Textbook of Medicine

flexneri 234
infections 234
sonnei 234
Shirokampam 1391
Shock 125, 814
classification of 814
distributive 814
hypovolemic 814, 816
therapy 1579
wave lithotripsy 564
Shohl's solution 461, 1248
Short course chemotherapy 304
Short stature, causes of 655
Short wavelength automated test 1317
Shoulder pad sign 1145
Shoulder-hand syndrome 763, 903
Shunt lesions, left-to-right 823
Shy-Drager syndrome 895
SIADH
causes of 645
diagnosis of 468
Sialadenitis 480
Sialidosis 1383
Sialorrhea 1435
Sick sinus syndrome 879
Sickle cell
anemia 786, 1082, 1494
disease 1082
Sickling crises 1083
Sideroblastic anemia 1093
Siderosis 183
Sigmoidoscopy 512
Sildenafil 702, 752, 835, 1015
Silicosis 1006
Silver
beaten appearance 1424
sulfadiazine 52
Sinecatechins 286
Single-chain antibodies 1117
Sinoatrial block 874
Sinus
arrest 874
arrhythmia 862, 1463
bradycardia 863
of Valsalva, aneurysms of 932
tachycardia 863
venosus type of defect 823
Sinusitis 974
complications of 975
Sister-Joseph's nodules 520
Sitagliptin 591
Situation-related seizures 1381
Sixth cranial nerve palsy 1323
Sjögren's syndrome 738, 1262
secondary 739
Sjögren-Larsson syndrome 1444
SK therapy, complications of 905
Skeletal abnormalities-renal osteodystrophy 1238
Skeletal fluorosis 147
Skeletal manifestations 637, 679
Skeletal muscle 453
changes in 666
Skeletal survey 1060
Skeletal symptoms 1084
Skeleton-fusimotor fibers 1290
Skin 730, 749, 1496, 1544, 1587, 1591, 1592
blood vessels 1461
care of 1337
changes 537, 636
in pregnancy, biological 1544
decontamination of 125
functions of 1498
glands of 1497
infected 860
infection of 238, 1500
infestations 1507
involvement purpura above eyelids 1146
lesions 106, 275, 740
snip 231
structure of 860, 1496
tumors 1542
benign 1542
Skull, salt pattern in 1239
Slapping gait 234
Sleep apnea 457
mild 1016
severe 1016

Sleep disorders 1571
Sleep disturbances 1589
Sleep walking (somnambulism) 1572
Sleeping sickness 402
Slow channel syndrome 1468
Slow-rising pulse 794
Small intestine, diseases of 499
Smallpox 330
Smokeless tobacco 151
Smoking 150, 727
and women 151
cessation of 951, 999
on asthma, effect of 992
Smooth-muscle antibodies 526
Smouldering multiple myeloma 1143
Smudge cells 1128
Snake bite 96
Snake venom, composition of 97
Sneeze 955
Snout 1301
Social phobia 1561
Sodium 442
nitroprusside 891
valproate 1372
Soft chancre 283
Soft neurological signs 1555
Soft sore 283
Soft tissue infections 236
Solar urticaria 1526
Solitary thyroid nodule 675
Somatic complaints, multiple 1596
Somatic symptoms 1559
Somatoform disorders 1563, 1564
Somatomammotropin group of hormones 646
Somatomedin-C 647
Somatosensory evoked
potentials 1338
responses 1305
Somatostatin 474, 549, 642
receptor ligands 652
Somatotropin-mammotropin group 646
Somatotropin-releasing inhibiting hormone 642
Somnambulism 1564
Soothing agents 1499
Sorafenib 77, 561
Soroche, chronic 113
Sotalol 868
South American hemorrhagic fevers 359
Sparfloxacin 54
Sparganosis 441
Sparganum mansoni 441
Sparse hair 1539
Spastic dysarthria 1300
Spastic gait 1302
Special senses 1592
Specific fungal infections, treatment of 59
Spectinomycin 53
Spectrum of disease 553, 1016
Spectrum penicillins, extended 48
Speech
and language 1299
disorders 1300
Spelling dyslexia 1298
Spherocytes 1200
Spider angioma 1545
Spider nevi 537
Spinal accessory nerve 1331
Spinal artery, anterior 1442
Spinal cord
diseases of 1439
injury 457, 1482
parts of 1288
syndromes 1441
Spinal epidural abscess 1444
Spinal muscular atrophy 1434
Spinal shock 1447
Spinal subarachnoid hemorrhage 1415
Spine X-ray 1445
Spinocerebellar ataxia 1436
Spinothalamic tract involvement 1440
Spiramycin 51, 52, 413
Spiroindolone 393
Spironolactone 448
Spleen 857, 1145
disorders 1167
functions of 1167
Splenectomy 1179

Splenic sequestration syndrome 1083
Spondyloarthritis, undifferentiated 769
Spondyloarthropathies 935
Spontaneous bacterial peritonitis 532
Spontaneous hypotension headache 1343
Spontaneous pneumothorax 1032
Spontaneous subarachnoid hemorrhage 1176
Sporadic goiter 664
Sporadic motor system disorders, classification of 1430
Sports injury 783
Spotted fever group 266
Spurious hemoptysis 962
Sputum 962, 966
examination 302, 966, 1023
Squamous cell 1020
carcinoma 487
St. Louis encephalitis virus 1360
Stable angina
chronic 910
pectoris 910
Stamping gait 1302
Standard nutrition tables 158
Staphylococcal bacteremia 215
Staphylococcal food poisoning 142, 215
Staphylococcal infections, diagnosis of 215
Staphylococcal pneumonia 215, 978
Staphylococcus aureus 142, 214
Staphylococcus epidermidis 216
Staphylococcus saprophyticus 216
Stasis eczema 1520
Stasis ulcer 1531
Statin myopathy 1479
Statistical manual of mental disorders 1551
Status epilepticus 457, 1381, 1383, 1389
Steatorrhea 500
Steinert's dystrophy 1478
Stein-Leventhal syndrome 709
Stem cell 1292
transplantation 1088, 1102, 1428, 1143
peripheral 1112
Stent thrombosis 900
Stenting of coarctation 822
Step-down therapy 889
Stereotactic limbic leucotomy 1580
Stereotactic tractotomy 1580
Stereotypy 1405, 1549
Sternberg's cells 1148
Steroid 992, 1470
courses of 1428
hormone secretion 685
synthesis pathway 685
therapy 100
management of 65
striae, female long-term 1181
withdrawal syndrome 65
Steroid-resistant asthma 993
Stevens-Johnson syndrome 1529
Stiff person syndrome 1405
Still's disease 737
Stimulatory hypersensitivity, type V 30
Stinging fishes 95
Stokes-Adams attacks 793
Stomach 470
abnormalities of 499
carcinoma of 495
diseases of 489
Stone disease 1259
Storage pool disease 1181
Strachan's syndrome 1348
Straight back syndrome 1035
Stransky sign 1301
Stratum basale 1496
Stratum corneum 1497
Stratum granulosum 1497
Stratum spinosum 1496
Street virus 361
Streptococcal bacteremia 208
Streptococcal gangrene 208
Streptococcal impetigo 208
Streptococcal infections 207
Streptococcal myositis 208
Streptococcal pharyngitis 208
Streptococcal toxic shock syndrome 209
Streptococcus agalactiae 209
Streptococcus pneumoniae 216, 1363

Streptococcus viridans 209
Streptococcus, group B 209
Streptomycin 50
Stress 1461, 1555
    disorder, acute 1565
    dosing 693
    reaction to 1563
    reticulocytes 1083
    test 799
Stretch reflex 1290
Striae distensae 1538
Striae gravidarum 1545
Strict bed rest 213
String of pearl 1525
Stroke 933, 1084, 1406, 1408
    anterior circulation 1409
    classification of 1406
    diagnosis of 1408
    posterior circulation 1409
    prevention of 1416
    syndromes 1409
Stroke-related complications, treatment of 1412
Strongyloides stercoralis 419
Strongyloidiasis 419
Strontium ranelate 772
Struvite stones 1258
Stupor 1333, 1578
Subarachnoid hemorrhage 1414
Subclinical hypothyroidism 672
Subcortical aphasia 1300
Subcortical dementia 1372
    mixed 1372
Subcutaneous nodules 210, 212
Subdiaphragm cistern 657
Subdural hematoma 1422
    chronic 1369
Subjective vertigo 1329
Sublingual dose 904
Sublingual mucosa 40
Subsultus tendinum 229
Subtle facial palsy 1328
Sucking 1301
Suicide 1577
    attempted 1577
Sulfadoxine 52
Sulfasalazine 735, 766
Sulfinpyrazone 776
Sulfisoxazole 410
Sulfonamides 52
Sulfonylurea compounds 589
Sulkowitch test 678
Sumatriptan 1341
Summation gallop 797
Sunatinib 77
Sunburn 1522
Sunscreens 1500
Sunstroke, first aid for 104
Superior sulcus tumor 1022
Supportive psychotherapy 1584
Suppression tests 678
Suppressive therapy 286
Suppressor cells 1051
Suppressor function 26
Suppurative infections 215
Supranuclear palsy, progressive 1396
Supraventricular tachycardia, management of 867
Sural nerve biopsy 1313
Suramin 439
Surgery, emergency 494, 498
Surgery, timing of 829
Surgical lung biopsy, absence of 1012
Surgically active stone disease 1257
Swan neck deformity 729
Sweat glands 1461
Sweat test 1463
Sweating 1462
Sweet syndrome 1132
Swimmer's itch 431
Swinging flashlight test 1319
Sycosis barbae 214, 1501
Sycosis nuchae 1501
Sydenham's chorea 211, 1401
Sylvian fissure 1299
Symmetrical neuropathy, distal 1456
Symmetrical polyneuropathy 730
Sympathetic nervous system 1266

Sympathetic system 1460
    activation 587
Sympathomimetic drugs 990
Symptomatic hemolytic anemia 1076
Symptomatic hyponatremia, acute 469
Symptomatic iron deficiency anemia 1065
Symptomatic management during attack 627
Symptomatic myoclonus 1403
Symptomatic purpura 1184
Synacthen stimulation 692
Syncope 793
Syndrome X 619
Synesthetic hallucination 1548
Synovial biopsy 726
Synovial fluid 779
    analysis 726
    aspiration 731
    examination 724
Syphilis 274, 278, 936
    clinical types of 274
    congenital 274, 275
    infective endocarditis 1075
    late 275, 277
    secondary stage of 275
    serodiagnosis of 276
    stage of 274
    treatment regimen for 277
Syphilitic deafness 1354
Syphilitic pemphigus 275
Syphilitic pseudoparalysis 276
Syphilitic wig 276
Syringobulbia 1446
Syringoma 1543
Syringomyelia 1446
Systemic corticosteroids 311, 735
Systemic disease 120, 709, 784, 1027, 1260,
    1270, 1334, 1456
    cardiac manifestations of 933
Systemic fungal infections 377
Systemic hypertension 881, 883
Systemic illness 1009
Systemic immune complex disease 33
Systemic lupus erythematosus 448, 739, 745,
    788, 935, 1274
    symptomatology in 742
Systemic manifestations 750
Systemic medical disorders 1574
Systemic reactions 93
Systemic responses in fever 195
Systemic rheumatologic disorders 935
Systemic sclerosis, progressive 748, 1263
Systemic steroid-sparing therapies 994
Systemic vasculitis 752
Systolic heart failure 805

T

T- and B-cells, interaction between 1053
Tabes dorsalis 1354
Tabes mesenterica 508
Tabetic crises 1354
Tachycardia
    atrioventricular
        junctional 865
        nodal reentrant 865
        reentrant 866
    prevention of 868
Tacrine 1371
Taenia solium 425
Taeniasis saginata 423
Taeniasis solium 424
Tafenoquine 392
Takayasu's arteritis 755, 929, 935, 1264
Takotsubo cardiomyopathy 919, 920
Takotsubo syndrome 939
Tall stature, causes of 651
Tamoxifen 78
Tandem mass spectrometry 1487
Tandem transplantation in myeloma 1143
Tapir's mouth 1473
Taspoglutide 598
Tauopathies 1395
Taxene group 75
T-cell
    function and migration 1052
    origin 1149

T-cell-mediated hypersensitivity reaction, type IV 30
Teardrop heart 936
Tecarfarin 1196
Teicoplanin 53
Telbivudine 57, 348
Teletherapy 73
Telmisartan 892
Telogen 1535
Temporal arteritis 754
Temporal encoding 1482
Temporal lobe 1318
    epilepsies 1380
Temporomandibular arthritis 729
Tenecteplase 906
Tennis elbow 763
Tenofovir 57
    disoproxil fumarate 348
Tensilon test 1469
Tension headaches 1342
Tension pneumothorax 1032
Tenth cranial nerve 1330
Tentorium cerebelli 1435
Teratospermia 706
Terazosin 890
Terbinafine 58, 59
Teriparatide 789
Terlipressin 549
Terry's nails 1540
Testicular failure, adult 699
Testicular leukemia 1114
    treatment of 1117
Tetanus 268, 269
    antitoxin 271
    local 270
    neonatorum 270
Tetany 171, 638
    treatment of 684
Tetracycline 51
Tetralogy of Fallot 831
Thalamic hemorrhage 1416
Thalamotomy 1394
Thalassemia 1085
    facies 1086
    intermedia 1085
    major 1085
    minima 1085
    minor 1085
    pathophysiology of 1085
    syndromes 1081, 1088
Thalidomide 766, 1142
Theophylline 1000
Therapeutic foods 165
Therapeutic index 40
Therapeutic modalities in rheumatology 787
Thermal injury 118
Thermoregulation 1461
Thiabendazole 420, 440
Thiamine 174, 1344
    deficiency, diagnosis of 175
Thiazide 459
    diuretics 645
Thiazolidinediones 555, 591
Thinking, disturbance of 1546
Thiocarbamides 667
Third-generation drugs 905
Thomsen's disease 1478
Thoracic cage, injuries to 1036
Thoracoscopy 968
Thorborn's sign 1441
Thought
    and speech 1559
    block 1547
    broadcast 1548, 1555
    deprivation 1548
    insertion 1548, 1555
    stopping 1585
    withdrawal 1555
Thought/talk 1558
Threadworm 420
Thrombin time 1174
Thrombocythemia, essential 1166
Thrombocytopathy 1181
Thrombocytopenia 231, 332, 337, 1494
    causes of 1175
    secondary 1181

Textbook of Medicine

Thrombocytosis 1494
causes of 1166
Thromboembolic pulmonary hypertension, chronic 925, 1013
Thrombolytic agents 906
classification of 905
Thrombolytic therapy 905, 906, 926
Thrombophilia 1204
Thromboplastin time, partial 1174
Thrombopoiesis-stimulating 1179
agents 1179
Thrombopoietin 1054
stimulating protein 1055
Thrombotic thrombocytopenic purpura 1202, 1494
Thunderclap headache 1343
Thyroid 658
acropachy 666
autoantibodies, demonstration of 661
crisis 669
disorders 658, 785, 1539
function 660
tests 660
tests abnormalities 661
hormone
actions of 659
resistance syndrome 673
medullary carcinoma of 676
peroxidase antibody 1374
scintiscanning 661
storm 668
tumor of 675
Thyroid-associated eye disease 665
Thyroiditis 673
acute suppurative 673
chronic 674
drug-induced 673
subacute 673
Thyroid-stimulating hormone 646
Thyrotoxic
crisis 668
ophthalmopathy 1473
Thyrotropin releasing hormone 474, 642
Thyroxine deficiency 1070
Tiagabine 1388
Tic douloureux 1325
Ticagrelor 913, 1185
Tick 94
paralysis 94
Tick-borne
relapsing fever 258
typhus 266
Ticlopidine 1185
Tidal percussion 965
Tidal volume 959
Tigecycline 51
Tiger snake 96
Tinea barbae 1504
Tinea capitis 1504
Tinea corporis 1504
Tinea cruris 1504
Tinea faciale 1504
Tinea manuum 1505
Tinea pedis 1505
Tinea unguium 1505
Tinea versicolor 1507
Tinidazole 55, 408
Tirofiban 913
Tissue
factor pathway inhibitor 1172
invasion 428
myiasis, deep 91
nematodes 432
plasminogen activator 906
alterations in 952
polypeptide specific antigen 71
serrulatus 92
Tizanidine 1428
T-lymphocytes 25, 1052
TNM descriptors 1024
Tobacco
chewing 151
workers 153
Tobacco-related diseases 150
Tobramycin 50, 51
Tocilizumab 736

Tocopherol 1347
Todd's paralysis 1386
Tofacitinib 736
Tolcapone, dose of 1394
Tongue
atrophy of 484
diseases of 480, 483
Tonic-clonic seizures 1381
Tonsillitis
acute 974
chronic 974
Tophaceous gout, chronic 774
Topiramate 1387
Topographagnosia 1298
Toremifene 78
Torsade-de-pointes 872
Torsemide 459
Torture 1566
Torulosis 380
Total dose infusion 1066
Total health value of food 158
Toxic 1456
adenomas 669
chemicals 1090
diffuse goiter 664
effect 1110
epidermal necrolysis 215, 1529
megacolon 512, 513
shock syndrome 215
Toxic/metabolic 1425
Toxicity
acute 169
chronic 169
Toxin 142, 1392
of staphylococci 214
reduce absorption of 125
Toxin-mediated lesions 214
Toxoplasma gondii 411
Toxoplasmosis 405, 411, 1356
congenital 411
in AIDS 412
in pregnancy 412
treatment of 413
Tracheal obstruction 977
Tracheostomy 272
Tractus solitarius 1326
Tranexamic acid 1188, 1193
Tranquilizers, minor 1582
Transarterial chemoembolization 561
Transarterial radioembolization 561
Transbronchial needle aspiration 1009
Transcellular fluid 442
Transcobalamin II, congenital deficiency of 1070
Transcranial Doppler 1306
test 1338
Transcranial magnetic stimulation 1304
Transcriptase inhibitors, reverse 295
Transcriptase polymerase chain reaction, reverse 329
Transesophageal echo 82
Transference neurosis 1584
Transferrin 182
receptor 182
Transformed bladder 1465
Transformed migraine 1341
Transfusion
indications for 1098
therapy, hazards of 1100
transmitted infections 1101
Transient erythroblastopenia of childhood 1093
Transient ischemic attack 1406
Transient myeloid disorder of infancy 1122
Transient proteinuria 1214
Transjugular intrahepatic portosystemic shunt 1490
Translocational hyponatremia 443
Transmagnetic stimulation 1579
Transmission
electron microscopy 1216
mode of 243
prevention of 1375
Transmyocardial laser revascularization 912
Transplacental transfer 42
Transplacental transmission 411
Transretinoic acid 77, 1110
Transthyretin-related amyloidosis 1147
Trans-tubular K+ gradient 446
Transudate, causes of 1030
Transudative effusion 1030

Transverse myelitis 1443
Trasylol 1194
Trazodone 1372
Treatment failure, management of 549
Trematode infections 428
Tremors, essential 1404
Trench fever 254
Treponema pallidum 274
immobilization 276
pertenue 255
Treprostinil 751
Triatoma 404
magista 404
Trichinellosis 421
Trichinosis 421
Trichoepithelioma 1543
Trichomonas vaginalis 283
Trichomoniasis 283
Trichuriasis 418
Triclabendazole 429
Tricuspid atresia 834
Tricuspid regurgitation 854
causes of primary 854
Tricuspid stenosis 853
Tricuspid valve lesions 853
Tricyclic antidepressants 935, 1581
Trifluridine 56, 57
Trigeminal autonomic cephalalgias 1341
Trigeminal nerve 1324
Trigeminal neuralgia 1325, 1343
Trigeminal neuropathy, bilateral 1326
Trimethoprim 52
Triose-phosphate deficiency 1081
Triplet repeat expansion disorders 15
Triradiate pelvis 171
Trisomy 16
13 17
18 17
Trochlear nerve palsy 1323
Trombicula deliensis 266
Trombone tremor 1353
Tropheryma whipplei 503, 767, 1376
Trophic factors 1402
Trophy sign, calf head on 1474
Tropical pancreatitis 615
Tropical pulmonary eosinophilia 995
Tropical pyomyositis 215
Tropical splenomegaly syndrome 390, 1169
Tropical sprue 503, 1490
Trotter's triad 1326
True hermaphroditism 707
True precocious puberty 704
Trypanids 402
Trypanosoma brucei 402
gambiense 402
Trypanosoma gambiense 402
Trypanosomiasis 384
Tryponosomal chancre 402
Trypsin 473
TSH-receptor antibodies 661
Tsutsugamushi fever 266
Tubeless pancreatic function tests 566
Tuberculin skin test 304
Tuberculoid leprosy 313
Tuberculosis 298, 508, 614, 936
abdominal 507
in HIV positive patients, treatment of 308
of mesenteric lymph nodes 508
prevention of 309
primary 300
Tuberculous 1352
disease 1351
exposure 1351
meningitis 310, 1351, 1352
pleural effusion 1031
Tubular necrosis, acute 1273
Tubular obstruction 1232
Tubular proteinuria 1214, 1221
Tubulointerstitial nephritis 1242
chronic 1243
Tumor 72, 658
benign 1019, 1369
cells, destruction of 26
demonstration of 679
in thorax 1022
kinetics 72

localization of 695
lysis syndrome 1265
malignant 1019
markers 70
necrosis factor 1000
primary 1420
secondary 1420
suppressor genes 11
Tumorigenesis 70
Tunga penetrans 95
Turiya avastha 1333
Turner's syndrome 18, 939
Twelfth cranial nerve 1331
Twenty-nail dystrophy 1537
Typhoid
cholecystitis 564
fever 228
nodules 229
state 229
Typhus exanthematicus 263
Tyrosine kinase inhibitors 1117
Tzanck smear 333

U

Udenafil 703
Ulcerohypertrophic forms 508
Ulcers 490
Ulcus molle 283
Ullrich congenital
muscular dystrophy 1474
myopathy 1474
Unarmed tapeworm 423
Undernutrition, types of 164
Underweight 164
mild 164
moderate 164
severe 164
Undulant fever 243
Uninhibited bladder 1465
Universal health coverage 3
Unstable angina pectoris 912
Unstable diabetes 598
Unverricht-lundborg disease 1383
Upper respiratory tract, diseases of 973
Urea cycle disorders 1437
Ureaplasma urealyticum 284
Uremic acidosis 452, 460
Uremic bleeding, treatment of 1241
Uremic encephalopathy 1492
Uremic lung 1239
Uremic renal osteodystrophy 1239
Uremic toxins, circulating 1238
Ureteric bud 1207
Ureterosigmoidostomy 460
Urethra, distal 1250
Urethritis, nonspecific 280
Uric acid 1218
stones 1257
Uricolytic drugs 775
Uricostatic drugs 775
Uricosuric agents 775
Urinary
anion gap 452, 455, 456
bladder, control of 1461
calcium 678
calculi 637
casts 1216
cyclic adenosine-3', 5'-monophosphate 678
hydroxyproline 678, 771
myiasis 91
phosphate 678
system 1207
tract 1207
anatomy of 1250
defense mechanisms of 1250
fungal infections of 1256
infection 236, 612, 1243, 1250, 1273
infection, complicated 1250, 1253
obstruction 1213, 1274
Urinary-free cortisol 687
Urine
avoids stasis, unobstructed flow of 1250
culture 231
role of 1250
examination 1140, 1213

Urokinase 906
Urologic investigations 1220
Ursodeoxycholic acid 564
Urticaria 1526
Urticarial
acute 1526
drug reactions 1530
treatment of 1527
vasculitis 1526
Ustekinumab 1515
Uterine bleeding, dysfunctional 710
Uterine dysfunction 706

V

Vaccination 250, 251, 325, 337, 360, 1187
indications for 351
Vaccine 233, 297, 339
against hepatitis E virus 351
immune globulin 332
Vaccinia gangrenosum 332
Vaccinology 38
Vacuolar myelopathy 293
Vagabond's disease 94
Vagal nerve 1330
stimulation in epilepsy 1390
Vagus nerve 1330
Valganciclovir 376
Valley sign 1473
Valproate 1582
Valsalva test 1463
Valsartan 892
Valvulae conneventes 471
Valvular heart disease 938, 946
causes of chronic 839
chronic 838
Valvular pneumothorax 1032
Vancomycin 53, 252
Vanillyl mandelic acid 71
Vanishing pulmonary tumor 1029
Vaptans 468
Vaquez's disease 1163
Vardenafil 703
Varenicline 152
Variable vessel vasculitis 759
Variant angina 914
Variceal bleeding, management of 548
Varicella 332, 1075, 1377
during pregnancy 333
gangrenosa 333
pneumonia, primary 333
Varicella-zoster
immune globulin 334
virus 1359
Varicose ulcer 1531
Variegate porphyria 626
Varilrix 334
Variola major 330
Variola minor 330, 331
Variola sine eruption 331
Vascular access
for hemodialysis 1277
routes for coronary interventions 945
Vascular changes 583
Vascular cognitive impairment 1416
Vascular dementia 1373, 1416
Vascular disease 294
peripheral 609
Vascular disorders 509, 1174
Vascular endothelial growth factor 1311
Vascular lesions of cerebellum 1438
Vascular phenomena 537
Vascular purpura 1183
drug-induced 1184
Vasculitic disorders, frequency distribution of 753
Vasculitic neuropathy 1456
Vasculitis 749, 935, 1531
causes of secondary 753
Vasoactive intestinal polypeptide 71, 471, 474
Vasodilator 891
drugs 816
Vasogenic cerebral edema 1363
Vasomotor
dysfunction 814
rhinitis 973
symptoms 710, 1462

Vasopressin 549, 1464
analogues 645
excess 645
Vasopressor drugs 816
Vegetable oil increases bioavailability 1348
Vein of Galen 1289
Vein thrombosis, deep 122, 1412
Velcade 1143
Vena cava
filter, inferior 947
obstruction, superior 938
Venezuelan hemorrhagic fever 359
Venom 97
Veno-occlusive disease of Jamaica 145
Venous drainage 1289, 1440
Venous filters 928
Venous pulsation 1320
Venous strokes 1406
Venous thromboembolism 513, 924
Venous thrombosis 938, 1095
Ventilation 327
assistance to 970
imaging 967
imbalance in 958
perfusion abnormalities 958
regulation of 956
Ventilator-associated pneumonia 977
Ventilatory assistance 992
indications for 993
Ventilatory impairment, severe 987
Ventricular assist devices 812
Ventricular asystole 878
Ventricular encephalitis 1359
Ventricular fibrillation 873
Ventricular premature beats 864
Ventricular septal defect 825, 947
Ventricular standstill 878
Ventricular tachycardia 872
Ventriculectomy, partial left 812
Venturi mask 970
VEP abnormalities, basis of 1305
Verapamil 868, 892
Vergence system 1322
Vernet syndrome 1331
Verocytotoxin 236
Verruca 1501
plana 1502
Verruga peruana 253
Vertebral column causing neurological lesions, diseases of 1448
Vertebrobasilar ischemia 1451
Vertebroplasty 1143
Vertigo 1329, 1595
causes of 1329
Vesiculobullous 1528
disorders 1523
Vessel vasculitides, small 756
Vessel vasculitis, large 754
Vestibular system 1328
Vestibulocochlear nerve 1328
Vibrio fetus 251
Vibrio parahaemolyticus 143
Vidarabine 56, 57
Vigabatrin 1388
Vigorous achalasia 487
Vildagliptin 591
Villus adenoma 509
Vim-Silverman needle 968
Vinca alkaloids 75
Vincent's angina 483
Vincent's spirochetes 483
Vincristine 1142
Viper 96
bites 98
Viperidae 96
Viral
antigens 322
diarrhea, causes of 251
diseases, prevention of 322
hepatitis 339
B in pregnancy 349
B, acute 349
diagnosis of 346
inclusions, demonstration of 322
infections 321, 323, 1075, 1501

Index

Textbook of Medicine

morphology 341
multiplication 321
spread 321
Virtual neck exploration 680
Virus 70, 322, 360
fixed 362
isolation 324
Visceral larva migrans 422
Visceral leishmaniasis 397
Visceral pain 475
Visceral syphilis 275
Viscosupplementation 779
Vision 1588
poor 1320
Visual evoked potential 649, 1305
Visual field 1317
defect 1367
Visual illusion 1298
Visual or cerebellar disturbance 1377
Visuospatial function 1366
Vital capacity 960
Vital signs 1334, 1587
Vitamin 473
A 168, 1348
deficiency, causes of 168
toxicity 169
B_1 174
deficiency 1344
B_{12} 177, 1347
absorption 501
B_2 175
B_3 175, 1345
B_5 1346
B_6 1346
B_7 176, 1346
B_9 1346
C 1347
adverse effects of 179
deficiency 1070
in health, major roles of 178
D 169, 1348
dependent rickets type i 172
metabolites 170, 1211
resistant rickets 172
E 173, 1347
deficiency 1437
H 176
K 173
antagonists 1196
deficiency 173, 1192
Vitiligo 636, 1534
Vivax malaria, uncomplicated 392
Vocal cord paralysis, causes of 976
Voglibose 592
Voltage gated potassium channel 1374
Voltage-dependent channels 861
Vomiting 475, 485
von Graefe's sign 1328
von Hippel-Lindau syndrome 1438

von Willebrand's disease 1190
genetic transmission of 1190
Voriconazole 58, 59
Voyeurism 1573
Vulpian-Bernhardt syndrome 1433
Vulvovaginal candidiasis 1506

W

Waddling gait 1303
Waldenstrom's macroglobulinemia 71, 1075
Warfarin 1196
administration 1197
effects 1196
reduce 1196
Warthin Finkeldey cells 328
Warts 1501
common 1501
Wasps 92
Water
abnormalities of 442
and electrolytes 473
balance 442
depletion heat exhaustion 105
deprivation test 467, 1214
loading test 1214
Waterhouse-Friderichsen syndrome 220, 221
Watering-can scrotum 279
Water-soluble vitamins 174
Waxy casts 1216
Waxy flexibility/catalepsy 1555
Weakness 636
Weber's syndrome 1410
Weber's test 1329
Wechsler adult intelligence scale 1551
Wechsler memory scale 1551
Wegener's granulomatosis 757, 1027, 1263
Weight and body composition 1587
Weight, loss of 475, 636
Weil-Felix reaction 266
Weingarten's syndrome 995
Wenckebach phenomenon 875
Wernicke's aphasia 1300
Wernicke's encephalopathy 174, 1345
Wernicke's hemianopic pupillary 1297
Wernicke-Korsakoff syndrome 1344, 1345
West Nile encephalitis 1360
West syndrome 1381
Westermark's sign 925
Western blotting 19
Westphal-Strumpell pseudosclerosis 624
Wet beriberi 174
Wet drowning 113
Wet purpura 1176
Whipple's disease 503, 767, 1375, 1376, 1490
Whipworm infection 418
Whispering pectoriloquy 966
White dermographism 1519
White hand 120
White pulp 1167

White-coat 882
Whitmore's disease 244
Whooping cough 225
Wickham's striae 1515
Widal test 231
Widow's hump 770
Wilson's disease 535, 624, 1396, 1438
Winterbottom's sign 402
Wire loop lesions 742
Withdrawal syndromes 1350
Wohlfahrtia 90, 91
Wolbachia 267
in lymphatic filariasis 434
Wolff-Parkinson-White syndrome 867
Woody thyroiditis 674
Woolsorter's disease 240
World Federation of Neurological Surgeons Scale 1415
World Health Organization classification 1133
World Hepatitis Day 339
World Malaria Day 394
Wound, surgical toilet of 271
Wuchereria bancrofti 432

X

Xanthine oxidase 773
inhibitors 912
Xanthochromia 1309
Xanthogranulomatous pyelonephritis 1255
Xeno diagnosis 405
Xenopsylla cheopis 265
Xerophthalmia 738
Xerostomia 738
Xylose absorption test 501

Y

Yawning sign 1467
Yaws 253, 255
Yellow fever 369, 936
Yellow mexican poppy 145
Yersinia enterocolitica 143
Yersinia pestis 241
Y-linked diseases 15
Yoga exercises 588
Young female arteritis 929

Z

Zanamivir 57, 324
Zenker's degeneration 229
Zika virus infections 373
Zinc 185, 1349
Zoledronate 682
Zollinger-Ellison syndrome 715, 494
Zonisamide 1388
Zoom endoscopes 478
Zoonoses 193
Zoster sine herpete 335
Zovirax 57
Zulu Dancer's hip 721
Zygomycetes 1362